INCLUDES 2 CD-ROMs.

OF01032

PEDIATRIC SURGERY

4 th EDITION

PEDIATRIC SURGERY

KEITH W. ASHCRAFT, MD

Emeritus Professor of Surgery
University of Missouri–Kansas City
Former Surgeon-in-Chief
The Children's Mercy Hospital
Kansas City, Missouri

GEORGE WHITFIELD HOLCOMB, III, MD

The Katharine B. Richardson Endowed Chair in Pediatric Surgery
University of Missouri–Kansas City
Surgeon-in-Chief and Director
Center for Minimally Invasive Surgery
The Children's Mercy Hospital
Kansas City, Missouri

J. PATRICK MURPHY, MD

Professor
University of Missouri–Kansas City
Staff Surgeon
Section Chief
Urologic Surgery
The Children's Mercy Hospital
Kansas City, Missouri

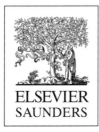

ELSEVIER
SAUNDERS

ELSEVIER
SAUNDERS

170 S. Independence Mall W 300 E
Philadelphia, Pennsylvania 19106

PEDIATRIC SURGERY   ISBN 0-7216-0222-3
Copyright © 2005, 2000, 1993, 1980 by Elsevier Inc.
All rights reserved

NOTICE

Medicine is an ever-changing field. Standard safety precautions must be followed, but as new research and clinical experience broaden our knowledge, changes in treatment and drug therapy may become necessary or appropriate. Readers are advised to check the most current product information provided by the manufacturer of each drug to be administered to verify the recommended dose, the method and duration of administration, and contraindications. It is the responsibility of the licensed prescriber or the health care provider, relying on experience and knowledge of the patient, to determine dosages and the best treatment for each individual patient. Neither the Publisher nor the authors assume any liability for any injury and/or damage to persons or property arising from this publication.

The Publisher

Previous editions copyrighted 2000, 1993, 1980 by Elsevier Inc.

Library of Congress Cataloging-in-Publication Data

Pediatric surgery/[edited by] Keith W. Ashcraft, George Whitfield Holcomb, J. Patrick
   Murphy.—4th ed.
      p. ; cm.
   Includes bibliographical references and index.
   ISBN 0-7216-0222-3
      1. Children—Surgery. I. Ashcraft, Keith W. II. Holcomb, Geroge W. III.
   Murphy, J. Patrick.
      [DNLM: 1. Surgical Procedures, Operative—Child. 2. Surgical Procedures,
   Operative—Infant. WO 925 P3715 2005]
   RD137.P43 2005
   617.9'8—dc22

                                                              2004051420

Printed in the United States of America

Last digit is the print number: 9 8 7 6 5 4 3 2 1

CONTRIBUTORS

William T. Adamson, MD
Assistant Professor, Division of Pediatric Surgery,
Department of Surgery, University of North Carolina–Chapel Hill;
Attending Surgeon, Pediatric Surgery, North Carolina Children's
Hospital, Chapel Hill, North Carolina
Tracheal Obstruction and Repair

John J. Aiken, MD
Assistant Professor of Surgery, Department of Pediatric Surgery,
Medical College of Wisconsin; Assistant Professor of Surgery,
Department of Pediatric Surgery, Children's Hospital of
Wisconsin, Milwaukee, Wisconsin
Malrotation

Craig T. Albanese, MD
Professor and Chief of Pediatric Surgery, Director of Pediatric
Surgical Services, Department of Surgery, Division of Pediatric
Surgery, Stanford University, Stanford, California
Bronchopulmonary Malformations

Uri S. Alon, MD
Professor of Pediatrics, University of Missouri–Kansas City School
of Medicine; Pediatric Nephrologist, The Children's Mercy
Hospital, Kansas City, Missouri
Renal Impairment

Maria H. Alonso, MD
Assistant Professor of Surgery, University of Cincinnati College
of Medicine; Assistant Professor of Surgery; Surgical Associate
Director of Liver Transplant; Surgical Director of Kidney
Transplant, Cincinnati Children's Hospital Medical Center,
Cincinnati, Ohio
Solid Organ Transplantation in Children

Richard J. Andrassy, MD
Denton A. Cooley Professor and Chairman, Department of
Surgery, Dean for Clinical Affairs, University of Texas Medical
School at Houston; Executive Vice-President for Clinical Affairs,
University of Texas Health Sciences Center, Houston, Texas
Rhabdomyosarcoma

Walter S. Andrews, MD
Professor of Pediatric Surgery, University of Missouri–Kansas City;
Chief, Transplant Surgery, Children's Mercy Hospital,
Kansas City, Missouri
Lesions of the Liver

Robert M. Arensman, MD
Professor of Surgery and Pediatrics, Departments of Surgery and
Pediatrics, Northwestern University; Lydia J. Frederickson
Professor of Pediatric Surgery, Department of Surgery, Division of
Pediatric Surgery, Children's Memorial Hospital, Chicago, Illinois
Congenital Diaphragmatic Hernia and Eventration

Keith W. Ashcraft, MD
Emeritus Professor of Surgery, University of Missouri–Kansas City;
Former Surgeon-in-Chief, The Children's Mercy Hospital,
Kansas City, Missouri
The Esophagus
Gastroesophageal Reflux
Acquired Anorectal Disorders

Daniel A. Bambini, MD
Attending Pediatric Surgeon, Pediatric Surgical Associates, P.A.;
Clinical Instructor, Department of General Surgery,
Carolinas Medical Center, Charlotte, North Carolina
Congenital Diaphragmatic Hernia and Eventration

**Osama A. Bawazir, MD, FRSCI, FRCS(Ed), FRCSC,
FRCS (Glas)**
Fellow, Department of Surgery, University of Calgary;
Fellow, Department of Pediatric General Surgery,
Alberta Children's Hospital, Calgary, Alberta, Canada
Mediastinal Tumors

Robert E. Binda, Jr., MD
Associate Professor, University of Missouri–Kansas City, School of
Medicine; Assistant Clinical Professor, University of Kansas
School of Medicine; Staff Anesthesiologist, Children's Mercy
Hospital, Kansas City, Missouri
Anesthetic Considerations

Martin L. Blakely, MD
Associate Professor, Department of Medicine, University of
Tennessee; Surgeon, Division of Pediatric Surgery, Le Bonheur
Children's Medical Center, Memphis, Tennessee
Rhabdomyosarcoma

Jose Boix-Ochoa, MD
Professor of Pediatric Surgery; Chair and Chief of Division of
Pediatric Surgery, Department of Pediatric Surgery, Children's
Hospital "Vall d'Hebron," Universidad Autônoma de Barcelona,
Barcelona, Spain
Gastroesophageal Reflux

Scott J. Boley, MD
Professor of Surgery and Pediatrics, Departments
of Surgery and Pediatrics, Albert Einstein College of
Medicine/Montefiore Medical Center, Bronx, New York
Anorectal Continence and Management of Constipation

Patrick C. Cartwright, MD
Professor of Surgery and Pediatrics, University of
Utah Health Sciences, Primary Children's Medical Center,
Salt Lake City, Utah
Bladder and Urethra

Michael G. Caty, MD
Associate Professor of Surgery and Pediatrics, Department of Surgery, State University of New York at Buffalo; Attending Surgeon, Division of Pediatric Surgery, Children's Hospital of Buffalo, Buffalo, New York
Meconium Disease

Bill Chiu, MD
Resident General Surgery, Department of Surgery, Northwestern University Feinberg School of Medicine; Department of Surgery, McCaw Medical Center, Chicago, Illinois
Congenital Diaphragmatic Hernia and Eventration

Dai H. Chung, MD
Associate Professor of Surgery, Department of Surgery, The University of Texas Medical Branch, Galveston, Texas
Burns

Arthur Cooper, MD
Professor of Surgery, Columbia University College of Physicians and Surgeons; Director of Trauma and Pediatric Surgical Services, Harlem Hospital Center, New York City, New York
Early Assessment and Management of Trauma

Douglas E. Coplen, MD
Associate Professor, Washington University School of Medicine; Director of Pediatric Urology, St. Louis Children's Hospital, St. Louis, Missouri
Ureteral Obstruction and Malformations

Daniel P. Croitoru, MD, FAAP, FACS
Associate Professor of Clinical Surgery and Pediatrics, Eastern Virginia Medical School; Pediatric Surgeon, Children's Hospital of the King's Daughters, Norfolk, Virginia
Congenital Chest Wall Deformities

Sidney Cywes, MMed(Surg), FRCS, FRCS(Edin)
Emeritus Professor of Pediatric Surgery, University of Cape Town and Red Cross War Memorial Children's Hospital, Cape Town, South Africa
Intestinal Atresia and Stenosis

Stephen R. Daniels, MD, MPH, PhD
Professor of Pediatrics and Environmental Health, University of Cincinnati; Professor of Pediatrics and Environmental Health, Cincinnati Children's Hospital Medical Center, Cincinnati, Ohio
Bariatric Surgical Procedures in Adolescence

Jack S. Elder, MD
Carter Kissell Professor of Urology, Professor of Pediatrics, Case Western Reserve University; Director of Pediatric Urology, Rainbow Babies and Children's Hospital, Cleveland, Ohio
Posterior Urethral Valves

Mary E. Fallat, MD
Professor of Surgery, Department of Surgery, Division of Pediatric Surgery, University of Louisville; Attending Surgeon, Department of Surgery, Kosair Children's Hospital, Louisville, Kentucky
Intussusception

Diana L. Farmer, MD
Professor of Clinical Surgery, Pediatrics, Obstetrics, Gynecology, and Reproductive Science; Chief, Division of Pediatric Surgery, University of California San Francisco; Surgeon-in-chief, University of San Francisco Children's Hospital, San Francisco, California
Prenatal Diagnosis and Surgical Intervention

Steven J. Fishman, MD
Assistant Professor of Surgery, Department of Surgery, Harvard Medical School; Assistant in Surgery, Department of Surgery, Children's Hospital Boston, Boston, Massachusetts
Vascular Anomalies

Dominic C. Frimberger, MD
Assistant Professor, Department of Urology, The University of Oklahoma Health Sciences Center, Oklahoma City, Oklahoma
Bladder and Cloacal Exstrophy

Jason S. Frischer, MD
Research Fellow in Pediatric Surgery, Department of Surgery, Columbia University College of Physicians and Surgeons; ECMO Fellow, Division of Pediatric Surgery, Children's Hospital of New York, New York City, New York
Extracorporeal Membrane Oxygenation

Alan S. Gamis, MD, MPH
Associate Professor of Pediatrics, University of Missouri–Kansas City School of Medicine; Chief, Section of Oncology, Children's Mercy Hospitals and Clinics, Kansas City, Missouri
Lymphomas

Victor F. Garcia, MD, FACS, FAAP
Professor, Pediatric Surgery and Clinical Pediatrics, University of Cincinnati College of Medicine; Professor of Surgery and Director of Trauma Services, Division of Pediatric Surgery, Cincinnati Children's Hospital Medical Center, Cincinnati, Ohio
Umbilical and Other Abdominal Wall Hernias
Bariatric Surgical Procedures in Adolescence

John M. Gatti, MD
Assistant Professor, University of Missouri–Kansas City School of Medicine; Staff Surgeon, Children's Mercy Hospital, Kansas City, Missouri
Intersex

John P. Gearhart, MD
Professor and Director, Pediatric Urology, Johns Hopkins University School of Medicine; Professor and Director, Pediatric Urology, Johns Hopkins Hospital, Baltimore, MD
Bladder and Cloacal Exstrophy

Keith E. Georgeson, MD
Professor of Surgery, Director, Division of Pediatric Surgery, University of Alabama at Birmingham; Surgeon-in-Chief, The Children's Hospital of Alabama, Birmingham, Alabama
Laparoscopy

Brian F. Gilchrist, MD
Associate Professor of Surgery, Department of Surgery, Tufts University School of Medicine; Surgeon-in-Chief, The Boston Floating Hospital for Children; Medical Director, Kiwanis Pediatric Trauma Institute, Boston, Massachusetts
Lesions of the Stomach

George K. Gittes, MD
Associate Professor of Surgery, Division of Pediatric Surgery, University of Missouri–Kansas City; Director, Surgical Research, Department of Pediatric Surgery, The Children's Mercy Hospital, Kansas City, Missouri
Lesions of the Pancreas and Spleen

Michael J. Goretsky, MD
Assistant Professor of Clinical Surgery and Pediatrics, Eastern Virginia Medical School; Pediatric Surgeon, Children's Hospital of the King's Daughters, Norfolk, Virginia
Congenital Chest Wall Deformities

Neil E. Green, MD
Professor of Orthopaedics, Director of Pediatric Orthopaedics, Vanderbilt University Medical Center, Nashville, Tennessee
Pediatric Orthopedic Trauma

Gerald M. Haase, MD
Clinical Professor of Surgery, Department of Surgery, University of Colorado School of Medicine; Attending Surgeon and Former Chairman, Department of Surgery, The Children's Hospital, Denver, Colorado
Adjuvant Therapy in Childhood Cancer

Michael R. Harrison, MD
Professor of Clinical Surgery, Pediatrics, Obstetrics, Gynecology, and Reproductive Sciences, University of California, San Francisco; Attending Pediatric Surgeon, University of California, San Francisco Medical Center, San Francisco, California
Prenatal Diagnosis and Surgical Intervention

Matthew T. Harting, MD
Resident/Research Fellow, Division of Pediatric Surgery, University of Texas Medical School at Houston; Research Fellow, M.D. Anderson Cancer Center, Houston, Texas
Rhabdomyosarcoma

Stanley Hellerstein, MD
Professor of Pediatrics, University of Missouri–Kansas City School of Medicine; The Ernest L. Glasscock Chair in Pediatric Research, Pediatric Nephrologist, The Children's Mercy Hospital, Kansas City, Missouri
Renal Impairment

Marion C. W. Henry, MD
General Surgery Resident, Yale University School of Medicine, New Haven, Connecticut
Surgical Infectious Disease

David N. Herndon, MD
Professor, Jesse H. Jones Distinguished Chair, Department of Surgery, The University of Texas Medical Branch; Chief of Staff, Shriners Burns Hospital for Children–Galveston, Galveston, Texas
Burns

Barry A. Hicks, MD
Professor of Pediatric Surgery, Acting Chief, Division of Pediatric Surgery, Department of Surgery, University of Texas Southwestern Medical Center; Chief of Surgical Services, Children's Medical Center, Dallas, Texas
Abdominal and Renal Trauma

M. John Hicks, MD, DDS, PhD
Professor of Pathology, Baylor College of Medicine; Medical Director of Surgical Pathology and Ultrastructural Pathology, Medical Director of Cytogenetics, Texas Children's Hospital, Houston, Texas
Nevus and Melanoma

Ronald B. Hirschl, MD
Professor, Department of Surgery, Section of Pediatric Surgery, University of Michigan Health System, Ann Arbor, Michigan
Mechanical Ventilation in Pediatric Surgical Disease

George W. Holcomb III, MD, MBA
The Katharine B. Richardson Endowed Chair in Pediatric Surgery, University of Missouri–Kansas City; Surgeon-in-Chief and Director, Center for Minimally Invasive Surgery, The Children's Mercy Hospital, Kansas City, Missouri
Alimentary Tract Duplications
Laparoscopy

Celeste Hollands, MD
Associate Professor of Surgery and Pediatrics, Department of Surgery, University at Buffalo; Director, Miniature Access Surgery Center, Department of Pediatric Surgery, Women's and Children's Hospital at Buffalo, Buffalo, New York
Robotic Surgery

Alexander Holschneider, MD, PhD
Professor of Pediatric Surgery, University of Cologne; Physician, Children's Hospital of the City of Cologne, Cologne, Germany
Hirschsprung's Disease

Gregory W. Hornig, MD
Clinical Assistant Professor, University of Missouri–Kansas City; Chief, Section of Neurosurgery, Children's Mercy Hospitals and Clinics, Kansas City, Missouri
Pediatric Head Trauma

Thomas H. Inge, MD, PhD
Assistant Professor of Surgery and Pediatrics, University of Cincinnati; Surgical Director, Comprehensive Weight Management Center, Cincinnati Children's Hospital Medical Center, Cincinnati, Ohio
Bariatric Surgical Procedures in Adolescence

Michael S. Irish, MD
Assistant Professor, The University of Iowa, Iowa City, Iowa; Pediatric Surgeon, Raymond Blank Children's Hospital, Iowa Methodist Medical Center, Des Moines, Iowa
Meconium Disease

Tom Jaksic, MD, PhD
Associate Professor of Surgery, Harvard Medical School; Department of Surgery, Children's Hospital Boston, Boston, Massachusetts
Nutritional Support of the Pediatric Patient
Nevus and Melanoma

Patrick J. Javid, MD
Research Fellow, Department of Surgery, Children's Hospital Boston, Harvard Medical School, Boston, Massachusetts
Nutritional Support of the Pediatric Patient

Sidney Johnson, MD
Research Fellow, Harvard Medical School; Children's Hospital,
Boston, Massachusetts
Inflammatory Bowel Disease and Intestinal Cancer

Stephanie A. Kapfer, MD
Research Fellow, Department of Surgery, University at Buffalo;
Research Fellow, Department of Pediatric
Surgery, Women's and Children's Hospital of Buffalo,
Buffalo, New York
Robotic Surgery

Michael A. Keating, MD, FAAP
Clinical Professor of Urology in Surgery, University of South Florida
School of Medicine, Tampa, Florida; Nemours Children's Clinic,
Orlando, Florida
Prune-belly Syndrome

Martin S. Keller, MD
Assistant Professor of Surgery, Department of Surgery, Division
of Pediatric Surgery, St. Louis University Medical School;
Assistant Professor of Surgery, Department of Surgery,
Division of Pediatric Surgery, Cardinal Glennon Children's
Hospital, St. Louis, Missouri
Groin Hernias and Hydroceles

Robert E. Kelly, Jr., MD
Associate Professor of Clinical Surgery and Pediatrics,
Eastern Virginia Medical School; Chief, Department of Surgery,
Children's Hospital of the King's Daughters,
Norfolk, Virginia
Congenital Chest Wall Deformities

E. M. Kiely, MD
Consultant Pediatric Surgeon, Great Ormond Street
Hospital for Children, London, England
Neuroblastoma

Philip A. King, MMBS, FRCS, FRACS†
Chairman, Surgical Services Clinical Care Unit; Consultant
Pediatric Surgeon and Pediatric Urologist, Princess Margaret
Hospital for Children, Subiaco, West Australia
The Acute Scrotum

Michael D. Klein, MD
The Alvin A. Philippart, M.D., Endowed Chair in Pediatric
Research, Wayne State University School of Medicine and
Children's Hospital of Michigan; Surgeon-in-Chief, Department
of Surgery, Children's Hospital of Michigan; Professor of
Surgery, Wayne State University; Active Staff, Department
of Surgery, St. John Hospital and Medical Center, Detroit,
Michigan
Congenital Abdominal Wall Defects

Susan G. Kreissman, MD
Associate Professor, Department of Pediatrics, Duke University;
Section of Pediatric Hematology/Oncology, Department of
Pediatrics, Duke University Medical Center,
Durham, North Carolina
Adjuvant Therapy in Childhood Cancer

Thomas M. Krummel, MD
Emile Holman Professor and Chair, Department of Surgery,
Stanford University School of Medicine, Stanford, California;
Professor of Surgery, Department of Surgery, Stanford Hospitals
and Clinics; Susan B. Ford Surgeon-in-Chief, Lucile Packard
Children's Hospital, Palo Alto, California
Surgical Infectious Disease

Jean-Martin Laberge, MD, FACS, FRCSC
Professor of Surgery, McGill University; Director, Division
of Pediatric General Surgery, The Montreal Children's
Hospital of the McGill University Health Centre, Montreal,
Quebec, Canada
Teratomas, Dermoids, and Other Soft Tissue Tumors

Hanmin Lee, MD
Assistant Professor of Surgery, Pediatrics, and Ob-Gyn and
Reproductive Services, University of California, San Francisco;
Attending Surgeon, University of California, San Francisco
Medical Center, San Francisco, California
Prenatal Diagnosis and Surgical Intervention

Keith L. Lee, MD
Chief Resident, Department of Urology, Stanford University
Medical Center, Stanford, California
Undescended Testis and Testicular Tumors

Joseph L. Lelli, Jr., MD
Instructor, Wayne State University School of Medicine;
Pediatric Surgeon, Children's Hospital of Michigan, Detroit,
Michigan; Pediatric Surgeon, Toledo Children's Hospital,
Toledo, Ohio
Foreign Bodies

Marc S. Lessin, MD
Attending Pediatric Surgeon, Scottish Rite Children's Hospital,
Atlanta, Georgia
Lesions of the Stomach

Marc A. Levitt, MD
Assistant Professor of Surgery and Pediatrics, Albert Einstein
College of Medicine, Bronx, New York; Attending Pediatric
Surgeon, Schneider Children's Hospital, North Shore–Long Island
Jewish Medical Center, New Hyde Park, New York
Imperforate Anus and Cloacal Malformations

Daniel Little, MD
Instructor in Surgery, University of Missouri–Kansas City;
Critical Care Fellow, Children's Mercy Hospital, Kansas City,
Missouri
Meconium Disease

Gary K. Lofland, MD
Professor of Surgery, University of Missouri–Kansas City; Chief,
Thoracic and Cardiovascular Surgery, Joseph Boon Gregg
Endowed Chair, Children's Mercy Hospitals and Clinics,
Kansas City, Missouri
Thoracic Trauma in Children

Charles W. McGill, MD
Pediatric Surgeon, Marshfield Clinic, Marshfield, Wisconsin
Bites

†Deceased

Sheilendra S. Mehta, MD
Pediatric Surgery Research Fellow, Department of Pediatric Surgery, The Children's Mercy Hospital, Kansas City, Missouri
Lesions of the Pancreas and Spleen

Gregory A. Mencio, MD
Associate Professor, Department of Orthopaedic Surgery, Vanderbilt University Medical Center, Nashville, Tennessee
Pediatric Orthopedic Trauma

Peter H. Mestad, MD
Associate Professor, University of Missouri–Kansas City School of Medicine; Assistant Clinical Professor, University of Kansas School of Medicine, The Children's Mercy Hospital System; Staff Anesthesiologist; Director, Anesthesia Services, Children's Mercy South, Kansas City, Missouri
Anesthetic Considerations

Marc P. Michalsky, MD
Assistant Professor of Surgery, Ohio State University School of Medicine and Public Health; Columbus Children's Hospital, Columbus, Ohio
Acquired Lesions of the Lung and Pleura

Alastair J. W. Millar, MBChB, FRCS, FRCS(Edin)
Professor of Pediatric Surgery, Red Cross War Memorial Children's Hospital and University of Cape Town; Principal Specialist, Department of Pediatric Surgery, Red Cross War Memorial Children's Hospital, Cape Town, South Africa
Intestinal Atresia and Stenosis

Eugene A. Minevich, MD, FACS, FAAP
Assistant Professor of Surgery, Department of Surgery, University of Cincinnati; Assistant Professor of Surgery, Department of Surgical Services, Division of Pediatric Urology, Cincinnati Children's Hospital Medical Center, Cincinnati, Ohio
Urinary Tract Infection and Vesicoureteral Reflux

Takeshi Miyano, MD
Professor and Head, Department of Pediatric Surgery, Chairman, Department of Surgery, School of Medicine, Juntendo University; Director, Juntendo University Hospital, Tokyo, Japan
Biliary Tract Disorders and Portal Hypertension

Stephen E. Morrow, MD
Assistant Professor of Surgery and Pediatrics, Uniformed Services University of the Health Sciences, School of Medicine; Chief, Pediatric Surgery, National Naval Medical Center, Bethesda, Maryland; Chief, Pediatric Surgery, Walter Reed Army Medical Center, Washington, DC
Appendicitis

J. Patrick Murphy, MD
Professor, University of Missouri–Kansas City School of Medicine; Staff Surgeon, Section Chief of Urologic Surgery, Children's Mercy Hospital, Kansas City, Missouri
Hypospadias

Don K. Nakayama, MD
Professor of Surgery and Pediatrics, University of North Carolina at Chapel Hill, Chapel Hill, North Carolina; Program Director, Residency in General Surgery, New Hanover Regional Medical Center, Wilmington, North Carolina
Breast Diseases in Children

Kurt D. Newman, MD
Professor of Surgery and Pediatrics, George Washington University School of Medicine; Surgeon in Chief and Executive Director of the Joseph E. Robert, Jr., Center for Surgical Care, Children's National Medical Center, Washington, DC
Appendicitis

Luong T. Nguyen, MD, FRCSC
Associate Professor of Pediatrics, McGill University; The Montreal Children's Hospital of the McGill University Health Centre, Montreal, Quebec, Canada
Teratomas, Dermoids, and Other Soft Tissue Tumors

James F. Nigro, MD
Volunteer Faculty, Dermatology, Baylor College of Medicine, Houston, Texas
Nevus and Melanoma

Kerilyn K. Nobuhara, MD
Assistant Professor of Clinical Surgery, Pediatrics, Obstetrics, Gynecology, and Reproductive Sciences, University of California, San Francisco; Attending Pediatric Physician, University of California, San Francisco Medical Center, San Francisco, California
Prenatal Diagnosis and Surgical Intervention

Donald Nuss, MB, ChB, FRCS(C), FACS, FAAP
Professor of Clinical Surgery and Pediatrics, Eastern Virginia Medical School; Surgeon-in-Chief and Vice President for Surgical Affairs, Children's Hospital of the King's Daughters, Norfolk, Virginia
Congenital Chest Wall Deformities

James E. O'Brien, Jr., MD
Assistant Professor of Surgery, University of Missouri–Kansas City; Attending Surgeon, Section of Cardiac Surgery, Children's Mercy Hospitals and Clinics, Kansas City, Missouri
Thoracic Trauma in Children

Keith T. Oldham, MD
Interim Chairman, Professor and Chief, Division of Pediatric Surgery, Department of Surgery, Medical College of Wisconsin; Surgeon-in-Chief, Department of Pediatric Surgery, Children's Hospital of Wisconsin, Milwaukee, Wisconsin
Malrotation

James A. O'Neill, Jr., MD
J. C. Foshee Distinguished Professor of Surgery and Chairman Emeritus, Department of Surgery, Vanderbilt University Medical Center; Surgeon-in-Chief Emeritus, Vanderbilt University Hospital, Nashville, Tennessee
Renovascular Hypertension

Daniel J. Ostlie, MD
Assistant Professor of Surgery, Department of Surgery, University of Missouri–Kansas City Medical School; Assistant Professor of Surgery, Department of Surgery, Children's Mercy Hospital, Kansas City, Missouri
Necrotizing Enterocolitis

H. Biemann Othersen, Jr., MD
Emeritus Professor of Surgery and Pediatrics, Medical University of South Carolina; Emeritus Chief of Pediatric Surgery, Medical University of South Carolina Children's Hospital, Charleston, South Carolina
Tracheal Obstruction and Repair

Alberto Peña, MD
Professor of Surgery and Pediatrics, Albert Einstein College of Medicine, Bronx, New York; Chief of Pediatric Surgery, Schneider Children's Hospital, North Shore–Long Island Jewish Medical Center, New Hyde Park, New York
Imperforate Anus and Cloacal Malformations

Kathy M. Perryman, MD
Assistant Professor, University of Missouri–Kansas City; Assistant Clinical Professor, University of Kansas School of Medicine; Chief, Department of Anesthesiology, Children's Mercy Hospital, Kansas City, Missouri
Anesthetic Considerations

Craig A. Peters, MD
Associate Professor, Department of Surgery, Division of Urology, Harvard Medical School; Associate in Urology, Department of Urology, The Children's Hospital of Boston, Boston, Massachusetts
Urologic Laparoscopy

Stephen C. Raynor, MD
Clinical Associate Professor, Department of Surgery, University of Nebraska; Staff Surgeon, Department of Surgery, Children's Hospital, Omaha, Nebraska
Circumcision

Mark A. Rich, MD, FACS
Clinical Associate Professor, University of South Florida School of Medicine, Tampa, Florida; Nemours Children's Clinic, Orlando, Florida
Prune-belly Syndrome

Heinz Rode, MBChB, MMed(Surg), FRCS(Edin)
Professor, University of Cape Town; Chief Pediatric Surgeon, Red Cross War Memorial Children's Hospital, Cape Town, South Africa
Intestinal Atresia and Stenosis

Bradley M. Rodgers, MD
Professor and Chief, Division of Pediatric Surgery, University of Virginia School of Medicine; Chief, Pediatric Surgery, University of Virginia Children's Hospital, Charlottesville, Virginia
Acquired Lesions of the Lung and Pleura

Michael T. Rohmiller, MD
Pediatric Orthopaedic Fellow, Children's Hospital of San Diego, San Diego, California
Pediatric Orthopedic Trauma

Stephen Rothenberg, MD
Associate Clinical Professor of Surgery, University of Colorado; Chief of Pediatric Surgery, Vice Chair of Surgery, The Mother and Child Hospital at Presbyterian/St. Luke's, Denver, Colorado
Thoracoscopy in Infants and Children

Frederick C. Rykman, MD
Professor of Surgery, University of Cincinnati College of Medicine; Professor of Surgery, Director of Liver Transplant, Cincinnati Children's Hospital Medical Center, Cincinnati, Ohio
Solid Organ Transplantation in Children

Shawn D. Safford, MD
Chief Resident in General Surgery, Duke University Medical Center, Durham, North Carolina
Endocrine Disorders and Tumors

Shawn D. St. Peter, MD
Clinical Instructor, Department of Surgery, University of Missouri–Kansas City School of Medicine; Senior Resident in Pediatric Surgery, Department of Surgery, Children's Mercy Hospitals and Clinics, Kansas City, Missouri
Necrotizing Enterocolitis

Daniel A. Saltzman, MD, PhD
Assistant Professor of Surgery and Pediatrics, Section of Pediatric Surgery, Department of Surgery, University of Minnesota, Minneapolis, Minnesota
Physiology of the Newborn

Kurt P. Schropp, MD
Associate Professor of Surgery, Department of Pediatric Surgery, Kansas University Medical Center, Kansas City, Kansas
Meckel's Diverticulum

Robert C. Shamberger, MD
Robert E. Gross Professor of Surgery, Harvard Medical School; Chief of Surgery, Children's Hospital, Boston, Massachusetts
Renal Tumors

Ellen Shapiro, MD, FACS, FAAP
Professor of Urology, Chief of Pediatric Urology, Department of Urology, New York University School of Medicine, New York, New York
Posterior Urethral Valves

Kenneth S. Shaw, MD, FRCSC
Assistant Professor of Surgery, McGill University; Pediatric General Surgeon, Director, Surgical Emergency Room, The Montreal Children's Hospital of the McGill University Health Centre, Montreal, Quebec, Canada
Teratomas, Dermoids, and Other Soft Tissue Tumors

Curtis A. Sheldon, MD, FACS, FAAP
Professor of Surgery, Department of Surgery, University of Cincinnati; Director and Professor, Surgical Services, Division of Pediatric Urology, Cincinnati Children's Hospital Medical Center, Cincinnati, Ohio
Urinary Tract Infection and Vesicoureteral Reflux

Stephen B. Shew, MD
Assistant Professor of Surgery, Division of Pediatric Surgery, University of California, Los Angeles, School of Medicine; Attending Pediatric Surgeon, UCLA Medical Center, Mattel Children's Hospital, Los Angeles, California
Alimentary Tract Duplications

Linda D. Shortliffe, MD
Professor and Chair, Department of Urology, Stanford University School of Medicine; Chief of Urology, Stanford University Medical Center (Stanford University Hospital and Lucile Packard Children's Hospital), Stanford, California
Undescended Testis and Testicular Tumors

David L. Sigalet, MD, PhD, FRCSC, FACS
Professor, Department of Surgery, University of Calgary; Regional Director, Pediatric General Surgery, Alberta Children's Hospital, Calgary, Alberta, Canada
Mediastinal Tumors

Michael A. Skinner, MD
Associate Professor and Chief, Division of Pediatric Surgery, Duke University School of Medicine, Durham, North Carolina
Endocrine Disorders and Tumors

Samuel D. Smith, MD
Boyd Family Professor and Chief, Department of Pediatric Surgery, Arkansas Children's Hospital, University of Arkansas for Medical Services, Little Rock, Arkansas
Physiology of the Newborn

C. Jason Smithers, MD
Research Fellow, Surgical Resident, Children's Hospital Boston, Boston, Massachusetts
Vascular Anomalies

Brent W. Snow, MD, FACS, FAAP
Professor of Surgery, University of Utah School of Medicine; Staff, Primary Children's Medical Center, Salt Lake City, Utah
Bladder and Urethra

Howard M. Snyder, III, MD
Professor of Urology, University of Pennsylvania School of Medicine; Associate Director, Pediatric Urology, Children's Hospital of Philadelphia, Philadelphia, Pennsylvania
Developmental and Positional Anomalies of the Kidneys

Lewis Spitz, MD, PhD
Nuffield Professor of Paediatric Surgery, Department of Paediatric Surgery, Institute of Child Health, University College; Consultant Paediatric Surgeon, Great Ormond Street Hospital, London, England
Esophageal Atresia and Tracheoesophageal Malformations

V. Sripathi, MS, MCh, FRACS
Sundaram Medical Foundation, Dr. Rangarajan Memorial Hospital, Chennai, Tamil Nadu, India
The Acute Scrotum

Charles J. H. Stolar, MD
Professor of Surgery and Pediatrics, Departments of Surgery and Pediatrics, Columbia University College of Physicians and Surgeons; Chief, Pediatric Surgery, Children's Hospital of New York, New York City, New York
Extracorporeal Membrane Oxygenation

Julie Strickland, MD
Associate Professor, University of Missouri–Kansas City; Attending Physician, Division of Gynecologic Surgery, Children's Mercy Hospital, Kansas City, Missouri
Pediatric and Adolescent Gynecology

Steven Stylianos, MD
Arnold P. Gold Foundation Associate Professor of Clinical Surgery and Pediatrics, Columbia University College of Physicians and Surgeons; Director, Regional Pediatric Trauma Program, Children's Hospital of New York, New York City, New York
Abdominal and Renal Trauma

Karl G. Sylvester, MD
Assistant Professor, Department of Surgery, Division of Pediatric Surgery, Stanford University; Assistant Professor, Department of Surgery, Division of Pediatric Surgery, Lucile Salter Packard Children's Hospital at Stanford, Stanford, California
Bronchopulmonary Malformations

Edward P. Tagge, MD
Professor of Surgery and Pediatrics, Medical University of South Carolina; Chief, Pediatric Surgery, Medical University of South Carolina, Charleston, South Carolina
Tracheal Obstruction and Repair

Joselito Tantoco, MD
Research Fellow, Department of Surgery, University at Buffalo; Research Fellow, Department of Pediatric Surgery, Women's and Children's Hospital of Buffalo, Buffalo, New York
Robotic Surgery

David Tapper, MD[†]
Professor of Surgery and Vice-Chair, Department of Surgery, University of Washington School of Medicine; Surgeon-in-Chief and Director, Department of Surgery, Children's Hospital and Regional Medical Center, Seattle, Washington
Head and Neck Sinuses and Masses

Gregory M. Tiao, MD
Assistant Professor of Surgery, University of Cincinnati; Assistant Professor of Surgery, Cincinnati Children's Hospital Medical Center, Cincinnati, Ohio
Solid Organ Transplantation in Children

Thomas F. Tracy, Jr., MD
Professor of Surgery and Pediatrics, Vice Chairman, Department of Surgery, Brown Medical School; Pediatric Surgeon-in-Chief, Hasbro Children's Hospital, Providence, Rhode Island
Groin Hernias and Hydroceles

[†]Deceased

Charles S. Turner, MD
Associate Professor of Pediatrics and Surgery, Wake Forest
University Medical Center; Chief of Pediatric Surgery,
Brenner Children's Hospital, Winsont-Salem, North Carolina
  Vascular Access

Benno M. Ure, MD, PhD
Consultant Pediatric Surgeon, Wilhelmina Children's Hospital,
University Medical Center–Utrecht, Utrecht, The Netherlands
  Hirschsprung's Disease

Daniel von Allmen, MD
Assistant Professor of Surgery, Department of General and
Thoracic Surgery, University of Pennsylvania; Attending Surgeon,
Department of Pediatric General and Thoracic Surgery,
Children's Hospital of Philadelphia, Philadelphia, Pennsylvania
  Adjuvant Therapy in Childhood Cancer

John H. T. Waldhausen, MD
Associate Professor of Surgery, Department of Surgery, University
of Washington School of Medicine; Attending Pediatric General
and Thoracic Surgeon, Department of Surgery, Children's
Hospital and Regional Medical Center, Seattle, Washington
  Head and Neck Sinuses and Masses

Bradley A. Warady, MD
Professor of Pediatrics, University of Missouri–Kansas City School
of Medicine; Chief, Section of Pediatric Nephrology; Director,
Dialysis and Transplantation, The Children's
Mercy Hospital, Kansas City, Missouri
  Renal Impairment

Masayo Watanabe, MD
Assistant Professor of Pediatrics, Department of Pediatrics,
University of Missouri–Kansas City School of Medicine;
Hematologist/Oncologist, Department of Hematology/Oncology,
The Children's Mercy Hospital and Clinics, Kansas City, Missouri
  Coagulopathies and Sickle Cell Disease

Thomas R. Weber, MD
Professor of Surgery and Pediatrics, Chief, Division of Pediatric
Surgery, St. Louis University School of Medicine; Director,
Division of Pediatric Surgery, Cardinal Glennon Children's
Hospital, St. Louis, Missouri
  Groin Hernias and Hydroceles

Gerard T. Weinberg, MD
Professor of Clinical Surgery and Pediatrics, Departments
of Surgery and Pediatrics, Albert Einstein College of
Medicine/Montefiore Medical Center, Bronx,
New York
  Anorectal Continence and Management of Constipation

Brian M. Wicklund, MD, CM, MPH
Associate Professor of Pediatrics, University of Missouri–Kansas
City School of Medicine; Director, Hemophilia Treatment Center,
Pediatric Hematologist/Oncologist, Children's Mercy Hospital,
Kansas City, Missouri
  Coagulopathies and Sickle Cell Disease

Gerald M. Woods, MD
Professor of Pediatrics, University of Missouri–Kansas City School
of Medicine; Chief, Division of Hematology/Oncology; Director,
Sickle Cell Program, Children's Mercy Hospital, Kansas City,
Missouri
  Coagulopathies and Sickle Cell Disease

Hsi-Yang Wu, MD
Assistant Professor, Department of Urology, University of
Pittsburgh; Attending Physician, Department of Pediatric
Urology, Children's Hospital of Pittsburgh,
Pittsburgh, Pennsylvania
  Developmental and Positional Anomalies of the Kidneys

Edmund Y. Yang, MD, PhD
Assistant Professor of Surgery, Department of Pediatric
Surgery, Vanderbilt School of Medicine; Assistant Professor
of Surgery, Department of Pediatric Surgery, Vanderbilt
University Medical Center, Vanderbilt Children's Hospital,
Nashville, Tennessee
  Inflammatory Bowel Disease and Intestinal Cancer

Moritz M. Ziegler, MD
Professor of Surgery, University of Colorado School of
Medicine; Surgeon-in-Chief, The Children's Hospital, Denver,
Colorado
  Inflammatory Bowel Disease and Intestinal Cancer

PREFACE

This volume represents the 25th anniversary of Holder and Ashcraft's *Pediatric Surgery*. I certainly never expected a 4th edition. The mission of this book has not changed: It is to provide for the student, resident, and pediatric surgeon who has but one book the information necessary to understand the basis and practice of pediatric surgery.

The evolution of pediatric surgery over these last 25 years has been truly amazing. Where we once talked about a disease possibly having a "familial" tendency we now are able to localize the genetic basis for the inheritance of the malformation with some accuracy. From a personal point of view, the progress in the treatment of childhood malignancies has been the most impressive change in pediatric surgery. This change reflects the accumulated knowledge of genetics and of molecular biology—both of which were barely on the scene when the first edition came off the press. Although children suffer the ravages of cancer and its treatment far too often, the current rate of "cure" offers so much more hope than in years gone by.

When I was a medical student and became acquainted with the wonderful world of surgery involving infants and children, an old urologist was fond of asking the budding surgeon if they could build a birdhouse. If you cannot, you have no business wanting to be a surgeon, he would say. It is hard to imagine what technical skills are necessary for the pediatric surgeon of the 21st century. Perhaps an electronic background is helpful, but I continue to maintain that the epitome of pediatric surgical skill resides in the ability to repair hypospadias. Most of the mechanization that has been interposed between the surgeon and the tissue cannot substitute for plain old surgical skill.

This time, I promise, is my last. Whit Holcomb and Pat Murphy will carry this load from now on. The combination of their vision and technical capabilities will provide a good basis for future editions. I only hope that they continue to have the help of Kathy Smith, who has seen the preparation of all four editions go from the typewriter to the word processor and beyond. Without her help this truly could not have been done.

Keith W. Ashcraft, MD
January, 2005

TABLE OF CONTENTS

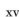

PEDIATRIC SURGERY

CHAPTER 1

Physiology of the Newborn

Daniel A. Saltzman, MD, PhD, and Samuel D. Smith, MD

Of all pediatric patients, the neonate possesses the most distinctive and rapidly changing physiologic characteristics. These changes are due to the newborn's adaptation from placental support to the extrauterine environment, early organ maturation, and the demands of rapid growth and development. Because of these dynamic physiologic alterations, this chapter emphasizes the neonate.

Newborns may be classified based on gestational age and weight. Preterm infants are those born before 37 weeks of gestation. Term infants are those born between 38 and 42 weeks of gestation, whereas post-term infants have a gestation that exceeds 42 weeks. Babies whose weight is below the 10th percentile for age are considered small-for-gestational-age (SGA), whereas those whose weight is at or above the 98th percentile are large-for-gestational-age (LGA). The babies whose weight falls between these extremes are appropriate-for-gestational-age (AGA).

SGA newborns are thought to suffer intrauterine growth retardation as a result of placental, maternal, or fetal abnormalities. Conditions associated with deviation in intrauterine growth are shown in Figure 1-1. SGA infants have a body weight below what is appropriate for their age, yet their body length and head circumference are age appropriate. To classify an infant as SGA, the gestational age must be estimated by the physical findings summarized in Table 1-1.

Although SGA infants may weigh the same as premature infants, they have different physiological characteristics. Due to intrauterine malnutrition, body fat levels are frequently less than 1% of the total body weight. This lack of body fat increases the risk of cold stress with SGA infants. Hypoglycemia develops earlier in SGA infants because of higher metabolic activity and reduced glycogen stores. The red blood cell (RBC) volume and the total blood volume are much higher in the SGA infant compared with the preterm average for gestational age or the non-SGA term infant. This increase in RBC volume frequently leads to polycythemia, with an associated increase in blood viscosity. Because of the adequate length of gestation, the SGA infant has pulmonary function approaching that of an AGA or a term infant.

Infants born before 37 weeks of gestation, regardless of birth weight, are considered premature. The physical examination of the premature infant reveals that the skin is thin and transparent with an absence of plantar creases. Fingers are soft and malleable; ears have poorly developed cartilage. In girls, the labia minora appear enlarged, but the labia majora are small. In boys, the testicles are usually undescended, and the scrotum is undeveloped. Special problems with the preterm infant include the following:

1. Weak suck reflex
2. Inadequate gastrointestinal absorption
3. Hyaline membrane disease (HMD)
4. Intraventricular hemorrhage
5. Hypothermia
6. Patent ductus arteriosus
7. Apnea
8. Hyperbilirubinemia

SPECIFIC PHYSIOLOGICAL PROBLEMS OF THE NEWBORN

Fetal levels of glucose, calcium, and magnesium are carefully maintained by maternal regulation. The transition to extrauterine life can have profound effects on the physiological well-being of the newborn.

Glucose Metabolism

The fetus maintains a blood glucose value 70% to 80% of maternal value by facilitated diffusion across the placenta. A buildup of glycogen stores occurs in the liver, skeleton, and cardiac muscles during the later stages of fetal development but with little gluconeogenesis. The newborn must depend on glycolysis until exogenous glucose is supplied. After delivery, the baby depletes its hepatic glycogen stores within 2 to 3 hours. Glycogen stores are more rapidly reduced in premature and SGA babies. The newborn is severely limited in his or her ability to use fat and protein as substrates to synthesize glucose.

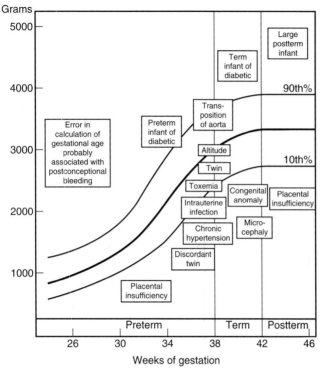

FIGURE 1-1. Graphic representation of conditions associated with deviations in intrauterine growth. The boxes symbolize the approximate birth weight and gestational age at which the condition is likely to occur. (Adapted from Avery ME, Villee D, Baker S, et al: Neonatology. In Avery ME, First LR [eds]: Pediatric Medicine. Baltimore, Williams & Wilkins, 1989, p 148.)

Hypoglycemia

Clinical signs of hypoglycemia are nonspecific and may include a weak or high-pitched cry, cyanosis, apnea, jitteriness, apathy, seizures, abnormal eye movements, temperature instability, hypotonia, and weak suck. Some infants, however, exhibit no signs, despite extremely low blood glucose levels.

Neonatal hypoglycemia is generally defined as a glucose level less than 40 mg/dL. After 72 hours of age, plasma glucose levels should be 40 mg/dL or more.[1] Infants who are at high risk for hypoglycemia developing require frequent glucose monitoring. Because most newborns who require surgical procedures are at risk for hypoglycemia development, a 10% glucose infusion is usually started on admission to the hospital, and blood glucose levels are measured at the bedside and confirmed by periodic laboratory determinations. If the blood glucose level is less than 40 mg/dL or if any signs of hypoglycemia are present, an hourly bolus infusion of 1 to 2 mL/kg (4 to 8 mg/kg/min) of 10% glucose is given intravenously (IV). If central venous access is present, concentrations of up to 50% glucose may be used. During the first 36 to 48 hours after a major surgical procedure, it is not uncommon to see wide variations in serum glucose levels; thus frequent blood and urine glucose determinations should be performed. Rarely, hydrocortisone, glucagon, or somatostatin is used to treat persistent hypoglycemia.

Hyperglycemia

Hyperglycemia is a common problem with the use of total parenteral nutrition (TPN) in very immature infants who are less than 30 weeks' gestation and less than 1.1 kg birth weight. These infants are usually younger than 3 days and are frequently septic.[2] The etiology of the hyperglycemia appears to be an inadequate insulin response to glucose. Hyperglycemia may cause intraventricular hemorrhage and water and electrolyte losses from glucosuria. The glucose concentration and infusion rate of the TPN must be adjusted based on serum glucose levels. Full parenteral caloric support is achieved with incremental increases in glucose, usually over a period of several days. Occasionally, IV insulin at 0.001 to 0.01 U/kg/min is needed to maintain normoglycemia.

Calcium

Calcium is continuously delivered to the fetus by active transport across the placenta. Of the total amount of calcium transferred across the placenta, 75% occurs after 28 weeks' gestation.[3] This observation partially accounts for the high incidence of hypocalcemia in extremely preterm infants. Any neonate has a tendency for hypocalcemia because of limited calcium stores, renal immaturity, and relative hypoparathyroidism secondary

TABLE 1-1			
CLINICAL CRITERIA FOR CLASSIFICATION OF LOW-BIRTH-WEIGHT INFANTS			
Criteria	36 Wk (Premature)	37–38 Wk (Borderline Premature)	39 Wk (Term)
Plantar creases	Rare, shallow	Heel remains smooth	Creases throughout sole
Size of breast nodule	Not palpable to <3 mm	4 mm	Visible (7 mm)
Head hair	Cotton wool quality		Silky; each strand can be distinguished
Earlobe	Shapeless, pliable with little cartilage		Rigid with cartilage
Testicular descent and scrotal changes	Small scrotum with rugal patch; testes not completely descended	Gradual descent	Enlarged scrotum creased with rugae; fully descended testes

Adapted from Avery ME, Villee D, Baker S, et al: Neonatology. In Avery ME, First LR (eds): Pediatric Medicine. Baltimore, Williams & Wilkins, 1989, p 148.

to suppression by high fetal calcium levels. Newborn calcium levels usually reach their nadir 24 to 48 hours after delivery, when parathyroid hormone responses become effective. Hypocalcemia is defined as an ionized calcium level of less than 1 mg/dL. At greatest risk for hypocalcemia are preterm infants, newborn surgical patients, and infants of complicated pregnancies, such as those of diabetic mothers or those receiving bicarbonate infusions. Calcitonin, which inhibits calcium mobilization from the bone, is increased in premature and asphyxiated infants.

Exchange transfusions or massive transfusions of citrated blood can result in the formation of calcium citrate complexes, reducing the ionized serum calcium levels to dangerous or even fatal levels. Late-onset (older than 48 hours) hypocalcemia is less frequent now that most formulas are low in phosphate.

Signs of hypocalcemia may include jitteriness, seizures, cyanosis, vomiting, and myocardial depression, some of which are similar to the signs of hypoglycemia. Hypocalcemic infants have increased muscle tone, which helps differentiate infants with hypocalcemia from those with hypoglycemia. Ionized calcium levels are easily determined in most intensive care settings. Symptomatic hypocalcemia is treated with 10% calcium gluconate administered IV at a dosage of 1 to 2 mL/kg over a 10-minute period while monitoring the electrocardiogram. Asymptomatic hypocalcemia is best treated with calcium gluconate in a dose of 50 mg of elemental calcium/kg/day added to the maintenance fluid: 1 mL of 10% calcium gluconate contains 9 mg of elemental calcium. Calcium mixed with sodium bicarbonate forms an insoluble precipitate. If possible, parenteral calcium should be given through a central venous line.

Magnesium

Magnesium is actively transported across the placenta. Half of total body magnesium is in the plasma and soft tissues. Hypomagnesemia is observed with growth retardation, with maternal diabetes, after exchange transfusions, and with hypoparathyroidism. Magnesium and calcium metabolism are interrelated. The same infants at risk for hypocalcemia also are at risk for hypomagnesemia. Whenever an infant who has seizures that are believed to be associated with hypocalcemia does not respond to calcium therapy, magnesium deficiency should be suspected and confirmed by obtaining a serum magnesium level. Emergency treatment consists of magnesium sulfate solution, 25 to 50 mg/kg IV every 6 hours, until normal levels are obtained.

Blood Volume

Total RBC volume is at its highest point at delivery. Estimation of blood volume for premature infants, term neonates, and infants are summarized in Table 1-2. By about 3 months of age, total blood volume per kilogram is nearly equal to adult levels. The newborn blood volume is affected by shifts of blood between the placenta and the baby before clamping the cord. Infants with delayed cord

TABLE 1-2 ESTIMATION OF BLOOD VOLUME	
Group	Blood Volume (mL/kg)
Premature infants	85–100
Term newborns	85
>1 mo	75
3 mo–adult	70

Adapted from Rowe PC (ed): The Harriet Lane Handbook (11th ed). Chicago, Year Book Medical, 1987, p 25.

clamping have higher hemoglobin levels.[4] A hematocrit greater than 50% suggests that placental transfusion has occurred.

Polycythemia

A central venous hemoglobin level greater than 22 g/dL or a hematocrit value greater than 65% during the first week of life is defined as polycythemia. After the central venous hematocrit value reaches 65%, further increases result in rapid exponential increases in blood viscosity. Neonatal polycythemia occurs in infants of diabetic mothers, infants of mothers with toxemia of pregnancy, or SGA infants. Polycythemia is treated by using a partial exchange of the infant's blood with fresh whole blood or 5% albumin. This is frequently done for hematocrit greater than 65%. Capillary hematocrits are poor predictors of viscosity; therefore decisions to perform exchange transfusions should be based on central hematocrits only.

Anemia

Anemia present at birth is due to hemolysis, blood loss, or decreased erythrocyte production.

HEMOLYTIC ANEMIA. Hemolytic anemia is most often a result of placental transfer of maternal antibodies that are destroying the infant's erythrocytes. This can be determined by the direct Coombs' test. The most common severe anemia is Rh incompatibility. Hemolytic disease in the newborn produces jaundice, pallor, and hepatosplenomegaly. The most severely affected infants manifest hydrops. This massive edema is not strictly related to the hemoglobin level of this infant. ABO incompatibility frequently results in hyperbilirubinemia but rarely causes anemia.

Congenital infections, hemoglobinopathies (sickle cell disease), and thalassemias produce hemolytic anemia. In a severely affected infant with a positive-reacting direct Coombs' test result, a cord hemoglobin level of less than 10.5 g/dL, or a cord bilirubin level of greater than 4.5 mg/dL, immediate exchange transfusion is indicated. For less severely affected infants, exchange transfusion is indicated when total indirect bilirubin level is greater than 20 mg/dL.

HEMORRHAGIC ANEMIA. Significant anemia can develop from hemorrhage that occurs during placental abruption.

Internal bleeding (intraventricular, subgaleal, mediastinal, intra-abdominal) in infants also can often lead to severe anemia. Usually, hemorrhage occurs immediately during delivery, and the baby occasionally requires transfusion. Twin-twin transfusion reactions can produce polycythemia in one baby and profound anemia in the other. Severe cases can lead to death in the donor and hydrops in the recipient.

ANEMIA OF PREMATURITY. Decreased RBC production frequently contributes to anemia of prematurity. Erythropoietin is not released until a gestational age of 30 to 34 weeks has been reached. These infants, however, have large numbers of erythropoietin-sensitive RBC progenitors. Research has focused on the role of recombinant erythropoietin (Epogen) in treating anemia in preterm infants.[5-7] Successful increases in hematocrit levels with Epogen may obviate the need for blood transfusions and reduce the risk of blood-borne infections and reactions. Studies suggest that routine use of Epogen is probably helpful for the very low-birth-weight infant (< 750 g), but its regular use for other preterm infants is not likely to reduce the transfusion rate significantly.

Hemoglobin

At birth, nearly 80% of circulating hemoglobin is fetal ($a_2{}^A\gamma_2{}^F$). When infant erythropoiesis resumes at about age 2 to 3 months, most new hemoglobin is adult. When the oxygen level is 27 mm Hg, 50% of the bound oxygen is released from adult hemoglobin (P-50). Therefore the P-50 of adult hemoglobin is 27 mm Hg. Reduction of hemoglobin's affinity for oxygen allows more oxygen to be released into the tissues at a given oxygen level.

Fetal hemoglobin has a P-50 value 6- to 8-mm Hg higher than that of adult hemoglobin. This higher P-50 value allows more efficient oxygen delivery from the placenta to the fetal tissues. In this situation, the hemoglobin equilibrium curve is considered to be shifted to the left of normal. This increase in P-50 is thought to be due to the failure of fetal hemoglobin to bind 2,3-diphosphoglycerate to the same degree as does adult hemoglobin.[8] This is something of a disadvantage to the newborn because lower peripheral oxygen levels are needed before oxygen is released from fetal hemoglobin. By age 4 to 6 months in a term infant, the hemoglobin equilibrium curve gradually shifts to the right, and the P-50 value approximates that of a normal adult.

Jaundice

In the hepatocyte, bilirubin created by hemolysis is conjugated to glucuronic acid and rendered water soluble. This conjugated or direct bilirubin is excreted in bile. Without this mechanism of conjugation, unconjugated bilirubin acts as a neural cell poison, interfering with cellular respiration. This neural damage is termed *kernicterus* and produces athetoid cerebral palsy, seizures, sensorineural hearing loss, and, rarely, death.

The newborn's liver has a metabolic excretory capacity for bilirubin that is not equal to its task. Even healthy

TABLE 1-3
CAUSES OF PROLONGED INDIRECT HYPERBILIRUBINEMIA

Breast milk jaundice	Pyloric stenosis
Hemolytic disease	Crigler-Najjar syndrome
Hypothyroidism	Extravascular blood

Data from Maisels MJ: Neonatal jaundice. In Avery GB (ed): Neonatology. Pathophysiology and Management of the Newborn. Philadelphia, JB Lippincott, 1987, p 566.

term infants usually have elevated unconjugated bilirubin levels. This peaks about the third day of life at approximately 6.5 to 7.0 mg/dL and does not return to normal until the tenth day of life. A total bilirubin level greater than 7 mg/dL in the first 24 hours or greater than 13 mg/dL at any time in term newborns often prompts an investigation for the cause. Breast-fed infants usually have serum bilirubin levels 1 to 2 mg/dL greater than formula-fed babies. The common causes of prolonged indirect hyperbilirubinemia are listed in Table 1-3.

Pathologic jaundice within the first 36 hours of life is usually due to excessive production of bilirubin. Hyperbilirubinemia is managed based on the infant's weight. Phototherapy is initiated for newborns (1) weighing less than 1500 g, when the serum bilirubin level reaches 5 mg/dL; (2) 1500 to 2000 g, when the serum bilirubin level reaches 8 mg/dL; or (3) 2000 to 2500 g, when the serum bilirubin level reaches 10 mg/dL. Formula-fed term infants without hemolytic disease are treated with phototherapy when levels reach 13 mg/dL. For hemolytic-related hyperbilirubinemia, phototherapy is recommended when the serum bilirubin level exceeds 10 mg/dL by 12 hours of life, 12 mg/dL by 18 hours, 14 mg/dL by 24 hours, or 15 mg/dL by 36 hours.[9] An absolute bilirubin level that triggers exchange transfusion is still not established, but most exchange-transfusion decisions are based on the serum bilirubin level and its rate of increase.

Retinopathy of Prematurity

Retinopathy of prematurity (ROP) develops during the active phases of retinal vascular development in the first 3 or 4 months of life. The exact causes are unknown, but oxygen exposure and extreme prematurity are the only risk factors that have been repeatedly and convincingly demonstrated. The risk of ROP is probably related to the degree of immaturity, length of exposure, and oxygen concentration. ROP is found in 1.9% of premature infants in large neonatal units.[10] Retrolental fibroplasia (RLF) is the pathologic change observed in the retina and overlying vitreous after the acute phases of ROP subside. A study conducted by the National Institutes of Health found that cryotherapy was effective in preventing retinal detachment, macular fold, and RLF.[11]

American Academy of Pediatrics guidelines recommend that all infants who received oxygen therapy who weigh less than 1800 g and are fewer than 35 weeks' gestation and any infants who weigh less than 1300 g and are fewer than 30 weeks' gestation should undergo an ophthalmologic examination to rule out ROP.[12] Babies younger than 4 to 6 weeks often have a vitreous haze that may obscure the view of the retina. An examination at age 7 to 9 weeks is more likely to be reliable.

Thermoregulation

A homeotherm is a mammal that can maintain a constant deep body temperature. Although human beings are homeothermic, newborns have difficulty maintaining constant deep body temperature because of their relatively large surface area, poor thermal regulation, and small mass to act as a heat sink. Heat loss may occur owing to (1) evaporation (a wet baby or a baby in contact with a wet surface), (2) conduction (direct skin contact with a cool surface), (3) convection (air currents blowing over the baby), and (4) radiation (the baby radiates heat to a cooler surface not in contact with him or her).

Of these, radiation is the most difficult to control. Infants produce heat by increasing metabolic activity, either by shivering like an adult or by nonshivering thermogenesis, by using brown fat. Brown-fat thermogenesis may be rendered inactive by vasopressors, by anesthetic agents, and through nutritional depletion.[13-15] *Thermoneutrality* (the optimal thermal environment for the newborn) is the range of ambient temperatures in which the newborn with a normal body temperature and a minimal metabolic rate can maintain a constant body temperature by vasomotor control. The *critical temperature* is the temperature below which a metabolic response to cold is necessary to replace lost heat. The appropriate incubator temperature is determined by the patient's weight and postnatal age (Figs. 1-2 and 1-3). For low-birth-weight infants, thermoneutrality is approximately 34°C to 35°C up to age 6 weeks and 31°C to 32°C until

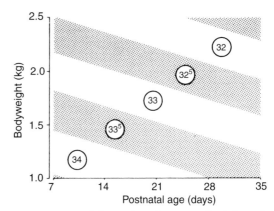

FIGURE 1-3. Neutral thermal environment (°C) from day 7 to 35. Dew point of air, 18°C; flow, 10 L/min. Body weight is current weight. Values for body weight > 2.0 kg are calculated by extrapolation. (From Sauer PJJ, Dane HJ, Visser HKA: New standards for neutral thermal environment of healthy very low birthweight infants in week one of life. Arch Dis Child 59:18–22, 1984.)

age 12 weeks. Infants who weigh 2 to 3 kg have a thermoneutrality zone of 31°C to 34°C on the first day of life and 29°C to 31°C until 12 days. Double-walled incubators offer the best thermoneutral environment. Radiant warmers cannot prevent convection heat loss and lead to higher insensible water loss.

Failure to maintain thermoneutrality leads to serious metabolic and physiological consequences. Special care must be exercised to maintain the body temperature within normal limits in the operating room.

Fluids and Electrolytes

At 12 weeks of gestation, the fetus has a total body water content that is 94% of body weight. This amount decreases to 80% by 32 weeks' gestation and 78% by term (Fig. 1-4). A further 3% to 5% reduction in total body water content occurs in the first 3 to 5 days of life. Body water continues to decline and reaches adult levels (approximately 60% of body weight) by age 1½ years. Extracellular water also declines by age 1 to 3 years. These water-composition changes progress in an orderly fashion in utero. Premature delivery requires the newborn to complete both fetal and term water-unloading tasks. Surprisingly, the premature infant can complete fetal water unloading by 1 week after birth. Postnatal reduction in extracellular fluid volume has such a high physiological priority that it occurs even in the presence of relatively large variations of fluid intake.[16]

Glomerular Filtration Rate

The glomerular filtration rate (GFR) of newborns is slower than that of adults.[17] From 21 mL/min/1.73 m² at birth in the term infant, GFR quickly increases to 60 mL/min/1.73 m² by age 2 weeks. GFR reaches adult levels by age 1½ to 2 years. A preterm infant has a GFR that is only slightly slower than that of a term infant. In addition to this difference in GFR, the concentrating

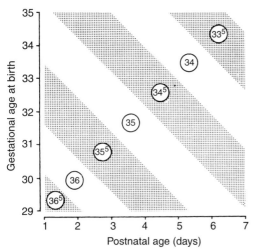

FIGURE 1-2. Neutral thermal environment (°C) during the first week of life calculated from these measurements: dew point of the air, 18°C; flow, 10 L/min. (From Sauer PJJ, Dane HJ, Visser HKA: New standards for neutral thermal environment of healthy very low birthweight infants in week one of life. Arch Dis Child 59:18–22, 1984.)

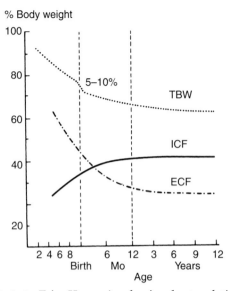

% Body weight

FIGURE 1-4. Friss-Hansen's classic chart relating total body weight (TBW) and extracellular (ECF) and intracellular fluid (ICF) to percentage of body weight, from early gestation to adolescence. (Adapted from Welch KJ, Randolph JG, Ravitch MM, et al. (eds): Pediatric Surgery, 4th ed. Chicago, Year Book Medical, 1986, p 24.)

capacity of the preterm and the term infant is well below that of the adult. An infant responding to water deprivation increases urine osmolarity to a maximum of only 600 mOsm/kg. This is in contrast to the adult, whose urine concentration can reach 1200 mOsm/kg. It appears that the difference in concentrating capacity is due to the insensitivity of the collecting tubules of the newborn to antidiuretic hormone. Although the newborn cannot concentrate urine as efficiently as the adult, the newborn can excrete very dilute urine at 30 to 50 mOsm/kg. Newborns are unable to excrete excess sodium, an inability thought to be due to a tubular defect. Term babies are able to conserve sodium, but premature infants are considered "salt wasters" because they have an inappropriate urinary sodium excretion, even with restricted sodium intake.

Insensible Water Loss

Insensible water loss from the lungs can be essentially eliminated by humidification of inspired air. Transepithelial water loss occurs by the diffusion of water molecules through the stratum corneum of the skin. Because of the immature skin, preterm infants of 25 to 27 weeks' gestation can lose more than 120 mL H_2O/kg/day by this mechanism. Transepithelial water loss decreases as age increases.

Neonatal Fluid Requirements

To estimate fluid requirements in the newborn requires an understanding of (1) preexisting fluid deficit or excess, (2) metabolic demands, and (3) losses.

Because these factors change quickly in the critically ill newborn, frequent adjustments in fluid management are necessary. Hourly monitoring of intake and output allows early recognition of fluid balance that will affect treatment decisions. This dynamic approach requires two components: an initial hourly fluid intake that is safe and a monitoring system to detect the patient's response to the treatment program selected. A table of initial volumes expressed in rates of milliliters per kilogram per 24 hours for various surgical conditions has been developed as a result of a study of a large group of infants monitored during their first 3 postoperative days (Table 1-4). The patients were divided into three groups, according to conditions: moderate surgical conditions, such as colostomies, laparotomies, and intestinal atresia; severe surgical conditions, such as midgut volvulus or gastroschisis; and necrotizing enterocolitis with perforation of the bowel or bowel necrosis requiring exploration.

No "normal" urine output exists for a given neonate. Ideal urine output can be estimated by measuring the osmolar load presented to the kidney for excretion and calculating the amount of urine necessary to clear this load, if the urine is maintained at an isotonic level of 280 mOsm/dL (Table 1-5).

After administering the initial hourly volume for 4 to 8 hours, depending on the patient's condition, the newborn is reassessed by observing urine output and concentration. With these two factors, it is possible to determine the state of hydration of most neonates and their responses to the initial volume. In more difficult cases, changes in serial serum sodium (Na), blood urea nitrogen (BUN), creatinine, and osmolarity, along with urine Na, creatinine, and osmolarity, make it possible to assess the infant's response to the initial volume and to use fluid status to guide the next 4 to 8 hours' fluid intake.

Illustrative Examples

INSUFFICIENT FLUID. A 1-kg premature infant, during the first 8 hours after surgery, has 0.3 mL/kg/hr of urine output. Specific gravity is 1.025. Previous initial volume was 5 mL/kg/hr. Serum BUN has increased from 4 mg/dL to 8 mg/dL; hematocrit value has increased from 35%

TABLE 1-4			
NEWBORN FLUID VOLUME REQUIREMENTS (mL/kg/24 h) FOR VARIOUS SURGICAL CONDITIONS			
Group	Day 1	Day 2	Day 3
Moderate surgical conditions (e.g., colostomies, laparotomies for intestinal atresia, Hirschsprung's disease)	80 ± 25	80 ± 30	80 ± 30
Severe surgical conditions (e.g., gastroschisis, midgut volvulus, meconium peritonitis)	140 ± 45	90 ± 20	80 ± 15
Necrotizing enterocolitis with perforation	145 ± 70	135 ± 50	130 ± 40

TABLE 1-5

MINIMUM NEWBORN IDEAL URINE OUTPUT (mL/kg/h) FOR VARIOUS SURGICAL CONDITIONS

Group	Day 1	Day 2	Day 3
Moderate surgical conditions (e.g., colostomies, laparotomies for intestinal atresia, Hirschsprung's disease)	2 ± 0.96	2.63 ± 1.71	2.38 ± 0.92
Severe surgical conditions (e.g., gastroschisis, midgut volvulus, meconium peritonitis)	2.67 ± 0.92	2.96 ± 0.54	2.96 ± 1.0
Necrotizing enterocolitis with perforation	2.58 ± 1.04	3.17 ± 1.67	3.46 ± 1.46

to 37%, without transfusion. This child is dry. The treatment is to increase the hourly volume to 7 mL/kg/hr for the next 4 hours and to monitor the subsequent urine output and concentration to reassess fluid status.

INAPPROPRIATE ANTIDIURETIC HORMONE RESPONSE. A 3-kg newborn with congenital diaphragmatic hernia during the first 8 hours after surgery has a 0.2 mL/kg/hr of urine output, with a urine osmolarity of 360 mOsm/L. The previous initial volume was 120 mL/kg/day (15 mL/hr). The serum osmolarity value has decreased from 300 mOsm before surgery to 278 mOsm/L; BUN, from 12 mg/dL to 8 mg/dL. The inappropriate antidiuretic hormone response requires reduction in fluid volume from 120 mL/kg/day to 90 mL/kg/day for the next 4 to 8 hours. Repeated urine and serum measurements will allow the further adjustment of fluid administration.

OVERHYDRATION. A 3-kg baby, 24 hours after operative closure of gastroschisis, had an average urine output of 3 mL/kg/hr for the past 4 hours. During that period, the infant received fluids at a rate of 180 mL/kg/day. The specific gravity of the urine has decreased to 1.006; serum BUN is 4 mg/dL; hematocrit value is 30%, down from 35% before surgery. The total serum protein concentration is 4.0 mg/dL, down from 4.5 mg/dL. This child is being overhydrated. The treatment is to decrease the fluids to 3 mL/kg/hr for the next 4 hours and then to reassess urine output and concentration.

RENAL FAILURE. A 5-kg infant with severe sepsis secondary to Hirschsprung's enterocolitis has had a urine output of 0.1 mL/kg/hr for the past 8 hours. The specific gravity is 1.012; serum sodium, 150; BUN, 25 mg/dL; creatinine, 1.5 mg/dL; urine sodium, 130; and urine creatinine, 20 mg/dL.

Fractional Na Excretion (FE Na)

$$\frac{Ur\ Na \times Pl\ Cr}{Pl\ Na \times Ur\ Cr} = \frac{130 \times 1.5}{150 \times 20}$$

FE Na = 193/3000 × 100

FE Na = 6.5% (normal = 2% to 3%)

FE Na less than 2% usually indicates a prerenal cause of oliguria, whereas greater than 3% usually implies a renal cause (acute tubular necrosis; ATN). This patient is in acute renal failure. The plan is to restrict fluids to insensible losses plus measured losses for the next 4 hours and to then reassess the plan by using both urine and serum studies.

PULMONARY SYSTEM OF THE NEWBORN

The dichotomous branching of the bronchial tree is usually completed by 16 weeks' gestation. No actual alveoli are seen until 24 to 26 weeks' gestation. Therefore the air–blood surface area for gas diffusion is limited should the fetus be delivered at this age. Between 24 and 28 weeks, the cuboidal and columnar cells become flatter and start differentiating into type I (lining cells) and/or type II (granular) pneumocytes. Between 26 and 32 weeks of gestation, terminal air sacs begin to give way to air spaces. From 32 to 36 weeks, further budding of these air spaces occurs, and alveoli become numerous. At the same time, the phospholipids that constitute pulmonary surfactant begin to line the terminal lung air spaces. Surfactant is produced by type II pneumocytes and is extremely important in maintaining alveolar stability.

The change in the ratio of the amniotic phospholipids, lecithin, and sphingomyelin is used to assess fetal lung maturity. A ratio greater than 2 is considered compatible with mature lung function. Absence of adequate surfactant leads to HMD or respiratory distress syndrome. HMD is present in nearly 10% of all premature infants and is the leading cause of morbidity and mortality (30%) among premature infants in the United States. Other conditions associated with pulmonary distress in the newborn include delayed fetal lung absorption (wet lung syndrome), intrauterine aspiration pneumonia (meconium aspiration), and intrapartum pneumonia. In all of these conditions, endotracheal intubation and mechanical ventilation may be required for hypoxia, CO_2 retention, or apnea. Ventilator options and management are discussed in Chapter 7.

Surfactant

Surfactant deficiency is believed to be the major cause of HMD. Surfactant-replacement therapy improves effective oxygenation. Three surfactant preparations have been under investigation: (1) surfactant derived from bovine or porcine lung, (2) human surfactant extracted from amniotic fluid, and (3) artificial surfactant. Multicenter-based, randomized trials for modified bovine surfactant (Survanta)[18] and artificial surfactant (Exosurf Neonatal)[19] have been published.

In one study in 1990, Survanta was given as a single dose via an endotracheal tube an average of 12 minutes after birth. The patients who received this bovine surfactant demonstrated less severe radiographic changes at age 24 hours compared with infants who received placebo. No difference occurred in clinical status 7 and 28 days after treatment compared with placebo.

In the Exosurf Neonatal study of 1991, the premature infants were randomized to receive one dose of the artificial surfactant or air placebo. In this study, a significant reduction was noted in the surfactant-treated infants compared with the control group in all of the following: number of deaths attributed to HMD, incidence of pulmonary air leaks, oxygen requirements, and mean airway pressure.

An uncontrolled case series also was reported in which surfactant was given to term newborns with pneumonia and meconium aspiration, with a significant improvement in oxygenation after treatment.[20] Although these and other reports are promising, more studies are needed to determine the most effective dose, the number of doses, and the best timing for surfactant treatment. Surfactant therapy is an important addition to the pulmonary care of the preterm newborn.

One recent multicenter study reported that surfactant therapy early in the course of term newborn respiratory failure resulted in a significantly lower requirement for extracorporeal membrane oxygenation and produced no additional morbidity. Several recent multicenter studies compared the efficacy and complication rates of synthetic versus calf-lung cannula surfactant therapies for neonatal respiratory failure.[21–24]

Results from one study suggest that a calf-lung surfactant preparation (Infasurf) is preferred to synthetic, owing to reduced incidence of RDS, severity of early pulmonary disease, development of air leaks, and overall mortality from RDS. However, calf-lung surfactant was associated with a greater risk of developing an intraventricular hemorrhage. Other studies reported that calf-lung surfactants produce more rapid onset of effects but noted no significant difference in the rate of complications compared with those with synthetic surfactants. However, support exists for the synthetic surfactant preparations. This support is based on the theoretical advantage of a possibly reduced risk of intraventricular hemorrhage, less exposure to animal antigen with subsequent reactions, and lower overall cost. Future studies may provide additional insight into the appropriate applications of the available agents.

Monitoring

Continuous monitoring of physiological indices provides data that assist in assessing response to therapy and trends that may be used to predict catastrophe. Many episodes of "sudden deterioration" in critically ill patients are viewed, in retrospect, as changes in clinical condition that had been occurring for some time.

Arterial Blood Gases and Derived Indices

Arterial oxygen tension (Pa_{O_2}) is measured, most commonly, by obtaining an arterial blood sample and by measuring the partial pressure of oxygen with a polarographic electrode. Defining normal parameters for Pa_{O_2} depends on the maturation and age of the patient. In the term newborn, the general definition for hypoxia is a Pa_{O_2} less than 55 mm Hg, whereas hyperoxia is greater than 80 mm Hg.

Capillary blood samples are "arterialized" by topical vasodilators or heat to increase blood flow to a peripheral site. Blood must be freely flowing and collected quickly to prevent exposure to the atmosphere. Blood flowing sluggishly and exposed to atmospheric oxygen falsely increases the Pa_{O_2} from a capillary sample, especially in the 40- to 60-mm Hg range.[25] Capillary blood pH and carbon dioxide tension (Pc_{O_2}) correlate well with arterial samples, except when perfusion is poor. Pa_{O_2} is the least reliable of all capillary blood gas determinations. In patients receiving oxygen therapy in whom arterial Pa_{O_2} exceeds 60 mm Hg, the capillary Pa_{O_2} correlates poorly with the arterial measurement.[26,27]

In newborns, umbilical artery catheterization provides arterial access. The catheter tip should rest at the level of the diaphragm or below L3. The second frequently used arterial site is the radial artery. Complications of arterial blood sampling include repeated blood loss and anemia. Changes in oxygenation are such that intermittent blood gas sampling may miss critical episodes of hypoxia or hyperoxia. Because of the drawbacks of ex vivo monitoring, several in vivo monitoring systems have been used.

Pulse Oximetry

The noninvasive determination of oxygen saturation (Sa_{O_2}) gives moment-to-moment information regarding the availability of O_2 to the tissues. If the Pa_{O_2} is plotted against the oxygen saturation of hemoglobin, the S-shaped hemoglobin dissociation curve is obtained (Fig. 1-5). Referring to this curve, hemoglobin is 50% saturated at 25 mm Hg Pa_{O_2} and 90% saturated at 50 mm Hg. Pulse oximetry has a rapid (5- to 7-second) response time, requires no calibration, and may be left in place continuously.

Pulse oximetry is not possible if the patient is in shock, has peripheral vasospasm, or has vascular constriction due to hypothermia. Inaccurate readings may occur in the presence of jaundice, direct high-intensity light, dark skin pigmentation, and greater than 80% fetal hemoglobin. Oximetry is not a sensitive guide to gas exchange in patients with high Pa_{O_2} because of the shape of the oxygen dissociation curve. On the upper horizontal portion of the curve, large changes in Pa_{O_2} may occur with little change in Sa_{O_2}. An oximeter reading of 95% could represent a Pa_{O_2} between 60 and 160 mm Hg.

A study to compare pulse oximetry with Pa_{O_2} determined from indwelling arterial catheters has shown that Sa_{O_2} greater than or equal to 85% corresponds to a Pa_{O_2} greater than 55 mm Hg, and saturations less than or equal to 90% correspond with a Pa_{O_2} less than 80 mm Hg.[28] Guidelines for monitoring infants by using pulse

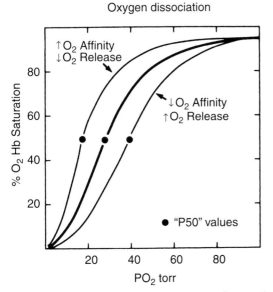

Oxygen dissociation

↑O$_2$ Affinity
↓O$_2$ Release

↓O$_2$ Affinity
↑O$_2$ Release

● "P50" values

PO$_2$ torr

FIGURE 1-5. The oxygen dissociation curve of normal adult blood. The P-50, the oxygen tension at 50% oxygen saturation, is ~27 mm Hg (torr). As the curve shifts to the right, the oxygen affinity of hemoglobin decreases, and more oxygen is released at a given oxygen tension. With a shift to the left, the opposite effects are observed. A decrease in pH or an increase in temperature reduces the affinity of hemoglobin for oxygen. (From Blancette V, Zipursky A: Neonatal hematology. In Avery GB [ed]: Neonatology. Philadelphia, JB Lippincott, 1987, p 663.)

oximetry have been suggested for the following three conditions:

1. In the infant with acute respiratory distress without direct arterial access, saturation limits of 85% (lower) and 92% (upper) should be set.
2. In the older infant with chronic respiratory distress who is at low risk for ROP, the upper saturation limit may be set at 95%; the lower limit should be set at 87% to avoid pulmonary vasoconstriction and pulmonary hypertension.
3. Because the concentration of fetal hemoglobin in newborns affects the accuracy of pulse oximetry, infants with arterial access should have both PaO$_2$ and SaO$_2$ monitored closely. A graph should be kept at the bedside documenting the SaO$_2$ each time the PaO$_2$ is measured. Limits for the SaO$_2$ alarm can be changed because the characteristics of this relation change.

Carbon Dioxide Tension

Arterial carbon dioxide tension (PaCO$_2$) is a direct reflection of gas exchange in the lungs and of the metabolic rate. In most clinical situations, changes in PaCO$_2$ are due to changes in ventilation. For this reason, serial measurement of PaCO$_2$ is a practical method to assess the adequacy of ventilation. The discrepancy among venous, capillary, and arterial carbon dioxide tensions is not great under most conditions, although one study noted a significant increase in PaCO$_2$ in venous samples compared with simultaneous arterial samples.[29]

Because it is possible to monitor PaCO$_2$ and pH satisfactorily with venous or capillary blood samples and because pulse oximetry is now commonly used to assess oxygenation, many infants with respiratory insufficiency no longer require arterial catheters for monitoring.

End-Tidal Carbon Dioxide

Measuring expired CO$_2$ by capnography provides a non-invasive means of continuously monitoring alveolar PCO$_2$. Capnometry measures CO$_2$ by an infrared sensor placed either in line between the ventilator circuit and the endotracheal tube, or off to the side of the air flow, both of which are applicable only to the intubated patient. A comparative study of end-tidal carbon dioxide in critically ill neonates demonstrated that both side-stream and mainstream end-tidal carbon dioxide measurements approximated PaCO$_2$.[30] When the mainstream sensor was inserted into the breathing circuit, the PaCO$_2$ increased an average of 2 mm Hg. Although this is not likely to affect significantly infants who are ventilated, it might create fatigue in weaning infants from mechanical ventilation. The accuracy of the end-tidal carbon dioxide is diminished with small endotracheal tubes.

Central Venous Catheter

Indications for central venous catheter placement include (1) hemodynamic monitoring, (2) inability to establish other venous access, (3) TPN, and (4) infusion of inotropic drugs or other medications that cannot be given peripherally. Measuring central venous pressure (CVP) to monitor volume status is frequently used in the resuscitation of a critically ill patient. A catheter placed in the superior vena cava or right atrium measures the filling pressure of the right side of the heart, which usually reflects left atrial and filling pressure of the left ventricle. Often a wide discrepancy exists between left and right atrial pressure when pulmonary disease, overwhelming sepsis, or cardiac lesions are present. To use the monitor effectively, continuous measurements must be taken with a pressure transducer connected to a catheter accurately placed in the central venous system. Positive-pressure ventilation, pneumothorax, abdominal distention, or pericardial tamponade all elevate CVP.

Pulmonary Artery

The pulmonary artery pressure catheter has altered the care of the child with severe cardiopulmonary derangement by allowing direct measurement of cardiovascular variables at the bedside. The indications for pulmonary catheter placement are listed in Table 1-6. With this catheter, it is possible to monitor CVP, pulmonary artery pressure, pulmonary wedge pressure, and cardiac output. A 4F, double-lumen catheter and a 5F to 8F, triple-lumen catheter are available. The catheter is usually placed by percutaneous methods (as in the adult), except in the smallest pediatric patient, in whom a cutdown is sometimes required.

Adapted from Perkin RM: Invasive monitoring in the pediatric intensive care unit. In Nussbaum E (ed): Pediatric Intensive Care (2nd ed). Mt. Kisco, NY, Futura Publishing, 1989, p 259.

TABLE 1-6
INDICATIONS FOR PULMONARY ARTERY CATHETER PLACEMENT
Inadequate systemic perfusion in the presence of elevated central venous pressure
Fluid management in noncardiogenic pulmonary edema
Evaluation of therapeutic interventions, such as changes in positive end-expiratory pressure, use of vasoactive drugs, or assisted circulation
Hemodynamic evaluation in children with pulmonary hypertension
Severe pulmonary disease with profound hypoxemia

When the tip of the catheter is in a distal pulmonary artery and the balloon is inflated, the resulting pressure is generally an accurate reflection of left atrial pressure because the pulmonary veins have no valves. This pulmonary "wedge" pressure represents left ventricular filling pressure, which is used as a reflection of preload. The monitors display phasic pressures, but treatment decisions are made based on the electronically derived mean CVP. A low pulmonary wedge pressure suggests that blood volume must be expanded. A high or normal pulmonary wedge pressure in the presence of continued signs of shock suggests left ventricular dysfunction.

Cardiac output is usually measured in liters per minute. When related to body surface area, the output is represented as the *cardiac index,* which is simply the cardiac output divided by the body surface area. The normalized cardiac index allows the evaluation of cardiac performance without regard to body size. The usual resting value for cardiac index is between 3.5 and 4.5 $L/min/m^2$. The determination of cardiac output by the thermodilution technique, which is possible with a Swan-Ganz pulmonary artery catheter, is widely used and has a good correlation with other methods. Accurate cardiac output determination depends on rapid injection, accurate measurement of the injectant temperatures and volume, and absence of shunting. Because ventilation affects the flow into and out of the right ventricle, three injections should be made at a consistent point in the ventilatory cycle, typically at end-expiration.

Doppler measurement of aortic flow velocity allows measurement of cardiac output by the following formula:

$$\text{Cardiac output (mL/min)} = \text{Mean aortic blood flow velocity (cm/sec)} \times \text{Aortic cross-sectional area (cm}^2) \times 60$$

Aortic cross-sectional area is determined with standard ultrasonographic techniques. With this cross-sectional measurement, pulsed Doppler aortic flow velocity is measured by a transducer placed at the suprasternal notch, in the esophagus, or in the trachea, with a specially modified endotracheal tube, to derive cardiac output. Studies are under way to determine whether cardiac output measured by this technique correlates well with thermodilution or the Fick method in critically ill pediatric patients. Previous studies have shown that cardiac output measured with intermittent Doppler measurement at the suprasternal notch was not of sufficient reliability to be used for hemodynamic monitoring in critically ill children.[31]

Impedance cardiography (bioimpedance) is another noninvasive technique that measures stroke volume on a beat-by-beat basis.[32] Bioimpedance uses a low-level current applied to the thorax, where changes in the volume and velocity of blood flow in the thoracic aorta result in detectable changes in thoracic conductivity. Previous application of this technique in critically ill patients met with only limited success.[33] Late refinements in electrode configuration, algorithms, and microprocessors have produced more acceptable results. A 1990 study in pigs demonstrated a good correlation of bioimpedance-derived cardiac output with thermodilutional cardiac output over a wide hemodynamic range.[34] These techniques have yet to be proved effective in children.

Another study concluded that using right heart catheters in treating critically ill adult patients resulted in an increased mortality.[35] However, a consensus committee report documented the continued safety and efficacy of right heart catheters in the care of critically ill children.[36]

Venous Oximetry

Mixed venous oxygen saturation (Svo_2) is an indicator of the adequacy of oxygen supply and of the demand in perfused tissues. Oxygen consumption is defined as the amount of oxygen consumed by the tissue, as calculated by the Fick equation:

$$O_2 \text{ Consumption} = \text{Cardiac output} \times \text{Arterial-venous oxygen content difference}$$

Reflectance spectrophotometry is currently used for continuous venous oximetry. Multiple wavelengths of light are transmitted at a known intensity by means of fiberoptic bundles in a special pulmonary artery or right atrial catheter. The light is reflected by RBCs flowing past the tip of the catheter. The wavelengths of light are chosen so that both oxyhemoglobin and deoxyhemoglobin are measured to determine the fraction of hemoglobin saturated with oxygen. The system requires either in vitro calibration by reflecting light from a standardized target that represents a known oxygen saturation or in vivo calibration by withdrawing blood from the pulmonary artery catheter and measuring the saturation by laboratory co-oximetry.

Mixed venous oxygen saturation values within the normal range (68% to 77%) indicate a normal balance between oxygen supply and demand, provided that vasoregulation is intact and distribution of peripheral blood flow is normal. Values greater than 77% are most commonly associated with syndromes of vasoregulation, such as sepsis. Uncompensated changes in O_2 saturation, hemoglobin level, or cardiac output lead to a decrease in $Svo_2.$ A sustained decrease in Svo_2 greater than 10% should lead to measuring SaO_2, hemoglobin level, and cardiac output to determine the cause of the decline.[37] The most common sources of error in measuring SvO_2 are calibration and catheter malposition. The most important concept in SvO_2 monitoring is the advantage of continuous monitoring, which allows early warning of a developing problem.[38]

Although most clinical experience has been with pulmonary artery catheters, right atrial catheters are more easily placed and may thus provide better information to detect hemodynamic deterioration earlier and permit more rapid treatment of physiological derangements.[39] A study has shown that, when oxygen consumption was monitored and maintained at a consistent level, the right atrial venous saturation was thought to be an excellent monitoring device.[40]

SHOCK

Shock is a state in which the cardiac output is insufficient to deliver adequate oxygen to meet metabolic demands of the tissues. Cardiovascular function is determined by preload, cardiac contractility, heart rate, and afterload. Shock may be classified broadly as hypovolemic, cardiogenic, or septic.

Hypovolemic Shock

Preload represents the volume of blood presented to the ventricles. Preload is a function of blood volume. Due to the impracticality of measuring volume, preload is commonly monitored by atrial pressure measurements. In most clinical situations, right atrial pressure or CVP is the index of cardiac preload. In situations in which left ventricular or right ventricular compliance is abnormal or in certain forms of congenital heart disease, right atrial pressure may not correlate well with left atrial pressure. In infants and children, most shock situations are the result of reduced preload secondary to fluid loss, such as from diarrhea, vomiting, or trauma.

Virtually all forms of pediatric shock have significant intravascular and functional interstitial fluid deficits. Hypovolemia results in decreased venous return to the heart. Preload is reduced, cardiac output decreases, and the overall result is a decrease in tissue perfusion. Invasive infection and hypovolemia are the most common causes of shock in both children and adults. The first step in treating all forms of shock is to correct existing fluid deficits. Inotropic drugs should not be initiated until adequate intravascular fluid volume has been established. The speed and volume of the infusate are determined by the patient's responses, particularly changes in blood pressure, pulse rate, urine output, and CVP. Shock resulting from acute hemorrhage is treated with the administration of 10 to 20 mL/kg of Ringer's lactate solution or normal saline as a fluid bolus. If the patient does not respond, a second bolus of crystalloid is given. Type-specific or cross-matched blood is given, when available.

The choice of resuscitation fluid in shock that results from sepsis or from loss of extracellular fluid (conditions such as peritonitis, intestinal obstruction, and pancreatitis) is less clear. Our initial resuscitation fluids include Ringer's lactate or normal saline in older infants and children and half-strength Ringer's or half-normal saline in the newborn. In spite of our reluctance to use colloid-containing solutions for shock, we make an exception in the desperately ill newborn or premature infant with septicemia. To replace the reduced serum factors, for example, in those children with a coagulopathy, we provide fresh frozen plasma or specific factors as the resuscitation fluid.

The rate and volume of resuscitation fluid given is adjusted based on feedback data obtained from monitoring the effects of the initial resuscitation. After the initial volume is given, the adequacy of replacement is assessed by monitoring urine output, urine concentration, plasma acidosis, oxygenation, arterial pressure, CVP, and pulmonary wedge pressure, if indicated. When cardiac failure is present, continued vigorous delivery of large volumes of fluid may cause further increases in preload to the failing myocardium and accelerates the downhill course. In this setting, inotropic agents are given while monitoring cardiac and pulmonary function, as outlined previously.

Cardiogenic Shock

Myocardial contractility is usually expressed in terms of the proportion of ventricular volume pumped, the ejection fraction. Myocardial contractility is reduced with hypoxemia and acidosis. Inotropic drugs increase cardiac contractility but have their best effect when hypoxemia and acidosis are corrected.

Adrenergic receptors are important in regulating calcium flux, which, in turn, is important in controlling myocardial contractility. α and β Receptors are proteins present in the sarcolemma of myocardial and vascular smooth muscle cells. β_1 Receptors are predominantly in the heart and, when stimulated, result in increased contractility of myocardium. β_2 receptors are predominantly in respiratory and vascular smooth muscle. When stimulated, these receptors result in bronchodilation and vasodilation. α_1-Adrenergic receptors are located on vascular smooth muscle and result in vascular constriction when stimulated. α_2 Receptors are found mainly on prejunctional sympathetic nerve terminals. The concept of dopaminergic receptors also has been used to account for the cardiovascular effects of dopamine not mediated through α or β receptors. Activation of dopaminergic receptors results in decreased renal and mesenteric vascular resistance and, usually, increased blood flow. The most commonly used inotropic drugs are listed in Table 1-7.

Epinephrine

Epinephrine is an endogenous catecholamine with α- and β-adrenergic effects. At low doses, the β-adrenergic effect predominates. These effects include an increase in heart rate, cardiac contractility, cardiac output, and bronchiolar dilation. Blood pressure increases, in part, not only because of increased cardiac output but also because of increased peripheral vascular resistance, which is noted

TABLE 1-7

VASOACTIVE MEDICATIONS COMMONLY USED IN THE NEWBORN

Vasoactive Agent	Principal Modes of Action	Major Hemodynamic Effects	Administration and Dosage	Indications
Epinephrine	α- and β-agonist	Increases heart rate and myocardial contractility by activating β_1 receptors	0.1 mL/kg of 1:10,000 solution given IV intracardial; *OR* Endotracheal 0.05–1.0 µg/kg/min IV	Cardiac resuscitation; short-term use when severe heart failure resistant to other drugs
Dopamine, low dose	Stimulates dopamine receptors	Decrease in vascular resistance in splanchnic, renal, and cerebral vessels	<2 µg/kg/min IV	Useful in managing cardiogenic or hypovolemic shock or after cardiac surgery
Dopamine, intermediate dose	Stimulates β_1 receptors; myocardial norepinephrine release	Inotropic response	2–10 µg/kg/min IV	Blood pressure unresponsive to low dose
Dopamine, high dose	Stimulates α receptors	Increased peripheral and renal vascular resistance	>10 µg/kg/min IV	Septic shock with low systemic vascular resistance
Dobutamine	Synthetic β_1-agonist in low doses; α and β_2 effects in higher doses	Increased cardiac output, increased arterial pressure; less increase in heart rate than with dopamine	1–15 µg/kg/min IV	Useful alternative to dopamine if increase in heart rate undesirable
Isoproterenol	β_1- and β_2-agonist	Increased cardiac output by positive inotropic and chronotropic action and increase in venous return; systemic vascular resistance generally reduced; pulmonary vascular resistance generally reduced	0.05–2.0 µg/kg/min IV	Useful in low-output situations, especially when heart rate is slow
Sodium nitroprusside	Direct-acting vasodilator that relaxes arteriolar and venous smooth muscle	Afterload reduction; reduced arterial pressure	1–10 µg/kg/min IV (for up to 10 min); 0.5–2 µg/kg/min IV	Hypertensive crisis; vasodilator therapy
Milrinone	Phosphodiesterase inhibitor relaxes arteriolar and venous smooth muscle via calcium/cyclic AMP	Increased cardiac output, slight decreased blood pressure, increased oxygen delivery	75 µg/kg bolus IV, then 0.75–1.0 mg/kg IV	Useful as an alternative or in addition to dopamine (may act synergistically) if increased HR undesirable

IV, intravenous; AMP, adenosine monophosphate; HR, heart rate.
Adapted from Lees MH, King DH: Cardiogenic shock in the neonate. Pediatr Rev 9:263, 1988.

with higher doses in which α-adrenergic effects become predominant. Renal blood flow may increase slightly, remain unchanged, or decrease, depending on the balance between greater cardiac output and changes in peripheral vascular resistance, which lead to regional redistribution of blood flow. Cardiac arrhythmias can be seen with epinephrine, especially with higher doses. Dosages for treating compromised cardiovascular function range from 0.05 to 1.0 µg/kg/min. Excessive doses of epinephrine can cause worsening cardiac ischemia and dysfunction from increased myocardial oxygen demand.

Isoproterenol

Isoproterenol is a β-adrenergic agonist. It increases cardiac contractility and heart rate, with little change in systemic vascular resistance (SVR). The peripheral vascular β-adrenergic effect and lack of a peripheral vascular α-adrenergic effect may allow reduction of left ventricular afterload. The intense chronotropic effect of isoproterenol produces tachycardia, which can limit its usefulness. Isoproterenol is administered IV at a dosage of 0.05 to 2.0 μg/kg/min.

Dopamine

Dopamine is an endogenous catecholamine with β-adrenergic, α-adrenergic, and dopaminergic effects. It is both a direct and an indirect β-adrenergic agonist. Dopamine elicits positive inotropic and chronotropic responses by direct interaction with the β receptor (direct effect) and by stimulating the release from the sympathetic nerve endings of norepinephrine, which interacts with the β receptor (indirect effect). At low dosages (< 3 μg/kg/min), the dopaminergic effect of the drug predominates, resulting in reduced renal and mesenteric vascular resistance and further blood flow to these organs. The β-adrenergic effects become more prominent at intermediate dosages (3 to 10 μg/kg/min), producing a higher cardiac output. At relatively high dosages (> 15 to 20 μg/kg/min), the α-adrenergic effects become prominent with peripheral vasoconstriction.

Experience with the use of dopamine in pediatric patients suggests that it is effective in increasing blood pressure in neonates, infants, and children. The precise dosages at which the desired hemodynamic effects are maximized are not known. The effects of low dosages of dopamine on blood pressure, heart rate, and renal function were studied in 18 hypotensive, preterm infants.[41] The blood pressure and diuretic effects were observed at 2, 4, and 8 μg/kg/min. Elevations in heart rate were seen only at 8 μg/kg/min. Further work is needed the better to characterize the pharmacokinetics and pharmacodynamics of dopamine in children, especially in newborns.

Recent clinical evidence has demonstrated some beneficial effects from orally administered levodopa for treating cardiac failure in pediatric patients. Because enteral medications for heart failure are currently limited to digoxin and diuretics, using levodopa may improve our ability to treat heart failure without using parenteral ionotropes.[42]

Dobutamine

Dobutamine, a synthetic catecholamine, has predominantly β-adrenergic effects with minimal α-adrenergic effects. The hemodynamic effect of dobutamine in infants and children with shock has been studied.[43] Dobutamine infusion significantly increased cardiac index, stroke index, and pulmonary capillary wedge pressure, and it decreased SVR. The drug appears more efficacious in treating cardiogenic shock than septic shock. The advantage of dobutamine over isoproterenol is its lesser chronotrophic effect and its tendency to maintain systemic pressure. The advantage over dopamine is the lesser peripheral vasoconstrictor effect of dobutamine. The usual range of dosages for dobutamine is 2 to 15 μg/kg/min. The combination of dopamine and dobutamine has been increasingly used. Little information regarding their combined advantages or effectiveness in pediatric patients has been published.

Milrinone

Milrinone, a phosphodiesterase inhibitor, is a potent positive inotrope and vasodilator that has been shown to improve cardiac function in infants and children.[44-46] The proposed action is due, in part, to an increase in intracellular cyclic adenosine monophosphate and calcium transport secondary to inhibition of cardiac phosphodiesterase. This effect is independent of β-agonist stimulation and may act synergistically with β-agonist to improve cardiac performance. Milrinone increases cardiac index and oxygen delivery without affecting heart rate, blood pressure, or pulmonary wedge pressure. Milrinone is administered as a 75-μg/kg bolus followed by infusion of 0.75 to 1.0 μg/kg/min.

Septic Shock

Afterload represents the force against which the left ventricle must contract to eject blood. It is related to SVR and myocardial wall stress. SVR is defined as the systemic mean arterial blood pressure minus right arterial pressure divided by cardiac output. Cardiac contractility is affected by SVR and afterload. In general, increases in afterload reduce cardiac contractility, and decreases in afterload increase cardiac contractility.

Septic shock is a distributive form of shock that differs from other forms of shock. Cardiogenic and hypovolemic shock lead to increased SVR and decreased cardiac output. Septic shock results from a severe decrease in SVR and a generalized maldistribution of blood and leads to a hyperdynamic state.[47] The pathophysiology of septic shock begins with a nidus of infection. Organisms may invade the bloodstream, or they may proliferate at the infected site and release various mediators into the bloodstream. Evidence now supports the finding that substances produced by the microorganism, such as lipopolysaccharide, endotoxin, exotoxin, lipid moieties, and other products can induce septic shock by stimulating host cells to release cytokines, leukotrienes, and endorphins.

Endotoxin is a lipopolysaccharide found in the outer membrane of gram-negative bacteria. Functionally, the molecule is divided into three parts: (1) the highly variable O-specific polysaccharide side chain (conveys serotypic specificity to bacteria and can activate the alternate pathway of complement); (2) the R-core region (less variable among different gram-negative bacteria; antibodies to this region could be cross protective); and (3) lipid-A (responsible for most of the toxicity of endotoxin). Endotoxin stimulates tumor necrosis factor (TNF) and can directly activate the classic complement pathway in the absence of antibody. Endotoxin has been implicated as an important factor in the pathogenesis of human septic shock and gram-negative sepsis.[48] Therapy has focused on developing antibodies to endotoxin to treat septic shock. Antibodies to endotoxin have been used in clinical trials of sepsis with variable results.[49-51]

Cytokines, especially TNF, play a dominant role in the host response. Endotoxin and exotoxin both induce TNF release in vivo and produce many other toxic effects through this endogenous mediator.[52-54] TNF is released primarily from monocytes and macrophages; however, it also is released from natural killer cells, mast cells, and some activated T lymphocytes. Antibodies against TNF protect animals from exotoxin and bacterial challenge.[55,56] Other stimuli for its release include viruses, fungi, parasites, and interleukin-1 (IL-1). In sepsis, the effects of TNF release may include cardiac dysfunction, disseminated intravascular coagulation, and cardiovascular collapse. TNF release also causes the release of granulocyte-macrophage colony-stimulating factor (GM-CSF), interferon-α, and IL-1.

IL-1 is produced primarily by macrophages and monocytes. IL-1, previously known as the endogenous pyrogen, plays a central role in stimulating a variety of host responses, including fever production, lymphocyte activation, and endothelial cell stimulation, to produce procoagulant activity and to increase adhesiveness. IL-1 also causes the induction of the inhibitor of tissue plasminogen activator and the production of GM-CSF. These effects are balanced by the release of platelet-activating factor and arachidonic metabolites.

IL-2, also known as *T-cell growth factor,* is produced by activated T lymphocytes and strengthens the immune response by stimulating cell proliferation. Its clinically apparent side effects include capillary leak syndrome, tachycardia, hypotension, increased cardiac index, decreased SVR, and decreased left ventricular ejection fraction.[57,58]

Studies done on dogs have suggested that in immature animals, septic shock is more lethal and has different mechanisms of tissue injury.[59] These include more dramatic aberrations in blood pressure (more constant decline), heart rate (progressive, persistent tachycardia), blood sugar level (severe, progressive hypoglycemia), acid-base status (severe acidosis), and oxygenation (severe hypoxemia). These changes are significantly different from those seen in the adult animals that also experience improved survival of almost 600% (18.5 vs. 3.1 hours) compared with the immature animal.

The neonate's host defense can usually respond successfully to ordinary microbial challenge. However, defense against major challenges appears limited, which provides an explanation for the high mortality rate with major neonatal sepsis. As in adults, the immune system consists of four major components: cell-mediated immunity (T cells), complement system, antibody-mediated immunity (B cells), and macrophage-neutrophil phagocytic system. The two most important deficits in newborn host defenses that seem to increase the risk of bacterial sepsis are the quantitative and qualitative changes in the phagocytic system and the defects in antibody-mediated immunity.

The proliferative rate of the granulocyte-macrophage precursor has been reported to be at near-maximal capacity in the neonate. However, the neutrophil storage pool is markedly reduced in the newborn compared with that in the adult. After bacterial challenge, newborns fail to increase stem cell proliferation and deplete their already reduced neutrophil storage pool. Numerous in vitro abnormalities have been demonstrated in neonatal polymorphonuclear neutrophils, especially in times of stress or infection.[60] These abnormalities include decreased deformability, chemotaxis, phagocytosis, C3b receptor expression, adherence, bacterial killing, and depressed oxidative metabolism. Chemotaxis is impaired in neonatal neutrophils in response to various bacterial organisms and antigen-antibody complexes.[61] Although phagocytosis has additionally been demonstrated to be abnormal in neonatal phagocytes, it appears that this phenomenon is most likely secondary to decreased opsonic activity rather than an intrinsic defect of the neonatal polymorphonuclear neutrophils.[62,63]

Preterm and term newborns have poor responses to various antigenic stimuli, reduced gamma globulin levels at birth, and reduced maternal immunoglobulin (Ig) supply from placental transport. In almost 33% of infants with a birth weight less than 1500 g, substantial hypogammaglobulinemia develops.[64] IgA and IgM are also low because of the inability of these two immunoglobulins to cross the placenta. Neonates, therefore, are usually more susceptible to pyogenic bacterial infections because most of the antibodies that opsonize pyrogenic bacterial capsular antigens are IgG and IgM. In addition, neonates do not produce type-specific antibodies, which appears to be secondary to a defect in the differentiation of B lymphocytes into immunoglobulin-secreting plasma cells and T lymphocyte–mediated facilitation of antibody synthesis. In the term infant, total hemolytic complement activity, which measures the classic complement pathway, constitutes approximately 50% of adult activity.[65] The activity of the alternative complement pathway, secondary to lowered levels of factor B, also is decreased in the neonate.[66] Fibronectin, a plasma protein that promotes reticuloendothelial clearance of invading microorganisms, is deficient in neonatal cord plasma.[67]

Using IV immunoglobulins (IVIGs) for the prophylaxis and treatment of sepsis in the newborn, especially the preterm, low-birth-weight infant, has been studied in numerous trials with varied outcomes. In one study, a group of infants weighing 1500 g was treated with 500 mg/kg of IVIG each week for 4 weeks and compared with infants who were not treated with immunoglobulin.[68] The death rate was 16% in the IVIG-treated group compared with 32% in the untreated control group. Another recent analysis examined the role of IVIG to prevent and treat neonatal sepsis.[69] A significant, but only marginal, benefit was noted from prophylactic use of IVIG to prevent sepsis in low-birth-weight premature infants. However, using IVIG to treat neonatal sepsis produced a greater than 6% decrease in the mortality rate.

No prospective trials have examined the routine use of IVIG to prevent neonatal sepsis. Until data are available, its prophylactic use cannot be recommended.

Colony stimulating factors (CSFs) are a family of glycoproteins that stimulate proliferation and differentiation of hematopoietic cells of various lineages. GM-CSF and G-CSF have similar physiologic actions. Both stimulate the proliferation of bone marrow myeloid progenitor cells, induce the release of bone marrow neutrophil storage pools, and enhance mature neutrophil effect or function.[69,70] Preliminary studies of GM-CSF in neonatal animals demonstrate enhancement of neutrophil oxidative metabolism, as well as priming of neonatal neutrophils for enhanced chemotaxis and bacterial killing. Both GM-CSF and G-CSF induce peripheral neutrophilia within 2 to 6 hours of IP administration. This enhanced affinity for neutrophils returns to normal baseline level by 24 hours.[71] Recent studies confirm the efficacy and safety of G-CSF therapy for neonatal sepsis and neutropenia.[72] Other studies have demonstrated no long-term adverse hematologic, immunologic, or developmental effects from G-CSF therapy in the septic neonate. The current recommended daily pediatric dose is 5 µg/kg/dose given subcutaneously.

Unique to the newborn in septic shock is the persistence of fetal circulation and resultant pulmonary hypertension.[73] The rapid administration of fluid can further exacerbate this issue by causing left-to-right shunting through a patent ductus arteriosus and subsequent congestive heart failure from ventricular overload. Infants in septic shock with a new heart murmur should be given indomethacin and a cardiac echo to evaluate the situation. A single-institution randomized trial demonstrated an improved outcome from ventricular overload with pentoxifylline in extremely premature infants.[74]

The critical care of a patient in septic shock can be challenging. Septic shock has a distinctive clinical presentation and is characterized by an early compensated stage in which one can see a decreased SVR, an increase in cardiac output, tachycardia, warm extremities, and an adequate urine output. Later in the clinical presentation, septic shock is characterized by an uncompensated phase in which one will see a decrease in intravascular volume, myocardial depression, high vascular resistance, and a decreasing cardiac output.[75] Care of these patients is based on the principles of source control, antibiotics, and supportive care. Patients with severe septic shock often do not respond to conventional forms of volume loading and cardiovascular supportive medications. Recently, the administration of arginine vasopressin has been shown to decrease mortality in adult patients with recalcitrant septic shock.[76–78] Vasopressin, also known as antidiuretic hormone (ADH), is made in the posterior pituitary and plays a primary role in water regulation by the kidneys. Food and Drug Administration (FDA)-approved uses of vasopressin and its derivatives are in diabetes insipidus; however, other non-FDA approved uses include its use in gastrointestinal hemorrhage and in bleeding disorders such as type I von Willebrand disease.[78] In septic shock, vasopressin has profound effects on increasing blood pressure in intravascular depleted states. The mechanisms behind this observation appear to be mediated by the ability of vasopressin to potentiate the catecholamine effects on blood vessels. Only one randomized, double-blinded, placebo-controlled study has been conducted and demonstrated a beneficial effect of vasopressin in recalcitrant septic shock.[79]

REFERENCES

1. Cornblath M, Schwartz R: Disorders of Carbohydrate Metabolism in Infancy, 2nd ed. Philadelphia, WB Saunders, 1976.
2. Dweck HS, Cassady G: Glucose intolerance in infants of very low birth weight, I: Incidence of hyperglycemia in infants of birth weights 1,110 grams or less. Pediatrics 53:189–195, 1974.
3. Ziegler EE, O'Donnell AM, Nelson SE, et al: Body composition of reference fetus: Growth 40:329, 1976.
4. Colozzi AE: Clamping of the umbilical cord: Its effect on the placental transfusion. N Engl J Med 250:629, 1954.
5. Asch J, Wedgwood JF: Optimizing the approach to anemia in the preterm infant: Is there a role for erythropoietin therapy? J Perinatol 17:276–282, 1997.
6. Doyle JJ: The role of erythropoietin in the anemia of prematurity. Semin Perinatol 21:20–27, 1997.
7. King PJ, Sullivan TM, Leftwich ME, et al: Score for neonatal acute physiology and phlebotomy blood loss predict erythrocyte transfusions in premature infants. Arch Pediatr Adolesc Med 151:27–31, 1997.
8. Bauer C, Ludwig I, Ludwig M: Different effects of 2,3-diphosphoglycerate and adenosine triphosphate on the oxygen affinity of adult and fetal human hemoglobin. Life Sci 7:1339, 1968.
9. Osborn LM, Lenarsky C, Oakes RC, et al: Phototherapy in full-term infants with hemolytic disease secondary to ABO incompatibility. Pediatrics 73:520–526, 1984.
10. Biglan AW, Cheng KP, Brown DR: Update on retinopathy of prematurity. Int Ophthalmol Clin 29:2–4, 1989.
11. National Institutes of Health: Cryotherapy for Retinopathy of Prematurity Cooperative Group: Multicenter trial of cryotherapy for retinopathy of prematurity. Arch Ophthalmol 106:471–479, 1988.
12. Ferson WM, et al: Retinopathy of prematurity guidelines [letter]. Pediatrics 101:1093, 1998.
13. Karlberg P, Moore RE, Oliver TK: The thermogenic response of the newborn infant to noradrenaline. Acta Paediatr Scand 51:284, 1962.
14. Stein J, Cheu H, Lee M, et al: Effects of muscle relaxants, sedatives, narcotics and anesthetics on neonatal thermogenesis. In Pannell M (ed): Surgical Forum, Vol 38, Chicago, American College of Surgeons, 1987, p 76.
15. Landsberg L, Young JB: Fasting, feeding and regulation of the sympathetic nervous system. N Engl J Med 198:1295, 1978.
16. Lorenz JM, Kleinman LI, Kotagal UR, et al: Water balance in very low birth weight infants: Relationship to water and sodium intake and effect on outcome. J Pediatr 101:423–432, 1982.
17. Aperia A, Broberger O, Herin P, et al: Postnatal control of water and electrolyte homeostatis in pre-term and full-term infants. Acta Paediatr Scand 305:61–65, 1983.
18. Soll RF, Holkstra RE, Fangman JJ, et al: Multicenter trial of single-dose modified bovine surfactant extract (Survanta) for prevention of respiratory distress syndrome. Pediatrics 85:1092–1102, 1990.
19. Corbet A, Bucciarelli R, Goldman S, et al: Decreased mortality rate among small premature infants treated at birth with a single dose of synthetic surfactant: A multicenter controlled trial. J Pediatr 118:277–284, 1991.
20. Auten RL, Notter RH, Kendig JW, et al: Surfactant treatment of full-term newborns with respiratory failure. Pediatrics 87:101–107, 1991.
21. Hudak ML, Martin DJ, Egan EA, et al: A multicenter randomized masked comparison trial of synthetic surfactant versus calf lung surfactant extract in the prevention of neonatal respiratory distress syndrome. Pediatrics 100:39–50, 1997.
22. Bloom BT, Kattwinkel J, Hall RT, et al: Comparison of Infasurf (calf lung surfactant extract) to Survanta (Beractant) in the treatment and prevention of respiratory distress syndrome. Pediatrics 100:31–38, 1997.
23. Halliday HL: Controversies: Synthetic or natural surfactant: The case for natural surfactant. J Perinat Med 24:417–426, 1996.

24. Whitelaw A: Controversies: Synthetic or natural surfactant treatment for respiratory distress syndrome? The case for synthetic surfactant. J Perinat Med 24:427–435, 1996.

25. Garg AK: "Arterialized" capillary blood [letter]. CMAJ 107:16, 1972.

26. Glasgow JF, Flynn DM, Swyer PR: A comparison of descending aortic and "arterialized" capillary blood in the sick newborn. CMAJ 106:660, 1972.

27. Siggaard-Andersen O: Acid-base and blood gas parameters: Arterial or capillary blood? Scand J Clin Lab Invest 21:289, 1968.

28. Reynolds GJ, Yu VYH: Guidelines for the use of pulse oximetry in the non-invasive estimation of oxygen saturation in oxygen-dependent newborn infants. Aust Paediatr J 24:346–350, 1988.

29. Weil MH, Rackow EC, Trevino R, et al: Difference in acid-base state between venous and arterial blood during cardiopulmonary resuscitation. N Engl J Med 315:153–156, 1986.

30. McEvedy BAB, McLeod ME, Kirpalani H, et al: End-tidal carbon dioxide measurements in critically ill neonates: A comparison of sidestream capnometers. Can J Anaesth 37:322–326, 1990.

31. Notterman DA, Castello FV, Steinberg C, et al: A comparison of thermodilution and pulsed Doppler cardiac output measurement in critically ill children. J Pediatr 115:554–560, 1989.

32. Pianesi P: Comparison of impedance cardiopathy with indirect FiO_2 (CO_2) method of measuring cardiac output in healthy children during exercise. Am J Cardiol 77:745–749, 1996.

33. Van de Water JM, Phillips PA, Thouin LG, et al: Bioelectric impedance: New developments and clinical application. Arch Surg 102:541, 1971.

34. Spinale FG: Relationship of bioimpedance to thermodilution and electrocardiographic measurements of cardiac function. Crit Care Med 18:414–418, 1990.

35. Connors A: The effectiveness of right heart catheterization in the initial care of critically ill patients. JAMA 276:889–897, 1996.

36. Thompson AE: Pulmonary artery catheterization in children. New Horiz 5:244–250, 1997.

37. Nelson LD: Application of venous saturation monitoring. In Civetta JM, Taylor RW, Kirby RR (eds): Critical Care. Philadelphia, JB Lippincott, 1988, pp 327–334.

38. Norfleet EA, Watson CB: Continuous mixed venous oxygen saturation measurement: A significant advance in hemodynamic monitoring? J Clin Monit Comput 1:245–258, 1985.

39. Ko WJ, Chang CI, Chiu IS: Continuous monitoring of venous oxygen saturation in critically-ill infants. J Formos Med Assoc 95:258–262, 1996.

40. Hirschl RB, Palmer P, Heiss KF, et al: Evaluation of the right atrial venous oxygen saturation as a physiologic monitor in a neonatal model. J Pediatr Surg 28:901–905, 1993.

41. DiSessa TG, Leitner M, Ti CC, et al: The cardiovascular effects of dopamine in the severely asphyxiated neonate. J Pediatr 99:772–776, 1981.

42. Mendelson AM, Johnson CE, Brown CE, et al: Hemodynamic and clinical effects of oral levodopa in children with congestive heart failure. J Am Coll Cardiol 30:237–242, 1997.

43. Perkin RM, Levin DL, Webb R, et al: Dobutamine: A hemodynamic evaluation in children with shock. J Pediatr 100:977–983, 1982.

44. Ramamoorthy C, Anderson GD, Williams GD, et al: Pharmacokinetics and side effects of milrinone in infants and children after open heart surgery. Anesth Analg 86:283–289, 1998.

45. Barton P, Garcia JK, Kitchen A, et al: Hemodynamic effects of i.v. milrinone lactate in pediatric patients with septic shock: A prospective double-blinded, randomized, placebo-controlled interventional study. Chest 109:1302–1312, 1996.

46. Chang AC, Am A, Wernovsky G, et al: Milrinone: Systemic and pulmonary hemodynamic effects in neonates after cardiac surgery. Crit Care Med 23:1907–1914, 1995.

47. Parrillo JE: Septic shock in humans. Advances in the understanding of pathogenesis, cardiovascular dysfunction, and therapy. Ann Intern Med 113:227–242, 1990.

48. Danner R, Elin RJ, Hosline KM, et al: Endotoxin determinations in 100 patients with septic shock. Clin Res 36:453A, 1988.

49. McCloskey RV, Straube KC, Sanders C, et al: Treatment of septic shock with human monoclonal antibody HA-1A: A randomized, double-blind, placebo-controlled trial, CHESS Trial Study Group. Ann Intern Med 121:1–5, 1994.

50. Rogy MA, Moldawer LL, Oldenburg HS, et al: Anti-endotoxin therapy in primate bacteremia with HA-1A and BPI. Ann Surg 220:77–85, 1994.

51. Ziegler EJ, Fisher CJ Jr, Sprung CL, et al: Treatment of gram-negative bacteremia and septic shock with HA-1A human monoclonal antibody against endotoxin: A randomized, double-blind, placebo-controlled trial: The HA-1A Sepsis Study Group. N Engl J Med 324:429–436, 1991.

52. Tracey KJ, Lowry SF, Cerami A: Chachectin: A hormone that triggers acute shock and chronic cachexia. J Infect Dis 157:413–420, 1988.

53. Nedwin GE, Svedersky LP, Bringman TS: Effect of interleukin-2, interferon-gamma and mitogens on the production of tumor necrosis factors alpha and beta. J Immunol 135:2492–2497, 1985.

54. Jupin C, Anderson S, Damais C, et al: Toxic shock syndrome toxin 1 as an inducer of human tumor necrosis factors and gamma interferon. J Exp Med 167:752–761, 1988.

55. Tracey KJ, Fong Y, Hesse DG, et al: Anti-cachectin/TNF mono-clonal antibodies prevent septic shock during lethal bacteraemia. Nature 330:662–664, 1987.

56. Beutler B, Milsaark IW, Cerami AC: Passive immunization against cachectin/tumor necrosis factor protects mice from the lethal effects of endotoxin. Science 229:869–871, 1981.

57. Rosenstein M, Ettinghausen SE, Rosenberg SA: Extravasation of intravascular fluid mediated by the systemic administration of recombinant interleukin-2. Immunology 137:1735, 1986.

58. Ognibene FP, Rosenberg SA, Lotze M, et al: Interleukin-2 admin-istration causes reversible hemodynamic changes and left ventricular dysfunction similar to those seen in septic shock. Chest 94:750, 1988.

59. Pryor RW, Hinshaw LB: Sepsis/septic shock in adults and children. Pathol Immunopathol Res 8:222–230, 1989.

60. Hill HR: Biochemical, structural and functional abnormalities of polymorphonuclear leukocytes in the neonate. Pediatr Res 22:375–382, 1987.

61. Miller M: Chemotactic function in the human neonate: Humoral and cellular aspects. Pediatr Res 5:487–492, 1971.

62. Miller ME: Phagocytosis in the newborn: Humoral and cellular factors. J Pediatr 75:255–259, 1969.

63. Forman ML, Stiehm ER: Impaired opsonic activity but normal phagocytosis in low-birth-weight infants. N Engl J Med 281:926–931, 1969.

64. Cates KL, Rowe JC, Ballow M: The premature infant as a compromised host. Curr Probl Pediatr 13:1–63, 1983.

65. Anderson DC, Hughes J, Edwards MS, et al: Impaired chemotaxigenesis by type III group B streptococci in neonatal sera: Relationship to diminished concentration of specific anticapsular antibody and abnormalities of serum complement. Pediatr Res 17:496–502, 1983.

66. Stossel TP, Alper CH, Rosen F: Opsonic activity in the newborn: Role of properidin. Pediatrics 52:134–137, 1973.

67. Gerdes JS, Yoder MC, Douglas SD, et al: Decreased plasma fibronectin in neonatal sepsis. Pediatrics 72:877–881, 1983.

68. Chirico G, Rondini G, Plebani A, et al: Intravenous gamma globu-lin therapy for prophylaxis of infection in high-risk neonates. J Pediatr 110:437–442, 1987.

69. Clark SC, Kamen R: The human hematopoietic colony-stimulating factors. Science 236:1229–1237, 1987.

70. Sieff CA: Hematopoietic growth factors. J Clin Invest 79:1549, 1987.

71. Barak Y, Leibovitz E, Mogilner B, et al: The in vivo effect of recombinant human granulocyte-colony stimulating factor in neutropenic neonates with sepsis. Eur J Pediatr 156:643–646, 1997.

72. Wolach B: Neonatal sepsis: Pathogenesis and supportive therapy [review]. Semin Perinatol 21:28–38, 1997.

73. Carcillo JA, Fields AI, Task Force Committee Members: Clinical practice parameters for hemodynamic support of pediatric and neonatal patients septic shock. Crit Care Med 30:1365–1377, 2002.

74. Lauterback R, Pawlik D, Kowalczyk A, et al: The effect of the immunomodulatory agent, pentoxifylline in the treatment of sepsis in prematurely delivered infants: Placebo-controlled, double-blinded trial. Crit Care Med 27:807–814, 1999.

75. Tobin JR, Wetzel RC: Schock and multi-organ system failure. In Rogers, Helfaer (eds.): Handbook of Pediatric Intensive Care. 1999, pp 324–351.

76. Ruokonen E, Parviainen I, Usuaro A: Treament of impaired perfusion in septic shock. Ann Med 34:590–597, 2002.

77. Dellinger RP: Cardiovascular management of septic shock. Crit Care Med 31:946–955, 2003.

78. Kaplan NM, Palmer BF, Chen P: Vasopressin: New uses in critical care. Am J Med Sci 324:146–154, 2002.

79. Malay MB, Ashton RC, Landry DW, et al: Low-dose vasopressin in the treatment of vasodilatory septic shock. J Trauma 47:699–703, 1999.

CHAPTER 2

Nutritional Support of the Pediatric Patient

Patrick J. Javid, MD, and Tom Jaksic, MD, PhD

The metabolic alterations in the child after operation, critical illness, or traumatic injury are well established. In general, the changes are catabolic in nature and incorporate the mobilization of host substrate to facilitate the healing process. Although the metabolic stress response is beneficial in the short term, the consequences are significant, as the child has limited tissue stores and substantial nutrient requirements for growth. Thus the prompt institution of nutritional support is a priority in ill neonates and children.

The basis for the metabolic response to injury in the human was first described by Cuthbertson in the 1930s.[1,2] He was the first investigator to realize the primary role that *whole body* protein plays in the *systemic* response to injury. By studying patients with long bone fractures, he determined that the body's response to injury incorporates a mobilization of tissue protein not only from the site of injury but also from muscle stores throughout the body. It was later realized that the provision of additional dietary protein could slow the rate of net protein loss, but not eliminate the overall negative protein balance associated with injury.[3] Two decades later, Francis Moore[4] carefully studied the hormonal and substrate mechanisms responsible for the body's response to surgery by using isotopic techniques. More recently, the advent of laboratory methods that facilitate the purification and identification of molecular structures has introduced a new class of small peptides termed cytokines. These agents act as the mediators of the unified inflammatory and metabolic stress response to injury.

An understanding of the metabolic events that accompany critical illness and surgery in the child is the first step in implementing nutritional support. The goal of nutrition in this setting is to augment the short-term benefits of the pediatric metabolic response while minimizing any long-term consequences.

BODY COMPOSITION AND ENERGY REQUIREMENTS

The body composition of the young child contrasts with that of the adult in several ways that significantly affect nutritional requirements. Table 2-1 lists the macronutrient stores of the neonate, child, and adult as a percentage of total body weight.[5-7] Carbohydrate stores are limited in all age groups and provide only a short-term supply of glucose when utilized. Despite this fact, neonates have a high demand for glucose and have shown elevated rates of glucose turnover when compared with those of the adult.[8] This is thought to be related to the neonate's increased brain–to–body mass ratio, because glucose is the primary energy source for the central nervous system. Neonatal glycogen stores are even more limited in the early postpartum period, especially in the preterm infant.[9] In the clinical setting, short periods of fasting can predispose the newborn to hypoglycemia. Thus when infants are burdened with critical illness, they must turn to the breakdown of protein stores to generate glucose through the process of gluconeogenesis.

Lipid reserves also are reduced in the neonate and gradually increase with age. Premature infants have the lowest proportion of lipid stores, as the majority of polyunsaturated fatty acids accumulate in the third trimester.[10] This renders lipid less useful as a potential fuel source in the young child.[11] However, the most dramatic difference between adult and pediatric patients is in the relative quantity of stored protein. The protein reserve of the adult is nearly twofold that of the neonate. Thus infants cannot afford to lose significant amounts of protein during the course of protracted critical illness or injury.

Neonates and children also share much higher baseline energy requirements. Studies have demonstrated that the resting energy expenditure for neonates is

TABLE 2-1

THE BODY COMPOSITION OF NEONATES, CHILDREN, AND ADULTS AS A PERCENTAGE OF TOTAL BODY WEIGHT

Age	Protein (%)	Fat (%)	Carbohydrate (%)
Neonates	11	14	0.4
Children (age 10 yr)	15	17	0.4
Adults	18	19	0.4

2 to 3 times that of adults when standardized for body weight.[12-14] Clearly, the child's need for rapid growth and development is a large component of this increase in energy requirement. Moreover, the relatively large body surface area of the young child may increase heat loss and further contribute to elevations in energy expenditure.

The basic requirements for protein and energy in the healthy neonate, child, and adult, based on recent recommendations by the National Academy of Sciences, are listed in Table 2-2.[15] As illustrated, the recommended protein provision for the neonate is almost 3 times that of the adult. In premature infants, a minimum protein allotment of 2.8 g/kg/day is required to maintain in utero growth rates.[16] Taken together, the increased metabolic demand and limited nutrient reserves of the infant mandate early nutritional support in times of traumatic injury and critical illness.

MEASUREMENT OF PEDIATRIC ENERGY METABOLISM

For children with critical illness or undergoing operative intervention, knowledge of energy requirements is important for the design of appropriate nutritional strategies. Dietary regimens that both under- and overestimate energy needs are associated with injurious consequences.

For all patients, the total energy requirement represents the sum of the resting energy expenditure, energy allotted to physical activity, and diet-induced thermogenesis. By definition, resting energy expenditure includes the body's energy requirement for growth. In general, resting energy expenditure rates decline with age from infancy to young adulthood, at which time the rate becomes stable. This occurs because the energy requirement for growth and the relative body surface area are

TABLE 2-2

ESTIMATED REQUIREMENTS FOR ENERGY AND PROTEIN IN HEALTHY HUMANS OF DIFFERENT AGE GROUPS

Age	Protein (g/kg/day)	Energy (kcal/kg/day)
Neonates	2.2	120
Children (age 10 yr)	1.0	70
Adults	0.8	35

both greater in the young child. In the critically ill patient, the remaining factors in the determination of total energy requirement are of reduced significance, as physical activity is low and diet-induced thermogenesis (the heat generated by the consumption of food products) is not significant. Thus the resting energy expenditure provides useful information as to the general energy requirement of the sick child.

The measurement of resting energy expenditure can be performed by using direct and indirect calorimetry as well as recently validated stable isotopic techniques. In direct calorimetry, a subject is placed in a thermally isolated chamber, and precise changes in temperature are measured with the subject at rest and performing various activities. The method is based on the principle that all energy is ultimately converted to heat.[17] The changes in temperature of the chamber are used to calculate the energy discharged, and therefore fuel oxidized, during the study period. Although precise, this method is not practical for most critically ill patients.[18]

The most commonly used technique to measure resting energy expenditure is indirect calorimetry. This involves the measurement of the volumes of O_2 consumed (Vo_2) and CO_2 produced (Vco_2), and the determination of a correction factor based on urinary nitrogen excretion to calculate the overall rate of energy exenditure.[19] A "metabolic cart," composed of a leak-free system with a microcomputer-controlled gas exchange measurement device, is usually used, and a 24-hour urine collection for nitrogen balance is obtained. The measurement of energy production, and thus the amount of energy required by the subject, is "indirect" because it uses O_2 consumption and CO_2 production instead of direct temperature assessment to evaluate the overall change in energy. Indirect calorimetry provides a measurement of the respiratory quotient (RQ) which is defined as the ratio of CO_2 produced to O_2 consumed. In general, oxidation of carbohydrate yields an RQ of 1.0, whereas fatty acid oxidation gives an RQ of 0.7. RQ values greater than 1.0 are associated with lipogenesis secondary to excessive caloric intake. Although this method is frequently used in the metabolic management of the adult patient, its accuracy is impaired in the pediatric population. Intubated infants with uncuffed endotracheal tubes may be susceptible to the leakage of CO_2, whereas babies who are not breathing calmly can render false RQ readings.[20,21] Finally, indirect calorimetry is difficult to use in babies on extracorporeal membrane oxygenation (ECMO) because a large proportion of the patient's oxygenation and ventilation is performed through the membrane oxygenator.

Two innovative, nonradioactive stable isotope techniques have recently been developed to measure resting energy expenditure more accurately in the pediatric patient. The ^{13}C-labeled bicarbonate method allows the calculation of resting energy expenditure solely on the basis of infusion rate and the ratio of labeled to unlabeled tracer in expired breath samples.[22] In a similar fashion, the intravenous administration of doubly labeled water ($^2H_2{}^{18}O$) requires only the assessment of hydrogen and oxygen enrichment most often in serial urine samples to measure energy expenditure.[23] Both the labeled bicarbonate and the doubly labeled water techniques have been validated and effectively studied in surgical neonates. Stable isotope tracer techniques also are being used to study protein, carbohydrate, and lipid metabolism in the neonatal and pediatric population.[24,25]

THE NUTRITIONAL MANAGEMENT OF THE CRITICALLY ILL CHILD

Overview of the Metabolic Response

Children undergo profound yet predictable changes in metabolism with the onset and continuation of critical illness. The initial response after severe injury is termed the "ebb phase" and consists of a decrease in cardiac output and metabolic rate. After adequate resuscitation, this stage quickly converts to the "flow phase," which is characterized by a marked catabolic state. The metabolic alterations that occur in children during the flow phase of illness are illustrated in Figure 2-1. Turnover rates of all nutrients increase substantially, and net protein breakdown is greatly accelerated. Despite a modest increase in protein synthesis, net protein balance (defined as the difference between protein synthesis and protein degradation) is considerably negative. Muscle protein is broken down, and amino acids are sent to the liver, which can use the amino acids to produce inflammatory mediators and acute phase reactants. The remaining amino acids are used to manufacture glucose through the process of gluconeogenesis. Glucose can subsequently be used as an energy substrate in a diverse array of tissues. Although these changes represent excellent short-term adaptations in the child, the persistent metabolic stress response can become injurious if left unrestrained, as it depletes body protein stores, dampens growth, and contributes to multiple organ failure.

Protein Metabolism

Amino acids are the key building blocks required for growth and tissue repair. The vast majority (98%) are found in existing proteins, and the remainder reside in the free amino acid pool. Proteins are continually degraded into their constituent amino acids and resynthesized through the process of protein turnover. The reutilization of amino acids released by protein breakdown is extensive; synthesis of proteins from the recycling of amino acids is more than 2 times greater than that from dietary protein intake. An advantage of high protein turnover is that a continuous flow of amino acids is available for the synthesis of new proteins. This allows the body tremendous flexibility in meeting ever-changing physiologic needs.

However, the process of protein turnover requires the input of energy to power both protein degradation and synthesis. At baseline, infants are known to have higher rates of protein turnover than adults. Healthy newborns have a protein-turnover rate of 6 to 12 g/kg/day compared with 3.5 g/kg/day in adults.[26] Even greater rates of protein turnover have been measured in premature and low-birth-weight infants.[27] For example, it has been demonstrated that extremely low–birth–weight infants receiving no dietary protein can lose in excess of 1.2 g/kg/day of endogenous protein.[21] At the same time, infants must maintain a positive protein balance to attain

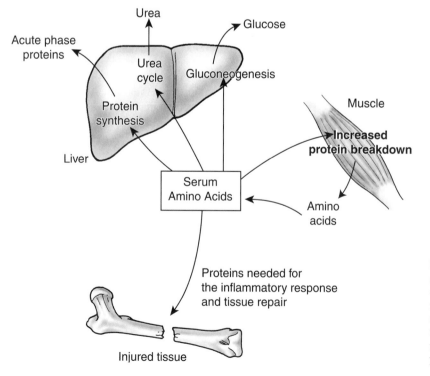

FIGURE 2-1. The metabolic changes associated with the pediatric stress response to critical illness and injury are illustrated. In general, net protein catabolism predominates, and amino acids are transported from muscle stores to the liver, where they are converted to inflammatory proteins and glucose through the process of gluconeogenesis.

normal growth and development, whereas the healthy adult can subsist with a neutral protein balance.

In the metabolically stressed patient, such as the child with severe burn injury or cardiorespiratory failure requiring ECMO, protein turnover is doubled when compared with that in normal subjects.[28,29] A recent study of critically ill infants and children found an 80% increase in protein turnover, which correlated with the duration of the critical illness.[30] This process redistributes amino acids from skeletal muscle to the liver, wound site, and tissues taking part in the inflammatory response. The mediators of the inflammatory response—acutely needed enzymes, serum proteins, and glucose—are thereby synthesized from degraded body protein stores. The well-established increase in hepatically derived acute phase proteins (including C-reactive protein, fibrinogen, transferrin, and α-1-acid glycoprotein), along with the concomitant decrease in transport proteins (albumin and retinol-binding protein), is evidence of this protein redistribution.

As substrate turnover is increased during the stress response, rates of both whole body protein degradation and whole body protein synthesis are accelerated. However, protein breakdown predominates, thereby leading to a hypercatabolic state with ensuing net negative protein and nitrogen balance.[31] Protein loss is evident in elevated levels of excreted urinary nitrogen during critical illness. For example, infants with sepsis demonstrate a severalfold increase in the loss of urinary nitrogen that directly correlates with the degree of illness.[32] Clinically, severe protein loss can be manifested by skeletal muscle wasting, weight loss, delayed wound healing, and immune dysfunction.[33]

The increased protein breakdown inherent in the metabolic stress response takes place for two primary reasons. Undoubtedly, the body needs to redistribute its amino acid utilization from structural proteins to those required for the inflammatory response and wound healing. In addition, the body appears to have an increased need for glucose production during times of metabolic stress.[34] Accelerated rates of gluconeogenesis are known to occur during illness and injury in both children and adults, and this process appears to be accentuated in infants with low body weight.[35,36] The increased production of glucose in times of illness is necessary, as glucose represents a versatile energy source for tissues taking part in the inflammatory response. It has been shown, for example, that glucose utilization by leukocytes is significantly increased in settings of inflammation.[37] Unfortunately, the provision of additional dietary glucose does not suppress the body's need for increased glucose production, and therefore net protein breakdown continues to predominate.[35,38,39]

Specific amino acids are transported from muscle to the liver to facilitate hepatic glucose production. The initial step of amino acid catabolism involves removal of the toxic amino group (NH_3). Through transamination, the amino group is transferred to α-ketoglutarate, thereby producing glutamate. The addition of another amino group converts glutamate to glutamine, which is subsequently transported to the liver. Here, the amino groups are removed from glutamine and detoxified to urea through the urea cycle. The amino acid carbon skeleton can then enter the gluconeogenesis pathway. Alternatively, in skeletal muscle, the amino group can be transferred to pyruvate, thereby forming the amino acid alanine. When alanine is transported to the liver and detoxified, pyruvate is reformed and can be converted to glucose through gluconeogenesis. The transport of alanine and pyruvate between peripheral muscle tissue and the liver is termed the glucose-alanine cycle.[40] Hence the transport amino acid systems involving glutamine and alanine provide carbon backbones for gluconeogenesis, while facilitating the hepatic detoxification of ammonia by the urea cycle.

Increased muscle protein catabolism is a successful short-term adaptation during critical illness, but it is limited and ultimately harmful to the pediatric patient with reduced protein stores and elevated protein demands. Without elimination of the inciting stress, the progressive breakdown of diaphragmatic, cardiac, and skeletal muscle can lead to respiratory compromise, fatal arrhythmia, and loss of lean body mass. Moreover, a prolonged negative protein balance may have a significant impact on the child's growth and development. Healthy, nonstressed neonates require a positive protein balance of nearly 2 g/kg/day.[41,42] In contrast, critically ill, premature neonates requiring mechanical ventilation have a negative protein balance of −1 g/kg/day.[43,44] Critically ill neonates who require ECMO have exceedingly high rates of protein loss, with a net negative protein balance of −2.3 g/kg/day.[28] It has been well established that the extent of protein catabolism correlates with the ultimate morbidity and mortality of the surgical patient.

Fortunately, amino acid supplementation tends to promote increased nitrogen retention and positive protein balance in critically ill patients.[39,45] The mechanism appears to be an increase in protein synthesis while rates of protein degradation remain constant.[46,47] Therefore the provision of dietary protein sufficient to optimize protein synthesis, facilitate wound healing and the inflammatory process, and preserve skeletal muscle mass is the single most important nutritional intervention in critically ill children. However, the quantity of protein needed to enhance protein accrual is greater in critically ill than in healthy children. Table 2-3 lists recommended quantities of dietary protein provision for critically ill children. Extreme cases of physiologic stress, including the child with extensive burn injury or the neonate on ECMO, may necessitate additional protein supplementation to

TABLE 2-3

RECOMMENDED PROTEIN REQUIREMENTS FOR CRITICALLY ILL INFANTS AND CHILDREN

Age (yr)	Estimated Protein Requirement (g/kg/day)
0–2	2.0–3.0
2–13	1.5–2.0
13–18	1.5

meet metabolic demands. It should be noted that toxicity from excessive protein administration has been reported, particularly in children with impaired renal and hepatic function. The provision of protein at levels greater than 3 g/kg/day is rarely indicated and is often associated with azotemia. Studies using protein provisions of 6 g/kg/day in children have demonstrated significant morbidity, including azotemia, pyrexia, strabismus, and lower IQ scores.[48,49]

Protein Quality

In addition to the sufficient quantity of dietary protein, an increased focus has been placed on the protein *quality* of nutritional provisions. The specific amino acid formulation to best increase whole-body protein balance has yet to be fully determined, although numerous clinical and basic science research projects are actively investigating this topic. It is known that infants have an increased requirement per kilogram for the essential amino acids compared to the adult.[50] In particular, neonates have immature biosynthetic pathways that may temporarily alter their ability to synthesize specific amino acids. One example is the amino acid histidine, which has been shown to be a conditionally essential amino acid in infants up to age 6 months. Recent data suggest that cysteine, taurine, and proline also may be of limited capacity in the premature neonate.[51-55] Interest has also been expressed in the use of arginine as an "immunonutrient" to enhance the function of the immune system in critically ill patients. Although preliminary studies show that arginine supplementation may reduce the risk of infectious complications, its safety and efficacy in the pediatric population have yet to be established.[56]

The restricted availability of the amino acid cysteine may have clinical relevance in the critically ill child. Cysteine is a required substrate for the production of glutathione, the body's major antioxidant. In critically ill children, cysteine turnover is increased significantly, whereas rates of glutathione synthesis are decreased by 60%.[57] In this way, cysteine may become a conditionally essential amino acid in the sick child. Recent experiments have demonstrated that the enteral feeding of cysteine in small quantities to rats dependent on total parenteral nutrition (TPN) significantly increases the hepatic concentration of glutathione.[58] The enteral supplementation of cysteine in a pediatric nutritional regimen warrants further basic science and clinical investigation.

Glutamine is another amino acid that has been studied extensively in both pediatric and adult patients in the intensive care unit. Glutamine is an important amino acid source for gluconeogenesis, intestinal energy production, and ammonia detoxification. In healthy subjects, glutamine is a nonessential amino acid, although it has been hypothesized that glutamine may become conditionally essential in critically ill patients. Because it is difficult to keep glutamine soluble in solution, standard TPN formulations do not include glutamine in the amino acid mixture. Although the preliminary data on glutamine supplementation in the clinical setting are encouraging, numerous problems with study methodology have

been noted.[59] Additional prospective, randomized trials are needed to define its utility fully in both the adult and pediatric population.

Current Research in Protein Metabolism

The dramatic increase in protein breakdown during critical illness, coupled with the known association between protein loss and patient mortality and morbidity, has stimulated a wide array of research efforts. The measurement of whole body nitrogen balance through urine and stool was once the only way to investigate changes in protein metabolism, but new and validated stable isotope tracer techniques now exist to measure the precise rates of protein turnover, breakdown, and synthesis.[24] However, the modulation of protein metabolism in critically ill patients has proved difficult. Dietary supplementation of amino acids does increase protein synthesis, but appears to have no effect on protein-breakdown rates. Thus investigators have recently focused on the use of alternative anabolic agents to decrease protein catabolism. Studies have used various pharmacologic tools to achieve this goal, including growth hormone, insulin-derived growth factor I (IGF-I), and testosterone, with varying degrees of success.[60-62] One of the most promising agents, however, may be the anabolic hormone insulin.

Multiple studies have used insulin to reduce protein breakdown in healthy volunteers and adult burn patients.[63-65] In children with extensive burns, intravenous insulin has been shown to increase lean body mass and mitigate peripheral muscle catabolism.[66] A recent prospective, randomized trial of more than 1500 adult postoperative patients in the intensive care unit demonstrated significant reductions in mortality and morbidity with the use of intravenous insulin.[67] Preliminary stable isotopic studies demonstrate that an intravenous insulin infusion may reduce protein breakdown by over 30% in critically ill neonates on ECMO.[68] The use of intensive insulin therapy for critically ill children and adults continues to be another active and interesting area of clinical investigation.

Carbohydrate Metabolism

Glucose production and availability are a priority in the pediatric metabolic stress response. Glucose is the primary energy source for the brain, erythrocyte, and renal medulla and also is used extensively in the inflammatory response. Injured and septic adults demonstrate a threefold increase in glucose turnover, glucose oxidation, and gluconeogenesis.[14] This increase is of particular concern in neonates who have an elevated glucose turnover at baseline.[8] Moreover, glycogen stores provide only a limited endogenous supply of glucose in adults and an even smaller reserve in the neonate. Thus the critically ill neonate has a greater glucose demand and reduced glucose stores. During illness, the administration of exogenous glucose does *not* halt the elevated rates of gluconeogenesis, and thus net protein catabolism continues unabated.[35] It is clear, however, that a combination of dietary glucose and amino acids can effectively improve protein balance during critical illness, primarily through an augmentation of protein synthesis.

In the past, nutritional support regimens for critically ill patients used large amounts of glucose in an attempt to reduce endogenous glucose production. Unfortunately, excess glucose increases CO_2 production, engenders fatty liver, and results in no reduction in endogenous glucose turnover.[69] Thus a surplus of carbohydrate may increase the ventilatory burden on the critically ill patient. Adult patients in the intensive care unit fed with high-glucose TPN demonstrate a 30% increase in oxygen consumption, a 57% increase in CO_2 production, and a 71% elevation in minute ventilation.[70] In critically ill infants, the conversion of excess glucose to fat has also been correlated with increased CO_2 production and higher respiratory rates.[71] In addition, excessive carbohydrate provision may play a role in the genesis of TPN-associated cholestatic liver injury. Finally, some data in critically ill neonates have shown that excess caloric allotments of carbohydrate are paradoxically associated with an increased rate of net protein breakdown.[72]

When designing a nutritional regimen for the critically ill child, excessive carbohydrate calories should be avoided. A mixed fuel system, with both glucose and lipid substrates, should be used to meet the patient's caloric requirements. When the postoperative neonate is fed a high-glucose diet, the corresponding RQ is approximately 1.0, and may be higher than 1.0 in selected patients, signifying increased lipogenesis.[73] A mixed dietary regimen of glucose and lipid (at 2 to 4 g/kg/day) lowers the effective RQ in neonates to 0.83.[74] This approach will provide the child with full nutritional supplementation while alleviating an increased ventilatory burden and difficulties with hyperglycemia. A mixed fuel system in theory also reduces the risk of TPN-associated cholestasis.

Lipid Metabolism

Along with protein and carbohydrate metabolism, the turnover of lipid is generally increased by critical illness, major surgery, and trauma in the pediatric patient.[75] During the early ebb phase, triglyceride levels may initially increase as the rate of lipid metabolism decreases. However, this process reverses itself in the predominant flow phase, and during this time, critically ill adult patients have demonstrated two- to fourfold increases in lipid turnover.[76,77] Recently it was shown that critically ill children on mechanical ventilation have increased rates of fatty acid oxidation.[31] The increased lipid metabolism is thought to be proportional to the overall degree of illness.

The process of lipid turnover involves the conversion of free fatty acids and their glycerol backbone into, and hydrolytic cleavage from, triglycerides. Approximately 30% to 40% of free fatty acids are oxidized for energy. RQ values may decline during illness, reflecting an increased utilization of fat as an energy source.[78] This suggests that fatty acids are a prime source of energy in metabolically stressed pediatric patients. In addition to the rich energy supply from lipid substrate, the glycerol moiety released from triglycerides may be converted to pyruvate and used to manufacture glucose. As seen with the other catabolic changes associated with illness and trauma, the provision of dietary glucose does not decrease fatty acid turnover in times of illness.

The increased demand for lipid utilization in critical illness coupled with the limited lipid stores in the neonate puts the metabolically stressed child at high risk for the development of essential fatty acid deficiency.[79,80] Preterm infants have been shown to develop biochemical evidence of essential fatty acid deficiency 2 days after the initiation of a fat-free nutritional regimen.[81] In the human, the polyunsaturated fatty acids linoleic and linolenic acid are considered essential fatty acids because the body cannot manufacture them by desaturating other fatty acids. Linoleic acid is used by the body to synthesize arachidonic acid, an important intermediary in prostaglandin synthesis. The prostaglandin family includes the leukotrienes and thromboxanes, all of which serve as mediators in such wide-ranging processes as vascular permeability, smooth muscle reactivity, and platelet aggregation. If the body lacks dietary linoleic acid, the formation of arachidonic acid (a tetraene, with four double bonds) cannot take place, and eicosatrienoic acid (a triene, with three double bonds) accumulates in its place. Clinically, a fatty acid profile can be performed on human serum, and an elevated triene-to-tetraene ratio greater than 0.4 is characteristic of biochemical essential fatty acid deficiency. Symptoms of this condition include dermatitis, alopecia, thrombocytopenia, increased susceptibility to infection, and overall failure to thrive. To avoid essential fatty acid deficiency in neonates, the allotment of linoleic and linolenic acid is recommended at concentrations of 4.5% and 0.5% of total calories, respectively.[82] In addition, some evidence exists that the long-chain fatty acid docosahexaenoic acid (DHA), a derivative of linolenic acid, also may be deficient in preterm and formula-fed infants. At present, clinical trials are actively seeking to determine whether supplementation with long-chain polyunsaturated fatty acids will be of clinical benefit in this population.

Parenterally delivered lipid solutions also limit the need for excessive glucose provision. These lipid emulsions provide a higher quantity of energy per gram than does glucose (9 kcal/g vs. 4 kcal/g). This reduces the overall rate of CO_2 production, the RQ value, and the incidence of hepatic steatosis.[83] Furthermore, the adequate provision of lipid eliminates the risk of essential fatty acid deficiency. Studies have shown that lipid and carbohydrate feeding appear to be equally efficacious in ameliorating net protein catabolism in surgical neonates.[74]

Some risks must be considered when starting a patient on intravenous lipid administration. These include hypertriglyeridemia, a possible increased risk of infection, and decreased alveolar oxygen-diffusion capacity.[84-86] Most institutions, therefore, initiate lipid provisions in children at 0.5 to 1.0 g/kg/day and advance over a period of days to 2 to 4 g/kg/day. During this time, triglyceride levels are monitored closely. Lipid administration is generally restricted to 30% to 40% of total caloric intake in ill children in an effort to obviate immune dysfunction, although this practice has not been validated in a formal clinical trial.

In settings of prolonged fasting or uncontrolled diabetes mellitus, the accelerated production of glucose depletes the hepatocyte of needed intermediaries in the citric acid cycle. When this occurs, the acetyl-coenzyme A (CoA) generated from the breakdown of fatty acids cannot enter the citric acid cycle and instead forms the ketone bodies, acetoacetate, and β-hydroxybutyrate. These ketone bodies are released by the liver to extrahepatic tissues, in particular, skeletal muscle and the brain, where they can be used for energy production in place of glucose. During surgical illness, however, ketone body formation is relatively inhibited secondary to elevated serum insulin levels.[87] Thus in critically ill surgical patients, ketone bodies do not significantly supplant the need for glucose and do not play a major role in the metabolic management of the pediatric stress response.

Energy Metabolism

As described earlier, the pediatric metabolic response is characterized by dramatic increases in the turnover of protein, carbohydrate, and lipid substrates. In the adult patient, these changes have been associated with an elevated resting energy expenditure.[88] Clearly, the increase in substrate turnover requires the input of energy and therefore provides an increased basal energy expenditure for the critically ill patient. However, the question of whether total energy requirements are actually increased in critically ill *children* has drawn much interest and is an expanding area of pediatric clinical research. The question is imperative because caloric provisions have significant consequences in the child's overall course of illness. For example, whereas protein balance can be optimized by providing adequate amino acid supplementation, the dietary provision of excess glucose in parenteral nutrition can result in an increased production of CO_2 and a higher risk for hepatic steatosis.[70,89] Hence, these consequences of nutritional support may increase the overall risk of mortality and morbidity in the critically ill patient.

From the use of both traditional and stable isotopic techniques to measure energy expenditure, it is known that the energy needs of the child are governed by the severity and duration of the critical illness. In general, however, any increase in resting energy expenditure during illness or after operation in the child is variable, and recent studies suggest that the increase in energy requirement is far less than originally hypothesized. In children with severe burn injuries, the resting energy expenditure during the initial flow phase of injury is increased by 50% but then returns to normal during convalescence.[90] Multiples studies have shown that newborns who undergo major surgery have a variable and transient increase in energy expenditure of 3% to 20%, which returns to baseline within 24 hours of operation.[78,91,92] At 5 days after a surgical procedure, no discernible difference is found in energy expenditure rates between stable, extubated surgical neonates and normal infants.[93] Energy expenditure measurements of children in the first 3 days after a cardiac operation are comparable to basal levels.[94] The energy expenditure of critically ill neonates on ECMO is nearly identical to that of age- and diet-matched nonstressed controls.[95]

Effective surgical intervention with adequate analgesia may prevent any increase in the neonate's energy expenditure. With fentanyl analgesia, patent ductus arteriosus ligation in the neonate causes no change in energy expenditure.[96] In this same group of patients, whole-body protein turnover and breakdown were significantly *reduced* postoperatively when compared with preoperative values.[92] The overall stress of the underlying illness may influence energy requirements more than the actual surgical intervention. A retrospective stratification of surgical infants into low- and high-stress cohorts based on the severity of underlying illness found that high-stress infants undergo moderate short-term elevations in energy expenditure after surgical intervention, whereas low-stress infants do not manifest any increase in energy expenditures during the course of illness.[97]

Taken together, the data suggest that critically ill and postoperative infants have only a small and transient increase in energy expenditure. Interestingly, this pattern occurs in the setting of a concomitant increase in energy-dependent substrate turnover and is in sharp contrast to the adult patient who demonstrates increased energy requirements during critical illness. The explanation for this apparent inconsistency is thought to involve changes in the overall growth of the child. It is known that growth in the ill child is halted or delayed during periods of physiological stress. In addition, levels of physical activity are low secondary to sedative agents and the nature of intensive care treatment. Thus it is possible that any increase in the energy requirement brought about by accelerated substrate turnover is alleviated by a decrease in energy utilization for purposes of growth and development. Hence, in general, energy (and caloric) requirements for the critically ill child are the same as those for the nonstressed child of similar age. The practice of providing high-calorie nutritional regimens to the child with critical illness may result in overfeeding and its untoward consequences.[98]

Therefore, in construction of an appropriate nutritional regimen for the sick child, the recommended dietary caloric intake for age-matched healthy children represents a reasonable starting point for caloric provisions. Table 2-4 outlines safe caloric provisions for

TABLE 2-4	
ESTIMATED ENERGY REQUIREMENTS FOR CRITICALLY ILL NEONATES, CHILDREN, AND NON-OBESE ADOLESCENTS	
Age (yr)	Estimated Energy Requirement (kcal/kg/day)
0–4	100
4–6	90
6–8	80
8–10	70
10–12	60
12–18	50

injured and ill children of various ages. This quantity of caloric allotment should afford adequate weight gain while optimizing positive protein balance. For example, postoperative parenterally fed neonates given adequate amino acid intake require a total of only 85 to 90 kcal/kg/day of energy to achieve sufficient protein-accretion rates during the first 3 days after surgery.[46] Children fed enterally require an additional caloric allotment of 10% because of obligate intestinal malabsorption. In children with a high work of breathing such as those with bronchopulmonary dysplasia or congenital diaphragmatic hernia, increased caloric allotments may be necessary during the convalescent period.[99] In general, caloric provision during convalescence should be guided by the attainment of adequate growth parameters.

Energy-expenditure measurements in critically ill children have demonstrated high individual variability in numerous studies. Therefore the actual measurement of resting energy expenditure (by using indirect calorimetry or stable isotopic techniques) is recommended when prolonged nutritional support is required in critically ill patients. Serial measurements of energy expenditure may be necessary to determine the individual child's pattern throughout a course of illness and into convalescence. Predictive equations for energy expenditure used in conjunction with factors to account for physiological stress have proven inaccurate and should not be relied on when determining caloric provisions.[100,101]

Electrolyte Metabolism

The basic electrolytes (Na^+, K^+, Cl^-, HCO_3^-, Ca^{2+}) must be evaluated frequently in the critically ill child. Fluid shifts, increased insensible losses, drainage of bodily secretions, and renal failure can complicate electrolyte management in these patients. In sick patients with significant gastrointestinal fluid loss (gastric, pancreatic, small intestinal, or bile), the actual measurement of electrolytes from the drained fluid is recommended. The daily measurement of serum electrolytes is routine in the unstable child on TPN, so that parenteral solution formulations can be adjusted accordingly. However, urgent changes in serum electrolytes should not be managed by changes in TPN infusion rate or composition because these represent imprecise methods to treat a potentially serious electrolyte abnormality. In addition, careful attention to phosphate and magnesium levels is recommended. Hypophosphatemia may lead to hemolytic anemia, respiratory muscle dysfunction, and cardiac failure. A significant decrease in serum phosphate also may be seen with the refeeding syndrome. In contrast, renal failure can result in the retention of phosphate and potassium, and nutritional allotments must be reduced accordingly. Deficiency of magnesium can cause fatal cardiac arrhythmia in children and adults alike.

Abnormalities of acid-base physiology also can influence the nutritional regimen of the critically ill child. If a metabolic alkalosis from active diuresis or gastric suction occurs, chloride (Cl^-) administration should be used to correct the alkalosis. Severe, untreated alkalemia may inhibit the patient's respiratory drive, shift potassium intracellularly, decrease ionized calcium concentrations by increasing the affinity of albumin for calcium, and promote refractory cardiac arrhythmias. Metabolic acidosis is often seen in critically ill children and may be associated with hypotension, ischemia, or renal failure. In this case, the provision of acetate instead of Cl-/// in the parenteral nutrition regimen may be of use.[102]

Vitamins and Trace Mineral Metabolism

Vitamin and trace mineral metabolism in ill and postoperative children has not been extensively studied. In the neonate and child, required vitamins include the fat-soluble vitamins (A, D, E, and K) as well as water-soluble vitamins, ascorbic acid, thiamine, riboflavin, pyridoxine, niacin, pantothenate, biotin, folate, and vitamin B_{12}. All of these vitamins are routinely administered. Because vitamins are not consumed stoichiometrically in biochemical reactions but instead act as catalysts, the administration of large vitamin supplements in metabolically stressed states is not logical from a nutritional standpoint.

The trace minerals required for normal growth and development include zinc, iron, copper, selenium, manganese, iodide, molybdenum, and chromium. Trace minerals are usually used in the synthesis of the active sites of a ubiquitous and extraordinarily important class of enzymes called metalloenzymes. More than 200 zinc metalloenzymes alone exist, and both DNA and RNA polymerase are included in this group. As with vitamins, the role of metalloenzymes is to act as catalytic agents. Unless excessive and specific mineral losses occur, such as enhanced zinc loss with severe diarrhea, large nutritional requirements would not be anticipated during critical illness. The vitamin and trace mineral needs of healthy children and neonates are well defined in the literature.[15] These levels have been used in critically ill pediatric patients; little evidence demonstrates that these provisions are nutritionally inadequate. In children with severe hepatic failure, copper and manganese accumulation occurs. Thus parenteral supplementation of trace minerals should be limited to once per week.

The pharmacologic use of vitamins and trace minerals in pediatric illness remains controversial. Reviews of both vitamin and trace mineral toxicity clearly demonstrate that excessive dosage is a health risk.[103,104]

ROUTES OF NUTRITIONAL PROVISION

In the critically ill child with a functioning gastrointestinal tract, the enteral route of nutrient provision is preferable to parenteral nutrition. Enteral nutrition is physiologic and has been shown to be more cost-effective without the added risk of nosocomial infection inherent in parenteral nutrition.[105,106] The institution of enteral nutrition is usually delayed until the patient is hemodynamically stable and without evidence of bowel ischemia. When enteral feedings are used, a postpyloric feeding tube may help to decrease the risk of aspiration. Diarrhea can be minimized by carefully controlling the infusion rate and avoiding bolus feedings until full absorptive tolerance is established. Before extubation, tube feeds are held for 6 to 12 hours to reduce the risk of aspiration.

The use of early enteral feedings is strongly advocated in the pediatric surgical patient with short bowel syndrome. Many of these patients are chronically dependent on TPN for full nutritional support, and in a significant percentage, TPN-associated cholestatic liver injury develops. In a recent review of a 12-year experience with pediatric short bowel patients, early enteral feeding (as measured at 6 weeks after initial surgical intervention) was associated with a reduced duration of TPN dependence and a reduced incidence of cholestasis.[107] Other salutary factors in averting TPN-associated liver disease in this cohort included the early restoration of bowel continuity and the provision of breast milk.

If the gastrointestinal tract is not functional and parenteral nutrition is necessary, central venous access is obtained to facilitate the administration of concentrated nutritional solutions. This obviates potential fluid overload and avoids the risk of sclerosis of smaller peripheral veins. Percutaneously placed peripheral intravenous lines that are threaded centrally and standard central venous catheters are the preferred routes of TPN administration. Intravenous lines in the groin are to be avoided because of their propensity for infection, although they may become necessary on a temporary basis in children with chronic venous access difficulties. Once gastrointestinal function has been reestablished, the patient can usually be converted to an enteral nutrition regimen.

REFERENCES

1. Cuthbertson DP: Further observations on the disturbance of metabolism caused by injury, with particular reference to the dietary requirements of fracture cases. Br J Surg 23:505–520, 1996.
2. Cuthbertson DP: Post-shock metabolic response. Lancet 1:433–437, 1942.
3. Munro HN, Chalmers MI: Fracture metabolism at different levels of protein intake. Br J Exp Pathol 26:396–404, 1945.
4. Moore FD: Metabolic Care of the Surgical Patient. Philadelphia, WB Saunders, 1959.
5. Forbes GB, Bruining GJ: Urinary creatinine excretion and lean body mass. Am J Clin Nutr 29:1359–1366, 1976.
6. Foman SJ, Haschke F, Zeigler EE, et al: Body composition of reference children from birth to age 10 years. Am J Clin Nutr 35:1169–1175, 1982.
7. Munro HN: Nutrition and muscle protein metabolism. Fed Proc 37:2281–2282, 1998.
8. Long CL, Spencer JL, Kinney JM, et al: Carbohydrate metabolism in normal man and effect of glucose infusion. J Appl Physiol 31:102–109, 1971.
9. Ogata ES: Carbohydrate metabolism in the fetus and neonate and altered neonatal glucoregulation. Pediatr Clin North Am 33:25–45, 1986.
10. Herrera E, Amusquivar E: Lipid metabolism in the fetus and the newborn. Diabet/Metab Res Rev 16:202–210, 2000.
11. Hamosh M. Lipid metabolism in pediatric nutrition. Pediatr Clin North Am 42:839–859, 1995.
12. Reichman B, Chessex P, Vercellen G, et al: Dietary composition and macronutrient storage in preterm infants. Pediatrics 72:322–328, 1983.
13. Schulze KF, Stefanski M, Masterson J, et al: Energy expenditure, energy balance and composition of weight gain in low birth weight infants fed diets of different protein and energy content. J Pediatr 110:753–759, 1987.
14. Whyte RK, Haslam R, Vlainic C, et al: Energy balance and nitrogen balance in growing low birthweight infants fed human milk or formula. Pediatr Res 18:891–898, 1983.
15. Food and Nutrition Board: Recommended Dietary Allowances, 10th ed Washington, DC., National Academy of Science–National Research Council, 1989.
16. Kashyap S, Schulze KF, Forsyth M, et al: Growth, nutrient retention, and metabolic response in low birth weight infants fed varying intakes of protein and energy. J Pediatr 113:713–721, 1988.
17. Seale JL, Rumpler WV: Synchronous direct gradient layer and indirect room calorimetry. J Appl Physiol 83:1775–1778, 1997.
18. Meis SJ, Dove EL, Bell EF, et al: A gradient layer calorimeter for measurement of energy expenditure in infants. Am J Physiol 266:R1052–R1062, 1994.
19. Ferrannini E: The theoretical basis of indirect calorimetry: a review. Metabolism 37:287–301, 1988.
20. Bauer K, Pasel K, Urhig C, et al: Comparison of face mask, head hood, and canopy for breath sampling in flow-through indirect calorimetry to measure oxygen consumption and carbon dioxide production of preterm infants < 1500 grams. Pediatr Res 41:139–144, 1997.
21. Hay WW, Lucas A, Heird WC, et al: Workshop summary: nutrition of the extremely low birth weight infant. Pediatrics 104:1360–1368, 1999.
22. Shew SB, Beckett PR, Keshen TH, et al: Validation of a [^{13}C]-bicarbonate technique to measure neonatal energy expenditure. Pediatr Res 47:787–791, 2000.
23. Jones PJ, Winthrop AL, Schoeller DA, et al: Validation of double labeled water for assessing energy expenditure in infants. Pediatr Res 21:242–246, 1987.
24. Liu Z, Barrett EJ: Human protein metabolism: its measurement and regulation. Am J Physiol 238:E1105–E1112, 2002.
25. Demmelmair H, Sauerwald T, Koletzko B, et al. New insights into lipid and fatty acid metabolism via stable isotopes. Eur J Pediatr 156(suppl 1):S70–S74, 1997.
26. Beaufrere B: Protein turnover in low-birth-weight infants. Acta Pediatr Suppl 405:86–92, 1994.
27. Denne SC, Karn CA, Ahlrichs JA, et al: Proteolysis and phenylalanine hydroxylation in response to parenteral nutrition in extremely premature and normal newborns. J Clin Invest 97:746–754, 1996.
28. Keshen T, Miller RG, Jahoor F, et al: Stable isotopic quantitation of protein metabolism and energy expenditure in neonates on and post extracorporeal life support. J Pediatr Surg 32:958–963, 1997.
29. Jaksic T, Wagner DA, Burke JF, et al: Proline metabolism in adult male burned patients and healthy control subjects. Am J Clin Nutr 54:408–413, 1991.
30. Cogo PE, Carnielli VP, Rosso F, et al: Protein turnover, lipolysis, and endogenous hormonal secretion in critically ill children. Crit Care Med 30:65–70, 2002.
31. Coss-Bu JA, Klish WJ, Walding D, et al: Energy metabolism, nitrogen balance, and substrate utilization in critically ill children. Am J Clin Nutr 74:664–669, 2001.
32. Mrozek JD, Georgieff MK, Blazar BR, et al: Effect of sepsis syndrome on neonatal protein and energy metabolism. J Perinatol 2:96–100, 2000.
33. Bilmazes C, Klein CL, Rorbaugh DK, et al: Muscle protein catabolism after injury in man, as measured by urinary excretion of 3-methyl-histidine. Clin Sci 52:527–533, 1977.
34. Pierro A: Metabolism and nutritional support in the surgical neonate. J Pediatr Surg 37:811–822, 2002.
35. Long CL, Kinney JM, Geiger JW: Non-suppressibility of gluconeogenesis by glucose in septic patients. Metabolism 25:193–201, 1976.
36. Keshen T, Miller R, Jahoor F, et al: Glucose production and gluconeogenesis are negatively related to body weight in mechanically ventilated, very low birth weight neonates. Pediatr Res 31:132–138, 1997.
37. Meszaros K, Bojta J, Bautista AP, et al: Glucose utilization by Kupffer cells, endothelial cells, and granulocytes in endotoxemic rat liver. Am J Physiol 267:G143, 1994.

38. Denne SC, Karn CA, Wang J, et al: Effect of intravenous glucose and lipid on proteolysis and glucose production in normal newborns. Am J Physiol 269:E361–E366, 1995.

39. Mitton SG, Garlick PJ: Changes in protein turnover after the introduction of parenteral nutrition in premature infants: Comparison of breast milk and egg protein-based amino acid solutions. Pediatr Res 32:447–454, 1992.

40. Felig P: The glucose-alanine cycle. Metabolism 22:179–207, 1973.

41. Pencharz P, Beesley J, Sauer P, et al: Total-body protein turnover in parenterally fed neonates: Effects of energy source studied by using [^{15}N]glycine and [$^{1\text{-}13}$C]leucine. Am J Clin Nutr 50: 1395–1400, 1989.

42. Beaufrere B, Fournier V, Salle B, et al: Leucine kinetics in fed low-birth-weight infants: Importance of splanchnic tissues. Am J Physiol 263:E214–E220, 1992.

43. Mitton SG, Calder AG, Garlick PJ: Protein turnover rates in sick, premature neonates during the first few days of life. Pediatr Res 30:418–422, 1991.

44. Rivera A Jr, Bell EF, Bier DM: Effect of intravenous amino acids on protein metabolism of preterm infants during the first three days of life. Pediatr Res 33:106–111, 1993.

45. Thureen PJ, Anderson AH, Baron KA, et al: Protein balance in the first week of life in ventilated neonates receiving parenteral nutrition. Am J Clin Nutr 68:1128–1135, 1998.

46. Duffy B, Pencharz P: The effects of surgery on the nitrogen metabolism of parenterally fed human neonates. Pediatr Res 20:32–35, 1996.

47. Poindexter BB, Karn CA, Leitch CA, et al: Amino acids do not suppress proteolysis in premature neonates. Am J Physiol 281:E472–E478, 2001.

48. Goldman HI, Freundenthal R, Holland B, et al: Clinical effects of two different levels of protein intake on low birth weight infants. J Pediatr 74:881–889, 1969.

49. Goldman HI, Liebman OB, Freundenthal R, et al: Effects of early dietary protein intake on low-birth-weight infants: Evaluation at 3 years of age. J Pediatr 78:126–129, 1971.

50. Imura K, Okada A: Amino acid metabolism in pediatric patients. Nutrition 14:143–148, 1998.

51. Miller RG, Jahoor F, Jaksic T: Decreased cysteine and proline synthesis in parenterally fed premature infants. J Pediatr Surg 30:953–958, 1995.

52. Miller RG, Keshen TH, Jahoor F, et al: Compartmentation of endogenously synthesized amino acids in neonates. J Surg Res 63:199–203, 1996.

53. Reeds PJ, Berthold HK, Boza JJ, et al: Integration of amino acid and carbon intermediary metabolism: studies with uniformly labeled tracers and mass isotopomer analysis. Eur J Pediatr 156:S50–S58, 1997.

54. Zlotkin SH, Anderson GH: The development of cystathionase activity during the first year of life. Pediatr Res 16:65–68, 1982.

55. Keshen TH, Jahoor F, Jaksic T: De novo synthesis of cysteine in premature neonates. Surg Forum 48:639–641, 1997.

56. Heyland DK, Novak F, Drover JW, et al: Should immunonutrition become routine in critically ill patients? JAMA 286:944–953, 2001.

57. Lyons J, Rauh-Pfeiffer A, Ming-Yu Y, et al: Cysteine metabolism and whole body glutathione synthesis in septic pediatric patients. Crit Care Med 29:870–877, 2001.

58. Dzakovic A, Eshach-Adiv O, Perez-Atayde A, et al: Trophic enteral nutrition increases hepatic glutathione and protects against peroxidative damage after exposure to endotoxin. J Pediatr Surg 28:844–848, 2003.

59. Duggan C, Gannon J, Walker WA: Protective nutrients and functional foods for the gastrointestinal tract. Am J Clin Nutr 75:789–808, 2002.

60. Takala J, Ruokonen E, Webster NR, et al: Increased mortality associated with growth hormone treatment in critically ill adults. N Engl J Med 341:785–792, 1999.

61. Yarwood GD, Ross RJ, Medbak S, et al: Administration of recombinant insulin-like growth factor-I in critically ill patients. Crit Care Med 25:1352–1361, 1997.

62. Demling RH, Orgill DP: The anticatabolic and wound healing effects of the testosterone analog oxandrolone after severe burn injury. J Crit Care 15:12–17, 2000.

63. Denne SC, Liechty EA, Liu YM, et al: Proteolysis in skeletal muscle and whole body in response to euglycemic hyperinsulinemia in normal adults. Am J Physiol 261:E809–E814, 1991.

64. Farrag HM, Nawrath LM, Healey JE, et al: Persistent glucose production and greater peripheral sensitivity to insulin in the neonate vs. the adult. Am J Physiol 272:E86–E93, 1997.

65. Sakurai Y, Aarsland A, Herndon DN, et al: Stimulation of muscle protein synthesis by long-term insulin infusion in severely burned patients. Ann Surg 222:283–297, 1995.

66. Thomas SJ, Morimoto K, Herndon DN, et al: The effect of prolonged euglycemic hyperinsulinemia on lean body mass after severe burn. Surgery 132:341–347, 2002.

67. van den Berghe G, Wouters P, Weeks F, et al: Intensive insulin therapy in critically ill patients. N Engl J Med 345:1359–1367, 2001.

68. Javid PJ, Agus MSDA, Dzakovic A, et al: Intravenous insulin improves protein breakdown in infants on extracorporeal membrane oxygenation [abstract]. J Am Col Surg 197 Suppl 1: 548, 2003.

69. Tappy L, Schwarz J-M, Schneiter P, et al: Effects of isoenergetic glucose-based or lipid-based parenteral nutrition on glucose metabolism, de novo lipogenesis, and respiratory gas exchanges in critically ill patients. Crit Care Med 26:860–867, 1998.

70. Askhanazi J, Rosenbaum SH, Hyman AI, et al: Respiratory changes induced by the large glucose loads of total parenteral nutrition. JAMA 243:1444–1447, 1980.

71. Jones MO, Pierro A, Hammond P, et al: Glucose utilization in the surgical newborn infant receiving total parenteral nutrition. J Pediatr Surg 28:1121–1125, 1993.

72. Shew SB, Keshen TH, Jahoor F, et al: The determinants of protein catabolism in neonates on extracorporeal membrane oxygenation. J Pediatr Surg 34:1086–1090, 1999.

73. Forsyth JS, Murdock N, Crighton A: Low birthweight infants and total parenteral nutrition immediately after birth, III: Randomised study of energy substrate utilization, nitrogen balance, and carbon dioxide production. Arch Dis Child Fetal Neonatal Ed 73:F13–F16, 1995.

74. Jones MO, Pierro A, Garlick PJ, et al: Protein metabolism kinetics in neonates: Effect of intravenous carbohydrate and fat. J Pediatr Surg 30:458–462, 1995.

75. Jeenvanandam M, Young DH, Schiller WR: Nutritional impact on energy cost of fat fuel mobilization in polytrauma victims. J Trauma 30:147–154, 1990.

76. Weiner M, Rothkop M, Rothkop G, et al: Fat metabolism in injury and stress. Crit Care Clin 3:25–56, 1987.

77. Nordenstrom J, Carpentier YA, Askanazi J, et al: Metabolic utilization of intravenous fat emulsion during total parenteral nutrition. Ann Surg 196:221–231, 1982.

78. Powis MR, Smith K, Rennie M, et al: Effect of major abdominal operations on energy and protein metabolism in infants and children. J Pediatr Surg 33:49–53, 1998.

79. Paulsrud JR, Pensler L, Whitten CF, et al: Essential fatty acid deficiency in infants induced by fat-free intravenous feeding. Am J Clin Nutr 25:897–904, 1972.

80. Friedman Z, Danon A, Stahlman MT, et al: Rapid onset of essential fatty acid deficiency in the newborn. Pediatrics 58:640–649, 1976.

81. Giovannini M, Riva E, Agostoni C. Fatty acids in pediatric nutrition. Pediatr Clin North Am 42:861–877, 1995.

82. Committee on Nutrition: European Society of Pediatric Gastroenterology and Nutrition: Comment on the content and composition of lipids in infant formulas. Acta Paediatr Scand 80:887–889, 1991.

83. Van Aerde JE, Sauer PJ, Pencharz PB, et al: Metabolic consequences of increasing energy intake by adding lipid to parenteral nutrition in full-term infants. Am J Clin Nutr 59:659–662, 1994.

84. Cleary TG, Pickering LK: Mechanisms of intralipid effect on polymorphonuclear leukocytes. J Clin Lab Immun 11:21–26, 1983.

85. Perriera GR, Fox WW, Stanley CA, et al: Decreased oxygenation and hyperlipidemia during intravenous fat infusions in premature infants. Pediatrics 66:26–30, 1980.

86. Freeman J, Goldmann DA, Smith NE, et al: Association of intravenous lipid emulsion and coagulase-negative staphylococcal

bacteremia in neonatal intensive care units. N Engl J Med 323:301–308, 1990.

87. Birkhahn RH, Long CL, Fitkin DL, et al: A comparison of the effects of skeletal trauma and surgery on the ketosis of starvation in man. J Trauma 21:513–519, 1981.

88. Blackburn GL, Bistrian BR, Mani BS, et al: Nutritional and metabolic assessment of the hospitalized patient. J Parenter Enteral Nutr 1:11–22, 1977.

89. Hart DW, Wolf SE, Herndon DN, et al: Energy expenditure and caloric balance after burn: Increased feeding leads to fat rather than lean mass accretion. Ann Surg 235:151–161, 2002.

90. Jahoor F, Desair M, Herndon DN, et al: Dynamics of the protein metabolic response to burn injury. Metabolism 37:330–337, 1988.

91. Jones MO, Pierro A, Hammond P, et al: The metabolic response to operative stress in infants. J Pediatr Surg 28:1258–1263, 1993.

92. Shew SB, Keshen TH, Glass NL, et al: Ligation of a patent ductus arteriosus under fentanyl anesthesia improves protein metabolism in premature neonates. J Pediatr Surg 35:1277–1281, 2000.

93. Pierro A, Carnielli V, Filler RM, et al: Partition of energy metabolism in the surgical newborn. J Pediatr Surg 26:581–586, 1991.

94. Gebara BM, Gelmini M, Sarnaik A: Oxygen consumption, energy expenditure, and substrate utilization after cardiac surgery in children. Crit Care Med 20:1550–1554, 1992.

95. Jaksic T, Shew SB, Keshen TH, et al: Do critically ill surgical neonates have elevated energy expenditure? J Pediatr Surg 36:63–67, 2001.

96. Garza JJ, Shew SB, Keshen TH, et al: Energy expenditure in ill premature neonates. J Pediatr Surg 37:289–293, 2002.

97. Chwals WJ, Letton RW, Jamie A, et al: Stratification of injury severity using energy expenditure response in surgical infants. J Pediatr Surg 30:1161–1164, 1995.

98. Letton RW, Chwals WJ, Jamie A, et al: Early postoperative alterations in infant energy use increase the risk of overfeeding. J Pediatr Surg 30:988–993, 1995.

99. Weinstein MR, Oh W: Oxygen consumption in infants with bronchopulmonary dysplasia. J Pediatr 99:958–961, 1981.

100. Briassoulis G, Venkataraman S, Thompson AE: Energy expenditure in critically ill children. Crit Care Med 28:1166–1172, 2000.

101. Coss-Bu JA, Jefferson LS, Walding D, et al: Resting energy expenditure in children in a pediatric intensive care unit: comparison of Harris-Benedict and Talbot predictions with indirect calorimetry values. Am J Clin Nutr 67:74–80, 1998.

102. Peters O, Ryan S, Matthew L, et al. Randomised controlled trial of acetate in preterm neonates receiving parenteral nutrition. Arch Dis Child 77:F12–F15, 1997.

103. Marks J: The safety of vitamins: An overview. Int J Vitam Nutr Res 30:S12–S20, 1989.

104. Foldin NW: Micronutrient supplements: Toxicity and drug interactions. Prog Food Nutr Sci 14:277–331, 1990.

105. de Lucas C, Moreno M, Herce JL, et al: Transpyloric enteral nutrition reduces the complication rate and cost in the critically ill child. J Pediatr Gastroenterol Nutr 30:175–180, 2000.

106. Kawagoe JY, Segre CA, Pereira CR, et al: Risk factors for nosocomial infections in critically ill newborns: A 5-year prospective cohort study. Am J Infect Control 29:109–114, 2001.

107. Andorsky DJ, Lund DP, Lillehei CW, et al: Nutritional and other postoperative management of neonates with short bowel syndrome correlates with clinical outcomes. J Pediatr 139:27–33, 2001.

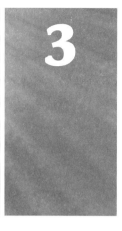

CHAPTER 3

Anesthetic Considerations

Robert E. Binda, Jr., MD, Peter H. Mestad, MD, and
Kathy M. Perryman, MD

PREANESTHETIC EVALUATION

Pediatric surgical procedures are frequently performed on an outpatient basis, or the patients are admitted from the postanesthetic care unit (PACU). As a consequence, information that can be used in evaluating the patient's readiness for surgery is often limited to that obtained in a telephone interview or on the day of surgery. This amount of information is generally adequate, but at times, clarification of complicating factors may necessitate postponement or delay of the procedure. In our experience, seeing more-complicated patients in our preanesthesia testing clinic before the day of surgery results in more thorough evaluation and fewer delays on the day of surgery. Exposure that pediatric patients and parents have to the healthcare facility can be abrupt and intimidating. "Preop parties" acquaint the children and parents with the surgical environment before the day of surgery and often alleviate many of these concerns.

A focused history provides valuable information. A history of pseudocholinesterase deficiency, malignant hyperthermia, or porphyria in family members or the patient is important, although the absence of these complications does not exclude them from consideration. Approximately 33% of patients in whom malignant hyperthermia develops, for example, have had a previous uneventful anesthetic. Drug allergies and adverse reactions are common. Focused questions often reveal an allergy that was previously denied or has been forgotten. Allergy to latex is an increasing problem that can result in life-threatening complications during a surgical procedure. Extensive exposure to latex is usually related in the history. Institutional protocols that deal with the prevention and treatment of latex allergy and latex susceptibility can be helpful in minimizing confusion and optimizing the care of this problem. The preanesthetic interview should include a short review of major organ systems and recent illnesses.

The preanesthetic physical examination should be appropriate for the surgical procedure and the patient's physical status. Frequently, children have evidence of upper respiratory infection. Common sense should dictate whether these patients should undergo an anesthetic. If the rhinorrhea and cough are chronic problems, and no other signs of acute illness are present, it is appropriate to proceed with the operation. However, if onset of the "runny nose" is recent or if the child has other signs of illness, such as decreased activity or appetite or an elevated temperature, it is best to postpone the procedure until the illness has run its course. Fever cannot be ignored, and unless a satisfactory alternative explanation for the temperature elevation is present, the operation should be postponed. Children who have an acute upper respiratory infection have a two- to sevenfold greater risk of having an adverse respiratory event during the anesthetic and recovery period.[1]

Routine laboratory testing is not indicated. Little new or useful information is gained from routine testing, and in most cases, management decisions are not changed as a result of the testing.[2,3] In 1987, the American Society of Anesthesiologists (ASA) House of Delegates stated that routine laboratory or diagnostic screening test is not necessary for the preanesthetic evaluation of patients. Decisions regarding the need for laboratory tests should be based on the individual patient and the proposed operative procedure. Trauma to the pediatric patients and indirectly to their parents is lessened, and healthcare costs are decreased by eliminating venipuncture.

Many children being operated on have preexisting illnesses for which they are taking medication. In general, medications, including oral as well as aerosolized medications, should be continued up to the time of operation. By doing this, we hope that exacerbations of illness will be avoided, making the anesthetic course smoother and safer. The possible exception is digoxin (Lanoxin) for cardiac surgery patients.

Frequently children who have cardiac anomalies must undergo extracardiac operations. Some of these patients are at risk for subacute bacterial endocarditis. Recommendations for prophylaxis of this disease have been clarified and simplified.[4] Only one preoperative antibiotic dose is now recommended. Young children often have a heart murmur that can be heard during a physical examination. It may be difficult to differentiate significant from innocent murmurs. The type of procedure that is planned as well as the physical status of the child dictates whether a more thorough evaluation is necessary before performing the surgical procedure.

Aspiration pneumonitis can be a serious complication to any anesthetic. However, the incidence and morbidity of aspiration may be decreasing.[5-7] Prolonged preoperative fasting may result in dehydration and hypoglycemia and thereby add to parental and patient stress.[8] ASA guidelines on fasting allow ingestion of clear liquids up to 2 hours, breast milk up to 4 hours, and formula, milk, and a light solid meal up to 6 hours before surgery.[9] The incidence of aspiration has not increased after the adoption of these policies, and the patients and parents have been more satisfied. Because of the low incidence of significant aspiration, the routine use of gastric antisecretory medications is not justified. The use of these agents in emergency procedures may be warranted, however.

Preoperative medication is another controversial issue. Preoperative medications were initially intended to make a safer anesthetic by shortening the excitation period of anesthetic induction. Anesthetics that are used today have a short induction time and therefore have a short excitation period. However, preoperative medication also may be used to lessen the psychological trauma that children may experience before their operation. Although a calm environment and a well-presented preanesthetic visit decrease anxiety in many cases, many medications have been administered by various routes. One technique that should be abandoned in most instances is the intramuscular injection, because oral medication has the same effect with less trauma to the patient.[10] Midazolam, 0.3 to 0.5 mg/kg given orally, is effective in decreasing patient anxiety without demonstrable delay in awakening time or the time to discharge from the facility.[11] During induction, preoperative medication appears to be more effective in relieving a child's anxiety than is parental presence.[12] In addition, parental presence is no added benefit to preoperative medication alone in relieving patient anxiety.[13] Regardless of the medication used, 30 to 45 minutes is required for peak effectiveness. In addition, it is prudent to monitor the oxygen saturation after administration and before the induction of anesthesia.

MANAGEMENT OF OUTPATIENT SURGERY

Ambulatory surgery composes 70% or more of the case load in most pediatric centers. Multiple factors should be considered when evaluating whether a child is suitable for outpatient surgery. Communication between surgeons and anesthesiologists is essential in this evaluation. Individual circumstances vary, and no set of rules can be applied to all situations. In most cases, the child should be free of severe systemic disease. However, a well-controlled systemic illness should not adversely affect the postoperative course. Operative procedures in which

major organ systems are significantly affected may not be suitable in an outpatient facility. Other factors that may determine the suitability of a child for outpatient surgery are family and social dynamics. For instance, will this child be cared for by a responsible and capable adult? Is the child to be cared for by a single parent who must work? How far must the child travel to receive appropriate medical attention, if needed? These and other individual factors should be considered when evaluating a pediatric patient for outpatient surgery.

Today's ideal anesthetic should have a rapid onset of action, allow a rapid recovery with minimal or no side effects, and be maximally effective at reasonable cost. The emphasis is on minimizing anesthetic time and hospital exposure. These demands present challenges to the anesthesiologist and have required re-evaluation of the type of care given to patients during the perioperative period as well as the way effectiveness is evaluated.[14] Routine admission to the PACU, for example, may no longer be required with newer anesthetics. Indeed, controlling admissions to the PACU may be the only way to decrease anesthetic costs significantly.[15] This issue is being actively investigated.

Anesthesiologists have at their disposal a wide choice of anesthetics suitable for outpatient use. Because of children's fear of needles, most pediatric hospitals use inhalation agents for induction of anesthesia. Sevoflurane has replaced halothane and isoflurane as the inhalation of choice in many institutions. Sevoflurane has the advantages of smelling somewhat less offensive to children, exhibiting faster induction and emergence times, and having less myocardial depression than does halothane.[16] However, emergence in the PACU is accompanied more frequently by agitation than it is with halothane, adding to the recovery care required of PACU personnel.[17] Medication given preoperatively, or in the PACU, lessens the incidence of emergence agitation, but it still remains a problem. Additionally, time to discharge from the hospital is similar regardless of the agent used. As a result, traditional volatile agents such as halothane remain useful to the pediatric anesthesiologist.

Newer drugs have made intravenous anesthesia more attractive in pediatrics. Opioids such as fentanyl and alfentanil are frequently used as adjuncts to inhalation anesthetics. Remifentanil, an ultra-short-acting opioid with a half-life of 11 minutes, is being used more frequently because of its rapid emergence time. Propofol is used as an induction and maintenance agent for operative and diagnostic procedures requiring deep sedation.[18] It has a short half-life, apparent lack of significant side effects, and antiemetic properties.

Fear of needles has limited the use of intravenous agents. Preoperative medication may mitigate this fear to some extent. In addition, the use of local anesthetics such as lidocaine and prilocaine (EMLA) cream has been effective in reducing the pain of needle insertions. Intravenous agents will certainly continue to play a role in pediatric anesthesia, and techniques are constantly being developed that will ensure their use to the greatest advantage.

Regional anesthetics, in particular spinal or caudal blocks, are used in some institutions for outpatient surgical procedures.[19] The regional technique may be used alone with sedation or in association with a general anesthetic. Personal preference will control how the procedure is performed.

To maximize safety, outpatients should be given the same consideration as inpatients when deciding on monitoring and postoperative care. It is often helpful to establish venous access after induction to rehydrate the patient partially, provide an avenue for intraoperative drug administration, and provide an avenue for postoperative pain relief in the recovery room. We try to administer at least 30 mL/kg of crystalloid while the intravenous line is in place. This amount provides adequate hydration if oral intake is diminished postoperatively and may help decrease nausea after an operation.

Recovery of Outpatients

The recovery period for pediatric patients may be more crucial than that for adult patients. Although the risks of intraoperative problems are similar in adults and children, 3% to 4% of infants and children experience major complications in the recovery period, whereas only 0.5% of adults experience these complications.[20, 21]

Because of the increased use of same-day surgery and because of the frequency of postoperative complications in children, clinicians must readdress some of the problems common in children who are recovering from surgery.

The outpatient who is experiencing pain can be managed in much the same manner as the inpatient. Local anesthetic blocks have proved to be extremely valuable in managing the postoperative pain of pediatric outpatients.[22] Bupivacaine may give a patient 12 to 24 hours of reasonable pain relief, thereby reducing the need for narcotics during the postoperative period.

Vomiting occurs in about 2% to 5% of all pediatric surgical patients.[20] Its incidence is much higher in adolescent patients, in whom it may be twice as high without regard to the procedure[20]; in patients with a history of motion sickness; and in patients undergoing certain procedures, such as eye muscle surgery, in whom it may occur with a frequency of 80%.[23] Guidelines developed within our department assist our treatment of postoperative nausea and vomiting. We no longer require that children be free from vomiting and be able to tolerate liquids before discharge from the hospital, because it is now recognized that oral intake before discharge may cause vomiting.[24] We make certain that the patients are well hydrated before discharge, typically by providing intravenous fluids intraoperatively. We also provide antiemetic therapy to children who have had a history of postoperative vomiting and to those who are undergoing a procedure that is associated with a high incidence of nausea and vomiting (e.g., strabismus surgery, dental rehabilitation, tonsillectomy, orchiopexy, and middle ear surgery). Preferred antiemetic agents include the serotonin 5-HT3 blocking agents and dexamethasone, and secondarily, metoclopropamide.[25] Ondansetron appears to be the treatment of choice in many centers,

but expense limits its use.[26] Combining drugs with differing actions may be more effective than using single medications.[27]

Airway problems are common in the pediatric age group, and they account for many of the problems in the recovery room. In a large study of pediatric perioperative problems, airway obstructions occurred in 3% of cases overall. Our incidence is similar, occurring in 2% of all our patients. This problem usually occurs in patients who arrive in the recovery room still deeply anesthetized, without mechanical airway support.

Another common airway problem in children is postintubation croup. When outpatient surgery was first offered for pediatric patients, many centers went to great lengths to avoid intubating outpatients because of the concern for this complication. If intubation was necessary, it often precluded that patient from being treated as an outpatient. With experience, it was noted that this type of croup, unlike viral croup, had a somewhat defined time course and was not associated with rebound edema when treated with racemic epinephrine.[28] It gradually became routine to provide endotracheal intubations wherever indicated and to exclude the need for intubation from the criteria for admission to the hospital after surgery.

Postintubation croup occurs in about 1% to 6% of all pediatric patients and is most common after surgery involving the head and neck region, in children between the ages of 1 and 4 years, in traumatic or repeated attempts at intubation, and after excessive coughing or straining on the endotracheal tube.[29] Treatment is usually limited to nebulized racemic epinephrine (0.5 mL in 2.5 mL of saline), although some investigators have recommended steroids.[30] Currently, our practice is to observe patients who require racemic epinephrine for 2 hours and then allow them to leave the hospital. The parents are instructed about signs and symptoms of increasing stridor or respiratory distress and whom to contact in the event that either occurs.

The final complication we have noted in the recovery room is oxygen desaturation. Reduction in oxygen saturation occurs in approximately 3% of patients. The most common cause for this complication is the admission to the PACU with a marginal airway because of still being deeply anesthetized. However, some patients have difficulty in maintaining adequate (95%) oxygen saturations on room air for no discernible reason. These patients are observed on oxygen, with the saturation monitored in the hospital for several hours postoperatively. If they improve, they are discharged; if not, they are admitted to the hospital overnight for oxygen therapy.

Care of the Former Preterm Infant

The potential dangers in performing outpatient surgery on former premature infants were first published in 1982.[31] The most life-threatening hazard is apnea after the surgical procedure, normally within the first 12 to 18 hours. Factors that contribute to the increased risk are not completely understood but may include immature neurologic development, particularly in the brainstem respiratory center, and less developed diaphragmatic musculature that leads to easier fatigability.[32] The age after birth at which this increased risk of apnea disappears is still being debated, despite numerous studies of this issue. A meta-analysis of pertinent studies was reported in 1995.[33] The results of this analysis indicated that a significant reduction occurred in the incidence of apnea at 52 to 54 weeks postconceptional age, depending on the gestational age. A hematocrit less than 30% was identified as a risk factor, and it was recommended that infants with this degree of anemia be hospitalized postoperatively for observation no matter what the age. However, conclusions drawn from meta-analysis have been challenged for their validity, and the sample size of this study may not have been large enough to draw valid conclusions.[34]

No anesthetic technique appears to be clearly superior to other techniques, although some evidence has suggested an advantage to spinal anesthesia.[35] General anesthesia is still the preferred anesthetic in most institutions.[36] Likewise, no medications can predictably prevent apnea, although caffeine may hold some promise.[37] Until more patients are systematically studied, the choice of when former preterm infants can be operated on as outpatients is up to the discretion and personal bias of the anesthesiologist and surgeon. Institutional policies most commonly mention ages of 44 to 46 weeks, 50 weeks, or 60 weeks postconceptual age. Indeed, a recent survey of surgical practices showed that approximately one-third of the surgeons chose to wait until 50 weeks, and that one-third waited until 60 weeks postconceptual age.[36] Legal issues direct such practices in some institutions. More important, regardless of the postconceptual age at time of surgery, an infant should be hospitalized if any safety concerns arise during the operative or PACU period.

Monitoring

In 1954, Beecher and Todd[38] were the first to analyze factors leading to anesthetic mortality. They assumed that the major risk of anesthetic mishaps was the use of dangerous and potent drugs, in this case, the muscle relaxant curare. Although their conclusions have subsequently been proved to be wrong, their methodology was sound and continues as the basis for most medical outcome studies. For instance, they were the first investigators to use a denominator when expressing mortality statistics.

Little change occurred in the thinking about anesthetic mishaps until the 1970s. It was then that experts began to attribute the majority of anesthetic mishaps to human error[38–43] and not to the anesthetic drugs or the equipment used to deliver them. These findings led to a precedent that all individuals administering anesthetics maintain a heightened awareness and vigilance. One study reported that 50% of the errors were the result of inexperience, haste, inattention, or fatigue on the part of the anesthetist.[42] It was a logical conclusion that increasing the monitoring of the patient might prevent many of these mishaps by alerting the anesthesia provider(s) to changes in the patient's condition.

It soon became evident that the major problems, although human in origin, most often resulted in respiratory events. Hypoventilation and hypoxemia were the most frequently noted complications. A landmark study of the Harvard hospitals, which looked at their malpractice losses, reported that 82% of all alleged anesthesia claims were respiratory in origin and that 90% of these were thought to be preventable.[44] These findings therefore began two decades of technologic advances directed at providing more intraoperative information to the anesthetist in the hopes of reducing adverse outcomes.

Prior to 1970, intraoperative monitoring consisted mainly of noninvasive blood pressure and heart-rate measurements. Invasive monitoring of arterial, central venous, pulmonary arterial, and intracranial pressures began to be used during prolonged anesthetics or when the patient's medical condition(s) dictated that more careful monitoring would be beneficial. The noninvasive monitors that were heralded as providing the most valuable information (with the least risk) were oxygen saturation and exhaled carbon dioxide (capnography).

What is often overlooked in reviews of anesthetic safety is that the anesthetic experience was actually becoming safer before the introduction of high-technology monitoring.[45] The improvement in anesthesia safety has not been critically evaluated and instead is offered simply as evidence that increased monitoring was responsible. Thus the anesthetic experience was becoming not only safer but also much more expensive because of increased monitoring.

In 1985 and 1986, standards for monitoring (which attempted to codify monitoring use in the United States) were proposed by Harvard University and the ASA. Insurance carriers assumed, as did the majority of physicians, that increased monitoring would produce increased safety. As anesthetic outcomes subsequently improved, malpractice premiums dropped dramatically for anesthesiologists. Once again, this was taken as evidence that the anesthetic experience had become safer solely because of increased monitoring. No critical scientific studies were undertaken to test the relation between improved outcome and monitoring.

Several recent studies, however, examined the impact that monitors have had on the safety of anesthesia. One of the first was a retrospective study claiming that the major difference in outcomes between cases performed at Harvard University hospitals before and after 1985 must have resulted from the impact of monitoring introduced in 1985.[46] As with most retrospective studies, many variables such as newer anesthetics, new anesthetic techniques, better preoperative and postoperative care, and different surgical techniques were not considered in this study. A recent prospective study of 20,000 anesthetics concluded that although the detection of hypoxia increased 19-fold in the group whose oxygen saturation was monitored, the overall incidence of complications was no different in the nonmonitored control group.[47] The relatively small numbers involved in this study may compromise its value.

Although no one would advocate the return to premonitoring days, we must guard against assuming that the more technologic information we have, the better the care will be for the patient. A risk also exists that false information or false interpretation of correct information can lead to bad decisions and bad patient consequences.[48]

Having offered this long disclaimer, we have to accept the fact that monitoring of infants and children during a surgical procedure is here to stay. Those monitors and their basis for use are now briefly summarized.

The electrocardiogram (ECG) monitor has been used primarily to determine abnormal cardiac rhythms and the presence or absence of myocardial ischemia. Significant arrhythmias are usually bradyarrythmias and extrasystoles that may portend a serious cardiac event. It is not uncommon to have healthy children become bradycardic during various procedures. On rare occasions, in healthy children, complete heart block has developed after they were anesthetized. In these children, subsequent cardiology evaluations often reveal previously undetected conduction defects. The other common use for ECG monitoring is the detection of myocardial ischemia. This condition is not often an important consideration in the pediatric population, and even in the adult age group, it is estimated that standard ECG monitors detect only 30% of ischemic events.

Because most (90%) pediatric anesthetic mishaps[49] are the result of respiratory events, the detection of hypoxemia and its correction have become the basis for most quality-improvement efforts of anesthesia departments. The advent of reliable practical oxygen saturation technology has been hailed as a major advance in pediatric anesthesia. When anesthetists were allowed to view the saturation monitor, only 14% of cases were associated with hypoxemia at any time during the anesthsia.[50] The control group, in which the anesthetist was blinded to the oxygen monitor, experienced saturations less than 90% in 42% of the cases.

The other part of respiratory monitoring is capnography or mass spectrometry. The purported advantages of capnography include its ability to confirm endotracheal intubation, to measure $Paco_2$ indirectly, and, when minute ventilation is controlled, to indicate changes in pulmonary blood flow (i.e., cardiac output).

Automated noninvasive blood pressure monitors have improved anesthetic care mainly by freeing the anesthetist from manual measurements of blood pressure, especially in critical situations.

The final part of monitoring is the use of multiple alarms to alert the anesthetist to changes in the patient's condition that exceed predetermined limits. All vital sign monitors, along with most aspects of the anesthesia machine (including ventilators), are now equipped with alarms. Again, in theory, these should increase the safety of anesthesia functioning as an early warning system. Unfortunately, as with the rest of the monitors discussed, the benefits of alarms are largely unproved. One study reported that these alarms sounded an average of 10 times per case.[51] In addition, 75% were false, and only 3% indicated a possible risk to the patient. Most of the time, they served as distractions to the anesthetists and other members of the surgical team. Alarms were often ignored and many times were turned off.

If monitors are to warrant their added expense, their reliability and true benefit to the care of the patient must be critically proved. Unfortunately, however, in our litigious society, the use of expensive monitoring, no matter how unproved, is here to stay.

Pain

The incidence of postoperative pain in the pediatric population, although difficult to evaluate objectively, is probably similar to that in the adult population. It is reasonable, therefore, to assume that about 75% of children will report significant pain on the first postoperative day.[52]

Ineffective treatment of postoperative discomfort in children is most often the result of four factors:

1. Individuals involved in the care of children are working with an evolving knowledge of the mechanisms of pain and its transmission in children. Attitudes toward the management of pain in children have often been biased by several observations made on newborns. It has been known for many years that newborns may cry for relatively short periods after experiencing noxious stimuli and then settle down and sleep without the use of analgesics.[53] In addition, microscopic examination of thalamocortical tracts in the newborn has shown a lack of myelin, leading investigators and clinicians to postulate that the pain perception of neonates is immature and rudimentary.[54] Finally, higher concentrations of endogenous opioids are present in the plasma and cerebrospinal fluid of neonates when compared with those of older children.[55] This type of information has led to the erroneous conclusion that babies do not have a normal sensation of pain and therefore do not require postoperative pain therapy. Evidence now indicates that neonates do experience pain in a manner similar to that of adults. Sophisticated observations of cry patterns, facial expressions, movements, and cardiovascular variables allow reproducible documentation of painful experiences in these smallest of patients.
2. Misconceptions remain regarding the pharmacokinetics of pain medications in children. Clearly, the neonate presents differences from older children and adults that must be taken into account. For instance, neonates appear to have a greater sensitivity to the respiratory depressant effects of narcotics. This may be explained by the fact that relatively fewer μ_1 narcotic receptors (mediating analgesia) exist relative to the μ_2 receptors (mediating respiratory depression) in neonates when compared with older individuals.[56] Evidence also suggests that for some narcotics, the volume of distribution is larger and the elimination half-life prolonged in premature infants. The elimination half-life of fentanyl is 129 minutes in the adult and 230 minutes in

the neonate. As a result of these two differences, higher levels of narcotics persist in the cerebrospinal fluid for longer periods. Many experts believe that narcotics should be used in neonates to 6-month-olds only in patients for whom observation in an intensive care setting is possible or postoperative ventilation is planned.[57]

3. The management of pain in the pediatric population is hampered by the difficulty that exists in assessing pain. Many children may respond to pain by emotionally withdrawing from their surroundings, and this may be misinterpreted by the medical and nursing staffs as evidence that they have no pain. In addition, when questioned as to their degree of pain, children may not volunteer useful information for fear of painful interventions. To circumvent these difficulties, several visual and verbal scales have been developed for quantifying painful sensations or describing typical painful behaviors. These have met with varying degrees of success because they are difficult to implement, time consuming to use, and still rely on patient comprehension and cooperation.

4. Individual biases exist in medical professionals caring for children. These biases run from the belief that pain is a natural consequence of surgery to the beliefs that the risks of respiratory depression and narcotic addiction outweigh the benefits that are associated with aggressive pain management.

Given these difficulties in managing the child who is in pain, what options are available to the clinician? The mainstay in pain control remains the use of narcotics. Not only is a bewildering array of narcotics available, but the methods of their administration also are changing.

Dose-dependent respiratory depression is common to the use of all narcotics and goes hand in hand with their analgesic properties. Other side effects that vary from drug to drug and patient to patient are somnolence, nausea and vomiting, pruritus, constipation, and urinary retention. Given time, patients develop tolerance to most, if not all, of these side effects while they continue to experience their analgesic properties. The side effects may be treated symptomatically while tolerance is developing, thereby making the patient much more comfortable and manageable. Often changing the narcotics reduces or eliminates the side effects.

Morphine remains the standard by which most pain therapy is measured. Some pharmacologic differences between morphine and other analgesics must be appreciated to use this narcotic well. Although morphine has roughly the same plasma elimination half-life as other narcotics, its effect and duration of action may have considerable variability because of the drug's low lipid solubility. A fourfold variation has been measured in the plasma concentration of morphine at which patients medicate themselves for pain.

Because a poor correlation exists between the plasma concentration of morphine and its desired analgesic effect, many clinicians believe that morphine is best administered in a patient-controlled device, patient-controlled analgesia (PCA). As the patient experiences changes in the level of morphine in the central nervous system, he or she is able to administer supplemental doses.

PCA dosing recommendations for morphine include a loading dose ranging from 0.04 to 0.06 mg/kg followed by use of intermittent PCA doses of 0.01 to 0.03 mg/kg. A lockout interval of 6 to 15 minutes and 0.2 to 0.4 mg/kg every 4 hours is the limit generally used with morphine.

When PCA devices are not used, the intermittent administration of morphine to opioid-naive children should be started at 0.05 to 0.1 mg/kg every 2 to 4 hours. If the treatment of pain is undertaken in a recovery room or intensive care setting, similar doses may be administered every 5 to 10 minutes until the child is comfortable.

The efficacy of a continuous background infusion of narcotics along with PCA would theoretically make sense by maintaining a consistent blood level of drug, especially during sleep. However, studies of continuous infusions in both children[58] and adults[59] have failed to show any documented improvement in pain scores. If any benefit is seen in sleep patterns, it might occur only on the first postoperative night.[58] Therefore, although in theory, continuous infusions in addition to PCA would seem beneficial, in reality, they serve only to increase the complications and dosages of narcotics used.[60]

It appears that the only indication for continuous infusion of narcotics may be for pain control in children who are unable to manage the PCA techniques because of age or mental capacity. The recommended dose for continuous infusion of morphine is 0.015 to 0.03 mg/kg/hr. Because feedback controls are not present with continuous infusions of narcotics, close observation and careful respiratory monitoring are mandatory.

Fentanyl is a synthetic narcotic that usually has a relatively short duration of action as a result of rapid distribution into fat and muscle because of its high lipid solubility. With repeated dosing, the duration of action appears to increase.[61] When compared with morphine, fentanyl is about 100 times more potent. (Fentanyl dosages are calculated in micrograms rather than milligrams.) In controlled comparisons with equipotent dosages, morphine is generally found to provide better analgesia than fentanyl but with more side effects, such as pruritus, hypotension, nausea, and vomiting.[62–64]

When using fentanyl for procedures, incremental dosing of 0.25 to 0.5 µg/kg every 5 minutes is safe. All of the respiratory depression from a single dose of fentanyl is evident within 5 minutes because of its rapid equilibration across the blood-brain barrier. The elimination rate of a single dose of fentanyl is reported to be about 1 µg/kg/hr.[65] A safe cumulative dose for procedures is 4 to 5 µg/kg.[66]

Other formulations of fentanyl have clinical applications in pain management. Although not approved for pediatrics at present, transdermal fentanyl, in doses of 25 to 100 µg/hr, has proved more efficacious in the treatment of chronic pain than some of the more traditional modalities.[67] Fentanyl has more recently been released in a transmucosal Oralet formulation that can be used for sedation and analgesia in pain of short duration. Dosage recommended is 10 to 15 µg/kg.[66]

Hydromorphone is a well-tolerated alternative to morphine and fentanyl and is associated with less pruritis and sedation than is morphine, and has a longer duration of action than that of fentanyl. It is 5 to 7 times more potent than morphine. The dosing schedule for PCA hydromorphone uses a loading dose of 5 to 15 µg/kg, a lockout of 6 to 15 minutes, supplemental PCA doses of 3 to 5 µg/kg, and a 4-hour limit of 100 µg/kg.

As more and more of pediatric surgery is being performed on an outpatient basis, significant interest has been expressed in the role of non-narcotic analgesics for the management of postoperative pain.

Many physicians have questioned the efficacy of acetaminophen for significant pain relief, although this may be more a question of the dosage used. Recent investigators have challenged established dosing recommendations for rectal acetaminophen.[68,69] Dosages for analgesia were based on recommendations for fever control (10 to 20 mg/kg), but these doses failed to produce serum levels shown to be effective even in reducing temperature. To achieve adequate serum levels for analgesia, doses of 30 to 40 mg/kg rectally are required. A dose of 30 mg/kg of acetaminophen rectally has proved to have analgesic properties similar to 1 mg/kg of ketorolac.[70] Further controlled studies are needed to delineate the benefits and doses of acetaminophen in the management of postoperative analgesia.

Ketorolac is an oral and parenteral nonsteroidal anti-inflammatory drug shown to have excellent pain-control characteristics with few side effects. Dosage recommendations are 0.5 mg/kg intravenously every 6 to 8 hours for 48 hours. One of the drawbacks associated with ketorolac is its inhibition of platelet aggregation, which has been associated with increased bleeding after a tonsillectomy.[71]

Regional anesthetic techniques used concomitant with general anesthesia have had a resurgence in both adult and pediatric patients. These techniques include local infiltration of the wound, peripheral nerve blocks (i.e., ilioinguinal blocks), and epidural or spinal blocks. The intent of these techniques is to prevent sensitization of the peripheral and central nervous systems, which could result in prolonged or excessive postoperative pain. This approach is often referred to as pre-emptive analgesia. Whether pre-emptive analgesia exists in children is still unresolved.[72] Anecdotal reports of improved, prolonged analgesia during the postoperative period when regional anesthetic techniques are used pre-emptively still await scientific validation.

Pediatric patients, whether undergoing an operation on an inpatient or an outpatient basis, should be afforded maximal pain relief. Recent developments in and understanding of pain-relieving techniques place this goal within the reach of all clinicians caring for children during the postoperative period.

LAPAROSCOPIC SURGERY

The successful application of minimally invasive surgical techniques in adults has spawned a multitude of like surgical procedures in the pediatric population. The cardiopulmonary effects of laparoscopic insufflation in adults and infants have been studied and published and deserve discussion here.

Laparoscopic fundoplication has gained in popularity in infants and children compared with open fundoplication because this technique has been shown to reduce both short-term postoperative morbidity and long-term complications such as intestinal obstruction. In a comparison study of these two techniques in 212 children over a 5-year period, the laparoscopic operative time was longer, but the average hospital stay was reduced to 3.5 days from 8.1 days with the open method.[73] The systemic stress response to laparoscopy and laparotomy was studied in children, and no significant differences were found between the two groups.[74]

The choice of the surgical and anesthetic perioperative plan requires close communication between the anesthesiologist and surgeon before a procedure. An appreciation of the physiologic cardiocirculatory and pulmonary consequences during and after laparoscopic fundoplication is an important part of careful patient selection. The widely varying nature of coexistent disease mandates close inspection of the potential impact of these laparoscopy-induced physiologic changes on each patient.

Two critical factors create unique considerations for the anesthetic management of infants and children undergoing laparoscopic procedures: (1) the creation of a pneumoperitoneum (PP) with the resulting elevation of intra-abdominal pressure (IAP), and (2) the extremes of patient positioning that may be required for optimal exposure of intra-abdominal structures.[75]

Carbon dioxide (CO_2) is now the insufflation gas of choice because it does not support combustion, as does air, nitrous oxide, and oxygen. CO_2 is cleared more rapidly than are other possible choices. The cardiovascular consequences of intravascular gas embolism are relatively less risky than with an insoluble gas, such as helium. CO_2 uptake may be significantly greater in children, because of the greater absorptive area of peritoneum in relation to body weight and the small distance between capillaries and peritoneum. Hypercarbia has been demonstrated in adult and pediatric studies during CO_2 insufflation for laparoscopy. Increases in minute ventilation by as much as 60% may be required to maintain baseline end-tidal CO_2 ($ETCO_2$). Potentially deleterious consequences of hypercarbia are sympathetic nervous system activation with resultant increases in blood pressure and heart rate, along with increases in myocardial contractility and oxygen consumption. Hypercarbia sensitizes the myocardium to catecholamines and can predispose to cardiac arrhythmias.[75]

Some physiologic responses to hypercarbia are uniquely hazardous to infants, particularly neonates.

Hypercarbia is a potent cerebrovascular dilator that, coupled with increased venous pressure due to increased IAP, can result in increased intracranial pressure.[75,76] This presents the risk of intracranial hemorrhage in infants. Newborns also are at risk for reactive pulmonary hypertension when exposed to the stress of surgery, hypoxia, or hypercarbia. Infants with many forms of congenital heart disease (CHD) are particularly vulnerable to the development of pulmonary hypertension.

The IAP increase seen with laparoscopy results in well-documented cardiorespiratory changes. Respiratory derangements occur because of cephalad displacement of the diaphragm. This results in reduction in lung volume, ventilation/perfusion mismatch, and altered gas exchange. Statistically significant decreases in pH and PAO_2 and increased $PACO_2$ after 30 minutes of PP have been demonstrated.[76] A 20% reduction in functional residual capacity (FRC) occurs with induction of general anesthesia, and an additional 20% decrease in FRC has been reported during laparoscopic surgery in adults.[76] Pediatric patients have a lower FRC relative to oxygen consumption than do the adults studied and a higher closing volume. Accordingly, infants have a smaller margin of safety and are less likely to tolerate the adverse respiratory effects of increased IAP.

Significant cardiovascular changes have been demonstrated in response to increased IAP and patient position. In the supine or Trendelenberg position, the venous return is augmented when the IAP is kept below 15 mm Hg. The position required for upper abdominal procedures is reverse Trendelenberg or supine. The head-up position reduces venous return and cardiac output (CO).[77] Several pediatric studies have used echocardiography (supine),[78] impedance cardiography (15 degrees head-down),[79] and continuous esophageal aortic blood flow echo-Doppler (supine)[80] to assess hemodynamic changes during laparoscopic surgery. These studies demonstrated significant reductions of stroke volume (SV) and cardiac index (CI) along with a significant increase in systemic vascular resistance (SVR). PP was found to be associated with significant increases in left ventricular end-diastolic volume, left ventricular end-systolic volume, and left ventricular end-systolic meridional wall stress. All three studies demonstrated a decrease in cardiac performance and increase in vascular resistance in healthy patients undergoing laparoscopy for lower abdominal procedures. The cardiovascular changes seen with PP occur immediately with the creation of the PP and resolve on exsufflation. However, study of laparoscopic Nissen fundoplication in a pig model also showed a significant decrease in CO that remained significantly altered after the release of the PP.[81] This study demonstrated a concomitant increase in mediastinal and pleural pressures thought to be due to dissection around the gastroesophageal junction. These parameters have not been examined in infants and children during upper abdominal procedures.

In a study of cardiorespiratory function in 25 children undergoing laparoscopic Nissen fundoplication, in six children, postoperative hypoxemia developed, defined as an oxygen saturation of less than 95%. This desaturation

has not been seen after laparoscopic surgery for inguinal hernia repair, leading the authors to conclude that interference with diaphragmatic function due to the surgical dissection may be the etiology of the impaired oxygenation. Several of the children in the study had preexisting respiratory disease, presumably secondary to aspiration, which also could account for the desaturation.[82]

In summary, studies of the cardiopulmonary consequences of PP for laparoscopic surgery have demonstrated a consistent and significant decrease in CI and increase in SVR and PVR. The reverse Trendelenberg position results in further reductions in preload and CI. Postoperative diaphragmatic dysfunction may be a result of surgical dissection around the esophageal hiatus. Healthy infants and children without significant comorbid conditions tolerate the cardiopulmonary effects of PP well. Infants and children with significant cardiopulmonary disease require advanced planning and may need invasive monitoring during prolonged insufflation. Close monitoring of IAP to ensure the use of minimally effective IAP can minimize the adverse cardiopulmonary effects of PP.

REFERENCES

1. Cohen M, Cameron C: Should you cancel the operation when a child has an upper respiratory tract infection? Anesth Analg 72:282–288, 1991.
2. Roizen MF: Preoperative laboratory testing-what is necessary? Int Anesth Res Soc Rev Course Lect 29–35, 1989.
3. Leonard JV, Clayton BE, Colley JRT: Use of biochemical profile in children's hospital: Results of two controlled trials. Br Med J 21:662–665, 1975.
4. Dajan A, Taubert K, Wilson W, Bolger A, et al: Prevention of bacterial endocarditis: Recommendations of the American Heart Association. Circulation 96:358–366, 1997.
5. Warner MA, Warner ME, et al: Perioperative pulmonary aspiration in infants and children. Anesthesiology 90:66–71, 1999.
6. Tiret L, Hivoche Y, Halton F, et al: Complications related to anesthesia in infants and children: A prospective survey of 40,240 anaesthetics. Br J Anaesth 61:263–269, 1988.
7. Borland L, Woelfel S, Saitz M, et al: Pulmonary aspiration in pediatric patients under general anesthesia: Frequency and outcome [abstract]. Anesthesiology 83:A1150, 1995.
8. Welborn LG, McCail WA, Hannallah RS, et al: Perioperative blood glucose concentrations in pediatric outpatients. Anesthesiology 65:543–547, 1986.
9. American Society of Anesthesiologists Task Force on Preoperative Fasting: Practice guidelines for preoperative fasting and the use of pharmacologic agents to reduce the risk of pulmonary aspiration: Application to healthy patients undergoing elective procedures. Anesthesiology 90:896–905, 1999.
10. Nicholson S, Betts E, Jobes D, et al: Comparison of oral and intramuscular preanesthetic medication for pediatric inpatient surgery. Anesthesiology 71:8–10, 1989.
11. Weldon B, Watcha M, White P: Oral midazolam in children: Effect of time and adjunctive therapy. Anesth Analg 75: 51–55, 1992.
12. Kain ZN, Mayes LC, et al: Parental presence during induction of anesthesia versus sedative premedication: Which is more effective? Anesthesiology 89:1147–1156, 1998.
13. Kain ZN, Mayes LC, et al: Parental presence and a sedative premedicant for children undergoing surgery. Anesthesiology 92:939–946, 2000.
14. Fisher D: Surrogate end points: Are they meaningful? Anesthesiology 81:795–796, 1994.
15. Dexter F, Tinker J: Analysis of strategies to decrease postanesthesia care unit costs. Anesthesiology 82:94–101, 1995.
16. Lerman J, Davis P, Welborn l, et al: Induction, recovery, and safety characteristics of sevoflurane in children undergoing ambulatory

surgery: A comparison with halothane. Anesthesiology 84:1332–1340, 1996.

17. Voepel-Lewis T, Malviya S, et al: A prospective cohort study of emergence agitation in the pediatric postanesthesia care unit. Anesth Analg 96:1625–1630, 2003.

18. Hanannallah R, Bulton J, Schaefer P, et al: Propofol anesthesia in pediatric ambulatory patients: A comparison with thiopental and halothane. Can J Anaesth 41:12–18, 1994.

19. Broadman LM: Regional anesthesia for the pediatric outpatient. Anesth Clin North Am 5:53–72, 1987.

20. Cohen MM, Duncan P, Pope W, Wolkenstein C: A survey of 112,000 anesthetics at one teaching hospital (1975-1983). Can Anaesth Soc J 33:22–31, 1986.

21. Cohen MM, Cameron C, Duncan P: Pediatric morbidity and mortality in the perioperative period. Anesth Analg 70:160–167, 1990.

22. Shandling B, Steward DJ: Regional analgesia for postoperative pain in pediatric outpatient surgery. J Pediatr Surg 15:477, 1980.

23. Abramowitz MD, Elder P, Friendly D, et al: Antiemetic effectiveness of intraoperatively administered droperidol in pediatric strabismus outpatient surgery. Anesthesiology 53:S323, 1980.

24. Schreiner M, Nicholsen S, Martin T, Whitney L: Should children drink before discharge from day surgery? Anesthesiology 76:528–533, 1992.

25. Domino KB, Anderson EA, et al: Comparative efficacy and safety of ondansetron, droperidol and metoclopramide for preventing postoperative nausea and vomiting: A meta-analysis. Anesth Analg 88:1379, 1999.

26. Watcha M, Smith I: Cost effectiveness analysis of antiemetic therapy for ambulatory surgery. J Clin Anesth 6:370–377, 1994.

27. Splinter WM, Elliot JR: Low dose ondansetron with dexamethasone more effectively decreases vomiting after strabismus surgery in children than does high dose ondansetron. Anesthesiology 88:72–75, 1998.

28. Koka BY, Jean I, Andre J, et al: Postintubation croup in children. Anesth Analg 56:501, 1977.

29. Gregory G (ed): Pediatric Anesthesia, 2nd ed. New York, Churchill Livingstone, 1989, p 635.

30. Goddard JE: Betamethasone for prophylaxis of postintubation inflammation. Anesth Analg 46:348, 1967.

31. Steward DJ: Preterm infants are more prone to complications following minor surgery than are term infants. Anesthesiology 56:304–306, 1982.

32. Rigatto H, Brady JP: Periodic breathing and apnea in preterm infants: Evidence for hypoventilation possibly due to central respiratory depression. Pediatrics 50:202–218, 1972.

33. Cote C, Zaslavsky A, Downe J, et al: Postoperative apnea in former preterm infants after inguinal herniorrhaphy: A combined analysis. Anesthesiology 82:809–822, 1995.

34. Fisher D: When is the ex-premature infant no longer at risk for apnea? Anesthesiology 82:807–808, 1995.

35. Welborn L, Rice L, Hannallah R, et al: Postoperative apnea in former preterm infants: Prospective comparison of spinal and general anesthesia. Anesthesiology 72:838–842, 1990.

36. Wiener E, Touloukian R, Rodgers B, et al: Hernia survey of the section on surgery of the American Academy of Pediatrics. J Pediatr Surg 31:1166–1169, 1996.

37. Welborn LG, Hannallah RS, Fiwle R, et al: High-dose caffeine suppresses postoperative apnea in former premature infants. Anesthesiology 71:347–349, 1989.

38. Beecher HK, Todd DP: A study of the deaths associated with anesthesia and surgery based on a study of 599,458 anesthesias in ten institutions, 1948-1952, inclusive. Ann Surg 140:2–35, 1954.

38. Dripps RD, Lamont A, Eckenhoff J: The role of anesthesia in surgical mortality. JAMA 178:261–266, 1961.

39. Macintosh RR: Deaths under anesthetics. Br J Anaesth 21:107–136, 1948.

40. Wylie WD: "There, but for the grace of God . . ." Ann R Coll Surg Engl 56:171–180, 1975.

41. Marx G, Mateo C, Orkin L: Computer analysis of postanesthetic deaths. Anesthesiology 39:54–58, 1973.

42. Cooper JB, Newbower RS, Long CD, McPeek B: Preventable anesthesia mishaps. Anesthesiology 49:399–406, 1978.

43. Green WA, Taylor TH: An analysis of anesthesia medical liability claims in the United Kingdom 1977-1982. Int Anesthiol Clin 22:73–90, 1984.

44. Eichhorn JH: Standards for patient monitoring during anesthesia at Harvard Medical School. JAMA 256:1017–1020, 1986.

45. Orkin FK: Practice standards: The Midas touch or the emperor's new clothes? Anesthesiology 70:567–571, 1989.

46. Eichhorn JH: Prevention of intraoperative anesthesia accidents and related severe injury through safety monitoring. Anesthesiology 70:572–577, 1989.

47. Moller JT, Johannessen NW, Espersen K, et al: Randomized evaluation of pulse oximetry in 20,802 patients: Perioperative events and postoperative complications clinical investigation. Anesthesiology 78:445–453, 1993.

48. Keats A: What do we know about anesthetic mortality? Anesthesiology 50:387–392, 1979.

49. Morray JP, Geiduschek JM, Caplan RA: A comparison of pediatric and adult anesthesia closed malpractice claims. Anesthesiology 78:461–467, 1993.

50. Cote CJ, Goldstein EA, Cote MA, et al: A single-blind study of pulse oximetry in children. Anesthesiology 68:184–188, 1988.

51. Kestin IG, Miller BR, Lockhart CH: Auditory alarms during anesthesia monitoring. Anesthesiology 69:106–109, 1988.

52. Mather L, Mackie J: The incidence of postoperative pain in children. Pain 15:271–282, 1983.

53. Hatch DJ: Analgesia in the neonate [editorial]. Br Med J 294:920, 1987.

54. Tilney F, Rossett J: The value of brain lipoids in an index of brain development. Bull Neurol Inst NY 1:28–71, 1931.

55. Orlowski JP: Cerebrospinal fluid endorphins and the infant apnea syndrome. Pediatrics 78:233–237, 1986.

56. Pasternak GW, Zhang A, Tecott L: Developmental differences between high and low affinity opiate binding sites: Their relationship to analgesia and respiratory depression. Life Sci 27:1185–1190, 1980.

57. Lloyd-Thomas AR: Pain management in paediatric patients. Br J Anaesth 64:85–104, 1990.

58. Doyle E, Harper I, Morton NS: Comparison of patient-controlled analgesia with and without a background infusion after lower abdominal surgery in children. Br J Anesth 71:670–673, 1993.

59. Parker RK, Holtmann B, White PF: Patient-controlled analgesia: Does a concurrent opioid improve pain management after surgery? JAMA 266:1947–1952, 1991.

60. McNeely JK, Trentadue NC: Comparison of patient-controlled analgesia with and without nighttime morphine infusion following lower extremity surgery in children. J Pain Symptom Manage 13:268–273, 1997.

61. Kay B, Rolly G: Duration of action of analgesia supplement of anesthesia: A double-blind comparison between morphine, fentanyl, and sufentanil. Acta Anaesthesiol Belg 28:25–32, 1977.

62. Claxton AR, McGuire G, Chung F, et al: Evaluation of morphine versus fentanyl for postoperative analgesia after ambulatory surgical procedures. Anesth Analg 84:509–514, 1997.

63. Sanford TJ Jr, Smith NT, Dec-Silver H, Harrison WK: A comparison of morphine, fentanyl, and sufentanil anesthesia for cardiac surgery: Induction, emergence, and extubation. Anesth Analg 65:259–266, 1986.

64. Lejus C, Roussiere G, Testa S, et al: Postoperative extradural analgesia in children: Comparison of morphine with fentanyl. Br J Anesth 72:156–159, 1994.

65. Kastrup EK, Hebel SK, Rivard R, et al: Narcotic Agonist Analgesics: Drug Facts and Comparisons, 1997 ed. St. Louis, Facts and Comparisons, 1997, pp 1316–1318.

66. Hill K, Anderson C: Pediatric pain management: Clinical aspects for the nineties. Semin Anesth 16:136–151, 1997.

67. Ahmedzai S, Brooks D: Transdermal fentanyl versus sustained release morphine in cancer pain: Preference, efficacy, and quality of life: The TTS-Fentanyl Comparative Trial Group. J Pain Symptom Manage 13:254–261, 1997.

68. Birmingham PK, Tobin MJ, Henthom TK, et al: Twenty-four hour pharmacokinetics of rectal acetaminophen in children. Anesthesiology 87:244–252, 1997.

69. Montgomery CJ, McCormack JP, Reichert CC, et al: Plasma concentrations after high-dose (45 mg•kg^{-1}) rectal acetaminophen in children. Can J Anaesth 42:982–986, 1995.

70. Rusy LM, Houck CS, Sullivan LJ, et al: A double-blind evaluation of ketorolac tromethamine versus acetaminophen in pediatric tonsillectomy: Analgesia and bleeding. Anesth Analg 80:226–229, 1995.

71. Gunter JB, Varughese AM, Harrington JF, et al: Recovery and complications after tonsillectomy in children: A comparison of ketorolac and morphine. Anesth Analg 81:1136–1141, 1995.

72. Ho JW, Khambatta HJ, Pang LM, et al: Preemptive analgesia in children: Does it exist? Reg Anesth 22:12–130, 1997.

73. Boix-Ochoa J, Marhuenda C: Gastroesophageal reflux. In Ashcraft KW, Murphy J, Sharp R, et al. (eds): Pediatric Surgery, 3rd ed. Philadelphia, WB Saunders, 2000, pp 370–380.

74. Bozkurt P, Kaya G, Altintas F, et al: Systemic stress response during operations for acute abdominal pain performed via laparoscopy or laparotomy in children. Anaesthesia 55:5–9, 2000.

75. Pennant JH: Anesthesia for laparoscopy in the pediatric patient. Anesth Clin North Am 19:69–74, 2001.

76. Bozkurt G, Kaya G, Yeker Y: The cardiorespiratory effects of laparoscopic procedures in infants. Anesthesia 54:831–834, 1999.

77. Joris JL, Noirot DP, Legrand MJ, et al: Hemodynamic changes during laparoscopic cholecystectomy. Anesth Analg 76:1067–1071, 1993.

78. Gentili A, Iannettone CM, Pigna A, et al: Cardiocirculatory changes during videolaparoscopy in children: An echocardiographic study. Paediatr Anaesth 10:399–406, 2000.

79. Kardos A, Vereczkey G, Pirot L, et al: Use of impedance cardiography to monitor haemodynamic changes during laparoscopy in children. Paediatr Anaesth 11:175–179, 2001.

80. Gueugniaud P, Abisseror M, Moussa M, et al: The hemodynamic effects of pneumoperitoneum during laparoscopic surgery in healthy infants: Assessment by continuous esophageal aortic blood flow echo-Doppler. Anesth Analg 86:290–293, 1998.

81. Talamini MA, Mendoza-Sagaon M, Gitzelmann CA, et al: Increased mediastinal pressure and decreased cardiac output during laparoscopic Nissen fundoplication. Surgery 122:345–353, 1997.

82. Sfez M, Guerard A, Desruelle P: Cardiorespiratory changes during laparoscopic fundoplication in children. Paediatr Anaesth 5:89–95, 1995.

CHAPTER 4

Renal Impairment

Stanley Hellerstein, MD, Uri S. Alon, MD, and
Bradley A. Warady, MD

BODY FLUID REGULATION

Effective kidney function maintains the normal volume
and composition of body fluids even though wide variation
exists in dietary intake and nonrenal expenditures of
water and solute. Water and electrolyte balance is maintained by the excretion of urine, with the volume and
composition defined by physiologic needs. Fluid balance
is accomplished by glomerular ultrafiltration of plasma
coupled with modification of the ultrafiltrate by tubular
reabsorption and secretion.[1,2] The excreted urine, the
modified glomerular filtrate, is the small residuum of the
large volume of nonselective ultrafiltrate modified by
transport processes operating along the nephron. The
glomerular capillaries permit free passage of water and
solutes of low molecular weight while restraining formed
elements and macromolecules. The glomerular capillary
wall functions as a barrier to the filtration of macromolecules based on their size, shape, and charge characteristics. The glomerular filtrate is modified during passage
through the tubules by the active and passive transport
of certain solutes into and out of the luminal fluid and
the permeability characteristics of specific nephron
segments. The transport systems in renal epithelial cells
serve to maintain global water, salt, and acid-base homeostasis rather than to regulate local cellular processes,
such as volume and metabolic substrate uptake, as do
nonrenal epithelial cells.

An adequate volume of glomerular filtrate is essential
for the kidney to regulate water and solute balance
effectively. Blood flow to the kidneys accounts for 20%
to 30% of cardiac output. Of the total renal plasma flow,
92% passes through the functioning excretory tissue and
is known as the *effective renal plasma flow* (ERPF).
Glomerular filtration rate (GFR) is usually about one
fifth of the ERPF, giving a filtration fraction of about 0.2.

The rate of ultrafiltration across the glomerular capillaries is determined by the same forces that allow the transmural movement of fluid in other capillary networks.[3]
These forces are the transcapillary hydraulic and osmotic
pressure gradients and the characteristics of capillary

wall permeability. A renal autoregulatory mechanism
enables the kidney to maintain relative constancy of
blood flow in the presence of changing systemic arterial
and renal perfusion pressures.[1] This intrinsic renal
autoregulatory mechanism appears to be mediated in
individual nephrons by tubuloglomerular feedback
involving the macula densa (a region in the early distal
tubule that juxtaposes the glomerulus) and the afferent
and efferent arterioles. A decrease in arteriolar resistance
in the afferent arteriole, with maintenance of the resistance in the efferent arteriole, sustains glomerular
hydraulic pressure despite a decrease in systemic and
renal arterial pressures.

Under normal conditions, the reabsorption of water
and the reabsorption and secretion of solute during passage of the filtrate through the nephron are subservient
to the maintenance of body fluid homeostasis. In
the healthy, nongrowing individual, the intake and
the expenditure of water and solute are equal, and the
hydrogen-ion balance is zero. Renal function may be
impaired by systemic or renal disease and by medications
such as vasoactive drugs, nonsteroidal anti-inflammatory
drugs, diuretics, and antibiotics. Hypoxia and renal
hypoperfusion appear to be the events most commonly
associated with postoperative renal dysfunction.

RENAL FUNCTION EVALUATION

The evaluation of kidney function begins with history,
physical examination, and laboratory studies. Persistent
oliguria or significant impairment in renal concentrating
capacity should be evident from the history. Examination
of the urinary sediment may provide evidence of renal
disease if proteinuria and/or cellular casts are present.
Normal serum concentrations of sodium, potassium,
chloride, total CO_2, calcium, and phosphorus indicate
appropriate renal regulation of the concentration of electrolytes in body fluids. Serum creatinine concentration is
the usual parameter for GFR. Important limitations and
caveats must be observed when using creatinine to
estimate GFR. Urinary creatinine excretion reflects both

filtered and secreted creatinine because creatinine not only is filtered by the glomerular capillaries but also is secreted by renal tubular cells. As a consequence, creatinine clearance, which is calculated by using serum creatinine concentration and the urinary excretion of creatinine, overestimates true GFR measured by using inulin clearance by 10% to 40%.[4] Serum creatinine concentration and the rate of urinary creatinine excretion are affected by diet. The ingestion of meat, fish, or fowl, substances containing preformed creatinine and creatinine precursors, causes an increase in serum creatinine concentration and in urinary creatinine excretion.[5] The effect of diet on serum creatinine concentration is more marked and sustained in individuals with decreased GFR.

During the last 10 years, the serum concentration of cystatin C, a nonglycosylated 13.3-kd basic protein, has been shown to correlate with GFR as well as or better than serum creatinine.[6-9] From about 12 months and up until age 50 years, normal serum cystatin C concentrations are similar in children and adults (0.70 to 1.38 mg/L). Beginning at about age 50 years, serum cystatin C concentrations increase, related to the decline in GFR associated with age. Serum cystatin C concentrations are not affected by gender, inflammatory conditions, or diet. Accurate automated systems allow the measurement of cystatin C.[10] Serum cystatin C, which has been widely used in Europe, is not yet generally available in North America.

Urine Volume

The appropriate urine volume in any situation depends on the status of body fluids, fluid intake, extrarenal losses, the obligatory renal solute load, and renal concentrating and diluting capacity. Patients with impaired renal concentrating capacity require a larger minimal urinary volume for excretion of the obligatory renal solute load than do those with normal renal concentrating ability. Patients with elevated levels of antidiuretic hormone (ADH) retain water out of proportion to solute and are prone to hyponatremia. Increased levels of ADH may occur because of physiologic factors such as hypertonicity of body fluids or decrease in the effective circulatory volume (as encountered with low levels of serum albumin or with generalized vasodilatation as in the sepsis syndrome). Recently some authors have expressed concern that "usual maintenance fluids," providing 2 to 3 mEq/L of sodium, potassium, and chloride per 100 calories metabolized, may contribute to development of hyponatremia in children hospitalized with conditions likely to be associated with ADH excess.[11] The children at risk are those with nonosmotic stimuli for ADH release such as central nervous system disorders, the postoperative state, pain, stress, nausea, and emesis.

The urinary volume making the diagnosis of oliguric renal failure likely is based on an estimate of the minimal volume needed to excrete the obligatory renal solute load. The reference base for the calculation of urine volume is per 100 mL of maintenance water, not per kilogram of body weight (Table 4-1).[12] The minimal urinary volume

TABLE 4-1

USUAL MAINTENANCE WATER REQUIREMENTS

Weight Range (kg)	Maintenance Water
2.5–10	100 mL/kg
10–20	1000 mL + 50 mL/kg > 10 kg
20	1500 mL + 20 mL/kg > 20 kg

for excretion of the obligatory renal solute load is derived by using the following assumptions:

1. The obligatory renal solute load in a patient being evaluated for ischemic acute renal failure (ARF) is more than the minimum endogenous renal solute load of 10 to 15 mOsm/100 mL of maintenance water and is probably less than 40 mOsm/100 mL of maintenance water generated by the usual diet.[12] Approximately 30 mOsm of obligatory renal solute/100 mL of usual maintenance water is taken as the obligatory renal solute load in children aged 2 months and older.

2. Urinary concentrating capacity increases rapidly during the first year of life and reaches the adult level of 1200 to 1400 mOsm/L at about the second year.[13,14] The maximum urinary concentrating capacity of the term infant from 1 week to 2 months is about 800 mOsm/L; from 2 months to 2 years, about 1000 mOsm/L; and beyond that age, about 1200 mOsm/L. Table 4-2 provides an estimate of the minimal urinary volumes that permit excretion of the obligatory renal solute load, assuming an appropriate physiologic response to renal hypoperfusion. The minimal urinary volumes have been calculated by dividing the expected obligatory renal solute load by the maximal urinary concentrating capacity. Significantly lower urinary volumes are present among patients with oliguric ARF.

3. The presence of oliguric renal failure, based on urine volume, can be diagnosed only in the hydrated patient who has adequate blood pressure for renal perfusion and has no urinary tract obstruction. Oliguric ARF is probably not present in an infant as old as 2 months with a urinary volume equal to or greater than 1.3 mL/hr /100 mL maintenance water or in an older patient with a urinary volume equal to or greater than 1.0 mL/hr/100 mL of maintenance water. Urine output less than these levels requires further evaluation for oliguric ARF.

4. Nonoliguric ARF occurs about as frequently as oliguric ARF. It is diagnosed when an adequately hydrated patient with normal blood pressure and urine volume has elevated serum creatinine and urea nitrogen concentrations. Usually the infant or child with nonoliguric ARF also has decreased serum bicarbonate concentration and may have increased serum potassium. Serum phosphorus concentration may be increased, and serum calcium decreased.

TABLE 4-2

MINIMAL URINARY VOLUMES FOR EXCRETION OF OBLIGATORY RENAL SOLUTE

Age	Assumptions		Urinary Volume	
	Renal Solute Load (mOsm/100 cal)	Maximum Urine Concentration (mOsm/kg)	Urine (mL) per 100 mL (Per 24 hr)	Maintenance Water (Per hr)
1 wk to 2 mo	25 (?)	800	31.3	1.3
2 mo to 2 yr	30 (?)	1000	25.0	1.0
2 yr	30	1200	20.8	1.0

Glomerular Filtration Rate

Glomerular filtration rate is the most useful index of renal function because it reflects the volume of plasma ultrafiltrate presented to the renal tubules. Decline in GFR is the principal functional abnormality in both acute and chronic renal failure. Assessment of GFR is important not only for evaluating the patient with respect to renal function but also for guiding the administration of antibiotics and other drugs. Inulin clearance, which is the accepted standard for measurement of GFR, is too time consuming and inconvenient to be used in the clinical evaluation of most patients. Serum urea nitrogen concentration shows so much variation with dietary intake of nitrogen-containing foods that it is not a satisfactory index of GFR. Serum creatinine concentration and creatinine clearance have become the usual clinical measures for estimation of GFR. However, precautions should be taken when creatinine is used for estimation of GFR because of the effect of diet and common medications on serum creatinine concentration and excretion rate. Ingestion of a meal containing a large quantity of animal protein increases serum creatinine levels about 0.25 mg/dL in 2 hours and increases creatinine excretion rate about 75% over the next 3- to 4-hour period.[5] Serum creatinine concentrations are increased by ingestion of commonly used medications such as salicylate and trimethoprim.[15,16] These agents compete with creatinine for tubular secretion through a base-secreting pathway. They do not alter GFR but elevate serum creatinine concentration.

Serum creatinine concentration in the neonate reflects the maternal level for approximately the first week of life. After this time, serum creatinine concentration should decrease. If it does not, a more in-depth evaluation of kidney function is warranted. Creatinine is formed by the nonenzymatic dehydration of muscle creatine, which accounts for 98% of the total body creatine pool.[4] From age 2 weeks to 2 years, serum creatinine concentration averages about 0.4 ± 0.04 mg/dL (35 ± 3.5 μM).[17] Serum creatinine concentration is relatively constant during this period of growth because the increase in endogenous creatinine production, which is directly correlated with muscle mass, is matched by the increase in GFR. During the first 2 years of life, GFR increases from 35 to 45 mL/min/1.73 m² to the normal adult range of 90 to 170 mL/min/1.73 m². The normal range for serum creatinine concentration increases from 2 years through puberty, although the GFR remains essentially constant when expressed per unit of surface area. This occurs because growth during childhood is associated with increased muscle mass, and therefore, increased creatinine production, which is greater than the increased GFR per unit of body weight.[17] Table 4-3 shows the mean values and ranges for plasma or serum creatinine levels at different ages.[18]

Fractional Excretion of Sodium (FE_{Na}) and Bicarbonate (FE_{HCO3})

Fractional excretions are indexes of renal function that are helpful in evaluating specific clinical conditions. Conceptually, a fractional excretion is the fraction of the filtered substance that is excreted in the urine. Fractional excretions are calculated by using creatinine clearance to estimate GFR and the serum and urine concentrations of the substance studied. The quantity of the substance filtered is taken as the creatinine clearance multiplied by the serum concentration of the substance being evaluated, and the quantity excreted is taken as the concentration in the urine multiplied by the urine volume. The fractional excretion of sodium is derived as follows:

$$\% FE_{Na} = \frac{Na\ Excreted}{Na\ Filtered} \times (100)$$
$$= \frac{(U_{Na} \times V)\,(100)}{(P_{Na})\,\dfrac{(U_{Cr} \times V)}{(P_{Cr})}}$$
$$= \frac{U_{Na}}{P_{Na}} \times \frac{P_{Cr}}{U_{Cr}} \times 100$$

where U_{Na} and U_{Cr} are the urine sodium and creatinine, respectively, and P_{Na} and P_{Cr} are the plasma sodium and creatinine, respectively. Volumes cancel out. So the fractional excretion is calculated from the measurement of sodium and creatinine concentrations in samples of blood and urine obtained at approximately the same time.

Fractional Excretion of Sodium (FE_{Na})

The normal FE_{Na} is usually less than 1% but may be elevated with high salt intake, adaptation to chronic renal failure, and diuretic administration.[19] When a decrease in renal perfusion pressure occurs, which is common in extracellular volume depletion or congestive heart failure, the normal renal response results in a marked increase in the tubular resorption of sodium and water and in the excretion of a small volume of concentrated urine. This physiologic response to decreased renal perfusion is a FE_{Na} less than 1%. FE_{Na} is usually greater than 2% in ischemic ARF.

PLASMA CREATININE LEVELS AT DIFFERENT AGES

Age	Height (cm)	True Plasma Creatinine* (mg/dL)	
		Mean	Range (±2 SD)
Fetal cord blood		0.75	0.15–0.99
0–2 wk	50	0.50	0.34–0.66
2–26 wk	60	0.39	0.23–0.55
26 wk–1 yr	70	0.32	0.18–0.46
2 yr	87	0.32	0.20–0.44
4 yr	101	0.37	0.25–0.49
6 yr	114	0.43	0.27–0.59
8 yr	126	0.48	0.31–0.65
10 yr	137	0.52	0.34–0.70
12 yr	147	0.59	0.41–0.78
Adult male	174	0.97	0.72–1.22
Adult female	163	0.77	0.53–1.01

*Conversion factor: $\mu mol/L = mg/dL \times 88.4$.
Adapted from Changler C, Barratt TM: Laboratory evaluation. In Holliday MA (ed): Pediatric Nephrology (2nd ed). Baltimore, Williams & Wilkins, 1987, pp 282–299.

When using FE_{Na} to aid in differentiating prerenal azotemia from ARF, it is essential that no recent diuretic therapy has been given. Prerenal azotemia may occur in patients with preexisting chronic renal disease who have FE_{Na} levels more than 1% as a consequence of the adaptation to chronic renal failure. When these patients are volume deficient, the elevated serum levels of urea nitrogen and creatinine and the high FE_{Na} may be partially volume responsive. The FE_{Na}, as well as the other diagnostic indices used to help differentiate prerenal azotemia from ischemic ARF, are not pathognomonic for either disorder. However, FE_{Na} provides helpful information when integrated into the overall clinical evaluation.

Fractional Excretion of Bicarbonate (FE_{HCO3})

Renal tubular acidosis (RTA) describes a group of disorders in which metabolic acidosis occurs as a result of an impairment in the reclamation of filtered HCO_3^- or as a result of a defect in the renal hydrogen-ion excretion, in the absence of significant reduction in GFR.[20] Renal tubular acidosis is considered in the differential diagnosis of the patient with metabolic acidosis, a normal serum anion gap (hyperchloremic metabolic acidosis), and a urinary pH above 6.0. A patient with proximal RTA, due to the decreased reclamation of filtered HCO_3^-, may have a urinary pH below 6.0 when the plasma HCO_3^- concentration is below the lowered renal threshold for HCO_3^- reabsorption. Another exception with respect to the presence of an elevated urinary pH in RTA occurs in type IV RTA, a form of distal RTA in which the normal serum anion gap metabolic acidosis is associated with hyperkalemia (*vide infra*).

The diagnosis of a defect in proximal tubular reabsorption of HCO_3^- is made by showing that the FE_{HCO3} is greater than 15% when the plasma HCO_3^- concentration is normalized by sufficient alkalinization. This results in flooding of the distal nephron with HCO_3^-, so the urine becomes highly alkaline. The FE_{HCO3} is calculated just as is the FE_{Na}, but with serum and urine HCO_3^- substituted for Na. A normal individual ingesting a usual diet reabsorbs all the filtered HCO_3^-, and the FE_{HCO3} is zero. A urinary pH of 6.2 or less indicates that urinary HCO_3^- excretion is negligible.

Urinary P_{CO2} or Urine Minus Blood P_{CO2}

Classic distal RTA is caused by a defect in the secretion of H^+ by the cells of the distal nephron. It is characterized by hyperchloremic metabolic acidosis, urine with a pH greater than 6.0 at normal as well as at low serum HCO_3^- concentrations, and an FE_{HCO3} less than 5% when serum HCO_3^- is normal.[20,21] Normally, the cells of the distal nephron secrete H^+ into the lumen where, in the presence of filtered HCO_3^-, carbonic acid (H_2CO_3) is formed. Slow dehydration of the H_2CO_3 into $CO_2 + H_2O$ in the medullary collecting ducts, renal pelvis, and urinary bladder results in urinary P_{CO2} greater than 80 mm Hg or urine minus blood (U–B) P_{CO2} greater than 30 mm Hg. Urinary P_{CO2} is evaluated after administering a single dose of $NaHCO_3$ (2 to 3 mEq/kg) or acetazolamide (17 ± 2 mg/kg) to flood the distal nephron with HCO_3^-. Sodium bicarbonate, rather than acetazolamide, should be used in a patient with significantly reduced serum HCO_3^- levels at the time of the test. Urinary P_{CO2} should be measured only after urinary pH exceeds 7.4 or urinary HCO_3^- concentration exceeds 40 mEq/L or both. A defect in distal nephron secretion of H^+ is diagnosed if U–B P_{CO2} is less than 20 mm Hg or urine P_{CO2} is below 60 mm Hg.

Type IV RTA, a form of distal RTA associated with low urinary pH (< 6.0) and hyperkalemia, is a result of decreased H^+ and K^+ secretion in the distal tubule and is related to a failure to reabsorb sodium.[20,21] Type IV RTA is probably the most commonly recognized type of RTA in both adults and children. The hyperkalemia inhibits ammonia synthesis, resulting in decreased ammonia to serve as a urinary buffer. Therefore a low urinary pH occurs despite decreased H^+ secretion ($NH_3 + H^+ = NH_4^+$). Type IV RTA is physiologically equivalent to aldosterone deficiency, which is one cause of the disorder. In children it may reflect true hypoaldosteronism but it is much more common as a consequence of renal parenchymal damage, especially that due to obstructive uropathy. In pediatric patients, the physiologic impairment of type IV RTA resolves in a few weeks to months after relief of an obstructive disorder.

MEDICAL ASPECTS OF MANAGING THE CHILD WITH POSTOPERATIVE IMPAIRMENT OF RENAL FUNCTION

Pathophysiology of Acute Renal Failure

ARF is characterized by an abrupt decrease in renal function. Because ARF is caused by a decrease in the GFR, the initial clinical manifestations are elevations in serum urea nitrogen and creatinine concentrations and, frequently, reduction in urine output. With improved standards of neonatal and pediatric care, the incidence of ARF associated with medical diseases and with surgery has been reduced. Among pediatric surgical patients, an impairment in renal function is most common in those who are undergoing cardiopulmonary procedures.[22,23]

The most important factor in the pathogenesis of postoperative renal failure is decreased renal perfusion. In the early phase, the reduction in renal blood flow results in a decline in GFR. Intact tubular function results in enhanced resorption of sodium and water. This clinical condition is recognized as prerenal azotemia. Analysis of the patient's urine reveals a high urinary osmolality of greater than 350 mOsm/kg H_2O and a urine sodium concentration less than 10 mEq/L (20 mEq/L in the neonate).[24] The most useful index of the tubular response to renal hypoperfusion with intact tubular function is FE_{Na}. The FE_{Na} test is invalid if the patient received diuretics before giving the urine sample. When kidney function is intact in the hypoperfused state, FE_{Na} is less than 1% in term infants and children and below 2.5% in premature infants.[25] In most patients with prerenal azotemia, intravascular volume depletion is clinically evident. However, in patients with diminished cardiac output (pump failure), clinical appreciation of reduced renal perfusion can be obscured because body weight and central venous pressure may suggest fluid overload. Similarly, assessment of volume status is difficult in patients with burns, edema, ascites, or anasarca. The reduced effective intra-arterial volume might be evident from the reduced systemic blood pressure, tachycardia, and prolonged capillary refill time.

Prerenal azotemia can be alleviated by improving renal perfusion either by repleting the intravascular fluid volume or by improving the cardiac output. The improved kidney function is recognized by increased urine output and normalization of serum urea nitrogen and creatinine concentrations. However, if renal hypoperfusion persists for a significant period or if other nephrotoxic factors are present, parenchymal renal failure can ensue. Factors that may predispose the patient to ARF include preexisting congenital urinary anomalies, septicemia, hypoxemia, hemolysis, rhabdomyolysis, hyperuricemia, drug toxicity, and use of radiocontrast agents. On rare occasions, abdominal compartment syndrome causing tense ascites may impair renal perfusion. Renal failure may be alleviated by abdominal decompression.[26]

Medical Management

The child with postoperative oliguria and elevated serum creatinine concentration should be assessed for possible prerenal azotemia. If the child is found to be hypovolemic, an intravenous (IV) fluid challenge of 20 mL/kg of isotonic saline or plasma is commonly infused. In most instances, however, it may be physiologically advantageous to provide a solution in which bicarbonate accounts for 25 to 40 mEq/L of the anions in the fluid bolus (½ isotonic NaCl in 5% glucose, to which is added 25 to 40 mEq/L of 1 M NaHCO$_3$). If no response is observed and the child is still dehydrated, the dose can be repeated. When the urine output is satisfactory after fluid replenishment, the child should receive appropriate maintenance and replacement fluids and should be monitored. Body weight, urinary volume, and serum concentrations of urea nitrogen, creatinine, and electrolytes also should be monitored.

If urinary output is inadequate after the fluid challenge, an IV infusion of furosemide, 1 mg/kg, may be given in a bolus. Patients with renal failure may require higher doses, up to 5 mg/kg. If no response occurs after the initial infusion of furosemide, a second, higher dose can be repeated after 1 hour. Some patients may require furosemide every 4 to 8 hours to maintain satisfactory urinary volume. A protocol with constant furosemide infusion has been successfully used in oliguric children after cardiac surgery.[27] Furosemide is infused at 0.1 mg/kg/hr, with the dose increased by 0.1 mg after 2 hours if the urinary volume remains less than 1 ml/kg/hr. The maximum dose is 0.4 mg/kg/hr. Urine output can at times be increased by the use of vasoactive agents such as dopamine; however, their efficacy in otherwise altering the course of ARF is not well established.[28]

Careful monitoring of the patient's fluid and electrolyte status is essential. Those children who fail to respond to furosemide are at risk for fluid overload. Overzealous fluid administration during anesthesia and surgery and for the management of persistent hypoperfusion along with decreased urinary output can result in hypervolemia, hypertension, heart failure, and pulmonary edema. In extreme cases, fluid administration must be decreased to the minimum necessary to deliver essential medications. In less severe instances, and in euvolemic patients with impaired kidney function, total fluid intake should equal insensible water loss, urine volume, and any significant extrarenal fluid losses. Urine output must be monitored hourly, and fluid management must be re-evaluated every 4 to 12 hours, as clinically indicated. Valuable information about the patient's overall fluid status can be obtained by carefully monitoring blood pressure, pulse, and body weight. The preoperative values of these parameters help serve as a baseline for postoperative evaluation. Ideally, the patient's hemodynamic status should be assessed continuously by using central venous pressure monitoring. In patients with complicated cardiac problems, a Swan-Ganz catheter that monitors pulmonary wedge pressure should be used.

Fluid overload can lead to hyponatremia. Because, in most cases, total body sodium remains normal or high, the best way to normalize serum sodium concentration is by restriction of fluid intake and enhancement of urinary volume.[29] In patients with acute symptomatic hyponatremia, careful infusion of NaCl 3% solution (512 mEq Na/L or 0.5 mEq/mL) may be given to correct hyponatremia. Rapid correction at a rate of 1 to 2 mEq/hr over a 2- to 3-hour period, with an increase of serum sodium level by 4 to 6 mEq/L, is usually well tolerated and adequate. Infusion of 6 mL/kg of 3% NaCl increases serum sodium concentration by about 5 mEq/L. Hyponatremia that is present more than 24 to 48 hours should not be corrected at a rate more rapid than 0.5 mEq/L/hr.

In children with ARF, hyperkalemia often develops. The early sign of potassium cardiotoxicity is peaked T waves on the electrocardiogram. Higher levels of serum potassium can cause ventricular fibrillation and cardiac asystole. The treatment for hyperkalemia is shown in Table 4-4. Emergency treatment of hyperkalemia is indicated when serum potassium concentration reaches 7.0 mEq/L or when electrocardiographic changes are noted.

In children with ARF, metabolic acidosis rapidly develops. Owing to decreased kidney function, fewer hydrogen ions are excreted. Organic acids then accumulate in the body, causing a reduction in the serum bicarbonate concentration. Although a child with uncompromised ventilatory capacity is able to hyperventilate and achieve partial compensation, a child with compromised pulmonary function or a hypercatabolic state is at risk for profound acidosis. Metabolic acidosis is usually treated by administering sodium bicarbonate. However, attention should be directed toward the excess sodium load associated with this mode of therapy. Because hypocalcemia develops in many patients with ARF, treatment with alkali should be done with care to protect them from hypocalcemic tetany. It is not necessary to correct the metabolic acidosis completely to prevent the untoward effects of acidemia. Increasing the serum bicarbonate concentration to 15 mEq/L is usually satisfactory.[30]

Dialysis

The inability to control medically the fluid-and-electrolyte or acid-base disorders caused by renal failure necessitates the initiation of dialysis therapy.

Indications for Urgent Dialysis

The indications for urgent dialysis follow:

Persistent oligoanuria
Hyperkalemia
Metabolic acidosis
Fluid overload
Severe electrolyte and mineral disturbances
Uremic syndrome

The most common indication for postoperative dialysis in a child is the hypervolemia caused by repeated attempts at fluid resuscitation, administration of medications, and total parenteral nutrition. Repeated IV catheter flushes and endotracheal tube lavages can add a significant amount of water and solute to the total intake.[31] Fluid overload in the postoperative patient can cause pulmonary edema and, less commonly, hypertension.

Dialysis Therapy

The three modes of therapy include hemodialysis, hemofiltration, and peritoneal dialysis. The last of these is used most commonly in children. The intrinsic factors that affect the efficacy of peritoneal dialysis include peritoneal blood flow, peritoneal vascular permeability, and peritoneal surface area.[32] Although removal of up to 50% of the peritoneal surface area does not seem to interfere with dialysis efficacy,[33] hypoperfusion of the peritoneal membrane vasculature renders dialysis ineffective.[34] Dialysis in the postoperative patient is feasible even in the presence of peritonitis or immediately after major abdominal procedures.[35,36] Increased intra-abdominal pressure caused by the administration of peritoneal fluid can cause respiratory embarrassment and contribute to fluid leakage from the sites of the surgical incisions and the entrance of the peritoneal catheter. Under such circumstances, the smallest effective dialysis fluid volume is used. It can be gradually increased with time after surgery. Common complications associated with peritoneal dialysis are peritonitis, exit-site infection, leaking dialysate, catheter obstruction, and abdominal wall hernia. A rare complication is abdominal organ perforation.[37] In children in whom prolonged peritoneal dialysis is anticipated, placement of Tenckhoff

---

TABLE 4-4

TREATMENT OF HYPERKALEMIA

Cardiac Protection
Calcium gluconate, 10%, 0.5–1.0 mL/kg body weight injected intravenously and slowly over 5–10 min, with continuous monitoring of heart rate

Shift of Potassium into the Intracellular Compartment
Sodium bicarbonate, 1–2 mEq/kg body weight intravenously over 10–20 min, provided that salt and water overload is not a problem
Glucose, 1 g/kg body weight, and insulin, 1 unit per every 4 g of glucose, intravenously over 20–30 min
Stimulants of β_2-adrenergic receptors, such as salbutamol, intravenously or by inhalation

Elimination of Excess Potassium
Cation exchange resin, sodium polystyrene sulfonate, 1 g/kg body weight, administered orally or rectally in 20% to 30% sorbitol or 10% glucose, 1 g resin/4 mL. Additional 70% sorbitol syrup may be given if constipation occurs
Dialysis, peritoneal or hemodialysis

catheter was shown to be advantageous over the placement of Cook catheter.[38]

Dialysate solution with a 1.5 % glucose concentration has an osmolality of 350 mOsm/kg H_2O, which is moderately hypertonic to normal plasma (280 to 295 mOsm/kg H_2O). With increased glucose concentration in the dialysate solution, the tonicity of the solution increases, reaching 490 mOsm/kg H_2O with 4.25 % glucose, the highest concentration commercially available. Other factors being equal, the higher the tonicity of the dialysate, the greater the ultrafiltrate (fluid removed from the body). Owing to the rapid movement of water and glucose across the peritoneal membrane, the effect of peritoneal dialysis on fluid removal is maximal when short dialysis cycles of 20 to 30 minutes are used. When solutions containing glucose concentrations higher than 1.5 % are given, close monitoring of the serum glucose concentration is necessary. If hyperglycemia greater than 200 mg/dL develops, it can be controlled by the addition of insulin to the dialysate solution or by IV insulin drip. The volume of fluid removed by dialysis in a 24-hour period should be limited to 500 mL in the neonate, range from 500 to 1000 mL in infants and 1000 to 1500 mL in young children, and be limited to 3000 mL in children weighing more than 30 kg.[28] The effect of dialysis on the removal of solutes depends mainly on the length of the dwell time in the peritoneal cavity and the molecular weight of the solute. The following are the relative rates of diffusion of common substances.[39]

Urea > Potassium > Sodium > Creatinine > Phosphate > Uric Acid > Calcium > Magnesium

Standard dialysate solutions do not contain potassium. Hyperkalemia therefore may be controlled with a few hours of effective peritoneal dialysis.

In children in whom peritoneal dialysis is not feasible, hemodialysis and hemofiltration are options. The latter may be preferred, especially in those patients who are hemodynamically unstable.[40] The most common mode of hemofiltration is the pump-assisted continuous venovenous hemofiltration. When indicated, it can be combined with dialysis. In children at risk for hemorrhage, a protocol using citrate instead of heparin as anticoagulant has been developed.[41]

ACUTE RENAL FAILURE IN THE NEONATE

ARF occurs in as many as 24 % of all patients admitted to the neonatal intensive care unit.[42,43] The definition of ARF in a term neonate is most often considered to be a serum creatinine level above 1.5 mg/dL for more than 24 hours in the setting of normal maternal renal function. On occasion, it may be diagnosed in the term infant with a serum creatinine less than 1.5 mg/dL when it fails to decrease in a normal manner over the initial days/weeks of life.[44-46] The limited availability of cystatin C data from the neonatal population currently precludes its routine use to define ARF.[47,48]

ARF is of the oliguric variety when the elevated serum creatinine is accompanied by a urine output below 1 mL/kg/hr after the initial 24 hours of life and when urine output fails to improve in response to a fluid challenge.[45] In contrast, in some patients, solute retention develops, as evidenced by an elevated serum creatinine level, with a normal (> 1.0 mL/kg/hr) urine flow rate: they are diagnosed as having nonoliguric ARF.[49] The nonoliguric form is particularly common in neonates with ARF secondary to perinatal asphyxia and appears to be associated with a better prognosis than does the oliguric form.[46,49] The diagnosis of nonoliguric ARF can be overlooked if patients at risk for developing renal insufficiency are monitored solely by the evaluation of urine output without repeated assessments of the serum creatinine.

The causes of ARF traditionally have been divided into three categories: prerenal, intrinsic, and postrenal (Table 4-5). This division, based on the site of the lesion, has important implications because the evaluation, treatment, and prognosis of the three groups can be quite different.

Prerenal Acute Renal Failure

Impairment of renal perfusion is the cause of 70 % of ARF during the neonatal period.[42-46] Prerenal ARF may occur in any patient with hypoperfusion of an otherwise

TABLE 4-5
MAJOR CAUSES OF ACUTE RENAL FAILURE IN THE NEWBORN

Prerenal Failure
Systemic hypovolemia: fetal hemorrhage, neonatal hemorrhage, septic shock, necrotizing enterocolitis, dehydration
Renal hypoperfusion: perinatal asphyxia, congestive heart failure, cardiac surgery, cardiopulmonary bypass–extracorporeal membrane oxygenation, respiratory distress syndrome, pharmacologic (tolazoline, captopril, enalapril, indomethacin)

Intrinsic Renal Failure
Acute tubular necrosis
Congenital malformations: bilateral agenesis, renal dysplasia, polycystic kidney disease, glomerular maturational arrest
Infection: congenital (syphilis, toxoplasmosis), pyelonephritis
Renal vascular: renal artery thrombosis, renal venous thrombosis, disseminated intravascular coagulation
Nephrotoxins: aminoglycosides, indomethacin, amphotericin B, contrast media, captopril, enalapril, vancomycin
Intrarenal obstruction: uric acid nephropathy, myoglobinuria, hemoglobinuria

Postrenal (Obstructive) Renal Failure
Congenital malformations: imperforate prepuce, urethral stricture, posterior urethral valves, urethral diverticulum, primary vesicoureteral reflux, ureterocele, megacystis megaureter, Eagle-Barrett syndrome, ureteropelvic junction obstruction, ureterovesicle obstruction
Extrinsic compression: sacrococcygeal teratoma, hematocolpos
Intrinsic obstruction: renal calculi, fungus balls
Neurogenic bladder

Adapted from Karlowicz MG, Adelman RD: Acute renal failure in the neonate. Clin Perinatol 19:139–158, 1992.

normal kidney. Although prompt correction of the low perfusion state usually reverses kidney-function impairment, delay in fluid resuscitation may result in renal parenchymal damage.

Intrinsic Acute Renal Failure

Intrinsic ARF occurs in 6% to 8% of admissions to the neonatal intensive care unit and implies the presence of renal cellular damage associated with impaired kidney function.[44] Intrinsic ARF usually falls into one of the following categories: ischemic (acute tubular necrosis), nephrotoxic (aminoglycoside antibiotics, indomethacin), congenital renal anomalies (autosomal recessive polycystic kidney disease), and vascular lesions (renal artery or vein thrombosis, especially with a solitary kidney).[50]

Postrenal Acute Renal Failure

Postrenal ARF results from obstruction of urine flow from both kidneys or from a solitary kidney. The most common causes of postrenal ARF in neonates are posterior urethral valves, bilateral ureteropelvic junction obstruction, and bilateral ureterovesicle junction obstruction.[51,52] Although these types of obstructions are characteristically reversible, neonates with long-standing intrauterine obstruction have varying degrees of permanent impairment of renal function.[53,54] This impairment may be due not only to the presence of renal dysplasia, but also to cellular damage secondary to ARF.

Clinical Presentation

Clinical presentation of the neonate with ARF often reflects the condition that has precipitated development of the renal insufficiency. Accordingly, sepsis, shock, dehydration, severe respiratory distress syndrome, and other related conditions may be present. Nonspecific symptoms related to uremia, such as poor feeding, lethargy, emesis, seizures, hypertension, and anemia, also are frequently present.

DIAGNOSTIC EVALUATION

Evaluation of the neonate with ARF should include a thorough patient and family history and a physical examination. Suspected prerenal causes of acute oliguria are usually addressed diagnostically and therapeutically by volume expansion, with or without furosemide. If this approach does not result in increased urine output, a more extensive evaluation of renal function is indicated.

Laboratory studies are an important component of the evaluation and should include the following measures: complete blood count and serum concentrations of urea nitrogen, creatinine, electrolytes, uric acid, calcium, glucose, and phosphorus. The serum creatinine value during the first several days of life is a reflection of the maternal value. In term infants, a value of 0.4 to 0.5 mg/dL is expected after the first week of life. In contrast, the expected value in preterm infants is related to their gestational age, with an initial increase followed by a gradual decrease.[55,56] In all cases, a urinalysis should be obtained to check for the presence of red blood cells, protein, and casts suggestive of intrinsic renal disease.

Urine indices can help distinguish intrinsic renal failure from prerenal azotemia in the oliguric patient. The index usually found to be the most useful is FE_{Na}. This factor is based on the assumption that the renal tubules of the poorly perfused kidney reabsorb sodium avidly, whereas the kidney with intrinsic renal disease and tubular damage is unable to do so. Accordingly, in most cases of neonatal oliguric renal failure secondary to intrinsic disease, the FE_{Na} is greater than 2.5% to 3.0%.[43,57] The FE_{Na} should be measured before administering furosemide. In addition, the results should be interpreted with caution in the very premature infant who normally has a high (i.e., >5%) FE_{Na}.[57,58]

Ultrasonography is commonly the initial imaging study performed.[59] The urinary tract should be evaluated for the presence of one or two kidneys and for their size, shape, and location. Dilation of the collecting system and the size and appearance of the urinary bladder should be evident. A voiding cystourethrogram (VCUG) also may be necessary, specifically when the diagnosis of posterior urethral valves or vesicoureteral reflux is entertained. In most cases, a VCUG is deemed preferable to radionuclide cystography in this setting because of its superior ability to provide reliable anatomic information about the grading of vesicoureteral reflux or the appearance of the urethra.[60] Antegrade pyelography or diuretic renography with either technetium[99m]-dimercaptosuccinic acid or technetium[99m]-MAG-3 as the radiopharmaceutical agent may be needed to evaluate for ureteral obstruction, because the limited GFR and renal tubular function of the neonate result in poor visualization of the kidneys and urinary tract with IV pyelography during the first several weeks of life. Radiocontrast agents may be nephrotoxic, as well.[61] Finally, radiologic assessment of the differential renal function may be performed with radioisotope scanning.

Management

The treatment of neonatal ARF should proceed simultaneous with the diagnostic workup. A fluid challenge, with or without subsequent furosemide therapy, usually enhances urine flow and fosters improved renal function in an infant with prerenal oliguria. Bladder catheter placement is good immediate therapy for posterior urethral valves, whereas high surgical drainage may be needed for other obstructive lesions in the neonate. The fluid challenge for the neonate should consist of 20 mL/kg of an isotonic solution containing 25 mEq/L of sodium bicarbonate infused over a 1- to 2-hour period. In the absence of a prompt diuresis of 2 mL or more of urine per kilogram during 1 to 2 hours, intravenous furosemide at 2 to 5 mg/kg may be helpful. The role of dopamine as therapy for neonatal oliguric ARF, owing to its ability to cause renal vasodilation via activation of DA1 and DA2 receptors, remains unclear.[45,62] The effects of dopamine are dose dependent. If used, the initial dose should be

1 μg/kg/min and should not exceed 5 μg/kg/min owing to its potential to induce vasoconstriction at the higher doses as a result of stimulation of the alpha receptors.[63] It also may be beneficial to combine its use with furosemide. The failure to achieve increased urinary output after volume expansion in the neonate with an adequate cardiac output (i.e., renal perfusion) and an unobstructed urinary tract indicates the presence of intrinsic renal disease and the need to manage oliguric or anuric renal failure appropriately.

Maintenance of normal fluid balance is of primary concern in the management of the patient with ARF. Daily fluid intake should equal insensible water loss, urine output, and fluid losses from nonrenal sources. In term infants, insensible water losses amount to 30 to 40 mL/kg/day, whereas premature infants may require as much as 50 to 100 mL/kg/day.[58,64] A frequent assessment of the neonate's body weight is essential for fluid management. The electrolyte content of the fluids administered should be guided by frequent laboratory studies. Insensible water losses are electrolyte free and should be replaced by using glucose in water.

Important systemic disturbances that may arise secondary to ARF include hyperkalemia, hyponatremia, hypertension, hypocalcemia, hyperphosphatemia, and metabolic acidosis. All exogenous sources of potassium should be discontinued in patients with ARF. Despite this restriction, elevated serum potassium levels develop in many and must be treated aggressively owing to the potential for cardiac toxicity.[25,45] Treatment should be initiated by correction of metabolic acidosis with sodium bicarbonate, 1 to 2 mEq/kg body weight (BW) provided intravenously over a 10- to 20-minute period, provided that salt and water balance is not problematic. The quantity of sodium bicarbonate to be prescribed also can be calculated in the following manner: ($0.3 \times$ BW [kg] $\times$ Base deficit [mM]).[45] Associated hypocalcemia should be treated with the intravenous administration of 10% calcium gluconate at a dose of 0.5 to 1.0 mL/kg injected slowly over a 5-minute period with continuous monitoring of the heart rate. If a progressive increase in the serum potassium is noted, additional treatment measures may include the use of a sodium-potassium exchange resin (sodium polystyrene sulfonate in 20% to 30% sorbitol, 1 g/kg by enema), with recognition of its frequent ineffectiveness and/or associated complications when used in low-birth-weight infants.[65] The use of glucose (0.5 to 1.0 g/kg) followed by insulin (0.1 to 0.2 units regular insulin per gram glucose over a 1- to 2-hour period), or either IV salbutamol or inhaled albuterol are additional therapeutic options.[66,67] Dialysis should be considered if these measures prove unsuccessful.

Hyponatremia and systemic hypertension are most often related to overhydration in the infant with oliguria and initially should be treated with fluid restriction. The addition of high-dose IV furosemide (5 mg/kg) may be beneficial. Serum sodium levels below 125 mEq/L can be associated with seizures, and values less than 120 mEq/L should be treated promptly with hypertonic (3%) saline. The approximate amount of sodium needed to correct symptomatic hyponatremia in neonates is calculated as follows:

$$Na^+ \text{ (mEq)} = ([Na^+] \text{ Desired} - [Na^+] \text{ Actual}) \times \text{Weight (kg)} \times 0.8$$

The treatment of persistent hypertension may include parenterally administered hydralazine (0.15 to 0.6 mg/kg/dose or 0.75 to 5.0 μg/kg/min infusion), labetalol (0.20 to 1.0 mg/kg/dose or 0.25 to 3.0 mg/kg/hr infusion), or enalaprilat (15 $\pm$ 5 μg/kg/dose) for the patient without symptoms. Treatment of the patient with marked or refractory hypertension can include IV diazoxide (2 to 5 mg/kg/dose), sodium nitroprusside (0.5 to 10 μg/kg/min infusion), nicardipine (1 to 3 μg/kg/min infusion), or labetalol. Caution should be exercised when initiating therapy with captopril (initial oral dose, 0.01 to 0.05 mg/kg) owing to the profound hypotension that can occur in neonates in association with higher doses.[45,68,69]

Hyperphosphatemia (serum phosphorus level, >7 mg/dL), which is often the cause of associated hypocalcemia, necessitates the use of a low-phosphorus infant formula (Similac PM 60/40) and calcium carbonate (50 to 100 mg/kg/day) as a phosphate binder.[70] The use of aluminum hydroxide as a binder is contraindicated, owing to its association with aluminum toxicity in infants and children with renal insufficiency.[71] No experience has been published about the use of newer phosphate-binding agents such as sevelemer in the neonatal population.[72]

Hypocalcemia, as reflected by a low total serum calcium level, often occurs in ARF in association with hypoalbuminemia. Less commonly, the ionized calcium level is low, and the patient is symptomatic. In these cases, IV 10% calcium gluconate, 0.5 to 1.0 mL/kg over a 5-minute period with cardiac monitoring should be given until the ionized calcium level is restored to the normal range.[45]

Metabolic acidosis may arise as a result of retention of hydrogen ions and may require sodium bicarbonate for correction. The dose of sodium bicarbonate to be given can be calculated as follows:

$$\text{Sodium bicarbonate (mEq)} = (\text{Desired bicarbonate} - \text{Observed bicarbonate}) \times \text{Weight (kg)} \times 0.5$$

This dose may be given orally or added to parenteral fluids and infused during several hours.

Adequate nutrition should be provided, with the goal of 100 to 120 calories and 1 to 2 g of protein/kg/day, provided via IV or orally. For neonates who can tolerate oral fluids, a formula containing low levels of phosphorus and aluminum, such as Similac PM 60/40, is recommended. An aggressive approach to nutrition may well contribute to renal recovery by providing necessary energy at the cellular level.[25]

Although most neonates with ARF can be managed conservatively, occasional patients require peritoneal dialysis or continuous renal replacement therapy (CRRT) for the treatment of the metabolic complications and fluid overload.[28,73–75] The mortality rate in this group of patients commonly exceeds 60%. Twenty-three patients who received peritoneal dialysis at Children's Mercy Hospital during the neonatal period had a mortality rate of 35% at 1 year.[76] The somewhat lower mortality rate in our center probably reflects the improved outcome of neonates with renal structural abnormalities leading to renal failure (17% mortality rate) compared with those infants with multisystem disease. In a report of 12 neonates in whom ARF developed after cardiac surgery and who received continuous venovenous hemofiltration (CVVH), seven (59%) of the infants survived, and no complications were noted related to the hemofiltration procedure.[77] In the most recent such report,[75] on the use of CRRT in 85 children weighing less than 10 kg, 16 of whom were less than 3 kg, the procedure was well tolerated, other than for the need of pressor support, with survival rates of 25% and 41% for those less than 3 kg and 3 to 10 kg, respectively.

OBSTRUCTIVE UROPATHY

Obstructive uropathy in the neonate is the most common renal abnormality diagnosed prenatally and is most often the result of ureteropelvic junction obstruction or posterior urethral valves or ureterovesicle obstruction.[51] Obstruction also represents a significant cause of end-stage renal disease (ESRD) in children, accounting for 16% of all cases, and is the underlying cause of ESRD in nearly 90% of affected boys younger than 4 years.[78,79] Accordingly, early recognition and treatment of these lesions are desirable, because of the adverse effects obstruction can have on renal function.[29,30,53,54,80] Regardless, after surgical intervention and relief of obstruction, alterations of GFR, renal blood flow, and renal tubular function may occur.[54,80,81] Specifically, injury to the renal tubule may result in an impaired capacity to reabsorb sodium, to concentrate urine, and to secrete potassium and hydrogen, all of which may have profound clinical implications. The resorption of other solutes, such as magnesium, calcium, and phosphorus, also may be affected.[54,81]

The ability of the renal tubule to reabsorb salt and water after relief of obstruction typically depends on whether the obstruction is unilateral or bilateral. In unilateral obstruction, the proximal tubules of the juxtamedullary nephrons are unable to reabsorb salt and water maximally, whereas the fractional reabsorption of salt and water is increased in the superficial nephrons.[81] However, the amount of sodium excreted by the previously obstructed kidney is not different from that of the contralateral kidney, because tubuloglomerular balance is maintained. In contrast, relief of bilateral obstruction or, on occasion, unilateral obstruction in neonates[82] results in a postobstructive diuresis characterized by a marked elevation in the absolute amount of sodium and water lost. In part, these changes are a result of an osmotic diuresis secondary to retained solutes, such as urea.[82,83] Some contribution also may occur from atrial natriuretic factor, the plasma level of which is elevated during obstruction, as well as from enhanced synthesis of prostaglandins.[81,84] Decreased renal medullary tonicity and decreased hydraulic water permeability of the collecting duct in response to ADH, the latter a result of reduced aquaporin channels, contribute to the impaired concentrating ability of the kidney.[27,80,85]

The clinical conditions associated with prolonged salt wasting are severe volume contraction and circulatory impairment, whereas conditions associated with the concentrating abnormalities are secondary nephrogenic diabetes insipidus and hypernatremic dehydration. Accordingly, management must ensure the provision of adequate amounts of fluid and salt. Sodium intake should be monitored by serum and urine electrolyte determinations. Fluid intake should equal insensible losses, urine output, and nonrenal losses, and should be guided by frequent assessments of body weight.

Ureteral obstruction also can result in the impairment of hydrogen and potassium secretion and the syndrome of hyperkalemic hyperchloremic metabolic acidosis, or type IV renal tubular acidosis.[86-88] This clinical situation appears to be the result of the impaired turnover of the sodium-potassium pump or a decreased responsiveness of the distal renal tubule to the actions of aldosterone. In a portion of the patients with this presentation, FE_{Na} is normal, and FE_K is inappropriately low, relative to the elevated serum level. Treatment is directed toward correcting the underlying obstructive abnormality with surgery as well as providing sodium bicarbonate to alleviate the metabolic acidosis and hyperkalemia.

Finally, the outcome of obstructive uropathy in the neonate in terms of preservation of GFR is, in part, related to how promptly surgical intervention and relief of obstruction take place. In these patients, the serum creatinine value obtained at age 12 months has been shown to be predictive of long-term kidney function.[29,30,54,80]

REFERENCES

1. Brenner BM, Dworkin LD, Kchikawa L: Glomerular ultrafiltration. In Brenner BM, Rector FC (eds): The Kidney, Vol.1, 3rd ed. Philadelphia, WB Saunders, 1986, pp 124–144.
2. Hogg RJ, Stapleton FB: Renal tubular function. In Holliday MA, Barratt TM, Vernier RL (eds): Pediatric Nephrology, 2nd ed. Baltimore, Williams & Wilkins, 1987, pp 59–77.
3. Yared A, Ichikawa I: Renal blood flow and glomerular filtration rate. In Holliday MA, Barratt TM, Vernier RL (eds): Pediatric Nephrology, 2nd ed. Baltimore, Williams & Wilkins, 1987, pp 45–58.
4. Perrone RD, Madias NE, Levey AS: Serum creatinine as an index of renal function: New insights into old concepts. Clin Chem 38:1933–1953, 1992.
5. Hellerstein S, Hunter JL, Warady BA: Creatinine excretion rates for evaluation of kidney function in children. Pediatr Nephrol 2:419–424, 1988.
6. Newman DJ, Thakkar H, Edwards RG, et al: Serum cystatin C measured by automated immunoassay: A more sensitive marker of changes in GFR than serum creatinine. Kidney Int 47:312–318, 1995.
7. Bökenkamp A, Domanetzki M, Zinck R, et al: Cystatin C serum concentrations underestimate glomerular filtration rate in renal transplant recipients. Clin Chem 45:1866–1868, 1999.
8. Finney H, Newman DJ, Price CP: Adult reference ranges for serum cystatin C, creatinine and predicted creatinine clearance. Ann Clin Biochem 37:49–59, 2000.

9. Fischbach M, Graff V, Terzie J, et al: Impact of age on reference values for serum concentration of cystatin C in children. Pediatr Nephrol 17:104–106, 2002.
10. Kyhse-Anderson J, Schmidt C, Nordin G, et al: Serum cystatin C, determined by a rapid, automated particle-enhanced turbidimetric method, is a better marker than serum creatinine for glomerular filtration rate. Clin Chem 40:1921–1926, 1994.
11. Mortiz ML, Ayus JC: Prevention of hospital-acquired hyponatremia: A case for using isotonic saline. Pediatrics 111:227–230, 2003.
12. Holliday MA, Segar WE: The maintenance need for water in parenteral fluid therapy. Pediatrics 19:823–832, 1957.
13. Edelmann CM Jr, Barnett HL: Role of the kidney in water metabolism in young infants. J Pediatr 56:154–179, 1960.
14. Polacek B, Vocel J, Neugebauerova L, et al: The osmotic concentrating ability in healthy infants and children. Arch Dis Child 40:291–295, 1965.
15. Burry HC, Dieppe PA: Apparent reduction of endogenous creatinine clearance by salicylate treatment. BMJ 2:16–17, 1976.
16. Berglund F, Killander J, Pompeius R: Effect of trimethoprim-sulfamethoxazole on the renal excretion of creatinine in man. J Urol 114:802–808, 1975.
17. Hellerstein S, Holliday MA, Grupe WE, et al: Nutritional management of children with chronic renal failure: Summary of the Task Force on Nutritional Management of Children with Chronic Renal Failure. Pediatr Nephrol 1:195–211, 1987.
18. Chantler C, Barratt TM: Laboratory evaluation. In Holliday MA, Barratt TM, Vernier RL (eds): Pediatric Nephrology, 2nd ed. Baltimore, Williams & Wilkins, 1987, pp 282–299.
19. Steiner RW: Interpreting the fractional excretion of sodium. Am J Med 77:699–702, 1984.
20. Halperin ML, Goldstein MB, Stinebaugh BJ, et al: Renal tubular acidosis. In Maxwell MH, Kleeman CR, Narins RG (eds): Clinical Disorders of Fluid and Electrolyte Metabolism, 4th ed. New York, McGraw-Hill, 1987, pp 675–689.
21. Rodriguez-Soriano J, Vallo A: Renal tubular acidosis. Pediatr Nephrol 4:268–275, 1990.
22. Gomez-Campdera FJ, Maroto-Alvaro E, Galinanes M, et al: Acute renal failure associated with cardiac surgery. Child Nephrol Urol 9:138–143, 1988.
23. Rigden SP, Barratt TM, Dillon MJ, et al: Acute renal failure complicating cardiopulmonary bypass surgery. Arch Dis Child 57:425–430, 1982.
24. Cohen ML, Rifkind D: The Pediatric Abacus. Boca Raton, Fla, The Parthenon Publishing Group, 2002.
25. Gaudio KM, Siegel NJ: Pathogenesis and treatment of acute renal failure. Pediatr Clin North Am 34:771–787, 1987.
26. Bailey J, Shapiro MJ: Abdominal compartment syndrome. Crit Care 4:23–29, 2000.
27. Singh N, Kissoon N, Al-Mofada S, et al: Furosemide infusion versus furosemide bolus in the postoperative pediatric cardiac patient. Pediatr Res 27:35A, 1990.
28. Chan JCM: Peritoneal dialysis for renal failure in childhood: Clinical aspects and electrolyte changes as observed in 20 cases. Clin Pediatr 17:349–354, 1978.
29. Trachtman H: Sodium and water homeostasis. Pediatr Clin North Am 42:1343–1363, 1995.
30. Feld LG, Cachero S, Springate JE: Fluid needs in acute renal failure. Pediatr Clin North Am 37:337–350, 1990.
31. Noble-Jamieson CM, Kuzmin P, Airede KI: Hidden sources of fluid and sodium intake in ill newborns. Arch Dis Child 61:695–696, 1986.
32. Gruskin AB, Morgenstern BZ, Perlman S: Kinetics of peritoneal dialysis in children. In Fine RN, Gruskin AB (eds): End Stage Renal Disease in Children. Philadelphia, WB Saunders, 1984, pp 95–117.
33. Alon U, Bar-Maor JA, Bar-Joseph G: Effective peritoneal dialysis in an infant with extensive resection of the small intestine. Am J Nephrol 8:65–67, 1988.
34. Erbe RW, Greene JA Jr, Weller JM: Peritoneal dialysis during hemorrhagic shock. J Appl Physiol 22:131–135, 1967.
35. Fine RN: Peritoneal dialysis update. J Pediatr 100:1–7, 1982.
36. Tzamaloukas AH, Garella S, Chazan JA: Peritoneal dialysis for acute renal failure after major abdominal surgery. Arch Surg 106:639–643, 1973.
37. Matthews DE, West KW, Rescorla FJ, et al: Peritoneal dialysis in the first 60 days of life. J Pediatr Surg 25:110–115, 1990.
38. Chadha V, Warady BA, Blowey DL, et al: Tenckhoff catheters prove superior to Cook catheters in pediatric acute peritoneal dialysis. Am J Kidney Dis 35:1111–1116, 2000.
39. Miller RB, Tassistro CR: Peritoneal dialysis. N Engl J Med 281:945–949, 1969.
40. Evans ED, Greenbaum LA, Ettenger RB: Principles of renal replacement therapy in children. Pediatr Clin North Am 42:1579–1602, 1995.
41. Chadha V, Garg U, Warady BA, et al: Citrate clearance in children receiving continuous venovenous renal replacement therapy. Pediatr Nephrol 17:819–824, 2002.
42. Norman ME, Asadi FK: A prospective study of acute renal failure in the newborn infant. Pediatrics 63:475–479, 1979.
43. Chan JC, Williams DM, Roth KS: Kidney failure in infants and children. Pediatr Rev 23:47–60, 2002.
44. Stapleton FB, Jones DP, Green RS: Acute renal failure in neonates: incidence, etiology and outcome. Pediatr Nephrol 1:314–320, 1987.
45. Gouyon JB, Guignard JP: Management of acute renal failure in newborns. Pediatr Nephrol 14:1037–1044, 2000.
46. Drukker A, Guignard JP: Renal aspects of the term and preterm infant: A selective update. Curr Opin Pediatr 14:182, 2002.
47. Finney H, Newman DJ, Thakkar H, et al: Reference ranges for plasma cystatin C and creatinine measurements in premature infants, neonates, and older children. Arch Dis Child 82:71–75, 2000.
48. Harmoinen A, Ylinen E, Ala-Houhala M, et al: Reference intervals for cystatin C in pre- and full-term infants and children. Pediatr Nephrol 15:105–108, 2000.
49. Karlowicz MG, Adelman RD: Nonoliguric and oliguric acute renal failure in asphyxiated term neonates. Pediatr Nephrol 9:718–722, 1995.
50. Blowey DL, Ben DS, Koren G: Interactions of drugs with the developing kidney. Pediatr Clin North Am 42:1415–1431, 1995.
51. Elder JS, Duckett JW: Management of the fetus and neonate with hydronephrosis detected by prenatal ultrasonography. Pediatr Ann 17:19–28, 1988.
52. Saphier CJ, Gaddipati S, Applewhite LE, et al: Prenatal diagnosis and management of abnormalities in the urologic system. Clin Perinatol 27:921–945, 2000.
53. Chevalier RL: Obstructive uropathy: State of the art. Pediatr Med Chir 24:95–97, 2002.
54. Kemper MJ, Müller-Wiefel DE: Renal function in congenital anomalies of the kidney and urinary tract. Curr Opin Urol 11:571–575, 2001.
55. Feldman H, Guignard JP: Plasma creatinine in the first month of life. Arch Dis Child 57:123–126, 1982.
56. Gallini F, Maggio L, Romagnoli C, et al: Progression of renal function in preterm neonates with gestational age < 32 weeks. Pediatr Nephrol 15:119–124, 2000.
57. Karlowicz MG, Adelman RD: Acute renal failure in the neonate. Clin Perinatol 19:139–158, 1992.
58. Anand SK: Acute renal failure. In Taeusch HW, Ballard RA, Avery ME (eds): Diseases of the Newborn. Philadelphia, WB Saunders, 1991, pp 894–895.
59. Mercado-Deane MG, Beeson JE, John SD: US of renal insufficiency in neonates. Radiographics 22:1429–1438, 2002.
60. Kraus SJ: Genitourinary imaging in children. Pediatr Clin North Am 48:1381–1424, 2001.
61. Gruskin AB, Oetliker OH, Wolfish NM, et al: Effects of angiography on renal function and histology in infants and piglets. J Pediatr 76:41–48, 1970.
62. Tulassay T, Seri I, Machay T, et al: Effects of dopamine on renal functions in premature neonates with respiratory distress syndrome. Int J Pediatr Nephrol 4:19–23, 1983.
63. Roberts RJ: Drug Therapy in Infants: Pharmacologic Principles and Clinical Experience. Philadelphia, WB Saunders, 1984.
64. Roy RN, Sinclair JC: Hydration of the low birth-weight infant. Clin Perinatol 2:393–417, 1975.
65. Ohlsson A, Hosking M: Complications following oral administration of exchange resins in extremely low-birth-weight infants. Eur J Pediatr 146:571–574, 1987.

66. Singh BS, Sadiq HF, Noguchi A, et al: Efficacy of albuterol inhalation in treatment of hyperkalemia in premature neonates. J Pediatr 141:16–20, 2002.

67. Mildenberger E, Versmold HT: Pathogenesis and therapy of non-oliguric hyperkalaemia of the premature infant. Eur J Pediatr 161:415–422, 2002.

68. Tack ED, Perlman JM: Renal failure in sick hypertensive premature infants receiving captopril therapy. J Pediatr 112:805–810, 1988.

69. Flynn JT: Neonatal hypertension: Diagnosis and management. Pediatr Nephrol 14:332–341, 2000.

70. Alon U, Davidai G, Bentur L, et al: Oral calcium carbonate as phosphate-binder in infants and children with chronic renal failure. Miner Electrolyte Metab 12:320–325, 1986.

71. American Academy of Pediatrics: Aluminum toxicity in infants and children. Pediatr 97:412–416, 1996.

72. Slatopolsky EA, Burke SK, Dillon MA, et al: RenaGel, a nonabsorbed calcium- and aluminum-free phosphate binder, lowers serum phosphorus and parathyroid hormone. Kidney Int 55:299–307, 1999.

73. Flynn JT: Choice of dialysis modality for management of pediatric acute renal failure. Pediatr Nephrol 17:61–69, 2002.

74. Golej J, Kitzmueller E, Hermon M, et al: Low-volume peritoneal dialysis in 116 neonatal and paediatric critical care patients. Eur J Pediatr 161:385–389, 2002.

75. Symons JM, Brophy PD, Gregory MJ, et al: Continuous renal replacement therapy in children up to 10 kg. Am J Kidney Dis 41:984–989, 2003.

76. Blowey DL, McFarland K, Alon U, et al: Peritoneal dialysis in the neonatal period: Outcome data. J Perinatol 13:59–64, 1993.

77. Leyh RG, Notzold A, Kraatz EG, et al: Continuous venovenous haemofiltration in neonates with renal insufficiency resulting from low cardiac output syndrome after cardiac surgery. Cardiovasc Surg 4:520–525, 1996.

78. Minoja M, Hirschman G, Jones C. Incidence and causes of ESRD in children in the USA [abstract]. J Am Soc Nephrol 6:396, 1995.

79. Neu AM, Ho PL, McDonald RA, et al: Chronic dialysis and renal insufficiency in children and adolescents: The 2001 NAPRTCS annual report. Pediatr Nephrol 17:656–663, 2002.

80. Chevalier RL, Kim A, Thornhill BA, et al: Recovery following relief of unilateral ureteral obstruction in the neonatal rat. Kidney Int 55:793–807, 1999.

81. Klahr S, Harris K, Purkerson ML: Effects of obstruction on renal functions. Pediatr Nephrol 2:34–42, 1988.

82. Boone TB, Allen TD: Unilateral postobstructive diuresis in the neonate. J Urol 147:430–432, 1992.

83. Harris RH, Yarger WE: The pathogenesis of post-obstructive diuresis: The role of circulating natriuretic and diuretic factors, including urea. J Clin Invest 56:880–887, 1975.

84. Peters CA: Obstruction of the fetal urinary tract. J Am Soc Nephrol 8:653–663, 1997.

85. Hanley MJ, Davidson K: Isolated nephron segments from rabbit models of obstructive nephropathy. J Clin Invest 69:165–174, 1982.

86. Rodriguez-Soriano J, Vallo A, Oliveros R, et al: Transient pseudohypoaldosteronism secondary to obstructive uropathy in infancy. J Pediatr 103:375–380, 1983.

87. Yarger WE, Buerkert J: Effect of urinary tract obstruction on renal tubular function. Semin Nephrol 2:17–30, 1982.

88. Alon U, Kordoff MB, Broecker BH, et al: Renal tubular acidosis type IV in neonatal unilateral kidney diseases. J Pediatr 104:855–860, 1984.

CHAPTER 5

Coagulopathies and Sickle Cell Disease

Masayo Watanabe, MD, Brian M. Wicklund, MD, CM, MPh, and Gerald M. Woods, MD

The pediatric surgeon will encounter patients with various hematologic disorders, including children with hemophilia and sickle cell disease (SCD), who represent the largest populations that have been followed up by hematologists over an extended period. We discuss these two conditions because of the unique surgical challenges that these patients provide to the pediatric surgeon, pediatric hematologist, and other physicians involved.

BIOCHEMISTRY AND PHYSIOLOGY OF HEMOSTASIS

The hemostatic system arrests bleeding from injured blood vessels and prevents the loss of blood from intact vessels. It keeps unwanted clots from developing and dissolves blood clots that have served their purpose. A complex, three-part system of proteins, platelets, and vessels containing them has evolved to maintain hemostasis. Pathologic defects in this regulatory system result in either bleeding or thrombosis when too little or too much clot is formed or when dissolution of a clot is not properly controlled.

Obtaining a complete history about the patient and his or her family is essential to anticipating hemostatic disorders. Preoperative preparations can be made only if a good history is taken so that medications that interfere with coagulation or platelet function can be discontinued. Laboratory studies help identify and characterize the problems that are uncovered by the history. Anticipation and workup of potential genetic bleeding and platelet disorders are the result of establishing the bleeding histories of family members and by physical examination.

Three distinct structures are involved in the process of hemostasis: blood vessels, platelets, and circulating hemostatic proteins. Together, these components form the coagulation system, the naturally occurring anticoagulation system, and the fibrinolytic system. These systems serve to amplify the stimulus that activates the coagulation system and to control the amount of response to that initial stimulus. Coagulation must act rapidly to stop the loss of blood from an injured vessel, but the clot that is formed must remain localized so that it does not interfere with the passage of blood through the intact circulation. The anticoagulation system prevents the extension of the clot beyond the site of injury. The fibrinolytic system removes excess hemostatic material that has been released into the circulation and slowly lyses the clot once it is no longer needed.

The initial stimulus to the formation of a clot comes from the disruption of endothelial cells, exposing collagen and subendothelial tissues. The hemostatic response to tissue injury consists of four stages. First, vasoconstriction by the contraction of smooth muscle in the injured vessel wall reduces blood flow. Second, platelets adhere to the exposed endothelium, aggregate, and release their granular contents. This activity stimulates further vasoconstriction and recruits more platelets. Primary hemostasis results from platelets occluding the hole in the blood vessel and halting the escape of blood. Third, the extrinsic and intrinsic coagulation systems are activated to form fibrin, which stabilizes the platelets and prevents disaggregation. Fourth, fibrinolysis results from the release of plasminogen activators from the injured vessel wall. These activators limit the coagulation process and, once healing has taken place, begin the resolution of formed clot so that vascular patency can be restored.[1]

Endothelial Cells

Endothelial cells line the lumen of all blood vessels, maintain the integrity of the blood vessel, and prevent the egression of blood into the surrounding tissue.[1] When the vessel is intact, they provide a thromboresistant surface that prevents the activation of the coagulation system. Passive thromboresistance is provided by endothelial proteoglycans, primarily heparin sulfate. Heparin is an anticoagulant compound that acts as a cofactor in converting antithrombin to a potent inhibitor of activated clotting factors. Active thromboresistance is achieved through several mechanisms, including the synthesis and release of prostacyclin (PGI$_2$),[1,2] a potent vasodilator and an inhibitor of platelet adhesion and aggregation.

When endothelium is injured, tissue factor (thromboplastin) is produced and rapidly promotes local thrombin formation.[3] Tissue factor binds factor VII and converts it to factor VIIa. The production of factor VIIa is the first step in activation of the extrinsic coagulation pathway, which begins the activation of the common pathway. It also activates factor IX, which is the major activator of the common pathway, resulting in the formation of fibrin.[4] The contribution these processes make to the control of bleeding depends on the size of the interrupted vessel. Capillaries seal with little dependence on the hemostatic system, but arterioles and venules require the presence of platelets to form an occluding plug. In arteries and veins, hemostasis depends on both vascular contraction and clot formation around an occluding primary hemostatic plug.[5]

Platelets

In the resting state, platelets circulate as disk-shaped, anuclear cells that have been released from megakaryocytes in the bone marrow. They are 2 to 3 μm in size, have a volume of 10 fL, and remain in circulation for as many as 8 days unless they participate in coagulation reactions, bind to formed clot, or are removed by the spleen.[6] In the resting state, platelets do not bind to intact endothelium. Platelets release growth factors to facilitate the proliferation of vascular endothelial and smooth muscle cells. These cells play a significant role in restoring the structure of injured blood vessels.[6]

Platelet Adhesion

Once platelets bind to injured tissue and are activated, their diskoid shape changes; they spread on the subendothelial connective tissue and degranulate. Degranulation occurs when platelets internally contract and extrude storage granule contents into the open canalicular system. Dense granules release serotonin, adenosine diphosphate (ADP), calcium, and adenosine triphosphate (ATP). Alpha granules release factor V, fibrinogen, von Willebrand's factor (FVIII:vWF), fibronectin, platelet factor IV, β-thromboglobulin, and platelet-derived growth factor.[6,7] Lysosomal vesicles also are present within platelets. The material released from the granules recruits and aggregates more platelets from the circulation onto the already adherent platelets.[6]

When a vessel is disrupted, platelet adhesion occurs through the binding of collagen and vWF (found in the subendothelium) to the platelet membrane. For platelet adhesion to occur, platelets must express specific glycoprotein Iβ receptors on their surface to bind the vWF complex. If this specific glycoprotein is missing, platelets are unable to adhere to areas of injury.[8] Platelets in Bernard-Soulier syndrome lack glycoprotein Iβ and are unable to adhere and form the initial hemostatic plug.[9] If the vWF is defective or deficient in amount, platelets do not adhere to sites of vascular injury. The result is von Willebrand's disease, for which several specific types and subtypes have been defined.[10–12] If an operation is performed on a patient with either Bernard-Soulier syndrome or von Willebrand's disease without the transfusion of normal amounts and types of platelets or vWF, respectively, serious bleeding can result because of the inability to form an initial hemostatic platelet plug. Very high concentrations of PGI$_2$ also can inhibit platelet adhesion to exposed subendothelium.[5]

After platelet adhesion has occurred, in addition to degranulation and an increased local concentration of ADP, small amounts of thrombin are formed, and platelet membrane phospholipase is activated to generate thromboxane A$_2$. Thromboxane A$_2$ and serotonin released from the dense granules stimulate vasoconstriction and induce the exposure of membrane receptors for fibrinogen (glycoproteins IIβ/IIIα). Fibrinogen binding to stimulated platelets then induces aggregation.[6]

Platelet Aggregation

Aggregation is a complex reaction that involves platelet granule release, cleavage of membrane phospholipids by phospholipases A$_2$ and C, alterations in intracellular cyclic adenosine monophosphate (cAMP) levels, mobilization of intracellular calcium, and the expression of fibrinogen receptors on the platelet surface. If fibrinogen receptors (glycoproteins IIβ and IIIα) or fibrinogen are missing, platelets do not aggregate.[13] Glanzmann's thrombasthenia is a deficiency of glycoproteins IIβ and IIIα in which platelets adhere normally but do not aggregate. These patients have a serious, life-long bleeding disorder.[7]

After aggregation, platelets function to enhance thrombin formation. Platelet membrane provides specific binding sites for factors Xa and V. The result is an efficient site for the assembly of the prothrombinase complex, which converts prothrombin into thrombin.[6] Thrombin formation results in the formation of a stable hemostatic plug of adherent platelets surrounded by a network of fibrin strands.

Generation of Thrombin

Tissue injury induces activation of the plasma-based coagulation system, resulting in the generation of thrombin from prothrombin. Thrombin is the enzyme responsible for transforming liquid blood into a fibrin gel. The initial activation of factor VII by tissue factor results in the production of thrombin by the extrinsic system. Tissue factor is released after injury to the endothelial cells but is not expressed on the surface of the cells.[14]

The majority of thrombin production results from the activation of the intrinsic coagulation system, not the extrinsic system. Exposed subendothelium converts factor XII to factor XIIa and thereby activates the intrinsic pathway, although it is interesting to note that deficits in factor XII do not cause a bleeding disorder. Activation of factors XI and IX follows, and activated factor IX in combination with factor VIII, calcium, and platelet phospholipid activates factor X. Activated factor VII complexed with tissue factor activates factor IX, which also activates factor XI. Factor Xa with factor V then cleaves prothrombin into the active molecule thrombin. When thrombin is free of the platelet membrane, it can convert fibrinogen into fibrin.[4,14]

Formation of Fibrin

When thrombin acts on fibrinogen, fibrin monomers result after the proteolytic release of fibrinopeptides A and B. The monomeric fibrin then polymerizes into a gel.[4,14] With additional stabilization of the fibrin gel provided by factor XIII, fibrin surrounds and stabilizes the platelet plug. This process makes the multimeric fibrin more resistant to plasmin digestion and completes the formation and stabilization of the blood clot.[15]

Several regulatory proteins serve to localize thrombin formation to the surface of the blood vessel. Endothelial cells have receptors for protein C, an anticoagulant protein. Protein C from the plasma binds to these receptors. Protein S is a cofactor for the activation of protein C. Thrombomodulin is an endothelial surface protein that acts in combination with thrombin to activate the bound protein C. Activated protein C then degrades factors Va and VIIIa, which inhibit thrombin formation.[16]

Heparin-like anticoagulant molecules are present on endothelial cells. They act in combination with antithrombin III to inhibit factors XIIa, XIa, IXa, and Xa and thrombin. Inhibition of these factors prevents the spread of clot to uninjured adjacent vessels and the blockage of large vessels by excessive clot formation.[14,16] Endothelial cells, as mentioned previously, produce PGI_2, a potent vasodilator and inhibitor of platelet aggregation and adhesion.

Fibrinolysis

The regulatory system that dissolves fibrin and preserves vessel patency is called *fibrinolysis*. Circulating plasminogen is converted into plasmin by tissue plasminogen activators. These activators are released from the vessel walls at the site of blood clotting. They bind to the fibrin clot and convert plasminogen to plasmin. Plasmin enzymatically degrades fibrin, fibrinogen, and other plasma proteins, and this process results in the dissolution of formed clot.[14,16]

CLINICAL EVALUATION

Currently, no screening test to evaluate hemostasis is completely reliable in the preoperative evaluation of patients.[17] A careful history, including a full family history, is still the best means of uncovering mild bleeding problems, such as von Willebrand's disease or qualitative platelet abnormalities. These disorders may easily escape standard laboratory screening procedures, such as prothrombin time (PT), activated partial thromboplastin time (aPTT), platelet count, and bleeding time. However, patients with mild hemophilia who have not previously undergone surgical procedures may have no history of bleeding problems and might be identified preoperatively only if an aPTT is done. Any of the preceding clinical situations is associated with a risk of excessive bleeding

in a surgical procedure that is sufficient to recommend the completion of a reasonable combination of history, physical examination, and clinically indicated laboratory tests.[18,19] It is important to consider the history as the most sensitive of the three testing procedures and to investigate thoroughly any story of unusual bleeding, even if the screening tests are normal. Conversely, preoperative coagulation testing done in the absence of a suggestive history can result in false-positive results.[20] Several studies examined the utility of the preoperative PT and aPTT in patients undergoing tonsillectomy and adenoidectomy and concluded that routine screening with a PT and aPTT in all patients cannot be recommended.[21,22]

In obtaining a history from the patient and parents,[17,23] positive answers to any of the following questions should indicate the need for further evaluation:

Is there any history of easy bruising, bleeding problems, or an established bleeding disorder in the patient or any family members?

Has excessive bleeding occurred after any previous surgical procedure or dental work? Have the parents or any siblings had excessive bleeding after any surgical or dental procedures, specifically tonsillectomy or adenoidectomy?

Have frequent nosebleeds occurred, and has nasal packing or cautery been needed? Has bleeding without trauma occurred into any joint or muscle?

Does excessive bleeding or bruising occur after aspirin ingestion?

Does significant gingival bleeding occur after tooth brushing?

Has the patient been taking any medication that might affect platelets or the coagulation system?

If the patient is male and was circumcised, were any problems noted with prolonged oozing after the circumcision?

If the patient is a child, do the parents remember any bleeding problems when the umbilical cord separated?

If the patient is menstruating, does she have profuse menstruation?

Has the patient ever received any transfusions of blood or blood products? If so, what was the reason for the transfusion?

If there is a history of abnormal bleeding, the following points must be established. The type of bleeding (i.e., petechiae, purpura, ecchymosis, and single or generalized bleeding sites) can give an indication of the underlying defect. Petechiae and purpura are most frequently associated with platelet abnormalities, either of function or of numbers. Von Willebrand's disease is most frequently associated with mucosal bleeding, including epistaxis, whereas hemophilia is most often associated with bleeding into joints or soft tissue ecchymosis or both. Bleeding when the umbilical cord separates is most often associated with a deficiency in factor XIII.[15,24] A single bleeding site is frequently indicative of a localized problem and not a system-wide coagulation defect.

The course or pattern of the bleeding (i.e., spontaneous or after trauma) and its frequency, duration of problems, and severity can provide clues to the cause of the problem. A family history of bleeding is important to define, and the pattern of inheritance (i.e., X-linked or autosomal; recessive or dominant) can help narrow the differential diagnosis (e.g., hemophilia A and B are X-linked recessive diseases, whereas von Willebrand's disease is autosomal dominant).[25]

Any previous or current drug therapy must be fully documented, and a search is made for any over-the-counter medications that the patient might be taking but does not consider "medicine" and has therefore not mentioned. Aspirin, ibuprofen, cough medications containing guaifenesin, and antihistamines can uncover a preexisting bleeding disorder such as von Willebrand's disease, when in a normal patient, they would not cause sufficient platelet dysfunction to result in clinical bleeding.[26] The presence of other medical problems is important to establish, because renal failure with uremia, hepatic failure, malignancies, gastrointestinal malabsorption, vascular malformations, cardiac anomalies with or without repair, and autoimmune disorders may have associated coagulopathies.

The physical examination is used to help narrow the differential diagnosis and guide the laboratory investigation of hemostatic disorders. Certain physical findings may be associated with a specific coagulation abnormality, whereas others may be indicative of an underlying systemic disease with an associated coagulopathy. Petechiae and purpuric bleeding occur with platelet and vascular abnormalities. If the petechiae are raised, a vasculitis is likely, whereas petechiae due to thrombocytopenia are not elevated and initially occur on lower extremities or mucosa. Acquired coagulation defects usually result in widespread ecchymotic bleeding with or without gastrointestinal or urinary tract bleeding. Bleeding into joints and bleeding that stops and restarts are characteristic of congenital coagulation factor deficiencies. Hemophilia patients often have bruises with a raised central nodule, called *palpable purpura*. Findings compatible with a collagen disorder include the body habitus of Marfan's syndrome; blue sclera; skeletal deformities; hyperextensible joints and skin; and nodular, spider-like, or pinpoint telangiectasias. Hepatosplenomegaly and lymphadenopathy may suggest an underlying malignancy, and jaundice plus hepatomegaly may indicate hepatic dysfunction.

LABORATORY EVALUATION

At present, the usual tests for screening the hemostatic system are the platelet count, PT, and aPTT.[25,27] Additional tests can be done to measure fibrinogen levels, assess the thrombin time, screen for inhibitors of specific coagulation factors, measure specific factor levels, and test for platelet function. Patients also can be evaluated for evidence of disseminated intravascular coagulation (DIC) by using multiple assays to test for the presence of various fibrinopeptides and products from the breakdown of fibrin or fibrinogen.

Platelet Count

The platelet count measures the adequacy of platelet numbers to provide initial hemostasis. Platelet counts are usually performed by using an automated hematology counter. The normal range is 150,000 to 400,000 platelets/mL, and excess bleeding with surgical procedures usually does not occur until the count is below 50,000 platelets/mL.[6,20] At counts between 50,000 and 20,000 platelets/mL, increased bruising and petechiae are expected, and when the platelet count is below 20,000/mL, spontaneous bleeding may occur. It is the usual practice to transfuse the patient with platelet concentrates to increase the platelet count above 50,000/mL before a surgical procedure.[18,27]

Bleeding Time and PFA-100 Analyzer

The bleeding time is defined as the length of time required for a standardized incision to stop oozing blood that can be absorbed onto filter paper. A variety of procedures have been used, including the Duke method with a stab incision of the earlobe and the Ivy method with a standardized cut on the forearm, but both have been difficult to reproduce accurately. The cooperation of the child may be difficult to obtain in the school-age patient, but it is essential for accurate and reproducible results. At present, the *simplate* test, using a spring-load blade to make a controlled cut of a specific length and depth on the volar surface of the forearm, is the most frequently used procedure and provides a reasonable reproducibility. The normal values vary, depending on the procedure used and the individual laboratory, but are usually less than 10 minutes.[1,5] Because of concerns about this test's accuracy and reproducibility, it has seen much less use over the last 10-year period.[28]

The PFA-100 Analyzer is a potential in vitro replacement for the bleeding time. It creates a high shear stress condition that results in the activation of platelet-dependent and vWF-dependent attachment and aggregation of platelets to a collagen-ADP or collagen-epinephrine surface. In most cases, the PFA-100 closure time is superior to the bleeding time in the detection of von Willebrand's disease, aspirin effect, or platelet dysfunction.[29]

Prothrombin Time

The PT screens the function of the extrinsic and common coagulation pathways. It is the time required to clot platelet-poor plasma after the addition of tissue factor, calcium, and phospholipid, the tissue factor being the material that is "extrinsic" to the plasma-based coagulation system.[1] Isolated prolongations of the PT are seen in factor VII deficiency, mild hypofibrinogenemia, dysfibrinogenemia, and patients taking warfarin sodium anticoagulation. It also is considered the most sensitive screening test for liver dysfunction coagulopathies.[1]

Partial Thromboplastin Time

The aPTT screens the function of the intrinsic and common coagulation pathways. Platelet-poor plasma is incubated with kaolin, diatomaceous earth (Celite), or ellagic acid to form activated factor XII (factor XIIa). Calcium and phospholipid are then added, and the time to formation of clot is measured.[1] Factor levels below 30% to 50% of normal levels are needed to produce an abnormal test result; the level at which the test becomes abnormal depends on the reagents and testing equipment used. The aPTT detects deficiencies in factors XII, XI, IX, and VIII and in the common pathway, but mild factor deficiencies may be missed. The aPTT also is used to monitor anticoagulation with heparin.[1]

Several inherited disorders of coagulation are not detected by the preceding tests. Factor XIII deficiency is detected by a urea clot solubility test[1] or a specific factor assay.[15,24] von Willebrand's disease patients may have normal or prolonged aPTTs, and patients with a deficiency in α_2-antiplasmin have a normal aPTT. Both the PT and aPTT are prolonged in patients with deficiencies of factors X and V, prothrombin, and fibrinogen and in patients with DIC or severe liver disease.[1,25]

Fibrinogen

The standard method for fibrinogen determination measures clottable fibrinogen by using a kinetic assay. Normal levels of fibrinogen are 150 to 350 mg/dL. Because fibrinogen is the substrate for the final reaction in the formation of a clot, and all plasma-based screening tests depend on the formation of a clot as the end point of the reaction, fibrinogen levels below 80 mg/dL prolong the PT, aPTT, and thrombin time, and therefore make the results uninterpretable.[1,2] Large amounts of fibrin degradation products interfere with the formation of fibrin and cause an artificially low level of fibrinogen to be measured. Partially clotted samples also cause a low level of fibrinogen to be assayed. An immunologic-based assay for fibrinogen is used to measure both clottable and nonclottable fibrinogen. This test is most often used in identifying patients with a dysfibrinogenemia in whom the functional level of fibrinogen is low and the immunologic level is normal.[1,25]

Inhibitor Screening Tests

Repeating the PT or aPTT by using a 1:1 mix of patient plasma with normal plasma is a useful procedure for investigating a prolonged PT or aPTT. Normal plasma has, by definition, 100% levels of all factors. When mixed with an equal volume of patient plasma, a minimum of 50% of any given factor is present, which should normalize the PT or aPTT. If the test normalizes, it suggests the presence of a factor deficiency, whereas lack of normalization suggests the presence of an inhibitor that interferes with either thrombin or fibrin formation.[1]

Two types of acquired inhibitors prolong the aPTT. One blocks or inactivates one of the intrinsic factors, whereas the other is a lupus-like inhibitor that interferes with phospholipid-based clotting reactions. The first type of inhibitor occurs in 5% to 15% of hemophiliacs and can occur spontaneously, but it is extremely rare in nonhemophiliac children.[25] The lupus-like inhibitor is associated not with bleeding problems but rather with an increased risk of thrombotic problems in adults. Lupuslike inhibitors are mentioned because they commonly cause prolongations of the aPTT.[30] Specific investigation of either of these situations should be referred to a skilled coagulation reference laboratory.

Platelet Function Studies

Platelet function studies measure in vitro platelet aggregation. In this procedure, platelet-rich plasma is incubated with an agonist, and changes in the amount of light transmitted through the platelet suspension are recorded. Agonists used to induce platelet aggregation include collagen, epinephrine, ADP, thrombin, and ristocetin. Three distinct phases are seen in the reaction. The first is an initial change in the shape of the platelets, leading to a temporary decrease in light transmission. Next is the first wave of aggregation, which is a reversible platelet-platelet interaction. With additional stimulation, the final phase—the second wave of aggregation—occurs and produces irreversible platelet aggregation. The second wave of aggregation is due to the release reaction of the platelet granules and thromboxane A_2 synthesis. The release reaction is extinguished by aspirin and is absent in patients with an inherited storage pool defect, congenital deficiency in thromboxane A_2 synthesis, or cyclooxygenase deficiency.[6]

Specific Factor Assays

Specific factor assays are available for all known coagulation, fibrinolysis, and anticoagulation factors to quantify their levels in plasma. These tests are not indicated unless a screening test result is abnormal. The only exception involves the patient with a history that is suggestive of von Willebrand's disease. In this case, the aPTT may not be sensitive enough to detect the decreased level or activity of vWF. Further testing may be justified by clinical suspicion based on the patient's history and would consist of measuring factor VIII levels, factor VIII–related antigen levels, ristocetin cofactor activity, and ristocetin-induced platelet aggregation. Analysis of the distribution of vWF multimers can be useful to the hematologist in identifying the specific type of von Willebrand's disease.[10–12]

Tests for Disseminated Intravascular Coagulation

The usually available tests in most hospital laboratories for identification of DIC are semiquantitative fibrin or fibrinogen degradation product assays, which involve a slide agglutination procedure. An increased amount of these degradation products suggests that either plasmin has circulated to lyse fibrin and fibrinogen or the patient's hepatic function is insufficient to clear the small amounts of regularly produced degradation products. The D-dimer test also is a slide agglutination procedure that tests for the presence of two D subunits of fibrin that are crosslinked by factor XIII. This test provides specific evidence that plasmin has digested fibrin clot and not fibrinogen. It is positive in patients with DIC, in patients with resolving large intravascular clots, and in patients with hepatic insufficiency. Specific assays to demonstrate the presence of soluble fibrin monomer complexes or fibrinopeptides produced by the conversion of prothrombin to thrombin also are useful in some situations.[31]

HEMOPHILIA A AND B

Hemophilia A and B are X-linked recessive bleeding disorders caused by decreased levels of functional procoagulant factors VIII and IX, respectively. Approximately 80% of all hemophilia patients have factor VIII deficiency, which is *classic hemophilia.* The remaining 20% have factor IX deficiency, which is called *Christmas disease.* Until 1964, the treatment of hemophilia was limited by volume restrictions imposed by the use of whole blood or fresh frozen plasma. At that time, the factor VIII–rich fraction of fresh frozen plasma called cryoprecipitate was discovered.[32] Specific lyophilized factor VIII concentrates have since been developed, as have prothrombin-complex concentrates containing factors II, VII, IX, and X; concentrates containing only factor IX for the treatment of hemophilia B patients;[33–35] and factor VIII/vWF concentrates for the treatment of von Willebrand's disease.[36] The lyophilized factor concentrates have allowed storage of the clotting factor by using standard refrigeration and have permitted the outpatient treatment of bleeding episodes plus the development of home self-infusion programs.[37] This treatment, combined with the development of comprehensive hemophilia treatment centers, has produced a remarkable change in the outlook for these patients who previously began to notice significant joint deformities in their teens to twenties and were frequently wheelchair bound in adult life. Rapid home therapy has decreased the damage caused by hemarthroses, with hemophiliac children born since the mid-1970s having far fewer joint deformities than do older hemophiliacs. These factor concentrates have allowed surgical procedures to be performed with much less risk, even to the point that orthopedic procedures can be readily accomplished.[38]

Viral infections transmitted by cryoprecipitate and factor concentrates have become one of the major problems faced by hemophilia patients. Approximately 60% of all hemophilia patients became human immunodeficiency virus (HIV) positive in the 1980s, and more than 1200 have died of AIDS.[38,39] This number is out of a total population of only 17,000 hemophiliacs in the United States.[40] Hepatitis is the other major viral infection transmitted by the factor concentrates used to treat hemophilia. Estimates from the mid-1980s are that more than 90% of multiply transfused hemophiliacs were positive for non-A, non-B hepatitis and that more than 95% had been infected with hepatitis B.[41] A different study shows that 75% of HIV-negative hemophiliacs, treated with earlier plasma-derived factor concentrates, have evidence of hepatitis C infection.[42] All medical personnel working with hemophiliacs must strictly observe universal blood precautions, and all patients should be assumed to be positive for HIV or hepatitis. Special precautions are warranted in the operating room, such as wearing double gloves and a plastic apron under the surgical gown, and making special arrangements to deal with aerosolized material during orthopedic procedures.

Hemophilia patients are classified into three categories based on their level of circulating procoagulant. Those with factor levels below 1% are *severe hemophiliacs,* are at a high risk of bleeding, and usually require replacement therapy 2 to 4 times per month.[40,43] Bleeding occurs in areas subject to minor trauma. Hemarthroses, hematomas, and ecchymoses are common. Recurrent hemarthroses can cause pseudotumors of the bone, whereas hematomas can cause compression damage to tissue or nerves and even ischemic compartment syndromes. Bleeding episodes in severe hemophiliacs can be irregularly spaced, with periods of recurrent hemarthrosis requiring frequent replacement doses of factor concentrate, interspersed with periods during which little or no concentrate is used.[40]

In *moderate hemophiliacs,* who have procoagulant levels of 1% to 5%, spontaneous hemorrhage occurs infrequently, but relatively minor trauma can cause bleeding into joints or soft tissues.

Mild hemophiliacs, with levels greater than 5%, rarely have bleeding problems and typically have problems only with major trauma or surgical procedures.[25,40] Some mild hemophilias may not be diagnosed until late childhood or adulthood, and therefore a history may not be present to alert the pediatric surgeon to the risk of bleeding. Moreover, because one third of all cases of hemophilia are caused by new mutations, there may not be a family history to arouse suspicion of a bleeding problem.[25] Preoperative laboratory testing may provide the only point at which a mild hemophilia is diagnosed.

The indications for surgical intervention in hemophiliacs are the same as those for patients with a normal clotting system, but they most frequently center on areas of damage secondary to bleeding episodes. In 1985, the results of a review of 350 consecutive operations performed at Orthopedic Hospital in Los Angeles were published.[44] The study examined patients with hemophilia A between 1967 and 1983. Because the study group represented patients from before the start of home therapy and comprehensive care, the group was expected to have significant orthopedic problems secondary to multiple hemarthroses. Of the 350 procedures reviewed, 312 were characterized as serious, and 38, as of lesser intensity; 318 operations were on hemophiliacs with moderate and severe hemophilia, and 30, on patients with mild hemophilia. As expected, musculoskeletal procedures made up two thirds of all operations on moderate and severe hemophiliacs and half of all operations on mild hemophiliacs. Pseudotumors of the bone were removed in 15 operations. One death occurred in a child with a massive intracranial hemorrhage who did not survive an emergency craniotomy.[44]

Bleeding problems during operation were not observed, but 23% of all serious operations were complicated by postoperative hemorrhages. Only operations on the knee had significantly more postoperative hemorrhages (40%). Operations on other joints and soft tissue areas had similar rates of complications (15%). Hemophilia management changed during the time of the patient series, causing increased amounts of factor concentrate to be given to maintain higher minimum factor levels, but did not produce any decrease in the number of postoperative hemorrhages. Most of the postoperative hemorrhages occurred with plasma factor levels greater than 30%, which is the minimum level that is considered hemostatic. During the course of this patient series, intermittent infusions of factor concentrates were used. These infusions are wasteful in that they create unnecessarily high levels of factor immediately after infusion, yet factor levels may decrease to less than those required for hemostasis before the next dose. The authors were not sure what role this might have played, but they suggested the use of continuous infusion for factor VIII concentrate to avoid these problems and to provide greater physiologic stability of factor levels. The authors also noted that the incidence of postoperative hemorrhage decreased after postoperative day 11, although other studies have found that vigorous physical therapy may cause postoperative hemorrhage and have therefore recommended the continuation of factor replacement throughout the period of physical therapy.[44,45]

The management of the hemophilic patient requires close cooperation among surgeons, hematologists, personnel in the hemophilia center, the coagulation laboratory, and the pharmacy or blood bank. Careful preoperative planning is essential to the success of the procedure, and an adequate supply of clotting factor concentrate must be available to cover the patient's needs before the patient is admitted. The patient also must be screened for the presence of an inhibitor to either factor VIII or IX during the 2 to 4 weeks before operation. If an inhibitor is present, management of the patient becomes much more complex and depends on the strength of the inhibitor. A low-titer inhibitor may be overcome with increased doses of human clotting factor, but high-titer inhibitors may require the use of porcine factor VIII, prothrombin complex concentrates, activated prothrombin complex concentrates such as Feiba or Autoplex, or recombinant activated factor VII. These patients have been desensitized with daily doses of human factor concentrate over a period of several months, and extracorporeal antibody absorption has been used to augment immune-tolerance therapy.[38]

The hemophilia patient is seen in the hematology clinic on the morning of the scheduled operation. After a bolus dose of factor (usually 50 units/kg of factor VIII in hemophilia A patients), a continuous infusion of 4 to 6 units/kg/hr of factor VIII (for the hemophilia A patient) is started to maintain a factor level greater than 80% for the next 1 to 2 days.[46] The factor level is checked immediately before the operation and is the final screen for the presence of an inhibitor. The infusion is maintained throughout the procedure and is then reduced on the second or third postoperative day to allow the plasma levels to decrease to 50%. Replacement is continued for a full 10 to 14 days after operation. Daily measurement of factor levels is necessary to ensure maintenance of appropriate levels. For neurosurgical or orthopedic procedures, much longer periods of factor coverage—even 4 to 6 weeks—are needed if significant physical therapy is planned.[38,40]

Many hemophiliacs do their own factor infusions at home and are supported by home care pharmacies. With the advent of home nursing services, patients are being discharged home with prolonged periods of factor coverage. Hemophilia center personnel must be closely involved in the planning of these discharges to ensure that sufficient clotting factor is available at home and that close follow-up is maintained during periods of scheduled home therapy. Hemophilia patients should not receive any compounds that contain aspirin, and their charts should be clearly marked. They also should avoid propoxyphene (Darvon Compound) and oxycodone (Percodan), as these compounds contain aspirin. Intramuscular injections should be avoided, and any minor procedures that would require factor correction should be combined with the major procedure, if possible, to save on the use of factor concentrate.

PROBLEMS IN PATIENTS WITH HEMOPHILIA B

Previously, the hemophilia B patient undergoing a surgical procedure had specific problems because of the thrombogenic risk inherent in the use of older factor IX concentrates. Thromboembolic complications were seen postoperatively, particularly in orthopedic surgery patients. The risk was not limited solely to these patients, however, as thrombosis also had been seen in other hemophilia B patients.[38,43] Heparin in low doses was added to factor IX concentrate to reduce the risk of thrombosis. Since the advent of newer, more purified factor IX concentrates with a decreased risk of thrombosis, surgical procedures in hemophilia B patients have been performed without excess thrombotic problems.[35]

Factor VIII is dosed differently from factor IX, based on their half-lives. Factor VIII has an 8- to 12-hour half-life, and the infusion of one unit of factor per kilogram body weight increases the plasma level by 2%. Thus if a severe hemophilia A patient weighs 50 kg, an infusion of 25 units/kg, or 1250 units, of factor VIII will raise his factor level to 50%. Factor IX has a half-life of 24 hours and must be infused in larger amounts than factor VIII to raise the plasma level. Infusion of 1 unit/kg of factor IX will raise the plasma level only by 1%. Continuous infusion of highly purified factor IX, as well as factor VIII, has been shown to prevent excessive peaks and troughs of factor levels, is simpler to manage, and decreases the cost by decreasing the overall amount of factor used. It has not shown any problems with excess thrombosis.[47,48] Recombinant factor IX has a marked variability in dose response to infusions, and individual recovery studies may be needed before its use for surgical hemostasis.[49]

NEONATAL HEMOSTASIS

The newborn's coagulation system is not fully mature until 6 months after birth. The lower levels of procoagulant, fibrinolytic, and anticoagulant proteins in neonatal patients complicate both surgical procedures and the care of sick and preterm infants. Platelet counts are within the usual adult normal ranges of 150,000 to 450,000/mL in healthy term and preterm infants. These platelets have a lower function than those of adults, but they function properly in hemostasis and produce a normal bleeding time.[49] Circulating coagulation factors do not cross the placenta, and infants with inherited deficiencies of clotting factors, fibrinolytic proteins, or natural anticoagulants may initially be seen in the neonatal period. Levels of fibrinogen, factor V, factor VIII, and vWF are within the adult normal range at birth.[50] All other procoagulants are at reduced levels, depending on gestational age. Vitamin K–dependent factors may become further depressed in infants who are breast-fed and not given vitamin K at birth.[49]

Of more concern are the low levels of anticoagulant and fibrinolytic proteins. Very low levels of protein C have been associated with purpura fulminans in newborns. In sick infants, levels of antithrombin III and plasminogen may be inadequate to deal with increased levels of clot-promoting activity in the blood. Sick infants with indwelling catheters are at significant risk of thrombotic complications and may endanger their renal circulation when umbilical venous lines are used.[51]

DISSEMINATED INTRAVASCULAR COAGULATION

DIC is the inappropriate activation of both thrombin and fibrin. It may follow sepsis, hypotension, hypoxemia, trauma, malignancy, burns, and extracorporeal circulation. Hemorrhage due to the depletion of clotting factors as well as thrombosis due to the excess formation of clot are seen, and the end-organ damage caused by ischemia and impairment of blood flow causes irreversible disease and death.[31]

Acute DIC is associated with the consumption of factors II, V, VIII, X, and XIII, as well as fibrinogen, antithrombin III, plasminogen, and platelets. Review of the peripheral smear usually shows a microangiopathic hemolytic anemia. The PT and aPTT may both be prolonged, and the fibrinogen level may be initially elevated as an acute-phase reactant but ultimately decreases as the DIC worsens. In active DIC, the presence of soluble fibrin monomer complexes indicates the ongoing formation of new clot. The presence of D-dimers indicates the circulation of plasmin digesting formed fibrin. Antithrombin III levels may be low, and the use of antithrombin III concentrates in septic shock indicates that they may play a role in the future treatment of DIC. At present, the major therapy of DIC is correction of the underlying disorder, with fresh frozen plasma and platelet transfusions as indicated to support hemostasis.

Low-dose heparin infusions have been used to stop the ongoing consumption of clotting factors before starting replacement therapy but have not been shown to improve the outcome appreciably.[31]

MANAGEMENT OF QUANTITATIVE AND QUALITATIVE PLATELET DISORDERS

Thrombocytopenias are caused by either inadequate production of platelets by the bone marrow or increased destruction or sequestration of the platelets in the circulation. The history and physical examination may be suggestive of a diagnosis that can be confirmed by laboratory testing. Medication use, a family history of blood disorders, a history of recent viral infection, short stature, absent thumbs or radii, or a congenital malformation may indicate a platelet-production defect. The destruction may be immunologic, as in immune thrombocytopenic purpura; mechanical, as in septicemia; or drug induced, as in patients with sensitivity to heparin or cimetidine. Establishing the cause of the thrombocytopenia determines the therapy needed to restore the platelet count in preparing the patient for operation. A bone marrow aspirate or biopsy or both can establish the normal number and morphology of the megakaryocytes as well as rule out malignancy. The clinical response to therapeutic modalities, such as a platelet transfusion, also can be an important test and lead to the diagnosis. In patients with immune-based platelet consumptions such as immune thrombocytopenic purpura, usually no response is found to platelet transfusion, and only a very short response may be seen in patients with other causes of increased consumption. Management of the patient is then aimed at reducing the consumption and should involve consultation with a hematologist about the use of steroids, the use of intravenous immunoglobulin, the discontinuation of medications, and other treatment modalities.[6,52]

If the thrombocytopenia is caused by a lack of production of platelets, due to either aplastic anemia, malignancy, or chemotherapy, transfusion with platelet concentrate to increase the platelet count above a minimum of 50,000 cells/mL will allow minor surgical procedures to be performed safely. Most surgeons and anesthesiologists prefer for the platelet count to be greater than 100,000 cells/mL before undertaking major surgery. Continued monitoring of platelet counts is vital as further transfusions may be needed to keep the platelet count above 50,000 cells/mL for 3 to 5 days after operations.[52]

Qualitative platelet defects can be caused by rare congenital defects, such as Bernard-Soulier syndrome, Glanzmann's thrombasthenia, or platelet storage pool disease. Alternatively, they can be caused by drug ingestions such as an aspirin-induced cyclo-oxygenase deficiency. In these situations, transfusion of normal donor platelets provides adequate hemostasis for surgical procedures. Discontinuation of all aspirin-containing products

1 week before operation permits correction of the cyclo-oxygenase deficiency as new platelets are produced.[7,26]

DISORDERS OF THROMBIN GENERATION AND FIBRIN FORMATION

Patients with rare deficiencies of other clotting factors, such as factors XI, X, VII, and V and prothrombin and fibrinogen, can have clinical bleeding depending on the level of deficiency. Most of these disorders are inherited in an autosomal recessive manner and can therefore affect both male and female patients. Replacement therapy with fresh frozen plasma or, in certain situations, with prothrombin complex concentrates corrects the deficiency[38,53] and should be conducted under the direction of a hematologist.

Vitamin K deficiency, both in the neonatal period and due to malabsorption, can cause deficiencies of factors II, VII, IX, and X. Treatment with 1 to 2 mg of intravenous vitamin K may begin to correct the deficiencies within 4 to 6 hours, but if a surgical procedure is contemplated, fresh frozen plasma (15 mL/kg body weight) should be given with the vitamin K, and prothrombin times are monitored for correction of the coagulopathy before the operation. Laboratory monitoring should be maintained during the postoperative period to ensure continuation of the appropriate factor levels; repeated doses of fresh frozen plasma and vitamin K may be needed.[5]

Patients with factor XIII deficiency usually are initially seen with delayed bleeding from the umbilical cord, rebleeding from wounds that have stopped bleeding, intracranial hemorrhage, and poor wound healing. These problems may be treated with relatively small amounts of fresh frozen plasma (5 to 10 mL/kg). Because factor XIII has a half-life of 6 days, this treatment is usually needed only once to stop bleeding or at the time of operation.[15,38] Patients with dysfibrinogenemia or afibrinogenemia may be treated with fresh frozen plasma or cryoprecipitate. Because fibrinogen has a long half-life, repeated infusions are usually not required to treat individual bleeding episodes. Some patients may benefit from monthly prophylactic infusions to prevent repeated bleeding.[38]

FIBRINOLYTIC AND THROMBOTIC DISORDERS

Failure to control excess fibrinolysis correctly can result in a bleeding disorder, and deficiencies of the naturally occurring anticoagulants may result in excess clot formations. A severe hemorrhagic disorder due to a deficiency of α_2-antiplasmin has responded to treatment with aminocaproic acid or tranexamic acid, both antifibrinolytic agents.[25] Congenital antithrombin III, protein S, and protein C deficiencies are associated with recurrent thrombosis and are usually controlled with oral anticoagulants.[25] Factor V Leiden, thrombin G20210A, MTHFR

variants, and other activated protein C–resistance gene mutations will cause or add additional risk for thrombotic tendency in proportion to their homozygous or heterozygous states.[54-56] Operation requires discontinuation of the anticoagulation, and the patients will require replacement therapy during the procedure and the postoperative healing period until oral anticoagulants can be restarted. Depending on the deficiency, antithrombin III concentrate or fresh frozen plasma can be used for replacement therapy, which should be conducted under the guidance of a hematologist with ready access to a full coagulation laboratory.

RECOMBINANT ACTIVATED FACTOR VII

Recombinant activated factor VII (rFVIIa) was developed for the treatment of bleeding in patients with hemophilia A or B who had inhibitors and was approved by the Food and Drug Administration (FDA) for this indication in 1999.[57-59] Good hemostasis with few side effects was seen in patients with intracranial hemorrhage, postlaparotomy and postpartum hemorrhage, hemorrhage into the gluteal muscles (as a complication after cholecystectomy), and for surgical prophylaxis for major and minor procedures.[60-63] Home treatment programs for some patients who are hemophiliacs with inhibitors now use rFVIIa as front-line therapy for bleeding.[64] Children have a more rapid rate of clearance (elimination mean half-life, 1.32 hours in children vs. 2.74 hours in adults).[65] They also seem to have fewer side effects with this treatment.[57,63] Although various dosages and schedules have been studied, initial recommended therapy in hemophilia A or B with inhibitors is 90 µg/kg intravenously every 2 hours until the bleeding is controlled.[66]

The off-label use of rFVIIa has been reported in therapy-resistant severe bleeding from other conditions such as congenital factor VII deficiency, chronic liver disease, and inherited platelet disorders.[67-70] Successes in patients without a known bleeding disorder who have trauma or postoperative hemorrhage also are described.[63,68,71] These reports should be interpreted with caution, as rFVIIa is currently not the standard of care in any of these off-label uses, and exceptional circumstances impelled its use. It is highly recommended that rFVIIa be administered under the supervision of a physician experienced in its use who can anticipate the risks and respond to the complications, particularly risks of thrombosis, which are reported in fewer than 1% of patients.[68] rFVIIa shows great future promise, however, in the emergency treatment of uncontrolled hemorrhage for many situations.

SICKLE CELL DISEASE

SCD is caused by a genetic mutation that results in the production of sickle hemoglobin (Hg S) instead of normal hemoglobin (Hg A). Hg S is a β-globin defect. The sickle cell gene in combination with any other abnormal β-globin gene results in SCD. Sickle cell anemia (Hg SS) is the most common and in general the most severe form of SCD. Sickle β^0-thalassemia patients have clinical manifestations similar to those in patients with Hg SS disease. Sickle-C (Hg SC disease) is the second most common form of SCD and generally has a more benign clinical course than does Hg SS disease. Sickle β^+-thalassemia patients have clinical manifestations similar to those in patients with Hg SC disease. Many other forms of SCD are found, among which the sickle-hereditary persistence of fetal hemoglobin (S/H) is the most common. Patients with Hg SS disease and sickle β^+-thalassemia generally have lower hemoglobin levels and present a greater risk under general anesthesia than do patients with Hg SC disease and sickle β^+ thalassemia. Patients with sickle-hereditary persistence of fetal hemoglobin may actually have normal hemoglobin levels.

The red cell membrane is abnormal in patients with SCD, and the red cell life span is shortened by hemolysis. Intermittent episodes of vascular occlusion cause tissue ischemia, which results in acute and chronic organ dysfunction.[72] Patients with SCD require special considerations to prevent perioperative complications due to hemolysis and vaso-occlusion.

Children with SCD require surgical evaluation and treatment because of either complications of their SCD or an unrelated process. The differential diagnosis for acute abdominal pain in a patient with SCD includes uncomplicated sickle cell acute pain episode ("crisis"), cholelithiasis, appendicitis, pancreatitis, ulcer, constipation, pneumonia, pericarditis, and splenic sequestration. Previous episodes of similar pain point to a sickle cell acute painful episode. A study that reviewed the presentation and management of acute abdominal conditions in adults with SCD suggested that a surgical condition is more likely if the pain does not resemble previous painful episodes and if no precipitating event is found.[73] Sickle crisis acute painful episodes were relieved within 48 hours with hydration and oxygen in 97% of patients, whereas no patient with a surgical disease achieved pain relief over the same period with these modalities. The leukocyte count and serum bilirubin were not helpful in establishing the correct diagnosis.

Vaso-occlusive episodes produce bone pain and fever, symptoms that are difficult to differentiate from those of osteomyelitis. The majority of bone pain in SCD is due to vaso-occlusion, but osteomyelitis secondary to *Salmonella* species or *Staphylococcus aureus* is not infrequent.[74] The presence of an immature white blood cell count or elevation of the sedimentation rate, C-reactive protein, or leukocyte alkaline phosphatase points to a bone infection and may be an indication for aspiration of the bone lesion. Radiographic studies including simple plain films, bone scan, or magnetic resonance imaging are generally not helpful unless they are performed within 2 days of the onset of pain.

The patient with SCD may require an operation. The most common procedures according to one recent study were cholecystectomy; ear, nose, and throat procedures; orthopedic procedures; splenectomy; or herniorrhaphy.[75] Cholecystectomy, splenectomy, and orthopedic procedures are often required to treat complications of SCD.

PREOPERATIVE ASSESSMENT AND MANAGEMENT

The outcome of children with SCD requiring a surgical procedure is improved by careful attention to the cardiorespiratory, hemodynamic, hydration, infectious, neurologic, and nutritional status of the child.[76,77] If possible, the operation should be performed when the child is in his or her usual steady state in regard to the SCD. Particular attention should be directed toward any recent history of acute chest syndrome, pneumonia, wheezing, and alloimmunization. Special efforts must be made to avoid perioperative hypoxia, hypothermia, acidosis, and dehydration. Any of these events can result in serious complications.

The use of preoperative blood transfusions is somewhat controversial. Although most centers administer preoperative transfusions for sickle cell patients, no controlled trials documented the benefit of these transfusions.[78] An aggressive transfusion regimen would involve decreasing Hg S to less than 30%, whereas a conservative transfusion regimen would simply increase the Hg level to 10 µg/dL. A national cooperative preoperative sickle cell transfusion study concluded that the conservative transfusion regimen was as effective as the aggressive regimen in preventing preoperative complications. The conservative approach reduced the risk of transfusion-associated complications by 55%.[75] The authors of this study and others have suggested that surgical procedures can be performed more safely in sickle cell patients if a multidisciplinary team is used.[79,80]

INTRAOPERATIVE MANAGEMENT

Anesthestic considerations are based more on the type of surgical procedure planned than on the presence of SCD. Careful monitoring for hypoxia, hypothermia, acidosis, and dehydration is essential in any case. Monitoring should include arterial blood gases, digital oxygen saturation, end-tidal carbon dioxide, temperature, electrocardiogram, blood pressure, and urine output.[81]

POSTOPERATIVE MANAGEMENT

A critical phase in the postoperative management occurs when the patient is moved to the recovery room and then to the surgical floor. It is important to prevent hypothermia, hypoxia, and hypotension. Before extubation, the patient should be awake and oxygenating well. The extubated patient must be carefully monitored with a digital oxygen-saturation monitor and the pulmonary status critically assessed before transfer to the floor. Continuous pulse oximetry should be provided in the early postoperative period. Assessment of fluid status should continue until the patient has resumed adequate oral intake and is able to maintain hydration without intravenous supplementation.

Appropriate levels of analgesic (preferably by a continuous intravenous line and patient-controlled analgesia, if appropriate) should be provided so the patient is comfortable enough to cooperate with ambulation and maintain pulmonary toilet without oversedation. Experienced respiratory therapists should administer a vigorous program for pulmonary toilet. The patient must be monitored closely for the occurrence of pulmonary edema or atelectasis that can progress to acute chest syndrome.[82]

SPECIFIC SURGICAL CONDITIONS

Cholelithiasis and Cholecystectomy

At present, no clear consensus exists regarding the appropriate therapy for SCD children who have cholelithiasis. The reported prevalence of cholelithiasis varies from 4% to 55%.[83,84] This wide variation is dependent on the ages of the study population and the diagnostic modalities used. The higher prevalence figures were obtained by using ultrasonography. We routinely screen symptomatic children with ultrasonography and laboratory studies (e.g., total and direct bilirubin, serum glutamic-oxaloacetic transaminase, serum glutamate-pyruvate transaminase, alkaline phosphatase, and γ-glutamyl-transpeptidase). It is our practice to screen all SCD children for gallstones no later than age 12 years.

A child with SCD and cholelithiasis should undergo cholecystectomy after appropriate preoperative preparation to avoid the increased morbidity of an emergency operation on an unprepared patient.[85–89] Intraoperative cholangiography is recommended because of the high prevalence of common duct stones and the low sensitivity of preoperative ultrasonography.[90]

The utility of laparoscopic cholecystectomy in SCD was first reported in 1990.[91] Since that time, laparoscopic cholecystectomy has been performed with increasing frequency in children with SCD.[92–94] The advantages of laparoscopic cholecystectomy over open cholecystectomy are decreased pain, earlier feeding, earlier discharge, earlier return to school, and improved cosmesis. The presence of common duct stones at times complicates the laparoscopic approach and may require conversion to an open operation for removal. At present, the role of extracorporeal shock wave lithotripsy as a palliative therapeutic modality is uncertain.

Splenic Sequestration and Splenectomy

Before the advent of routine newborn screening for hemoglobinopathies, acute splenic sequestration was the second most common cause of mortality in children younger than 5 years with sickle cell anemia.[95] Splenic sequestration classically was first seen with the acute onset of pallor and listlessness, a precipitate decrease in hemoglobin, thrombocytopenia, and massive splenomegaly.[96] It now appears that parental education along with earlier recognition and immediate treatment with volume support (including red blood cell transfusions) has resulted in significantly decreased mortality in this condition. It is rare for an uncomplicated patient with Hg SS disease who is older than 6 years to develop an acute splenic sequestration syndrome. However, patients with Hg SC and sickle β$^+$-thalassemia disease can experience splenic sequestration at an older age.[97]

The management of the SCD child with splenic sequestration is a clinical dilemma. Options include immediate splenectomy, observation with delaying splenectomy until after two acute episodes, or a prophylactic transfusion protocol to prevent splenic sequestration. The current trend is toward earlier splenectomy.[98,99] The benefit of splenectomy must be balanced with the increased risk of overwhelming bacterial sepsis in the younger asplenic SCD patient.[100] Partial splenectomy[101,102] and especially laparoscopic splenectomy[103] are being performed more commonly as the number of experienced practitioners grows.

Other Surgical Conditions

Children with SCD may require various surgical procedures for which the same principles should be used. As a consequence of their disease, school-aged and adolescent patients are at higher risk for other medical complications such as priapism. If a patient with priapism is refractory to medical management, operative treatment may be required.[104] Ear, nose, and throat minor procedures, such as tonsillectomy, adenoidectomy, and myringotomy, seem to have the same complication rate despite the use of preoperative transfusion.[105]

REFERENCES

1. Thompson AR, Harker LA: Manual of Hemostasis and Thrombosis, 3rd ed. Philadelphia, FA Davis, 1983.
2. Moncada S, Gryglewski R, Bunting S, et al: An enzyme isolated from arteries transforms prostaglandin endoperoxides to an unstable substance that inhibits platelet aggregation. Nature 263:663, 1976.
3. Stern D, Nawroth P, Handley D, et al: An endothelial cell dependent pathway of coagulation. Proc Natl Acad Sci U S A 82:2523, 1985.
4. Esmon CT: Blood coagulation. In Nathan DG, Orkin SA (eds): Nathan and Oski's Hematology of Infancy and Childhood, 5th ed. Philadelphia, WB Saunders, 1998, p 1532.
5. Saito H: Normal hemostatic mechanisms. In Ratnoff OD, Forbes CD (eds): Disorders of Hemostasis, 2nd ed. Philadelphia, WB Saunders, 1991, p 18.
6. Marcus AJ: Platelets and their disorders. In Ratnoff OD, Forbes CD (eds): Disorders of Hemostasis, 2nd ed. Philadelphia, WB Saunders, 1991, p 57.
7. George JN, Nurden AT, Phillips DR: Molecular defects in interactions of platelets with the vessel wall. N Engl J Med 311:1084, 1984.
8. Turitto VT, Baumgartner HR: Platelet-surface interactions. In Coleman RW, Hirsh J, Marder VJ, et al (eds): Hemostasis and Thrombosis: Basic Principles and Clinical Practice, 2nd ed. Philadelphia, JB Lippincott, 1987, p 555.
9. Nurden AT, Didry D, Rosa JP: Molecular defects of platelets in Bernard-Soulier syndrome. Blood Cells 9:333, 1983.
10. Tuddenham EGD: von Willebrand factor and its disorders: An overview of recent molecular studies. Blood Rev 3:251, 1989.
11. Sadler JE. Appendix II: A revised classification of von Willebrand disease. Haemophilia 3(suppl 2):11, 1997.
12. Castaman G, Federici AB, Rodeghiero F, et al: von Willebrand's disease in the year 2003: Towards the complete identification of gene defects for correct diagnosis and treatment. Haematol J 88:94, 2003.

13. Colman RW, Walsh PN: Mechanisms of platelet aggregation. In Colman RW, Hirsh J, Marder VJ, et al (eds): Hemostasis and Thrombosis: Basic Principles and Clinical Practice, 2nd ed. Philadelphia, JB Lippincott, 1987, p 594.

14. Mackie IJ, Bull HA: Normal haemostasis and its regulation. Blood Rev 3:237, 1989.

15. Lorand L, Losowsky MS, Miloszewski KJM: Human factor XIII: Fibrin-stabilizing factor. Prog Hemost Thromb 5:245, 1980.

16. Rosenberg RD, Rosenberg JS: Natural anticoagulant mechanisms. J Clin Invest 74:1, 1984.

17. Rappaport S: Preoperative hemostatic evaluation: Which tests, if any? Blood 61:229, 1983.

18. Stockman JA III: Hematologic evaluations. In Raffensperger JG (ed): Swenson's Pediatric Surgery, 5th ed. Norwalk, Conn, Appleton & Lange, 1990, p 37.

19. Messmore HL, Godwin J: Medical assessment of bleeding in the surgical patient. Med Clin North Am 78:627, 1994.

20. Rohrer MJ, Michelotti MC, Nahrwold DL: A prospective evaluation of the efficacy of preoperative coagulation testing. Ann Surg 208:554, 1988.

21. Zwack GC, Derkay CS: The utility of preoperative hemostatic assessment in adenotonsillectomy. Int J Pediatr Otorhinolaryngol 39:75, 1997.

22. Close HL, Kryzer TC, Nowlin JH, et al: Hemostatic assessment of patients before tonsillectomy: A prospective study. Otolaryngol Head Neck Surg 111:737, 1994.

23. Sramek A, Eikenboom JCJ, Briet E, et al: Usefulness of patient interview in bleeding disorders. Arch Intern Med 155:1413, 1995.

24. Anwar R, Minford A, Gallivan L, et al: Delayed umbilical bleeding: A presenting feature for factor XIII Deficiency: Clinical features, genetics, and management. Pediatrics 109: http://www.pediatrics.org/cgi/content/full/109/2/e32, February, 2002. PDF file version retrieved February, 2002.

25. Lusher JM: Approach to the bleeding patient. In Nathan DG, Orkin SA (eds): Nathan and Oski's Hematology of Infancy and Childhood, 5th ed. Philadelphia, WB Saunders, 1998, p 1574.

26. George JN, Shattil SJ: The clinical importance of acquired abnormalities of platelet function. N Engl J Med 324:27, 1991.

27. Salzman EW: Hemostatic problems in surgical patients. In Coleman RW, Hirsh J, Marder VJ, et al (eds): Hemostasis and Thrombosis: Basic Principles and Clinical Practice, 2nd ed. Philadelphia, JB Lippincott, 1987, p 920.

28. Rodgers RP, Levin J: A critical reappraisal of the bleeding time. Semin Thromb Hemost 16:1, 1990.

29. Mammen EF, Comp PC, Gosselin R, et al: PFA-100 system: A new method for assessment of platelet dysfunction. Semin Thromb Hemost 24:195, 1998.

30. Thiagarjan P, Shapiro SS: Lupus anticoagulants. Prog Hemost Thromb 5:198, 1982.

31. Bick RL: Disseminated intravascular coagulation and related syndromes: A clinical review. Semin Thromb Hemost 14:299, 1988.

32. Pool JG, Hershgold EJ, Pappenhagen AR: High potency antihaemophilic factor concentrate prepared from cryoglobulin precipitate. Nature 203:312, 1964.

33. Tullis JL, Melin M, Jurigian P: Clinical use of prothrombin complexes. N Engl J Med 273:667, 1965.

34. Johnson AJ, Newman J, Howell MB, et al: Purification of antihemophilic factor (AHF) for clinical and experimental use. Thromb Diath Haemorrh 26(suppl):377, 1967.

35. Scharrer I: The need for highly purified products to treat hemophilia B. Acta Haematol 94(suppl 1):2, 1995.

36. Mannucci PM, Chediak J, Hanna W, et al.: Treatment of von Willebrand disease with a high-purity factor VIII/von Willebrand factor concentrate: A prospective, multicenter study. Blood 99:450, 2002.

37. Levine PH: Delivery of health care in hemophilia. Ann N Y Acad Sci 240:201, 1975.

38. Hilgartner MW: Factor replacement therapy. In Hilgartner MW, Pochedly C (eds): Hemophilia in the Child and Adult, 3rd ed. New York, Raven Press, 1989, p 1.

39. Centers for Disease Control: HIV/AIDS Surveillance Report. Atlanta, Ga, CDC, 1991, p 1.

40. Soucie JM, Evatt B, Jackson D: Occurrence of hemophilia in the United States: The Hemophilia Surveillance System Project Investigators. Am J Hematol 59:288, 1998.

41. Kernoff PB, Lee CA, Karayiannis P, et al: High risk of non-A non-B hepatitis after a first exposure to volunteer or commercial clotting factor concentrates: Effects of prophylactic immune serum globulin. Br J Haematol 60:469, 1985.

42. Troisi CL, Hollinger FB, Hoots WK, et al: A multicenter study of viral hepatitis in a United States hemophilic population. Blood 81:412, 1993.

43. Lusher JM, Warrier I: Hemophilia. Pediatr Rev 12:275, 1991.

44. Kasper CK, Boylen AL, Ewing NP, et al: Hematologic management of hemophilia A for surgery. JAMA 253:1279, 1985.

45. Nilsson IM, Hedner U, Ahlberg A, et al: Surgery of hemophiliacs: 20 years' experience. World J Surg 1:55, 1977.

46. Montgomery RR, Gill JC, Scott JP: Hemophilia and von Willebrand disease. In Nathan DG, Orkin SA (eds): Nathan and Oski's Hematology of Infancy and Childhood, 6th ed. Philadelphia, WB Saunders, 2003, p 1547.

47. Kobrinsky NL, Stegman DA: Management of hemophilia during surgery. In Forbes CD, Aledort LM, Madhok R (eds): Hemophilia. Oxford, UK, Chapman & Hall, 1997, p 242.

48. Shapiro AD, White GC II, Kim HC, et al: Efficacy and safety of monoclonal antibody purified factor IX concentrate in haemophilia B patients undergoing surgical procedures. Haemophilia 3:248, 1997.

49. Shapiro AD: Coagulation factor concentrates. In Goodnight SH, Hathaway WE (eds): Disorders of Hemostasis and Thrombosis: A Clinical Guide. New York, McGraw-Hill, 2001, p 505.

50. Andrew M, Paes B, Milner R, et al: Development of the human coagulation system in the full-term infant. Blood 70:165, 1987.

51. Gibson BES: Normal and disordered coagulation. In Hann IM, Gibson BES, Letsky EA (eds): Fetal and Neonatal Haematology. London, Baillière Tindall, 1991, p 123.

52. Jackson DP: Management of thrombocytopenia. In Colman RW, Hirsh J, Marder VJ, et al (eds): Hemostasis and Thrombosis: Basic Principles and Clinical Practice, 2nd ed. Philadelphia, JB Lippincott, 1987, p 530.

53. Greenberg CS: Hemostasis: Pathophysiology and management of clinical disorders. In Sabiston DC Jr (ed): Sabiston's Essentials of Surgery. Philadelphia, WB Saunders, 1987, p 79.

54. Whiteman T, Hassouna HI: Hypercoagulable States. Hematol/Oncol Clin North Am 14:355, 2000.

55. Nicolaes GAF, Dahlback B: Activated protein C resistance (FV[Leiden]) and thrombosis: Factor V mutations causing hypercoagulable states. Hematol Oncol Clin North Am 17:37, 2003.

56. Bick RL: Prothrombin G20210A mutation, antithrombin, heparin cofactor II, protein C, and protein S defects. Hematol Oncol Clin North Am17:9, 2003.

57. Hedner U, Bjoern S, Bernvil SS, et al: Clinical experience with human plasma-derived factor VIIa in patients with hemophilia A and higher titer inhibitors. Haemostasis 19:335, 1989.

58. Hay CRM: The treatment of bleeding in acquired haemophilia with recombinant factor VIIa: A multicentre study. Thromb Haemost 78:1463, 1997.

59. Hedner U: Recombinant coagulation factor VIIa: From the concept to clinical application in hemophilia treatment in 2000. Semin Thromb Hemost 26:363, 2000.

60. Arkin S, Cooper HA, Hutter JJ, et al: Activated recombinant human coagulation factor VII therapy for intracranial hemorrhage in patients with hemophilia A or B with inhibitors. Haemostasis 28:93, 1998.

61. Leibman HA, Chediak J, Fink KI, et al: Activated recombinant human coagulation factor VII (rFVIIa) therapy for abdominal bleeding in patients with inhibitory antibodies to factor VIII. Am J Hematol 63:109, 2000.

62. Shapiro AD, Gilchrist GS, Hoots KW, et al: Prospective, randomized trial of two doses of rFVIIa (NovoSeven) in haemophilia patients with inhibitors undergoing surgery. Thromb Haemost 80:773, 1998.

63. Lusher J, Ingerslev J, Roberts H, et al: Clinical experience with recombinant factor VIIa. Blood Coagul Fibrinolysis 9:119, 1998.

64. Santagostino E, Gringeri A, Mannucci PM: Home treatment with recombinant activated factor VII in patients with factor VIII inhibitors: The advantages of early intervention. Br J Haematol 104:22, 1999.

65. Erhardtsen E: Pharmacokinetics of recombinant activated factor VII (rFVIIa). Semin Thromb Hemost 26:385, 2000.

66. NovoSeven; Novo Nordisk; Package Insert, 2003. (FDA approved)
67. Mariani G, Testa MG, DiPaolantonio T, et al: Use of recombinant activated factor VII in the treatment of congenital factor VII deficiencies. Vox Sanguinis 77:131, 1999.
68. Hedner U, Erhardtsen E: Potential role for rFVIIa in transfusion medicine. Transfusion 42:114, 2002.
69. Poon M-C, d'Oiron R, and the International Registry on Recombinant Factor VIIa and Congenital Platelet Disorders Group: Recombinant activated factor VII (NovoSeven) treatment of platelet-related bleeding disorders. Blood Coagul Fibrinolysis 11:S55, 2000.
70. Monroe DM, Hoffman M, Allen GA, et al: The factor VII-platelet interplay: Effectiveness of recombinant factor VIIa in the treatment of bleeding in severe thrombocytopathia. Semin Thromb Hemost 26:373, 2000.
71. Martinowitz U, Kenet G, Segal E, et al: Recombinant activated factor VII for adjunctive hemorrhage control in trauma. J Trauma Injury Infect Crit Care 51:431, 2001.
72. Lane PA: Sickle cell disease. Pediatr Clin North Am 43:639, 1996.
73. Baumgartner F, Klein S: The presentation and management of the acute abdomen in the patient with sickle cell anemia. Am Surgeon 55:660, 1989.
74. Epps CH, Bryant DD, Coles MJ, et al: Osteomyelitis in patients who have sickle cell disease: Diagnosis and management. J Bone Joint Surg 73:1281, 1991.
75. Vichinsky EP, Haberkern CM, Neumayr L, et al: A comparison of conservative and aggressive transfusion regimens in the perioperative management of sickle cell disease. N Engl J Med 333:206, 1995.
76. Ware RE, Filston HC: Surgical management of children with hemoglobinopathies. Surg Clin North Am 72:1223, 1992.
77. Sutton JP, Farrer JJ, Rodning CB: Surgical management of patients with sickle cell syndromes. In Mankad VN, Moore RB (eds): Sickle Cell Disease: Pathophysiology, Diagnosis, and Management. Westport, Conn, Praeger, 1992, pp 364–386.
78. Griffin TC, Buchanan GR: Elective surgery in children with sickle cell disease without preoperative blood transfusion. J Pediatr Surg 28:681, 1993.
79. Wayne AS, Kevy SV, Nathan DG: Transfusion management of sickle cell disease. Blood 81:1109, 1993.
80. Koshy M, Weiner SJ, Miller ST, et al: Surgery and anesthesia in sickle cell disease. Blood 86:3676, 1995.
81. Mankad AV: Anesthetic management of patients with sickle cell disease. In Mankad VN, Moore RB (eds.): Sickle Cell Disease: Pathophysiology, Diagnosis, and Management. Westport, Conn, Praeger, 1992, pp 351–363.
82. Castro O, Brambilla DJ, Thorington B, et al: The acute chest syndrome in sickle cell disease: Incidence and risk factors. Blood 84:643, 1994.
83. Lachman BS, Lazerson J, Starshak RJ, et al: The prevalence of cholelithiasis in sickle cell disease as diagnosed by ultrasound and cholecystography. Pediatrics 64:601, 1979.
84. Sarnaik S, Slovis TL, Corbett DP, et al: Incidence of cholelithiasis in sickle cell anemia using the ultrasonic gray-scale technique. J Pediatr 96:1005, 1980.
85. Pappis CH, Galanakis S, Moussatos G, et al: Experience of splenectomy and cholecystectomy in children with chronic hemolytic anemia. J Pediatr Surg 24:543, 1989.
86. Stephens CG, Scott RB: Cholelithiasis in sickle cell anemia: Surgical or medical management. Arch Intern Med 140:648, 1980.
87. Ware R, Filston HC, Schultz WH, et al: Elective cholecystectomy in children with sickle hemoglobinopathies. Ann Surg 208:17, 1988.
88. Haberkern CM, Neumayr LD, et al: Cholecystectomy in sickle cell anemia patients: Perioperative outcome of 364 cases from the National Preoperative Transfusion Study. Blood 89:1533, 1997.
89. Miltenburg DM, Schaffer R III, Breslin T, et al: Changing indications for pediatric cholecystectomy. Pediatrics 105:1250, 2000.
90. Ware RE, Schultz WH, Filston HC, et al: Diagnosis and management of common bile duct stones in patients with sickle hemoglobinopathies. J Pediatr Surg 27:572, 1992.
91. Dubois F, Icard P, Berthelot G, et al: Coelioscopic cholecystectomy: Preliminary report of 36 cases. Ann Surg 211:60, 1990.
92. Gadacz TR, Talamini MA, Lillemoe KD, et al: Laparoscopic cholecystectomy. Surg Clin North Am 70:1249, 1990.
93. Tagge EP, Othersen HB Jr, Jackson SM, et al: Impact of laparoscopic cholecystectomy on the management of cholelithiasis in children with sickle cell disease. J Pediatr Surg 29:209, 1994.
94. Ware RE, Kinney TR, Casey JR, et al: Laparoscopic cholecystectomy in young patients with sickle hemoglobinopathies. J Pediatr 120:58, 1992.
95. Gill FM, Sleeper LA, Weiner SJ, et al: Clinical events in the first decade in a cohort of infants with sickle cell disease. Blood 86:776, 1995.
96. Emond AM, Collis R, Darvill D, et al: Acute splenic sequestration in homozygous sickle cell disease: Natural history and management. J Pediatr 107:201, 1985.
97. Aquino VM, Norvell JM, Buchanan GR: Acute splenic complications in children with sickle cell-hemoglobin C disease. J Pediatr 130:961, 1997.
98. Al-Salem AH, Qaisaruddin S, Nasserallah Z, et al: Splenectomy in patients with sickle cell disease. Am J Surg 172:254, 1996.
99. Kinney TR, Ware RE, Schultz WH, et al: Long-term management of splenic sequestration in children with sickle cell disease. J Pediatr 117:194, 1990.
100. Pegelow CH, Wilson B, Overturf GD, et al: Infection in splenectomized sickle cell patients. Clin Pediatr 19:102, 1980.
101. Svarch E, Vilorio P, Nordet I, et al: Partial splenectomy in children with sickle cell disease and repeated episodes of splenic sequestration. Hemoglobin 20:393, 1996.
102. Nouri A, de Montalembert M, Revillon Y, et al: Partial splenectomy in sickle cell syndromes. Arch Dis Child 66:1070, 1991.
103. Hicks BA, Thompson WE, Rogers ZR, et al: Laparoscopic splenectomy in childhood hematologic disorders. J Laparoendosc Surg 6:531, 1996.
104. Miller ST, Rao SP, Dunn EK, et al: Priapism in children with sickle cell disease. J Urol 154:844, 1995.
105. Waldron P, Pegelow C, Neumayr L, et al: Tonsillectomy, adenoidectomy, and myringotomy in sickle cell disease: Perioperative morbidity. J Pediatr Hemat Oncol 21:129, 1999.

CHAPTER 6

Extracorporeal Membrane Oxygenation

Jason S. Frischer, MD, and Charles J. H. Stolar, MD

Extracorporeal membrane oxygenation (ECMO) is a life-saving technology that uses partial heart/lung bypass for extended periods. It is not a therapeutic modality, but rather a supportive tool that provides sufficient gas exchange and perfusion for patients with acute, *reversible* cardiac or respiratory failure. This affords the patient's cardiopulmonary system a time to "rest," at which point the patient is spared the deleterious effects of high airway pressure, high Fio_2, traumatic mechanical ventilation, and perfusion impairment. Since the early anecdotal reports of neonatal and pediatric ECMO, the Extracorporeal Life Support Organization (ELSO) has registered approximately 25,000 neonatal and pediatric patients treated with ECMO for a variety of cardiopulmonary disorders.[1]

HISTORY

The initial effort to develop extracorporeal bypass was first led by cardiac surgeons. Their goal was to repair intracardiac lesions under direct visualization and therefore they needed to arrest the heart, divert and oxygenate the blood, and perfuse the patient so that repair could be performed. The first cardiopulmonary bypass circuits used in the operating room involved direct cross circulation between the patient and another subject (usually the patient's mother or father) acting as both the pump and the oxygenator.[2]

The first attempts at establishing cardiopulmonary bypass by complete artificial circuitry and oxygenation were constructed with disk-and-bubble oxygenators and were limited because of hemolysis encountered by direct mixing of oxygen and blood. The discovery of heparin and the development of semipermeable membranes (silicone rubber) capable of supporting gas exchange by diffusion were major advancements toward the development of ECMO.[3] During the 1960s and early 1970s, the silicone membrane was configured into a number of oxygenator models by a multitude of investigators.[4-7]

In 1972, the first successful use of prolonged cardiopulmonary bypass was reported.[8] The patient sustained a ruptured aorta after a motorcycle accident. Venoarterial extracorporeal bypass support was maintained for 3 days. A multicenter prospective randomized trial sponsored by The National Heart, Lung, and Blood Institute (branch of the National Institutes of Health; NIH) studied the efficacy of ECMO for adult respiratory distress syndrome. In 1979 they concluded that the use of ECMO had no advantage over that of conventional mechanical ventilation in this study, and the trial was stopped early.[9] Bartlett et al.[10] noted that all of the patients in the study had irreversible pulmonary fibrosis before the initiation of ECMO. In 1976, he reported the first series of infants treated with long-term ECMO, with a significant number of survivors. Six (43%) of 14 patients with respiratory distress syndrome survived. Many of these patients were premature and weighed less than 2 kg. They also reported that 22 patients with meconium aspiration syndrome (MAS) had a 70% survival. These neonates were noted to be larger in size.

Since then, three randomized control trials and a number of retrospective published reports have reported, despite study-design issues, the efficacy of ECMO versus conventional mechanical ventilation.[11-18] Other centers started to use ECMO, and by 1996, 113 centers were maintaining ECMO programs registered with ELSO. Currently 101 institutions are registered.[1] Over the next two decades, improvements in technology, a better understanding of the pathophysiology of pulmonary failure, and a greater experience in using ECMO have contributed to the improved outcomes for infants with respiratory failure. In 2003, the University of Michigan reported an association between ECMO volume and observed reduction in neonatal mortality seen in that state between 1980 through 1999.[19]

ELSO, formed in 1989, is a collaboration of physicians and scientists with an interest in ECMO. The organization provides the medical community with guidelines, training manuals and courses, and a forum in which these individuals can meet and discuss the future of extracorporeal life support. The group also provides investigators a registry that collects data from almost all centers that maintain an ECMO program throughout the world. This database provides valuable information for analysis of this life-saving biotechnology.[20,21]

CLINICAL APPLICATIONS OF ECMO

Neonates are the patients that benefit most from ECMO. Cardiopulmonary failure in this population secondary to MAS, congenital diaphragmatic hernia (CDH), persistent pulmonary hypertension of the newborn (PPHN), and congenital cardiac disease are the most common pathophysiologic processes requiring ECMO intervention. For the pediatric population, the most common disorders treated with ECMO are viral and bacterial pneumonia, acute respiratory failure (non–acute respiratory distress syndrome [ARDS]), ARDS, sepsis, and cardiac disease. The experience with cardiac ECMO has been increasing over the past few years. Its use for treating patients who are unweanable from bypass after cardiac surgical procedures and as a bridge to heart transplantation in patients with postsurgical or end-stage ventricular failure are areas in which ECMO use is increasing.[1,22] Some less frequently used indications for ECMO include respiratory failure secondary to smoke inhalation,[23] severe asthma,[24] rewarming of hypercoagulopathic/hypothermic trauma patients,[25] and maintenance of an organ donor pending liver allograft harvest and transplantation.[26]

PATHOPHYSIOLOGY OF NEWBORN PULMONARY HYPERTENSION

Pulmonary vascular resistance (PVR) is the hallmark and driving force of the fetal circulation. Normal fetal circulation is characterized by PVR that exceeds systemic pressures, resulting in higher right-sided heart pressures and therefore preferential right-to-left blood flow. The fetal umbilical vein carries oxygenated blood from the placenta to the inferior vena cava via the ductus venosus. Because of the high PVR, the majority of the blood that reaches the right atrium from the inferior vena cava is directed to the left atrium through the foramen ovale. The superior vena cava delivers deoxygenated blood to the right atrium that is preferentially directed to the right ventricle and pulmonary artery. This blood takes the path of least resistance and shunts from the main pulmonary artery directly to the descending aorta via the ductus arteriosus, bypassing the pulmonary vascular bed and the left side of the heart. Therefore as a consequence of these anatomic right-to-left shunts, the lungs are almost completely bypassed by the fetal circulation.

At birth, with the infant's initial breath, the alveoli distend and begin to fill with air. This is paralleled by relaxation of the muscular arterioles of the pulmonary circulation and the expansion of the pulmonary vascular bed. This causes a rapid decrease in PVR to below systemic levels. This activity causes the left atrial pressure to become higher than the right atrial pressure, leading to the closure of the foramen ovale, resulting in all venous blood flowing from the right atrium to the right ventricle

and into the pulmonary artery. The ductus arteriosus also closes at this time, and therefore all fetal right-to-left circulation ceases, completing separation of the pulmonary and systemic circulations. Anatomic closure of these structures takes several days to weeks. Thus maintaining the pressure gradient of systemic pressure greater than the pulmonary circulation is vital to sustaining normal circulation.

Failure of the transition from fetal circulation to newborn circulation is described as PPHN or persistent fetal circulation.[27] Clinically, PPHN is characterized by hypoxemia out of proportion to pulmonary parenchymal or anatomic disease. Normally, in fetal and term neonates, the pulmonary arterioles are muscular only as far as the terminal bronchioles. In hypoxic fetuses and infants, the proliferation of smooth muscle in the arterioles may extend far beyond the terminal bronchioles, resulting in thickened and more reactive vessels. In response to hypoxic conditions, these vessels undergo significant self-perpetuating vasoconstriction. Although sometimes idiopathic, PHN can occur secondary to a number of disease processes such as MAS, CDH, polycythemia, and sepsis.

Treatment for PPHN is directed at decreasing right-to-left shunts and increasing pulmonary blood flow. Previously, most patients were treated with hyperventilation with mechanical ventilation, induction of alkalosis, neuromuscular blockade, and sedation. Unfortunately, these therapies have not reduced morbidity, mortality, or the need for ECMO in the neonatal population. ECMO allows the interruption of the hypoxia-induced negative cycle of increased smooth muscle tone and vasoconstriction. ECMO provides richly oxygenated blood and allows pulmonary blood pressures to return to normal subsystemic values without the iatrogenic complications encumbered by overly aggressive "conventional" therapy. Recently, data recommending gentle ventilation and the use of inhaled nitric oxide for these children has been reported.[28] Hyperventilation and neuromuscular blockade were not part of the treatment strategy. The infants were allowed to breathe spontaneously. This strategy has decreased morbidity, mortality, and the use of ECMO.

PATIENT-SELECTION CRITERIA

The selection of patients as potential ECMO candidates continues to remain controversial. The selection criteria are based on data from multiple institutions, patient safety, and mechanical limitations related to the equipment. The risk of performing an invasive procedure that requires heparinization of a critically ill child must be weighed against the estimated mortality of the patient with conventional therapy alone. A predictive mortality of greater than 80% after exhausting all conventional therapies is the criterion most institutions follow to select patients for ECMO. Obviously, these criteria are subjective and will vary between facilities, based on local clinical experience and available technology. All ECMO centers must develop their own criteria and continually evaluate their patient selection based on ongoing outcomes data.

Recommended pre-ECMO studies are listed in Table 6-1. Indications for neonatal, cardiac, and pediatric ECMO all have their own modifiers. The definition of "conventional therapy" also is anything but consistent in any category. Nevertheless, ECMO is indicated when (1) a reversible disease process is present, (2) ventilator treatment is causing more harm than good, and (3) tissue oxygenation requirements are not being met. A discussion of generally accepted selection criteria for using neonatal ECMO follows.

Reversible Cardiopulmonary Disorders

The underlying principle of ECMO relies on the premise that the patient has a reversible disease process that can be corrected with either therapy or "rest," and that this reversal will occur in a relatively short period. Prolonged exposure to high-pressure mechanical ventilation with high concentrations of oxygen will frequently lead to the development of bronchopulmonary dysplasia (BPD).[29] It has been suggested that BPD can result from high levels of ventilatory support for as little as 4 days or less.[30] The pulmonary dysfunction that follows barotrauma and oxygen toxicity associated with mechanical ventilation typically requires weeks to months to resolve. Therefore patients that have been ventilated for a long period and in whom lung injury has developed are not amenable to a short course of therapy with ECMO. Most ECMO centers will not accept as candidates for ECMO patients who have had more than 10 to 14 days of mechanical ventilation, owing to the high probability of established, irreversible pulmonary dysfunction.

Echocardiography should be performed on every patient being considered for ECMO to determine cardiac anatomy and function. Treatable conditions such as total anomalous pulmonary venous return and transposition of the great vessels, which may masquerade initially as pulmonary failure, can be surgically corrected, but may require ECMO resuscitation initially. Infants with correctable cardiac disease should be considered on an individual basis. ECMO also provides an excellent bridge to cardiac transplantation. ECMO as a bridge to lung transplantation is controversial because the usual time needed to locate a suitable lung donor generally far exceeds the period during which the recipient can be maintained on bypass.

Coexisting Anomalies

Every effort should be made to establish a clear diagnosis before the initiation of ECMO. The baby should have no anomalies incompatible with life, as these infants do not benefit from ECMO. ECMO is not a resource that is intended to delay an inevitable death. Many lethal pulmonary conditions such as overwhelming pulmonary hypoplasia, congenital alveolar proteinosis, and alveolar capillary dysplasia may appear to be reversible conditions but are considered lethal.[31]

Gestational Age

The gestational age of an ECMO patient should be at least 34 to 35 weeks. In the early experience with ECMO, significant morbidity and mortality related to intracranial hemorrhage (ICH) was associated with prematurity (< 34 weeks of gestation).[32] Despite modification of ECMO technique over the past decade, premature infants continue to be at risk for ICH. In preterm infants, ependymal cells within the brain are not fully developed, thus making them susceptible to hemorrhage. Systemic heparinization necessary to maintain a thrombus-free circuit adds to the risk of hemorrhagic complications.

Birthweight

Technical consideration and limitation of cannula size restrict ECMO candidates to babies weighing at least 2000 g. The smallest single-lumen ECMO cannula is 8F, and flow through a tube is related to the radius of the tube by a power of 4. Small veins permit only small cannulas, resulting in flow that will be reduced by a power of 4. Babies that weigh less than 2 kg provide technical challenges in cannulation and in maintaining adequate blood flow through the small catheters.

Bleeding Complications

Babies with ongoing, uncontrollable bleeding or an uncorrectable bleeding diathesis pose a relative contraindication to ECMO.[20] Coagulopathy should be corrected before initiating ECMO because the need for continuous systemic heparinization adds an unacceptable risk of bleeding.

Intracranial Hemorrhage

Candidates for ECMO should not, as a rule, have had an ICH. A preexisting ICH may be exacerbated by the use of heparin and the unavoidable alterations in cerebral blood flow while receiving ECMO. Patients with small interventricular hemorrhages (grade I) or a small intraparenchymal hemorrhage can be successfully treated on ECMO by maintaining a lower than optimal activated clotting time (ACT) in the range of 180 to 200 seconds.

TABLE 6-1
RECOMMENDED PRE-ECMO STUDIES

Head ultrasound
Cardiac echocardiogram
Chest radiograph
Complete blood count, platelets
Type and cross
Electrolytes, calcium
Coagulation studies (PT, PTT, fibrinogen, fibrin
   degradation products)
Serial arterial blood gases

ECMO, extracorporeal membrane oxygenation; PT, prothrombin time; PTT, partial thromboplastin time.

These cases should be closely observed for extension of intracranial bleeding. Those patients posing a particularly high risk for ICH are those with a history of a previous ICH, cerebral infarction, prematurity, coagulopathy, ischemic central nervous system injury, or sepsis. Consideration of these patients for ECMO should be individualized.[31]

Failure of Medical Management

ECMO candidates are expected to have a reversible cardiopulmonary disease process, with a predictive mortality of greater than 80% to 90% with all available modalities short of ECMO. Because different institutions have varying technical capabilities, opinions, and expertise, "optimal" medical management is a subjective term that varies widely. Vasoconstrictive agents, inotropic agents, sedatives, and analgesia are all pharmacologic agents that are part of the medical management. Ventilatory management usually begins with conventional support but also may include the administration of surfactant, nitric oxide, inverse inspiration/expiration (I:E) ratios, or high-frequency ventilation. Ventilator/respiratory-care strategies that incur significant barotrauma and other morbidity should be rigorously avoided.

ECMO use has been obviated in patients who otherwise meet ECMO criteria because of recent innovations in medical management. These innovations include the use of permissive hypercapnea with spontaneous ventilation, avoidance of muscle paralysis, and the avoidance of chest tubes. In 1978, the Children's Hospital of New York developed a nontraditional approach to the management of patients with PPH, which has been successfully extended to infants with CDH.[33] Hyperventilation, hyperoxia, and muscle relaxants were not used, and permissive hypercapnea in conjunction with spontaneous ventilation was emphasized. We used low-pressure ventilator settings, tolerated persistent $PaCO_2$ of 50 to 80 mm Hg and a PaO_2 of 40 mm Hg. With careful attention to maintaining a *preductal* oxygen saturation greater than 90% or PaO_2 of 60 torr or greater, 15 infants who met ECMO criteria with PPHN and in severe respiratory failure were initially treated with this management and survived without ECMO.

Risk Assessment

Because of the invasive nature of ECMO and the potentially life-threatening complications, investigators have worked to develop an objective set of criteria to predict which infants have an 80% mortality without ECMO. The two most commonly used measurements for neonatal respiratory failure are the alveolar-arterial oxygen gradient ($AaDO_2$) and the oxygenation index (OI), which are calculated as follows:

Alveolar-Arterial Oxygen Gradient

$$AaDO_2 = (P_{ATM} - 47)(FiO_2) - [(PaCO_2)/0.8] - PaO_2$$

where P_{ATM} is the atmospheric pressure, and FiO_2 is the inspired concentration of oxygen.

Oxygenation Index

$$OI = \frac{MAP \times FiO_2 \times 100}{PaO_2}$$

where MAP is the mean airway pressure.

Although institutional criteria for ECMO vary, it is generally accepted that, in the setting of optimal management, an $AaDO_2$ greater than 625 mm Hg for more than 4 hours, or an $AaDO_2$ greater than 600 mm Hg for more than 12 hours, or an OI of greater than 40 establishes both a relatively sensitive and specific predictor of mortality. Other criteria used by many institutions include a preductal PaO_2 less than 35 to 50 mm Hg for 2 to 12 hours or a pH of less than 7.25 for at least 2 hours with intractable hypotension. These are sustained values measured over a period of time and are not accurate predictors of mortality.[14,20,34–36]

Older infants and children do not have as well-defined criteria for high mortality risk. The combination of a ventilation index

$$\frac{Respiratory\ rate \times PaCO_2 \times Peak\ inspiratory\ pressure}{1000}$$

greater than 40 and an OI more than 40 correlates with a 77% mortality risk. A mortality of 81% is associated with an $AaDO_2$ greater than 580 mm Hg and a peak inspiratory pressure of 40 cm H_2O. Indications for support in patients with cardiac pathology are based on clinical signs such as hypotension despite the administration of inotropes or volume resuscitation, oliguria (urine output < 0.5 mL/kg/hr), and decreased peripheral perfusion.

Congenital Diaphragmatic Hernia

Of most interest to surgeons are neonates with abdominal viscera in the thoracic cavity due to a CDH. These patients have pulmonary hypertension and have pulmonary hypoplasia that is more pronounced on the side of the hernia. Pulmonary insufficiency quickly leads to a vicious cycle of hypoxia, hypercarbia, and acidosis. Interruption of this cycle has vastly improved over the last two decades with the use of permissive hypercapnea/spontaneous respiration, and delayed elective repair.

High-frequency oscillation (HFOV) may have its major role in forestalling respiratory failure rather than as a "rescue therapy."[37] Nitric oxide and surfactant play no more than an anecdotal role. The primary indicator for ECMO in the patient with CDH is when tissue oxygen requirements are not being met, as evidenced by progressive metabolic acidosis, mixed venous oxygen desaturation, and multiple organ failure. The other indicator is mounting iatrogenic pulmonary injury.

Permissive hypercapnea with spontaneous respiration is initiated with intermittent mandatory ventilation (IMV) at 30 to 40 breaths per minute, equal I/E time, inspiratory gas flow of 5 to 7 L/min, peak inspiratory pressure (PIP) of 20 to 22 cm H_2O, and positive end-expiratory pressure (PEEP) of 5 cm H_2O. The FiO_2 is selected to maintain preductal SaO_2 greater than 90%. If this mode is not sufficient, as demonstrated by severe paradoxical chest movement, severe retractions, tachypnea, preductal O_2 saturations less than 80%, or $PaCO_2$ greater than 60 mm Hg, then a new mode of ventilation is needed.

High-frequency ventilation would be the next mode of ventilation to be considered. The ventilator is set to IMV with a rate of 100, the inspiratory time is 0.3, the inspiratory gas flow is 10 to 12 L, the PIP is 20, and the PEEP will be automatic. The PIP is adjusted as needed, based on chest excursion, maintaining PIP at less than 25 mm Hg.

HFOV can be instituted if the high-frequency ventilation alone does not maintain the parameters mentioned earlier. Improvement with HFOV may be no more than temporary. The goal is to maintain preductal oxygen saturations between 90% and 95%. Spontaneous breathing is preserved by rigorously avoiding administering muscle relaxants. Sedation is used only as needed. Meticulous attention to maintaining a clear airway and the well-being of the infant is critical.[38,39]

Before ECMO is initiated for an infant with CDH, the infant must first demonstrate some evidence of adequate lung parenchyma. This is assessed by having a recorded best $PaCO_2$ less than 50 mm Hg and a preductal oxygen saturation greater than 90% for a sustained period of at least 1 hour at any time in the clinical course. With these criteria, successful ECMO should yield an overall survival rate of 75%. If patients with lethal anomalies, overwhelming pulmonary hypoplasia, or neurologic complications are not included, survival approaches 85%.[38–40]

METHODS OF EXTRACORPOREAL SUPPORT

The goal of ECMO support is to provide oxygen delivery. Three different extracorporeal configurations are used clinically: venoarterial (VA), venovenous (VV), and double-lumen single-cannula venovenous (DLVV) bypass. The inception of ECMO and its early days were characterized by VA ECMO because it offered the ability to replace both cardiac and pulmonary function. Venous blood is drained from the right atrium (RA) through the right internal jugular vein (RIJ), and oxygenated blood is returned via the right common carotid artery (RCCA) to the aorta.

Potential disadvantages are associated with VA ECMO. A major artery must be cannulated and sacrificed; risk of gas and particulate emboli into the systemic circulation is substantial; pulmonary perfusion is reduced; decreased preload and increased afterload may reduce cardiac output, resulting in nonpulsatile flow; and the coronary arteries are largely perfused by left ventricular blood, which is relatively hypoxic.

VV and DLVV avoid these disadvantages and provide pulmonary support but do not provide cardiac support. VV bypass is established by draining the RA via the RIJ, with reinfusion into a femoral vein. DLVV is accomplished by means of a double-lumen catheter inserted into the RA via the RIJ. A major limitation of VV or

DLVV ECMO is that a fraction of the infused, oxygenated blood re-enters the pump and, at high flows, may limit oxygen delivery. A limitation specific to DLVV is catheter size, which confines use of this method of support to larger infants and smaller pediatric patients. VV and DLVV bypass have become the preferred method of extracorporeal support of all appropriate patients that do not require cardiac support.[20]

CANNULATION

Cannulation can be performed in the neonatal or pediatric intensive care units under adequate sedation and intravenous anesthesia, with proper monitoring. The infant is positioned with the head at the foot of the bed, supine, the head and neck hyperextended over a shoulder roll and turned to the left. Local anesthesia is administered over the proposed incision site. A transverse cervical incision is made along the anterior border of the sternomastoid muscle, one finger-breadth above the right clavicle. The platysma muscle is divided, and dissection is carried down with the sternomastoid muscle retracted to expose the carotid sheath. The sheath is opened, and the internal jugular vein, common carotid artery, and vagus nerve are identified (Fig. 6-1*A*). The vein is dissected first and mobilized over proximal and distal ligatures. Occasionally it is necessary to ligate the inferior thyroid vein. The common carotid artery lies medial and posterior, contains no branches, and is mobilized in a similar fashion. The vagus nerve should be identified and protected from injury.

The patient is then systemically given 50 to 100 U/kg of heparin, which is allowed to circulate for 2 to 3 minutes, which should produce an ACT of more than 300 seconds. The arterial cannula (usually 10F for newborns) is measured so that the tip will lie at the junction of the brachiocephalic artery and the aorta (2.5 to 3 cm or approximately one third the distance between the sternal notch and the xiphoid). The venous cannula (12 to 14F for neonates) is measured to have its tip in the RA (6 to 8 cm or approximately half the distance between the suprasternal notch and the xiphoid process). The arterial cannula is placed first with VA bypass. The carotid artery is ligated distally. Proximal control is obtained, and a transverse arteriotomy is made near the distal ligature (Fig. 6-1*B*). To help prevent intimal dissection, stay sutures are placed around the arteriotomy and used for retraction when placing the arterial cannula. The saline-filled cannula is inserted to its premeasured position and secured in the vessel with two silk ligatures (2-0 or 3-0). A small piece of vessel loop may be placed under the ligatures on its anterior aspect of the carotid to protect the vessel from injury during decannulation (Fig. 6-1*C*).

The patient must be paralyzed with succinylcholine before venous cannulation to prevent spontaneous respiration. The jugular vein is then ligated above the site selected for the venotomy. Gentle traction on this ligature helps during the venous catheter insertion. A venotomy is made close to the ligature. The saline-filled venous catheter is passed to the measured level of the RA

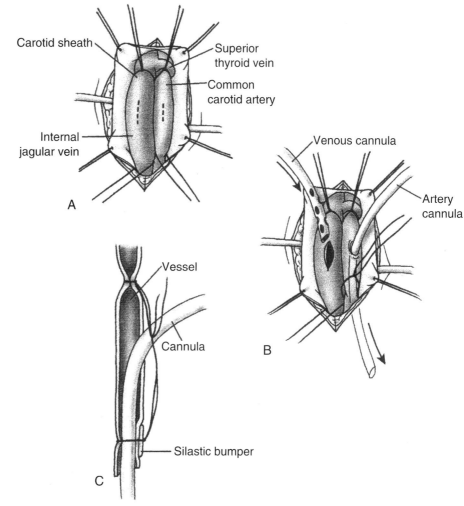

FIGURE 6-1. Details of the cannulation procedure. *A,* The carotid sheath is exposed, the sternocleidomastoid muscle is retracted laterally, and the common carotid artery and the internal jugular vein are dissected free. *B,* The patient is anticoagulated after the vessels are dissected and ligated cephalad. The arterial cannula is passed into the junction of the innominate artery and the aorta. The venous catheter is passed into the right atrium. *C,* A polymeric silicone (Silastic) bumper is used to facilitate ligation of the cannulas. The two ligatures on each vessel are then tied together.

and secured in a manner similar to that used for the arterial catheter. Any bubbles are removed from the cannulae as they are connected to the ECMO circuit. Bypass is initiated. The cannulae are then secured by sutures to the skin above the wound. The wound is closed in layers, ensuring that hemostasis is meticulous.

For VV and DLVV bypass, the procedure is exactly as described, including dissection of the artery, which is surrounded by a vessel loop to facilitate conversion to VA ECMO should that become necessary. The venous catheter tip should be positioned in the mid-right atrium with the arterial portion of the DLVV catheter oriented medially to direct the oxygenated blood flow toward the tricuspid valve.[41] Cannula position is confirmed by a chest radiograph or transthoracic echocardiogram or both.

ECMO CIRCUIT

Venous blood is drained from the infant by gravity into a small reservoir or bladder (Fig. 6-2). An in-line oxymetric probe is located between the venous-return cannula and the bladder. This continuously monitors blood pH, Pao_2, Pco_2, and O_2 saturation. The monitor provides the information equivalent to the mixed venous blood gas (excluding any recirculation in VV or DLVV ECMO) and is extremely useful in monitoring the patient's status. The bladder is a 30- to 50-mL reservoir that acts as a safety valve. In the event that venous drainage does not keep up with arterial flow from the pump, the bladder volume will be depleted, sounding an alarm and automatically shutting off the pump. The blood flow through the circuit ceases to prevent gas bubbles forming from solution or drawing air into the circuit. Hypovolemia is one of the common causes of decreased venous inflow into the circuit, but kinking with occlusion of the venous line should be suspected first. Raising the height of the patient's bed can improve venous drainage by gravity. An algorithm for managing pump failure due to inadequate venous return is shown in Figure 6-3.

A displacement roller pump pushes blood through the membrane oxygenator. The roller pumps are designed with microprocessors that allow calculation of the blood flow based on roller-head speed and tubing diameter of the circuit. The pumps are connected to continuous pressure monitoring throughout the circuit and are servoregulated if pressures within the circuit exceed preset parameters. Another safety device, a bubble detector (not depicted

ECMO Circuit

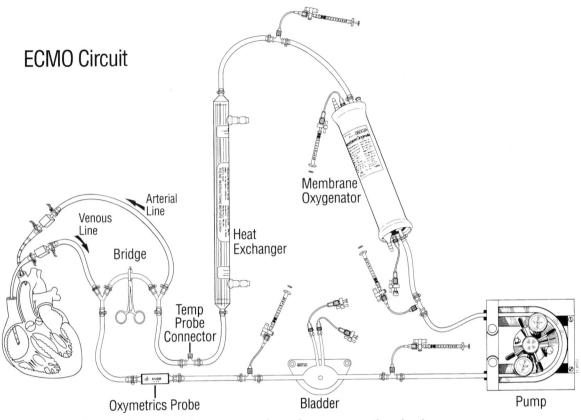

FIGURE 6-2. Diagram of venoarterial extracorporeal membrane oxygenation circuit.

in Fig. 6-2) is interposed between the pump and the membrane oxygenator that halts perfusion to the patient if air is detected within the circuit. The oxygenator consists of a long, two-compartment chamber composed of a spiral-wound silicone membrane and a polycarbonate core, with blood flow in one direction and oxygen flow in the opposite direction. Oxygen diffuses through the membrane into the blood circuit, and carbon dioxide and water vapor diffuse from the blood into the sweep gas. The size (surface area) of the oxygenator is based on the patient's size. Another oxymetric probe is located in the arterial return line distal to the oxygenator to provide information about the blood returning to the patient. The blood emerges from the upper end of the oxygenator and passes through the countercurrent heat exchanger and returns at body temperature to the aortic arch via the right common carotid artery.

PATIENT MANAGEMENT ON ECMO

Once the cannulas are connected to the circuit, bypass is initiated, and flow is slowly increased to 100 to 150 mL/kg/min, so that the patient is stabilized. Continuous in-line monitoring of the venous (prepump) SV_{O_2} and arterial (postpump) Pa_{O_2} as well as pulse oximetry is vital. The goal of VA ECMO is to maintain a mixed venous P_{O_2} (SV_{O_2}) of 37 to 40 mm Hg and saturation of 65% to 70%. VV ECMO is more difficult to monitor

because of recirculation, which may produce a falsely elevated SV_{O_2}. Inadequate oxygenation and perfusion are indicated by metabolic acidosis, oliguria, hypotension, elevated liver function tests, and seizures. Arterial blood gases should be monitored closely with Pa_{O_2} and Pa_{CO_2} maintained at as close to normal level as possible. The oxygen level of the blood returning to the patient should be maintained fully saturated. To increase a patient's oxygen level on ECMO, one can either increase the ECMO flow rate (~cardiac output), or increase the hemoglobin to maintain hemoglobin at 15 g/dL (~oxygen content). CO_2 elimination is extremely efficient with the membrane, and it is important to adjust the sweep (gas mixing) to maintain a Pa_{CO_2} in the range of 40 to 45 mm Hg. This is important, especially during weaning, because a low Pa_{CO_2} inhibits the infant's spontaneous respiratory drive. Vigilant monitoring allows timely adjustments. In addition to continuous blood gas monitoring, the arterial blood gas is directly measured every 4 hours. As soon as these parameters are met, all vasoactive drugs are weaned, and ventilator levels are adjusted to "rest" settings. Gastrointestinal prophylaxis (H_2 antagonists, antacids) is initiated, and mild sedation and analgesia are provided, usually with fentanyl and midazolam. Paralyzing agents are avoided. Ampicillin and either gentamicin or cefotaxime are administered for prophylaxis. Routine blood, urine, and tracheal cultures should be sent.[20,41] A daily chest radiograph is obtained. Opacification or "white-out" is often noted during the early ECMO

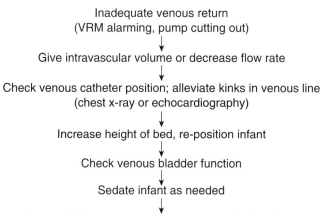

Inadequate venous return
(VRM alarming, pump cutting out)

↓

Give intravascular volume or decrease flow rate

↓

Check venous catheter position; alleviate kinks in venous line
(chest x-ray or echocardiography)

↓

Increase height of bed, re-position infant

↓

Check venous bladder function

↓

Sedate infant as needed

↓

Place additional venous drainage cannula if required

FIGURE 6-3. Suggested algorithm for the management of inadequate venous return during extracorporeal membrane oxygenation. VRM, venous return monitor. (Adapted from Zwischenberger JB, Upp JR Jr: Emergencies during extracorporeal membrane oxygenation and their management. In Zwischenberger JB, Bartlett RH [eds]: ECMO: Extracorporeal Cardiopulmonary Support in Critical Care. Ann Arbor, Mich, Extracorporeal Life Support Organization, 1995, pp 221–249.)

course. The reasons for this are multifactorial, including decreased ventilatory pressures (both PIP and PEEP), reperfusion of the injured lung, as well as the exposure of the blood to a foreign surface, causing an inflammatory response with the release of cytokines. A list of typical diagnostic tests ordered is shown in Table 6-2.

Heparin is administered (30 to 60 mg/kg/hr) throughout the ECMO course to preserve a thrombus-free circuit. ACTs should be monitored hourly and maintained at 180 to 220 seconds. A complete blood count should be obtained every 6 hours, and coagulation profiles, daily.

TABLE 6-2
GENERAL STUDIES OBTAINED DURING ECMO

Lab Study	General Frequency and Comments
Chest radiograph	Daily
Cranial ultrasound	Only for neonates, the first 3 days and then as needed
Activated clotting time	Every 1 hr, more often if outside of parameters
Preoxygenator blood gas	Every 4 hr
Postoxygenator blood gas	Every 4 hr
Patient blood gas	Every 6 hr
Glucose monitoring test	Every 4 hr
Complete blood count with platelets	Every 6 hr, include a differential daily
Chem-7	Every 6 hr, include a Mg, Ca, P daily
Fibrinogen	Daily and after infusion of cryoprecipitate and FFP, may also include PT and D-dimer

PT, prothrombin time; FFP, fresh frozen plasma; ECMO, extracorporeal membrane oxygenation.

To prevent a coagulopathy, platelets are transfused to maintain a platelet count greater than $100,000/mm^3$. The use of fibrinogen and other clotting factors is controversial. The hematocrit should remain above 40% by using red blood cell transfusions, so that oxygen delivery is maximized.[20]

Volume management of patients on ECMO is extremely important and very difficult. It is imperative that all inputs and outputs be diligently recorded and electrolytes monitored every 6 hours. All fluid losses should be repleted, and electrolyte abnormalities, corrected. All patients should receive maintenance fluids as well as adequate nutrition by using hyperalimentation. The first 48 to 72 hours of ECMO typically involve fluid extravasation into the soft tissues. The patient becomes edematous and may require volume replacement (crystalloid, colloid, or blood products) to maintain adequate intravascular and bypass flows, hemodynamics, and urine output greater than 1 mL/kg/hr. By the third day of bypass, diuresis of the excess extracellular fluid begins and can be facilitated with the use of furosemide, if necessary.[20,41]

Operative Procedures on ECMO

Surgical procedures, such as CDH repair, may be performed while the child remains on bypass, but one must account for the need for continued postoperative anticoagulation. Hemorrhagic complications are a frequent morbidity associated with this situation, and these complications increase mortality. To try to avoid these problems, before the procedure, the platelet count should be greater than $150,000/mm^3$, an ACT reduced to 180 to 200 seconds, and ECMO flow increased to full support. Moreover, it is imperative that meticulous hemostasis be obtained throughout the procedure. The fibrinolysis inhibitor, aminocaproic acid (100 mg/kg), is administered just before the incision and is followed by a continuous infusion (30 mg/kg/hr) until all evidence of bleeding ceases.[20,41]

Weaning and Decannulation

As the patient improves, less blood flow is required to pass through the ECMO circuit, and the flow may be weaned at a rate of 10 to 20 mL/hr as long as the patient maintains good oxygenation and perfusion. The most important guide to VA ECMO weaning is the Sv_{O_2}. For VV, it is the Sa_{O_2}. Flows should be decreased to 30 to 50 mL/kg/min, and the ACT should be at a higher level (200 to 220 seconds) to prevent thrombosis. Moderate conventional ventilator settings are used, but higher settings can be used if the patient needs to be weaned from ECMO urgently. If the child tolerates the low flow, all medications and fluids should be switched to vascular access on the patient, and the cannulas may be clamped with the circuit, bypassing the patient via the bridge. If the possibility remains that the child may need to be placed back on bypass, then the cannulas should be flushed with heparin (2 U/mL). The patient is then observed for 2 to 4 hours, and if this is tolerated, decannulation can be accomplished. Decannulation is performed in a near identical manner as cannulation. This should be executed under sterile conditions in the Trendelenburg position using a muscle relaxant to prevent air aspiration into the vein. The ventilator settings should be increased with the use of the muscle relaxant. The venous catheter is typically removed first to allow for better exposure, and the vessel is ligated. Repair of the carotid artery is controversial. Short-term results demonstrate acceptable patency rates and an equivalent short-term neurodevelopmental outcome when compared with those of children undergoing carotid artery ligation.[42,43] However, long-term follow-up of ECMO survivors is necessary to determine whether carotid artery repair is a necessary procedure. The wound should be irrigated and closed over a small drain, which is removed 24 hours later.[20,41]

COMPLICATIONS

Mechanical Complications

Membrane Failure

Failure of the membrane oxygenator is demonstrated by a decrease in oxygenation or retention of carbon dioxide. The cause of such complications includes either fibrin clot formation or water condensation, both of which diminish the membrane's ability to transfer oxygen and CO_2. An incidence of oxygenator failure or clot in the oxygenator is reported, requiring intervention in 9% of respiratory ECMO applications in the neonatal and pediatric population.[1] The membrane should not be subject to high pressures, which should be continuously monitored. Pressure limits are specific for different manufacturers of membranes and for the size of the membrane. Signs of clot formation within the membrane can be detected by direct visualization of the top or bottom of the membrane, but the extent of the clot cannot be determined. The progressive consumption of coagulation factors, such as platelets and fibrinogen, also indicates that the membrane may be progressively building clot, and the need to change the oxygenator should be considered. Another sign of impending membrane failure is the formation of water vapor exiting the exhaust port of the oxygenator along with climbing carbon dioxide levels. The oxygenator can easily be exchanged without coming off bypass if the circuit was built with a double-diamond tubing arrangement with dual connectors both before and after the membrane. Such an arrangement allows parallel placement of a new oxygenator without having to come off bypass.

Raceway Tubing Rupture

Tubing rupture has become a much less frequent event with the introduction of Super Tygon (Norton Performance Plastics, Inc., Akron, OH) tubing. The extra tubing between the bladder and the oxygen membrane can be used to rotate or "walk the raceway" tubing within the roller pump, which should be performed every 5 to 7 days and requires coming off pump for a matter of seconds. The tubing should be inspected repeatedly and all connections secured properly and replaced if defective. When a raceway rupture does occur, the pump must be turned off immediately, and the patient must be ventilated and perfused by conventional methods (increased ventilator pressures and oxygen, and cardiopulmonary resuscitation [CPR] performed if necessary). The raceway tubing should be replaced and the flow recalibrated.

Accidental Decannulation

Securing the cannulas properly and taping the tubing to the bed, with some motion of the patient's head still possible, will prevent accidental decannulation. Unexpected decannulation is a surgical emergency, and immediate pressure should be applied to the cannula site. Conventional ventilator settings should be increased simultaneously. The neck incision must be immediately re-explored to prevent further hemorrhage, and the cannulas replaced, if ECMO is still needed.

Patient Complications

Air Embolism

The ECMO circuit has several potential sources for entry of air. The initial cannulation procedure can be a source of air embolism. Thus all visible air bubbles should be removed by using heparinized saline. Other entry points throughout the circuit include all of the connectors, stopcocks, and the membrane oxygenator. Therefore the circuit must be continually inspected. Air on the arterial side requires the patient to be taken off bypass immediately. The air should be aspirated from a port and blood recirculated through the bridge until all air has been removed. Air on the venous side is not as urgent, and the air can often be "walked" into the bladder, where it can be aspirated without coming off bypass.

In the event that an air embolism reaches the patient, he or she should be immediately taken off ECMO, and conventional ventilator settings adjusted to best meet the child's needs. The patient should be placed in the Trendelenburg position to prevent air from entering the cerebral circulation. Next, an attempt should be made to aspirate any accessible air out of the arterial cannula. If air enters the coronary circulation, inotropic support may be necessary. Before reinstituting ECMO, identifying and repairing the cause of the embolus is essential. Prevention of air embolism is vital. When setting up the circuit, all air must be removed and all connections made tight and thoroughly inspected before initiating bypass.

Neurologic Complications

For respiratory ECMO in neonates and pediatric patients, neurologic complications have an overall incidence of 27%.[1] ICH, infarct, and seizure carry significant mortality when encountered in ECMO patients. Frequent neurologic examinations should be performed, and the use of paralytic agents avoided. The examination should include evaluation of alertness and interaction, spontaneous movements, eye findings, the presence of seizures, fullness of the fontanels, tone, and reflexes. A cranial sonogram should be performed on all neonates before initiating ECMO to identify those patients in whom a significant ICH already exists. A retrospective analysis revealed that birth weight and gestational age were the most significant correlating factors with ICH for neonates on ECMO.[32] Once the patient goes on ECMO, sonography is repeated during the first 3 days when indicated by clinical condition. If the examination reveals a new moderate (grade II) hemorrhage or an expanding ICH, ECMO is usually discontinued, and reversal of anticoagulation is advised.

In the event that an ICH is suspected or detected on cranial sonogram and deemed to be small, the heparin should should be reduced to maintain an ACT at 180 to 200 seconds with a platelet count greater than 125,000 to 150,000/mm^3. Serial head sonography should be used to monitor the progression of the hemorrhage.[20]

Cannula Site or Bleeding at Other Sites

The ECMO registry reports a 6.2% incidence of cannulation-site bleeding and a 7.5% incidence of other surgical-site bleeding.[1] Contact of blood with the foreign surface of the circuit activates the coagulation cascade. Platelet numbers and function also are affected, and in conjunction with anticoagulation, the risk of bleeding while undergoing operation on ECMO is considerable. To reduce this risk, meticulous hemostasis should be maintained during the procedure and before closure. If necessary, the surgeon should use topical hemostatic agents. Lowering the ACT parameters to 180 to 200 seconds and maintaining a platelet count of at least 125,000/mm^3 can assist in obtaining hemostasis. If bleeding from the cannula incision is greater than 10 mL/hr for 2 hours despite conservative treatment strategies, it should be explored.[20]

Bleeding into the site of previous surgical interventions occurs frequently and must be handled aggressively. Constant monitoring for bleeding by observing a decreasing hematocrit, an increasing heart rate, a decline in the blood pressure, or an inadequate venous return are signs of hemorrhage. Treatment includes replenishing lost blood products, including coagulation factors, if necessary. ACT parameters should be decreased to 180 to 200 seconds, and the platelet count maintained at least greater than 125,000/mm^3. The use of agents that inhibit fibrinolysis, such as aminocaproic acid, also can help prevent bleeding. Often one must evacuate hematoma and explore for surgical bleeding, if necessary, as is often the case in the post–cardiac operation patients left with an open chest and central cannulation.

Coagulation Abnormalities

ECMO patients can have a coagulopathy secondary to consumption by the circuit. The treatment for this coagulopathy is removal of the source; hence a circuit change is the logical approach.[20] Disseminated intravascular coagulation (DIC) occurs in approximately 1.2% of ECMO cases.[1] DIC is characterized by the consumption of plasma clotting factors and platelets, resulting in deposition of fibrin thrombi in the microvasculature. Once the factor levels and platelet count decrease below certain levels, bleeding will occur. Sepsis, acidosis, hypoxia, and hypotension are the most common causes of DIC, which is why ECMO patients are at risk for developing DIC. It is important to note that the most common cause of coagulopathy is consumption of clotting factors by the circuit, and only seldom is it due to sepsis or DIC.

Patent Ductus Arteriosus

The dramatic decrease in pulmonary hypertension seen usually in the first 48 hours of an ECMO run causes dramatic changes in the neonate's circulation. A left-to-right shunt through the patent ductus arteriosus (PDA) develops and causes less-efficient oxygenation, pulmonary edema, and poor peripheral perfusion. As a rule, the PDA closes spontaneously with the use of fluid restriction and diuresis. The use of indomethacin should be avoided because of its effects on platelet function. Rarely is PDA ligation required or indicated while on ECMO.

Renal Failure

Oliguria is common in ECMO patients and is often seen during the first 24 to 48 hours. The capillary leak that is seen after placing a child on ECMO may cause decreased renal perfusion, or it may be due to the nonpulsatile nature of blood flow seen in VA ECMO. Once the patient is considered to be adequately volume resuscitated, furosemide (1 to 2 mg/kg) can be used to improve urine output. If the creatinine level continues to increase, then renal sonography is recommended. The use of continuous hemofiltration, which is easily added in-line to the ECMO circuit, is another mechanism to assist in fluid balance, hyperkalemia, and azotemia. Hemofiltration removes plasma water and dissolved solutes while retaining proteins and cellular components of the intravascular space.[20,44]

Hypertension

The reported incidence of hypertension on ECMO varies from 28% to as high as 92%.[45] According to the ELSO registry, 12.2% of respiratory ECMO patients require pharmacologic intervention. One group reported that in 44% of their hypertensive patients, detectable ICH developed, and in 27%, clinically significant ICH developed.[46] The patient should initially be assessed for reversible causes of hypertension such as pain, hypercarbia, and hypoxia. Embolic renal infarction is another important cause of hypertension. Medical management includes the use of hydralazine, nitroglycerin, and captopril.

Infection

The incidence of nosocomial infections during ECMO has been reported as high as 30%. Associated risk factors include the duration of the ECMO run, the length of hospitalization, and surgical procedures performed before the initiation of ECMO or during the run.[47] The ELSO registry data from 2003 reports an 8.4% culture-proven infection rate in ECMO neonates and pediatric patients.[1] This is remarkably low, considering the large surface area of the circuit, the duration of bypass, and the frequency of access to the circuit. Fungal infections carry a significantly higher hospital mortality rate, and the onset of sepsis carries a higher morbidity and mortality rate in neonates, as would be expected.[48,49] Because of the large volume of blood products often transfused into ECMO patients, the risk of developing a bloodborne infectious disease is significant. One study states that approximately 8% of a group of children who were treated with ECMO as neonates were seropositive for antibodies to hepatitis C virus.[50]

RESULTS

Extracorporeal membrane oxygenation is a prime example of the evolution of an experimental technique to a commonly used therapeutic technique. The ELSO registry has accumulated data since the early 1980s from all registered centers throughout the world, allowing analysis of this technique. At its peak, in 1996, 113 centers were reporting to ELSO. Currently 101 centers are registered. This trend follows the number of overall cases, which also is declining. In 1992, more than 1500 neonatal respiratory cases were reported and, in 2002, only 649 cases were reported. In contrast, the number of cardiac cases has steadily increased over the last 15 years, with the exception of 2002. The decline in case volume is likely due to improvements in ventilation-management strategies and the addition of new agents to our armamentarium for respiratory failure (inhaled nitric oxide, surfactant, and HFOV).

Overall survival to discharge for neonates and pediatric patients is 68.4% for all diagnoses.[1] Higher survival rates are seen in neonates with respiratory diseases (78%) versus pediatric patients with respiratory failure (55%) (Table 6-3).[1] According to the 2003 ELSO Registry data, newborns with MAS that require ECMO have the best survival rate at 94%, whereas ECMO survival for infants with CDH is 53% (Table 6-4).[1]

TABLE 6-3

ECMO CASES BY PATIENT GROUP (ELSO REGISTRY, 1980–2002)

Indication	No. of Cases	Survival to Discharge (%)
Neonatal respiratory failure	17,878	78
Neonatal cardiac failure	1,828	37
Pediatric respiratory failure	2,408	55
Pediatric cardiac failure	2,550	42

ECMO, extracorporeal membrane oxygenation; ELSO, Extracorporeal Life Support Organization.

TABLE 6-4

NEONATAL RESPIRATORY ECMO CASES (ELSO REGISTRY, 1980–2002)

Indication	No. of Cases	Survival to Discharge (%)
Meconium aspiration syndrome	6263	94
Respiratory distress syndrome	1357	84
PPHN/PFC	2649	79
Sepsis	2307	75
Congenital diaphragmatic hernia	4101	53

ECMO, extracorporeal membrane oxygenation; ELSO, Extracorporeal Life Support Organization; PPHN, persistent pulmonary hypertension of the newborn; PFC, persistent fetal circulation.

The pediatric population of ECMO patients represents a diverse group with regard to patient age as well as diagnosis. Almost an equal number of respiratory cases (2408) and cardiac cases (2550) have been reported. This is in stark contrast to the neonatal population, in which an almost 10:1 ratio of respiratory versus cardiac primary diagnosis is found.[1] A higher complication rate exists with the pediatric patients, reflecting the longer duration of bypass required for reversal of the respiratory failure.

Feeding and Growth Sequelae

Approximately one third of ECMO-treated infants have feeding problems.[51-53] The possible causes for the poor feeding are numerous and include tachypnea, generalized central nervous system depression, poor hunger drive, soreness in the neck from the surgical procedure, manipulation or compression of the vagus nerve during the cannulation, sore throat from prolonged intubation, and poor oral-motor coordination.[53,54] CDH babies have a higher incidence of feeding difficulties as compared with infants with MAS. CDH children often have foregut dysmotility, which leads to significant gastroesophageal reflux, delayed gastric emptying, and obvious feeding difficulties. Respiratory compromise and chronic lung disease add to the problem.[54-56]

Normal growth is most commonly reported in ECMO-treated patients, yet these children are more likely to experience problems with growth than are normal controls. Head circumference below the fifth percentile occurs in 10% of ECMO-treated children.[57] Growth problems are most commonly associated with ECMO children who had CDH or residual lung disease.[55]

Respiratory Sequelae

Respiratory morbidity is more likely to be iatrogenic than a consequence of congenital lung disease. Nevertheless, approximately 15% of infants require supplemental oxygen at age 4 weeks in some series. At age 5 years, ECMO children were twice as likely to have reported cases of pneumonia as compared with controls (25% vs. 13%). These children with pneumonia are more likely to require hospitalization, and the pneumonia occurs at a younger age (half of the pneumonias were diagnosed before 1 year of life).[58,59] CDH infants, in particular, have been found to have severe lung disease after ECMO and may require supplemental oxygen at the time of discharge.[56,60–62]

Neurodevelopmental Sequelae

Probably the most serious post-ECMO morbidity is neuromotor handicap. The average rate of handicap noted in 540 patients from 12 institutions is 6%, with a range from 2% to 18%.[57,63–75] Nine percent of ECMO survivors have significant developmental delay, ranging from none to 21%. This is comparable to other critically ill, non–ECMO-treated neonates.[76] Auditory defects are reported in more than one fourth of ECMO neonates at discharge.[77] The deficits are detected by brainstem auditory evoked response (BAER) testing, are considered mild to moderate, and generally resolve over time. The cause of the auditory defects also may be iatrogenic, caused by induced alkalosis, diuretics, or gentamicin ototoxicity. As a result, all patients should have a hearing screening at the time of neonatal intensive care unit (NICU) discharge. Visual deficits are uncommon in the ECMO neonates that are larger than 2 kg.[78]

Seizures are widely reported among ECMO neonates, ranging from 20% to 70%.[79–82] However, by age 5 years, only 2% had a diagnosis of epilepsy. Seizures in the neonatal population are associated with neurologic disease and poorer outcomes, including cerebral palsy and epilepsy.[83] Severe nonambulatory cerebral palsy has an incidence of less than 5% and is usually accompanied by significant developmental delay.[57,63,68] Milder cases of cerebral palsy are seen in up to 20% of ECMO survivors. This morbidity reflects how desperately ill these children are and that these handicaps are not a direct effect of ECMO.

REFERENCES

1. Extracorporeal Life Support Organization: International Registry Report of the Extracorporeal Life Support Organization. Ann Arbor, Mich, University of Michigan Medical Center, 2003.
2. Lillehei CW, Cohen M, Warden HE, et al: The direct-vision intracardiac correction of congenital anomalies by controlled cross circulation. Surgery 38:11–29, 1955.
3. Clowes GHA Jr, Hopkins AL, Neville WE: An artificial lung dependent upon diffusion of oxygen and carbon dioxide through plastic membranes. J Thorac Surg 32:630–637, 1956.
4. Kolobow T, Zapol W, Pierce JE, et al: Partial extracorporeal gas exchange in alert newborn lambs with a membrane artificial lung perfused via an AV shunt for periods up to 96 hours. Trans Am Soc Artif Intern Organs 14:328–334, 1968.
5. Osborn JJ, Bramson ML, Main FB, et al: Clinical experience with a disposable membrane oxygenator. Bull Soc Int Chir 25:346–353, 1966.
6. Peirce EC II, Thebaut AL, Kent BB, et al: Techniques of extended perfusion using a membrane lung. Ann Thorac Surg 12:451–470, 1971.
7. Lande AJ, Edwards L, Block JH, et al: Prolonged cardio-pulmonary support with a practical membrane oxygenator. Trans Am Soc Artif Intern Organs 16:352–356, 1970.
8. Hill D, O'Brien TG, Murray JJ, et al: Extracorporeal oxygenation for acute post-traumatic respiratory failure (shock-lung syndrome): Use of the Bramson Membrane Lung. N Engl J Med 286:629–634, 1972.
9. Zapol WM, Snider MT, Hill JD, et al: Extracorporeal membrane oxygenation in severe respiratory failure. JAMA 242:2193–2196, 1979.
10. Bartlett RH, Gazzaniga AB, Jefferies MR, et al: Extracorporeal membrane oxygenation (ECMO) cardiopulmonary support in infants. Trans Am Soc Artif Intern Organs 22:80–93, 1976.
11. Bartlett RH, Roloff DW, Cornell RG, et al: Extracorporeal circulation in neonatal respiratory failure: A prospective randomized study. Pediatrics 76:479–487, 1985.
12. O'Rourke PP, Crone RK, Vacanti JP, et al: Extracorporeal membrane oxygenation and conventional medical therapy in neonates with persistent pulmonary hypertension of the newborn: A prospective randomized study. Pediatrics 84:957–963, 1989.
13. Firmin R: United Kingdom Neonatal ECMO Study, Presented at the 7th International ELSO Conference, Dearborn, Michigan, 1995.
14. Krummel TM, Greenfield LJ, Kirkpatrick BU, et al: Extracorporeal membrane oxygenation in neonatal pulmonary failure. Pediatr Ann 11:905–908, 1982.
15. Toomasion JM, Snedecor SM, Cornell RG, et al: National experience with extracorporeal membrane oxygenation for newborn respiratory failure: Data from 715 cases. Trans Am Soc Artif Intern Organs 34:140–147, 1988.
16. Stolar CJH, Snedecor SM, Bartlett RH: Extracorporeal membrane oxygenation and neonatal respiratory failure: Experience from the extracorporeal life support organization. J Pediatr Surg 26:563–571, 1991.
17. O'Rourke PP, Stolar CJ, Zwischenberger JB, et al: Extracorporeal membrane oxygenation: Support for overwhelming pulmonary failure in the pediatric population: Collective experience from the extracorporeal life support organization. J Pediatr Surg 28:523–528, 1993.
18. Galantowicz ME, Stolar CJ: Extracorporeal membrane oxygenation for perioperative support in pediatric heart transplantation. J Thorac Cardiovasc Surg 102:148–151, 1991.
19. Campbell BT, Braun TM, Schumacher RE, et al: Impact of ECMO on neonatal mortality in Michigan (1980–1999). J Pediatr Surg 38:290–295, 2003.
20. Zwischenberger JB, Steinhorn RH, Bartlett RH (eds): ECMO: Extracorporeal Cardiopulmonary Support in Critical Care, 2nd ed. Ann Arbor, Mich, Extracorporeal Life Support Organization, 2000.
21. Van Meurs K (ed): ECMO Specialist Training Manual, 2nd ed. Ann Arbor, Mich, Extracorporeal Life Support Organization, 1999.
22. Gajarski RJ, Mosca RS, Ohye RG, et al: Use of extracorporeal life support as a bridge to pediatric cardiac transplantation. J Heart Lung Transplant 22:28–34, 2003.
23. Lessin JS, el-Eid SE, Klein MD, et al: Extracorporeal membrane oxygenation in pediatric respiratory failure secondary to smoke inhalation injury. J Pediatr Surg 31:1285–1287, 1996.
24. Tobias JD, Garrett JS: Therapeutic options for severe, refractory status asthmaticus: Inhalational anesthetic agents, extracorporeal membrane oxygenation and helium/oxygen ventilation. Paediatr Anesth 7:47–57, 1997.
25. Travis JA, Pranikoff T, Chang MC, et al: Extracorporeal rewarming in trauma patients: Presented at the 13th Annual ELSO Conference, Scottsdale, Arizona, 2002.
26. Johnson LB, Plotkin JS, Howell CD, et al: Successful emergency transplantation of a liver allograft from a donor maintained on extracorporeal membrane oxygenation. Transplantation 63:910–911, 1997.
27. Gersony WM, Duc GV, Sinclair JC: "PFC" syndrome (persistence of the fetal circulation). Circulation 40(suppl 111):87, 1969.
28. Gupta A, Shantanu R, Rakesh S, et al: Inhaled nitric oxide and gentle ventilation in the treatment of pulmonary hypertension of the newborn: A single-center 5-year experience. J Perinatol 22:435–441, 2002.
29. Northway WH, Rosan RC, Porter DY: Pulmonary disease following respiratory therapy of hyaline membrane disease. N Engl J Med 276:357–368, 1967.
30. Kornhauser MS, Cullen JA, Baumgart S, et al: Risk factors for bronchopulmonary dysplasia after extracorporeal membrane oxygenation. Arch Pediatr Adolesc Med 148:820–825, 1994.
31. Kim ES, Stolar CJ: ECMO in the newborn. Am J Perinatol 17:345–356, 2000.

32. Cilley RE, Zwischenberger JB, Andrews AF, et al: Intracranial hemorrhage during extracorporeal membrane oxygenation in neonates. Pediatrics 78:699–704, 1986.
33. Wung JT, James LS, Kilchevsky E, et al: Management of infants with severe respiratory failure and persistence of the fetal circulation, without hyperventilation. Pediatrics 76:488–494, 1985.
34. Beck R, Anderson KD, Pearson GD, et al: Criteria for extracorporeal membrane oxygenation in a population of infants with persistent pulmonary hypertension of the newborn. J Pediatr Surg 21:297–302, 1986.
35. Marsh TD, Wilkerson SA, Cook LN: Extracorporeal membrane oxygenation selection criteria: Partial pressure of arterial oxygen versus alveolar-arterial oxygen gradient. Pediatrics 82:162–166, 1988.
36. Ortiz RM, Cilley RE, Bartlett RH: Extracorporeal membrane oxygenation in pediatric respiratory failure. Pediatr Clin North Am 34:39–46, 1987.
37. Azarow K, Messineo A, Pearl R, et al: Congenital diaphragmatic hernia: A tale of two cities: the Toronto experience. J Pediatr Surg 32:395–400, 1997.
38. Wung JT, Sahni R, Moffitt ST, et al: Congenital diaphragmatic hernia: Survival treated with very delayed surgery, spontaneous respiration, and no chest tube. J Pediatr Surg 30:406–409, 1995.
39. Boloker J, Bateman DA, Wung JT, et al: Congenital diaphragmatic hernia in 120 infants treated consecutively with permissive hypercapnea/spontaneous respiration/elective repair. J Pediatr Surg 37:357–366, 2002.
40. Stolar CJH, Dillon PW, Reyes C, et al: Selective use of extracorporeal membrane oxygenation in the management of congenital diaphragmatic hernia. J Pediatr Surg 23:207–211, 1988.
41. Frischer JS, Stolar CJH: Extracorporeal membrane oxygenation. In: Puri P (ed): Operative Pediatric Surgery (Springer Atlas Series) (in press).
42. Levy MS, Share JC, Fauza DO, et al: Fate of the reconstructed carotid artery after extracorporeal membrane oxygenation. J Pediatr Surg 30:1046–1049, 1995.
43. Cheung PY, Vickar DB, Hallgren RA, et al: Carotid artery reconstruction in neonates receiving extracorporeal membrane oxygenation: A 4-year follow-up study. J Pediatr Surg 32:560–564, 1997.
44. Sell LL, Cullen ML, Whittlesey GC, et al: Experience with renal failure during extracorporeal membrane oxygenation: Treatment with continuous hemofiltration. J Pediatr Surg 22:600–602, 1987.
45. Boedy RF, Goldberg AK, Howell CG, et al: Incidence of hypertension in infants on extracorporeal membrane oxygenation. J Pediatr Surg 25:258–261, 1990.
46. Sell LL, Cullen ML, Lerner GR, et al: Hypertension during extracorporeal membrane oxygenation: Cause, effect, and management. Surgery 102:724–730, 1987.
47. Coffin SE, Bell LM, Manning M, et al: Nosocomial infections in neonates receiving extracorporeal membrane oxygenation. Infect Control Hosp Epidemiol 18:93–96, 1997.
48. Douglass BH, Keenan AL, Purohit DM: Bacterial and fungal infection in neonates undergoing venoarterial extracorporeal membrane oxygenation: An analysis of the registry data of the Extracorporeal Life Support Organization. Artif Organs 20:202–208, 1996.
49. Meyer DM, Jessen ME, Eberhart RC: Neonatal extracorporeal membrane oxygenation complicated by sepsis: Extracorporeal Life Support Organization. Ann Thorac Surg 59:975–980, 1995.
50. Nelson SP, Jonas MM: Hepatitis C infection in children who received extracorporeal membrane oxygenation. J Pediatr Surg 31:644–648, 1996.
51. Grimm P: Feeding difficulties in infants treated with ECMO. Paper presented at CNMC ECMO Symposium 25, 1993.
52. Nield T, Hallaway M, Fodera C, et al: Outcome in problem feeders post ECMO. Paper presented at CNMC ECMO Symposium 79, 1990.
53. Glass P: Patient neurodevelopmental outcomes after neonatal ECMO. In: Arensman R, Cornish J (eds): Extracorporeal Life Support. Boston: Blackwell Scientific, 1993, pp 241–251.
54. Tarby T, Waggoner J: Are the common neurologic problems following ECMO related to jugular bulb thrombosis? Paper presented at CNMC ECMO Symposium 110, 1994.
55. Van Meurs K, Robbins S, Reed V, et al: Congenital diaphragmatic hernia: Long-term outcome of neonates treated with ECMO. Paper presented at CNMC ECMO Symposium 25, 1991.
56. Rajasingham S, Reed V, Glass P, et al: Congenital diaphragmatic hernia: Outcome post-ECMO at 5 years. Paper presented at CNMC ECMO Symposium 35, 1994.
57. Glass P, Wagner A, Papero P, et al: Neurodevelopmental status at age five years of neonates treated with extracorporeal membrane oxygenation. J Pediatr 127:447–457, 1995.
58. Gershan L, Gershan W, Day S: Airway anomalies after ECMO: Bronchoscopic findings. Paper presented at CNMC ECMO Symposium 65, 1992.
59. Wagner A, Glass P, Papero P, et al: Neuropsychological outcome of neonatal ECMO survivors at age 5. Paper presented at CNMC ECMO Symposium 31, 1994.
60. D'Agostino J, Bernbaum J, Gerdes M, et al: Outcome for infants with congenital diaphragmatic hernia requiring extracorporeal membrane oxygenation: the first year. J Pediatr Surg 30: 10–15, 1995.
61. Van Meurs K, Robbins S, Reed V, et al: Congenital diaphragmatic hernia: Long-term outcome in neonates treated with extracorporeal membrane oxygenation. J Pediatr 122:893–899, 1993.
62. Atkinson J, Poon M: ECMO and the management of congenital diaphragmatic hernia with large diaphragmatic defects requiring a prosthetic patch. J Pediatr Surg 27:754–756, 1992.
63. Adolph V, Ekelund C, Smith C, et al: Developmental outcome of neonates treated with ECMO. J Pediatr Surg 25:43–46, 1990.
64. Andrews A, Nixon C, Cilley R, et al: One-to-three year outcome for 14 neonatal survivors of extracorporeal membrane oxygenation. Pediatrics 78:692–698, 1986.
65. Flusser H, Dodge N, Engle W, et al: Neurodevelopmental outcome and respiratory morbidity for ECMO survivors at 1 year of age. J Perinatol 13:266–271, 1993.
66. Glass P, Miller M, Short BL: Morbidity for survivors of extracorporeal membrane oxygenation: Neurodevelopmental outcome at 12 years of age. Pediatrics 83:72–78, 1989.
67. Griffin M, Minifee P, Landry S, et al: Neurodevelopmental outcome in neonates after ECMO: Cranial magnetic resonance imaging and ultrasonography correlation. J Pediatr Surg 27:33–35, 1992.
68. Hofkosh D, Thompson A, Nozza R, et al: Ten years of ECMO: Neurodevelopmental outcome. Pediatrics 87:549–555, 1991.
69. Krummel T, Greenfield L, Kirkpatrick B, et al: The early evaluation of survivors after ECMO for neonatal pulmonary failure. J Pediatr Surg 19:585–590, 1984.
70. Schumacher R, Palmer T, Roloff D, et al: Follow-up of infants treated with ECMO for newborn respiratory failure. Pediatrics 87:451–457, 1991.
71. Towne B, Lott I, Hicks D, et al: Long-term follow-up of infants and children treated with ECMO: A preliminary report. J Pediatr Surg 20:410–414, 1985.
72. Wildin S, Landry S, Zwischenberger J: Prospective, controlled study of developmental outcome in survivors of ECMO: The first 24 months. Pediatrics 93:404–408, 1994.
73. Stolar CJ, Crisafi MA, Driscoll YT: Neurocognitive outcome for neonates treated with extracorporeal membrane oxygenation: Are infants with congenital diaphragmatic hernia different? J Pediatr Surg 30:366–372, 1995.
74. Davis D, Wilkerson S, Stewart D: Neurodevelopmental follow-up of ECMO survivors at 7 years. CNMC ECMO Symposium 34, 1995.
75. Stanley C, Brodsky K, McKee L, et al: Developmental profile of ECMO survivors at early school age and relationship to neonatal EEG status. CNMC ECMO Symposium 33, 1995.
76. Hack M, Taylor H, Klein N, et al: School-age outcomes in children with birthweights under 750 g. N Engl J Med 331:753–759, 1994.
77. Desai S, Stanley C, Graziani L, et al: Brainstem auditory evoked potential screening (BAEP) unreliable for detecting sensorineural hearing loss in ECMO survivors: A comparison of neonatal BAEP and follow-up behavioral audiometry. CNMC ECMO Symposium 62, 1994.
78. Haney B, Thibeault D, Sward-Comunelli S, et al: Ocular findings in infants treated with ECMO. CNMC ECMO Symposium 63, 1994.
79. Hahn J, Vaucher Y, Bejar R, et al: Electroencephalographic and neuroimaging findings in neonates undergoing extracorporeal membrane oxygenation. Neuropediatrics 24:19–24, 1993.

80. Graziani L, Streletz L, Baumgart S, et al: Predictive value of neonatal electroencephalograms before and during extracorporeal membrane oxygenation. J Pediatr 125:969–975, 1994.
81. Campbell L, Bunyapen C, Gangarosa M, et al: The significance of seizures associated with ECMO. CNMC ECMO Symposium 26, 1991.
82. Kumar P, Bedard M, Delaney-Black V, et al: Post-ECMO electroencephalogram (EEG) as a predictor of neurological outcome. CNMC ECMO Symposium 65, 1994.
83. Scher M, Kosaburo A, Beggerly M, et al: Electrographic seizures in preterm and full-term neonates: Clinical correlates, associated brain lesions, and risk for neurologic sequelae. Pediatrics 91:128–134, 1993.

CHAPTER 7

Mechanical Ventilation in Pediatric Surgical Disease

Ronald B. Hirschl, MD

HISTORY

Amazingly, ventilation via tracheal cannulation was performed as early as 1543, when Vesalius demonstrated the ability to maintain the beating heart in animals with open chests.[1] Such techniques were first applied to humans in 1780, but little progress in the development of positive-pressure ventilation was achieved until the Fell-O'Dwyer apparatus, which provided translaryngeal ventilation via a bellows, was used in 1887 in both adults and children (Fig. 7-1). [2,3] The Drinker-Shaw iron lung, which allowed piston-pump cyclic ventilation of a metal cylinder and associated negative-pressure ventilation, became available in 1928 and was followed by a simplified design built by Emerson in 1931.[4] Such machines were the mainstays in the ventilation of victims of polio epidemics that occurred in the 1930s through 1950s.

In 1928, the technique of tracheal intubation was refined by Magill and Rowbotham, and in World War II, the Bennett valve, which allowed cyclic application of high pressure, was devised to allow pilots to tolerate high-altitude bombing missions.[5-7] Subsequently, the use of translaryngeal intubation and mechanical ventilation became common in the operating room as well as in the treatment of respiratory insufficiency. However, application of mechanical ventilation to newborns, both in the operating room and in the intensive care unit, lagged behind its pediatric and adult counterparts. The use of positive-pressure mechanical ventilation in the management of respiratory distress syndrome (RDS) was described in 1962.[8] However, it was the death of Patrick Bouvier Kennedy at 32 weeks' gestation in 1963 that resulted in additional National Institutes of Health funding for research in the management of newborns with respiratory failure.[9] The discovery of surfactant deficiency as the etiology of RDS in 1959, documentation of the ability to provide positive-pressure ventilation in newborns with respiratory insufficiency in 1965, and demonstration of the effectiveness of continuous positive airway pressure (CPAP) in enhancing lung volume and ventilation in patients with RDS in 1971 set the stage for the development of continuous-flow ventilators specifically designed for neonates.[10-12] The development of neonatal intensive care units, hyperalimentation, and neonatal invasive and noninvasive monitoring enhanced the care of newborns with respiratory failure and increased survival in preterm newborns from 50% in the early 1970s to more than 90% today.[13]

GAS EXCHANGE DURING MECHANICAL VENTILATION

The approach to mechanical ventilation is best understood if the two variables of oxygenation and carbon dioxide elimination are considered separately.[14]

Carbon Dioxide Elimination

The primary purpose of ventilation is to eliminate CO_2. This is accomplished by delivering tidal volume (V_T) breaths at a designated rate. The product, V_T rate, determines the minute volume ventilation (V_E). Although CO_2 elimination is proportional to V_E, it is, in fact, directly related to the volume of gas ventilating the alveoli. This is true because part of the V_E resides in the conducting airways or in nonperfused alveoli. As such, this portion of the ventilation does not participate in CO_2 exchange and is termed the *dead space* (V_D).[15] In the patient with healthy lungs, this dead space is fixed or "anatomic" and consists of about one third of the tidal volume ($V_D/V_T = 0.33$). The dead space can unwittingly be increased through the presence of extensions of the trachea such as the endotracheal tube, a pneumotachometer to measure tidal volume, an end-tidal carbon dioxide monitor, or an extension of the ventilator tubing beyond the "Y." It is critical, therefore, that endotracheal tubes be shortened as much as is reasonable and that other safeguards be applied to ensure that the V_D is minimized. In the setting of respiratory insufficiency, the proportion of dead space (V_D/V_T) may be augmented by the presence of nonperfused alveoli and a reduction in tidal volume.

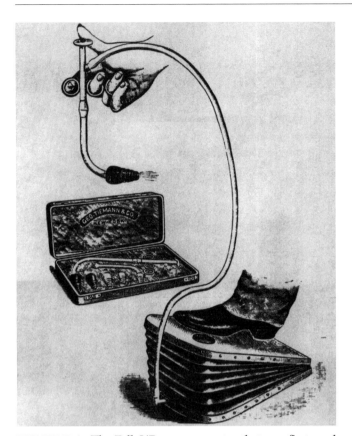

FIGURE 7-1. The Fell-O'Dwyer apparatus that was first used to perform positive pressure ventilation in newborns. (Reprinted with permission from Matas R: Intralaryngeal insufflation. JAMA 34:1468–1473, 1900.)

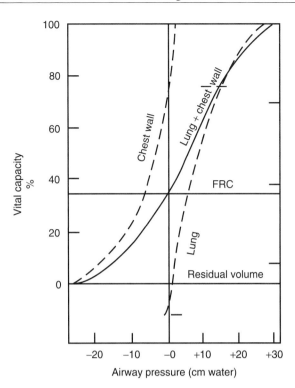

FIGURE 7-2. Pulmonary function as a function of chest-wall and lung compliance in healthy patients. At functional residual capacity, the tendency for the chest wall to expand and the lung to collapse are balanced. (Adapted with permission from West JB: Respiratory Physiology: The Essentials. Baltimore, Williams & Wilkins, 1985.)

The tidal volume is a function of the applied ventilator pressure and the volume/pressure relation (compliance), which describes the distensibility of the lung and chest. At the functional residual capacity (FRC), which is the static point of end-expiration, the tendency for the lung to collapse (elastic recoil) is in balance with the forces that promote chest-wall expansion (Fig. 7-2).[15] As each breath develops, however, the elastic recoil of both the lung and chest wall work in concert to oppose lung inflation. Therefore pulmonary compliance is a function of both the lung elastic recoil (lung compliance) and the distensibility of the rib cage and diaphragm (chest-wall compliance).

The compliance can be determined in a dynamic or static mode. Figure 7-3 demonstrates the dynamic volume/pressure relation for a normal patient. Note that application of 25 cm H_2O of inflating pressure (ρP) above static FRC at positive end-expiratory pressure (PEEP) of 5 cm H_2O generates a tidal volume of 40 mL/kg. The lung, at an inflating pressure of 30 cm H_2O when compared with ambient (transpulmonary pressure), is considered to be at total lung capacity (TLC) (Table 7-1). Note that the loop observed during both inspiration and expiration is curvilinear. This is due to the resistance that is present in the airways and describes the work required to overcome airflow resistance. As a result, at any given point of active

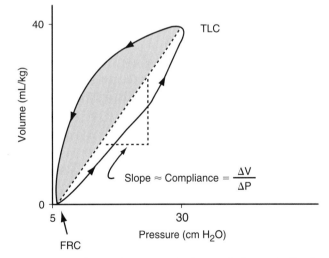

FIGURE 7-3. Dynamic pressure/volume relation and effective pulmonary compliance (C_{eff}) in the normal lung. The volume at 30 cm H_2O is considered total lung capacity (TLC). C_{eff} is calculated by $\Delta V/\Delta P$. (Adapted from Bhutani VK, Sivieri EM: Physiological principles for bedside assessment of pulmonary graphics. In Donn SM (ed): Neonatal and Pediatric Pulmonary Graphics: Principles and Applications. Armonk, NY, Futura Publishing, 1998.)

TABLE 7-1

THE DEFINITIONS AND NORMAL VALUES FOR RESPIRATORY PHYSIOLOGIC PARAMETERS

Variable	Definition	Normal Value
TLC	Total lung capacity	80 mL/kg
FRC	Functional residual capacity	40 mL/kg
IC	Inspiratory capacity	40 mL/kg
ERV	Expiratory reserve volume	30 mL/kg
RV	Residual volume	10 mL/kg
T_V	Tidal volume	5 mL/kg
V_E	Minute volume ventilation	100 mL/kg/min
V_A	Alveolar ventilation	60 mL/kg/hr
V_D	Dead space	mL = wt in lbs
V_D/V_T	% Dead space	0.33
C_{St}	Static Compliance	2 mL/cmH$_2$O/kg
C_{EFF}	Effective compliance	1 mL/cm H$_2$O/kg

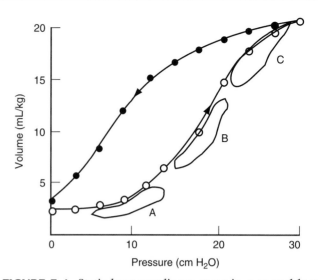

FIGURE 7-4. Static lung-compliance curve in a normal lung. Effective compliance would be altered depending on whether functional residual capacity were to be at a level resulting in lung atelectasis (*A*) or overdistention (*C*). Optimal lung mechanics are observed when FRC is set on the steepest portion of the curve (*B*). (Adapted from West JB: Respiratory Physiology. Baltimore, Williams & Wilkins, 1985.)

flow, the measured pressure in the airways is higher during inspiration and lower during expiration than at the same volume under zero-flow conditions. Therefore pulmonary-compliance measurements, as well as alveolar-pressure measurements, can be effectively performed only when no flow is present in the airways (zero flow), which occurs at FRC and TLC. The line drawn between the two points describes the "effective" compliance. The change observed is a volume of 40 mL/kg and pressure of 25 cm H$_2$O pressure or 1.6 mL/kg/cm H$_2$O. It is termed *effective compliance* because this analysis provides assessment of compliance only between the two arbitrary points of end-inspiration and end-expiration. As can be seen from Figure 7-4, the volume/pressure relation is not linear over the range of most inflating pressures when a static compliance curve is developed. Such static compliance assessments are most commonly performed via a large syringe in which aliquots of 1 to 2 mL/kg of oxygen, up to a total of 15 to 20 mL/kg, are instilled sequentially with 3- to 5-second pauses between each. At the end of each pause, zero-flow pressures are measured. By graphing the data, a *static* compliance curve may be generated, which demonstrates how the calculated compliance can change depending on the arbitrary points used for assessment of the *effective* compliance.[16] Alternatively, the pulmonary pressure/volume relations can be assessed by administration of a slow constant flow of gas into the lungs with simultaneous determination of airway pressure.[17,18] A curve may be fit to the data points to determine the optimal compliance and FRC.[19] The compliance will change as the FRC or end-expiratory lung volume (EELV) increases or decreases. For instance, as can be seen in Figure 7-4, at low FRC (point A), atelectasis is present, and a given ρP will not optimally inflate alveoli. Likewise, at a high FRC (point C), because of air trapping or application of high PEEP, the lung is already distended, and application of the same ρP will result only in overdistention and potential lung injury with little benefit in terms of added tidal volume. Thus optimal compliance is provided when the pressure/volume range

is on the linear portion of the static compliance curve (point B). Clinically, the compliance at a variety of FRC or PEEP values can be monitored to establish optimal FRC.[20]

Typical ventilator-rate requirements in patients with healthy lungs range from 10 breaths/minute in an adult to 30 breaths/minute in a newborn. Tidal volume is maintained at 5 to 10 mL/kg. This affords a minute volume ventilation of up to 100 mL/kg/min in adolescents and 150 mL/kg/min in newborns. These settings should provide sufficient ventilation to maintain normal Paco$_2$ levels of approximately 40 mm Hg and should generate peak inspiratory pressures of between 15 and 20 cm H$_2$O above an applied PEEP of 5 cm H$_2$O. Clinical assessment by observing chest-wall movement, auscultation, and evaluation of gas exchange determines the appropriate tidal volume.

It is important to recognize that a portion of the tidal volume generated by the ventilator is actually compression of gas within both the ventilator tubing and the airways (Fig. 7-5). The ratio of gas compressed in the ventilator tubing to that entering the lungs is a function of the compliance of the ventilator tubing and the lung. The compliance of the ventilator tubing is 0.3 to 4.5 mL/cm H$_2$O.[21] A ΔP of 15 cm H$_2$O in a 3-kg newborn with respiratory insufficiency and a pulmonary compliance of 0.4 mL/cm H$_2$O/kg would result in a lung tidal volume of 18 mL and an impressive ventilator-tubing gas-compression volume of 15 mL if the tubing compliance were 1.0 mL/cm H$_2$O. The relative ventilator-tubing gas-compression volume would not be as striking in an adult. The ventilator-tubing compliance is characterized for all current ventilators and should be factored when

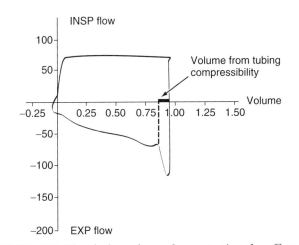

FIGURE 7-5. Flow/volume loops demonstrating the effect of ventilator-tubing gas-compression volume in the ventilator tubing of a patient with respiratory insufficiency. The high flow during expiration results from gas decompressing from the ventilator tubing. (Adapted with permission from Pilbeam SP: Mechanical Ventilation: Physiological and Clinical Applications. St . Louis, MO, CV Mosby, 1998.)

considering tidal volume data. The software in many ventilators corrects for ventilator-tubing compliance when displaying tidal volume values.

Oxygenation

In contrast to carbon dioxide determination, oxygenation is determined by the fraction of inspired oxygen (FiO_2) and the degree of lung distention or alveolar recruitment that is determined by the level of PEEP and the mean airway pressure (P_{aw}) during each ventilator cycle. Were CO_2 not to be a competing gas at the alveolar level, oxygen absorbed by pulmonary capillary blood would simply be replaced by that provided at the airway, as long as alveolar distention were maintained. Such apneic oxygenation has been used in conjunction with extracorporeal carbon dioxide removal ($ECCO_2R$) or arteriovenous CO_2 removal ($AVCO_2R$), in which oxygen is delivered at the carina, whereas lung distention is maintained through application of PEEP.[22,23] Under normal circumstances, however, alveolar ventilation serves to remove carbon dioxide from the alveolus and to replenish the partial pressure of oxygen, thereby maintaining the alveolar/pulmonary capillary blood oxygen gradient.

Rather than depending on the degree of alveolar ventilation, oxygenation predominantly is a function of the appropriate matching of pulmonary blood flow to inflated alveoli (ventilation/perfusion matching, $\dot{V}/\dot{Q}$).[15] Areas of ventilation but no perfusion (high $\dot{V}/\dot{Q}$), such as in the setting of pulmonary embolus, do not contribute to oxygenation. Hypoxemia supervenes in this situation once the average residence time of blood in the remaining perfused pulmonary capillaries exceeds that necessary for complete oxygenation; normal residence time is threefold that required for full oxygenation of pulmonary

capillary blood. The common pathophysiology observed in the setting of respiratory insufficiency is that of minimal or no ventilation, with persistent perfusion (low $\dot{V}/\dot{Q}$), resulting in right-to-left shunt and hypoxemia. Patients with the acute respiratory distress syndrome (ARDS) have collapse of the posterior, or dependent, regions of the lungs when supine.[24, 25] As the majority of blood flow is distributed to these dependent regions, one can easily imagine the limited oxygen transfer, large shunt, ventilation/perfusion mismatch, and resulting hypoxemia that occurs in patients with ARDS. Attempts to inflate the alveoli in these regions, with interventions such as the application of PEEP, can reduce $\dot{V}/\dot{Q}$ mismatch and enhance oxygenation. In normal lungs, the PEEP should be maintained at 5 cm H_2O, an expiratory pressure which allows maintenance of alveolar inflation at end-expiration. An FiO_2 of 0.50 should be administered initially. However, one should be able to wean the FiO_2 rapidly in the patient with healthy lungs and normal $\dot{V}/\dot{Q}$ matching. The arterial oxygen (PaO_2) and arterial oxygen saturation (SaO_2) levels are measured most frequently to evaluate oxygenation. Lung-oxygenation capabilities are frequently assessed as a function of the difference between the ideal alveolar and the measured systemic arterial oxygen levels [$(A - a)DO_2 = (FiO_2 \times (P_B - P_{H_2O}) - PaCO_2 \times RQ) - PaO_2$], the ratio of the PaO_2 to the FiO_2 (P/F ratio), the physiologic shunt ($Qps/Qt = \dfrac{CiO_2 - CaO_2}{CiO_2 - CvO_2}$), and the oxygen index (O.I. $= \dfrac{PaO_2 \times FiO_2 \times 100}{P_{aw}}$) where P_B is the barometric pressure, P_{H_2O} is the partial pressure of water, R.Q. is the respiratory quotient or the ratio of the oxygen consumption (VO_2) and the CO_2 production (VCO_2), and $CvO_2/CaO_2/CiO_2$ is the oxygen content of venous, arterial, and expected pulmonary capillary blood, respectively.[15]

The overall therapeutic goal of optimizing parameters of oxygenation is to maintain oxygen delivery (DO_2) to the tissues. Three variables ascertain oxygen delivery: cardiac output (Q), hemoglobin concentration (Hgb), and arterial blood oxygen saturation (SaO_2). The product of these three variables determines oxygen delivery by the relation:

$$DO_2 = Q \times CaO_2,$$
$$\text{where } CaO_2 = [(1.36 \times Hgb \times SaO_2) + (0.003 \times PaO_2)].$$

Note that the contribution of the PaO_2 to oxygen delivery is minimal and, therefore may be disregarded in most circumstances. If the hemoglobin concentration of the blood is normal (15 g/dL) and the hemoglobin is fully saturated with oxygen, the amount of oxygen bound to hemoglobin is 20.4 mL/dL (Fig. 7-6). In addition, approximately 0.3 mL of oxygen is physically dissolved in each deciliter of plasma, which makes the oxygen content of normal arterial blood equal to approximately 20.7 mL O_2/dL. Similar calculations reveal that the normal venous blood oxygen content is approximately 15 mL/O_2/dL.

Typically oxygen delivery is 4 to 5 times greater than the associated oxygen consumption. As DO_2 increases or oxygen consumption (VO_2) decreases, more oxygen remains in the venous blood. The result is an increase in

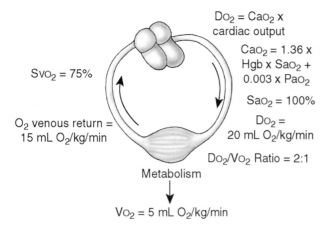

$$Do_2 = Cao_2 \times \text{cardiac output}$$

$$Cao_2 = 1.36 \times Hgb \times Sao_2 + 0.003 \times Pao_2$$

$$Sao_2 = 100\%$$

$$Do_2 = 20 \text{ mL } O_2/\text{kg/min}$$

$$Do_2/Vo_2 \text{ Ratio} = 2:1$$

SvO_2 = 75%

O_2 venous return = 15 mL O_2/kg/min

Metabolism

$$Vo_2 = 5 \text{ mL } O_2/\text{kg/min}$$

FIGURE 7-6. Oxygen consumption (Vo_2) and delivery (Do_2) relations. (Adapted with permission from Hirschl RB: Oxygen delivery in the pediatric surgical patient. Opin Pediatr 6:341–347, 1994.)

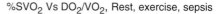

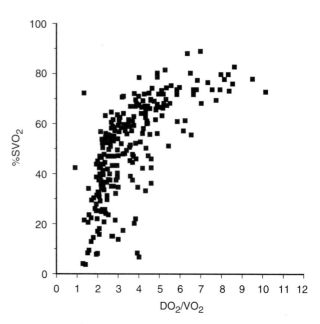

%SVO_2 Vs DO_2/VO_2, Rest, exercise, sepsis

FIGURE 7-7. The relation of the mixed venous oxygen saturation (Svo_2) and the ratio of oxygen delivery to oxygen consumption (Do_2/Vo_2) in normal eumetabolic, hypermetabolic septic, and hypermetabolic exercising canines. (Reprinted with permission from Hirschl RB: Cardiopulmonary Critical Care and Shock: Surgery of Infants and Children: Scientific Principles and Practice. Philadelphia, Lippincott-Raven, 1997.)

the oxygen hemoglobin saturation in the mixed venous pulmonary artery blood (Svo_2). In contrast, if the Do_2 decreases or Vo_2 increases, relatively more oxygen is extracted from the blood, and therefore less oxygen remains in the venous blood. A decrease in Svo_2 is the result. In general, the Svo_2 serves as an excellent monitor of oxygen kinetics because it specifically assesses the adequacy of oxygen delivery in relation to oxygen consumption (Do_2/Vo_2 ratio; Fig. 7-7).[26] Many pulmonary arterial catheters contain fiberoptic bundles that provide continuous mixed venous oximetry data. Such monitoring provides a means for assessing the adequacy of oxygen delivery, rapid assessment of the response to interventions such as mechanical ventilation, and cost savings due to a diminished need for sequential blood gas monitoring.[26,27] If a pulmonary artery catheter is unavailable, the central venous oxygen saturation ($Scvo_2$) may serve as a surrogate of the Svo_2.[28]

Four factors are manipulated in an attempt to improve the Do_2/Vo_2 ratio: cardiac output, hemoglobin concentration, Sao_2, and Vo_2. The result of various interventions designed to increase cardiac output, such as volume administration, infusion of inotropic agents, administration of afterload-reducing drugs, and correction of acid/base abnormalities, may be assessed by the effect on the Svo_2 (Fig. 7-8). One of the most efficient ways to enhance oxygen delivery is to increase the oxygen-carrying capacity of the blood. For instance, an increase in hemoglobin from 7.5 to 15 g/dL will be associated with a twofold increase in oxygen delivery at constant cardiac output. However, blood viscosity is increased with blood transfusion, which may result in a reduction in cardiac output.[29]

The Sao_2 can often be enhanced through application of supplemental oxygen and mechanical ventilation. The use of PEEP and mechanical ventilation are, however, limited by the adverse effects observed on cardiac output, the incidence of barotrauma, and the risk for ventilator-induced lung injury with application of peak inspiratory

pressures greater than 30 to 40 cm H_2O.[30,31] Assessment of the "best PEEP" identifies the level at which oxygen delivery and Svo_2 are optimal without compromising compliance.[32,33] Evaluation of the best PEEP should be performed in any patient requiring an Fio_2 greater than 0.60 and may be determined by continuous monitoring of the Svo_2 as the PEEP is sequentially increased from 5 to 15 cm H_2O over a short period. The point at which the Svo_2 is maximal indicates optimal oxygen delivery.

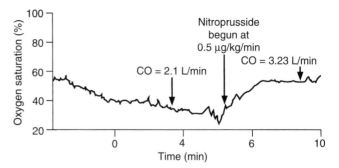

FIGURE 7-8. Alterations in mixed venous blood oxygen saturation are shown as sodium nitroprusside is administered to reduce left ventricular afterload in the setting of cardiac insufficiency. (Reprinted with permission from Hirschl RB: Cardiopulmonary Critical Care and Shock: Surgery of Infants and Children: Scientific Principles and Practice. Philadelphia, Lippincott-Raven, 1997.)

Oxygen consumption may be elevated because of sepsis, burns, agitation, seizures, hyperthermia, hyperthyroidism, and increased catecholamine production or infusion. A number of interventions may be applied to reduce oxygen consumption, such as sedation and mechanical ventilation. Paralysis may enhance the effectiveness of mechanical ventilation while simultaneously reducing oxygen consumption.[34,35] In the appropriate setting, hypothermia may be induced with an associated reduction of 7% in V_{O_2} with each 1°C decrease in core temperature.[36]

THE MECHANICAL VENTILATOR

The ventilator must overcome the pressure generated by the elastic recoil of the lung at end-inspiration plus the resistance to flow at the airway. To do so, most ventilators in the intensive care unit are pneumatically powered by gas pressurized at 50 p.s.i. Microprocessor controls allow accurate management of proportional solenoid-driven valves, which carefully control infusion of a blend of air or oxygen into the ventilator circuit while simultaneously opening and closing an expiratory valve.[37] Additional components of a ventilator include a bacterial filter, a pneumotachometer, a humidifier, a heater/thermostat, an oxygen analyzer, and a pressure manometer. A chamber for nebulizing drugs is usually incorporated into the inspiratory circuit. Tidal volume is not usually measured directly. Rather flow is assessed as a function of time, thereby allowing calculation of tidal volume.

The modes of ventilation are characterized by three variables: the parameter used to initiate or "trigger" a breath, the parameter used to "limit" the size of the breath, and the parameter used to terminate inspiration or "cycle" the breath (Fig. 7-9).[38] Gas flow in most ventilators is triggered either by time (controlled breath) or by patient effort (assisted breath). Controlled ventilation modes are time triggered: the inspiratory phase is concluded once a desired volume, pressure, or flow is attained, but the expiratory time (E_T) will form the difference between the inspiratory time (I_T) and the preset respiratory cycle time. In the assist mode, the ventilator is pressure or flow triggered. With the former, a pressure generated by the patient of approximately −1 cm H_2O will trigger the initiation of a breath. The sensitivity of the triggering device can be adjusted so that patient work is minimized. Other ventilators detect the reduction in constant ventilator tubing gas flow that is associated with patient initiation of a breath. Detection of this decrease in flow results in initiation of a positive-pressure breath.

The magnitude of the breath is controlled or limited by one of three variables: volume, pressure, or flow. When a breath is volume, pressure, or flow "controlled," it indicates that inspiration concludes once the limiting variable is reached. In contrast, a factor that limits inspiration suggests that the chosen value limits the level of the variable during inspiration, but the inspiratory phase does not conclude once this value is attained. For instance, during "pressure-limited" ventilation, gas flow continues until a given pressure limit is attained. However, the inspiratory phase does not necessarily conclude at that point. In contrast, during pressure-controlled ventilation, both gas flow and the inspiratory phase terminate once the preset pressure is reached.

Pressure-controlled or pressure-limited modes are the most popular for all age groups, although volume-control ventilation may be of advantage in preterm newborns.[39,40] In this mode, the respiratory rate, the inspiratory gas flow, the PEEP level, the I_T/E_T ratio, and the peak airway pressure (PIP) are determined. The ventilator infuses gas until the desired PIP is provided. Zero-flow conditions are realized at end-inspiration during pressure-limited ventilation Therefore in this mode, PIP is frequently equivalent to end-inspiratory pressure (EIP) or plateau pressure. In many ventilators, the gas flow rate is fixed, although some ventilators allow manipulation of the flow rate and therefore the rate of positive pressure development. Those with rapid flow rates will provide rapid ascent of pressure to the preset maximum, where it will remain for the duration of the inspiratory phase. This "square wave" pressure pattern results in decelerating flow during inspiration (Fig. 7-10). Airway pressure is "front loaded," which increases P_{aw}, alveolar volume,

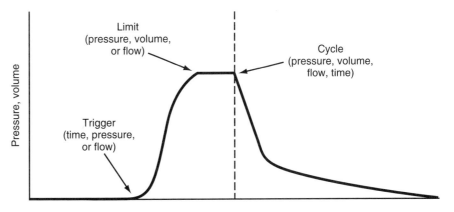

FIGURE 7-9. Variables that characterize the mode of mechanical ventilation.

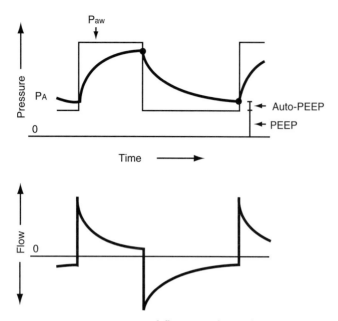

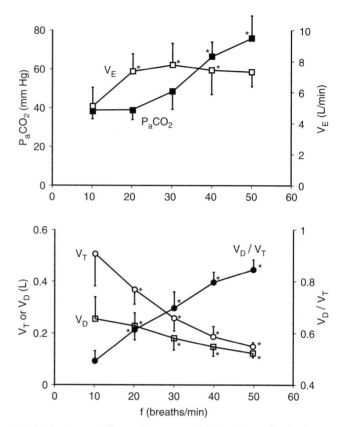

FIGURE 7-10. Pressure and flow waveforms during pressure-limited, time-cycled ventilation. Decelerating flow is applied, which "front loads" the pressure during inspiration. Auto-positive end-expiratory pressure is present when the expiratory time is inadequate for complete expiration. (Reprinted with permission from Marini JJ: New Horizons 1:489–503, 1993.)

FIGURE 7-11. Effect of rate on tidal volume (V_D/V_T) and minute ventilation (V_E) during pressure-limited ventilation. Note that V_E remains unchanged above 20 breaths per minute. Simultaneously, V_D/V_T and $Paco_2$ increase, despite an increase in respiratory rate. (Reprinted with permission from Nahum A, Burke WC, Ravenscraft SA: Lung mechanics and gas exchange during pressure-control ventilation in dogs. Augmentation of CO_2 elimination by an intratracheal catheter. Am Rev Resp Dis 146:965–973, 1992.)

and oxygenation without increasing PIP.[41] However, one of the biggest advantages of pressure-controlled or -limited ventilation is the ability to avoid lung overdistention and barotrauma/volutrauma (discussed later). The disadvantage of pressure-controlled or pressure-limited ventilation is that delivered volume varies with airway resistance and pulmonary compliance and may be reduced when short inspiratory times are applied (I_T; Fig. 7-11).[42] For this reason, tidal volume and minute volume ventilation both must be monitored carefully.

Volume-controlled or volume-limited ventilation requires delineation of the tidal volume, respiratory rate, and inspiratory gas flow. Gas will be inspired until the preset tidal volume is attained. The volume will remain constant despite changes in pulmonary mechanics, although the resulting EIP and PIP may be altered. Flow-controlled or flow-limited ventilation is similar in many respects to volume-controlled or volume-limited ventilation. A flow pattern is predetermined, which effectively results in a fixed volume as the limiting component of inspiration.

The ventilator breath is concluded based on one of four variables: pressure, flow, volume, or time. With volume-cycled ventilation, inspiration is terminated when a prescribed volume is obtained. Likewise, with time-, pressure-, or flow-cycled ventilation, expiration begins once a certain period has passed, the airway pressure reaches a certain value, or when the flow has decreased to a predetermined level, respectively.

MODES OF MECHANICAL VENTILATION

Controlled Mechanical Ventilation

Controlled mechanical ventilation (CMV) is time triggered, flow limited, and volume or pressure cycled. Spontaneous breaths may be taken between the mandatory breaths. However, no additional gas is provided during spontaneous breaths. Therefore the work of breathing is markedly increased in the spontaneously breathing patient. This mode of ventilation is no longer used.

Intermittent Mandatory Ventilation

Intermittent mandatory ventilation (IMV) is time triggered, volume or pressure limited, and either time, volume, or pressure cycled. A rate is set, as is a volume or pressure parameter. Additional inspired gas is provided by the ventilator to support spontaneous breathing when additional breaths are desired. This constitutes the difference between CMV and IMV: in the latter, inspired gases are provided to the patient during spontaneous breaths.[43]

IMV is useful in patients who do not have respiratory drive, for example, in those who are neurologically impaired or pharmacologically paralyzed. Work of breathing is still elevated in this mode in the awake and spontaneously breathing patient.

Synchronized Intermittent Mandatory Ventilation

In the SIMV mode, the ventilator synchronizes IMV breaths with the patient's spontaneous breaths (Fig. 7-12).

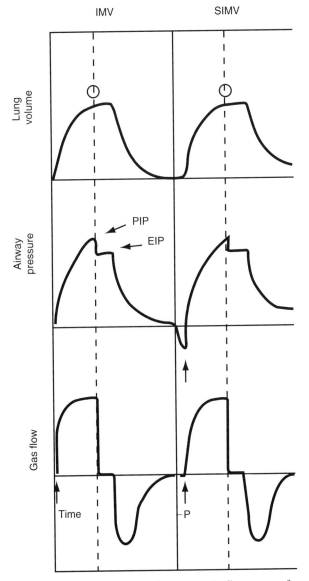

FIGURE 7-12. Pressure, volume, and flow waveforms observed during intermittent mandatory ventilation (IMV) and synchronized IMV (SIMV). In this case, an end-inspiratory pause has been added. Note the difference between peak (PIP) and end-inspiratory (EIP) or plateau pressure. *Arrows,* triggering variables; *open circles,* cycling variables. (Adapted with permission from Bartlett RH: Use of the mechanical ventilator: Surgery. New York, Scientific American, 1988.)

Small, patient-initiated negative deflections in airway pressure (pressure-triggered) or decreases in the constant ventilator gas flow (bias flow) passing through the exhalation valve (flow triggered) provide a signal to the ventilator that a patient breath has been initiated. Ventilated breaths are timed with the patient's spontaneous respiration, but the number of supported breaths each minute is predetermined and remains constant. Additional constant inspired gas flow is provided for use during any other spontaneous breaths. Advances in neonatal ventilators have provided the means for detecting small alterations in bias flow. As such, flow-triggered SIMV may now be applied to newborns, which appears to enhance ventilatory patterns and to allow ventilation with reduced airway pressures and FiO2.[44,45] SIMV may be associated with a reduction in the duration of ventilation and the incidence of air leak in newborns in general, as well as in those premature infants with bronchopulmonary dysplasia (BPD) and intraventricular hemorrhage (IVH) in preterm neonates.[46,47]

Assist Control Ventilation

In the spontaneously breathing patient, brainstem reflexes dependent on cerebral spinal fluid levels of carbon dioxide and pH can be harnessed to determine the appropriate breathing rate.[15] As in SIMV, the assisted breaths can be either pressure triggered or flow triggered. The triggering-mechanism sensitivity can be set in most ventilators. In contrast to SIMV, the ventilator supports all patient-initiated breaths. This mode is similar to IMV, but allows the patient inherently to control the ventilation needs and minimizes patient work of breathing in adults and neonates.[48,49] Occasionally patients may hyperventilate, such as when they are agitated or have neurologic injury. Heavy sedation may be required if agitation is present. A minimal ventilator rate below the patient's assist rate should be established in case of apnea.

Pressure-Support Ventilation or Volume-Support Ventilation

Pressure-support ventilation (PSV) is a pressure- or flow-triggered, pressure-limited, and flow-cycled mode of ventilation. It is similar in concept to assist control, in that mechanical support is provided for each spontaneous breath, and the patient determines ventilator rate. During each breath, inspiratory flow is applied until a predetermined pressure is attained.[50] As the end of inspiration approaches, flow decreases to a level below a specified value (2 to 6 L/min) or a percentage of peak inspiratory flow ($\cong$25%). At this point, inspiration terminates. Although it may apply full support, PSV is frequently used to support the patient partially by assigning a pressure limit for each breath that is less than that required for full support.[51] For example, in the spontaneously breathing patient, PSV can be sequentially decreased from full support to a PSV 5 to 10 cm H_2O above PEEP.[52,53] This allows weaning while providing partial support with each breath. Therefore during PSV, tidal volume may be dependent on patient effort.

PSV provides two advantages during ventilation of spontaneously breathing patients: (1) it provides excellent support and decreases the work of breathing associated with ventilation, and (2) lower PIP and Paw and higher V_T and cardiac output levels may be observed.[50,54,55]

Pressure-triggered SIMV and PSV may be applied to newborns. Inspiration is terminated when the peak airway flow decreases to a set percentage of between 5% and 25%. This flow cutoff for inspiration is known as the termination sensitivity, which may be adjusted: the higher the termination-sensitivity value, the shorter the inspiratory time. The termination-sensitivity function also may be disabled, at which point ventilation is time-cycled instead of flow-cycled. Studies have demonstrated a reduction in work of breathing and sedation requirements when SIMV with pressure support is applied to newborns.

Volume-support ventilation (VSV) is similar to PSV except that a volume, rather than a pressure, is assigned to provide partial support. Automation with VSV is enhanced because less need occurs for manual changes to maintain stable tidal and minute volume during weaning.[56] Both VSV and PSV are equally effective at weaning infants and children from the ventilator.[57]

Volume-Assured Pressure-Support Ventilation

This mode attempts to combine volume- and pressure-controlled ventilation to assure a desired tidal volume within the constraints of the pressure limit. Volume-assured pressure-support ventilation (VAPSV) has the advantage of maintaining inflation to a point below an injurious PIP level while maintaining tidal volume constant in the face of changing pulmonary mechanics. Work of breathing may be markedly decreased and C_{eff} increased during VAPSV.[58]

Proportional Assist Ventilation

Proportional assist ventilation (PAV) is an intriguing approach to the support of the spontaneously breathing patient. It relies on the concept that the combined pressure generated by the ventilator (P_{aw}) and respiratory muscles (P_{mus}) is equivalent to that required to overcome the resistance to flow of the endotracheal tube/airways (P_{res}) and the tendency for the inflated lungs to collapse (elastic recoil or elastance = 1/Compliance, P_{el}):

$$P_{aw} + P_{mus} = P_{el} + P_{res}$$

Elastance and resistance can be assessed in patients during periods of mechanical ventilation in which no spontaneous breaths occur with the following equations:

$$\text{Elastance} = \frac{\text{Plateau pressure} - \text{PEEP}}{V_T} \text{ and}$$

$$\text{Airway resistance} = \frac{\text{PIP} - \text{PEEP}}{\text{Flow}}$$

The pressure required to overcome lung elastic recoil is equivalent to the product of the current lung volume and the elastance (P_{el} = Volume × Elastance), and the pressure required to overcome airway resistance is equivalent to the product of the current flow and the resistance (P_{res} = Flow × Resistance). At any point during inspiration, therefore, instantaneous patient pressure generation (P_{mus}) may be assessed if elastance and resistance have already been calculated, and volume, flow, and P_{aw} are instantaneously measured: $P_{mus} = (V \times E + \text{Flow} \times R) - P_{aw}$.[59] With proportional-assist ventilation, airway-pressure generation by the ventilator is proportional at any instant to the respiratory effort (P_{mus}) generated by the patient. Small efforts, therefore, result in small breaths, whereas greater patient effort results in development of a greater tidal volume. Inspiration is patient triggered and terminates with discontinuation of patient effort. Rate, V_T, and I_T are entirely patient controlled. The predominant variable to be set on the ventilator is the proportional response between P_{mus} and the applied ventilator pressure. This proportional assist (P_{aw}/P_{mus}) can be increased until nearly all patient effort is provided by the ventilator.[60] Patient work of breathing, dyspnea, and PIP are reduced.[61,62] Elastance and resistance are set, as is applied PEEP. V_T is variable, and risk of atelectasis may be present. PAV produces similar gas exchange with lower airway pressures when compared with conventional ventilation in infants.[63] Compared with preterm newborns with the assist control mode of ventilation and IMV, preterm newborns managed with PAV maintained gas exchange with lower airway pressures and a decrease in the oxygenation index by 28%.[64] Chest-wall dynamics also are enhanced.[65] PAV represents an exciting first step in servoregulating ventilators to patient requirements.

Continuous Positive Airway Pressure

During continuous positive airway pressure (CPAP), pressures greater than those of ambient pressure are continuously applied to the airways to enhance alveolar distension and oxygenation.[66] Both airway resistance and work of breathing may be substantially reduced. However, no support of ventilation is provided. Therefore this mode requires that the patient provide all of the work of breathing. It is to be avoided in patients with hypovolemia, untreated pneumothorax, lung hyperinflation, or elevated intracranial pressure and in infants with nasal obstruction, cleft palate, tracheoesophageal fistula, or untreated congenital diaphragmatic hernia. CPAP is frequently applied via nasal prongs, although it can be delivered in adult patients with a nasal mask.

Inverse Ratio Ventilation

In the setting of respiratory failure, one would wish to enhance alveolar distention to reduce hypoxemia and shunt. One means to accomplish this is to maintain the inspiratory plateau pressure for a longer proportion of the breath.[67] The inspiratory time may be prolonged to the point at which the ratio of inspiratory time to expiratory time may be as high as 4:1.[68] In most circumstances, however, the I_T/E_T ratio is maintained at approximately 2:1. Inverse ratio ventilation (IRV) is usually performed during pressure-controlled ventilation (PC-IRV), although prolonged inspiratory times can be applied during volume-controlled ventilation by adding a decelerating flow pattern or an end-inspiratory pause to the volume-controlled ventilator breath.[69] One advantage of IRV is the ability to recruit alveoli that are associated with high-resistance airways and therefore inflate only with prolonged application of positive pressure.[70] Unfortunately, IRV is associated with a profound sense of dyspnea in patients who are awake and spontaneously breathing. Therefore heavy sedation and pharmacologic paralysis is required during this ventilator mode. One also must be cognizant of the risk for incomplete expiration as the E_T is reduced. This may be identified by the failure to achieve zero-flow conditions at end-expiration. The result is "auto-PEEP" or a total PEEP greater than that of the preset or applied PEEP. Care should be taken to recognize the presence of auto-PEEP and to incorporate it into the ventilation strategy to avoid barotrauma.[71] IRV also may affect cardiac output and therefore oxygen delivery.[72] Some studies using IRV revealed an increase in P_{aw} and oxygenation while protecting the lungs by reducing peak inspiratory pressure.[73-76] Likewise, others suggest that early implementation of IRV in severe ARDS enhances oxygenation and allows reduction in FiO_2, PEEP, and PIP.[77] On the contrary, a number of studies have failed to demonstrate enhanced gas exchange with this mode of ventilation. Some series have suggested that IRV is less effective at enhancing gas exchange than is application of PEEP to maintain the same mean airway pressure.[78] Overall, it appears that oxygenation is determined primarily by the mean airway pressure rather than specifically by application of IRV. As such, the usefulness of IRV remains in question.[79] Continuous monitoring of the SvO_2 may aid in determining whether the addition of IRV has enhanced DO_2 in addition to PaO_2 and SaO_2.

Airway Pressure–Release Ventilation

Airway pressure–release ventilation (APRV) is a unique approach to ventilation in which CPAP at high levels is used to enhance mean alveolar volume, while intermittent reductions in pressure to a "release" level provide a period of expiration (Fig. 7-13). Reestablishment of CPAP results in inspiration and return of lung volume back to the baseline level. The advantage of APRV is a reduction in PIP of approximately 50% in adult patients with ARDS supported with this technique when compared with other more conventional modes of mechanical ventilation.[80,81] Spontaneous ventilation also is allowed throughout the cycle, which may enhance cardiac function and renal blood flow.[82] Some data suggest that $\dot{V}/\dot{Q}$ matching may be improved and dead space reduced.[84,85] In performing APRV, tidal volume is altered by adjusting the release pressure. Conceptually, ventilator management during APRV is the inverse of other modes of PPV in that the peak inspiratory pressure, or CPAP, determines oxygenation, while the expiratory pressure (release pressure) is used to adjust tidal volume and CO_2 elimination. APRV is very similar to modes of ventilation that use prolonged I_T/E_T ratios, such as IRV. However, APRV appears to be better tolerated when compared with IRV in patients with acute lung injury (ALI)/ARDS, as demonstrated by a reduced need for paralysis and sedation, increased cardiac performance, decreased pressor use, and decreased PIP requirements.[86] The clinical experience with APRV is limited in the pediatric population.[87,88]

Bilevel Control of Positive Airway Pressure

Although sometimes used in the acute lung setting, bilevel control of PAP (BiPAP) is frequently used for home respiratory support by varying airway pressure between one of two settings: the inspiratory positive airway pressure (IPAP) and the expiratory positive airway pressure (EPAP).[89,90] With patient effort, a change in flow is detected, and the IPAP pressure level developed. With reduced flow at end-expiration, EPAP is reestablished. This device, therefore, provides both ventilatory support and airway distention during the expiratory phase. However, BiPAP ventilators should be used only to support the patient who is spontaneously breathing.

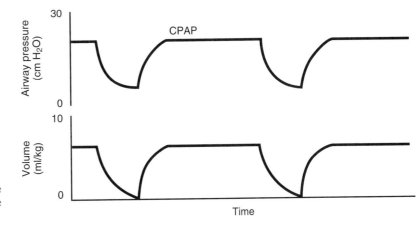

FIGURE 7-13. Typical pressure and volume waveforms observed during airway pressure release ventilation (APVR).

MONITORING DURING MECHANICAL VENTILATION

Current mechanical ventilators incorporate highly accurate solid-state pressure transducers that provide data on a variety of pressures and gas flows. Volume is not measured directly; rather, flow is integrated over time in the determination of volume. Low-pressure alarms are present to detect disconnection and leaks and are set at approximately 10 cm H_2O below the anticipated PIP, whereas high-pressure alarms are set approximately 10 cm H_2O above PIP to avoid incidental application of excessive pressure to the lungs. Apnea alarms typically are triggered if tidal volume is not delivered for more than 10 seconds. Alarms for numerous other parameters such as PEEP, low tidal volume, low and high rate, and low and high FiO_2 may be adjusted on various ventilators. Most ventilators also have an indicator that notifies the operator if the ventilator settings result in an I_T/E_T ratio that is greater than 1:1. Current ventilators can calculate and display a variety of pressure/volume, flow/volume, or volume/pressure waveforms as well as demonstrate volume, flow, and pressure over time. In the setting of respiratory insufficiency, mechanical ventilation should be used in conjunction with invasive monitoring, such as systemic arterial and pulmonary arterial (PA) catheters, as well as pulse oximetry and end-tidal CO_2 monitoring. Technology that allows frequent blood gas sampling without blood loss is now available for newborns and infants. It is likely that ventilators in the future will incorporate PA catheter-derived SvO_2, pulse oximeter–derived SaO_2, and oxygen-consumption data in determining online cardiac output and oxygen delivery values.[91] As online blood gas monitoring becomes more accurate, FiO_2, rate, PIP, and PEEP will be servoregulated on the basis of SaO_2, SvO_2, and $PaCO_2$.

MANAGEMENT OF THE MECHANICAL VENTILATOR

IMV and SIMV may suffice for patients with normal lungs, such as those after an operation.[92] If a patient is spontaneously breathing and is to be ventilated for more than a brief period, a flow- or pressure-triggered assist mode, pressure support, or PAV will result in maximal support and minimal work of breathing.[48,49] Ventilator modes that allow adjustment of specific details of pressure, flow, and volume are required in the patient with severe respiratory failure. With all these modes, the ventilator rate, tidal volume or PIP, PEEP, and either I_T alone or I_T/E_T (if ventilation is pressure limited) must be assigned. Other secondary controls such as the flow rate, the flow pattern, the trigger sensitivity for assisted breaths, the inspiratory hold, the termination sensitivity, and the safety pressure limit also are set on individual ventilators. The normal minute volume ventilation is 100 to 150 mL/kg/min. The FiO_2 is usually initiated at 0.50 and decreased based on pulse oximetry. All efforts should be made to maintain the FiO_2 less than 0.60 to avoid alveolar nitrogen depletion and the development of atelectasis.[93,94]

Oxygen toxicity likely is a result of this phenomenon, although free oxygen radical formation may play a role when an FiO_2 greater than 0.40 is applied for prolonged periods.[95] A short inspiratory phase with a low I_T/E_T ratio favors the expiratory phase and CO_2 elimination, whereas longer I_T/E_T ratios enhance oxygenation. In the normal lung, I_T/E_T ratios of 1:3 and I_T of 0.5 to 1 second are typical.

MECHANICAL VENTILATION IN THE PATIENT WITH RESPIRATORY FAILURE

Ventilator-Induced Lung Injury

One typically observes both a decrease in pulmonary compliance and functional residual capacity in the patient with ALI (PaO_2/FiO_2 ratio, 200 to 300) or ARDS (PaO_2/FiO_2 ratio, less than 200). These two parameters are related, as the loss of FRC associated with alveolar collapse results in a decrease in the volume of lung available for ventilation and therefore a decrease in pulmonary compliance. As a result, higher ventilator pressures are necessary to maintain tidal volume and minute volume ventilation. However, the use of high ventilator pressures in an attempt to ventilate the patient with respiratory insufficiency can result in compromise of cardiopulmonary function and the development of ventilator-induced lung injury (VILI).[96] The concept of VILI was first demonstrated in 1974 by demonstrating the detrimental effects of ventilation at PIP of 45 cm H_2O in rats.[97] Electron microscopy has been used to document an increased incidence of alveolar stress fractures in ex vivo, perfused rabbit lungs exposed to transalveolar pressures more than 30 cm H_2O (Fig. 7-14).[98] Other studies have demonstrated increases in albumin leak, elevation of the capillary leak coefficient, enhanced wet-to-dry lung weight, deterioration in gas exchange, and augmented diffuse alveolar damage on histology with application of increased airway pressure (45 to 50 cm H_2O) in otherwise normal rats and sheep over a 1- to 24-hour period.[31,99,100] It has been theorized that pulmonary exposure to high pressures may worsen nascent respiratory insufficiency and, ultimately, lead to the development of pulmonary fibrosis. Such injury may be prevented during application of high peak inspiratory pressures by strapping the chest, thereby preventing lung overdistention, suggesting that alveolar distention or "volutrauma" is the injurious element, rather than application of high pressures or "barotrauma."[101] A low-tidal-volume (6 mL/kg) approach to mechanical ventilation in rabbits with *Pseudomonas aeruginosa*–induced acute lung injury appears to be associated with enhancement in oxygenation, increase in pH, increase in arterial blood pressure, and decrease in extravascular lung water when compared with a high-tidal-volume group (15 mL/kg).[102] A relation may exist between ventilator gas flow rate and the development of lung injury.[103] Positive blood cultures have been seen in five of six animals exposed to high end-inspiratory pressure, but rarely in those with low end-inspiratory pressure.[104] Together, all

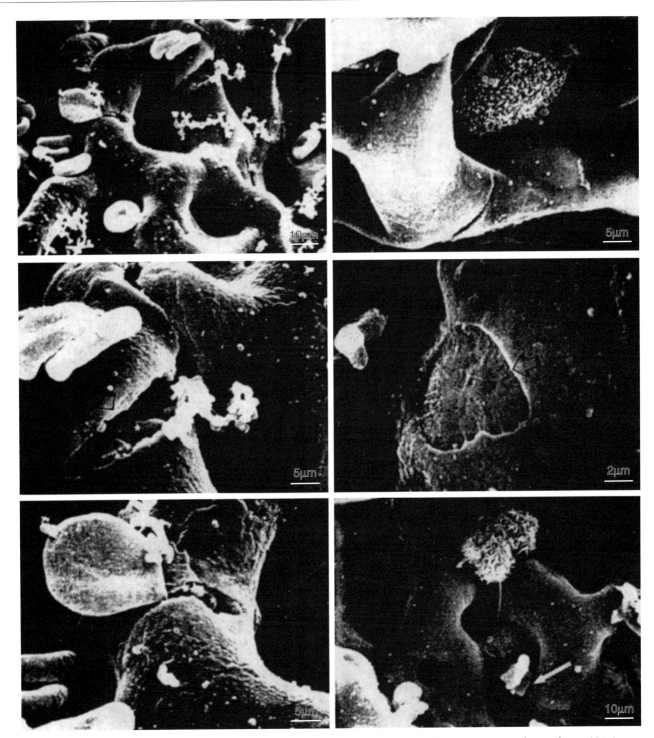

FIGURE 7-14. Scanning electron micrographs demonstrating disruptions in the blood-gas barriers (*arrows*) in rabbit lungs subjected to 20 cm H_2O airway pressure and 75 cm H_2O pulmonary arterial pressure. (Reprinted with permission from Fu Z, Costello ML, Tsukimoto K, et al: High lung volume increases stress failure in pulmonary capillaries. J Appl Physiol 73:123–133, 1992.)

of these data suggest that the method of ventilation has an effect on lung function and gas exchange as well as a systemic effect, which may include translocation of bacteria from the lungs. As such, avoidance of high PIPs and lung overdistention should be a primary goal of mechanical ventilation.

Although the animal data would suggest that high PIPs and volumes may be deleterious, two multicenter studies have attempted to randomize patients with ARDS to high and low peak pressure or volume strategies. The first failed to demonstrate a difference in mortality or duration of mechanical ventilation in patients randomized to either the low-volume (7.2 ± 0.8 mL/kg) or the high-volume (10.8 ± 1.0 mL) strategy, although the applied PIP was not elevated to what would commonly be considered injurious levels in either group (low, 23.6 ± 5.8 cm H_2O;

high, 34.0 ± 11.0 cm H₂O).[105] Another study revealed similar results but had similar design limitations.[106] A survival increase from 38% to 71% at 28 days, a higher rate of weaning from mechanical ventilation, and a lower rate of barotrauma has been demonstrated in patients in whom a lung-protective ventilator strategy was used, which consisted of lung distention to a level that prevented alveolar collapse during expiration (see later) and avoidance of high distending pressures.[107] One study identified a significant reduction over time in bronchoalveolar lavage concentrations of polymorphonuclear cells ($P < .001$), IL-1β ($P < .05$), tumor necrosis factor (TNF)-α ($P < .001$), interleukin (IL)-8 ($P < .001$), and IL-6 ($P < .005$), and in plasma concentration of IL-6 ($P < .002$) among 44 patients randomized to receive a lung-protective strategy rather than a conventional approach.[108] The mean number of ventilator-free days at 28 days (VFDs) in the lung-protective strategy group was higher than in the control group (12 ± 11 vs. 4 ± 8 days, respectively; $P < .01$). Mortality rates at 28 days from admission were 38% and 58% in the lung-protective strategy and control groups, respectively ($P = .19$). The National Institutes of Health (NIH) ARDSnet convincingly demonstrated that mortality was reduced with the use of a low volume (6 mL/kg, mortality of 31%) when compared with a high volume (12 mL/kg, mortality of 39%; $P = 0.005$) ventilator approach (Fig. 7-15).[109] Interestingly, no difference was found in gas exchange or pulmonary mechanics between groups to account for the difference in mortality. However, IL-6 levels were increased in the high-volume when compared with the low-volume ventilation group, as was the incidence of organ failure. Similarly, multisystem organ failure (MSOF) scores increased significantly 72 hours after admission only in patients who were ventilated with a conventional rather than a lung-protective strategy, with

renal failure being the most prevalent organ dysfunction.[110] Significant correlations were noted between changes in overall MSOF score and changes in plasma concentration of inflammatory mediators, including interleukin 6 ($P < .001$); TNFα ($P = .02$); IL-1β ($P = .02$); and IL-8 ($P = .001$). A significant correlation was seen between IL-6 level and the number of failing organs. Exposure of PMNs to bronchoalveolar lavage fluid from a control group of ARDS patients resulted in increased PMN activation as compared with those exposed to bronchoalveolar lavage fluid (BALF) from a group of patients managed with a lung-protective strategy.[111] The majority of clinicians are now convinced that avoidance of high PIP and support of lung recruitment through application of appropriate levels of PEEP (see later) should be a primary goal of any mechanical ventilatory program.

Permissive Hypercapnia

To avoid VILI, practitioners have applied the concept of permissive hypercapnia, in which arterial carbon dioxide is allowed to increase to levels as high as 120 mm Hg as long as the blood pH is maintained in the 7.1 to 7.2 range by administration of buffers.[112] Mortality was reduced to 26% when compared with that expected (53%; $P < .004$) based on APACHE II scores when low-volume, pressure-limited ventilation with permissive hypercapnia was applied in the setting of ARDS in adults.[113] For burned children, the mortality rate was only 3.7% despite a high degree of inhalation injury when a ventilator strategy used a PIP of 40 cm H₂O and accepted an elevated PaCO₂ as long as the arterial pH was greater than 7.20.[114] Other studies suggested that a strategy of high-frequency (40 to 120 breaths/minute) ventilation with low tidal volumes, low PIP, high PEEP (7 to 30 cm H₂O), and mild hypercapnia (PaCO₂ from 45 to 60 mm Hg) enhances the survival rate in children with severe ARDS.[115]

Protective Effects of Positive End-Expiratory Pressure

Although application of high, overdistending airway pressures appears to be associated with the development of lung injury, a number of studies have demonstrated that application of PEEP or high-frequency oscillatory ventilation (HFOV) may allow avoidance of lung injury by the following mechanisms: (1) recruitment of collapsed alveoli, which reduces the risk for overdistention of healthy units; (2) resolution of alveolar collapse, which in and of itself is injurious; and (3) avoidance of the shear forces associated with the opening and closing of alveoli.[116,117] In the older child with injured lungs, a pressure of 8 to 12 cm H₂O is required to open alveoli and to begin tidal volume generation.[107,118,119] Alveoli will subsequently close unless the end-expiratory pressure is maintained at such pressures. This cyclic opening and closing is thought to be particularly injurious because of application of large shear forces.[118] One way to avoid this process is through the application of PEEP to a point above the inflection pressure (P_{flex}), such that alveolar distention is maintained throughout the ventilatory cycle

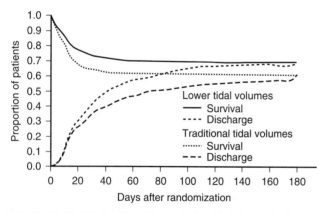

FIGURE 7-15. Probability of survival and of being discharged home and breathing without assistance during the first 180 days after randomization in patients with acute lung injury and the acute respiratory distress syndrome. The status at 180 days or at the end of the study was known for all but nine patients. (From The Acute Respiratory Distress Network: Ventilation with lower tidal volumes as compared with traditional tidal volumes for acute lung injury and the acute respiratory distress syndrome. N Engl J Med 342(18):1301–1308, 2000, with permission.)

(Fig. 7-16).[120,121] In addition, as mentioned previously, it has been demonstrated that the distribution of infiltrates and atelectasis in the supine patient with ARDS is predominantly in the dependent regions of the lung.[122] This is likely the result of compression due to the increased weight of the overlying edematous lung. It has been shown that when the superimposed gravitational pressure from the weight of the overlying lung exceeded the PEEP applied to a given region of the lung, end-expiratory lung collapse increased, resulting in derecruitment.[123] Thus application of PEEP may result in recruitment of these atelectatic lung regions, simultaneously enhancing pulmonary compliance and oxygenation. PEEP and the prone positioning (see later) are more effective if the need for ventilation is of extrapulmonary etiology rather than pulmonary etiology.[124]

Approach to the Patient with Respiratory Failure

As a result of these new data and concepts, the approach to mechanical ventilation in the patient with respiratory failure has changed drastically over the past few years (Table 7-2). Time-cycled, pressure-controlled ventilation has become favored because of the ability to limit EIP to noninjurious levels at a maximum of 35 cm H_2O.[119] In infants and newborns, this EIP limit is set lower at 30 cm H_2O. Tidal volume should be maintained in the range of 6 cc/kg.[109] A lung-protective approach also incorporates lung distention and prevention of alveolar closure. Pressure/volume (P/V) curves should be developed on each patient at least daily, so that the P_{flex} can be identified and the PEEP maintained above P_{flex}. If a P/V curve cannot be determined, then P_{flex} can be assumed to be in the 7 to 12 cm H_2O range, and PEEP at that level or up to

TABLE 7-2
CURRENT FAVORED APPROACHES TO THE TREATMENT OF ARDS

Pressure-limited ventilation
    TV ≈ 6 mL/kg
    IRV
    EIP <35 cm H_2O
    PEEP > P_{flex} or > 12 cm H_2O
Permissive hypercapnia
    FiO_2 ≤ 0.06
    SvO_2 ≥ 65%
    Sao_2 ≥ 80%–85%
Transfusion to Hgb >13 g/dL
Diuresis to dry weight
Prone positioning
Extracorporeal support

ARDS, acute respiratory distress syndrome; TV, tidal volume; IRV, inverse ratio ventilation; EIP, end-expiratory pressure.

2 cm H_2O higher applied.[119,125,126] Recruitment maneuvers that use intermittent sustained inflations of approximately 40 cm H_2O for up to 40 seconds can often be of benefit by initially inflating collapsed lung regions.[127] The inflation obtained with the recruitment maneuver is then sustained by maintaining PEEP greater than P_{flex}. As both PIP and PEEP are increased, enhancements in compliance and reductions in V_D/V_T and shunt are to be expected. If they are not observed, then one should suspect the presence of overdistention of currently inflated alveoli instead of the desired recruitment of collapsed lung units. Application of increased levels of PEEP also may result in a decrease in venous return and cardiac output. In addition, West's zone I physiology, which predicts diminished or absent pulmonary capillary flow in the nondependent regions of the lungs at end-inspiration, may be exacerbated with application of higher airway pressures. This may be especially detrimental, because it is the nondependent regions that are best inflated and to which one would wish to direct as much pulmonary blood flow as possible.[15] As a result, parameters of oxygen delivery should be carefully monitored during application of increased PEEP.[128] One means for doing so is by attention to the SvO_2 whenever the PEEP is increased to more than 5 cm H_2O. As mentioned, one approach is to increase the PEEP gradually in increments of 2.5 cm H_2O until the desired level of oxygenation or lung protection is achieved or a decrease in SvO_2 to below the maximum is observed. Effective lung compliance also should be monitored to ensure that alveolar recruitment is being achieved.

If oxygenation remains inadequate with application of higher levels of PEEP, FiO_2 should be increased to maintain an SaO_2 greater than 90%, although levels as low as 80% may be acceptable in patients with adequate oxygen delivery. As mentioned previously, one of the most effective ways to enhance oxygen delivery is with transfusion. All attempts should be made to avoid the atelectasis and oxygen toxicity associated with FiO_2 levels greater than 0.60.[93] Extending FiO_2 to levels more than 0.60 often has little effect on oxygenation, because severe respiratory

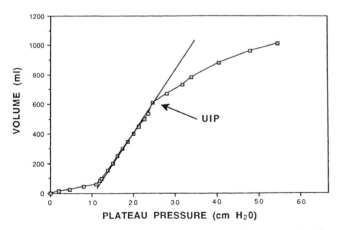

FIGURE 7-16. Static pressure/volume curve demonstrating the P_{flex} point in a patient with adult respiratory distress syndrome. Positive end-expiratory pressure should be maintained approximately 2 cm H_2O above that point. The upper inflection point (UIP) indicates the point at which lung overdistention is beginning to occur. Ventilation to points above the UIP should be avoided in most circumstances. (Reprinted with permission from Roupie E, Dambrosio M, Servillo G: Titration of tidal volume and induced hypercapnia in acute respiratory distress syndrome. Am J Respir Crit Care Med 152:121–128, 1995.)

failure is frequently associated with a large transpulmonary shunt. If inadequate oxygen delivery persists, a trial increase in PEEP level should be performed or institution of extracorporeal support considered.[129] Inflation of the lungs also can be enhanced by prolonging the inspiratory time by PC-IRV. Pharmacologic paralysis and sedation are required during performance of PC-IRV, although paralysis may have the additional benefit of decreasing oxygen consumption and enhancing ventilator efficiency.[35] PaO_2 may improve with application of PC-IRV.[130,131] However, monitoring the effect on oxygen delivery and the SvO_2 is critical to ensure the benefit of this intervention. The advantages of the alveolar inflation associated with a decelerating flow waveform during pressure-limited modes of ventilation also should be used.[41]

Altering the patient from the supine to the prone position appears to enhance gas exchange (Fig. 7-17).[132,133] Enhanced blood flow to the better-inflated anterior lung regions with the prone position would logically appear to account for the increase in oxygenation. However, data in oleic acid lung-injured sheep suggest that the enhancement in gas exchange may be due predominantly to more homogeneous distribution of ventilation, rather than to redistribution of pulmonary blood flow, because lung distention is more uniform in the prone position.[134–136] This effect may be reversed after a number of hours. However, enhanced posterior region lung inflation frequently accounts for persistent increases in oxygenation when the patient is replaced into the supine position.[122] Therefore benefit may be seen when the prone and supine positions are alternated, usually every 4 to 6 hours. A randomized, controlled, multicenter trial evaluating the effectiveness of the prone position in the treatment of patients with ARDS was recently completed.[137] The prone group was placed in the prone position for 6 or more hours daily for 10 days while the control group remained in the supine position. Although the PaO_2/FiO_2

ratio was greater in the prone when compared with the supine group (prone, 63.0 + 66.8, vs. supine, 44.6 + 68.2; P = 0.02), no difference in mortality was noted between groups. It is clear that some patients will not respond to altered positioning, in which case this adjunct should be discontinued. Attention to careful patient padding and avoidance of dislodgment of tubes and catheters is critical to successful implementation of this approach.

Another means for enhancing oxygenation may be through administration of diuretics and the associated reduction of left atrial and pulmonary capillary hydrostatic pressure.[138] Diuresis results in a decrease in lung interstitial edema. In addition, reduction of lung edema decreases compression of the underlying dependent lung.[139] Collapsed dependent lung regions are thereby recruited. Although this treatment approach has not been proven in randomized clinical trials, reduction in total body fluid in adult patients with ARDS appears to be associated with an increase in survival.[140] One must be cognizant of the risks of hypoperfusion and organ system failure, especially renal insufficiency, if overly aggressive diuresis is performed. Overall, however, a strategy of fluid restriction and diuresis should be pursued in the setting of ARDS, while monitoring organ perfusion and renal function.[141]

One protects the lung by applying noninjurious PIPs and enhancing PEEP levels, which limits the ΔP and V_T. This results in compromise of CO_2 elimination. Therefore the concept of permissive hypercapnia, which was discussed previously, is integral to the successful application of lung-protective strategies. $PaCO_2$ levels greater than 100 mm Hg have been allowed with this approach, although most practitioners prefer to maintain the $PaCO_2$ at less than 60 to 70 mm Hg.[113] Bicarbonate or trishydroxymethylaminomethane (THAM) may be used to induce a metabolic alkalosis to maintain the pH at greater than 7.20. Few significant physiologic effects are observed with elevated $PaCO_2$ levels as long as the pH is maintained at reasonable levels.[142] If adequate CO_2 elimination cannot be achieved while limiting EIP to noninjurious levels, then initiation of extracorporeal life support (ECLS) should be considered.

The one situation in which it may be acceptable to increase EIP to levels greater than 35 cm H_2O (30 cm H_2O in the infant and newborn) is in the patient with reduced chest-wall compliance and relatively normal pulmonary compliance. Because pulmonary compliance is a combination of lung compliance and chest-wall compliance, a decrease in chest-wall compliance, such as due to abdominal distention or chest-wall edema, can markedly reduce pulmonary compliance despite reasonable lung compliance. This situation is analogous to studies discussed previously in which the lungs remain uninjured despite application of high airway pressures because the chest is strapped to prevent lung overdistention.[101] This is a frequent problem in secondary respiratory failure due to trauma, sepsis, and other frequent disease processes observed among surgical patients. A cautious increase in EIP in such patients may be warranted. A simple intervention such as raising the head of the bed may have marked effects on FRC and gas exchange in such patients.

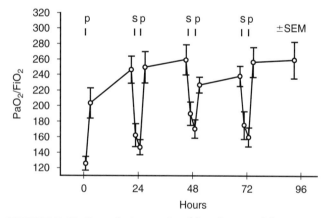

FIGURE 7-17. PaO_2 during supine (s) and prone (p) positioning. Note the increase in oxygenation when trauma patients with adult respiratory distress syndrome are in the prone position and a general trend toward increased PaO_2 with each return to the supine position. (Reprinted with permission from Fridrich P, Krafft P, Hochleuthner H, Mauritz W: The effects of long-term prone positioning in patients with trauma-induced acute respiratory distress syndrome. Anesth Analg 83:1206–1211, 1996.)

Weaning from Mechanical Ventilation

Once a patient is spontaneously breathing and able to protect the airway, consideration should be given to weaning from ventilator support. Weaning in the majority of children should take 2 days or less.[143] The FiO_2 should be decreased to less than 0.40 before extubation. Simultaneously, PEEP should be lowered to 5 cm H_2O. The pressure-support mode of ventilation is an efficient means for weaning, as the preset inspiratory pressure can be gradually decreased while partial support is provided for each breath.[144] Adequate gas exchange during a pressure support of 7 to 10 cm H_2O above PEEP in adults and newborns is predictive of successful extubation.[145] However, another study in adults demonstrated that simple transition from full ventilator support to a "T-piece," in which oxygen flow-by is provided, is as effective at weaning as is gradual reduction in rate during IMV or pressure during PSV.[146] In all circumstances, brief trials of spontaneous breathing before extubation should be performed with flow-by oxygen and CPAP. Prophylactic dexamethasone administration does not appear to increase the odds of a successful trial in infants.[147] Parameters during a T-piece trial that indicate readiness for extubation include the following: (1) maintenance of the pretrial respiratory and heart rates; (2) inspiratory force greater than 20 cm H_2O; (3) minute volume ventilation less than 1 cc/kg/min; and (4) SaO_2 greater than 95%. If the patient's status is in question, transcutaneous CO_2 monitoring, along with arterial blood gas analysis ($PaCO_2$ less than 40 mm Hg; PaO_2 greater than 60 mm Hg), may help to ascertain whether extubation is appropriate. The weaning trial should be brief and, under no circumstances, should last longer than 1 hour, because the narrow endotracheal tube provides substantial resistance to spontaneous ventilation. In most cases, the patient who tolerates spontaneous breathing through an endotracheal tube for only a few minutes will demonstrate enhanced capabilities once the airway access device is removed.

Frequent causes of failed extubation include persistent pulmonary parenchymal disease, interstitial fibrosis, and reduced breathing endurance. Pressure-support ventilation is ideal for use in the difficult-to-wean patient because it allows gradual application of spontaneous support to enhance respiratory strength and conditioning (Table 7-3).[144] Enteral and parenteral nutrition should be adjusted to maintain the total caloric intake to no more than 10% above the estimated caloric needs of the patient. Excess calories will be converted to fat, with a high respiratory quotient and increased CO_2 production. Nutritional support high in glucose will have a similar effect.[148] Manipulation of feedings along with treatment of sepsis may reduce VCO_2 and enhance weaning. Pulmonary edema should be treated with diuretics. Some patients will benefit from a tracheostomy to avoid ongoing upper airway contamination, to decrease dead space and airway resistance, and to provide airway access for evacuation of secretions during the weaning process. In addition, the issue of "extubating" the patient is removed by tracheostomy tube placement. Spontaneous breathing

TABLE 7-3
MANAGEMENT OF THE PATIENT FOR WHOM EXTUBATION ATTEMPTS HAVE FAILED
Frequent spontaneous breathing trails
Pressure support ventilation
Caloric intake ≤10% above expenditure
Minimize carbohydrate calories
Diuresis to dry weight
Treat infection
Tracheostomy

trials, therefore, are easy to perform, and the transition off the mechanical ventilator is a much more smooth and efficient process. Tracheostomy tube placement in older patients can be performed by percutaneous means at the bedside.[149] Long-term complications are fairly minimal in older patients, but in newborns and infants, the rate of development of stenoses and granulation tissue may be significant.[150,151]

NONCONVENTIONAL MODES AND ADJUNCTS TO MECHANICAL VENTILATION

High-frequency Ventilation

The concept of high-frequency jet ventilation (HFJV) was developed in the early 1970s to provide gas exchange during procedures performed on the trachea. HFJV uses small bursts of gas through a small "jet port" in the endotracheal tube typically at a rate of 420 per minute, with the range being 240 to 660 breaths per minute.[152] The expiratory phase is passive.[153] Tidal volume is adjusted by controlling the PIP, which is usually initiated at 90% of conventional PIP. CO_2 removal is most affected by the ΔP, or amplitude between the PIP and the PEEP. Therefore an increase in the PIP or decrease in the PEEP will result in enhanced CO_2 elimination. Adjusting the P_{aw}, PEEP, and FiO_2 alters oxygenation. HFJV is typically superimposed on background conventional tidal volume mechanical ventilation.

The utilization of HFJV has decreased in favor of high-frequency oscillatory ventilation (HFOV), which uses a piston pump–driven diaphragm and delivers small volumes at frequencies between 3 and 15 Hz.[152] Both inspiration and expiration are active. Oxygenation is manipulated by adjusting P_{aw}, which controls lung inflation similar to the role of PEEP in conventional mechanical ventilation. CO_2 elimination is controlled by manipulating the tidal volume, also known as the amplitude or power. In short, only four variables are adjusted during HFOV:

1. Mean airway pressure (P_{aw}) is typically initiated at a level 1 to 2 cm H_2O higher in premature newborns and 2 to 4 cm H_2O higher in term newborns and children than that used during conventional

mechanical ventilation.[154] For most disease processes, P_{aw} is adjusted thereafter to maintain the right hemidiaphragm at the rib 8 to 9 level on the anteroposterior chest radiographj.

2. Frequency (Hz) is usually set at 12 Hz in premature newborns and 10 Hz in term patients. Lowering the frequency tends to result in an increase in tidal volume and a decrease in $Paco_2$.
3. Inspiratory time (I_T), which may be increased to enhance tidal volume, is usually set at 33%.
4. Amplitude or power (ρP) is set to achieve good chest-wall movement and adequate CO_2 elimination.

Gas exchange during high-frequency ventilation is thought to occur by convection involving those alveoli located close to airways and, for others, by streaming, a phenomenon in which inspiratory gas, which has a parabolic profile, tends to flow down the center of the airways, whereas the expiratory flow, which has a square profile, takes place at the periphery (Fig. 7-18).[155] Other effects may play a role: (1) Pendelluft, in which gas exchange takes place between lung units with different time constants, as some are filling while others are emptying; (2) the movement of the heart itself may enhance mixing of gases in distal airways; (3) Taylor dispersion, in which convective flow and diffusion together function to enhance distribution of gas; and (4) local diffusion.[156]

High-frequency ventilation should be applied to the newborn and pediatric patient for whom conventional ventilation is failing, because of either parameters of oxygenation or carbon dioxide elimination. The advantage of high-frequency ventilation lies in the alveolar distention and recruitment that is provided while limiting exposure to potentially injurious high ventilator pressures.[157] Thus the approach during high-frequency ventilation should be to apply a mean airway pressure that will effectively recruit alveoli and maintain oxygenation while limiting the ρP to that which will provide chest-wall movement and adequate CO_2 elimination. Carbon dioxide elimination at lower peak inspiratory pressures may be a specific advantage in patients with air leak, especially those with bronchopleural fistulae.[158] Once again, the effect on oxygen delivery, rather than simply Pao_2, should be considered.

Although some studies with HFOV in preterm newborns suggested that the incidence of BPD was similar to that in the conventional ventilation group and that adverse effects were noted on intraventricular hemorrhage and periventricular leukomalacia, other trials noted an increase in the rescue rate and a reduction in BPD in this population.[159–163] One multicenter, randomized trial revealed that 56% of preterm newborns managed with HFOV were alive without the need for supplemental oxygen at 36 weeks postmenstrual age as compared with 47% of those receiving conventional ventilation ($P = .046$).[164]

In an additional pilot study, those preterm infants managed with HFOV were extubated earlier and had decreased supplemental oxygen requirements.[165] Thus although mixed, the data would suggest a reduction in pulmonary morbidity with use of HFOV when compared with conventional ventilation.

In term newborns and pediatric patients with respiratory insufficiency, studies suggested that the rescue rate and survival in those treated with HFOV is significantly increased when compared with conventional mechanical ventilation.[166–168] In a randomized controlled trial of HFOV and inspired nitrous oxide (iNO) in pediatric ARDS, HFOV with or without iNO resulted in greater improvement in the Pao_2/Fio_2 ratio than did conventional mechanical ventilation.[169] However, in contrast, one randomized controlled trial in term newborns failed to identify a significant difference in outcome between these treatment modalities.[170]

Reductions in oxygenation index and Fio_2 were observed during HFOV in 17 adult patients with ARDS.[171] A multicenter, randomized, controlled trial of HFOV for adults with ARDS demonstrated a nonsignificant trend toward improved 30-day mortality in the HFOV group when compared with the CV group (37% vs. 52%, respectively; $P = .102$).[172]

Intratracheal Pulmonary Ventilation or Tracheal Gas Insufflation

Intratracheal pulmonary ventilation (ITPV) involves infusion of fresh gas (oxygen) into the trachea via a cannula placed at the tip of the endotracheal tube. This gas flow effectively replaces the central airway dead space with fresh oxygen during the expiratory phase of the ventilatory cycle and functions to reduce dead space, which augments carbon dioxide elimination. For this purpose, a special "reverse thruster catheter" (RTC) was developed for gas insufflation that reverses the flow of gas at the tip such that it follows a retrograde path up the endotracheal tube (Fig. 7-19).[173] This provides a Venturi effect, which entrains gas, providing for more effective dead-space reduction during expiration. ITPV has been

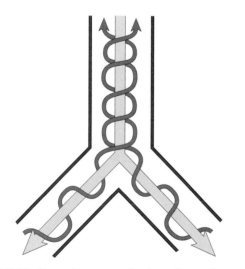

FIGURE 7-18. Streaming as a mechanism of gas exchange during high-frequency ventilation. Note that the parabolic wavefront of the inspiratory gas induces central flow in the airways, whereas expiratory gas flows at the periphery.

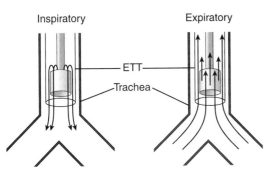

FIGURE 7-19. The reverse-thruster catheter used in performance of intratracheal pulmonary ventilation (ITPV). During inspiration, the exhalation valve on the ventilator closes, and gas flows prograde, filling the lung with a tidal volume of oxygen gas. During expiration, the gas flows retrograde, entraining and replacing the gas in the airways, thereby reducing dead space and Paco2. (Reprinted with permission from Wilson JM, Thompson JR, Schnitzer JJ, et al: Intratracheal pulmonary ventilation and congenital diaphragmatic hernia: a review of two cases. J Pediatr Surg 28:484–487, 1993.)

shown to maintain reasonable levels of ventilation in normal animals at PIPs one half to one third those required during conventional mechanical ventilation. This same group also demonstrated the ability to maintain adequate levels of CO_2 during ITPV, but not during CMV, in lambs in whom only 12.5% of the lung parenchyma remained available for gas exchange.[174] Others have demonstrated that PIPs could be reduced from 28.3 cm H_2O on CMV to 10.3 cm H_2O during ITPV ($P = .028$) in term lambs while maintaining gas exchange.[175] In the same study, initiation of ITPV in lambs resulted in a decrease in PIP from 44 to 32 cm H_2O ($P = .002$), with a simultaneous decrease in Paco2 from 52.2 to 31.9 mm Hg ($P = .029$). This same group also demonstrated that initiation of ITPV in newborn lambs with congenital diaphragmatic hernia led to a decrease in Paco2 from 110 ± 21 to 52 ± 24 ($P = .0014$).[176] The concept of reducing dead space by replacing upper airway gas during the expiratory phase also was applied by using a simple catheter, rather than the RTC, and has been termed *tracheal gas insufflation* (TGI).[42,177]

Clinical studies have demonstrated the ability of ITPV to reduce airway dead space and therefore the ventilator pressures required to achieve equivalent rates of CO_2 elimination when compared with those observed during conventional mechanical ventilation in adult patients with ARDS, pediatric patients on venoarterial ECLS, and newborns with congenital diaphragmatic hernia (CDH) after ECLS.[178–180] TGI was compared with conventional ventilation in a randomized, controlled trial in preterm newborns.[181] The PIP and PEEP were lower, while generating the same Paco2. Time to extubation also was reduced. In adult patients with ARDS, TGI allowed a reduction in PIP without an increase in Paco2.[182]

Inhaled Nitric Oxide Administration

Nitric oxide is an endogenous mediator that serves to stimulate guanylate cyclase in the endothelial cell to produce cyclic guanosine monophosphate (cGMP), which results in relaxation of vascular smooth muscle (Fig. 7-20).[183] NO is rapidly scavenged by heme moieties. As such, inhaled nitric oxide (iNO) serves as a selective vasodilator of the pulmonary circulation because it is inactivated before reaching the systemic circulation. It is diluted in nitrogen and then mixed with blended oxygen and air to administer it in doses of from 1 to 80 parts per million (ppm).

Initial studies in adults with ARDS who were treated with iNO demonstrated a decrease in pulmonary vascular resistance and an increase in Pao2, without change in systemic arterial pressure. In addition, a prospective, multicenter, randomized trial of iNO in 177 adults with ARDS demonstrated a significant improvement in oxygenation compared with placebo over the first 4 hours of treatment (Pao2 increase $\geq 20\%$: iNO, 60%; CMV, 24%; $P = .00002$).[184–186] This initial increase in oxygenation translated to a reduction in Fio2 over the first day and in the intensity of mechanical ventilation over the first 4 days of treatment. However, no differences were observed between the pooled iNO groups and placebo groups with respect to mortality rate and number of days alive and off mechanical ventilation. A subgroup of patients who received iNO at a dose of 5 ppm showed an improvement in the number of patients alive and off

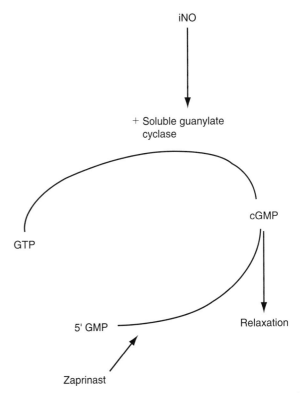

FIGURE 7-20. Mechanism of action of inhaled nitrous oxide (iNO) in inducing vascular smooth muscle relaxation. Aprinast is a phosphodiesterase inhibitor that may increase the potency and duration of the effect of iNO. (Reprinted with permission from Hirschl RB: Innovative therapies in the management of newborns with congenital diaphragmatic hernia. Semin Pediatr Surg 5:255–265, 1996.)

mechanical ventilation at day 28 (62% vs. 44%; $P < .05$). In another randomized and controlled trial in adults, iNO increased PaO_2/FiO_2 at 1 hour and 12 hours.[187] Beyond 24 hours, the two groups demonstrated an equivalent improvement in PaO_2/FiO_2. Pediatric patients with respiratory failure demonstrate increases in PaO_2 with iNO at 20 ppm.[188] Unfortunately, a prospective, randomized, controlled trial of the effects of iNO therapy in children with respiratory failure revealed that, although pulmonary vascular resistance and systemic oxygenation were acutely improved at 1 hour by administration of 10 ppm iNO, a sustained improvement at 24 hours was not identified.[189]

It has been observed that only 40% of the iNO-treated term infants with pulmonary hypertension required ECLS when compared with 71% of the control subjects.[190] These results were corroborated by demonstrating a reduction in the need for ECLS in control newborns (ECLS, 64%) when compared with iNO-treated newborns (ECLS, 38%; $P = 0.001$).[191] The incidence of chronic lung disease was decreased in newborns managed with iNO (7% vs. 20%). Similar results were noted for infants with persistent pulmonary hypertension of the newborn (PPHN) who were on HFOV: the need for ECLS was decreased from 55% in the control HFOV group to 14% in the combined iNO and HFOV group ($P = .007$).[192] In a clinical trial conducted by The Neonatal Inhaled Nitric Oxide Study (NINOS) Group, neonates born at 34 weeks or older gestational age with hypoxic respiratory failure were randomized to receive 20 ppm iNO or 100% oxygen as a control.[193] If a complete response, defined as an increase in PaO_2 of more than 20 mm Hg within 30 minutes after gas initiation, was not observed, then iNO at 80 ppm was administered. Sixty-four percent of the control group and 46% of the iNO group died within 120 days or were treated with ECLS ($P = .006$). No difference in death was found between the two groups (iNO, 14% vs. control, 17%), but significantly fewer neonates in the iNO group required ECLS (39% vs. 54%). Follow-up at age 18 to 24 months failed to demonstrate a difference in the incidence of cerebral palsy, rate of sensorineural hearing loss, and mental developmental index scores between the control and iNO patients.[194] Other studies have similarly failed to identify a difference in pulmonary, neurologic, cognitive, or behavioral outcomes between survivors managed with iNO and those in the conventional group.[195]

An associated, but separate, trial demonstrated no difference in death rates and a significant increase in need for ECLS when neonates with CDH were treated with 20 or 80 ppm of iNO versus 100% oxygen as control.[196] It should be noted, however, that some investigators have suggested that the efficacy of iNO in patients with CDH may be more substantial after surfactant administration or at the point at which recurrent pulmonary hypertension occurs.[197] iNO administration also may be helpful in the moribund CDH patient until ECLS can be initiated.

Some concern has been expressed for the development of intracranial hemorrhage in premature newborns treated with iNO. Although a more than 25% increase in the arterial/alveolar oxygen ratio (PaO_2/PAO_2) was observed

in 10 of 11 premature newborns with a mean gestational age of 29.8 weeks and severe RDS in response to administration of 1 to 20 ppm iNO, in 7 of these 11 newborns, intracranial hemorrhage developed during their hospitalization.[198] However, a meta-analysis of the three completed studies evaluating the efficacy of iNO in premature newborns suggests no significant difference in survival, incidence of chronic lung disease, or rate of development of intracranial hemorrhage between iNO and control patients.[199]

It should be recognized that NO is associated with the production of potentially toxic metabolites: when combined with O_2, iNO produces peroxynitrates, which can be damaging to epithelial cells and also can inhibit surfactant function.[200,201] Nitrogen dioxide, which is toxic, also can be produced, and hemoglobin may be oxidized to methemoglobin. Additional concerns exist about the immunosuppressive effects and the potential for platelet dysfunction.

Surfacant Replacement Therapy

The use of exogenous surfactant has been responsible for a 30% to 40% reduction in the odds of death among very low birth weight newborns with RDS (Fig. 7-21).[202,203] In addition, in those premature neonates with birthweight more than 1250 g, mortality in a controlled, randomized, blinded study decreased from 7% to 4%.[204] Two general forms of surfactant are available: synthetic surfactant (e.g., Exosurf; Burroughs Wellcome, Raleigh-Durham, NC), which is made of dipalmytoyl phosphatidylcholine and is protein free; and bovine surfactant extracts (e.g., Survanta; Ross Laboratories, Columbus, OH; or Infrasurf; ONY, Inc., Amherst, NY), which contains natural surfactants and associated proteins. Studies reveal a significantly

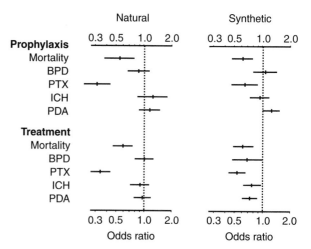

FIGURE 7-21. A meta-analysis of studies evaluating the outcome and complications of the prophylactic use and treatment approach to exogenous natural and synthetic surfactant administration in preterm newborns. (Adapted from Jobe AH: Pulmonary surfactant therapy. N Engl J Med 328:861–868, 1993, with permission.)

lower risk of chronic lung disease in Survanta (27%) when compared with the Exosurf (34%) infants with birth weights of 1001 to 1500 g.[205] Compared with that with Exosurf, Infasurf treatment results in a 62% decrease in the incidence of RDS (Infasurf, 16% vs. Exosurf, 42%) and a 70% decrease in death due to RDS (Infasurf, 1.7% vs. Exosurf, 5.4%).[206] However, IVH occurs more frequently in Infasurf-treated infants (Infasurf, 39.0% vs. Exosurf, 29.9%).

A randomized, prospective, controlled trial in term newborns with respiratory insufficiency demonstrated that the need for ECMO was significantly reduced in those managed with surfactant when compared with placebo.[207] The benefit of surfactant was greatest in those with a lower oxygenation index (<23). Another controlled, randomized study demonstrated the utility of surfactant in term newborns with the meconium aspiration syndrome.[208] The oxygen index minimally decreased with the initial dose, but markedly decreased with the second and third doses of surfactant from a baseline of 23.7 to 5.9 (Fig. 7-22). After three doses of surfactant, PPHN had resolved in all but one of the infants in the study group versus none of the infants in the control group. The incidence of air leaks and need for ECLS were markedly reduced in the surfactant group compared with the control patients.

Studies have concluded that surfactant phospholipid concentration, synthesis, and kinetics are not significantly deranged in infants with CDH compared with controls, although surfactant protein A concentrations may be reduced in CDH newborns on ECMO.[209–211] Animal and human studies have suggested that surfactant administration before the first breath is associated with enhancement in PaO$_2$ and pulmonary mechanics.[212,213] However, among CDH patients on ECLS, no difference between those randomized to receive surfactant ($n = 9$) and those control patients receiving air ($n = 8$) was noted in terms of lung compliance, time to extubation, period of oxygen requirement, and total number of hospital days.[209]

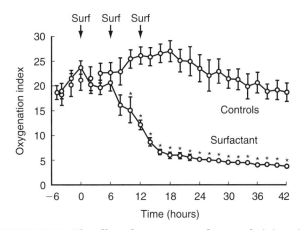

FIGURE 7-22. The effect of exogenous surfactant administration on oxygen index in term newborns with meconium-aspiration syndrome. (Reprinted with permission from Findlay RD, Taeusch HW, Walther FJ: Surfactant replacement therapy for meconium aspiration syndrome. Pediatrics 97:48–52, 1996.)

Liquid Ventilation with Perfluorocarbon

Perfluorocarbons are clear, colorless, odorless fluids that carry large amounts of oxygen (50 mL O$_2$/dL) and carbon dioxide (210 mL CO$_2$/dL).[214] They are relatively dense fluids (1.9 g/mL) and have low surface tension (19 din/cm). Liquid ventilation has been performed by one of two methods.[215] The first is *total* liquid ventilation (TLV), in which the lungs are filled with perfluorocarbon to a volume equivalent to FRC, on which a device is used to generate tidal volumes of perfluorocarbon in the perfluorocarbon-filled lung.[216] The second technique of liquid ventilation involves administration of intratracheal perfluorocarbon to a volume equivalent to FRC followed by standard gas mechanical ventilation of the perfluorocarbon-filled lung, otherwise known as *partial liquid ventilation* (PLV).[217] The former technique appears to be somewhat more effective at enhancing gas exchange, whereas the latter technique is more easily generalized to critical care clinicians managing patients with severe respiratory insufficiency.

A number of studies have demonstrated the efficacy of PLV in enhancing gas exchange in animal models of respiratory insufficiency.[218–221] It appears that intratracheal administration of perfluorocarbon acts as a surrogate surfactant, recruits atelectatic lung regions, and redistributes pulmonary blood flow toward the better-ventilated, nondependent regions of the lungs in the patient with ARDS.[22,222] Of great interest is the demonstration of enhanced gas exchange with aerosolized perfluorocarbon in saline-lavaged, surfactant-depleted piglets: PaO$_2$ was higher and PaCO$_2$ lower in the PLV and aerosolized perfluorocarbon group compared with that in the standard mechanical-ventilation animals.[223] This response was sustained after discontinuation of aerosolization, but not standard PLV. A number of phase I and II clinical studies have demonstrated the efficacy of PLV in enhancing oxygenation and pulmonary mechanics in adults, children, and newborns with respiratory insufficiency, including those with CDH and those that are premature.[224–227] Studies in pediatric and adult patients have demonstrated decreases in the (A-a)DO$_2$ from approximately 450 to 250 mm Hg within the first 48 hours after initiation of PLV.[228] However, prospective, controlled, randomized pilot studies evaluating the safety and efficacy of PLV in adult and pediatric patients with respiratory insufficiency have shown no differences between the PLV and CMV groups. A surprisingly low mortality of 20% among the pediatric patients with isolated respiratory failure prohibited successful completion of the study, and it was discontinued. Among adult patients with ALI or ARDS, no difference in ventilatory pulmonary mechanics, gas-exchange parameter, or in survival were noted between the PLV ($n = 65$) and CMV ($n = 25$) patients.[229] In May 2001, the results of a multicenter, prospective, randomized study comparing PLV and CMV in adults with ARDS revealed no significant difference in mortality or 28-day VFD in the PLV compared with those in the CMV group.[230] Although PLV may be further evaluated in subgroups of adult and pediatric patients with respiratory failure, it is unlikely that

PLV will play a general role in the treatment of adult or pediatric ARDS.

Premature newborns for whom surfactant therapy fails demonstrate a twofold increase in mean pulmonary compliance and a decrease in mean oxygen index from approximately 50 to 10 over the 24-hour period after initiation of partial liquid ventilation, although a pilot randomized study failed to reveal increased survival in the PLV compared with the CMV group.[231] Likewise a prospective, randomized, controlled pilot trial evaluating PLV in term newborns with respiratory failure did not demonstrate an increase in survival in the PLV compared with that in the CMV patients.

Studies have demonstrated the ability of in utero tracheal ligation to correct the structural and physiologic effects of pulmonary hypoplasia in the sheep fetus with CDH.[232,233] The ability to induce lung growth has been demonstrated by distention of the isolated right upper lobe in newborn sheep with perflubron (LiquiVent; Alliance Pharmaceutical Corp.; San Diego, CA) to a pressure of 7 to 10 mm Hg O.[234] These data demonstrated an increase in size and alveolar number in the right upper

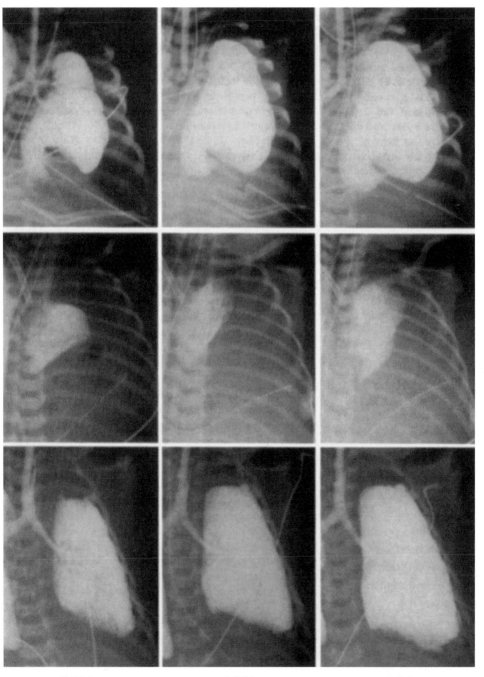

DAY 1   DAY 3   DAY 7

FIGURE 7-23. Progression of the distended lungs ipsilateral to the hernia with time (the perfluorocarbon is radiopaque) in the three patients that received 7 days of pulmonary distention with perfluorocarbon. Notice the evident increase in lung size, which was not observed in the contralateral lungs. (Reprinted with permission from Fauza DO, Hirschl RB, Wilson JM: Continuous intrapulmonary distension with perfluorocarbon accelerates lung growth in infants with congenital diaphragmatic hernia: initial experience. J Pediatr Surg 36:1237–1240, 2001.)

lobe while maintaining the air-space fraction, the protein/DNA ratio, and the alveolar/arterial ratio unchanged compared with those in nondistended control animals. This technique of perfluorocarbon-induced lung growth (PILG) would apply to patients with CDH who required ECLS. The use of PILG demonstrated radiologic evidence of an increase in ipsilateral lung size in CDH patients managed with PILG (Fig. 7-23).[235] A randomized, prospective, controlled pilot study demonstrated encouraging survival rates of six (75%) of eight in PILG-treated CDH patients on ECLS compared with two (40%) of five in conventionally treated patients on ECLS.[236]

In 1989, the first report of the use of TLV in humans was published.[234,237] Three moribund, preterm newborns, for whom surfactant therapy had failed, were managed with TLV. Pulmonary compliance increased during the period of TLV. The gas-exchange response was variable. However, this was the first demonstration of the ability to sustain gas exchange during TLV in humans. A multicenter study of TLV in pediatric models of ARDS demonstrated increased oxygenation and pulmonary function with enhancement in cardiac output and decrease in histologic parameters of lung injury in the TLV group.[238] Although not yet effectively tested in the clinical setting, these data suggest that TLV may play a significant role in lavaging, reinflating, and ventilating injured lungs.

REFERENCES

1. Baker AB: Artificial respiration, the history of an idea. Med Hist 15:336–351, 1971.
2. Matas R: Intralaryngeal insufflation. JAMA 34:1468–1473, 1900.
3. Daily WJR, Smith PC: Mechanical ventilation of the newborn infant. Curr Probl Pediatr 1:3–37, 1971.
4. Emerson JH: The evolution of iron lungs. Cambridge, JH Emerson, 1978.
5. Magill IW: Endotracheal anesthesia. Proc R Soc Med 22:83–88, 1928.
6. Rowbotham S: Intratracheal anesthesia by the nasal route for operation on the mouth and lips. Br Med J 1:590–591, 1920.
7. Eckman M, Barach B, Fox C, et al: An appraisal of intermittent pressure breathing as a method of increasing altitude tolerance. J Aviat Med 18:565–574, 1947.
8. Stahlman MT, Young WC, Payne G: Studies of ventilatory aids in hyaline membrane disease. Am J Dis Child 104:526, 1962.
9. Cassani VL: We've come a long way baby! Mechanical ventilation of the newborn. Neonatal Netw 13:63–68, 1994.
10. Avery ME, Mead J: Surface properties in relation to atelectasis and hyaline membrane disease. Am J Dis Child 97:517–523, 1959.
11. Thomas DV, Fletcher G, Sunshine P, et al: Prolonged respiratory use in pulmonary insufficiency of the newborn. JAMA 193:183, 1965.
12. Gregory GA, Kitterman JA, Phibbs RH, et al: Treatment of the idiopathic respiratory distress syndrome with continuous positive airway pressure. N Engl J Med 284:1333, 1971.
13. Kossel H, Versmold H: 25 years of respiratory support of newborn infants. J Perinat Med 25:421–432, 1997.
14. Bartlett RH: Use of the mechanical ventilator. In Douglas MD, Wilmore W (eds): Surgery. New York, Scientific American, 1988.
15. West JB: Respiratory Physiology: The Essentials. Satterfield TS (ed): Baltimore, Williams & Wilkins, 1990, pp 1–185.
16. Gattinoni L, Mascheroni D, Basilico E, et al: Volume/pressure curve of total respiratory system in paralysed patients: Artefacts and correction factors. Intens Care Med 13:19–25, 1987.
17. Gama AM, Meyer EC, Gaudencio AM, et al: Different low constant flows can equally determine the lower inflection point in acute respiratory distress syndrome patients. Artif Organs 25:882–889, 2002.
18. Kondili E, Prinianakis G, Hoeing S, et al: Low flow inflation pressure-time curve in patients with acute respiratory distress syndrome. Intens Care Med 26:1756–63, 2000.
19. Harris RS, Hess DR, Venegas JG: An objective analysis of the pressure-volume curve in the acute respiratory distress syndrome. Am J Respir Crit Care Med 161:432–439, 2000.
20. Putensen C, Baum M, Hormann C: Selecting ventilator settings according to variables derived from the quasi-static pressure/volume relationship in patients with acute lung injury. Anesth Analg 77:436–447, 1993.
21. Bartel LP, Bazik JR, Powner DJ: Compression volume during mechanical ventilation: comparision of ventilators and tubing circuits. Crit Care Med 13:851–854, 1985.
22. Gattinoni L, Pesenti A, Mascheroni D, et al: Low-frequency positive-pressure ventilation with extracorporeal CO_2 removal in severe acute respiratory failure. JAMA 256:881–886, 1986.
23. Zwischenberger J, Wang D, Lick SD, et al: The paracorporeal artificial lung improves 5-day outcomes from lethal smoke/burn-induced acute respiratory distress syndrome in sheep. Ann Thorac Surg 74:1011–1016, 2002.
24. Gattinoni L, D'Andrea L, Pelosi P, et al: Regional effects and mechanism of positive end-expiratory pressure in early adult respiratory distress syndrome. JAMA 269:2122–2127, 1993.
25. Maunder RJ, Shuman WP, McHugh JW, et al: Preservation of normal lung regions in the adult respiratory distress syndrome: Analysis by computed tomography. JAMA 255:2463–2465, 1986.
26. White KM: Completing the hemodynamic picture: Svo2. Heart Lung 14:272–280, 1985.
27. Nelson L: Continuous venous oximetry in surgical patients. Ann Surg 203:329–333, 1986.
28. Rivers EP, Ander DS, Powell D: Central venous oxygen saturation monitoring in the critically ill patient. Curr Opin Crit Care 7:204–211, 2001.
29. Jan K, Usami S, Smith JA: Effects of transfusion on rheological properties of blood in sickle cell anemia. Transfusion 22:17–20, 1982.
30. Marini JJ: Pressure-targeted, lung-protective ventilatory support in acute lung injury. Chest Suppl 105:109S–116S, 1994.
31. Parker JC, Townsley MI, Rippe B, et al: Increased microvascular permeability in dog lungs due to high peak airway pressures. J Appl Physiol 57:1809–1816, 1984.
32. Ranieri VM, Mascia L, Fiore T, et al: Cardiorespiratory effects of positive end-expiratory pressure during progressive tidal volume reduction (permissive hypercapnia) in patients with acute respiratory distress syndrome. Anesthesiology 83:710–720, 1995.
33. Michaels AJ, Wanek SM, Dreifuss BA, et al: A protocolized approach to pulmonary failure and the role of intermittent prone positioning. J Trauma Injury Infect Crit Care 52:1037–1047, 2002.
34. Palmisano BW, Fisher DM, Willis M, et al: The effect of paralysis on oxygen consumption in normoxic children after cardiac surgery. Anesthesiology 61:518, 1984.
35. Coggeshall JW, Marini JJ, Newman JH: Improved oxygenation after muscle relaxation in adult respiratory distress syndrome. Arch Intern Med 145:1718–1720, 1985.
36. Ganong WF: Energy Balance, Metabolism, & Nutrition, in Review of Medical Physiology. Los Altos, Calif, Lange Medical Publications, 1979.
37. Kacmarek RM, Hess D: Basic principles of ventilator machinery. In Tobin MJ (ed.): Principles and Practice of Mechanical Ventilation. New York, McGraw-Hill, 1994, pp 65-110.
38. Pilbeam SP: Physical aspects of mechanical ventilators. In Russell J (ed): Mechanical Ventilation: Physiological and Clinical Applications. St. Louis, Mosby, 1998, pp 62–91.
39. Piotrowski A, Sobala W, Kawczynski P: Patient-initiated, pressure-regulated, volume-controlled ventilation compared with intermittent mandatory ventilation in neonates: A prospective, randomised study. Intens Care Med 23:975–981, 1927.
40. Sinha SK, Donn SM: Volume-controlled ventilation: Variations on a theme. Clin Perinatol 28:547–560, 2001.
41. Abraham E, Yoshihara G: Cardiorespiratory effects of pressure controlled ventilation in severe respiratory failure. Chest 98:1445–1449, 1990.
42. Nahum A, Burke WC, Ravenscraft SA, et al: Lung mechanics and gas exchange during pressure-control ventilation in dogs: Augmentation of CO_2 elimination by an intratracheal catheter. Am Rev Respir Dis 146:965–973, 1992.

43. Kirby RR: Intermittent mandatory ventilation in the neonate. Crit Care Med 5:18–22, 1977.

44. Bernstein G, Mannino FL, Heldt HP, et al: Randomized multicenter trial comparing synchronized and conventional intermittent mandatory ventilation in neonates. J Pediatr 129:948–950, 1996.

45. Cleary JP, Bernstein G, Mannino FL, et al: Improved oxygenation during synchronized intermittent mandatory ventilation in neonates with respiratory distress syndrome: A randomized, crossover study. J Pediatr 126:407–411, 1995.

46. Chen JY, Ling UP, Chen JH: Comparison of synchronized and conventional intermittent mandatory ventilation in neonates. Acta Paediatr Jpn 39:578–583, 1997.

47. Greenough A, Milner AD, Dimitriou G: Synchronized mechanical ventilation for respiratory support in newborn infants. Cochrane Database Syst Rev 2001.

48. Leung P, Jubran A, Tobin MJ: Comparison of assisted ventilator modes on triggering, patient effort, and dyspnea. AJRCCM 155:1940–1948, 1997.

49. Jarreau PH, Moriette G, Mussat P, et al: Patient-triggered ventilation decreases the work of breathing in neonates. AJRCCM 153:1176–1181, 1996.

50. Dekel B, Segal E, Perel A: Pressure support ventilation. Arch Intern Med 156:369–373, 1996.

51. Banner MJ, Kirby RR, Blanch PB, et al: Decreasing imposed work of the breathing apparatus to zero using pressure-support ventilation. Crit Care Med 21:1333–1338, 1993.

52. Kacmarek RM: The role of pressure support ventilation in reducing the work of breathing. Respir Care 33:99–120, 1988.

53. Brochard L, Pluskwa F, Lemaire F: Improved efficacy of spontaneous breathing with inspiratory pressure support. Crit Care Med 136:411–415, 1987.

54. Gullberg N, Winberg P, Sellden H: Pressure support ventilation increases cardiac output in neonates and infants. Paediatr Anaesth 6:311–315, 1996.

55. Tokioka H, Kinjo M, Hirakawa M: The effectiveness of pressure support ventilation for mechanical ventilatory support in children. Anesthesiology 78:880–884, 1993.

56. Marraro GA: Innovative practices of ventilatory support with pediatric patients. Pediatr Crit Care Med 4:8–20, 2003.

57. Randolph AG, Wypij D, Venkataraman ST, et al: Effect of mechanical ventilator weaning protocols on respiratory outcomes in infants and children: a randomized controlled trial. JAMA 288:2561–2568, 2002.

58. Amato MB, Barbas CS, Bonassa J, et al: Volume-assured pressure support ventilation (VAPSV): A new approach for reducing muscle workload during acute respiratory failure. Chest 102:1225–1234, 1992.

59. Younes M: Proportional assist ventilation, a new approach to ventilatory support. Crit Care Med 149:268, 1994.

60. Younes M: Proportional assist ventilation and pressure support ventilation: similarities and differences. Intens Care Emerg Med 15:361–380, 1991.

61. Bigatello LM, Nishimura M, Imanaka H, et al: Unloading of the work of breathing by proportional assist ventilation in a lung model. Crit Care Med 25:267–272, 1997.

62. Younes M, Puddy A, Roberts D, et al: Proportional assist ventilation: Results of an initial clinical trial. Am Rev Respir Dis 145:121–129, 1992.

63. Schulze A, Bancalari E: Proportional assist ventilation in infants. Clin Perinatol 28:561–578, 2001.

64. Schulze A, Gerhardt T, Musante G, et al: Proportional assist ventilation in low birth weight infants with acute respiratory disease: A comparison to assist/control and conventional mechanical ventilation. J Pediatr 135:339–344, 1999.

65. Musante G, Schulze A, Gerhardt T, et al: Proportional assist ventilation decreases thoracoabdominal asynchrony and chest wall distortion in preterm infants. Pediatr Res 49:175–180, 2001.

66. Gittermann MK, Fusch C, Gittermann AR, Regazzoni BM, Moessinger AC: Early nasal continuous positive airway pressure treatment reduces the need for intubation in very low birth weight infants. Eur J Pediatr 156:384–388, 1997.

67. Lain DC, DiBenedetto R, Morris SL, et al: Pressure control inverse ratio ventilation as a method to reduce peak inspiratory pressure and provide adequate ventilation and oxygenation. Chest 95:1081–1088, 1989.

68. Tharratt RS, Allen RP, Albertson TE: Pressure controlled inverse ratio ventilation in severe adult respiratory failure. Chest 94:755–762, 1988.

69. Marcy TW, Marini JJ: Inverse ratio ventilation in ARDS: Rationale and implementation. Chest 100:494–504, 1991.

70. Porembka DT: Inverse ratio ventilation. Probl Respir Care 2:69–76, 1989.

71. McCarthy MC, Cline AL, Lemmon GW, et al: Pressure control inverse ratio ventilation in the treatment of adult respiratory distress syndrome in patients with blunt chest trauma. Am Surg 65:1027–1030, 1999.

72. Mercat A, Titiriga M, Anguel N, et al: Inverse ratio ventilation (I/E = 2/1) in acute respiratory distress syndrome: A six-hour controlled study. AJRCCM 155:1637–1642, 1997.

73. Armstrong BWJ, MacIntyre NR: Pressure-controlled, inverse ratio ventilation that avoids air trapping in the adult respiratory distress syndrome. Crit Care Med 23:279–285, 1995.

74. Mancebo J, Vallverdu I, Bak E, et al, Volume-controlled ventilation and pressure-controlled inverse ratio ventilation: A comparison of their effects in ARDS patients. Monaldi Arch Chest Dis 49:201–207, 1994.

75. Lessard MR, Guerot E, Lorino H, et al: Effects of pressure-controlled with different I:E ratios versus volume-controlled ventilation on respiratory mechanics, gas exchange, and hemodynamics in patients with adult respiratory distress syndrome. Anesthesiology 80:983–991, 1994.

76. Goldstein B, Papadokos PJ: Pressure-controlled inverse-ratio ventilation in children with acute respiratory failure. Am J Crit Care 3:11–15, 1994.

77. Wang SH, Wei TS: The outcome of early pressure-controlled inverse ratio ventilation on patients with severe acute respiratory distress syndrome in surgical intensive care unit. Am J Surg 183:151–155, 2002.

78. Huang CC, Shih MJ, Tsai YH, et al: Effects of inverse ratio ventilation versus positive end-expiratory pressure on gas exchange and gastric intramucosal PCO(2) and pH under constant mean airway pressure in acute respiratory distress syndrome. Anesthesiology 95:1182–1188, 2002.

79. McIntyre RC, Pulido EJ, Bensard DD, et al: Thirty years of clinical trials in acute respiratory distress syndrome. Crit Care Med 28:3314–3331, 2000.

80. Chiang AA, Steinfeld A, Cooper C, et al: Demand-flow airway pressure release ventilation as a partial ventilatory support mode: Comparison with synchronized intermittent mandatory ventilation and pressure support ventilation. Crit Care Med 22:1431–1437, 1994.

81. Rasanen J, Cane RD, Downs JV, et al: Airway pressure release ventilation during acute lung injury: A prospective multicenter trial. Crit Care Med 19:1234–1241, 1991.

82. Neumann P, Golisch W, Strohmeyer A, et al: Influence of different release times on spontaneous breathing pattern during airway pressure release ventilation. Intens Care Med 28:1742–1749, 2002.

83. Hering R, Peters D, Zinserling J, et al: Effects of spontaneous breathing during airway pressure release ventilation on renal perfusion and function in patients with acute lung injury. Intens Care Med 28:1426–1433, 2002.

84. Cane RD, Peruzzi WT, Shapiro BA: Airway pressure release ventilation in severe acute respiratory failure. Chest 100:460–463, 1991.

85. Valentine DD, Hammond MD, Downs JB, et al: Distribution of ventilation perfusion with different modes of mechanical ventilation. Am Rev Respir Dis 143:1262–1266, 1991.

86. Kaplan LJ, Bailey H, Formosa V: Airway pressure release ventilation increases cardiac performance in patients with acute lung injury/adult respiratory distress syndrome. Crit Care (Lond) 5:221–226, 2001.

87. Martin LD, Wetzel RC, Bilenki AL: Airway pressure release ventilation in a neonatal lamb model of acute lung injury. Crit Care Med 19:373–378, 1991.

88. Foland JA, Martin J, Novotny T, et al: Airway pressure release ventilation with a short release time in a child with acute respiratory distress syndrome. Respir Care 46:1019–1023, 2001.

89. Padman R, Lawless ST, Kettrick RG: Noninvasive ventilation via bilevel positive airway pressure support in pediatric practice. Crit Care Med 26:169–173, 1988.

90. Lofaso F, Brochard L, Hang T, et al: Home versus intensive care pressure support devices: Experimental and clinical comparison. AJRCCM 153:1591–1599, 1996.

91. Baxley WA, Cavender JB, Knoblock J: Continuous cardiac output monitoring by the Fick method. Cathet Cardiovasc Diagn 28:89–92, 1993.

92. Hollinger IB: Postoperative management: Ventilation. Int Anesth Clin 18:205–216, 1980.

93. Jenkinson SG: Oxygen toxicity. New Horizons 1:504–511, 1993.

94. Wolfe WG, DeVries WC: Oxygen toxicity. Annu Rev Med 26:203–217, 1975.

95. Gladstone IM Jr, Levine RL: Oxidation of proteins in neonatal lungs. Pediatrics 93:764–768, 1994.

96. Wung JT, James LS, Kilchevsky E, et al: Management of infants with severe respiratory failure and persistence of the fetal circulation without hyperventilation. Pediatrics 76:488, 1985.

97. Webb HH, Tierney DF: Experimental pulmonary edema due to intermittent positive pressure ventilation with high inflation pressures: Protection by positive end-expiratory pressure. Am Rev Respir Dis 110:556–565, 1974.

98. Fu Z, Costello ML, Tsukimoto K, et al: High lung volume increases stress failure in pulmonary capillaries. J Appl Physiol 73:123–133, 1992.

99. Kolobow T, Moretti MP, Fumagalli R, et al: Severe impairment in lung function induced by high peak airway pressure during mechanical ventilation. Am Rev Respir Dis 135:312–315, 1987.

100. Dreyfuss D, Basset G, Soler P, et al: Intermittent positive-pressure hyperventilation with high inflation pressures produces pulmonary microvascular injury in rats. Am Rev Respir Dis 132:880–884, 1985.

101. Hernandez LA, Peevy K, Moise AA, et al: Chest wall restriction limits high airway pressure-induced lung injury in young rabbits. J Appl Physiol 66:2364–2368, 1989.

102. Savel R, Yao E, Gropper M: Protective effects of low tidal volume ventilation in a rabbit model of *Pseudomonas aeruginosa*-induced acute lung injury. Crit Care Med 29:392–398, 2001.

103. Rich PB, Reickert CA, Sawada S, et al: Effect of rate and inspiratory flow on ventilator induced lung injury. J Trauma 49:903–911, 2000.

104. Nahum A, Hoyt J, Schmitz L, et al: Effect of mechanical ventilation strategy on dissemination of intratracheally instilled *Escherichia coli* in dogs. Crit Care Med 25:1733–1743, 1997.

105. Stewart TE, Meade M, Cook DJ, et al: Evaluation of a ventilation strategy to prevent barotrauma in patients at high risk for acute respiratory distress syndrome. N Engl J Med 338:355–361, 1998.

106. Brochard L: Low versus high tidal volumes. In Vincent JL (ed): Acute Lung Injury. Brussels, Springer-Verlag, pp 276–281, 1998.

107. Amato MB, Barbas CS, Mederios DM, et al: Effect of a protective-ventilation strategy on mortality in the acute respiratory distress syndrome. N Engl J Med 338:347–354, 1998.

108. Ranieri VM, Suter PM, Tortoralla T, et al: Effect of mechanical ventilation on inflammatory mediators in patients with acute respiratory distress syndrome. JAMA 282:54–61, 1999.

109. The Acute Respiratory Distress Syndrome Network: Ventilation with lower tidal volumes as compared with traditional tidal volumes for acute lung injury and the acute respiratory distress syndrome. New Engl J Med 342:1301–1308, 2000.

110. Ranieri V, Giunta F, Suter P, et al: Mechanical ventilation as a mediator of multisystem organ failure in acute respiratory distress syndrome [Letter]. JAMA 284:43–44, 2000.

111. Zach TL, Steinhorn RH, Georgieff MK, et al: Complications of neonatal extracorporeal membrane oxygenation [Letter]: Leukopenia associated with extracorporeal membrane oxygenation in newborn infants. J Pediatr 116:1005–1007, 1990.

112. Hickling KG: Low volume ventilation with permissive hypercapnea in the adult respiratory distress syndrome. Clin Intens Care 3:67–78, 1992.

113. Hickling KG, Walsh J, Henderson S, et al: Low mortality rate in adult respiratory distress syndrome using low-volume, pressure-limited ventilation with permissive hypercapnia: A prospective study. Crit Care Med 22:1568–1578, 1994.

114. Sheridan R, Kacmarek R, McEttrick M, et al: Permissive hypercapnia as a ventilatory strategy in burned children: Effect on barotrauma, pneumonia, and mortality. J Trauma 39:854–859, 1995.

115. Paulson TE, Spear RM, Silva PD, et al: High-frequency pressure-control ventilation with high positive end-expiratory pressure in children with acute respiratory distress syndrome. J Pediatr 129:566–573, 1996.

116. McCulloch PR, Forkert PG, Forese AB: Lung volume maintenance prevents lung injury during high frequency oscillatory ventilation in surfactant-deficient rabbits. Am Rev Respir Dis 137:1185–1192, 1988.

117. Dreyfuss D, Sjoer P, Basset G, et al: High inflation pressure pulmonary edema: Respective effects of high airway pressure, high tidal volume, and positive end-expiratory pressure. Am Rev Respir Dis 137:1159–1164, 1988.

118. Lachmann B: Open up the lung and keep the lung open. Intens Care Med 18:319–321, 1992.

119. Mancebo J: PEEP, ARDS, and alveolar recruitment. Intens Care Med 18:383–385, 1992.

120. Gattinoni L, Pesenti A, Avalli L, et al: Pressure-volume curve of total respiratory system in acute respiratory failure. Am Rev Respir Dis 136:730–736, 1987.

121. Roupie E, Dambrosio M, Servillo G, et al: Titration of tidal volume and induced hypercapnia in acute respiratory distress syndrome. AJRCCM 152:121–128, 1995.

122. Gattinoni L, Presenti A: Adult Respiratory Distress Syndrome: Computed Tomography Scanning in Acute Respiratory Failure. New York, Marcel Dekker, 1991.

123. Crotti S, Mascheroni D, Caironi P, et al: Recruitment and derecruitment during acute respiratory failure. AJRCCM 164:131–140, 2001.

124. Desai S, Wells A, Suntharalingam G, et al: Acute respiratory distress syndrome caused by pulmonary and extrapulmonary injury: A comparative CT study. Radiology 218:689–693, 2001.

125. DiRusso SM, Nelson LD, Safcsak K, et al: Survival in patients with severe adult respiratory distress syndrome treated with high-level positive end-expiratory pressure. Crit Care Med 23:1485–1496, 1995.

126. Nagano O, Tokioka H, Ohta Y, et al: Inspiratory pressure-volume curves at different positive end-expiratory pressure levels in patients with ALI/ARDS. Acta Anaesth Scand 45:1255–1261, 2001.

127. Valente Barbas CS: Lung recruitment maneuvers in acute respiratory distress syndrome and facilitating resolution. Crit Care Med 31:265–271, 2003.

128. Witte MK, Galli SA, Ghatburn RL, et al: Optimal positive end-expiratory pressure therapy in infants and children with acute respiratory failure. Pediatr Res 24:217–221, 1988.

129. Bartlett R, Roloff DW, Custer J, et al: Extracorporeal life support: The University of Michigan experience. JAMA 283:904–908, 2000.

130. Sjostrand UH, Lichtwarch-Aschoff M, Nielsen JB, et al: Different ventilatory approaches to keep the lung open. Intens Care Med 21:310–318, 1995.

131. Papadakos PJ, Halloran W, Hessney JI, et al: The use of pressure-controlled inverse ratio ventilation in the surgical intensive care unit. J Trauma 31:1211–1214, 1991.

132. Pappert D, Rossaint R, Slama K, et al: Influence of positioning on ventilation-perfusion relationships in severe adult respiratory distress syndrome. Chest 106:1511–1516, 1994.

133. Fridrich P, Krafft P, Hochleuthner H, et al: The effects of long-term prone positioning in patients with trauma-induced adult respiratory distress syndrome. Anesth Analg 83:1206–1211, 1996.

134. Langer M, Mascheroni D, Marcolin R, et al: The prone position in ARDS patients: A clinical study. Chest 94:103–107, 1988.

135. Albert R: Prone ventilation. Clin Chest Med 21:511–517, 2000.

136. Wiener CM, Kirk W, Albert RK: Prone position reverses gravitational distribution of perfusion in dog lungs with oleic acid-induced injury. J Appl Physiol 68:1386–1392, 1990.

137. Gattinoni L, Tognoni G, Pesenti A, et al: Effect of prone positioning on the survival of patients with acute respiratory failure. N Engl J Med 345:568–573, 2001.

138. Baltopoulos G, Zakynthinos S, Dimpoulos A, et al: Effects of furosemide on pulmonary shunts. Chest 96:494–498, 1989.

139. Gattinoni L: Decreasing edema results in improved pulmonary function and survival in patients with ARDS. Intens Care Med 12:137, 1986.

140. Simmons RS, Berdine GG, Seidenfeld JJ, et al: Fluid balance in the respiratory distress syndrome. Am Rev Respir Dis 135:924–929, 1987.

141. Schuster DP: The case for and against fluid restriction and occlusion pressure reduction in adult respiratory distress syndrome. New Horizons 1:478–488, 1993.

142. McIntyre RC Jr, Haenel JB, Moore FA, et al: Cardiopulmonary effects of permissive hypercapnia in the management of adult respiratory distress syndrome. J Trauma 37:433–438, 1994.

143. Randolph AG, Wypij D, Venkataraman ST, et al: Effect of mechanical ventilator weaning protocols on respiratory outcomes in infants and children: A randomized controlled trial. JAMA 288:2561–2568, 2002.

144. Brochard L, Rauss A, Benito SM, et al: Comparison of three methods of gradual withdrawal from ventilation support during weaning from mechanical ventilation. AJRCCM 150:896–903, 1995.

145. Leitch EA, Moran JL, Grealy B: Weaning and extubation in the intensive care unit: Clinical or index-driven approach? Intens Care Med 22:752–759, 1996.

146. Esteban A, Frutos F, Tobin MJ, et al: A comparison of four methods of weaning patients from mechanical ventilation. N Engl J Med 332:345–350, 1995.

147. Ferrara TB, Georgieff MK, Ebert J, et al: Routine use of dexamethasone for the prevention of postextubation respiratory distress. J Perinatol 9:287–290, 1989.

148. Dries DJ: Weaning from mechanical ventilation. J Trauma 43:372–384, 1997.

149. Holdgaard HO, Pedersen J, Jensen RH, et al: Percutaneous dilatational tracheostomy versus conventional surgical tracheostomy: A clinical randomised study. Acta Anaesth Scand 42:545–550, 1988.

150. Rosenbower TJ, Morris JA Jr, Eddy VA, et al: The long-term complications of percutaneous dilatational tracheostomy. Am Surg 64:82–87, 1998.

151. Citta-Pietrolungo TJ, Alexander MA, Cook SP, et al: Complications of tracheostomy and decannulation in pediatric and young patients with traumatic brain injury. Arch Phys Med Rehab 74:905–909, 1993.

152. Nicks JJ, Becker MA: High-frequency ventilation of the newborn: Past, present, and future. J Respir Care Pract 16–21.

153. Clark RH: High-frequency ventilation. J Pediatr 124:661–670, 1994.

154. Minton SD, Gerstmann DR, Stoddard RA: High-frequency oscillation: Ventilator strategies to interrupt pulmonary injury sequence. J Respir Care Pract 15–31, 1992.

155. Froese AB, Bryan AC: High frequency ventilation. Am Rev Respir Dis 135:1363–1374, 1987.

156. Krishnan JA, Brower RG: High-frequency ventilation for acute lung injury and ARDS. Chest 118:795–807, 2000.

157. Rouby JJ, Simonneau G. Benhamou D, et al: Factors influencing pulmonary volumes and CO_2 elimination during high-frequency jet ventilation. Anesthesiology 63:473–482, 1985.

158. Baumann MH, Sahn SA: Medical management and therapy of bronchopleural fistulas in the mechanically ventilated patient. Chest 97:721–728, 1991.

159. The HSG: High frequency oscillatory ventilation compared to conventional mechanical ventilation treatment of respiratory failure in preterm infants. N Engl J Med 320:88–93, 1989.

160. Clark RH, Gerstmann DR, Null DMJ, et al: Prospective randomized comparison of high-frequency oscillatory and conventional ventilation in respiratory distress syndrome. Pediatrics 89:5–12, 1992.

161. Keszler M, Donn SM, Bucciarelli RL, et al: Multicenter control trial comparing high frequency jet ventilation and conventional ventilation in newborn patients with pulmonary interstitial emphysema. J Pediatr 119:85–93, 1991.

162. Gerstmann DR, Minton SD, Stoddard RA, et al: The Provo multicenter early high-frequency oscillatory ventilation trial: Improved pulmonary and clinical outcome in respiratory distress syndrome. Pediatrics 98:1044–1057, 1996.

163. Moriette G, Paris-Llado J, Walti H, et al: Prospective randomized multicenter comparison of high-frequency oscillatory ventilation and conventional ventilation in preterm infants of less than 30 weeks with respiratory distress syndrome. Pediatrics 107:363–372, 2001.

164. Courtney SE, Durand DJ, Asselin JM, et al: High-frequency oscillatory ventilation versus conventional mechanical ventilation for very-low-birth-weight infants. N Engl J Med 347:643–652, 2002.

165. Durand DJ, Asselin LM, Hudak HL, et al: Early high-frequency oscillatory ventilation versus synchronized intermittent mandatory ventilation in very low birth weight infants: A pilot study of two ventilation protocols. J Perinatol 21:221–229, 2001.

166. Clark RH, Yoder BA, Sell MS: Prospective, randomized comparison of high-frequency oscillation and conventional ventilation in candidates for extracorporeal membrane oxygenation. J Pediatr 124:447–454, 1994.

167. Arnold JH, Hanson JH, Toro-Figuero LO, et al: Prospective, randomized comparison of high-frequency oscillatory ventilation and conventional mechanical ventilation in pediatric respiratory failure. Crit Care Med 22:1530–1539, 1994.

168. Rosenberg RB, Broner CW, Peters KJ, et al: High-frequency ventilation for acute pediatric respiratory failure. Chest 104:1216–1221, 1994.

169. Dobyns EL, Anas NG, Fortenberry JD, et al: Interactive effects of high-frequency oscillatory ventilation and inhaled nitric oxide in acute hypoxemic respiratory failure in pediatrics. Crit Care Med 30:2425–2429, 2002.

170. Bhuta T, Clark RH, Henderson-Smart DJ: Rescue high frequency oscillatory ventilation vs conventional ventilation for infants with severe pulmonary dysfunction born at or near term. Cochrane Database Syst Rev 2001.

171. Fort P, Farmer C, Westerman J, et al: High-frequency oscillatory ventilation for adult respiratory distress syndrome: A pilot study. Crit Care Med 25:937–947, 1997.

172. Derdak S: High-frequency oscillatory ventilation for acute respiratory distress syndrome in adult patients. Crit Care Med 31:S317–S323, 2003.

173. Kolobow T, Powers T, Mandava S, et al: Intratracheal pulmonary ventilation (ITPV): Control of positive end-expiratory pressure at the level of the carina through the use of a novel ITPV catheter design. Anesth Analg 78:455–461, 1994.

174. Muller EE, Kolobow T, Mandava S, et al: How to ventilate lungs as small as 12.5% of normal: The new technique of intratracheal pulmonary ventilation. Pediatr Res 34:606–610, 1993.

175. Schnitzer JJ, Thompson JE, Hedrick HL, et al: High-frequency intratracheal pulmonary ventilation: Improved gas exchange at lower airway pressures. J Pediatr Surg 32:203–206, 1997.

176. Schnitzer JJ, Thompson JE, Henrick HL: A new ventilator improves CO_2 removal in newborn lambs with congenital diaphragmatic hernia. Crit Care Med 27:109–112, 1999.

177. Ravenscraft SA, Burke WC, Nahum A, et al: Tracheal gas insufflation augments CO_2 clearance during mechanical ventilation. Am Rev Respir Dis 148:345–351, 1993.

178. Raszynski A, Hultquist KA, Latif H, et al: Rescue from pediatric ECMO with prolonged hybrid intratracheal pulmonary ventilation: A technique for reducing dead space ventilation and preventing ventilator induced lung injury. ASAIO 39:M681–M685, 1993.

179. Wilson JM, Thompson JR, Schnitzer JJ, et al: Intratracheal pulmonary ventilation and congenital diaphragmatic hernia: A report of two cases. J Pediatr Surg 28:484–487, 1993.

180. Rossi N, Musch G, Sangalli F, et al: Reverse-thrust ventilation in hypercapnic patients with acute respiratory distress syndrome: Acute physiological effects. Am J Respir Crit Care Med 162:363–368, 2000.

181. Dassieu G, Brochard L, Benani N, et al: Continuous tracheal gas insufflation in preterm infants with hyaline membrane disease: A prospective randomized trial. Am J Respir Crit Care Med 162:826–831, 2000.

182. Hoffman LA, Miro AM, Tasota FJ, et al: Tracheal gas insufflation: Limits of efficacy in adults with acute respiratory distress syndrome. Am J Respir Crit Care Med 162:387–932, 2000.

183. Murad F: Cyclic guanosine monophosphate as a mediator of vasodilation. J Clin Invest 78:1–5, 1986.

184. Rossaint R, Falke KJ, Lopez F, et al: Inhaled nitric oxide for the adult respiratory distress syndrome. N Engl J Med 328:399–405, 1993.

185. Rossaint R, Slama K, Steudel W, et al: Effects of inhaled nitric oxide on right ventricular function in severe acute respiratory distress syndrome [see comments]. Intens Care Med 21:197–203, 1995.
186. Dellinger RP, Zimmerman JL, R.W. Taylor, et al: Effects of inhaled nitric oxide in patients with acute respiratory distress syndrome: results of a randomized phase II trial. Crit Care Med 26:15–23, 1998.
187. Michael J, Barton R, Saffle J: Inhaled nitric oxide versus conventional therapy: Effect on oxygenation in ARDS. AJRCCM 157:1372–1380, 1998.
188. Abman SH, Griebel JL, Parker DK, et al: Acute effects of inhaled nitric oxide in children with severe hypoxemic respiratory failure. J Pediatr 124:881–888, 1994.
189. Day RW, Allen EM, Witte MK: A randomized, controlled study of the 1-hour and 24-hour effects of inhaled nitric oxide therapy in children with acute hypoxemic respiratory failure. Chest 112:1324–1331, 1997.
190. Roberts JJ, Fineman J, Morin F: Inhaled nitric oxide and persistent pulmonary hypertension of the newborn: The Inhaled Nitric Oxide Study Group. N Engl J Med 336:605–610, 1997.
191. Clark R, Kueser T, Walker M, et al: Low-dose nitric oxide therapy for persistent pulmonary hypertension of the newborn. N Engl J Med 342:469–474, 2000.
192. Christou H, Van Marter L, Wessel D, et al: Inhaled nitric oxide reduces the need for extracorporeal membrane oxygenation in infants with persistent pulmonary hypertension of the newborn. Crit Care Med 28:3722–3727, 2000.
193. (NINOS), T.N.I.N.O.S.G: Inhaled nitric oxide in full-term and nearly full-term infants with hypoxic respiratory failure. N Engl J Med 336:597–604, 1997.
194. (NINOS), T.N.I.N.O.S.G: Inhaled nitric oxide in term and near-term infants: Neurodevelopmental follow-up of the Neonatal Inhaled Nitric Oxide Study Group (NINOS). J Pediatr 136:611–617, 2000.
195. Ellington MJ, O'Reilly D, Allred E, et al: Child health status, neurodevelopmental outcome, and parental satisfaction in a randomized, controlled trial nitric oxide for persistent pulmonary hypertension of the newborn. Pediatrics 107:1351–1356, 2001.
196. (NINOS), T.N.I.N.O.S.G: Inhaled nitric oxide and hypoxic respiratory failure in infants with congenital diaphragmatic hernia. Pediatrics 99:838–845, 1997.
197. Karamanoukian HL, Glick PL, Wilcox DT, et al: Pathophysiology of congenital diaphragmatic hernia, VIII: Inhaled nitric oxide requires exogenous surfactant therapy in the lamb model of congenital diaphragmatic hernia. J Pediatr Surg 30:1–4, 1995.
198. Meurs KP, Rhine WD, Asselin JM, et al: Response of premature infants with severe respiratory failure to inhaled nitric oxide: Preemie NO collaborative group. Pediatr Pulmonol 24:319–323, 1997.
199. Hoehn T, Krause M, Buhrer C: Inhaled nitric oxide in premature infants: A meta-analysis. J Perinat Med 28:7–13, 2000.
200. Haddad IY, Ischiropoulos H, Holm BA, et al: Mechanisms of peroxynitrite-induced injury to pulmonary surfactants. Am J Physiol 265:L555–L564, 1993.
201. Beckman JS, Beckman T, Chen J, et al: Apparent hydroxyl radical production by peroxynitrite: Implications for endothelial injury from nitric oxide and superoxide. Proc Natl Acad Sci U S A 87:1620–1624, 1990.
202. Jobe AH: Pulmonary surfactant therapy. N Engl J Med 328:861–868, 1993.
203. Hallman M, Merritt TA, Jarvenpaa AL, et al: Exogenous human surfactant for treatment of severe respiratory distress syndrome: A randomized prospective clinical trial. J Pediatr 106:963–969, 1985.
204. Long W, Corbet A, Cotton R, et al: A controlled trial of synthetic surfactant in infants weighing 1250 g or more with respiratory distress syndrome: The American Exosurf Neonatal Study Group I, and the Canadian Exosurf Neonatal Study Group. N Engl J Med 325:1696–1703, 1991.
205. Vermont-Oxford NN: A multicenter, randomized trial comparing synthetic surfactant with modified bovine surfactant extract in the treatment of neonatal respiratory distress syndrome: Vermont-Oxford Neonatal Network. Pediatrics 97:1–6, 1996.
206. Hudak ML, Martin DJ, Egan EA, et al: A multicenter randomized masked comparison trial of synthetic surfactant versus calf lung surfactant extract in the prevention of neonatal respiratory distress syndrome. Pediatrics 100:39–50, 1997.
207. Lotze A, Mitchell BR, Bulas DI, et al: Multicenter study of surfactant (beractant) use in the treatment of term infants with severe respiratory failure: Survanta in Term Infants Study Group. J Pediatr 132:40–47, 1998.
208. Findlay RD, Taeusch HW, Walther FJ: Surfactant replacement therapy for meconium aspiration syndrome. Pediatrics 97:48–52, 1996.
209. Lotze A, Knight GR, Anderson KD, et al: Surfactant (beractant) therapy for infants with congenital diaphragmatic hernia on ECMO: Evidence of persistent surfactant deficiency [see comments]. J Pediatr Surg 29:407–412, 1994.
210. Cogo PE, Zimmermann LJ, Rosso F, et al: Surfactant synthesis and kinetics in infants with congenital diaphragmatic hernia. Am J Respir Crit Care Med 166:154–158, 2002.
211. IJsselstijn H, Zimmermann LJ, Bunt JE, et al: Prospective evaluation of surfactant composition in bronchoalveolar lavage fluid of infants with congenital diaphragmatic hernia and of age-matched controls. Crit Care Med 26:573–580, 1998.
212. Wilcox DT, Glick PL, Karamanoukian H, et al: Pathophysiology of congenital diaphragmatic hernia, V: Effect of exogenous surfactant therapy on gas exchange and lung mechanics in the lamb congenital diaphragmatic hernia model. J Pediatr 124:289–293, 1994.
213. Glick PL, Leach CL, Besner GE, et al: Pathophysiology of congenital diaphragmatic hernia, III: Exogenous surfactant therapy for the high-risk neonate with CDH. J Pediatr Surg 27:866–869, 1992.
214. Shaffer TH: A brief review: liquid ventilation. Undersea Biomed Res 14:169–179, 1987.
215. Shaffer TH, Wolfson MR, Clark L Jr: State of the art review: Liquid ventilation. Pediatr Pulmonol 14:102–109, 1992.
216. Hirschl RB, Merz S, Montoya P, et al: Development of a simplified liquid ventilator. Crit Care Med 23:157–163, 1995.
217. Fuhrman BP, Paczan PR, DeFrancisis M: Perfluorocarbon-associated gas exchange. Crit Care Med 19:712–722, 1991.
218. Hirschl RB, Tooley R, Parent AC, et al: Improvement of gas exchange, pulmonary function, and lung injury with partial liquid ventilation: A study model in a setting of severe respiratory failure. Chest 108:500–508, 1995.
219. Leach CL, Fuhrman BP, Morin FD, et al: Perfluorocarbon-associated gas exchange (partial liquid ventilation) in respiratory distress syndrome: A prospective, randomized, controlled study. Crit Care Med 21:1270–1278, 1993.
220. Major D, Cadenas M, Cloutier R, et al: Combined gas ventilation and perfluorochemical tracheal instillation as an alternative treatment for lethal congenital diaphragmatic hernia in lambs. J Pediatr Surg 30:1178–1182, 1995.
221. Wilcox DT, Glick PL, Karamanoukian HL, et al: Perfluorocarbon-associated gas exchange improves pulmonary mechanics, oxygenation, ventilation, and allows nitric oxide delivery in the hypoplastic lung congenital diaphragmatic hernia lamb model. Crit Care Med 23:1858–1863, 1995.
222. Hirschl RB, Overbeck MC, Parent A, et al: Liquid ventilation provides uniform distribution of perfluorocarbon in the setting of respiratory failure. Surgery 116:159–167, 1994.
223. Kandler M, von der Hardt K, Schoof E, et al: Persistent improvement of gas exchange and lung mechanics by aerosolized perfluorocarbon. Am J Respir Crit Care Med 164:31–35, 2002.
224. Greenspan JS, Wolfson MR, Rubenstein SD, et al: Liquid ventilation of human preterm neonates. J Pediatr 117:106–111, 1990.
225. Gauger PG, Pranikoff T Schreiner RJ, et al: Initial experience with partial liquid ventilation in pediatric patients with the acute respiratory distress syndrome. Crit Care Med 24:16–22, 1996.
226. Hirschl RB, Pranikoff P, Wise C, et al: Initial experience with partial liquid ventilation in adult patients with the acute respiratory distress syndrome. JAMA 275:383–389, 1996.
227. Pranikoff T, Gauger P, Hirschl RB: Partial liquid ventilation in newborn patients with congenital diaphragmatic hernia. J Pediatr Surg 31:613–618, 1996.

228. Toro-Figueroa LO, Melinoes JN, Curtis SE, et al: Perflubron partial liquid ventilation (PLV) in children with ARDS: A safety and efficacy pilot study. Crit Care Med 24:A150, 1996.

229. Hirschl RB, Croce M, Gore D, et al: Prospective, randomized, controlled pilot study of partial liquid ventilation in adult acute respiratory distress syndrome. AJRCCM 165:781–787, 2002.

230. Wiedemann H: Alliance Pharmaceutical Corp Announces Preliminary Results of LiquiVent Phase 2-3 Clinical Study. 2001.

231. Leach CL, Greenspan JS, Rubenstein SD, et al: Partial liquid ventilation with perflubron in premature infants with severe respiratory distress syndrome. N Engl J Med 335:761–767, 1996.

232. DiFiore JW, Fauza DO, Slavin R, et al: Experimental fetal tracheal ligation reverses the structural and physiological effects of pulmonary hypoplasia in congenital diaphragmatic hernia. J Pediatr Surg 29:248–256; discussion 256–257, 1994.

233. Hedrick MH, Estes JM, Sullivan KM, et al: Plug the lung until it grows (PLUG): A new method to treat congenital diaphragmatic hernia in utero. J Pediatr Surg 29:612–617, 1994.

234. Fauza D, Hine M, Fackler J, et al: Continuous positive airway pressure with perfluorocarbon accelerates postnatal lung growth. Surg Forum 46:666–669, 1995.

235. Fauza D, Hirschl R, Wilson J: Continuous intrapulmonary distension with perfluorocarbon accelerates lung growth in infants with congenital diaphragmatic hernias: initial experience. J Pediatr Surg 36:1237–1240, 2001.

236. Hirschl R, Philip WF, Glick P, et al: A prospective, randomized pilot trial of perfluorocarbon-induced lung growth (PILG) in newborns with congenital diaphragmatic hernia (CDH). J Pediatr Surg 38:283–289, 2003.

237. Greenspan JS, Wolfson MR, Rubenstein SD, et al: Liquid ventilation of preterm baby. Lancet 2:1095, 1989.

238. Wolfson M, Jackson J, Foley D, et al: Multi-center comparative study of conventional mechanical (CMV) to tidal liquid ventilation (TLV) in oleic acid (OA) injured sheep. AJRCCM 161:A46, 2000.

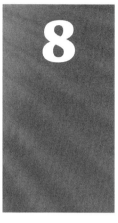
Vascular Access

Charles S. Turner, MD

Vascular access in infants and children is one of the most frustrating and exasperating aspects of pediatric surgical procedures. What is delegated to the role of an ancillary surgical procedure in adults might become a major task in children and might, in the operating arena, take as long as the surgical procedure itself. The least experienced physician is often given the task of starting the intravenous (IV) line.

Nowhere is this situation more critical than during attempted resuscitation of a child. In a study of 66 emergency department cardiac arrests in children, IV access required 10 or more minutes in 24% of the cases.[1] Indeed, in 6% of resuscitations, access was never established. When resuscitation was successful, access had been established significantly sooner than when resuscitation failed. Placing an IV catheter took the most time in children younger than 2 years.

In 1986, a prospective study was undertaken to determine the effectiveness of a protocol designed to standardize the route and site of pediatric IV access in an emergency situation.[2] This study found that resuscitations using the protocol achieved IV access more rapidly (median, 4.5 minutes) than did those deviating from the protocol (median, 10 minutes) (Fig. 8-1). Therefore surgeons must develop and maintain a high degree of expertise in vascular access in infants and children. Beyond the immediate need for IV access in resuscitative efforts, the surgeon must often establish arterial access lines for monitoring and central venous access lines for hemodialysis, parenteral nutrition, chemotherapy, critical care monitoring, and extracorporeal membrane oxygenation.

This chapter reviews the options available for vascular access so that this aspect of pediatric surgical care can be improved.

PERIPHERAL VENOUS ACCESS

Peripheral venous access in infants and children is usually accomplished by using the veins of the hand and forearm, the distal leg and foot, and the scalp (Table 8-1).

A thorough knowledge of anatomy is mandatory for successful access.

In infants, the superficial veins on the dorsum of the hand are most frequently selected. These veins are straight and flat on the metacarpals. They feed the larger dorsal branch of the distal cephalic vein, which also is stabilized for access without difficulty. The lateral branch of the distal cephalic vein is difficult to stabilize and is less accessible for venous puncture and catheter placement.

The median vein tributaries located on the ventral surface of the wrist are accessible, but they are small and acutely angulated. Therefore they require a small catheter, which is difficult to advance into the vein. These tributaries may be used during an operation, but they become unreliable in the awakened patient. The cephalic and basilic veins in the antecubital fossa are accessible, but advancement of the cannula may be difficult owing to the angulation of the veins across the fossa.

In the lower extremity, the tributaries of the dorsal venous arch on the dorsal aspect of the foot are useful. The largest reliable vein is the saphenous vein just anterior and lateral to the medial malleolus. This vein is always palpable, although it is only sometimes visible. A larger catheter can be accommodated.

Although the external jugular vein can be seen, cannulation is difficult. Once the catheter is in place, it serves well during anesthesia. However, the external jugular vein infuses poorly when the child awakens because of motion and the acute angulation of the external jugular as it enters the subclavian vein. The external jugular vein catheter also is difficult to stabilize and easy to dislodge.

EMERGENCY SITUATION

The next step for venous access, when percutaneous peripheral venous access is unsuccessful, depends on the speed with which access is needed. In an emergency situation, when difficult venous access is secondary to cardiac

TABLE 8-1

PERIPHERAL VEIN ACCESS PRIORITY IN INFANTS AND CHILDREN

1. Dorsal veins of the hands
2. Antecubital veins of the arms
3. Saphenous vein at the ankle
4. Dorsal veins of the foot
5. Median vein tributary at the wrist
6. External jugular veins
7. Scalp

arrest or hypovolemia, the options are tracheal instillation, intraosseous infusion,[3] venous cutdown,[4–6] and central venous access[6–8] (Fig. 8–1).

The sites for intraosseous infusion in infants and small children are the tibia, iliac crest, and femur. Access can be accomplished with a bone marrow aspiration needle or a 16- or 19-gauge butterfly needle. In the femur, the needle is introduced in a cephalad direction, 3 cm proximal to the condyles. Tibial introduction is 1 to 3 cm distal to the tibial tuberosity; the needle is placed in a distal direction. Most drugs, crystalloid solutions, and blood products can be given by interosseous infusion in an emergency. Infusion is as rapid as through IV routes. Intramedullary vessels do not collapse in the hypovolemic, "shocky" patient.[3]

In the past, the venous cutdown has been the mainstay of difficult venous access by the pediatric surgeon. An American Pediatric Surgical Association survey showed that an average of 56 cutdowns per pediatric surgeon per year was performed.[4]

The time required for venous cutdowns in neonates, children younger than 5 years, and children older than 5 years was 11, 8, and 6 minutes, respectively.

Access for Emergency Resuscitation

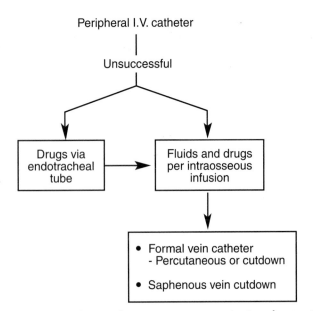

FIGURE 8-1. Access for emergency resuscitation (protocol example). I.V., intravenous.

The saphenous vein was preferred (79%) over the brachial and external jugular veins (21%). However, the time required even by the surgeons most experienced in the procedure made the cutdown in an emergency situation supplementary, at best. Alternative routes must be established to give medications (endotracheal instillation) and fluids (interosseous infusion) while cutdowns are being prepared.[3]

Now more experience has been acquired with polyethylene catheters, 3F to 6F sizes, including single-lumen and triple-lumen catheters, placed in the femoral vein in emergency situations. Likewise, the catheters are used with a subclavian approach and Seldinger technique. Multiple factors have made the use of these catheters more commonly accepted: (1) less thrombogenicity, (2) softer catheters and guidewires, (3) increased surgeon experience, and (4) safer sedation techniques for neonates.

NONEMERGENCY SITUATIONS

In nonemergency situations, are peripheral venous cutdowns necessary? The option is central venous catheterization. Two specific contraindications to central venous insertion exist: an uncorrected coagulopathy and an undefined major cardiac anomaly. Otherwise, percutaneous central venous lines are preferred when peripheral lines are unavailable or when long-term access is required.

A comparison study of percutaneous central venous catheterization versus peripheral venous cutdowns in children aged 1 day to 17 years was conducted. Within age groups, the children were similar in weight and size. More successful placements, fewer complications, and longer functional states were found in the patients with central venous catheters versus those with peripheral venous cutdowns.[6] Surgical cutdowns also carry a significantly greater risk of infectious complications than do percutaneous catheterizations.[7] Therefore percutaneous central venous catheterization is the method of choice when venous access other than routine peripheral IV access is required.

Butterfly needles are used now to introduce small polymeric silicone (Silastic) catheters percutaneously into neonates.[8] This needle enhances the ability to obtain central venous access in very small infants without cutdown. The catheter is Silastic medical grade tubing (0.012 mm inside diameter and 0.025 mm outside diameter)[8] (Fig. 8-2). The catheter is inserted into a peripheral vein (scalp, neck, or arm) through a 19-gauge scalp vein needle or through a 20-gauge angiocatheter.[8,9] The catheter is threaded centrally.

Owing to the small catheter size, the flow rate is limited to 25 mL/hr. An increased risk of calcium phosphate precipitation may exist if lipid emulsions are given simultaneously with parenteral nutrition.[9,10] For short-term use in a neonate who weighs less than 6 kg, these small-diameter catheters introduced percutaneously offer a good alternative to the large-diameter lines that require cutdown or subclavian insertion. Certainly, however, the surgeon must perfect the technique of peripheral venous

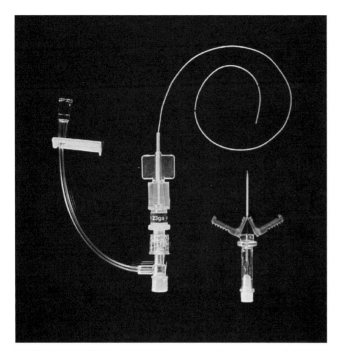

FIGURE 8-2. Butterfly peel-away angiocatheter with polymeric silicone (Silastic) catheter.

cutdown and use the newer Silastic catheters, which are less thrombogenic than the older polyethylene catheters.

Central Venous Access

Access to the central veins of the chest has altered the outcome of a multitude of pediatric surgical problems. With this access, the hemodynamics in a critically ill child can be monitored precisely. Children with problems such as short-gut syndrome, intestinal pseudo-obstruction, and gastroschisis can be kept alive with central parenteral nutrition. Survival among extremely premature babies has increased owing to the ability to provide adequate calories, protein, and fat via central venous catheters (Fig. 8-3).

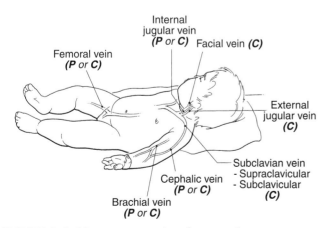

FIGURE 8-3. Most common sites for central venous access. *P*, percutaneous; *C*, cutdown.

Pediatric oncology patients require central venous access not only for reliable delivery of chemotherapeutic agents but also for nutritional support. Central venous access also has allowed catheters to be placed for both short-term and long-term hemodialysis and for plasmapheresis in the treatment of certain metabolic disorders. The special aspects of cannulation for extracorporeal membrane oxygenation are covered elsewhere in this text.

CATHETER TYPE

The first consideration is the type of catheter, which is dictated primarily by the intended use and by the size of the patient. Duration, patient compliance, and ability to care for the catheter also enter into the catheter-selection process. For short periods in the critical care or emergency situation, single- to triple-lumen polyethylene catheters are available. These can be inserted percutaneously into the internal jugular, subclavian, or femoral veins by Seldinger's technique.

For long-term application in parenteral nutrition or oncology, the silicone rubber catheters are preferred, owing to their pliability and decreased thrombogenicity.[11] Broviac or Hickman catheters are made of silicone rubber with a Dacron cuff around the nonvascular portion of the catheter. These catheters can be placed percutaneously into the subclavian, internal jugular, or femoral veins, by using Seldinger's technique and "peel-away" introducers.

The tip is advanced to the caval-atrial junction under fluoroscopy. The extravascular portion with its Dacron cuff is brought out through a long subcutaneous tunnel to the anterior chest wall or to the abdominal wall, if the femoral approach is taken. The Dacron cuff should be midway between the skin and the vein entrance sites.[11] Other veins for the cutdown technique include the external jugular, common facial, inferior thyroid, saphenous, and inferior epigastric. When those veins are exhausted, the azygos vein can be cannulated via the intercostal veins on the right, although this requires thoracotomy or thoracoscopy. The inferior vena cava also has been accessed through a percutaneous translumbar approach for central venous catheter placement.[12,13]

Implantable access devices consist of an injection reservoir connected to a silicone rubber catheter (Fig. 8-4). The port or reservoir is placed in a subcutaneous pocket on the anterior chest. The catheter is tunneled under the skin to the vein entrance site. The vein can be accessed with a percutaneous Seldinger's technique or a cutdown technique. The subcutaneous reservoirs have a Silastic diaphragm, which can be punctured by a side hole (Huber) needle, preventing a core of Silastic being taken with entrance of the needle.

The back and side walls of the reservoir are metal, so that it is known when the needle is completely inserted. This type of device allows access to the central venous system without the need to care for an external catheter. These implantable reservoirs also are available as double- and triple-lumen types and as low-profile types for infants. The ease of care, the absence of protruding tubes,

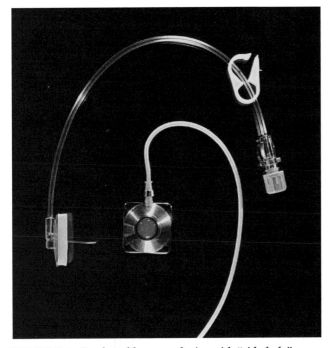

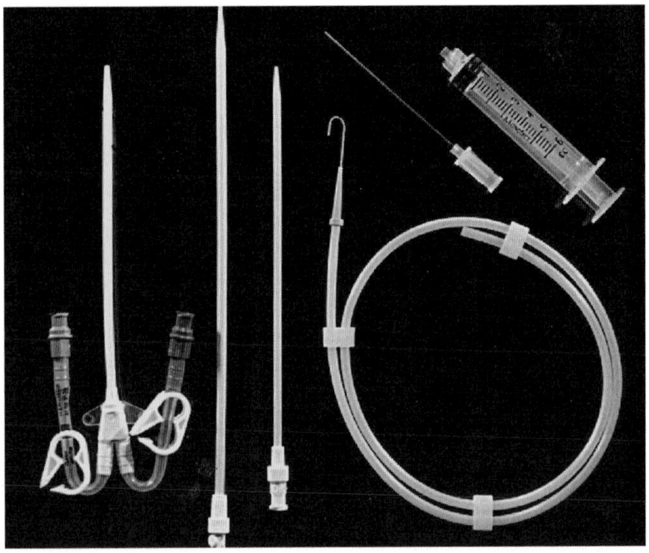

FIGURE 8-5. Hemodialysis catheter (*right*) with Seldinger introducer kit (*left*).

FIGURE 8-4. Implantable access device with "side-hole" access needle.

and the compatibility with normal activities are their major advantages.[14] The complication rate of central venous access is not increased with their use[15-17]; in fact, the infection rate is lower.[18,19] For patients who require intermittent but long-term central venous access (as for managing cancer, cystic fibrosis, and hemophilia),[20] an implantable system seems appropriate. Whether a continuous need, such as prolonged home parenteral nutrition, is better met with an implantable device or an external catheter is still unanswered.

Special catheters for hemodialysis allow a single-needle dialysis technique to be used. These catheters (Cook, Inc., Bloomington, IN), which have offset inflow and outflow ports, are made of polyurethane[21] (Fig. 8-5). They can be introduced percutaneously by using a peel-away catheter technique; they also have Dacron cuffs that are tunneled in, as described for Broviac catheters.[11] They can be used in children who weigh as little as 7 kg.[21]

Centrally placed Hickman (Evermed) catheters also have been used for hemodialysis with the single-needle dialysis technique. Various sizes, depending on the size of the patient, provide adequate hemodialysis in children as light as 7.7 kg.[22] These catheters are best suited for acute hemodialysis in children with acute renal failure without availability of peritoneal dialysis, in children with peritonitis that requires temporary removal of a peritoneal dialysis catheter, and in children with unsuccessful peritoneal dialysis outcome who are awaiting kidney transplant. Hemodialysis catheters inserted into the internal jugular vein or femoral vein might help avoid thrombosis of the subclavian vein, thus saving it to provide adequate runoff for an arteriovenous (A/V) fistula

later in life. These catheters also have been used for long-term dialysis,[21] although the best long-term dialysis for children is believed to be peritoneal.

If long-term hemodialysis is required because of chronic peritonitis and problematic transplant matching, a Brescia-Cimino A/V fistula is possible in children weighing at least 15 kg.[23]

The site of insertion of a central venous catheter in a child depends greatly on the expertise and training of the surgeon. The percutaneous route to the subclavian vein is feasible even in very small infants.[24,25] As mentioned earlier, long lines from the antecubital fossa by a cutdown technique or a percutaneous technique have been placed in neonates weighing as little as 0.5 kg.[9]

COMPLICATIONS

The femoral route for central line placement has been thought to be associated with increased thrombophlebitis of the ipsilateral leg and with wound infection due to proximity of the groin.[26-28] Gangrene of the lower extremity,[29] septic arthritis of the hip,[30] A/V fistula,[31] penetration of a viscus in an unrecognized femoral hernia, and infused fluid into the abdominal wall[32] also have been reported as complications of femoral vein cannulation. However, because the femoral approach has been the route of choice for cardiac catheterization,[27] the femoral approach for central venous catheter placement has been accepted for use in pediatric patients.[26-28,33,34] The advantages listed are the anatomy, the attained hemostasis, and the distance from other lifesaving maneuver sites in a multiply injured patient.

Therefore for rapid central venous access in cases of cardiac arrest, hypotension, respiratory arrest, and multiple trauma, the femoral vein approach, either by percutaneous or cutdown technique, is the route of choice.

In neonates, infants, and children who require long-term central venous lines, the femoral approach is acceptable and is available with the exit site or reservoir located on the lower abdominal wall.

Except for the complications listed earlier, those for central venous catheters are associated primarily with percutaneous placement of the catheter in the subclavian or internal jugular veins. Acute complications include aberrant location of the catheter; perforation of the vein or artery with resultant hemothorax, hydrothorax, or extravasation of fluid into surrounding tissues; perforation of the lung with pneumothorax; and perforation of the heart with resultant pericardial tamponade.[35-39] Misplacing the tip of the catheter into a small tributary can lead to phlebitis when hypertonic solutions are infused. Fluoroscopy and immediate postinsertion radiographs allow accurate placement of the catheter and early detection of these complications.

Long-term complications include tunnel infection, sepsis, venous thrombosis, superior vena caval obstruction, thrombosis of the catheter tip, and septic emboli.[10,36-40] A review of central venous catheter infections is available.[10] It should be studied by anyone who works with patients who require vascular access.

The overall rate of septic infections in central venous catheters is 1.7 cases per 1000 days of catheter use. This rate varies, depending on whether the patient is receiving total parenteral nutrition only or is also receiving chemotherapy, and whether more than one lumen is being used (not just being in position). The diagnosis of catheter-related sepsis is assumed in any case with fever. Quantitative blood cultures obtained centrally and peripherally that show a 5:1 or greater ratio of colonies per milliliter suggest the catheter as the most likely source.

Initial therapy should be removal of the catheter if the patient can get along without it. If the line is still needed, antibiotics can be given through the catheter. A thrombolytic agent is added if thrombus is seen on echocardiography or if flow is restricted.[40] If no clinical improvement is seen within 48 hours or if the patient's condition deteriorates sooner, the catheter must be removed. Although bacterial infections may be cured without removal of the catheter, fungal infections are unlikely to resolve unless the catheter is removed.[10]

TREATMENT OF INFECTION

The best treatment for infection is prevention. Strict aseptic technique at the time of insertion as well as following the protocols of meticulous aseptic care of the catheter site is essential. This care includes the iodoform ointments (most effective against *Candida* and gramnegative bacilli) at the entrance site and gauze and tape dressings[10] or transparent semipermeable adhesive dressings, which should be changed every 48 to 72 hours.[41]

Thrombosis of the Silastic catheter can be suggested before complete occlusion by difficulty in flushing, inability to withdraw blood, and measured increase in resistance to flow.[38] When partial or total occlusion occurs,

urokinase, 5000 international units/mL, can be administered.[39,40] The volume of urokinase depends on the size of the catheter (e.g., 1.8 to 2.0 mL for Hickman catheters and 0.8 mL for Broviac catheters). After 30 to 60 minutes, the catheter is aspirated and then flushed with heparinized saline. Regular administration of dilute heparin decreases thrombus formation and also may lead to a reduction in septic complications.[10,41] An intracardiac thrombus at the tip of the catheter can become infected.[40] The presence of such a thrombus usually causes symptoms (sepsis, respiratory or cardiac insufficiency, or catheter malfunction).[37] Detection is confirmed by echocardiography.

Various modes of treatment include thrombolytic agents (urokinase infusion at 2000 to 10,000 international units/kg/hr for 1 to 8 days) and heparin, with or without catheter removal; catheter removal only; observation only[37]; a regimen of aspirin, dipyridamole, and antibiotics[40]; and atriotomy.[37] On the basis of published reports, thrombolytic therapy through the catheter, with the addition of antibiotics in the case of sepsis, would be the first line of treatment. Atriotomy is saved for deteriorating sepsis or cardiac compromise due to the mechanical presence of the thrombus.

Arterial Access

Intra-arterial catheters in infants are frequently used to monitor blood pressure and to provide access to arterial blood for blood gas and other laboratory determinations, thereby eliminating the need for intermittent arterial puncture.[42,43] The arterial sites of cannulation include the umbilical,[44-46] radial,[47-50] femoral,[26,51] and posterior tibial arteries[42] (Fig. 8-6).

UMBILICAL ARTERY

The umbilical artery usually constricts minutes after birth, although this constriction is delayed by hypoxia and acidosis. The artery can usually be catheterized within 2 to 4 days of life. The usual approach is at the

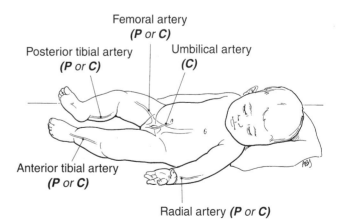

FIGURE 8-6. Sites for arterial access. *P*, percutaneous; *C*, cutdown.

umbilical stump itself, although the umbilical artery can be cannulated through a minilaparotomy.[45] The advantages of catheterizing the umbilical artery are the ease of access, the longer functional life for umbilical catheters than for peripheral arterial catheters, and the ability to infuse fluids, glucose, electrolytes, and drugs by such a direct route.[52] Its use also allows postductal blood gas evaluations, which are helpful in determining the amount of right-to-left shunting in neonates with persistent fetal circulation. The umbilical artery also can be used for access in cardiac catheterization.[46]

Complications from umbilical artery catheters include thrombosis, distal embolism, vasospasm, vascular perforation with hemoperitoneum, hemorrhage from catheter disconnection, and, after catheter removal, visceral infarction, paraplegia, hypertension, and sepsis.[43,46,48] All of these situations require immediate removal of the catheter. Additionally, thrombosis of the aorta may require thrombolytic or surgical therapy. Multiple aortic aneurysms in a neonate after umbilical artery catheter insertion have been reported.[53] The umbilical artery cannot be catheterized in 5% to 10% of patients, nor can it be catheterized after the neonatal period. Complications from the umbilical artery catheter may require premature removal. In these instances, 22- to 24-gauge catheters can be placed by percutaneous technique or by cutdown in the peripheral arteries.

RADIAL ARTERY

The most frequently used peripheral artery is the radial artery. It carries a low risk of infection (12% for catheters in place >48 hours) and of thrombosis. The catheter allows preductal gas determinations if it is in the right radial artery. The overall incidence of complications from peripheral artery catheters is approximately 7% compared with 27% from umbilical artery catheters.[48] The catheters in the artery are of 22- to 24-gauge Teflon. They can be placed either by percutaneous or cutdown technique. If placed by cutdown, the catheter can be inserted through the skin and then, under direct vision, into the artery without ligating the artery.[49] A palpable pulse usually returns within 3 to 5 days after removal of a radial artery catheter.[47]

Complications from radial artery catheters include skin ischemia, radial artery obstruction, and inability to withdraw blood through the catheter. In patients who need insertion via a cutdown technique, the interval to recanalization after catheter removal is longer than that in patients with percutaneously placed catheters.[49] The radial artery catheter must be flushed continuously. Catheters infused continuously with heparin, 1 U/mL of saline, last longer than those flushed intermittently,[50] and continuous slow flushing avoids the possible catastrophic complication of retrograde embolization of clot and air to the cerebral circulation.[54] If the patency of the ulnar artery is proved before placement of the radial artery catheter and if continuous flushing is done, few significant complications of radial artery catheterization will occur.[49]

The indications for arterial access must constantly be reassessed. With the increasing sophistication of noninvasive monitoring systems, often arterial access is not mandatory.[55] The needs of the patient rather than the convenience of the physician should determine the use of this approach.

REFERENCES

1. Rossetti V, Thompson BM, Aprahamian C, et al: Difficulty and delay in intravascular access in pediatric arrests [abstract]. Ann Emerg Med 13:406, 1984.
2. Kanter RK, Zimmerman JJ, Strauss RH, et al: Pediatric emergency intravenous access: Evaluation of a protocol. Am J Dis Child 140:132–134, 1986.
3. Orlowski JP: My kingdom for an intravenous line [editorial]. Am J Dis Child 138:803, 1984.
4. Iserson KV, Criss EA: Pediatric venous cutdowns: Utility in emergency situations. Pediatr Emerg Care 2:231–234, 1986.
5. Peter G, Lloyd-Still JD, Lovejoy FH Jr: Local infection and bacteremia from scalp vein needles and polyethylene catheters in children. J Pediatr 80:78–83, 1972.
6. Newman BM, Jewett TC Jr, Karp MP, et al: Percutaneous central venous catheterization in children: First-line choice for venous access. J Pediatr Surg 21:685–688, 1986.
7. Meignier M, Heloury Y, Roze J-C, et al: Surgical central venous access in low birth infants [letter]. J Pediatr Surg 23:596, 1988.
8. Durand M, Ramanathan R, Martinelli B, et al: Prospective evaluation of percutaneous central venous Silastic catheters in newborn infants with birth weights of 510 to 3,920 grams. Pediatrics 78:245–250, 1986.
9. Loeff DS, Matlak ME, Black RE, et al: Insertion of a small central venous catheter in neonates and young infants. J Pediatr Surg 17:944–949, 1982.
10. Decker MD, Edwards KM: Central venous catheter infections. Pediatr Clin North Am 35:579–612, 1988.
11. Broviac JW, Cole JJ, Scribner BH: A silicone rubber atrial catheter for prolonged parenteral alimentation. Surg Gynecol Obstet 136:602–606, 1973.
12. Robards JB, Jaques PF, Mauro MA, et al: Percutaneous translumbar inferior vena cava central line placement in a critically ill child. Pediatr Radiol 19:140–141, 1989.
13. Denny DF Jr, Greenwood LH, Morse SS, et al: Inferior vena cava: Translumbar catheterization for central venous access. Radiology 170:1013–1014, 1989.
14. Pegelow CH, Narvaez M, Toledano SR, et al: Experience with a totally implantable venous device in children. Am J Dis Child 140:69–71, 1986.
15. Krul EJ, van Leeuwen EF, Vos A, et al: Continuous venous access in children for long-term chemotherapy by means of an implantable system. J Pediatr Surg 21:689–690, 1986.
16. Kappers-Klunne MC, Degener JE, Stijnen T, et al: Complications from long-term indwelling central venous catheters in hematologic patients with special reference to infection. Cancer 64:1747–1752, 1989.
17. Guenier C, Ferreira J, Pector JC: Prolonged venous access in cancer patients. Eur J Surg Oncol 15:553–555, 1989.
18. Mirro J Jr, Rao BN, Kumar M, et al: A comparison of placement techniques and complications of externalized catheters and implantable port use in children with cancer. J Pediatr Surg 25:120–124, 1990.
19. Ross MN, Haase GM, Poole MA, et al: Comparison of totally implanted reservoirs with external catheters as venous access devices in pediatric oncologic patients. Surg Gynecol Obstet 167:141–144, 1988.
20. Schultz WH, Ware R, Filston HC, et al: Prolonged use of an implantable central venous access system in a child with severe hemophilia. J Pediatr 114:100–101, 1989.
21. Lally KP, Brennan LP, Sherman NJ, et al: Use of a subclavian venous catheter for short- and long-term hemodialysis in children. J Pediatr Surg 22:603–605, 1987.

22. Gibson TC, Dyer DP, Postlethwaite RJ, et al: Vascular access for acute haemodialysis. Arch Dis Child 62:141–145, 1987.
23. Matlak ME: Vascular access in pediatric patients. In Wilson SE, Owens ML (eds): Vascular Access Surgery. Chicago, Year Book Medical, 1980, pp 273–292.
24. Morgan WW Jr, Harkins GA: Percutaneous introduction of long-term indwelling venous catheters in infants. J Pediatr Surg 7:538–541, 1972.
25. Groff DB, Ahmed N: Subclavian vein catheterization in the infant. J Pediatr Surg 9:171–174, 1974.
26. Purdue GF, Hunt JL: Vascular access through the femoral vessels: Indications and complications. J Burn Care Rehabil 7:498–500, 1986.
27. Meland NB, Wilson W, Soontharotoke C-Y, et al: Saphenofemoral venous cutdowns in the premature infant. J Pediatr Surg 21:341–343, 1986.
28. Stenzel JP, Green TP, Fuhrman BP, et al: Percutaneous femoral venous catheterizations: A prospective study of complications. J Pediatr 114:411–415, 1989.
29. Nabseth DC, Jones JE: Gangrene of the lower extremities of infants after femoral venipuncture: Report of two cases. N Engl J Med 268:1003–1005, 1961.
30. Asnes RS, Arendar GM: Septic arthritis of the hip: A complication of femoral venipuncture. Pediatrics 38:837–841, 1966.
31. Fuller TJ, Mahoney JJ, Juncos LI, et al: Arteriovenous fistula after femoral vein catheterization [letter]. JAMA 236:2943–2944, 1976.
32. Bonadio WA, Losek JD, Melzer-Lange M: An unusual complication from a femoral venous catheter. Pediatr Emerg Care 4:27–29, 1988.
33. Kanter RK, Gorton JM, Palmieri K, et al: Anatomy of femoral vessels in infants and guidelines for venous catheterization. Pediatrics 83:1020–1022, 1989.
34. Kanter RK, Zimmerman JJ, Strauss RH, et al: Central venous catheter insertion by femoral vein: Safety and effectiveness for the pediatric patient. Pediatrics 77:842–847, 1986.
35. Dunbar RD, Mitchell R, Lavine M: Aberrant locations of central venous catheters. Lancet 1:711–715, 1981.
36. Stine KC, Friedman HS, Kurtzberg J, et al: Pulmonary septic emboli mimicking metastatic rhabdomyosarcoma. J Pediatr Surg 24:491–493, 1989.
37. Ross P Jr, Ehrenkranz R, Kleinman CS, et al: Thrombus associated with central venous catheters in infants and children. J Pediatr Surg 24:253–256, 1989.
38. Stokes DC, Rao BN, Mirro J Jr, et al: Early detection and simplified management of obstructed Hickman and Broviac catheters. J Pediatr Surg 24:257–262, 1989.
39. Ross P Jr, Seashore JH: Bilateral hydrothorax complicating central venous catheterization in a child: Case report. J Pediatr Surg 24:263–264, 1989.
40. Teitelbaum DH, Caniano DA, Wheller JK: Resolution of an infected intracardiac thrombus. J Pediatr Surg 24:1118–1120, 1989.
41. Chathas MK: Percutaneous central venous catheters in neonates. J Obstet Gynecol Neonatal Nurs 15:324–332, 1986.
42. Spahr RC, MacDonald HM, Holzman IR: Catheterization of the posterior tibial artery in the neonate. Am J Dis Child 133:945–946, 1979.
43. Randel SN, Tsang BHL, Wung J-T, et al: Experience with percutaneous indwelling peripheral arterial catheterization in neonates. Am J Dis Child 141:848–851, 1987.
44. Pourcyrous M, Korones SB, Bada HS, et al: Indwelling umbilical arterial catheter: A preferred sampling site for blood culture. Pediatrics 81:821–825, 1988.
45. Singer RL, Wolfson PJ: Experience with umbilical artery cutdowns in neonates. Pediatr Surg Int 5:295–297, 1990.
46. Kitterman JA, Phibbs RH, Tooley WH: Catheterization of umbilical vessels in newborn infants. Pediatr Clin North Am 17:895–912, 1970.
47. Adams JM, Rudolph AJ: The use of indwelling radial artery catheters in neonates. Pediatrics 55:261–265, 1975.
48. Barr PA, Sumners J, Wirtschafter D, et al: Percutaneous peripheral arterial cannulation in the neonate. Pediatrics 59(suppl 6, pt 2):1058–1062, 1977.
49. Miyasaka K, Edmonds JF, Conn AW: Complications of radial artery lines in the paediatric patient. Can Anaesth Soc J 23:9–14, 1976.
50. Sellden H, Nilsson K, Larsson LE, et al: Radial arterial catheters in children and neonates: A prospective study. Crit Care Med 15:1106–1109, 1987.
51. Taylor LM Jr, Troutman R, Feliciano P, et al: Late complications after femoral artery catheterization in children less than five years of age. J Vasc Surg 11:297–306, 1990.
52. Goetzman BW: Arterial access in the newborn [editorial]. Am J Dis Child 141:841, 1987.
53. Kirpekar M, Augenstein H, Abiri M: Sequential development of multiple aortic aneurysms in a neonate post umbilical arterial catheter insertion. Pediatr Radiol 19:452–453, 1989.
54. Lowenstein E, Little JW III, Lo HH: Prevention of cerebral embolization from flushing radial-artery cannulas. N Engl J Med 285:1414–1415, 1971.
55. Willard D, Messer J: Arterial access and monitoring in the newborn [letter]. Am J Dis Child 142:480, 1988.

Surgical Infectious Disease

Marion C. W. Henry, MD, and Thomas M. Krummel, MD

Despite advances in antimicrobial therapy and surgical and aseptic techniques, infection continues to be an enormous problem for the surgeon. Widespread antibiotic use has not significantly decreased the number of infections since the 1950s and has brought with it the deadly complication of resistant organisms.[1] Antibiotic selection also has become increasingly complex as newer antibiotics are continually developed.[2]

Two broad classes of infectious disease processes affect a surgical practice: those infectious conditions brought to the pediatric surgeon for treatment and cure[3] and those that arise in the postoperative period that are a complication of surgical intervention.

COMPONENTS OF INFECTION

The pathogenesis of infection involves a complex interaction between host and pathogens. Four components, present in varying degrees, are present in any infection: virulence of organism, size of inoculum, presence of nutrient source for the organism, and breakdown of host defense.

Virulence of Organism

The virulence of any microorganism depends on its ability to cause damage to the host. Exotoxins, such as streptococcal hyaluronidase, are digestive enzymes released locally that allow the spread of infection by breaking down host extracellular matrix proteins. Exotoxins also may be absorbed systemically by the host and cause remote damage. Endotoxins, such as lipopolysaccharides, are components of gram-negative cell walls that are released only after bacterial cell death. Endotoxin causes no local injury; rather, once systemically absorbed, endotoxin triggers a severe and rapid systemic inflammatory response.[4]

Infections are often polymicrobial; thus the concept of virulence requires an understanding of the types of interactions among species of microorganisms.[5] Different species may exist together within tissue through three separate mechanisms. *Species indifference* exists when a relatively stable balance exists between colonies of different species within the same environment. The best example of this is the complex flora of the human intestinal tract, which contains more than 100 species of bacteria.[6] *Species antagonism* is common and occurs when one or a few species emerge predominant from an initial large group as a result of external forces. A clinical example occurs when *Clostridium difficile* grows disproportionately owing to antibiotic disruption of the balance of colonic flora. *Species synergism* is seen when two or more species act in concert to allow continued growth of both species. In this mechanism, the observed damage to the host outweighs an additive affect of the individual organisms. The most common example of species synergism is seen in the mixed anaerobic and aerobic infections of an intra-abdominal abscess.[7] Anaerobic bacteria have high invasive potential but have difficulty propagating in an aerobic environment. However, when mixed with aerobic species, the oxygen content of the local tissues is consumed, allowing anaerobes to flourish, while aerobes benefit from the increased soft tissue invasion.

Size of Inoculum

The size of inoculum is the second component of an infection. The number of colonies of microorganisms per gram of tissue is a key determinant to infection. A minimal number of colonies is necessary for survival against host defenses. The smallest number of bacteria required to cause clinical infection varies from species to species, and, predictably, any decrease in host resistance decreases the absolute number of colonies necessary to cause clinical disease. In general, if the bacterial population in a wound exceeds 100,000 organisms per gram of tissue, invasive infection is present.[8]

Presence of Nutrient Source

For any inoculum, the ability for the organism(s) to find suitable nutrients is essential for their survival and comprises the third component of any clinical infection.

The only other requirement for most microorganisms is water; microorganisms do poorly in dry environments. Accumulation of necrotic tissue, hematoma, or other environmental contamination offers nutrient medium for continued growth and spread. Of special importance to the surgeon is the concept of necrotic tissue and infection. Retained necrotic tissue plays a dual role in the pathogenesis of infection. This tissue is recognized as a nutrient source for invading microorganisms,[9] and recent data also showed that necrotic tissue accumulates complement proteins.[10] Therefore necrotic tissue at a wound site attracts neutrophils and diverts them from invading microorganisms.

Breakdown of Host Defense

Finally, for a clinical infection to arise, the body's defenses must be broken. Even highly virulent organisms can be eradicated before clinical infection occurs if resistance is intact and nutrients are scarce. Evolution has equipped humans with redundant mechanisms of defense, both anatomic and systemic.

DEFENSE AGAINST INFECTION

Anatomic Barriers

Intact skin and mucous membranes provide an effective surface barrier to infection.[11] These tissues are not merely a mechanical obstacle; physiologic aspects of skin and mucous membranes provide additional protection. The constant turnover of keratinocytes leaves the uppermost surface of the skin dry, causing microorganisms to desiccate there. Skin temperature tends to be about 5°C less than physiologic, which inhibits bacterial growth. Acid secretion from sebaceous glands creates an environment on the skin surface with a pH of 5.5, further inhibiting bacterial cell growth. Finally, keratinocytes themselves can express the antigen responsible for recognition of cytotoxic T cells and can excrete proinflammatory cytokines in certain disease states.

Those mucosal surfaces that are exposed to the environment also have developed advanced defense mechanisms to prevent and combat microbial invasion. Specialized epithelial layers provide a defense to prevent bacterial invasion. The respiratory bronchial tree is protected by the mucociliary transport mechanism, which efficiently removes particulate contamination from inspired air. In the gastrointestinal (GI) tract, the harsh acidic environment of the stomach effectively kills most invading bacteria. Distally, the normal colonic flora competes with pathogenic organisms and prevents their emergence. In the urinary tract, the bladder also possesses an acidic environment and undergoes continuous and near-complete evacuation, diluting and eliminating organisms. In the eye, the surface of the cornea is continually bathed in the bactericidal enzyme lysozyme.[12]

Any pathologic situation affecting the normal function of these anatomic barriers increases the host's susceptibility to infection. A skin wound or a burn provides open access to soft tissues, tobacco damages the mucociliary transport system in the respiratory tree,[13] and antibiotic use disrupts normal colonic flora.[14] Such breakdowns in surface barriers are dealt with by the second line of defenses, the immune system.

Immune Response

The mammalian immune system involves complex pathways and many specialized effector responses.[15] Multiple overlapping mechanisms of intercellular communication (paracrine) act in concert with endocrine mechanisms to constitute this essential protective system.

The immune response is triggered by any infectious, traumatic, or foreign body invasion, resulting in inflammation (calor, rubor, dolor, and tumor). The components of acute inflammation are changes in local blood flow, presence of vascular permeability, and exudation of leukocytes. An initial vasoconstriction response is followed by vasodilation. Injury stimulates macrophages, production of proinflammatory cytokines, and microcirculation with activation of endothelial cells, blood elements, and a capillary leak. These processes are potentiated by ischemia, impaired oxygen delivery, and necrotic tissue, each of which exacerbates the inflammatory response. The classic hypothalamic-pituitary-adrenal axis, activated via neurologic afferent pathways, significantly influences inflammation by producing catecholamines and glucocorticoids.

Once initiated, the immune response operates by releasing cytokines and by receptors interacting on cell membranes.[16] Cytokines are endogenously produced proteins of low molecular weight and multiple biologic effects that are released locally by activated leukocytes. They exert both local and systemic responses. The best understood of these cytokines are tumor necrosis factor (TNF) and interleukin-1 (IL-1), which act to increase local synthesis of nitric oxide, prostaglandins, platelet-activating factor (PAF), and endothelial cell adhesion molecules. Cytokines also have the ability to exert control over the cells that produce them in an autocrine fashion. Sepsis, hemorrhage, ischemia, ischemia-reperfusion, and soft tissue trauma all share an ability to activate macrophages and produce proinflammatory cytokines that may progress to the uncontrolled systemic inflammatory response syndrome (SIRS).[17] Second-message compounds and effector molecules mediate the observed clinical phenomena (Fig. 9-1).

The local effect of these cytokines is chemotaxis, a targeted migration of the phagocyte toward an infectious focus. Most bacteria and fungi are destroyed by phagocytosis, the single most important process in the control of infection.[18] Three important aspects of microbe recognition exist before phagocytosis: receptor redundancy, receptor cooperation, and transduction of specific cellular signals after receptor binding. Multiple receptors on leukocytes often participate in a given microbial recognition event. This cooperation among multiple receptors often increases the apparent affinity of the receptors for their ligand, thereby increasing the killing power of the leukocyte. Further, the receptor may orchestrate

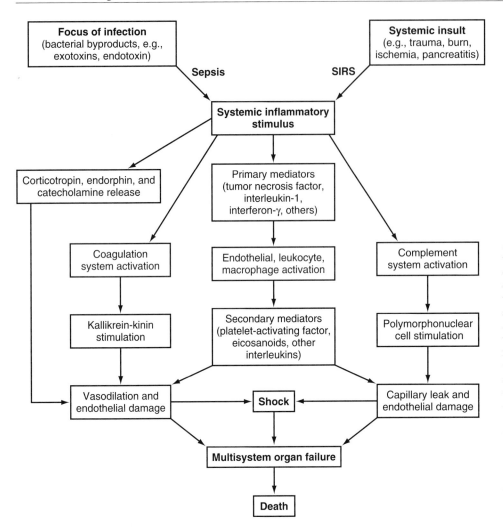

FIGURE 9-1. The parallel systemic inflammatory response that can result from infection, trauma, or critical illness. All of these types of insults may progress to shock, multisystem organ failure, and death. SIRS, systemic inflammatory response syndrome. (Data from Saez-Llorens X, McCracken GH Jr: Sepsis syndrome and septic shock in pediatrics: Current concepts of terminology, pathophysiology, and management. J Pediatr 123:497–508, 1993; and American College of Chest Physicians/Society of Critical Care Medicine Consensus Conference: Definitions for sepsis and organ failure and guidelines for the use of innovative therapies in sepsis. Crit Care Med 20:864–874, 1992.)

subsequent intracellular events during phagocytosis by transducing specific cellular signals. For example, the mannose and Fc γ-receptors direct particles to lysosomes and trigger a respiratory burst, whereas other receptors may not. Ingesting is an ameboid process in which the microbe is incorporated into the cytoplasm of the cell via endocytosis. Occasionally, however, ingested bacteria or their products are sufficiently potent to destroy the phagocyte before digestion. If this occurs, the release of contained lysozymes can lead to a destructive autodigestion of local host tissues. These defense mechanisms are nonspecific and do not rely on the host's targeted recognition of the invading organism.

Humoral and Cell-Mediated Immunity

Specific immunity has two major components. The *humoral mechanism* (B-cell system) is based on bursal cell lymphocytes and plasma cells and is independent of the thymus. The *cellular mechanism* (T-cell system) consists of the thymic-dependent lymphocytes.[19]

Humoral antibodies may neutralize toxins, tag foreign matter to aid phagocytosis (opsonization), or lyse invading cellular pathogens. Plasma cells and non–thymic-dependent lymphocytes that reside in the bone marrow and in the germinal centers and medullary cords of lymph nodes produce the reactive components of this humoral system. These components account for most of the human immunity against extracellular bacterial species.

Immunity provided by the B-cell system consists of both relatively specific antibodies, which are heat stable, and complement, which is heat labile and relatively nonspecific. Antibody receptor sites combine with antigen to form either soluble macromolecular compounds or insoluble complexes that precipitate or agglutinate. Human antibodies are classified into five basic types of immunoglobulins that vary considerably in concentration, diffusibility, size, and other properties. Complement is consumed whenever the humoral system has been activated, usually as a cascading system of at least nine complement components. Endotoxin and other proteins also are known to activate the sequence in what is called the *alternative pathway.*

The cellular or T-cell component of immunity is based on sensitized lymphocytes, probably of thymic origin, located in the subcortical regions of lymph nodes and in the periarterial spaces of the spleen; these lymphocytes form a part of the recirculating lymphocyte pool.

The T cells are specifically responsible for immunity to viruses, most fungi, and intracellular bacteria. They produce a variety of lymphokines, such as transfer factors, that activate further lymphocytes, chemotactic factors, leukotrienes, and interferons.

IMMUNODEFICIENCIES

Susceptibility to infection is increased when some component of the host defense mechanism is absent, reduced in absolute numbers, or significantly curtailed in function. Such derangements may have a congenital basis, although the majority are acquired as a direct result of drugs, radiation, endocrine disease, surgical ablation, tumors, or bacterial toxins.

Any alteration in the timing, magnitude, or quality of the host inflammatory response may permit the immediate invasion of pathogens. These defects, in local reaction to injury, are observed with extreme degrees of vasoconstriction, as in shock, and under certain other conditions. If the barrier has been injured (e.g., burns), fails to repair, or increases its permeability, microbial invasion can occur. Whenever a normal drainage system becomes obstructed (e.g., nephrolithiasis, cholelithiasis) or fails to function, infection may occur.

In diabetes mellitus, leukocytes often fail to respond normally to chemotaxis. Measurable reductions in the number of mature phagocytes occur in leukemia, agranulocytosis, and marrow dysplasia.[20] Tumors, drugs (e.g., chloramphenicol, steroids), radiation, or other agents that impair hematopoiesis may account for derangements in phagocytosis. Poor nutritional status has adverse effects on immune function. In general, cell-mediated and nonspecific immunity are more sensitive than humoral immunity.[21]

In patients with a primary immune defect, susceptibility to a specific infection is based on whether the defect is humoral, cellular, or a combination. Primary immunodeficiencies are rare but important, because prompt recognition can lead to life-saving treatment or significant improvement in the quality of life.[22] B-cell deficiencies are associated with sepsis from encapsulated bacteria, especially pneumococcus, *Haemophilus influenzae,* and meningococcus. Often a fulminating course rapidly ends in death, despite timely therapeutic measures. Although congenital agammaglobulinemia or dysgammaglobulinemia has been widely recognized, other causes of humoral defects include radiation, steroid and antimetabolite therapy, sepsis, splenectomy, and starvation.

Chronic granulomatous disease (CGD) is caused by a deficiency in the respiratory burst action of phagocytes. Genetic mutations in the genes encoding nicotinamide adenine dinucleotide phosphate (NADPH) oxidase result in a failure to produce superoxide and its reactive oxygen metabolites hydrogen peroxide and hypochlorous acid. This defect leads to a decreased ability to fight fungi and catalase-positive bacteria. Children with CGD are at risk for inflammatory and infectious syndromes because superoxide and its metabolites are necessary to downgrade inflammatory mediators such as leukotriene B$_4$ and C$_{5a}$ as well. Children with CGD are prone to develop hepatic abscesses, which may be first seen with fever and abdominal pain. Suppurative adenitis also is a common infection in this disease, with the involvement of a single node or multiple nodes. Surgical drainage is indicated in both of these infections, with accompanying long-term antibiotic treatment. Osteomyelitis and pneumonia also are common infections with CGD.[23-25]

T-cell deficiencies are responsible for many viral, fungal, and bacterial infections. Cutaneous candidiasis is a good example of a common infection seen with a T-cell deficiency. DiGeorge syndrome is a developmental anomaly in which both the thymus and the parathyroid glands are deficient, thus increasing the risk for infection and hypocalcemic tetany during infancy. Bacterial toxins, immunosuppressive drugs, malnutrition, and radiation also can produce defects in cellular immunity.[19]

HIV

Vertical transmission from mother to child is the dominant mode of human immunodeficiency virus (HIV) acquisition among infants and children. Most of this transmission is thought to occur during late pregnancy and the labor and delivery process. In the last decades, substantial epidemiologic changes have occurred in pediatric HIV infection with the increase in zidovudine administration to infected women during pregnancy. The vertical transmission of HIV infection can be decreased by two-thirds by maternal ingestion of zidovudine during the second and third trimesters of pregnancy, followed by neonatal administration of this medication.[26] Since 1995 when the American Academy of Pediatrics recommended documented HIV education and routine testing with consent for all pregnant women in the United States, a substantial decrease has occurred in the number of new cases of pediatric acquired HIV (acquired immunodeficiency syndrome; AIDS).[27]

Serologic tests are reliable diagnostic tests in children older than 18 months. Before this age, the presence of maternal antibodies acquired transplacentally preclude the possibility of a definitive diagnosis. These maternal antibodies can be present up to age 24 months. Anti-HIV immunoglobulin A (IgA) and IgM antibodies do not cross the placenta and can confirm the diagnosis if detected. However, these assays are not very sensitive. Thus in infants younger than 18 months, DNA polymerase chain reaction (PCR), HIV culture, or p24 antigen tests must be used to make the diagnosis.[28] Early recognition is crucial for early intervention, as early treatment has been shown to delay disease progression. Infants infected with HIV are at a particularly high risk for disease progression. The use of combination antiretroviral therapy in infants infected with HIV has been shown to slow the progression of the disease, leading to a more chronic illness rather than rapid progression and death.[29]

Children who have perinatally acquired HIV are more likely to have an early onset of symptoms, on average at age 12 months, than are children who have transfusion-acquired infection, closer to age 41 months. However, studies suggest that a bimodal distribution of disease progression is present, with the first peak at age 4 months and the second at age 6 years. Various models suggest a 14% to 20% incidence of AIDS in the first year, with an 8% to 10% incidence annually after that.[30]

Whereas almost two-thirds of children who are vertically infected with HIV remain asymptomatic until they attain school age, 20% to 30% have a more progressive course and manifest symptoms of serious opportunistic infections within the first year of life. Most infants who are diagnosed with AIDS have *Pneumocystis carinii* pneumonia (PCP) as their AIDS-defining condition. Encephalopathy and failure to thrive also are often seen in these infants.[29] The use of trimethoprim-sulfamethoxazole has led to significant decreases in the incidence of PCP.[31–33] Additionally, children are being treated with chemoprophylaxis to decrease the incidence of *Mycobacterium avium* complex.[34,35] The AIDS case definitions are similar for children and adults, except that lymphoid interstitial pneumonitis and multiple or recurrent bacterial infections are AIDS-defining conditions in children only.[36] Given that the risk of PCP is greatest in the first months of life, all HIV-exposed infants should begin prophylaxis treatment at age 4 to 6 weeks and continue this treatment through the first year. Given the high risk for rapid progression of the disease, antiretroviral therapy should be initiated. Combination antiretroviral therapy has been shown to reduce morbidity and mortality in adults and children.[37,38]

Unfortunately, only 25% to 40% of children receiving regimens of antiretrovirals experience suppression of their plasma HIV RNA levels to undetectable levels compared with 43% to 75% of adults.[39] Several factors may contribute to diminished response, including inadequate dosages and inadequate combinations of antiretrovirals. Effective suppression of the virus requires multiple drug therapy to which the virus is susceptible. Children have a higher baseline plasma RNA level, and their RNA levels appear to decrease more slowly; thus they may need more aggressive treatment.[39] Studies also have shown that children may need higher dosages of nelfinavir, ritonavir, saquinavir, and indinavir than previously thought. Children also may not be receiving adequate treatment because of problems with compliance. These treatments are difficult to administer because of their complexity with combination regimens as well as the number of pills, size of the capsules that must be taken, and the volume and poor taste of the medications. Adequate education may alleviate some problems with poor compliance. If the problem persists, gastrostomy tube placement for drug administration may be indicated.[39,40]

ANTIBIOTICS

The several classes of antibiotics are based on their molecular structure and site of action. The varying classes of antibiotics may be divided into bacteriostatic, which inhibit bacterial growth, and bacteriocidal, which destroy bacteria.

Penicillins

Penicillins were originally derived from molds and were the first major class of antibiotics developed. Penicillins are bacteriocidal and act by disrupting the cell wall of gram-positive organisms. They have a short half-life and a narrow spectrum, and they carry a significant risk of sensitivity. Penicillins are inactivated by β-lactamase. Synthetic derivatives have somewhat greater activity but are still susceptible to enzyme degradation. Penicillins plus β-lactamase inhibitors have increased the antimicrobial spectrum of penicillins by preventing the hydrolytic action of β-lactamase on the penicillin and increasing the antimicrobial activity of the penicillin by binding directly to the penicillin-binding proteins of the bacteria.[41]

Cephalosporins

Also bacteriocidal, cephalosporins are subdivided into generations based on increasing gram-negative activity. Adverse reactions include hypersensitivity reactions and alcohol intolerance. On the whole, they are less susceptible to β-lactamases and, like penicillins, act by inhibiting cell-wall synthesis. First-generation cephalosporins are effective against most aerobic gram-positive organisms. Second-generation drugs have increased gram-negative and anaerobic coverage. Third-generation cephalosporins have the broadest gram-negative coverage of the family, but they lose most of the gram-positive activity of the first generation. Fourth-generation cephalosporins are projected to have an extended spectrum of activity for gram-negative and gram-positive organisms and minimal β-lactamase susceptibility.

Aminoglycosides

Used to treat susceptible aerobic gram-negative bacteria, the aminoglycosides act by inhibiting protein synthesis. Aminoglycosides have a narrow margin of safety within the therapeutic dose range. Aminoglycosides can produce four types of dose-related adverse effects: (1) renal proximal tubular cell damage, (2) destruction of sensory cells in the cochlea, (3) destruction of sensory cells in the vestibular apparatus, and (4) neuromuscular paralysis.

Tetracyclines

Tetracyclines inhibit protein synthesis but are only bacteriostatic. They are active against gram-negative and gram-positive bacteria, mycoplasmas, chlamydiae, and protozoans. Tetracyclines remain a good first-line antibiotic in the penicillin-allergic patient. The use of tetracyclines has been limited, though, because they cause dental discoloration in children younger than 8 years. The severity and extent of discoloration appears to be related to total dosage of therapy.[42]

Quinolones

Quinolones are bacteriocidal. The fluoroquinolones destroy aerobic Enterobacteriaceae, staphylococci,

Pseudomonas aeruginosa, and some streptococci. The quinolones are excreted in the urine and are useful in treating urinary tract infections. Use of fluoroquinolones has been contradicted in children, according to Food and Drug Administration (FDA) labeling, because of concerns with cartilage damage in juvenile animal model testing. Ciprofloxacin, however, has been used and tolerated in children. Additionally, it is an oral agent that treats a number of infections that would otherwise require parenteral antibiotic treatment. Ciprofloxacin should be considered in situations in which no other oral agent is available and parenteral therapy would be required, or infection is caused by multidrug-resistant, gram-negative, enteric and other pathogens, such as certain *Pseudomonas* and *Mycobacterium* strains.[42]

Macrolides

The macrolides erythromycin, azithromycin, and clarithromycin are similar to each other in activity. They are primarily bacteriostatic agents active against aerobic and anaerobic gram-positive cocci and gram-negative anaerobes. Hypersensitivity reactions are rare, but pseudomembranous enterocolitis due to *C. difficile* does occur.

Imipenem

Imipenem is an extremely active bacteriocidal antibiotic with a spectrum against almost all gram-positive and gram-negative organisms, both aerobic and anaerobic. Enterococci, *Bacteroides fragilis,* and *Pseudomonas aeruginosa* are all susceptible. One of the carbapenem class of antibiotics, it is one of the most broadly active antibiotic available and should be reserved for the treatment of mixed infections not susceptible to other β-lactams.[43]

Aztreonam

Aztreonam is a parenteral antibiotic with excellent activity against *P. aeruginosa* equivalent to that of imipenem, ceftazidine, piperacillin, and azlocillin. Gram-positive organisms and anaerobes are resistant to aztreonam. Aztreonam is used primarily as an alternative to aminoglycosides for the treatment of aerobic gram-negative infections.[43]

Vancomycin

A bactericidal antibiotic active against all gram-positive cocci and bacilli, including *Staphylococcus aureus* and *Staphylococcus epidermidis* resistant to penicillins and cephalosporins, vancomycin also has bacteriostatic activity against enterococci. Vancomycin is the drug of choice for serious staphylococcal infection and endocarditis caused by *Streptococcus viridans* or enterococci or when penicillins or cephalosporins cannot be used because of drug allergy. Oral vancomycin is the drug of choice in *C. difficile* colitis, when it is resistant to metronidazole (Flagyl). Nephrotoxicity occurs occasionally, and deafness

may be associated with very high blood levels, usually in patients with renal insufficiency.

Linezolid

Linezolid is the first of the oxazolidinone antibiotics to receive FDA approval for the treatment of infections caused by resistant pathogens such as vancomycin-resistant enterococcus (VRE) and methicillin-resistant *Staphylococcus aureus* (MRSA). Pharmacokinetic studies in children demonstrated that children have a higher plasma clearance than do adults. More frequent dosing also is required in the younger children. The pediatric doses are not firmly established, but doses of 10 mg/kg every 12 hours for children younger than 12 years are recommended. Linezolid has been studied in pediatric populations and is a safe and effective antibiotic for the treatment of infections caused by gram-positive organisms resistant to more conventional agents or for patients intolerant of those agents. It also is an option for the oral treatment of serious infections caused by organisms such as VRE and MRSA.[44]

Trimethoprim and Sulfamethoxazole (Bactrim)

This bacteriostatic combination is active against most aerobic gram-positive and gram-negative organisms. Trimethoprim and sulfamethoxazole combined is the drug of choice to treat PCP. It also is effective in prophylaxis of this infection in children with AIDS or with malignancies. The side effects are nausea, vomiting, rash, and folate deficiency, resulting in macrocytic anemia.

Metronidazole

A bacteriocidal agent used primarily to treat protozoal infections and infections caused by anaerobes, particularly *B. fragilis,* metronidazole also has been used successfully in Hirschsprung's enterocolitis and for bowel preparation. It is the agent of choice in treatment of *C. difficile* colitis.

ANTIFUNGALS

Amphotericin B

Amphotericin B is a fungicidal and fungistatic antibiotic useful in any systemic fungal infection. Many attempts at reducing the toxicity of amphotericin have been investigated.[45] New lipid-encapsulated amphotericin formulations are available that allow increased dosing efficacy and decreased toxicity. Although these drugs reduce the toxicities of amphotericin B, their expense has led to restrictions on their use.

Fluconazole

A fungistatic agent useful against oropharyngeal and esophageal candidiasis, fluconazole has been successfully used in systemic fungal infections with *Candida* species not including *Candida glabrata*. Fluconazole has rarely been associated with hepatic toxicity, which is sometimes fatal in patients with serious comorbid conditions. Toxicity is most often related to coadministered drugs, which can alter the cytochrome P-450 system, leading to increased serum concentrations. Limited studies regard the safety and efficacy of azoles in pediatric patients; good comparison studies with amphotericin B do not exist.[42] Itraconazole may have a better spectrum of activity, but it is poorly absorbed in patients with GI disease, and cross-resistance has been reported across the azoles.

Azoles

Several new azoles with broader spectrum and increased potency are under investigation. The azoles inhibit the cytochrome p450–dependent 14-α-sterol demethylase, a critical step in the synthesis of ergesterol. These agents halt cell division, but do not cause membrane leakage or destroy the cell. Although these new azoles are more potent than fluconazole, cross-resistance may be found across the azoles. Voriconazole is under investigation for both PO and IV formulations. Its strengths are its strong activity against *Aspergillus* and *Cryptococcus*, its broad activity against *Candida* spp, and its low toxicity and good bioavailability. Posaconazole is being tested in an oral formulation and shows excellent activity against the zygomycetes. Ravuconazole also is being tested. Its advantage is a long half-life (83 to 145 hours).[46]

Flucytosine

Flucytosine is an antifungal agent with a limited spectrum of activity, a potential for toxicity, and when used alone, often leads to resistance. However, it is the only pyrimidine antifungal approved for use in children. It is best used in combination with amphotericin B in the treatment of cryptococcal meningitis and life-threatening candidal meningitis.[42] Patients with AIDS do not tolerate flucytosine.

Nystatin

Both fungistatic and fungicidal against a wide variety of yeast and yeast-like fungi, nystatin is passed unchanged in the stool. It is used to treat intestinal and oral cavity infections caused by *Candida albicans*. Large oral doses occasionally produce diarrhea, GI distress, nausea, or vomiting.

Caspofungin

Caspofungin is an echinocandin, the first of a new class of antifungals. These agents are β-1,3-glucan synthase inhibitors. These agents have high potency and broader activity. It is a good treatment for patients with *Aspergillus* refractory to or intolerant of other therapies. Given its few side effects, it tends to be better tolerated by patients as well. Unfortunately, safety and efficacy studies have not yet been carried out in children.[46]

ANTIVIRALS

Acyclovir

Acyclovir is an antiviral agent effective for preventing and treating viruses in the herpes family. Both IV and PO formulations are approved for use in children. Very little active drug accumulates in uninfected cells, which accounts for the low toxicity of the drug.

Ganciclovir

Related to acyclovir but with greater efficacy against cytomegalovirus, ganciclovir inhibits viral replication by interfering with cellular DNA. Adverse reactions include bone marrow suppression, mild nephrotoxicity, and transient hepatic enzyme elevation.

Valacyclovir, Penciclovir, and Famciclovir

Valacyclovir is a prodrug of acyclovir and is approved for the treatment of herpes zoster in adults. No specific safety data exist for the use of this medication in children. Penciclovir also has been studied in adults for the treatment of herpes labialis. It has a longer half-life intracellularly than acyclovir but is less potent in inhibiting viral DNA replication. It's safety in children has not been studied yet. Famciclovir is the oral prodrug of penciclovir and is approved in adults for the treatment of herpes zoster. Its efficacy is similar to that of acyclovir. No specific safety or pharmacologic data in children are available yet.[47]

Amantadine

Amantadine interferes with the replication mechanism of influenza A virus by blocking the M2 protein. In the pediatric population, it is approved for prophylaxis against influenza A. It does not have any activity against influenza B. In adults, amantadine has been used to treat active influenza A, leading to an amelioration of symptoms and reduction of viral titers. The efficacy of amantadine in treating active influenza A in children has not now been shown.[48]

Rimantadine

Structurally similar to amantadine, rimantadine also acts against influenza A by preventing the uncoding of the viral particles. This drug is less lipophilic than amantadine and does not cross the blood-brain barrier. It also is metabolized to a greater extent before renal excretion; thus it is safer in patients with renal insufficiency. Rimantadine is approved only for prophylaxis against influenza A.

Zanamivir

Zanamivir is the sialic acid analogue inhibitor of influenza A and B virus neuraminidases. Its action is to prevent release of the virus from infected cells. Currently it is approved for use in children older than 12 years. This drug is not used for prophylaxis against influenza A and B but can significantly reduce the severity and duration of infection.

Ribavirin

Ribavarin is a guanosine analogue with broad antiviral activity against both RNA and DNA viruses, including adenovirus. It has shown potential benefit against respiratory syncytial virus (RSV), influenza, parainfluenza, measles, and hantavirus. Ribavirin is excreted renally and thus high levels can be achieved in the kidneys and bladder for the treatment of adenovirus cystitis. Mild anemia is the most common side effect and is rarely symptomatic. Ribavirin is licensed in intravenous (IV), aerosol, and oral formulations.[49]

Antiretrovirals

Many antiretrovirals are approved for the treatment of HIV in adults in the United States, but the number approved for children is more limited. The following are approved for use in the pediatric population:

Nucleoside analogue reverse transcriptase inhibitor agents: didanosine (ddI), lamivudine (3TC), stavudine (d4T), zalcitabine (ddC), and zidovudine (ZDV, AZT)
Non-nucleoside reverse transcriptase inhibitor agents: delavirdine (DLV) and nevirapine (NVP)
Protease inhibitor agents: indinavir (IDV), nelfinavir (NFV), ritonavir (RTV), and saquinavir (SQV).[28,50]

Although antiretroviral combined therapy has significantly improved the prognosis for children with HIV infection, it also has introduced new complications. These medications cause a complete spectrum of metabolic complications, including fat maldistribution, hyperglycemia, insulin resistance, hyperlipidemia, lactic acidosis, and decreased bone mineral density. Additionally, growth retardation, due to both infection and the neurologic consequences of toxicity to the mitochondria caused by these medications, appears to be a unique complication to the pediatric population of HIV-infected patients. The unique position of children as growing and developing organisms and their longer exposure to antiretroviral therapy put them at increased risk for these metabolic side effects.[51]

PHARMACOKINETICS AND MONITORING

The efficacy and safety of many drugs have not been established in the pediatric patient, especially in the newborn.[52] Dosages based on pediatric pharmacokinetic data offer the most rational approach. The assumption that a child is a miniature adult as the basis for extrapolation of adult dosages to children is certainly not ideal. Dosage requirements constantly change as a function of age and body weight. Knowledge of a drug's pharmacokinetic profile allows manipulation of the dose to achieve and maintain a given plasma concentration. For example, penicillins and cephalosporins have a distribution in children that prolongs their half-life.[53] Many drugs exhibit a biexponential plasma disappearance curve in neonates and children, in that a certain fraction of the drug remaining in the body is eliminated per unit of time. Some drugs (e.g., gentamicin) exhibit saturation kinetics, in which a specific amount, not a fraction, of the drug is eliminated per unit of time.[54] The body surface area (BSA) method of calculating drug dosages

$$BSA = (Weight\ [kg] \div 1.73) \times Adult\ dose$$

approximates the pediatric dose of many drugs but does not always accurately determine dosage requirements in the premature and term newborn.

Newborns usually have extremely skewed drug-distribution patterns. Thus the entire body during the newborn period could be considered as if it were a single compartment for purposes of dose calculations. For the majority of drugs, dose adjustments can be based on plasma drug concentration. Administering a loading dose is advisable when rapid onset of drug action is required. For many drugs, loading doses (milligrams per kilogram) are generally greater in neonates and young infants than in older children or adults.[54] However, prolonged elimination of drugs in the neonate requires lower maintenance doses, given at longer intervals, to prevent toxicity. Monitoring serum drug concentrations is useful if the desired effect is not attained or if adverse reactions occur. In the sick premature newborn, almost all medications are administered IV because GI function and drug absorption are unreliable. Intramuscular injection is impractical because these neonates have little muscle mass. In older preterm neonates, term newborns, and older pediatric patients who do not have vomiting or diarrhea, oral drugs may be used. Drug absorption through the skin is enhanced in the neonate and is currently being evaluated.[55]

The neonate undergoing extracorporeal membrane oxygenation (ECMO) presents a special challenge to drug delivery and elimination. Because the ECMO circuit may bind drugs and make them unavailable to the patient, dosing of drugs requires careful attention to drug response and serum levels. In one in vitro study, drug levels of common medications were significantly lowered, depending, partially, on the age of the membrane.[56]

PREVENTION OF INFECTIONS

The most effective way to deal with surgical infectious complications is to avoid them. The clinician must recognize the variables that increase the risk of infection and eliminate them.

Patient Characteristics

In the adult surgical patient population, patient characteristics and comorbidities such as diabetes, systemic steroid use, obesity, extremes of age, poor nutritional status, and perioperative transfusion of certain blood products are associated with an increased risk of surgical-site infection. However, these chronic disease states are less frequently encountered in children. A recent study of surgical wound infections in the pediatric surgical population showed that wound infections are more related to factors at the operation. In a prospective multicenter study of more than 800 pediatric patients, the only factors associated with increased surgical-site infection were contamination at the time of operation and the duration of the procedure.[57]

Surgical Preparation

Preoperative preparation of the operative site and the hands of the entire surgical team is of utmost importance in reducing the risk of postoperative infection. Hand scrubbing remains the most important proactive mechanism to reduce infection. Although debated, a 5-minute first scrub followed by subsequent 2- or 3-minute scrubs for secondary cases with one of several different cleansing solutions is adequate.[58,59] By using either 5% povidone-iodine or 4% chlorhexidine gluconate, a consistent 95% decrease in skin flora can be achieved.

Hand washing is one of the most important measure to decrease nosocomial infections. However, studies have shown that compliance among medical personnel is unacceptably low, less than 50%.[60,61] Hand rubbing with alcohol-based hand antiseptic increases compliance with hand hygiene and has been shown in studies to be as effective as or even more effective than hand washing in decreasing bacterial contamination.[62,63]

Preoperative showering with an antiseptic such as chlorhexidine can reduce colony counts up to ninefold. Several applications are required to attain maximal antimicrobial benefit. Despite reducing the colony counts, though, no definitive data suggest that this actually reduces the risk of infection.

Similar reduction in the patient's skin flora can be achieved with aggressive preoperative cleansing and sterile draping. Shaving the operative field, if necessary, should be done only just before prepping the skin, and preferably with electric clippers.[64-66] Preoperative shaving the night before has been shown to increase rates of infection.[65,67]

Normothermia has been suggested as a means to decrease the incidence of surgical wound infections. A prospective randomized trial of 200 patients showed that intraoperative hypothermia caused delayed wound healing and a greater incidence of infections. Hypothermia during the decisive period for establishing an infection, the several hours after initial contamination, causes an increase in culture-positive wounds.[68]

Supplemental oxygen during the perioperative period also has been shown to decrease the rate of wound infection by as much as 50%.[69]

Antibiotic Prophylaxis

Operative procedures can be classified into one of four types, based on clinical situation and anatomic site, as

---

TABLE 9-1
DIAGNOSIS OF HIV INFECTION IN CHILDREN

Diagnosis: HIV Infected
a) A child <18 mo who is known to be HIV seropositive or born to an HIV-infected mother and
  - has positive results on two separate determinations (excluding cord blood) from one or more of the following HIV detection tests:
      HIV culture
      HIV polymerase chain reaction
      HIV antigen (p24)
              or
  - meets criteria for AIDS diagnosis based on the 1987 AIDS surveillance case definition
b) A child ≥18 mo born to an HIV-infected mother or any child infected by blood, blood products, or other known modes of transmission (e.g., sexual contact) who
  - is HIV-antibody positive by repeatedly reactive enzyme immunoassay (EIA) and confirmatory test (e.g., Western blot or immunofluorescence assay [IFA])
              or
  - meets any of the criteria in a) above

Diagnosis: Perinatally Exposed (Prefix E in Table 9-2)
A child who does not meet the criteria above who
  - is HIV seropositive by EIA and confirmatory test (e.g., Western blot or IFA) and is <18 mo at the time of test
              or
  - has unknown antibody status, but was born to a mother known to be infected with HIV

Diagnosis: Seroreverter (SR)
A child who is born to an HIV-infected mother and who
  - has been documented as HIV-antibody negative (i.e., two or more negative EIA tests performed at age 6–18 mo or one negative EIA test after age 18 mo)
              and
  - has had no other laboratory evidence of infection (has not had two positive viral detection tests, if performed)
              and
  - has not had an AIDS-defining condition

Adapted from Centers for Disease Control and Prevention: 1994 Revised classification system for human immunodeficiency virus infection in children less than 13 years of age. MMWR Morb Mortal Wkly Rep 43: RR-12, 1994.
AIDS, acquired immunodeficiency syndrome; HIV, human immunodeficiency virus.

---

outlined in Table 9-1. In adults, several well-designed prospective trials document decreased infection rates for all types of operative procedures with established antibiotic recommendations.[70] Timing of the perioperative antibiotic coverage is crucial; the first dose must be given within a time frame before the surgical incision to achieve bacteriocidal levels of antibiotic at the site of the incision, generally 30 minutes to 3 hours before. In cases that take more than 3 hours, a second dose of prophylactic antibiotics may be indicated to reachieve adequate serum levels.

Prophylaxis accounts for nearly 75% of antibiotic use on pediatric surgical services. Additionally, prophylaxis is a major cause of inappropriate use of antimicrobials in children. In one study of children younger than

6 years undergoing surgical procedures, prophylactic antibiotics were administered inappropriately to 42% of children receiving preoperative antibiotics, 67% of children receiving intraoperative antibiotics, and 55% of those receiving postoperative antibiotics.[71] In pediatric surgery, it is clear that antibiotic coverage is required during clean-contaminated, contaminated, or dirty cases. However, some disagreement exists concerning antimicrobial prophylaxis in clean operations. In clean cases in children with no other associated risk factors for infection, some pediatric surgeons still believe that preoperative antibiotics are necessary. Review of the pediatric surgical literature yields studies that advocate the use of antibiotics[72] and those that do not.[73] Antibiotic prophylaxis in a clean case in the pediatric population is now at the discretion of the operating surgeon.

Bowel Preparation

The efficacy of bowel preparation before elective colon operation has been established.[74] The three components of the technique, each with its own variations, include mechanical irrigation and flushing of the colon to remove stool; oral topical antibiotics against colonic aerobes and anaerobes; and preoperative IV antibiotics that cover both common skin and colonic flora.[75] The preparation can be started on an outpatient basis the day before operation, and the parenteral drugs are added to the regimen just before the procedure. One must be careful in the pediatric population, however, to avoid dehydration associated with bowel preps.

Drains and Irrigation

The use of drains varies widely; drains are indicated in those surgical procedures in which one expects accumulation of blood, serum, exudates from wounds, and potential dead space.[76] Drains also are indicated when closure of a hollow viscous is imperfect. When a drain is required, use a closed drainage system, and bring the drain out via a separate stab wound away from the operative incision. Drains should be removed as soon as possible because they are foreign bodies that can impede wound closure and because bacteria can colonize the wound via a drain or its exit site.[77]

Irrigating the operative field is an important component in preventing postoperative infectious complications.[78] Irrigation with copious amounts of sterile saline mechanically removes loose debris, necrotic tissue, serum, and excess clot. Use of antibiotics in the irrigation solution has not been proved to be efficacious,[79] but noxious solutions, such as povidone-iodine or hydrogen peroxide, are deleterious.[80]

TYPES OF INFECTION

Postoperative Soft Tissue Infection

Despite meticulous technique, perioperative antibiotics, and proper use of drains and irrigation, surgical infectious complications still occur. The fundamental principles of surgical treatment of an infectious process are straightforward: (1) drain pus, (2) débride the wound, (3) reestablish anatomic continuity, and (4) treat with appropriate antibiotic(s).

Postoperative soft tissue infections can be divided into confined local lesions and invasive, spreading ones. Early diagnosis and prompt intervention help to avoid morbidity and occasional mortality. Erythema, fever, leukocytosis, tenderness, crepitus, and suppuration in a wound are diagnostic signs that are not always present. When confronted with a suggestive wound, clinical judgments must be made. Treatment should be suited to the extent of the infection and may include oral or IV antibiotics, simple incision and drainage, or extensive surgical débridement. Fortunately, soft tissue infections are uncommon in the pediatric surgical population. The incidence of wound infection varies from 1% to 11% in clean wounds and from 6% to 20.7% in contaminated wounds.[81,82]

A localized surgical wound infection with seroma or pus requires drainage and packing to allow healing by secondary intention. Antibiotic therapy should be reserved for those infections with associated cellulitis. Localized cellulitis without fluid accumulation sometimes is amenable to antibiotic treatment only.

An abscess is a localized collection of pus in a cavity formed by an expanding infectious process. The pus is a combination of leukocytes, necrotic material, bacteria, and extracellular fluid. The usual cause is staphylococcal species in combination with one or more organisms; treatment is incision and drainage followed by antibiotic therapy. Streptococcus soft tissue infections are probably the most virulent and can arise in just a few hours after surgical procedures. High fever, irrational behavior, and leukocytosis are hallmarks of patient presentation. Penicillin in high doses is the appropriate initial management of streptococcal infections.

Bacillus infections are the next most virulent infections. Inspection of the wound will show dark, mottled areas, as opposed to the bright pink of a streptococcal cellulitis. Less than half of patients with bacillus infections have detectable gas crepitation. Severe pain is the most telling clinical symptom of this type of infection. Massive doses of penicillin also are the hallmarks of treatment for these patients. Hyperbolic oxygen has not been proven to improve outcomes.

Drainage must be complete, or the abscess will reform. A phlegmon is an area of diffuse inflammation with little pus and some necrotic tissue. A phlegmon usually progresses to an abscess if untreated.

Dehiscence

Dehiscence is defined as breakdown of the fascial components of a surgically closed wound. In any incision, the long-term tensile strength lies in the healing of the fascial component of the closure. By definition, dehiscence can occur in any surgically closed wound. Poor nutrition, renal failure, corticosteroid use, immune compromise, and poor wound-closure technique increase the chance of wound dehiscence.[83]

Nosocomial Infection

Nosocomial infections are defined as those infections that are hospital acquired.[84] As such, they are a potential threat to all hospitalized patients and increase morbidity and mortality significantly.[85] A recent report described a total of 676 operative procedures performed in 608 pediatric patients. Nosocomial infection occurred in 38 (6.2%). In total, 53 infectious complications were tabulated: wound, 17 (2.5%); septicemia, 14 (2.1%); pulmonary, 10 (1.5%); urinary tract, 5 (0.7%); abdominal, 5 (0.7%); and diarrhea, 2 (0.3%). Broviac catheter sepsis occurred in 7 (11.5%) of 61 lines. The highest overall occurrence of infection was in the infant group (1 month to 1 year; 13 [8.1%] of 161). The probability of septicemia was highest in neonates (4.2%) compared with infants (3.1%) and older children (1.2%) ($P < .05$). The most common isolates were *Staphylococcus epidermidis* (10 of 17) from septic patients, and gram-negative enteric bacteria (27 of 50) from organ and wound infections. Infection was associated with impaired nutrition, multiple disease processes, and multiple operations. The risk of nosocomial infection in this population was comparable to that reported in adult surgical patients. In one study, ECMO use correlated with increased incidence of nosocomial infection.[86] Two factors that increase the risk of nosocomial infection in surgical wounds as well as other sites are length of the preoperative stay and exposure to invasive medical devices.[87]

Pneumonia is the most lethal nosocomial infection, with mortality ranging from 20% to 70% and accounting for 10% to 15% of all pediatric hospital-acquired infections.[88] The mortality rate is dependent on the causative organism. The risk factors for nosocomial pneumonia in the pediatric population include serious underlying illness, immunosuppression, length of time on a ventilator, and nasopharyngeal floral changes with prolonged hospitalization.[6] An increased risk may be found in patients with gastric alkalinization, because use of antacids in the intensive care unit to prevent stress ulceration increases bacterial counts in the stomach and may predispose the patient to increased bacterial translocation.[89]

Clostridium difficile is a well-recognized cause of infectious diarrhea that develops after antibiotic therapy in many patients, although it likely only accounts for 20% of antibiotic-associated diarrhea. Furthermore, it is the most common nosocomial infection, infecting one-fifth of all hospitalized patients, and its incidence is on the increase. The best method of prevention is the judicious and appropriate use of antibiotics. Prolonged antibiotic use has an association with increased rates of *C. difficile* colitis. Some studies have suggested the use of probiotics for the prevention and treatment of antibiotic-associated diarrhea. However, these studies were performed in adults, and reports on the efficacy of *Lactobacillus GG* in children are conflicting. Until better evidence is available, the best method of prevention is the judicious and appropriate use of antibiotics.[90-92]

Catheter Infections

Central venous catheters (CVCs) are essential in managing critically ill pediatric patients. However, the complication of catheter-related infection prevails, despite a great deal of effort to reduce its occurrence. It is important to recognize the difference between colonization of the catheter and CVC infection. Colonization is defined as the presence of a positive culture without signs and symptoms of clinical infection. Five major factors are associated with the development of the following catheter-related nosocomial infections:

1. Sterility of the insertion technique
2. Type of solution being administered through the line
3. Care of the catheter once inserted
4. Proximity of the catheter to another wound
5. Presence of another infection elsewhere

Absolute sterile techniques should be maintained in all instances of line insertion except in a trauma or other emergency situation in which the need for expedient line placement may necessitate less-than-sterile technique. The use of maximal sterile barriers, including sterile gown and gloves and a large sterile sheet, has been shown to reduce greatly the risk of catheter-related infection.[93-96] Povidone-iodine has long been the standard for cleansing of the skin before catheter insertion, but recent studies suggest that chlorhexidine significantly reduces the incidence of microbial colonization compared with povidone-iodine.[96-100]

The use of CVCs in pediatric patients has increased as prolonged vascular access has become increasingly necessary to provide parenteral nutrition, chemotherapy, blood products, and antimicrobial therapy to an increasing number of children. A major complication of these catheters is infection, which can lead to serious morbidity and mortality. Many methods have been tried to decrease these infections. Location of the catheter is correlated with the risk of infection, as placement in the subclavian vein leads to fewer infections than that in the internal jugular vein or the femoral vein.[93,101-104] For catheters that will remain in place for a longer period, tunneling the catheter has been shown to reduce significantly the risk of catheter-related infection.[105-107]

The skin and catheter hub are the most common sources of colonization and infection, and thus various methods have been tried to combat these risks. Silver ions have broad antimicrobial activity, and catheters with silver-impregnated cuffs have been proposed as a preventive measure. Although these cuffs decreased the short-term risk for infection, their efficacy wears off with time.[108-111]

Antibiotics flushes were first shown to reduce complications 20 years ago and have been studied extensively since then. Studies have shown that this antibiotic flush can reduce the number of gram-negative catheter infections and decrease the number of catheter occlusions. Used daily, these flushes can decrease the risk of catheter-related infection.[112-114] However, significant concern exists that the routine use of vancomycin flushes will lead to an increased risk for the acquisition of vancomycin-resistant enterococcus,[115] as well as the development of vancomycin-resistant *Staphylococcus*.[116,117] These concerns are serious enough that the Centers for Disease Control (CDC) Guidelines for the prevention of intravascular catheter-related infections do not recommend the use of vancomycin flushes.[95]

A novel technique proposed to decrease the risk of catheter-related infections is a new antiseptic hub for the catheter. One study suggested that these new hubs can reduce the risk of infection fourfold,[118] but another study showed no benefit from these antiseptic hubs. Further clinical trials are needed before recommendation of an antiseptic hub.[119]

New technology also has been instrumental in the development of antimicrobial-coated catheters, which have been shown to decrease colonization of catheters and decrease the risk of catheter-related bloodstream infections. Catheters coated with chlorhexidine–silver sulfadiazine externally can cut colonization rates in half and reduce infection risks up to fourfold.[120–125] Several studies have not shown a benefit to these catheters, particularly if used longer than a few weeks.[102,126–128] It is likely that these catheters become less effective in reducing infection risks after being in place for longer than 3 weeks because of a decrease in their antimicrobial activity and their lack of luminal protection.[125]

Catheters with a combination of minocycline and rifampin coating both their internal and external surfaces have been shown to be even more effective in decreasing the risks of catheter-related infection.[123,128] Studies also have shown that no emergence of antimicrobial resistance occurs with the use of these catheters.[124,129] The current CDC recommendations include the use of an antimicrobial catheter if a CVC will be used for longer than 5 days in an adult.[95,124,125] The use of these catheters in children is still under investigation. Chlorhexidine has been absorbed into the bloodstream of newborns when used for cleansing and has been shown to cause bradycardia and local reactions. Minocycline has led to serum sickness in adolescents taking the medication. The reactions these medications might cause while coating a central catheter still require further investigation.[130]

The use of a chlorhexidine-impregnated polyurethane foam dressing on the catheter-insertion site has been shown to reduce colonization.[131] However, a multicenter study of neonatal intensive care units showed that this novel dressing has results comparable to those with gauze and tape with periodic disinfection with povidone-iodine. The chlorhexidine dressing, though, led to dermatotoxicity in low-birthweight neonates.[132]

OTHER INFECTIONS

Although the infections listed earlier are possibly preventable and occur after surgical procedures or hospitalization, some infections are seen by the pediatric surgeon for treatment and cure.

Soft Tissue Infection

Necrotizing fasciitis is a rapidly progressing infection of the fascial tissues and overlying skin. Although it can occur as a postoperative complication or as a primary infection, necrotizing fasciitis is more likely in immunocompromised patients.[133] Because the diagnosis is often not obvious, the clinician must look for clinical clues such as edema beyond the area of erythema, crepitus, skin vesicles, or cellulitis refractory to IV antibiotics. Prompt surgical intervention, including wide excision of all necrotic and infected tissue, along with the institution of antibiotics, is mandatory to avoid progression and mortality. Approximately half of pediatric cases occur in neonates. Combining the 47 patients reported in three series, the most common associated diagnosis was varicella infection (46%).[134–136] The mortality was 25% and was usually associated with delayed diagnosis. All survivors were operated on within 3 hours of diagnosis. Extensive débridement and triple antibiotic therapy were the hallmarks of survival.

Peritonitis

Peritonitis is defined as inflammation of the peritoneum.[137] Peritonitis is divided into primary, secondary, and tertiary, depending on the etiology. Spontaneous primary peritonitis is a bacterial infection without enteric perforation. In young girls, this is thought to arise from the genital tract, and in those with cirrhosis, from translocation.[138] Primary peritonitis is usually caused by a single organism of gut origin; however, if an invasive catheter is present, the most likely organism is grampositive.[139] Susceptible infants are those with ascites, indwelling peritoneal dialysis catheters, ventriculoperitoneal shunts, or compromised immunity. An infant with primary peritonitis usually does not exhibit signs of peritonitis but may have poor feeding, lethargy, distention, vomiting, and mild to severe abdominal tenderness. Definitive treatment may require only a course of broadspectrum antibiotics. Primary peritonitis in children now represents approximately 1% of all cases of peritonitis.

Secondary peritonitis is associated with GI tract disruption.[140] This can be caused directly by perforation, bowel-wall necrosis, or trauma, or postoperatively as a result of iatrogenic injury or anastomotic leak. Treatment of secondary peritonitis is a combination of surgical intervention and antibiotics and removal of any prosthetic device.

Tertiary peritonitis, also called recurrent peritonitis, is characterized by organ dysfunction and systemic inflammation in association with recurrent infection. The mortality rate is often very high, and treatment is very difficult.[138] Treatment consists of broader-spectrum antibiotics, as the infection often includes nosocomial organisms and multidrug-resistant bacteria.

Lymphangitis

Lymphangitis is often manifested by a red streak extending up an extremity. The causative organism is

TABLE 9-2

PEDIATRIC HIV CLASSIFICATION*

	Clinical Category			
Immunological Category	N: No Signs/ Symptoms	A: Mild Signs/ Symptoms	B: Moderate Signs/ Symptoms[†]	C[†]: Severe Signs/ Symptoms
1. No evidence of suppression	N1	A1	B1	C1
2. Evidence of moderate suppression	N2	A2	B2	C2
3. Severe suppression	N3	A3	B3	C3

*Children whose HIV infection status is not confirmed are classified by using the above grid with a letter E (for perinatally exposed) placed before the appropriate classification code (e.g., EN2).
[†]Both category C and lymphoid interstitial pneumonitis in category B are reportable to state and local health departments as AIDS.
Adapted from Centers for Disease Control and Prevention: 1994 Revised classification system for human immunodeficiency virus infection in children less than 13 years of age. MMWR Morb Mortal Wkly Rep 43:RR-12, 1994.
AIDS, acquired immunodeficiency syndrome; HIV, human immunodeficiency virus.

usually *Staphylococcus* or *Streptococcus* species. Prompt, aggressive therapy includes immobilization, elevation, and IV antibiotics. The infection worsens without treatment, and obliteration of the lymphatic channels can result.

Sepsis

Sepsis, by contemporary definition, distinguishes between the systemic derangements that are caused by the infectious organisms and their by-products and those that are caused by the host systemic inflammatory response.[141] In 1992, the Society of Critical Care Medicine published the results of a consensus conference to define accurately the terms regarding sepsis and the inflammatory response to injury and infection[142] (Tables 9-2, 9-3, and 9-4). Independent of the original infection, SIRS may progress to multiorgan dysfunction and death. Gram-negative organisms possess a lipopolysaccharide moiety on the cell wall that has been shown to incite most, if not all, of the toxic effects of end-organ failure. In animal models, injection of lipopolysaccharide can induce a septic response by both direct and indirect effects. Directly, it activates macrophages and neutrophils to release the cytokines, TNF, IL-1, and IL-6, which are the primary host mediators of end-organ failure.[143]

The indirect host responses to these cytokines include release of PAF, IL-8, prostaglandins, and nitric oxide. These secondary mediators induce vasodilation, more polymorphonuclear cell stimulation, endothelial cell damage and leak, as well as platelet activation. The systemic response to these derangements is hypotension, fever, hypoxia, and end-organ failure. The process is self-propagating. Figure 9-1 shows a schematic of the current understanding of the pathogenesis of the inflammatory response in sepsis.[144]

Therefore in addition to conventional surgical débridement and drainage, antibiotic treatment, and supportive intensive therapy, modulating the host inflammatory mediators as a therapeutic addition, have been explored since the mid-1980s. Although successful in animal models of sepsis, inhibiting host inflammatory response in human sepsis has not improved survival. New treatment modalities, such as granulocyte-stimulating factor, immunoglobulin infusion, and cytokine antagonists offer theoretical promise but so far have not improved the results of clinical trials.[145]

Neonatal sepsis is defined as a generalized bacterial infection accompanied by a positive blood culture within the first month of life.[146] Neonatal sepsis occurring during the first week of life is caused primarily by maternal organisms transferred during delivery. Maternal contamination of the neonate can be transmitted through the

TABLE 9-3

CLINICAL CATEGORIES FOR CHILDREN WITH HIV INFECTION

Category N: Not Symptomatic
Children who have no signs or symptoms considered to be the result of HIV infection or who have only one of the conditions listed in category A

Category A: Mildly Symptomatic
Children with two or more of the conditions listed below but none of the conditions listed in categories B and C
• Lymphadenopathy (≥0.5 cm at more than two sites; bilateral, one site)
• Hepatomegaly
• Splenomegaly
• Dermatitis
• Parotitis
• Recurrent or persistent upper respiratory infection, sinusitis, or otitis media

TABLE 9-3

CLINICAL CATEGORIES FOR CHILDREN WITH HIV INFECTION—cont'd

Category B: Moderately Symptomatic

Children who have symptomatic conditions other than those listed for category A or C that are attributed to HIV infection. Examples of conditions in clinical category B include but are not limited to

- Anemia (<8 g/dL), neutropenia (<1000/mm³), or thrombocytopenia (<100,000/mm³) persisting ≥30 d
- Bacterial meningitis, pneumonia, or sepsis (single episode)
- Candidiasis, oropharyngeal (thrush), persisting (>2 mo) in children age >6 mo
- Cardiomyopathy
- Cytomegalovirus infection, with onset before age 1 mo
- Diarrhea, recurrent or chronic
- Hepatitis
- Herpes simplex virus stomatitis, recurrent (more than two episodes within 1 yr)
- HSV bronchitis, pneumonitis, or esophagitis with onset before age 1 mo
- Herpes zoster (shingles) involving at least two distinct episodes or more than one dermatome
- Leiomyosarcoma
- Lymphoid interstitial pneumonia or pulmonary lymphoid hyperplasia complex
- Nephropathy
- Nocardiosis
- Persistent fever (lasting >1 mo)
- Toxoplasmosis, onset before age 1 mo
- Varicella, disseminated (complicated chickenpox)

Category C: Severely Symptomatic

Children who have any condition listed in the 1987 surveillance case definition for AIDS, with the exception of lymphocytic interstitial pneumonitis

- Serious bacterial infections, multiple or recurrent (i.e., any combination of at least two culture-confirmed infections within a 2-yr period), of the following types: septicemia, pneumonia, meningitis, bone or joint infection, or abscess of an internal organ or body cavity (excluding otitis media, superficial skin or mucosal abscesses, and indwelling catheter–related infections)
- Candidiasis, esophageal or pulmonary (bronchi, trachea, lungs)
- Coccidioidomycosis, disseminated (at site other than or in addition to lungs or cervical or hilar lymph nodes)
- Cryptococcosis, extrapulmonary
- Cryptosporidiosis or isosporiasis with diarrhea persisting >1 mo
- Cytomegalovirus disease with onset of symptoms at age >1 mo (at a site other than liver, spleen, or lymph nodes)
- Encephalopathy (at least one of the following progressive findings present for 2 mo in the absence of a concurrent illness other than HIV infection that could explain the findings: (a) failure to attain or loss of developmental milestones or loss of intellectual ability, verified by standard developmental goals or neuropsychological tests; (b) impaired brain growth or acquired microcephaly demonstrated by head circumference measurements or brain atrophy demonstrated by computerized tomography or magnetic resonance imaging (serial imaging is required for children age <2 yr); (c) acquired symmetrical motor deficit manifested by two or more of the following: paresis, pathologic reflexes, ataxis, or gait disturbance
- Herpes simplex virus infection causing a mucocutaneous ulcer that persists for >1 mo; or bronchitis, pneumonitis, or esophagitis for any duration affecting a child age >1 mo
- Histoplasmosis, disseminated (at a site other than or in addition to lungs or cervical or hilar lymph nodes)
- Kaposi's sarcoma
- Lymphoma, primary, in brain
- Lymphoma, small, noncleaved cell (Burkitt's), or immunoblastic or large cell lymphoma of B-cell or unknown immunologic phenotype
- *Mycobacterium tuberculosis*, disseminated or extrapulmonary
- *Mycobacterium*, other species or unidentified species, disseminated (at a site other than or in addition to lungs, skin, or cervical or hilar lymph nodes)
- *Mycobacterium avium* complex or *Mycobacterium kansasii*, disseminated (at site other than or in addition to lungs, skin, or cervical or hilar lymph nodes)
- *Pneumocystis carinii* pneumonia
- Progressive multifocal leukoencephalopathy
- *Salmonella* (nontyphoid) septicemia, recurrent
- Toxoplasmosis of the brain with onset at age >1 mo
- Wasting syndrome in the absence of a concurrent illness other than HIV infection that could explain the following findings: (a) persistent weight loss >10% of baseline, (b) downward crossing of at least two of the following percentile lines on the weight-for-age chart (e.g., 95th, 75th, 50th, 25th, 5th) in a child age ≥1 yr; (c) <5th percentile on weight-for-height chart on two consecutive measurements, ≥30 d apart plus (1) chronic diarrhea (i.e., at least two loose stools/d for ≥30 d); (2) documented fever (for ≥30 d, intermittent or constant)

Adapted from Centers for Disease Control and Prevention: 1994 Revised classification system for human immunodeficiency virus infection in children less than 13 years of age. MMWR Morb Mortal Wkly Rep 43:RR-12, 1994; and Centers for Disease Control: Revision of the CDC surveillance case definition for acquired immunodeficiency syndrome. MMWR Morb Mortal Wkly Rep 36:1S, 1987.
HSV, herpes simplex virus; AIDS, acquired immunodeficiency virus; HIV, human immunodeficiency virus.

TABLE 9-4

IMMUNOLOGIC CATEGORIES FOR CHILDREN WITH HIV INFECTION BASED ON AGE-SPECIFIC CD4+ T-LYMPHOCYTE COUNTS AND PERCENTAGE OF TOTAL LYMPHOCYTES

	Age of Child					
	<12 mo		1–5 yr		6–12 yr	
Immunologic Category	μL	(%)	μL	(%)	μL	(%)
1. No evidence of suppression	≥1500	(≥25)	≥1000	(≥25)	≥500	(≥25)
2. Evidence of moderate suppression	750–1499	(15–24)	500–999	(15–24)	200–499	(15–24)
3. Severe suppression	<750	(<15)	<500	(<15)	<200	(<15)

Adapted from Centers for Disease Control and Prevention: 1994 Revised classification system for human immunodeficiency virus infection in children less than 13 years of age. MMWR Morb Mortal Wkly Rep 43:RR-12,1994.

placenta, via the birth canal, or by direct contamination of the amniotic fluid. The mortality of this early-onset variety approaches 50%. Late-onset neonatal sepsis is primarily nosocomial, most often secondary to indwelling catheters or bacterial translocation from the gut. In the surgical neonate, three factors promote bacterial translocation and sepsis: (1) intestinal bacterial colonization and overgrowth, (2) compromised host defenses, and (3) disruption of the mucosal epithelial barrier.[147] The mortality of late-onset sepsis is 20%. The clinician must be alert for the subtle signs and symptoms of neonatal sepsis, which include lethargy, irritability, temperature instability, and change in respiratory or feeding pattern. Neonates may not demonstrate leukocytosis. Empirical triple-antibiotic coverage may be started, pending the results of blood and other cultures.

Mycotic Infection

Mycotic infections are an increasing problem in immunocompromised pediatric patients.[148] Successful management of fungal infections requires recognition of the potential for infection, understanding of the organisms that can cause infection, and identification of the organ system(s) affected. The immature immune system of neonates is partially responsible for some specific diseases and poses unique management problems. Hospitalized infants today are increasingly stressed to degrees not previously seen in intensive care nurseries and may be receiving long-term antibiotic therapy for other illnesses. Hyperalimentation, administration of fat emulsion, endotracheal intubation, and administration of antibiotic therapy are significant risks associated with the development of candidemia in children. Chemotherapy for malignancy, bone marrow transplant, trauma, and chronic illness increase the risk of immunocompromise and systemic fungal infection.[149] The frequent use of long-term intravascular catheters contributes to fungal infections. Therapy includes administration of topical and parenteral antifungal agents and supportive care.

REFERENCES

1. Neu HC: The changing ecology of bacterial infections in children. Compr Ther 2:47–52, 1976.
2. Liu HH: Antibiotics and infectious diseases. Prim Care 17:745–774, 1990.
3. Kosloske AM: Surgical infections in children. Curr Opin Pediatr 6:353–359, 1994.
4. DeLa Cadena RA, Majluf-Cruz A, Stadnicki A, et al: Activation of the contact and fibrinolytic systems after intravenous administration of endotoxin to normal human volunteers: Correlation with the cytokine profile. Immunopharmacology 33:231–237, 1996.
5. White RL, Burgess DS, Manduru M, et al: Comparison of three different in vitro methods of detecting synergy: Time-kill, checkerboard, and E test. Antimicrob Agents Chemother 40:1914–1918, 1996.
6. Jarvis WR: The epidemiology of colonization. Infect Control Hosp Epidemiol 17:47–52, 1996.
7. Brook I: Anaerobic infections in childhood. Rev Infect Dis 6(suppl 1): S187–S192, 1984.
8. Robson MC, Stenberg BD, Heggers JP: Wound healing alterations caused by infection. Clin Plast Surg 17:485–492, 1990.
9. Baxter CR: Immunologic reactions in chronic wounds. Am J Surg 167:12S–14S, 1994.
10. Harris BH, Gelfand JA: The immune response to trauma. Semin Pediatr Surg 4:77–82, 1995.
11. Forslind B, Lindberg M, Roomans GM, et al: Aspects on the physiology of human skin: Studies using particle probe analysis. Microsc Res Tech 38:373–386, 1997.
12. Bleacher JC, Krummel TM: Host resistance to infection. In Fonkalsrud EW, Krummel TM (eds): Infections and Immunologic Disorders in Pediatric Surgery. Philadelphia, WB Saunders, 1993, pp 63–75.
13. Brown R, Pinkerton R, Tuttle M: Respiratory infections in smokers. Am Fam Physician 36:133–140, 1987.
14. Godet AS, Williams RD: Postoperative *Clostridium difficile* gastroenteritis. J Urol 149:142–144, 1993.
15. Daynes RA, Araneo BA, Hennebold J, et al: Steroids as regulators of the mammalian immune response. J Invest Dermatol 105(suppl 1): 14S–19S, 1995.
16. del Guercio P: The self and the nonself: Immunorecognition and immunologic functions. Immunol Res 12:168–182, 1993.
17. Karzai W, Reinhart K: Immune modulation and sepsis. Int J Clin Pract 51:232–237, 1997.
18. Mosser DM: Receptors on phagocytic cells involved in microbial recognition. Immunol Ser 60:99–114, 1994.
19. Fleisher TA: Immune function. Pediatr Rev 18:351–356, 1997.
20. Bessman AN, Sapico FL: Infections in the diabetic patient: The role of immune dysfunction and pathogen virulence factors. J Diabet Complications 6:258–262, 1992.
21. Scrimshaw NS, San Giovanni JP: Synergism of nutrition, infection, and immunity: An overview. Am J Clin Nutr 66:464S–477S, 1997.
22. Puck JM: Primary immunodeficiency diseases. JAMA 278: 1835–1841, 1997.
23. Berescher ES: Infectious complications of dysfunction or deficiency of polymorphonuclear and mononuclear phagocytes. In Long SS, Pickering LK, Prober CG (eds): Principles and Practices of Pediatric Infectious Diseases, 2nd ed. New York: Churchill Livingstone, 2003, pp 635–642.
24. Holland SM: Update on phagocytic defects. Pediatr Infect Dis J 22:87–88, 2003.

25. Geiszt M, Kapus A, Ligeti E: Chronic granulomatous disease: More than the lack of superoxide? J Leukoc Biol 69:191–196, 2001.

26. Connor EM, Sperling RS, Gelber R, et al: Reduction of maternal-infant transmission of human immunodeficiency virus type 1 with zidovudine treatment. N Engl J Med 331:1173–1180, 1994.

27. Mofenson LM, and the Committee on Pediatric AIDS: Technical report: Perinatal human immunodeficiency virus testing and prevention of transmission. Pediatrics 106:88, 2000.

28. Khoury M, Kovacs A: Pediatric HIV infection. Clin Obstet Gynecol 44:243–275, 2001.

29. Melvin A, Mohan K, Manns Arcuino LA, et al: Clinical, virologic and immunologic responses of children with advanced human immunodeficiency virus type I disease treated with protease inhibitors. Pediatr Infect Dis 16:968–974, 1997.

30. Maldonado YA, Shetty A: Epidemiology of HIV Infection in children and adolescents. In Long SS, Pickering LK, Prober CG (eds): Principles and Practice of Pediatric Infectious Diseases, 2nd ed. New York, Churchill Livingstone, 2003, pp 658–662.

31. Simonds RJ, Oxtoby MJ, Caldwell B, et al: *Pneumocystis carinii* pneumonia among US children with perinatally acquired HIV infection. JAMA 270:470–473, 1993.

32. Thea DM, Lambert G, Weedon J, et al: Benefit of primary prophylaxis before 18 months of age in reducing the incidence of *Pneumocystis carinii* pneumonia and early death in a cohort of 112 human immunodeficiency virus-infected infants. Pediatrics 97:59–64, 1996.

33. Rigaud M, Pollack H, Leibovitz E, et al: Efficacy of primary prophylaxis against *Pneumocystis carinii* pneumonia during the first year of life in infants infected with human immunodeficiency virus type I. J Pediatr 125:476–480, 1994.

34. Hoyt L, Oleske J, Holland B, et al: Nontuberculous mycobacteria in children with acquired immunodeficiency syndrome. Pediatr Infect Dis J 11:354–360, 1992.

35. Centers for Disease Control: 1997 USPHS/IDSA guidelines for the prevention of opportunistic infections in persons infected with human immunodeficiency virus. MMWR Morb Mortal Wkly Rep 46:RR-12, 1997.

36. Hilmers DC, Kline MW: Clinical manifestations of human immunodeficiency virus infection. In Long SS, Pickering LK, Prober CG (eds): Principles and Practice of Pediatric Infectious Diseases, 2nd ed. New York, Churchill Livingstone, 2003, pp 664–669.

37. Palella FJ Jr, Delaney KM, Moorman AC, et al: Declining morbidity and mortality among patients with advanced human immunodeficiency virus infection: HIV Outpatient Study Investigators. N Engl J Med 338:853–860, 1998.

38. deMartino M, Tovo PA, Balducci M, et al: Reduction in mortality with availability of antiretroviral therapy for children with perinatal HIV-1 infection: Italian register for HIV infection in children and the Italian National AIDS Registry. JAMA 284:190–197, 2000.

39. Melvin AJ: Anti-retroviral therapy for HIV-infected children toward maximal effectiveness. Pediatr Infect Dis J 18:723–724, 1999.

40. Tobin NH, Frenkel LM: Human immunodeficiency virus drug susceptibility and resistance testing. Pediatr Infect Dis J 21:681–684, 2002.

41. Wright AJ. The penicillins. Mayo Clin Proc 74:290–307, 1999.

42. American Academy of Pediatrics: 2000 Red Book: Report of the Committee on Infectious Diseases, 25th ed. Evanston, Ill., AAP, 2000, pp 645–672.

43. Hellinger WC, Brewer NS. Carbapenems and monobactams: Imipenem, meropenem and aztreonam. Mayo Clin Proc 74: 420–434, 1999.

44. Kaplan SL: Use of linezolid in children. Pediatr Infect Dis 21: 869–872, 2002.

45. Leenders AC, de Marie S: The use of lipid formulations of amphotericin B for systemic fungal infections. Leukemia 10:1570–1575, 1996.

46. Wellington M, Gigliotti F: Update on antifungal agents. Pediatr Infect Dis 20:993–995, 2001.

47. Dekker CL, Prober CG: Pediatric uses of valacyclovir, penciclovir and famciclovir. Pediatr Infect Dis 20:1079–1082, 2001.

48. Arora A, Magee L, Peck J, et al: Antiviral therapeutics for the pediatric population. Pediatr Emerg Care 17:369–380, 2001.

49. Gavin PJ, Katz BZ: Intravenous ribavirin treatment for severe adenovirus disease in immunocompromised children. Pediatrics 110:e9, 2002.

50. Steele RW: AIDS. In Steele RW (ed): The Clinical Handbook of Pediatric Infectious Disease, 2nd ed. New York, Parthenon, 2000, pp 201–212.

51. Leonard EG, McComsey GA: Metabolic complications of antiretroviral therapy in children. Pediatr Infect Dis J 22:77–84, 2003.

52. Musoke RN: Rational use of antibiotics in neonatal infections. East Afr Med J 74:147–150, 1997.

53. Butler DR, Kuhn RJ, Chandler MH: Pharmacokinetics of anti-infective agents in paediatric patients. Clin Pharmacokinet 26:374–395, 1994.

54. Routledge P: Pharmacokinetics in children [review]. J Antimicrob Chemother 34(suppl A):19–24, 1994.

55. Amato M, Huppi P, Isenschmid M, et al: Developmental aspects of percutaneous caffeine absorption in premature infants. Am J Perinatol 9:431–434, 1992.

56. Dagan O, Klein J, Gruenwald C, et al: Preliminary studies of the effects of extracorporeal membrane oxygenator on the disposition of common pediatric drugs. Ther Drug Monit 15:263–266, 1993.

57. Horwitz JR, Chwals WJ, Doski JJ et al: Pediatric wound infections: A prospective multicenter study. Ann Surg 227:553–558, 1998.

58. Pereira LJ, Lee GM, Wade KJ: The effect of surgical handwashing routines on the microbial counts of operating room nurses. Am J Infect Control 18:354–364, 1990.

59. Wheelock SM, Lookinland S: Effect of surgical hand scrub time on subsequent bacterial growth. AORN J 65:1087–1092, 1094–1098, 1997.

60. Pittet D, Hugonnet S, Harbarth S, et al. Effectiveness of a hospital-wide programme to improve compliance with hand hygiene: Infection Control Programme. Lancet 14:1307–1312, 2000.

61. Naikoba S, Hayward A. The effectiveness of interventions aimed at increasing handwashing in healthcare workers: A systematic review. J Hosp Infect 47:173–180, 2001.

62. Girou E, Soyeau S, Legrand P, et al: Efficacy of handrubbing with alcohol based solution versus standard handwashing with antiseptic soap: Randomized clinical trial. BMJ 325:362, 2002.

63. Parienti JJ, Thibon P, Heller R et al: Hand-rubbing with an aqueous alcoholic solution vs traditional surgical hand-scrubbing and 30-day surgical site infection rates. JAMA 288:722–727, 2002.

64. Mishriki SF, Law DJ, Jeffery PJ: Factors affecting the incidence of postoperative wound infection. J Hosp Infect 16:223–230, 1990.

65. Kovach T: Nip it in the bud: Controlling wound infection with preoperative shaving. Todays OR Nurse 12:23–26, 1990.

66. Mangram AJ, Horan TC, Pearson ML, et al: Guideline for prevention of surgical site infection, 1999. Am J Infect Control 27:97–134, 1999.

67. Kjonniksen I, Andersen BM, Sondenaa V, et al. Preoperative hair removal: A systematic literature review. AORN J 75:928–936, 2002.

68. Benzer A, Sparr HJ, Kempen PM, et al: Perioperative normothermia and surgical-wound infection. N Engl J Med 335:747–750, 1996.

69. Greif R, Akca O, Horn EP, et al: Supplemental perioperative oxygen to reduce the incidence of surgical wound infection. N Engl J Med 342:161–167, 2000.

70. Nichols RL: Surgical antibiotic prophylaxis. Med Clin North Am 79:509–522, 1995.

71. American Academy of Pediatrics, AAP Red Book: Report of the Committee on Infectious Diseases, 25th ed. Evanston, Ill., AAP, 2000, pp 730–735.

72. Inserra A, Serventi P, Ciprandi G, et al: Antibioticoprofilassi con ceftazidime in chirurgia pediatrica. Clin Ter 136:393–398, 1996.

73. Kesler RW, Guhlow LJ, Saulsbury FT: Prophylactic antibiotics in pediatric surgery. Pediatrics 69:1–3, 1982.

74. Debo Adeyemi S, Tai da Rocha-Afodu J: Clinical studies of 4 methods of bowel preparation in colorectal surgery. Eur Surg Res 18:331–336, 1986.

75. Le TH, Timmcke AE, Gathright JB Jr, et al: Outpatient bowel preparation for elective colon resection. South Med J 90:526–530, 1997.

76. Samelson SL, Reyes HM: Management of perforated appendicitis in children, revisited. Arch Surg 122:691–699, 1987.

77. Raves JJ, Slifkin M, Diamond DL: A bacteriologic study comparing closed suction and simple conduit drainage. Am J Surg 148:618–620, 1984.

78. Badia JM, Torres JM, Tur C, et al: Saline wound irrigation reduces the postoperative infection rate in guinea pigs. J Surg Res 63:457–459, 1996.

79. Oestreicher M, Tschantz P: Prevention de l'infection de la plaie operatoire: Lavage par dérive iode, ou NaCl. Étude prospective et randomisée en chirurgie generale. Helv Chir Acta 56:133–137, 1989.

80. Kaysinger KK, Nicholson NC, Ramp WK, et al: Toxic effects of wound irrigation solutions on cultured tibiae and osteoblasts. J Orthop Trauma 9:303–311, 1995.

81. Davenport M, Doig CM: Wound infection in pediatric surgery: A study in 1,094 neonates. J Pediatr Surg 28:26–30, 1993.

82. Bhattacharyya N, Kosloske AM: Postoperative wound infection in pediatric surgical patients: A study of 676 infants and children. J Pediatr Surg 25:125–129, 1990.

83. Poon TS, Zhang AL, Cartmill T, et al: Changing patterns of diagnosis and treatment of infantile hypertrophic pyloric stenosis: A clinical audit of 303 patients. J Pediatr Surg 31:1611–1615, 1996.

84. Allen U, Ford-Jones EL: Nosocomial infections in the pediatric patient: An update. Am J Infect Control 18:176–193, 1990.

85. Bhattacharyya N, Kosloske AM, MacArthur C: Nosocomial infection in pediatric surgical patients: A study of 608 infants and children. J Pediatr Surg 28:338–343; discussion, 343–344, 1993.

86. Coffin SE, Bell LM, Manning M, et al: Nosocomial infections in neonates receiving extracorporeal membrane oxygenation. Infect Control Hosp Epidemiol 18:93–96, 1997.

87. Martin MA: Nosocomial infections in intensive care units: An overview of their epidemiology, outcome, and prevention. New Horiz 1:162–171, 1993.

88. Stein F, Trevino R: Nosocomial infections in the pediatric intensive care unit. Pediatr Clin North Am 41:1245–1257, 1994.

89. Avanoglu A, Herek O, Ulman I, et al: Effects of H_2 receptor blocking agents on bacterial translocation in burn injury. Eur J Pediatr Surg 7:278–281, 1997.

90. Yassin AF, Young-Fadok TM, Zein NN, et al: *Clostridium difficile*-associated diarrhea and colitis. Mayo Clin Proc 76:725–730, 2001.

91. Morris AM, Jobe BA, Stoney M, et al: *Clostridium difficile* colitis. Arch Surg 137:10916–11000, 2002.

92. Szajewska H, Mrukowicz JZ: Probiotics in prevention of antibiotic-associated diarrhea: Meta-analysis. J Pediatr 142:85, 2003.

93. Mermel LA, McCormick RD, Springman SR, et al: The pathogenesis and epidemiology of catheter-related infection with pulmonary artery Swan-Ganz catheters: A prospective study utilizing molecular subtyping. Am J Med 91(suppl 3B):1897–1905, 2001.

94. Raad I, Hohn DC, Gilbreath BJ, et al: Prevention of central venous catheter-related infections by using maximal sterile barrier precautions during insertion. Infect Control Hosp Epidemiol 15:231–238, 1994.

95. O'Grady NP, Alexander M, Dellinger EP, et al: Guidelines for the prevention of intravascular catheter-related infections. MMWR Recomm Rep 51 (RR-10):1–29, 2002.

96. Safdar N, Kluger DM, Maki DG: A review of risk factors for catheter-related bloodstream infection caused by percutaneously inserted, noncuffed central venous catheters. Medicine 81:466–479, 2002.

97. Maki DG, Ringer M, Alvarado CJ: Prospective randomized trial of povidone-iodine, alcohol, and chlorhexidine for prevention of infection associated with central venous and arterial catheters. Lancet 338:339–343, 1991.

98. Mimoz O, Pieroni L, Lawrence C, et al: Prospective, randomized trial of two antiseptics solutions for prevention of central venous or arterial catheter colonization and infection in intensive care unit patients. Crit Care Med 24:1818–1823, 1996.

99. Garland JS, Buck RK, Maloney P et al: Comparison of 10% povidone-iodine and 0.5% chlorhexidine gluconate for the prevention of peripheral intravenous catheter colonization in neonates: A prospective trial. Pediatr Infect Dis J 13:510–516, 1995.

100. Humar A, Ostromecki A, Direnfeld J, et al: Prospective randomized trial of 10% povidone-iodine versus 0.5% tincture of chlorhexidine as cutaneous antisepsis for prevention of central venous catheter infection. Clin Infect Dis 31:1001–1007, 2000.

101. Goetz AM, Wagener MM, Miller JM, et al: Risk of infection due to central venous catheters: Effect of site of placement and catheter type. Infect Control Hosp Epidemiol 19:842–845, 1998.

102. Heard SO, Wagle M, Vijayakumar E, et al: Influence of triple-lumen central venous catheters coated with chlorhexidine and silver sulfadiazine on the incidence of catheter-related bacteremia. Arch Intern Med 158:81–87, 1998.

103. Merrer J, De Jonghe B, Golliot F, et al: Complications of femoral and subclavian venous catheterization in critically ill patients: A randomized controlled trial. JAMA 286:700–707, 2001.

104. Richet H, Hubert B, Nitemberg G, et al: Prospective multi-center study of vascular-catheter-related complications and risk factors for positive central-catheter cultures in intensive care unit patients. J Clin Microbiol 28:2520–2525, 1990.

105. Randolph AG, Cook DJ, Gonzales CA, et al: Tunneling short-term central venous catheters to prevent catheter-related infection: a meta-analysis of randomized, controlled trials. Crit Care Med 26:1452–1457, 1998.

106. Timsit JF, Bruneel F, Cheval C, et al: Use of tunneled femoral catheters to prevent catheter-related infection: A randomized, controlled trial. Ann Intern Med 130:729–735, 1999.

107. Timsit JF, Sebille V, Farkas JC, et al: Effect of subcutaneous tunneling on internal jugular catheter-related sepsis in critically-ill patients: A prospective randomized multicenter study. JAMA 276:1416–1420, 1996.

108. Maki DG, Cobb L, Garman JK, et al: An attachable silver-impregnated cuff for prevention of infection with central venous catheters: A prospective randomized multicenter trial. Am J Med 85:307–314, 1988.

109. Bonawitz SC, Hammell JJ, Kirkpatrick JR, et al: Prevention of central venous catheter sepsis: A prospective randomized trial. Am Surg 57:518–523, 1991.

110. Dahlberg PJ, Agger WA, Singer JR, et al: Subclavian hemodialysis catheter infections: A prospective randomized trial of an attachable silver-impregnated cuff for prevention of catheter-related infections. Infect Control Hosp Epidemiol 15:506–511, 1995.

111. Groeger JS, Lucas AB, Colt D, et al: A prospective, randomized evaluation of the effect of silver impregnated subcutaneous cuff for preventing tunneled chronic venous access catheter infections in cancer patients. Ann Surg 218:206–210, 1993.

112. Schwartz C, Henrickson KJ, Roghmann K, et al: Prevention of bacteremia attributed to luminal colonization of tunneled central venous catheters with vancomycin-susceptible organisms. J Clin Oncol 8:591–597, 1990.

113. Henrickson KJ, Axtell RA, Hoover SM, et al: Prevention of central venous catheter-related infections and thrombotic events in immunocompromised children by the use of vancomycin/ciprofloxacin/heparin flush solution: A randomized, multicenter, double-blind trial. J Clin Oncol 18:1269–1278, 2000.

114. Rackoff WR, Weiman M, Jakobowski D, et al: A randomized controlled trial of the efficacy of heparin and vancomycin solution in preventing central venous catheter infections in children. J Pediatr 127:147–151, 1995.

115. Spatford PS, Sinkin RA, Cox C, et al: Recommendations for preventing the spread of vancomycin resistance: Recommendations of the Hospital Infection Control Practices Advisory Committee (HICPAC). MMWR Morb Mortal Wkly Rep 44:1–13, 1994.

116. Hiramatsu K, Aritaka AN, Hanaki H, et al: Dissemination in Japanese hospitals of *Staphylococcus aureus* heterogeneously resistant to vancomycin. Lancet 350:1670–1673, 1997.

117. Smith TL, Pearson ML, Wilcox KR, et al, for the Glycopeptide-Intermediate *Staphylococcus aureus* Working Group: Emergence of vancomycin resistance in *Staphylococcus aureus*. N Engl J Med 340:493–501, 1999.

118. Sequra M, Alvarez-Lerma F, Tellado JM, et al. Advances in surgical technique: A clinical trial on the prevention of catheter-related sepsis using a new hub model. Ann Surg 223:262–269, 1996.

119. Luna L, Masdeu G, Perez M, et al: Clinical trial evaluating a new hub device designed to prevent catheter-related sepsis. Eur J Clin Microbiol Infect Dis 19:655–662, 2000.

120. Maki DK, Stolz SM, Wheeler S, et al. Prevention of central venous catheter-related bloodstream infection by use of an antiseptic-impregnated catheter: A randomized, controlled trial. Ann Intern Med 127:257–266, 1997.

121. Kamal GD, Pfaller MA, Rempe LE, et al: Reduced intravascular catheter infection by antibiotic bonding. JAMA 265:2364–2368, 1991.

122. Greenfield JI, Sampath L, Posikis SJ, et al: Decreased bacterial adherence and biofilm formation on chlorhexidine and silver sulfadiazine impregnated central venous catheters implanted in swine. Crit Care Med 23:894–900, 1995.

123. Bach A, Bohrer H, Motsch J, et al: Prevention of bacterial colonization of intravenous catheters by antiseptic impregnation of polyurethane polymers. J Antimicrob Chemother 33:969–978, 1994.

124. Raad I, Darouiche R, Dupuis J, et al, and the Texas Medical Center Catheter Study Group: Central venous catheters coated with minocycline and rifampin for the prevention of catheter-related colonization and bloodstream infections: A randomized double-blind trial. Ann Intern Med 127:267–274, 1997.

125. Veenstra DL, Saint S, Saha S, et al: Efficacy of antiseptic-impregnated central venous catheters in preventing catheter-related bloodstream infection: A meta-analysis. JAMA 281:261–267, 1999.

126. Pemberton LB, Ross V, Cuddy P, et al: No difference in catheter sepsis between standard and antiseptic central venous catheters: A prospective randomized trial. Arch Surg 131:986–989, 1996.

127. Ciresi D, Albrecht RM, Volkers PA, et al: Failure of an antiseptic bonding to prevent central venous catheter-related infection and sepsis. Am Surg 62:641–646, 1996.

128. Logghe C, Van Ossel C, D'Hoore W, et al: Evaluation of chlorhexidine and silver-sulfadiazine impregnated central venous catheters for the prevention of bloodstream infection in leukemia patients: A randomized controlled trial. J Hosp Infect 37:145–156, 1997.

129. Darouiche RO, Raad II, Heard SO, et al, for the Catheter Study Group: A comparison of two antimicrobial-impregnated central venous catheters. N Engl J Med 240:1–8, 1999.

130. Schutze GE: Antimicrobial-impregnated central venous catheters. Pediatr Infect Dis J 21:63–64, 2002.

131. Hanazaki K, Shingu K, Adachi M, et al: Chlorhexidine dressing for reduction in microbial colonization of the skin with central venous catheters: A prospective randomized controlled trial. J Hosp Infect 42:165–168, 1999.

132. Garland JS, Alex CP, Mueller CD, et al: A randomized trial comparing povidone-iodine to a chlorhexidine gluconate-impregnated dressing for prevention of central venous catheter infections in neonates. Pediatrics 107:1431–1436, 2001.

133. Farrell LD, Karl SR, Davis PK, et al: Postoperative necrotizing fasciitis in children. Pediatrics 82:874–879, 1988.

134. Murphy JJ, Granger R, Blair GK, et al: Necrotizing fasciitis in childhood. J Pediatr Surg 30:1131–1134, 1995.

135. Moss RL, Musemeche CA, Kosloske AM: Necrotizing fasciitis in children: Prompt recognition and aggressive therapy improve survival. J Pediatr Surg 31:1142–1146, 1996.

136. Waldhausen JH, Holterman MJ, Sawin RS: Surgical implications of necrotizing fasciitis in children with chickenpox. J Pediatr Surg 31:1138–1141, 1996.

137. Heemken R, Gandawidjaja L, Hau T: Peritonitis: Pathophysiology and local defense mechanisms. Hepatogastroenterology 44:927–936, 1997.

138. Nathens AB, Rotstein OD, Marshall JC: Tertiary peritonitis: Clinical features of a complex nosocomial infection. World J Surg 22:158–163, 1998.

139. Levy M, Balfe JW, Geary D, et al: Exit-site infection during continuous and cycling peritoneal dialysis in children. Perit Dial Int 10:31–35, 1990.

140. Ohmann C, Hau T: Prognostic indices in peritonitis. Hepatogastroenterology 44:937–946, 1997.

141. Kelly JL, Osullivan C, Oriordain M, et al: Is circulating endotoxin the trigger for the systemic inflammatory response syndrome seen after injury. Ann Surg 225:530–541, 1997.

142. SCCM Consensus Committee, American College of Chest Physicians/Society of Critical Care Medicine Consensus Conference: Definitions for sepsis and organ failure and guidelines for the use of innovative therapies in sepsis. Crit Care Med 20:864–874, 1992.

143. Horn DL, Opal SM, Lomastro E: Antibiotics, cytokines, and endotoxin: A complex and evolving relationship in gram-negative sepsis. Scand J Infect Dis 101(suppl):9–13, 1996.

144. Shapiro L, Gelfand JA: Cytokines and sepsis: Pathophysiology and therapy. New Horiz 1:13–22, 1993.

145. Wexler LH, Weaver-McClure L, Steinberg SM, et al: Randomized trial of recombinant human granulocyte-macrophage colony-stimulating factor in pediatric patients receiving intensive myelosuppressive chemotherapy. J Clin Oncol 14:901–910, 1996.

146. Wolach B: Neonatal sepsis: Pathogenesis and supportive therapy. Semin Perinatol 21:28–38, 1997.

147. Jackson RJ, Smith SD, Wadowsky RM, et al: The effect of *E. coli* virulence on bacterial translocation and systemic sepsis in the neonatal rabbit model. J Pediatr Surg 26:483–485; discussion, 485–486, 1991.

148. Hilfiker ML, Azizkhan RG: Mycotic infections in pediatric surgical patients. Semin Pediatr Surg 4:239–244, 1995.

149. Barson WJ, Brady MT: Management of infections in children with cancer. Hematol Oncol Clin North Am 1:801–839, 1987.

CHAPTER 10

Prenatal Diagnosis and Surgical Intervention

Hanmin Lee, MD, Diana L. Farmer, MD,
Kerilyn K. Nobuhara, MD, and Michael R. Harrison, MD

Advances in radiology and sampling techniques have given clinicians increasingly accurate methods with which to make diagnoses of prenatal anomalies. Early in utero diagnosis allows families greater time to make informed decisions regarding their pregnancy. Most prenatally diagnosed anomalies are best treated by routine postnatal care, as further gestation will not adversely affect the developing fetus. Some are best treated by early delivery if the condition poses an imminent threat to the fetus and the fetus is of viable gestational age. In a small subset of pregnancies, fetuses with anomalies that cause progressive injury during gestation may respond favorably to fetal surgical intervention. The pathophysiology of these anomalies has been delineated over the past 25-year period by serial in utero examination and postnatal observation. Advances in ultrasonography (US), computerized tomography (CT) scanning, and magnetic resonance imaging (MRI) have increased the sensitivity and specificity of detecting fetal anomalies and observing the physiologic consequences to the fetus. Over this same time, techniques for open hysterotomy, minimal-access hysteroscopy, and image-guided percutaneous fetal access for purposes of in utero intervention have been established, first in animal models and subsequently in humans. With regard to all fetal interventions, maternal safety is of primary importance. In this chapter, we present an overview of fetal surgical procedures and then review specific diseases amenable to fetal surgical interventions and the techniques used to treat these anomalies.

GENERAL PRINCIPLES

The decisions regarding treatment of the fetus are complicated by the potential for harm to the mother. Perhaps the only parallel to fetal surgical procedures, in which a woman undergoes a significant operative intervention for the benefit of another without direct physical health benefits to herself, is that of living-related transplantation. The transplantation of kidneys and livers has now extended to living, nonrelated transplants. As with these transplant procedures, in the case of fetal surgery, the pregnant woman undergoes a significant surgical procedure for the potential benefit of the fetus without any direct health benefit to herself. For this reason, fetal surgical procedures should be considered only if the in utero anomaly has been shown by experimental animal models and clinical observation in humans to have severe irreversible consequences, and experimental animal data show that fetal surgical interventions could be beneficial.

Extensive research has been conducted to ascertain whether fetal operations can be performed safely while minimizing maternal risk. The initial investigation began with thousands of fetal surgical interventions in small and large animal models, including primates.[1-8] This resulted in the refinement of techniques, with the conclusion that fetal surgical procedures could be performed safely in humans.

The first open fetal surgical procedure was performed 20 years ago, at the University of California, San Francisco (UCSF).[9] Our initial review of maternal outcome after open fetal surgery showed no mortality and no detectable adverse sequelae on future fertility. The main complication was preterm labor, as gestational age at delivery ranged from 25 to 35 weeks. In more than 150 subsequent cases at UCSF, we have had no maternal mortality after fetal procedures and no known adverse effects on fertility. Midgestation hysterotomy is not performed in the lower uterine section, and thus all further deliveries of women undergoing open fetal operations should be by cesarean section because of the risk of uterine rupture with vaginal delivery. Fetal surgical intervention does not seem to have an adverse effect on future fertility.[10,11] A review of the first 50 fetal surgical cases performed at UCSF revealed no infections, but six patients required blood transfusions. With respect to open and minimally invasive fetal surgical intervention, preterm labor remains the most common complication of fetal operations.

A critical component to a successful fetal treatment program is a multidisciplinary approach. At UCSF, all cases with the potential for fetal intervention are discussed extensively at a multidisciplinary team meeting. Pertinent diagnostic studies are reviewed, and a consensus is reached regarding further evaluation or treatment or both. Families who are candidates for fetal intervention at our program routinely meet with fetal treatment coordinators, perinatologists, geneticists, neonatologists, anesthesiologists, obstetrical nursing staff, social workers, radiologists, and pediatric general surgeons, all of whom attend the weekly fetal treatment meeting. In addition, pediatric subspecialists (such as neurosurgeons for in utero myelomeningocele repair) are available for consultation when appropriate. Appropriate available treatment options including continued observation, termination, early delivery, and fetoscopic or open fetal intervention are discussed. Finally, an institutional fetal treatment oversight committee, comprising practitioners not directly involved in the fetal surgery enterprise, reviews all fetal surgical interventions on a monthly basis. This group serves a quality-assurance role as well as an ethical review function.

ACCESS TO THE FETUS

Access to the fetus can be gained by one of three general methods: (1) US-guided percutaneous intervention, (2) fetoscopically guided (FETENDO) intervention, and (3) directly visualized intervention via hysterotomy. With all three approaches, three factors are of utmost importance: the position of the placenta, uterine anatomy/anomalies, and the position of the fetus. All must be accurately identified by US before intervention. The presence of a skilled sonographer is particularly critical in minimal-access cases, as sonography serves as the only real-time intrauterine "visualization" in some procedures and augments the use of fetoscopy or direct visualization in others .

For all fetal surgical procedures, the mother is placed in either the supine position or in lithotomy position. The left side of the table should be tilted downward to minimize pressure on the inferior vena cava by the gravid uterus. Anesthesia ranges from local and sedation for some minimally invasive procedures to general and epidural for open fetal procedures. In most cases that require fetal sedation, narcotics and paralytics are given directly to the fetus as an intramuscular injection.

Percutaneous procedures are performed for a variety of fetal anomalies with real-time continuous US guidance, generally for drainage of a fetal fluid–filled structure to the amniotic space. We also have used percutaneous radiofrequency ablation for the treatment of a variety of fetal anomalies. Both the catheters and the radiofrequency devices have an outer diameter of 2.0 to 2.5 mm and can be introduced percutaneously with a relatively low risk for membrane separation and bleeding.

Fetoscopic procedures require initial port site placement under US guidance. The optimal site for this initial cannula is an area of the uterus, free of placenta, that will allow optimal visualization of the target structure. Fetendo can be performed either percutaneously or via a limited maternal laparotomy incision. Most clinicians have used warmed isotonic crystalloid solutions or amniotic fluid, rather than gas, to create a clear visual field and space for intervention. These fluids can be instilled through a side port on the cannula for the fetoscope. One- to five-millimeter endoscopes are generally used for fetoscopy; the smaller scopes in this range may be placed entirely percutaneously with minimal risk for uterine rupture. In general, we prefer minilaparotomy and uterine closure when using 5-mm or larger ports. Fetal interventions can then be performed through a working port on the telescope cannula or through accessory cannulas placed with US and fetoscopic guidance.[12,13]

Open fetal surgical procedures are performed through a low transverse abdominal incision. The rectus muscle and fascia are divided either transversely or vertically in the midline, depending on the degree of exposure necessary. The placenta is identified with US and marked so it can be avoided. If an open hysterotomy is used, specially designed uterine staplers and back-biting uterine clamps are essential for controlling myometrial bleeding. The fetus may be monitored with pulse oximetry on an exposed limb and with intermittent or continuous echocardiography. Exposure of the fetus is limited to the appropriate body part. After repair of the defect, the fetus is returned to the uterus, and the hysterotomy is closed with continuous sutures and fibrin glue. Monitoring for uterine irritability and adequate tocolysis is particularly important in open fetal procedures.[14] If an open hysterotomy is used, future deliveries should be accomplished through cesarean delivery to avoid the risk of uterine rupture during labor.

Potential complications may result from any procedure that violates the uterine integrity. Bleeding may result from any surgical intervention and, in instances of fetal surgery, may arise from the abdominal wall, the uterine wall, or the placenta. The lateral aspects of the uterus should be avoided, as the uterine vessels course laterally. Premature membrane rupture remains one of the greatest obstacles to successful fetal surgery and may occur whether a minimally invasive approach or an open technique is used. Contributing causes may include inadequate membrane closure, chorioamnionitis, membrane separation, and uterine contractions. Meticulous sterile technique, careful membrane and uterine closure, and adequate tocolysis are important considerations in minimizing the risk of membrane rupture. Tocolytic agents that are used perioperatively include halogenated inhalation agents, magnesium sulfate, β-sympathomimetics, indomethacin, and nitroglycerin.[15–17]

ANOMALIES AMENABLE TO FETAL SURGERY

Congenital Diaphragmatic Hernia

Despite advances in neonatal methods of respiratory support, survival for children born with congenital diaphragmatic hernia (CDH) remains only 60% to 70% throughout the United States.[18] Additionally, survival for all fetuses diagnosed with CDH may be as low as 20% to 27% due to in utero death of infants with unrecognized CDH.[19] We have studied fetal lung development extensively and have theorized that in utero intervention may allow increased antenatal lung growth with improved pulmonary function and postnatal survival. In a fetal lamb model, compression of the lungs during the last trimester, either with an intrathoracic balloon or by creation of a diaphragmatic hernia, results in fatal pulmonary hypoplasia. In addition, removal of the compressing lesion allows the lung to grow and develop sufficiently to permit survival at birth.[20]

Fetal surgery for CDH initially involved in utero diaphragmatic hernia repair. Analysis of this initial group of patients showed that open fetal surgery for CDH was feasible, but did not show an increase in survival.[21] However, the subset of fetuses with severe lung hypoplasia continues to have poor prognosis and is identifiable prenatally by US and MRI. The factors associated with poor outcome that can be assessed prenatally by US are (1) the presence of liver herniation into the chest, and (2) a low lung-to-head ratio (LHR). In our experience, survival was 100% in fetuses with CDH without liver herniation and 56% in fetuses with CDH and liver herniation into the chest. The LHR is calculated as the area of the contralateral lung at the level of the cardiac atria, divided by the head circumference. This LHR value has been shown to correlate in a statistically significant fashion with survival: 100% survival with an LHR greater than 1.35, 61% survival with an LHR between 0.6 and 1.35, and no survival with an LHR less than 0.6.[22] Sonography also is critical in identifying other anomalies associated with CDH, particularly cardiac anomalies, as those portend an extremely poor prognosis.[23] Magnetic resonance volumetric imaging of the lung for CDH is a promising modality for prognostic purposes.[24]

Over the last 20-year period, we have been able to stratify risk for fetuses with CDH. Over this same period, extensive animal studies and observation in fetuses born with congenital high airway obstruction have proven that lung growth may be driven by tracheal obstruction or occlusion, leading to pressurized fluid accumulating in the airway.[25,26] This has led to the study of lung distention either by tracheal occlusion or by partial or complete liquid ventilation as a method of achieving postnatal lung growth.[27,28] Our group has focused on in utero tracheal occlusion as a method of augmenting lung growth in fetuses with CDH[29,30] (Fig. 10-1). Our preliminary study examined the effect of extrinsic tracheal occlusion by the placement of an obstructing clip in utero by using both open and fetoscopic techniques. We found, in a small number of patients, that survival was increased in the Fetendo but not in the open group as compared with the control group, which consisted of patients undergoing standard postnatal care. This led to the current National Institutes of Health (NIH)-funded trial comparing in utero tracheal occlusion by using Fetendo with standard postnatal care by using minimal-access techniques for fetuses diagnosed with severe left-sided CDH and no other detectable anomalies. Results of the trial showed survival of 75% with no difference between the tracheal

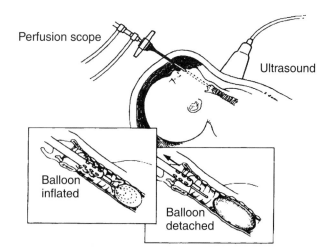

FIGURE 10-1. This schematic diagram shows the method of fetoscopic tracheal occlusion. A fetoscope is placed into the fetal mouth, the airway is identified, and a balloon is placed into the trachea by using both fetoscopic and ultrasonographic visualization.

occlusion group and the standard postnatal care group. The survival in the postnatal care group was considerably greater when compared with historic controls.[31] The results of this trial demonstrate the tremendous importance of proper randomized controlled trials for novel fetal surgical procedures. Currently, our group is offering fetal tracheal occlusion for fetuses with liver herniation in the chest and an LHR of less than 1.0, as these patients continue to have greater than 60% mortality.

Fetal Tumors

Although nearly all fetal tumors are benign and sometimes regress, some prenatally diagnosed solid tumors grow so large that they either obstruct central venous return by mass effect or create an arteriovenous fistula, causing high-output cardiac failure. These hemodynamic changes may result in hydrops fetalis, as exhibited by skin and scalp edema; fluid in the pleural, pericardial, and peritoneal cavities; and placentomegaly. The natural history of hydrops fetalis is fetal death in virtually all cases. The tumors that most commonly result in hydrops are congenital cystic adenomatoid malformation of the lung (CCAM) and sacrococcygeal teratoma (SCT).

CCAM is a cystic pulmonary lesion with a broad spectrum of initial presentation. It is characterized by overgrowth of respiratory bronchioles with the formation of cysts of various sizes. Classification of CCAM has centered around the sizes of the cysts.[32,33] Children and infants diagnosed with CCAM with a paucity of symptoms undergo elective resection. A fetus diagnosed with a CCAM should undergo serial surveillance studies. A small subset of fetuses with large lesions will develop nonimmune hydrops fetalis. The natural history of the vast majority of these fetuses is that of rapidly progressive deterioration and in utero death.

If the fetus is of a viable gestational age in the presence of hydrops, early delivery should be considered.

In instances in which one dominant macrocystic lesion is present in a previable fetus, a thoracoamniotic shunt may reverse the hydrops. Needle drainage has not proven to be an effective option, as rapid reaccumulation of fluid usually occurs. Fetal thoracotomy with resection is an option in the previable fetus without the presence of a dominant cyst. The fetal thoracic space is exposed through a fifth intercostal space thoracotomy after maternal hysterotomy. The lobe containing the CCAM is identified and exteriorized through the incision. The pulmonary hilar structures are then mass ligated by using an endoloop or a vascular endostapling device (Fig. 10-2) The thoracotomy is then closed in layers.[32,34]

The experience with CCAM at UCSF and the Children's Hospital of Philadelphia was recently reviewed. One hundred thirty-four women pregnant with fetuses with CCAM diagnosed in utero were seen at the two institutions. Of this group, 120 elected to continue their pregnancies. Seventy-nine fetuses had no evidence of hydrops. Of these, 76 were followed up expectantly, and all survived. Three fetuses without evidence of hydrops with large dominant cysts underwent thoracoamniotic shunt placement, and all three of these patients survived. Twenty-five hydropic fetuses were followed up with no intervention. All mothers delivered prematurely, and all fetuses died perinatally. Sixteen fetuses with hydrops underwent intervention: 13 underwent open fetal surgery, whereas 3 underwent thoracoamniotic shunting placement. Two of three survived in the group that underwent shunting, whereas 8 of 13 survived in the open fetal surgery group.

Sacrococcygeal teratoma is a rare tumor that is being diagnosed in utero with increasing frequency, allowing observation of the prenatal natural history of the disease and appropriate perinatal management. As with CCAM, fetuses with SCT are susceptible to in utero death. SCT tumors can grow to a tremendous size in relation to the fetus, resulting in a vascular shunt and, in the extreme form, high-output cardiac failure and nonimmume hydrops. Rarely, these tumors bleed either within the tumor or externally and may cause fetal anemia and hypovolemia. Other potential problems with a fetus with a large SCT are those of dystocia and preterm labor. Delivery can be particularly difficult when the diagnosis has not been made prenatally. Traumatic delivery may result in hemorrhage or tumor rupture. Most clinicians would favor cesarean delivery for fetuses with known large SCTs. Thus prenatal diagnosis and careful obstetric planning are critical in the appropriate management of the fetus with an SCT.

The UCSF experience with prenatally diagnosed SCT was reviewed recently.[35] Of the 17 fetuses that have been cared for, hydrops developed in 12 but not in 5. All 5 of the nonhydropic fetuses were delivered near term and survived. Of the 12 hydropic fetuses, 7 underwent fetal intervention, with three survivors. Five hydropic fetuses were followed up without fetal intervention, and none of this group survived. Hydrops in fetuses with SCTs has been shown by other groups to correlate with an exceedingly high rate of fetal death.[36-38] The most common method of fetal intervention is hysterotomy with resection of the tumor (Fig. 10-3). A predominantly cystic

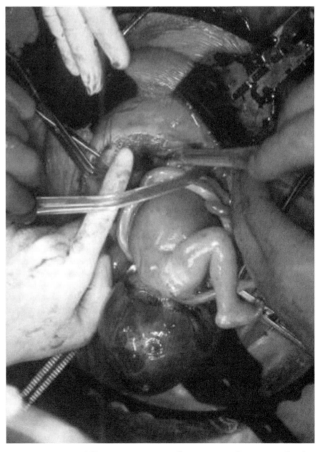

FIGURE 10-3. The sacrococcygeal teratoma is exposed after maternal laparotomy and excised in standard fashion.

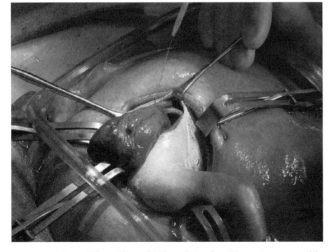

FIGURE 10-2. The affected lobe of the fetal lung is exposed by a standard posterolateral thoracotomy after maternal hysterotomy. The lobe is then mass ligated at its hilum and excised.

lesion may be amenable to percutaneous drainage or placement of a shunt. Effectively debulking the tumor with percutaneous coagulation, such as with radiofrequency ablation to decrease the vascular shunt, is a minimally invasive alternative to open resection that warrants further investigation.

Twin Anomalies

Complications of monochorionic twin pregnancies are relatively common, occurring in 10% to 15% of twin pregnancies.[39] The most common anomaly is twin/twin transfusion syndrome (TTTS), a condition in which the twin/twin vasculature communicates via placental vessels. These vascular connections are often multiple, and flow may occur in either direction. Complications arise when net flow of blood from one twin (donor) to the other (recipient) occurs. As a result of the transfusion, both twins have hemodynamic compromise. The donor twin has diminished cardiac output and may sustain low-flow injuries, particularly to the brain and the kidneys. The recipient twin, conversely, has increased cardiac output and may sustain congestive heart failure. Clinically, early TTTS is manifested by size discordance in the midtrimester. Progressive disease is evidenced by oligohydramnios in the donor twin and polyhydramnios in the recipient twin. Advanced disease is evidenced by the absence of urine in the bladder of the donor twin and hydrops fetalis in one or both twins. The mortality of TTTS diagnosed in the midtrimester is greater than 80% and may occur in the donor twin, recipient twin, or both twins.[40] Additionally, when one monozygotic twin dies in utero, significant risk exists in the other twin, including ischemic brain or renal injury or death.[41,42]

Clinicians have attempted a variety of management strategies aimed at achieving improved outcome in one or both twins. The most commonly used treatment is high-volume amnioreduction in the polyhydramniotic sac. Because polyhydramnios may incite labor, the initial aim of amnioreduction is to reduce uterine volume to decrease the risk of preterm labor. High-volume amnioreduction has resulted in the survival of 58% of twins registered in the International Amnioreduction Registry.[40]

Several groups have used fetoscopic guidance to laser ablate twin/twin vascular connections. This can be accomplished either nonselectively, by ablating all twin/twin connections or, selectively, by ablating only vascular connections with flow in the causative direction. Fetoscopic laser ablation can be performed either percutaneously by using 1.0- to 3.0-mm endoscopes or by maternal laparotomy with 4.0- to 5.0-mm endoscopes. A maternal laparotomy is favored, with the use of the larger scopes, to close the uterine defect created by placement of these devices. All telescopes are inserted through ports that have side channels for irrigation and insertion of the laser. Survival for TTTS with laser ablation of vascular connections is reported to be 50% to 67%.[43-47] Several multi-institutional trials are currently under way to compare the efficacy of large-volume amnioreduction and laser ablation in the treatment of TTTS.

Myelomeningocele

Myelomeningocele (MMC) is a relatively common birth defect that is associated with significant neurologic deficits. Neurologic sequelae include loss of hindlimb function, loss of bowel and bladder function, hydrocephalus, and the development of hindbrain herniation (Chiari II malformation). The degree of neurologic injury is dependent on a variety of factors, prominently, the extent and location of the open neural tube defect, with more cephalad and larger lesions generally leading to more extensive debilitation. Current therapy consists of postnatal closure of the open neural tube defect and extensive rehabilitation. However, most of the neurologic deficits are relatively fixed by birth and are not reversible. With advances in fetal diagnosis and therapy, researchers hypothesized that prenatal intervention for MMC might prevent or lessen some of the neurologic consequences of the disease. Fetal models of MMC were created and repaired in rats, lambs, and monkeys.[5-7,48-50] The data from these experiments showed that animals undergoing prenatal correction of the MMC defect had improved neurologic function, including hindlimb movement, as compared with control animals who did not undergo repair.[5,7]

These animal experiments led to pilot trials of in utero MMC repair in humans. MMC is the first nonlethal anomaly for which fetal surgery was performed (Fig. 10-4). Repair has been approached via both open hysterotomy and fetoscopy by using primary repair and skin allografts.[51-53] Several groups, including ours, reported successful technical repair, primarily with open fetal surgery.[31,53,54] Unfortunately, to date, in utero repair has not shown improvement of lower extremity function or improved bowel or bladder function as compared with historical controls. However, some evidence indicates that hindbrain herniation and hydrocephalus may be lessened by prenatal repair as compared with historical

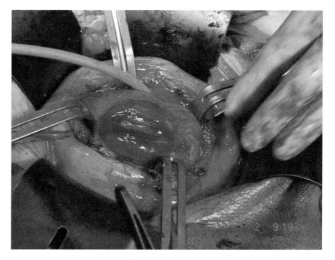

FIGURE 10-4. The myelomeningocele is exposed after maternal hysterotomy. The defect is closed by pediatric neurosurgeons under an operating microscope.

controls undergoing postnatal surgery. Based on these results as well as the animal studies, the NIH is currently funding a prospective, multi-institutional, randomized trial to investigate the effectiveness of in utero MMC repair.

THE FUTURE

Fetal surgery is a promising novel therapy for a variety of prenatally diagnosed conditions. Fetal intervention for anomalies that have a high mortality has shown improved survival compared with that of historical controls. Currently, NIH-funded trials comparing fetal surgery with standard therapy are either under way or soon to be started for congenital diaphragmatic hernia, twin/twin transfusion syndrome, and MMC. Until recently, only fetal malformations that were likely to result in an in utero or postnatal death were considered for fetal surgery because of the inherent risks to the mother. MMC was the first nonlethal anomaly for which fetal surgery was undertaken.

As minimal-access techniques improve and are applied to fetal surgery, resulting in decreasing morbidity to the mother, indications for in utero intervention will continue to broaden. Future procedures will likely be accomplished through a minimal-access approach. In utero gene therapy for metabolic deficiencies and tissue engineering for organ and tissue deficits will become a reality. In utero procedures performed in humans should be grounded in basic science research and animal models that show the likelihood of benefit for the fetus. As the field of fetal surgery evolves, maternal safety must continue to be of highest priority. The prospect of performing fetal surgery for nonfatal lesions opens a whole new area of ethical dilemmas for this evolving field, and places particular importance on randomized, prospective trials.

REFERENCES

1. Adzick NS, Harrison MR, Glick PL, et al: Fetal surgery in the primate, III: Maternal outcome after fetal surgery. J Pediatr Surg 21:477–480, 1986.
2. Adzick NS, Harrison MR: Fetal surgical therapy. Lancet 343:897–902, 1994.
3. Harrison MR, Adzick NS: The fetus as a patient: Surgical considerations. Ann Surg 213:279–291, 1991.
4. Rice HE, Estes JM, Hedrick MH, et al: Congenital cystic adenomatoid malformation: A sheep model of fetal hydrops. J Pediatr Surg 29:692–696, 1994.
5. Meuli M, Meuli-Simmen C, Hutchins GM, et al: In utero surgery rescues neurological function at birth in sheep with spina bifida. Nat Med 1:342–347, 1995.
6. Meuli M, Meuli-Simmen C, Yingling CD, et al: Creation of myelomeningocele in utero: A model of functional damage from spinal cord exposure in fetal sheep. J Pediatr Surg 30:1028–1032, 1995.
7. Meuli M, Meuli-Simmen C, Yingling CD, et al: In utero repair of experimental myelomeningocele saves neurological function at birth. J Pediatr Surg 31:397–402, 1996.
8. Michejda M: Intrauterine treatment of spina bifida: primate model. Z Kinderchir 39:259–261, 1984.
9. Harrison MR, Golbus MS, Filly RA, et al: Fetal surgery for congenital hydronephrosis. N Engl J Med 306:591–593, 1982.
10. Farrell JA, Albanese CT, Jennings RW, et al: Maternal fertility is not affected by fetal surgery. Fetal Diagn Ther 14:190–192, 1999.
11. Longaker MT, Golbus MS, Filly RA, et al: Maternal outcome after open fetal surgery: A review of the first 17 human cases. JAMA 265:737–741, 1991.
12. VanderWall KJ, Meuli M, Szabo Z, et al: Percutaneous access to the uterus for fetal surgery. J Laparoendosc Surg 1:S65–S67, 1996.
13. VanderWall KJ, Bruch SW, Meuli M, et al: Fetal endoscopic ("Fetendo") tracheal clip. J Pediatr Surg 31:1101–1103, 1996.
14. Harrison MR, Adzick NS: Fetal surgical techniques. Semin Pediatr Surg 2:136–142, 1993.
15. Cauldwell CB, Rosen MA, Jennings R: Anesthesia and monitoring for fetal intervention. In Harrison MR, Evans AN, Hozgreve MIW (eds): The Unborn Patient. Philadelphia, WB Saunders, 2001, pp 149–169.
16. Rosen MA: Anesthesia for procedures involving the fetus. Semin Perinatol 15:410–417, 1991.
17. Rosen MA: Anesthesia for fetal procedures and surgery. Yonsei Med J 42:669–680, 2001.
18. Clark RH, Hardin WD Jr, Hirschl RB, et al: Current surgical management of congenital diaphragmatic hernia: A report from the Congenital Diaphragmatic Hernia Study Group. J Pediatr Surg 33:1004–1009, 1998.
19. Harrison MR, Bjordal RI, Langmark F, et al: Congenital diaphragmatic hernia: The hidden mortality. J Pediatr Surg 13:227–230, 1978.
20. Adzick NS, Outwater KM, Harrison MR, et al: Correction of congenital diaphragmatic hernia in utero, IV: An early gestational fetal lamb model for pulmonary vascular morphometric analysis. J Pediatr Surg 20:673–680, 1985.
21. Harrison MR, Adzick NS, Flake AW, et al: Correction of congenital diaphragmatic hernia in utero, VI: Hard-earned lessons. J Pediatr Surg 28:1411–1417, 1993.
22. Metkus AP, Filly RA, Stringer MD, et al: Sonographic predictors of survival in fetal diaphragmatic hernia. J Pediatr Surg 31:148–151, 1996.
23. Sharland GK, Lockhart SM, Heward AJ, et al: Prognosis in fetal diaphragmatic hernia. Am J Obstet Gynecol 166:9–13, 1992.
24. Coakley FV, Lopoo JB, Lu Y, et al: Normal and hypoplastic fetal lungs: Volumetric assessment with prenatal single-shot rapid acquisition with relaxation enhancement MR imaging. Radiology 216:107–111, 2000.
25. DiFiore JW, Fauza DO, Slavin R, et al: Experimental fetal tracheal ligation and congenital diaphragmatic hernia: A pulmonary vascular morphometric analysis. J Pediatr Surg 30:917–923, 1995.
26. DiFiore JW, Fauza DO, Slavin R, et al: Experimental fetal tracheal ligation reverses the structural and physiological effects of pulmonary hypoplasia in congenital diaphragmatic hernia. J Pediatr Surg 29:248–256, 1994.
27. Wilson JM, DiFiore JW, Peters CA: Experimental fetal tracheal ligation prevents the pulmonary hypoplasia associated with fetal nephrectomy: Possible application for congenital diaphragmatic hernia. J Pediatr Surg 28:1433–1439, 1993.
28. Nobuhara KK, Fauza DO, DiFiore JW, et al: Continuous intrapulmonary distension with perfluorocarbon accelerates neonatal (but not adult) lung growth. J Pediatr Surg 33:292–298, 1998.
29. Hedrick MH, Ferro MM, Filly RA, et al: Congenital high airway obstruction syndrome (CHAOS): A potential for perinatal intervention. J Pediatr Surg 29:271–274, 1994.
30. Hedrick MH, Estes JM, Sullivan KM, et al: Plug the lung until it grows (PLUG): A new method to treat congenital diaphragmatic hernia in utero. J Pediatr Surg 29:612–617, 1994.
31. Harrison MR, Keller RL, Hawgood SB, et al: A randomized trial of fetal endoscopic tracheal occlusion for severe fetal congenital diaphragmatic hernia. N Engl J Med 349:1916–1924, 2003.
32. Adzick NS, Harrison MR, Flake AW, et al: Fetal surgery for cystic adenomatoid malformation of the lung. J Pediatr Surg 28:806–812, 1993.
33. Adzick NS, Harrison MR, Glick PL, et al: Fetal cystic adenomatoid malformation: Prenatal diagnosis and natural history. J Pediatr Surg 20:483–488, 1985.
34. Adzick NS, Harrison MR, Crombleholme TM, et al: Fetal lung lesions: Management and outcome. Am J Obstet Gynecol 179:884–889, 1998.

35. Westerburg B, Feldstein VA, Sandberg PL, et al: Sonographic prognostic factors in fetuses with sacrococcygeal teratoma. J Pediatr Surg 35:322–325, 2000.
36. Flake AW, Harrison MR, Adzick NS, et al: Fetal sacrococcygeal teratoma. J Pediatr Surg 21:563–566, 1986.
37. Flake AW: Fetal sacrococcygeal teratoma. Semin Pediatr Surg 2:113–120, 1993.
38. Bond SJ, Harrison MR, Schmidt KG, et al: Death due to high-output cardiac failure in fetal sacrococcygeal teratoma. J Pediatr Surg 25:1287–1291, 1990.
39. Sebire NJ, Snijders RJ, Hughes K, et al: The hidden mortality of monochorionic twin pregnancies. Br J Obstet Gynaecol 104:1203–1207, 1997.
40. Fisk N: The fetus with twin-twin transfusion syndrome. In Harrison MR, Adzick N, Evans MI, Hozgreve W (eds): The Unborn Patient. Philadelphia, WB Saunders, 2001, pp 341–355.
41. Fusi L, Gordon H: Twin pregnancy complicated by single intrauterine death: Problems and outcome with conservative management. Br J Obstet Gynaecol 97:511–516, 1990.
42. Fusi L, McParland P, Fisk N, et al: Acute twin-twin transfusion: A possible mechanism for brain-damaged survivors after intrauterine death of a monochorionic twin. Obstet Gynecol 78:517–520, 1991.
43. Quintero RA, Comas C, Bornick PW, et al: Selective versus non-selective laser photocoagulation of placental vessels in twin-to-twin transfusion syndrome. Ultrasound Obstet Gynecol 16:230–236, 2000.
44. Quintero RA, Bornick PW, Allen MH, et al: Selective laser photocoagulation of communicating vessels in severe twin-twin transfusion syndrome in women with an anterior placenta. Obstet Gynecol 97:477–481, 2001.
45. Ville Y, Hecher K, Gagnon A, et al: Endoscopic laser coagulation in the management of severe twin-to-twin transfusion syndrome. Br J Obstet Gynaecol 105:446–453, 1998.
46. Feldstein VA, Machin GA, Albanese CT, et al: Twin-twin transfusion syndrome: The 'Select' procedure. Fetal Diagn Ther 15:257–261, 2000.
47. Deprest JA, Van Schoubroeck D, Evrard VA, et al: Fetoscopic Nd:YAG laser coagulation for twin-twin transfusion syndrome in cases of anterior placenta. J Am Assoc Gynecol Laparosc 3:S9, 1996.
48. Meuli-Simmen C, Meuli M, Hutchins GM, et al: The fetal spinal cord does not regenerate after in utero transection in a large mammalian model. Neurosurgery 39:555–556, 1996.
49. Heffez DS, Aryanpur J, Hutchins GM, et al: The paralysis associated with myelomeningocele: Clinical and experimental data implicating a preventable spinal cord injury. Neurosurgery 26:987–992, 1990.
50. Heffez DS, Aryanpur J, Rotellini NA, et al: Intrauterine repair of experimental surgically created dysraphism. Neurosurgery 32:1005–1010, 1993.
51. Bruner JP, Tulipan NE, Richards WO: Endoscopic coverage of fetal open myelomeningocele in utero. Am J Obstet Gynecol 176:256–257, 1997.
52. Bruner JP, Tulipan NB, Richards WO, et al: In utero repair of myelomeningocele: A comparison of endoscopy and hysterotomy. Fetal Diagn Ther 15:83–88, 2000.
53. Bruner JP, Tulipan N, Paschall RL, et al: Fetal surgery for myelomeningocele and the incidence of shunt-dependent hydrocephalus. JAMA 282:1819–1825, 1999.
54. Adzick NS, Sutton LN, Crombleholme TM, et al: Successful fetal surgery for spina bifida. Lancet 352:1675–1676, 1998.

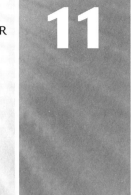

CHAPTER 11

Foreign Bodies

Joseph L. Lelli, Jr., MD

Infants and young children are naturally curious about themselves and their environment. Such inclinations by children for exploration have resulted in the serious problem of aspiration, insertion, and ingestion of foreign bodies (FBs). The complications of FBs in the upper and lower airway, the gastrointestinal tract, and the ears carry a significant morbidity and mortality. FB aspiration has been the cause of 160 annual deaths in children younger than 14 years in the United States.[1] In 2001, the Annual Report of the American Association of Poison Control Centers noted 115,320 cases of ingestion of a foreign body by a minor. More than 70% of these cases (82,614) involved a child younger than 6 years.[2] The Centers for Disease Control (CDC) reported an estimated 17,537 children, 14 years of age or younger, who were treated in emergency departments in 2001 for choking-related episodes.[3] Although many of these events are benign, significant complications ensue from FB entrapment, including but not limited to infection, obstruction, erosion, fistula formation, hemorrhage, and nerve injury. FBs are not always a primary dilemma but may be a secondary sign of underlying disorder such as pica, otalgia, rhinitis, neurologic dysfunction, and even child abuse. Despite significant advances in prevention, first aid, and intervention, FBs in the pediatric patient will always remain a problem as long as "kids will be kids."

Other factors contribute to ingestion and aspiration of FBs besides age. Contributing factors include the male gender, immature coordination of swallowing, lack of molars before age 4 years, mental retardation, seizure disorders, anatomic or functional esophageal disorders, immature laryngeal sphincter control, and an unsafe environment.[4,5] Children who are neglected or abused have been found to have an increased risk for FB ingestion or aspiration. The suspicion of child abuse should be raised if a very young child has a history of multiple previous episodes or is found to have multiple FBs on evaluation.[6,7]

We have found a plethora of publications describing different and unique ways to remove FBs, both in and out of the operating room. Many of the distinctive articles describe the techniques being performed by a medical specialist in the conscious, sedated patient.

These articles describe using magnets, Foley and Fogarty catheters, and ring forceps, as well as small-diameter flexible endoscopes. Many of these bedside techniques are performed in a manner such that the foreign body and the surrounding tissue are indirectly or not at all visualized. The complexity of some FBs and the tissue reaction that is generated by their presence makes removal of these materials difficult, if not impossible, in such settings. Evaluating a patient with the suspicion of foreign body should mandate the most effective and safest method for diagnosis and removal.

Prior to 1930, the mortality rate associated with FBs was reported to be 24%. Largely due to the work of Chevalier Jackson,[8] the mortality rate was reduced significantly to 2%. Jackson has been credited for the development of appropriate preparation of the patient and optimal supine positioning, the techniques, and the equipment that made endoscopic removal of foreign bodies safe and successful. This was done successfully under distal illumination.[9] In 1968, Harold Hopkins[10,11] made the next significant evolution in endoscopy. The Hopkins rod-lens telescope was added to the endoscope, bringing vastly improved illumination and visualization. As extraction devices progressed, the visualization during removal improved, and so did the rate of complications associated with the procedure. During this same period, the ability to make better diagnoses of FB complications improved, reducing the mortality and complication rates overall in these patients.[12]

Chevalier Jackson initiated the Federal Caustic Act of 1927 in response to the high mortality rate from FB obstruction of the aerodigestive tract. This was the first child environment safety act, which was followed 50 years later by the 1979 Consumer Product Safety Act of the Federal Hazardous Substance Act (U.S. Code of Federal Registrations §1500.18 [a] [9]), which bans from interstate commerce any toy or other article intended for use by children younger than 3 years that presents a choking, aspiration, or ingestion hazard because of small parts.

Food items compose 50% to 80% of FBs removed by endoscopy from children's aerodigestive tracts.[13-16] In the

2001 CDC annual report, 60% of choking episodes treated in emergency departments were due to food substances, and 30% were due to a nonfood substance.[1] Sixty-five percent of food-based choking episodes were due to candy or gum. The list of foods causing choking injury was similar in many published reports: hot dogs, nuts, seeds, and vegetable or fruit pieces.[14–17] Coins account for a significant portion of nonfood substances causing choking events in children.[1,16,18,19] Sixty-eight percent of the deaths in children younger than 14 years reported to the Consumer Product Safety Commission (CPSC), between 1972 and 1992, were due to nonfood items. The cause of fatal choking episodes was often balloons, balls, and other toys intended for children's use. The remaining 32% of causes of fatal choking episodes were household items. Two deaths in the CPSC database were due to choking on latex examination gloves given to children in clinicians' offices. The majority of choking deaths occur in children age 3 years and older with balloons and other conforming objects.[16]

The diagnosis of an FB in the aerodigestive tract of a small child may be challenging because of the difficulty in obtaining a reliable history from children. The timely recognition of aspiration or ingestion relies heavily on clinical suspicion. Symptoms are mild or even absent in 40% to 60% of patients. Eighty percent of the asymptomatic patients have a normal physical examination. Twenty to twenty-five percent of FB events are not witnessed.[18,20,21] In one report, 15% of children evaluated by an emergency medicine physician for choking were not recognized as FB victims. FBs persisted undetected in these children for 7 or more days, not suspected by caretakers, parents, or the physician.[21] The clinician has a limited amount of data available when evaluating these patients; therefore a high index of suspicion for FB ingestion and aspiration must always be maintained.

AIRWAY FOREIGN BODIES

Approximately 75% of FB aspiration events in the pediatric age group occur in children younger than 3 years. Boys are affected 2 times more frequently than are girls. A predominant number of factors make young children much more susceptible to aspiration (Table 11-1). Most FBs are small enough to pass through the larynx and enter the trachea. The narrowest point in the child's airway is the cricoid ring. The 1% to 7% of airway FBs that become lodged in the laryngeal inlet are most commonly seen in infants younger than 1 year (Fig. 11-1). Because the trachea is relatively large compared with the cricoid, FBs that lodge within it account for only an additional 3% to 12% of cases. These usually occur in cases of tracheomalacia, in the patient who has poor respiratory effort, or when previous postoperative stricture has occurred. In majority of cases, the FB will pass easily through the trachea and lodge in the primary or secondary bronchi. A predominance of right bronchial involvement is somewhat dependent on age (Fig. 11-2). The prevalence of right-sided FBs is due to the greater diameter of the right bronchus, smaller angle of divergence

TABLE 11-1
FACTORS THAT MAKE YOUNG CHILDREN SUSCEPTIBLE TO ASPIRATION
Age younger than 3 years
Male sex
Often cry, shout, run, and play with objects in their mouths
Do not have molars to chew certain foods adequately
Immature coordination of swallowing and airway protection
Oral exploration of their environment
Immature laryngeal sphincter control

from the tracheal axis, greater airflow to the right lung, and the position of the carina to the left of the midline. In one anatomic study, the position of the carina was thought to be the only determining factor in the distribution of an FB.[22] The angle of the left bronchus and therefore the position of the carina is determined by the development of the aortic knob. The aortic knob reaches adult size by the age of about 15 years, at which time it displaces the left main-stem bronchus downward, creating a more obtuse angle at the carina, changing the more symmetrical bronchial angles in young children. This may explain the increased propensity for right bronchial FBs in young children compared with those in older children and adults.

Children the world over will put almost any object into their mouths, making it a candidate for aspiration. The type of airway FB varies from generation to generation and country to country. For instance, in the United States as diapers became disposable, the incidence of aspirated safety pins declined dramatically. Fifty years ago, a safety pin, usually opened, was an extremely common FB, but now accounts for less than 10% in most reports.

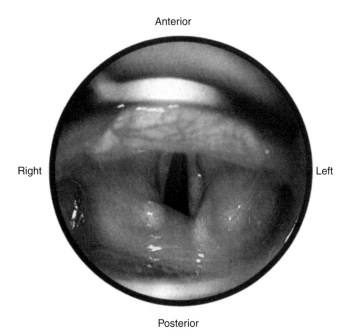

FIGURE 11-1. Coin entrapped between the tongue and epiglottis in the vallecular region.

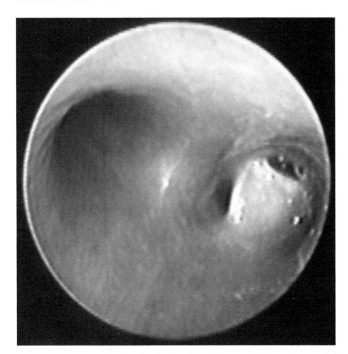

FIGURE 11-2. Foreign body in the right main bronchus of a 3-year-old girl after aspiration.

Small plastic products are now significant items in childhood FB aspiration. Nevertheless, food matter is still the most commonly aspirated FB for all generations and nations (Table 11-2).

The most important factor in evaluating a child who has possibly aspirated an FB is an accurate history and physical examination. The common signs and symptoms will be present in 50% to 90% of children who aspirate an FB. In a series of 100 FB aspiration cases, a choking crisis occurred in 95% and was the most sensitive clinical parameter.[23] FBs that lodge in the larynx or trachea can be completely obstructive, causing sudden death. Partial obstruction by an FB can lead to sufficient inflammatory reaction in the surrounding tissue to produce total, or near total, obstruction (Figs. 11-3 and 11-4). A history of choking without initial physical findings of reduced air exchange requires a high degree of suspicion if a timely diagnosis is to be made. The larynx, trachea, and bronchi can initially accommodate foreign objects with minimal

physical findings. The easy diagnosis is apparent only when complications arise. This may account for the fact that 20% to 50% of FBs are detected more than 1 week after aspiration.[24]

The complications that develop as a result of aspiration are obstruction due to granulation tissue formation or strictures, atelectasis, bronchiectasis, pneumonia, empyema, lung abscess, perforation with pneumothorax, and systemic sepsis. Clinical findings that develop in a previously asymptomatic patient include croup, persistent cough, hemoptysis, fever, malaise, and respiratory compromise.[21,24,25] Obviously it is more difficult and dangerous to remove an FB in a sick patient. Because an unwitnessed choking event may not produce initial symptoms of physical findings, radiographic evaluation is essential to timely diagnosis and treatment.

Radiographic examination consists of anteroposterior and lateral views of the extended neck and posteroanterior and lateral radiographs of the chest. Chest radiographs in inspiration and expiration are beneficial in demonstrating unilateral air trapping that is present in up to 62% of patients when the bronchial FB acts as a one-way valve.[27] Air moves past the FB as the bronchus expands during inhalation, but the air is trapped, producing obstructive emphysema. Hyperinflation of the obstructed lobe or lung produces mediastinal shift to the contralateral or unobstructed side. For evaluation of the young patient who cannot cooperate with inspiration and expiration radiograms, left and right lateral decubitus radiographs may be helpful because the obstructed lung will not deflate while in the dependent position. Although 56% of patients will exhibit a normal chest radiograph within 24 hours of aspiration, others will demonstrate mediastinal shift (55%), pneumonia (26%),

TABLE 11-2	
COMMONLY ASPIRATED FOREIGN BODIES	

Food Products	Nonfood Products
Candy/gum	Coins
Peanuts and other nuts	Toy parts
Seeds	Crayons
Popcorn	Pen tops
Hot dogs	Tacks, nails, needles, pins
Vegetable matter	Beads
Meat matter	Screws
Fish bones	

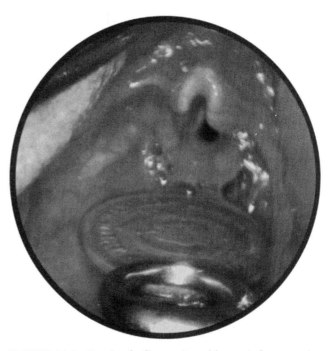

FIGURE 11-3. Foreign bodies aspirated by an infant, causing partial obstruction of the child's airway.

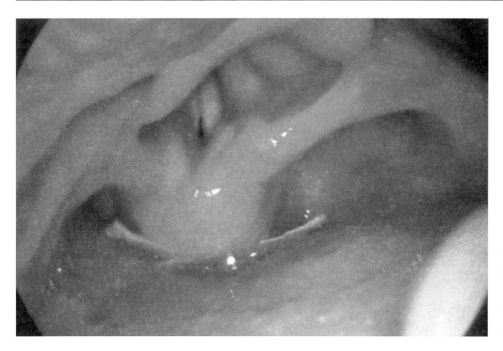

FIGURE 11-4. Chicken bone trapped behind the epiglottis of a 5-year-old boy with a history of choking and drooling. The laryngoscopic examination is complicated because of bleeding in the area from mucosal laceration of the bone.

atelectasis (18%), or a radiopaque object (3%). FBs that are present for a long time will develop complete obstruction and atelectasis secondary to local inflammatory reaction. A radiolucent FB often is evident only because of the ball-valve effect. The benefit of the radiographic assessment is dependent on location of the FB. Laryngotracheal FBs can be evaluated radiographically with a high yield, about 90%. In cases of bronchial FBs, chest radiography is less diagnostic, with a sensitivity and specificity of 65% to 75%.[14,25–28]

Radiographic evaluation is helpful in evaluating the patient with a choking history, but the definitive diagnostic assessment is still surgical intervention, bronchoscopy. A unified surgical team is a must when dealing with FB removal. Each member of the team, from the surgeon to the circulating nurse, must be trained and experienced in dealing with endoscopy of the pediatric patient. A plan is always delineated before the procedure, and the members of the team act as one integrated unit to perform the procedure. Such preparation can significantly shorten the duration and enhance the accuracy and safety of the procedure.

General anesthesia provides a controlled environment for removal of most airway FBs. Only in the small group of patients with laryngeal FBs can removal be accomplished at times without anesthesia. Spontaneous ventilation, with the patients generating their own negative intrathoracic pressure, is the preferred technique. Positive-pressure ventilation is avoided because it may force the FB further into the airway or may produce complete occlusion. Induction is preformed as in any standard operation, with precautions taken to minimize secretions, laryngospasm, and hypoxia. After induction, the patient's head is extended and placed in the "sniffing" position. A laryngoscope is used to expose the larynx for insertion of the bronchoscope and to ensure that the FB is not within easy grasp of McGill forceps. When the laryngeal inlet is deemed clear, the endoscopy is performed.

The endoscopic extraction of FBs from children is a technique requiring a gentle, experienced hand. Great care is taken to protect the eyes, lips, teeth, tongue, and other laryngeal structures on insertion of the bronchoscope. The tongue is always swept to the left side with a laryngoscope to expose the glottis. The bronchoscope is passed into the upper trachea, and ventilation is performed through the side arm. The tracheobronchial tree is then completely inspected, and the FB is removed (Fig. 11–5).

The rigid bronchoscope is the primary instrument for evaluating the tracheobronchial tree. The instruments most commonly used are the Doesel-Huzly bronchoscope with Hopkins rod-lens telescope (Karl Storz) and the Holinger ventilating fiber-illuminated bronchoscope (Pilling). They come in a range of sizes. Both have the benefit of good exposure and the ability to shield FBs within the tube during extraction. The rigid instruments also allow the use of diverse numbers of forceps. The length and diameter of the endoscope used is dictated by the patient's age and size, but in general, one should use the largest scope possible that will not cause trauma. The forceps used in most pediatric surgical practices are the positive-action, "center-action," or passive action forceps. The combination optical/illumination system with the forceps allows the greatest visibility. More than 60 variations of FB forceps are on the market designed for grasping a wide variety of foreign material from easily fragmented peanuts to very difficult to grasp beads.

The primary causes of unsuccessful FB removal are inexperience, an impacted FB obscured by granulation tissue, and inadequate equipment. Many endoscopists describe the use of a Fogarty catheter for extraction of FBs inaccessible to grasping instruments. Removal may be limited by poor visualization, associated with bleeding granulation tissue and edema. In cases with significant granulation tissue and bleeding or multiple FB fragments that migrate distally and become impacted, a second

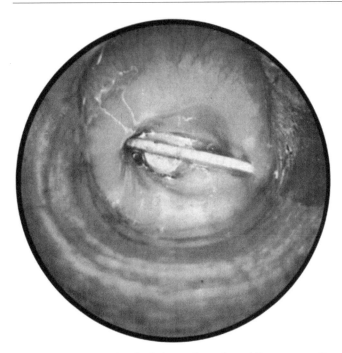

FIGURE 11-5. Foreign body in trachea of a toddler, present for longer than 2 days. Mucosal edema and reactive vascularization can be appreciated, which can make removing the foreign body from the airway difficult.

procedure may be required. Postinstrumentation laryngeal edema can result and may require respiratory therapy intervention before a second procedure. The postinstrumentation edema responds well to inhaled epinephrine (Vaponephrine) and intravenous steroid treatment.[29,30] The second procedure may include repeated endoscopy or thoracotomy with bronchotomy, segmentectomy, or lobectomy, as required. In an attempt to minimize the complications associated with delay of diagnosis of FB aspiration in young children, bronchoscopy based on the history of choking alone has been advocated.[12,14,17,21,24] A negative bronchoscopy rate of 10% to 15% has been deemed acceptable to prevent the morbidity associated with the delayed diagnosis.[31] Individual patient circumstances, including access to expert care, will enter into decisions for this more aggressive approach.

ESOPHAGEAL FOREIGN BODIES

The esophagus is a muscular tube that has two shallow curves as it descends through the diaphragm to its termination at the gastric cardia. It is the narrowest portion of the alimentary tract and is protected at its upper end by the cricopharyngeus muscle, where many ingested FBs will lodge. The esophagus is narrowed somewhat at the aortic arch, left main bronchus, and at the diaphragm, areas where FBs will be stopped (Table 11–3).

Most swallowed objects, once they pass the cricopharyngeus, will pass into the stomach. Congenital and acquired esophageal anomalies may contribute to FB obstruction of the esophagus. The middle and lower esophageal motility is abnormal in patients born with esophageal

TABLE 11-3

LEVEL OF RETENTION OF ASPIRATED ESOPHAGEAL FOREIGN BODIES

Cricopharyngeus muscle	63%–84%
Aortic crossover mid-esophagus	10%–17%
Lower esophagus sphincter	5%–20%

From Stack LB, Munter DW. Foreign bodies in the gastrointestinal tract. Emerg Med Clin North Am 14:493, 1996, with permission.

atresia malformations, even if expertly repaired. It is relatively common for young children to swallow soft, rubbery foods and have them lodge firmly near the area of esophageal anastomosis. FB obstruction may be seen in patients with an unsuspected vascular ring, ectopic salivary gland, cartilaginous rest, middle mediastinal mass, an esophageal stricture, achalasia, or duplication cyst. Twenty-two percent of patients older than five years with esophageal FBs were noted to have anatomic abnormalities.[32,33] In a series of patients with an impacted esophageal food bolus, up to 70% had esophageal abnormalities.[34] In most cases in which the level is reported, ingested FBs lodge at the normal anatomic narrowing of the cricopharyngeal muscle or the level of the aortic arch (see Table 11-3).

Coins and smooth blunt objects are the most commonly ingested items in large pediatric series. The patients are most commonly between ages 18 and 48 months.[35] In one review of almost 200 patients, 89% of foreign bodies were coins.[36] A well-documented cultural and geographic difference is found in the types of FBs aspirated. In a review of 343 Chinese children, 42% had ingested fish bones, and only 39% had ingested coins.[33] In a report from Belgium, only 89 (27%) of 325 patients were found to have ingested coins, but 16% had ingested sharp objects, a significantly higher percentage when compared with other nations (Fig. 11-6). In older children, food boluses and school supplies—parts of pencils and pens—are most common.

The ingestion of an FB is often unrecognized and without symptoms, as the FB passes uneventfully through the gut. Swallowed FBs are not considered as dangerous as aspirated foreign bodies, yet up to 1500 deaths per year have been documented from esophageal FB ingestion.[37] Clinical symptoms of a patient with an FB that obstructs the esophagus include the sudden onset of acute and severe coughing, pain in the pharyngeal or retrosternal region, gagging, poor feeding, drooling, nausea, vomiting, ptyalism, dysphagia, respiratory distress, laryngeal irritation, and choking. Periesophageal inflammation from an unsuspected esophageal FB can cause airway symptoms such as wheezing, stridor, and coughing (Fig. 11-7). Significant respiratory symptoms are seen with esophageal FBs because the distensibility of the esophagus allows impingement on the airway.

The ingestion of small batteries creates a different set of serious FB problems. A 7-year review reported 2320 cases of battery ingestion, and only 9.9% of these patients were symptomatic.[38] Because of the prevalence of small electronic devices, the rate of disk and button

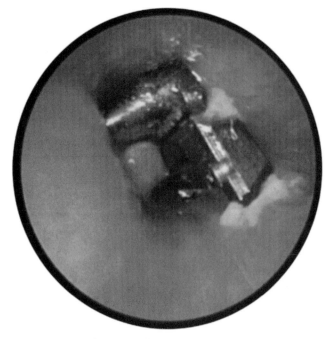

FIGURE 11-6. Sharp metallic toy ingested by a toddler; the toy is trapped in the proximal esophagus.

battery ingestion has grown significantly over recent decades. Batteries can cause unique injuries not seen with other FBs. These include direct caustic injury, pressure necrosis, tissue necrosis from electrical discharge, and toxin release (mercury poisoning). The main chemical ingredients of disk batteries include alkaline corrosive agents or heavy metals. Battery size and type may affect management and outcome. Lithium batteries cause more adverse effects because of their size and greater voltage.

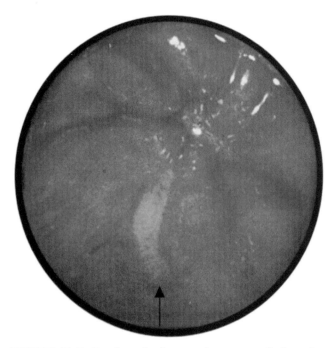

FIGURE 11-7. Esophageal edema and an area of ulceration (*arrow*) from entrapped foreign body.

Even batteries discarded because they contain insufficient voltage to operate an electronic device may contain enough voltage to produce a very significant tissue injury. A 3-volt lithium battery is enough to cause local cellular electrolyte flux, releasing intracellular potassium, resulting in cell death and tissue necrosis. Complications caused by esophageal impaction of button batteries include tracheo-esophageal fistula, esophageal burn with and without perforation, aortoesophageal fistula, esophageal stricturing, and death. Emergency endoscopy must be performed for batteries retained in the esophagus because of the propensity for serious injury.[39]

Chevalier Jackson recognized decades ago that in some of the most severely complicated cases of esophageal FBs, the diagnosis was often never considered until late complications had developed. FB ingestion is extremely common, and in this area, prolonged retention is rare. Permanently retained esophageal FBs can produce hematemesis, chronic dysphagia, chronic cough, stridor, and aspiration pneumonitiis. Other more severe complications include true and false esophageal diverticulum, lobar atelectasis, esophageal-airway fistula, esophageal perforation with migration of the FB outside the esophagus, an aorto-esophageal fistula, and acute mediastinitis.

Radiologic evaluation for possible FB ingestion must include lateral view and anteroposterior views of both the neck and the chest. The radiologic evaluation of a child with a history of possibly swallowing a coin or a radiopaque object is highly sensitive and specific (Fig.11-8). In a review of the preoperative radiographs of 182 children with a history of FB ingestion (primarily coins), 96.7% had a positive radiologic finding that was confirmed on endoscopy.[35] Objects that are only faintly radiopaque, such as bones or small items of aluminum, are often seen on lateral views because the "end-on" view increases their radiodensity. Totally radiolucent foreign bodies such as plastic beads or toys present a much more difficult radiographic challenge. In these cases, suspicion must be high enough to use contrast studies for the diagnosis. An esophagogram may demonstrate a radiolucent FB as a filling defect and also may reveal such anomalies as compression by a vascular ring or an intrinsic stricture. Even though preoperative radiographic evaluation is accurate in demonstrating an FB in a child, the clinical situation should prevail in the decision to perform an esophagoscopy. Small coins, for example, lodged at the gastroesophageal junction, are likely to pass if given a chance. In an attempt to minimize the complications associated with the delay in diagnosis, endoscopy for suggestive cases with or without radiologic confirmation has been advocated. A negative esophagoscopy rate of 6.2% has been quoted as acceptable to prevent the morbidity associated with the missed diagnosis of an esophageal FB.[35]

Rapid diagnosis and prompt treatment of FBs in the esophagus will decrease morbidity. The three common techniques for FB removal from the esophagus are Foley catheter extraction, bougienage to push the FB into the stomach, and endoscopic retrieval.

Foley catheter retrieval is generally easy and successful for removing smooth objects located in the upper two thirds of the esophagus. The procedure is cost efficient

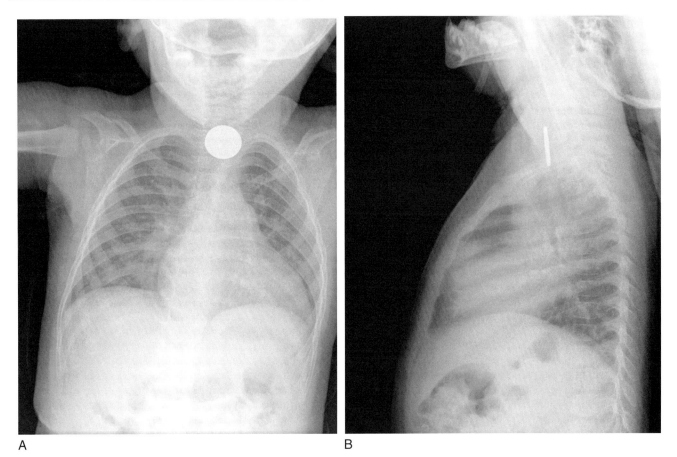

A   B

FIGURE 11-8. Coin, ingested by a child, has become trapped in the proximal esophagus.

and can be done without anesthesia. The procedure often is performed under fluoroscopic guidance. The risks of the procedure are potential airway compromise, risk of esophageal injury, inability to visualize the esophageal reaction to the FB, and the discomfort of the awake child. The success rate of 84% to 96% with Foley catheter extraction is less than that of endoscopy.[40-43] Objects that have been retained in the esophagus for longer than 24 hours may have produced significant tissue reaction that significantly increases the risk of catheter extraction as well as the risk of failure to retrieve the FB. The Foley catheter insertion has, on occasion, resulted in pushing foreign objects into the stomach. Bougienage has been shown to be successful in selected cases. The patient has usually ingested a single coin within 24 hours of presentation, is stable, and has no history of esophageal abnormalities or FB aspiration. Blunt-tipped, weighted esophageal bougies are passed to advance the coin or other smooth object into the stomach, with the expectation the object will be passed per rectum. Roughly 90% to 95% of these objects will be evacuated spontaneously.[44] The concern with bougienage is that the nonevacuated FBs can lead to obstruction or perforation of the small intestine, requiring much more difficult endoscopic retrieval or surgical exploration.

Rigid endoscopy is the most reliable and successful method used in retrieval of esophageal FBs. The safety and success rate with rigid endoscopy has approached 100%, with minimal complications, in the hands of a trained experienced endoscopist. The procedure is performed in a controlled environment with the same precautions that apply to the use of the rigid bronchoscope. The patient is placed in the supine position with the head in the neutral sniffing position with the cervical spine straight, allowing passage of the endoscope over the cervical kyphosis. Esophagoscopes differ from bronchoscopes in that they have a smooth, flared leading edge. This difference allows the endoscopist to lift the larynx with minimal trauma to expose and open the cricopharyngeus "sphincter." These instruments come in a variety of lengths and sizes appropriate to the wide range of patient sizes in pediatric surgical practice. The appropriate size is the largest that can be accommodated without forcing the esophagoscope. These systems come with an array of grasping forceps suitable to the wide range of materials to be retrieved.

GASTROINTESTINAL FOREIGN BODIES

The vast majority of foreign bodies that are ingested by children are not retained in the esophagus. Sixty percent of patients who were evaluated for FB ingestion were found to have the FB in their stomach at the time of evaluation.[45] With the exception of some sharp objects and batteries, most gastric FBs do not have to be removed because they are eliminated spontaneously.[39,46,47] In a study of 1481 children, 97% of ingested FBs that passed through the esophagus on radiographic study were spontaneously evacuated. The incidence of operative retrieval of ingested FBs first found to be in the stomach is 1%, whereas the rate for ingested sharp objects is 15% to 30%. Some surgeons recommend early endoscopic retrieval of sharp FBs.[48] Commonly ingested sharp FBs include bones, nails, safety pins, needles, sharp toys, and toothpicks. Toothpicks and bones are the most commonly ingested objects that require retrieval. If either of these objects becomes impacted in the intestinal mucosa, erosion may develop, which then can lead to visceral perforation and peritonitis. Objects larger than 2 cm or longer than 3 cm swallowed by infants have been shown to have difficulty traversing the pyloric channel. In older children and adults, objects thicker than 2 cm and longer than 5 cm tend to have difficulty passing through the duodenal loop, causing functional gastric outlet obstruction. These objects also warrant endoscopic retrieval. Rarely do foreign objects become lodged distal to the ligament of Trietz. The ileocecal valve is the only natural narrowing in the lower intestinal tract, but it is rarely the site for FB retention.

Bezoars are FBs that have accumulated over time in the alimentary tract (see Chapter 29). These can cause obstructive symptoms, bleeding, failure to thrive, weight loss due to early satiety, abdominal pain, anorexia, halitosis, and nausea. Common concentrations include plant and vegetable matter (phytobezoar), hair (trichobezoar), persimmons (disopyrobezoar), and neonatal casein curd (proteinaceous) aggregations. Bezoars may be retrieved endoscopically or eliminated by enzymatic fragmentation. Laparotomy may be warranted with large obstructing bezoars.

EAR AND NOSE FOREIGN BODIES

FBs may be the cause of mouth breathing and rhinorrhea in children. Identification and removal require appropriate suspicion and adequate instrumentation. Although most foreign objects recently inserted are easily removed from the nose, those of long standing may not be as simple. Nasal mucosal reaction with edema and granulation tissue develops rather quickly. The mucosal lining of the nose is a dynamic surface that requires uninterrupted mucociliary flow to remain free of crusting and inflammation. Interruption of the flow pattern by an FB readily produces inflammation and infection. FBs placed in the anterior nares may be inert or reactive. Common objects placed in the nares are dried beans, plastic objects, buttons, metals, food, erasers, nuts, seeds, and button batteries. Presenting signs and symptoms with nasal FBs include rhinorrhea, crusting, airflow obstruction, rhinitis, sinusitis, lymphadenopathy, epistaxis, otitis media, and adenoiditis. Otitis media is a potential sequela of a posterior nasal reaction from an FB, causing eustachian tube obstruction. Plastic and other inert materials may be

tolerated for relatively long intervals, while granulation tissue develops to produce an obstruction. More reactive objects are seen earlier with more acute symptoms. Button batteries may lead to septal perforation and destruction of cartilage, leading to a saddle-nose deformity. The site of maximal damage from button batteries has been shown to correspond to the negative pole of the battery. Successful removal of a nasal FB in a child requires visualization and appropriate instrumentation. Usually this is a simple bedside procedure. The primary or emergency physician, by using a tweezer, cerumen curette, or a cotton-tip applicator, can often remove most FBs. Long-standing objects may be more complicated, requiring assistance from a surgical specialist. Tools that can be helpful in visualizing the object are Frazier tip suction, the optic headlight, and the nasal speculum. The Hartmann forceps, wire loop, flexible cerumen curette, alligator forceps, and right-angled hook are tools that will increase the likelihood of recovering the foreign object. It is beneficial to place the instrument alongside or behind the object for successful removal. Great care must be taken not to impact the FB or to push it through the nose and risk aspiration.

The external ear canal is another orifice of interest to the curious child. The child can place a multitude of FBs in the ear canal. Symptoms may vary, depending on the nature of the FB, the size of the FB, and the duration that the FB has been present. Local trauma can occur, with bleeding and difficulty with hearing. The child may describe a fullness sensation. Complications may arise with inflammatory changes. Secondary infection may cause canal wall skin to bleed and slough, producing otorrhea and severe granulation tissue formation. The presence of a secondarily infected ear canal from an FB may mimic a chronic mastoid infection that will not respond to antibiotics. Disc batteries, as in the nose and gastrointestinal tract, are extremely caustic and can cause extensive damage to the external auditory canal, tympanic membrane, and middle ear. The removal of an FB requires that the patient be extremely cooperative. Therefore the use of anesthetic should be considered to minimize iatrogenic injury.

REFERENCES

1. Centers for Disease Control: MMWR 51:945–948, 2001.
2. American Association of Poison Control Centers: 2001 Annual Report of the American Association of Poison Control Centers.
3. Nonfatal choking-related episodes among children: Unites States. JAMA 288:2400–2402, 2001.
4. Mazzadi S, Salis GB, Garcia A, et al: Foreign body impaction in the esophagus: Are there underlying motor disorders? Dis Esophagus 11:51, 1998.
5. Wiseman N: The diagnosis of foreign body aspiration in childhood. J Pediatr Surg 19:531, 1984.
6. Binder L, Anderson WA: Pediatric gastrointestinal foreign body ingestions. Ann Emerg Med 13:61, 1984.
7. Nolte KB: Esophageal foreign bodies as child abuse: Potential fatal mechanisms. Am J Forensic Med Pathol 14:323, 1993.
8. Jackson C, Jackson CL: Diseases of the Air and Food Passage of Foreign Body Origin. Philadelphia, WB Saunders, 1936.
9. Jackson C: Foreign bodies in the trachea, bronchi and oesophagus: The aids of oesophagus, bronchoscopy and magnetism in their extraction. Laryngoscope 15:257, 1905.

10. Hopkins HH: Endoscopy. New York, Appleton Century Crofts, 1976, p 17.
11. Marsh BR: Historic development of broncho-esophagology. Otolaryngol Head Neck Surg 114:689, 1996.
12. Inglis AF, Wagner DV: Lower complication rates associated with bronchial foreign bodies over the last 20 years. Ann Otol Rhinol Laryngol 101:61, 1992.
13. Blazer S, Naveh Y, Friedman A: Foreign body in the airway. Am J Dis Child 134:68–71, 1980.
14. Mu L, He P, Sun D: Inhalation of foreign bodies in Chinese children: A review of 400 cases. Laryngoscope 101:657–660, 1991.
15. Wolach B, Raz A, Weinberg J, et al: Aspirated foreign bodies in the respiratory tract of children. Int J Pediatr Otorhinolaryngol 30:1–10, 1994.
16. Rimell FL, Thome A, Stool S, et al: Characteristics of objects that cause choking in children. JAMA 274:1763–1766, 1995.
17. Aytac A, Yurdakul Y, Ikizler C, et al: Inhalation of foreign bodies in children: Report of 500 cases. J Thorac Cardiovasc Surg 74:145–151, 1977.
18. Hawkins DB: Removal of blunt foreign bodies from the esophagus. Ann Otol Rhinol Laryngol 99:935–940, 1990.
19. Binder L, Anderson WA: Pediatric gastrointestinal foreign body ingestions. Ann Emerg Med 13:112–117, 1984.
20. Crysdale WS, Sendi KS, Yoo J: Esophageal foreign bodies in children: 15-year review pf 484 cases. Ann Otol Rhinol Laryngol 100:320, 1991.
21. Reilly J, Thompson J, MacArthur C, et al: Pediatric aerodigestive foreign body injuries are complications related to timeliness of diagnosis. Laryngoscope 107:17–20, 1997.
22. Lowe D, Russell RI: Tracheobronchial foreign bodies: The position of the carina. J Laryngol Otol 98:499, 1984.
23. Barrios-Fontoba JE, Gutierrez C, Lluna J, et al: Bronchial foreign body: Should bronchoscopy be performed in all patients with a choking crisis? Pediatrc Surg Int 12:118, 1997.
24. Baharloo F, Veyckemans F, Francis C, et al: Tracheobronchial foreign bodies: Presentation and management in children and adults. J Laryngol Otol 102:1029, 1988.
25. Metrangolo S, Monetti C, Meneghini L, et al: Eight years' experience with foreign body aspiration in children: What is really important for a timely diagnosis? J Pediatr Surg 34:1229, 1999.
26. Oguz F, CItak A, Unuvar E, et al: Airway foreign bodies in childhood. Intl J Pediatr Otorhinolaryngol 52:11, 2000.
27. Zerella JT, Dimler M, McGill LC, et al: Foreign body aspiration in children: Valve of radiography and complications of bronchoscopy. J Pediatr Surg 33:1651, 1998.
28. Karakoc F, Karadag B, Akbenglioglu C, et al: Foreign body aspiration: What is the outcome? Pediatr Pulmonol 34:30–36, 2002.
29. Ritter FN: Questionable methods of foreign body treatment. Ann Otol 83:729, 1974.
30. Black RE, Johnson DG, Matlak ME: Bronchoscopic removal of aspirated foreign bodies in children. J Pediatr Surg 29:682–684, 1994.
31. Mantor PC, Tuggle DW, Tunell WP: An appropriate negative bronchoscopy rate in suspected foreign body aspiration. Am J Surg 158:622, 1989.
32. Crysdale WS, Sendi KS, Yoo J: Esophageal foreign bodies in children: 15-year review of 484 cases. Ann Otol Rhinol Laryngol 100:320, 1991.
33. Nandi P, Ong GB: Foreign body in the esophagus: Review of 2394 cases. Br J Surg 65:5–9, 1978.
34. Lemberg PS, Darrow DH, Hollinger LD: Aerodigestive tract foreign bodies in the older child and adolescent. Ann Otol Rhinol Laryngol 105:267, 1996.
35. Stack LB, Munter DW: Foreign bodies in the gastrointestinal tract. Emerg Med Clin North Am 14:493, 1996.
36. Shinhar S, Strabbing R, Madgy D: Esophagoscopy for removal of foreign bodies in the pediatric population. Int J Pediatr Otorhinolaryngol (in press).
37. Webb WA: Management of foreign bodies of the upper gastrointestinal tract. Gastroenterology 94:204–216, 1988.
38. Litovitz T, Schmitz BF: Ingestion of cylindrical and button batteries: An analysis of 2382 cases. Pediatrics 89:747–757, 1992.
39. Pellerin D, Fortier-Beaulieu M, Gueguen F: The fate of swallowed foreign bodies: Experience of 1250 instances of sub-diaphragmatic foreign bodies in children. Progr Pediatr Radiol 2:286–302, 1969.
40. Harned RK, Strain JD, Hay TC, et al: Esophageal foreign bodies: Safety and efficacy of Foley catheter extractions of coins. AJR Am J Roentgenol 168:443–446, 1997.
41. Schunk JE, Harrison AM, Corneli HM: Fluoroscopic Foley catheter removal of esophageal foreign bodies in children: experience with 415 episodes. Pediatrics 94:709, 1994.
42. Hawkins DB: Removal of blunt foreign objects from the esophagus. Ann Otol Rhinol Laryngol 99:935–940, 1990.
43. Morrow SE, Bickler SW, Kennedy AP, et al: Balloon extraction of esophageal foreign bodies in children. J Pediatr Surg 14:323, 1998.
44. Calkins CM, Christians KK, Sell LL: Cost analysis in the management of esophageal coins: Endoscopy versus bougienage. J Pediatr Surg 34:412, 1999.
45. Conners GP, Chamberlain JM, Ochsenschlager DW: Symptoms and spontaneous passage of esophageal coins. Arch Pediatr Adolesc Med 149:36–39, 1995.
46. Gross RE: The Surgery of Infancy and Childhood. Philadelphia, WB Saunders, 1953.
47. Caravsti EM, Bennett DL, McElwee NE: Pediatric coin ingestion: A prospective study on the utility of routine roentgenograms. Am J Dis Child 143:549, 1989.
48. Chen MK, Beierle EA. Gastrointestinal foreign bodies. Pediatr Ann 30:736–742, 2001.

CHAPTER 12

Bites

Charles W. McGill, MD

Bite injuries are common trauma for children and adolescents. In the United States, annual reports are made of tens of thousands of bites of various mammalian and insect species, and perhaps thousands of snakebites, no more than one third of which are poisonous.[1,2] The incidence of various bites is very likely under-reported.

TETANUS

Most bite injuries are bacteriologically contaminated, and the ubiquity of *Clostridium tetani* requires that treatment include consideration of this organism. Patients with clean wounds and little devitalized tissue seen promptly have low risk of tetanus. Dirty wounds, those with nonviable tissue, and those delayed in getting treatment for 24 hours or more have greater risk of tetanus. Equally important to these risk factors is the immunization status of the patient before injury. Children who are current with their immunizations have usually received three diphtheria, pertussis, and tetanus (DPT) injections 2 months apart during the first year of life. A booster is given 1 year after completion of the immunizing doses and again 4 to 5 years later when the child begins school. Afterward, boosters are required every 10 years for routine tetanus prophylaxis.

The patient with a low-risk wound and incomplete or uncertain immunization record should receive a dose of tetanus toxoid or a diphtheria/tetanus (DT) injection, if younger than 6 years. The immunization course is completed with two more doses of toxoid. The patient with a high-risk wound and an incomplete immunization history should receive 3000 to 6000 U of tetanus immune globulin (TIG) in addition to the previously outlined regimen. Tetanus toxoid and TIG should be given at separate sites so as not to neutralize each other. Half the volume of TIG may be injected around the wound.

A person who has been fully immunized and has had a booster within 10 years is probably well protected. If the wound is high risk, and it as been more than 5 years

since the last booster, one dose of toxoid is advisable. If the wound is more than 24 hours old, 3000 to 6000 U of TIG also should be given.

A patient with a low-risk wound who is fully immunized but has not had a booster within 10 years should be given a dose of tetanus toxoid. The same patient with a high-risk wound should receive both TIG and toxoid. The antibiotic of choice to reduce the number of vegetative forms is metronidazole or penicillin G. A 10- to 14-day course should be used if antibiotics are started.[3]

DOG AND OTHER MAMMALIAN BITES

Children between ages 5 and 14 years account for 40% of dog-bite victims reported annually. The peak incidence is in warm weather months. Reported deaths from dog-bite injuries were all from hemorrhage; none was from rabies.[1,2]

Tetanus coverage should be provided as outlined earlier. These wounds should be copiously irrigated with saline or soap and water. The use of quaternary ammonium compounds offers no extra protection. Devitalized tissue should be debrided, and areas that are not cosmetically important should be left open. Puncture wounds anywhere should be left open. The wound should be reexamined in 24 to 48 hours.

A dog's oral flora includes streptococci, staphylococci, actinomycetes, and species of *Pasteurella,* gram-negative bacteria, plus anaerobes. Penicillin or cephalosporin will cover most, but amoxicillin plus clavulanic acid may be preferable because of its activity on *Pasteurella multocida* and *Staphylococcus aureus.*[4–7]

RABIES AND POSTEXPOSURE PROPHYLAXIS

A major source of concern with any mammalian bite is the risk of exposure to rabies. Since enforced vaccinations have been undertaken in the United States, the risk of rabies exposure from domestic dogs is small. Still decisions on whether to treat should be made quickly. Rabies treatment with vaccines should be considered prophylactic. If it is to have the desired effect, it must be started as soon as possible after exposure. The mortality of human rabies is exceedingly high.[4,8]

The decision to administer postexposure prophylaxis is based on an assessment of risks, the most important of which is the likelihood the animal was rabid. Of particular importance is an understanding of which animals are more likely to carry the virus. No transmission of rabies to humans by any rodent has been reported. Therefore the bites of rats, mice, squirrels, chipmunks, and the like are low-risk incidents.[4,8,9] Wild animals carry the highest risk in the United States. Local knowledge of rabies carriers is important, and such information should be available from Departments of Public Health as well as Department of Natural Resources wildlife personnel. Risks of rabies animals such as skunks have been estimated to be as high as 1 in 3; bats, 1 in 10; wild dogs, 1 in 100; and cats, 1 in 200.[8]

Abnormal behavior by the biting animal, such as unusual aggression, can be a symptom of rabies and thus is indicative of a high-risk situation. Most bites by pet dogs are actually provoked, but in instances in which such behavior is in question, the vaccination status becomes important. A bite from a vaccinated pet should represent a low-risk case. However, observation of the animal for 10 days is advised. No cases of human rabies infection have been reported from animals that were not symptomatic within this period.[4] If the animal is to be killed to look for rabies infection, the brain must not be damaged in doing so. The presence of rabies is confirmed by studying the brain with fluorescent antibody techniques.

Wound characteristics also figure in the assessment of risk. The virus is transmitted in saliva. Therefore scratch wounds, unless contaminated by saliva, are a low-risk situation. Clinical rabies is more likely to progress in children. Wounds that are in densely innervated areas and close to the central nervous system are more likely to produce clinical rabies because of transmission of virus via nerve elements. Wounds of the head and neck are of particular concern. The greater the amount of tissue destruction, the more likely the inoculation. Any patient having two of the four significant risk factors should have postexposure prophylaxis. They are (1) younger than 10 years, (2) head and neck wounds, (3) deep lacerations, and (4) a bite by an animal whose vaccination status is in doubt.[10] High-risk cases call for simultaneous active and passive immunization. In the United States, human diploid cell vaccine (HDCV) is used for active immunization. This is a series of intramuscular 1 mL injections given on days 0, 3, 7, 14, and 28. Deltoids are the preferred site. Boosters are not recommended except for repeated exposures or for those who expect to become repeatedly exposed to the virus.

Passive immunization is done with human rabies immune globulin (HRIG). This would be omitted only if the patient were previously immunized. HRIG should be given simultaneously with HDCV if available. Two doses should be given on days 0 and 3, each 20 international units per kilogram body weight. Half should be injected around the wound, and half elsewhere intramuscularly and distant from the HDCV sites.[4]

SNAKE BITES

The estimated 8 thousand poisonous snake bites occurring in the United States annually result in about 12 to 15 deaths. More than half of these are in children younger than 12 years.[1,11,12]

Four genera of venomous snakes are found wild in the United States and are medically the most important. They are in the families Elapidae, *Micrurus* (five species of coral snakes), and Crotalidae, the pit vipers, *Crotalus* (large rattlesnakes), *Sistrurus* (pigmy rattlesnakes and ground rattlesnakes), and *Agkistrodon* (cottonmouth moccasin and copperheads).

Pit vipers have two needle-like fangs through which venom is injected. Their heads are triangular, and the characteristic "pit" lies between the nostril and the eye. Venomous snakes have vertically elliptical pupils. Nonpoisonous snakes have round pupils.[13]

Coral snakes are not pit vipers. They have short, fixed fangs, and they must chew the victim to envenomate.[14] They are colorful, with transversely oriented alternating bands of black and yellow or white, red, yellow, and black. The nose is black. The nonpoisonous scarlet king snake has alternating bands also. The king snake's bands, however, run red, black, yellow, black, and red. Thus the rhyme: "red on yellow kills a fellow" and "red on black won't hurt Jack."[15]

General Care and First Aid

General care of a suspected poisonous snakebite victim should begin with as rapid as possible transport to an adequate medical facility. The patient should be kept calm and as still as possible. This simple first aid is the best. Although writings on incision and suction go back thousands of years, this practice is inefficient in removing venom and may cause more injury or risk of infection than if the wound is left alone.[16] Tourniquets do little to impede venom spread and, if applied too tightly, may cause more injury from vascular compromise. More effective than a tourniquet is not allowing the victim to walk and move about.[17] Cooling with ice packs *is not* indicated.[4,11] Excision of snakebite wounds, if done very quickly after the bite, can remove venom.[18] Excision in the field by inexperienced hands is more likely to add to problems than to solve them. Situations that call for this should be rare.

All snakebite patients should follow the previously mentioned tetanus guidelines. Nonvenomous snakebites do not require antibiotics, and data suggest that neither do venomous ones.[19,20] Many persons caring for victims of a poisonous snakebite, however, do recommend antibiotic coverage. Ampicillin or cephalothin should be adequate.[11,13,21]

Pit-Viper Envenomation

Crotalids or pit-viper venoms are not identical from species to species, but they share much, and the polyvalent horse serum antivenin (ACP equine) prepared in the United States will cover pit vipers found there. These venoms are multiple poisons, a complex of enzymes, nonenzymatic proteins, and peptides. The nonenzymatic polypeptides are the neurotoxins, cardiotoxins, and hemorrhagins. Their cumulative effect is quite toxic.

Cardiotoxin can depolarize membranes, particularly in cardiac muscle. The neurotoxins are chiefly nondepolarizing, like curare. The hemorrhagins inhibit platelet aggregation and disrupt endothelial cell junctions. Enzymes such as phospholipase A cause lyses of cells locally and within the bloodstream. Proteases are fibrinolytic and antithromboplastic. Amino acid esterases cause intravascular clotting by releasing procoagulant and activating factor X. Esterases do not activate or destroy factors V or VIII; therefore heparin is of little value in this form of disseminated intravascular clotting (DIC). Esterases also may release bradykinin, the mediator of shock seen early after envenomation.[13,16,21]

The effect of envenomation is directly proportional to the dose delivered. This is a function of the volume of venom delivered (bigger snake, more venom), the site of bite (soft tissue vs. direct vascular puncture), and the size of the victim. The smaller the victim, the greater the relative dose. This explains the higher mortality in young children and the fact that small children will require more antivenin than a similarly envenomated adult.

Pit vipers leave fang marks. No puncture wound means no bite. Not all bites envenomate. Local reaction will include swelling that is painful at a minimum, and may be seen with bleb formation, necrosis, and bleeding around the wound site. The progression of swelling is a key observation in determining the grade of envenomation. If no swelling is seen around the wound within 4 hours, likely no envenomation occurred.

Systemic symptoms often begin with nausea and vomiting and progress to more life-threatening problems. Hypotension may develop from decrease in vascular tone or from fluid shifts. Hemorrhage can be both local and, later, intrapulmonary. Hemolysis and cardiac arrhythmias also may occur.

Treatment decisions require an orderly and rapid clinical assessment followed by appropriate action. Pain and swelling around fang marks identify a patient envenomated by a pit viper. Such patients should be observed in the hospital up to 24 hours after the bite. If no swelling or pain has been noted around the fang mark within 4 hours of the bite, likely no envenomation occurred. Local care is enough, and hospitalization may not be required.

An envenomated victim should have baseline complete blood count with platelet count, electrolytes, blood urea nitrogen, fibrinogen levels, and prothrombin time done on admission. Type and cross-match should be done with this blood drawing, because systemic effects of the venom may make typing and cross-matching difficult later. A urinalysis also should be done. Laboratory tests do not tell you the grade of envenomation, but will help in assessing treatment later in the severely envenomated.[16,22]

Intravenous fluids should be started. Two intravenous lines should be started on the more severely envenomated, one for antivenin, and another for volume support and other drugs. The patient should not be allowed to eat or drink for the first 24 hours because nausea and vomiting are among the earliest systemic symptoms. Careful input and output monitoring should be done. An electrocardiogram is not always required for children.

Treatment of the envenomated patient must be modified according to its severity. The system of grading illustrated in Table 12-1 is probably the most commonly used for the use of ACP equine antivenin.[22,23] Local swelling may become extensive. Some impressive swelling can be seen from snakes such as copperheads. Their venom is not usually so toxic that it causes systemic symptoms. Antivenin should rarely be needed for these bites.[24] Extremity swelling can proceed to the extent that blood flow is impeded. Aggressive antivenin use should prevent this problem. Fasciotomy may have a role in extreme cases, but for the most part, more antivenin is the required treatment. Measuring compartment pressures is

TABLE 12-1			
GRADING SEVERITY OF ENVENOMATION			
Grade	Local Characteristics	Systemic Signs	ACP (Equine) Antivenin
0	No envenomation: fang marks but no edema	None	None
1	Fang marks with edema of 1 to 5 inches within 12 hr	None	None
2	Fang marks with edema of 6 to 12 inches within 12 hr	Early systemic symptoms (nausea and vomiting)	2 to 5 vials
3	Fang marks with edema greater than 12 inches	Systemic symptoms and measurable defects in coagulation	5 to 10 vials
4	Fang marks with necrosis and bleb formation; edema to ipsilateral trunk	Hypotension; severe coagulation defects	10 to 20 vials

Adapted from McCollough NC, Gennaro JF: Clin Toxicol 3:483, 1970; Wood JJ, Hoback WW, Green TW: Va Mo 82:130, 1955.

not helpful. The swelling is not restricted to muscle compartments, and if a fasciotomy is required, the skin and subcutaneous tissues also must be opened. Such wounds done with alterations in local and systemic coagulation processes can bring on a whole new order of difficulties with hemorrhage.[16]

Antivenin Crotalidae Polyvalent (ACP) Equine Use

Grades 2, 3, or 4 envenomation require treatment with antivenin. The amount suggested in Table 12-1 is a beginning estimate for ACP equine antivenin. Doses may have to be repeated depending on how local and systemic symptoms respond. As stated earlier, the small child will require more antivenin than will a similar-grade envenomation in an adult. A case was reported in which a 3-year-old required 60 vials in the first 11 hours of treatment.[25]

Once it is determined that a patient should receive antivenin, the required test for sensitivity to horse serum is done. Instructions for this are supplied with the antivenin. Usually a skin test, this is a reasonable screening for anaphylaxis but is not foolproof. It does not address serum sickness risks. Anyone given more than five vials has at least a 50% chance of some serum sickness symptoms developing in the weeks after treatment. Some authorities advocate the prophylactic use of antihistamines and steroids in postdischarge planning.[26,27] A patient sensitive to horse serum may still receive antivenin, but in such cases, experts in handling anaphylaxis should be part of the treating team.

Overtreatment should obviously be avoided, but once the need for antivenin is clear, no benefit is found from proceeding slowly. In the presence of a coagulopathy, it is antivenin and not fresh frozen plasma or heparin that is required to reverse this form of DIC.[12] The goal is to neutralize the venom quickly. After skin testing, an initial test-strength dose of one vial in 500 mL of normal saline (a 1:50 dilution) is begun. If no allergic reactions are seen after 5 minutes, the concentration should be increased by adding to the original mixture, not to exceed a 1:4 concentration. The initial dose estimate should be given within the first 2 hours if possible. All antivenin is administered intravenously; none is infiltrated around the wound. Response will include cessation of tissue swelling, elimination of systemic symptoms, and return of abnormal laboratory values to normal.

Fab (Ovine) Polyvalent Antivenin

ACP equine (antivenin Crotalidae polyvalent), an immunoglobulin G (IgG) antivenin prepared from horse serum, has been used in the United States since the 1950s. It has been effective, and although serum sickness is very common, and risk of more acute allergic reactions require skin testing before use, it remains the only antivenin stocked in many hospitals.

Fab (ovine) polyvalent crotalid antivenin is a sheep-serum product. The serum is digested with papain to yield Fab and Fc antibody fragments. The Fc fragment is removed because it is more allergenic. Pooled Fab components to various species of pit vipers make up the polyvalent antivenin. Packaged as powder, it is reconstituted in sterile water. It has had Food and Drug Administration (FDA) approval since 2000. The preapproval trials excluded children.[28–31]

Fab (ovine) polyvalent antivenin in animal models was shown to be more potent than ACP antivenins in neutralizing venoms. It has been shown to be quite effective in human use as well. It is less allergenic for both acute hypersensitivity reactions and serum sickness than are ACP antivenins. Skin testing is not recommended by the manufacturer.

Reports of the use of Fab (ovine) antivenin continue to show effectiveness in neutralizing venoms. Its use in children shows similar results. The cases of acute hypersensitivity reactions seen may be particularly related to rate of infusion. Overall frequency of allergic responses is lower than that seen with ACP (equine) antivenins.[29]

Criteria for using Fab antivenin are similar to those for ACP (equine) antivenins, but the titration of dosing does not follow the same pattern, as seen in Table 1. Any envenomation resulting in grades 2, 3, or 4, as described in Table 12-1, also would be considered an indication to begin Fab antivenin.

The initial dose of Fab antivenin calls for four to six vials of reconstituted antivenin to be added to 250 mL of normal saline. A beginning rate of 25 to 50 mL per hour for about 10 minutes serves as a test for hypersensitivity reactions. If no acute reactions are noted, then the remainder should go in during about 1 hour; the rate should not exceed 250 mL/hr.[29,30]

The initial dose is not repeated if control is established. Control is defined as stopping the spread of edema and any systemic symptoms, and at least stabilizing any abnormal laboratory studies. If control is not obtained after 1 hour, then the initial dose is repeated with four to six vials in another 250 mL of normal saline. Recent experience has shown control to be achieved in nearly 60% of cases with the initial dose. The mean number of vials used was 16, and the range was 10 to 47.[30]

After initial control is established, the patient must remain hospitalized and observed. The risk of re-emergent symptoms and/or abnormalities in coagulation profiles calls for repeated doses of two vials every 6 hours for three additional doses.[31] After the last three doses, no further antivenin is given unless symptoms appear or laboratory abnormalities emerge. In envenomations in which coagulopathy develops, some debate is found on what constitutes adequate treatment. Delayed return to normal coagulation profiles is seen after both ACP and Fab antivenins. Clinical bleeding certainly calls for more active treatment. Abnormalities of one component of a profile without clinical problems can safely be observed. It is recommended that patients who experienced coagulation defects should be monitored after discharge with laboratory studies at 48 to 72 hours.[30]

Fab (ovine) polyvalent antivenin has yet to have the thousands of exposures that ACP (equine) antivenin has had. It does, however, seem to be both safe and effective.[29–31] For patients with known sensitivity to horse serum, it offers a significant benefit.

Coral Snake Bites

The venom of coral snake species has virtually no cytotoxins. Minimal local tissue reaction will occur, by which to judge envenomation. Pain at the site is minimal also. A patient with sufficient local injury to suggest chewing by the snake must be assumed to have been envenomated. The clinical symptoms of envenomation may well be delayed for between 4 and 12 hours.

Coral snake venom consists mainly of neurotoxic peptides and enzymes. It will have curare-like action. None of the baseline studies done for pit-viper victims will be abnormal and so are not needed. The initial symptoms may be drowsiness or even euphoria. Urine and blood alcohol and toxic screens may be appropriate studies, if the clinical situation dictates. As symptoms progress, weakness, local fasciculations, diplopia, and slurred speech may indicate bulbar paralysis. Respiratory depression and respiratory muscle paralysis may last days. Total recovery may take weeks. Once symptoms begin, progression may take place rapidly.

Any patient suspected to have been envenomated by a coral snake must be observed for a minimum of 12 hours. Respiratory-depressant drugs should be avoided. A patient with high suspicion of envenomation, such as the history that the snake was difficult to remove from the bite site, should be observed for 24 hours. Some would advocate beginning antivenin in such a patient even if initial systemic symptoms were absent.[32]

Respiratory and neurologic function must be monitored closely. Peak flows and tidal volume are important parameters, and the patient should be intubated early if progression of respiratory symptoms becomes worrisome. Antivenin is absolutely indicated at the first sign of symptoms. A grading scheme such as used for pit vipers does not work as well for coral snake bites. The antivenin also is horse serum, and similar skin testing should be done before administration. The initial dose should be five vials, even with mild signs of envenomation. This dose can be diluted in 250 mL of normal saline and delivered at 3 to 4 mL/hr initially to test for allergic reactions. If no signs of allergy appear, the infusion should be increased slowly to 120 mL/hr, which will deliver two to three vials per hour. Additional dosing will be dictated by symptom response. The response will not be as rapid or predictable as in pit-viper envenomation.[14]

HUMAN BITES

Human bites are the third most common after dog and cat bites.[33] The human mouth harbors a variety of pathogens including staphylococci, streptococci, spirochetes, spirilla of Vincent, and others. Human-bite injuries are generally of three varieties. An outright bite from another person, a hand injury from striking another person's mouth, and a self-inflicted bite, such as a tongue injury.

All these wounds should be carefully examined for deep tissue injury, cleansed, and debrided as necessary. Tetanus coverage should be administered. Antibiotics are required. The combination of penicillin and dicloxacillin should provide good coverage.[34,35]

Exposure to viral infections by human bites is rare, but possible. Hepatitis B can be transmitted by the bite of a carrier. Hepatitis B immune globulin and hepatitis B vaccine are recommended. The reverse situation of biting a carrier should not require treatment unless a mucosal lesion is found in the mouth of the biter.[36]

Transmission of human immunodeficiency virus (HIV) by human bite has been debated.[37] Reports of transmission by human bites are seen in the literature, so some risk should be assumed to exist.[33,38,39]

SPIDER BITES

Brown Recluse Spider

Loxosceles reclusa, the North American brown recluse spider, is a medium-sized spider of 8 to 9 mm in body length, with a distinguishing dark violin-shaped spot located dorsally on the carapace. This fuses with a thin line extending forward to the abdomen. This marking accounts for the name "fiddleback" often given to this spider. The brown recluse is common in the southern and central United States. It is frequently found indoors in dry, dark areas. It may be less well known than the black widow, but may present a greater medical problem.[40]

The venom is a composite poison containing proteases, hyaluronidase, hemolysin, and other cytotoxins that mediate cell wall destruction. These effects may extend beyond local tissue to injure red blood cells and glomeruli.[41-43] "Systemic loxoscelism" refers to these distant effects such as hemolysis, hemoglobinuria, renal failure, and DIC. Systemic effects are more likely to be seen in small children whose degree of envenomation is greater.[42] Systemic symptomatic therapy is mainly supportive. Intravenous fluids to provoke a brisk diuresis may lessen the risk of tubular injury from hemoglobinuria. Blood or frozen plasma may be needed for DIC.[43]

The wound may go unnoticed initially, but within 3 to 4 days, the progression of erythema to vesiculation to central necrosis will be seen. An eschar will form by 5 to 7 days. Treatment of these wounds usually involves local cleansing, antibiotics to cover staphylococci and streptococci, and pain medication. Debriding of the wound is done only if tissue destruction is significant and begun only after the wound is well demarcated.[42] The use of dapsone and hyperbaric oxygen are mentioned in the literature, but animal model studies have shown no significant utility of these.[44] The diagnosis may be in question because of the delay between injury and symptoms. A passive hemagglutination test may diagnose brown recluse bites,[45] and an older thymidine uptake by lymphocytes can be done.[46] Either of these may be particularly helpful clinically.

Black Widow Spider

Black widow spiders, *Latrodectus mactans,* "the murderer," are web spinners found throughout the United States.

Only the female of these five species of widow spiders is dangerous. A red hourglass-shaped spot on the abdomen identifies the spider. The venom is mainly neurotoxic, causing both local and generalized spasm. This is mediated by acetylcholine depletion at motor nerve endings and catecholamine release at adrenergic nerve endings. The bite is immediately painful. The wound will demarcate with a wheal and erythema, piloerection, and local cyanosis. This causes the so-called "target lesion."

The progression of generalized cramping and pain may be rapid, and the chief complaint often is more directed at abdominal pain than at wound pain. Smaller children again are more likely to have a greater systemic response. Treatment is usually symptomatic, with narcotics for pain relief and muscle relaxants such as diazepam to deal with the muscle spasm. The relief from diazepam is superior to that from calcium gluconate.[42] An antivenin, another horse serum preparation, is used for black widow envenomation. It works rapidly to relieve symptoms, and one vial is usually all that is required. It is delivered in 50 to 100 mL of dextrose and water over a 30-minute period. It should be noted, however, that in a large review series of black widow cases, the only mortality occurred from a bronchospasm reaction to antivenin.[47]

REFERENCES

1. Litovitz TL, Felberg L, Soloway RA, et al: Annual report of American Poison Control Centers Toxic Exposure Surveillance System. Am J Emerg Med 13:551–597, 1995.
2. American Academy of Pediatrics: Report of the Committee on Infectious Diseases, 25th ed. American Academy of Pediatrics, Elk Grove Village, Ill, 2002, p 255.
3. American Academy of Pediatrics: Report of the Committee on Infectious Diseases, 25th ed American Academy of Pediatrics, Elk Grove Village, Ill, 2002, pp 563–568.
4. American Academy of Pediatrics: Report of the Committee on Infectious Diseases, 25th ed American Academy of Pediatrics, Elk Grove Village, Ill, 2002, pp 475–482.
5. Winkler WG: Human deaths induced by dog bites: United States 1974-75. Public Health Rep 92:425, 1977.
6. Cummings P: Antibiotics to prevent infection in patients with dog bite wounds: Meta-analysis of randomized trials. Ann Emerg Med 23:535–540, 1994.
7. Tan JS: Human zoonotic infections transmitted by dogs and cats. Arch Intern Med 157:1933–1943, 1997.
8. Cantor SB, Clover RD, Thompson RF: A decision-analytic approach to post exposure rabies prophylaxis. Am J Public Health 84:1144–1148, 1994.
9. Anonymous: Rabies prevention: United States, 1991. Recommendations of the Immunization Practices Advisory Committee (ACIP). Morb Mortal Wkly Rep 40(RR-3):1-19, 1991.
10. Robinson DA: Dog bites and rabies: An assessment of risk. Br Med J 1:1066, 1976.
11. Forks TP: Evaluation and treatment of poisonous snakebites. Am Fam Physician 50:123–130, 1994.
12. Gold BS, Dart RC, Barish RA: Bites of venomous snakes. N Engl J Med 347:347–352, 2002.
13. Van Mierop LHS: Poisonous snakebite: A review. J Fla Med Assoc 63:191–201, 1976.
14. Gaar GG: Assessment and management of coral and other exotic snake envenomations. J Fla Med Assoc 83:178–182, 1996.
15. Strickland NE: Snakebites: A review. J Ark Med Soc 73:69–77, 1976.
16. Wingert WA: Rattlesnake bites in Southern California and rationale for recommended treatment. West J Med 148:37–44, 1988.
17. Howarth DM, Southee AE, Whyte IM: Lymphatic flow rates and first aid in simulated peripheral snake or spider envenomation. Med J Aust 16:700–701, 1994.
18. Huang TT, Lynch JB, Larson K, et al: The use of excisional therapy in the management of snakebites. Ann Surg 179:598–607, 1974.
19. Weed HG: Nonvenomous snakebite in Massachusetts: Prophylactic antibiotics are unnecessary. Ann Emerg Med 22:220–224, 1993.
20. Clark RF, Selden BS, Furbee B: The incidence of wound infection following Crotalid envenomation. J Emerg Med 11:583–586, 1993.
21. Nelson BK: Snake envenomation: Incidence, clinical presentation and management. Med Toxicol Adverse Drug Exp 4:17–31, 1989.
22. Wood JT, Hoback WW, Green TW: Treatment of snake venom poisoning with ACTH and cortisone. Va Med Mon 82:130, 1955.
23. McCollough NC, Gennaro JF: Treatment of venomous snakebites in the United States. Clin Toxicol 3:483–500, 1970.
24. White BD, Rodgers GC, Matyunas NJ, et al: Copperhead snakebites reported to the Kentucky Regional Poison Center 1986: Epidemiology and treatment suggestions. J Ky Med Assoc 86: 61–66, 1988.
25. Buntain WL: Successful venomous snakebite neutralization with massive antivenin infusions in child. J Trauma 23:1012–1014, 1983.
26. Jurkovich GJ, Lutherman A, McCullar K, et al: Complications of Crotalid antivenin therapy. J Trauma 28:1032–1037, 1988.
27. Holstege CP, Miller MB, Wermuth M, et al: Crotalid snake envenomations. Crit Care Clin 13:889–921, 1997.
28. Jucket G, Hancox JG: Venomous snakebite in the United States: Management review and update. Am Fam Physician 65:1367–1374, 2002.
29. Dart RC, McNally J: Efficacy, safety, and use of snake antivenoms in the United States. Ann Emerg Med 37:181–188, 2001.
30. Ruha AM, Curry SC, Beuhler M, et al: Initial post marketing experience with Crotalidae polyvalent immune Fab for treatment of rattlesnake envenomation. Ann Emerg Med 39:609–615, 2002.
31. Dart RC, Seifert SA, Boyer LV et al: A randomized multicenter trial of Crotalinae polyvalent immune Fab (ovine) antivenom for the treatment for Crotaline snakebite in the United States. Arch Intern Med 161:2030–2036, 2001.
32. Weisman RS, Lizarralde SS, Thompson V: Snake and spider antivenin: risks and benefits of therapy. J Fla Med Assoc 83:192–195, 1996.
33. Pretty IA, Anderson GS, Sweet DJ: Human bites and risk of human immunodeficiency virus transmission. Am J Forens Med Pathol 20:232–239,1999.
34. Ruskin JD, Laney TJ, Wendt SV, et al: Treatment of mammalian bite wounds of maxillofacial area. J Oral Maxillofac Surg 51:174–176, 1993.
35. Stewart GM, Quan L, Horton MA: Laceration management. Pediatr Emerg Care 9:247–250, 1993.
36. American Academy of Pediatrics: Report of the Committee on Infectious Diseases, 24th ed American Academy of Pediatrics, Elk Grove Village, Ill, 1997, p 259.
37. Rickman KM, Rickman LS: The potential for transmission of human immunodeficiency virus through human bite. J Acquir Immune Defic Syndr 6:402–406, 1993.
38. Vidmar L, Poljak M, Tomazic J, et al: Transmission of HIV-1 by human bite [letter]. Lancet 347:1762–1763, 1996.
39. Khajotia FF, Lee E: Transmission of human immunodeficiency virus through saliva after lip bite. Arch Intern Med 157:1901, 1997.
40. Young VL, Pin P: The brown recluse spider bite. Ann Plast Surg 20:447–452, 1988.
41. Anderson PC: Missouri brown recluse spider: A review and update. Mo Med 95:318–322, 1998.
42. Carbonaro PA, Janniger CK, Schwartz RA: Spider bite reactions. Cutis 56:256–259, 1995.
43. Arnold RE: Brown recluse spider bites: Five cases with a review of the literature. J Am Coll Emerg Physicians 5:262–264, 1976.

44. Hobbs GD, Anderson AR, Greene TJ, et al: Comparison of hyperbaric oxygen and dapsone therapy for *Loxosceles* envenomation. Acad Emerg Med 3:758–761, 1996.
45. Barrett SM, Romine-Jenkins M, Blick KE: Passive hemagglutination inhibition test for diagnosis of brown recluse spider bite. Clin Chem 39:2104–2107, 1993.
46. Majeski JA, Durst GG: Necrotic arachnidism. South Med J 69:887–891, 1976.
47. Clark RF, Wethern-Kestner S, Vance MV, et al: Clinical presentation and treatment of black widow spider envenomation: A review of 163 cases. Ann Emerg Med 21:782–787, 1992.

CHAPTER 13

Burns

Dai H. Chung, MD, and David N. Herndon, MD

GENERAL CONSIDERATIONS

Major advances in burn care have occurred in the past 5 decades. In 1944, the Lund and Browder diagram was developed to draw the burned areas, allowing a quantifiable assessment of percentage of total body surface area (TBSA) burned.[1] In 1946, Oliver Cope and Francis Moore[2] were able to quantify the appropriate amount of fluid required to maintain central electrolyte composition after burn shock while treating victims of the Coconut Grove fire in Boston. In the 1960s, the discovery of efficacious topical antimicrobial agents, such as 0.5% silver nitrate,[3] mafenide acetate (Sulfamylon),[4] and silver sulfadiazine (Silvadene),[5] made a significant impact on the survival of burn patients. Recently, better understanding and improvement in the areas of fluid resuscitation, infection control, support of the hypermetabolic response, treatment of inhalation injury, and early surgical excision and grafting of the burn wound have all contributed to a 50% decline in burn-related deaths and hospital admissions in the United States.[6] Today, this overall increase in survival is most evident in the pediatric patient population, in which a predictable 50% mortality rate that was associated with 75% TBSA burns now is the risk for 98% TBSA burns in children aged 14 years and younger.[7]

Approximately 2 million burn injuries occur every year in the United States. Although most cases are minor, approximately 50,000 patients have moderate to severe burns, requiring hospitalization for treatment. Of these cases, two thirds are young males and 40% are children younger than 15 years.[8] As the second leading cause of accidental death in children younger than 5 years, burns result in approximately 2,500 childhood deaths each year. In 1997, an estimated 83,000 children younger than 14 years were treated in hospital emergency departments for burn-related injuries. Of these, 59,000 were thermal burns, and 24,000, scald burns.[9] Of the children age 4 years and younger who are hospitalized for burn-related injuries, 65% have scald burns, 20% contact burns, and the remainder, flame burns. The majority of

scald burns in infants and toddlers are from hot foods and liquids. Hot grease spills are notorious for causing deep burns. Hot tap-water burns, which can easily be prevented by installing special faucet valves that restrict the delivery of water above 120°F (48.8°C), frequently result in large burns to children.[10] Children also frequently have contact burns from curling irons, ovens, steam irons, and fireworks. The insertion of metallic objects into wall outlets results in electrical injuries, as also result from playing with electrical cords. Child abuse accounts for a significant number of burns in children. Burns that are bilaterally symmetrical, of stocking/glove distribution, and burns to the dorsum of hands, accompanied by delay in seeking medical attention should raise suspicion of child abuse. In the adolescent age group, flame burns are more common, frequently occurring as a result of experimenting with fire and volatile agents.

PATHOPHYSIOLOGY

As the largest organ of the body, the skin guards against harmful environmental insults, prevents entry of microorganisms, and maintains fluid and electrolyte homeostasis. Other important functions include thermoregulation, the production of vitamin D, and processing neurosensory inputs. The surface area of skin ranges from 0.2 to 0.3 m² in an average newborn and 1.5 to 2.0 m² in an adult. The skin makes up nearly 15% of total body weight. The epidermis is composed primarily of epithelial cells, specifically keratinocytes. The cells from basal layer of keratinocytes, stratum germinativum, divide and migrate outward to stratum spinosum, granulosum, lucidum, and eventually to stratum corneum, which is impervious and eventually desquamates. This entire process of epidermal growth and maturation from the basal layer to desquamation generally takes about 2 to 4 weeks. The basement membrane at the dermoepidermal junction, composed of mucopolysaccharides rich in fibronectin, functions as a barrier to passage of macromolecules. The dermis is made up of fibroblasts producing collagen and elastin and is subdivided into a

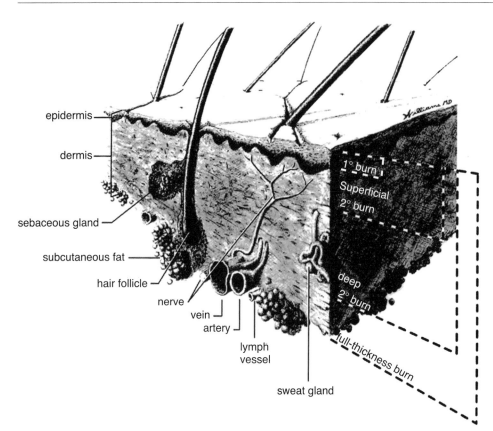

FIGURE 13-1. Anatomy of the skin. (Adapted from Williams WG: Pathophysiology of the burn wound. In Herndon DN [ed]: Total Burn Care, 2nd ed. Philadelphia, WB Saunders, 2002, p 515.)

superficial papillary dermis and a deep reticular dermis. The papillary and reticular layers of the skin are separated by a plexus of nerves and blood vessels. The reticular dermis and fatty layer contain skin appendages, such as hair follicles, sweat glands, and sebaceous glands (Fig. 13-1).

Thermal injury results in coagulation necrosis of the epidermis and the varying degree of injury to the underlying tissue. The extent of burn injury depends on the temperature, duration of exposure, skin thickness, tissue conductance, and specific heat of the causative agent. For example, the specific heat of fat is higher than that of water; therefore grease burns often result in much deeper burns than does a scald burn from water with the same temperature and duration of exposure. Thermal energy is

easily transferred from high-energy molecules to those of lower energy during contact, through a process of heat conduction. The skin generally provides a barrier to transfer of energy to deeper tissues; therefore much of the burn injury is confined to this layer. However, local tissue response to the zone of initial burn injury can lead to progression of burn-induced destruction of surrounding tissue. The area of cutaneous burn injury is divided into three zones: zone of coagulation, zone of stasis, and zone of hyperemia (Fig. 13-2). The zone of coagulation comprises the initial burn eschar where cells become irreversibly damaged and necrotic at the time of injury. The area immediately surrounding the necrotic area is a zone of stasis, where most cells are initially viable, but

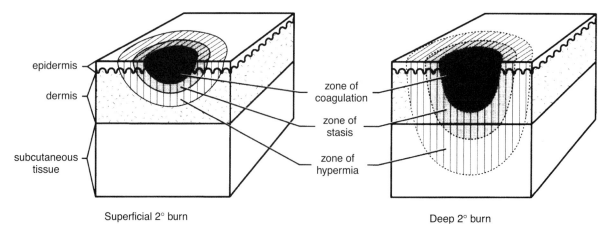

FIGURE 13-2. Three zones of burn injury: coagulation, stasis, and hyperemia.

tissue perfusion becomes progressively impaired from local release of inflammatory mediators, such as thromboxane A_2, arachidonic acid, oxidants, and cytokines.[11] Their influence on the microcirculation results in the formation of platelet thrombus, neutrophil adherence, fibrin deposition, and vasoconstriction, which lead to cell necrosis. Thromboxane A_2 inhibitors can significantly improve the dermal blood flow to decrease zone of stasis.[12] Antioxidants as well as bradykinin antagonists also improve local blood flow.[13,14] Inhibition of neutrophil adherence to endothelium with anti–CD-18 or anti-intercellular adhesion molecules to monoclonal antibodies improves tissue perfusion in animal models.[15,16] Peripheral to the zone of stasis lies the zone of hyperemia, which is characterized by vasodilation with increased blood flow as part of inflammatory response.

The burn-induced inflammatory response is not limited to the local burn wounds. A massive systemic release of thromboxane A_2, along with other inflammatory mediators (bradykinin, leukotrienes, catecholamines, activated complements, and vasoactive amines), induces major physiologic burden on cardiopulmonary, renal, and gastrointestinal tract organ systems.[17] Decreased plasma volume due to increased capillary permeability and subsequent plasma leak into the interstitial space can lead to depressed cardiac functions. As a result of low cardiac output, renal blood flow can decrease, leading to diminished glomerular filtration rate. Activation of other stress-induced hormones and mediators, such as angiotensin, aldosterone, and vasopressin, can further compromise renal blood flow, resulting in oliguria.[18] If not properly treated, this condition can progress to acute tubular necrosis and renal failure, which is associated with reduced survival for burn patients.[19] The gastrointestinal tract also is affected by cutaneous burn injury. Atrophy of small bowel mucosa occurs as a result of increased epithelial apoptosis and decreased epithelial proliferation.[20–22] Intestinal permeability to macromolecules, which are normally repelled by an intact mucosal barrier, increases after a burn injury.[23–25] Transient mesenteric ischemia is thought to be an important contributing factor to increases in intestinal permeability, which can result in more frequent incidence of bacterial translocation and subsequent endotoxemia. Burn injury also causes a global depression of immune function. Macrophage production is decreased; neutrophils are impaired in terms of their functions, such as diapedesis, chemotaxis, and phagocytosis; cytotoxic T-lymphocyte activity is decreased. These impaired functions of neutrophils, macrophages, and T lymphocytes contribute to increased risks for infectious complications after burns.[26–31]

MANAGEMENT OF BURNS

Initial Evaluation

A burn patient must be immediately removed from the source of burn injury. Burning clothing articles as well as metal jewelry are removed. Immediate cooling by, for example, pouring cool water, can minimize the depth of the burn, but it must be used with caution to prevent hypothermia. After the removal of clothing articles, the patient should be kept warm with sterile blankets to prevent hypothermia. With chemical burns, patients should be quickly separated from the chemical agent, and the wound irrigated with copious amounts of water, while being cautious to not spread any residual chemical to adjacent uninvolved areas. Attempts to neutralize chemicals are contraindicated, as this process may produce additional heat, producing further injury.

As with any trauma patients, burn patients are quickly assessed through primary and secondary surveys. In the primary survey, airway, breathing, and circulation are assessed, and any potential life-threatening conditions are quickly identified. Symptoms such as wheezing, tachypnea, and hoarseness indicate impending major airway problems and call for ensuring the patency of the airway and the administration of 100% oxygen. Oxygen saturation is monitored by using pulse oximetry. It is important to observe chest expansion to ensure equal air movement. Circumferential full-thickness burns to the chest can significantly restrict respiratory movement. If necessary, escharotomy should be performed to allow better chest expansion and improve ventilation. Cuff blood pressure measurement may be difficult in patients with burned extremities. The pulse rate can be used as an indirect measure of intravascular volume; the presence of tachycardia is an indication for aggressive fluid resuscitation.

Burn depth is categorized by estimation of injury to the layers of the skin: epidermis, papillary dermis, reticular dermis, subcutaneous fat, and underlying structures (see Fig. 13-1). First-degree burns are confined to the epidermis. The epidermis appears intact, erythematous, and is painful to touch. The application of topical ointment containing aloe vera, along with oral nonsteroidal anti-inflammatory agents, constitutes the standard treatment therapy. First-degree burns (e.g, sunburn) heal spontaneously without scarring in 7 to 10 days. The second-degree burns are divided into superficial and deep, based on the depth of dermal involvement. Superficial second-degree burns are limited to papillary dermis and are typically erythematous and painful, with blisters. These burns spontaneously re-epithelialize in a period of 10 to 14 days from retained epidermal structures and may only leave some slight skin discoloration. Deep second-degree burns extend into reticular layer of the dermis. The deep epidermal appendages allow some of these wounds to heal slowly over a period of several weeks, usually with significant scarring. Third-degree burns are full-thickness injuries resulting in complete destruction of the epidermis, dermis, and dermal appendages and are characterized by dry, leathery eschar that is insensate to any stimuli. Without any residual epidermal or dermal appendages, ungrafted third-degree burn wounds heal by re-epithelialization from the edges. Fourth-degree burns involve organs beneath the layers of the skin, such as muscle and bone.

Accurate and rapid determination of burn depth is vital to the proper management of burn injury. In particular, distinction between superficial and deep dermal burns is critical, as this dictates whether the burns can be managed with or without surgical procedures. Evaluation by an experienced surgeon as to whether an apparent deep dermal burn is likely to heal in 3 weeks is only about 50% accurate. In many of these cases, early excision and grafting provides better results than does expectant therapy for such "indeterminate" burns. More-precise objective methods to determine the burn depth include techniques such as multisensor heatable laser Doppler flowmeter and fluorescein to determine blood flow, ultrasonography to detect denatured collagen, and light reflectance of the wound.[32-35] Ultimately, burn-wound biopsy would seem to be the most precise diagnostic tool[36]; however, it is not clinically useful because it is invasive and provides only static information about the burn wound. It also requires an experienced pathologist to interpret the histologic findings. Despite these modern technologies, clinical observation still remains the standard and the most reliable method of determining the burn depth.

Full-thickness circumferential burns to the extremities produce a constricting eschar, which potentially results in vascular compromise to the distal tissues, including nerves. Accumulation of tissue edema beneath the nonelastic eschar impedes venous outflow first and eventually affects arterial flow. When distal pulses are absent by palpation or Doppler examination, escharotomies of the extremities must immediately be performed to avoid ischemic damage to the limb tissues. With either a scalpel or an electrocautery unit, the physician performs escharotomies at the bedside along the lateral and medial aspects of the involved extremity (Fig. 13-3). When the hands are involved, escharotomy incisions should be carried out on the thenar and hypothenar eminences, and/or along the dorsolateral aspects of the digits.

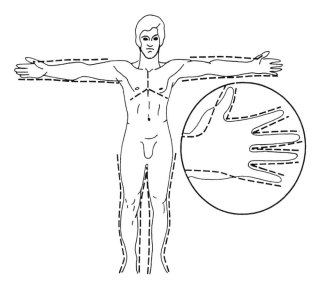

FIGURE 13-3. Escharotomies. The incisions are made on the medial and lateral aspects of the extremity. Hand escharotomies are performed on the medial and lateral digits and on the dorsum of the hand. (From Eichelberger MR [ed]: Pediatric Trauma: Prevention, Acute Care, Rehabilitation. St. Louis, Mosby, 1993.)

Because of the full-thickness burn injury, minimal bleeding should be encountered. If vascular compromise has been prolonged, reperfusion after an escharotomy may cause reactive hyperemia and further edema formation in the muscle compartments. Ischemia-reperfusion injury also releases free oxygen radicals, resulting in transient hypotension. If increased compartment pressures are noted, fasciotomy should be performed immediately to avoid permanent ischemic injuries to nerves and soft tissues.

Intravenous (IV) access should be established immediately for the administration of lactated Ringer's solution according to the resuscitation formula. Peripheral IV access is preferred, but femoral venous access is an ideal alternative in patients with massive burns. When vascular access is problematic in small children (younger than 6 years) with burned extremities, the intraosseous route is an option. A nasogastric tube is placed in all patients with major burns, anticipating gastric ileus. Almost immediate enteral nutrition can be initiated via a transpyloric feeding tube. A Foley catheter is placed to monitor urine output accurately as a measure of end-organ perfusion. Admission laboratory studies should include complete blood count, type and cross-match for packed red cell blood, chemistry profile, coagulation profile, urinalysis, and chest radiograph. If inhalation injury is suspected, arterial blood gas analysis with carboxyhemoglobin level should be obtained.

Burn size is generally assessed by the "rule of nines" in adolescents and adults. Each upper extremity and the head are 9% of the TBSA. The lower extremities and the anterior and posterior trunks are 18% each. The perineum, genitalia, and neck each measures 1% of the TBSA. A quick estimate of the burn size also can be obtained by the use of palm of the hand to represent 1% TBSA and transposing this measurement onto the wound. However, the general use of this rule can be misleading in children because of different body proportions. Children have a relatively larger portion of the BSA in the head and neck, and smaller surface area in the lower extremities. For example, an infant's head constitutes 19% of TBSA compared with 9% in an adult. Thus a modified rule of nines based on anthropomorphic differences of infancy and childhood is generally used to assess pediatric burn size (Fig. 13-4). Table 13-1 demonstrates the chart used to calculate the burn size, based on the age of the patient.

Fluid Resuscitation

Appropriate fluid resuscitation should begin immediately on securing IV access. Peripheral IV access is sufficient in the majority of small- to moderate-size burns. Saphenous vein cutdowns are useful in cases of difficult access, but in children, percutaneous femoral central venous access may be easier and more reliable. Many guidelines exist as fluid-resuscitation formulas, delivering various concentrations of colloid and crystalloid solutions. The Parkland formula (4 mL of lactated Ringer's per kilogram of body weight per percentage of TBSA burned) is most widely used, but the pediatric fluid-resuscitation formula should

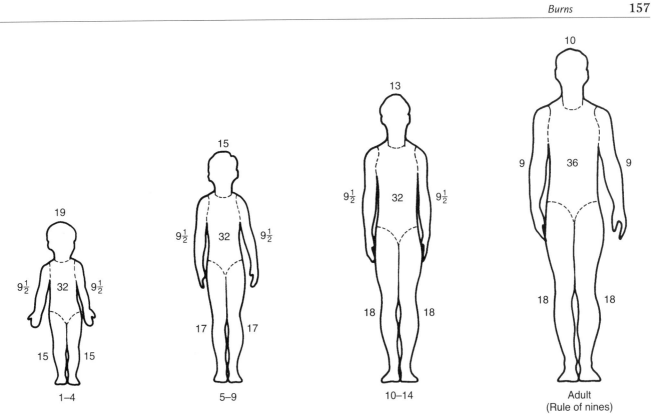

FIGURE 13-4. Modified "rule of nines" for pediatric patients. (Adapted from Benjamin D, Herndon DN: Special consideration of age: The pediatric burned patient. In Herndon DN [ed]: Total Burn Care, 2nd ed. Philadelphia, WB Saunders, 2002, p 429.)

TABLE 13-1
BURN SIZE ESTIMATE: AGE VERSUS AREA

Area	Birth–1 yr	1–4 yr	5–9 yr	10–14 yr	15 yr	Adult	Second Degree	Third Degree	TBSA%
Head	19	17	13	11	9	7			
Neck	2	2	2	2	2	2			
Ant. Trunk	13	13	13	13	13	13			
Post. Trunk	13	13	13	13	13	13			
R. Buttock	2.5	2.5	2.5	2.5	2.5	2.5			
L. Buttock	2.5	2.5	2.5	2.5	2.5	2.5			
Genitalia	1	1	1	1	1	1			
R.U. Arm	4	4	4	4	4	4			
L.U. Arm	4	4	4	4	4	4			
R.L. Arm	3	3	3	3	3	3			
L.L. Arm	3	3	3	3	3	3			
R. Hand	2.5	2.5	2.5	2.5	2.5	2.5			
L. Hand	2.5	2.5	2.5	2.5	2.5	2.5			
R. Thigh	5.5	6.5	8	8.5	9	9.5			
L. Thigh	5.5	6.5	8	8.5	9	9.5			
R. Leg	5	5	5.5	6	6.5	7			
L. Leg	5	5	5.5	6	6.5	7			
R. Foot	3.5	3.5	3.5	3.5	3.5	3.5			
L. Foot	3.5	3.5	3.5	3.5	3.5	3.5			
						Total			

TBSA, total body surface area.

be based on burned BSA and TBSA because of the disparity of the BSA-to-weight ratio. Children have greater BSA in relation to their weight, and as a result, weight-based formulas can under-resuscitate children with minor burns and may grossly over-resuscitate children with extensive burns.[37] TBSA can be easily calculated by using the child's height and weight and a standard nomogram (Fig. 13-5). The Galveston formula calls for the administration of 5000 mL/m^2 of burned BSA plus 2000 mL/m^2 of TBSA of lactated Ringer's solution administered at a rate to deliver half the calculated volume during the first 8 hours and the remaining half over the following 16 hours (Table 13-2).

TABLE 13-2

BURN RESUSCITATION FORMULAS

Formula	First 24 hr	Fluid Solution
Parkland	4 mL/kg/% TBSA burn	Lactated Ringer's (LR)
Brooke	1.5 mL/kg/% TBSA burn	LR + colloid 0.5 mL/ kg/% TBSA burn
Shriners-Galveston	5000 mL/m^2 burned + 2000 mL/m^2 total	LR + 12.5 g albumin

TBSA, total body surface area.

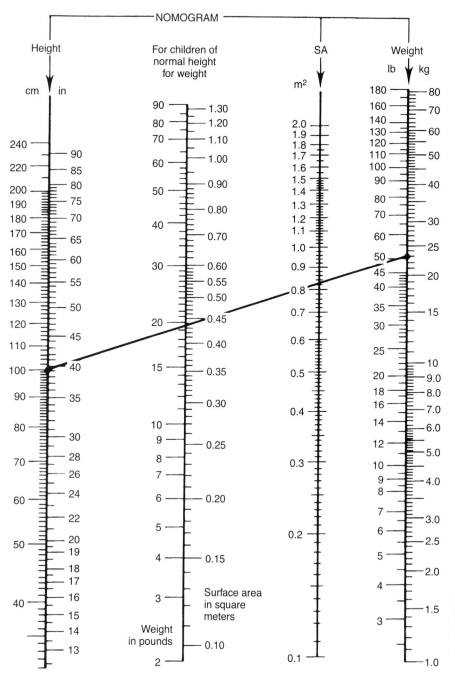

FIGURE 13-5. Standard nomogram for the determination of body surface area based on height and weight. A straight line drawn between the height and weight measurements determines the total body surface area in square meters.

The primary goal of fluid resuscitation is to achieve adequate organ tissue perfusion. Fluid administration should be titrated to maintain a urine output of 1 mL/kg/hr. Approximately 50% of the administered fluid will be sequestered in nonburned tissues in a patient with a 50% TBSA burn because of increased capillary permeability that occurs, particularly in the first 6 to 8 hours after injury.[38] During this period, large molecules leak into the interstitial space to increase extravascular colloid osmotic pressure. Therefore to maintain intravascular osmotic pressure, albumin is added 12 hours after the injury. After the first 24 hours, the volume is reduced to 3750 mL/m^2 for the burn area plus 1500 mL/m^2 TBSA delivered in equal hourly portions. Dextrose, 5%, should be added to the solution at this time in either quarter- or half-normal saline. Children younger than 2 years are susceptible to hypoglycemia because of limited glycogen stores, and the initial 24-hour resuscitation fluid should be lactated Ringer's solution with 5% dextrose.

Children often do not exhibit clinical signs of hypovolemia until more than 25% of their circulating volume is depleted and complete cardiovascular collapse is imminent. Tachycardia reflects a compensatory response to hypovolemia, but reflex tachycardia due to postinjury catecholamine release also is common. A lethargic child with decreased capillary refill and cool, clammy extremities needs prompt attention to blood volume. Measurement of arterial blood pH and base deficit values also can reflect on the adequacy of fluid resuscitation. Hyponatremia also is a frequent complication in pediatric burn patients after aggressive fluid resuscitation. Frequent monitoring of serum chemistry with appropriate correction is required to avoid electrolyte imbalance. A serious complication such as central pontine myelinolysis can occur as a result of overly rapid correction of hypernatremia.[39]

Hypertonic saline resuscitation may be beneficial, however, in treating burn-induced shock.[40,41] It will enhance intravascular volume by osmosis of fluid from the interstitial space and therefore decrease generalized tissue edema. However, it is not widely used because of its potential risks for hypernatremia, hyperosmolarity, renal failure, and alkalosis.[17,42] Some favor the use of modified hypertonic solution by adding sodium bicarbonate to each liter of lactated Ringer's solution during the first 24 hours of resuscitation.[43]

Burn units with experienced multidisciplinary team members are best prepared and experienced to handle major burns. As defined by the American Burn Association, patients who sustain major burn injury should be transferred promptly to a nearby burn center to receive optimal care (Table 13-3).

WOUND CARE

The proper wound-care plan is guided by the accurate assessment of the burn depth and size. First-degree burns require no dressing, but the involved areas should be kept out of direct sunlight. They are generally treated with topical ointments for symptomatic pain relief. Superficial

TABLE 13-3
MAJOR BURN INJURY CRITERIA (AMERICAN BURN ASSOCIATION)

Second-degree burns >10% TBSA in patients younger than 10 yr
Third-degree burns >5% TBSA
Burns involving the face, hands, feet, genitalia, perineum, and major joints
Chemical burns
Electrical burns including lightning injury
Inhalation injury
Burns with significant concomitant trauma
Burns with significant preexisting medical disorders

TBSA, total body surface area.

second-degree burns are treated with daily dressing changes with topical antimicrobials. They also can be treated with simple application of petroleum gauze or synthetic dressings to allow rapid spontaneous re-epithelialization. Deep second- and third-degree burns require excision of the eschar with skin grafting.

Antimicrobials

Table 13-4 lists various topical antimicrobial agents used in the management of burn wounds. None of these agents effectively prevent colonization of organisms in the eschar, but they limit bacterial quantity to less than 10^2 to 10^5 colonies/g of tissue. Standardized routine punch biopsy of burned areas can provide quantitative culture counts and alert the care team to impending burn-wound sepsis.

Silver sulfadiazine (Silvadene) is the most commonly used topical agent for burn-wound dressings. Although it does not penetrate eschar, it has a broad spectrum of efficacy and soothes the pain associated with second-degree burns. Silver sulfadiazine on fine-mesh gauze can be used separately or in combination with other antimicrobial agents, such as nystatin. This combination, providing antifungal coverage, has significantly reduced the incidence of *Candida* infection in burned patients.[44,45] The most common side effect is leukopenia; however, this is caused by margination of white blood cells and is only transient.[46] When the leukocyte count is less than 3000 cells/mm^3, changing to another topical antimicrobial quickly resolves this complication.

Mafenide acetate (Sulfamylon) is more effective in penetrating eschar and is frequently used in third-degree burns. Fine-mesh gauze impregnated with Sulfamylon (10% water-soluble cream) is applied directly onto the burn wound. Sulfamylon has a broad spectrum of efficacy, including *Pseudomonas* and *Enterococcus*. It also is available in 5% solution to soak burn wounds, eliminating a need to perform frequent dressing changes. Sulfamylon is a potent carbonic anhydrase inhibitor and can cause metabolic acidosis. This side effect can usually be avoided by limiting its use to only 20% TBSA at any one time and rotating application sites every several hours with another topical agent. Additionally, it is painful when applied, therefore limiting its use in an outpatient setting, especially with children.

TABLE 13-4

TOPICAL ANTIMICROBIAL AGENTS

Agent	Advantages	Disadvantages
Silver sulfadiazine (Silvadene)	Painless; broad-spectrum; rare sensitivity	Leukopenia; some gram-negative resistance; mild inhibition of epithelialization
Mafenide acetate (Sulfamylon)	Broad-spectrum; penetrates eschar; effective against *Pseudomonas*	Painful; metabolic acidosis; mild inhibition of epithelialization
Silver nitrate	Painless; broad-spectrum; rare sensitivity	Does not penetrate eschar; discolor contacted areas; electrolyte imbalance; methemoglobinemia
Bacitracin/Polysporin Neomycin	Painless; transparent; use on face	Minimal antimicrobial activity
Nystatin	Effective in inhibiting fungal growth; use in combination with Silvadene, Bacitracin	Cannot be used in combination with Sulfamylon
Mupirocin (Bactroban)	More effective against *Staphylococcus*	
Providone-iodine	Broad-spectrum	Painful; systemic absorption

In addition to 5% Sulfamylon solution, other agents are available as a soak solution: 0.5% silver nitrate and 0.025% sodium hypochloride (Dakins solution). These soak solutions are generally poured onto gauze dressings on the wound, avoiding frequent dressing changes with potential loss of grafts or healing cells. Silver nitrate is painless on application and has broad coverage, but its side effects include electrolyte imbalance (hyponatremia, hypochloremia) and dark gray or black stains. A new commercially available dressing containing biologically active silver ions (Acticoat) holds promise to retain the effectiveness of silver nitrate without the side effects. Dakins (0.025%) solution is effective against most microbes, including *Pseudomonas*. However, it requires frequent application because of inactivation of hypochlorite when in contact with wound protein. It also can retard healing cells.[47]

Petroleum-based antimicrobial ointments, such as polymyxin B, bacitracin, and polysporin, are painless and transparent, allowing easier monitoring of burn wounds. These agents are mostly effective against gram-positive organisms, and their use is limited to facial burns, small areas of partial-thickness burns, and healing donor sites. As with Silvadene, these petroleum-based agents also can be used in combination with nystatin to suppress *Candida* colonization.

The use of perioperative IV antibiotics has made a tremendous impact on the improvement of survival of major burn patients in the last two decades. Bacteria colonized in burn eschar can be disseminated systemically at the time of eschar excision, contributing to sepsis. It is a general practice to administer IV antibiotics against *Streptococcus, S. aureus,* and *Pseudomonas* perioperatively until quantitative cultures of excised eschar are finalized. The antibiotic therapy regimen should be guided by culture results and used for specific indications to reduce the risk of emergence of resistant organisms.

Wound Dressings

Superficial second-degree burns can be managed by using a variety of methods. Topical antimicrobial dressing with Silvadene may be used, but synthetic dressings, such as Biobrane and Opsite, offer unique advantages of eliminating frequent painful dressing changes and potential tissue fluid loss. The general principle of these synthetic products is to provide sterile coverage of superficial second-degree burn wounds to allow rapid spontaneous re-epithelialization of the involved areas.

Biobrane is a thin synthetic material made of silicone and collagen, supplied in simple sheets or preshaped gloves (Fig. 13-6).[48] After being placed onto clean fresh superficial second-degree burn wounds by using Steri-strips and bandages, the Biobrane dressing dries, becoming closely adherent to the burn wound within 24 to 48 hours. Once adherent, the covered areas are kept open to air and examined closely for the first few days to detect any signs and symptoms of infection. As the epithelialization occurs beneath the Biobrane sheet, it is easily peeled off the wound. Sterile aspiration of serous fluid from beneath the Biobrane can prolong its use, but once foul-smelling exudate is detected, it should be removed, and topical antimicrobial dressings applied. Alternatively, Opsite or Tegaderm can be used to cover superficial second-degree burn wounds. Commonly used as postoperative dressings in surgical patients, they are

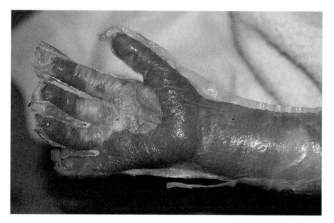

FIGURE 13-6. Biobrane glove.

easy to apply and provide an impervious barrier to the environment. They are also relatively inexpensive, and their transparent nature allows easier monitoring of covered second-degree burn wounds. Despite lacking any special biologic factors (collagen and growth factors) to enhance wound healing, they promote the spontaneous re-epithelialization process. Biobrane and Opsite are preferred to topical antimicrobial dressings when dealing with small superficial second-degree burn wounds, especially in the outpatient settings.

Synthetic and biologic dressings also are available to provide coverage for full-thickness burn wounds. Integra, which is made of a collagen matrix with an outer silicone sheet, is a synthetic dermal substitute for treatment of full-thickness burn wounds. After the collagen matrix engrafts into the wound in approximately 2 weeks, the outer silicone layer is replaced with epidermal autografts. Epidermal donor sites heal rapidly without significant morbidity. Integra-covered wounds heal with less scar formation; however, they also are susceptible to wound infection and must be monitored carefully. Alloderm is another dermal substitute with decellularized preserved cadaver dermis. These synthetic dermal substitutes have a tremendous potential for minimizing scar contractures and improving cosmetic and functional outcome. Biologic dressings, such as xenografts from swine and allografts from cadaver donors, also can be used to cover full-thickness burn wounds as a temporary dressing. Particularly useful when dealing with large TBSA burns, biologic dressings can provide immunologic and barrier functions of normal skin. The areas of xenograft and allograft are eventually rejected by the immune system and sloughed off, leaving healthy recipient beds for subsequent autografts. Although extremely rare, the transmission of viral diseases from allograft is a potential concern.

Excision and Grafting

Early excision with skin grafting has shown to decrease operative blood loss, length of hospital stay, and ultimately to improve overall survival of burn patients.[7,49] Typically, tangential excision of full-thickness burn wound is performed 1 to 3 days after burn injury when a relative hemodynamic stability has occurred. Eschar is sequentially shaved by using a powered dermatome (Zimmer) and/or knife blades (Watson, Weck) until a viable tissue plane is achieved (Fig. 13-7). Early excision of eschar (usually < 24 hours after burns) generally decreases operative blood loss because of the actions of vasoconstrictive substances, such as thromboxane and catecholamines, in the burn wounds. Once the burn wounds become hyperemic 48 hours after burns, bleeding at this time of excision of eschar can be excessive. Tourniquets and subcutaneous injections of dilute epinephrine solutions also can lessen the blood loss, but these techniques can potentially hinder the surgeon's ability to differentiate viable from nonviable tissues.[50] Topical hemostatic agents such as thrombin may be used, but are expensive and not very effective against excessive bleeding from an open wound. In patients with deep

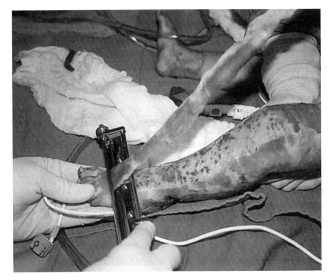

FIGURE 13-7. Tangential excision of eschar. The excision of eschar is performed to the depth of a viable, bleeding tissue plane (From Herndon DN [ed]: Total Burn Care, 2nd ed. Philadelphia, WB Saunders, 2002, plate 2.)

full-thickness burns, electrocautery is used to excise eschar rapidly with minimal blood loss. More important, the earlier the excision, the less blood loss is anticipated in burns greater than 30% TBSA.[51] Scald-burn depth is more difficult to assess initially, and the treatment requires a more conservative approach, perhaps with delayed excision.

The excised burn wound ideally is covered with autografts. Burns wounds less than 20% to 30% TBSA can be excised and closed at one operation with split-thickness autografts. Split-thickness autografts are harvested by using a dermatome, and the donor sites are dressed with petroleum-based gauze, such as Xeroform or Scarlet-red. Opsite also is used to cover donor sites. It is preferred to use sheet autografts for better long-term aesthetic outcome, but narrowly meshed autografts (1:1 or 2:1) also have the advantages of limiting the total surface area of donor harvest and allowing better drainage of fluid at the grafted sites. With massive burns, the closure of burn wounds is achieved by a combination of widely meshed autografts (4:1 to 6:1) with allograft (2:1) overlay (Fig. 13-8).

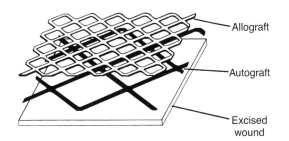

FIGURE 13-8. Schematic diagram of wound covering with 4:1 meshed autograft with 2:1 meshed allograft overlay. (From Eichelberger MR [ed]: Pediatric Trauma: Prevention, Acute Care, Rehabilitation. St. Louis, Mosby, 1993, p 581.)

Repeated grafting is required for large burns, with sequential harvesting of split-thickness autografts from limited donor sites until the entire burn wound is closed. As the meshed autografts heal, allografts slough off, and formation of significant scar remains the major disadvantage of this technique. To prevent scarring in the face and hands, the use of wide-meshed grafts is avoided. Full-thickness grafts that include both dermal and epidermal components provide the best outcome in wound coverage with diminished contracture and better pigment match. However, their use is generally limited to small areas because of lack of abundant full-thickness donor skin.

The limitation of donor site in massive-burn patients is partially addressed with the use of systemic recombinant human growth hormone. Administration of growth hormone has resulted in accelerated donor-site healing, allowing more frequent donor-site harvest in a given period.[52,53] Growth hormone decreases donor-site healing time by an average of 2 days, which ultimately reduces the overall length of hospital stay from 0.8 to 0.54 days per % TBSA burned.[52] These effects of growth hormone are thought to be due to stimulation of insulin-like growth factor (IGF)-1 release along with induction of IGF-1 receptors in the burn wound.[53] Insulin given alone also can decrease donor-site healing time from 6.5 to 4.7 days.[54] The decrease in donor-site healing by 1 day between each harvest can significantly affect the overall length of hospital stay in massively burned patients who require multiple grafting procedures. The administration of growth hormone in burned children has produced up to a 23% reduction in total cost of hospital care for a typical 80% TBSA burn.[52]

Recently, the use of cultured keratinocytes from the patient's own skin has generated considerable interest as a potential solution for massively burned patients with limited donor sites.[55-57] The concept of using cultured skin to provide complete coverage is appealing, but several problems must be overcome before its use will become widespread. Cultures of keratinocytes grow slowly, and once grafted, they are very susceptible to mechanical trauma, resulting in only 50% to 70% graft take. A recent report shows that patients with greater than 80% TBSA burns receiving conventional treatment had shorter hospital stays than did patients receiving cultured epithelial grafts.[58] Yet the use of cultured epithelial graft holds promise for the treatment of massively burned patients in the future.

HYPERMETABOLIC RESPONSE

Burn patients demonstrate a dramatic increase in metabolic rate. This hypermetabolic response, which generally increases with increasing burn size, reaching a plateau at a 40% TBSA burn,[59] is characterized by increased energy expenditure, oxygen consumption, proteolysis, lipolysis, and nitrogen losses. These physiologic changes are induced by upregulation of catabolic agents, such cortisol, catecholamine, and glucagons, which act synergistically to increase the production of glucose, a principal fuel during acute inflammation.[60] Cortisol stimulates

gluconeogenesis and proteolysis and sensitizes adipocytes to lipolytic hormones. Catecholamines stimulate the rate of glucose production through hepatic gluconeogenesis and glycogenolysis, as well as promotion of lipolysis and peripheral insulin resistance, in which serum insulin levels are elevated, but cells become resistant.[61] The increase in glucagon, which is stimulated by catecholamines, further promotes gluconeogenesis.

A significant protein catabolism occurs in severe burns. Cortisol is catabolic and is partially responsible for loss of tissue protein and negative nitrogen balance. In addition, burn injury is associated with decreased levels of anabolic hormones, such as growth hormone and IGF-1, and contributes significantly to net protein loss. The synthesis of protein, which is essential for the production of collagen for wound healing and antibodies and leukocytes for immune responses, requires a net positive nitrogen balance. Exogenous administration of recombinant human growth hormone, which increases protein synthesis, has been shown to improve nitrogen balance, preserve lean muscle mass, and increase the rate of wound healing.[53,62]

Excessive catecholamines in patients with burns also contribute to persistent tachycardia and lipolysis. The consequences of these physiologic insults are cardiac failure and fatty infiltration of the liver. The use of the beta-blocker, propranolol, has been shown to reduce the resting heart rate and left ventricular work and decrease peripheral lipolysis without adversely affecting cardiac output or the ability to respond to cold stress.[63-65]

NUTRITION

The metabolic rate of patients with burns increases from 1.5 times the normal rate in a patient with 25% TBSA burns to 2 times the normal rate in 40% TBSA burns.[66] Children are particularly vulnerable to protein-calorie malnutrition because of their proportionately less body fat and smaller muscle mass in addition to increased metabolic demands associated with growth. The malnutrition associated with burn injury results in dysfunction of various organ systems, including the immune system, and delays wound healing. Therefore optimal nutrition support must be provided to maintain and improve vital organ functions. Feeding tubes are generally placed under fluoroscopy immediately after the initial evaluation of the burn, and enteral nutrition is started within hours of injury. Early enteral feedings have been shown to decrease the level of catabolic hormones, improve nitrogen balance, maintain gut mucosal integrity, and decrease overall hospital stay.[67-69] Although parenteral hyperalimentation can deliver sufficient calories, its use in burn patients has been associated with deleterious effects on the immune system, small bowel mucosal atrophy with increased incidence of bacterial translocation, and decreased survival.[70,71] Enteral nutrition provided via a feeding tube placed in the stomach or duodenum is always preferable to parenteral nutrition and is associated with reduction of the metabolic rate and reduction of the incidence of sepsis in burn patients.

TABLE 13-5

NUTRITIONAL REQUIREMENTS FOR BURNED CHILDREN (SHRINERS BURNS HOSPITAL–GALVESTON)

Age Group	Daily Caloric Requirements
Infant and Toddler	2100 kcal/m^2 total + 1000 kcal/m^2 burn
Child	1800 kcal/m^2 total + 1300 kcal/m^2 burn
Adolescent	1500 kcal/m^2 total + 1500 kcal/m^2 burn

Several formulas are available to estimate caloric requirement in burn patients. Both Curreri (25 kcal/kg plus 40 kcal/% TBSA burned) and modified Harris-Benedict (calculated or measured resting metabolic rate × injury factor) formulas use the principle of providing maintenance caloric needs plus additional calories related to the burn size. Similar to fluid-resuscitation formulae, caloric requirement formulae that are based on total BSA and burned BSA are more appropriate for pediatric burn patients (Table 13-5).[72-74] The exact nutrient requirements of burn patients are not clear, but it is generally accepted that maintenance of energy requirement and replacement of protein losses are vital. The recommended enteral tube feedings should have 20% to 40% of the calories as protein, 10% to 20% as fat, and 40% to 70% as carbohydrates. Milk is one of the least expensive and best-tolerated nutritional preparations, but sodium supplementation may be needed to avoid dilutional hyponatremia. Numerous commercial enteral mixtures are available.

PAIN MANAGEMENT

Burn-wound treatment and rehabilitation therapy produce pain for patients of all age groups. Infants and children do not express their pain in the same way as do adults and may display pain through behaviors of fear, anxiety, agitation, tantrums, depression, and withdrawals. In older children, allowing the child to participate in wound care can provide the child some control and will help alleviate both fear and pain. Various combinations of analgesics with antianxiety medications are used effectively during procedures and wound-dressing changes. Successful pain management of burned children requires understanding by all the burn team members on how pain is related to burn depth and the phase of wound healing. Pain-management protocols should be tailored to control background pain as well as procedure-related painful stimuli (Table 13-6). Physical therapy treatment, which is vital to optimize good functional outcome, can more effectively be provided with appropriate pain control; however, caution must be exercised to prevent potential injury due to overmedication at the time of exercise therapy. Burn injuries are traumatic for the burned child as well as for the family. Burn-care professionals must do everything possible to make the experience as tolerable as possible in assisting burn patients to a successful recovery.

INHALATION INJURY

Inhalation injury is the major cause of death in burn patients. The mortality rate of children with isolated cutaneous burns is 1% to 2%, but it increases to approximately 40% in the presence of inhalation injury.[75,76] Inhalation injury is caused primarily by inhaled toxins such as fumes, gases, and mists. Although the supraglottic region can be injured by both thermal and chemical insults, tracheobronchial and lung parenchymal injuries rarely occur as a result of direct thermal damage because the heat is dispersed rapidly in the larynx. Hypoxia, increased airway resistance, decreased pulmonary compliance, increased alveolar epithelial permeability, and increased pulmonary vascular resistance may be triggered by the release of vasoactive substances (thromboxanes A$_2$, C$_{3a}$ and C$_{5a}$) from the damaged epithelium.[77] Neutrophil activation plays a critical role in this process, in which pulmonary function has been shown to improve with the use of a ligand binding to E-selectins (inhibiting neutrophil adhesion) and anti–interleukin-8 (inhibiting neutrophil chemotaxis). Another significant respiratory tract event is the sloughing of ciliated epithelial cells from the basement membrane, resulting in the formation of exudates. The exudates, which consist of lymph proteins,

TABLE 13-6

PAIN MEDICATION GUIDELINES

Background Pain	Acetaminophen, 15 mg/kg, PO q4h; if not adequate:
	a. (<3 yr) MSO$_4$ 0.1 mg/kg, PO q4h or 0.03 mg/kg, IV q4h
	b. (>3 yr) MSO$_4$ 0.3 mg/kg, PO q4h
Postoperative	1. MSO$_4$, 0.3 mg/kg, PO, and midazolam (Versed), 0.5 mg/kg, PO q3–4h
	2. MSO$_4$, 0.03 mg/kg, IV, and Versed, 0.03 mg/kg IV q2–4h
	3. PCA if patient older than 5 years: MSO$_4$, 0.05 mg/kg basal rate; 6- to 15-min lockout interval; 0.2–0.3 mg/kg, 4-hr limit
Dressing Changes and Procedures	1. MSO$_4$, 0.3 mg/kg, PO, and Versed, 0.3 mg/kg, PO
	2. MSO$_4$, 0.03 mg/kg, IV, and Versed, 0.03 mg/kg IV
	3. Ketamine, 0.5–2 mg/kg IV
Rehabilitation Therapy	1. MSO$_4$, 0.1–0.3 mg/kg, PO
	2. MSO$_4$, 0.03 mg/kg, IV

PCA, patient-controlled anesthesia.

coalesce to form fibrin casts. These fibrin casts are frequently resistant to removal by routine pulmonary toilet and can create a "ball-valve" effect to areas of the lung, eventually causing barotrauma.

The diagnosis is usually made on clinical history and physical findings at initial evaluation. Victims trapped in a house fire with excessive smoke and fumes are likely to have sustained severe inhalation injury. Facial burns with singed hair and carbonaceous sputum suggest inhalation injury. Hoarseness and stridor are signs of significant airway obstruction. The airway should immediately be secured with endotracheal intubation in this circumstance. Patients who are disorientated and obtunded are likely to have an elevated carbon monoxide level (carboxyhemoglobin > 10%). The fiberoptic bronchoscopy remains the best way to confirm the presence of inhalation injury.[78] It can demonstrate the presence of airway edema and inflammatory changes of the tracheal mucosa such as edema, hyperemia, mucosal ulceration, and sloughing. Ventilation scan with xenon 133 also can identify regions of inhalation injury by assessing respiratory exchange and excretion of xenon by the lungs.[79] The use of these complementary diagnostic tools, bronchoscopy and xenon-133 scanning, is more than 90% accurate in the diagnosis of inhalation injury. Bronchoscopic examination of the airway at the bedside, without having to transport critically ill burn patients to nuclear medicine, is frequently sufficient to establish the diagnosis of inhalation injury.

The treatment of inhalation injury begins at the scene of burn accident. The administration of 100% oxygen rapidly decreases the half-life of carbon monoxide. Immediate intubation should be done in patients with signs and symptoms of imminent respiratory failure.

Aggressive pulmonary toilet with physiotherapy and frequent suctioning is vital to prevent any serious respiratory complications. High-flow delivery of humidified air, bronchodilators, and racemic epinephrine are used to treat bronchospasm. Intravenous heparin has been shown to reduce tracheobronchial cast formation and peak inspiratory pressures after smoke inhalation. Inhalation treatments with nebulized 2% acetylcystine solution (3 mL every 4 hours) plus nebulized heparin (5000 to 10,000 units with 3 mL normal saline every 4 hours) are effective in improving the clearance of tracheobronchial secretions, minimizing bronchospasm and significantly reducing reintubation rates and mortality.[80,81]

The presence of inhalation injury generally requires an increased amount of fluid resuscitation, up to 2 mL/kg/% BSA burn more than would be required for an equal-size burn without an inhalation injury. The pulmonary edema that is associated with inhalation injury is not prevented by fluid restriction, but rather, inadequate resuscitation may increase the severity of pulmonary injury by sequestration of polymorphonuclear cells.[82] Steroids have not been shown to be of benefit in inhalation injury. Prophylactic intravenous antibiotics are not indicated, but are started with the clinical suspicion of pneumonitis. Early pneumonitis is usually the result of gram-positive organisms such as methicillin-resistant *Staphylococcus aureus*, whereas later infection is caused by gram-negative

organism, such as *Pseudomonas*. Antibiotic therapy should be guided by sputum cultures and bronchial washings.

NONTHERMAL INJURIES

Chemical Burns

Children accidentally come in contact with various household cleaning products. Treatment of chemical burns involves immediate removal of the causative agent and lavage with copious amounts of water, with caution regarding potential hypothermia and care that the effluent does not contact uninjured areas. After completion of irrigation, wounds should be covered with topical antimicrobial dressing, and appropriate surgical plans made. The rapid recognition of the offending chemical agent is crucial to the proper management.[83] When in doubt, the nearest poison control center should be contacted for identification of chemical composition of the product involved. The common offending chemical agents can be classified as alkali or acid. Alkali, such as lime, potassium hydroxide, sodium hydroxide, and bleach, are among the most common agents involved in chemical injury. Mechanisms of alkali-induced burns are saponification of fat, resulting in increased cell damage from heat, extraction of intracellular water, and formation of alkaline proteinates with hydroxyl ions. These ions induce further chemical reaction into the deeper tissues. Attempts to neutralize alkali are not recommended, as the chemical reaction can generate more heat and add to injury. Acid burns are not as common. Acids induce protein breakdown by hydrolysis, resulting in formation of eschar, and therefore, do not penetrate as deeply as do the alkali burns. Formic acid injuries are rare but can result in multiple systemic organ failures, such as metabolic acidosis, renal failure, intravascular hemolysis, and acute respiratory distress syndrome. Hydrofluoric acid burns are managed differently from other acid burns in general.[84] After copious local irrigation with water, fluoride ion must be neutralized with the topical application of 2.5% calcium gluconate gel. If not appropriately treated, the free fluoride ion causes liquefaction necrosis of the soft tissues, including bones with which it comes into contact. Because of potential hypocalcemia, patients should be closely monitored for prolonged QT intervals.

Electrical Burns

Three percent to 5% of all admitted burn patients are injured from electrical contact, but fortunately, electrical burns are rare in children. Electrical burns are categorized into high- and low-voltage injuries.[85] High-voltage injuries are characterized by varying degrees of local burns with destruction of deep tissues.[85, 86] Electrical current enters a part of the body and travels through tissues with lowest resistance, such as nerves, blood vessels, and muscles. The heat generated by the transfer of electrical current damages deep tissues that are not readily visible. The skin is mostly spared because of its high resistance to electrical current. Primary and secondary surveys, including electrocardiography, should be completed. If the initial electrocardiogram is normal, no further monitoring is necessary; however, any abnormal findings require continued monitoring for 48 hours and appropriate treatment of dysrhythmias when detected.[87] The key to management of electrical burns lies in the appreciation and proper treatment of injuries to deep structures. Edema formation and subsequent vascular compromise is common to extremities. Fasciotomies are frequently necessary to avoid potential limb loss. If myoglobin is present in urine, vigorous intravenous hydration with added sodium bicarbonate and mannitol are indicated. Low-voltage injury is similar to thermal injury without transmission of electrical current to deep tissues and usually requires only local wound care.

OUTPATIENT BURNS

A majority of all pediatric burns are minor, often resulting from scald of less than 10% TBSA or thermal injuries isolated to hands from touching hot objects. Such injuries are usually limited to a partial thickness of the skin and can be treated on an outpatient basis. After the initial assessment, the burn wound is gently washed with water and a mild bland soap with appropriate pain control. Blisters should be left intact, especially in the palm of the hand, because they provide a natural barrier against the environment and obviate the need for daily dressing changes. Spontaneous resorption of the blister fluid occurs in approximately 1 week with the re-epithelialization process. Larger areas or disrupted blisters should be debrided, and topical antimicrobial dressings applied. Silvadene is the most commonly used topical agent with the fewest side effects. However, because silver sulfadiazine can impede epithelialization, its use should be discontinued when evidence of re-epithelialization is noted. Alternatively, antimicrobial dressings with triple antibiotic ointment (neomycin, bacitracin and polymyxin B sulfate) and polysporin, which do not have any negative effects on epithelialization, are commonly used. For small superficial partial-thickness burns, nonmedical white petrolatum–impregnated fine-mesh or porous-mesh gauze (Adaptic), or fine-mesh absorbent gauze impregnated with 3% bismuth tribromophenate in nonmedicinal petrolatum blend (Xeroform) is usually sufficient without using topical antimicrobials.

The frequency of dressing change varies from twice daily to once a week, depending on the size, the depth of the burn, and the amount of drainage. Those who advocate twice-daily dressing changes base their care on the use of topical antimicrobials whose half-life is about 8 to 12 hours. Others who use petrolatum-based or bismuth-impregnated gauze recommend less frequent, once every 3 to 5 days, dressing changes. The use of synthetic wound dressings also is ideal for treatment of superficial partial-thickness burns as an outpatient.[88] Biobrane is a bilayer fabric composed of an inner layer of nylon coated with porcine collagen and an outer layer of rubberized silicone, pervious to air but not to fluids. When applied appropriately to fresh, partial-thickness wounds, Biobrane adheres to the wounds rapidly and is very effective in promoting re-epithelialization in 1 to 2 weeks (see Fig. 13-6). Although daily dressing changes are eliminated, Biobrane-covered wounds should still be monitored closely for signs of infection.

Superficial burns to the face can be treated with application of triple antibiotic ointment only, without any dressings.

REHABILITATION

Rehabilitation therapy is a vital component of burn care. During the acute phase of burn care, splints are used to prevent joint deformities and contractures. With thermoplastic materials, which are amendable to heat manipulation, splints are fitted individually to each patient. Continuous splinting except during an exercise period can help prevent the severe contractures that occur in patients with large burns. Early mobilization of the patient after the graft has taken and aggressive physical therapy should be provided.

After the acute phase, hypertrophic scar formation is a major concern. Burn depth, patient's age, and genetic factors all play an important role in hypertrophic scar formation. In general, deep second-degree burn wounds, requiring 3 weeks or more to heal, will produce hypertrophic scarring. Children are more prone to hypertrophic scar formation than are adults, probably because of the high rate of cell mitosis associated with growth. Using dressings that exert constant pressure on the healing wound is the most effective way of decreasing the incidence of hypertrophic scar formation. These pressure garments should be worn until scars are mature. Scar maturation usually occurs 6 to 18 months after injury, although in younger patients, scars mature at a much slower rate. In addition to splints and pressure garments, long-term exercise therapy is a crucial component of rehabilitation therapy. Families should be thoroughly instructed on a program of range-of-motion exercises and muscle strengthening.

REFERENCES

1. Lund CC, Browder NC: The estimation of areas of burns. Surg Gynecol Obstet 79:352–258, 1944.
2. Cope O, Moore FD: The redistribution of body water. Ann Surg 126:1016, 1947.
3. Moyer CA, Brentano L, Gravens DL, et al: Treatment of large human burns with 0.5 per cent silver nitrate solution. Arch Surg 90:812–867, 1965.
4. Lindberg RB, Moncrief JA, Switzer WE, et al: The successful control of burn wound sepsis. J Trauma 5:601–616, 1965.
5. Fox CL Jr, Rappole BW, Stanford W: Control of Pseudomonas infection in burns by silver sulfadiazine. Surg Gynecol Obstet 128:1021–1026, 1969.
6. Brigham PA, McLoughlin E: Burn incidence and medical care use in the United States: Estimates, trends, and data sources. J Burn Care Rehabil 17:95–107, 1996.
7. Herndon DN, Gore D, Cole M, et al: Determinants of mortality in pediatric patients with greater than 70% full-thickness total body surface area thermal injury treated by early total excision and grafting. J Trauma 27:208–212, 1987.

8. Barillo DJ, Goode R: Fire fatality study: Demographics of fire victims. Burns 22:85–88, 1996.
9. National Safe Kids Program: Burn Injury Fact Sheet. Washington, DC.
10. Baptiste MS, Feck G: Preventing tap water burns. Am J Public Health 70:727–729, 1980.
11. Vo LT, Papworth GD, Delaney PM, et al: A study of vascular response to thermal injury on hairless mice by fibre optic confocal imaging, laser Doppler flowmetry and conventional histology. Burns 24:319–324, 1998.
12. DelBeccaro EJ, Robson MC, Heggers JP, et al: The use of specific thromboxane inhibitors to preserve the dermal microcirculation after burning. Surgery 87:137–141, 1980.
13. Demling RH, LaLonde C: Early postburn lipid peroxidation: Effect of ibuprofen and allopurinol. Surgery 107:85–93, 1990.
14. Nwariaku FE, Sikes PJ, Lightfoot E, et al: Effect of a bradykinin antagonist on the local inflammatory response following thermal injury. Burns 22:324–327, 1996.
15. Bucky LP, Vedder NB, Hong HZ, et al: Reduction of burn injury by inhibiting CD18-mediated leukocyte adherence in rabbits. Plast Reconstr Surg 93:1473–1480, 1994.
16. Mileski W, Borgstrom D, Lightfoot E, et al: Inhibition of leukocyte-endothelial adherence following thermal injury. J Surg Res 52:334–339, 1992.
17. Warden GD: Fluid resuscitation and early management. In: Herndon DN (ed): Total Burn Care. Philadelphia, WB Saunders, 1996, pp 53–60.
18. Myers SI, Minei JP, Casteneda A, et al: Differential effects of acute thermal injury on rat splanchnic and renal blood flow and prostanoid release. Prostaglandins Leukot Essent Fatty Acids 53:439–444, 1995.
19. Jeschke MG, Barrow RE, Wolf SE, et al: Mortality in burned children with acute renal failure. Arch Surg 133:752–756, 1998.
20. Chung DH, Evers BM, Townsend CM Jr, et al: Role of polyamine biosynthesis during gut mucosal adaptation after burn injury. Am J Surg 165:144–149, 1993.
21. Chung DH, Evers BM, Townsend CM Jr, et al: Burn-induced transcriptional regulation of small intestinal ornithine decarboxylase. Am J Surg 163:157–163, 1992.
22. Wolf SE, Ikeda H, Matin S, et al: Cutaneous burn increases apoptosis in the gut epithelium of mice. J Am Coll Surg 188:10–16, 1999.
23. Carter EA, Gonnella A, Tompkins RG: Increased transcellular permeability of rat small intestine after thermal injury. Burns 18:117–120, 1992.
24. LeVoyer T, Cioffi WG Jr, Pratt L, et al: Alterations in intestinal permeability after thermal injury. Arch Surg 127:26–30, 1992.
25. Ryan CM, Yarmush ML, Burke JF, et al: Increased gut permeability early after burns correlates with the extent of burn injury. Crit Care Med 20:1508–1512, 1992.
26. Bjerknes R, Vindenes H, Laerum OD: Altered neutrophil functions in patients with large burns. Blood Cells 16:127–143, 1990.
27. Klimpel GR, Herndon DN, Stein MD: Peripheral blood lymphocytes from thermal injury patients are defective in their ability to generate lymphokine-activated killer (LAK) cell activity. J Clin Immunol 8:14–22, 1988.
28. Bjerknes R, Vindenes H, Pitkanen J, et al: Altered polymorphonuclear neutrophilic granulocyte functions in patients with large burns. J Trauma 29:847–855, 1989.
29. Gamelli RL, He LK, Liu H: Macrophage suppression of granulocyte and macrophage growth following burn wound infection. J Trauma 37:888–892, 1994.
30. Hunt JP, Hunter CT, Brownstein MR, et al: The effector component of the cytotoxic T-lymphocyte response has a biphasic pattern after burn injury. J Surg Res 80:243–251, 1998.
31. Zedler S, Faist E, Ostermeier B, et al: Postburn constitutional changes in T-cell reactivity occur in CD8+ rather than in CD4+ cells. J Trauma 42:872–881, 1997.
32. Park DH, Hwang JW, Jang KS, et al: Use of laser Doppler flowmetry for estimation of the depth of burns. Plast Reconstr Surg 101:1516–1523, 1998.
33. Jerath MR, Schomacker KT, Sheridan RL, et al: Burn wound assessment in porcine skin using indocyanine green fluorescence. J Trauma 46:1085–1088, 1999.
34. Brink JA, Sheets PW, Dines KA, et al: Quantitative assessment of burn injury in porcine skin with high-frequency ultrasonic imaging. Invest Radiol 21:645–651, 1986.
35. O'Reilly TJ, Spence RJ, Taylor RM, et al: Laser Doppler flowmetry evaluation of burn wound depth. J Burn Care Rehabil 10:1–6, 1989.
36. Ho-Asjoe M, Chronnell CM, Frame JD, et al: Immunohistochemical analysis of burn depth. J Burn Care Rehabil 20:207–211, 1999.
37. Graves TA, Cioffi WG, McManus WF, et al: Fluid resuscitation of infants and children with massive thermal injury. J Trauma 28:1656–1659, 1988.
38. Demling RH, Mazess RB, Witt RM, et al: The study of burn wound edema using dichromatic absorptiometry. J Trauma 18:124–128, 1978.
39. Ayus JC, Arieff AI: Hyponatremia and myelinolysis. Ann Intern Med 127:163, 1997.
40. Monafo WW: The treatment of burn shock by the intravenous and oral administration of hypertonic lactated saline solution. J Trauma 10:575–586, 1970.
41. Warden GD: Burn shock resuscitation. World J Surg 16:16–23, 1992.
42. Huang PP, Stucky FS, Dimick AR, et al: Hypertonic sodium resuscitation is associated with renal failure and death. Ann Surg 221:543–557, 1995.
43. Du GB, Slater H, Goldfarb IW: Influences of different resuscitation regimens on acute early weight gain in extensively burned patients. Burns 17:147–150, 1991.
44. Desai MH, Herndon DN: Eradication of *Candida* burn wound septicemia in massively burned patients. J Trauma 28:140–145, 1988.
45. Desai MH, Rutan RL, Heggers JP, et al: *Candida* infection with and without nystatin prophylaxis: An 11-year experience with patients with burn injury. Arch Surg 127:159–162, 1992.
46. Jarrett F, Ellerbe S, Demling R: Acute leukopenia during topical burn therapy with silver sulfadiazine. Am J Surg 135:818–819, 1978.
47. Heggers JP, Sazy JA, Stenberg BD, et al: Bactericidal and wound-healing properties of sodium hypochlorite solutions: The 1991 Lindberg Award. J Burn Care Rehabil 12:420–424, 1991.
48. Lal S, Barrow RE, Wolf SE, et al: Biobrane improves wound healing in burned children without increased risk of infection. Shock 14:314–319, 2000.
49. Herndon DN, Parks DH: Comparison of serial debridement and autografting and early massive excision with cadaver skin overlay in the treatment of large burns in children. J Trauma 26:149–152, 1986.
50. Marano MA, O'Sullivan G, Madden M, et al: Tourniquet technique for reduced blood loss and wound assessment during excisions of burn wounds of the extremity. Surg Gynecol Obstet 171:249–250, 1990.
51. Desai MH, Herndon DN, Broemeling L, et al: Early burn wound excision significantly reduces blood loss. Ann Surg 211:753–762, 1990.
52. Herndon DN, Barrow RE, Kunkel KR, et al: Effects of recombinant human growth hormone on donor-site healing in severely burned children. Ann Surg 212:424–431, 1990.
53. Herndon DN, Hawkins HK, Nguyen TT, et al: Characterization of growth hormone enhanced donor site healing in patients with large cutaneous wounds. Ann Surg 221:649–659, 1995.
54. Pierre EJ, Barrow RE, Hawkins HK, et al: Effects of insulin on wound healing. J Trauma 44:342–345, 1998.
55. Sheridan RL, Tompkins RG: Cultured autologous epithelium in patients with burns of ninety percent or more of the body surface. J Trauma 38:48–50, 1995.
56. Gallico GG 3rd, O'Connor NE, Compton CC, et al: Permanent coverage of large burn wounds with autologous cultured human epithelium. N Engl J Med 311:448–451, 1984.
57. Rue LW III, Cioffi WG, McManus WF, et al: Wound closure and outcome in extensively burned patients treated with cultured autologous keratinocytes. J Trauma 34:662–668, 1993.
58. Barret JP, Wolf SE, Desai MH, et al: Cost-efficacy of cultured epidermal autografts in massive pediatric burns. Ann Surg 231:869–876, 2000.
59. Herndon DN, Hart DW, Wolf SE, et al: Reversal of catabolism by beta-blockade after severe burns. N Engl J Med 345:1223–1229, 2001.

60. Shamoon H, Hendler R, Sherwin RS: Synergistic interactions among antiinsulin hormones in the pathogenesis of stress hyperglycemia in humans. J Clin Endocrinol Metab 52:1235–1241, 1981.

61. Jahoor F, Herndon DN, Wolfe RR: Role of insulin and glucagon in the response of glucose and alanine kinetics in burn-injured patients. J Clin Invest 78:807–814, 1986.

62. Wilmore DW, Moylan JA Jr, Bristow BF, et al: Anabolic effects of human growth hormone and high caloric feedings following thermal injury. Surg Gynecol Obstet 138:875–884, 1974.

63. Chance WT, Nelson JL, Foley-Nelson T, et al: The relationship of burn-induced hypermetabolism to central and peripheral catecholamines. J Trauma 29:306–312, 1989.

64. Drost AC, Burleson DG, Cioffi WG, et al: Plasma cytokines following thermal injury and their relationship with patient mortality, burn size, and time postburn. J Trauma 35:335–339, 1993.

65. Honeycutt D, Barrow R, Herndon DN: Cold stress response in patients with severe burns after beta-blockade. J Burn Care Rehabil 13:181–186, 1992.

66. Goran MI, Peters EJ, Herndon DN, et al: Total energy expenditure in burned children using the doubly labeled water technique. Am J Physiol 259:E576–585, 1990.

67. Chiarelli A, Enzi G, Casadei A, et al: Very early nutrition supplementation in burned patients. Am J Clin Nutr 51:1035–1039, 1990.

68. Saito H, Trocki O, Alexander JW, et al: The effect of route of nutrient administration on the nutritional state, catabolic hormone secretion, and gut mucosal integrity after burn injury. JPEN J Parenter Enteral Nutr 11:1–7, 1987.

69. Mochizuki H, Trocki O, Dominioni L, et al: Mechanism of prevention of postburn hypermetabolism and catabolism by early enteral feeding. Ann Surg 200:297–310, 1984.

70. Herndon DN, Stein MD, Rutan TC, et al: Failure of TPN supplementation to improve liver function, immunity, and mortality in thermally injured patients. J Trauma 27:195–204, 1987.

71. Herndon DN, Barrow RE, Stein M, et al: Increased mortality with intravenous supplemental feeding in severely burned patients. J Burn Care Rehabil 10:309–313, 1989.

72. Hildreth MA, Herndon DN, Desai MH, et al: Caloric requirements of patients with burns under one year of age. J Burn Care Rehabil 14:108–112, 1993.

73. Hildreth MA, Herndon DN, Desai MH, et al: Current treatment reduces calories required to maintain weight in pediatric patients with burns. J Burn Care Rehabil 11:405–409, 1990.

74. Hildreth MA, Herndon DN, Desai MH, et al: Caloric needs of adolescent patients with burns. J Burn Care Rehabil 10:523–526, 1989.

75. Herndon DN, Thompson PB, Traber DL: Pulmonary injury in burned patients. Crit Care Clin 1:79–96, 1985.

76. Thompson PB, Herndon DN, Traber DL, et al: Effect on mortality of inhalation injury. J Trauma 26:163–165, 1986.

77. Traber DL, Herndon DN, Stein MD, et al: The pulmonary lesion of smoke inhalation in an ovine model. Circ Shock 18:311–323, 1986.

78. Hunt JL, Agee RN, Pruitt BA Jr: Fiberoptic bronchoscopy in acute inhalation injury. J Trauma 15:641–649, 1975.

79. Moylan JA Jr, Wilmore DW, Mouton DE, et al: Early diagnosis of inhalation injury using 133 xenon lung scan. Ann Surg 176:477–484, 1972.

80. Kimura R, Traber LD, Herndon DN, et al: Treatment of smoke-induced pulmonary injury with nebulized dimethylsulfoxide. Circ Shock 25:333–341, 1988.

81. Brown M, Desai M, Traber LD, et al: Dimethylsulfoxide with heparin in the treatment of smoke inhalation injury. J Burn Care Rehabil 9:22–25, 1988.

82. Herndon DN, Barrow RE, Linares HA, et al: Inhalation injury in burned patients: Effects and treatment. Burns Incl Therm Inj 14:349–356, 1988.

83. Fitzpatrick KT, Moylan JA: Emergency care of chemical burns. Postgrad Med 78:189–194, 1985.

84. Trevino MA, Herrmann GH, Sprout WL: Treatment of severe hydrofluoric acid exposures. J Occup Med 25:861–863, 1983.

85. Laberge LC, Ballard PA, Daniel RK: Experimental electrical burns: Low voltage. Ann Plast Surg 13:185–190, 1984.

86. Robson MC, Murphy RC, Heggers JP: A new explanation for the progressive tissue loss in electrical injuries. Plast Reconstr Surg 73:431–437, 1984.

87. Robson MC, Smith DJ: Care of the thermal injured victim. In: Jurkiewicz MJ, Krizek TJ, Mathes, SJ Ariyan S (eds). Plastic Surgery: Principles and Practice. St. Louis, CV Mosby, 1990, pp 1355–1410.

88. Gerding RL, Emerman CL, Effron D, et al: Outpatient management of partial-thickness burns: Biobrane versus 1% silver sulfadiazine. Ann Emerg Med 19:121–124, 1990.

Early Assessment and Management of Trauma

Arthur Cooper, MD, MS

Trauma is the leading cause of mortality and morbidity in children from ages 1 to 14 years and results in more death and disability than all other childhood diseases combined.[1] It is defined as forceful disruption of bodily homeostasis. Moreover, this term encompasses those injuries whose severity poses a demonstrable threat to life, which corresponds to an Injury Severity Score (ISS) of 10 or higher in children, or a Pediatric Trauma Score (PTS) of 8 or lower.[2] The term *first trauma* refers to the anatomic and physiologic disruption that results from acute injury, whereas the term *second trauma,* recently defined and described by the American Trauma Society, refers to the social and familial dislocation associated with first trauma, which in pediatric patients is often considerable. Pediatric trauma remains a major public health problem of childhood in the United States, killing more than 10,000 pediatric patients annually nationwide[1] and causing some 10% of all pediatric hospitalizations,[3] about 15% of all pediatric intensive care unit admissions,[4] approximately 25% of pediatric emergency department visits,[5] and 50% or more of all pediatric ambulance runs.[6] Moreover, it also represents nearly 20% of all hospitalizations for serious injury among all age groups.[7]

TRAUMA EPIDEMIOLOGY

The incidence of serious traumatic injury, with hospitalization as the indicator of injury severity, is approximately 420/100,000.[8] Although the hospital-based fatality rate is 2.4/100,000, the population-based mortality rate is 11.8/100,000, indicating that 78% of fatally injured children die before hospital admission, demonstrating the need for effective injury prevention and prehospital care. The mortality rate for pediatric injuries serious enough to require hospitalization approximates 0.5%, but, for injuries severe enough to warrant pediatric trauma center care, it approximates 2.5%.[9] Intracranial injuries are the cause of most pediatric trauma deaths because of the untoward effects of traumatic coma on airway patency, breathing control, and cerebral perfusion. Intrathoracic and intra-abdominal injuries are the cause of few pediatric trauma deaths, because they are seldom associated with hypotensive shock, which occurs in only 6% to 8% of pediatric patients with demonstrable mortality risk.

Most blunt trauma in childhood is sustained unintentionally (during the course of family, play, or sports activities), but 7% of serious injuries are due to intentional physical assault (of which nearly half, or 3%, are due to physical abuse).[9] Blunt injuries outnumber penetrating injuries in children by a ratio of 12:1, a ratio that has decreased significantly in recent years. Whereas blunt injuries are more common, penetrating injuries are more lethal. The leading killer of children is the motor vehicle, responsible for approximately 75% of all childhood deaths, which are evenly split between those resulting from pedestrian trauma and those resulting from occupant injuries (Table 14-1).

INJURY PREVENTION

Injuries are not accidents, but rather are predictable events that respond to harm-reduction strategies similar to those applied to other diseases. The Haddon Factor Phase Matrix neatly depicts these in graphic form (Fig. 14-1).[10] It demonstrates how strategies to lessen the burden of injury can be applied to the host, agent, and environment before, during, and after the traumatic event—the latter corresponding to the primary, secondary, and tertiary phases of injury control aimed, respectively, at **A**voidance, **A**lteration, and **A**melioration of injury occurrence, severity, and consequences. Recently modified through addition of a third dimension to articulate key values that might be considered when choosing intervention strategies (effectiveness, equity, freedom, cost, stigmatization),[11] it has lately been further refined to demonstrate the four fundamental tactics used by public health professionals for illness and injury control (**E**ngineering, automation, and technologic innovation; **E**nactment and **E**nforcement of legislation and regulations; **E**ducation of the public in safe behaviors; and **E**conomic incentives and disincentives for healthy and

TABLE 14-1		
INCIDENCE AND MORTALITY OF PEDIATRIC TRAUMA		
By Injury Mechanism	Incidence (%)	Mortality (%)
Blunt	92.0	3
Fall	27.2	0.4
Motor vehicle injury: occupant	21.2	4.2
Motor vehicle injury: pedestrian	11.9	4.8
Bicycle	8.6	1.9
Sport	7.5	0.7
Struck	4.2	2.9*
Beating	3.2	9.0
Animal bite	2.8	2.9*
All terrain/recreational vehicle	2.0	2.5+
Motorcycle	1.2	2.5+
Machine	1.0	2.9*
Caught	0.7	2.9*
Penetrating	7.7	5
Gunshot wound	2.3	10.2
Stabbing	2.8	2.9*
Crush	0.1	2.9*
Other	3.2	2.9*
By Body Region	Incidence (%)	Mortality (%)
Multiple	46.3	5
Extremities	21.9	0
Head and neck	14.5	5
External	10.2	0
Abdomen	3.6	1
Face	1.8	0
Thorax	0.7	3
By Anatomic Diagnosis	Incidence (%)	Mortality (%)
Head injury	25.8	10
Fracture	25.9	4
Abrasion/contusion	19.6	3
Open wound	14.2	3
Thoracic/abdominal injury	9.1	14
Spine injury	2.0	9
Other	3.6	9

*Collective mortality of these seven categories.
+Collective mortality of these two categories.
From Discala C: National Pediatric Trauma Registry Annual Report. Boston, Tufts University Rehabilitation and Childhood Trauma Research and Training Center, 2002, with permission.

unhealthy activities) and serves as the model for effective injury-control planning at the national, regional, and local levels.[12]

Effective injury-prevention programs are community based and require extensive collaboration with civic leaders, governmental agencies, and neighborhood coalitions. Programs such as the National Safe Kids Campaign (*www.safekids.org*) and the Injury Free Coalition for Kids (*www.injuryfree.org*) have proven highly successful in reducing the burden of childhood injury in many communities.[13,14] Such programs require ongoing collaboration between trauma programs and local public health entities

so the incidence of injury can be tracked by locality, and specific plans made to target high-frequency risks. Thus they require major personal and institutional commitment on the part of trauma professionals and trauma centers, including the commitment of necessary resources.

INJURY MECHANISMS

The effects of injury on the pediatric patient are related to the laws of physics and biomechanics. The kinetic energy transferred is equal to one half of the mass of the impacting object times its velocity squared, but because the child's body is smaller, it is compacted into a smaller space. In blunt trauma, the forces of impact are dependent on factors such as the size and speed of the vehicle or the vertical displacement after a fall. These impact forces can be mitigated through use of design elements such as roll bars and crumple zones in automobiles, active and passive restraint devices such as lap belts, shoulder harnesses, air bags, and age-specific and properly fitted infant car seats or child booster seats for young passengers, helmets for bicycle riders, safety surfaces beneath playground equipment, and window guards in medium- and high-rise buildings. In penetrating trauma, the forces of violation are dependent on the weapon used (specifically, the size of the missile it discharges and the muzzle velocity with which it is delivered).

Injury mechanism is the main predictor of injury pattern. Pedestrian–motor vehicle trauma results in the Waddell triad of injuries to the head, torso, and pelvis, femur, or tibia (Fig. 14-2), whereas occupant injuries may cause head, face, and neck injuries in unrestrained passengers and cervical spine injuries, bowel disruption or hematoma, and Chance fractures in restrained passengers (Fig. 14-3). Bicycle trauma results in head injury in unhelmeted riders as well as upper extremity and upper abdominal injuries, the latter the result of contact with the handlebar (Fig. 14-4). Low falls, the most common cause of childhood injury, rarely produce significant trauma, but high falls from the second story or higher are associated with serious head injuries, with the addition of long-bone fractures at the third story, and intrathoracic and intra-abdominal injuries at the fifth story (the height from which 50% of children can be expected to die after a high fall)[15] (Table 14-2).

INJURY PATTERNS

The injured child is subject to different mechanisms of injury than the adult, which, when coupled with the immature anatomic features and physiologic responses of the child, produces distinct patterns of injury that are unique to childhood. The body regions most frequently injured in major childhood trauma are the lower extremities, head and neck, and abdomen, whereas in minor childhood injury, soft tissue and upper extremity injuries predominate. Because most pediatric trauma is blunt trauma involving the head, it is primarily a disease of airway and breathing rather than of circulation, bleeding, and shock. Even so, although neuroventilatory derangements

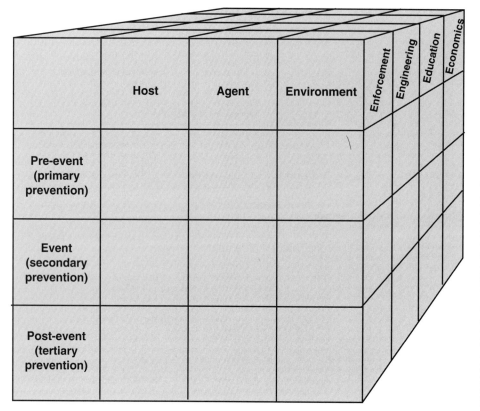

FIGURE 14-1. The Haddon Factor Phase Matrix, as modified and refined to include a third strategic dimension, integrates all phases of injury control into a single system. (From DiScala C: National Pediatric Trauma Registry Annual Report. Boston, Tufts University Rehabilitation and Childhood Trauma Research and Training Center, 2002; Haddon W: Advances in the epidemiology of injuries as a basis for public policy. Public Health Rep 95:411–421, 1980; Runyan CW: Using the Haddon Matrix: Introducing the third dimension. Inj Prev 4:302–307, 1998; and Cooper G, Dawson D, Kaufmann C, et al: Trauma Systems Planning and Evaluation: A Model Approach to a Major Public Health Problem. Rockville, Md, Health Resources and Services Administration, in press.)

(abnormalities in Glasgow Coma Scale score and respiratory rate) are 5 times more common than hemodynamic derangements, the latter are twice as lethal as the former.[16]

Injuries to specific body regions give rise to specific anatomic diagnoses (see Table 14-1). Because multiple injuries usually involve the head and neck, brain injury constitutes a major cause of injury mortality in childhood. Precise estimates of injury mortality by anatomic diagnosis cannot presently be calculated, owing to lack of population-based databases and inability to determine with accuracy the relative contribution of individual diagnoses to injury mortality in multisystem trauma. Despite these constraints, brain injuries are directly (primary tissue injury) or indirectly (secondary hypoxic injury due to respiratory failure and shock) responsible for 75% of childhood trauma deaths.[17,18]

Head

Head injuries are potentially more dangerous in children than in adults for several reasons. Developing neural tissue is delicate, and the softer bones of the skull allow impacting forces to be transmitted directly to the underlying brain, especially at points of bony contact. Intracranial bleeding in infants in whom the fontanelles and sutures remain open may, on rare occasions, be severe enough to cause hypotensive shock. Most important, the proportionately larger size of the head, when coupled with the injury mechanisms commonly observed in children, virtually guarantees that most serious blunt trauma in childhood will involve the brain and produce loss of consciousness.

As a consequence, the voluntary muscles of the neck lose their tone, promoting development of soft tissue obstruction in the upper airway (which leads to hypoxia). It follows that diffuse brain injuries, particularly cerebral swelling (which results chiefly from cerebral hypoxia, loss of cerebral pressure autoregulation, and subsequent cerebral hyperemia, instead of vasogenic edema), are more common in childhood than in later years. Focal areas of cerebral contusion or laceration may occur adjacent to bony prominences in a coup-contrecoup pattern (typically in the frontal and temporal lobes), but major intracranial hemorrhage is uncommon and usually does not warrant surgical evacuation. Bilateral subdural hematomas in infants are indicative of child abuse (particularly when associated with retinal hemorrhages) and result from tearing of the bridging meningeal veins associated with the whiplash shaken impact syndrome.

Neck

Cervical spine injury is an uncommon event in pediatric trauma, occurring at a rate of 1.8/100,000 population, in contrast to closed head injury, which occurs at a rate of 185/100,000 population.[19] When such injury does occur, it is more frequent at levels (C2, C1, and the occipitoatlantal junction) above those whose nerve roots give rise to diaphragmatic innervation (C4), predisposing the child to respiratory arrest as well as muscular paralysis. The increased angular momentum produced by movement of the proportionately larger head, the greater elasticity of the interspinous ligaments, and the more horizontal

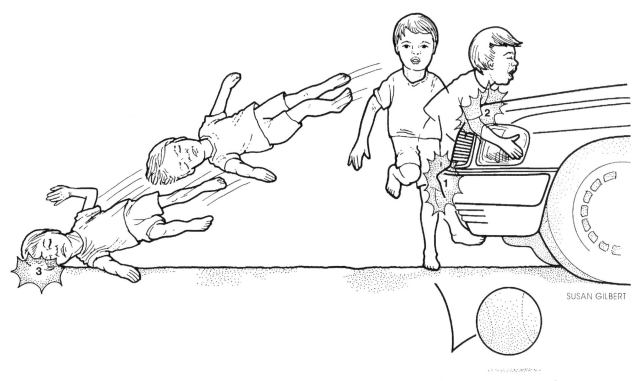

SUSAN GILBERT

FIGURE 14-2. The Waddell Triad of injuries to head, torso, and lower extremity is shown in this diagram. (From Foltin G, Tunik M, Cooper A, et al. [eds]: Teaching Resource for Instructors of Prehospital Pediatrics. New York, Center for Pediatric Emergency Medicine, 1998.)

apposition of the cervical vertebrae are responsible for this spectrum of injuries, in which "locking" of facet joints in lower cervical vertebrae is quite rare, whereas subluxation (with or without dislocation) and odontoid fractures are more common. Subluxation without dislocation causes spinal cord injury without radiographic abnormality (SCIWORA), from lateral shearing or axial stretching, and accounts for up to 20% of pediatric spinal cord injuries as well as a number of prehospital deaths previously attributed to head trauma.[21,22] The greater elasticity of the interspinous ligaments also gives rise to a normal anatomic variant known as pseudosubluxation, which affects up to 40% of children younger than 7 years. The most common finding is a short (2 to 3 mm) anterior displacement of C2 on C3, although anterior displacement of C3 on C4 also may be seen. The condition is accentuated when the pediatric patient is placed in a supine position, which forces the cervical spine of the young child into mild flexion because of the forward displacement of the head by the more prominent occiput. The greater elasticity of the interspinous ligaments also is responsible for the increased distance between the dens and the anterior arch of C1 that is found in up to 20% of children.

Chest

Serious intrathoracic injuries occur in 6% of pediatric blunt trauma victims[23] and rarely require thoracotomy, although thoracostomy is needed in about 50%.

Lung injuries (52%), pneumothorax and hemothorax (42%), and rib and sternal fractures (32%) occur most frequently (Table 14-3). Injuries to the heart (6%), diaphragm (4%), great vessels (2%), bronchi (<1%), and esophagus (<1%) occur the least frequently. Because blunt trauma is nearly 10 times more deadly when associated with major intrathoracic injury, this condition serves as a marker of injury severity, even though it is the proximate cause of death in fewer than 1% of all pediatric blunt trauma.[24]

The child compensates poorly for respiratory derangements associated with serious thoracic injury because of (1) larger oxygen consumption but smaller functional reserve capacity (which makes the child more susceptible to hypoxia), (2) lesser pulmonary compliance yet greater chest wall compliance (which dictate chiefly a tachypneic response to hypoxia), and (3) horizontally aligned ribs and rudimentary intercostal musculature (which make the small child a diaphragmatic breather). The thorax of the child usually escapes major harm because the pliable nature of the cartilaginous ribs allows the kinetic energy associated with forceful impacts to be absorbed without significant injury, either to the chest wall itself or to underlying structures. Pulmonary contusions are the typical result but seldom are life-threatening. Pneumothorax and hemothorax, due to lacerations of the lung parenchyma and intercostals vessels, occur less commonly but place the child in grave danger of sudden, marked ventilatory and circulatory compromise as the mediastinum shifts.

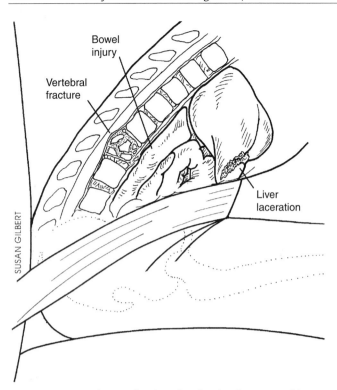

SUSAN GILBERT

FIGURE 14-3. The mechanism for the development of intestinal and vertebral injuries from lap belts is depicted. (From Foltin G, Tunik M, Cooper A, et al. [eds]: Teaching Resource for Instructors of Prehospital Pediatrics. New York, Center for Pediatric Emergency Medicine, 1998.)

Abdomen

Serious intra-abdominal injuries occur in 8% of pediatric blunt trauma victims[23] and are caused by crushing of solid upper abdominal viscera against the vertebral column, sudden compression and bursting of hollow upper abdominal viscera against the vertebral column, or shearing of the posterior attachments or vascular supply of the upper abdominal viscera after rapid deceleration (see Table 14-3).[25] Injuries to the liver (27%), spleen (27%), kidneys (25%), and gastrointestinal tract (21%) occur most frequently and account for most of the deaths that result from intra-abdominal injury, because of irreversible hemorrhagic shock. Injuries to the great vessels (5%), genitourinary tract (5%), pancreas (4%), and pelvis (<1%) occur less frequently and account for few of the deaths that result from intra-abdominal injury. Most solid visceral injuries are successfully treated nonoperatively, especially those involving kidneys (98%), spleen (95%), and liver (90%).[26-28]

The abdomen of the child is vulnerable to injury for several reasons. Flexible ribs cover only the uppermost portion of the abdomen; thin layers of muscle, fat, and fascia provide little protection to the large solid viscera; and the pelvis is shallow, lifting the bladder into the abdomen. Moreover, the overall small size of the abdomen predisposes the child to multiple rather than single injuries, as

energy is dissipated from the impacting force. Finally, gastric dilatation due to air swallowing (which often confounds abdominal examination by simulating peritonitis) leads to ventilatory and circulatory compromise by (1) limiting diaphragmatic motion, (2) increasing risk of aspiration, and (3) causing vagally mediated dampening of the normal tachycardic response to hypovolemia.

Skeleton

Although they are the leading cause of disability, fractures are rarely an immediate cause of death in blunt trauma, but they occur in 26% of serious blunt-injury cases and constitute the principal anatomic diagnosis in 22%.[9] Upper extremity fractures outnumber lower extremity fractures by 7:1, although, in serious blunt trauma, this ratio is 2:3. The most common long-bone fractures sustained during childhood pedestrian–motor vehicle crashes are fractures of the femur and tibia, whereas falls typically are associated with both upper and lower extremity fractures if the fall height is significant (from the top of a bunk bed,[29] or the window of a high-rise dwelling,[15] not from falls from beds[30] or down stairs[31]). Because isolated long-bone and pelvic fractures are rarely associated with significant hemorrhage,[32] a diligent search must be made for another source of bleeding if signs of hypotensive shock are observed. This source is usually found in the abdomen.

The pediatric skeleton is susceptible to fractures because cortical bone in childhood is highly porous, whereas the periosteum is more resilient, elastic, and vascular. This results in higher percentages both of incomplete (torus and greenstick) fractures and complete but nondisplaced fractures. Other factors make skeletal trauma in children unique: (1) a rapid rate of healing and freedom from nonunion; (2) a tendency to remodel in the plane of the fracture (although not in the rotational plane); (3) a high incidence of ischemic vascular injuries, particularly about the elbow (which may threaten the limb and cause disfiguring contracture); and (4) a low incidence of associated ligamentous injuries. Long-term growth disturbances also may complicate childhood fractures: diaphyseal fractures of the long bones cause significant overgrowth (2 to 3 centimeters in those aged 2 to 10 years), whereas physeal (growth plate) fractures, particularly if severe (Salter-Harris types 3 and 4), cause significant undergrowth.

PREHOSPITAL CARE

Basic life support of the pediatric trauma patient consists of oxygen administration, airway adjuncts, bleeding control, and spine stabilization, providing assisted ventilation and fracture immobilization as needed. Spinal immobilization requires both neutral positioning (which cannot be achieved without placing a thin layer of padding beneath the torso from shoulders to hips)[33] and careful strapping (because forced vital capacity may be decreased by 4% to 59%).[34] One recent study suggested that cervical spine immobilization can be safely avoided in most pediatric trauma patients with minor injuries,

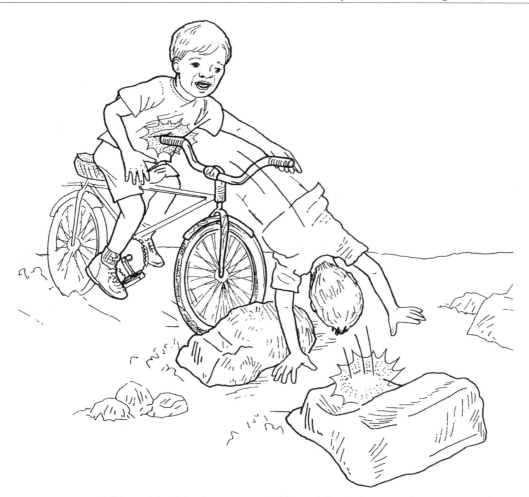

FIGURE 14-4. Children riding bicycles can sustain blunt abdominal trauma after contact with handlebars or head trauma from falling off the bicycle. (From Foltin G, Tunik M, Cooper A, et al. [eds]: Teaching Resource for Instructors of Prehospital Pediatrics. New York, Center for Pediatric Emergency Medicine, 1998.)

but caution was urged in view of the known risks of SCIWORA and atlantoaxial instability.[35] Advanced life support of the pediatric trauma patient theoretically adds endotracheal intubation and volume resuscitation to this armamentarium, but neither intervention appears to improve outcome.[36-38]

Field triage of pediatric trauma patients to pediatric trauma centers is now well established, and regional protocols should direct ambulance transports to such centers where available. Although both the PTS[39] and the Revised Trauma Score (RTS)[40] reliably predict the need for pediatric trauma care, neither is optimally sensitive or specific (Table 14-4). Good results also have been achieved by using checklists to identify anatomic, physiologic, and mechanistic criteria rather than calculated scores (Table 14-5).[41,42] Ambulance transport is inherently unsafe, because of both the nature of the vehicle and driving at high speeds, but risks can be minimized by properly strapping the infant car seat to the ambulance gurney and following established defensive-driving techniques.[43,44]

EMERGENCY CARE

Primary Survey

Early management of childhood trauma begins in the field and continues in the emergency department.[45] Attention is first directed to a "primary survey" of the **A**irway, **B**reathing, **C**irculation, and neurologic **D**isabilities, the purpose of which is to identify and correct deficits in ventilation, oxygenation, perfusion, and mentation, as well as conditions of the thorax and abdomen (such as tension pneumothorax and gastric dilatation) that pose an immediate threat to life (Table 14-6). The primary survey continues with complete **E**xposure of the patient to ensure that no injuries are missed, taking care to avoid hypothermia (through the use of blankets, overbed radiant warmers, and warmed intravenous fluids). It concludes with placement of adjuncts, such as a **F**oley catheter and a **G**astric tube (unless contraindicated, respectively, by evidence of pelvic, or basilar skull or oromaxillofacial fractures), which together with other adjuncts (such as pulse

TABLE 14-2
COMMON INJURY MECHANISMS AND CORRESPONDING INJURY PATTERNS IN CHILDHOOD TRAUMA

Injury Mechanism		Injury Pattern
Motor vehicle injury: occupant	Unrestrained	Head/neck injuries
		Scalp/facial lacerations
	Restrained	Internal abdomen injuries
		Lower spine fractures
Motor vehicle injury: pedestrian	Single	Lower extremity fractures
	Multiple	Head/neck injuries
		Internal chest/abdomen injuries
		Lower extremity fractures
Fall from height	Low	Upper extremity fractures
	Medium	Head/neck injuries
		Scalp/facial lacerations
		Upper extremity fractures
	High	Head/neck injuries
		Scalp/facial lacerations
		Internal chest/abdomen injuries
		Upper/lower extremity fractures
Fall from bicycle	Unhelmeted	Head/neck injuries
		Scalp/facial lacerations
		Upper extremity fractures
	Helmeted	Upper extremity fractures
	Handlebar	Internal abdomen injuries

From American College of Surgeons Committee on Trauma: Advanced Trauma Life Support for Doctors: Student Manual, 2004 edition. Chicago, American College of Surgeons (in press).

TABLE 14-3
INCIDENCE AND MORTALITY OF INJURIES TO THORACIC AND ABDOMINAL ORGANS

Thoracic Organ	Incidence (%)	Mortality (%)
Lung	52	18
Pneumothorax/hemothorax	42	17
Ribs/sternum	32	11
Heart	6	40
Diaphragm	4	16
Great vesssels	2	51
Bronchi	<1	20
Esophagus	<1	43
Abdominal Organ		
Liver	27	13
Spleen	27	11
Kidneys	25	13
Gastrointestinal tract	21	11
Great vessels	5	47
Genitourinary tract	5	3
Pancreas	4	7
Pelvis	<1	7

From Cooper A, Barlow B, Discala C, et al: Mortality and truncal injury: The pediatric perspective. J Pediatric Surg 29:33–38,1994.

oximetry and the trauma series of plain chest, pelvic, and lateral cervical spine radiographs that is obtained for all seriously injured patients) facilitate the early recognition and treatment of immediate threats to vital functions.

Resuscitation

Resuscitation of the child trauma victim is conducted concurrent with the primary survey in a continuous cycle of assessment, intervention, and reassessment. An **A**irway obstructed by soft tissues and secretions is opened (by using the modified jaw-thrust maneuver with or without an oropharyngeal airway to displace the mandibular block forward) while taking proper cervical spine precautions (maintaining the cervical spine in a neutral position with bimanual cervical spine stabilization followed by application of a semirigid cervical extrication collar and long backboard), then cleared (by using a large-bore Yankauer-type suction device) before its patency can be confirmed and assessment can proceed to the next step (Table 14-7). Abnormalities of **B**reathing (ventilation and oxygenation) are next addressed with supplemental oxygen or assisted ventilation, if needed. Finally, the integrity of the **C**irculation is assured through control of bleeding and administration of fluid.

Any child initially seen with major trauma should receive high-concentration oxygen by the most appropriate means (Table 14-8). For the child with simple respiratory distress (increased work of breathing), a nonrebreather mask normally will suffice, provided the airway is open and breathing is spontaneous. For the child with frank respiratory failure (labored or inadequate work of breathing), assisted ventilation via face mask or an endotracheal tube attached to a bag valve device should be initiated in preparation for endotracheal intubation. Orotracheal intubation with rapid-sequence induction techniques (etomidate and succinylcholine are now the preferred pharmacologic agents) and uncuffed endotracheal tubes (equivalent in diameter to the size of the naris or tip of the small finger, selected by using either a length-based resuscitation tape[46] or the formula 4 + age in years/4) is mandatory for all cases of respiratory failure and traumatic coma.

The child with major trauma will require volume resuscitation if signs of hypovolemic shock are present (Table 14-9). This is best carried out by means of large-bore peripheral catheters placed percutaneously in median cubital veins at the elbow or saphenous veins at the ankle, or by cutdown in the saphenous veins at the ankle or groin. Intraosseous access may be necessary if intravenous access is not rapidly obtained. Simple hypovolemia usually responds to 20 to 40 mL/kg of warmed lactated Ringer's solution, but frank hypotension (clinically defined by a systolic blood pressure less than 70 mm Hg plus twice the age in years) typically requires 40 to 60 mL/kg of warmed lactated Ringer's solution followed by 10 to 20 mL/kg warmed packed red blood cells (using type-specific blood in an urgent situation, if available, or type O negative blood, if not). Insertion of central venous catheters, except in rare cases in which venous access cannot otherwise be obtained, is not indicated, but urinary output should be measured in all seriously injured children as an indication of tissue perfusion.

TABLE 14-4			
TRAUMA SCORES COMMONLY USED IN CHILDREN			
	+2	+1	−1
Pediatric Trauma Score			
Size (kg)	>20	10–20	<10
Airway	Normal	Maintained	Unmaintained
Systolic blood pressure (mm Hg)	>90	50–90	<50
Central nervous system	Awake	Obtunded	Coma
Open wound	None	Minor	Major
Skeletal trauma	None	Closed	Open-Multiple
Glasgow Coma Scale	Systolic Blood Pressure (mm Hg)	Respiratory Rate (breaths/min)	Code Value
Revised Trauma Score			
13–15	>89	10–29	4
9–12	76–89	>29	3
6–8	50–75	6–9	2
4–5	1–49	1–5	1
3	0	0	0

Fom Tepas JJ, Mollitt DL, Talbent JL, et al: The pediatric trauma score as a predictor of trauma severity in the injured child. J Pediatr Surg 22:14–18, 1987; and Champion HR, Sacco WJ, Copes WS, et al: A revison of the trauma score. J Trauma 29:623–629, 1989.

Due to the ability of a child's blood vessels to compensate vigorously for hypovolemia by intense vasoconstriction, frank hypotension is a late sign of shock and may not develop until 30% to 35% of circulating blood volume is lost.[47] Thus any child who cannot be stabilized after 40 to 60 mL/kg of lactated Ringer's solution and 10 to 20 mL/kg of packed red blood cells likely has internal bleeding and needs emergency operation. If a child initially is in shock, has no signs of intrathoracic, intra-abdominal, or intrapelvic bleeding, but fails to improve despite seemingly adequate volume resuscitation, other forms of shock (obstructive, cardiogenic, neurogenic) should be considered: (1) has tension pneumothorax or cardiac tamponade developed? (2) is an unrecognized myocardial contusion present? or (3) was a possible spinal cord injury missed on physical examination? Yet it must be emphasized that most children in hypotensive shock are victims of unrecognized hemorrhage that can be reversed only if promptly recognized and appropriately treated by means of rapid blood transfusion and immediate surgical intervention.

Assessment of disability (neurologic status) relies on use of the Glasgow Coma Scale (GCS) score (for level of consciousness) and evaluation of bilateral papillary responses (to exclude mass lesions) and serves as a critical indicator of core organ function (Table 14-10). Traumatic coma (GCS score, 8) and pupillary asymmetry mandate immediate involvement of neurosurgical consultants. Further resuscitation is guided by findings on complete exposure of the patient (Table 14-11). The resuscitation phase concludes with use of adjuncts selected expressly to warn of conditions likely to affect the integrity of the airway, breathing, and circulation (Table 14-12).

Secondary Survey

Once the "primary survey" has been performed, "resuscitation" has commenced, and stabilization is assured, a secondary survey is undertaken for definitive evaluation of the injured child. This consists of a "SAMPLE" history (**S**ymptoms, **A**llergies, **M**edications, **P**ast illnesses, **L**ast meal, **E**vents, and **E**nvironment) and a complete head-to-toe examination, addressing all body regions and organ systems. The examination should be targeted particularly to the head and neck (for any history of blunt injury above the clavicles, alteration in level of consciousness, or neck pain or swelling), to the chest (for any history of chest pain, noisy or rapid breathing, respiratory insufficiency, or hemoptysis), and to the abdomen (for any history of abdominal pain, bruising or tenderness, distention, or vomiting, especially if the emesis is stained with blood or bile). In examining the child, the physician's first responsibility is to identify life-threatening injuries that may have been overlooked during the primary survey, such as tension pneumothorax (unilaterally decreased breath sounds with hyper-resonance to percussion and contralateral tracheal shift), massive hemothorax (unilaterally decreased breath sounds with dullness to percussion and a midline trachea), and gastric dilatation (upper abdominal distention with hyper-resonance to percussion).

Drainage from the nose or ears, or any evidence of midface instability, suggests the presence of a basilar skull fracture (which precludes passage of a nasogastric tube) or an oromaxillofacial fracture (which may threaten the airway). Evidence of neck tenderness, swelling, torticollis, or spasm suggests the presence of a cervical spine fracture (which may not be detected on

TABLE 14-5
POSSIBLE INDICATIONS FOR TRANSFER TO A PEDIATRIC TRAUMA CENTER

History of Injury
Patient thrown from a moving vehicle
Falls from >15 feet
Extrication time >20 min
Passenger cabin invaded >12 inches
Death of another passenger
Accident in a hostile environment (heat, cold water, etc.)

Anatomic Injuries
Combined system injury
Penetrating injury of the groin or neck
Three or more long-bone fractures
Fractures of the axial skeleton
Amputation (other than digits)
Persistent hypotension
Severe head trauma
Maxillofacial or upper airway injury
CNS injury with prolonged loss of consciousness, posturing, or paralysis
Spinal cord injury with neurologic deficit
Unstable chest injury
Blunt or penetrating trauma to the chest or abdomen
Burns, flame, or inhalation

System Considerations
Necessary service or specialist not available
No beds available
Need for pediatric ICU care
Multiple casualties
Family request
Paramedic judgment
Severity scores: Trauma Score ≤12; or
    Revised Trauma Score ≤11; or
    Pediatric Trauma Score ≤8

CNS, central nervous system; ICU, intensive care unit.
From Harris BH, Barlow BA, Ballantine TV, et al: American Pediatric Surgical Association: Principles of pediatric trauma care. J Pediatr Surg 27:423–426, 1992.

---

lateral cervical spine films in cases of SCIWORA). On chest examination, point tenderness, palpable bony deformity, crepitus or subcutaneous emphysema on inspection or palpation, or inadequate chest rise or air entry on auscultation or percussion suggests the presence of a rib fracture. Air or blood in the hemithorax indicates the need to search for an associated or subclinical pneumothorax or hemothorax. An abdomen that remains distended after gastric decompression suggests the presence of intra-abdominal bleeding (most often from the spleen or liver) or a disrupted hollow viscus (especially if fever, tenderness, or guarding is found together with abdominal distention or nasogastric aspirate stained with blood or bile).

All skeletal components should be palpated for evidence of instability or discontinuity, especially bony prominences such as the anterior superior iliac spines, which commonly are injured in major blunt trauma. In the absence of obvious deformities, fractures should be suspected if bony point tenderness, hematoma, spasm of overlying muscles, an unstable pelvic girdle, or perineal

TABLE 14-6
PRIMARY SURVEY, RESUSCITATION, AND SECONDARY SURVEY

Primary Survey
Airway: clear and maintain, protect cervical spine
Breathing: ventilate and oxygenate, fix chest wall
Circulation: control bleeding, restore volume
Disability: GCS and pupils, call the neurosurgeon
Exposure: disrobe, logroll, avoid hypothermia
Foley catheter unless contraindicated*
Gastric tube unless contraindicated†

Secondary Survey
History and physical: SAMPLE history, complete examination
Imaging studies: plain radiographs,‡ special studies§

---

*Meatal blood, scrotal hematoma, high-riding prostate.
†CSF oto-rhinorrhea, basilar skull fracture, midface instability.
‡Chest, pelvis, lateral cervical spine; others as indicated.
§FAST, CT as indicated.
GCS, Glasgow Coma Scale; CSF, cerebrospinal fluid; FAST, focused assessment by sonography in trauma; CT, computed tomography.
From American College of Surgeons Committee on Trauma: Advanced Trauma Life Support for Doctors: Student Manual, 2004 edition. Chicago, American College of Surgeons (in press).

---

swelling or discoloration is found. The integrity of the pelvic ring may be tested in two ways: (1) by auscultating over one anterior superior iliac spine, while gently tapping over the other, to see if bone conduction is preserved, which will be the case only if the ring is intact; and (2) by pressing simultaneously on the anterior superior iliac spines to see if the pelvic wings "spring" apart because of separation of the pubic symphysis. Most long-bone fractures will be self-evident, but such injuries are occasionally missed during the secondary survey, which emphasizes the (1) assumption that a fracture is present on the basis of history alone (even if no obvious deformity is seen) until proven otherwise; and (2) performance of ongoing evaluation of all injured extremities for evidence of pain, pallor, pulselessness, paresthesias, and paralysis (the classic signs of associated neurovascular trauma).

Laboratory evaluation is an integral part of the secondary survey. Arterial blood gases are of paramount importance in determining the adequacy of ventilation

TABLE 14-7
AIRWAY/CERVICAL SPINE

Open: jaw thrust/spinal stabilization
Clear: suction/remove particulate matter
Support: oropharyngeal/nasopharyngeal airway
Establish: orotracheal/nasotracheal intubation*
Maintain: primary/secondary confirmation†
Bypass: needle/surgical cricothyroidotomy

---

*RSI technique: etomidate then succinylcholine.
†1°, chest rise, air entry; 2°, exhaled CO_2 detector, esophageal detector device; watch for DOPE: **D**islodgement, **O**bstruction, **P**neumothorax, **E**quipment failure.
From Amercian College of Surgeons Committee on Trauma: Advanced Trauma Life Support for Doctors: Student Manual, 2004 edition. Chicago, American College of Surgeons (in press).

TABLE 14-8

BREATHING/CHEST WALL

Ventilation: chest rise/air entry/effort/rate
Oxygenation: central color/pulse oximetry
Support: distress — NRB/failure — BVM
Chest wall: ensure integrity/expand lungs
   Tension pneumothorax: needle, chest tube*
   Open pneumothorax: occlude, chest tube
   Massive hemothorax: volume, chest tube

NRB, nonrebreather mask; BVM, bag valve mask
*Do not wait for confirmatory chest radiograph!
From Amercian College of Surgeons Committee on Trauma: Advanced Trauma Life Support for Doctors:Student Manual, 2004 edition. Chicago, Amercian College of Surgeons (in press).

($Paco_2$), oxygenation (Pao_2), and perfusion (base deficit).[48] However, the critically important determinant of blood oxygen content, hence tissue oxygen delivery (assuming the Pao_2 exceeds 60 mm Hg), is the blood hemoglobin concentration. Serial hemoglobin values better reflect the extent of blood loss than does the initial value. Elevations in serum transaminases or amylase and lipase suggest injury to the liver or pancreas, but the infrequency of pancreatic injury makes the latter cost ineffective versus the former.[49,50] Urine that is grossly bloody or is positive for blood by dipstick or microscopy (≥20 red blood cells per high-power field) suggests kidney trauma. Damage to adjacent organs due to the high incidence of associated injuries should be suspected.[51]

Radiologic evaluation is another important part of the secondary survey. Arrangements should be made, before other plain films are ordered, to obtain computed tomography (CT) of the head (without contrast) and abdomen (double contrast), as indicated. Once these are completed, whatever plain films are required may be obtained. However, at no time should imaging studies take precedence over resuscitation for life-threatening injuries, nor should an unstable patient be taken to the radiology department, nor should the physician fail to accompany and continuously monitor the child.

TABLE 14-9

CIRCULATION/EXTERNAL BLEEDING

Stop bleeding: direct pressure, avoid clamps
Shock evaluation: pulse, skin CRT, LOC
Blood pressure: avoid over/undercorrection
   Infant/child: low normal, 70 + (age × 2) mm Hg
   Adolescent: low normal, 90 mm Hg
Volume resuscitation: Ringer's lactate → packed cells
   Infant/child: 20 mL/kg RL, repeat × 1–2 → 10 mL/PRBCs
   Adolescent: 1–2 L, repeat × 1–2 → 1–2 U PRBCs

CRT, capillary refill time; LOC, level of consciousness; PRBCs, packed red blood cells. Consider obstructive and neurogenic as well as hypovolemic shock: exclude tension pneumothorax, cardiac tamponade, spinal shock. From American College of Surgeons Committe on Trauma: Advanced Trauma Life Support for Doctors: Student Manual, 2004 edition. Chicago, American College of Surgeons (in press).

TABLE 14-10

DISABILITY/MENTAL STATUS

Pupils: symmetry, reaction
LOC: GCS
   Track and trend as a vital sign
   Significant change, 2 points
   Intubate for coma, GCS ≤8
Motor: strength, symmetry
Abnormality/deterioration: call neurosurgeon
   Mild TBI (GCS 14–15): observe, consider CT for history of LOC
   Moderate TBI (GCS 9–13): admit, obtain CT, repeat CT 12–24 hr
   Severe TBI (GCS 3–8): intubate, ventilate, obtain CT, repeat CT 12–24 hr

LOC, loss of consciousness; GCS, Glasgow Coma Scale; CT, computed tomography; TBI, traumatic brain injury.
From Amercian College of Surgeons Committee on Trauma: Advanced Trauma Life Support for Doctors: Student Manual, 2004 edition. Chicago, American College of Surgeons (in press).

CT of the head should be obtained whenever loss of consciousness has occurred. CTs of the abdomen should be obtained whenever signs of internal bleeding (abdominal tenderness, distention, bruising, or gross hematuria)[52] or a history of hypotensive shock (which has responded to volume resuscitation) is noted. **F**ocused **A**ssessment by **S**onography in **T**rauma (FAST) may be useful in detecting intra-abdominal blood, but it is not sufficiently reliable to exclude blunt abdominal injury in hemodynamically stable children. Like diagnostic peritoneal lavage, which it has largely supplanted, FAST adds little to the management of pediatric abdominal trauma, as unstable patients with suspected intra-abdominal injuries are candidates for immediate operation, whereas stable patients are managed nonoperatively without regard to the presence of intra-abdominal blood.[53,54] However, FAST has been successfully used in screening for intra-abdominal injuries.[55] Moreover, a detailed sonographic examination may be useful for those cases in which intra-abdominal injury is suspected and CT cannot be obtained, whether because of lack of equipment or a history of allergy to iodinated contrast agents.

Critical Care

Definitive management of childhood trauma begins once sustentative care (the primary survey and resuscitation

TABLE 14-11

EXPOSURE AND ENVIRONMENT

Disrobe: cut off clothes
Logroll: requires four people
Screening examination: front and back
Avoid hypothermia: keep patient warm!

From American College of Surgeons Committee on Trauma: Advanced Trauma Life Support for Doctors: Student Manual, 2004 edition. Chicago, American College of Surgeons (in press).

FAST, focused assessment by sonography in trauma; DPL, diagnostic peritoneal lavage.
From American College of Surgeons Committee on Trauma: Advanced Trauma Life Support for Doctors: Student Manual, 2004 edition. Chicago, American College of Surgeons (in press).

TABLE 14-12

PRIMARY SURVEY ADJUNCTS

Vital signs/pulse oximetry
Chest/pelvis/lateral cervical spine radiographs
Foley catheter/gastric tube
FAST/DPL

phases) has concluded. This care is the responsibility not of a single individual or specialty, but of a multidisciplinary team of pediatric-capable health professionals led by a surgeon with experience and commitment to the care of both trauma and children. It begins with the secondary survey and re-evaluation of vital functions, concludes with rehabilitation, and encompasses the operative, critical, acute, and convalescent phases of care. Avoidance of secondary injury (injury due to persistent or recurrent hypoxia or hypoperfusion) is a major goal of definitive management and mandates reliance on continuous monitoring of vital signs, GCS score, oxygen saturation, urinary output, and, when necessary, arterial and central venous pressure.

Definitive management of childhood trauma also depends on the type, extent, and severity of the injuries sustained. Any child requiring resuscitation should be admitted to the hospital under the care of a surgeon experienced in the management of childhood injuries. Such a child should initially not receive oral intake (because of the temporary paralytic ileus that often accompanies major blunt abdominal trauma, and because general anesthesia may later be required), but intravenous fluid at a maintenance rate (assuming both normal hydration at the time of the injury and normalization of both vital signs and perfusion status after resuscitation). Soft tissue injuries also should receive proper attention, including wound closure and tetanus prophylaxis, and intravenous lines inserted under substerile circumstances should be replaced to prevent the development of thrombophlebitis.

Brain

The overall mortality and morbidity of major pediatric trauma are closely linked with the functional outcome of the brain injury that typically occurs after significant blunt impact. The results of treatment of severe closed head trauma are somewhat better in children age 3 to 12 years than in adults, an advantage that is ablated in the presence of hypotension, but are worse in children younger than 3 years. Although the general principles of definitive management of traumatic brain injury are similar in children and adults, nonoperative management predominates because diffuse brain injuries are more common than focal injuries in pediatric patients. Surgically remediable causes of intracranial hypertension must be treated if found, but medically remediable causes are addressed aggressively. The goal of treatment is to

optimize cerebral blood flow through maintenance of cerebral perfusion pressure (by concomitant restoration of mean arterial pressure and reduction of intracranial pressure) and avoidance of prolonged hyperventilation, which causes cerebral ischemia.

Current management of traumatic brain injury in children should adhere to evidence-based consensus guidelines (see Chapter 17).[56] Conservative treatment, including discharge to home care under the supervision of responsible adult caretakers who have been instructed to return if signs of increased intracranial pressure (nausea, vomiting, increasing lethargy) develop, suffices for management of mild head injury (GCS score, 14 to 15). At the same time, noncontrast CT is indicated for all patients who have a documented loss of consciousness or are amnestic. Expectant management, consisting of hospital admission, CT, and continuous neurologic observation, is used for all patients with moderate head injury (GCS, score 9 to 13). Controlled ventilation is initiated after endotracheal intubation via rapid-sequence technique for all patients with severe head injury (GCS score, 3 to 8, or a rapid deterioration in GCS score of ≥ 2 points). Hyperventilation (P_aCO_2, 25 to 30 mm Hg) and mannitol (0.5 mg/kg) are reserved for patients with evidence of transtentorial (papillary asymmetry, neurologic posturing) or cerebellar (ataxic breathing) herniation.

Immediate operation is necessary for all acute collections of intracranial (epidural, subdural, intracerebral) blood of sufficient size to cause mass effect, for all open skull fractures, and for all depressed skull fractures that invade the intracranial vault by more than the thickness of the adjacent skull. Intravenous antibiotics are used only for patients with open skull fractures. Anticonvulsants (phenytoin preceded by diazepam, as needed) are indicated for all patients with active seizures, impact seizures, or moderate or severe brain injury, but should be discontinued after 2 weeks of therapy, as no benefit accrues after this treatment interval.[57] Corticosteroids are not advantageous in traumatic brain injury. Moreover, nitrogen losses may be accelerated.[58,59]

Acute complications of severe traumatic brain injury include hyperglycemia, diabetes insipidus, the syndrome of inappropriate antidiuretic hormone secretion, and brain death. The first three are managed, respectively, through the use of insulin, desamino-D-arginine vasopressin (DDAVP), and water restriction. Brain death results from uncontrolled intracranial hypertension and is manifested in a normothermic patient by total absence of brainstem function on neurologic examination, a positive apnea test, isoelectric activity on electroencephalogram on two successive occasions (preferably 24 hours apart), or complete absence of cerebral perfusion on nuclear scan or cerebral arteriography. Due consideration should be given to organ preservation and donation under such circumstances.

Spine

The cervical region is most often injured. High-dose methylprednisolone (30 mg/kg/15 min loading dose immediately on diagnosis, followed by 5.4 mg/kg/hr constant infusion for 24 hours) may hold some promise in mitigating the effects of spinal cord injury and should be administered to all patients with suggestive neurologic findings.[60] Early care with volume resuscitation followed by vasopressor agents as needed should focus on management of neurogenic shock and immobilization of associated fractures (extrication collar and backboard followed by skeletal traction with Gardner-Wells tongs), realizing that SCIWORA is more common in children than in adults. Later care addresses repair of associated vertebral fractures through use of halo traction with or without surgical fusion.

Critical care of patients with spinal cord injury is chiefly supportive. Alternating-pressure or air-fluidizing mattresses should be used whenever available to prevent the development of decubitus ulcers. Indwelling urinary catheterization, followed by intermittent clean catheterization, should be used to prevent the development of urinary stasis and subsequent infection. Aggressive pulmonary toilet, including bronchoscopy as needed, should be used to prevent the development of pulmonary infections, especially in patients with intercostal or diaphragmatic muscle paralysis.

Chest

Most life-threatening chest injuries can be managed expectantly, or by tube thoracostomy inserted via the fifth intercostal space on the midaxillary line, provided that a tunnel of adequate length is created, because the thinner chest wall provides a less effective seal around the catheter (Table 14-13). Indications for resuscitative

TABLE 14-13

EARLY ASSESSMENT AND MANAGEMENT OF CHEST INJURIES IN CHILDHOOD

	Clinical Signs	Emergency Treatment
Immediate Threats		

Upper airway obstruction	Incomplete: noisy breathing
	  Snoring (soft tissue collapse)
	  Gurgling (secretions, blood)
	  Stridor (edema, foreign body)
	  Hoarseness (larnygeal fracture)
	Complete: rocking chest-wall motions
	  unrelieved by simple measures
		Incomplete: clear obstruction
		  Jaw thrust, oral airway
		  Oropharyngeal suction
		  Foreign body retrieval
		  Tracheostomy and repair
		Complete: needle or surgical
		  cricothyroidotomy

Tension pneumothorax	Ipsilaterally decreased breath sounds,
	  contralaterally shifted trachea,
	  hyper-resonance to percussion
		Needle decompression without waiting
		  for chest radiograph followed
		  by urgent tube thoracostomy

Open pneumothorax	Chest-wall defect, sucking chest
	  wound
		Occlusive dressing followed by
		  urgent tube thoracostomy

Massive hemothorax	Ipsilaterally decreased breath sounds,
	  midline trachea, dullness to
	  percussion
		Volume resuscitation together
		  with urgent tube thoracostomy

Cardiac tamponade	Muffled heart tones, distended neck
	  veins, narrowed pulse pressure,
	  Focused Assessment by Sonography
	  in Trauma (FAST)
		Pericardiocentesis followed by
		  urgent operative repair

Flail chest	Paradoxical chest-wall motions,
	  bony crepitus
		Endotracheal intubation for
		  respiratory failure

Potential Threats		
Pulmonary contusion	Rales, rhonchi	Supplemental oxygen
Myocardial contusion	Cardiac arrhythmias	Monitoring, antiarrhythmics
Diaphragmatic rupture	Elevated hemidiaphragm, nasogastric tube in hemithorax	Urgent operative repair
Aortic rupture	Murmur radiating to back, widened mediastinum	Urgent operative repair
Bronchial disruption	Persistent large air leak, persistent pneumothorax despite thoracostomy	Urgent operative repair
Esophageal disruption	Food or saliva draining from thoracostomy, pneumomediastinum	Urgent operative repair
Possible Threats		

Simple pneumothorax	Ipsilaterally decreased breath sounds,
	  midline trachea, hyper-resonance to
	  percussion
		Urgent tube thoracostomy

Simple hemothorax	Ipsilaterally decreased breath sounds, midline trachea, dullness to percussion	Urgent tube thoracostomy
Rib fractures	Bony crepitus	Analgesics
Traumatic asphyxia	Multiple petechiae of head and neck	Supportive and expectant

thoracotomy are limited to patients with physical or electrocardiographic signs of life in the field or emergency department after penetrating chest trauma. The universally dismal results bar its use in blunt chest or abdominal trauma,[61] even though cardiopulmonary resuscitation by itself is associated with a 23.5% survival rate.[62] Emergency thoracotomy is reserved for injured patients with massive hemothorax (20 mL/kg) and ongoing hemorrhage (2 to 4 mL/kg/hr), massive air leak, and food or salivary drainage from the chest tube. Severe pulmonary contusions, if complicated by aspiration, overhydration, or infection, can predispose the patient to development of adult respiratory distress syndrome (ARDS) or post-traumatic pulmonary insufficiency (PTPI). These complications require aggressive ventilatory support and, occasionally, extracorporeal membrane oxygenation. Traumatic asphyxia, characterized by facial and conjunctival petechiae, requires no specific treatment but serves to indicate the considerable severity of the impacting force.

Critical care of the respiratory insufficiency that accompanies severe chest injury also is expectant. To avoid both oxygen toxicity and resorption atelectasis, it is best to use the least amount of artificial respiratory support necessary to maintain the Pao_2 at 70 to 80 mm Hg (hence the Spo_2 at 90% to 100%) and the $Paco_2$ (or the $Petco_2$) at 35 to 45 mm Hg. Continuous positive airway pressure (CPAP) or positive end expiratory pressure (PEEP) should be used for maintenance of functional residual capacity whenever the Fio_2 exceeds 40%, but adverse effects on the circulation should be avoided. Peak inspiratory pressure should be kept below 20 to 25 cm H_2O whenever positive-pressure ventilation is required, especially if pneumothoraces, or fresh bronchial or pulmonary suture lines, are present. Pulmonary contusions uncomplicated by aspiration, overhydration, or infection can be expected to resolve in 7 to 10 days. Thus the judicious use of pulmonary toilet, crystalloid fluid, loop diuretics, and therapeutic (not prophylactic) antibiotics to preclude the development of ARDS or PTPI is required.

Abdomen

Immediate management of intra-abdominal and genitourinary injuries in children is chiefly nonoperative, although not nonsurgical, as mature surgical judgment is needed to determine whether, or when, operation may be required. Bleeding from renal, splenic, and hepatic injuries is mostly self-limited and resolves spontaneously in most cases, unless the patient is in hypotensive shock or the transfusion requirement exceeds 40 mL/kg of body weight (half the circulating blood volume) within 24 hours of injury.[26-28] Laparotomy for management of renal, pancreatic, gastrointestinal, and genitourinary injuries is performed as indicated, by using damage-control methods for patients in extremis and staged closure for patients with abdominal compartment syndrome (Table 14-14). Pancreatic pseudocyst is heralded by the development of a tender epigastric mass 3 to 5 days after upper abdominal trauma and mandates 4 to 6 weeks of

TABLE 14-14
INDICATIONS FOR EARLY OPERATION IN ABDOMINAL TRAUMA IN CHILDHOOD

Blunt
Hemodynamic instability despite adequate volume resuscitation
Transfusion requirement >50% of estimated blood volume
Physical signs of peritonitis
Endoscopic evidence of rectal tear
Radiologic evidence of intraperitoneal or retroperitoneal gas
Radiologic evidence of gastrointestinal perforation
Radiologic evidence of renovascular pedicle injury
Radiologic evidence of pancreatic transection
Bile, bacteria, stool, or >500 WBC/mm³ on peritoneal lavage

Penetrating
All gunshot wounds
All stab wounds associated with evisceration; blood in stomach, urine, or rectum; physical signs of shock or peritonitis; radiologic evidence of intraperitoneal or retroperitoneal gas
All suspected thoracoabdominal injuries (unless excluded by thoracoscopy or laparoscopy)
Bile, bacteria, stool, or >500 WBC/mm³ on peritoneal lavage

WBCs, white blood cells.

bowel rest along with parenteral nutrition in preparation for an internal drainage procedure.

Critical care of hemodynamically stable children with solid visceral injuries should follow consensus guidelines (see Chapter 16).[63] If respiratory care is required, incentive spirometry is preferred, as clots that are organizing may be disturbed by vigorous chest physiotherapy. The stomach should be kept decompressed after splenic injury to prevent reactivation of bleeding due to stretching of the short gastric vessels that can accompany gastric dilatation. Serial hematocrit determination should be obtained regularly until stable. Elevated serum enzyme determinations should be repeated at intervals until normal, as should urinalyses that are positive for blood or myoglobin. Dilutional coagulopathies should be anticipated when the transfusion requirement exceeds 80 mL/kg (the entire circulating blood volume) and may require administration of platelet concentrates, fresh frozen plasma, and intravenous calcium supplements.

Skeleton

Because long-bone fractures are rarely life threatening unless associated with major bleeding (bilateral femur fractures, unstable pelvic fractures), the general care of the injured patient takes precedence over orthopedic care. At the same time, early stabilization will serve both to decrease patient discomfort and to limit the amount of hemorrhage. Closed treatment predominates for fractures of the clavicle, upper extremity, tibia, and femur (infants and preschoolers), although fractures of the femur increasingly involve use of external fixation and intramedullary rods (school-age children and adolescents).

Operative treatment is required for open fractures, displaced supracondylar fractures (because of their association with ischemic vascular injury), and major or displaced physeal fractures (which must be reduced anatomically). Owing to the ability of most long-bone fractures to remodel, reductions need not be perfectly anatomic. However, remodeling is limited in torus and greenstick fractures, as the hyperemia typical of complete fractures is unlikely to occur.

Critical care of skeletal injuries consists of careful immobilization, as appropriate, with emphasis on prevention of immobilization-related complications (such as friction burns and bed sores) through use of supportive and assistive devices (such as egg-crate or similar mattresses and a trapeze to permit limited freedom of movement). Fracture-associated arterial insufficiency is recognized by the presence of a pulse deficit on serial observation. Detection of compartment syndrome may require measurement of tissue pulp pressure, which mandates fasciotomy when greater than 40 cm H_2O. Traumatic fat embolism after long-bone fracture and rhabdomyolysis after severe crush injury are rare but require aggressive respiratory support and crystalloid diuresis. Early rehabilitation is vital to optimal recovery and mandates routine physiatric consultation on admission.

Physical Support

The care of children with major traumatic injury also involves nutritional support, of nitrogen even more than energy.[64] In patients who are not eating, antiacid therapys with both topical and systemic agents to avoid gastric stress ulcer bleeding, is recommended. In children with hematomas of the liver, spleen, or pelvis, low-grade fever may develop as these are resorbed, but high spiking fevers should prompt investigation for a source such as infected hematomas or effusions or pelvic osteomyelitis. In children with large retroperitoneal hematomas, hypertension may develop on rare occasions, presumably due to pressure on the renal vessels. The temporary use of antihypertensive agents may be required, but the hematomas usually resolve without the need for surgical decompression. Children with chest tubes or long-term indwelling urinary catheters are at risk for systemic infection and should receive prophylactic or suppressive antibiotics as long as the tube is required.

Emotional Support

Efforts must be made to attend to the emotional needs of the child and family, especially for those families facing the death of a child or a sibling.[65] In addition to loss of control over their child's destiny, parents of seriously injured children also may feel enormous guilt, whether or not these feelings are warranted. The responsible surgeon should attempt to create as normal an environment as possible for the child and allow the parents to participate meaningfully in postinjury care. In so doing, treatment interventions will be facilitated as child perceives that parents and staff are working together to assure an optimal recovery.

SPECIAL CONSIDERATIONS

Child Abuse

Child abuse is the underlying cause of 3% of major traumatic injuries in childhood.[9] A detailed review of the mechanisms, patterns, presentations, and findings of physical abuse is beyond the scope of this chapter, but child abuse may be suspected whenever unexplained delay occurs in obtaining treatment, when the history is vague or otherwise incompatible with the observed physical findings, when the caretaker blames siblings or playmates or other third parties, or when the caretaker protects other adults rather than the child. Although the recognition and sociomedicolegal management of suspected cases of child abuse require a special approach, assessment and medical treatment of physical injuries is no different from that for any other mechanism of injury. Most important, confrontation and accusation hinder treatment and rehabilitation and have no place in the surgical management of any pediatric patient, regardless of the nature of the injury (although reports of suspected child abuse must be filed with local child protective services in every state and territory).

Penetrating Injuries

Early involvement of social services, psychiatric support, pastoral care, and responsible law enforcement and child protective agencies is mandatory, especially in cases of nonaccidental injury for which the initial history is rarely accurate and the potential for recidivism is significant. All penetrating wounds are contaminated and must be treated as infected. Accessible missile fragments should be removed (once swelling has subsided) to prevent the development of lead poisoning (especially those in contact with bone or joint fluid).[66] Thoracotomy is usually not required except for massive hemothorax (20 mL/kg) or ongoing hemorrhage (2 to 4 mL/kg/hr) from the chest tube, persistent massive air leak, or food or salivary drainage from the chest tube. Laparotomy is always required for gunshot wounds as well as stab wounds associated with hemorrhagic shock, peritonitis, or evisceration. Thoracoabdominal injury should be suspected whenever the torso is penetrated between the nipple line and the costal margin, if peritoneal irritation develops after thoracic penetration, if food or chyle is recovered from the chest tube, or if injury-trajectory imaging studies suggest the possibility of diaphragmatic penetration. Tube thoracostomy, followed by laparotomy or laparoscopy for repair of diaphragm and damaged organs, is mandated with such signs.

Systems Issues

Pediatric patients at high risk of death from multiple and severe injuries are best served by a fully inclusive trauma system (each component of which is pediatric capable) that incorporates all appropriate health care facilities and personnel to the level of their resources and capabilities. Moreover, collaboration with local public health agencies (in programs for injury prevention and control), as well as local public health, public safety, and emergency-management agencies (in regional disaster-planning efforts) is necessary.[67] Although the regional trauma center is at the hub of the system (and ideally also is the regional pediatric trauma center), area trauma centers may be needed in localities distant from the regional trauma center. These distant centers must be capable of surgical management of pediatric trauma. All other hospitals in the region should participate as they are able, but must be fully capable of initial resuscitation, stabilization, and transfer of pediatric trauma patients. Finally, a regional trauma advisory committee should include pediatric representation that has the authority to develop and implement guidelines for triage of pediatric trauma within the system.

Transport Issues

Pediatric victims of multisystem trauma should undergo direct primary transport from the injury scene to a pediatric-capable trauma center.[68–75] If this proves impossible, additional secondary transport from the initial trauma receiving hospital to the pediatric-capable trauma center may be needed. Transport providers must be capable of critical pediatric assessment and monitoring and skilled in the techniques of endotracheal intubation and vascular access, as well as drug and fluid administration in children.[76,77] Specialized pediatric-transport teams staffed by physicians and nurses with advanced training in pediatric trauma and critical care treatment and transport should be used whenever possible, because complications related to endotracheal intubation and vascular access are the leading causes of adverse events during transport, occurring at twice the rate of those in the pediatric intensive care unit, and 10 times more frequently when specialized teams are not used.[78,79]

Hospital Preparedness

Regional pediatric trauma centers should be located in trauma hospitals with comprehensive pediatric services (such as a full-service general, university, or children's hospital) that demonstrates an institutional commitment to pediatric trauma care, including child abuse.[67] Pediatric medical and surgical subspecialty services and units must be present, as well as pediatric nursing and allied health professionals. Adult trauma centers can achieve results comparable to those of pediatric trauma centers if pediatric subspecialty support (pediatric emergency and critical care medicine) is used.[80–87] Finally, an organized pediatric trauma service must be available within the regional pediatric trauma center that, in addition to exemplary patient care, supports education and research in pediatric trauma and provides leadership in pediatric trauma system coordination.

Emergency Preparedness

Recent literature describing pediatric disaster management has focused on multiple casualty incidents involving children that resulted from motorized transport crashes, natural disasters, and terrorist incidents, underscoring the need for meaningful involvement of pediatric-capable trauma surgeons and trauma hospitals in regional disaster-planning efforts for pediatric patients. Airplane crashes predominantly cause severe traumatic brain injuries, severe intrathoracic hemorrhage, and femur fractures, whereas bus crashes predominantly cause closed head injuries, soft tissue damage, and superficial lacerations.[88,89] Major hurricanes appear to result chiefly in open wounds, gastroenteritis, skin infections, and, to a lesser extent, hydrocarbon and bleach ingestions, whereas earthquakes appear to result chiefly in orthopedic and soft tissue injuries as well as burns.[90–92] Building collapses after massive bomb explosions are associated with high fatality rates (due chiefly to lethal head and torso injuries, as well as traumatic amputations).[93] In the aftermath of the April 19, 1995, bombing of the Alfred P. Murrah Federal Building in Oklahoma City, Oklahoma, and the September 11, 2001, suicide airliner attacks on the World Trade Center in New York and the Pentagon near Washington, DC, thoughtful approaches to pediatric disaster planning as well as dissemination of policy and practice guidelines from key professional organizations and experts in pediatric emergency and disaster medicine have evolved.[94–100]

REFERENCES

1. National Center for Injury Prevention and Control: Injury Fact Book 2000-2002. Atlanta, Centers for Disease Control and Prevention, 2001.
2. Tepas JJ, Ramenofsky ML, Mollitt DL, et al: The pediatric trauma score as a predictor of injury severity: An objective assessment. J Trauma 28:425–429, 1988.
3. Graves EJ: Detailed Diagnoses and Procedures, National Hospital Discharge Survey, 1989. Hyattsville, Md, National Center for Health Statistics, Vital Health Stat 13, 1991.
4. Klem SA, Pollack MM, Glass NL, et al: Resource use, efficiency, and outcome prediction in pediatric intensive care of trauma patients. J Trauma 30:32–36, 1990.
5. Krauss BS, Harakal T, Fleisher GR: The spectrum and frequency of illness presenting to a pediatric emergency department. Pediatr Emerg Care 7:67–71, 1991.
6. Tsai A, Kallsen G: Epidemiology of pediatric prehospital care. Ann Emerg Med 16:284–292, 1987.
7. Hale GC, Caudill SA, Hicks-Waller CM, et al: The New York State Trauma System: A Special Report on Pediatric Trauma. Albany, NY, New York State Department of Health, 2002.
8. Cooper A, Barlow B, Davidson L, et al: Epidemiology of pediatric trauma: Importance of population-based statistics. J Pediatr Surg 27:149–154, 1992.
9. DiScala C: National Pediatric Trauma Registry Annual Report. Boston, Tufts University Rehabilitation and Childhood Trauma Research and Training Center, 2002.
10. Haddon W: Advances in the epidemiology of injuries as a basis for public policy. Public Health Rep 95:411–421, 1980.
11. Runyan CW: Using the Haddon Matrix: Introducing the third dimension. Inj Prev 4:302–307, 1998.
12. Cooper G, Dawson D, Kaufmann C, et al: Trauma Systems Planning and Evaluation: A Model Approach to a Major Public Health Problem. Rockville, Md, Health Resources and Services Administration (in press).
13. Davidson LL, Durkin MS, Kuhn L, et al: The impact of the safe kids/health neighborhoods injury prevention program in Harlem 1988 to 1991. Am J Public Health 84:580–596, 1992, 1994.
14. Laraque D, Barlow B, Davidson L, et al: Central Harlem playground injury project: A model for change. Am J Public Health 84:1691–1692, 1994.

15. Barlow B, Niemirska M, Gandhi R: Ten years of experience with falls from a height in children. J Pediatr Surg 18:509–511, 1983.

16. Cooper A, Barlow B, DiScala C: Vital signs and trauma mortality: The pediatric perspective. Pediatr Emerg Care 16:66, 2000.

17. Gennarelli TA, Champion HR, Sacco WJ, et al: Mortality of patients with head injury and extracranial injury treated in trauma centers. J Trauma 29:1193–1201, 1989.

18. Pigula FA, Wald SL, Shackford SR, et al: The effect of hypotension and hypoxia on children with severe head injuries. J Pediatr Surg 28:310–316, 1993.

19. Kewalramani LS, Kraus JF, Sterling HM, et al: Acute spinal-cord lesions in a pediatric population: Epidemiological and clinical features. Paraplegia 18:206–219, 1980.

20. Kraus JF, Fife D, Cox P: Incidence, severity, and external causes of pediatric brain injury. Am J Dis Child 140:687–693, 1986.

21. Pang D, Wilberger E: Spinal cord injury without radiographic abnormality in children. J Neurosurg 57:114–129, 1982.

22. Bohn D, Armstrong A, Becker L, et al: Cervical spine injuries in children. J Trauma 30:463–469, 1990.

23. Cooper A, Barlow B, DiScala C, String D: Mortality and truncal injury: The pediatric perspective. J Pediatr Surg 29:33–38, 1994.

24. Peclet MH, Newman KD, Eichelberger MR, et al: Thoracic trauma in children: An indicator of increased mortality. J Pediatr Surg 25:961–966, 1990.

25. Haller JA: Injuries of the gastrointestinal tract in children: Notes on recognition and management. Clin Pediatr 5:476–480, 1966.

26. Bass DH, Semple PL, Cywes S: Investigation and management of blunt renal injuries in children: A review of 11 years' experience. J Pediatr Surg 26:196–200, 1991.

27. Pearl RH, Wesson DE, Spence LJ, et al: Splenic injury: A 5-year update with improved results and changing criteria for conservative management. J Pediatr Surg 24:121–125, 1989.

28. Galat JA, Grisoni ER, Gauderer MWL: Pediatric blunt liver injury: Establishment of criteria for appropriate management. J Pediatr Surg 25:1162–1165, 1990.

29. Selbst SM, Baker MD, Shames M: Bunk bed injuries. Am J Dis Child 144:721–723, 1990.

30. Helfer RE, Slovis TL, Black M: Injuries resulting when small children fall out of bed. Pediatrics 60:533–535, 1977.

31. Joffe M, Ludwig S: Stairway injuries in children. Pediatrics 82:457–461, 1988.

32. Barlow B, Niemirska M, Gandhi R, et al: Response to injury in children with closed femur fractures. J Trauma 27:429–430, 1987.

33. Herzenberg JE, Hensinger RN, Dedrick DK, et al: Emergency transport and positioning of young children who have an injury of the cervical spine. J Bone Joint Surg Am 71:15–22, 1989.

34. Schafermeyer RW, Ribbeck BM, Gaskins J, et al: Respiratory effects of spinal immobilization in children. Ann Emerg Med 20:1017–1019, 1991.

35. Viccellio P, Simon H, Pressman BD, et al: A prospective multicenter study of cervical spine injury in children. Pediatrics 108:e20, 2001.

36. Gausche M, Lewis RJ, Stratton SJ, et al: Effect of out-of-hospital pediatric endotracheal intubation on survival and neurological outcome: A controlled clinical trial. JAMA 283:783–790, 2000.

37. Cooper A, DiScala C, Foltin G, et al: Prehospital endotracheal intubation for severe head injury in children: A reappraisal. Semin Pediatr Surg 10:3–6, 2001.

38. Teach SJ, Antosia RE, Lund DP, et al: Prehospital fluid therapy in pediatric trauma patients. Pediatr Emerg Care 11:5–8, 1995.

39. Tepas JJ, Mollitt DL, Talbert JL, et al: The pediatric trauma score as a predictor of injury severity in the injured child. J Pediatr Surg 22:14–18, 1987.

40. Champion HR, Sacco WJ, Copes WS, et al: A revision of the trauma score. J Trauma 29:623–629, 1989.

41. Harris BH, Barlow BA, Ballantine TV, et al: American Pediatric Surgical Association: Principles of pediatric trauma care. J Pediatr Surg 27:423–426, 1992.

42. Hannan E, Farrell L, Meaker P, et al: Predicting inpatient mortality for pediatric blunt trauma patients: A better alternative. J Pediatr Surg 35:155–159, 2000.

43. Levick NR, Li G, Yannaccone J: Biomechanics of the patient compartment of ambulance vehicles under crash conditions: Testing countermeasures to mitigate injury. Soc Automotive Eng Australasia 01:73, 2001.

44. National Highway Traffic Safety Administration/Emergency Medical Services for Children/Health Resources and Services Administration: Do's and Don'ts of Transporting Children in an Ambulance: Fact Sheet. Washington, DC, National Highway Traffic Safety Administration/Emergency Medical Services for Children/ Health Resources and Services Administration, 1999.

45. American College of Surgeons Committee on Trauma: Advanced Trauma, Life Support for Doctors Student Manual 2004 Edition. Chicago: American College of Surgeons (in press).

46. Lubitz DS, Seidel JS, Chameides L, et al: A rapid method for estimating weight and resuscitation drug doses from length in the pediatric age group. Ann Emerg Med 17:576–581, 1988.

47. Schwaitzberg SD, Bergman KS, Harris BH: A pediatric model of continuous hemorrhage. J Pediatr Surg 23:605–609, 1988.

48. Kincaid EH, Chang MC, Letton RW, et al: Admission base deficit in pediatric trauma: A study using the National Trauma Data Bank. J Trauma 51:332–335, 2001.

49. Oldham KT, Guice KS, Kaufman RA, et al: Blunt hepatic injury and elevated hepatic enzymes: A clinical correlation in children. J Pediatr Surg 19:457–461, 1984.

50. Adamson WT, Hebra A, Thomas PB, et al: Serum amylase and lipase alone are not cost-effective screening methods for pediatric pancreatic trauma. J Pediatr Surg 38:354–357, 2003.

51. Lieu TA, Fleisher GR, Mahboubi S, et al: Hematuria and clinical findings as indications for intravenous pyelography in pediatric blunt renal trauma. Pediatrics 82:216–222, 1988.

52. Taylor GA, Eichelberger MR, O'Donnel R, et al: Indications for computed tomography in children with blunt abdominal trauma. Ann Surg 213:212–218, 1991.

53. Coley BD, Mutabagani KH, Martin LC, et al: Focused abdominal sonography for trauma (FAST) in children with blunt abdominal trauma. J Trauma 48:902–906, 2000.

54. Emery KH, McAneney CM, Racadio JM et al: Absent peritoneal fluid on screening trauma ultrasonography in children: A prospective comparison with computed tomography. J Pediatr Surg 36:565–569, 2001.

55. Filiatrault D, Longpre D, Patriquin H, et al: Investigation of childhood blunt abdominal trauma: A practical approach using ultrasound as the initial diagnostic modality. Pediatr Radiol 17:373–379, 1987.

56. Adelson PD, Bratton SL, Carney NA, et al: Guidelines for the acute medical management of severe traumatic brain injury in infants, children, and adolescents. J Trauma 54:S235–S310, 2003.

57. Temkin NR, Dimken SS, Wilensky AJ, et al: A randomized, double-blind study of phenytoin for the prevention of post-traumatic seizures. N Engl J Med 323:673–680, 1990.

58. Fanconi S, Klotio J, Meuli M, et al: Dexamethasone and endogenous cortisol production in severe pediatric head injury. Intens Care Med 14:163–166, 1988.

59. Ford EG, Jennings LM, Andrassy RJ: Steroid administration potentiates nitrogen losses in head-injured children. J Trauma 27:1074–1077, 1987.

60. Bracken MB, Shepard MJ, Collins WF, et al: A randomized, controlled trial of methylprednisolone or naloxone in the treatment of acute spinal cord injury. N Engl J Med 322:1405–1411, 1990.

61. Rothenberg SS, Moore EE, Moore FA, et al: Emergency department thoracotomy in children: A critical analysis. J Trauma 29:1322–1325, 1989.

62. Li G, Tang N, DiScala C, et al: Cardiopulmonary resuscitation in pediatric trauma patients: Survival and functional outcome. J Trauma 47:1–7, 1999.

63. Stylianos S, APSA Trauma Committee: Evidence-based guidelines for resource utilization in children with isolated spleen or liver injury. J Pediatr Surg 35:164–169, 2000.

64. Winthrop AL, Wesson DE, Pencharz PB, et al: Injury severity, whole body protein turnover, and energy expenditure in pediatric trauma. J Pediatr Surg 22:534–537, 1987.

65. Oliver RC, Sturtevant JP, Scheetz JP, et al: Beneficial effects of a hospital bereavement intervention program after traumatic childhood death. J Trauma 50:440–448, 2001.

66. Selbst SM, Henretig F, Fee MA, et al: Lead poisoning in a child with a gunshot wound. Pediatrics 77:413–416, 1986.

67. American College of Surgeons Committee on Trauma: Resources for Optimal Care of the Injured Patient: 2004. Chicago, American College of Surgeons (in press).

68. Pollack MM, Alexander SR, Clarke N, et al: Improved outcomes from tertiary center pediatric intensive care: A statewide comparison of tertiary and nontertiary care facilities. Crit Care Med 19:150–159, 1991.

69. Nakayama DK, Copes WS, Sacco WJ: Differences in pediatric trauma care among pediatric and nonpediatric centers. J Pediatr Surg 27:427–431, 1992.

70. Cooper A, Barlow B, DiScala C, et al: Efficacy of pediatric trauma care: Results of a population-based study. J Pediatr Surg 28:299–305, 1993.

71. Hall JR, Reyes HM, Meller JT, et al: Outcome for blunt trauma is best at a pediatric trauma center. J Pediatr Surg 31:72–77, 1996.

72. Hulka F, Mullins RJ, Mann NC, et al: Influence of a statewide trauma system on pediatric hospitalization and outcome. J Trauma 42:514–519, 1997.

73. Potoka DA, Schall LC, Gardner MJ, et al: Impact of pediatric trauma centers on mortality in a statewide system. J Trauma 49:237–245, 2000.

74. Potoka DA, Schall LC, Ford HR: Improved functional outcome for severely injured children treated at pediatric trauma centers. J Trauma 51:824–834, 2001.

75. Farrell LS, Hannan EL, Cooper A: Severity of injury and mortality associated with pediatric blunt injuries: Hospitals with pediatric intensive care units vs. other hospitals. Pediatr Crit Care Med (in press).

76. Smith DF, Hackel A: Selection criteria for pediatric critical care transport teams. Crit Care Med 11:10–12, 1983.

77. MacNab AJ: Optimal escort for interhospital transport of pediatric emergencies. J Trauma 31:205–209, 1991.

78. Kanter RK, Boeing NM, Hannan WP, et al: Excess morbidity associated with interhospital transport. Pediatrics 90:893–898, 1992.

79. Edge WE, Kanter RK, Weigle CGM, et al: Reduction of morbidity in interhospital transport by specialized pediatric staff. Crit Care Med 22:1186–1191, 1994.

80. Knudson MM, Shagoury C, Lewis FR: Can adult trauma surgeons care for injured children? J Trauma 32:729–739, 1992.

81. Fortune JM, Sanchez J, Graca L, et al: A pediatric trauma center without a pediatric surgeon: A four year outcome analysis. J Trauma 33:130–139, 1992.

82. Rhodes M, Smith S, Boorse D: Pediatric trauma patients in an "adult" trauma center. J Trauma 35:384–393, 1993.

83. Bensard DD, McIntyre RC, Moore EE, et al: A critical analysis of acutely injured children managed in an adult level I trauma center. J Pediatr Surg 29:11–18, 1994.

84. D'Amelio LF, Hammond JS, Thomasseau J, et al: "Adult" trauma surgeons with pediatric commitment: A logical solution to the pediatric trauma manpower problem. Am Surg 61:968–974, 1995.

85. Partrick DA, Moore EE, Bensard DD, et al: Operative management of injured children at an adult level I trauma center. J Trauma 48:894–901, 2000.

86. Osler TM, Vane DW, Tepas JJ, et al: Do pediatric trauma centers have better survival rates than adult trauma centers? An examination of the National Pediatric Trauma Registry. J Trauma 50:96–101, 2001.

87. Sherman HF, Landry VL, Jones LM: Should level I trauma centers be rated NC-17? J Trauma 50:784–791, 2001.

88. vanAmerongen RH, Fine JS, Tunik MG, et al: The Avianca plane crash: An emergency medical system's response to pediatric survivors of the disaster. Pediatrics 92:105–110, 1993.

89. Wass AR, Williams MJ, Gibson MF: A review of the management of a major incident involving predominantly pediatric casualties. Injury 25:371–374, 1994.

90. Quinn B, Baker R, Pratt J: Hurricane Andrew and a pediatric emergency department. Ann Emerg Med 23:737–741, 1994.

91. Iskit SH, Aplay H, Tugtepe H, et al: Analysis of 33 pediatric trauma victims in the 1999 Marmara, Turkey, earthquake. J Pediatr Surg 36:368–372, 1999.

92. Jain V, Noponen V, Smith BM: Pediatric surgical emergencies in the setting of a natural disaster: Experiences from the 2001 earthquake in Gujarat, India. J Pediatr Surg 38:663–667, 2003.

93. Quintana DA, Jordan FB, Tuggle DW, et al: The spectrum of pediatric injuries after a bomb blast. J Pediatr Surg 32:307–311, 1997.

94. American Academy of Pediatrics Committee on Pediatric Emergency Medicine: The pediatrician's role in disaster preparedness. Pediatrics 99:130–133, 1997.

95. Committee on Pediatric Emergency Medicine: Pediatricians' liability during disasters. Pediatrics 106:1492–1493, 2000.

96. American Academy of Pediatrics Committee on Pediatric Emergency Medicine: Chemical-biological terrorism and its impact on children: A subject review. Pediatrics 105:662–670, 2000.

97. Henretig FM, Cieslak TJ: Bioterrorism and pediatric emergency medicine. Clin Pediatr Emerg Med 2:211–222, 2001.

98. American Academy of Pediatrics Committee on Environmental Health: Radiation disasters in children. Pediatrics 111:1455–1466, 2003.

99. Rotenberg JS, Newmark J: Nerve agent attacks on children: Diagnosis and management. Pediatrics 112:648–658, 2003.

100. Foltin G, Tunik M, Cooper A, et al. (eds): Teaching Resource for Instructors of Prehospital Pediatrics. New York, Center for Pediatric Emergency Medicine, 1998.

CHAPTER 15

Thoracic Trauma in Children

Gary K. Lofland, MD, and James E. O'Brien, Jr., MD

In North America, trauma is the leading cause of death in patients younger than 35 years, the leading cause of death in children older than 1 year, and the third leading cause of death overall. A study by the Institute of Medicine verified that for 30 years, the number 1 cause of death between the ages of 1 and 16 years is unintentional injury.[1] Although thoracic injury accounts for only 5% to 12% of admissions to a trauma center, it is associated with greater lethality. In isolation, thoracic trauma in children carries a 5% mortality; however, this increases to 25% when head or abdominal injuries are superimposed.[2,3] The majority of these patients die before reaching a patient care facility.

EPIDEMIOLOGIC OVERVIEW

When the lethal nature of thoracic injury in children became more apparent, an increased interest arose in the epidemiology of this issue. Prior to 1979, only two comprehensive studies of this subject existed in the English literature. However, since then, at least a dozen additional reports published with the report of the National Pediatric Trauma Registry contain the greatest amount of information.[4] The overall incidence of thoracic injury in children sustaining blunt trauma was measured at 29% of 230 children in one study.[5] In another study of 110 patients, 25% of the patients had major thoracic injury requiring therapy, and an additional 33% had minor to moderate chest injury not requiring therapy.[6] Blunt trauma accounts for approximately 85% of chest injuries serious enough to warrant treatment in a pediatric trauma center. Of these, nearly three fourths are attributable to motor vehicle trauma, with the remainder caused by falls or bicycle- or motorcycle-related trauma. Penetrating injuries account for 15% of the pediatric patients sustaining major chest trauma. Of these, three-fifths are caused by gunshots, and two fifths, by stabbings or injuries from other sharp objects.

Fifteen percent of the children with thoracic injuries will not survive their trauma. This is true for both blunt and penetrating trauma. In patients with blunt trauma, approximately half of these deaths are caused by the associated neurologic injury, whereas nearly 100% of the mortality resulting from penetrating injuries is caused by the chest injury. Multiple injuries involving the thorax are about twice as common as is isolated injury to this region and also are about twice as lethal. Data from the National Pediatric Trauma Registry show that whereas the incidence of injury to the thoracic region is measured at only 1%, the mortality associated with injury to thoracic organs is higher than any other type of injury including traumatic brain injury.[4] Major blunt trauma to the chest is associated with a mortality rate of about 20% if only the lung and pleural spaces are involved; however, this increases dramatically as other organs are involved, increasing to 50% if great vessels are involved. For major penetrating injuries, lung injuries are associated with a mortality rate approaching 30%, yet with injuries to the heart and blood vessels, predictable mortality rates approach 50%. If two body systems are injured, as assessed by the Abbreviated Injury Scale (AIS), the mortality rate is 28.6%. For injuries to three body regions, the mortality rate is 33%. Combined injuries to the head, chest, and abdomen produce a mortality rate of 38%.[7]

In summary, despite its low overall incidence, chest trauma is among the most serious of childhood injuries, second only to severe head injury in lethal potential. Although thoracic injuries themselves are the cause of death in fewer than 1% of all cases of major pediatric blunt trauma, multisystem trauma is about 10 times more deadly when it is associated with a chest injury. The presence of a major thoracic trauma therefore serves as a marker of injury severity.

UNIQUE FEATURES OF PEDIATRIC THORACIC INJURIES

The pattern of injury and resultant physiologic derangement is somewhat different in a child than in an adult. Some of this difference relates to body size and proportions, and some relates to elasticity. Biomechanically, the smaller body mass of a child means

185

that transferred energy from a traumatic impact results in a greater force applied per unit body area. This focused intense energy is applied to a body with less fat, less elastic connective tissue, and a close proximity of vital organs, especially in the thoracic region. In addition, the blood volume of the small patient is 7% to 8% of total body weight. A relatively small blood-volume loss can lead to hypovolemia and shock.

The child's thorax is remarkably compliant. The bony and cartilaginous structures are pliable and will absorb kinetic energy that must be dissipated by intrathoracic structures. The child might have significant intrathoracic injury without any injury to bony structures of the chest wall. Flail-chest injury is rarely seen until the child reaches adolescence.

Children sustaining trauma of any form may experience aerophagia. Gastric dilation may become massive, may compromise diaphragmatic excursion, and may compress intrathoracic structures. Nasogastric decompression of the stomach is necessary in the injured child to decrease the size of the air-filled stomach, allowing better ventilation and protection against aspiration.

It is unusual for children sustaining thoracic injury to have preexisting disease involving other organ systems. As a result, the potential for recovery is tremendous if the pathophysiology that accompanies those injuries can be reversed.

Although one usually associates injury with blunt or penetrating mechanisms, other causes of injury to intrathoracic organs exist. Injuries to the esophagus may occur as a result of foreign body ingestion or as a result of ingestion of corrosive agents. Iatrogenic injury to the esophagus may occur at the time of esophageal intubation occurring with nasogastric intubation, transesophageal echocardiography (TEE), or esophagogastroduodenoscopy (EGD).

Bronchopulmonary injuries may be caused by blunt and penetrating trauma. Mechanical ventilation predisposes babies to barotrauma. This is especially true in the premature neonate.

Finally, because of the proportionately smaller size of the chest when compared with the abdomen or head in a young child, significant thoracic trauma is almost always accompanied by injury to other organ systems, which is associated with a markedly increased mortality. These systems must be evaluated concurrent with evaluation of the potentially life-threatening intrathoracic injury.

HISTORICAL ASPECTS

The management of thoracic trauma has evolved over a period of 5000 years. The Smith Papyrus (3000 BC) contains notations about chest injuries treated by Imhotep.[8] These were simple injuries treated with relatively simple techniques.

Hippocrates,[9] writing in the 4th century BC, associated rib fractures with hemoptysis and prescribed rest and bloodletting for patients with broken ribs. He also advocated stabilization of the chest wall with binding, an appropriate therapy in an age of inadequate pain control. The ancient Egyptians, Romans, and Greeks considered penetrating injuries of the chest almost uniformly fatal. In the 3rd century BC, Aristotle[10] wrote, "The heart alone of all the viscera cannot withstand injury." Galen,[11] writing in the 2nd century AD, described packing open chest wounds suffered by gladiators in Rome. Ambrose Paré[12] in the 16th century described subcutaneous emphysema associated with chest-wall injury and recommended debriding segments of broken ribs. In the 17th century, Riolanus[13] treated cardiac injuries in animals. Riolanus and Scultetus[14] described empyema as a complication of penetrating thoracic injury. Scultetus also advocated drainage tubes and irrigation for established intrapleural infections, with the drainage tubes functioning largely as passive conduits. The importance of suction was recognized, however, especially in the treatment of infection. In the absence of an efficient mechanical means of aspiration, oral aspiration of wounds by professional "wound suckers" arose as a means of treating chest infections (Fig. 15-1). Anel,[15] a military surgeon who wrote a treatise entitled The Art of Sucking Wounds in 1707, noted that professional wound suckers had (not surprisingly) frequent oral infections.

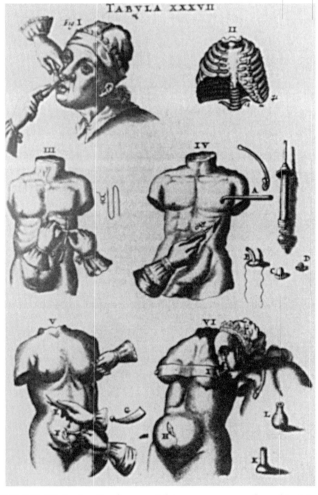

FIGURE 15-1. In the lower right corner, wound sucking is demonstrated. Also illustrated are incisions for the drainage of empyema and irrigation devices. (From a 17th century text, Scultetus J: The Surgeon's Storehouse. London, Starkey, 1674, p 159, with permission.)

Playfair[16] developed a rudimentary water seal device to drain the pleural cavity in the 19th century. Thoracentesis, however, was associated with a high mortality rate. Dupuytren of Paris, one of the leading surgeons of the day, reportedly performed thoracentesis on 50 patients, with only two long-term survivors. When Dupuytren[17] subsequently developed an empyema himself, he refused thoracentesis, saying that he would "rather die by the hand of God than by that of surgeons."

Considerable debate occurred about the treatment of injuries to the heart, with no less a figure than Theodore Billroth[18] stating in 1885, "The surgeon who should attempt to suture a wound to the heart would lose the respect of his colleagues." Despite these sentiments expressed by otherwise erudite figures, the first repairs of a penetrating cardiac wound in a human were performed in 1896 by Rehn of Frankfurt, Germany,[19] and shortly thereafter by Lucius Hill of Montgomery, Alabama.

Many of the advances in the treatment of thoracic trauma in the 20th century are the result of improvements in anesthesia, imaging, and respiratory supportive care. Positive-pressure ventilation permitted more aggressive surgical management of thoracic wounds. Refinements in equipment and technique allowed radiography of the chest, which rapidly became widely available.[20] As an outgrowth of experience with casualties during World War I, drainage of the chest for empyema became routine.[21] The development of antibiotics, which began in the 1930s, and widespread acceptance of the importance of drainage of the pleural cavity for noninfectious complications, markedly improved the prognosis for both penetrating and blunt injuries. Experience with mass casualties during World War II demonstrated the efficacy of aggressive management of thoracic injuries.

Since the Korean War, the availability of cardiopulmonary bypass has allowed treatment of cardiac injuries. More recently, the development of computed tomography (CT) and MRI has allowed better understanding of thoracic injuries and their management. In critical care, prolonged survival of patients with injuries that had previously been fatal has led to the formal description of the adult respiratory distress syndrome. Increasing organization of trauma care delivery, much of which was based on experience in Korea and Vietnam, and efforts at injury prevention also have reduced morbidity and mortality.[22]

Pediatric patients with thoracic injuries have benefited immensely from the military experience in the management of adults with thoracic injuries. The establishment of pediatric advanced life support and of designated pediatric trauma centers has resulted in better definition of thoracic injuries and expedited management of these injuries.

INITIAL EVALUATION AND MANAGEMENT

The initial resuscitation of patients with thoracic injuries follows the same principles as the resuscitation of any trauma patient or any patient for whom advanced cardiac life support is required. These principles are known as the "ABCs," a popular acronym for airway, breathing, and circulation.[23,24] Some elements of the ABCs are of particular significance for patients with thoracic injuries.

The first priority is ensuring an adequate airway.[25–27] The goal of airway management in the injured pediatric patient is optimal ventilation and oxygenation while simultaneously protecting the cervical spine. One should assume that any child who sustains significant trauma has a cervical spine injury until proven otherwise. A 42% mortality rate is associated with traumatic spinal injuries in children.[28] The cervical spines of all injured children should be managed with cervical in-line immobilization with the head in a neutral position. One should assume that cervical spine injury exists until a roentgenogram of a lateral cervical spine clearly delineates all seven cervical vertebrae to be intact. In a hemodynamically unstable child, however, when cervical radiographs cannot be obtained immediately, the neck should be immobilized both for transport and for ensuring airway patency.

The pediatric airway is easily obstructed, especially in the child with multiple injuries and an altered level of consciousness. A loss of muscle tone in the oropharynx may cause the tongue to fall posteriorly, contributing to airway obstruction. Another cause of airway obstruction is the presence of blood, vomitus, secretions, or foreign objects in the oropharynx, larynx, or trachea. Severe injuries of the mandible or facial bones or crush injuries of the larynx or trachea also may contribute to airway obstruction. Compared with that of the adult, the child's tongue is proportionately larger in a smaller oral cavity, the glottic opening is more anterior and cephalad, and the trachea is shorter and narrower. These anatomic differences make the pediatric airway somewhat more difficult to manage and also more prone to iatrogenic injury by inexperienced personnel. Symptoms of upper airway obstruction are dyspnea, diminished breath sounds despite respiratory effort, retractions, dysphagia, drooling, and dysphonia.

Acute management of the obstructed airway consists first of a jaw-thrust maneuver and the administration of supplemental oxygen. The jaw-thrust maneuver is accomplished by placing fingers behind the angles of the mandible and lifting. The neck should remain in a neutral position; both hyperextension and flexion should be avoided. Any foreign materials in the mouth or oropharynx should be removed, either manually or by strong suction. Oral or nasopharyngeal airways are very poorly tolerated by the semiconscious child, and they may induce gagging and vomiting. Any child who tolerates an oral or nasopharyngeal airway should be assumed to have compromised protective reflexes and therefore requires definitive airway management with an endotracheal tube. The child should be ventilated by bag/valve/mask with 100% oxygen until intubation is accomplished. Orotracheal intubation is the preferred approach in the injured child, as opposed to the adult, who may tolerate nasotracheal intubation. Unlike in adults, cricothyroidotomy or tracheostomy is rarely necessary in children, except when severe maxillofacial or laryngeal injury has occurred. Even in these circumstances, an oral airway can usually be established. In children younger than 12 years, the cricothyroid cartilage is the major support structure for the upper airway, and thus cricothyroidotomy should be avoided in children if at all possible.[23]

Tension pneumothorax may profoundly affect ventilation and perfusion. Physical signs of tension pneumothorax include acute respiratory distress or cyanosis despite adequate airway, tracheal deviation, unilateral absence of breath sounds, or diffuse breath sounds over the chest and abdomen. Both penetrating and blunt injuries also may cause hemothorax or pulmonary contusion.

Resuscitation of the child with chest trauma begins with a survey for immediate life-threatening injury by using the Oslerian principles of observation, inspection, palpation, and auscultation. To assess for adequate ventilation, observe symmetrical chest expansion, auscultate equal breath sounds bilaterally, and evaluate the entire chest wall for signs of contusion or chest-wall penetration. If ventilation or oxygenation is inadequate, reassess airway and breathing. Check for correct placement and patency of the endotracheal tube, and consider the presence of pneumothorax, hemothorax, or other thoracic injury. These can be confirmed radiographically. Adequate oxygenation is present if the skin is pink centrally and oxygen saturation is 85% or greater by pulse oximetry.

Cardiovascular collapse after the institution of positive pressure ventilation is usually indicative of a major tracheobronchial injury. These injuries can carry mortality as high as 30%, and rapid recognition and treatment are required.

When breathing remains inadequate after positive pressure ventilation, needle thoracentesis to exclude pneumothorax should be considered. One should keep in mind, however, that diagnosis by needle thoracentesis requires tube thoracostomy for definitive treatment. If an open pneumothorax is present, petrolatum-impregnated gauze in a sterile dressing will suffice to cover the defect, thereby reestablishing chest-wall integrity. Once this is accomplished, however, a tube thoracostomy is necessary, because it is likely that the visceral pleura would have been injured, creating the potential for development of a tension pneumothorax. In the unlikely event of an unstable chest wall from flail chest, the management of any degree of respiratory compromise is endotracheal intubation and mechanical ventilation. Flail chest will usually be seen only in older children or adolescents who sustain substantial crush injuries to the chest.

Once ventilation and oxygenation are established, circulation is the next priority. Early signs of shock may be subtle in children. Normal blood volume in a child varies from 7% to 8% or 70 to 80 mL/kg body weight.[28] A volume loss that might be considered small in an adult may induce shock in a child, although hypotension may not occur until 25% of blood volume is lost. Fluid management should be aggressive and instituted early during resuscitation. An initial bolus of 20 mL/kg of lactated Ringer's solution is appropriate for any signs of shock. This volume may be repeated as necessary, even in the event of concomitant head injury. The goal of aggressive fluid resuscitation is the prevention of irreversible hypotension resistant to any resuscitative efforts, leading to multiple organ system failure and death.

If prompt improvement in the circulatory status does not occur or if signs of venous obstruction appear, the possibility of a cardiac tamponade must be entertained. In children, cardiac tamponade may result from the usual hemopericardium or also from trapped air in the pericardial space from a bronchial injury. Needle aspiration in the pericardial space is life saving in the presence of a pericardial tamponade. However, all patients with a positive pericardiocentesis will require urgent thoracotomy or a median sternotomy for inspection of the heart. Quite frequently the pericardiocentesis will allow stabilization of the patient and alleviate the need for an emergency thoracotomy.

The indications for proceeding with urgent thoracotomy are as follows[7]:

1. Penetrating wound to the heart or great vessels
2. Massive or continuous interpleural hemorrhage
3. Open pneumothorax with major chest-wall defect
4. Aortogram confirming aortic transection
5. Massive pleural air leak suggestive of bronchial or tracheal disruption
6. Positive results from pericardiocentesis or subxyphoid window
7. Rupture of the esophagus
8. Rupture of the diaphragm
9. No palpable pulse despite cardiac massage

Whereas the need for emergency department thoracotomy is rare, the presence of a penetrating wound in the area of the midsternum or left sternal border and failure of the child to respond promptly to resuscitation efforts are the usual indications. Emergency department thoracotomies for blunt trauma are rarely successful and should be avoided.

THE MANAGEMENT OF SPECIFIC INJURIES

Traumatic Asphyxia

Traumatic asphyxia is an entity observed in children because of a flexible thorax and absence of valves in the venous system of the inferior and superior vena cava. Direct compression of the chest wall is sustained when the child is run over by a vehicle or otherwise crushed. At the time of injury, if the glottis is closed and the thoracoabdominal muscles are tensed, the increased intrathoracic pressure is transmitted through the central venous system to solid organs such as the brain, liver, spleen, and kidneys. The patient is usually disoriented, with tachypnea, hemoptysis, and respiratory insufficiency. The face and neck are cyanotic, with petechiae on the head, neck, and chest. Subconjunctival and retinal hemorrhages are often present. Acute hepatomegaly secondary to transmitted caval pressure may be seen. If the patient exhibits a significant degree of pulmonary contusion, endotracheal intubation and mechanical ventilation with positive end-expiratory pressure (PEEP) may be necessary. Traumatic asphyxia is rarely life threatening, although mortality may result from the associated injuries.[29,30]

Subcutaneous Emphysema

Subcutaneous emphysema occurs when the air is forced into the tissue planes of the chest. It is primarily a sign of underlying injury to ribs, pleura, intercostal muscles, bronchus, trachea, or pulmonary parenchyma. Treatment of children with subcutaneous emphysema is directed toward the primary injury, because the subcutaneous air has no physiologic effect and is spontaneously absorbed.

Rib Fractures

The thorax of the child is quite compliant because of the elasticity of the ribs, resulting from their having greater cartilage content than those in adults. This compliance diffuses the force of impact, leading to fewer rib fractures than would result from a similar injury to an adult. Although splinting from the discomfort is common in children, atelectasis rarely occurs because of the propensity of children to cry.

Diagnosis of acute rib fractures is by roentgenogram or by roentgenogram plus bone scan to detect healing rib fractures in the child thought to be a victim of abuse. Multiple rib fractures should always raise the suspicion of child abuse. Rib fractures often result in intrapleural injury. Children with rib fractures are twice as likely to have a pneumothorax or hemothorax as are those without. Whereas some of this may be attributable to the sharp edges of the bony fragments tearing the visceral and parietal pleura, the force required to produce a rib fracture is frequently sufficient to produce intrathoracic injury (Fig. 15-2).

Oral analgesics are usually sufficient to control pain, and only rarely is an intercostal nerve block necessary.

Pneumothorax

Pneumothorax may result from puncture of the lung by a rib, by a penetrating chest wall injury, by disruption of the pulmonary parenchyma, or by injury to the tracheobronchial tree.

Sucking chest wounds are relatively rare in children. When they do occur, they are most commonly associated with blast injuries, severe avulsion injuries, or close-range shotgun wounds. Sucking chest wounds can be urgently treated by covering them with an occlusive dressing, which prevents further ingress of air from the outside. Because a pneumothorax or hemopneumothorax may develop, tube thoracostomy drainage also should be done. Definitive treatment is dictated by the mechanism of injury and the response to simple therapeutic methods.

Pneumothorax is more commonly caused by air entering the pleural space via a hole in the lung. The lung is often injured on its surface by broken ribs. When the patient inspires, the hole in the lung surface opens as the lung expands, but with expiration, the hole closes. As pressure in the pleural space increases, the hole in the pulmonary surface is less and less likely to open with inspiratory effort. In most cases, the lung collapses to the point at which intrapleural air no longer accumulates with inspiration, and the pneumothorax is stable.

Sometimes, however, air continues to accumulate in the pleural space with each inspiratory effort. The fact that the hole opens with inspiration and closes with expiration produces a valvelike mechanism that causes the pneumothorax to increase in size with each respiratory cycle, producing a tension pneumothorax. Although tension pneumothorax is possible during spontaneous ventilation, it is more commonly seen when a patient is undergoing positive-pressure ventilation. Accordingly, when a patient deteriorates hemodynamically with institution of positive-pressure ventilation, the possibility of a tension pneumothorax should be considered and urgently treated.

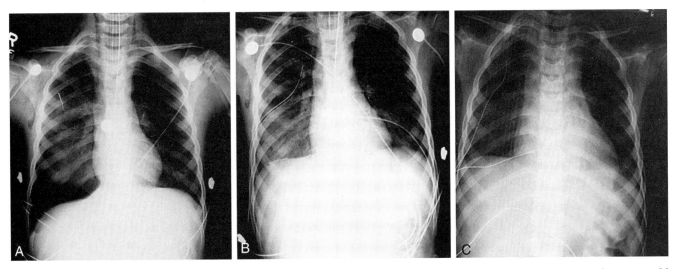

FIGURE 15-2. *A*, Multiple rib fractures and a pneumothorax are clearly apparent in this chest roentgenogram of a 7-year-old patient involved in a motor vehicle accident. The patient was not wearing restraints at the time of injury and had multiple other injuries. *B*, Complete re-expansion of the lung after chest tube insertion. *C*, Persistent complete expansion of the right lung and resolution of pulmonary contusion after chest tube removal.

If the pressure in the pleural space with tension pneumothorax becomes high enough, both respiration and hemodynamics are impaired. High intrapleural pressures on the side of injury minimize effective expansion of the lungs. As the pressure in the ipsilateral pleural cavity increases, the heart is pushed toward the contralateral side of the chest, venous return is compromised, and cardiac output decreases. This pathophysiology is easily and quickly reversed with decompression of the pneumothorax. Some of the physical findings associated with tension pneumothorax are identical to those seen with any pneumothorax but may be more pronounced. No breath sounds are observed on the injured side, subcutaneous air may develop, and the trachea may be deviated away from the site of injury. Shock also may be present and, because of interference with venous return to the right atrium, neck veins may be distended. Neck vein distention is not a particularly sensitive sign, however, because it may not be present in patients who also are hypovolemic.

It is almost always necessary to treat a pneumothorax resulting from blunt injury with a chest tube, particularly in patients who also are being treated with positive-pressure ventilation (Fig. 15-3). The presence of unexpanded

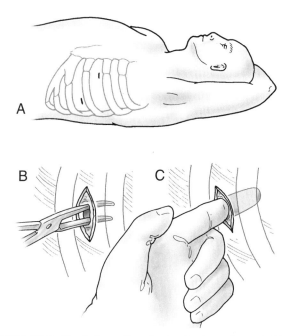

FIGURE 15-3. Technique for chest tube insertion. *A,* Two potential sites for chest tube insertion. The upper site is in the anterior axillary line in the fourth intercostal space. The lower site is in the fifth or sixth intercostal space in the midaxillary line. Either site allows the chest tube to be directed either anteriorly or posteriorly. An anterior direction is preferred for pneumothorax, whereas a more posterior placement is preferred for fluid or hemothorax. *B,* After a small skin incision has been made, a Crile or Kelly clamp may be used to enlarge the incision slightly, dissect subcutaneously, and penetrate the pleural space on the anterior surface of a rib. *C,* Placement of a finger through the incision into the pleural space ensures that no pleural adhesions are present and that the pleural space has indeed been entered. Such a maneuver helps prevent placement of the tube into pulmonary parenchyma.

lung and fluid in the chest can predispose the patient to the development of empyema. In addition, some element of lung function may be permanently lost if the lung is not re-expanded.

Tubes that are large enough to drain any associated hemothorax adequately should generally be placed in the fourth or fifth intercostal space in the midaxillary line. Small catheters, such as pigtail catheters, should be avoided. Careful insertion with an open technique should be used, especially as the hemidiaphragm is sometimes quite elevated in the chest or may even be ruptured.

Hemothorax

Like pneumothorax, hemothorax is a common finding after chest trauma and frequently accompanies pneumothorax. Physical findings are not usually helpful, and the diagnosis is usually established radiographically. Hemothorax may be missed if the radiograph is taken with the patient in the supine position. A fluid level is not always appreciated, and even a large hemothorax can appear as simple elevation of the hemidiaphragm if the radiograph is taken in the upright position.

As with pneumothorax, a small traumatic hemothorax is sometimes missed on the initial chest radiograph and is seen later on the upper cuts of a computerized tomographic study or MRI study of the abdomen. One should maintain a very low threshold for tube thoracostomy. Persistent blood in the chest increases the risk of empyema and loss of lung function and may sometimes necessitate decortication later.

Early placement of a thoracostomy tube can help greatly in the drainage of blood from the pleural cavity, but blood has a natural tendency to clot, and small amounts of residual hemothorax in a chest film taken shortly after placement of a chest tube are therefore fairly common. Usually this clot will lyse over the next several days.

When drainage from the tube is minimal and the radiographic findings demonstrate persistent hemothorax, continued attempts at drainage are rarely successful. Definitive treatment of significant hemothorax that persists beyond several days involves evacuation of the clot, removal of whatever organized peel has developed on the pleural surfaces, and placement of a new thoracostomy tube.

The increased use of thoracoscopy and refinement of video thoracoscopic equipment has led to a resurgence in the use of thoracoscopy in the trauma patient. Thoracoscopy can be used as both a diagnostic and therapeutic modality. Factors that dissuade the surgeon from using video-assisted thoracic surgery (VATS) in acute situations include the time required for setup, the lack of access to the great vessels and the heart, as well as the need to collapse the lung partially. Conversely, VATS is less invasive and is associated with less morbidity than is thoracotomy. Thus, VATS will be useful in the acute trauma patient when vital signs are stable and in subacute cases when signs are yet too ambiguous to warrant thoracotomy. Use of thoracoscopy as a diagnostic tool is appropriate in the acute or subacute hemodynamically stable patient with a hemothorax, particularly from penetrating trauma. In certain patients with a large initial drainage or continuing blood loss from the chest injury, it may aid in avoiding thoracotomy by visualizing a nonbleeding injury, evacuating hematoma, and allowing tamponade by a fully expanded lung or cauterizing or endoclipping intercostal vessels. It also has been used to diagnose correctly the presence or absence of diaphragmatic injury.[31]

In addition to the acute setting, thoracoscopy can be useful as a therapeutic tool in subacute trauma patients and in patients who have retained hemothorax. By alleviating the need for a thoracotomy in a patient with a retained hemothorax, thoracoscopy can lead to a more aggressive drainage of a retained hemothorax, decreasing the incidence of empyema. In a series of patients with empyema after penetrating chest injury, thoracoscopy also was found to be effective in completely draining the pleural space and is used as definitive therapy for empyema after penetrating chest injury.[32] One study found that 18% of patients with hemothorax treated mostly with tube thoracostomy developed a clotted hemothorax, and approximately 39% of these patients eventually required decortication.[33] The use of VATS would allow a more aggressive management of these patients without the morbidity of a thoracotomy.

Pulmonary Contusion

Some of the damage in a contused lung is the result of hemorrhage into the pulmonary parenchyma. In other areas, injury is more subtle, with damage to the pulmonary microvasculature but no extravasation of red blood cells. This range of injury is analogous to contusion in other areas of the body. Part of the fluid accumulation associated with a contusion is related to hemorrhage, but much of it is caused by extravasation of fluid from the intravascular to the extravascular space as a consequence of the increased pulmonary microvascular permeability seen with a generalized inflammatory reaction. Increased permeability promotes diapedesis of inflammatory cells and diffusion of inflammatory mediators necessary to combat infection and begin repair.

In the lungs, as well as in other areas of the body, accumulation of edema fluid is a natural consequence of increased permeability. Although edema formation may help with resisting infection and initiating repair, edema certainly harms organ function. Alveoli are rendered poorly functional or nonfunctional, interfering with oxygenation and ventilation. In areas such as skeletal muscle and soft tissue, these functional side effects are of minimal importance. In the lungs, however, interstitial and alveolar edema cause arteriovenous shunting and hypoxemia.

The diagnosis of pulmonary contusion, established on the basis of radiography and blood gas analysis, can be difficult. Radiographically, pulmonary contusion appears as patchy areas of pulmonary infiltrate and is usually localized to areas of the lung that underlie obvious chest-wall injury. The radiographic appearance may lag behind the loss of pulmonary function. A higher resolution of CT makes it more sensitive to the detection of pulmonary contusion immediately after injury.[34,35] Its usefulness may be to predict the need for ventilatory support in these patients. According to one study, when CT showed a contusion involving 28% of the total lung volume, those patients eventually required mechanical ventilation, whereas no patient required mechanical ventilation when less than 18% of the lung volume was involved.[36] Blood gas analyses, in the presence of an established contusion, are manifested by hypoxemia. Although other entities such as aspiration can still be confused with contusion, the distinction between the two is largely insignificant in the emergency setting because the initial treatments of the two are identical.

Because pulmonary capillary membrane integrity is part of the pathogenesis of pulmonary contusion, the radiographic abnormalities may increase over the first 24- to 48-hour period after injury as extravasation and edema formation occur. It may be extremely difficult to distinguish contusion from respiratory distress syndrome or from pneumonia.

Whether patients with pulmonary contusion should receive prophylactic antibiotics is controversial. The evidence that antibiotics help prevent pneumonia is not particularly convincing, and antibiotics should not be given routinely unless aspiration has occurred.

An equally contentious issue in the treatment of pulmonary contusion is fluid management. Theoretically, colloid-containing fluids should maintain intravascular osmotic pressure and discourage movement of fluid from the intravascular to the extravascular space. In actuality, the damaged pulmonary microvasculature cannot maintain a colloid osmotic gradient, and contusion is not effectively treated with this approach. Furthermore, the use of diuretics and overly stringent restriction of fluids in the acutely traumatized patient can compromise intravascular volume and perfusion, leading to dysfunction of other organ systems. Patients with pulmonary contusion should be carefully monitored, the goal being the assurance of adequate perfusion. In larger patients, pulmonary artery catheters can be placed, but this is virtually impossible in patients weighing less than 10 kg. Therefore, a balance must be struck between adequate oxygenation and tissue perfusion through careful volume administration.

Injuries to the Trachea and Major Bronchi

Blunt injuries of the trachea and major bronchi are rare.[37–39] The trachea can be injured anywhere along its course, but the most common locations are the neck and near the carina. Injuries to the major bronchi are usually within 2.5 cm of the carina.[40] It is thought in adults that right-sided injuries may be more common than are those on the left, but this is not proven to be true in children (Fig. 15-4).

In the neck, the pathophysiology of blunt injury to the trachea is a "clothesline" mechanism, in which sudden and violent tracheal compression occurs. Sometimes associated injury to the larynx or esophagus is noted.

Several theories about the mechanism of airway injury within the chest have been proposed. One is that the chest is flattened in its anterior/posterior dimension, and

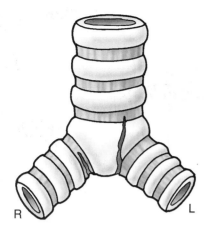

FIGURE 15-4. Complex injury to the trachea and main-stem bronchi secondary to blunt trauma. Of note is that most such injuries are located within 2.5 cm of the carina. (From Millham FH, Rajii-Khorasani A, Birkett DF, et al: Carinal injury: Diagnosis and treatment-case report. J Trauma 31:1420, 1991.)

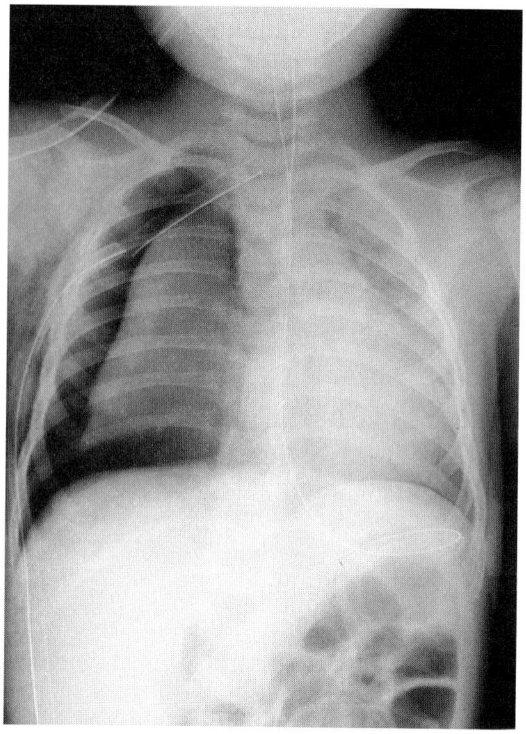

FIGURE 15-5. Chest roentgenogram of a 2-year-old patient who was run over by an automobile. Note the persistent large right pneumothorax despite the adequate placement of a chest tube. This patient was found to have a complete disruption of the right main-stem bronchus at the level of the right upper lobe takeoff.

the lungs, in contact with the parietal pleural of the chest wall, are stretched transversely, with disruption of the carina secondary to the stretching mechanism. Another theory is that chest compression against a closed glottis disrupts the airway from increased intraluminal pressure, creating a "blow-out." Because wall tension is directly proportional to the diameter of the airway, it is greatest in the larger airways, keeping with the empirical observation that most blunt injuries to thoracic trachea or bronchi occur near the carina. A final theory about the pathogenesis of tears of the thoracic trachea and bronchi is similar to the theory for pathogenesis of tears of the thoracic aorta. According to this theory, the trachea is fixed relative to the lungs. With sudden deceleration, shear forces are generated near the carina that can disrupt the airway.

The diagnosis of blunt injury to the trachea or bronchi is sometimes missed initially because many of the associated findings are nonspecific[41] and would be identical to those findings in a patient with a pneumothorax due to pulmonary parenchymal injury. Patients who can communicate often describe dyspnea. If a laryngeal injury is present, speech may be altered or impossible. Most patients have subcutaneous emphysema, but this finding is not always present and may not become manifest until after the institution of positive-pressure ventilation.[42]

Pneumomediastinum may be present. A large pneumothorax is another finding that can aid diagnosis. The likelihood of a major tracheobronchial injury increases if the pneumothorax is not relieved by a tube thoracostomy or if a massive air leak is present after chest tube placement (Fig. 15-5). Although the previously mentioned clinical and radiographic findings suggest a major airway injury, definitive diagnosis should be made with bronchoscopy. Most patients who are stable enough to reach the hospital are stable enough to permit bronchoscopy. Both rigid and fiberoptic bronchoscopy can be used, but injuries can be missed if the bronchoscopist is not experienced.[43]

The first aim of therapy is to stabilize the airway.[44] Nonoperative management may be attempted for small injuries that are seen to encompass less than a third of the airway circumference. Short longitudinal tears of a single airway are particularly likely to be managed successfully in this way. Nonoperative management should not be attempted, even if the injury is less than a third of the circumference of the airway, if the air leak is massive and ventilation is difficult. If nonoperative treatment is attempted, ventilator management must be designed to minimize airway pressures.

Injuries to the cervical trachea should be approached via a transverse neck incision. Tears to the thoracic trachea and major bronchi can be transverse or longitudinal, simple or complex. If the injury is to the distal trachea or right main-stem bronchus, it should be approached via a right thoracotomy. If the injury is limited to the left main-stem bronchus, a left posterior lateral thoracotomy should be used. If injury to only one main-stem bronchus is present, the endotracheal tube should be positioned in the contralateral main-stem bronchus to allow ventilation of the patient while the injured side is repaired. Positioning of the endotracheal tube should be guided by flexible bronchoscopy. Flexible bronchoscopy also will allow an evaluation of the bronchial injury, which will assist in preparation for the surgical repair. Sometimes it is necessary to manipulate placement of the distal end of the endotracheal tube under direct vision after the chest has been opened and the airway has been visualized. Relatively simple repair techniques suffice in most patients, but some patients with complex injury involving the carina or both mainstem bronchi can be safely controlled and repaired with only cardiopulmonary bypass.[44]

Major airway injuries generally should be closed with interrupted sutures, but a continuous suture can be used for longitudinal tears. Although the choice of suture is variable, evidence exists that an absorbable suture reduces the development of granulation tissue and subsequent stricture.[45,46] After closure of the airway defect, the endotracheal tube should be positioned so that the cuff of the tube does not press against the repair. Whenever possible, a tissue flap of pleura, pericardium, or muscle should be placed over the suture line. Postoperative ventilator management should minimize airway pressures. Before extubation, the integrity of the repair can be assessed with fiberoptic bronchoscopy.

Injuries to Great Vessels

Blunt trauma can injure the aorta or the branches of the aortic arch. Approximately 95% of patients with blunt tears of the thoracic aorta die before reaching the hospital.[47] In the small percentage who survive the initial postinjury period, bleeding is limited by the adventitia and other mediastinal tissues.[48,49] Aortic transection in children is extraordinarily rare and does not truly begin to appear until children are of sufficient age to begin riding motorized vehicles, thereby subjecting themselves to potential deceleration injuries.

Pseudoaneurysms of the innominate, common carotid, and subclavian arteries are rare and probably related to a stretch injury. One of the more common of these injuries is disruption of a vessel at its origin from the aorta. The thoracic aorta can tear at a variety of locations, including its ascending portion and at the diaphragm. In patients who survive to reach the hospital, the most common site of disruption is just distal to the origin of the left subclavian artery at the ligamentum arteriosum. This site is the juncture of the mobile aortic arch and the immobile descending thoracic aorta tethered by the intercostal arteries. The aorta is further tethered by the ligamentum arteriosum. In sudden deceleration, the descending aorta stops with the rest of the body, whereas the heart and aortic arch continue moving forward. Shear force develops at the juncture of these two segments of the aorta, creating a tear.[47] Tears range from partial to complete disruption. When partial, the tear usually includes the posteriomedial aorta in the vicinity of the ligamentum arteriosum.

In most patients with tears of the thoracic aorta, no specific physical findings are seen. Occasionally, blood from the aortic tear dissects distally along the course of the left subclavian artery and causes compression and spasm of that artery. The result on physical examination is diminished blood pressure in the left arm as compared with the right. Similar pathophysiology of the descending aorta can lead to differential pulses and blood pressures in the lower as compared with the upper extremities. However, these findings are uncommon and occasionally occur in the absence of a thoracic aorta tear.

Radiographic findings are often more helpful than physical examination. A widened superior mediastinal silhouette should certainly raise suspicions, but the definition of "widened" varies (Fig. 15-6*A*). Only 10% to

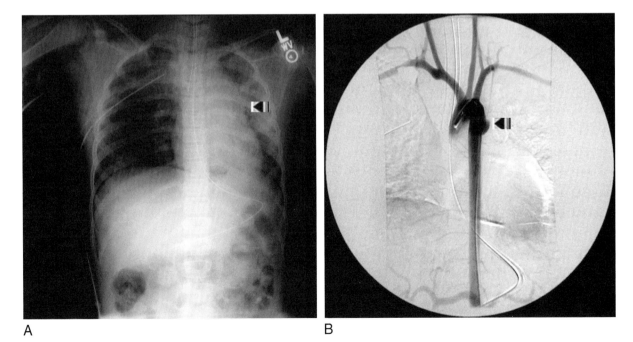

A   B

FIGURE 15-6. Chest radiograph and an aortogram from an 8-year-old patient who was an unrestrained passenger in a motor vehicle accident. On the chest radiograph *(A)* note the widened superior mediastinum and loss of definition of the aortic knob *(arrow)*. Patient also had a right hemothorax that was treated with tube thoracostomy. The aortogram *(B)* shows the pseudoaneurysm at the location of the ligamentum arteriosum just distal to the left subclavian artery, representing the partial transaction of the descending aorta at this point *(arrow)*.

20% of adult patients have what is perceived to be a widened mediastinum. The low specificity can be attributed to mediastinal hematomas that occur in association with venous bleeding, a poor inspiratory effort, and supine views. In a young child, the persistence of a large thymus also may contribute to superior mediastinal widening. Perhaps a more sensitive radiographic indicator is deviation of the esophagus, as visualized on chest roentgenogram after passage of a nasogastric tube.

It is sometimes difficult to decide, on the basis of the initial chest radiograph, which patients require further study.[50] If further investigation is warranted, a decision must be made about what imaging procedure should be used. Angiography is the commonly accepted approach to the definitive diagnosis of a torn thoracic aorta (Fig. 15-6*B*). Aortography is expensive, labor intensive, and invasive, especially in younger patients. For these reasons, a less costly, less invasive, and simpler diagnostic imaging study is desirable. CT is one possibility whose advantages as an alternative to angiography are obvious.[51-53] It can be performed more quickly and is less invasive. It also is more available in more hospitals. Potential disadvantages also exist. If the CT study is not definitive and the patient requires angiography anyway, more contrast agent is necessary, with a delay in diagnosis. Some series also have a disturbingly high percentage of false-negative results.[51,54,55]

Other imaging alternatives for traumatic aortic transection include MRI and TEE. Diagnostic accuracy of MRI is quite acceptable; however, the disadvantage of using this modality revolves around the availability and expediency of obtaining an MRI in an emergency situation. Similarly, TEE also has been shown to have good diagnostic accuracy.[56-58] It has the advantage of being done at the bedside in either the intensive care unit or the trauma bay; however, the availability of TEE will be institution specific and may limit its usefulness in an emergency situation.

Because of their propensity for rupture, traumatic pseudoaneurysms of the thoracic aorta should be treated surgically. A major complication of such repairs is the development of paraplegia as a result of spinal chord ischemia during aortic cross-clamping. Several methods have been developed to prevent this complication, and all of these methods are designed to maintain distal perfusion. None of these methods is foolproof.[59-61] A heparin-bonded Gott shunt may be used to shunt blood without an interposed pump from the proximal aorta to the distal aorta or to the femoral artery. Although this technique is relatively simple and avoids systemic heparinization, it can be cumbersome to work around, and control of the amount of distal perfusion is lacking. Partial left heart bypass uses a centrifugal pump with a draw of oxygenated blood from the left atrium that is reinfused into the femoral artery or the distal thoracic aorta. The advantages of this technique are again the avoidance of systemic heparinization. However, the cannula again can interfere with the operative field. This is especially true in small children. Femoral/femoral cardiopulmonary bypass by using an oxygenator will maintain the lower body perfusion and is relatively easy to institute. In addition, the cannulae are remote from the operative field, and bypass may be instituted before dissection around the

aorta, should rapid aortic cross-clamping become necessary. With modern high-flow, thin-wall cannulae, more than adequate bypass rates can be achieved. In addition, body temperature can be increased or decreased, and hypertension proximal to the cross-clamp can be more easily controlled. This technique does require systemic anticoagulation, and thus may be relatively contraindicated in patients with unstable associated injuries, especially cerebral hemorrhage. The method of femoral/femoral bypass for spinal cord protection is preferred in children. It is relatively easy to institute, and the cannulae do not interfere with the operative field. The bypass cannulae may be placed before dissection around the aorta so that if rapid aortic cross-clamping is necessary, bypass can be instituted immediately.

Thoracic aortic pseudoaneurysm generally should be approached via a left-sided posterolateral thoracotomy. If the pseudoaneurysm is not actively bleeding, and some form of bypass is planned, the thoracotomy incision should be in place so that if aortic cross-clamping is subsequently necessary, bypass can be instituted rapidly. The aorta distal to the pseudoaneurysm should be dissected and encircled with tapes or loops. Proximal control is then obtained, first with the encirclement of the proximal left subclavian artery, and then with encirclement of the aorta between the left common carotid and left subclavian arteries. This technique of proximal control is preferred because it gives the best chance of obtaining control without entering the pseudoaneurysm and because often a very short cuff exists between the origin of the left subclavian artery and the tear. Obtaining proximal control is the most difficult part of the operation. The left recurrent laryngeal nerve loops beneath the ligamentum arteriosum or ductus arteriosus and should be protected. After proximal and distal control have been obtained, the bypass should be started, the pseudoaneurysm entered, and the free edges of the aorta defined. Most patients require placement of a graft, but in occasional cases of partial tears, a primary repair can be done. If a graft is used, woven Dacron is the graft material of choice.

Perioperative antibiotics appropriate for skin flora are used. With an associated pulmonary injury with an air leak, broad-spectrum antibiotics are required. Hypertension should be rigorously controlled with cardioactive β-blocker agents rather than peripheral vasodilators.

Occasionally, patients with a remote history of trauma demonstrate an abnormal mediastinal silhouette on a chest roentgenogram or other symptoms such as airway compression, left recurrent laryngeal nerve compression, or compression of the left subclavian artery. Surgical repair of the chronic aortic pseudoaneurysm is indicated, as outlined previously, even in asymptomatic patients. Repair of the mature aneurysm is considerably more difficult secondary to chronic scarring and the exuberant inflammatory reaction that accompanies extravasation of blood into the mediastinum.

Although most blunt injuries to the great vessels involve the descending thoracic aorta, penetrating injuries of the great vessels can occur in any location. Entrance sites for the wounds to the intrathoracic great vessels can occur in the upper thoracic region, but many will actually be found at the base of the neck. Patients with injuries that are not contained by the surrounding structures or adventitia will have massive bleeding and are in shock on presentation. These patients require emergency thoracotomy, and the definitive diagnosis will be made at the time of surgery. Patients with traumatic pseudoaneurysms of the major intrathoracic vessels are stable, and immediate angiography is used to evaluate the vascular injuries (Fig. 15-7).

The key surgical decision to be made once an injury has been identified is the approach to the great vessels. Injuries to the descending aorta should be approached through a left-sided thoracotomy. Injuries to the proximal aortic arch, the innominate artery, and the proximal left common carotid artery should be approached via median sternotomy. Supraclavicular and/or anterior sternocleido-mastoid extensions are usually necessary for control of the distal carotid or subclavian vessels. Injuries to the left subclavian artery can be exposed by several methods; a left thoracotomy will usually provide adequate exposure to the length of the left subclavian artery. This can be extended in a "trap door" incision, in which a supracla-vicular incision is connected by a partial sternotomy to the thoracotomy. Once the decision regarding the approach has been made, the principles of arterial repair remain the same regardless of the vessel injured. Principles of proximal and distal control should be adhered to and the repairs done by using standard vascular techniques.

Cardiac Injury

Of the nearly 1300 children with blunt thoracic trauma in the National Pediatric Trauma Registry (accumulated from 1985 to 1991), 4.6% had blunt cardiac injury.[62]

Most injuries in this series resulted from children being struck by motor vehicles. Fortunately, cardiac injuries are uncommon in children, the most common being a myocardial contusion. Both blunt and penetrating cardiac trauma are, not surprisingly, more common in boys than in girls. Eighty-eight percent of the patients in the registry multicenter study had at least one other organ system injured in addition to their cardiac injury. Neurologic injury is a common cause of death in these children.[63]

Blunt injuries of the myocardium range from mild asymptomatic contusion to cardiac rupture.[64,65] Nonmyocardial cardiac injuries also are possible. Rupture of the pericardium can occur with or without associated cardiac injury. Laceration or thrombosis of the coronary arteries from blunt trauma is rare but possible. Diagnosis is best made with electrocardiogram and, if time permits, with coronary angiography. Treatment is selective. Repair is indicated if ischemia and myocardial dysfunction are severe and salvageable myocardium is found.

Most patients with rupture of the heart do not survive to reach medical attention. Occasionally, however, bleeding is controlled by tamponade, in which case the patient is initially seen in shock from a combination of hemorrhage and cardiac tamponade.[66] However, in some patients, the admission blood pressure is normal. An admission chest radiograph reveals a wide cardiac shadow.

The mechanism of injury is probably sudden severe compression of the chest at the end of diastole. The site of traumatic rupture from autopsy series are, in order of decreasing frequency: right ventricle, left ventricle, right atrium, and left atrium (Fig. 15-8).[67,68] The prognosis of left atrial and right ventricular injuries is intermediate. Survivors of left ventricular rupture are rare.

Blunt cardiac rupture should be treated surgically (Fig. 15-9). Either sternotomy or thoracotomy can be used, with left-sided thoracotomy being the best approach for left-sided lesions, particularly of the left

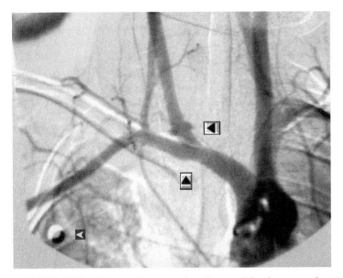

FIGURE 15-7. The angiogram of a 7-year-old who was shot with a BB gun. The entrance wound was in the neck. Note the pseudoaneurysm at the base of the right carotid artery and take-off of the right subclavian artery (*solid triangles*). The BB can be seen in the apex of the right thorax (*open arrow*). The repair was performed via a median sternotomy with a cervical extension.

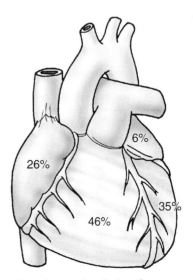

FIGURE 15-8. Location and relative frequency of various cardiac injuries from Baylor College of Medicine.

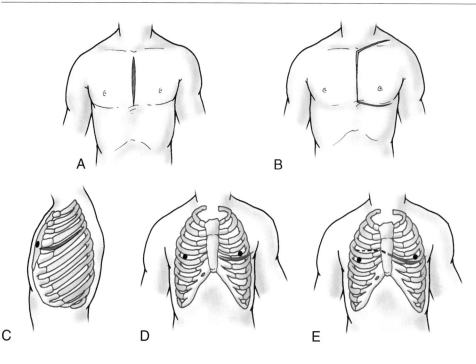

FIGURE 15-9. Incisions that may be used for exposure of intrathoracic injuries.

atrium, and sternotomy, the best approach for right atrial and right ventricular lesions. Most injuries can be repaired without cardiopulmonary bypass. Ruptures of the atria, particularly at the atrial appendage, can initially be controlled with a vascular clamp. Bleeding from rupture of the ventricle sometimes can be temporarily controlled with balloon tamponade by using a urinary catheter placed through the defect.

Blunt trauma more frequently produces contusion of the myocardium. In experimental animals, this can lead to serious arrhythmias and cardiac pump failure. In most animals, these effects occur within seconds to minutes of the blunt injury, but the possibility of delayed manifestation of myocardial contusion is a concern.[69] No reliable standard exists for diagnosis. A number of different diagnostic tests have been proposed.[70–74] Troponin 1 has been found to be elevated (> 2.0 ng/mL) in children with cardiac injury. Levels of greater than 8 ng/mL are associated with a fatal outcome in a group of children with dramatic injury.[75] For many other of these tests, however, establishment of a diagnosis does not correlate with outcome in the vast majority of patients. Creatinine phosphocreatine levels and echocardiography are examples of such low-sensitivity, low-specificity tests and are not helpful in either diagnosis or treatment planning.

Sequelae of myocardial contusion are uncommon in patients who demonstrate hemodynamic and cardiac stability on admission.[70,76] Obviously unstable patients declare the severity of their illness early in the emergency department course and are transferred to a intensive care setting, where they receive treatment for possible myocardial contusion with monitoring, antiarrhythmic drugs, and cardiac support as needed.

One of the most sensitive indicators of significance of contusion appears to be rhythm disturbances. In several series in adults and children, no patients without

dysrhythmias or shock in the emergency department progressed to dysrhythmia, shock, or death during their hospitalization. Patients without a rhythm disturbance on admission can be admitted to an unmonitored bed. In the presence of a cardiac contusion, rhythm disturbances will usually result within 48 hours. However, a significant incidence occurs of developing shock during their hospitalization if the patient has dysrhythmias in the emergency department.[77]

Penetrating wounds of the heart are managed in a manner similar to that for blunt injury. If the heart is perforated by a knife, bullet, or other penetrating object, one of two pathophysiologic events may occur. Blood may leak from the heart into the adjacent pleural cavity and form a hemothorax. This diagnosis is suspected when hemodynamic instability occurs from hemorrhagic shock or persistent bleeding from a chest tube. The other possibility is that blood will accumulate in the pericardial space. For this to occur, the hole in the pericardial space must tamponade. The pericardial membrane is thick and elastic, and the hole created in it often becomes occluded, which prevents the patient from exsanguinating. Unfortunately, continued pericardial blood accumulation also leads to pericardial tamponade.

Penetrating injuries to the heart can involve any of the four chambers but are most common in the right ventricle. The right ventricle is anteriorly located and therefore more vulnerable. Because right-sided pressures are lower than left-sided pressures, the bleeding of injuries to the right side of the heart is more likely to tamponade and allow patients to survive to reach medical attention.

Many patients with penetrating injuries to the heart have obvious hemodynamic compromise from blood loss, pericardial tamponade, or a combination of the two. When the compromise is severe enough, no vital signs are present, and the patient is a candidate for emergency department thoracotomy. Regardless of whether tamponade is present, the pericardium should be opened, and the heart should be visualized. This maneuver relieves tamponade, if present, and allows digital control of the cardiac wound. Attempts at suture of the heart in an emergency setting should be avoided. If sutures are not carefully placed and pledgeted, they can tear through the myocardium, enlarge the traumatic defect, and convert a salvageable wound into one that cannot be repaired.

Although many patients with penetrating cardiac injuries are first seen in extremis, some are hemodynamically stable on presentation. In most patients, bleeding within the pericardial space produces some element of tamponade, and venous return to the right heart is compromised. Administration of intravenous fluids only temporarily improves the situation.

In children, transthoracic echocardiography is extraordinarily sensitive in detecting even small amounts of pericardial fluid. Pericardiocentesis is a more invasive approach to the diagnosis of intrapericardial blood. A needle is placed in the subxyphoid position and directed toward the left shoulder at a 30- to 45-degree angle from the skin surface. While the needle is advanced, constant aspiration is maintained. If blood is aspirated, the result is positive. It is important to observe the aspirated blood for clot formation. Blood that has been aspirated from a cardiac chamber will clot, whereas blood aspirated from the pericardial sac is defibrinated and will not clot.

Pericardiocentesis is controversial and not without risk of injuring the heart. If the result is positive, nothing definitive can be done if surgical expertise is not immediately present.[78–80] Removal of only a small amount of blood from the pericardial sac may temporarily improve the hemodynamic status, but repeated aspirations may be necessary.

In a stable patient, creation of a subxyphoid pericardial window is another approach to treating a wound that may have injured the heart.[81,82] A small subxyphoid incision is made, through which the diaphragmatic portion of the pericardial surface is grasped and incised. If a small amount of normal serous pericardial fluid is seen, the wound is closed. Hemopericardium is an indication that the patient should undergo sternotomy or thoracotomy for repair of the cardiac injury. Subxyphoid pericardial windows are both sensitive and highly specific. Emergency conversion of the subxyphoid pericardial window into a sternotomy or thoracotomy may be necessary, and thus the window should not be performed until the appropriate personnel and environment are available.

One must keep in mind that many of the wounds that raise the possibility of cardiac injury also suggest underlying abdominal injury. The abdominal viscera, depending on the patient's positioning and phase of respiration at the time of injury, can rise as high as the fourth or fifth intercostal space. In many cases of penetrating precordial trauma, a diagnostic peritoneal lavage or abdominal exploration is necessary. If a laparotomy is performed, and concern exists about the possibility of a penetrating injury to the heart, it is simple to make a small hole in the diaphragmatic surface of the pericardium via laparotomy incision. Extension of the midline laparotomy into a sternotomy facilitates repair of the cardiac injury.

Either thoracotomy or sternotomy can be used to repair cardiac injuries, but sternotomy affords access to all cardiac chambers, even if some cardiac manipulation is required, whereas left thoracotomy precludes effective repair of injuries to the right side of the heart.

Repair of most cardiac injuries is straightforward. Nonabsorbable sutures should be used for repair. The type of suture is less important than the size and type of needle. An atraumatic needle should be used and should be big enough to take moderately large bites of the myocardium for approximation but not so large that large needle holes remain after the repair is done. Pledget material should be used to reinforce the repair and to prevent the sutures from pulling through the myocardium. Some reports exist on the use of staples and/or biologic glue for temporary control of the bleeding; however, this should not be considered a definitive repair of a ventricular injury. In some wounds of the atria, a side-biting vascular clamp can be used for control during repair. Alternatively, the area of injury can be compressed with a finger while it is being sutured. Precise location of each initial suture is difficult in a bleeding, beating heart and is not so important as getting some degree of control of the bleeding, so that refinements of the repair can be performed in a relatively bloodless field. Care always must be taken to avoid injury to coronary arteries.

Commotio Cordis

Commotio cordis is a disorder found in the pediatric population resulting from sudden impact on the anterior chest wall that results in cessation of normal cardiac function. The precordial blows that trigger commotio cordis are often not perceived as unusual for the sporting event involved or of sufficient magnitude to cause death. This disorder is most common in young children and adolescents, because these age groups characteristically have compliant chest walls that probably facilitate the transmission of the energy from the chest blow to the myocardium.[83,84] Survival after commotio cordis is uncommon, as low as 15% in one study, and is most likely when cardiopulmonary resuscitation and defibrillation are prompt. The availability of automatic external defibrillators at schools and athletic facilities will certainly result in increased survival for many athletes who have a cardiac arrest as a result of blows to the chest.

Diaphragm

Blunt injuries of the diaphragm are becoming more common with higher automotive speeds and increased use of seat-belt restraints.[85–87] When a seat belt is in place, sudden deceleration can lead to a marked increase in intra-abdominal pressure, which is transmitted to the diaphragm.

Blunt rupture of the diaphragm occurs more commonly on the left than on the right.[85] Teleologically, the liver protects the right hemidiaphragm and helps dissipate kinetic energy throughout its substance. It also is easier to make the diagnosis on the left side because radiographic findings are more obvious. Right-sided ruptures are therefore more likely to be missed because the liver prevents abdominal visceral herniations, and small tears in the right side are of minimal consequence. Rarely, both hemidiaphragms are ruptured. The diaphragm can rupture in any location, but ruptures of the central tendon and the lateral attachments of the torso wall are most common. The size varies, but most of the tears that are diagnosed are at least several centimeters long. On the left side, abdominal viscera can herniate through the diaphragmatic defect, but this does not universally occur, and herniation is unlikely in patients on controlled positive-pressure ventilation.

The diagnosis of diaphragmatic rupture is usually made with either radiographic findings or incidentally discovered at the time of an operation. Herniation of hollow abdominal viscera is usually easily recognized on the radiograph, whereas solid viscera such as the liver or spleen may be interpreted as elevation of the hemidiaphragm. Bleeding from associated intra-abdominal injuries is common, and when this blood leaks into the pleural cavity, it may appear as a hemothorax. Subtle blunting of the costophrenic angle and a fuzzy quality to the hemidiaphragm are common radiographic findings. Persistence of the blunting after chest tube placement and drainage of the ipsilateral pleural cavity is a clue to differentiating diaphragmatic rupture from simple hemothorax.

The incidence of associated abdominal injuries in patients with diaphragmatic rupture is quite high. For this reason, in patients with a diagnosed diaphragmatic rupture, a laparotomy should be considered as the surgical approach to allow simultaneous repair of any abdominal injuries. In some patients, bleeding from associated intra-abdominal injuries is severe and manifests itself as a large hemothorax with persistent bleeding. In the absence of a definitive diagnosis of diaphragmatic rupture, the decision about whether to perform thoracotomy or laparotomy is difficult. Although thoracotomy may be appropriate on rare occasions when an intrathoracic source of hemorrhage is most likely, it is prudent to position the patient so that a laparotomy also can be done if the chest is opened and bleeding is seen to be coming through a ruptured hemidiaphragm.

It is important to inspect the diaphragm closely during exploratory laparotomy, regardless of whether the diagnosis of diaphragmatic rupture has been made preoperatively. Some of the tears are subtle and hidden by folds of the diaphragm, which can balloon and collapse with the cycle of positive pressure ventilation. When the tear is located, any herniated viscera should be returned to the abdomen and inspected for bleeding or ischemia. The rent should then be repaired. Both monofilament nonabsorbable sutures and large continuous absorbable sutures are appropriate for the repair. If not already present, a chest tube should be placed on the affected side. Drainage over the first several postoperative days is often considerable until the diaphragmatic tear has healed and become watertight.

Occasionally, the diagnosis of blunt rupture of the diaphragm is initially missed. If the hemidiaphragm is elevated in the early postinjury period and the diagnosis is suspected, computed tomography of the lower chest and upper abdomen sometimes aids diagnosis. Detection of visceral herniation can be delayed, appearing even years after the traumatic event. Herniation may be asymptomatic and appear on a chest roentgenogram obtained only incidentally, or the herniated viscera may become strangulated and cause symptoms. If the diagnosis is delayed and the patient is asymptomatic, repair can be effected by either an abdominal or a thoracic approach. If the patient is symptomatic and a possibility exists of visceral ischemia or perforation, the approach should always be through the abdomen.

REFERENCES

1. Institute of Medicine: Reducing the Burden of Injury. Washington, DC, National Academic Press, 1999.
2. Peclet MH, Newman KD, Eichelberger MR, et al: Thoracic trauma in children: An indicator of increased mortality. J Pediatr Surg 25:961–965, 1990.
3. Black TL, Snyder CL, Miller JP, et al: Significance of chest trauma in children. South Med J 89:494–496, 1996.
4. Cooper A, Barlow B, DiScala C, et al: Mortality and truncal injury: The pediatric perspective. J Pediatr Surg 29:33–38, 1994.
5. Drew R, Perry JF, Fisher R: The expediency of peritoneal lavage for blunt trauma in children. Surg Gynecol Obstet 145:885, 1977.
6. Mayer T, Matlak M, Johnson D, et al: The modified injury severity scale in pediatric multiple trauma patients. J Pediatr Surg 15:422, 1980.
7. Newman KD, Eichelberger MR: The child with thoracic trauma. In Fallis JC, Filler RM, Lemoine M (eds): Current Topics in General Thoracic Surgery: An International Series. New York; Elsevier Science, 1991, pp 277–285.
8. Breasted JH: The Edwin Smith Papyrus, Vol 1. Chicago, University of Chicago Press, 1930.
9. Hippocrates: Works, Vol. III. Withington ET (trans). Cambridge, MA, Harvard University Press, 1959, p 307.
10. Aristotle: De Partibus Animalum. Peck A, (trans). Cambridge, MA, Harvard University Press, 1937.
11. Pickard LR, Mattox KL: Thoracic Trauma: General Considerations and Indications for Thoracotomy in Trauma, 2nd ed. Norwalk, CT, Appleton & Lange, 1991, p 319.
12. Paré A: Collected Works (AD 1582). Johnson I (trans). London, Cotes and Young, 1634, p 571.
13. Riolanus J: En cheiridium anatomicum et pathologicum, in quo ex naturali constituione partium, recessus, a naturale statu demonstratur: Ad usum theatri anatomici adornatum. Lugd Bat, A Wynedaerden, 1649.
14. Scultetus J: The Surgeon's Storehouse. London, Starkey, 1674, p 159.
15. Anel D: L'Art de Succer les Plaies. Amsterdam, Francois Vander Plaats, 1707.
16. Playfair WS: On the treatment of empyema in children. Obstet Soc London Trans 14:4, 1872.
17. Guthrie GJ: On Wounds and Injuries of the Chest. London, Rensaw & Churchill, 1848.
18. Jeger E: Die Chirurgie der Blutgefass und des Herzens. Berlin, Hirschwal, 1913, p 295.
19. Rehn L: Veber penetrierende Herzwunder und Herznaht. Arch Klin Chir 55:315, 1897.
20. Graham EA: A brief account of the development of thoracic surgery and some of its consequences. Surg Gynecol Obstet 104:241, 1957.
21. Graham EA, Bell RD: Open pneumothorax: Its reaction to the treatment of empyema. Am J Med Sci 156:839, 1918.
22. West JG, Williams MJ, Trunkey DD, et al: Trauma systems: Current status, future challenges. JAMA 259:3597, 1988.
23. American College of Surgeons: Advanced Trauma Life Support Course. Chicago, American College of Surgeons, 1997.

24. Wood PR, Lawler PGP: Managing the airway in cervical spine injury: A review of the Advanced Trauma Life Support protocol. Anaesthesia 47:792, 1992.

25. Barone JE, Pizzi WF, Nealon TF Jr, et al: Indications for intubation in blunt chest trauma. J Trauma 26:334, 1986.

26. Grande CM, Stene JK, Bernhard WN: Airway management: Considerations in the trauma patient. Crit Care Clin 6:37, 1990.

27. Rhee KJ, Green W, Holcroft JW, et al: Oral intubation in the multiply injured patient: The risk of exacerbating spinal cord injury. Ann Emerg Med 19:511, 1990.

28. Young G, Eichelberger, MR: Initial Resuscitation of the Child with Multiple Injuries: Pediatric Emergency Medicine. Philadelphia, JB Lippincott, 1991.

29. Landercasper S, Cogbill TH: Long-term follow up after traumatic asphyxia. J Trauma 25:838–841, 1985.

30. Sarihan H, Abes M, Akyazici R, et al: Traumatic asphyxia in children. J Cardiovasc Surg 38:93–95, 1997.

31. Ochsner MG, Rozycki GS, Lucente F, et al: Prospective evaluation of thoracoscopy for diagnosing diaphragmatic injury in thoracoabdominal trauma: A preliminary report. J Trauma 34:704, 1993.

32. O'Brien J, Cohen M, Solit R, et al: Thoracoscopic drainage and decortication as definitive treatment for empyema thoracis following penetrating chest injury. J Trauma 36:536–540, 1994.

33. Helling TS, Gyles NR, Eisenstein CL, et al: Complications following blunt and penetrating injuries in 216 victims of chest trauma requiring tube thoracostomy. J Trauma 29:1367, 1989.

34. Shin B, McAlslan TC, Hankins JR: Management of lung contusion. Am Surg 45:168–179, 1979.

35. Schild HH, Strunk H, Weber W: Pulmonary contusion: CT vs plain radiograms. J Comput Assist Tomogr 13:417–420, 1989.

36. Wagner RB, Jamieson PM: Pulmonary contusion: Evaluation and classification by computed tomography. Surg Clin North Am 69:211–220, 1990.

37. Flynn AE, Thomas AN, Schecter WP: Acute tracheobronchial injury. J Trauma 29:1326, 1989.

38. Grover FL, Ellestad C, Arom KV, et al: Diagnosis and management of major tracheobronchial injuries. Ann Thorac Surg 28:384, 1979.

39. Symbas PN, Diorio DA, Tyras DH, et al: Penetrating cardiac wounds: Significant residual and delayed sequelae. J Thorac Cardiovasc Surg 66:526, 1973.

40. Kiser AC, O'Brien SM, Detterbeck FC: Blunt tracheobronchial injuries: Treatment and outcomes. Ann Thorac Surg 71:2059–2065, 2001.

41. Jones WS, Mavroudis C, Richardson JD, et al: Management of tracheobronchial disruption resulting from blunt trauma. Surgery 95:319, 1984.

42. Grant WJ, Meyers RL, Jaffe RL, et al: Tracheobronchial injuries after blunt chest trauma in children-hidden pathology. J Pediatr Surg 33:1707–1711, 1998.

43. Baumgartner F, Sheppard B, de Virgilio C, et al: Tracheal and main bronchial disruptions after blunt chest trauma: Presentations and management. Ann Thorac Surg 50:569, 1990.

44. Symbas PN, Justicz AG, Ricketts RR: Rupture of the airways from blunt trauma: Treatment of complex injuries. Ann Thorac Surg 54:177, 1992.

45. Gibbons JA, Peniston RL, Diamond SS, et al: A comparison of synthetic absorbable suture with synthetic nonabsorbable suture for construction of tracheal anastomoses. Chest 79:340, 1981.

46. Urschel HC, Razzuk MA: Management of acute traumatic injuries of tracheobronchial tree. Surg Gynecol Obstet 136:113, 1973.

47. Feczko JD, Lynch L, Pless JE, et al: An autopsy case review of 148 nonpenetrating (blunt) injuries of the aorta. J Trauma 33:846, 1992.

48. Parmley LF, Mattingly TW, Manlow WC: Non-penetrating traumatic injury to the aorta. Circulation 17:1096, 1958.

49. Pickard LR, Mattox KL, Espada R, et al: Transection of the descending thoracic aorta secondary to blunt trauma. J Trauma 17:749, 1977.

50. Gundry SR, Burney RE, MacKenzie JR, et al: Assessment of mediastinal widening associated with traumatic rupture of the aorta. J Trauma 23:293, 1983.

51. Agee CK, Metzler MH, Churchill RJ, Mitchell FL: Computer tomographic evaluation to exclude traumatic aortic disruption. J Trauma 33:876, 1998.

52. Heiberg E, Wolverson MK, Sundaram M, Shields JB: CT in aortic trauma. Am J Roentgenol 140:1119, 1983.

53. Ishikawa T, Nakajima Y, Kaji T: The role of CT in traumatic rupture of the thoracic aorta and its proximal branches. Semin Roentgenol 24:38, 1989.

54. McLean TR, Olinger GN, Thorsen MK: Computed tomography in the evaluation of the aorta in patients sustaining blunt chest trauma. J Trauma 31:254, 1991.

55. Miller FB, Richardson JD, Thomas HA: Role of CT in the diagnosis of major arterial injury after blunt thoracic trauma. Surgery 106:596, 1989.

56. Goarin JP, Catoire P, Jacquens Y, et al: Use of transesophageal echocardiography for diagnosis of traumatic aortic injury. Chest 112:71–80, 1997.

57. Minard G, Schurr MJ, Croce MA, et al: Prospective analysis of transesophageal echocardiography in the diagnosis of traumatic disruption of the aorta. J Trauma 40:225–230, 1996.

58. Cohn SM, Burns GA, Jaffe C, et al: Exclusion of aortic tear in the unstable trauma patient: The utility of transesophageal echocardiography. J Trauma 39:1087–1090, 1995.

59. McCroskey BL, Moore EE, Moore FA, et al: A unified approach to the torn thoracic aorta. Am J Surg 162:473, 1991.

60. Merrill WH, Lee RB, Hammon JW Jr, et al: Surgical treatment of acute traumatic tear of the thoracic aorta. Ann Surg 207:699, 1988.

61. Van Norman GA, Pavlin EG, Eddy AC, et al: Hemodynamic and metabolic effects of aortic unclamping following emergency surgery for traumatic thoracic aortic tear in shunted and unshunted patients. J Trauma 31:1007, 1991.

62. Cooper A, Foltin GL: Thoracic trauma. In: Barkin A (ed): Pediatric Emergency Medicine: Concepts and Clinical Practice. St. Louis, Mosby, 1992, pp 261–275.

63. Scorpio RJ, Wesson DE, Smith CR, et al: Blunt cardiac injuries in children: A postmortem study. J Trauma 41:306–309, 1996.

64. Brathwaite CEM, Rodriguez A, Turney SZ, et al: Blunt traumatic cardiac rupture. Ann Surg 212:701, 1990.

65. Fulda G, Brathwaite CEM, Rodriguez A, et al: Blunt traumatic rupture of the heart and pericardium: A ten-year experience (1979-1989). J Trauma 31:167, 1991.

66. Pevec WC, Udekwu AO, Peitzman AB: Blunt rupture of the myocardium. Ann Thorac Surg 48:139, 1989.

67. Calhoon JH, Hoffmann TH, Trinkle JK, et al: Management of blunt rupture of the heart. J Trauma 26:495–502, 1986.

68. Ivatury RR, Rohman M, Steichen FN, et al: Penetrating cardiac injuries: Twenty-year experience. Am Surg 53:310–317, 1987.

69. Tenzer ML. The spectrum of myocardial contusion: A review. J Trauma 25:620, 1985.

70. Fabian TC, Mangiante EC, Patterson CR, et al: Myocardial contusion in blunt trauma: Clinical characteristics, means of diagnosis, and implications for patient management. J Trauma 28:50, 1988.

71. Mattox KL, Flint LM, Carrico CJ, et al: Blunt cardiac injury [editorial]. J Trauma 33:649, 1992.

72. Shapiro MJ, Yanofsky SD, Trapp J, et al: Cardiovascular evaluation in blunt thoracic trauma using transesophageal echocardiography (TEE). J Trauma 31:835, 1991.

73. Miller FB, Shumate CR, Richardson JD: Myocardial contusion. Arch Surg 124:805, 1989.

74. Sturaitis M, McCallum D, Sutherland G, et al: Lack of significant long-term sequelae following traumatic myocardial contusion. Arch Intern Med 146:1765, 1986.

75. Hirsch R, Landt Y, Porter S, et al: Cardiac troponin 1 in pediatrics: Normal values and potential use in the assessment of cardiac injury. J Pediatr 130:872–877, 1997.

76. Wisner DH, Reed WH, Riddick RS: Suspected myocardial contusion: Triage and indications for monitoring. Ann Surg 212:82, 1990.

77. Dowd MD, Krug S. Pediatric blunt cardiac injury: Epidemiology, clinical features, and diagnosis. J Trauma 40:61–67, 1996.

78. Demetriades D: Cardiac penetrating injuries: Personal experience of 45 cases. Fr J Surg 71:95, 1984.

79. Ivatury RR, Rohman M, Steichen RM, et al: Penetrating cardiac injuries: Twenty-year experience. Am Surg 53:310, 1987.

80. Marshall WG Jr, Bell JL, Kouchoukos NT: Penetrating cardiac trauma. J Trauma 24:147, 1984.

81. Jimenez E, Martin M, Krukenkamp I, et al: Subxiphoid pericardiotomy versus echocardiography: A prospective evaluation of the

diagnosis of occult penetrating cardiac injury. Surgery 108:676, 1990.

82. Mayor-Davies, JA, Britz RS: Subxiphoid pericardial windows-helpful in selected cases. J Trauma 30:1399, 1990.

83. Maron BJ, Poliac LC, Kaplan JA, et al: Blunt impact to the chest leading to sudden death from cardiac arrest during sports activities. N Engl J Med 333:337–342, 1995.

84. Maron BJ, Gohman TE, Kyle SB, et al: Clinical profile and spectrum of commotio cordis. JAMA 287:1142–1146, 2002.

85. Beal SL, McKennan M: Blunt diaphragm rupture: A morbid injury. Arch Surg 123:828, 1988.

86. Ilgenfritz FM, Stewart DD: Blunt trauma of the diaphragm: A 15-county, private hospital experience. Am Surg 6:334, 1992.

87. Kearney PA, Rouhana SW, Burney RE: Blunt rupture of the diaphragm: Mechanism, diagnosis and treatment. Ann Emerg Med 18:1326, 1989.

CHAPTER 16

Abdominal and Renal Trauma

Steven Stylianos, MD, and Barry A. Hicks, MD

The management of children with major abdominal injuries has changed significantly in the past two decades. An increased awareness of the anatomic patterns and physiologic responses characteristic of pediatric trauma has resulted in the successful nonoperative treatment of most abdominal solid organ injuries. Our colleagues in adult trauma care have acknowledged this success and applied many of the principles learned in pediatric trauma to their patients.[1] A recent review of the National Pediatric Trauma Registry (NPTR) indicates that 8% to 12% of children with blunt trauma have an abdominal injury.[2] Fortunately, more than 90% of them survive. Only 22% of the deaths in the NPTR were related to the abdominal injury. Although abdominal injuries are 30% more common than thoracic injuries, they are 40% less likely to be fatal.

Historically, trauma surgeons unfamiliar with the nonoperative management of solid organ injuries often raised doubts about the wisdom of this approach. Their concerns included the potential for increased transfusion requirements, increased length of hospitalization, and missed associated injuries. Some even questioned the need for involvement of pediatric surgeons in pediatric trauma care. The clinical experience accumulated over the past 20- to 30-year period, which has settled this controversy, is reviewed.

Few surgeons have extensive experience with massive abdominal solid organ injury requiring immediate surgery. It is imperative that surgeons familiarize themselves with current treatment algorithms for life-threatening abdominal trauma. Important contributions have been made in the diagnosis and treatment of children with abdominal injury by radiologists and endoscopists. The resolution and speed of computed tomography (CT), screening capabilities of focused abdominal sonography for trauma (FAST), and the percutaneous, angiographic, and endoscopic interventions of nonsurgeon members of the pediatric trauma team have all enhanced patient care and improved outcomes. Each section of this chapter focuses on the more common blunt injuries and unique aspects of care in children.

DIAGNOSTIC MODALITIES

The initial evaluation of the acutely injured child is similar to that of the adult. Plain radiographs of the cervical spine, chest, and pelvis are obtained after the initial survey and evaluation of A (airway), B (breathing), and C (circulation). Plain abdominal radiographs offer little in the urgent evaluation of the pediatric trauma patient. In a child with a suspected intra-abdominal injury, treatment algorithms have changed significantly as imaging modalities have improved. Prompt identification of potentially life-threatening injuries is now possible in the vast majority of children.

Computerized Tomography

Computerized tomography (CT) has become the imaging study of choice for the evaluation of injured children because of several advantages. CT is now readily accessible in most health care facilities, is noninvasive, and is a very accurate method of identifying and qualifying the extent of abdominal injury, which has reduced the incidence of nontherapeutic exploratory laparotomy (Fig. 16-1). Intravenous contrast is essential, and utilization of "dynamic" methods of scanning have optimized vascular and parenchymal enhancement. The finding of a contrast "blush" on CT in children with blunt liver injury has been associated with larger transfusion requirements and a higher mortality rate in a small series.[3] A head CT, if indicated, should be performed first without contrast to avoid contrast concealing a hemorrhagic brain injury. Enteral contrast for enhancement of the gastrointestinal (GI) tract is generally not required in the acute trauma setting and can lead to aspiration.[4]

Not all children with potential abdominal injuries are candidates for CT evaluation. Obvious penetrating injury often necessitates immediate operative intervention. The hemodynamically unstable child should not be transported from an appropriate resuscitation room for a CT. These children may benefit from an alternative diagnostic

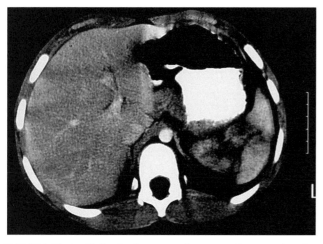

FIGURE 16-1. Abdominal computed tomography scan showing major (grade III) spleen injury and hemoperitoneum.

TABLE 16-1	
POSITIVE PERITONEAL LAVAGE CRITERIA

10 mL gross blood return with lavage catheter insertion
>100,000 RBC/mm³
>500 WBC/mm³
Bile, bacteria, or vegetable matter on microscopic examination
Amylase, >175 IU/dL

RBC, red blood cell; WBC, white blood cell.

study, such as a diagnostic peritoneal lavage, focused abdominal sonogram, or urgent operative intervention. The greatest limitation of abdominal CT scanning in trauma is the lack of ability to reliably identify intestinal rupture.[5,6] Findings suggestive but not diagnostic of intestinal perforation are pneumoperitoneum, bowel wall thickening, free intraperitoneal fluid, bowel wall enhancement, and dilated bowel.[7] A high index of suspicion should exist for the presence of a bowel injury in the child with intraperitoneal fluid and no identifiable solid organ injury on CT scanning.[8]

Focused Abdominal Sonography for Trauma

Clinician-performed sonography for the early evaluation of the injured child is currently being evaluated to determine its optimal use. Examination of Morrison's pouch, the pouch of Douglas, the left flank to include the perisplenic region, and a subxiphoid view to visualize the pericardium is the standard four-view FAST examination. This bedside examination may be useful as a rapid screening study, particularly in those patients too unstable to undergo an abdominal CT scan. Early reports have found FAST to be a useful screening tool in children, with a high specificity (95%) but a low sensitivity (33%) in identifying intestinal injury.[9] A lack of identifiable free fluid does not exclude a significant injury. FAST may be very useful in decreasing the number of CT scans performed for "low-likelihood" injuries. The study may have to be repeated, depending on clinical correlation, and the finding of free fluid in itself is not an indication for surgical intervention. Recently, a simple scoring system for quantifying the amount of hemoperitoneum was shown to be predictive of the need for laparotomy in a small series of children after blunt abdominal trauma.[10] Prospective validation of such a FAST score is necessary.

Diagnostic Peritoneal Lavage

Since its description in 1965, the use of diagnostic peritoneal lavage (DPL) has diminished significantly,

especially in the pediatric trauma population, as the availability of high-resolution CT scanners and the use of nonoperative treatment have increased. Although very accurate for intra-abdominal hemorrhage, retroperitoneal injuries may be missed. Perhaps more important, a positive DPL may lead to a nontherapeutic laparotomy. Because the majority of solid organ injuries do not require surgical intervention, intraperitoneal blood identified by DPL has little clinical significance. The need for operative management is determined by clinical instability and the requirement for ongoing blood replacement. Incisional pain also may interfere with serial examinations in a child being managed nonoperatively after a negative DPL.

In some clinical situations, a DPL may prove to be very useful. A hemodynamically unstable child may have a rapid DPL to exclude the abdomen as a source of hemorrhage. Children with lap-belt injury pose diagnostic challenges, particularly if a concomitant neurologic injury is present. The initial abdominal CT is frequently normal in those with lap-belt injury, but a DPL may document the presence of an occult hollow visceral injury with the return of bile, bacteria, feculent matter, or an increased leukocyte count. Infusion of 10 mL/kg normal saline into the peritoneal cavity is followed by allowing the infusate to drain. The criteria for a positive lavage are listed in Table 16-1.

Diagnostic and Therapeutic Laparoscopy

Laparoscopy of the injured child may have its place in the evaluation of the hemodynamically stable patient. The sensitivity is comparable to that of DPL, but the specificity is higher, as would be expected by actually visualizing the injury.[11] A decrease in the number of nontherapeutic laparotomies has been demonstrated in adult series.[12] Studies also have shown that not only may the traumatic injury be identified with laparoscopy, but the definitive repair also may frequently be performed (Fig. 16-2).[13]

SOLID ORGAN INJURY

Spleen and Liver

The spleen and liver are the organs most commonly injured in blunt abdominal trauma, with each accounting for one third of the injuries. Nonoperative treatment of isolated splenic and hepatic injuries in stable children is now standard practice. Although nonoperative treatment

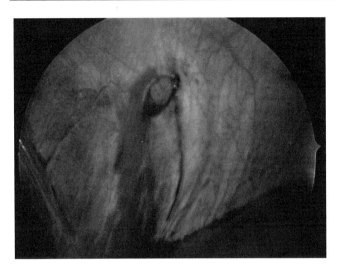

FIGURE 16-2. Diagnostic laparoscopy in a stable patient after a stab wound to the upper abdomen revealed this diaphragmatic injury. Repair was performed by using minimal-access techniques.

of children with isolated, blunt spleen or liver injury has been universally successful, great variation is seen in the management algorithms used by individual pediatric surgeons. Review of the NPTR and recent surveys of the American Pediatric Surgical Association (APSA) membership confirm the wide disparity in practice.[14,15] Controversy also exists regarding the utility of CT grading as a prediction of outcome in liver and spleen injury.[16-19] Recently the APSA Trauma Committee defined consensus guidelines for resource utilization in hemodynamically stable children with isolated liver or spleen injury, based on CT grading, by analyzing a contemporary, multi-institution database of 832 children treated nonoperatively at 32 centers in North America from 1995 to 1997 (Table 16-2).[20] Consensus guidelines on intensive care unit (ICU) stay,

TABLE 16-2

RESOURCE UTILIZATION AND ACTIVITY RESTRICTION IN 832 CHILDREN WITH ISOLATED SPLEEN OR LIVER INJURY

CT Grade	I	II	III	IV
Admitted to ICU	55.0%	54.3%	72.3%	85.4%
No. hosp days (mean)	4.3 days	5.3 days	7.1 days	7.6 days
No. hosp days (range)	1-7 days	2-9 days	3-9 days	4-10 days
Transfused	1.8%	5.2%	10.1%*	26.6%*
Laparotomy	none	1.0%	2.7%†	12.6%†
Follow-up imaging	34.4%	46.3%	54.1%	51.8%
Activity restriction (mean)	5.1 wk	6.2 wk	7.5 wk	9.2 wk
Activity restriction (range)	2-6 wk	2-8 wk	4-12 wk	6-12 wk

*Grade III vs. grade IV, $P < .014$; †Grade III vs. grade IV, $P < .0001$.
CT, computed tomography; ICU, intensive care unit.
From Stylianos S and the APSA Trauma Committee: Evidence-based guidelines for resource utilization in children with isolated spleen or liver injury. J Pediatr Surg 35:164-169, 2000.

TABLE 16-3

PROPOSED GUIDELINES FOR RESOURCE UTILIZATION IN CHILDREN WITH ISOLATED SPLEEN OR LIVER INJURY[20]

CT Grade	I	II	III	IV
ICU days	None	None	None	1 day
Hospital stay	2 days	3 days	4 days	5 days
Predischarge imaging	None	None	None	None
Postdischarge imaging	None	None	None	None
Activity restriction*	3 wk	4 wk	5 wk	6 wk

*Return to full-contact, competitive sports (i.e., football, wrestling, hockey, lacrosse, mountain climbing) should be at the discretion of the individual pediatric trauma surgeon. The proposed guidelines for return to unrestricted activity include "normal" age-appropriate activities.

length of hospitalization, use of follow-up imaging, and physical activity restriction for clinically stable children with isolated spleen or liver injuries (grades I to IV) were defined by analysis of this database (Table 16-3).

The guidelines were then applied prospectively in 312 children with liver or spleen injuries treated nonoperatively at 16 centers from 1998 to 2000.[21] Patients with other minor injuries such as nondisplaced, noncomminuted fractures or soft tissue injuries were included as long as the associated injuries did not influence the variables in this study. The patients were grouped by severity of injury, defined by CT grade. Compliance with the proposed guidelines was analyzed for age, organ injured, and injury grade. All patients were followed up for 4 months after injury. *(It is imperative to emphasize that these proposed guidelines assume hemodynamic stability.)* The extremely low rates of transfusion and operation document the stability of the study patients.

Specific guideline compliance was 81% for ICU hospitalization, 82% for length of hospital stay, 87% for follow-up imaging, and 78% for activity restriction. A significant improvement in compliance was noted from year 1 to year 2 for ICU stay (77% vs. 88%; $P < .02$) and activity restriction (73% vs. 87%; $P < .01$). No differences in compliance were found by age, gender, or organ injured. Deviation from guidelines was the surgeon's choice in 90% and patient related in 10%. Six (1.9%) patients were readmitted, although none required operation. Compared with the previously studied 832 patients, the 312 patients managed prospectively under the proposed guidelines had a significant reduction in ICU stay ($P < .0001$), total hospitalization ($P < .0006$), follow-up imaging ($P < .0001$), and interval of physical activity restriction ($P < .04$) within each grade of injury.

From these data, it was concluded that prospective application of specific treatment guidelines based on injury severity resulted in conformity in patient management, improved utilization of resources, and validation of guideline safety. Significant reduction of ICU care, hospital stay, follow-up imaging, and activity restriction was achieved without adverse sequelae when compared with our retrospective database.

The attending surgeon's decision to operate for spleen or liver injury is best based on evidence of continued blood loss, such as hypotension, tachycardia, decreased urine output, and decreasing hematocrit unresponsive to crystalloid and blood transfusion. The rates of successful nonoperative treatment of isolated blunt splenic and hepatic injury now exceed 90% in most pediatric trauma centers and adult trauma centers with a strong pediatric commitment.[20-23] A recent study of more than 100 patients from the NPTR indicated that nonoperative treatment of spleen or liver injury is indicated even in the presence of associated head injury, if the patient is hemodynamically stable.[24] Rates of operative intervention for blunt spleen or liver injury were similar with or without an associated closed head injury.

Surgeons unfamiliar with current treatment algorithms for blunt splenic injuries in children occasionally question the nonoperative approach. This is important because the majority of seriously injured children are treated outside of dedicated pediatric trauma centers. Although several adult trauma services have reported excellent survival rates for pediatric trauma patients, analysis of treatment for spleen and liver injuries reveals an alarmingly high rate of operative treatment.[22,25-27] It is possible that trauma surgeons, influenced by their past experience with adult patients, are more likely to favor operative treatment than are their pediatric surgical colleagues. Adult trauma surgeons caring for injured children must consider the anatomic, immunologic, and physiologic differences between pediatric and adult trauma patients and incorporate these differences into their treatment protocols. The major concerns regarding nonoperative management are related to the potential risks of increased transfusion requirements, missed associated injuries, and increased length of hospital stay. Each of these concerns has been shown to be without merit.[15,28-33]

Missed Associated Abdominal Injuries

Advocates of surgical intervention for splenic trauma cite their concern about missing associated abdominal injuries if an operation is not performed. One study reported successful nonoperative treatment in 110 (91%) of 120 children with blunt splenic trauma, of whom 22 (18%) had associated abdominal injuries.[30] Only 3 (2.5%) of these 120 patients had GI injuries, and each was found at early celiotomy performed for a specific indication. No morbidity occurred from missed injuries or delayed surgical intervention. Similarly, a review of the NPTR from 1988 through 1998 revealed 2977 patients with solid abdominal visceral injury; only 96 (3.2%) had an associated hollow viscus injury.[31] Higher rates of hollow viscus injury were observed in assaulted patients and those with multiple solid visceral injury or pancreatic injury. Differences in mechanism of injury may account for the much lower incidence of associated abdominal injuries in children with splenic trauma. No justification exists for an exploratory celiotomy solely to avoid missing potential associated injuries in children.

Complications of Nonoperative Treatment

Nonoperative treatment protocols have been the standard for most children with blunt liver and spleen injury during the past two decades. The cumulative experience gained allows us to evaluate both the benefits and risks of the nonoperative approach. Fundamental to the success of the nonoperative strategy is the early, spontaneous cessation of hemorrhage. Transfusion rates for children with isolated spleen or liver injury have decreased to less than 10%, confirming the lack of continued blood loss in the majority of patients.[18-23,34] Despite many favorable observations, isolated reports of significant delayed hemorrhage with adverse outcome continue to appear.[35-38] Two children with delayed hemorrhage 10 days after blunt liver injury have been reported.[37] Both children had persistent right upper quadrant (RUQ) and right shoulder pain despite having normal vital signs and stable hematocrits. The authors recommended continued in-house observation for injured patients until symptoms resolve. Recent reports described patients with significant bleeding 38 days after grade II spleen injury and 24 days after grade IV liver injury.[36,38] These rare occurrences create anxiety in identifying the minimal safe interval before resuming unrestricted activities.

Routine follow-up imaging studies have identified pseudocysts and pseudoaneurysms after splenic injury.[23,39,40] Splenic pseudoaneurysms often cause no symptoms and appear to resolve with time. The true incidence of self-limited, post-traumatic splenic pseudoaneurysms is unknown, as routine follow-up imaging after successful nonoperative treatment has been largely abandoned. Once it is identified, the actual risk of splenic pseudoaneurysm rupture also is unclear. Angiographic embolization techniques can be used to treat these lesions successfully, obviating the need for operation and loss of splenic parenchyma (Fig. 16-3).[23] Splenic pseudocysts may reach enormous size, leading to pain and GI disturbance (Fig. 16-4). Simple percutaneous aspiration leads to a high recurrence rate. Laparoscopic excision and marsupialization is highly effective (Fig. 16-5).

Sequelae of Damage Control Strategies

Even the most severe solid organ injuries can be treated nonoperatively if a prompt response to resuscitation occurs.[41] In patients who are hemodynamically unstable, despite fluid and packed red blood cell transfusion, emergency laparotomy is indicated. Most spleen and liver injuries requiring operation are amenable to simple methods of hemostasis, using a combination of manual compression, direct suture, and topical hemostatic agents. In young children with significant hepatic injury, the sternum can be divided rapidly to expose the suprahepatic or intrapericardial inferior vena cava (IVC). Children will tolerate clamping of the IVC above the liver as long as their blood volume is replenished. With this exposure, the liver and major perihepatic veins can be isolated and the bleeding controlled to permit direct suture repair or ligation of the injured vessel.

The early morbidity and mortality of severe hepatic injuries are related to the effects of massive blood loss and replacement with large volumes of cold blood products. The consequences of prolonged operations with massive blood-product replacement include hypothermia, coagulopathy, and acidosis. Although the surgical team

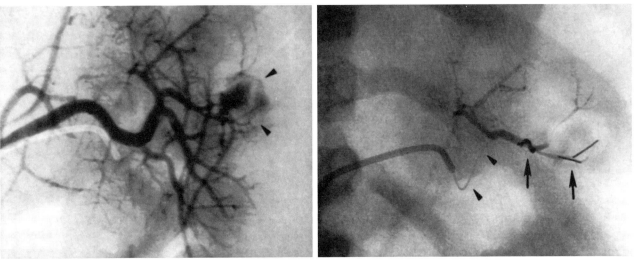

A   B

FIGURE 16-3. *A,* Splenic pseudoaneurysm (*arrows*) has developed after non-operative treatment of blunt splenic injury. *B,* Successful angiographic embolization has been accomplished.

may keep pace with blood loss, serious physiologic and metabolic consequences are inevitable, and many of these critically ill patients are unlikely to survive. A multi-institutional review identified exsanguination as the cause of death in 82% of 537 intraoperative deaths at 8 academic trauma centers.[42] The mean serum pH was 7.18, and the mean core temperature was 32°C before death. Survival in only 5 (40%) of 12 consecutive operative cases of retrohepatic vascular or severe parenchymal liver injury in children has been reported.[43]

Maintenance of physiologic stability during the struggle for surgical control of severe bleeding is a formidable challenge even for the most experienced operative team, particularly when hypothermia, coagulopathy, and acidosis occur. This triad creates a vicious cycle in which each derangement exacerbates the others, and the physiologic and metabolic consequences of the triad often preclude completion of the procedure. Lethal coagulopathy from dilution, hypothermia, and acidosis can rapidly occur.[44]

Increased emphasis on physiologic and metabolic stability in emergency abdominal operations has led to

the development of staged, multidisciplinary treatment plans including abbreviated laparotomy, perihepatic packing, temporary abdominal closure, angiographic embolization, and endoscopic biliary stenting.[45–47] In a series of 22 reported patients with grade IV or V hepatic injuries treated between 1992 and 1997, mean blood loss was estimated at 4.6 L, and mean packed red cell transfusion was 15 units.[48] Ten patients underwent packing of the hepatic injuries at the first operation. Fifteen patients had postoperative angiographic embolization in an attempt to control hemorrhage (Fig. 16-6). Survival was 92% in 13 grade IV patients and 78% in 9 grade V patients.

Abbreviated laparotomy with packing for hemostasis allowing resuscitation before planned reoperation is an alternative in unstable patients in whom further blood loss would be untenable. This "damage control" philosophy is a systematic, phased approach to the management of the exsanguinating trauma patient.[49–51] The three phases of damage control are detailed in Table 16-4. Although controversial, several resuscitative end points have been proposed beyond the conventional vital signs and urine output, including serum lactate, base deficit, mixed venous oxygen saturation, and gastric mucosal pH. Once patients become normothermic, coagulation factors replaced, and oxygen delivery optimized, a second procedure is done for pack removal and definitive repair of injuries. A review from several institutions of nearly 700 adult patients treated with abdominal packing demonstrated hemostasis in 80%, survival of 32% to 73%, and abdominal abscess rates of 10% to 40%.[52,53] Although abdominal packing (PACKS) with planned reoperation has been used with increasing frequency in adults during the past two decades, little published experience has been reported in children.[54–61] Nevertheless, this technique has a place in the management of children with massive intra-abdominal bleeding, especially after blunt trauma.

A 3-year-old child required PACKS for a severe liver injury, making closure of the abdomen impossible.[55] A polymeric silicone (Silastic) "silo" was constructed to

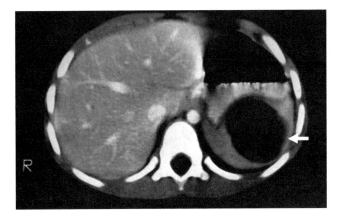

FIGURE 16-4. This computed tomography scan shows a post-traumatic splenic pseudocyst (*arrow*).

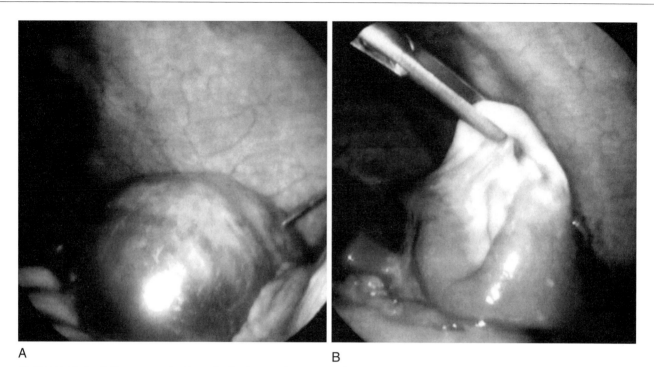

A   B

FIGURE 16-5. *A,* Laparoscopic view of splenic pseudocyst capsule. *B,* Appearance of cyst wall after laparoscopic aspiration and before marsupialization.

accommodate the bowel until the PACKS could be removed. The patient made a complete recovery. The combined technique of PACKS and a silo allowed time for correction of the hypothermia, acidosis, and coagulopathy without compromise of respiratory mechanics. A recent review reported 22 infants and children with refractory hemorrhage (ages 6 days to 20 years) who were treated with PACKS.[56] The anatomic site of hemorrhage was the liver and/or hepatic veins in 14,

retroperitoneum and/or pelvis in 7, and the pancreatic bed in 1. Primary fascial closure was accomplished in 12 (55%) patients, and temporary skin closure or prosthetic material was used in the other 10. PACKS controlled hemorrhage in 21 (95%) of 22 patients. Removal of PACKS was possible within 72 hours in 18 (82%) patients. No patient rebled after PACKS removal; however, two patients died with PACKS in place. In 7 (32%) patients, an abdominal or pelvic abscess developed. All were successfully drained by laparotomy (6 patients) or percutaneously (1 patient). Six of the 7 patients with abdominal sepsis survived. Overall, 18 (82%) patients survived. Two deaths were due to multisystem organ failure, one succumbed to cardiac failure from complex cardiac anomalies, and one death was from exsanguination after blunt traumatic liver injury. No differences were noted in the volume of intraoperative blood product transfusion, time to

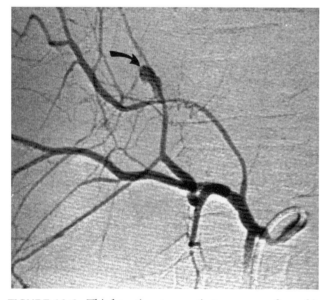

FIGURE 16-6. This hepatic artery angiogram was performed in a patient with persistent hemorrhage after initial damage-control laparotomy. The site of hemorrhage is identified (*curved arrow*), and embolization was successfully performed.

TABLE 16-4	
"DAMAGE CONTROL" STRATEGY IN THE EXSANGUINATING TRAUMA PATIENT	
Phase 1	Abbreviated laparotomy for exploration
	Control of hemorrhage and contamination
	Packing and temporary abdominal wall closure
Phase 2	Aggressive ICU resuscitation
	Core rewarming
	Optimize volume and oxygen delivery
	Correction of coagulopathy
Phase 3	Planned reoperation for packing change, evacuation, and definitive repair of injuries
	Abdominal-wall closure

ICU, intensive care unit.

initiate PACKS, physiologic status, or type of abdominal closure between survivors and nonsurvivors.

Although the success of abdominal packing is encouraging, it may contribute to significant morbidity such as intra-abdominal sepsis, organ failure, and increased intra-abdominal pressure. Fluid samples taken from 28 patients with abdominal packing found peritoneal endotoxin and mediator accumulation even when cultures were sterile.[62] The assumption was that fluid accumulating after damage-control laparotomy can contribute to neutrophil dysfunction by enhancing neutrophil respiratory burst and inhibiting neutrophil responses to specific chemotactic mediators needed to fight infection. Thus the known propensity of such patients for both intra-abdominal and systemic infection may be related to changes in neutrophil receptor status and effector function related to accumulation of inflammatory mediators in the abdomen. Early washout, repetitive packing, and other efforts to minimize mediator accumulation deserve consideration.

It is essential to emphasize that the success of the abbreviated laparotomy and planned reoperation depends on a decision to use this strategy before irreversible shock. Abdominal packing, when used as a desperate, last-ditch resort after prolonged attempts at hemostasis have failed, has been uniformly unsuccessful. Physiologic and anatomic criteria have been identified as indications for abdominal packing. Most of these have focused on intraoperative parameters including pH (~7.2), core temperature (< 35°C), and coagulation values (prothrombin time, > 16 seconds) in the patient with profuse hemorrhage requiring large volumes of blood-product transfusion.

The optimal time for re-exploration is controversial because neither the physiologic end points of resuscitation nor the increased risk of infection with prolonged packing is well defined. The obvious benefits of hemostasis provided by packing also are balanced against the potential deleterious effects of increased intra-abdominal pressure on ventilation, cardiac output, renal function, mesenteric circulation, and intracranial pressure. Timely alleviation of the secondary "abdominal compartment syndrome" may be a critical salvage maneuver for patients. Temporary abdominal wall closure at the time of packing can prevent the abdominal compartment syndrome. We recommend temporary abdominal wall expansion in all patients requiring packing until the hemostasis is obtained and visceral edema subsides.

A staged operative strategy for unstable trauma patients represents *advanced* surgical care and requires sound judgment and technical expertise. Intra-abdominal packing for control of exsanguinating hemorrhage is a life-saving maneuver in highly selected patients in whom coagulopathy, hypothermia, and acidosis render further surgical procedures unduly hazardous. Early identification of patients likely to benefit from abbreviated laparotomy techniques is crucial for success.

Abdominal Compartment Syndrome

The abdominal compartment syndrome is a term used to describe the deleterious effects of increased intra-abdominal pressure.[63] The "syndrome" includes respiratory insufficiency from worsening ventilation/perfusion mismatch, hemodynamic compromise from preload reduction due to IVC compression, impaired renal function from renal vein compression as well as decreased cardiac output, intracranial hypertension from increased ventilator pressures, splanchnic hypoperfusion, and abdominal wall overdistention. The causes of intra-abdominal hypertension in trauma patients include hemoperitoneum, retroperitoneal and/or bowel edema, and use of abdominal/pelvic packing. The combination of tissue injury and hemodynamic shock creates a cascade of events including capillary leak, ischemia-reperfusion, and release of vasoactive mediators and free radicals, which combine to increase extracellular volume and tissue edema. Experimental evidence indicates significant alterations in cytokine levels in the presence of sustained intra-abdominal pressure elevation.[64,65] Once the combined effects of tissue edema and intra-abdominal fluid exceed a certain level, abdominal decompression must be considered.

The adverse effects of abdominal compartment syndrome have been acknowledged for decades; however, abdominal compartment syndrome has only recently been recognized as a life-threatening yet potentially treatable entity.[46,66] The measurement of intra-abdominal pressure can be useful in determining the contribution of abdominal compartment syndrome to altered physiologic and metabolic parameters.[67–69] Intra-abdominal pressure can be determined by measuring bladder pressure. This involves instilling 1 mL/kg of saline into the Foley catheter and connecting it to a pressure transducer or manometer via a three-way stop-cock. The symphysis pubis is used as the zero reference point, and the pressure measured in centimeters of H_2O or millimeters of mercury. Intra-abdominal pressures in the range of 20 to 35 cm H_2O or 15 to 25 mm Hg have been identified as an indication to decompress the abdomen. Many surgeons prefer to intervene according to alterations in other physiologic and metabolic parameters rather than a specific pressure measurement. One series reported 11 adult trauma patients with abdominal compartment syndrome in whom abdominal decompression improved preload, pulmonary function, and visceral perfusion by using pulmonary artery catheters and gastric tonometry.[68]

Experience with abdominal decompression for abdominal compartment syndrome in children is limited.[56,66,69-71] Nonspecific abdominal CT findings in children with abdominal compartment syndrome include narrowing of the IVC, direct renal compression or displacement, bowel wall thickening with enhancement, and a rounded appearance of the abdomen.[70] One study reported the use of patch abdominoplasty in 23 infants and children, of whom only three were trauma patients.[71] These authors found that patch abdominoplasty for abdominal compartment syndrome effectively decreased airway pressures and oxygen requirements. Failure to respond with a decrease in airway pressures or FIO_2 was an ominous sign in their series. Several authors found that abdominal decompression resulted in decreased airway pressures, increased PO_2, and increased urine output in children with abdominal compartment syndrome.[66,69,71]

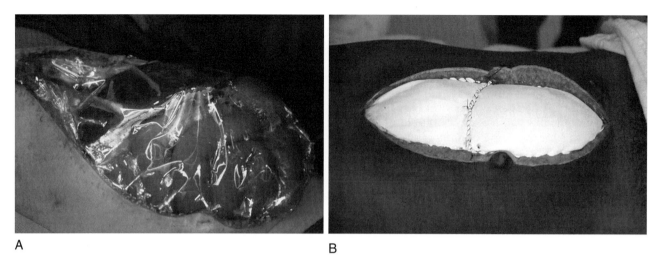

A   B

FIGURE 16-7. *A,* Abdominal wall expansion was performed in this patient with a bowel bag. *B,* Abdominal wall expansion in this patient was accomplished with a polytetrafluoroethylene patch.

Many materials have been suggested for use in temporary patch abdominoplasty including Silastic sheeting, polytetrafluoroethylene (PTFE) sheeting, intravenous bags, cystoscopy bags, ostomy appliances, and various mesh materials (Fig. 16-7). The vacuum pack technique, recently used in adults, seems promising.[50,61]

Biliary Duct Injury

Nonoperative management of pediatric blunt liver injury is highly successful but is complicated by a 4% risk of persistent bile leakage.[72,73] Radionuclide scanning is recommended when biliary tree injury is suspected.[74] Delayed views may show a bile leak even if early views are normal. Several reports have highlighted the benefits of endoscopic retrograde cholangiopancreatography (ERCP) with placement of transampullary biliary stents for biliary duct injury after blunt hepatic trauma, acknowledging that whereas ERCP is invasive and requires conscious sedation, it can pinpoint the site of injury and allow treatment of the injured ducts without laparotomy (Fig. 16-8). Endoscopic transampullary biliary decompression is a recent addition to treatment for patients with persistent bile leakage. The addition of sphincterotomy during ERCP for persistent bile leakage after blunt liver injury has been advocated to decrease intrabiliary pressure and promote internal decompression.[75-77] It is important to note that endoscopic biliary stents may migrate or clog and require specific treatment.

PANCREAS

With blunt abdominal trauma, injury to the pancreas occurs infrequently in children but is commonly very difficult to diagnose and to characterize. It is estimated that injuries to the pancreas compose 3% to 12% of intra-abdominal injuries in children sustaining blunt trauma.[78] The lack of surrounding fat planes and the small size of the retroperitoneal gland make it challenging to

document even a major ductal injury by routine CT screening.[79] A dynamic CT pancreatogram, with multiple thin slices while infusing IV contrast, gives much more detail than routine abdominal CT. Magnetic resonance cholangiopancreatography also is a useful diagnostic modality but is not appropriate in the acute resuscitative phase of the multiply injured child.[80] Elevations in serum amylase and lipase levels are very common in abdominal trauma but are not indicative of the extent of injury or

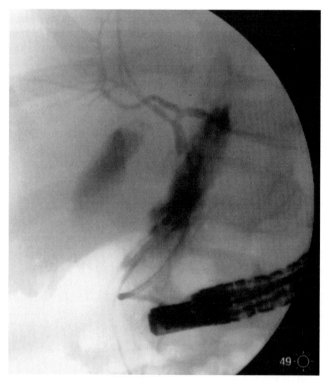

FIGURE 16-8. This endoscopic retrograde cholangiopancreatography demonstrated several areas of bile leaks after blunt liver injury.

need for surgical intervention. Hyperamylasemia also may occur with salivary gland injury, bowel perforation or obstruction, intracranial hemorrhage, or other nonspecific mesenteric injuries.[81] In contrast, ERCP is a very accurate technique in evaluating potential injury to the pancreatic ductal system.[82] It is not widely used in the early evaluation of the acutely injured child because of the highly specialized skills required, the need for general anesthesia, and the likelihood of significant need for treatment of head and thoracic injuries as a result of the blunt force incurred.

Nonoperative management of blunt injuries to the liver, spleen, and kidney in children is accepted as the standard of care in the majority of cases. Controversy exists when discussing management of the child with a significant pancreatic injury. Those with a pancreatic contusion without major ductal disruption will heal spontaneously. Direct visualization of the pancreas is very important when exploring a child's abdomen for a traumatic injury. The lesser sac is entered above the transverse colon, and the body and tail of the gland are carefully inspected. A Kocher maneuver is then used to inspect the duodenum and head of the pancreas. The posterior surface of the gland may be accessed by mobilization of the spleen along with the tail of the pancreas from a lateral to medial direction.

In the child with a major pancreatic ductal injury (Fig. 16-9), early operative intervention has been reported to shorten hospitalization and lessen total parenteral nutrition (TPN) dependence compared with those children who were initially managed nonoperatively.[83,84] Pseudocyst formation occurs in 45% to 100% of ductal injuries managed nonoperatively.[85,86] Of these, a significant number, up to 60%, may resolve with time. Percutaneous or cystenteric drainage procedures may be initiated if resolution does not occur spontaneously. These children have an increased length of hospitalization as well as an increased TPN dependence compared with those undergoing early distal pancreatectomy.

ERCP as a diagnostic and therapeutic option has recently gained some favor in selected centers with pediatric ERCP expertise. Documentation of a ductal injury, sphincterotomy, and possible stenting of the injury are all maneuvers used to assist in ductal drainage and healing.[82,87,88]

HOLLOW VISCUS INJURY

GI tract injuries in children may occur by either blunt or penetrating mechanisms. Penetrating injuries to the abdomen require minimal diagnostic evaluation before operative management. Blunt injury may be seen with obvious indications for surgical intervention, or may have a more subtle, insidious presentation. The mechanism may be from a compressive force (child abuse), a deceleration shearing force (fall from a height), or a combination of the two (lap-belt injury).

CT diagnosis of a bowel injury is often quite difficult. Nonspecific findings of free fluid within the peritoneal cavity are frequently the only sign of a hollow viscus injury. Pneumoperitoneum often is not present, even with a full-thickness bowel wall disruption. Virtually all neurologically intact patients have findings or symptoms suggestive of peritoneal contamination from a perforated viscus, such as pain, rebound tenderness, or guarding.[89] The unconscious patient with multiple injuries presents a significant diagnostic challenge, and a high index of suspicion must be maintained.

Children who have a visible contusion of the abdominal wall from a seat belt–lap restraint have been documented to have an increased incidence of abdominal injuries, both solid and hollow organs, as well as fractures of the lower thoracic and lumbar spine (Fig. 16-10). These children must have frequent in-hospital assessments, serial physical examination by the same surgeon, and diagnostic imaging to assess for abdominal and spinal injuries.

Stomach

Injuries to the stomach due to penetration are variable in the amount of tissue destruction, dependent primarily on the velocity of the offending missile or penetrating object.

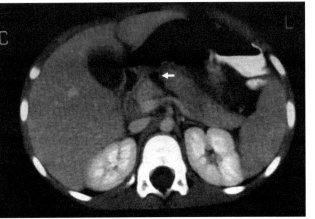

FIGURE 16-9. This abdominal computed tomography scan demonstrates blunt pancreatic transection (*arrow*).

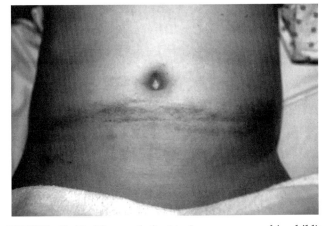

FIGURE 16-10. The seatbelt sign is seen across this child's lower abdomen.

Blunt injury to the stomach occurs when a compressive force causes a burst injury in a patient with a full stomach. Gastric injuries are relatively infrequent, but nearly always occur after a meal.

The diagnosis of a gastric injury from blunt force is often problematic. Free air often is not seen. A nasogastric tube lying outside the stomach contour on a roentgenogram or CT is diagnostic. The child with abdominal ecchymosis, tenderness, and/or free fluid in the peritoneal cavity should prompt the suspicion of hollow viscus injury.

Surgical exploration for a suspected gastric injury is initiated with an upper midline incision. The stomach and duodenum should be adequately mobilized, and hemorrhage controlled. Particular attention should be paid to the lesser curve and to the posterior stomach near the gastroesophageal junction, sites of possible missed injuries. The lesser sac should always be opened to explore the posterior wall of the stomach adequately.

Duodenum

Duodenal injuries may be extremely difficult to manage because of the intimate association with the pancreas, extrahepatic biliary system, and intra-abdominal vascular systems. Thorough mobilization is key to identifying injuries, both blunt and penetrating. The procedure required to repair a duodenal injury is dependent on the location and amount of tissue destruction encountered. Extravasation of air or enteral CT contrast material into the paraduodenal, pararenal, or retroperitoneal space is the key finding in those patients with a duodenal perforation. This is not seen in patients sustaining a duodenal hematoma.[90]

An intramural duodenal hematoma due to blunt force applied to the epigastrium (kick, fist, handlebar) may be managed nonoperatively if the child has no evidence of full-thickness injury or peritonitis.[91] The CT scans or upper GI contrast studies typically reveal duodenal narrowing, spiraling, or partial obstruction of the duodenum, and no contrast or air extravasating from the duodenal lumen. When managed nonoperatively, nasogastric decompression and TPN may be required for an average of 1 to 3 weeks. If a duodenal hematoma is encountered during exploration for additional abdominal trauma, the serosa may be incised and the clot carefully evacuated, taking care not to enter the duodenal lumen.

Full-thickness duodenal injuries may be closed primarily if tissue destruction is not excessive and if the closure will not compromise the duodenal lumen. Adequate drainage is important if a pancreatic injury or major duodenal tissue devitalization has occurred. Duodenal closure may be obtained with the aid of a Roux limb of jejunum sewn to a debrided duodenal injury. A duodenal drainage tube for decompression is left in place. Temporary pyloric exclusion with an absorbable suture via a gastrotomy also may aid in management of a complex duodenal repair, allowing healing of the duodenum before spontaneous recanalization of the pylorus. A gastrostomy tube for decompression also is placed for gastric drainage. A third enteral tube, a feeding jejunostomy, also is introduced for enteral nutritional support. Drains are placed near the injured tissue at the time of initial repair so that a controlled fistula will result from any enteric leak. Somatostatin analogues may be helpful in decreasing pancreatic and intestinal secretions and are useful in management of a fistula if one occurs. Rarely is a pancreaticoduodenectomy required in blunt trauma in children.[92]

Small Bowel

Penetrating injury to the abdomen frequently injures the small intestine. Identification of mesenteric and bowel wall injuries must be carefully and systematically performed. Extensive injuries should be managed by resection and anastomosis. Isolated perforations and lacerations may be repaired with debridement and closure, with care to avoid luminal narrowing.

Hematomas to the mesentery should be explored, and control of bleeding vessels should be meticulously performed. If a segment of bowel is in jeopardy because of a mesenteric injury, resection and primary anastomosis should be performed to avoid stricture formation. Injuries to the superior mesenteric artery or vein should be repaired with a vein patch as needed to avoid stenosis of the affected vessel. Delayed injuries also may be seen secondary to rapid deceleration and avulsion of the bowel from its mesentery (Fig. 16-11).

Colon

Colon injuries in children may occur by the same mechanisms as small bowel injuries, but the consequences may be more significant. The serious septic complications that result from delayed treatment of a colon injury can be life threatening. If isolated colonic injuries are identified and repaired early, a primary bowel anastomosis with appropriate perioperative antibiotic coverage is safe and avoids the potential complications of stomas and reoperation for stoma closure. Once a colonic injury has

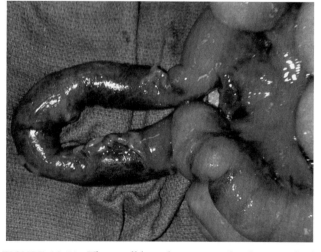

FIGURE 16-11. The small bowel mesentery has been avulsed, resulting in ischemic bowel.

been identified, multiple factors influence management of the wound. In the absence of shock and/or significant fecal contamination, many colon injuries may be repaired primarily. A proximal diverting stoma may be necessary if extensive repair or resection of a segment of colon with fecal soiling has been required. If extensive damage to the abdominal wall has occurred, requiring prosthetic material to be placed for wound closure, care must be taken to place the colostomy in a location that will minimize soiling of the wound.

Rectal Injuries

The etiology of the majority of perineal and rectal injuries in children is either accidental falls in a straddle fashion onto sharp or blunt objects, or sexual abuse. Typically, rectal perforations require proximal diversion with an end colostomy and drainage of the distal injured rectum. Identification of these injuries may be difficult. The ability to ascertain the extent of the injury will frequently require a formal examination under anesthesia. Proctosigmoidoscopy in a nonprepped colon may not clearly localize a perforation, but endoluminal blood must be assumed to be evidence of injury. After colostomy and presacral drainage, rectal washout should be performed to empty the distal rectum of feces. Meticulous repair of the injured anal sphincter musculature must be performed. The nonviable tissue should be debrided, and closure of the rectal injury may be accomplished transanally if the injury is low enough to permit this approach.

DIAPHRAGM

Traumatic injury to the diaphragm is infrequently observed, even at the largest pediatric trauma centers. These injuries are caused by massive compressive forces to the abdomen, which create acceleration of abdominal contents cephalad followed by rupture of the diaphragmatic muscle. Occasionally, penetrating trauma will cause this injury; however, in these cases, it is often found incidentally at exploration for other injuries. In one reported series, 13 of 15 patients had diaphragmatic rupture from blunt trauma; the mean age was 7.5 years, with the right and left diaphragm equally involved.[93] The diagnosis was made frequently by chest radiograph (53%), with other studies infrequently required.[94] The plain radiographic findings include

- Obscured hemidiaphragm
- Elevated hemidiaphragm
- Gas in herniated viscus above the diaphragm
- Tip of nasogastric tube in thorax
- Atypical pneumothorax
- Platelike atelectasis adjacent to the diaphragm

In this series, three injuries were missed at the initial evaluation. Because of the force required to cause this injury, multiple associated injuries were observed (and should be expected). In this report, 81% of patients had multiple injuries, which included liver lacerations (47%), pelvic fractures (47%), major vascular injuries (40%),

bowel perforations (33%), long bone fractures (20%), renal lacerations (20%), splenic lacerations (13%), and closed head injuries (13%). As would be expected, many complications were noted, five deaths, and a mean length of stay of 20 days. Emergency operation with minimal diagnostic testing is often necessary in patients with multiple abdominal injuries. Therefore when operating on children with this constellation of associated injuries, observation and palpation of both diaphragms must be a routine part of the abdominal exploration. Direct suture repair is usually possible after debridement of any devitalized tissue. We use pledgets to buttress the repair, to prevent tearing of the muscle, and to make the closure more secure. If sufficient diaphragm tissue is destroyed, a tension-free closure with a 2-mm polypropylene patch can be used in the manner of repairing congenital diaphragmatic hernias in newborns. Reports of laparoscopic or thoracoscopic repair of diaphragm injury included stable patients without associated injuries and delayed repairs.[95,96] Delayed diagnosis of this injury has been reported, as has renal avulsion into the chest through a traumatically ruptured diaphragm.[97–99] Because of the rarity of this injury, a high index of suspicion must be maintained when the mechanism of injury and degree and location of other injured body systems suggest the possibility of this injury occurring.

RENAL TRAUMA

The kidney is the most commonly injured organ in the urogenital system. Children appear to be more susceptible to major renal trauma than are adults.[100] Several unique anatomic aspects contribute to this observation, including less cushioning from perirenal fat, weaker abdominal musculature, and a less-well-ossified thoracic cage. The child's kidney also occupies a proportionately larger space in the retroperitoneum than does an adult kidney. In addition, the pediatric kidney may retain fetal lobulations, permitting easier parenchymal disruption.

Renal trauma is broadly classified as being blunt or penetrating. Blunt trauma is more common, accounting for more than 90% of injuries in some series.[101] The kidney, which is relatively mobile within Gerota's fascia, can be crushed against the ribs or vertebral column, resulting in parenchymal lacerations or contusions. The kidney also can be lacerated by fractured ribs. Penetrating trauma accounts for only 10% to 20% of renal injuries, yet is responsible for the majority of renal injuries that require operation.[102] Penetrating injuries to the chest, abdomen, flank, and lumbar regions should be assumed to have caused renal injury until proven otherwise.

Preexisting or congenital renal abnormalities, such as hydronephrosis, tumors, or abnormal position, make the kidney vulnerable to relatively mild traumatic forces. Historically, congenital abnormalities in injured kidneys have been reported to vary from 1% to 21%, although recent reviews have shown that the incidence rates are more nearly 1% to 5%.[103,104] Renal abnormalities, particularly hydronephrosis, may be discovered as a result of minor blunt abdominal trauma. Rarely the child may be seen with an acute abdomen secondary to intraperitoneal rupture of a hydronephrotic kidney.[105]

Major deceleration/flexion injuries may produce renal arterial or venous injuries due to stretching of a normally fixed vascular pedicle. This type of injury may be more common in children because of their increased flexibility and relatively increased renal mobility.[106–108] Post-traumatic thrombosis of the renal artery follows an intimal tear that occurs because the media and adventitia of the renal artery are more elastic than the intima. The intimal tear produces thrombosis that results in renal ischemia. A high index of suspicion must be maintained to identify these injuries in a timely fashion.

Diagnosis of Renal Injury

Once the patient has been resuscitated and life-threatening injuries have been addressed, evaluation of the genitourinary system can be undertaken. After any blunt injury, the presence of hematuria (microscopic or gross), a palpable flank mass, or flank hematomas are indications for urologic evaluations. Most major blunt renal injuries occur in association with other major injuries of the head, chest, and abdomen. Urologic investigations should be undertaken when trauma to the lower chest is associated with rib, thoracic, or lumbar spine fractures. It also should be performed in all crush injuries to the abdomen or pelvis when the patient has sustained a severe deceleration injury. Because a renal pedicle injury or ureteropelvic junction (UPJ) disruption may not be associated with one of the classic signs of renal injury such as hematuria, radiologic evaluation to demonstrate bilateral renal function should always be considered in patients with a mechanism of injury that could potentially injure the upper urinary tract.

Gross hematuria is the most reliable indicator for serious urologic injury.[109] The need for imaging in the patient with blunt trauma and microscopic hematuria is not so clear. Moreover, the degree of hematuria does not always correlate with the degree of injury.[110] Renal vascular pedicle avulsion or acute thrombosis of segmental arteries can occur in the absence of hematuria, whereas mild renal contusions can appear with gross hematuria.[111] In adults, the vast majority of patients with blunt trauma with microscopic hematuria and no evidence of shock (systolic blood pressure, < 90 mm Hg) have minor renal injuries and thus do not need to be studied radiographically.[111,112] Guidelines for evaluating the pediatric population are not so clearly defined. All children with any degree of microscopic hematuria after blunt trauma have traditionally undergone renal imaging. Recently, a meta-analysis of all reported series of children with hematuria and suspected renal injury revealed that only 11 (2%) of 548 of patients with insignificant microscopic hematuria [< 50 red blood cells per high-power field (RBC/HPF)] had a significant renal injury.[113] However, it is important to note that all 11 of these patients were found to have multiple organ trauma, and renal imaging would have been performed in the course of evaluation despite the relatively minor amount of microscopic hematuria. Detection of significant renal injury was

found to increase to 8% with significant microhematuria (> 50 RBC/HPF), and to 32% in those with gross hematuria after blunt trauma. The presence of multisystem trauma significantly increases the risk for significant renal damage. Thus it seems reasonable to consider observation without renal imaging in children with microscopic hematuria of less than 50 RBC/HPF that are stable unless they have multiple organ system injuries.

Historically, excretory urography (intravenous pyelogram; IVP) has been the radiographic imaging study of choice in suspected renal trauma. Sensitivity has been reported as high as 90% in diagnosing renal injury. Unfortunately, IVP misses other intra-abdominal injuries and may miss or understage renal injury in children by 50% compared with CT scan.[114,115] CT scans are now used almost exclusively as the imaging study of choice for suspected renal trauma in hemodynamically stable adults and children.[116] CT is both sensitive and specific for demonstrating parenchymal laceration or urinary extravasation, for delineating segmental parenchymal infarcts, for determining the size and location of the surrounding retroperitoneal hematoma, and/or for diagnosing associated intra-abdominal injury (Fig. 16-12). CT also allows accurate staging of the renal injury.

The most commonly used staging system for renal trauma is from the American Association for the Surgery of Trauma. This classification categorizes renal trauma into five grades that have predictive value in the subsequent management strategy of these injuries.[117] The ultimate goal of complete staging is to provide sufficient information for management that results in the preservation of renal parenchyma and the salvage of injured kidneys.

Ultrasonography (US) also has been used to assess renal trauma. However, its sensitivity in demonstrating renal injury in comparison to CT is only 25% to 70%. It also may miss associated intra-abdominal injuries. Unfortunately, FAST has been shown to have a low sensitivity for solid-organ injury in children. It also provides poor information concerning renal function or pedicle injuries. At present, renal US is not currently

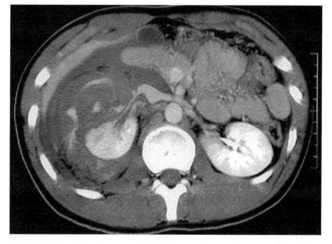

FIGURE 16-12. Severe right kidney disruption, resulting in a large perirenal hematoma, is seen on this computed tomography scan with intravenous contrast.

recommended as a useful screening tool for urologic evaluation in the setting of blunt renal trauma.[118]

It is imperative to acknowledge that major renal injuries such as UPJ disruption or segmental arterial thrombosis may occur without the presence of hematuria or hypotension. Therefore a high index of suspicion is necessary to diagnose these injuries. Nonvisualization of the injured kidney on IVP or failure of contrast uptake with a large associated perirenal hematoma on CT are hallmark findings for renal artery thrombosis. UPJ disruption is classically seen as perihilar extravasation of contrast with nonvisualization of the distal ureter.[119]

Treatment of Renal Injury

In most patients, attempts should be made to manage all renal injuries non-operatively.[120–122] Minor renal injuries constitute the majority of blunt renal injuries and usually resolve without incident.[123] The management of major renal parenchymal lacerations, although accounting for only 10% to 15% of all renal trauma patients, is currently controversial. Operative intervention is not always mandatory, and many major renal injuries due to blunt trauma may be managed without operation.[124–126] When necessary, the goals of surgical renal exploration are either to treat major renal injuries definitively with preservation of renal parenchyma when possible or to evaluate thoroughly a suspected renal injury. The need for surgical exploration is much higher in patients with penetrating trauma as opposed to blunt trauma.

The indications for renal exploration vary greatly between individual trauma centers. Most centers expectantly manage grade I to III injuries with bed rest and observation. Controversies arise in the management of grade IV to V injuries. The majority of blunt renal injuries sustained are minor contusions and lacerations. Even in the presence of gross hematuria, most blunt renal injuries will not require exploration and will have excellent long-term outcomes.[126] Absolute indications for renal exploration include persistent life-threatening bleeding; an expanding, pulsatile, or uncontained retroperitoneal hematoma; or suspected renal pedicle avulsion. Relative indications for exploration include substantial devitalized renal parenchyma or urinary extravasation. Injuries with significant (>25%) nonviable renal tissue associated with parenchymal laceration that are managed nonoperatively have a complication rate of more than 75%.[127] When such renal injuries are associated with an intraperitoneal organ injury, the postinjury complication rate is much higher unless the kidney is surgically repaired. By surgically repairing such injuries, surgeons reduced the overall morbidity from 85% to 23%. Urinary extravasation in itself does not demand surgical exploration. In patients with major renal injury and urinary extravasation who are managed non-operatively, urinary extravasation resolved spontaneously in 87%.[121] Extravasation persisted in 13% and was successfully managed endoscopically. Incomplete staging of the renal injury demands either further imaging or renal exploration and reconstruction. Most commonly these patients undergo renal exploration because they are bleeding persistently or because they have an associated injury that requires laparotomy.

When the nonoperative approach is chosen, supportive care with bed rest, hydration, antibiotics, and serial hemoglobin and blood pressure monitoring is required. After the gross hematuria resolves, limited activity is advised for 2 to 4 weeks until microscopic hematuria ceases. Complications can occur during the period of observation within the first 4 weeks of injury and include delayed bleeding, abscess, sepsis, urinary fistula, urinary extravasation, urinoma, and hypertension. The greatest risk is life-threatening hemorrhage occurring within the first 2 weeks of injury. Immediate surgical exploration or angiographic embolization is indicated. Angiographic embolization is an alternative to exploration in a hemodynamically stable patient in whom persistent gross hematuria signifies persistent low-grade hemorrhage from the injured kidney. Persistent urinary extravasation has successfully been managed by percutaneous drainage. Hypertension in the early posttrauma period is uncommon. Hypertension may develop in the ensuing months and, in most instances, is treated with medical management.

Renal Exploration and Reconstruction

If operation is required, early control of the vessels increases the rate of renal salvage.[128] When proximal vascular control is initially achieved before any renal exploration, nephrectomy is required in fewer than 12% of cases.[129] When primary vascular control is not achieved and massive bleeding is encountered, in the rush to control bleeding, a kidney that could have been salvaged may be sacrificed unnecessarily. The surgeon must carefully identify the kidney's relations with the posterior abdomen and the posterior parietal peritoneum. The colon is lifted from the abdomen and placed on the anterior chest to allow mobilization of the small bowel. The inferior mesenteric vein and the aorta are identified at this point, and the posterior peritoneum is incised medial to the inferior mesenteric vein. The aorta is dissected superiorly to the ligament of Treitz, where the left renal vein is found crossing anterior to the aorta. Retraction of the left renal vein exposes both renal arteries beneath it. These arteries may now be isolated and controlled with vessel loops. Once vessel isolation is complete, an incision is made in the peritoneum just lateral to the colon. The colon is reflected medially to expose the retroperitoneal hematoma in its entirety, and the kidney may be exposed. If significant bleeding is encountered, the ipsilateral renal vessels may be occluded. Warm ischemia time should not surpass 30 minutes.[129]

Renal vascular injuries must be addressed promptly. Major lacerations to the renal vein are repaired directly with venorrhaphy. Repair of renal arterial injuries may require a variety of techniques including resection with end-to-end anastomosis, bypass graft with autogenous vein or a synthetic graft, and arteriorrhaphy. Traumatic renal artery occlusion requires many of the same techniques for repair. However, this must be performed in the first 12 hours from the time of injury; otherwise, the kidney is usually nonviable after this length of ischemia.

REFERENCES

1. Malhotra AK, Fabian TC, Croce MA, et al: Blunt hepatic injury: A paradigm shift from operative to nonoperative management in the 1990s. Ann Surg 231:804–813, 2000.
2. Cooper A, Barlow B, DiScala C, et al: Mortality and truncal injury: The pediatric perspective. J Pediatr Surg 29:33–38, 1994.
3. Eubanks JW, Meier DE, Hicks BA, et al: Significance of "blush" on computed tomography scan in children with liver injury. J Pediatr Surg 38:363–366, 2003.
4. Clancy TV, Ragozzino MW, Ramshaw D, et al: Oral contrast is not necessary in the evaluation of blunt trauma by computed tomography. Am J Surg 166:680–685, 1993.
5. Bensard DD, Beaver BL, Besner GE, et al: Small bowel injury in children after blunt abdominal trauma: Is diagnostic delay important? J Trauma 41:476–483, 1996.
6. Bulas DI, Taylor GA, Eichelberger MR: The value of CT in detecting bowel perforation in children after blunt abdominal trauma. Am J Roentgenol 153:561–564, 1989.
7. Jamieson DH, Babyn PS, Pearl R: Imaging gastrointestinal perforation in pediatric blunt abdominal trauma. Pediatr Radiol 26:188–194, 1996.
8. Sivit CJ, Taylor GA, Bulas DI, et al: Blunt trauma in children: Significance of peritoneal fluid. Radiology 178:185–188, 1991.
9. Patel JC, Tepas JJ: The efficacy of focused abdominal sonography for trauma (FAST) as a screening tool in the assessment of injured children. J Pediatr Surg 34:44–47, 1999.
10. Ong AW, McKenney MG, McKenney KA, et al: Predicting the need for laparotomy in pediatric trauma patients on the basis of the ultrasound score. J Trauma 54:503–508, 2003.
11. Cuschieri A, Hennessy TP, Stephens RB, et al: Diagnosis of significant abdominal trauma after road traffic accidents: Preliminary results of a multicentre clinical trial comparing mini-laparoscopy with peritoneal lavage. Ann R Coll Surg Engl 70:153–155, 1988.
12. Simon RJ, Rabin J, Kuhls D: Impact of increased use of laparoscopy on negative laparotomy rates after penetrating trauma. J Trauma 53:297–302, 2002.
13. Smith RS, Fry WR, Morabito DJ, et al: Therapeutic laparoscopy in trauma. Am J Surg 170:632–636, 1995.
14. Fallat ME, Casale AJ: Practice patterns of pediatric surgeons caring for stable patients with traumatic solid organ injury. J Trauma 43:820–824, 1997.
15. Stylianos S: Controversies in abdominal trauma. Semin Pediatr Surg 4:116–119, 1995.
16. Potoka DA, Schall LC, Ford HR: Risk factors for splenectomy in children with blunt splenic trauma. J Pediatr Surg 37:294–299, 2002.
17. Hackam DJ, Potoka D, Meza M, et al: Utility of radiographic hepatic injury grade in predicting outcome for children after blunt abdominal trauma. J Pediatr Surg 237:386–389, 2002.
18. Mehall JR, Ennis JS, Saltzman DA, et al: Prospective results of a standardized algorithm based on hemodynamic status for managing pediatric solid organ injury. J Am Coll Surg 193:347–353, 2001.
19. Moore EE, Cogbill TH, Jurkovich GJ: Organ injury scaling: Spleen and liver (1994 Revision). J Trauma 38:323–324, 1995.
20. Stylianos S, APSA Trauma Committee: Evidence-based guidelines for resource utilization in children with isolated spleen or liver injury. J Pediatr Surg 35:164–169, 2000.
21. Stylianos S, APSA Trauma Study Group: Prospective validation of evidence-based guidelines for resource utilization in children with isolated spleen or liver injury. J Pediatr Surg 37:453–456, 2002.
22. Mooney DP, Birkmeyer NJO, Udell JV: Variation in the management of pediatric splenic injuries in New Hampshire. J Pediatr Surg 33:1076–1080, 1998.
23. Lovvorn HN: Unpublished communication.
24. Keller MS, Sartorelli KH, Vane DW: Associated head injury should not prevent nonoperative management of spleen or liver injury in children. J Trauma 41:471–475, 1996.
25. Frumiento C, Vane DW: Changing patterns of treatment for blunt splenic injuries: An 11-year experience in a rural state. J Pediatr Surg 35:985–989, 2000.
26. Rhodes M, Smith S, Boorse D: Pediatric trauma patients in an "adult" trauma center. J Trauma 35:384–393, 1993.
27. Keller MS, Vane DW: Management of pediatric blunt splenic injury: Comparison of pediatric and adult trauma surgeons. J Pediatr Surg 30:221–225, 1995.
28. Pearl RH, Wesson DE, Spence LJ: Splenic injury: A five year update with improved results and changing criteria for conservative management. J Pediatr Surg 24:428–431, 1989.
29. Lynch JM, Ford H, Gardner MJ: Is early discharge following isolated splenic injury in the hemodynamically stable child possible? J Pediatr Surg 28:1403–1407, 1993.
30. Morse MA, Garcia VF: Selective nonoperative management of pediatric blunt splenic trauma: Risk for missed associated injuries. J Pediatr Surg 29:23–27, 1994.
31. Nance ML, Keller MS, Stafford PW: Predicting hollow visceral injury in the pediatric blunt trauma patient with solid visceral injury. J Pediatr Surg 35:1300–1303, 2000.
32. Shafi S, Gilbert JC, Carden S: Risk of hemorrhage and appropriate use of blood transfusions in pediatric blunt splenic injuries. J Trauma 42:1029–1032, 1997.
33. Miller K, Kou D, Stallion A, et al: Pediatric hepatic trauma: Does clinical course support intensive care unit stay? J Pediatr Surg 33:1459–1462, 1998.
34. Leinwand MJ, Atkinson CC, Mooney DP: Application of the APSA evidence-based guidelines for isolated liver or spleen injuries: a single-institution experience. J Pediatr Surg 39:487–490, 2004.
35. Goettler CE, Stallion A, Grisoni ER, et al: Delayed hemorrhage after blunt hepatic trauma. J Trauma 52:556–559, 2002.
36. Fisher JC, Moulton SL: Nonoperative management and delayed hemorrhage following pediatric liver injury. J Pediatr Surg 39:619–622, 2004.
37. Shilyansky J, Navarro O, Superina RA, et al: Delayed hemorrhage after nonoperative management of blunt hepatic trauma in children: A rare but significant event. J Pediatr Surg 34:60–64, 1999.
38. Brown RL, Irish MS, McCabe AJ, et al: Observation of splenic trauma: When is a little too much? J Pediatr Surg 34:1124–1126, 1999.
39. Norotsky MC, Rogers FB, Shackford SR: Delayed presentation of splenic artery pseudoaneurysms following blunt abdominal trauma: Case reports. J Trauma 38:444–447, 1995.
40. Frumiento C, Sartorelli K, Vane DW: Complications of splenic injuries: Expansion of the nonoperative theorem. J Pediatr Surg 35:788–791, 2000.
41. Pryor JP, Stafford PW, Nance ML: Severe blunt hepatic trauma in children. J Pediatr Surg 36:974–979, 2001.
42. Hoyt DB, Bulger EM, Knudson MM: Death in the operating room: An analysis of a multi-center experience. J Trauma 37:426–432, 1994.
43. Moulton SL, Lynch FP, Canty TG: Hepatic vein and retrohepatic vena caval injuries in children: Sternotomy first? Arch Surg 126:1262–1266, 1991.
44. Watts DD, Trask A, Soeken K, et al: Hypothermic coagulopathy in trauma: Effect of varying levels of hypothermia on enzyme speed, platelet function, and fibrinolytic activity. J Trauma 44:846–854, 1998.
45. Denton JR, Moore EE, Codwell DM: Multimodality treatment for grade V hepatic injuries: Perihepatic packing, arterial embolization, and venous stenting. J Trauma 42:964–968, 1997.
46. Yang EY, Marder SR, Hastings G, et al: The abdominal compartment syndrome complicating nonoperative management of major blunt liver injuries: Recognition and treatment using multimodality therapy. J Trauma 52:982–986, 2002.
47. Kushimoto S, Arai M, Aiboshi J, et al: The role of interventional radiology in patients requiring damage control laparotomy. J Trauma 54:171–176, 2003.
48. Asensio JA, Demetriades D, Chahwan S: Approach to the management of complex hepatic injuries. J Trauma 48:66–69, 2000.
49. Shapiro MB, Jenkins DH, Schwab CW, et al: Damage control: Collective review. J Trauma 49:969–978, 2000.
50. Barker DE, Kaufman HJ, Smith LA, et al: Vacuum pack technique of temporary abdominal closure: A 7-year experience with 112 patients. J Trauma 48:201–207, 2000.

51. Vargo D, Sorenson J, Barton R: Repair of grade VI hepatic injury: Case report and literature review. J Trauma 53:823–824, 2002.
52. Cogbill TH, Moore EE, Jurkovich GJ: Severe hepatic trauma: A multicenter experience with 1,335 liver injuries. J Trauma 28:1433–1438, 1988.
53. Hirshberg A, Mattox KL: Planned re-operation for severe trauma. Ann Surg 222:3–8, 1995.
54. Rotondo MF, Schwab CW, McGonigal MD: Damage control: An approach for improved survival in exsanguinating penetrating abdominal injury. J Trauma 35:375–383, 1993.
55. Stylianos S, Jacir NN, Hoffman MA, et al: Pediatric blunt liver injury and coagulopathy managed with packs and silo. J Trauma 30:1409–1410, 1990.
56. Stylianos S: Abdominal packing for severe hemorrhage. J Pediatr Surg 33:339–342, 1998.
57. Evans S, Jackson RJ, Smith SD: Successful repair of major retro-hepatic vascular injuries without the use of shunt or sternotomy. J Pediatr Surg 28:317–320, 1993.
58. Horwitz JR, Black T, Lally KP: Venovenous bypass as an adjunct for the management of a retrohepatic venous injury in a child. J Trauma 39:584–585, 1995.
59. Davies MRQ: Iatrogenic hepatic rupture in the newborn and its management by pack tamponade. J Pediatr Surg 32:1414–1419, 1997.
60. Strear CM, Graf JL, Albanese CT, et al: Successful treatment of liver hemorrhage in the premature infant. J Pediatr Surg 33:849–851, 1998.
61. Markley MA, Mantor PC, Letton RW, et al: Pediatric vacuum packing wound closure for damage-control laparotomy. J Pediatr Surg 37:512–514, 2002.
62. Adams JM, Hauser CJ, Livingston DH, et al: The immunomodulatory effects of damage control abdominal packing on local and systemic neutrophil activity. J Trauma 50:792–800, 2001.
63. Saggi BH, Sugerman HJ, Ivatury RR, et al: Abdominal compartment syndrome. J Trauma 45:597–609, 1998.
64. Oda J, Ivatury RR, Blocher CR, et al: Amplified cytokine response and lung injury by sequential hemorrhagic shock and abdominal compartment syndrome in a laboratory model of ischemia-reperfusion. J Trauma 52:625–632, 2002.
65. Rezende-Neto JB, Moore EE, de Andrade MVM, et al: Systemic inflammatory response syndrome secondary to abdominal compartment syndrome: Stage for multiple organ failure. J Trauma 53:1121–1128, 2002.
66. Sharpe RP, Pryor JP, Gandhi RR, et al: Abdominal compartment syndrome in the pediatric blunt trauma patient treated with paracentesis: Report of two cases. J Trauma 53:380–382, 2002.
67. Hobson KG, Young KM, Ciraulo A, et al: Release of abdominal compartment syndrome improves survival in patients with burn injury. J Trauma 53:1129–1134, 2002.
68. Chang MC, Miller PR, D'Agostino R, et al: Effects of abdominal decompression on cardiopulmonary function and visceral perfusion in patients with intra-abdominal hypertension. J Trauma 44:440–445, 1998.
69. DeCou JM, Abrams RS, Miller RS, et al: Abdominal compartment syndrome in children: Experience with three cases. J Pediatr Surg 35:840–842, 2000.
70. Epelman M, Soudack M, Engel A, et al: Abdominal compartment syndrome in children: CT findings. Pediatr Radiol 32:319–322, 2002.
71. Neville HL, Lally KP, Cox CS: Emergent abdominal decompression with patch abdominoplasty in the pediatric patient. J Pediatr Surg 35:705–770, 2000.
72. Bass BL, Eichelberger MR, Schisgall MR: Hazards of non-operative therapy of hepatic trauma in children. J Trauma 24:978–982, 1984.
73. Scioscia PJ, Dillon PW, Cilley RE: Endoscopic sphincterotomy in the management of posttraumatic biliary fistula. J Pediatr Surg 29:3–6, 1994.
74. Sharif K, Pimpalwar AP, John P, et al: Benefits of early diagnosis and preemptive treatment of biliary tract complications after major blunt liver trauma in children. J Pediatr Surg 37:1287–1292, 2002.
75. Sharpe RP, Nance ML, Stafford PW: Nonoperative management of blunt extrahepatic biliary duct transection in the pediatric patient. J Pediatr Surg 37:1612–1616, 2002.
76. Church NG, May G, Sigalet DL: A minimally invasive approach to bile duct injury after blunt liver trauma in pediatric patients. J Pediatr Surg 37:773–775, 2002.
77. Moulton SL, Downey EC, Anderson DS: Blunt bile duct injuries in children. J Pediatr Surg 28:795–797, 1993.
78. Lane MJ, Mindelzun RE, Jeffery RB: Diagnosis of pancreatic injury after blunt abdominal trauma. Semin Ultrasound CT MR 17:177–182, 1996.
79. Canty TG, Weinman D: Management of major pancreatic duct injuries in children. J Trauma 50:1001–1007, 2001.
80. Soto JA, Alvarez O, Munera F, et al: Traumatic disruption of the pancreatic duct: Diagnosis with MR pancreatography. Am J Roentgenol 176:175–178, 2001.
81. Moosa AR: Diagnostic tests and procedures in acute pancreatitis. N Engl J Med 311: 639–643, 1984.
82. Rescorla FJ, Plumkey DA, Sherman S, et al: The efficacy of early ERCP in pediatric pancreatic trauma. J Pediatr Surg 30:336–340, 1995.
83. Meier DE, Coln CD, Hicks BA, et al: Early operation in patients with pancreas transaction. J Pediatr Surg 36:341–344, 2001.
84. McGahren ED, Magnuson D, Schauer RT, et al: Management of transection of the pancreas in children. Aust N Z J Surg 65: 242–246, 1995.
85. Shilyansky J, Sena LM, Kreller M, et al: Nonoperative management of pancreatic injuries in children. J Pediatr Surg 33:343–349, 1998.
86. Kouchi K, Tanabe M, Yoshida H, et al: Nonoperative management of blunt pancreatic injury in childhood. J Pediatr Surg 34:1736–1739, 1999.
87. Harrell DJ, Vitale GC, Larson GM: Selective role for endoscopic retrograde cholangiopancreatography in abdominal trauma. Surg Endosc 12:400–404, 1998.
88. Kim HS, Lee DK, Kim IW, et al: The role of retrograde pancreatography in the treatment of traumatic pancreatic duct injury. Gastrointest Endosc 54:45–55, 2001.
89. Jerby BL, Attorri RJ, Morton K: Blunt intestinal injury in children: The role of the physical examination. J Pediatr Surg 32:580–584, 1997.
90. Shilyansky J, Pearl RH, Kroutouro M, et al: Diagnosis and management of duodenal injuries in children. J Pediatr Surg 32: 880–886, 1997.
91. Winthrop AL, Wesson DE, Filler RM: Traumatic duodenal hematoma in the pediatric patient. J Pediatr Surg 21:757–760, 1986.
92. Ladd AP, West KW, Rouse TM, et al: Surgical management of duodenal injuries in children. Surgery 132:748–753, 2002.
93. Ramos CT, Koplewitz BZ, Babyn PS, et al: What have we learned about traumatic diaphragmatic hernias in children? J Pediatr Surg 35:601–604, 2000.
94. Koplewitz BZ, Ramos C, Manson DE, et al: Traumatic diaphragmatic injuries in infants and children: Imaging findings. Pediatr Radiol 30:471–479, 2000.
95. Pitcher G: Fiber-endoscopic thoracoscopy for diaphragmatic injury in children. Semin Pediatr Surg 10:17–19, 2000.
96. Meyer G, Huttl TP, Hatz RA, et al: Laparoscopic repair of traumatic diaphragmatic hernias. Surg Endosc 14:1010–1014, 2000.
97. Sola JE, Mattei P, Pegoli W Jr, et al: Rupture of the right diaphragm following blunt trauma in an infant: Case report. J Trauma 36: 417–420, 1994.
98. Cohen Z, Gabriel A, Izrachi S, et al: Traumatic avulsion of kidney into the chest through a ruptured diaphragm in a boy. Pediatr Emerg Care 3:180–181, 2000.
99. Stylianos S, Bergman KS, Harris BH: Traumatic renal avulsion into the chest: Case report. J Trauma 31:301–302, 1991.
100. Brown SL, Elder JS, Spirnak JP: Are pediatric patients more susceptible to major renal injury from blunt trauma? A comparative study. J Urol 160:138–140, 1998.
101. Medica J, Caldamone A: Pediatric renal trauma: Special considerations. Semin Urol 13:73–76, 1995.
102. Nash PA, Bruce JE, McAninch JW: Nephrectomy for traumatic renal injuries. J Urol 153:609–611, 1995.
103. Abou-Jaoude WA, Sugarman JM, Fallat ME: Indicators of genitourinary tract injury or anomaly in cases of pediatric blunt trauma. J Pediatr Surg 31:86–89, 1996.

104. Brower P, Paul J, Brosman SA: Urinary tract abnormalities presenting as a result of blunt abdominal trauma. J Trauma 18: 719–722, 1978.

105. Ekwueme O, Adibe SO: Intraperitoneal rupture of hydronephrotic kidney. Br J Surg 63:637–638, 1976.

106. Smith EM, Elder JS, Spirnak JP: Major blunt renal trauma in the pediatric population: Is a nonoperative approach indicated? J Urol 149:546–548, 1993.

107. McAleer IM, Kaplan GW: Pediatric genitourinary trauma. Urol Clin North Am 22:177–188, 1995.

108. Smith SD, Gardner MJ, Rowe MI: Renal artery occlusion in pediatric blunt abdominal trauma: Decreasing the delay from injury to treatment. J Trauma 35:861–864, 1993.

109. Quinlan DM, Gearhart JP: Blunt renal trauma in childhood: Features indicating severe injury. Br J Urol 66:526–531, 1990.

110. Stein JP, Kaji DM, Eastham J, et al: Blunt renal trauma in the pediatric population: Indications for radiographic evaluation. Urology 44:406–410, 1994.

111. Miller KS, McAninch JW: Radiographic assessment of renal trauma: Our 15-year experience. J Urol 154:352–355, 1995.

112. Eastham JA, Wilson TG, Ahlering TE: Radiographic evaluation of adult patients with blunt renal trauma. J Urol 148:266–267, 1992.

113. Morey AF, Bruce JE, McAninch JW: Efficacy of radiographic imaging in pediatric blunt renal trauma. J Urol 156:2014–2018, 1996.

114. Hashmi A, Klassen T: Correlation between urinalysis and intravenous pyelography in pediatric abdominal trauma. J Emerg Med 13: 255–258, 1995.

115. Middlebrook PF, Schillinger JF: Hematuria and intravenous pyelography in pediatric blunt renal trauma. Can J Surg 36:59–62, 1993.

116. Taylor GA, Eichelberger MR, O'Donnell R, et al: Indications for computed tomography in children with blunt abdominal trauma. Ann Surg 213:212–218, 1991.

117. Moore EE, Shackford SR, Pachter HL, et al: Organ injury scaling: spleen, liver, and kidney. J Trauma 29:1664–1666, 1989.

118. Mutabagani KH, Coley BD, Zumberge N, et al: Preliminary experience with focused abdominal sonography for trauma (FAST) in children: Is it useful? J Pediatr Surg 34:48–52, 1999.

119. Boone TB, Gilling PJ, Husmann DA: Ureteropelvic junction disruption following blunt abdominal trauma. J Urol 150:33–36, 1993.

120. Husmann DA, Gilling PJ, Perry MO, et al: Major renal lacerations with a devitalized fragment following blunt abdominal trauma: A comparison between nonoperative (expectant) versus surgical management. J Urol 150:1774–1777, 1993.

121. Matthews LA, Smith EM, Spirnak JP: Nonoperative treatment of major blunt renal lacerations with urinary extravasation. J Urol 157:2056–2058, 1997.

122. Bass DH, Semple PL, Cywes S: Investigation and management of blunt renal injuries in children: A review of 11 years' experience. J Pediatr Surg 26:196–200, 1991.

123. Haller JA, Papa P, Drugas G, et al: Nonoperative management of solid organ injuries in children: Is it safe? Ann Surg 219:625–628, 1994.

124. Partrick DA, Bensard DD, Moore EE, et al: Nonoperative management of solid organ injuries in children results in decreased blood utilization. J Pediatr Surg 34:1695–1699, 1999.

125. Altman AL, Haas C, Dinchman KH, et al: Selective nonoperative management of blunt grade 5 renal injury. J Urol 164:27–30, 2000.

126. Baumann L, Greenfield SP, Aker J, et al: Nonoperative management of major blunt renal trauma in children: In-hospital morbidity and long-term followup. J Urol 148:691–693, 1992.

127. Husmann DA, Morris JS: Attempted nonoperative management of blunt renal lacerations extending through the corticomedullary junction: The short-term and long-term sequelae. J Urol 143: 682–684, 1990.

128. McAninch JW, Carroll PR, Klosterman PW, et al: Renal reconstruction after injury. J Urol 145:932–937, 1991.

129. Carroll PR, Klosterman P, McAninch JW: Early vascular control for renal trauma: A critical review. J Urol 141:826–829, 1989.

CHAPTER 17

Pediatric Head Trauma

Gregory W. Hornig, MD

Pediatric head trauma is a major medical problem. The incidence of traumatic brain injury (TBI) is approximately 200 per 100,000 children in the United States. Four hundred thousand children aged 0 to 14 years are seen every year in the emergency department for evaluation of head trauma.[1] Many of these children have relatively minor trauma with Glasgow Coma Scale scores (GCSs) of 14 to15 (maximum score is 15 in an intact individual). However, 6% of pediatric admissions with brain injury have severe injuries and require extensive medical assistance, including invasive diagnostic procedures and surgical intervention. About 5% of pediatric head injuries are fatal, with death often occurring at the scene of the accident. Approximately 3000 children die annually of TBI. In children younger than 1 year, the most common cause of fatal traumatic head injury is nonaccidental trauma secondary to abuse. Even in children up to the age of 2 years, one-fourth of head injuries are caused by adults in abusive encounters.

In the entire American population, more than 1.5 million TBI patients are treated and released from emergency departments, and almost a quarter of a million adults and children are placed in inpatient care. Approximately 50,000 of the persons with TBI die, and about 80,000 leave the hospital with some disability.[2] The economic costs of TBI have been estimated to be $56.3 billion in 1995 dollars.[3] The morbidity created by head injury is a major public health problem that victimizes all segments of our society, with lower socioeconomic class members having a disproportionate number of head injuries. In general, a trend is found toward improvement in outcome from severe head injuries, mainly because of improved diagnostic tools such as computed tomographic (CT) scanning, better prehospitalization care, early surgical evacuation of mass lesions, and advances in the intensive care of patients to provide comprehensive care of patients with severe head injury.

BRAIN INJURY MECHANISMS

Axonal Shearing

Sudden abrupt changes in the angular momentum of the head can cause diffuse brain damage, as the components of brain tissue rotate in relation to one another, resulting in shearing of axonal bundles that constitute white matter. Axonal shearing also may occur between white matter bundles and deeper subcortical neuronal structures such as the basal ganglia and the thalamus, and within the upper brainstem, where the cerebrum rotates on its axis. The result of these shearing forces on vascular and parenchymal tissues is unpredictable; the neurologic outcome can be as little as transient loss of consciousness (LOC) or as much as profound and persistent neurologic deficits and death. After the initial injury, important secondary events often are associated with cerebral ischemia, in which the initial axonal and cellular damage is further aggravated. Swelling in areas adjacent to the primary injury often occurs for several days after the initial trauma. Moreover, it is a common clinical observation that patients with severe head injury have progressive neurologic deterioration for 4 to 6 days after injury, despite aggressive and appropriate treatment.

Nonpenetrating Cranial Trauma

Direct impact against the brain and calvarium produces focal damage to the involved brain. In some instances, *contrecoup* damage occurs from the rebound movement of the viscoelastic brain within its rigid encasement. The predominant *contrecoup* damage occurs on the side opposite the impact, as is commonly seen with subdural hemorrhages with associated cortical contusion, when the brain rebounds off the skull, causing disruption of delicate surface vessels. The inner surface of the skull at its base is irregular, ridged, and restrictive at its anterior margins. As a result, the anterior and inferior portions of temporal and frontal lobes are often injured by abrupt brain acceleration or deceleration in a sagittal plane.

Penetrating Injury

Penetrating injury causes cerebral lacerations with deleterious effects on the underlying neurons, their functional interconnections, and the cerebral vasculature at the surface of the brain. Such primary brain trauma leads to additional delayed events such as global and regional ischemia, which, in turn, produce a variety of abnormal cellular and metabolic events: the release of excitatory neurotransmitters (glutamate, aspartate, and catecholamines), cellular breakdown with disruption of cytoskeleton, disruption of the blood-brain barrier, release of cytokines (interleukins and tumor necrosis factor), massive efflux of calcium into extracellular spaces, lipolysis, proteolysis, the breakdown of cellular membranes, and the induction of several classes of genes that contribute to programmed cell death (apoptosis). Destruction of cerebral tissue incites an inflammatory response along with the formation of oxygen free radicals that causes further membrane peroxidation and disruption of the key enzymes necessary for normal neuronal function. Given the multiplicity and complexity of events after head trauma and the relative vulnerability of the central nervous system, normalization of brain function is difficult to achieve in the context of any significant brain injury, including nonpenetrating injuries.

PATHOPHYSIOLOGY

The intracranial contents include brain parenchymal tissue, cerebrospinal fluid, and blood. The adult brain weighs approximately 1400 g and is composed of 80% water. Twenty percent of brain water is extracellular. Cerebrospinal fluid (CSF) occupies about 140 mL. The majority of the CSF is in subarachnoid spaces, with about 40 mL of CSF residing in the ventricles. Finally, about 150 mL of blood is in the brain, mostly in the postcapillary circulation. According to the Monro-Kellie hypothesis, the total bulk of these incompressible elements is at all times constant, and any increase in the volume of one must be at the expense of the others, assuming that intracranial volume also is constant. However, in children with distensible skulls, the Monro-Kellie hypothesis does not apply. In children, as in adults, elevation of intracranial pressure (ICP) results from a combination of pathophysiologic states, generally limited to mass lesions (including clots), vascular engorgement, cerebral edema, and hydrocephalus.

The brain of most individuals after age 5 years is encased in a relatively nonexpansile skull. Any volumetric loading of the intracranial space displaces or loads normal intracranial contents and usually results in an abrupt increase in ICP. Even though the Monro-Kellie doctrine indicates that the intracranial contents are constant in volume, a tolerance is found for approximately 100 mL of additional volume within the skull before a significant increase of pressure occurs. This happens mainly as the result of displacement of blood out of the intracranial venous circulation and movement of CSF out of the head. The ability to accommodate increased intracranial volume is age and time dependant: older and very young people can accept greater loading, and gradual increases in mass volume over a longer period are better tolerated. When ICP increases, compression of vascular and parenchymal tissues is particularly deleterious. When ICP reaches or exceeds 33 mm Hg, cerebral blood flow (CBF) is seriously impeded, and cerebral ischemia begins to occur.

The human brain is especially oxygen avid, using approximately 20% of total body oxygen consumption and receiving about 15% of cardiac output. Even brief episodes of oxygen and CBF deprivation are destructive to neuronal and vascular tissues. Of the vascular tissues, the capillary endothelial cells that constitute the blood-brain barrier are especially vulnerable to the effects of ischemia and hypoxia; damage to the barrier causes significant problems in terms of deleterious leakage across the usual barrier between blood plasma and extracellular spaces, and damage furthermore precludes normal transportation of necessary hexoses and amino acids into the brain.

CBF is defined as the velocity of blood through the cerebral circulation. Usually this is in the range of 50 mL/100 g/min. In infants, this figure is about 40 mL/100 g/min, and, in older children, the CBF can increase to the level of 100 mL/100 g/min. Flow is inversely related to vascular resistance, with resistance increasing as vessel diameter becomes smaller. CBF is proportional to the pressure gradient and, in accordance to Poiseuille's law, inversely proportional to blood viscosity.

In practical terms, the interventions available to a clinician to improve flow include manipulations of systemic BP and alterations of blood viscosity by the use of mannitol. Even in the intact individual, changes in the caliber of impedance vessels cannot be done: the effect of α-adrenergic vasoconstriction on pial vessels is comparatively small when compared with the response seen in other peripheral vessels (it is < 1% of the effect seen in cremasteric vessels). In patients with TBI, no practical way exists to manipulate sympathetic tone of cerebral vessels in an attempt to improve flow selectively at the level of intact arterioles or capillaries. Furthermore, relaxation of vasoconstriction (to augment flow) via a variety of exogenous agents may have undesired effects. For example, carbon dioxide, papaverine, nitric oxide, and prostaglandins can increase flow but also can cause acute systemic hypertension, disruption of the blood-brain barrier, and increased ICP and volume.[4]

Cerebral perfusion pressure (CPP) is the differential pressure of arterial inflow and venous outflow. Intracranial venous pressure is usually slightly less than ICP and CSF pressure. CPP is considered the transmural pressure gradient, which is the driving force required for supplying tissue metabolic needs. Formally, CPP is defined as the differential mean pressure within the arterial vessel (MAP) and the pressure surrounding the vessel wall (ICP).

As ICP increases from head injury, the difference between perfusion pressure and ICP narrows, and at a perfusion pressure of 10 mm Hg, blood vessels collapse and blood flow ceases.

Because CPP is easily determined in the clinical situation in which ICP monitoring is done, it has become a critical parameter for defining treatment options. A generation ago, treatment protocols were principally directed toward reducing ICP, and hyperventilation and fluid restriction were important components in older protocols. Current treatment goals seek to enhance perfusion pressure while reducing ICP, with little reliance on either hyperventilation or fluid restriction. Maintenance of a perfusion pressure greater than 70 mm Hg has been associated with a substantial reduction in mortality and improvement in quality of survival. No evidence exists that this treatment is deleterious: the incidence of intracranial hypertension (ICH), morbidity, or mortality is not increased by the active maintenance of CPP above 70 mm Hg, even if this means normalizing the intravascular volume or inducing systemic hypertension.[5]

After head trauma, cerebral edema becomes a significant factor in increasing ICP. Direct damage to or ischemia of brain tissue can cause cytotoxic and vasogenic edema. Cytotoxic edema results from disruption of cell membranes that normally regulate intracellular and extracellular ionic and fluid balances; vasogenic edema results from disruption of the blood-brain barrier with extravasation of fluids into the extravascular (interstitial) spaces. The edematous brain tissue that is seen in early post-traumatic CT scans represents tissue that is both reversibly and irreversibly damaged and that has excess water in cellular and extracellular spaces. This excess fluid forms as a result of cell membrane damage and direct damage to brain cells. The distinction between cellular and vascular sources of edema is often subtle. The intact blood-brain barrier depends on the cellular integrity of the cerebral capillary vasculature. Capillary endothelial mitochondria are very sensitive to oxygen deprivation, and injury to these organelles results in barrier leakiness. Hypoxic injury to the brain causes diffuse damage to cellular organelles including endothelial mitochondria, resulting in edema that is both cytotoxic and vasogenic.

In children, rapid formation of edema is commonly seen on serial CT scans after trauma. In early (<24 hours after injury), fatal, closed head injury in children, CT scans demonstrate little or no significant parenchymal bleeding, but diffuse brain swelling is seen with obliteration of the ventricles and loss of the perimesencephalic cisterns and subarachnoid space (Fig. 17-1). Some have interpreted this as meaning that the brain is "hyperemic," with increased blood flow as opposed to increased brain water. The meaning of hyperemia in this context refers to increased blood flow in excess of metabolic demand, sometimes termed "luxury perfusion," which can often occur in the areas of the brain surrounding an area of focal contusion. However, the term *luxury perfusion* is probably not accurate when used in the context of acute trauma and does not reflect the reality of CBF in TBI, in which flow is typically lowest in the first 24 hours after

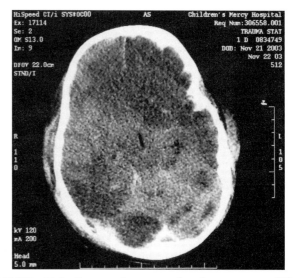

FIGURE 17-1. Computed tomography demonstrates diffuse cerebral swelling with obliteration of the basilar cisterns. The low attenuation of the brain parenchyma suggests diffuse edema. This moribund 3-year-old had fallen approximately 20 feet the day before this scan. At the time of this scan, her pupils had become fixed and dilated despite a ventriculostomy and aggressive management of her intracranial pressure. (Photograph courtesy of Dr. Lisa Lowe.)

injury, particularly in brain regions that have been the most damaged. After head injury in patients with a GCS of less than 8, blood flow is typically low for the first 24 hours. This is followed by a transient hyperemic phase for several days in about 40% of patients, in whom CBF increases above 55 mL/100 g/min, particularly in those patients with elevated ICP. After day 3 after head trauma, vasospasm can occur in up to 50% of patients, causing additional ischemic damage and resulting in a strong association of poor outcome with low CBF.[6] Hyperemia is a distinct problem because it signifies perfusion at the upper limits of vessel compliance, particularly in children who have higher physiologic CBF and who typically have a higher incidence of hyperemic changes after head trauma. Leakage and microaneurysm formation in pial arterioles occur in cats subjected to induced hypertension greater than 200 mm Hg.[7]

In areas of brain injury, blood flow is initially depressed, and brain cells are deprived of oxygen and essential nutrients. If blood flows between 10 and 12 mL/100 g/min are prolonged for more than several hours, a threshold is reached that permits a toxic cascade of lactic acid, lipid peroxidase, free radicals, intracellular calcium and sodium, and extracellular potassium, which results in further breakdown of cell membranes and a pattern of diffuse edema, as seen on CT scans. If an acute Cushing hypertensive reflex is superimposed in this setting of elevated ICP, and this is further exacerbated by a phasic hyperemic response 24 hours after injury, it is not surprising to see clinical deterioration for several days after initial trauma. In the extensive literature concerning the relation of CBF and head trauma, poor outcomes occur in settings of both hypoperfusion and hyperperfusion.

Currently it is possible to qualitatively measure CBF at the bedside with techniques such as thermal diffusion flowmetry and laser Doppler flowmetry, which require placement of intracerebral monitors that measure regional flow continuously in areas immediately adjacent to the probe. Additionally, the Kety-Schmidt/nitrous oxide method permits global CBF measurements, and xenon-133 gives global values with marginal spatial resolution. These techniques are not universally available nor are they commonly used in clinical practice. Newer radiographic techniques such as magnetic resonance diffusion perfusion imaging, xenon-CT, single-photon emission tomography (SPECT), and positron emission tomography (PET) are used in clinical practice, particularly the magnetic resonance techniques.

The correlation between flow and cerebral metabolism is complicated, as often states of mismatch exist between flow and metabolism. Some therapies, such as hypothermia and barbiturate coma, also can result in uncoupling by decreasing brain metabolism, whereas other agents, such as nitric acid and adenosine, can cause true hyperemia. Nonetheless, information in a particular individual about CBF and its relation to cerebral metabolism can be useful in pinpointing the optimal perfusion and hyperventilation therapies necessary to avoid ischemia. Because the distinction between cerebral edema and vascular engorgement is not obvious from the usual clinical and radiologic findings, CBF studies might suggest a way to treat the underlying pathology directly. As an example, if cerebral edema is the main culprit in a particular patient with high ICP and normal or low CBF, hyperosmolar treatment with mannitol would be indicated. If, in another patient, CBF does not change in response to carbon dioxide—suggesting impaired pressure autoregulation—then induced systemic hypertension might increase ICP, and pressors used to drive up perfusion pressure would be relatively contraindicated. Finally, in another patient, if the cause of elevated pressure is mainly from vascular engorgement (as suggested by elevated jugular oxygen saturation, which measures global CBF), then barbiturate therapy might be a more effective treatment than mannitol.[8]

In general, maintenance of a physiologic level of CBF is associated with improved clinical outcomes. Moderately increased CBF is often associated with lowered ICP, decreased vasospasm and vasoconstriction in areas of damaged microcirculation, improved utilization of oxygen, and improved GCS outcomes. Very high flow rates, particularly when associated with ICH and poor metabolic use of oxygen, predict poor clinical outcomes. The currently accepted concept of moderate support of blood flow is particularly important in children, in whom the normal CBF is double that of adults (100 mL/100 g/min in infants), thereby increasing the vulnerability of the infant brain to flow perturbations associated with trauma. In general, consensus is found that moderately increased blood flow is associated with positive outcomes in TBI. Deliberate manipulation to increase systemic BP and cardiac output (and hence blood flow to the brain) are ways of increasing perfusion and flow. Because CBF is not easily quantified in the normal clinical setting, perfusion pressures become the focus of therapeutic decisions. The implicit assumption is that increased perfusion pressure causes increased flow, and that the increased flow protects against ischemia, particularly in those areas where autoregulatory function is lost, and achieves this without significantly increasing blood volume or ICP. Normally a 2% change in cerebral blood volume occurs with each unit change of flow, and because vascular volumes account for a small percentage of total intracranial volume, the increased flow is tolerable.

Blood flow, perfusion pressure, and blood volume are theoretically linked at the level of autoregulation, where arterial vessels can dilate or constrict in response to various physiologic changes including ICP and systemic arterial pressure to maintain normal flow and normal brain metabolism. Autoregulation of flow is considered to be "functional" within perfusion limits of 50 and 140 mm Hg. Normally, reflexive vasoconstriction in the face of elevated systemic BP will impede ICH; an increase in systemic pressure (and an increase in perfusion pressure) will cause reflex vasoconstriction and a volume reduction within the arterioles, causing a relative decrease in ICP. A moderate decrease in systemic BP will paradoxically result in increased ICP because reflex vasodilatation will occur in compensation. When perfusion pressures fall below 50 mm Hg, cerebral ischemia occurs, and compensatory cerebral arteriole vasodilatation is exhausted. When perfusion exceeds 140 mm Hg, cerebral arteriolar impedance is overcome, and the affected vessels passively dilate as fluid is forced through a damaged endothelium into the brain, causing diffuse "vasogenic" edema. Autoregulatory processes occur mainly at the level of conductance vessels, which is the arteriolar bed that is responsive to vasodilatory and vasoconstrictive agents. The actual events causing changes in cerebral blood volume and flow are likely more complicated and, in the acute phases of post-traumatic ischemia, include obstructive changes inside and outside the microvasculature of damaged areas caused by plugging of vessels with leukocytes and astrocystic swelling.[9]

A second hypothesis explaining rapid formation of brain swelling in head trauma of children is mechanical: with expansion of a viscoelastic brain, mechanical compression occurs at bridging veins and venous sinuses. In this setting, blood flow is blocked by compression of the venous system. The surgical experience in which the traumatized brain suddenly becomes engorged and begins to herniate through a craniotomy opening suggests a rapid increase in intracranial blood volume as opposed to cytotoxic edema, which would predictably occur and regress in a slower fashion. The partial or complete reversibility of this condition by a combination of surgical tactics such as elevation of the head above the heart, removal of a hematoma, decompression of venous sinuses, or hyperventilation would argue against regional edema formation alone as the cause of engorgement.

The relation between brain tissue pressure and brain volume is called *brain compliance*. Compliance is a measure of stiffness of the brain, and it is defined as the change in volume divided by the change in pressure, and its inverse is referred to as elasticity. As a technical item called the pressure–volume index (PVI), brain compliance can be measured on a logarithmic scale of pressure versus volume, with a resulting linear slope that reflects the amount of volume required to increase ICP tenfold. The PVI for a normal child is below 10 mL. More practically, brain compliance can be roughly estimated by looking at the waveform of a continuous ICP monitor. If the amplitude of the waveform is relatively high, then it is reasonable to assume that brain compliance is poor and that marginal changes in volume result in greater displacement of ICP. With pathologic elevations of ICP and loss of autoregulatory tone in impedance vessels, the transmission of the pulse from the vascular system to the veins and then to the CSF is more obvious.[10]

INITIAL EVALUATION AND MANAGEMENT OF HEAD INJURY

The fundamentals of resuscitation apply to children with head injury and include restoration of an adequate circulating blood volume, BP support, appropriate ventilation, and adequate oxygenation. Patients with severe head injury often have multisystem failure, and a multidisciplinary collaboration is usually undertaken at trauma centers. The trauma surgeon should initiate maneuvers that serve to lower ICP and do not interfere with the ABCs (airway, breathing, circulation) of resuscitation of any patient with a head injury. A strong caveat remains: treatment modalities such as hyperventilation and mannitol administration that have the potential of exacerbating intracranial ischemia or interfering with resuscitation should be reserved for patients who show signs of ICH such as evidence of herniation or neurologic deterioration.[5]

The following algorithm remains a reasonable approach to resuscitation and treatment of patients with severe head injury (Fig. 17-2). It is comparable to the guidelines issued by the Brain Trauma Foundation.[5] Initial evaluation of patients with head injury includes the establishment of level of consciousness at the time of presentation and the identification of focal neurologic deficits. In children with TBI, assessment is best obtained before delivery of drugs for sedation and paralysis. However, the process of transporting children with head trauma is often complicated by the confusion and agitation of even moderate head injury. These children will arrive after orotracheal intubation and pharmacologic sedation and paralysis; a meaningful neurologic assessment is nearly impossible in such children. Unenhanced cranial CT scanning becomes the initial and most critical diagnostic tool, particularly for the identification of bleeding. If certain neurologic tests are possible at this early stage, it is important to document and then repeat the examination as many times as needed to establish a consistent trend in neurologic status. A decline in neurologic status is an ominous finding, often associated with an expanding lesion such as an intracranial hematoma.

The most common classification now used to grade the severity of head injury is the GCS (Table 17-1). The GCS is useful for guiding initial and subsequent

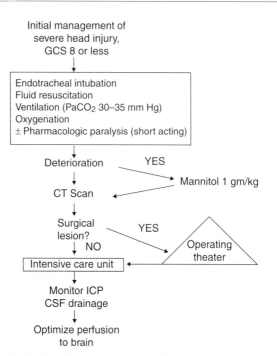

FIGURE 17-2. This algorithm describes a reasonable approach for treatment of patients with severe head trauma.

patient evaluation, management, and prognosis for recovery. The GCS often serves as the basis for communication between treating physicians; for this reason, it should be part of the objective scoring when treating trauma patients.

Limitations occur in using the GCS: preverbal children are often too young to converse or use words; pharmacologic sedation and paralysis will depress all neurologic functions; orbital swelling can make eye opening impossible; preexisting conditions such as spina bifida and spasticity associated with cerebral palsy will alter the baseline motor function; and endotracheal intubation will make verbal responses impossible.

Despite these limitations, head injury severity is often graded by combining clinical information including

TABLE 17-1		
GLASGOW COMA SCALE (GCS)		
Eye Opening	None	1 point
	To pain	2
	To voice	3
	Spontaneously	4
Vocalization	None	1 point
	Incomprehensible sounds	2
	Incomprehensible words	3
	Confused speech	4
	Normal speech	5
Motor Examination	Flaccid bilaterally	1 point
	Extensor posturing	2
	Flexion posturing	3
	Withdrawal from pain	4
	Localizes pain	5
	Follows commands	6

amnesia for the traumatic event and LOC along with the GCS. The maximum GCS score is 15, and the minimal score is 3. "Minimal" head injury has an initial GCS score of 15 with no associated LOC or amnesia. These patients do not require prolonged observation in hospital.

"Mild" head trauma has a GCS of 14 to 15 and brief LOC of less than 5 minutes, along with amnesia for the period before or after the event; some disturbance of sensorium is found, including disorientation, confusion, or somnolence. No focal neurologic findings (such as hemiparesis or cranial nerve deficits) are present in patients designated in this category of mild head trauma. Nonetheless, this group will often have some definite structural abnormality such as a cranial fracture or parenchymal contusion or hematoma; as such, patients with so-called mild injury are at risk for delayed complications and require appropriate observation.

"Moderate" head injury is defined in children having an initial GCS of 9 to 13, with impairment in their level of consciousness and a history of LOC longer than 5 minutes at the time of the traumatic event. These children require hospitalization to exclude the possibility of subsequent intracranial bleeding or the development of pathologically elevated ICP or both. Moderate head injury is often associated with skull fractures, lacerations, and cerebral contusions. Diffuse axonal injury occurs within this group.

"Severe" head injury is defined by a GCS of 8 or less. Most of these patients are considered comatose, as defined by an inability to follow commands, speak words, or open their eyes. All these patients require hospitalization in an intensive care unit (ICU) with vigorous supportive treatment.

The assessment of an initial GCS score is often done arbitrarily in patients intubated and paralyzed before scoring, giving these patients a score of 1 (i.e., no verbal ability) and possibly overestimating the severity of injury. In those patients with a very depressed GCS score of 3 to 5, the mortality remains high, ranging between 65% and 88%.[11] The GCS score does have significant correlation with outcome, as studies have demonstrated a predicted poor outcome (dead, vegetative, or severely disabled) in 77% patients with a GCS score of 3 to 5 and a poor outcome in 26% of persons with a GCS score of 6 to 8.[12]

From these data, it is clear that even small positive differences on the initial examination correlate with a much improved outcome. In comatose patients with acute subdural hematomas, the ability to withdraw from pain versus an abnormal flexion response gives only one additional point, boosting the total score to 6 points. This additional point in the GCS score reduces the likelihood of death by nearly 50%.[13] A note of caution must be added regarding the strength of prediction in individuals with severe head trauma: when predictions based on GCS scores, CT scans, and vital signs were made by experienced neurosurgeons, the ability to make a correct prognosis was less than 60%.[14]

Respiratory Monitoring and Management

Most severely head-injured patients require respiratory support. A 1989 English study revealed that 44% of brain-injured patients were hypoxemic in the field, with documented O_2 saturations less than 75% in 16% of the patients.[15] Because head trauma is often associated with multiple organ injury or neurogenic pulmonary edema, maintenance of adequate oxygenation is not simple. Two parameters that can be manipulated in the ventilated patient are the positive end-expiratory pressure (PEEP) and the fraction of inspired oxygen content (FiO_2). FiO_2 levels persistently greater than 0.6 are associated with oxygen toxicity. PEEP in excess of 7.5 cm H_2O can elevate venous pressure and ICP and furthermore can depress venous return and cardiac output. In the setting of acute respiratory distress syndrome (ARDS) and poor lung compliance, the use of PEEP becomes necessary despite the potentially deleterious effects on brain physiology.

Adequacy of ventilation is determined by the partial pressure of carbon dioxide in arterial blood. Arterial $PaCO_2$ is determined by the respiratory rate and the tidal volume, and can be readily reduced by increasing the rate of ventilation. In the head-injured patient, hypercapnia (excess $PaCO_2 > 45$ mm Hg) can cause a significant elevation in ICP because of CO_2-induced dilatation of the cerebral vasculature, with increased cerebral blood volume and flow.

The immediate effect of hyperventilation is a reduction of ICP, although this response is neither universal nor sustained. Hyperventilation reduces ICP by causing cerebral vasoconstriction, with a subsequent reduction in CBF in reactive vascular beds. Research has demonstrated that CBF after injury is less than 50% of that of normal individuals. Moreover, the risk of cerebral ischemia is very high and likely compounded by the further decrements in flow caused by deliberate hyperventilation done to control ICP. Even in healthy individuals who do not have cerebral tissue at or below the threshold perfusion needed to sustain normal brain metabolism, hyperventilation ($PaCO_2$ of 26) leads to a 7% decrease in cerebral volume but a 31% decrease in CBF, a far greater change in flow than in blood volume. In a prospective, randomized study of 77 patients with severe head injury, groups were randomized to prolonged prophylactic hyperventilation for 5 days after injury or to a group with $PaCO_2$ in a more normal range (35 mm Hg), and the outcome for the hyperventilation group was significantly worse than that for the normocapneic group.[16]

In conclusion, prolonged, aggressive prophylactic hyperventilation therapy ($PaCO_2 < 25$ mm Hg) should be avoided during the first 5 days after severe brain trauma, particularly in the first 24 hours when CBF is at its nadir. Hyperventilation causes a reduction in CBF but will not consistently cause a reduction of ICP. Because local variability in perfusion occurs in the damaged brain, the cerebral response to hypocapnia is unknown, and loss of perfusion may be greatest at relatively normal sites, putting even these areas at risk for hypoperfusion. A goal of management to control ICP is mild hyperventilation with $PaCO_2$ in the 33 to 37 mm Hg range.

Cardiovascular Management

Cardiovascular management is important to maintain perfusion of vital structures, and electrocardiogram (ECG) and BP monitoring is mandatory for head-injured patients. Maintenance of urine output greater than 1 mL/kg/hr in children and 0.5 mL/kg/hr in adults usually excludes hypovolemia. Hypotension after head trauma requires intravenous administration of crystalloid or colloid solutions. The use of hypertonic solutions appears to be justified but is not proven to extend survival in a statistically significant way. In a prospective, randomized, and double-blind study involving 194 patients with severe head injury (GCS ≤ 8), initial administration of either 250 mL of 7.5% saline solution or normal saline appeared to give a higher survival rate to the group with hypertonic saline.[17] In addition, a meta-analysis of studies regarding TBI patients who received hypertonic saline-dextran demonstrated that they were about twice as likely to survive as the comparison groups receiving standard therapy.[18] Despite these optimistic studies, a lack of class I evidence-based data exists to justify or negate the use of hypertonic solutions during initial resuscitation. Until further evidence can better correlate good outcomes with the use of hypertonic solutions, the recommendation of the American College of Surgeons regarding the use of crystalloid solutions (either Ringer's lactate or normal saline) is reasonable. In patients with severe TBI, dextrose-containing crystalloid solutions are often not initially given because of the concern that dextrose can promote lactic acidosis and anaerobic glycolysis in ischemic brain tissue.

Cardiac preload refers to right ventricular filling pressure or right-sided end-diastolic volume, which is usually equal to central venous pressure. Manipulation of preload volumes is usually accomplished with proper intravenous infusions in head-injured patients, as mentioned earlier, although management is complicated by elevated pulmonary vascular resistance (from ARDS or acute lung injury). In general, all patients with severe brain injury are optimally treated with either central venous pressure or pulmonary capillary wedge pressure monitoring in the ICU to assure normovolemia and normal cardiac output.

Afterload management to decrease vascular resistance is often difficult but critical to achieving adequate resuscitation, because BP must be maintained at a point above tissue vascular resistance to allow proper perfusion. Left ventricular afterload becomes the focus of treatment because output from the left side of the heart determines cerebral perfusion. To elevate pressure, pressors with α_1-receptor selectivity (e.g., phenylephrine, high-dose dopamine) are preferred because cerebral arterioles lack significant α_1-receptors, and systemic BP can be elevated without causing significant cerebral vasoconstriction. Afterload-reducing agents used in treating systemic hypertension, including sodium nitroprusside, labetolol, and oral nifedipine, are important medications used in the ICU to decrease afterload.

Intracranial Hypertension Monitoring and Management in the Acute Setting

ICH is a common cause of progressive or secondary injury to the brain after trauma. The designation of ICH is arbitrary, but most centers define ICH as a sustained pressure of 20 mm Hg or higher, because a normal adult ICP is approximately 10 mm Hg (136 mm H_2O). The patients most at risk for elevated pressures developing include comatose patients with an initial GCS of 8 or less. For patients in coma with an abnormal CT scan, the incidence of ICH is 53% to 63%.[19] Sustained elevation of ICP is especially deleterious in comatose patients (GCS, 3 to 8). Therefore ICP monitoring has become a common practice in many trauma centers for these patients. ICP monitors have been studied extensively, and the published clinical experience suggests several reasons for their use: (1) they effectively discriminate between therapies most useful for treating ICH, (2) they can provide earlier detection of intercranial hemorrhage or progressive hydrocephalus, (3) they can be used in conjunction with drainage of CSF and thereby directly reduce ICP, and (4) they may improve outcome and prognosis.[20]

Intracranial Pressure Monitoring

The use of ICP devices has become standard in the United States in the treatment of severe head injury, even in the absence of a prospective, randomized clinical trial to establish efficacy in improving outcome from TBI. Coagulation abnormalities are a relative contraindication to the insertion of these devices. Intraventricular devices (with either a fluid-coupled catheter or a catheter-tip pressure transducer) are effective monitors that allow drainage of CSF and treatment of ICP. Their placement is complicated when damaged brain and cerebral edema have effaced the normal ventricle. Intraparenchymal monitors have fiberoptic or strain-gauge transducers that provide continuous pressure readings and can be placed, with relative ease, in any region of the brain. Newer monitors can measure brain tissue oxygen and permit manipulations to optimize regional oxygenation, including adjustments in FiO_2 and blood transfusion.[21] As a practical matter, placement of an ICP monitor should be discouraged in a patient who can localize and dislodge the device, because additional sedation and paralysis are then needed in a patient who already has neurologic compromise.

Surgical Treatment to Control Intracranial Hypertension

Management of ICH requires direct treatment of the cause of the problem, if this is possible, while preserving cerebral perfusion. Several efficacious surgical methods are used to control the ICP, including removal of large mass lesions such as extra-axial hematomas or large intraparenchymal clots, drainage of trapped CSF, and decompression of venous sinuses. However, even when surgical evacuation has been achieved, secondary brain swelling remains a problem.

The decision regarding evacuation of intracerebral hematomas and hemorrhagic contusions is often difficult and depends on many factors, including the size of the lesion, the extent of brain shift caused by single or multiple lesions, the depth and position of the lesion relative to the adjacent normal brain, and the presence of other problems such as depressed bone fragments and CSF leaks that require surgical intervention. Even if an initial conservative attitude is maintained and the surgical evacuation of focal hemorrhagic lesions is considered excessive or harmful, placement of ICP monitors and CSF drainage devices is often done in a surgical suite. In some patients, decompressive craniectomies can be considered either as a primary procedure or as a secondary operation, done after the removal of an intracranial mass lesion. The effect of craniectomy on the biomechanics of a hypertensive brain is immediately decreased ICP and increased tissue compliance, allowing greater volumes without concomitant elevation of pressure.[22] Not unlike the medical management by using barbiturates for treatment of refractory elevated ICP, the surgical treatment of bifrontal craniectomy with dural expansion grafts is reserved for extremely sick patients, and the outcome results from case-controlled studies are not conclusive, particularly for patients with GCS scores of 3 or 4, even with reasonable control of ICP.[22]

Osmotic Diuretics

Osmotic diuretics such as mannitol have become the mainstay of ICP treatment. Mannitol is usually infused in intermittent bolus form every 4 to 6 hours, with effective doses ranging from 0.25 to 1.0 g/kg body weight. Serum osmolarity is usually kept below 320 mOsm because of concern for renal failure. Mannitol has a rapid rheologic effect and reduces blood viscosity, increases cerebral oxygen delivery, and increases CBF. The osmotic effect of mannitol is delayed for up to 30 minutes, as gradients occur between blood plasma and brain tissue. Thus intermittent bolus administration is preferred because of the possibility that, as mannitol accumulates in the brain after being in the circulation for long periods (after continuous IV infusion), it can cause a reverse osmotic shift with movement of fluid into brain cells.

Corticosteroids

The use of corticosteroids has been extensively investigated, and the majority of clinical evidence indicates that steroids do not improve outcome or reduce ICP in patients with head trauma. Therefore steroids are not recommended in the treatment of ICH.

Anticonvulsant Prophylaxis

Anticonvulsants are used routinely in patients with severe head injury, either for prophylaxis or for treatment. The most commonly used drug is phenytoin, given with an initial loading dose of 10 to 15 mg/kg, with a maintenance dose of 5 mg/kg daily. The incidence of seizures after penetrating head injury is about 50% in a follow-up period of 15 years. In a class 1 study investigating the incidence of early and late post-traumatic seizures in 404 patients randomized to use of phenytoin, a significant reduction in the incidence of early post-traumatic seizures was observed in the treated group, without any reduction in late post-traumatic seizures.[24] Routine seizure prophylaxis later than 1 week after head injury is therefore not recommended, but the option to use phenytoin or carbamazepine during the first week after head injury appears to be justified. Such prophylaxis reduces the early incidence of seizures in the treated group to 4% versus the placebo group of 14%.

Barbiturate Coma/Hypothermia

About 10% of patients hospitalized with severe head injury experience intractable, elevated ICP, with an associated mortality of 84% to 100%. High-dose barbiturate, usually pentobarbital, has been used with success to depress cerebral metabolism and decrease noxious levels of brain glutamate, aspartate, and lactate. Barbiturates exert a protective effect on the brain ICP by reducing metabolic demand and decreasing regional blood flow and blood volume. Barbiturates create systemic hypotension and hemodynamic instability, and their use is not recommended as a prophylactic measure for anticipated ICH. Barbiturate coma should not be used in hemodynamically unstable patients. Volume and vasopressor therapy are usually used in conjunction with barbiturate coma, and overall management is both intensive and complex. The patients are generally extremely sick, and their clinical outcomes are often marginal. Nonresponders to this treatment modality had a high risk of death (83%) compared with that of responders (8%).[25] It appears that only those patients who had preserved autoregulation were significant "responders," again suggesting a coupling of CBF to regional metabolic demands. The uncoupling achieved by induced coma in these individuals permits reduction in cerebral metabolism, with concomitant decreased blood volume and reduction of ICP.[26]

Moderate hypothermia to temperatures of 32°C to 35°C improves outcome in patients with GCS scores in the 5 to 7 range by decreasing cerebral basal metabolism and oxygen consumption, reducing glutamate, and reducing the post-traumatic inflammatory response. It remains a second-tier therapy for treatment of moderately elevated ICP and is often used in conjunction with barbiturate coma.[27]

Primary Injuries

Skull fractures are very common in the pediatric population and are readily diagnosed with a combination of plain radiographs and CT scanning. Decisions regarding medical and surgical management often depend on the nature of the fracture and its involvement with the underlying brain and vascular structures. Linear skull fractures are often associated with damage to major vascular structures and carry an increased risk of ICH, particularly when they occur through the temporal squamosa near the middle meningeal artery. Fractures overriding the sagittal and lambdoid sutures may be associated with laceration of the superior sagittal sinus and the transverse sinus. Hemorrhage into these intracranial areas will be easily visualized on axial views with CT scanning, and the resulting bleeding is often epidural. Diastatic fractures involve separation of the bone at the edge of the fracture line. "Growing" fractures represent a distinctly different kind of diastatic fracture that results from laceration of the dura with gradual herniation of brain tissue through dura and bone. They are identified by gradual expansion of the fracture line as seen on serial plain radiographs, usually over several weeks, and they all require surgical repair of both the dura and the calvarium.

Depressed skull fracture is often associated with dural tear, CSF leak, contusion of the brain parenchyma, and ICH. Because depressed fractures are often associated with a scalp laceration and the introduction of foreign bodies, including devitalized skin and bone, a much higher risk exists of contamination of the intracranial space. Thus more aggressive management is appropriate, including surgical debridement of the involved areas, dural repair, cranioplasty, and use of appropriate antibiotics. Criteria for surgical elevation of depressed skull fractures include a depression exceeding the thickness of the skull, neurologic insult related to compression of the underlying brain, and CSF leak. When a depressed cranial fracture overlies and depresses a major dural sinus, particularly the posterior aspect of the superior sagittal sinus, surgical intervention is contraindicated unless evidence is noted of persistent CSF leak, persistent hemorrhage, or progressive neurologic problems caused by venous hypertension.

Basilar skull fractures are seen in 8% to 14% of children with head trauma and are often suspected because of the physical findings of Battle's sign (retroauricular ecchymosis), hemotympanum, and periorbital ecchymosis ("raccoon eyes"). Rhinorrhea and otorrhea frequently are seen, but this CSF leak usually clears without specific treatment other than elevation of the head of bed. When the CSF drainage is identified as a persistent problem in a patient hospitalized for several days, continuous lumbar drainage for 5 to 7 days is often used in an effort to divert fluid away from the intracranial defect and permit healing of the meningeal disruption. Lumbar drainage can introduce air and infection into the central nervous system, and "overdrainage" headaches are not uncommon. In the roughly 5% of children with persistent CSF leaks, despite this treatment, more-direct surgical interventions become necessary. Antibiotics are often used in conjunction with elective drainage. The use of antibiotics on a prophylactic basis in patients with untreated post-traumatic CSF leaks is controversial: treatment with antibiotics appears to be neither harmful nor beneficial in patients with CSF leak.[28]

Basilar skull fractures can cause damage to various cranial nerves. The olfactory tract is permanently damaged in 3% to 10% of children who later report anosmia because of fractures running through the cribriform plate. Ocular problems also are reported in 1% to 10%; oculomotor, trochlear, and abducens nerve injuries are usually treated conservatively. Bony disruption of the optic nerve at the level of the optic foramen usually causes irreversible ipsilateral blindness. Facial nerve injury results from disruption of the petrous bone. The facial paralysis resulting from acute disruption of the peripheral facial nerve (and resulting in paralysis of the entire face, the inability to close the eye, and the inability to taste in the anterior tongue) may require surgical decompression in addition to the use of steroids.

POST-TRAUMATIC INTRACRANIAL HEMORRHAGE

Subarachnoid bleeding in acutely traumatized children is common and is rarely the result of aneurysmal bleeding (Fig. 17-3). Bleeding occurs from disruption of the somewhat fragile pia-arachnoidal vasculature. If subarachnoid bleeding is an isolated finding resulting from minor trauma, no specific therapies are indicated except symptomatic amelioration of chemical meningitis, meningismus, and photophobia. In cases with severe TBI, subarachnoid hemorrhage is associated with poor outcomes and may be further associated with cerebral vasospasm. When vasospasm occurs as a result of subarachnoid bleeding, the calcium-blocking drug nimodipine has been useful in providing protection to marginally ischemic neurons from the harmful effects of calcium influx, particularly in the setting of postaneurysmal bleeding, in which the volume of subarachnoid blood correlates with the severity of subsequent vasospasm. Nimodipine is not often used in the context of TBI, in part because of its hypotensive effects, and in part because vasospasm is considered a relatively minor factor in the totality of pathophysiologic troubles resulting from head trauma.

Epidural Hematomas

Epidural hematomas have both arterial and venous sources of bleeding, and most occur in the context of skull fractures (Fig. 17-4). Some epidural hemorrhages result from laceration of a dural sinus or disruption of diploic vessels. When the force of impact has caused a laceration of a meningeal vessel, often a progressive accumulation of blood has a classic lentiform shape (like a

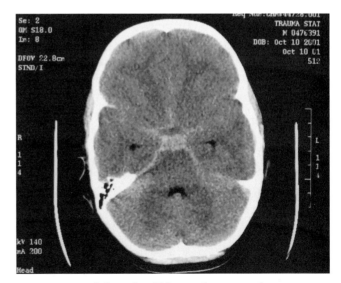

FIGURE 17-3. Subarachnoid hemorrhage secondary to trauma is present on this cranial computed tomography scan without contrast. Blood is seen in the perimesencephalic, prepontine, and suprasellar cisterns. The patient was involved in motor vehicle accident and complained of headache. He was neurologically normal. (Photograph courtesy of Dr. Lisa Lowe.)

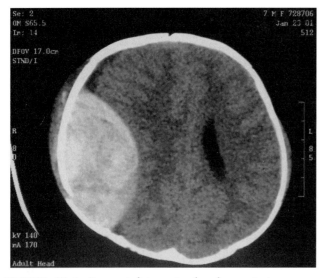

FIGURE 17-4. Computed tomography demonstrates a very large epidural hematoma that compresses the right hemisphere and causes midline shift. The 7-month-old patient reportedly fell and became obtunded, and on examination she had a fixed and dilated right pupil. She had a good recovery after immediate surgical evacuation of her epidural bleed, with persistent partial third nerve and facial palsies on the side ipsilateral to the bleed. (Photograph courtesy of Dr. Lisa Lowe.)

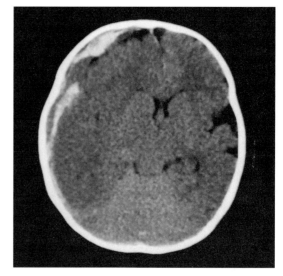

FIGURE 17-5. Hyperacute subdural bleeding on the right side on this cranial computed tomography scan. Compression of right-sided cerebral structures is seen with no intraparenchymal bleeding. Despite immediate craniotomy and evacuation of the subdural blood, the patient had a prolonged convalescence. He is hemiparetic on the left side and has significant developmental and cognitive delay. (Photograph courtesy of Dr. Lisa Lowe.)

biconvex lens) on axial CT scan. Clot formation under the calvarium compresses the dura underneath and can cause rapid neurologic depression as the brain becomes further displaced. In more than 50% of children with epidural hematomas, no disturbance of consciousness is seen at the time of injury; only after the hematoma enlarges is clinical evidence of elevated ICP noted. These symptoms include headache, lethargy, emesis, irritability, confusion, and a decreased level of consciousness. The so-called lucid interval is absent in more than half of children. Progressive deterioration results in seizures, changes in vital signs with hypertension and respiratory instability, papillary changes, posturing, and cardiovascular abnormalities. Operative intervention is always indicated once neurologic deterioration occurs; evacuation of extremely large clots (> 40 mL) in children often results in very good long-term results, provided that surgical interventions are timely.

Subdural Hematoma

Subdural hematomas are classified as acute (< 3 days old), subacute (3 to 10 days old), and chronic. Acute and subacute subdural hematomas are not infrequent in infants, usually the result of either birth injury or abuse (Fig. 17-5). The mechanism for subdural bleeding is most likely the shearing of bridging veins from the superior cortical surface to the midline sinus. This occurs when a differential movement of the brain occurs relative to the skull, caused by rapid translational (anterior to posterior) movement, which predominantly causes surface damage but spares the deeper brain matter. The superficial cortical veins in small children lack any reinforcement from

arachnoidal trabeculae and are susceptible to inertial loading. Infants are particularly susceptible to subdural hemorrhage developing, unlike older children.

The subdural hemorrhage occurs most frequently over the cerebral convexities and can extend over the entire hemisphere because, unlike the epidural space, the subdural space is not tethered to the cranial sutures. CT scan demonstrates hyperdense crescent-shaped blood collections at the surface of the brain, often associated with mass effect and cortical edema. On CT, particularly when anemia is present, acute subdurals may have an isodense appearance that belies their actual hemorrhagic character later found at the time of operation.

Surgical intervention is indicated when neurologic deterioration occurs as a result of the combined effect of subdural hemorrhage and parenchymal injury, either from the compressive effect of subdural blood or from the combined effect of impact forces on the entire cerebrum and diffuse bleeding. In infants it is possible to tap the subdural space at the level of the fontanel and produce rapid decompression. Large subdural hematomas with significant mass effect require more extensive craniotomies.

Subacute subdural hematomas, in the context of the trauma, are much less frequent in the pediatric population. However, they will be seen in emergency settings when they are the cause of neurologic problems, and when they are considered a manifestation of previous or recurrent nonaccidental head trauma. As with acute hematomas, the subacute subdural hematoma patient will have a nonspecific presentation. These children have both the symptoms of increased ICP (coma, irritability, lethargy, emesis, seizures) and the signs of elevated ICP (frontal bossing, enlarged heads, dilated scalp veins, sun-setting eyes, papilledema, and bulging fontanelles). CT scan often shows isodense or hypodense fluid collections at the cerebral convexities. MRI studies are often valuable in making the diagnosis of these bleeding events. As with the acute subdural hematoma, surgical intervention is often necessary.

Chronic subdural hematomas can cause pathologic elevation of ICP and can require surgical interventions to control cranial growth and CSF pressure. Interventions include serial percutaneous drainage, limited craniotomies to drain and irrigate the subdural space, and subdural/peritoneal shunts.

Hydrocephalus

Ventriculostomies are performed either at the bedside or in the operating room, often in conjunction with other operative procedures. Most ventricular catheters are placed in the right frontal horn of the nondominant right hemisphere. In addition to draining CSF, ventricular catheters provide direct measurement of CSF pressure, which reflects parenchymal pressures. Because the ventricles are often small in post-traumatic patients as a result of diffuse swelling, intermittent rather than continuous drainage may be recommended, thus allowing more accurate pressure measurements and avoiding collapse of the ventricular walls against the ventriculostomy catheter and causing occlusion of CSF drainage.

REFERENCES

1. Centers for Disease Control (2002). http://www.cdc.gov/ncipc/factsheets/tbi.htm. Accessed November 13, 2003.
2. Centers for Disease Control (2002): Traumatic brain injury in the United States: Available at: http://www.cdc.gov/ncipcpub-res/tbi_congress/index.htm. Accessed November 12, 2003.
3. Centers for Disease Control (2002): http://www.cdc.gov/ncipc/factsheets/tbi.htm. Accessed November 13, 2003.
4. Davson H, Welch K, Segal MB (eds): Physiology and Pathophysiology of the Cerebrospinal Fluid. Edinburgh, Churchill Livingston, 1987, pp 445–451.
5. Bullock R, Chestnut RM, Clifton G, et al: Guidelines for the management of severe traumatic brain injury. New York, Brain Trauma Foundation, 2000, p 94.
6. Martin NA, Patwardhan RV, Alexander MJ, et al: Characterization of cerebral hemodynamic phases following severe head trauma: Hypoperfusion, hyperemia, and vasospasm. J Neurosurg 87:9–19, 1997.
7. Kontos HA, Wei EP, Navari R, et al: Responses of cerebral arteries and arterioles to acute hypotension and hypertension. Am J Physiol 234:H371–H383, 1978.
8. Miller JD, Piper IR, Dearden NM: Management of intracranial hypertension in head injury: matching treatment with cause. Acta Neurochir Suppl 57:152–159, 1993.
9. Schroder M, Muizelaar JP, Fatouros PP: Regional cerebral blood volume after severe head injury in patients with regional cerebral ischemia. Neurosurgery 42:1276–1281, 1998.
10. Davson H, Welch K, Segal MB (eds): Physiology and Pathophysiology of the Cerebrospinal Fluid. Edinburgh, Churchill Livingston, 1987, p 758.
11. Gale JL, Dikmen S, Wyler A, et al: Head injury in the Pacific Northwest. Neurosurgery 12:487–491, 1983.
12. Narayan RK, Greenberg RP, Miller JD, et al: Improved confidence of outcome prediction in severe head injury. J Neurosurg 54:751–762, 1981.
13. Phuenpathom N, Choomuang M, Ratanalert S: Outcome and outcome prediction in acute subdural hematoma. Surg Neurol 40:22–25, 1993.
14. Kaufmann MA, Buchmann B, Scheidegger D, et al: Severe head injury: Should expected outcome influence resuscitation and first-day decisions? Resuscitations 23:199–206, 1992.
15. Silverston P: Pulse oximetry at the roadside: A study of pulse oximetry in immediate care. BMJ 298:711–713, 1989.
16. Muizelaar JP, Marmarou Al, Ward JD, et al: Adverse effects of prolonged hyperventilation in patients with severe head injury: A randomized clinical trial. J Neurosurg 75:731–739, 1991.
17. Vassar MJ, Fischer RP, O'Brien PE, et al: A multicenter trial for resuscitation of injured patients with 7.5% sodium chloride: The effect of added dextran 70: The Multicenter Group for the Study of Hypertonic Saline in Trauma Patients. Arch Surg 128:1003–1011, 1993.
18. Wade CE, Grady JJ, Kramer GC, et al: Individual patient cohort analysis of the efficacy of hypertonic saline/dextran in patients with traumatic brain injury and hypotension. J Trauma 42:561–565, 1997.
19. Narayan RK, Kishore PR, Becker DP, et al: Intracranial pressure: To monitor or not to monitor? A review of our experience with severe head injury. J Neurosurg 56:650–659, 1982.
20. Davson H, Welch K, Segal MB (eds): Physiology and Pathophysiology of the Cerebrospinal Fluid. Edinburgh, Churchill Livingston, 1987, p 53.
21. Zauner A, Daugherty WP, Bullock R, et al: Brain oxygenation and energy metabolism, I: biological function and pathophysiology. Neurosurgery 51:289–302, 2002.
22. Hatashita S, Hoff JT: The effect of craniectomy on the biomechanics of normal brain. J Neurosurg 67:573–578, 1987.
23. Polin RS, Shaffrey ME, Bogaev CA: Decompressive bifrontal craniectomy in the treatment of severe refractory post traumatic cerebral edema. Neurosurgery 41:84–94, 1997.
24. Temkin NR, Dikmen SS, Wilkensy AJ, et al: A randomized, double-blind study of phenytoin for the prevention of post-traumatic seizures. N Engl J Med 323:497–502, 1990.
25. Eisenberg HM, Frankowski RF, Contant CF, et al: High-dose barbiturate control of elevated intracranial pressure in patients with severe head injury. J Neurosurg 69:15–23, 1988.
26. Nordstrom GH, Messeter K, Sundberg B, et al: Cerebral blood flow, vasoreactivity, and oxygen consumption during barbiturate therapy in severe traumatic brain lesions. J Neurosurg 68:424–431, 1988.
27. Marion DW, Penrod LE, Kelsey SF, et al: Treatment of traumatic brain injury with moderate hypothermia. N Engl J Med 336:540–546, 1997.
28. Eljamel MS: Antibiotics prophylaxis in unrepaired CSF fistulae. Br J Neurosurg 7:501, 1993.

CHAPTER 18

Pediatric Orthopedic Trauma

Michael T. Rohmiller, MD, Gregory A. Mencio, MD, and Neil E. Green, MD

Musculoskeletal trauma is the most common medical emergency in children.[1] In children age 1 to 14 years, accidents are the leading cause of death.[2] However, most orthopedic injuries sustained by children are not life threatening. It has been estimated that between 1% and 2% of children sustain a fracture each year.[3] As participation in sporting and recreational activities increases, the number of fractures is likely to increase.

Patient gender, age, climate, time of day, and social situation in the home have been shown to affect the frequency of orthopedic injuries. In children, boys sustain fractures at 2.7 times the rate of girls.[4] However, as girls become involved in more athletic events, the margin may narrow. It has been shown that fracture location varies with chronologic age, a finding that is probably due to a combination of the anatomic maturation of the child and the age-specific activities of childhood.[5] Several authors have shown that fractures are more common during the summer months when children are out of school.[3,4–6] It also has been shown that a strong association exists between sunshine and fractures, and a negative association, between rainy weather and fractures.[7] Likewise, two studies have documented that the afternoon is the most frequent time for fractures to occur; this correlates with the time of peak activity for children.[8,9] Injuries in the home during the late afternoon and evening account for the majority of all injuries to children.[10] Moreover, the overall incidence of fractures occurring at home increases with age of the child.[3,11] In a Swedish study, the physical quality of the home environment did not correlate well with the fracture incidence. The major correlation was with the degree of social handicaps such as welfare dependence or alcoholism in the family.[12] Similarly, a recent Canadian study elicited the social situation at home as a major influence of children's injuries.[13]

Unfortunately, nonaccidental trauma occurs to children. The incidence of physical abuse to children is estimated to be 4.9 per 1000, and of those abused, 1 of every 1000 will ultimately die.[14] Early recognition and reporting of abuse is essential, as children who return home after a case of unrecognized abuse have a 25% risk of

serious injury and a 5% risk of death.[15] Children at highest risk for abuse include first-born infants, premature infants, stepchildren, and handicapped children.[16] Most cases of abuse involve children younger than 3 years.[17]

PATHOPHYSIOLOGY

Regarding the nature of musculoskeletal trauma, the major difference between children and adults is that children are growing. In the immature skeleton, longitudinal and appositional growth occurs through the physes (growth plates) that are located at the ends of the long bones, in the endplates of the vertebral bodies, or at the periphery of the round bones in the feet and hands. Therefore the physis is essential for normal skeletal growth but is the weakest portion of the bone in children. Consequently, fractures in children frequently involve this region. It is estimated that approximately 30% of children's long bone fractures include an injury to the physis.[18–20] Most fractures that involve the growth plates heal without consequence. However, some injuries can result in permanent damage with significant sequelae such as angular deformity or complete cessation of growth.

The ends of every long bone consist of an epiphysis (near the joint), the physis, and metaphysis (area of newly formed bone). At the time of skeletal maturity, the physis closes, and longitudinal growth ceases. Fracture healing in children is rapid, and the potential for remodeling is great, because of the growth and dynamism of the immature skeleton. These characteristics allow nonoperative treatment in children of some fractures that demand operative treatment in skeletally mature patients. Remodeling after a fracture occurs primarily in the plane of motion of the adjacent joint (flexion/extension) and, to a lesser degree, with varus and valgus deformities but is virtually nonexistent for rotational malalignment.[21]

Classification of fractures is done to predict outcome and to guide treatment. Fractures in children are classified according to the pattern of involvement. Currently, most orthopedic surgeons use the classification designed by Salter and Harris in 1963 (Fig. 18-1).[22] Type I injuries

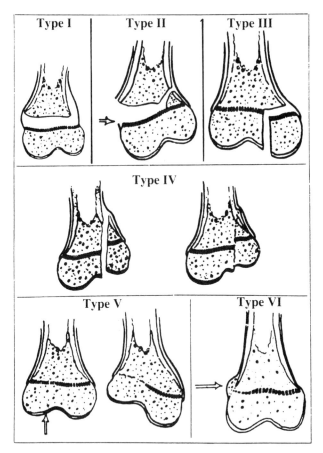

FIGURE 18-1. Salter classification of physeal injuries with Rang modification. (From Rang ML [ed]: The Growth Plate and Its Disorders. Edinburgh, E&S Livingston, 1969, p 139.)

involve the physis only and may be missed on radiographs if they are not displaced. Type II injuries start in the physis and exit the metaphysis. Type III injuries involve the physis and epiphysis, exiting into the joint, and type IV fractures involve both the epiphysis and metaphysis. Classic teaching states that type I and II injuries, if reduced, heal without adverse growth sequelae. However, more recent studies dispute this previously reported optimism.[23-25] Types III and IV injuries usually occur in older children and require anatomic realignment with open reduction to restore congruity of the joint to minimize the risk of arthritis and also to restore continuity of the physis to decrease the risk of growth disturbance. Type V injuries are crush injuries and are not usually recognized at presentation, although the injury carries a high risk of growth arrest.[26]

COMPLEX INJURIES

Children sustain injuries that are different from those of adults because of the child's size and activities. A common example is a pedestrian struck by a car. In such an event, an adult will frequently sustain an injury to the

tibia or knee from the car's bumper. However, the same mechanism in a child will result in a fracture of the femur or pelvis and, in small children, a chest or head injury.[27] Motor vehicle accidents are the most common cause of multiple injuries to children, as both occupants and pedestrians.[27,28] Although not restricted to motor vehicle accidents, spinal trauma is frequently seen in the multiply injured child. Awareness of the possibility of a cervical spine injury is mandatory in any child first seen with facial injuries.[29,30] Likewise, ecchymosis in the lower abdomen from the lap-belt portion of a seat belt should alert the physician to the possibility of significant intra-abdominal and/or spine injury.[31,32] Frequently seen with the use of lap belts without shoulder restraint, the lap-belt syndrome consists of flexion-distraction injuries to the lumbar spine (Chance fracture), hollow viscus rupture, and traumatic pancreatitis (Fig. 18-2).[33]

Open fractures are considered one of the true orthopedic emergencies in children. These injuries usually involve a high-energy force and may involve multiple injuries. Open fractures in children and adults are classified according to the system of Gustilo-Anderson (Table 18-1).[34] The four goals of treatment of open fractures are prevention of infection, bony union, prevention of malunion, and return to function of limb and patient.[35] To attain these goals, open fractures must be treated with early irrigation and debridement along with administration of broad-spectrum antibiotics.[34,36] In one study, the early treatment of tibial shaft fractures in children resulted in fewer cases of osteomyelitis compared with those treated late.[37] However, recent data from our institution demonstrated no difference in infection or nonunion rates in 346 open fractures of the lower extremities in adults.[38]

FRACTURES OF THE PELVIS AND LOWER EXTREMITY

Because of the high energy required, fractures of the pelvis and proximal femur are rare but serious injuries in children. Approximately two thirds of patients with pelvic fractures have associated injuries, and approximately one third have residual, long-term morbidity.[39] Pelvic fractures rank second to head injuries in terms of complications, including life-threatening visceral injuries. The mortality rate for children with pelvic fractures ranges from 9% to 18%, which is lower than that in adults.[40] Children with multiple injuries should be examined carefully to exclude fractures of the pelvis. Some common findings of fractures of the pelvis are the presence of a hematoma beneath the inguinal ligament (Desot's sign); decreased distance between the greater trochanter and anterior superior iliac spine on the affected side in lateral compression injuries (Roux's sign); and the presence of a bony prominence or hematoma on rectal examination (Earl's sign). An anteroposterior radiograph of the pelvis is usually sufficient as the initial screening radiograph, although these injuries are being increasingly diagnosed with spiral tomography that is performed as part of the initial trauma evaluation. Most pediatric pelvic fractures, even those in which the

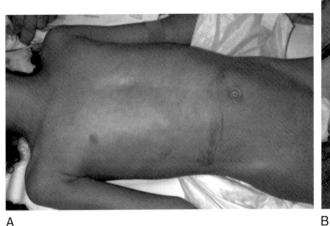

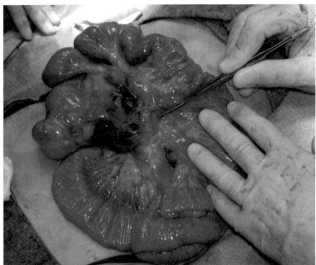

A   B

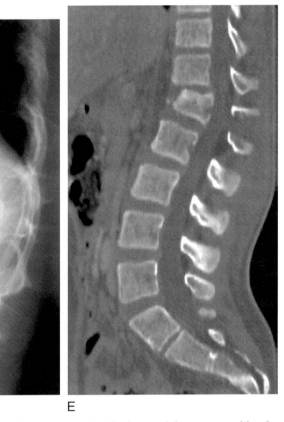

C   D   E

FIGURE 18-2. Twelve-year-old girl involved in a motor vehicle accident with ecchymosis in the lower abdomen caused by the lap-belt portion of a three-point restraint (*A*). This child had a laceration of the omentum discovered at laparotomy (*B*) and a flexion distraction fracture of L1 with disruption of all three columns of the spine (*C–E*) that required surgical stabilization.

pelvic ring is disrupted, can be treated nonoperatively with good outcomes.[41]

Fractures of the femoral neck are serious injuries that typically require operative treatment. Osteonecrosis, caused by disruption of the vascular supply to the femoral epiphysis, is a significant complication of this fracture that occurs in up to 75% of children after this injury.[42] The risk of developing osteonecrosis correlates with a higher anatomic location of the fracture in the femoral neck, the extent of displacement, and the length of delay

TABLE 18-1

SEVERITY CLASSIFICATION FOR OPEN FRACTURES

Grade	Description
I	Wound <1 cm
II	Transitional wound (1–10 cm)
III	Wound >10 cm
IIIA	Extensive soft tissue injury
IIIB	Reconstructive soft tissue injury
IIIC	Vascular injury

From Gustilo RB, Mendoza RM, Williams DN: Problems in the management of type III (severe) open fractures: A new classification of type III open fractures. J Trauma 24:747–796, 1984; Gustilo RB, Anderson T: Prevention of infection in the treatment of 1025 open fractures of long bones. Retrospective and prospective analyses. J Bone Joint Surg Am 50:453–458, 1976.

in reducing the fracture. Thus fractures and dislocations of the proximal femur are treated as orthopedic emergencies. They require immediate anatomic reduction, which may be achieved by closed or open techniques, and internal fixation (Fig. 18-3).

Pediatric femoral shaft fractures are common injuries. The incidence and mechanism of these femoral shaft fractures varies with patient age and gender. Child abuse accounts for up to 67% of femur fractures in children younger than 1 year, but only 11% of fractures in children between ages 1 and 2 years.[43] Classic teaching states that spiral fractures in preambulatory children are pathognomonic for abuse; however, other studies have demonstrated that any fracture pattern can occur as the result of abuse.[44] Falls are the leading cause of femur fractures in children age 2 to 3 years, and motor vehicle accidents are the most common cause in older children.[43] Treatment of femur fractures also varies with age. Younger children (younger than 4 to 5 years) are usually treated nonoperatively with closed reduction and immediate spica cast immobilization; older children (ages 4 to 10 years) are treated with flexible nails or plates; and adolescents and teenagers (older than 10 years) may be treated as adults with solid, reamed, femoral nails.

Knee injuries in children also differ from those in adults. In children, the cartilage of the physes, apophyses, menisci, and articular surfaces are weaker than the knee ligaments and thus more prone to injury.[45] Therefore fractures about the knee occur more commonly than ligamentous injuries in skeletally immature individuals.[46,47] The distal femoral physis is the largest and fastest-growing physis. It is often injured as a result of a direct blow and is a common injury in American football players. Most fractures are Salter-Harris type I or II injuries. These fractures can usually be treated with closed reduction and percutaneous, cross-pin stabilization. Fractures extending into the articular surface (type III and IV injuries) require open reduction and internal fixation if displacement of the articular surface is greater than 2 mm. Because of the size of this growth plate, its complex undulating anatomy, and the forces required for displacement, fractures of the distal femoral physis, even type I and II injuries, may result in permanent growth disturbance in up to 50% of cases.[48] All of these fractures should be followed up for a minimum of 1 year to exclude sequelae of permanent (limb-length inequality) or partial (angular deformity) growth arrest.

Proximal tibial physeal injuries are uncommon because of the reinforcement provided by the capsule and collateral ligaments. However, vascular compromise of the lower leg due to popliteal artery injury is possible with displaced fractures of the proximal tibial physis, particularly with extension-type injuries in which the proximal portion of the tibial metaphysis is displaced posteriorly, tenting the popliteal artery at the level of the physis and proximal to its trifurcation (Fig. 18-4). Close attention to the vascular examination of the lower extremity is critical after injuries to the proximal tibia. Intra-articular injuries, including patellar fractures, tibial spine/plateau fractures, osteochondral fractures, and ligamentous/meniscal injuries exhibit an hemarthrosis at presentation. These fractures are not typically emergencies and can be splinted initially and then treated definitively on a delayed basis.

Nonphyseal fractures of the tibia and fibula are among the most common injuries involving the lower extremity in children.[49,50] Fortunately, most of these injuries are low energy and can be treated nonoperatively with good long-term results and few complications. However, one must always be cognizant of the possibility of compartment syndrome after closed or open fractures of the tibial shaft.[51] Indications for operative treatment of tibial shaft fractures include open fractures, fractures with neurovascular injury or impending compartment syndrome, those with unacceptable alignment after closed reduction, and fractures occurring in the setting of polytrauma.

Foot and ankle fractures are typically caused by indirect, torsional forces. Injuries to the distal tibial and fibular physes account for 25% to 38% of all children's physeal injuries.[52,53] Sports injuries account for up to 58% of physeal fractures about the ankle.[54] Nonoperative treatment has historically been the treatment of choice except for intra-articular fractures and those that cannot be adequately reduced by closed means. Newer data suggest improved results with open reduction of distal tibial physeal injuries.[23] Computed tomography (CT) is very useful in defining the pathoanatomy of fractures with intra-articular involvement or unusual patterns and has proven to be very helpful in making management decisions and in preoperative planning.[55] Fractures of the foot are uncommon and infrequently cause problems for the child. Most foot fractures can be treated nonoperatively with immobilization and restricted weight bearing and produce good functional results. More complex problems that require operative intervention include fractures of the talar neck and calcaneus, fractures or dislocations of the tarsometatarsal (Lisfranc) joint, and open fractures and lawn-mower injuries.[55]

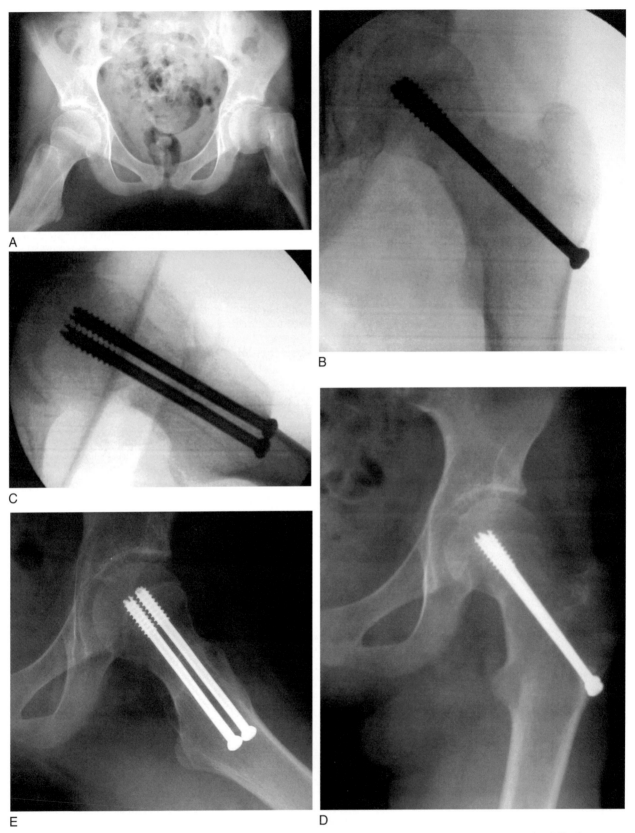

FIGURE 18-3. Anteroposterior radiograph of the pelvis of a 12-year-old girl injured as the result of a fall, showing a displaced transcervical fracture of the left femoral neck (*A*). Fracture was treated as an emergency with closed reduction and internal fixation with two cannulated screws. Intraoperative fluoroscopic images demonstrate anatomic reduction of the fracture (*B, C*). Radiographs 1 year later show healing of the fracture and no evidence of osteonecrosis (*D, E*).

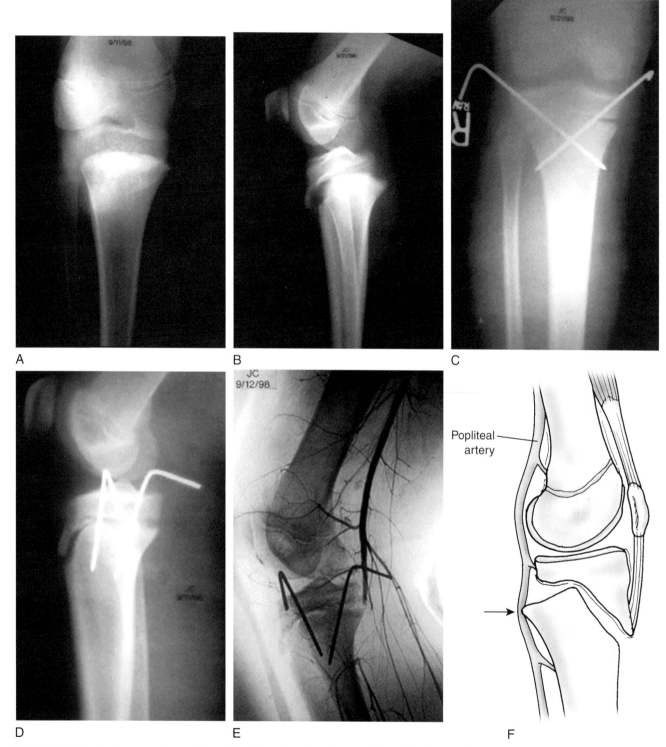

FIGURE 18-4. Anteroposterior and lateral radiographs of a 13-year-old boy showing a Salter-Harris type I fracture of the prox-imal tibial physis with posterior displacement of the distal fragment after an extension-type injury (*A, B*). Distal pulses were diminished before and after closed reduction and stabilization of the fracture (*C, D*). Arteriogram shows occlusion of the popliteal artery at the level of the fracture (*E*). Vascular repair with an interposition graft was performed successfully. Drawing shows the relation of the popliteal artery to the proximal tibial physis and the mechanism of vascular injury in this fracture (*F*). (From Green NE: Fractures and dislocations about the elbow. In Green NE, Swiontkowski MF (eds): Skeletal Trauma in Children, Vol 3. Philadelphia, WB Saunders, 2003.)

SPINE INJURIES

Cervical

Cervical spine injuries (CSIs) in children are relatively uncommon but potentially catastrophic. Accurate diagnosis requires an awareness of the injury patterns, anatomic characteristics, and radiographic variants of the immature cervical spine. CSIs account for approximately 1% of all pediatric fractures, yet only 2% of all spine fractures.[56–58] Pediatric CSIs are quite different from their adult counterparts due to the anatomic characteristics of the immature spine and, to a lesser extent, to differences in the mechanisms of injury between adults and children.[59] The cervical spine in children is inherently mobile because of the presence of generalized laxity of the interspinous ligaments and joint capsules, underdeveloped neck musculature, thick cartilaginous endplates, incomplete vertebral ossification (wedge-shaped vertebral bodies), and shallow-angled facet joints, particularly in the upper segments (between the occiput and C4).[59]

In infants and young children, injuries to the upper cervical spine (above C3) predominate because the head is disproportionately large and creates a large bending movement in the upper cervical spine. In an 11-year experience with 122 pediatric neck injuries, none of the 21 patients age 8 years or younger had evidence of injury below C3.[60] Multilevel spinal injuries also are more common, occurring in approximately 25% of children with cervical spine fractures.[61] Moreover, spinal cord injury without radiographic abnormality (SCIWORA) occurs more frequently in children than in adults.[57,59] After age 8 to 10 years, the anatomic and biomechanical characteristics of the cervical spine are more like those in an adult, and injuries to the cervical spine are much more likely to occur in the subaxial region (below C3). Evaluation and treatment of these injuries is essentially the same as those in an adult.[57,59,62]

Mechanisms of injury vary somewhat with age. In neonates, birth trauma is the most common cause of CSI, and occult spinal cord injury (SCI) has been demonstrated at necropsy in 30% to 50% of stillborns. Excessive distraction and/or hyperextension of the cervical spine is thought to be the most common mechanism of injury and may be associated with abnormal intrauterine position (transverse lie) or a difficult cephalic or breech delivery.[63,64] In infants and young children, nonaccidental trauma is a significant cause of injury to the cervical spine. Avulsion fractures of the spinous processes, fractures of the pars or pedicles (most commonly C2), or compression fractures of multiple vertebral bodies are the most common patterns of injury and are thought to result from severe shaking or battering.[65,66] These injuries may be associated with other signs of child abuse, including fractures of the skull, ribs, or long bones, and cutaneous lesions. In older children up to about 10 years old, the most common causes are pedestrian–motor vehicle accidents and falls. In children older than 10 years, the most common etiologies are passenger-related motor vehicle accidents, sports-related injuries, and diving accidents.

Appropriate methods of immobilizing children for transport and evaluating them clinically and radiographically are crucial to avoid detrimental outcomes. The goal of immobilization during transport of the injured child with potential spine trauma is to prevent excessive angulation of the spinal column to avoid causing or exacerbating SCI. Immobilization of children younger than 8 years on a standard spine board during emergency transportation has been shown to cause excessive flexion of the cervical spine because of the disproportionately large diameter of the head relative to the torso. It has been recommended that the child's spine board be modified by building up the area under the torso with padding to allow the head to fall back slightly or by creating a cutout in the area under the occiput to accept the skull (Fig. 18-5).[67] In addition to proper spine-board immobilization, an appropriately fitting cervical collar is necessary to achieve neutral alignment of the cervical spine after injury.[68]

Clinical evaluation of a child suspected of having an injury to the cervical spine is often hampered by the inability to obtain accurate historical information and the unreliability of the physical examination.[62] Historically, overt or occult injury to the cervical spine is more likely to occur as a result of falls from a height of more than 4 feet, pedestrian or cyclist versus motor vehicle accidents, and unrestrained occupant–motor vehicle accidents. Head or facial trauma, altered mental status, and/or loss of consciousness also are risk factors. Neck pain, guarding, and torticollis are the most reliable signs of an injury to the cervical spine in children. Extremity weakness, sensory changes (numbness or tingling), bowel and bladder dysfunction, and, less frequently, headaches, seizures, syncope, and respiratory distress are all signs of possible injury to the spinal cord (Table 18-2). When these conditions are present or when any question exists, the cervical spine should be immobilized until imaging studies can be completed and the spine cleared of injury.

Radiographic evaluation of the cervical spine in children is hampered by the presence of normal anatomic variants that can be mistaken for traumatic injury. Synchondroses and incompletely ossified, wedge-shaped vertebral bodies can simulate fractures.[69,70] Anterior angulation of the odontoid is a normal variant in approximately 5% of children and may be mistaken for a Salter-Harris type I fracture of the dens. Physiologic subluxation of C2 on C3 or C3 on C4 of up to 3 mm is a normal variant (pseudo-subluxation) in about 40% of children younger than 8 years that is often misinterpreted as pathologic instability.[71,72] Focal kyphosis of the midcervical spine is a normal variant in about 15% of children younger than 16 years that can also be misinterpreted as abnormal.

Initial radiographic evaluation should include cross-table lateral and anteroposterior radiographs. On the lateral view, it is essential to see the C7-T1 disc space. Oblique views are additionally helpful to define the detail of the pedicles and facet joints. Open-mouth odontoid radiographs are technically difficult to perform and rarely helpful. CT is a very good modality with which to evaluate the upper cervical spine and also provides excellent definition of known fractures, confirmation of suggestive areas, and excellent visualization of the cervicothoracic levels, which can be difficult to evaluate

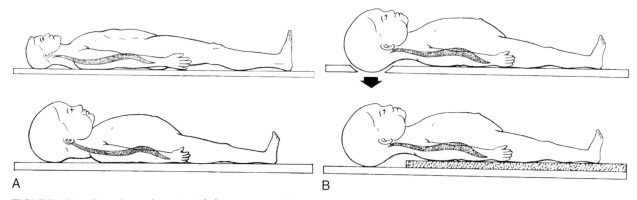

A   B

FIGURE 18-5. Drawings of an adult (*A*) and a child (*B*) on a normal spine board contrasting the differences in position of the head and neck during emergency transport. Because of the disproportionate head-to-body ratio in children, the child's cervical spine is flexed. *B,* Two methods of modifying the traditional spine board for pediatric patient transport. In (*A*), a cutout in the board allows the occiput to be recessed, and in (*B*), the area under the thorax is built up with padding. Both methods effectively allow the head to translate posteriorly, creating more normal alignment of the cervical spine. (Reprinted from Herzenberg JE, Hensiger RN, Dedrick DK: Emergency transport and positioning of young children who have an injury to the cervical spine. J Bone Joint Surg Am 71:15–21, 1989.)

adequately on plain radiography. Magnetic resonance imaging (MRI) is the study of choice to evaluate the spinal cord and soft-tissue structures including ligaments, cartilage, and intervertebral discs.

Once a cervical collar has been placed on a child or the neck immobilized, either at the scene of an accident or in the emergency department, formal clearance of the cervical spine is necessary before immobilization may be discontinued. In general, the cervical spine may be cleared based on clinical examination alone if the child is awake, alert, and cooperative; if no signs of cervical injury are found; and if the mechanism of injury is not consistent with cervical trauma.[73] For children younger than 8 to 10 years who are obtunded or otherwise unable to be examined, and all those with a profile suggestive of injury to the cervical spine, clearance may be based on a five-view cervical spine series consisting of anteroposterior, lateral, open-mouth odontoid, two oblique views, and CT of the axial region of the spine from the occiput to C2. The rationales for CT include the predisposition for injuries to occur in the upper cervical region in children younger than 8 years and the technical difficulty

imaging this area with plain radiographs. In a study in which this protocol was followed, 8 of 112 children were diagnosed with CSIs. Two (33%) of six children with bony injuries had them diagnosed only with CT scan. No injuries were missed, and cervical immobilization was discontinued in a timely fashion.[73]

Others have advocated the definitive role of MRI as an adjunct to plain radiographs and CT, particularly in identifying soft-tissue pathology. In one study of 79 children, MRI revealed injuries in 15 patients with normal radiographs and excluded injuries suspected on plain radiographs and CT scans in 7 and 2 patients, respectively. In 25 obtunded or uncooperative children, MRI demonstrated three with significant injuries.[74]

Halo-vest immobilization is being used with increasing frequency in children with CSIs. It affords superior immobilization when compared with a rigid cervical collar and is easier to apply and more versatile than a Minerva cast. It permits access for skin and wound care while avoiding the skin problems (maceration, ulceration) typically associated with both hard collars and casts. However, complication rates associated with pediatric halo use have been reported as high as 68%.[75] Pin-site infections are the most common problems, but pin perforation, cerebrospinal fluid leaks, and brain abscesses also have been reported.[62,75] In children younger than 6 years, a CT scan of the skull to measure calvarial thickness can be helpful in determining the optimal sites for pin placement.[76] In children older than 6 years, the standard adult halo construct with four pins (two anterolaterally, two posterolaterally) inserted at standard torques of 6 to 8 inch-pounds generally works (Fig. 18-6A). In younger children, more pins (up to 12) placed with lower insertional torques (2 to 4 inch-pounds) have been advocated (Fig. 18-6B).[75,76] Standard pediatric halo rings fit most children, but infants and toddlers usually require customized rings. Although standard pediatric halo vests are available, custom vests or body casts generally provide superior immobilization.[77]

TABLE 18-2
RISK FACTORS FOR CERVICAL SPINE INJURY

Mechanism of injury
    Pedestrian- or cyclist–motor vehicle accident
    Unrestrained occupant–motor vehicle accident
    Fall >4 feet
Loss of consciousness
Neck pain, limited range of motion, torticollis
Abnormal neurologic examination
    Numbness, tingling
    Extremity weakness
Head or facial trauma

From Weiser ER, Mencio GA: Pediatric cervical spine injuries: Assessment and treatment. Semin Spine Surg 13:142–151, 2001.

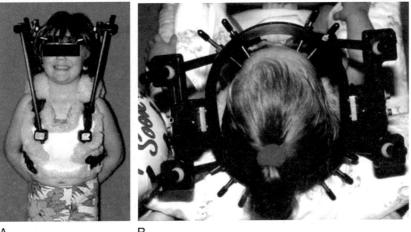

A   B

FIGURE 18-6. *A,* Six-year-old immobilized in standard halo construct with four pins (two anterolateral, two posterolateral) inserted at torques of 6 to 8 inch-pounds. *B,* Three-year-old child with halo ring with 10 pins inserted at low torque, in contrast to the usual four-pin configuration used in older children and adults. (From Weiser ER, Mencio GA. Pediatric cervical spine injuries: Assessment and treatment. Sem Spine Surg 13:142–151, 2001.)

The possibility of SCI without radiographic abnormality should be considered in children, particularly in those younger than 8 years. SCIWORA is defined as an SCI in a patient in whom no fracture is visible on plain radiographs or CT scan.[78–80] MRI may be diagnostic in demonstrating spinal cord edema or hemorrhage, soft-tissue or ligamentous injury, or apophyseal or disc disruption but is completely normal in approximately 25% of cases. SCIWORA is the cause of paralysis in approximately 20% to 30% of children with injuries of the spinal cord. Potential mechanisms of SCIWORA include hyperextension of the cervical spine (which can cause compression of the spinal cord by the ligamentum flavum) followed by flexion (which can cause longitudinal traction); transient subluxation without gross failure; or unrecognized cartilaginous end plate failure (Salter-Harris type I fracture).

Regardless of the specific mechanism, injury to the spinal cord occurs because of the variable elasticity of the elements of the spinal column in children.[81] Experimentally, it has been shown that the bone, cartilage, and soft tissue in the spinal column can stretch about 2 inches without disruption, but that the spinal cord ruptures after one-fourth inch.[64,80,82] Injury occurs when deformation of the musculoskeletal structures of the spinal column exceeds the physiologic limits of the spinal cord.[81] The injury may be complete or incomplete. Partial spinal cord syndromes reported in SCIWORA include Brown-Sequard, anterior, and central cord syndromes, as well as mixed patterns of injury.[78,79,81]

The prognosis after SCIWORA is correlated to MRI findings, if any are present, and to the severity of neurologic injury.[79] Effective management demands careful evaluation of the cervical spine to exclude osseous injury, cartilaginous injury, or mechanical instability, along with stabilization of the spine to prevent recurrent injury.[79,80] Immobilization with a rigid cervical collar for 2 to 3 months is usually adequate treatment for SCIWORA. There are no reports of recurrent spinal cord injury when the cervical spine has been immobilized in this manner. Surgery is occasionally necessary for unstable injury patterns. The prevalence of scoliosis after infantile quadriplegia is more than 90%. Long-term follow-up to monitor for spinal deformity is necessary.

Administration of high-dose corticosteroids within the first 8 hours of SCI has been shown to improve the chances of neurologic recovery in adults.[83] Methylprednisolone is administered as an intravenous bolus of 30 mg/kg over a 15-minute period followed by a continuous infusion of 5.4 mg/kg/hr over the next 23-hour period. Although the effect on younger children is not known, this protocol is used in all patients with SCIs at our institution.

Thoracic, Lumbar, and Sacral Fractures

Thoracic, lumbar, and sacral fractures are relatively uncommon in children. The majority of these injuries are caused by motor vehicle accidents or falls. The most common injuries are compression fractures and flexion-distraction injuries. Compression fractures are caused by a combination of hyperflexion and axial compression. Because the disk in children is stronger than cancellous bone, the vertebral body is the first structure to fail. It is common for children to sustain multiple compression fractures, but the compression rarely exceeds more than 20% of the vertebral body. These fractures are managed with rest, analgesics, and bracing.

Flexion/distraction injuries occur in the upper lumbar spine in children wearing a lap belt.[31,33,84–91] With sudden deceleration, the belt slides up on the abdomen where it acts as an axis about which the spine rotates, with disruption of the posterior column with variable patterns of extension into the middle and anterior column. A lateral radiograph showing widening of the interspinous space posteriorly is helpful in diagnosing this fracture (Fig, 18-2D). Approximately two thirds of patients have intra-abdominal injuries that may be life-threatening,[33] but neurologic injury is unusual. Less than 20% of lap-belt injuries with mostly bony involvement and kyphosis can be treated with hyperextension casting. Those with posterior ligamentous disruption and soft-tissue injury require surgical stabilization with compression instrumentation and posterior arthrodesis.

Although rare, fracture-dislocations of the spine are unstable injuries that usually occur at the thoracolumbar junction and often are associated with neurologic deficits. These fractures require surgical stabilization and fusion.

Burst fractures also are uncommon injuries in children, resulting from axial compression, and typically occur at the thoracolumbar junction or in the lumbar spine.[92] The need for operative treatment is determined by the stability of the fracture and the presence of neurologic deficits. Fractures of the sacrum are usually associated with pelvic fractures. Fractures that involve the sacral foramina or central sacral canal are associated with neurologic deficits in 28% and 50% of patients, respectively. Decompression of the sacral nerve root(s) and stabilization of the sacral fracture may be necessary to improve neurologic function. In most instances, however, fractures of the sacrum may be treated nonoperatively.

FRACTURES OF THE CLAVICLE

Fractures of the clavicle are among the most common injuries in children. They are usually uncomplicated and require little, if any, treatment, other than sling immobilization for comfort. Distal clavicular fractures in the immature child may mimic acromioclavicular separation, but the trauma surgeon should be aware of this injury and should not mistake this for a true acromioclavicular dislocation. The periosteal sleeve of the distal clavicle remains intact with the coracoclavicular ligaments attached.[20,93-95] The fracture heals very rapidly with an enormous amount of callus and does not require treatment other than sling immobilization for comfort. Complete remodeling of the bone will occur.

Injuries to the medial end of the clavicle are somewhat rare but potentially problematic from the standpoint of recognition and neurovascular complications. The medial clavicle consists of the clavicle and its medial growth plate plus the ligaments of the sternoclavicular joint. The physis of the medial clavicle is the last one in the body to close and frequently does not close until after age 21 years.[20,95,96] The so-called "dislocation of the sternoclavicular joint" in the teenager and young adult is almost always a type I physeal fracture. It is important to recognize this distinction because a true dislocation would likely be unstable, whereas a type I fracture of the physis is a stable injury once reduced.

Anterior or posterior displacement of the medial end of the clavicle may occur as a result of indirect trauma to the shoulder with a secondary force vector that determines the final resting position of the bone. Posterior displacement almost always occurs by a direct mechanism such as occurs when one falls on a football and others land on top of him. The medial portion of the clavicle is pushed posteriorly, resulting in an injury directly through the growth plate of the medial clavicle. The patient appears in the emergency department with pain and swelling about the sternoclavicular joint. The shoulder is usually held forward. No pain occurs about the distal clavicle or the shoulder joint. Although uncommon, compression of mediastinal structures is the most devastating complication of this injury. The diagnosis of this injury requires awareness of the possibility of the injury and a CT scan for confirmation. Radiographs may show the posterior dislocation, but it is most clearly seen on CT scan with thin cuts through the medial clavicle and sternoclavicular joint (Fig. 18-7).

FRACTURES OF THE UPPER EXTREMITY

Because the shoulder has essentially a full arc of rotation, fractures about the proximal humerus in the younger child will remodel very quickly, with no need for treatment other than immobilization for comfort.[97,98]

Markedly displaced fractures in the teenager, however, will not remodel because insufficient growth potential remains.[98-100] These fractures are usually type II fractures of the proximal humeral physis and, if significantly angulated and displaced, should be reduced. Moreover, the reduction is usually not stable, and some form of fixation is necessary. Generally these fractures can be stabilized with percutaneous Steinmann pins or cannulated screws inserted from the distal fragment into the proximal fragment by using fluoroscopy.[101,102] Internal fixation should be supplemented with a sling and swathe. If pins are used, they should remain for 3 to 4 weeks, after which gentle range of motion may begin. The fracture should heal very quickly. Permanent injury to the

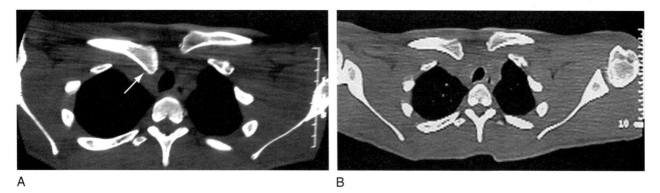

A   B

FIGURE 18-7. Sixteen-year-old boy injured his right clavicle when he was checked into the board while playing hockey. He complained of difficulty swallowing. Anteroposterior radiograph of the right clavicle appeared normal. Computed tomography scan with thin cuts through the sternoclavicular joint shows posterior displacement of the medial end of the clavicle (*arrow*) (*A*) and restoration of alignment after closed reduction (*B*).

growth plate is not an issue because this fracture generally occurs very close to the completion of skeletal growth.

Fractures about the elbow in children can be difficult to diagnose because the anatomy of the immature elbow is confusing because of the presence of numerous centers of ossification. Knowledge of the sequence of appearance and maturation of the secondary ossification centers is mandatory, and a comparison radiograph of the contralateral elbow is often helpful in correctly identifying the nature of the injury.[103]

The most common fracture about the distal humerus in the child is a supracondylar fracture. It is classified according to the amount of displacement. The type III fracture is the most devastating, with both fragments completely displaced. The injury usually occurs from a fall on the outstretched hand. In children who are ligamentously lax, the elbow will hyperextend and shear off the distal portion of the humerus through the olecranon fossa.[104]

The major problems with this injury are soft-tissue swelling along with nerve and vascular injury. In the past, it was thought that this fracture should be treated immediately; however, it is now recognized that this fracture does not need immediate operative stabilization unless other extenuating circumstances are found, such as compartment syndrome, significant vascular compromise, or an open wound. The general policy is to delay treatment of these fractures if they occur in the middle of the night until the next day and to operate on them during the daylight hours with familiar operating room personnel. The patients are admitted to the hospital after the injury and watched carefully. The elbow is splinted in less than 90 degrees of flexion with a loose bandage over a posterior splint.[105,106] These fractures can usually be reduced by closed manipulation and stabilized with percutaneous pins (Fig. 18-8). Occasionally open reduction and pinning of this fracture is necessary if one is unable to obtain a perfect anatomic reduction or if other

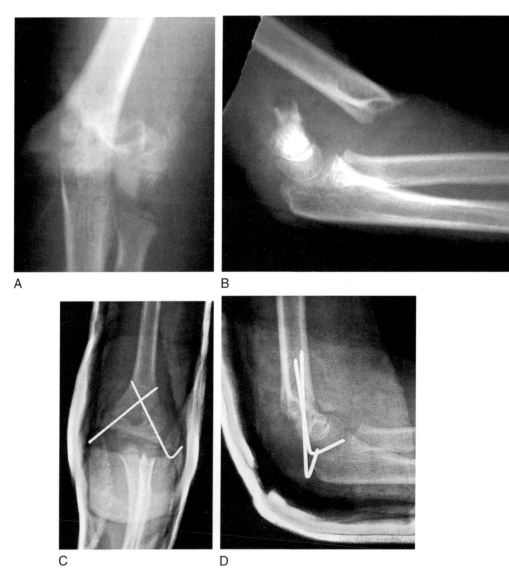

FIGURE 18-8. Six-year-old fell while horseback riding and landed on his outstreched left arm. Anteroposterior and lateral radiographs show completely displaced (type III) supracondylar humerus fracture (*A, B*). Neurovascular status of the extremity was intact. The child was treated with closed reduction and percutaneous fixation with smooth Steinmann pins (*C, D*).

extenuating circumstances exist, such as an open fracture or a vascular injury that requires exploration.

The treatment of the pulseless extremity has been controversial for some time in patients who have sustained a supracondylar fracture. Absence of the pulse with this fracture is not uncommon. It is postulated that the absence of the pulse may be the result of either vascular spasm and/or direct vascular injury; however, the collateral circulation about the elbow is so rich that the circulation to the forearm and hand remains normal. Treatment of the vascular injury has been debated for decades in the orthopedic and vascular surgery literature.

The current practice is observation as long as circulation to the hand and forearm is normal.[104,107,108] It has been shown by longitudinal studies that vein grafting of vascular injuries will frequently thrombose because of the excellent collateral circulation.[108] The only true indication for vascular exploration is the pulseless, ischemic extremity, and this is a true surgical emergency. In this instance, the fracture should be reduced and stabilized with crossed pins before vascular repair.[109,110] Compartment syndrome is a feared complication that is actually quite uncommon in the modern era of treatment of this fracture. Stabilizing the fracture with internal fixation

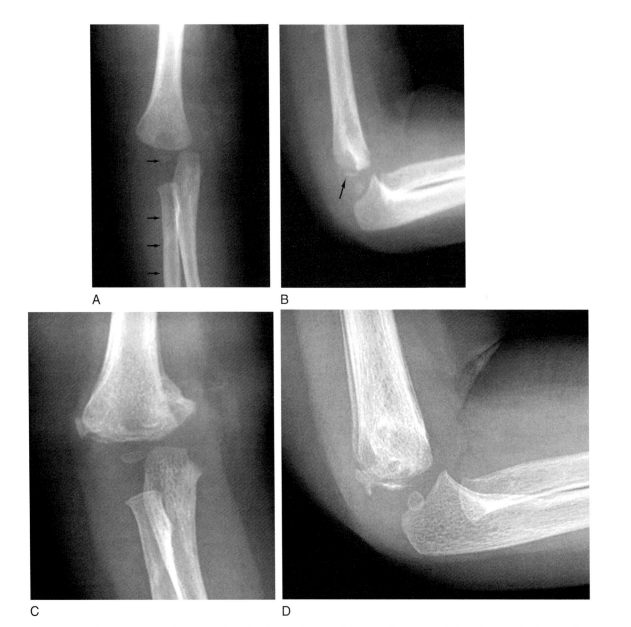

FIGURE 18-9. Eleven-month-old child, ultimately determined to have been the victim of abuse, had a swollen arm. On the anteroposterior radiograph of the elbow, the capitellum, the proximal radius, and the ulna are displaced from their normal positions relative to the distal humerus (*arrows*), consistent with a fracture/separation of the distal humeral epiphysis (*A*). In an elbow dislocation, the radius and ulna are displaced relative to the distal humerus, but the capitellum is not displaced from its normal position in the distal humerus. The lateral radiograph of the elbow shows a small metaphyseal fragment (*arrow*), also consistent with a fracture of the distal humeral physis and not with dislocation of the elbow (*B*). This fracture was treated with cast immobilization. Note the exuberant fracture callus 3 weeks after the injury (*C, D*).

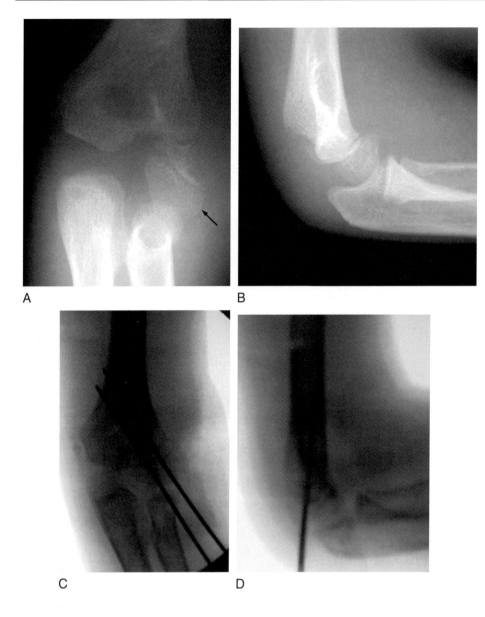

A   B

C   D

FIGURE 18-10. Seven-year-old child fell from a bunk-bed, resulting in a fracture of the lateral condyle of the humerus. Anteroposterior (AP) and lateral radiographs show displacement of the capitellum (*arrow*), whereas the radius and ulna remain aligned with the humerus (*A, B*). Even if they were minimally displaced, the risk of joint incongruity and nonunion is high after nonoperative treatment of this fracture. AP and lateral radiographs of the elbow after open reduction and pin fixation show anatomic alignment (*C, D*).

obviates the need to immobilize the elbow in hyperflexion, which has been shown to increase the risk of vascular compression and forearm compartment swelling.[104]

The signs of compartment syndrome are well known, but the primary sign that one should look for is pain out of proportion to the fracture itself. Once this fracture is stabilized, the child should be comfortable and not have significant pain. Passive extension of the fingers should be possible to a neutral position and, if not, suggests the need for investigation of a compartment syndrome by removal of the splint, palpation of the forearm compartment, and pressure measurement, if necessary. If the pressures are elevated consistent with a forearm compartment syndrome, then fasciotomy should be performed immediately.

Salter-Harris type I fractures of the distal humerus are less common than other injuries about the elbow. Moreover, they are frequently misdiagnosed (Figs. 18-9 and 18-10). Equally important is the recognition that, in very young children, this fracture often occurs as the

result of nonaccidental trauma, and its occurrence should trigger investigation into the possibility of child abuse as the mechanism of injury.[111] This fracture also may occur in newborns as a result of birth trauma.[104] In this instance, it is usually a stable fracture that will heal in a matter of days and requires only splint immobilization for comfort. In the child, this fracture may require closed manipulation and pinning if the fracture is expediently diagnosed before some healing has occurred. Unfortunately, especially in instances of nonaccidental trauma, the child is seen long after this injury has already begun to heal, and manipulation of the fracture is either not possible or ill advised.

Forearm fractures have traditionally been treated with closed manipulation and casting. In most instances, especially with distal fractures, this treatment is highly successful and results in normal function of the extremity. Our preference is to perform closed reduction of these fractures in the emergency department by using ketamine (2 to 4 mg/kg) or another method of conscious sedation.

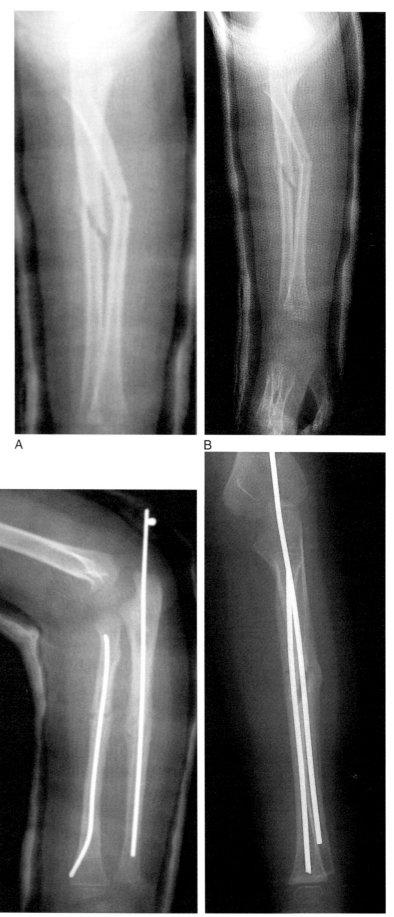

FIGURE 18-11. Anteroposterior and lateral radiographs show diaphyseal fractures of the radius and ulna in a 6-year-old, with angulation after closed treatment (*A, B*). Fractures were treated with internal fixation by using flexible titanium nails inserted via 1-cm incisions, distally in the radius and proximally in the ulna, and advanced across the fracture under fluoroscopic visualization (*C, D*).

A

B

C

D

Versed also is frequently given to prevent emergence reactions that are sometimes seen with this drug, especially in the older child.[112,113]

The use of a portable fluoroscopy unit is essential in treating pediatric forearm fractures, both to guide reduction of the fracture and to confirm alignment after immobilization. After manipulation of the fracture, the extremity is immobilized in a sugar-tong splint, which allows swelling. When swelling is no longer a concern, the sugar-tong splint is incorporated into a long-arm, fiberglass cast. In general, the child should be seen weekly for the first 3 weeks to ensure that the alignment of the fracture is maintained. Three weeks after the injury, the cast may be changed to a short-arm cast, which remains for another 3 weeks, after which progressive use and motion is begun.

Fractures of the shaft of both bones of the forearm, especially proximal to the midportion of the forearm, are poorly treated with cast immobilization alone, especially in children older than 8 or 9 years. It is difficult to maintain reduction of these fractures in cast or splint, and angulation or malrotation in the diaphysis of either the radius or ulna will result in loss of rotation in the forearm. For this reason, fractures of the shafts of the radius and ulna are increasingly being treated with internal fixation by using flexible titanium nails (Fig. 18-11). These fractures can usually be reduced with closed manipulation although open reduction may occasionally be required.

REFERENCES

1. Smith MD, Burrington JD, Woolf AD: Injuries in children sustained in free falls: An analysis of 66 cases. J Trauma 15:987–991, 1975.
2. Starfield B: Childhood morbidity: Comparisons, clusters, and trends. Pediatrics 88:519–527, 1991.
3. Worlock P, Stower M: Fracture patterns in Nottingham children. J Pediatr Orthop 6:656–662, 1986.
4. Cheng JC, Shen WY: Limb fracture pattern in different pediatric age groups: A study of 3350 children. J Orthop Trauma 7:15–20, 1993.
5. Landin LA: Fracture patterns in children. Acta Orthop Scand 54:1–23, 1983.
6. Reed MH: Fractures and dislocations of the extremities in children. J Trauma 17:351–355, 1977.
7. Masterson E, Borton D, Foster BK: Victims of our climate. Injury 24:247–251, 1993.
8. Shank LP, Bagg RJ, Wagnon J: Etiology of pediatric fractures: The fatigue factors in children's fractures. National Conference of Pediatric Trauma, Indianapolis, Indiana, 1992.
9. Westfelt JARN: Environmental factors in childhood accidents: A prospective study in Goteborg, Sweden. Acta Paediatr Scand Suppl:291, 1982.
10. Izant RJ, Hubay CA: The annual injury of 15,000,000 children: A limited study of childhood accidental injury and death. J Trauma 6:65–69, 1966.
11. Ong ME, Ooi SB, Manning PG: A review of 2,517 childhood injuries seen in a Singapore emergency department in 1999: Mechanisms and injury prevention suggestions. Singapore Med J 44:12–19, 2003.
12. Wilkins KE: The Incidence of Fractures in Children, Vol 3. Philadelphia, Lippincott-Raven, 1996.
13. Brownell M, Friesen D, Mayer T: Childhood injury rates in Manitoba: Socioeconomic influences. Can J Public Health 93(suppl 2):S50–S56, 2002.
14. Johnson CF: Inflicted injury versus accidental injury. Pediatr Clin North Am 37:791–814, 1990.
15. Schmitt BD, Gray JD, Britton HL: Child Abuse in Pediatrics III. Philadelphia, WB Saunders, 1984.
16. Akbarnia B, Akbarnia NO: The role of the orthopedist in child abuse and neglect. Orthop Clin North Am 7:733–742, 1976.
17. Galleno H, Oppenheim WL: The battered child syndrome revisited. Clin Orthop 62:11–19, 1982.
18. Mann DC, Rajmatra S: Distribution of physeal and non-physeal fractures of long bones in children aged 0 to 16 years. J Pediatr Orthop 10:719–722, 1990.
19. Marcus RE, Mills MF, Thompson GH: Multiple injury in children. J Bone Joint Surg 65:1290–1295, 1983.
20. Ogden JA: Skeletal Injury in the Child. Philadelphia, Lea & Febiger, 1990.
21. Ogden JA: Complications of Fractures. Philadelphia, JB Lippincott, 1995.
22. Salter RB, Harris WR: Injuries involving the epiphyseal plate. J Bone Joint Surg [Am] 45:587–596, 1963.
23. Barmada A, Gaynor T, Mubarak S: Premature physeal closure following distal tibia physeal fractures: A new radiographic predictor. J Pediatr Orthop 23:733–739, 2003.
24. Kling TF Jr, Bright RW, Hensinger RN: Distal tibial physeal fractures in children that may require open reduction. J Pediatr Orthop 66:647–657, 1984.
25. Spiegel PG, Mast JW, Cooperman DR, et al: Epiphyseal fractures of the distal ends of the tibia and fibula: A retrospective study of two hundred and thirty-seven cases in children. J Bone Joint Surg [Am] 60:1046–1050, 1978.
26. Mendez AA, Bartal E, Grillot MB, et al: Compression (Salter-Harris type V) physeal fracture: An experimental model in the rat. J Pediatr Orthop 12:29–32, 1992.
27. Wilber JH, Thompson GH: The multiply injured child. In Green NE, Swiontkowski MF (eds): Skeletal Trauma in Children, Vol 3. Philadelphia, WB Saunders, 2003, pp 73–104.
28. Morrison A, Stone DH, Redpath A, et al: Childhood injury mortality in Scotland, 1981–95. Health Bull (Edinb) 57:241–246, 1999.
29. Kim LH, Lam LK, Moore MH: Associated injuries in facial fractures: Review of 839 patients. Br J Plastic Surg 46:635–638, 1993.
30. Lewis VL, Manson PN, Morgan RF: Facial injuries associated with cervical fractures: Recognition patterns and management. J Trauma 25:90–93, 1985.
31. Atlas H, Allard M, Denis R, et al: Seat belt syndrome: A new abdominal pathology. Can J Surg 27:464–465, 1984.
32. Sivit CJ, Taylor GA, Newman KD, et al: Safety-belt injuries in children with lap-belt ecchymosis: CT findings in 61 patients. AJR Am J Roentgenol 157:111–114, 1991.
33. Newman KD, Bowman LM, Eichelberger MR, et al: The lap belt complex: Intestinal and lumbar spine injury in children. J Trauma 30:1133–1138, 1990.
34. Gustilo RB, Anderson JT: Prevention of infection in treatment of 1025 open fractures of long bones: Retrospective and prospective analysis. J Bone Joint Surg [Am] 58:453–458, 1976.
35. Chapman MW: The use of immediate internal fixation in open fractures. Orthop Clin North Am 11:579–591, 1980.
36. Gustilo RB, Merkow RL, Templeman D: Current concepts review: The management of open fractures. J Bone Joint Surg Am 72:299–304, 1990.
37. Kindsfater K, Jonassen EA: Osteomyelitis in grade II and III open tibia fractures with late debridement. J Orthop Trauma 9:121–127, 1995.
38. Rohmiller MT, Kusuma S, Blanchard GM, et al: Management of open fractures of the lower extremity: Does time to debridement and primary wound closure really matter? Toronto, Ontario, Canada, Othopaedic Trauma Association, 2002.
39. Hensinger RN: Operative treatment of lower extremity fractures. J Bone Joint Surg 74:1439–1440, 1992.
40. Demetriades D, Karaiskakis M, Velmahos GC, et al: Pelvic fractures in pediatric and adult trauma patients: Are they different injuries? J Trauma 54:1146–1151, 2003.
41. Grisoni N, Connor S, Marsh E, et al: Pelvic fractures in a pediatric level I trauma center. J Orthop Trauma 16:458–463, 2002.
42. Mirdad T: Fractures of the neck of femur in children: An experience at the Aseer Central Hospital, Abha, Saudi Arabia. Injury 33:823–827, 2002.
43. Nork SE, Bellig GJ, Woll JP, et al: Overgrowth and outcome after femoral shaft fracture in children younger than 2 years. Clin Orthop 186–191, 1998.

44. Scherl SA, Miller L, Lively N, et al: Accidental and nonaccidental femur fractures in children. Clin Orthop 376:96–105, 2000.

45. Zobel MS, Borrello JA, Siegel MJ, et al: Pediatric knee MR imaging: Pattern of injuries in the immature skeleton. Radiology 190:397–401, 1994.

46. Close BJ, Strouse PJ: MR of physeal fractures of the adolescent knee. Pediatr Radiol 30:756–762, 2000.

47. Poland J: Traumatic Separation of the Epiphysis. London, Elder, 1898.

48. Riseborough EJ, Barrett IR, Shapiro F: Growth disturbances following distal femoral physeal fracture-separation. J Bone Joint Surg Am 65:885–893, 1983.

49. Karholm J, Hansson LI, Svensonn K: Incidence of tibio-fibular shaft and ankle fractures in children. J Pediatr Orthop 2:386–392, 1982.

50. Shannak AO: Tibial fractures in children: Follow-up study. J Pediatr Orthop 8:306–310, 1988.

51. Hope PG, Cole WG: Open fractures of the tibia in children. J Bone Joint Surg Br 74:546–553, 1992.

52. Hynes D, O'Brien T: Growth disturbance lines after injury to the distal tibial physis. J Bone Joint Surg Br 70:231–233, 1988.

53. Rogers LF: The radiography of epiphyseal injuries. Radiology 96:289–297, 1970.

54. Goldberg VM, Aadalen R: Distal tibial epiphyseal injuries: The role of athletics in fifty-three cases. Am J Sports Med 6:263–268, 1978.

55. Vanhoenacke FM, Bernaerts A, Gielen J, et al: Trauma of the pediatric ankle and foot. J Bone Joint Surg Br 85:212–218, 2002.

56. Eleraky MA, Theodore N, Adams M: Pediatric cervical spine injuries: Report of 102 cases and review of the literature. J Neurosurg 92:12–17, 2000.

57. Jones ET, Haid R: Injuries to the Pediatric Subaxial Cervical Spine, Vol 3. WB Saunders, 1991.

58. McGrory BJ, Klassen RA, Chao E: Acute fractures and dislocations of the cervical spine in children and adolescents. J Bone Joint Surg Am 75:988–995, 1993.

59. Givens TG, Polley KA, Smith GF: Pediatric cervical spine injury: A three-year experience. J Trauma 41:310–314, 1996.

60. Hill SA, Miller CA, Kosnik EJ: Pediatric neck injuries: A clinical study. J Neurosurg 60:700–704, 1984.

61. Hadden WA, Gillepsie WJ: Multiple level injuries of the cervical spine. Injury 16:628–633, 1985.

62. Jones ET, Hensinger RN: Injuries of the Cervical Spine. In Rockwell W, Beaty J (eds): Fractures in Children, Vol 3. Philadelphia, Lippincott-Raven, 1996.

63. Bresnam J, Adams F: Neonatal spinal cord transection secondary to intrauterine neck hyperextension in breech presentation. Fetal Neonat Med 84:734–741, 1971.

64. Leventhal HR: Birth injuries of the spinal cord. J Pediatr Orthop 56:447–453, 1960.

65. Caffey J: The whiplash shaken infant syndrome. Pediatrics 54:396, 1974.

66. Swischuck LE: Spine:spinal cord trauma in the battered child syndrome. Radiology 92:733–735, 1977.

67. Herzenberg JE, Hensiger RN, Dedrick DK: Emergency transport and positioning of young children who have an injury to the cervical spine. J Bone Joint Surg Am 71:15–21, 1989.

68. Curran C, Dietrich A, Bowman M: Pediatric cervical-spine immobilization: achieving neutral position? J Trauma 39:729–732, 1995.

69. Smith T, Skinner SR, Shonnard NH: Persistent synchondrosis of the second cervical vertebra simulating a hangman's fracture in a child. J Bone Joint Surg Am 75:892–893, 1993.

70. Swischuck LE, Swischuck PN, John SD: Wedging of C3 in infants and children: Usually a normal finding, not a fracture. Radiology 188:523–526, 1993.

71. Cattell HS, Filtzer DL: Pseudosubluxation and other normal variations of the cervical spine in children. J Bone Joint Surg Am 47:1295–1309, 1965.

72. Swischuck LE: Anterior displacement of C2 in children. Physiologic or pathologic? Radiology 122:759–763, 1977.

73. Hartley W, Mencio GA, Green NE: Clinical and radiographic algorithm for acute management of pediatric cervical spine trauma in Scoliosis Research Society, 32nd Annual Meeting, St. Louis, Missouri, 1997.

74. Dormans JP: The role of MRI in the assessmzent of pediatric cervical spine injuries in evaluation and management of pediatric spine trauma. American Academy of Orthopedic Surgeons,

67th Annual Meeting. Instructional Course Lecture 321, Orlando, Florida, 2000.

75. Dormans JP, Criscitiello AA, Drummond DS, et al: Complications in children managed with immobilization in a halo vest. J Bone Joint Surg Am 77:1370–1373, 1995.

76. Letts M, Kaylor D, Gouw G: A biomechanical analysis of halo fixation in children. J Bone Joint Surg Br 70:277–279, 1988.

77. Mubarak SJ, Camp JF, Vueltich W: Halo application in the infant. J Pediatr Orthop 9:612–616, 1989.

78. Pang D, Wilberger JE: Spinal cord injury without radiographic abnormalities in children. J Neurosurg 57:114–129, 1982.

79. Pang D, Pollack I: Spinal cord injury without radiographic abnormality in children: The SCIWORA syndrome. J Trauma 29:654–664, 1989.

80. Sullivan A: Fractures of the spine in children. In Green N, Swiontowski M (eds): Skeletal Trauma in Children. Philadelphia, WB Saunders, 1996, pp 343–368.

81. Kriss VM, Kriss TC: SCIWORA (spinal cord injury without radiographic abnormality) in infants and children. Clin Pediatr 35:119–124, 1996.

82. Copley LA, Dormans JP: Pediatric cervical spine problems: Developmental evaluation and congenital anomalies. J Am Acad Orthop Surg 6:204–214, 1998.

83. Bracken MB, Shepard MJ, Collins WF: A randomized, controlled trial of methylprednisolone or naloxone in the treatment of acute spinal cord injury: Results of the Second National Spinal Cord Injury study. N Engl J Med 322:1405–1411, 1990.

84. Akbarnia B: Pediatric spine fractures. Orthop Clin North Am 30:521–536, 1999.

85. Banerian KG, Wang AM, Samberg LC, et al: Association of vertebral end plate fracture with pediatric lumbar intervertebral disk herniation: value of CT and MR imaging. Radiology 177:763–765, 1990.

86. Greenwald TA, Mann DC: Pediatric seatbelt injuries: Diagnosis and treatment of lumbar flexion-distraction injuries. Paraplegia 32:743–751, 1994.

87. Griffet J, Bastiani-Griffet F, El-Hayek T, et al: Management of seat-belt syndrome in children: Gravity of 2-point seat-belt. Eur J Pediatr Surg 12:63–66, 2002.

88. Johnson DL, Falci S: The diagnosis and treatment of pediatric lumbar spine injuries caused by rear seat lap belts. Neurosurgery 26:434–441, 1990.

89. Raney EM, Bennett JT: Pediatric Chance fracture. Spine 17:1522–1524, 1992.

90. Reid AB, Letts RM, Black GB: Pediatric Chance fractures: Association with intra-abdominal injuries and seatbelt use. J Trauma 30:384–391, 1990.

91. Smith MD, Camp E, James H, et al: Pediatric seat belt injuries. Am Surg 63:294–298, 1997.

92. Lalonde F, Letts M, Yang JP, et al: An analysis of burst fractures of the spine in adolescents. Am J Orthop 30:115–120, 2001.

93. Golthamer CR: Duplication of the clavicle ("os claviculare"). Radiology 68:576–578, 1957.

94. Twigg HL: Duplication of the clavicle. Skeletal Radiol 6:281–283, 1981.

95. Webb LX, Mooney JF: Fractures and dislocations about the shoulder. In Green NE, Swiontkowski (eds): Skeletal Trauma in Children. Philadelphia, WB Saunders, 2003, pp 322–343.

96. Gray H: Anatomy of the Human Body. Philadelphia, Lea & Febiger, 1985.

97. Baxter MP, Wiley JJ: Fractures of the proximal humeral epiphysis: Their influence on humeral growth. J Bone Joint Surg Br 68:570–573, 1986.

98. Beaty JH: Fractures of the proximal humerus and shaft in children. Instr Course Lect 41:369–372, 1992.

99. Dameron TB, Reibel DB: Fractures involving the proximal humeral epiphyseal plate. J Bone Joint Surg Am 51:289–297, 1969.

100. Smith FM: Fracture-separation of the proximal humeral epiphysis. Am J Surg 91:627–635, 1956.

101. Beebe A, Bell DF: Management of severely displaced fractures of the proximal humerus in children. Tech Orthop 4:1–4, 1989.

102. Loder RT: Pediatric polytrauma: Orthopedic care and hospital course. J Orthop Trauma 1:48–54, 1987.

103. Haraldsson S: On osteochondrosis deformans juvenilis capituli humeri including investigation of intra-osseous vasculature in distal humerus. Acta Orthop Scand Suppl 38, 1959.

104. Green NE: Fractures and dislocations about the elbow. In Green NE, Swiontkowski MF (eds): Skeletal Trauma in Children, Vol 3. Philadelphia, WB Saunders, 2003, pp 257–321.

105. Green NE: Overnight delay in the reduction of supracondylar fractures of the humerus in children. J Bone Joint Surg Am 93:321–322, 2001.

106. Mehlman CT, Strub WM, Roy DR: The effect of surgical timing on the perioperative complications of treatment of supracondylar humeral fractures in children. J Bone Joint Surg Am 83:323–327, 2001.

107. Luhmann SJ, Gordon JE, Schoenecker PL: Intramedullary fixation of unstable both-bone forearm fractures in children. J Pediatr Orthop 18:451–456, 1998.

108. Sabharwal S, Tredwell SJ, Beauchamp RD: Management of pulseless pink hand in pediatric supracondylar fractures of the humerus. J Pediatr Orthop 17:303–310, 1997.

109. Copley LA, Dormans JP, Davidson RS: Vascular injuries and their sequelae in pediatric supracondylar humeral fractures: Toward a goal of prevention. J Pediatr Orthop 16:99–103, 1996.

110. Schoenecker PL, Delgado E, Rotman M: Pulseless arm in association with totally displaced supracondylar fracture. J Orthop Trauma 10:410–415, 1996.

111. DeLee JC, Wilkins KE, Rogers LF: Fracture separation of the distal humerus epiphysis. J Bone Joint Surg Am 62:46–51, 1980.

112. McCarty EC, Mencio GA, Green NE: Anesthesia and analgesia for the ambulatory management of fractures in children. J Am Acad Orthop Surg 2:81–91, 1999.

113. McCarty EC, Mencio GA, Green NE: Ketamine sedation for the reduction of children's fractures in the emergency department. J Bone Joint Surg Am 82:912–918, 2000.

Congenital Chest Wall Deformities

Donald Nuss, MB, ChB, Daniel P. Croitoru, MD,
Robert E. Kelly, Jr., MD, and Michael J. Goretsky, MD

Congenital chest wall deformities fall into two groups—those with overgrowth of the rib cartilages causing either a depression or protuberance, and those with varying degrees of either aplasia or dysplasia.

Pectus excavatum, an "excavated, sunken, or funnel chest," constitutes about 88% of the deformities and is by far the most common. Pectus carinatum, a chest wall protuberance, constitutes approximately 5% of chest wall deformities. Combined excavatum/carinatum deformities constitute 6% of the total. Jeune's syndrome, or asphyxiating chondrodystrophy, is an extreme form of mixed pectus excavatum/carinatum and is very rare. Poland's syndrome (0.8%) and bifid sternum represent different forms of aplasia of the anterior chest wall. In Poland's syndrome, there are varying degrees of dysplasia of the breast, of the pectoralis muscles, and of ribs. In bifid sternum, partial or complete failure of midline fusion of the sternum is noted, which may result in ectopia cordis if the sternal fissure is complete, or it may result in varying degrees of sternal dysplasia and deficiencies of associated structures such as the heart, pericardium, diaphragm, and anterior abdominal wall (pentalogy of Cantrell).

Many of these deformities are present at birth. In some cases, such as ectopia cordis, they are incompatible with life and have rarely been successfully repaired. Chest wall deformities are frequently associated with systemic weakness of the connective tissues and with poor muscular development of the abdominal region, thorax, and spine. There is, therefore, a markedly increased association with Marfan syndrome, Ehlers-Danlos syndrome, and scoliosis, as well as with omphalocele in the case of bifid sternum, all of which complicate the management of these patients (Table 19-1).

The surgical management has undergone major changes over the last 15 years. In the 1960s and 1970s, radical surgical operations were in vogue, even in very young children. However, it came to be realized that pulmonary function actually decreased over time because of the scarring of the anterior chest wall, and in some patients, "acquired asphyxiating chondrodystrophy" developed from extensive and too early resections. As a result, surgeons stopped operating on prepubertal patients and reverted to "modified" resections of the deformed cartilages. Recently a minimally invasive procedure with no resection, only internal bracing, was introduced.

PECTUS EXCAVATUM

Introduction

Pectus excavatum is a depression of the anterior chest wall of variable severity, which may be mild, moderate, or severe. All variations of depth, symmetry, and breadth of the deformity may be seen. The deformities may be small in diameter and deep, "cup-shaped" (Fig. 19-1A), or of large diameter and shallow, "saucer-shaped" (Fig. 19-1B), or eccentric (Fig. 19-1C). The depth and extent of the depression determine the degree of cardiac and pulmonary compression, which in turn determines the degree of incapacitation. The deformity is frequently noted at birth and progresses with growth.

Progression may be especially pronounced during puberty, a fact apparently unknown to many pediatricians, who mistakenly advise younger patients that the condition will resolve spontaneously. We have seen many families who were given this advice and missed the opportunity to have the deformity repaired before puberty while the chest was still soft and malleable and before it interfered with physical performance. Approximately one third of patients have a deformity severe enough to require surgical correction.

History of Pectus Excavatum

Pectus excavatum was recognized as early as the 16th century. Johan Schenck (1531–1590) collected literature on the subject, as cited in Ebstein.[1] A classic article by Bauhinus[2] in 1594 described the clinical features of pectus excavatum in a patient who had pulmonary compression with dyspnea and paroxysmal cough, attributed to severe pectus excavatum. The genetic predisposition was first noted by Coulson[3] in 1820, who cited a family of

TABLE 19-1
INCIDENCE AND ETIOLOGY

	Number of Patients
Total evaluated	1009
Total with pectus excavatum only	883 (87.5%)
Total with mixed pectus excavatum/	
pectus carinatum	62 (6.1%)
Total with pectus carinatum only	51 (5.1%)
Total with Poland's syndrome	8 (0.8%)
Total with other deformities	5 (0.5%)
Male-to-female ratio	4:1
Family history of pectus excavatum	45.3%
Incidence of scoliosis	29.8%
Incidence of Marfan diagnosed	3%
Marfanoid (presumed Marfan)	19%
Patients with Ehlers-Danlos	2.2%

three brothers with pectus excavatum, and by Williams[4] in 1872, who described a 17-year-old patient who was born with a pectus excavatum and whose father and brother also had the condition.

Numerous other case reports appeared in the 19th century, including a five-case report by W. Ebstein in 1882,[5] which covered the clinical spectrum of the condition. Treatment at that time was limited to "fresh air, breathing exercises, aerobic activities and lateral pressure."[6,7]

Thoracic surgery remained forbidden territory until the early years of the 20th century. The first attempt at surgical correction was a tentative approach in 1911 by Meyer,[8] who removed the second and third costal cartilages on the right side without improvement of the deformity. Sauerbruch,[7] one of the pioneers of thoracic surgery, used a more aggressive approach in 1913 by excising a section of the anterior chest wall, which included the left fifth to ninth costal cartilages as well as a segment of the adjacent sternum. Before his operation, the patient was incapacitated by severe dyspnea and palpitations, even at rest, and was unable to work in his father's watch factory. After recovery, the heart could be seen to pulsate under the muscle flap, but the patient was able to work without dyspnea and even was married 3 years later.

In the 1920s, Sauerbruch performed the first pectus repair that used the bilateral costal cartilage resection and sternal osteotomy technique[9] later popularized by Ravitch. He also advocated external traction to hold the sternum in its corrected position for 6 postoperative weeks. His technique was soon used by others in Europe and rapidly gained popularity in the United States. In 1939, Ochsner and DeBakey[10] published their experience with the procedure and reviewed the entire surgical literature on the subject. Also in 1939, Lincoln Brown[11] published his experience with the procedure in two patients and reviewed the literature with particular reference to the etiology of pectus excavatum. He was impressed with

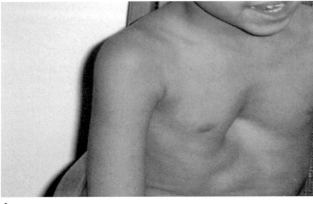

A

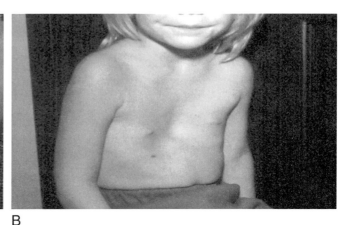

B

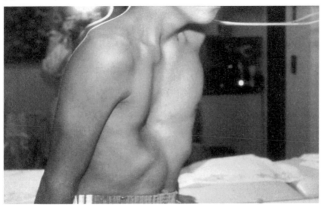

C

FIGURE 19-1. *A,* Localized or "cup-shaped" pectus excavatum. *B,* Diffuse or "saucer-shaped" deformity. *C,* Eccentric deformity.

the theory that short diaphragmatic ligaments and the pull of the diaphragm were the causative factors.

Ravitch,[12] having read Brown's article, also believed this theory and as a result advocated even more radical mobilization of the sternum, with transection of all sternal attachments, including the intercostal bundles, rectus muscles, diaphragmatic attachments, and excision of the xiphisternum. In 1949, he published his experience with eight patients by using this radically extended modification of Sauerbruch's technique of bilateral cartilage resection and sternal osteotomy. In addition, Ravitch did away with external traction.

However, the abolition of external traction led to increased recurrence. As a result, Wallgren and Sulamaa[13,14] introduced the concept of internal support in 1956 by use of a slightly curved stainless steel bar, which was pushed through the caudal end of the sternum from side to side and bridged the newly created gap between the sternum and ribs. In 1961, Adkins and Blades[15] took internal bracing one step further by passing a straight stainless steel bar behind the sternum rather than through the sternum. This form of pectus repair became a widely used technique for patients of all ages.

As early as 1958, Welch[16] already advocated a less radical approach than that of Ravitch. He produced excellent results in 75 cases without cutting through all the intercostal bundles and did not cut through the rectus muscle attachments. However, he still advocated doing the procedure in young patients. Pena,[17] conversely, was very disturbed by the idea of resecting the rib cartilages from very young patients, and his article showed the development of asphyxiating chondrodystrophy in baby rabbits after cartilage resection during their growth phase. Later, Haller[18] also drew attention to the risk of *acquired asphyxiating chondrodystrophy* in his article entitled, "Chest Wall Constriction After Too Extensive and Too Early Operations for Pectus Excavatum." As a result, many surgeons stopped performing open pectus repair in young children and waited until after puberty. They also decreased the amount of cartilage resected and spoke about a "modified Ravitch procedure."

In 1997, we published[19,20] our 10-year experience with a minimally invasive technique that required no cartilage incision, no resection, and no sternal osteotomy, but instead relied on internal bracing made possible by the flexibility and malleability of the costal cartilages.

The rationale for this technique was based on the three following observations.

1. Malleability of the chest. Children have a soft and malleable chest. In young children, the chest is so soft that even minor respiratory obstruction can cause severe sternal retraction. Trauma rarely causes rib fractures, flail chest, etc., because "the chest is so soft and malleable."[21-23] The American Heart Association recommends "using only two fingers" when performing cardiac resuscitation in young children and "only one hand in older children" for fear of crushing the heart.
2. Chest reconfiguration. Even in middle-aged and older adults, a barrel-shaped chest configuration develops in response to chronic obstructive respiratory diseases such as emphysema. If older adults are able to reconfigure the chest wall, children and teenagers should be able to do the same, given the increased malleability of their anterior chest wall.
3. Bracing. The role of braces and serial casting in successfully correcting skeletal anomalies such as scoliosis, clubfoot, and maxillomandibular malocclusion by orthopedic and orthodontic surgeons is well established. The anterior chest wall, being even more malleable than the previously mentioned skeletal structures, is therefore ideal for this type of correction.

Incidence and Etiology

Pectus excavatum occurs in approximately 1 in 1000 children and constitutes 88% of all the chest wall deformities (see Table 19-1). However, this is not the case in all countries. In Argentina, pectus carinatum is more common than excavatum.[24] Pectus excavatum also is very rare in blacks, and we have seen only ten African-American patients out of more than 1000 patients with pectus excavatum. Genetic predisposition, already noted in the 19th century,[3,4] was present in 45% of our patients. We have seen families with three siblings as well as cousins and other family members who had a pectus deformity severe enough to require correction. We also have seen patients whose fathers and grandfathers have the deformity. The male-to-female ratio of 4:1 in our series of pectus excavatum patients is similar to that of other large series.[25] Male patients have an increased risk of this deformity, whereas female patients have an increased risk of associated scoliosis.

The association with connective tissue disorder is higher than that in the normal population. A definitive diagnosis of Marfan syndrome was present in 3.0% of our patients, and an additional 19% had clinical features suggestive of Marfan syndrome. Mild scoliosis was noted in 18.4% of the patients, and severe scoliosis was noted in an additional 11.4%. Because severely asymmetric pectus excavatum tends to aggravate the postural abnormality of scoliosis, early correction of the pectus excavatum has improved mild scoliosis in some patients. Ehlers-Danlos syndrome was present in another 2.2%. The vast majority of our patients had an asthenic build and resembled basketball players; very few had an endomorphic or mesomorphic builds.

Clinical Features

Pectus excavatum is most frequently noted in infancy[25] and usually progresses slowly as the child grows. Because young children have significant cardiac and pulmonary reserves and their chest wall is still very pliable, the majority of young children are asymptomatic. However, as they become older, the deformity becomes more severe, and the chest wall, more rigid. They find that they have difficulty keeping up with their peers when playing aerobic sports. A vicious cycle may develop: patients stop participating in aerobic activities because of their inability to keep up, so their exercise capacity diminishes even more. The downward spiral is given added impetus by the fact that these patients, already embarrassed by their deformity, will avoid situations in which they have to take their shirts off in front of other children, further inhibiting participation in school and team activities.

By withdrawing from participation in activities with their peers, they also become depressed, which may affect their schoolwork. Most pectus patients have a typical geriatric or "pectus posture" that includes thoracic kyphosis, forward-sloping shoulders, and a protuberant abdomen (Fig. 19-2). A sedentary "couch potato" lifestyle may aggravate this posture, and the poor posture depresses the sternum even further. For this reason, we recommend an aggressive pectus posture exercise and breathing program.

Many patients have a relatively mild deformity during childhood. Because pediatricians are unaware of the potential for marked progression of the deformity with growth, they reassure the parents that it will resolve spontaneously. Although the deformity may not always deepen, it is unlikely that it will resolve spontaneously. When the patients grow rapidly during puberty, the deformity often suddenly accelerates, and a mild deformity may become severe in as little as 6 to 12 months. These patients have a history that "my chest suddenly caved in." It is the rapid progression that alarms parents and induces them to seek surgical consultation despite their pediatrician's reassurance. Patients with a rapid progression of their deformity exhibit the most pronounced symptom complex.

The earliest complaints are shortness of breath and lack of endurance with exercise. As the deformity progresses, chest pain and palpitations with exercise may occur, giving rise to exercise intolerance. Other symptoms include frequent and prolonged respiratory tract infections, which may lead to the development of asthma (Table 19-2).

A recent study showed[26] that patients have a poor body image, which has a major impact on self-worth. Therefore it is important to correct the deformity before it affects their ability to function normally. One of our

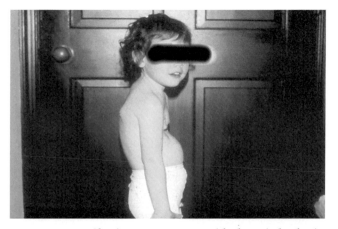

FIGURE 19-2. Classic pectus posture with thoracic kyphosis, forward sloping shoulders, and lumbar lordosis.

TABLE 19-2		
PRESENTING SYMPTOMS OF 503 SURGICAL PATIENTS		
Shortness of breath, lack of endurance, exercise intolerance	87.3%	(439)
Chest pain, with or without exercise	51.1%	(246)
Frequent respiratory infections	36.2%	(182)
Asthma/Asthma-like symptoms	35.4%	(178)
Cardiology Indicators		
Cardiac compression (by CT, Echo)	91%	(428/471)
Cardiac displacement (by CT, Echo)	81%	(366/452)
Murmur on examination	22%	(110/503)
Mitral valve prolapse	17%	(67/394)
Other anomalies (BBB, aortic insufficiency, regurgitation, hypertrophy, malformations)	16%	(63/394)
Pulmonary Indicators (N = 454)		
▪ FVC <80%	25.5%	(116)
▪ FEV1% <80%	32.8%	(149)
▪ FEF25–75% <80%	43.2%	(196)

CT, computed tomography; BBB, bundle branch block; FVC, forced vital capacity; FEV, forced expiratory volume; FEF, forced expiratory flow.

patients, a 35-year-old lawyer, confided that he had not married because he was too ashamed of his chest abnormality to have a serious relationship. A 16-year-old patient left a note for his parents, before attempting suicide, detailing the harassment and abuse that he had received from children at school. Just as one would not consider leaving a child with a cleft lip untreated, one should not leave a child with a severe pectus untreated. Both have a physiologic and psychological impact on the patient.

Cardiac and Pulmonary Effects of Pectus Excavatum

A great deal has been written about cardiopulmonary function in patients with pectus excavatum.[27] Some authors have shown significant compromise of cardiac or pulmonary function or both,[28,29] whereas others have been unable to demonstrate significant variation from predicted values.[30] Several factors play a role when testing cardiopulmonary function. These include the severity of the deformity, the inherent physical fitness of the individual patient, the patient's age, associated conditions, whether the tests are done supine or erect, and whether they are done at rest or during exercise.

Cardiac effects fall into three categories: decreased cardiac output, mitral valve prolapse, and arrhythmias (see Table 19-2). Compression of the heart results in incomplete filling and decreased stroke volume, which in turn results in decreased cardiac output.[28,29] Second, the compression interferes with normal valve function. Mitral valve prolapse was present in 17% of our patients and in up to 65% of those in other published series,[31,32] compared with only 1% in the normal pediatric population.[33] Dysrhythmias including first-degree heart block, right bundle branch block, Wolff-Parkinson-White syndrome,[34] etc., were present in 16 % of our patient series.

Pulmonary effects also fall into three categories: restrictive lung disease, atelectasis due to lung compression, and paradoxical respiration, in severe cases. The result is varying degrees of pulmonary compromise, prolonged respiratory infections, and even the development of asthma (see Table 19-2). Children with a severe deformity from birth tend to compensate by increasing the diaphragmatic component of their respiration. This partly compensates for their deformity and is seen in patients who, despite a severe deformity, are able to achieve low-normal pulmonary function studies at rest. However, they demonstrate a lack of endurance during exercise because they have little or no reserve. Stress testing has shown an increase in oxygen consumption for a given exercise when compared with that of normal patients.[35] This shows that the work of breathing is increased and explains why they lack endurance.

Evaluation and Indications for Operation

A complete history and physical examination is done for all patients and includes documenting photographs. Patients who have a mild to moderate deformity are treated with a posture and exercise program in an attempt to halt the progression and are followed up at 6-month intervals (Fig. 19-3).

Patients who have a severe deformity or who have a documented progression also are treated with the exercise and posture program, but in addition, they undergo objective studies to see whether their condition is severe enough to warrant surgical correction. These studies include pulmonary function tests (PFTs), a thoracic computed tomography (CT) scan, and a cardiac evaluation that includes an electrocardiogram (ECG) and an echocardiogram.

PFTs are done in all patients old enough to cooperate with testing. They are best done while the patient is exercising but also are helpful in the resting state.

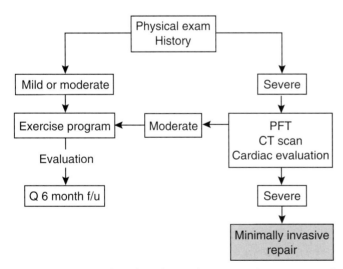

FIGURE 19-3. Algorithm for evaluation and treatment of patients with pectus deformities.

The cardiology evaluation includes an ECG, an echocardiogram, and an examination by a pediatric cardiologist to determine the presence of cardiac compression, murmurs, mitral valve prolapse, conduction abnormalities, or other structural abnormalities.

CT scans are very helpful because they clearly show the degree of cardiac compression and displacement, the degree of pulmonary compression and atelectasis, asymmetry of the chest, sternal torsion, compensatory development of a barrel-chest deformity in long-standing deformities, and ossification of the cartilages in patients with previous repairs (Fig. 19-4A, B). They also are used to calculate the CT index, which gives an objective measurement for comparing the severity between different patients. The CT index is calculated by dividing the transverse diameter by the anteroposterior diameter[36] (Fig 19-4C).

Determination of a severe pectus excavatum and the need for repair include two or more of the following criteria: (1) a CT index greater than 3.25; (2) pulmonary function studies that indicate restrictive or obstructive airway disease or both; (3) a cardiology evaluation in which the compression is causing murmurs, mitral valve prolapse, cardiac displacement, or conduction abnormalities on the echocardiogram or ECG tracings; (4) documentation of progression of the deformity with associated physical symptoms other than isolated concerns of body image; (5) a failed Ravitch procedure; or (6) a failed minimally invasive procedure. With these criteria, fewer than 50 % of patients are found to have a deformity severe enough to warrant surgical correction.[19,20,37]

The age parameters for surgical correction depend on the type of procedure selected. Unlike the more invasive procedures (Ravitch procedure, sternal turnover, etc.), no interference with growth plates occurs with the minimally invasive procedure[17,18]; therefore it can be done at any age, as evidenced by the fact that we have successfully operated on patients from ages 17 months to 29 years (Fig. 19-5). However, the concern with patients younger than 6 years is that if the procedure is done at too young an age, many years of subsequent growth remain during which the pectus excavatum may recur.

Our experience has shown that the optimal age is 7 to 14 years, because, before puberty, the patients' chests are still soft and malleable, they show quick recovery with a rapid return to normal activities, and they have excellent results (Fig. 19-6). After puberty, the flexibility of the chest wall is decreased, requiring the insertion of two bars, making the procedure more difficult. It also takes the patients longer to recover. However, all our patients older than 20 years have been extremely pleased with their results. Several other university centers have reported success with patients up to age 44 years.[38–40]

Surgical Technique

Minimally Invasive Pectus Repair

The minimally invasive pectus repair (Fig. 19-7A–J) involves making incisions on each side of the chest and creating a skin tunnel from the lateral thoracic incision to the top of the pectus ridge on each side. At the top of the

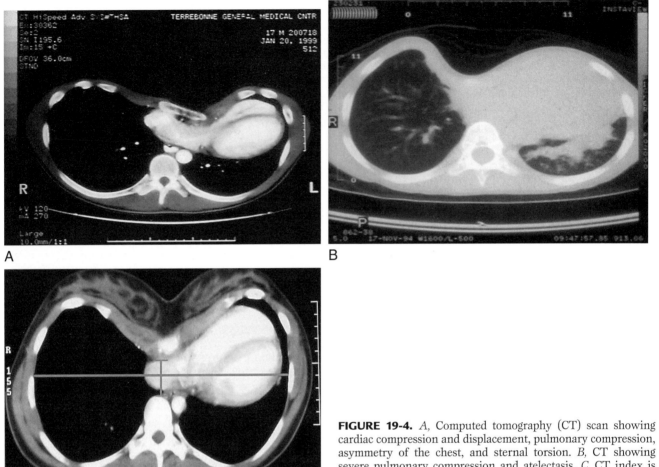

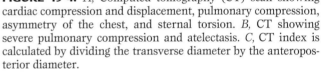

FIGURE 19-4. *A,* Computed tomography (CT) scan showing cardiac compression and displacement, pulmonary compression, asymmetry of the chest, and sternal torsion. *B,* CT showing severe pulmonary compression and atelectasis. *C,* CT index is calculated by dividing the transverse diameter by the anteroposterior diameter.

NUMBER OF PRIMARY OPERATIONS BY AGE

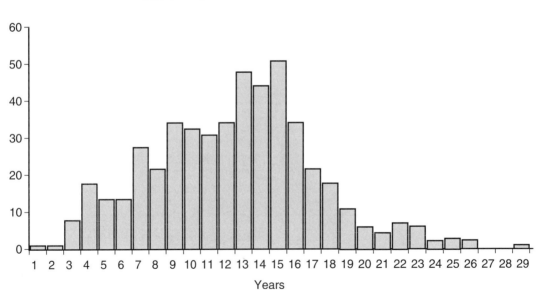

FIGURE 19-5. Distribution of our primary pectus repairs by age.

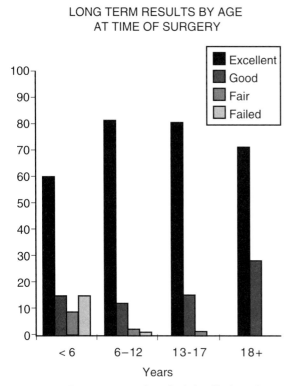

FIGURE 19-6. Long-term results of minimally invasive pectus repair by age groups.

ridge, bilateral thoracostomy incisions are made, and then a large introducer is inserted into the chest under thoracoscopic guidance. Very carefully with the thoracoscope in place and under good vision, the pleura and pericardium are dissected off the undersurface of the sternum, and the introducer is slowly advanced across the mediastinum and then brought out through the thoracostomy incision on the contralateral side. When the introducer is in place, it is elevated by lifting on each end and thereby correcting the pectus excavatum. The sternum is lifted out of its depressed position by the introducer. Once the sternal depression has been corrected, an umbilical tape is attached to the introducer, and the introducer is slowly withdrawn from the chest. A pectus support bar is then attached to the umbilical tape and slowly guided through the substernal tunnel, with its convexity facing posteriorly until it merges on the contralateral side. The length of the bar is determined by measuring the distance from midaxillary line to midaxillary line and subtracting 2.5 cm (1 inch). The bar is then bent to the desired configuration. Once the bar is in position inside the chest with the convexity facing posteriorly, it is turned over by using specially designed bar flippers. This gives instant correction of the pectus excavatum. The bar is stabilized by wiring a stabilizer to one end of the bar. In addition, sutures may be placed around the bar and underlying ribs. The sutures are usually placed with thoracoscopic guidance by using an autosuture needle. It is essential that the bar be adequately stabilized, or it will become displaced. Once the bar is in

position, the incisions are closed. The thoracoscope is removed, and the pneumothorax is evacuated by using a water-seal system. The patient is kept on thoracic epidural analgesia for 3 postoperative days and is then discharged from the hospital, usually on the fourth or fifth day. Patients need to refrain from sporting activities for 6 weeks after surgery. All patients are started on an exercise and posture program to facilitate chest expansion and to maintain a good posture.

Open Technique

The preoperative preparation and evaluation are the same as those for the minimally invasive technique. However, because there is a risk of interference with growth plates in young children and of the development of asphyxiating chondrodystrophy,[17,18] the procedure should be reserved for patients who have completed their growth. The open procedure is better suited to the older patients, especially those who have asymmetric or eccentric deformities and patients with carinatum deformities.

The open technique involves making an anterior thoracic incision, elevating skin and muscle flaps until all the costal cartilages from T3 to T6 are exposed. The perichondrium is incised longitudinally, and the deformed cartilages are either partially or completely removed. An anterior table, wedge-shaped, sternal osteotomy is performed at the angle of Louis. The sternum is elevated, and the osteotomy closed with nonabsorbable sutures. A pectus bar is inserted under the sternum to bridge the gap between the ribs and the sternum and to prevent the sternum from sinking back into the chest. The perichondrial "sleeves" are resutured, drains are inserted, the muscle flaps sutured back into position, and the incisions are closed. Postoperative management is similar to that with the open technique, except that patients are required to refrain from contact-sports activities for at least 3 months.

Results

Demographics

The minimally invasive technique for the repair of pectus excavatum received rapid acceptance by the surgical community because the technique requires neither rib incision or resection, nor sternal osteotomy. The blood loss is minimal, operating time short, and the patient rapidly returns to regular activity.[40-47]

Although the initial article presented a 10-year experience,[19] the numbers were limited (42 patients), the long-term results were affected by the early learning experience of using a support bar that was too soft, and in some patients, the bar was removed too soon. Our experience, as of December 2002, encompasses 503 patients who had their primary operation at our institution, with 268 patients after pectus bar removal. Since the original presentation, numerous important modifications have been made both to the surgical technique (e.g., routine use of thoracoscopy) and to the instruments to minimize the risks of the procedure and to facilitate insertion and

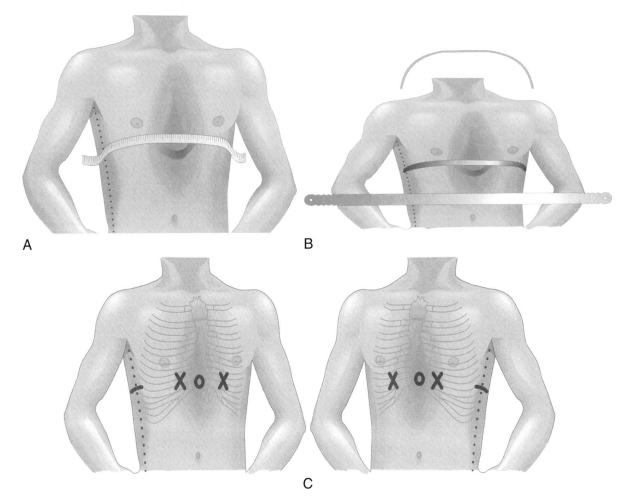

FIGURE 19-7. *A,* To calculate the length of the pectus bar, measure the distance from right to left midaxillary line, and subtract 1 to 2 cm (1 inch). *B,* Bend the Lorenz pectus support bar to conform to the desired chest wall curvature. *C,* Mark the deepest point of the pectus excavatum with a circle by using a marking pen. If this point is inferior to the sternum, then move the circle superiorly to the lower end of the sternum just above the xiphoid. This point sets the horizontal plane bar for insertion.

stabilization of the substernal support bar. These have markedly reduced the risks and complications and have been well documented in recent publications.[37]

One thousand and nine (1,009) patients were evaluated for chest wall deformities in the 15-year period from 1987 through January 2003, and 548 were judged to be severe enough to require correction (Table 19-3). Five-hundred three had their initial minimally invasive procedure done at our facility, and 45 had redo operations.

Of these 503 patients, 496 (97.6%) had pectus excavatum, and 7 (2.3%) had mixed pectus excavatum and carinatum. One (0.3%) patient had associated Poland's syndrome, and one (0.3%) had an associated complex cardiac anomaly (atrioventricular canal). Marfan syndrome was confirmed or suspected in 110 (22%) patients, and Ehlers-Danlos syndrome was noted in 11 (2.2%) patients. The male-to-female ratio in patients undergoing repair was more than 4:1. The median age

was 13 years, with a range from 19 months to 29 years. Preoperative evaluation included CT scan in 451 patients, with a median CT index of 4.8 (range, 2.4 to 21). Cardiac compression was noted on echocardiography or CT scan or both in 428 (91%) of 471 patients. Mitral valve prolapse was noted in 67 (17%) patients. Resting PFT was completed in 454 patients and demonstrated abnormalities in 43% of the patients.

Operative Procedure, Analgesia, and Length of Stay

In 429 (85.3%) patients, a single bar was inserted. Two bars were inserted in 74 (14.7%) patients. Blood loss in most patients was minimal (± 10 mL), with the exception of one patient in whom a hemothorax developed. Epidural analgesia was used for 3 days in the vast majority of patients. The median length of stay (LOS) was 5 days.

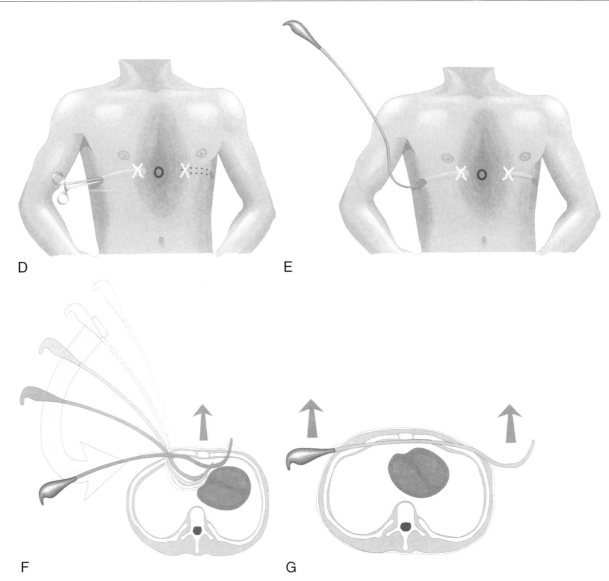

FIGURE 19-7, Cont'd *D,* After confirming by thoracoscopy that the internal and external anatomy match up well, make lateral thoracic skin incisions, and raise skin flaps anteriorly toward the X marked on the external skin at the top of the pectus ridge. *E,* Retract skin incision anteriorly to allow visualization of the intercostal space previously marked with an X, and under thoracoscopic control, insert the appropriate size Lorenz introducer through the right intercostal space at the top of the pectus ridge and at the previously marked X. *F,* When the substernal tunnel has been completed, gently push the tip of the introducer through the contralateral intercostal space at the previously marked X, medial to the top of the pectus ridge on the left side. *G,* Use the introducer to elevate the sternum. The surgeon lifts on the right side, and the assistant, on the left.

Continued

Complications

Early Complications

No deaths or cardiac perforations occurred during the 503 repairs. Pneumothorax requiring chest-tube drainage occurred in 11 (2.18%) repairs and required only percutaneous aspiration in 3 (0.6%) repairs. Hemothorax requiring drainage occurred after 1 (0.2%) repair. Four (0.8%) pleural effusions required treatment with either chest tube or aspiration (Table 19-4).

Pericarditis requiring treatment with indomethacin occurred after six (1.2%) repairs, one requiring pericardiocentesis. Pneumonia occurred after two (0.4%) repairs, and medication reactions have occurred after 11 (2.2%) repairs. Wound infection occurred after four (0.8%) repairs, resulting in bar infection and eventual early bar removal in two (0.4%) patients. One hundred fifty-five patients had a transient Horner's syndrome at varying times during the thoracic epidural administration.

Late Complications

Of 61 bar displacements, 42 (8.3%) required repositioning. Of these 42 displacements, 16 (15.2%) of 105 occurred

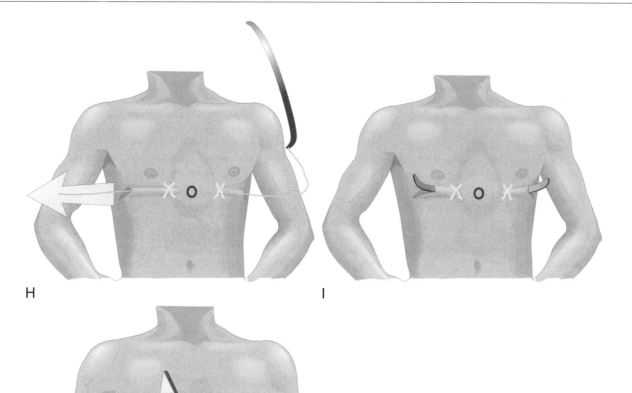

H

I

J

FIGURE 19-7, Cont'd *H,* Attach the previously prepared pectus bar to the umbilical tape, and slowly guide the bar through the tunnel by using the umbilical tape for traction. *I,* The bar is inserted with the convexity facing posteriorly. *J,* When the bar is in position, use the specially designed Lorenz bar rotational instrument (bar flipper) to turn the bar over.

before stabilizers were available, a time period covering our first 105 repairs. After the introduction of stabilizers, the incidence of bar displacement decreased from 15.2% to 6.5% or 26 of 398 patients. When the bar and stabilizers were wired together, the incidence of bar displacement decreased to 4.3% or 14 of 322 patients. No bar displacements occurred since we combined placing a stabilizer on the left and polydioxanone (PDS) sutures around the bar and underlying rib on the right.

In two patients, late hemothorax developed secondary to trauma. Both underwent thoracoscopy with drainage of the hemothorax. No active bleeding was found, with a presumed etiology therefore being an injury to an intercostal vessel. Whether hemothoraces would have developed in these patients as a result of their thoracic trauma if they had not had a pectus bar in situ is unknown. We do have several patients who were involved in major automobile accidents who sustained head and musculoskeletal trauma but no chest injuries.

Three (0.06%) of 503 patients had unsuspected allergies to the metal in the bars. These were initially seen as rashes in the area of the bar or stabilizer and required

revision to custom-made bars of other alloys. Of 503 patients, in 27 (5.3%), a mild overcorrection of their deformity developed, and in 4 (0.8%), a true carinatum deformity. Of the patients in whom a true carinatum deformity developed, 3 had Marfan syndrome, and the other had Ehlers-Danlos syndrome. In no patient did thoracic chondrodystrophy develop.

Overall Results and Long-Term Follow-Up

Patients are followed up at 6 months after the operation, and then yearly. Long-term assessments classified the results into excellent, good, fair, or failed categories.

An excellent repair indicates that the patient experienced total repair of the pectus and resolution of associated symptoms. A good repair is distinguished by a markedly improved but not totally normal chest wall appearance and resolution of associated symptoms. A fair result indicates a mild residual pectus excavatum without complete resolution of symptoms. A failed repair is marked by a recurrence of the pectus deformity and associated symptoms or need for additional surgery or both after final removal of the bar.

TABLE 19-3
MINIMALLY INVASIVE TECHNIQUE MATERIALS AND METHODS

1009 patients were evaluated for chest wall deformity
548 patients had minimally invasive pectus repair
503 patients underwent primary operations
73 patients evaluated had prior pectus repairs
45 have had redo operations
    25 failed Ravitch procedures
    19 failed Nuss procedures*
    2 failed Leonard procedures†

Minimally Invasive Technique Operation and Length of Stay

Single pectus bar	85.3%	(429/503)
Double pectus bar	14.7%	(74/503)
No stabilizers	21%	(105/503)
Stabilizers	79%	(398/503)
Wired	81%	(322/398)
Not wired	19%	(76/398)
Median age (yr)	13.2	(2–29)
Median Haller CT Index	4.8	(2.4–21)
Epidural	3 days	(2–5)
Length of stay	5 days	(3–10)

*16 done elsewhere.
†One patient was both a prior Ravitch and a prior Leonard; counted once.

In addition, patients with ECG conduction abnormalities or mitral valve prolapse (MVP) had follow-up assessments. Patients old enough to have PFT studies were reassessed with repeated studies.

It has been noted that patients who are sedentary and who do not perform the pectus breathing exercises tend to have mild recurrence over the long term. We therefore strongly emphasize the importance of aerobic activities and deep-breathing exercises.

TABLE 19-4
EARLY POSTOP COMPLICATIONS

Deaths	0	
Cardiac perforations	0	
Pneumothorax (<20%)	296	(59%)
Chest tube	11	(2.2%)
Aspiration	3	(.6%)
Hemothorax	1	(.2%)
Pleural effusion requiring drainage	4	(.8%)
Pericarditis	6	(1.2%)
Wound/bar infection	4/2	(0.8%)/(0.4%)
Pneumonia	2	
Transient Horner's	155	
Late complications	61/503	(12.1%)
Bar displacement requiring revision	42/503	(8.3%)
Before stabilizer	16/105	(15.2%)
With stabilizer	26/398	(6.5%)
With wired stabilizer	14/322	(4.3%)
Hemothorax (post-traumatic)	2	(0.4%)
Bar allergy	3	(0.6%)
Overcorrection	27/503	(5.3%)
Skin erosion	1	(0.2%)

The initial cosmetic and functional results are excellent in 438 (87%) patients, good in 64 (13%) patients, and failed in 1 (0.2%) patient overall. The bars have been removed in 268 (53%) patients, with 33 (12.3%) patients more than 5 years after bar removal, 110 (41.0%) patients 1 to 5 years after bar removal, and 125 (47%) patients less than 1 year after bar removal. In the group whose bar had been out for less than 1 year, the results were excellent in 85.6%, good in 13%, and fair in 1.6%; and in the group whose bar had been removed more than 1 year ago, the results were excellent in 73.2%, good in 19%, fair in 2.8%, and failed in 5% (Fig. 19-8). The long-term results were affected by the length of time the bar was left in place (Fig. 19-9) and by the age of the patients at the time of surgery.

Bar Removal

We advise that the pectus bar be left in place for 2 to 4 years, with 3 years being the optimal time. We evaluate patients on an annual basis and monitor their growth, their activity level, their PFTs, and encourage them to do their pectus exercises and to participate in aerobic sports. Patients between ages 6 and 10 years often do not grow rapidly. Therefore they tolerate the bar well for 3 or even 4 years. Conversely, we have had teenagers who have had a massive growth spurt, growing 14 cm a year. They completely outgrow the bar and require bar removal after only 2 years. We consider the exercise programs to be just as important as the surgery. Many children and

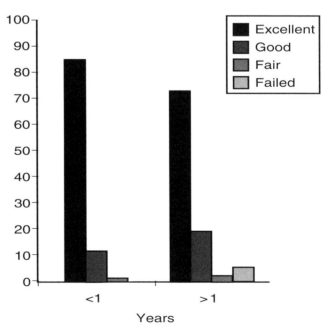

FIGURE 19-8. Our outcomes evaluated over time since bar removal.

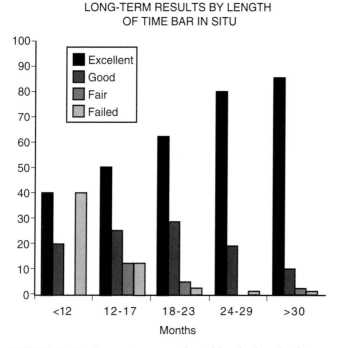

FIGURE 19-9. Our outcomes evaluated by the length of time the bar was left in situ.

adults lead sedentary lifestyles and never perform aerobic activities. Therefore their lungs never expand beyond the resting tidal volume, or approximately 10% of total lung capacity. Deep breathing with breath holding for 10 to 15 seconds and aerobic activities like running (e.g., soccer, basketball) and swimming are vigorously encouraged. We have seen mild recurrence over the long term in patients who do not follow our exercise protocol.

Pectus excavatum can be corrected with excellent long-term results without necessitating costal cartilage incision or resection, or sternal osteotomy. A significant number of patients have been safely and effectively managed at long-term follow-up. Pectus excavatum repair without cartilage resection is a simpler operation with tolerable morbidity. As a result, it has received rapid acceptance by the surgical community.

PECTUS CARINATUM

Pectus carinatum, or protrusion deformity of the chest, occurs less frequently than does pectus excavatum. It composes about 5% of patients with chest wall deformities.[48] The prominence may be in the upper manubrium of the sternum,[49] which is called a chondromanubrial deformity. The most common protrusion occurs in the lower or body of the sternum (the gladiolus) and is called chondrogladiolar. The protrusion may be unilateral, bilateral, or mixed.[50] About 80% of patients are boys. Although the etiology is unknown,[51] a genetic component of causation is suggested by the approximately one-fourth of patients with a family history of chest wall defect.[48]

Pectus carinatum has been reported to occur after treatment for pectus excavatum.[52]

The natural history of the condition differs from that of pectus excavatum. Pectus carinatum is usually noted in childhood, especially around the time of a growth spurt, rather than at birth, as generally happens with pectus excavatum. Symptoms are confined to tenderness at the site of the protrusion.[50,53] Associated mitral valve disease has been reported.[54,55] In patients without congenital heart disease, cardiopulmonary limitation due to the condition has not been reported. Other associations include Marfan syndrome and scoliosis (in 15%).[48]

Limited experience has been noted with orthotic bracing. Two reports have described correction or improvement in the condition by means of a brace analogous to that used for treatment of scoliosis, but exerting pressure in the anteroposterior direction.[53] Our group has had limited success with bracing.

Surgical treatment is by costochondral resection with sternotomy.[25,50,57,58] These studies emphasize the importance of performing a bilateral cartilage resection, even with unilateral deformity of the cartilages, to prevent recurrence.

Postoperative problems are uncommon, and recurrence is reported to be rare by centers with a large experience.

POLAND'S SYNDROME

Poland's syndrome affects 1 in 30,000 live births and is sporadic in occurrence.[59] It is a constellation of anomalies, apparent in a variety of ways. Clinical manifestations include the absence of the pectoralis major, pectoralis minor, serratus anterior, rectus abdominis, and latissimus dorsi muscles (Fig. 19-10). Athelia or amastia, nipple deformities, limb deformities (syndactyly, brachydactyly), absent axillary hair, and limited subcutaneous fat can occur.

In 1841, Alfred Poland, an English medical student, published a partial description of the deformity.[60]

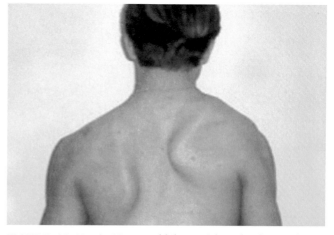

FIGURE 19-10. A 12-year-old boy with Poland's syndrome and absence of the serratus anterior muscles, leading to a winged scapula.

However, the syndrome was initially described in the French and German literature in 1826 and 1839.[61,62]

Poland's syndrome does not appear to be genetic, although rare family occurrences have been reported. The right side is more commonly affected and is present in boys 70% of the time.[63] One of six patients with breast hypoplasia/aplasia has Poland's syndrome. The etiology is unclear, but some theories include abnormal migration of the embryonic tissues forming the pectoralis muscles, hypoplasia of the subclavian artery, or in utero injury.

No correlation is found between the extent of hand deformities and chest wall deformities. Varying degrees of either can occur with mild hypoplasia to total aplasia of muscles, ribs, and cartilage. The latter can lead to major depressions and paradoxical respiratory motion.

Surgical repair is rarely required. Except in those patients with aplasia of the ribs or a major depression deformity,[64] chest wall reconstruction with correction of contralateral carinatum-type protrusions can usually be performed at the same time (Fig. 19-11). Autologous rib grafts, or a variety of bioprosthetic agents, can be used with or without a latissimus dorsi flap. The use of custom-made chest wall prostheses has been associated with significant problems such as migration, erosion of local tissues, and adverse cosmesis.[65] Chest wall reconstruction

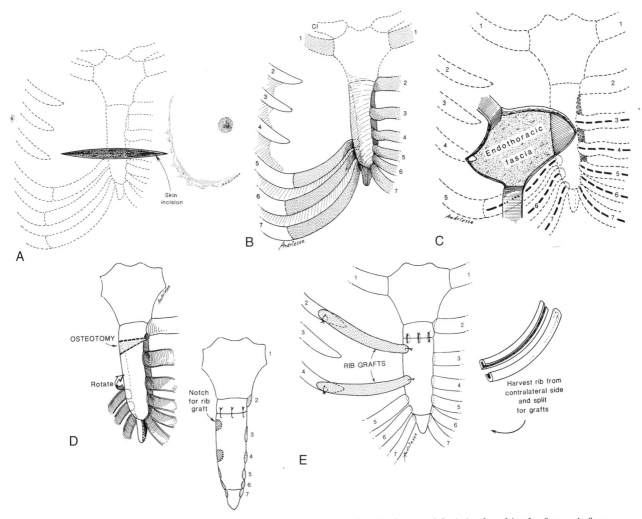

FIGURE 19-11. *A,* The transverse incision is placed below and within the nipples. In girls, it is placed in the future inframammary crease. *B,* A schematic depiction of the deformity with rotation of the sternum, depression of the cartilages of the involved side, and carinate protrusion of the contralateral side. *C,* In cases with aplasia of the ribs, the endothoracic fascia is encountered directly below the attenuated subcutaneous tissue and pectoral fascia. The pectoral muscle flap is elevated on the contralateral side, with the pectoral fascia, if present, on the involved side. Subperichondrial resection of the costal cartilages is carried out as shown (*dashed line*), preserving the costochondral junction. Rarely this resection must be carried to the level of the second costal cartilage. *D,* A transverse, offset, wedge-shaped sternal osteotomy is created below the second costal cartilage. Closure of this defect with heavy silk sutures or elevation of the sternum with a strut corrects both the posterior displacement and the rotation of the sternum. *E,* In cases with rib aplasia, rib grafts are harvested from the contralateral fifth or sixth ribs, split and secured medially with wire sutures into notches created in the sternum and with wire to the native ribs laterally. Ribs are split as shown, along their short axes, to maintain maximal mechanical strength. (From Shamberger RC, Welch KJ, Upton J III: Surgical treatment of thoracic deformity in Poland's syndrome. J Pediatr Surg 24:760–766, 1989.)

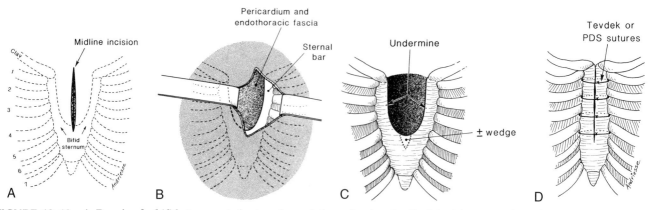

FIGURE 19-12. *A,* Repair of a bifid sternum is best performed through a longitudinal incision extending the length of the defect. These defects are characteristically cleft superiorly, as shown. *B,* Directly beneath the subcutaneous tissues, the sternal bars are encountered, with the origin of the pectoral muscles on the lateral aspect of the bars. The endothoracic fascia and pericardium are just below these structures. *C,* The endothoracic fascia is mobilized off the sternal bars posteriorly with blunt dissection to allow safe placement of the sutures. Approximation of the sternal bars may be facilitated by excising a wedge of cartilage inferiorly. Repair is best accomplished in the neonatal period because of the flexibility of the chest wall. *D,* Closure of the defect is achieved with 2-0 Tevdek or polydioxanone sutures. (From Shamberger RC, Welch KJ: Sternal defects. Pediatr Surg Int 5:156-164, 1990.)

should take place before breast reconstruction in a female with hypoplasia or aplasia of the breast.

STERNAL DEFECTS

Sternal defects are midline defects of the upper torso that range from the relatively benign sternal cleft (sternal defect without displacement of the heart) to the very rare and almost uniformly fatal thoracic ectopia cordis (the heart is out of the chest without a skin covering).

Cleft sternum (bifid sternum, partial ectopia cordis) is a rare malformation (0.15% of all chest wall malformations in some series) due to partial or total failure of sternal fusion at an early stage of embryonic development. Sternal clefts can be classified as either complete (the rarest form) or superior or inferior.[66] Superior clefts are either U-shaped (proximal to the fourth cartilage) or V-shaped (reaching the xiphoid process) and are most often isolated, with only minor associated lesions such as vascular dysplasias and superumbilical raphe.

The heart is in a normal position, and cardiac anomalies are rare. Surgical repair, which is very successful, is warranted once the diagnosis is made and can be done electively. Optimally it is done in the neonatal age when the sternal bars can be approximated easily because of flexibility and minimal compression of mediastinal structures (Fig. 19-12). After age 1 year, primary repair is difficult, and more intensive techniques may be needed such as use of autologous (costal cartilage, ribs) or prosthetic materials (Marlex mesh, Teflon).[67]

Thoracic ectopia cordis (true ectopia cordis) are lesions in which the heart has no overlying somatic structures. It is very rare and usually occurs with some form of an abdominal wall defect, with the heart sitting on the chest and the apex pointed toward the chin (Fig. 19-13). Intrinsic cardiac anomalies are frequent, especially tetralogy of Fallot, pulmonary artery stenosis, transposition of the great arteries, and ventricular septal defects.[68]

Survival is rare, and only three survivors have been reported. Very few survive because the return of the heart to the thorax is poorly tolerated. Most die because of torsion of the great vessels and compression of the heart on attempt to reduce it back in the chest. The goals of therapy are to cover the heart; preserve cardiac output by preventing kinking of the great vessels; repair the associated abdominal wall defect; and stabilize the thoracic cavity so that spontaneous ventilation can be effective.[69,70]

Thoracoabdominal ectopia cordis (Cantrell's pentalogy) involves lesions in which the heart is covered by an omphalocele-like membrane (Fig. 19-14). Intrinsic cardiac anomalies also are common in these patients, with tetralogy of Fallot and ventricular septal defects being the most common.[68] Cantrell's pentalogy consists of inferior sternal cleft, ectopia cordis, midline abdominal

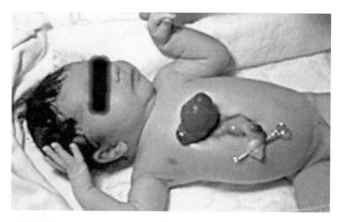

FIGURE 19-13. An infant with thoracic ectopia cordis with no significant abdominal wall defect present. The infant also demonstrates the characteristic high insertion of the umbilicus and anterior projection of the apex of the heart.

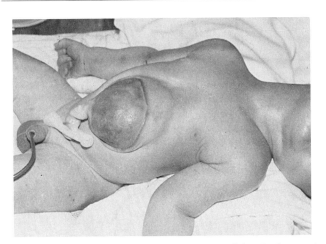

FIGURE 19-14. A newborn with thoracoabdominal ectopia cordis (Cantrell's pentalogy). Flaring of the lower thoracic cavity is present, with a large epigastric omphalocele. The transverse septum of the diaphragm and the inferior portion of the pericardium are absent. The patient also has tetralogy of Fallot.

wall defects or omphalocele, pericardial defects, and one or more cardiac defects. Repair is much more successful than that in thoracic ectopia cordis. Initial surgical management addresses the lack of skin overlying the heart and abdominal cavity. After initial stabilization and echocardiogram (ECHO), the goal of the initial operation is to provide coverage of the midline defects, separate the abdominal and pericardial compartments, and repair the diaphragm. Various techniques to gain closure include flap mobilization, skin closure only, and a variety of bioprosthetic agents. The congenital heart defect is repaired at a later date.

THORACIC INSUFFICIENCY SYNDROME ASSOCIATED WITH DIFFUSE SKELETAL DISORDERS

Thoracic insufficiency syndrome may be defined as any disorder that produces the inability of the thorax to support normal respiration or lung growth.[71] It includes a spectrum of disorders including asphyxiating thoracic

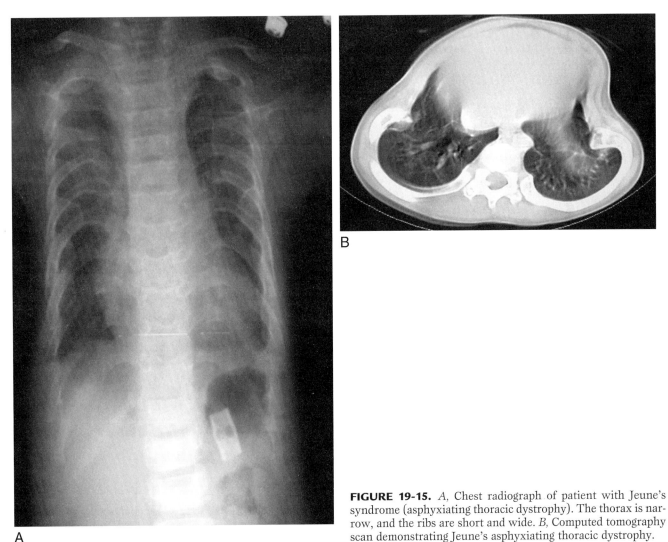

A

B

FIGURE 19-15. *A,* Chest radiograph of patient with Jeune's syndrome (asphyxiating thoracic dystrophy). The thorax is narrow, and the ribs are short and wide. *B,* Computed tomography scan demonstrating Jeune's asphyxiating thoracic dystrophy.

dystrophy (Jeune syndrome), acquired asphyxiating thoracic dystrophy (after open techniques for pectus repair), spondylothoracic dysplasia (Jarcho-Levin syndrome), congenital scoliosis with multiple vertebral anomalies with fused or absent ribs (jumbled spine), and severe kyphoscoliosis.

These disorders have been viewed and treated as separate entities, with little coordinated effort between specialties. They are best addressed with a unified approach integrating pediatric general and orthopedic surgeons as well as the pulmonologist.

Jeune's syndrome[72] is an autosomal recessive inherited osteochondrodystrophy with variable expressions. In mild forms, the chest may support adequate respiration. In more severe cases, the thorax is narrowed both transversely and in height, with short, wide horizontal ribs and irregular costochondral junctions (Fig. 19-15 *A, B*). This chest wall configuration produces a rigid chest with

very little intercostal excursion for normal respiration.[73] This leads to ventilatory dependence and death of respiratory failure.[74]

Pathologic examination varies, with some findings of pulmonary hypertension, but most cases have normal bronchial development with variable alveolar density.[75] This suggests that the extrinsic chest wall plays a significant role in the underlying hypoplasia.[76]

Other associated skeletal abnormalities in Jeune's syndrome include short stubby extremities, fixed elevated clavicles, hypoplastic iliac wings,[77,78] and a high incidence of C1 spinal stenosis.[79] These patients also have varying degrees of renal dysplasia.[80]

Spondylothoracic dysplasia (Jarcho-Levin) syndrome occurs in two forms with different inheritance patterns. Type I is an autosomal recessive deformity characterized by multiple vertebral hemivertebrae and posterior rib fusions.[81] This produces a marked shortening of the thoracic spine and a crab-like appearance of the chest on standard radiograph[82] (Fig. 19-16).

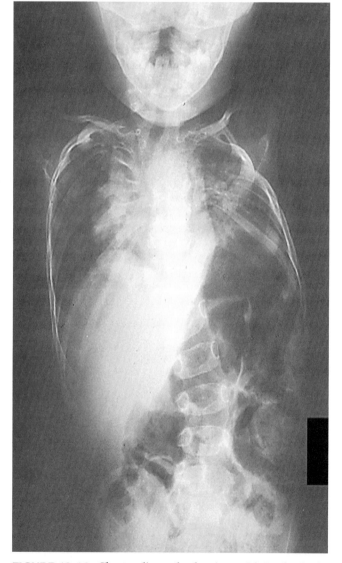

FIGURE 19-16. Chest radiograph of patient with Jarcho-Levin syndrome with markedly shortened thoracic spine producing crab-like appearance.

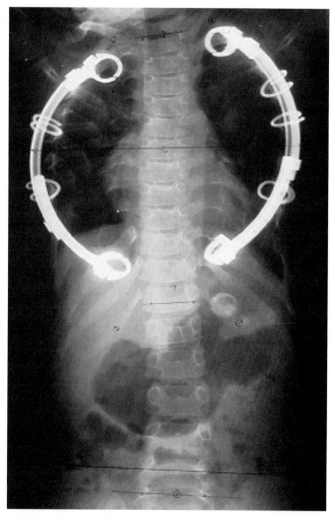

FIGURE 19-17. Bilateral vertical expandable prosthetic titanium rib (VEPTR) fixed with titanium rings to ribs of the patient from Fig. 19-15A with Jeune's asphyxiating thoracic dystrophy.

Associated malformations are noted in 30% and include cardiac and renal anomalies. The type I form is often fatal by age 15 months, and a high incidence of this disorder is reported in Puerto Rican families.[83] Type II spondylothoracic dysplasia has an autosomal dominant inheritance pattern and is associated with near-normal longevity. It is seen mostly in white children.[83]

Thoracic insufficiency also may arise secondary to too early or too extensive pectus operations.[18] Complex spine anomalies producing the so-called "jumbled spine"; unilateral thoracic hypoplasia seen with the VACTERL association (**V** [vertebral anomalies], **A** [anal atresia], **C** [cardiac anamolies], **TE** [tracheoesophageal fistula or esophageal atresia], **R** [renal or urinary anomolies], and **L** [limb defect]), and kyphoscoliosis also may be a cause for thoracic insufficiency.[84–88]

Surgical techniques to correct the spectrum of these complex disorders have attempted to address the issue of thoracic volume by various approaches. In both congenital (Jeune's) and acquired (postpectus) thoracic dystrophy, one approach has been an anterior longitudinal sternal split with widening of the sternum.

This has been done with methylmethacrylate, bone grafts or rib, and metal plates.[89–91] A staged approach with a methylmethacrylate plate followed by secondary removal of the plate and latissimus dorsi flaps to cover the created sternal cleft also has been described.[92] Sternal elevation also has been done in cases of acquired thoracic dystrophy by both open technique[18] and the minimally invasive technique used for standard pectus repair.[37] A lateral staged approach with staggered rib osteotomies, staggered division of the chest wall, intercostal muscles, and pleura, with transposition of alternating ribs by using metal plate fixation also has been described.[93]

These approaches have had variable results because they are not easily revised to allow continued growth of the chest wall to allow lung expansion. The lateral thoracic expansion may also interfere with intercostal muscle function after division of multiple intercostal muscles and nerves.

In regard to patients with Jarcho-Levin syndrome, jumbled spine, and kyphosis, pediatric general surgeons have done little to approach these problems that they considered either lethal or solely in the domain of the orthopedic surgeon.

A promising technique to address patients with the spectrum of causes for thoracic insufficiency syndrome rejoins the discipline of pediatric general, thoracic, and orthopedic surgery. Expansion thoracoplasty and use of a vertical expandable prosthetic titanium rib (VEPTR) developed by Campbell (pediatric orthopedic surgeon) and Smith (pediatric surgeon) address many problems in the spectrum of these disorders. This technique allows serial expansion of the chest wall to allow continued growth of the thorax and spine until skeletal maturity is achieved.[94]

More than 300 patients with various disorders have been treated with this technique. In Jeune's asphyxiating thoracic dystrophy, 14 patients have undergone staged bilateral expansions. Anterior rib osteotomies adjacent to the costochondral junction and posterior osteotomies adjacent to the transverse process of the spine in ribs

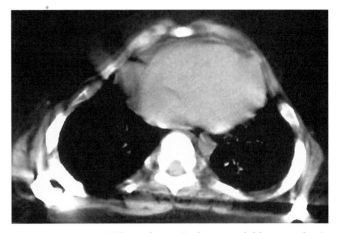

FIGURE 19-18. Bilateral vertical expandable prosthetic titanium rib in patient from Fig. 19-17 with Jarcho-Levin syndrome.

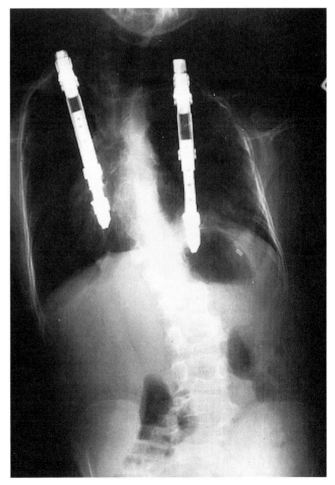

FIGURE 19-19. Postoperative computed tomography scan of patient from Fig. 19-15*B* after vertical expandable prosthetic titanium rib, demonstrating expansion of thorax.

3 to 9 are performed, creating a mobilized segment of chest wall that is distracted posterolaterally and anchored to a curved VEPTR that is attached to the second and tenth ribs (Fig. 19-17). The segment is anchored to the VEPTR with 2-mm titanium rings stabilizing the segment and allowing reossification of the multiple osteotomies (Fig. 19-18). The second stage is done 3 months later, and then the devices are expanded every 6 months.

In patients with fused or absent ribs and scoliosis, a wedge thoracostomy through the fused segment of ribs not only allows expansion of the chest, but also will correct the scoliosis and the rotational spinal deformity (producing a windswept thorax).[88] It also stimulates increased spinal height in both congenital scoliosis and Jarcho-Levin syndrome, in which bilateral devices are placed (Fig. 19-19).

REFERENCES

1. Ebstein E: Die Trichterbrust in ihren Beziehungen zur Konstitution. Z Konstitutionslehre 8:103, 1921.
2. Bauhinus J: Observationum Medicariam. Liber II, Observ. 264, Francfurti 1600, p 507.
3. Coulson W: Deformities of the chest. London Med Gaz 4:69–73, 1820.
4. Williams CT: Congenital malformation of the thorax: Great depression of the sternum. Trans Pathol Soc London 24:50, 1872.
5. Ebstein W: Ueber die Trichterbrust. Deutsches Arch 30: 411, 1882.
6. Meade RH: A History of Thoracic Surgery. Springfield, Ill, Thomas, 1961.
7. Sauerbruch F: Die Chirurgie der Brustorgane. Vol 1:437, Berlin, Springer, 1920.
8. Meyer L: Zurchirurqishen Behandlung der augeborenen Trichterbrust. Verh Bel Med Gest 42:364, 1911.
9. Sauerbruch F: Operative Beseitigung der Angeborenen Trichterbrust. Deutsche Z Chir 234:760, 1931.
10. Ochsner A, DeBakey M: Chone-Chondrosternon. J Thorac Surg 8:469–511, 1939.
11. Brown AL: Pectus excavatum. J Thorac Surg 9:164–184, 1939.
12. Ravitch MM: The operative treatment of pectus excavatum. Ann Surg 129:429–444, 1949.
13. Wallgren GR, Sulamaa M: Surgical treatment of funnel chest. Exhib. VIII, presented at the International Congress of Paediatrics, 1956, p 32.
14. Paltia V, Parkkulainen KV, Sulamaa M, et al: Operative technique in funnel chest. Acta Chir Scand 116:90–98, 1958/1959.
15. Adkins PC, Blades BA: Stainless steel strut for correction of pectus excavatum. Surg Gynecol Obstet 113:111–113, 1961.
16. Welch KJ: Satisfactory surgical correction of pectus excavatum deformity in childhood. J Thorac Surg 36:697–713, 1958.
17. Martinez D, Juame J, Stein T, et al: The effect of costal cartilage resection on chest wall development. Pediatr Surg Int 5:170–173, 1990.
18. Haller JA, Colombani PM, Humphries CT, et al: Chest wall constriction after too extensive and too early operations for pectus excavatum. Ann Thorac Surg 61:1618–1625, 1996.
19. Nuss D, Kelly RE Jr, et al: A 10-year review of a minimally invasive technique for the correction of pectus excavatum. J Pediatr Surg 33:545–552, 1998.
20. Nuss D, Kelly RE Jr, et al: Repair of pectus excavatum. Pediatr Endosurg Innovat Techniq 2:205–221, 1998.
21. Kelley SW: Surgical Diseases of Children: Dislocations, Congenital and Acquired. Vol 1, 3rd ed. St. Louis, Mo; CV Mosby, 1929, p 537.
22. Haller JA Jr: Thoracic injuries. In Welch KJ, Randolph JG, Ravitch MM, et al (eds): Pediatric Surgery, Vol 1, 4th ed. Chicago, Year Book Medical Publishers, 1986, p 147.
23. Wesson DE: Thoracic injuries. In O'Neill JA Jr, Rowe MI, Grosfeld JL, et al (eds): Pediatric Surgery, Vol 1, 5th ed. St. Louis, Mo, Mosby Grosfeld, 1998, p 245.
24. Martinez-Feno M: Personal communication.
25. Shamberger RC: Congenital chest wall deformities. In Pediatric Surgery, 5th ed. Philadelphia, Elsevier, 1998, pp 787–817.
26. Lawson ML, Cash TF, Akers RA, et al: A pilot study of the impact of surgical repair on disease-specific quality of life among patients with pectus excavatum. J Pediatr Surg 38:916–918, 2003.
27. Shamberger RC: Cardiopulmonary effects of anterior chest wall deformities. Chest Surg Clin North Am 10:245–251, 2000.
28. Zhao L, Fenberg MS, et al: Why is exercise capacity reduced in subjects with pectus excavatum? J Pediatr 136:163–167, 2000.
29. Mocchegiani R, Badano L, et al: Relation of right ventricular morphology and function in pectus excavatum to the severity of the chest wall deformity. Am J Cardiol 76:941–946, 1995.
30. Haller JA Jr, Peters GN, Mazur D, et al: Pectus excavatum: A 20-year surgical experience. J Thorac Cardiovasc Surg 60:375–383, 1970.
31. Shamberger RC, Welch KJ, Sanders SP: Mitral valve prolapse associated with pectus excavatum. J Pediatr 111:404–407, 1987.
32. Saint-Mezard G, Duret JC, Chanudet X, et al: Mitral valve prolapse and pectus excavatum. Presse Med 15:439, 1986.
33. Warth DC, King ME, Cohen JM, et al: Prevalence of mitral valve prolapse in normal children. J Am Coll Cardiol 5:1173–1177, 1985.
34. Park JM, Farmer AR: Wolff-Parkinson-White syndrome in children with pectus excavatum. J Pediatr 112:926–928, 1988.
35. Haller JA Jr, Loughlin GM: Cardiorespiratory function is significantly improved following corrective surgery for severe pectus excavatum. J Cardiovasc Surg 41:125–130, 2000.
36. Haller JA Jr, Kramer SS, Lietman SA: Use of CT scans in selection of patients for pectus excavatum surgery: A preliminary report. J Pediatr Surg 22:904–908, 1987.
37. Croitoru DP, Kelly RE Jr, Nuss D, et al: Experience and modification update for the minimally invasive Nuss technique for pectus excavatum repair in 303 patients. J Pediatr Surg 37:437–445, 2002.
38. Coln D, Gunning T, Ramsay M, et al: Early experience with the Nuss minimally invasive correction of pectus excavatum in adults. World J Surg 26:1217–1221, 2002.
39. Columbani, P: Personal communication.
40. Park HJ, Lee SY, Lee CS, et al: The Nuss procedure for pectus excavatum: An evolution of techniques and results on 322 patients. Presented at the 39th annual meeting of the Society of Thoracic Surgeons, San Diego, Calif, January 31 to February 2, 2003.
41. Azizkhan RG: What's new in pediatric surgery? J Am Coll Surg 186:203–211, 1998.
42. Adzick NS, Nance ML: Pediatric surgery. N Engl J Med 342:1651–1657, 2000.
43. Hebra A, Swoveland B, Egbert M, et al: Outcome analysis of minimally invasive repair of pectus excavatum: Review of 251 cases. J Pediatr Surg 35:252–258, 2000.
44. Miller KA, Woods RK, Sharp RJ, et al: Minimally invasive repair of pectus excavatum: A single institution's experience. Surgery 130:652–659, 2001.
45. Molik KA, Engum SA, Rescoda FJ, et al: Pectus excavatum repair: Experience with standard and minimally invasive techniques. J Pediatr Surg 36:324–328, 2001.
46. Wu PC, Knauer EM, McGowan GE, et al: Repair of pectus excavatum deformities in children: A new perspective of treatment using minimal access surgical technique. Arch Surg 136:419–424, 2001.
47. Hosie S, Sitkiewicz T, Peterson C, et al: Minimally invasive repair of pectus excavatum: The Nuss procedure: A European Multicenter Experience. Eur J Pediatr Surg 12:235–238, 2002.
48. Shamberger RC, Welch KJ: Surgical correction of pectus carinatum. J Pediatr Surg 22:48–53, 1987.
49. Chin EF: Surgery of funnel chest and congenital sternal prominence. Br J Surg 44:360–376, 1957.
50. Robisek F, Cook JW, Daugherty HK, et al: Pectus carinatum. J Thorac Cardiovasc Surg 78:52–61, 1979.
51. Pena A, Perez L, Nurka S, et al: Pectus carinatum and pectus excavatum: Are they the same disease? Am Surg 47:215–218, 1981.
52. Hebra A, Thomas PB, Tagge EP, et al: Pectus carinatum as a sequela of minimally invasive pectus excavatum repair. Pediatr Endosurg Innovat Techn 6:41–44, 2002.
53. Haje SA, Bowen JR: Preliminary results of orthotic treatment of pectus deformities in children and adolescents. J Pediatr Orthop 12:795–800, 1992.

54. Currarino G, Silverman FN: Premature obliteration of the sternal sutures and pigeon-breast deformity. Radiology 70:532–540, 1958.
55. Shamberger RC, Welch KJ: Surgical correction of pectus excavatum. J Pediatr Surg 23:615–622, 1988.
56. Chidambaram B, Mehta AV: Currarino-Silverman syndrome (pectus carinatum type 2 deformity) and mitral valve disease. Chest 102:780–782, 1992.
57. Ravitch MM: The operative correction of pectus carinatum (pigeon breast). Ann Surg 151:705–714, 1960.
58. Welch KJ, Vos A: Surgical correction of pectus carinatum (pigeon breast). J Pediatr Surg 8:659–667, 1973.
59. Amato U, Zelen J, Talwalker NG: Single-stage repair of thoracic ectopia cordis. Ann Thorac Surg 59:518–520, 1995.
60. Freire-Maia N, Chautard EA, Opitz JM: The Poland syndrome: Clinical and genealogical data, dermatoglyphic analysis, and incidence. Hum Hered 23:97–104, 1973.
61. Froriep R: Beobachtung eines Falles Von Mangel der Brustdrauuse. 10:9–14, 1839.
62. Golladay ES: Pectus carinatum and other deformities of the chest wall. In Zeigler MM, Azizkhan RG, Weber TR (eds): Operative Pediatric Surgery. New York, McGraw-Hill, 2003, pp 269–278.
63. Groner JI: Ectopia cordis and sternal defrects. In Zeigler MM, Azizkhan RG, Weber TR (eds): Operative Pediatric Surgery. New York, McGraw-Hill, 2003, pp 279–293.
64. Knox L, Tuggle D, Knott-Craig CJ: Repair of congenital sternal clefts in adolescence and infancy. J Pediatr Surg 29:1513–1516, 1994.
65. Lallemand LM: Ephermerides Medicales de Montpellier. 1:144–147, 1826.
66. Poland A: Deficiency of the pectoralis muscles. Guys Hosp Rep 6:191–193, 1841.
67. Samarrai AR, Charmockley HA, Attr AA: Complete cleft sternum: Classification and surgical repair. Int Surg 70:71–73, 1985.
68. Seyfer AE, Icochea R, Graber GM: Poland's anomaly: Natural history and long-term results of chest wall reconstruction in 33 patients. Ann Surg 208:776–782, 1988.
69. Shamberger RC, Welch KJ, Upton J III: Surgical treatment of thoracic deformity in Poland's syndrome. J Pediatr Surg 24:760–765, 1989.
70. Shamberger RC, Welch KJ: Sternal defects. Pediatr Surg Int 5:156–164, 1990.
71. Campbell RM, Smith M: Treatment of thoracic insufficiency syndrome associated with congenital scoliosis. J Bone Joint Surg Br 79:82, 1997.
72. Jeune M, Carron R, Beraud C, et al: Polychondrodystrophie avec blocage thoracique d'evolution fatale. Pediatriq :390–392, 1954.
73. Borland LM: Anesthesia for children with Jeune's syndrome (asphyxiating thoracic dystrophy). Anesthesiology 66:86–88, 1987.
74. Tahernia AC, Stamps P: Jeune's syndrome (asphyxiating thoracic dystrophy). Chin Pediatr 16:903–907, 1977.
75. Williams AJ, Vawter G, Reid LM: Lung structure in asphyxiating thoracic dystrophy. Arch Pathol Lab Med 108:658–661, 1984.
76. Finegold J, Katzew H, Genieser NB, et al: Lung structure in thoracic dystrophy. Am J Dis Child 122:153–159, 1971.
77. Langer LO: Thoracic pelvic phalangeal dystrophy: Asphyxiating thoracic dystrophy of the newborn, infantile thoracic dystrophy. Radiology 91:447–456, 1968.
78. Oberklaid F, Danks DM, Mayne V, et al: Asphyxiating thoracic dysplasia. Arch Dis Child 52:758–765, 1977.
79. Campbell RM: The incidence of proximal cervical spine stenosis in Jeune's asphyxiating dystrophy. Paper presented at the Scoliosis Research Society, 2001.
80. Herdman RC, Langer LO: The thoracic asphyxiant dystrophy and renal disease. Am J Dis Child 52:192–201, 1977.
81. Jarcho S, Levin PM: Hereditary malformations of the vertebral bodies. Bull Johns Hopkins Hosp 62:216–226, 1938.
82. Roberts AP, Conner AN, Tolmie JL, et al: Spondylothoracic and spondylocostal dysostosis: Hereditary forms of spinal deformity. J Bone Joint Surg Br 70:123–126, 1988.
83. Heilbronner DM, Renshaw TS: Spondylothoracic dysplasia. J Bone Joint Surg Am 66:302–303, 1984.
84. McMaster MJ: Congenital scoliosis. In Weinstein SL (ed): The Pediatric Spine: Principles and Practice. New York, Raven Press, 1994.
85. McMaster MJ: Congenital scoliosis caused by unilateral failure of vertebral segmentation with contralateral hemivertebrae. Spine 23:998–1005, 1998.
86. McMaster MJ, David C: Hemivertebrae as a cause of scoliosis: A study of 104 patients. J Bone Joint Surg Br 68:588–595, 1986.
87. Campbell RM: Congenital scoliosis due to multiple vertebrae anomalies associated with thoracic insufficiency syndrome. Spine 14:209–218, 2000.
88. Campbell RM, Smith MD, Mayes T, et al: The characteristics of thoracic insufficiency syndrome associated with fused ribs and congenital scoliosis. J Bone Joint Surg 85:399–408, 2003.
89. Todd DW, Tinguely ST, Norberg WJ: A thoracic expansion technique for Jeune's asphyxiating thoracic dystrophy. J Pediatr Surg 21:161–163, 1986.
90. Barnes ND, Hall D, Milner AD, et al: Chest reconstruction in asphyxiating thoracic dystrophy. Arch Dis Child 46:833–837, 1971.
91. Weber TR, Kurkchubasche AG: Operative management of asphyxiating thoracic dystrophy after pectus repair. J Pediatr Surg 33:262–265, 1998.
92. Sharoni E, Erez E, Chorer G, et al: Chest reconstruction in asphyxiating thoracic dystrophy. J Pediatr Surg 33:1578–1581, 1998.
93. Davis JT, Heistein JB, Castile RG, et al: Lateral thoracic expansion for Jeune's syndrome: Mid-term results. Ann Thorac Surg 72:872–878, 2001.
94. Campbell RM, Hell-Vocke AK: Growth of the thoracic spine in congenital scoliosis after expansion thoracoplasty. J Bone Joint Surg Am 85:409–419, 2003.

CHAPTER 20

Tracheal Obstruction and Repair

H. Biemann Othersen, Jr., MD, William T. Adamson, MD, and Edward P. Tagge, MD

INTRODUCTION

The pediatric surgeon is often involved in the management of acute or chronic airway obstruction. More often than not, the obstruction is located in the subglottic airway, and unfortunately, many of the obstructing lesions are either of iatrogenic etiology or are congenital defects amplified by inappropriate medical care. These obstructive lesions are, by implication, largely preventable, yet iatrogenic injury of the pediatric airway is so common that anyone who inserts an endotracheal tube or who cares for any intubated child must know how to prevent iatrogenic laryngeal and tracheal injury and subsequent airway stenosis.[1,2] Even if the reader does not perform airway reconstructive procedures or airway endoscopy, he or she should be conversant with the sections of this chapter dealing with *injuries* and *endotracheal intubation*. A trachea, and a life, may be saved if these admonitions are observed.

This chapter addresses primarily the recognition of airway problems and prevention of permanent injury to the child's trachea. General principles and initial therapy are stressed. Some of the open tracheoplasties are briefly presented, but details of the myriad procedures for reconstruction of the pediatric airway are not within the scope of this chapter. The large number of operative techniques for the treatment of tracheal stenosis suggests that no single procedure or technique is universally applicable and successful. Prevention of, or prompt therapy for, injury is all important.

PRACTICAL EMBRYOLOGY AND ANATOMY

Some knowledge of the embryonic development of mediastinal structures aids in understanding the etiology of both congenital and acquired laryngeal and tracheal obstruction. With our present knowledge of the subject, embryology does not improve the clinical care of patients with congenital tracheal anomalies. Associated anomalies must be considered when a narrowed airway is discovered

to be caused by complete tracheal rings. Malformations of the great vessels (vascular rings) should be suspected and investigated when evaluating a child with complete tracheal rings, the most common of which is a pulmonary vascular sling. Pulmonary vascular sling occurs when the left pulmonary artery passes to the right of the trachea just above the carina and then passes between the trachea and esophagus before reaching the left lung[3] (Fig. 20-1). Other vascular ring malformations may produce varying degrees of tracheal, bronchial, and esophageal compression. The developmental defects leading to laryngeal webs, laryngomalacia, and vocal cord paralysis are not covered in this chapter.

TRACHEAL MALFORMATIONS

Congenital Subglottic Stenosis

The most common gross morphologic abnormality, congenital subglottic stenosis, is a narrowing of the airway at the distal end of the larynx, just at the beginning of the trachea. This subglottic region lies at the junction of the cricoid cartilage and trachea and is the narrowest point of the child's airway. The cricoid cartilage is the only normally complete cartilaginous ring in the airway. In young children, the anatomy of the trachea and larynx differs from that of the adult as follows: (1) the child's epiglottis is short and small, and the valleculae are very shallow; (2) the larynx points posteriorly toward the nasopharynx, and the arytenoid apparatus is large in relation to the lumen of the larynx; (3) the narrowest point of the normal pediatric airway is the cricotracheal junction, whereas in the adult, it is the glottis (Fig. 20-2). The anatomy of the pediatric airway has been compared with an inverted cone, in which the trachea fits telescopically into the cricoid above it; the cricoid into the thyroid cartilage; and then the thyroid into the hyoid space, as illustrated in Figure 20-3.[4] Congenital abnormalities of this subglottic area consist of narrowing or malformation of the cricoid cartilage, the nature of which is not truly known. Cricoid stenosis is exceeded only by

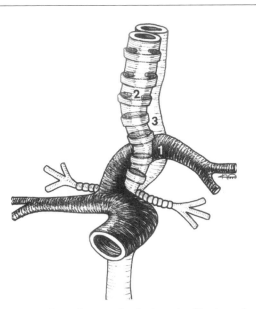

FIGURE 20-1. Complete tracheal rings in distal trachea and pulmonary vascular sling. 1, Left pulmonary artery. 2, trachea. 3, esophagus.

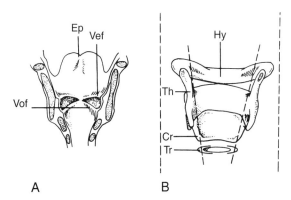

A   B

FIGURE 20-3. *A,* Ventral area of the larynx in the neonate viewed from behind. The ventricle, or "third cavity," is bounded above by the ventricular folds (Vef) and below by the vocal folds (Vof). Ep, epiglottis. *B,* Laryngeal cartilages (without arytenoids). Th, thyroid; Cr, cricoid; Tr, trachea; and Hy, hyoid viewed from behind. *Inner dotted line* shows telescopic configuration in the neonate as opposed to the rectangular shape in the adult (*outer dotted line*). (From Othersen HB, Jr. [ed.]: The Pediatric Airway. Philadelphia, WB Saunders, 1991.)

laryngomalacia and vocal cord paralysis in frequency of congenital airway anomalies.

Acquired Subglottic and Tracheal Stenosis

Acquired airway malformations usually result from intrinsic injury with subsequent inflammation, ulceration, and scarring, leading to severe subglottic or tracheal stenosis. Occasionally external trauma will produce the injury,[2] but an iatrogenic component can create a really difficult situation. For example, a child with a congenitally small airway might be asymptomatic until an endotracheal tube is inserted. The tube may be of an appropriate size but, because of the congenital stenosis, will fit tightly and can

lead to ulceration and stricture. Particularly difficult to treat are those injuries that occur well below the subglottic region, usually produced by an endotracheal balloon that has caused compression and ulceration in the trachea. Frequently these areas of injury are below the usual site for a tracheostomy. The cuff may even erode into overlying vessels (Fig 20-4).

VASCULAR COMPRESSIONS

Compression and partial obstruction of the trachea may be caused by abnormalities of the aortic arch that impinge on or encircle the trachea or esophagus or both.[5,6] When both trachea and esophagus are encircled and constricted, swallowing frequently produces acute airway compression and respiratory distress.

Vascular rings are often asymptomatic in babies and infants and yet lead to significant airway obstruction

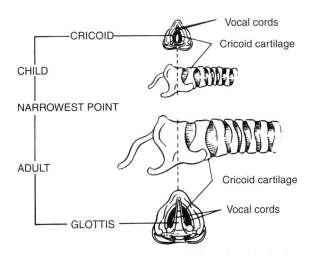

FIGURE 20-2. Difference between adult and pediatric airway. (Reprinted from Othersen HB, Jr: Intubation injuries of the trachea in children: Management and prevention. Ann Surg 189:601–606, 1979.)

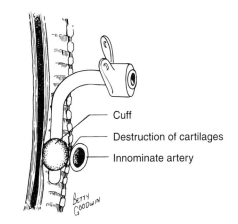

FIGURE 20-4. An inflated cuff of a tracheostomy tube may erode anteriorly into the innominate artery. (From Othersen HB, Jr. [ed.]: The Pediatric Airway. Philadelphia, WB Saunders, 1991.)

in a child. Various deviations of embryonic development of the aortic arch can lead to vascular rings, which may or may not appear with airway-compression symptoms.[7]

The physiologic impingement on the trachea by a vascular ring is similar to that seen frequently in patients after repair of esophageal atresia. The persistently distended upper esophageal pouch can displace the trachea anteriorly, producing tracheomalacia or softened tracheal rings (Fig. 20-5). Particularly with swallowing, the distended esophageal pouch may collapse the trachea against the innominate artery (Figs. 20-6 and 20-7). This sequence of events is thought responsible for reflex apnea. Consequently, surgical correction of this problem consists of anterior mobilization and suspension of the innominate artery[8-11] (Fig. 20-8). The treatment of pulmonary vascular sling usually requires not only relocation and reimplantation of the pulmonary artery but also tracheal repair for the stenotic distal trachea.[7,12,13]

Stridor and dyspnea are symptoms that may be produced by vascular impingement on the trachea. Patients with severe compression by a double aortic arch are usually symptomatic, but their manifestations are variable (Fig. 20-9). Some patients are first seen with frequent coughing and stridor accompanied by dyspnea and cyanosis, whereas small infants may have reflex apnea. The symptoms of vascular impingement on the trachea are usually more dramatic than those of compression of the esophagus. The diagnosis of vascular ring anomalies has classically been made or suspected by barium esophagram with observation of indentations on the esophageal column of barium and a decrease in the tracheal air column. Offset of the axis of the barium column above and below the indentation is diagnostic of a double aortic arch.

Occasionally a child will appear with acute airway obstruction or other medical problems requiring intensive care, during which endotracheal intubation and a concomitant nasogastric tube are inserted. The presence of tubes in both airway and esophagus makes detection of a vascular ring difficult and also can generate complications. However, in a child who is already intubated, performance of contrast radiographic procedures may not be possible.

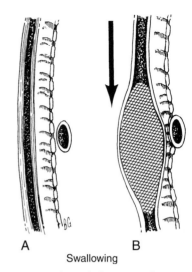

FIGURE 20-6. An enlarged diagram of Fig. 20-7 illustrates how the compression is increased by ingestion of a feeding. (From Othersen HB, Jr. [ed.]: The Pediatric Airway. Philadelphia, WB Saunders, 1991.)

Ultrasonography (US) or computed tomography (CT) scan and magnetic resonance imaging (MRI), with contrast, may delineate the vascular abnormality. When both tracheal and esophageal intubation are necessary in a patient with double aortic arch, the encircling vessels may sustain pressure necrosis. Erosion into the aortic arch produces an acute aortoesophageal fistula, which may not be manifest until either the endotracheal or the esophageal tube is removed. A sentinel bleed may occur before massive, and often fatal, hemorrhage into the esophagus. The passage of a Sengstaken-Blakemore tube with inflation of the esophageal balloon can be lifesaving by tamponade of the fistula.[14] Because no reliable diagnostic study is available to demonstrate an aortoesophageal fistula, the observation of a sentinel bleed in such a patient with US confirmation of double aortic arch is a clear indication for cardiopulmonary bypass and open repair.[14]

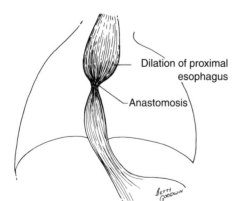

FIGURE 20-5. After repair of esophageal atresia, the proximal esophagus, which is already enlarged, is further dilated by anastomotic stricture. (From Othersen HB, Jr. [ed.]: The Pediatric Airway. Philadelphia, WB Saunders, 1991.)

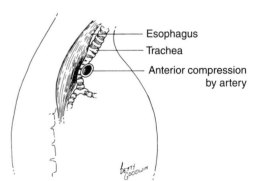

FIGURE 20-7. A lateral view shows how the dilated proximal esophagus displaces the trachea and compresses it against the overlying innominate artery. (From Othersen HB, Jr. [ed.]: The Pediatric Airway. Philadelphia, WB Saunders, 1991.)

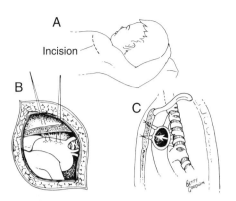

FIGURE 20-8. The operative technique for aortopexy. *A,* Anterior left thoracotomy in the third interspace. *B,* Sutures placed into the wall of the innominate artery and the aortic arch. *C,* Sutures passed through the sternum and tied to elevate the compressing vessels. Tracheal attachments pull the anterior wall of the trachea forward. (From Othersen HB, Jr. [ed.]: The Pediatric Airway. Philadelphia, WB Saunders, 1991.)

Operative correction of a vascular ring consists of division of the ring and suspension of the compressing vessel. It must be emphasized that vascular compression produces primarily airway problems rather than vascular problems. Simple division of the vascular ring is often enough to relieve tracheal compression. A vessel that continues to compress the airway must not be dissected away from the trachea but suspended anteriorly to the back of the sternum so that the vascular-tracheal attachment will lift the anterior trachea, thereby enlarging the tracheal lumen. Flexible endoscopic observation of the trachea during these maneuvers can corroborate relief of the compression[5] (see Fig. 20-8).

INFLAMMATORY OBSTRUCTIONS

Viral laryngotracheitis (croup), bacterial or membranous tracheitis, and epiglottitis are inflammatory conditions that may require surgical intervention. The acute inflammatory airway process may progress rapidly to life-threatening obstruction and require emergency tracheostomy. However, in all cases of inflammatory obstruction, endotracheal intubation before tracheostomy is advisable, if at all possible. Croup and bacterial tracheitis should be distinguished from epiglottitis, because treatment is so different. Children with epiglottitis characteristically tolerate endotracheal intubation without airway injury because the inflammation and edema are supraglottic and not circumferential. They do, however, present more risks of intubation failure because of the severe edema of the epiglottis. Some hospitals have strict protocols requiring diagnostic laryngoscopy in the operating room, with anesthesia standby, for suspected cases of epiglottitis in case an emergency tracheostomy is necessary. Conversely, when the inflammatory process, as with viral or bacterial laryngotracheitis, involves the entire circumference of the airway, prolonged intubation may lead to permanent scarring.[1,15] Thus it is crucial to differentiate these processes (Table 20-1).

Croup characteristically occurs during viral seasons in children age 3 months to 3 years. Children in whom the classic "croupy" cough develops frequently have a history of an antecedent respiratory infection, usually with high fever.[16]

Bacterial tracheitis, a nonviral infectious disease, is seen with high fever and rapid development of upper airway obstruction, characterized by copious mucopurulent secretions.

Epiglottitis typically affects children who are age 2 to 6 years and who have sore throat and dysphagia. Consequently, speech may be slurred, and drooling of saliva is prominent. Lateral roentgenograms of the neck may show an edematous epiglottis.[17]

Fortunately, most of these inflammatory processes are controlled with antibiotics and respiratory care without surgical intervention. Treatment includes oxygen with increased humidification and inhalation of racemic epinephrine. Endotracheal intubation is well tolerated in epiglottitis and usually causes no further injury, while antibiotic therapy produces resolution of the epiglottic edema. However, in cases of viral or bacterial tracheitis, intubation, often only 24 to 48 hours in duration, may cause ulceration in a trachea that is already acutely inflamed and swollen. Therefore endotracheal intubation may best be used only to establish a definitive diagnosis, to be followed by a temporary tracheostomy.

A recent review of inflammatory disorders of the airway confirms these statements.[18] The same authors pointed out that the decreasing incidence of epiglottitis is probably due to the increasing use of immunization against *Haemophilus influenzae* type B, the most common causative organism. Other infectious organisms, however, may produce the typical epiglottic swelling. Intubation is usually not necessary for more than 24 to 48 hours until antibiotics can control the infection. Croup also is now more easily treated without intubation with racemic epinephrine inhalation combined with administration of dexamethasone 0.6 mg/kg, either orally, intramuscularly or intravenously.

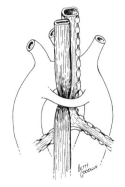

FIGURE 20-9. Both trachea and esophagus are compressed by vascular rings. (From Othersen HB, Jr. [ed.]: The Pediatric Airway. Philadelphia, WB Saunders, 1991.)

TABLE 20-1

CHARACTERISTICS OF LARYNGOTRACHEOBRONCHITIS AND EPIGLOTTITIS

Characteristic	Layngotracheobronchitis	Epiglottitis
Incidence	Common	Uncommon
Etiology	Viral	*Haemophilus influenzae* type B
Age	6 months to 3 years	2–6 years
Clinical picture	Gradual onset; preceding upper respiratory infection, barking cough	Rapid onset; fever; drooling; dysphagia
Physical examination	Respiratory distress, inspiratory stridor, low-grade temperature	Anxious; muffled voice, chin forward, drooling, high temperature
Laboratory	WBC usually <10,000/mm with lymphocytosis; x-ray shows narrowing of subglottic region	WBC often >10,000/mm with band cells increased; x-ray shows swollen epiglottis

Adapted from McLain LG: Croup syndrome. Am Fam Physican 36(4):213, 1987.

Regardless of the cause of the inflammatory process, rapid obstruction of the airway can occur in a small child. The surgeon must be prepared to work with anesthesiologist and pediatrician to establish an airway by endotracheal intubation, bronchoscopy, or tracheostomy.

INJURIES

Intrinsic

Most intrinsic laryngotracheal injuries are iatrogenic and produced by inappropriate introduction of an endotracheal tube or instrumentation of the airway. Endotracheal intubation is covered in the following section. Benign laryngeal tumors, such as subglottic hemangioma and lymphangioma, require repeated endoscopic treatments that can be injurious to the larynx. It is wise to consider a preliminary tracheostomy. Therapy consists of removal of the obstruction with the CO_2 or KTP lasers. Laser therapy of these lymphovascular malformations can be painstaking and tedious, requiring frequent retreatments.

Other techniques such as sclerotherapy have been applied to these same intrinsic airway lesions. Intralesional steroid injection has been reported to promote rapid involution of a subglottic hemangioma.[19] A relatively new agent, OK-432, has shown promise when injected into lymphovascular lesions around the head and neck.[20,21] OK-432, derived from group A *Streptococcus pyogenes*, stimulates a local inflammatory reaction that leads to involution of the lymphovascular mass. This compound has been used extensively in Japan and Europe.[22] One such series of children with lymphangioma described a case of partial airway obstruction resulting from OK-432 injection and cautioned against use of this agent around the airway.[23] Controlling the depth of injection of this agent and others is difficult and may result in producing damage to the airway in an area where treatment is difficult.

Another injury which, although not usually iatrogenic, can be considered intrinsic is a tracheal burn.

The inhalation of hot gases, steam, and toxic smoke produces acute injury that can lead to inflammation and edema in addition to actual burn necrosis. These individuals require special considerations in their management.[24,25] However, general principles should be followed. Whenever an endotracheal tube passes through an inflamed glottis and upper trachea, early tracheostomy should be considered. With more extensive involvement, prolonged stenting with a T-shaped tracheostomy or T-tube with open proximal and distal limbs may be required.[25]

Extrinsic

Extrinsic injury to the larynx and trachea may occur when an unrestrained child in an automobile strikes his or her neck on the dashboard or the back of the front seat (Fig. 20-10). A blow directly to the neck from a wire when falling or from riding a bicycle ("clothesline injury") (Fig. 20-11) may damage the larynx or trachea. Transection of trachea and esophagus may occur without

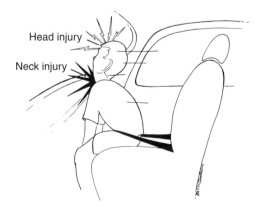

FIGURE 20-10. Mechanism of head injury. With a padded dashboard, external evidence of injury is minimal. (Reprinted from Othersen HB, Jr: Cardiothoracic injuries. In Touloukian RJ [ed.]: Pediatric Trauma. New York, John Wiley & Sons, 1978.)

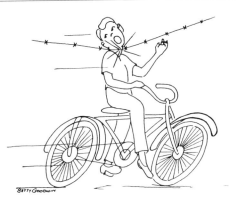

FIGURE 20-11. This neck injury may produce fracture or transection of the airway with little evidence of skin injury. (Reprinted from Othersen HB, Jr: Cardiothoracic injuries. In Touloukian RJ [ed.]: Pediatric Trauma. New York, John Wiley & Sons, 1978.)

visible external neck injuries beyond slight erythema. Crepitus may be present. A good history is essential in determining the mechanism of injury. In these instances, and particularly in conjunction with severe craniofacial injuries, a tracheostomy performed under general anesthesia but without endotracheal intubation is usually advisable, because attempts at intubation may further compromise a critical airway. Penetrating injuries in children are infrequent, but the same general principles used in adults, emphasizing rapid diagnosis and early repair, should be followed.[26]

ENDOTRACHEAL INTUBATION

Endotracheal intubation may be difficult in small children. The best laryngoscopic blade for children is a straight blade, either Miller or Wis-Hipple, which is a straight blade that allows passage of a bronchoscope or endotracheal tube through the blade. The child's head should be in the neutral position and not extended. Because the larynx is anterior in small infants, extension of the head draws the airway even farther anteriorly and makes visualization of the larynx difficult. With the infant's head in neutral, or "sniffing" position and not extended, the laryngoscope blade is introduced, and the tongue and floor of the mouth lifted to expose the epiglottis. Once the epiglottis is seen, extension or flexion of the head and neck may be required to improve visualization. Although many elect to stiffen the endotracheal tube with a curved stylette for all intubations, frequently the use of a stylette makes introduction of the tube somewhat more difficult in a child. The stylette may be curved slightly at the tip, and when the tube is inserted through the glottis, it may impinge on the narrow anterior subglottic region. A tube without stylette tends to follow the lumen more easily.

Usually a tube that approximates the size of the child's little finger will be appropriate. The size of the external nares also may be used as a guide (Fig. 20-12). For pediatric patients, a commonly applied formula to determine appropriate endotracheal tube size is (age + 16)/4.

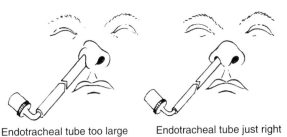

Endotracheal tube too large   Endotracheal tube just right

FIGURE 20-12. An endotracheal tube should fit through the external naris without deforming it. (From Othersen HB, Jr. [ed.]: The Pediatric Airway. Philadelphia, WB Saunders, 1991.)

If a child must be rapidly intubated with a tube that fits snugly and allows no air leak, this fact should be noted and documented. Then at the earliest possible opportunity, the snugly fitting tube should be changed to a smaller size. If intubation is required for a long period (usually > 2 weeks), tracheostomy should be considered, and if it is not performed, an entry in the chart should explain. Daily notes should document whether the cuff is inflated and whether an air leak with an uninflated cuff is present. An air leak is generally an indication that the tube is not too snug.

Ordinarily a cuffed endotracheal tube is not necessary in children because compensation for air leaks can be accomplished by increasing the volume of air delivered by a ventilator. However, with massive craniofacial injuries and bleeding or severe gastroesophageal reflux, a cuff may be necessary to prevent aspiration of blood or gastric contents. Otherwise it is best not to use a cuff for fear of damage to the trachea below the cricoid region. The mechanism for production of tracheal injury by endotracheal tubes has been known for some time,[27] and the steps necessary for prevention have been suggested.[1,28] Although many surgeons elect to intubate the patient initially via the mouth, it is easier to overestimate the endotracheal tube size and produce a subglottic injury than if the tube is passed through the nose. Additionally, the conscious or unconscious movement of the tongue will produce a shearing injury to the glottis and subglottis with prolonged orotracheal intubation. The considerations in determining whether endotracheal intubation should be continued or tracheostomy performed are summarized in Table 20-2.

TRACHEOSTOMY

It has been well established now that tracheostomy with a linear tracheal incision through the second, third, and fourth rings without excising any of the anterior wall of the trachea is the preferred technique in children (Fig. 20-13). Cruciate incisions should not be used because the flaps created may be inverted and narrow the lumen. Tracheostomy is best performed with an endotracheal tube in place so that the procedure is unhurried. A transverse incision made in the lower neck is deepened to allow lateral retraction of the strap muscles after the midline is opened. This dissection is then carried down to the trachea. In small children, palpation of the ridges

TABLE 20-2

INDICATIONS FOR ENDOTRACHEAL INTUBATION AND TRACHEOSTOMY

Clinical Situation	Endotracheal Intubation	Tracheostomy
Emergencies	Always, except →	Severe craniofacial or head and neck injuries
Neonates and infants <6 months	Oral intubation unless no hope of extubation →	When long-term intubation is required or when there is difficulty in maintaining intubation because of activity
Infants >6 months and children	Maintain for 7–14 days and then →	When long-term intubation or ventilatory support is required for conditions such as severe head injuries
Epiglottitis	Until infection has cleared	Usually not necessary
Croup or other severe glottic inflammatory diseases	If does not respond to inhalations of racemic epinephrine or with airway obstruction as a temporary measure before →	When glottic edema and inflammation are severe

of the tracheal cartilages is frequently more valuable than visualization for determining the appropriate level of tracheotomy. The assistant places a retractor on either side of the trachea to retract the strap muscles and to stabilize the trachea. The incision in the trachea is made below the thyroid isthmus, no higher than the second ring. The tracheostomy tube specifications are as illustrated in Table 20-3. Traction sutures of polypropylene (Prolene), left long and labeled Left and Right, allow easier reintubation in the event of accidental dislodgement within the first week. The tube is left in place only as long as necessary, and if the tracheostomy has been in place for longer than 2 weeks, bronchoscopy can be helpful during decannulation. A large granuloma frequently develops at the superior rim of the tracheostomy stoma and may need endoscopic excision.

TRACHEAL REPAIR

Congenital Stenosis

Most congenital obstructions have a cartilaginous base but also have a fibrous tissue component. As explained earlier, many congenital stenotic lesions in the airway are asymptomatic until an acute event, such as an injury, an acute tracheal inflammation, or endotracheal intubation occurs. At that point, the constriction of the airway is manifest. Complete tracheal rings may first be suspected when the child requires an anesthetic, and an endotracheal tube meets a tracheal obstruction.[29]

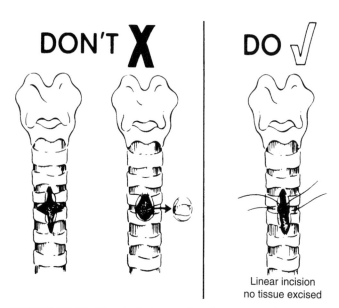

FIGURE 20-13. Two techniques of tracheostomy to be avoided in children and the preferred linear incision. (Reprinted from Othersen HB Jr: Intubation injuries of the trachea in children. Management and prevention. Ann Surg 189:601–606, 1979.)

TABLE 20-3

TRACHEOSTOMY TUBE SPECIFICATIONS

Tube Type	French Size	I.D.	O.D.	Length (mm)
Shiley				
Neonatal	00			
	0	3.4	5.0	32
	1	3.7	5.5	34
Pediatric	00	3.1	4.5	39
	0	3.4	5.0	40
	1	3.7	5.5	41
	2	4.1	6.0	42
	3	4.8	7.0	44
	4	5.5	8.0	46
Argyle (Dover)	000	2.5	4.0	32
	00	3.0	4.7	34
	0	3.5	5.4	36
	1	4.0	6.0	36
	2	4.5	6.6	40
	3	5.0	7.3	46
	4	5.5	7.8	50
	5	6.0	8.5	54
Silastic	1	3.0	5.5	35
(Dow Corning)	3	4.0	7.0	40
	4½	5.0	8.0	43
	6	7.0	10.0	46

Note: I.D. = inside diameter, O.D. = outside diameter.

For treatment of long-segment obstruction from complete tracheal rings, we have devised a procedure in which either the KTP or CO_2 laser is used to divide each complete cartilaginous ring in the posterior midline.[30] With endoscopic balloons, the trachea is gradually dilated as the rigid bronchoscope is advanced. When all complete rings have been divided, a tube is inserted to serve as a stent. If long-term stenting is required, a T-tube is used (see later). If this procedure is done carefully without forceful dilation, no air leak should occur because the esophagus posteriorly fills the gap in the posterior tracheal wall. With a short segment of complete rings, resection and anastomosis has been accepted as effective therapy, but few surgeons have a large series of patients.[31] Other groups have used resection for long and short lesions but are now considering slide tracheoplasty.[32]

An improvement on standard resection techniques is the procedure of *slide tracheoplasty,* a technique that allows reconstruction without tension.[33] The narrowed segment is transected in its midportion, and the remaining stenotic segments incised—one end of the trachea opened in the posterior midline, and the other, in the anterior midline. Long-term evaluation has been satisfactory.[34] The diameter of the resulting anastomosis is broad enough to avoid airway narrowing. Some have compared laryngotracheal reconstruction with cricotracheal resection and attempted to categorize the indications for each procedure.[35] The surgical therapy for these patients continues to evolve, as evidenced by a recent review of 50 patients treated for congenital tracheal stenosis at a single institution over an 18-year span (1982 to 2000).[36] Although the operation originally preferred was pericardial tracheoplasty,[37] four procedures were compared: pericardial-patch tracheoplasty ($n = 28$); tracheal autograft ($n = 12$); tracheal resection ($n = 8$); and slide tracheoplasty ($n = 2$). These authors concluded that their operation of choice for short segments would be resection, and for long-segment stenoses (more than eight rings), resection with tracheal autograft was preferred.[38] In this latter procedure, the stenotic trachea is incised anteriorly, and the midportion excised. A primary anastomosis is made posteriorly, and the anterior defect closed with a free autograft fashioned from the excised portion. Others have used human cadaver tracheal allografts[39,40] for reconstruction. The ideal surgical treatment for congenital tracheal stenosis has not yet been found.

Anterior cricoid split is a procedure that is useful in treating moderate subglottic stenosis in neonates and young infants. Infants selected for the anterior cricoid split procedure should not weigh less than 1500 g or require assisted ventilation or inspired oxygen more than 35%. They should also not be in cardiac failure. This technique is illustrated in Figure 20-14.[41] Proper selection of patients for anterior cricoid split is crucial. After anterior cricoid split, those infants that can be successfully extubated have excellent long-term outcomes, whereas those that cannot will require tracheostomy. This procedure was originally described in 1980 and updated in 1991.[42,43]

Acquired Stenosis

When an endotracheal tube is removed, tracheal injury may be manifest by stridor and dyspnea. Prompt therapy may allow the trachea to heal without cicatricial stenosis. An endotracheal tube of a size that allows a slight air leak is carefully inserted to serve as a temporary stent. The polyvinyl (Portex) tube is pliable, softens at body temperature, and is preferred. This soft tube can be left in place while the patient is treated with high doses of systemic steroids (0.8 to 1 mg dexamethasone/kg/day, IV) in an attempt to abort dense scar. Before insertion of the stent, the trachea may require gentle dilation by using balloon dilators. Rigid dilators may produce more injury, because while they dilate, they also impart a shearing force to the tracheal mucosa. Balloons dilate with only radial forces. Dexamethasone is continued in the dose of 0.8 to 1 mg/kg/day divided into four doses (0.2 to 0.25 mg/kg per dose) for at least 72 hours. Longer treatment may be necessary for more severe injuries. The steroids are then rapidly tapered, and the endotracheal tube is removed once the patient is stable and spontaneously breathing without ventilatory assistance.

If dense stenosis has already occurred, this technique will not be effective. Acquired tracheal obstruction can be classified as granulomatous, inflammatory, fibrous, or calcific. Congenital obstructions are usually cartilaginous. With dense fibrous and calcific strictures, open resection or reconstruction is usually necessary. However, endoscopic laser incision with gradual and gentle balloon expansion of the lumen combined with insertion of an endotracheal stent may allow a functional airway to remodel over a period of time. Some authors advocate treatment of tracheal granulation tissue with mitomycin C. Topical application of mitomycin C during endoscopic surgery can reduce recurrence of granulation tissue.[44] If stenosis recurs whenever the stent is removed, the stent can be reinserted and a balloon tracheoplasty performed with the stent in situ.

T-tubes have been used effectively as stents in the past for both children and adults.[25] Newer expandable metal stents are frequently used in adults. Some of these nickel-titanium (Nitinol)-coated stents have been used in children in selected cases.[45] However, these stents may not be appropriate for children for the following reasons:

1. The child may grow, and the metal stent does not. Removal of the stent is then necessary and may be hazardous.
2. The ingrowth of granulation tissue through the interstices of the metal stent may produce obstruction in itself and lead to severe hemorrhage when removal is attempted.
3. The medical conditions for which stents are placed in children are different from those in adults. Many adult placements are due to neoplastic conditions that are associated with a short life expectancy; thus the stent is not required for long periods. However, in children, a stent may be required for years.

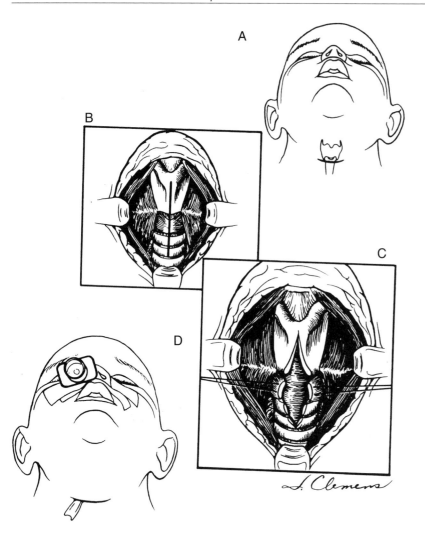

FIGURE 20-14. The anterior cricoid split procedure. *A,* Make a horizontal incision over the cricoid cartilage. *B,* Use a combination of sharp and blunt dissection to expose the larynx and upper trachea. *C,* Split the lower portion of the thyroid cartilage, the cricoid cartilage, and upper tracheal rings. *D,* Close the wound loosely over a drain with the airway stented by a nasotracheal tube. (From Othersen HB, Jr. [ed.]: The Pediatric Airway. Philadelphia, WB Saunders, 1991.)

Straight tracheal stents of silicone rubber have been successfully used in adults, but fixation by projections from the circumference of the tube is necessary to prevent migration when it is not used as a T-tube.[46,47] The small diameter of a child's trachea makes these stents impractical. A T-shaped tube inserted through a tracheotomy with proximal and distal tracheal extensions can be readily inserted in a child's airway and will not migrate.

We have preferred modification of the Montgomery T-tubes for the following reasons:

1. The tubes are made of silicone rubber and are pliable yet rigid enough to serve as a stent.
2. The tubes can be constructed to the exact dimensions necessary to fit the individual child's trachea.
3. The proximal limb can be placed below the cords, and the distal limb can be made as long as necessary for bridging the obstruction.
4. The cervical tube can be used for suctioning or for insufflation in an emergency. If these measures do not improve the airway obstruction, the T-tube can be removed by the parents and replaced

with an endotracheal tube inserted through the cervical stoma.
5. The T-tube allows normal laryngeal breathing and phonation when the side-arm is plugged.

Our technique for insertion of a T-tube is shown in the composite drawings (Fig. 20-15).

Open Laryngotracheoplasty

Many variations exist in the operative techniques of procedures available for tracheal reconstruction for a scarred and stenotic trachea.[48] First, an open procedure can be done with or without cardiopulmonary bypass. An increasing tendency is seen to avoid bypass and use only endotracheal anesthesia. Second, the repair can be performed with or without an augmentation graft. The grafts may include tracheal autografts, costal cartilage, cartilage from other sites such as thyroid or alar cartilage, autologous or allogeneic pericardium, skin, and tracheal allografts. Third, a stent may be used to maintain the lumen and to remain in place for hours, days, months, or years.

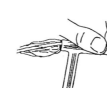
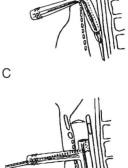
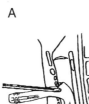
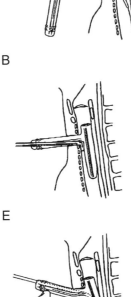
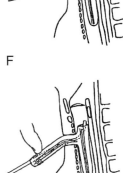

A B C

D E F

FIGURE 20-15. T-tube stent insertion with aid of dilating balloon to stiffen T-tube during insertion.

G H I

Without Cartilage

This procedure is essentially a cricoid split or the expansion of the lumen with the use of a castellated incision.[49] These procedures are often performed with an internal stent.

With Cartilage

This procedure is the classic cartilage laryngotracheoplasty (Fig. 20-16). The cartilage is inserted anteriorly after incision of the stenotic segment.[35,50] Cartilage inserts also can be placed posteriorly and laterally in sites where the stenotic cricoid is incised. Ciliated mucosa can be demonstrated on the surface of a mature costal cartilage graft in some studies, if the perichondrium faces the airway lumen.[51]

Resection and Anastomosis

The stenotic portion of the trachea is excised, and an end-to-end anastomosis is performed. The principles of tracheal operations, devised for adult patients, should be strictly followed.[35,52–54]

Slide Tracheoplasty

This innovative technique uses autologous trachea by dividing the trachea in the midportion of the stenotic segment. The upper and lower portions of the stenosis are then incised in the midline, one anteriorly and the other posteriorly.[34,55,56]

Patch Autograft

Early experience in repairing congenital tracheal stenosis by anterior incision and closure of the defect with pericardium. All pericardial patch operations were done with cardiopulmonary bypass.[36] Experience at other centers with this procedure was not good because of complications secondary to patch collapse.[57] The original proponents of pericardial patching have now reported improved results with a free tracheal autograft, in which the excised stenotic segment is flattened and used as a free anterior autograft to expand the lumen at the anastomosis.[38,58]

T-tubes

Silicone T-tubes are used as internal stents to maintain the tracheal lumen and allow tracheal remodeling.[59] These tubes can be placed temporarily to allow for growth of the airway or to maintain the lumen while the airway heals after tracheoplasty. Alternatively, T-tubes can be effective as a permanent stent for the difficult pediatric airway or in cases of failed tracheoplasty.

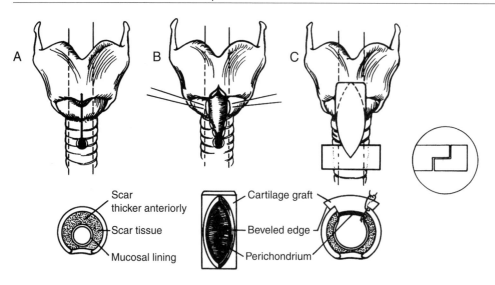

FIGURE 20-16. An autogenous costal cartilage graft reconstruction. *A,* Expose the larynx and upper trachea. *B,* Incise the aforementioned region, remaining superior to the tracheostomy stoma if the stenosis does not involve this site. *C,* Sew the costal cartilage to the incised edges of the larynx and trachea, placing the perichondrium internally. (From Othersen HB, Jr. [ed]: The Pediatric Airway. Philadelphia, WB Saunders, 1991.)

THE FUTURE

One group has attempted to set up a foundation to develop a "disease-based and operation-specific model" to predict the outcome of airway reconstruction.[60] They have concluded that operations for pediatric laryngotracheal reconstruction are challenging and that multiple procedures may be required. We agree. For all of the foregoing reasons, we continue to stress **PREVENTION.**

The following principles are essential in treating the pediatric airway.

1. Be gentle. Endotracheal tube insertion should be atraumatic and of a size that allows an air leak.
2. If injury occurs and dilation is necessary, use balloon, not rigid, dilators.
3. Stents may aid in the healing process by maintaining the lumen.
4. Immediate high-dose and short-term steroid therapy may be helpful in acute injuries, and their use may prevent dense cicatrix.
5. In all children with an endotracheal tube in place, document:
   a. The size of the tube
   b. Presence or absence of an air leak
   c. Cuff inflation
   d. Considerations regarding possible tracheostomy

REFERENCES

1. Othersen HB Jr: Intubation injuries of the trachea in children: Management and prevention. Ann Surg 189:601, 1979.
2. Weber TR, Connors RH, Tracy TF Jr: Acquired tracheal stenosis in infants and children. J Thorac Cardiovasc Surg 102:29, 1991.
3. Macpherson RI: Radiologic aspects of airway obstruction. In Othersen HB (ed): The Pediatric Airway. Philadelphia, WB Saunders, 1991, pp 30–65.
4. De Vries PA, De Vries CR: Embryology and development. In Othersen HB (ed): The Pediatric Airway. Philadelphia, WB Saunders, 1991, pp 3–16.
5. Roberts CS, Othersen HB Jr, Sade RM, et al: Tracheoesophageal compression from aortic arch anomalies: Analysis of 30 operatively treated children. J Pediatr Surg 29:334, 1994.
6. Erwin EA, Gerber ME, Cotton RT: Vascular compression of the airway: Indications for and results of surgical management. Int J Pediatr Otorhinolaryngol 40:155, 1997.
7. Braunstein PW, Sade RM: Vascular malformations with airway obstruction. In Othersen HB (ed): The Pediatric Airway. Philadelphia, WB Saunders, 1991, pp 81–96.
8. Clevenger FW, Othersen HB Jr, Smith CD: Relief of tracheal compression by aortopexy. Ann Thorac Surg 50:524, 1990.
9. Adler SC, Isaacson G, Balsara RK: Innominate artery compression of the trachea: Diagnosis and treatment by anterior suspension: A 25-year experience. Ann Otol Rhinol Laryngol 104:924, 1995.
10. Kamerkar DR, Gladstone D J: Innominate artery compression of the trachea: A simplified technique for anterior suspension of the innominate artery. J Cardiovasc Surg 35:549, 1994.
11. Corbally MT, Spitz L, Kiely E, et al: Aortopexy for tracheomalacia in oesophageal anomalies. Eur J Pediatr Surg 3:264, 1993.
12. Ziemer G, Heinemann M, Kaulitz R, et al: Pulmonary artery sling with tracheal stenosis: Primary one-stage repair in infancy. Ann Thorac Surg 54:971, 1992.
13. Pasic M, von Segesser L, Carrel T, et al: Anomalous left pulmonary artery (pulmonary sling): Result of a surgical approach. Cardiovasc Surg 1:608, 1993.
14. Othersen HB Jr, Khalil B, Zellner J, et al: Aortoesophageal fistula and double aortic arch: Two important points in management. J Pediatr Surg 31:594, 1996.
15. Othersen HB: Medical diseases of the airway: A surgeon's role. In Othersen HB (ed): The Pediatric Airway. Philadelphia, WB Saunders, 1991, pp 64–70.
16. Mauro RD, Poole SR, Lockhard CH: Differentiation of epiglottitis from laryngotracheitis in the child with stridor. Am J Dis Child 142:679, 1988.
17. Sendi K, Crysdale WS: Acute epiglottitis: A decade of change: A 10-year experience with 242 children. J Otolaryngol 16:196, 1987.
18. Stroud RH, Friedman NR: An update on inflammatory disorders of the pediatric airway: Epiglottitis, croup, and tracheitis. Am J Otolaryngol 22:268, 2001.
19. Wang LY, Hung HY, Lee KS: Infantile subglottic hemangioma treated by intralesional steroid injection: Report of one case. Acta Paediatr Taiwanica 44:35, 2003.
20. Laranne J, Keski-Nisula L, Rautio R, et al: OK-432 (Picibanil) therapy for lymphangiomas in children. Eur Arch Oto Rhino Laryngol 259:274, 2002.
21. Giguere CM, Bauman NM, Sato Y, et al: Treatment of lymphangiomas with OK-432 (Picibanil) sclerotherapy: A prospective multi-institutional trial. Arch Otolaryngol Head Neck Surg 128:1137, 2002.
22. Suzuki Y, Obana A, Gohto Y, et al: Management of orbital lymphangioma using intralesional injection of OK-432. Br J Ophthalmol 84:614, 2000.

23. Hall N, Ade-Ajayi N, Brewis C, et al: Is intralesional injection of OK-432 effective in the treatment of lymphangioma in children? Surgery 133:238, 2003.

24. Gaissert HA, Lofgren RH, Grillo HC: Upper airway compromise after inhalation injury: Complex strictures of the larynx and trachea and their management. Ann Surg 218:672, 1993.

25. Gaissert HA, Grillo HC, Mathisen DJ, et al: Temporary and permanent restoration of airway continuity with the tracheal T-tube. J Thorac Cardiovasc Surg 107:600, 1994.

26. Huh J, Milliken JC, Chen JC: Management of tracheobronchial injuries following blunt and penetrating trauma. Am Surgeon 63:896, 1997.

27. Cooper JD, Grillo HG: The evolution of tracheal injury due to ventilatory assistance through cuffed tubes: A pathologic study. Ann Surg 169:334, 1969.

28. Othersen HB Jr: Subglottic tracheal stenosis. Semin Thorac Cardiovasc Surg 6:200, 1994.

29. Andrews TM, Cotton RT, Bailey WW, et al: Tracheoplasty for congenital complete tracheal rings. Arch Otolaryngol Head Neck Surg 120:1363, 1994.

30. Othersen HB Jr, Hebra A, Tagge EP: A new method of treatment for complete tracheal rings in an infant: Endoscopic laser division and balloon dilation. J Pediatr Surg 35:262, 2000.

31. Brown JW, Bando K, Sun K, et al: Surgical management of congenital tracheal stenosis. Chest Surg Clin North Am 6:837, 1996.

32. Acosta AC, Albanese CT, Farmer DL, et al: Tracheal stenosis: The long and the short of it. J Pediatr Surg 35:1612, 2000.

33. Grillo HC: Slide tracheoplasty for long-segment congenital tracheal stenosis. Ann Thorac Surg 58:613, 1994.

34. Grillo HC, Wright CD, Vlahakes GJ, et al: Management of congenital tracheal stenosis by means of slide tracheoplasty or resection and reconstruction, with long-term follow-up of growth after slide tracheoplasty. J Thorac Cardiol Surg 123:145, 2002.

35. Gustafson LM, Hartley BE, Liu JH, et al: Single-stage laryngotracheal reconstruction in children: A review of 200 cases. Otolaryngol Head Neck Surg 123:430, 2000.

36. Backer CL, Mavroudis C, Gerber ME, et al: Tracheal surgery in children: An 18-year review of four techniques. Eur J Cardiothorac Surg 19:777, 2001.

37. Backer CL, Mavroudis C, Dunham ME, et al: Reoperation after pericardial patch tracheoplasty. J Pediatr Surg 32:1108, 1997.

38. Backer CL, Mavroudis C, Dunham ME, et al: Repair of congenital tracheal stenosis with a free tracheal autograft. J Thorac Cardiovasc Surg 115:869, 1998.

39. Elliott MJ, Haw MP, Jacobs JP, et al: Tracheal reconstruction in children using cadaveric homograft trachea. Eur J Cardiol Thorac Surg 10:707, 1996.

40. Kunachak S, Kulapaditharom B, Vajaradul Y, et al: Cryopreserved, irradiated tracheal homograft transplantation for laryngotracheal reconstruction in human beings. Otolaryngol Head Neck Surg 122:911, 2000.

41. Myer CM 3rd, Cotton RT: Cricoid split and cartilage tracheoplasty. In Othersen HB (ed): The Pediatric Airway. Philadelphia, WB Saunders, 1991, pp 117–124.

42. Cotton R, Seid AB: Management of the extubation problem in the premature child: Anterior cricoid split as an alternative to tracheotomy. Ann Otol Rhinol Laryngol 89:508, 1980.

43. Silver FM, Myer CM 3rd, Cotton RT: Anterior cricoid split: Update 1991. Am J Otolaryngol 12:343, 1991.

44. Ward RF, April MM: Mitomycin-C in the treatment of tracheal cicatrix after tracheal reconstruction. Int J Pediatr Otorhinolaryngol 44:221, 1998.

45. Prasad M, Bent JP, Ward RF, et al: Endoscopically placed nitinol stents for pediatric tracheal obstruction. Int J Pediatr Otorhinolaryngol 66:155, 2002.

46. Puma F, Ragusa M, Avenia N, et al: The role of silicone stents in the treatment of cicatricial tracheal stenoses. J Thorac Cardiovasc Surg 120:1064, 2000.

47. Vergnon JM, Costes F, Polio JC: Efficacy and tolerance of a new silicone stent for the treatment of benign tracheal stenosis: Preliminary results. Chest 118:422, 2000.

48. Matute JA, Villafruela MA, Delgado MD, et al: Surgery of subglottic stenosis in neonates and children. Eur J Pediatr Surg 10:286, 2000.

49. Evans JN: Laryngeal disorders in children. In Wilkinson AW (ed): Recent Advances in Pediatric Surgery. Edinburgh, Churchill Livingston, 1975, p 174.

50. Forsen JW, Lusk RP, Huddleston CB: Costal cartilage tracheoplasty for congenital long-segment tracheal stenosis. Arch Otolaryngol Head Neck Surg 128:1165, 2002.

51. Oue T, Kamata S, Usui N, et al: Histopathologic changes after tracheobronchial reconstruction with costal cartilage graft for congenital tracheal stenosis. J Pediatr Surg 36:329, 2001.

52. Grillo HC, Donahue DM, Mathisen DJ, et al: Postintubation tracheal stenosis: Treatment and results. J Thorac Cardiovasc Surg 109:486, 1995.

53. Har-El G, Shaha A, Chaudry R, et al: Resection of tracheal stenosis with end-to-end anastomosis. Ann Otol Rhinol Laryngol 102:670, 1993.

54. Rutter MJ, Hartley BE, Cotton RT: Cricotracheal resection in children. Arch Otolaryngol Head Neck Surg 127:289, 2001.

55. Lipshutz GS, Jennings RW, Lopoo JB, et al: Slide tracheoplasty for congenital tracheal stenosis: A case report. J Pediatr Surg 35:259, 2000.

56. Lang FJ, Hurni M, Monnier P: Long-segment congenital tracheal stenosis: Treatment by slide-tracheoplasty. J Pediatr Surg 34:1216, 1999.

57. Houel R, Serraf A, Macchiarini P, et al: Tracheoplasty in congenital tracheal stenosis. Int J Pediatr Otorhinolaryngol 44:31, 1998.

58. Backer CL, Mavroudis C, Dunham ME, et al: Intermediate-term results of the free tracheal autograft for long segment congenital tracheal stenosis. J Pediatr Surg 35:813, 2000.

59. Huang CJ: Use of silicone T-tube to treat tracheal stenosis or tracheal injury. Ann Thorac Cardiol Surg 7:192, 2001.

60. Hartnick CJ, Hartley BE, Lacy PD, et al: Surgery for pediatric subglottic stenosis: Disease-specific outcomes. Ann Otol Rhinol Laryngol 110:1109, 2001.

Bronchopulmonary Malformations

Karl G. Sylvester, MD, and Craig T. Albanese, MD

INTRODUCTION

A variety of developmental abnormalities of the tracheo-bronchial tree and pulmonary parenchyma are found in the newborn. Some of these have a genetic basis and, as such, produce more widespread maladies. Many of these, such as surfactant protein deficiencies, alveolar capillary dysplasias, and generalized pulmonary hypoplasia, are newly described, are not formally in the traditional scope of care of the pediatric surgeon, and are therefore not addressed in this chapter. For pediatric surgeons, the more focal abnormalities of the foregut and its anlagen, traditionally termed *bronchopulmonary malformations* (BPMs), are covered. Although these lesions have been recognized for years and grouped as related for discussion purposes, no uniform pathologic or embryologic reason exists for this clustering. Rather, this grouping remains appropriate to facilitate an understanding of the common clinical presentation and management of BPMs.

With the advent of near-routine prenatal ultrasonography (US), a great deal has been learned about the natural history and pathophysiology of BPMs. Currently US findings are altering many of the conventional beliefs and understanding of these lesions. Moreover, prenatal identification and a more accurate understanding of their natural history have given rise to advanced fetal interventions. The lessons learned from prenatal US also have affected the postnatal management of cystic lung lesions, as previously unrecognized and likely clinically silent malformations are being detected with ever greater frequency. Still, despite these advances, BPMs defy a common embryologic classification and, as a whole, their pathophysiology remains varied.

EMBRYOLOGY AND CLASSIFICATION

The traditional understanding is that the tracheo-bronchial tree and proximal gastrointestinal tract arise from common foregut anlagen.[1-3] At the end of the third week of gestation, the laryngotracheal groove or diverticulum can be seen in the caudal end of the embryonic foregut. This groove arises as a ventral enlargement of the foregut and then grows caudally to form the primordium of the trachea and lung bud. This outgrowth of endoderm is ventral and in parallel with the more dorsal portion of the foregut or future esophagus. Next the lateral walls of the foregut, now called longitudinal ridges, begin to approximate in the midline, forming the tracheoesophageal septum. The separation of the dorsal esophagus and more ventral tracheobronchial tree is thought to be caused by this tracheoesophageal septum and is complete by the sixth week of gestation. If this process fails or is incomplete, congenital defects affecting the trachea, conducting airways, or esophagus may result.

Some now question this traditional embryologic description.[4] Several lines of evidence tend to refute these long-held beliefs. Findings in chick embryos by using scanning electronic microscopy at various stages of development have described a paired caudal "lung bud" diverticulum with no identifiable tracheal primordium.[4] Even more elusive is the developmental program of the lung primordia after separation from the foregut anlagen, which occurs between 6 and 16 weeks of gestation. Current advances in molecular biologic technique including conditional mutants and transgenic mice have allowed a more in-depth investigation and understanding of the molecular regulators of airway and pulmonary parenchymal development. In more generalized terms, the epithelium of the trachea, bronchi, and alveoli originate from endoderm, whereas muscle and cartilage originate from mesoderm.[2] Subsequent epithelial mesenchymal interactions result in the changes of branching morphogenesis and yield site-specific specialized epithelia for air conduction and gas exchange.[5,6] Studies in mice have established nonoverlapping cell lineages of conducting airways (trachea and bronchi) as being distinct from those of peripheral airways (bronchioles, acini, and alveoli), well before formation of the definitive lung buds.[7,8] Similarly, studies in knockout mice and conditional mutants have revealed the involvement of many of the

TABLE 21-1

BRONCHOPULMONARY MALFORMATIONS: CLASSIFICATION BY SITE OF ORIGIN

Trachea and Bronchi	Pulmonary Parenchyma	Vascular
Agenesis	Congenital cystic adenomatoid malformation	Hemangioma
Atresia, stenosis	Bronchopulmonary sequestration	Arterio-venous malformation
Tracheal bronchus	Congenital lobar emphysema	Scimitar syndrome
Esophageal bronchus/lung (communicating broncho-pulmonary malformation)	Agenesis	Congenital pulmonary lymphangiectasia
Bronchogenic cyst	Aplasia	Lymphangioma
Enteric duplication cyst	Hypoplasia	Congenital chylothorax
Neuroenteric cyst	Bronchiolar cysts (cystic bronchiectasis-multiple)	
Bronchial cysts (peripheral)	Lobulation anomalies	

secreted protein morphogens involved in organogenesis throughout mammalian development, such as members of the BMP, FGF, Hhh and Wnt families.[8-11]

Knowledge of this embryology serves to elucidate the reasons for the frequent consideration of the close relation between anomalies of the proximal gastrointestinal tract and pulmonary system. Congenital BPMs comprise a broad spectrum of clinical lesions from both systems, including esophageal duplications, cystic lung lesions, and anomalies of solid pulmonary parenchyma with abnormal vascular supply. Classification of congenital BPMs therefore is not easy from either a morphologic or embryologic standpoint. A more simplified listing of BPMs by location becomes the most useful classification system for the clinician charged with managing the myriad presentations and diagnoses (Table 21-1).

PRENATAL DIAGNOSIS AND THERAPY

The widespread use of prenatal US has expanded our understanding of the natural history and pathophysiology of some of the more common BPMs.[12] With ever-increasing sophistication in prenatal imaging, a wide range of lesions including bronchogenic and enteric cysts, mediastinal cystic teratomas, congenital lobar emphysema, bronchial atresia, and the cystic lung masses of congenital cystic adenomatoid malformation (CCAM) and bronchopulmonary sequestration (BPS) are now identified with regularity.[13] Confusion still can occur, particularly in the fetus with a basilar cystic lung lesion in which a diagnosis of diaphragmatic hernia also is entertained. More recently, ultrafast magnetic resonance imaging (MRI) of many of these same lesions has allowed an even more detailed distinction based on an assessment of their anatomic variability.[14] Overall, prenatal imaging of BPMs also has demonstrated the rarity of other associated anomalies, a fact of importance when therapeutic options are considered.[15]

The most commonly identified prenatal pulmonary anomaly remains the cystic lung lesion (Fig. 21-1).[12,16] An irregularity in the US echogenicity of lung parenchyma has become the initial diagnostic hallmark of the congenital cystic lung masses.[17] CCAMs, which are manifest histologically by an adenomatoid increase in terminal respiratory bronchioles, can be classified according to their prenatal US findings.[13,17,18] Microcystic lesions appear as a solid echodense mass.[17] Macrocystic lesions, which comprised either a single dominant cyst or several daughter cysts measuring more than 5 mm in diameter, appear more echolucent and less dense.[15] In contradistinction to a CCAM, a BPS is defined by its morphologic characteristics of nonfunctioning lung parenchyma without communication to the tracheobronchial tree and with an anomalous systemic blood supply.[18] These characteristics are the clinically relevant diagnostic findings both grossly and by prenatal US. BPS appears, like some CCAMs, as an echodense homogeneous mass.[13,17] The finding on

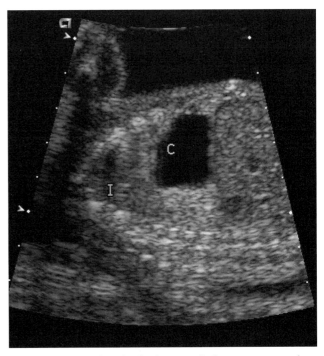

FIGURE 21-1. This fetal ultrasound demonstrates a large unilocular cystic lesion above the fetal liver in the chest. C, cystic lesion; I, inferior vena cava.

color Doppler of a systemically derived feeding arterial vessel, as opposed to bronchial circulation, is pathognomonic of BPS.[12,17] Microcystic CCAM and BPS can have an otherwise identical sonographic appearance if the anomalous blood supply is not identified. Ultrafast fetal MRI can aid in the distinction between these two lesions.[13,14,19] However, in the majority of cases without definitive in utero pathologic manifestations, the distinction is perhaps irrelevant.

Cystic fetal lung lesions may manifest several alternative outcomes. The overall prognosis of cystic lung masses relates to size, although with great variability.[13,20] Small pulmonary masses as an incidental finding may be entirely asymptomatic both in utero and after birth. Very large masses can have reproducible physiologic effects on the developing fetus. Compression of the fetal esophagus may impede the normal swallowing of amniotic fluid that may result in polyhydramnios. Simple mass effect can displace normal or unaffected lung, producing pulmonary hypoplasia. Through a similar mechanism of extreme vena caval obstruction and cardiac compression, low-output cardiac failure and fetal hydrops may be produced. Either polyhydramnios or hydrops can occur in isolation, as they do not represent a continuum of pathophysiology. Hydrops is manifest by fetal ascites, pleural and pericardial effusions, and skin or scalp edema or both. These findings have historically been viewed as a harbinger of fetal or neonatal death.[13,15] The ability to identify a lesion and witness its pathophysiologic evolution has produced a management scheme based on prognosis that now includes fetal intervention, as outlined in Figure 21-2.

In 2003, an extensive 7-year experience with 350 prenatally diagnosed cystic fetal lung lesions was reported.[15] In this experience, 15% of CCAMs and 68% of BPS lesions were observed to decrease in size during gestation. Other groups have reported similar involution of

fetal cystic lung masses.[21–23] The mechanism by which these lesions involute remains unknown. Despite the strong association of hydrops from a cystic lung mass with fetal death, a recent series of three cases of hydrops resolution with fetal survival were reported after the administration of prenatal steroids.[21] Although the occasional case of fetal hydrops has been documented to resolve with spontaneous tumor shrinkage, it remains the collective experience that hydrops portends a poor either pre- or postnatal outcome.[12,13,15,17,21–23] Overall, caution should be exercised when discussing the prognosis of the fetus, as an understanding of which lesions will shrink remains elusive.

In an effort to derive a more objective prognostic tool, measurements of overall cyst size relative to the remainder of the fetus were compared. The index of cystic adenomatoid malformation volume ratio (CVR) is obtained by dividing the CCAM volume by the fetal head circumference.[20] This index was found to be predictive of fetal hydrops when the ratio is greater than 1.6. Through these and similar serial US observations, it has been shown that most CCAMs do not increase in size relative to overall fetal size past 28 weeks of gestation. Based on these data, the authors' recommendations for fetuses of less than 28 weeks of gestation are twice-weekly US examinations, given a CVR greater than 1.6, and weekly scans for those with smaller indices.[15,20]

The reproducible finding on prenatal US that fetuses with very large cystic lung lesions and hydrops remain at risk has led to the development of fetal therapeutic options. Fetal thoracentesis and thoracoamniotic shunting has been performed with some success in fetuses with large, space-occupying pleural effusions, usually associated with BPS, or for the dominant cyst in a principally macrocystic CCAMs.[15,24,25] Thoracentesis alone has proven ineffective because of the rapid reaccumulation of fluid and should therefore be considered as only a

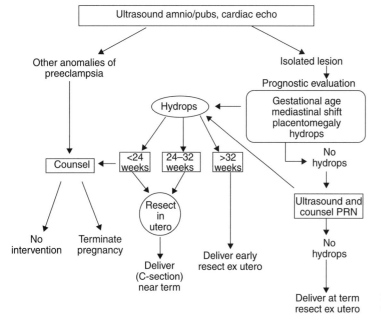

FIGURE 21-2. A proposed algorithm for the management of a fetus found by prenatal ultrasound to have a thoracic mass.

temporizing measure. Shunt placement for the continuous decompression of large single-cyst–predominant masses has resulted in the consistent resolution of hydrops in several centers.[24,25] In one report, nine fetuses were successfully treated for macrocystic CCAM with thoracoamniotic shunting, all with complete hydrops resolution, and with eight survivors.[15,26] Given an average time to delivery of 13 weeks, it seems that percutaneously placed shunts are well tolerated by the gravid uterus with respect to preterm labor after therapeutic fetal intervention. Of course, microcystic CCAMs associated with hydrops would not be amenable to shunting, based on knowledge of their microscopic anatomy and subsequent behavior. Somewhat paradoxically, the rare BPS with hydrops also has been treated successfully with shunting.[13] In BPS with hydrops, fluid accumulates in the pleural and peritoneal spaces and is believed to produce tension hydrothorax from the obstructed flow of either fluid or lymph. All surviving fetuses should undergo more definitive postnatal resection after delivery and stabilization.

Numerous well-documented studies in the fetal lamb model to simulate a large thoracic mass with the mechanisms of compression, hydrops, and subsequent resolution, have been studied.[12,27–29] The techniques of fetal surgical resection, anesthetic, and tocolytic management were extensively investigated in nonhuman primates before the first clinical application of open fetal therapy.[12] Based on these collective experiences, guidelines for the gestational age of the fetus, size of the lesion, maternal health and well-being, and the presence of hydrops has allowed selected fetuses with life-threatening lesions to be surgically approached (see Fig. 21-2). Open fetal surgery is offered at a few selected centers after a comprehensive multidisciplinary screening process.[16] Extensive prenatal US and echocardiography is done to exclude associated anomalies.[12,16] In addition, amniocentesis or percutaneous umbilical blood sampling is performed to confirm a normal karyotype. With the knowledge that prenatal hydrops from mass effect is highly predictive of fetal death, massive multicystic or predominantly solid CCAMs associated with hydrops can be resected in utero before 32 weeks of gestation. The largest reported series to date comprised 22 cases, with 11 healthy survivors of procedures performed between 21 and 31 weeks of gestation.[15] Findings at operation in the original 22 cases necessitated 16 single lobectomies, 4 double lobectomies, and 2 pneumonectomies. In the 11 survivors, histologic confirmation of CCAM was acquired, and all survivors had postresection resolution of hydrops within 1 to 2 weeks. In addition, compensatory fetal lung growth was noted as the mediastinum returned to a more anatomic configuration. In this same series, 11 failures were noted from a variety of causes. The same lessons of advanced fetal hydrops or maternal pre-eclampsia, also known as the *maternal mirror syndrome,* were causative in several cases. Mirror syndrome is a maternal hyperdynamic state that remains poorly understood.[30] It seems that there is a rationale for the belief that close US follow-up is warranted to identify fetuses before the complications of hydrops render the fetus unsalvageable. Preterm labor precipitated fetal delivery and death in several others.

Thus it seems that the lessons learned about the indications and limitations of the open operative fetal cases are reproducible.

For fetuses that have reached 32 weeks of gestation or more at the time of presentation, early elective delivery is recommended to effect ex utero resection (see Fig. 21-2).[15,16] However, the outcome remains dismal for hydropic fetuses, even with advanced postnatal support, including extracorporeal membrane oxygenation (ECMO). The combined results and experience cited earlier have demonstrated that fetal CCAM resection is a viable option for selected fetuses with otherwise fatal BPMs and hydrops.

POSTNATAL MANAGEMENT OF BRONCHOPULMONARY MALFORMATIONS

Several fetal anomalies can be confused with CCAMs and BPS.[3] Chief among these are congenital diaphragmatic hernias, bronchogenic and enteric cysts, mediastinal cystic teratomas, congenital lobar emphysema, and bronchial atresia.[31–34] In addition, the majority of these lesions are amenable to postnatal treatment. Smaller lesions may be asymptomatic at birth. Many of these lesions, before the increased use of prenatal US, may have gone unnoticed, even by perinatal chest radiography. Current practice is to obtain computed tomography (CT) of the chest before neonatal discharge in those infants previously diagnosed with a cystic lung lesion prenatally. Planned elective resection of asymptomatic CCAMs and BPS is recommended, given the accumulating evidence of the risks of either infection or occult malignant transformation.[3,35–38] Moderate-sized lesions may cause some respiratory embarrassment at birth, either from hyperinflation or from the secondary mass effects on normal lung. The traditional postnatal management of planned delivery with multidisciplinary neonatal evaluation, stabilization, and eventual excision has produced an excellent overall prognosis. On rare occasions when severe perinatal respiratory distress is anticipated, a strategy with ECMO has been used.[13,15]

CONGENITAL CYSTIC ADENOMATOID MALFORMATION

CCAM is traditionally described as a multicystic lung mass resulting from a proliferation of terminal bronchiolar structures with an associated suppression of alveolar growth. On histologic examination, these cysts are lined by cuboidal or columnar epithelium.[18] A pathologic classification system adopted by Stocker[39] is important to note for historic purposes, but does not currently represent a helpful designation clinically to predict the natural history.

The Stocker classification system subdivided cysts based on cyst size into three major subtypes (Table 21-2).[39] Type I lesions have large multiple cysts of varying size, each measuring at least 2 cm and lined by a ciliated pseudostratified columnar epithelium. Type II cysts were also

TABLE 21-2

COMPARISON OF CCAM CLASSIFICATION SCHEMES

	Stocker (Classic)	Anatomic (Current)
Cyst Size	I, >2 cm	Macrocystic, >5 mm
	II, <2 cm	Microcystic, <5 mm
	III, solid	
Associated Anomalies	II	Microcystic
Prognosis		
Favorable	I	Macrocystic
Unfavorable	III	Microcystic
Echogenicity		
Solid (echogenic)	III	Microcystic
Cystic (echolucent)	I, II	Macrocystic

multilocular, but of smaller and more uniform daughter cyst size less than 2 cm and lined by ciliated cuboidal to columnar epithelium. Type III lesions are macroscopically and microscopically solid, without cystic components. Many problems of overlap with hybrid lesions and atypical cysts that do not fit this classification system have subsequently been identified.[40,41] One published report documented a complex lesion with elements of CCAM, BPS, and bronchogenic cyst, prompting speculation about a previously unidentified common ontogeny.[41]

Currently a more generalized classification of cysts into macrocystic (>5 mm diameter) and microcystic (<5 mm diameter) subtypes is more commonly used and seems more clinically relevant (see Table 21-2).[42] The macrocystic lesions are not true cysts, as they do communicate with the more proximal conducting airways. These lesions therefore typically are first seen in early infancy with progressive respiratory distress, as air trapping leads to cystic expansion and compression of normal lung. These lesions are being identified prenatally with increasing frequency; they are only infrequently associated with hydrops or pulmonary hypoplasia. Therefore macrocystic lesions have a generally favorable prognosis and are frequently asymptomatic at birth.

Microcystic CCAM lesions can be distinguished from the macrocystic type radiographically, pathologically, and clinically.[16,42] These lesions appear more homogeneous and solid on imaging. Similar to the macrocystic lesions, they are not true cysts. The microcystic lesions, however, are currently believed to be more frequently associated with other developmental abnormalities, and therefore the patients have a poorer prognosis.[16,42] The small-cyst CCAMs may be seen in association with developmental airway obstruction due to bronchial atresia or stenosis. The pathologic features are consistent and demonstrate focal areas of increased bronchiolar proliferation, variable alveolar development, and regional displacement of unaffected lung parenchyma.

Macrocystic CCAMs most typically affect only one lobe and may have one or more very large dominant cyst-like structures with multiple smaller daughter cysts. All cysts have some respiratory epithelial lining, whereas some also contain mucigenic epithelium resembling stomach. In some series, at least 25% of these lesions have an associated systemic, nonpulmonary, arterial supply. Confusion between macrocystic and microcystic lesions may exist shortly after birth, with both appearing as solid on early imaging. The cystic nature of the macrocystic lesions becomes apparent within a few postnatal days as amniotic fluid is replaced by air (Fig. 21-3). When very large cystic changes occur on imaging, other diagnoses to be considered include pulmonary interstitial emphysema (PIE), pneumatocele, pleuropulmonary blastoma, and intraparenchymal lymphangioma.

BRONCHOPULMONARY SEQUESTRATION

Sequestrations should be distinguishable from CCAMs by their pathologic, radiologic, and clinical characteristics.[16] A pulmonary sequestration is classically described as a cystic mass of nonfunctioning lung parenchyma that lacks a demonstrable connection to the tracheobronchial tree. In addition, this sequestered mass of lung tissue receives its blood supply anomalously from the systemic circulation. However, as with many of these lesions, the exceptions are as much the rule, with a wide variety of arterial supply and venous drainage combinations being described. Because of the anomalous blood supply, many believe the true embryologic derivation of these lesions should classify them as vascular anomalies. Because the majority of the clinical symptoms are respiratory, we will continue the more traditional classification of these lesions as lung lesions. Sequestrations are largely solid lesions. Pathologically these lesions demonstrate parenchymal maldevelopment, reflected as microcystic abnormalities similar to type II or microcystic CCAMs.

Sequestrations are typically classified as either intralobar or extralobar (Fig. 21-4). If the lesion is contained within the same investing pleura as normal lung, it is intralobar. Extralobar lesions are found outside the investing parietal pleura of frequently adjacent normal lung. Intralobar sequestrations are usually found in the lower lobe basilar segments and more commonly in the patient's left hemithorax. Extralobar lesions have a more variable occurrence pattern; however, their typical location is basilar, below the more normally formed lung (Fig. 21-5A). Extralobar lesions also have been found in the upper thorax, below the diaphragm in the upper abdomen, throughout the mediastinum, and within the pericardium[16,34,43-47] (Fig. 21-5B).

Many sequestrations are asymptomatic. Given the lack of communication to the tracheobronchial tree, infectious complications develop most likely from hematogenous seeding. Extralobar sequestrations are frequently identified as an incidental finding, with approximately 15% occurring below the diaphragm and, not infrequently, in association with a left-side congenital diaphragmatic hernia (CDH).[46] The radiographic findings for either intralobar or extralobar sequestrations are usually that of an opacified solid lung mass or a cystic parenchymal lesion with an air-fluid level secondary to infection.

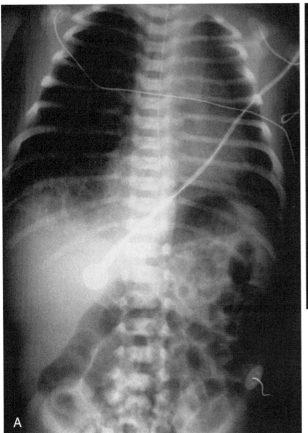

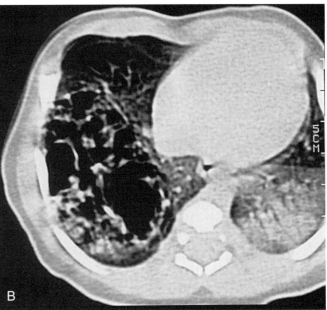

FIGURE 21-3. *A,* A chest radiograph of a neonate with mild respiratory distress and oxygen requirement; note the small cystic appearance of the right lower lung field overlying the diaphragm and the shifting of the mediastinum to the left. *B,* A chest computed tomography scan demonstrates multiple small and larger cysts suggestive of a type II congenital cystic adenomatoid malformation of the right lower lobe.

Intralobar BPS accounts for the majority of lesions overall, yet extralobar lesions are more likely to have other associated anomalies in as many as 50% to 65% of cases.[47,48] The most commonly recognized anomalies associated with BPS, in addition to CDH, include diaphragmatic eventration, and other foregut malformations such as tracheoesophageal fistula and esophageal duplication.[43,44,48]

Historically, angiography was performed to confirm the anomalous systemic blood supply and to help in planning surgical management. Currently, the hallmark anomalous vascular supply can be identified by Doppler US, CT, or MR angiography or a combination of these. Typically a single large feeding vessel arising from the abdominal aorta is found (Fig. 21-6). This vessel can be typically found within a pedicle or stalk. However, not infrequently, more than one major vessel is found to supply the sequestration. The venous anatomy may be even more variable, with systemic, bronchial, and azygous system involvement. If a bronchus is found within the pedicle, communication with the gastrointestinal tract should be sought.

SURGICAL MANAGEMENT OF CONGENITAL CYSTIC ADENOMATOID MALFORMATION AND BPS

The presence of a CCAM or a BPS, regardless of symptoms, is an indication for resection, given the risk of either infection or malignant transformation. Either pleuropulmonary blastoma in infants or bronchoalveolar carcinoma have been reported in older children and perhaps adults with known CCAMs.[35-38] The preoperative CT of the chest can help in planning the operative approach. Traditionally, a lateral thoracotomy is performed, depending on the exact location of the target lesion.

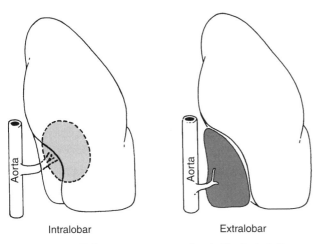

Intralobar   Extralobar

FIGURE 21-4. Pulmonary sequestration is illustrated. It occurs either within the lung or outside the visceral pleura.

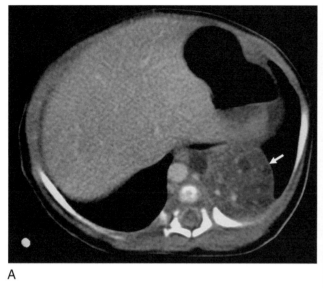

A

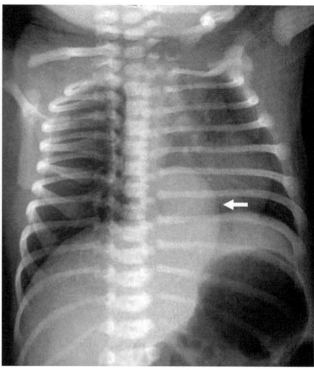

B

FIGURE 21-5. *A,* This computed tomography scan demonstrates an extralobar sequestration in the typical basilar location of the left chest (*arrow*). *B,* This chest radiograph shows a large transdiaphragmatic extralobar sequestration (*arrow*).

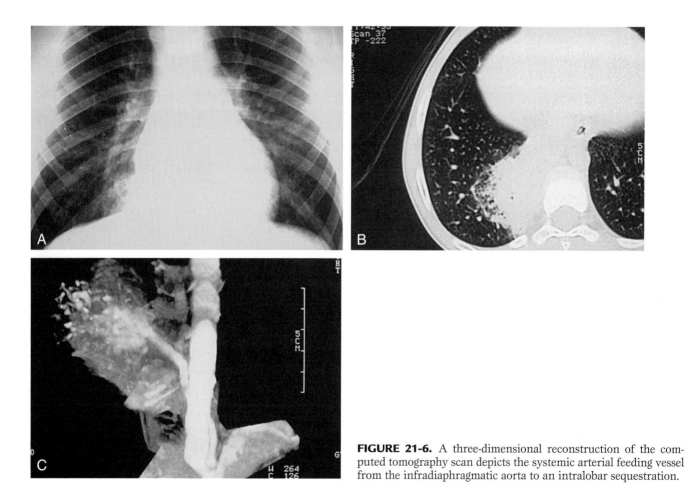

FIGURE 21-6. A three-dimensional reconstruction of the computed tomography scan depicts the systemic arterial feeding vessel from the infradiaphragmatic aorta to an intralobar sequestration.

Either a lobectomy, or less frequently, a segmentectomy allows the complete extirpation of the majority of these lesions. For extralobar sequestrations, the preoperative imaging and localizing studies are even more important, given the potential for various lesions to be located below the diaphragm. Obviously, for extralobar lesions, a nonanatomic resection is possible and is facilitated by the stalk or pedicle-like nature of the feeding vessel.

Recently the thoracoscopic approach to the resection of CCAMs and BPSs has been described.[49] This approach was driven by the experience with prenatally diagnosed asymptomatic lesions at birth. If the perinatal chest radiograph fails to demonstrate the lesion and the child is asymptomatic, an elective CT scan of the chest is performed within the first 2 to 3 months. If the CT scan demonstrates the lesion, an elective thoracoscopic resection is planned. The first reported large series of thoracoscopic pulmonary procedures in infants and children was in 2000.[50] The vast majority of the 113 cases reported were pulmonary biopsies and wedge resections. Lobectomies were performed with a hybrid technique of directed thoracoscopy and minithoracotomy. Most of these procedures were accomplished with instruments such as the endoscopic stapler, which were adopted from the adult surgical practice of video-assisted thoracoscopic surgery. These instruments were subsequently found to be too large for use in the neonate's chest, because the cartridges routinely span the infant's entire hemithorax. This experience pre-dated many of the instruments that are currently used for hemostasis and tissue sealing. The Ligasure (Tyco, Inc., Norwalk, CT), for example, also can be used to seal neonatal lung parenchyma when an incomplete fissure is encountered.

In 2003, two series of totally thoracoscopic lobectomies, performed mostly for congenital lung lesions, were reported.[49,51] The majority of these were lower lobe resections, which are technically less difficult than upper lobectomies. In the larger series of 44 patients, all but one were completed thoracoscopically, and all infants survived.[51] The other reported 14 patients, all of whom had a prenatal diagnosis of CCAM (12 cases) or BPS (2) and underwent operation at a mean age of 6 months.[49] In this series, no conversions were made to an open procedure, and no intraoperative complications occurred. The results of these studies compared quite favorably with the more standard open technique. An obvious benefit is the avoidance of an early thoracotomy, which is known to be associated with a higher incidence of shoulder girdle weakness and scoliosis.[52]

With further evolution of technique, a broader range of lesions, such as bilateral disease and very large lesions, can be approached. Our current thoracoscopic technique includes chest insufflation to 4 torr, while the smallest of infants are maintained on double-lung ventilation. Most procedures can be completed intracorporally with a combination of 3-mm instruments, hook cautery, and the Ligasure device.[49] A 4-mm telescope and slight enlargement of this port site facilitates removal of the lesion. Three cannulas are usually all that is necessary to complete most thoracoscopic cases. However, it is important to position the camera port in line with the fissure

for dissection. An incomplete fissure is dissected and sealed with the Ligasure. Pulmonary vessels, including both arteries and veins that measure less than 7 mm, can be sealed before division with the Ligasure. Larger pulmonary vessels either may be suture ligated or may be clipped with 5- or 10-mm endoclips. Operations on very small infants necessitate intracorporeal suturing of the bronchus, because the current-generation endostaplers are too large for the infant's hemithorax.

Postoperative hospitalization is usually 1 to 2 days. It may be best to stage bilateral cases to give the remaining normal lung a period of accommodation between elective resections. Currently, the main limiting factor for the thoracoscopic approach is the child who is unstable because of the mass effect, which also may eliminate the effective working space for thoracoscopic resection. On occasion, intraoperative cyst rupture has provided the necessary working space for resection by minimal-access techniques. An exceedingly large lesion requiring pneumonectomy also will require additional plans for managing potential pulmonary hypertension or the temporary respiratory insufficiency that can result from pulmonary hypoplasia. ECMO can be used as a temporizing measure for each of these potential complications.

EMPHYSEMATOUS LESIONS

On occasion, congenital lobar emphysema (CLE) can be confused with macrocystic CCAM.[31,32] Radiographically, CLE appears as overdistention involving one or more lobes (Fig. 21-7A). This is believed to be caused by a variant of bronchomalacia with focal cartilaginous deficiency of the tracheobronchial tree, leading to regional airway collapse with expiration.[2,3] With postnatal air exchange, air trapping behind a structurally inadequate conducting airway leads to emphysematous changes. Other rare causes include extrinsic compression from anomalous pulmonary vessels or by a very large ductus arteriosus[3,53] (Fig. 21-7B). In the premature infant with significant respiratory distress syndrome, pulmonary interstitial emphysema (PIE), in its more chronic form, can evolve into a variant of CLE. One-third of cases remain classified as idiopathic.[2,3,54]

The clinical presentation of CLE can be as varied as its numerous etiologies. With massive lobar overdistention (Fig. 21-7C), compression of the normal lung and the mediastinum can cause respiratory and cardiovascular collapse. In these cases, emergency thoracotomy is necessary and life saving. In less dramatic presentations, progressive tachypnea and expansion lead to assisted ventilation and radiographic identification of the offending lesion. Plain chest radiographs and CT scans have been used both for diagnosis and for determining the appropriateness of surgical resection and the boundaries of normal lung. In most cases, resection of the abnormal lung allows re-expansion and compensatory growth of the normal lung. Expectant management is acceptable for the largely asymptomatic lesion.[54] However, complete resolution of the radiographic findings is rare, and for this reason, surgical resection is indicated.[54-56]

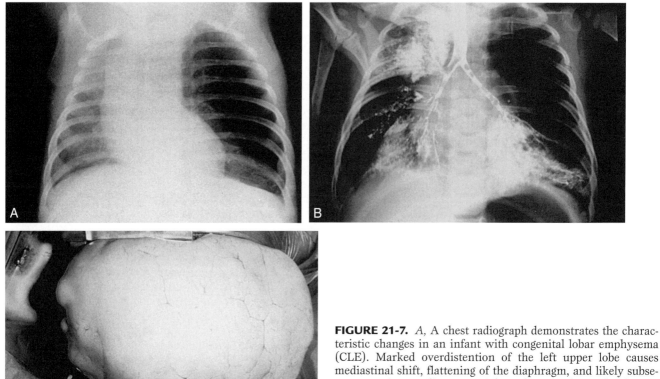

FIGURE 21-7. *A,* A chest radiograph demonstrates the characteristic changes in an infant with congenital lobar emphysema (CLE). Marked overdistention of the left upper lobe causes mediastinal shift, flattening of the diaphragm, and likely subsequent respiratory distress. *B,* A bronchogram shows the absence or occlusion of the left upper lobe bronchus, producing the typical findings in CLE. *C,* This operative photograph demonstrates the dramatic herniation of an emphysematous lobe through the thoracotomy.

The aforementioned concerns of retained secretions as a nidus for infection exist with CLE as for CCAMs.

The acquired forms of emphysematous pulmonary lesions generally are first seen in a more time-dependent fashion than are the lesions caused purely by congenital structural defects.[54-56] A history of chronic ventilation of a poorly compliant premature lung precedes the development of PIE and its sequelae of lobar emphysema or parenchymal cysts. Many of these lesions will resolve spontaneously. However, if the mass effect produces some of the same clinical symptoms of compression of the normal lung and mediastinum, then surgical intervention is indicated. In the most chronic forms of CLE, operative therapy for cystic pulmonary lesions from prolonged ventilator barotrauma can be quite difficult, because little residual normal lung will be available for continued gas exchange.

PNEUMATOCELE AND POST-TRAUMATIC PULMONARY CYST

Two other cystic pulmonary lesions that resemble CLE and CCAMs are post-traumatic pulmonary cysts and pneumatocele. Pneumatoceles are postinfectious pulmonary cysts that most typically occur after lobar pneumonia caused by *Staphylococcus aureus* (Fig. 21-8*A* and *B*).[3,57]

This lesion can radiographically resemble CLE. However, the timing and history of a consolidating pneumonia with cavitation makes the diagnostic distinction. These lesions have a very thin wall left from the destruction of normal parenchyma due to the bacterial infection, but they frequently regress. Post-traumatic lesions occur in areas of contused parenchyma or bronchial disruption.[58-60] Like many other post-traumatic cystic lesions, these cysts are pseudocysts without an epithelial lining.[58-60] Unlike other traumatic pseudocysts, pulmonary traumatic cysts may resolve with observation alone if infection does not supervene.[61]

LOBULATION ANOMALIES AND ISOMERISM

Significant variations of lung anatomy occur with respect to the pattern of lung lobulation. The most common variability is an absent or incomplete fissure separating the anatomic lobes. Absent fissures occur in 30% of individuals, whereas incomplete fissures can be seen in more than half of the general population.[2,3] Despite this variability, these variations do not indicate disordered lobulation and, as such, have no clinical significance, other than to the operating surgeon. True lobulation and segmentation abnormalities can result in extra lobes such as a cardiac lobe (division of the left lower lobe into two

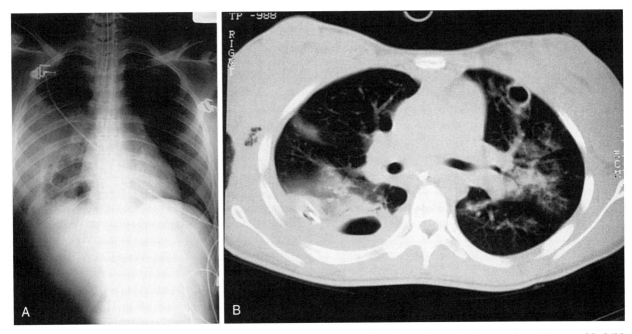

FIGURE 21-8. *A,* This chest radiograph shows right lower lobe consolidation with cystic changes in a 10-year-old child with staphylococcal pneumonia. *B,* The computed tomography scan of the same patient demonstrates the emergence of changes consistent with pneumatoceles in both right and left hemithoraces.

separate lobes) or supersegmentation of the lower lobes.[2,3] The majority of these anomalies are without clinical relevance. Lobulation anomalies can occur with abnormal bronchial patterns, as seen with accessory tracheal lobes with direct airway connection to the trachea.

The azygous lobe is a malformation usually of the right upper lobe that is caused by an aberrant azygous vein, suspended by pleura, which acts as a mesentery and produces the defect.[2] These lesions also most likely are clinically silent. Reports have mentioned esophageal lung, also termed *communicating bronchopulmonary foregut malformation,* in which a tract is preserved between the respiratory and alimentary system.[62] These anomalies are almost always seen in association with esophageal atresia and tracheal stenosis or fistula.

Pulmonary isomerism is the mirror-image reversal of pulmonary lobar sidedness, in which the left lung has three lobes, and the right has two.[2] This abnormality may or may not be associated with *situs inversus,* but nearly always involves other organ system abnormalities, most notably congenital cardiac lesions. In addition, asplenia and polysplenia have been described with relative frequency. The associated cardiac lesions are usually responsible for the majority of the clinically relevant morbidity.

PULMONARY AGENESIS, APLASIA, AND HYPOPLASIA

Pulmonary agenesis is the complete failure of both airway and parenchymal development. Pulmonary aplasia is used to describe the incomplete development of lung parenchyma supplied by a rudimentary bronchus. Pulmonary hypoplasia is distinguished by a normal tracheobronchial tree and underdeveloped pulmonary parenchyma. Agenesis can occur either unilaterally or bilaterally; in the latter case, this would be incompatible with life. In cases of unilateral agenesis, frequently other associated severe developmental abnormalities are seen.[2] Most commonly, these include the elements of the VACTERL syndrome (nonrandom association of malformations including V [vertebral anomalies], A [anal atresia], C [cardiac anomalies], TE [tracheoesophageal fistula or esophageal atresia], R [renal/urinary anomalies], and L [limb defect]) anomalies. The etiology and embryonic pathophysiology of aplasia and agenesis remain largely unknown.

Pulmonary hypoplasia is the most commonly encountered anomaly of underdeveloped lung parenchyma, with a variety of known causes. The compressive effects of lung, mediastinal, or cardiac masses or herniated abdominal viscera, as seen with CDH, can result in arrested pulmonary parenchymal development. Other causes include the abnormal mechanical effects of fetal diaphragmatic excursion or fetal lung and amniotic fluid volume. Specifically, abnormal or absent fetal breathing or oligohydramnios, with or without renal dysgenesis or obstructive uropathy, can be causative of pulmonary hypoplasia.[63]

The diagnosis and treatment of pulmonary hypoplasia is dependent on the underlying etiology. For example, severe respiratory impairment can be seen with pulmonary hypoplasia from a CDH.[63] In these cases, stabilization of the underlying physiologic impairment is the priority. In cases of aplasia or agenesis, the chest radiographs may demonstrate opacification of the ipsilateral hemithorax and ipsilateral mediastinal shift with volume loss. In addition, asymmetry of the chest with obviously impaired respiratory movement of the affected side is seen. Treatment is initially directed at any associated anomalies, with particular focus on congenital cardiac lesions. If surgery is indicated to remove a nonfunctioning lobe or lung, every effort is made to preserve functional parenchyma. In cases that render an empty hemithorax, consideration should be given to the intrathoracic placement of a tissue expander to prevent significant musculoskeletal disfigurement from the eventual mediastinal and skeletal shift toward the volume loss side (Fig. 21-9).

BRONCHIAL LESIONS

As has been discussed, many of the commonly recognized congenital bronchial malformations, such as bronchial agenesis, atresia, or stenosis, produce parenchymal abnormalities that distinguish these lesions clinically. However, a subset of congenital malformations is unique to the bronchial tree, traditionally grouped under the nomenclature of bronchogenic cysts or foregut duplication cysts. As discussed earlier, the embryologic derivation of these from common foregut anlagen, their occurrence in the chest, and their most frequent clinical symptoms make their inclusion appropriate in a discussion of BPMs. The nomenclature in common usage remains confusing. In general, the term foregut duplication cyst appropriately links these lesions embryologically as arising from a common developmental structure. When one considers their histologic architecture, these lesions can be divided into three subdivisions: (1) bronchogenic cysts, (2) enteric duplication cysts, and (3) neuroenteric cysts, all of which reveal their common endodermal origins.[64]

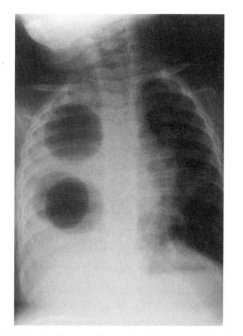

FIGURE 21-9. A chest radiograph of a 3-year-old who underwent right pulmonary plumbage with three Ping-Pong balls 1 year earlier.

Bronchogenic cysts are lined by respiratory bronchial epithelium, are mucus filled, and may contain cartilage in their walls.[2,64] Enteric duplication cysts are lined by intestinal epithelium (either esophageal or gastric) and may contain smooth muscle. Most commonly, enteric cysts occur within the muscular wall of an otherwise intact esophagus without communication with the lumen. Neuroenteric cysts are the embryologic exception, arising from a failure of separation of notochord and foregut. These lesions contain gastrointestinal mucosa with well-developed smooth muscle walls and communicate with the central nervous system (CNS), spinal cord, and perhaps dura. This association explains their frequent coexistence with congenital vertebral defects, most commonly hemivertebrae.[65] Neuroenteric cysts are, however, much rarer than either bronchogenic or enteric cysts. (Enteric duplication cysts and neuroenteric cysts are discussed further in Chapter 39.)

Foregut duplications must be considered in the differential diagnosis of a cystic mediastinal lesion (Fig. 21-10). Bronchogenic cysts can be diagnosed prenatally, perinatally, or in an older child. The lesion may be seen in the newborn with acute respiratory distress because a large lesion can compress adjacent normal lung tissue. They may be totally asymptomatic in an older child or may occur with infection in an occult lesion. Occasionally, the lesion is discovered incidentally on chest radiograph performed for unrelated reasons. Further studies should include CT of the chest to identify the lesion and its relation to surrounding structures. Mediastinal cysts also have been identified on prenatal US and are followed up perinatally with these same imaging modalities. Close scrutiny of the mediastinal structures is indicated, as all bronchogenic cysts, whether symptomatic or not, should be excised, given their propensity for expansion, infection, and hemorrhage.[66] As bronchogenic cysts are most commonly discrete lesions, they can be successfully approached thoracoscopically. Care must be taken to avoid injury to either the bronchial or esophageal wall, particularly when they share a common wall. The development of intracorporeal suturing techniques has enhanced our ability to excise these lesions completely endoscopically. Previous infection makes their removal more difficult by either means, given the fibrovascular reaction that occurs surrounding infected lesions.

Bronchogenic cysts also may occur within the pulmonary parenchyma separate from the hilar structures. Peripheral bronchogenic cysts may be multiple, in which case, they are more appropriately termed bronchiolar cysts or cystic bronchiectasis.[2] The more peripheral bronchogenic or pulmonary cysts are lined by ciliated respiratory epithelium and likely result from abnormalities during the latter portion of the pseudoglandular stage of lung development, as contrasted with the more central lesions that are true foregut abnormalities.[2] These lesions invariably communicate with the airway and often create obstruction of accompanying bronchi. Peripheral lesions may initially be seen early from the accumulation of mucus that leads to obstruction, or they may be seen later as infected peripheral lesions. They may be confused with necrotizing pneumonia. Diagnostic evaluation

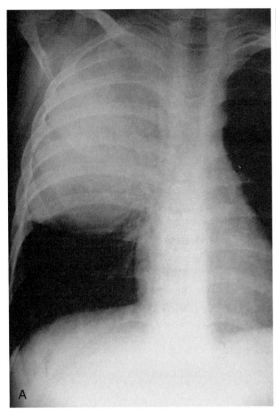

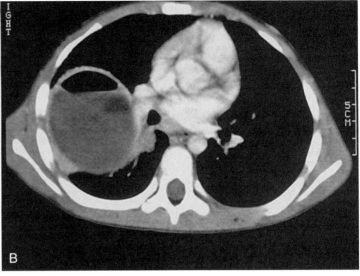

FIGURE 21-10. *A,* A chest radiograph of a 10-year-old child with a right upper lobe infiltrate. *B,* A chest computed tomography scan demonstrates a large bronchogenic cyst with an air-fluid level indicating bronchial communication.

almost always includes CT. The treatment is surgical resection, given the natural history of persistence with recurring symptoms.

VASCULAR ANOMALIES

Although the majority of pulmonary vascular anomalies are more appropriately discussed with congenital cardiac defects, several vascular malformations of the peripheral pulmonary parenchyma are within the scope of treatment for most pediatric surgeons. Arteriovenous malformations (AVMs) of the lung typically are initially seen with a triad of symptoms including dyspnea on exertion, cyanosis, and clubbing of the digits. The symptoms are produced because of pathologic right-to-left shunting produced by these lesions. Radiographically, pulmonary AVMs appear as solid, frequently peripheral, lobulated masses of varying size. CT scanning reveals the tortuous nature of the involved vessels, leading to more specific diagnostic testing by angiography and with therapeutic capability offered by embolization. Complications of pulmonary AVMs include cardiac failure and, less commonly, rupture and hemorrhage, either into a neighboring bronchus or into the pleura. Treatment options include segmental surgical resection or catheter-directed embolization (which may be the preferred approach for the emergently bleeding AVM).

A rare entity known commonly as *scimitar syndrome* is a distinct variation of both BPS and the AVM anomalies. Also known as congenital venolobar syndrome, scimitar syndrome consists of a hypoplastic and malformed right lung with anomalous venous return directly to the vena cava.[2] Similarly, the arterial supply is variable and normally includes a hypoplastic right pulmonary artery and a systemic arterial branch from the aorta to the right lower lobe. Occasionally confused with BPS, this lesion always involves the right lung and maintains its bronchial connection to the airway. The syndrome takes its name from the scimitar appearance on a plain radiograph, arising as the lateral outline of the abnormal pulmonary venous connection with the right atrium. This constellation of anatomic abnormalities produces a left-to-right shunt. Associated intracardiac anomalies frequently occur. Treatment options include redirecting the venous drainage to the left atrium or a right lower lobectomy.

Lymphatic malformations of the thorax are rare but, when present, can take one of two different forms. Congenital pulmonary lymphangiectasia is an anomaly with diffuse dysplasia and dilation of the pulmonary lymphatics. This can be seen in association with generalized lymphangiectasia; it may be secondary to pulmonary venous hypertension; or it can be seen as an isolated finding. With generalized lymphangiectasia, the treatment is supportive, whereas the less frequent focal abnormalities may be amenable to surgical excision. Congenital chylothorax is the accumulation of chyle in the pleural space. In the newborn, this results either from a congenital abnormality of the thoracic duct or from birth trauma. Frequently, an exact etiology cannot be identified, rendering the label "idiopathic." For the majority of congenital chylothoraces, treatment is supportive, with enteral diet modification or total parenteral nutrition. Serial thoracenteses or tube thoracostomy or both are the mainstays of therapeutic interventions that are largely temporizing and not curative. Recalcitrant cases may necessitate interventional radiology-guided attempts at embolization, thoracoscopic thoracic duct ligation, or placement of a thoracoabdominal shunt. These lesions may be fatal.

REFERENCES

1. Kluth D, Steding G, Seidl W: The embryology of foregut malformations. J Pediatr Surg 22:389–393, 1987.
2. Skandalakis JE: The trachea and lungs. In Wood Gray S (ed): Embryology for Surgeons. Baltimore, Williams & Wilkins, 1994, pp 414–490.
3. Hebra A, Othersen HB, Tagge EP: Bronchopulmonary malformations. In Ashcraft KW (ed): Pediatric Surgery. New York, WB Saunders, 2000, pp 273–286.
4. Kluth D, Fiegel H: The embryology of the foregut. Semin Pediatr Surg 12:3–9, 2003.
5. Chuang PT, McMahon AP: Branching morphogenesis of the lung: New molecular insights into an old problem. Trends Cell Biol 13:86–91, 2003.
6. Weaver M, Batts L, Hogan BL: Tissue interactions pattern the mesenchyme of the embryonic mouse lung. Dev Biol 258:169–184, 2003.
7. Perl AK, Wert SE, Nagy A, et al: Early restriction of peripheral and proximal cell lineages during formation of the lung. Proc Natl Acad Sci U S A 99:10482–10487, 2002.
8. Mucenski ML, Wert SE, Nation JM, et al: Beta-catenin is required for specification of proximal/distal cell fate during lung morphogenesis. J Biol Chem 278:40231–40238, 2003.
9. Perl AK, Hokuto I, Impagnatiello MA, et al: Temporal effects of Sprouty on lung morphogenesis. Dev Biol 258:154–168, 2003.
10. Reynolds PR, Mucenski ML, Whitsett JA: Thyroid transcription factor (TTF)-1 regulates the expression of midkine (MK) during lung morphogenesis. Dev Dyn 222:227–237, 2003.
11. Izvolsky KI, Shoykhet D, Yang Y, et al: Heparan sulfate-FGF10 interactions during lung morphogenesis. Dev Biol 258:185–200, 2003.
12. Harrison MR, Evans MI, Adzick NS, et al (eds): The Unborn Patient. Philadelphia, WB Saunders, 2001.
13. Adzick NS, Harrison MR, Crombleholme TM, et al: Fetal lung lesions: Management and outcome. Am J Obstet Gynecol 179:884–889, 1998.
14. Quinn TM, Hubbard AM, Adzick NS: Prenatal magnetic resonance imaging enhances prenatal diagnosis. J Pediatr Surg 33:312–316, 1998.
15. Adzick NS, Flake AW, Crombleholme TM: Management of congenital lung lesions. Semin Pediatr Surg 12:10–16, 2003.
16. Tsao K, Albanese CT, Harrison MR: Prenatal therapy for thoracic and mediastinal lesions. World J Surg 27:77–83, 2003.
17. Gushiken BJ, Filly RA: Sonography for fetal thoracic intervention. In Harrison MR, Evans MI, Adzick NS, et al (eds): The Unborn Patient. Philadelphia, WB Saunders, 2001, pp 95–109.
18. Langston C: New concepts in the pathology of congenital lung malformations. Semin Pediatr Surg 12:17–37, 2003.
19. Hubbard AM, Adzick NS, Crombleholme TM, et al: Congenital chest lesions: Diagnosis and characterization with prenatal MR imaging. Radiology 212:43–48, 1999.
20. Crombleholme TM, Coleman B, Hedrick H, et al: Cystic adenomatoid malformation volume ratio predicts outcome in prenatally diagnosed cystic adenomatoid malformation of the lung. J Pediatr Surg 37:331–338, 2002.
21. Tsao K, Hawgood S, Vu L, et al: Resolution of hydrops fetalis in congenital cystic adenomatoid malformation after prenatal steroid therapy. J Pediatr Surg 38:508–510, 2003.
22. MacGillivray TE, Harrison MR, Goldstein RB: Disappearing fetal lung lesions. J Pediatr Surg 28:1321–1325, 1993.
23. daSilva O, Ramanan R, Romano W: Nonimmune fetal hydrops fetalis, pulmonary sequestration, and favorable neonatal outcome. Obstet Gynecol 88:681–683, 1996.
24. Bernaschek G, Deutinger J, Hansmann M: Feto-amniotic shunting: Report of the experience of four European centers. Prenat Diagn 14:821–833, 1994.
25. Chao SL, Vitale DJ, Minton SD: Successful fetal therapy for cystic adenomatoid malformation associated with second trimester hydrops. Am J Obstet Gynecol 157:294–297, 1987.
26. Baxter JK, Johnson MP, Woilson RD: Thoracoamniotic shunts: Pregnancy outcome for congenital cystic adenomatoid malformation and pleural effusion. Am J Obstet Gynecol 185:S245, 1998.
27. Harrison MR, Bressack MA, Churg AM, et al: Correction of congenital diaphragmatic hernia in utero, II: Simulated correction permits fetal lung growth with survival at birth. Surgery 88:260–268, 1980.
28. Harrison MR, Jester JA, Ross NA: Correction of congenital diaphragmatic hernia in utero, I: The model: Intrathoracic balloon produces fatal pulmonary hypoplasia. Surgery 88:174–182, 1980.
29. Rice HE, Estes JM, Hedrick MH, et al: Congenital cystic adenomatoid malformation: A sheep model of fetal hydrops. J Pediatr Surg 29:692–696, 1994.
30. Midgley DY, Harding K: The Mirror syndrome. Eur J Obstet Gynecol Rep Biol 88:201–202, 2000.
31. Richards DS, Langham MR, Dolson LH: Antenatal presentation of a child with congenital lobar emphysema. J Ultrasound Med 11:165–168, 1992.
32. Albright EB, Crane JP, Shackelford GD: Prenatal diagnosis of a bronchogenic cyst. J Ultrasound Med 7:90–95, 1988.
33. DeBustamante TD, Azpeitia J, Miralles M, et al: Prenatal sonographic detection of pericardial teratoma. J Clin Ultrasound 28:194–198, 2000.
34. Bromley B, Parad R, Estroff JA, et al: Fetal lung masses: prenatal course and outcome. J Ultrasound Med 14:927–936, 1995.
35. Benjamin DR, Cahill JL: Bronchoalveolar carcinoma of the lung and congenital cystic adenomatoid malformation. Am J Pathol 95:889–892, 1991.
36. d'Agostino S, Bonoldi E, Dante S: Embryonal rhabdomyosarcoma of the lung arising in cystic adenomatoid malformation. J Pediatr Surg 32:1381–1383, 1997.
37. Murphy JJ, Blair GK, Fraser GC: Rhabdomyosarcoma arising within congenital pulmonary cysts: Reports of three cases. J Pediatr Surg 27:1364–1367, 1992.
38. Ribet ME, Copin MC, Soots JG: Bronchioalveolar carcinoma and congenital cystic adenomatoid malformation. Ann Thorac Surg 60:1126–1128, 1995.
39. Stocker TJ, Manewell JE, Drake RM: Congenital cystic adenomatoid malformation of the lung: Classification and morphologic spectrum. Hum Pathol 8:155–171, 1977.
40. Cass DL, Crombleholme TM, Howell L, et al: Cystic lung lesions with systemic arterial blood supply: A hybrid of congenital cystic adenomatoid malformation and bronchopulmonary sequestration. J Pediatr Surg 32:986–990, 1997.
41. MacKenzie TC, Guttenberg ME, Nisenbaum HL, et al: A fetal lung lesion consisting of bronchogenic cyst, bronchopulmonary sequestration and congenital cystic adenomatoid malformation: The missing link? Fetal Diagn Ther 6:193–195, 2001.
42. Adzick NS, Harrison MR, Glick PL: Fetal cystic adenomatoid malformation: Prenatal diagnosis and natural history. J Pediatr Surg 20:483–488, 1985.
43. Gerle RD, Jaretzki A, Ashley CA, et al: Congenital bronchopulmonary foregut malformation: Pulmonary sequestration communicating with the gastrointestinal tract. N Engl J Med 278:1413–1419, 1968.
44. Buntain WL, Woolley MM, Mahour GH, et al: Pulmonary sequestration in children: A twenty-five year experience. Surgery 81:413–420, 1977.
45. Levi A, Findler M, Dolfin T, et al: Intrapericardial extralobar pulmonary sequestration in a neonate. Chest 98:1014–1015, 1990.
46. Lager DJ, Kuper KA, Haake GK: Subdiaphragmatic extralobar pulmonary sequestration. Arch Pathol Lab Med 115:536–538, 1991.
47. Piccione W, Burt ME: Pulmonary sequestration in the neonate. Chest 97:244–246, 1990.
48. Stocker JT: Sequestrations of the lung. Semin Diagn Pathol 3:106, 1986.
49. Albanese CT, Sydorak R, Tsao K, et al: Thoracoscopic lobectomy for prenatally diagnosed lung lesions. J Pediatr Surg 38:553–555, 2003.

50. Rothenberg SS: Thoracoscopic lung resection in children. J Pediatr Surg 35:271–275, 2000.
51. Rothenberg SS: Experience with thoracoscopic lobectomy in infants and children. J Pediatr Surg 38:102–104, 2003.
52. Rothenberg SS, Pokorny WJ: Experience with muscle sparing approach for thoracotomies in neonates, infants and children. J Pediatr Surg 27:1157–1159, 1992.
53. Hishitani T, Ogawa K, Hoshino K, et al: Lobar emphysema due to ductus arteriosus compressing right upper bronchus in an infant with congenital heart disease. Ann Thorac Surg 75:1308–1310, 2003.
54. Al-Bassam A, Al-Rabeeah A, Al-Nassar S, et al: Congenital cystic disease of the lung in infants and children (experience with 57 cases). Eur J Pediatr Surg 9:364–368, 1999.
55. Horak E, Bodner J, Gassner I, et al: Congenital cystic lung disease: Diagnostic and therapeutic considerations. Clin Pediatr 42: 251–261, 2003.
56. Ozcelik U, Gocmen A, Kiper N, et al: Congenital lobar emphysema: Evaluation and long-term follow-up of thirty cases at a single center. Pediatr Pulmonol 35:384–391, 2003.
57. Caksen H, Ozturk MK, Uzum K, et al: Pulmonary complications in patients with staphylococcal sepsis. Pediatr Int 42:268–271, 2000.
58. Crestanello JA, Samuels LE, Kaufman MS, et al: Posttraumatic pulmonary pseudocyst [comment]. J Trauma Injury Infect Crit Care 44:401–403, 1998.
59. Evans DA, Bokulic RE: Radiological case of the month: Posttraumatic pseudocysts. Arch Pediatr Adolesc Med 151:47–49, 1997.
60. Schimpl G, Schneider U: Traumatic pneumatoceles in an infant: Case report and review of the literature. Eur J Pediatr Surg 6:104–106, 1996.
61. Gincherman Y, Luketich JD, Kaiser LR: Successful nonoperative management of secondarily infected pulmonary pseudocyst: Case report. J Trauma Inj Infect Crit Care 38:960–963, 1995.
62. Saydam TC, Mychaliska GB, Harrison MR: Esophageal lung with multiple congenital anomalies: Conundrums in diagnosis and management. J Pediatr Surg 34:615–618, 1999.
63. Sydorak RM, Hedrick MH, Longaker MT, et al: Pathophysiologic patterns influencing fetal surgery. World J Surg 27:45–53, 2003.
64. Philippart AI, Farmer DL: Benign mediastinal cysts and tumors. In Coran AG (ed): Pediatric Surgery. Philadelphia, Mosby, 1988, pp 839–851.
65. Azzie G, Beasley S: Diagnosis and treatment of foregut duplications. Semin Ped Surg 12:46–54, 2003.
66. Wilkinson CC, Albanese CT, Jennings RW, et al: Fetal neuroenteric cyst causing hydrops: Case report and review of the literature. Prenatal Diag 19:118–121, 1999.

CHAPTER 22

Acquired Lesions of the Lung and Pleura

Marc P. Michalsky, MD, and Bradley M. Rodgers, MD

Acquired pulmonary and pleural lesions in the pediatric age group continue to pose a significant challenge for the medical community. Despite dramatic advances in antibiotic therapy and the implementation of widespread immunization protocols, the emergence of opportunistic infections and resultant changes in disease patterns have led to increasing complexity with regard to adequate treatment modalities. The widespread and often inappropriate use of antibiotics, along with an increased incidence of immunocompromised children, as a result of better chemotherapeutic regimens and emergence of human immunodeficiency virus (HIV) infections, has led to recent increases in several acquired pulmonary and pleural entities previously regarded as being uncommon. Infectious diseases as a result of multiple drug-resistant bacterial organisms and, specifically, the recent re-emergence of tuberculosis, necessitate a multidisciplinary approach to the treatment of such disorders. The treatment of such disorders poses a significant challenge and necessitates that the surgeon caring for such children be well versed in the varied and often complex therapeutic options.

EMPYEMA

Empyema is the accumulation of infected fluid within the thoracic cavity. In the pediatric population, this pathophysiologic process is typically associated with severe pneumonia and an associated parapneumonic effusion. Although pneumonia remains the leading cause of thoracic empyema in both the pediatric and adult populations, other potential sources of infection resulting in the development of empyemas include the extension of mediastinal, retropharyngeal, and/or paravertebral infectious processes. In addition, empyema formation also has been shown to be associated with an immunocompromised state and also may be the consequence of direct trauma to the thoracic cavity.[1] Although the incidence of this disease process is reported to be as low as 0.6% in hospitalized pediatric patients,[1] the associated mortality may be as high as 8%,[2-6] making it a diagnostic

and therapeutic challenge for pediatric pulmonologists, infectious disease specialists, and surgeons alike.

Pathogenesis

The American Thoracic Society characterized three pathologic stages of empyema in the early 1960s that remain in use today.[7] Stage one, commonly referred to as the "exudative stage," generally consists of thin fluid (with minimal cells), which moves freely within the thoracic cavity and is associated with mobile lung parenchyma. This phase, often referred to as a "parapneumonic effusion" lasts for approximately 24 to 72 hours and is typically amenable to thoracentesis or chest-tube drainage without difficulty. Stage two, or the "fibrinopurulent stage," lasts for approximately 7 to 10 days and is marked by the presence of fibrinous debris and cell-laden fluid (large numbers of polymorphonuclear cells). At this phase, the fluid is often acidic, in comparison with fluid collected during the exudative stage. A notable difference, compared with the earlier disease process, is demonstrated by the fact that the fluid is often compartmentalized as a result of multiple loculations. The presence of organized loculations makes effective tube drainage more difficult to achieve. With this limitation in mind, the use of computed tomography becomes an invaluable tool when planning the placement of chest tubes in the hopes of establishing adequate drainage of the thoracic cavity. Stage three, or the "organizing stage," typically occurs 2 to 4 weeks after the initial process has begun and is marked by thickening of the visceral and parietal pleura as a consequence of significant fibroblast deposition. The result of this process is the establishment of an organized peel or rind, which is intimately associated with the visceral pleura and serves to entrap the underlying lung parenchyma.

The bacteriologic characteristics associated with thoracic empyemas have changed significantly over the past half century. Although pneumococcal species were the predominant organisms associated with the development of thoracic empyemas in the mid-20th century, the introduction of penicillin and pneumococcal vaccine resulted in *Staphylococcus aureus* now being the leading bacterial pathogen.[8] *Staphylococcus aureus* has been reported to be cultured in the majority of pediatric patients and in approximately 50% of adult patients with documented empyema.[8] Additional organisms include *Streptococcus pneumoniae, Haemophilus influenzae, Pseudomonas aeruginosa,* and several Bacteroides species. Recently, however, the effective treatment of *S. aureus* has resulted in the emergence of a variety of other species with a greater proportion of organisms from the gram-negative family.[7] Interestingly, more contemporary series cite a predominance of *H. influenzae* and streptococcal species among pediatric patients,[9–11] although it has been speculated that the increasing use of vaccination against *H. influenzae* may further affect the current trends.

Tube thoracostomy is rarely capable of completely evacuating the pleural space in a child that has progressed to an advanced disease stage (i.e., stages two and three). Most often, more invasive surgical techniques are required to ensure complete re-expansion of the affected lung.

Clinical Presentation and Diagnosis

Because the most common cause of empyema in children is infection related to a severe underlying pneumonia, the typical clinical presentation consists of a recent history of upper respiratory tract infection, high fevers, malaise, and cough. This clinical scenario often progresses to a state of respiratory distress, accompanied by severe malaise, fever, and pleuritic chest pain.[3,8,13,14] The typical appearance often includes lethargy with pronounced tachycardia, shallow and rapid breathing, and decreased breath sounds with dullness to percussion on the affected side. Dehydration requires aggressive resuscitation with intravenous fluids. Paralytic ileus is commonly encountered at the initial presentation.

A chest radiograph obtained at the time of presentation often reveals the presence of a moderate to large pleural effusion in conjunction with pleural thickening and underlying parenchymal disease (Fig. 22-1). The ability to differentiate between a simple parapneumonic effusion and an empyema lies in the ability to analyze the fluid. Thoracentesis may reveal thin fluid or turbid, foul-smelling fluid depending on the stage of the disease process. An initial Gram stain is satisfactory to confirm the diagnosis and may be the only analysis required. In instances in which the Gram stain is negative, in the face of a clinically suggestive diagnosis, evaluation of the fluid for specific gravity, lactate dehydrogenase (LDH), protein, and pH can provide support for the diagnosis. Laboratory analysis suggestive of empyema typically shows a specific gravity greater than 1.016, protein greater than 3 g/dL, LDH greater than 200 U/L, white blood cell (WBC) count greater than 15,000/mm^3, and a pleural fluid protein–to–serum protein ratio greater than 0.6.[14]

CT and/or ultrasonography (US) of the chest are not required during the initial diagnosis and/or treatment phase of patients with a thoracic empyema, but they may help in assessing the condition of underlying lung parenchyma during advanced stages of the disease process and in allowing identification of loculated fluid

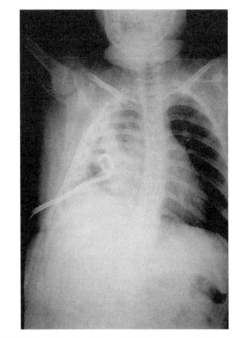

FIGURE 22-1. Chest radiograph of a 6-year-old boy with left-sided empyema.

collections that have not been adequately drained. The identification of complex and undrained loculations suggests the need for more aggressive surgical management (Fig. 22-2).

Therapy

The optimal course of therapy for children with empyema has been the topic of much debate over the past several decades. The mainstay of treatment is often dictated by the stage at which the individual patient is first seen. Several authors have proposed treatment pathways encompassing several clinical and radiologic factors

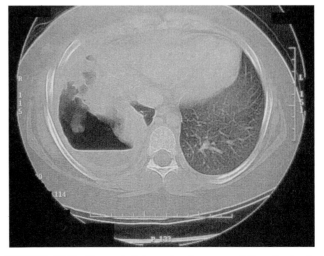

FIGURE 22-2. Computed tomography scan of the chest of a 6-year-old boy with a left-sided empyema.

in an effort to help define optimal therapeutic management of this patient population.[6]

For patients initially seen during stage I disease, the fluid is usually very thin and communicates freely throughout the thoracic cavity. The optimal treatment for empyema diagnosed in the exudative phase consists of drainage of the infected fluid to obliterate the empyema space. This can be accomplished through the use of paracentesis or chest-tube drainage. This type of intervention, in combination with the use of empiric antibiotics, guided by results of the initial Gram stain analysis, often results in rapid improvement in the clinical picture. The early clinical effects (24 to 48 hours) of closed chest-tube drainage and antibiotic therapy are often quite dramatic and include deffervescence of persistent fevers, decrease in the serum WBC count, and improved respiratory status. Failure to demonstrate rapid improvement often indicates the presence of residual, loculated fluid. A typical uncomplicated course involves removal of the chest tube(s) within 1 to 2 weeks' time, with subsequent discharge from the hospital soon thereafter.

Although serial chest radiographs are often used to guide the effectiveness of therapy in patients with early disease, the complete resolution of many radiologic findings may take weeks to months despite clinical improvement. The persistence of such radiographic abnormalities during the convalescent phase must be carefully considered. Specifically, when presented with a patient whose overall clinical picture continues to improve, one must consider the potential "lag time" encountered for resolution of radiographic abnormalities and thereby avoid the mistake of misinterpreting such radiologic findings as being consistent with a diagnosis of chronic empyema.

Advancement of the disease process to stage II is marked by a change in the consistency of the pleural fluid. During this stage, the fluid is often thick and turbid. In addition, the free communication, typically noted in the earlier disease process, is hindered by the presence of fibrinous strands within the fluid itself, as well as organized loculations. This results in the formation of multiple, noncommunicating compartments within the pleural space. When patients are encountered in the later stages of the disease process, or in those for whom initial therapy fails, with chest tube drainage and intravenous antibiotics, the use of more-invasive procedures must be considered.[9,10,15,16]

Although many authors have advocated the use of formal thoracotomy and decortication as the optimal treatment for patients at more advanced stages of the disease process, more recent series have promoted the use of video-assisted thoracoscopy (VAT) as a treatment modality in the case of thoracic empyema.[18] This minimally invasive technique allows complete evacuation, irrigation, and debridement of the involved hemithorax during the fibropurulent stage (stage II) but is less effective during the more advanced, or organized, stage (stage III). The overall inflammatory process often results in marked thickening of the parietal and visceral pleura (Fig. 22-3).

In addition to the use of VAT as a treatment modality for advanced-stage empyemas, variable reports exist on

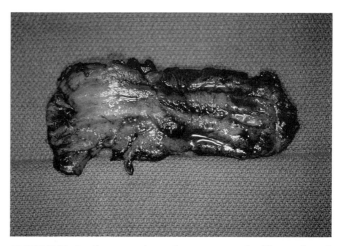

FIGURE 22-3. Gross specimen demonstrates significant pleural thickening encountered in the latter stages of thoracic empyema.

the use and effectiveness of fibrinolytic therapy in an effort to avoid the need for more-invasive procedures.[5] In a recent randomized trial comparing pleural drainage in combination with fibrinolytic therapy versus VAT in patients in the fibrinopurulent phase, investigators reported that a primary treatment strategy using VAT was associated with a higher efficacy, shorter hospitalization, and lower cost when compared with catheter-directed drainage and administration of fibrinolytic agents.[18]

Outcomes

Despite the complex nature of this disease process, and the need to individualize patient care, the overall morbidity and mortality is relatively low. Patients rarely have significant sequelae if treated successfully, although some reports relate long-term pleural scarring and restrictive pulmonary pathophysiology as the result of a prior history of empyema. The recent acceptance of VAT as an effective tool in the case of patients with more advanced disease or in patients whose early disease process progresses despite closed-tube drainage (with or without concomitant fibrinolytic therapy) has made an important impact in the overall cost and time of hospitalization, without sacrificing treatment efficacy.[18]

BRONCHIECTASIS

First described by Laenec,[19] in 1819, bronchiectasis is defined as a permanent dilatation of segmental airways and has been sited as the cause for a significant number of deaths due to respiratory insufficiency seen in the century and a half since its initial description. Reid,[20] in 1950, described three pathologic forms of bronchiectasis: saccular, cylindrical, and fusiform or varicose. Saccular bronchiectasis tends to occur in third- and fourth-order bronchioles, whereas cylindrical bronchiectasis occurs in sixth- to seventh-order bronchioles. The fusiform variety has an intermediate type of pathology and involvement.

Many forms of cylindrical bronchiectasis are completely reversible with control of the underlying infection and probably should be referred to as "pseudobronchiectasis." As better treatment paradigms have been established, the frequency of bronchiectasis has decreased significantly in the industrialized world, although it continues to be a major problem in developing nations.

Pathogenesis

Bronchiectasis should not be thought of as a diagnostic entity in itself. Rather, the term refers to the morphologic abnormalities that represent the final common pathway of a variety of conditions, causing long-standing pulmonary inflammation. The etiologies of bronchiectasis can be divided into congenital or acquired, depending on the source and etiology of the inflammation (Table 22-1). Most patients with congenital causes of bronchiectasis are found to have bilateral disease, whereas most patients with acquired bronchiectasis will have unilateral disease. Bronchiectasis can involve any of the pulmonary segments, but it is generally most common in the left lower lobe or lingula and in the right middle lobe. A specific cause for the development of bronchiectasis is found in less than 40% of patients, but most modern series indicate that about 50% of those patients in whom a specific etiology is determined developed their first pulmonary insult before age 14 years.[21,22]

The dilatation of the bronchi in bronchiectasis is secondary to destruction of the elastic lamina and muscularis of the bronchial walls, secondary to recurrent infection. The pathologic process usually begins with impaired pulmonary clearance of mucus and bacteria, resulting in an increased endoluminal pressure. Migration of WBCs into the bronchial lumen leads to degranulation and release of tissue-damaging oxidants, neutrophil elastase, and myeloperoxidases, in addition to the inflammatory cytokines tumor necrosis factor-α (TNF-α), interleukin (IL)-8, and IL-6.[23] The ciliated epithelium in this region is destroyed, leading to an increased propensity for recurrent infection. Repeated localized infection leads to replacement of the ciliated epithelium by squamous epithelium and loss of the supporting cartilage, allowing further bronchial inflammation and dilatation.

Clinical Presentation and Diagnosis

Patients with active bronchiectasis initially appear with systemic signs of infection such as fever, fatigue, and anorexia. The scenario is often accompanied by the presence of a productive cough, pleuritic chest pain, and hemoptysis. Physical examination usually reveals coarse inspiratory crackles and expiratory wheezes. Because few specific signs of bronchiectasis exist, the diagnosis often is delayed. The initial diagnostic workup should include a chest radiograph. Although this is sensitive for the diagnosis of bronchiectasis in only 50% of patients, it may show focal increase and "crowding" of interstitial markings. In diffuse, long-standing disease, a coarse honeycomb appearance may be seen (Fig. 22-4*A, B*). For many years, the specific diagnosis of bronchiectasis depended on the performance of bronchography, a relatively invasive test for pediatric patients. In the past decade, high-resolution CT scans have replaced bronchography for this purpose. Modern thin-section CT scans have more than 90% correlation with bronchographic findings.[24] The characteristic changes on thin-section CT include focal regions of volume loss and vascular crowding, "ring shadows" of dilated bronchi sectioned on end, broncho-arteriolar ratios less than 1, loss of bronchial tapering, and visualization of bronchi within 1 cm of the pleural surface. Of these findings, the presence of bronchi within 1 cm of the pleural surface appears to correlate best with bronchographic findings.[25] Additional types of CT studies that may be useful in evaluating patients with bronchiectasis include inspiratory-expiratory CT, which may give insights into the pathophysiologic processes involved; spiral CT and virtual bronchoscopy, which may allow better visualization of peripheral bronchi; and CT angiography, which may demonstrate neovascularization of the chronically inflamed bronchus.

The incidence of bronchiectasis in the United States has declined progressively since the 1950s. This has been attributed to the widespread use of bacterial and viral immunizations in childhood and the near elimination of tuberculosis in this country. Conversely, some suggestion has been made that the frequency of bronchiectasis is beginning to increase as children are being less uniformly vaccinated and as resistant strains of tuberculosis are encountered. An accelerated form of bronchiectasis has been described in patients with HIV infections.[26]

Therapy

The best therapy for bronchiectasis involves prevention of the disease by promptly treating recurrent pulmonary infections. The development of bronchiectasis may be inevitable in children with congenial etiologies such as cystic fibrosis or ciliary dyskinesia, but the disease in those patients with acquired etiologies should, for the most part, be preventable. Aggressive treatment of children with recurrent pulmonary infections should be accomplished with targeted antibiotic therapy and pulmonary physical

TABLE 22-1	
THE CONGENITAL AND ACQUIRED CONDITIONS ASSOCIATED WITH THE DEVELOPMENT OF BRONCHIECTASIS	
Congenital	Acquired
Cystic fibrosis	Pneumonia
Kartagener's syndrome	Repeated aspiration (GERD)
Immunodeficiency states	Sequestration
Ciliary dyskinesia states	Tuberculosis
	Airway foreign body
	Endobronchial tumor
	Smoking
	HIV Infection

GERD, gastroesophageal reflux disease; HIV, human immunodeficiency virus.

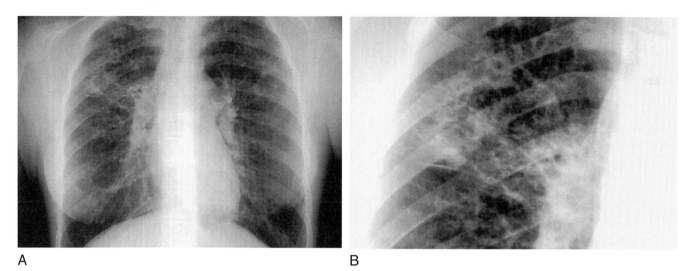

A   B

FIGURE 22-4. *A,* Chest radiograph demonstrating the classic appearance of bronchiectasis in a pediatric patient with cystic fibrosis. *B,* Magnified view of patient in *(A)* demonstrating honeycombed appearance.

therapy. A high index of suspicion must be maintained for bronchial obstruction, either by foreign body or endobronchial tumors, and bronchoscopy should play a role in the early management of these children. Pulmonary resection is reserved for those children who have repeated localized involvement despite adequate medical therapy. The criteria of perfusion or nonperfusion of involved segments are suggested as defining an operative candidate.[27] Absence of vascular perfusion, as determined by either angiography or perfusion nuclear scans, is an indication of end-stage disease, and those patients will generally experience excellent operative results. Patients with perfused segments may have reversible, cylindrical bronchiectases and should be subjected to continued medical therapy. Occasionally, massive hemoptysis will be the indication for surgical resection, although interventional radiology with embolization of bronchial vessels may eliminate resection as an emergency procedure. The principles of surgical therapy should be to preserve noninvolved pulmonary tissue by liberal use of segmental pulmonary resection and resection of all diseased segments, including staged bilateral thoracotomy, if necessary. Care must be taken to avoid contamination of the dependent lung while the patient is in the lateral decubitus position. The use of bifurcated endotracheal tubes or cuffed tubes with main-stem intubation is recommended. Although no recent series looked at the results of surgery for bronchiectasis in children, larger series, which included adults and children, would indicate that about 75% to 80% of the patients have complete relief of symptoms after excision.[28] It is generally conceded that the outcomes are better in the younger patients.

LUNG ABSCESS

Lung abscesses in the pediatric population are considered to be relatively rare and are typically the result of an infection with mixed aerobic and anaerobic flora.

The treatment of a lung abscess in an infant or child follows the same basic principles of postural drainage and pulmonary toilet used in adults, but it is often ineffectual secondary to the small airway size.[29]

Pathogenesis

The etiologic conditions associated with formation of a primary pulmonary abscess are not clearly identified in many cases. Associated events include aspiration of gastric contents, operations involving the upper respiratory tract, foreign-body inhalation, and prolonged unconsciousness.[30,31] In addition, formation of a lung abscess may be associated with a preceding pneumonic process (i.e., bacterial pneumonia) characterized by a significant degree of necrosis.[31] Resulting inflammation leads to the formation of a spherical cavity surrounded by a thick fibrous wall.

As in the adult population, the development of a lung abscess is the result of contamination with a mixed spectrum of both aerobic and anaerobic organisms. Specifically, one or more species of anaerobic oral bacteria, along with staphylococci, streptococci, or gramnegative enteric organisms are recovered from culture of the airway and/or abscess fluid. The most commonly recovered organisms include *S. aureus, Streptococcus viridans,* group A hemolytic streptococcus, *Pneumococcus* and *H. influenzae.* Less commonly encountered species include *Escherichia coli, Pseudomonas, Klebsiella, Peptococcus* and *Peptostreptococcus.*

Clinical Presentation and Diagnosis

The presentation of a pediatric patient with a lung abscess is characterized by tachycardia, fever, malaise, pleuritic chest pain, and a productive, often foul-smelling cough. Underlying disorders include an immunocompromised state, severe neurologic impairment, chronic lung disease, and poor oral hygiene. When a lung abscess is encountered in infants, underlying conditions such as congenital cystic adenomatoid malformation, bronchogenic cysts, or airway foreign bodies should be suspected. In older children, the existence of an intralobar pulmonary sequestration should be ruled out as a potential etiologic factor.

Most primary lung abscesses are located in the posterior segment of the right upper lobe and the superior segments of the right and left lower lobes. In contrast, secondary and/or recurrent collections may be found in multiple locations with no specific anatomic predilection. Chest radiographs are often nondiagnostic during the early phase of development but can go on to reveal striking abnormalities, including cavitary lesions with or without associated air/fluid levels. Recent evidence has shown that etiologic organisms can be identified in most cases of lung abscess (82%) despite prior use of antiotics.[32]

Therapy

As with any abscess cavity, the therapeutic goal is centered on the establishment of adequate drainage. Unlike in the adult patient, however, the use of postural drainage in the treatment of lung abscesses in infants and children, along with coughing and chest physiotherapy, is considered to be less effective. This observation is thought to be the consequence of smaller airways and less effective patient-driven pulmonary toilet (i.e., purposeful coughing and patient-directed incentive spirometry). In addition to the therapeutic maneuvers described, fiberoptic bronchoscopy, with direct drainage and irrigation of the cavity, has been recommended as a diagnostic and therapeutic modality often producing excellent results.[28]

Despite implementation of the various drainage procedures discussed earlier, an adequate therapeutic regimen is not fully complete unless a prolonged course (2 to 3 weeks' duration) of broad-spectrum antibiotics is administered (even in instances in which an infectious organism has not been identified). Bacterial organisms recovered from most cases of lung abscesses are susceptible to penicillin. Increased therapeutic effect can usually be achieved by using a combination of ampicillin and metronidazole or clindamycin. Although the typical antibiotic regimen is administered intravenously throughout the hospital stay, completion of the prescribed course in an outpatient setting, by using oral antibiotics, is often successful and has not been shown to result in an increased incidence of recurrent disease.

In cases of medical failure, more-invasive surgical intervention may be required. The procedure of choice for a solitary abscess located directly beneath the visceral pleura is pneumonostomy. Alternatively, thoracotomy and wedge resection may be required for abscesses that are more centrally located, involving multiple sites of fungal etiology.[28]

Outcome

As described earlier, successful management of a lung abscess is based on adequate drainage in combination with long-term antibiotic therapy. Resolution of the infectious and inflammatory processes can be seen over a period of several weeks. Although unusual, recurrence of a lung abscess at the site of the primary lesion can occur if the underlying cause persists (e.g., poorly treated gastroesophageal reflux in a nonambulatory patient). The mortality associated with primary lung abscess among children is very low. Increased complications and overall worse outcomes are seen, however, in immunocompromised individuals and in the neonatal population.

CHYLOTHORAX

Chylothorax is a rare condition defined as an abnormal collection of lymphatic fluid within the pleural space and may be encountered at any age. First described as a clinical entity by Asellius,[33] in the 17th century, chylothorax typically occurs during the neonatal and childhood periods, and is seen less often during adulthood.

Pathogenesis

Although the exact course of events responsible for the development of many chylous effusions remains uncertain, related pathophysiologic factors are often subcategorized as being traumatic or nontraumatic in origin. Potential traumatic events related to this disease process include a multitude of potential iatrogenic causes secondary to surgical procedures (i.e., operations involving structures in proximity to the mediastinum and major lymphatic vessels), penetrating injuries or crush wounds, as well as injuries related to the birth process (presumably secondary to hyperextension of the spine). Nontraumatic causes associated with chylous effusions include various congenital abnormalities (i.e., lymphangiomatosis) (see Chapter 72), venous thrombosis (which also may be associated with traumatic etiologies), and mediastinal and thoracic infections or malignancies.

During the neonatal period, the presence of chylous effusion has been commonly referred to as spontaneous and/or congenital in nature. Although presentation during this early period has been associated with various dysmorphic syndromes, most cases have no identifiable etiologic factor. In these cases, it is presumed that the formation of a chylous effusion is the result of a structural defect involving the lymphatic vessels.[34,35] Although reports of nontraumatic chylous effusions in the postneonatal period have been reported, traumatic causes as described earlier are far more common. Injury to the main thoracic duct as well as to the tributaries has been reported as a result of both blunt and penetrating thoracic trauma, with an incidence of as high as 0.9% after cardiac surgery among children.[36]

Clinical Presentation and Diagnosis

Chylothorax typically begins with significant respiratory distress; however, it may be encountered as an incidental finding during routine prenatal US or while obtaining a thoracic imaging study. In the case of postoperative chylothorax, a seemingly unremarkable postoperative effusion may rapidly increase once enteral nutrition is resumed, raising the suspicion of an injury to the thoracic duct and/or the network of intrathoracic lymphatic vessels. In addition to the obvious respiratory embarrassment that can occur as a result of the accumulation of significant volumes of fluid within the thoracic cavity, prolonged loss of chyle results in severe nutritional deficiencies, immunologic disturbances, and electrolyte derangement.

The diagnosis of chylothorax is established by using direct fluid analysis. The gross appearance is typically described as "milky," although straw-colored fluid is often encountered in the case of a patient whose gastrointestinal tract is at rest. Fluid should be considered highly suggestive if noted to contain a total fat content greater than 400 mg/dL, triglycerides greater than 200 mg/dL, and a specific gravity greater than 1.012. In addition, Gram stain analysis demonstrates the presence of more than 90% lymphocytes, and Sudan red staining may reveal the presence of chylomicrons.[37]

The term *pseudochylorthorax* refers to the circumstance of a prolonged (i.e., several weeks) nonchylous effusion, which may have a milky appearance, with elevated triglyceride levels. In the patient with no obvious risk factors for true chylothorax, this entity may be differentiated by using lipoprotein electrophoresis.[38]

Therapy

Treatment for chylothorax has traditionally been nonoperative, with as many as 80% of patients responding to conservative measures.[37] Most treatment algorithms are based on adequate drainage of the pleural fluid in combination with attempted trials of dietary modifications. Although no strict guidelines exist, many authors recommend one or several attempts to drain chylous fluid by using simple thoracentesis. When presented with a scenario of persistent reaccumulation, however, formal chest-tube drainage is then recommended.

The use of medium-chain triglyceride (MCT)–based formulas, with high protein content, have been shown to promote spontaneous resolution of persistent chest-tube drainage and/or reaccumulation of chylous fluid after multiple attempts at percutaneous drainage. The success of this intervention is thought to be the result of effectively reducing the amount of chyle produced while still providing adequate nutrition. This is the result of preferential absorption of MCT-based formulas into the portal venous system, rather than into the intestinal lymphatic network. The reduction in resultant chyle formation is thought to improve the likelihood of achieving a spontaneous resolution. In cases in which this therapeutic approach fails to result in resolution of the chyle drainage, or as an alternative initial therapy, many investigators have promoted a therapeutic algorithm consisting of complete cessation of enteral feeds, with concurrent administration of total parenteral nutrition (TPN). The results of both interventions are varied, and a clear consensus does not presently exist.

Because considerable volumes of pleural fluid can be lost on a daily basis (representing large amounts of protein and lymphocytes), extensive efforts to replace lost volume (typically with albumin) must be made to avoid the development of severe nutritional and hemodynamic derangements. In addition to drainage of the pleural space in combination with dietary interventions and/or TPN, recent literature supports the use of somatostatin in the treatment of ongoing chylous effusions. Although the exact mechanisms are not understood, such reports cite the reduced need for surgical intervention, potential for early return to enteral feeding, and shorter overall hospitalization with minimal side effects.[39,40] Although the majority of such reports cite the use of somatostatin analogues in the treatment of postsurgical chylous effusions, recent experience, including that of the authors, suggests a potential role for its use in the case of spontaneous chylothorax as well.[41,42]

If nonoperative therapy fails to stop the lymphatic drainage, several surgical options are available. The best timing of such operative interventions remains uncertain, with some authors advocating a trial of nonoperative therapy for 5 to 21 days before consideration of surgical intervention.[37] The principles of operative intervention focus on attempts to obliterate the thoracic duct or areas of leakage either directly (if visualized) or by pleurodesis[43] and are dictated by the nature of the chylothorax being treated (i.e., traumatic or nontraumatic). Most of these patients may now be managed by using thoracoscopic techniques rather than the open thoracotomy used in the past. Right thoracoscopy with ligation of the thoracic duct as it crosses the diaphragm has been shown to be a useful technique in patients with traumatic disruption of the thoracic duct as a result of surgical intervention.[44,45] Still others described direct suture of the area of chylous leak with the concurrent application of fibrin glue.[46] More recent reports described the highly successful technique of pleuroperitoneal-shunt devices to treat refractory chylothorax[47] (Fig. 22-5*A–H*).

Outcomes

Because of the relatively small number of cases in the current literature, the natural course of childhood chylothorax and the exact success rate of nonsurgical therapy in the pediatric age group remains unclear. Despite this, however, most patients appear to be successfully treated with pleural drainage and a combination of dietary intervention and/or TPN and somatostatin. Most authors agree that a relatively short period of nonsurgical therapy should be used, beyond which more aggressive therapy, in the form of surgical intervention, should be offered.

TUBERCULOSIS

Tuberculosis is a virulent pulmonary infection caused by *Mycobacterium tuberculosis* organisms. Primary pulmonary infection with atypical mycobacterial organisms is rare in children. After several decades of dramatic

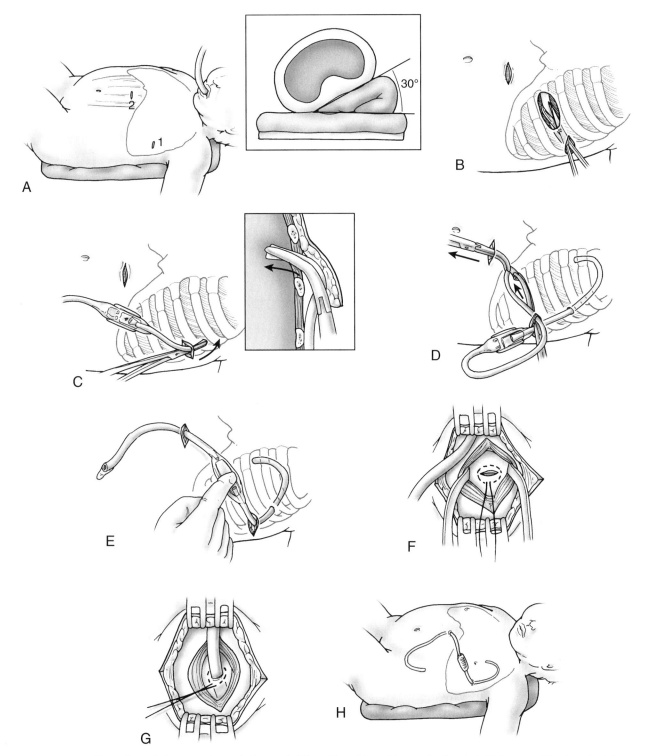

FIGURE 22-5. Insertion of pleuroperitoneal shunt. *A,* The affected hemithorax is elevated 30 degrees. The two incisions are planned to allow the pump chamber to rest on the costal margin. *B,* A small incision is made over the rib in the anterior axillary line, and a deep subcutaneous pocket is created inferiorly. *C,* Insertion of pleuroperitoneal shunt into the pleural space is done with a large curved clamp. The pleural catheter is tunneled 2 to 3 cm and bluntly passed through the intercostal space. The catheter must be carefully passed through the intercostal muscle at an angle to avoid kinking. *D,* A second small incision is made overlying the rectus muscle, and the peritoneal catheter is tunneled through this incision. The distal end of the shunt device is delivered to the second incision, as shown. Insertion of pleuroperitoneal shunt: The pumping chamber is drawn into the subcutaneous pocket by traction on the peritoneal catheter. *E,* The flow of chyle is confirmed before the distal catheter is inserted into the peritoneum. *F, G,* A pursestring suture is used to secure the peritoneal catheter at the level of the posterior rectus fascia. *H,* Both incisions should be closed with an absorbable suture, leaving a totally implanted system. (From Murphy M, Newman B, Rodgers B: Pleuroperitoneal shunts in the management of persistent chylothorax. Ann Thorac Surg 48:195–200, 1989.)

reduction of the frequency of pulmonary tuberculosis, particularly in the United States, a worldwide increase is now seen in the incidence, sufficient that the World Health Organization declared pulmonary tuberculosis "a global emergency" in 1993.[48] Pulmonary tuberculosis in 1995 caused more fatalities worldwide than did any other infectious disease. It is currently estimated that about one third of the world's population is infected with tuberculosis.

The incidence of pulmonary tuberculosis in the United States has shown a progressive increase over the past two decades because of a multitude of factors, including immigration of individuals from countries with a high incidence of infection, increasing incidence of HIV infection, increasing intravenous drug abuse, and a general worsening of social conditions in many of our larger cities.[49] Children, particularly in the younger age groups, are at high risk, often living in close contact with infected adults. Pulmonary tuberculosis in young children is usually the primary form of the disease, whereas adolescents tend to have reinfection tuberculosis, with cavitation.

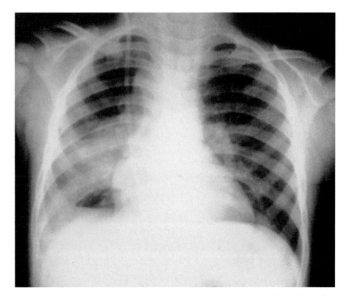

FIGURE 22-6. Chest radiograph of a 12-year-old girl with pulmonary tuberculosis demonstrates bilateral hilar infiltrates.

Clinical Presentation and Diagnosis

The diagnosis of pulmonary tuberculosis in children is often quite difficult. The patient may remain asymptomatic throughout much of the early phase of the disease, and bacteriologic confirmation may be quite difficult. Adequate sputum collection in young children is difficult to obtain, and gastric washings demonstrate tuberculosis organisms in only about 30% of the cases. Primary diagnosis is highly dependent on abnormalities noted on chest radiographs and by surveying patients living in close contact with infected adults. Approximately 75% to 90% of these patients will be noted to have pulmonary opacities from parenchymal involvement. These tend to be more heavily concentrated in the subpleural location. Approximately 85% to 90% of these children will be noted to have hilar or subcarinal lymphadenopathy on plain chest radiographs[50] (Fig. 22-6). Calcification of these nodes is rarely seen. Liberal use of CT scans may facilitate identification of these pathologic changes. Cavitary disease, so common in adult patients with pulmonary tuberculosis, is rarely seen in infected children in the first 5 years of life, but becomes much more common in adolescents, presumably from reinfection. Approximately 60% of adolescents with tuberculosis will be noted to have cavitary disease in one or the other of the upper lobes on chest radiograph.[51,52] Bacterial confirmation of pulmonary tuberculosis also is easier in the older adolescent. A suggestion of pulmonary tuberculosis on radiograph should be supported by a skin test.

The incidence of pulmonary tuberculosis is greatest in patients with compromised immunity, such as bone marrow transplant patients, diabetics, and those with HIV infection.[53] Symptoms may be more variant, and radiologic changes more dramatic among the immunocompromised subpopulation. The mortality of HIV-infected patients with pulmonary tuberculosis is approximately 70%.[53]

Therapy

First-line therapy for patients with pulmonary tuberculosis consists of multidrug antibiotic therapy. A 6-month course of isoniazid and rifampin forms the basis for most antibiotic regimens. This may be supplemented with 2 months of pyrazinamide. These drugs appear to have an acceptable toxicity spectrum in children. Isoniazid causes changes in liver enzymes in children much less commonly than in adults. In otherwise normal children who are compliant with this regimen, a 100% cure rate should be found. Drug treatment should be initiated as soon as the diagnosis is confirmed, as delay in treatment has been linked to an increased risk of death.[53]

Surgery for pulmonary tuberculosis in children is generally performed to treat the complications of the disease and to reduce the bacillary load.[54] In the younger patients, enlargement of hilar and subcarinal lymph nodes can cause bronchial obstruction with distal atelectasis. In these patients, in addition to adding a fourth antibiotic, usually streptomycin or ethambutol, a short course of prednisone (2 mg/kg/day) may be beneficial.[55] Serial chest CT scans may be used to monitor the progress of this disease and its response to therapy. These scans also can identify those patients with endobronchial extension of their disease who may be helped by bronchoscopy. If steroids and antibiotics fail to relieve the bronchial compression, these patients should have a thoracotomy and partial resection of the hilar and subcranial nodes to relieve the compression of the airway.[56] Actual pulmonary resection should be avoided in these young children. Indications for surgical treatment in adolescents with cavitary disease include continued positive sputum cultures after 6 months of appropriate antibiotic therapy or massive hemoptysis. Surgery in all of these patients can be very challenging because of the degree of scarring from the chronic infection, and blood loss may be substantial.[57]

In the past decade, the emergence of antibiotic-resistant strains of *M. tuberculosis* organisms has become a problem. By definition, these organisms are resistant to isoniazid and rifampin, significantly limiting options for therapy. Currently, drug-resistant *M. tuberculosis* is the primary indication for tuberculosis surgery in the United States.[58] Although primary infection with drug-resistant organisms in young children has not yet been reported, secondary infection in adolescents has been encountered.

HISTOPLASMOSIS

The lung is the most commonly involved site of clinical infection as a result of endemic fungal organisms in North America and typically includes *Histoplasma capsulatum, Blastomyces dermatitidis,* and *Coccidiodes.*[59] Histoplasmosis, a thermal dimorphic fungus found in mold form within the soil, has a nearly worldwide distribution with endemic concentrations in the eastern half of the United States (e.g., Ohio and Mississippi River Valleys) and a large proportion of Latin America.[59] The presence of a large concentration of bird and bat feces within the soil of these areas appears to be associated with endemic or hyperendemic rates of infection.

Manipulation of infected soil can result in airborne dissemination and infection of individuals with no other obvious source of exposure. Although outbreaks of histoplasmosis have been attributed to specific point sources in the past, the fact that airborne spores can travel considerable distances is thought to be responsible for the majority of current cases having no obvious source of exposure.[60, 61]

Pathogenesis

The majority of infections are mild or completely asymptomatic and associated with patchy infiltrates on chest radiographs. After being inhaled into the lungs, *H. capsulatum* spores germinate into yeast forms, which results in an influx of macrophages, neutrophils, and T cells. T-cell immunity typically develops 10 to 14 days after the initial exposure and is a crucial component responsible for the typically self-limiting process observed among immunocompetent individuals. Although primary infection and subsequent T-cell immunity does provide some degree of protection, reinfection and/or reactivation may occur.[59]

Clinical Presentation and Diagnosis

The incubation period ranges from 1 to 3 weeks and may result in an acute clinical infection or the patient may be completely asymptomatic. The majority of symptomatic patients have a "flu-like" illness consisting of general myalgia, malaise, a nonproductive cough, headache, and fever. Progressive or diffuse disease is encountered in patients with some element of immunocompromise. Chest radiographs during acute infection typically show diffuse, often bilateral, infiltrates, whereas cavitations

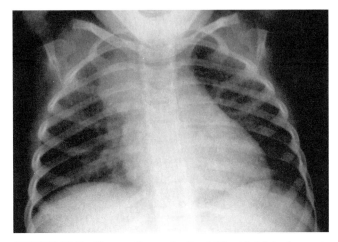

FIGURE 22-7. Chest radiograph of a child with histoplasmosis demonstrates hilar lymphadenopathy.

and miliary processes may be observed as a result of chronic infection. As seen in Figures 22-7 and 8, hilar adenopathy may be observed in both acute and chronic disease states. Intraoperative specimens often appear to be firm and rubbery, making them grossly indistinguishable from lymphadenopathy secondary to other infectious and noninfectious causes.

Less common manifestations include acute overwhelming pulmonary infections, fibrosing mediastinitis, pericarditis, and enlargement of mediastinal lymph nodes. These processes may result in dysphagia, pleuritic chest pain, airway obstruction, and superior vena caval syndrome. Surgical intervention in the cases of major vascular and airway obstruction are rare, hazardous, and should be considered only in severe cases in which medical therapy has failed to improve the clinical picture.

Therapy

As previously mentioned, the majority of immunocompetent patients experience a self-limiting process and

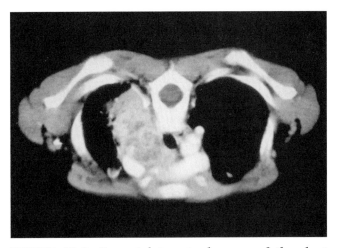

FIGURE 22-8. Computed tomography scan of the chest demonstrating hilar lymphadenopathy secondary to pulmonary histoplasmosis.

therefore require only supportive therapy. Treatment with antifungal agents is typically reserved for patients who have persistent symptoms (longer than 2 to 3 weeks), or demonstrate progressive disease based on serial radiologic examinations. Itraconazole has been used for treatment of mild persistent disease. Amphotericin B is strongly recommended for patients with more severe manifestations of histoplasmosis and is followed by oral itraconazole or ketoconazol after achieving an adequate clinical response. Surgical intervention may be required for constrictive pericarditis or to relieve obstructive airway and/or vascular complications of the disease process.

DIFFUSE INTERSTITIAL DISEASE

Chronic interstitial lung disease may result from infectious as well as noninfectious processes (Table 22-2). It is characterized by restrictive lung physiology and abnormal gas exchange that produce considerable morbidity and mortality. The list of differential diagnoses to consider in the etiology of diffuse interstitial lung disease comprises more than 100 separate conditions in both adults[62] and children.[63,64] The clinical disease patterns range from a chronic, slowly progressive picture in a relatively stable patient, to one of acute pulmonary decompensation, requiring emergency life-saving maneuvers. Because sorting through the potential causes may delay treatment, and the ability to establish a specific diagnosis is often time consuming and difficult, it is not uncommon for pediatric surgeons to be involved in such cases to help establish the correct diagnosis through lung biopsy. In addition, surgical intervention may be required to deal with respiratory failure. In severe cases of acute respiratory compromise, a pediatric surgeon may be asked to provide cannulae for the patient for extracorporeal life support (ECMO). In addition, the need for long-term ventilatory and prolonged airway management may require the creation of a tracheostomy. Prompt diagnosis, especially in the case of immunocompromised or otherwise debilitated patients, may require an urgent lung biopsy to guide further therapeutic interventions. The importance of such information cannot be overemphasized, and, in the case of an extremely unstable patient, should warrant the use of thoracoscopy and/or thoracotomy, even in the intensive care unit (ICU) setting, to obtain the necessary tissue specimens.

Pathogenesis

Although the precise pathophysiology responsible for the development of interstitial lung disease remains poorly understood, current evidence suggests that the process responsible for its development is related to inflammation at the level of the interstitial and perialveolar tissues. This common feature appears to explain the presence of similar histologic, radiologic, and clinical characteristics among an heterogeneous group of pulmonary disorders.[63] Histologic evidence suggests that the establishment and subsequent progression of the interstitial process involves injury to both the epithelial and endothelial structures.[65] Furthermore, recent studies have focused on the potential genetic determination in interstitial lung disease, hypothesizing the existence of an aberrant immunologic defect(s), which results in a failure of the normal immunomodulatory and mucociliary functions. This paradigm results in a predisposition for development of a pathologic interstitial pulmonary process.[66]

Clinical Presentation and Diagnosis

As discussed earlier, the spectrum of disease can be quite varied. Studies have attempted to correlate survival with associated symptoms and physical examination characteristics. Determinants evaluated for correlation with survival include the patient's age, weight, duration of symptoms, presence of crackles on auscultation of the lung fields, clubbing of fingernails, and severity-of-illness score[66] (Table 22-3).

TABLE 22-2

INFECTIOUS AND NONINFECTIOUS PROCESSES ASSOCIATED WITH THE DEVELOPMENT OF CHRONIC INTERSTITIAL LUNG DISEASE

Infectious	Noninfectious
Pneumocystis	Hypersensitivity pneumonitis
Cryptococcus	Sarcoidosis
Aspergillis	Neoplasms
Streptococcus	Systemic lupus erythematosus
Chlamydia	Graft vs. host disease
Mycoplasma pneumonia	Radiation pneumonitis
Rickettsia	Adult respiratory distress syndrome
Adenovirus	Aspiration pneumonitis (GERD)
Parainfluenza virus	Chemotherapeutic agents
Respiratory syncytial virus	Fat embolism
Cytomegalovirus	Allergic alveolitis
Varicella zoster virus	Pulmonary hemosiderosis
Herpes simplex virus	

GERD, gastroesophageal reflux disease.

TABLE 22-3

SEVERITY-OF-ILLNESS SCORE CORRELATES DEGREE OF ILLNESS WITH OVERALL SURVIVAL RATES AMONG PATIENTS WITH DIFFUSE INTERSTITIAL LUNG DISEASE

Score	Severity of Illness
1	Asymptomatic
2	Symptomatic: room air oxygen saturation normal under all conditions
3	Symptomatic: room air oxygen saturation normal during resting but abnormal (<90%) with sleep or exercise
4	Symptomatic: abnormal resting room air oxygen saturation (<90%)
5	Symptomatic: pulmonary hypertension

The task of establishing the correct diagnosis relies on the combined results of several modalities (e.g., radiologic studies, bronchoalveolar lavage [BAL], and lung biopsy). Although the use of plain chest radiographs can offer the ability to follow disease progression, it offers little specific diagnostic and/or prognostic information. One recent study of 39 adult patients with pulmonary fibrosis demonstrated a possible correlation between disease severity (as measured by standard pulmonary-function testing) and high-resolution CT images.[67] Practical applications of such observations are less clear in the pediatric population.

The results of BAL are disappointing. In a recent prospective analysis of children with interstitial lung disease undergoing BAL, a definitive primary diagnosis was made in only 5 (17%) of 29 patients. Although the use of BAL provided important information overall, its ability to determine the primary cause of diffuse interstitial lung disease was limited.[68]

Several other invasive techniques have been outlined as useful in obtaining lung tissue in an effort to establish the diagnosis. These techniques are generally well tolerated and include percutaneous needle biopsy, transbronchial lung biopsy, open lung biopsy, and VAT. Although the use of lung biopsy has been considered the most definitive, it has been cited as being nondiagnostic in as many as 30% of patients.[68] In addition to the modalities described, more-focused diagnostic modalities, such as radiologic evaluation for gastroesophageal reflux disease (GERD) should always be considered in newly diagnosed cases because GERD has been cited as an important contributory process that should not be overlooked.[69]

Therapy

The treatment of chronic interstitial lung disease is often challenging and necessitates an extremely detailed and systematic review of all historic, physical, and environmental factors that may help lead to a specific diagnosis. Because pediatric interstitial lung disease is relatively rare, controlled clinical studies addressing treatment algorithms do not presently exist. The paucity of reliable diagnostic guidelines often leaves the physician with little choice but to initiate a treatment regimen based on what appears to be the most likely diagnosis. Therapeutic interventions can range from simple expectant therapy for mild or self-limited cases to the initiation of complex rescue therapy requiring high-frequency oscillating ventilation (HFOV) and/or ECMO in the most severe cases. Pharmacologic first-line therapy with various immunosuppressants, administered after confirming the absence of a responsible bacteriologic organism, also is a common practice. Corticosteroids are the most commonly used first-line agents in noninfectious disease, followed by hydroxychloroquine. Less commonly used agents include chloroquine, cyclosporin, colchicines, and methotrexate.[66] In all cases, supportive measures in the form of nutritional and psychosocial support and environmental modification (i.e., avoiding identified irritants or allergens) are important tools in the treatment armamentarium.

Outcomes

The natural history of chronic interstitial lung disease that is unresponsive to therapy appears to be progressive fibrosis and resultant failure of the normal gas-exchange mechanisms. The morbidity and mortality as well as the long-term outcome associated with chronic interstitial lung disease vary depending on the associated etiologic factors and existing comorbid conditions. Despite several attempts to identify reliable means with which to monitor the progression of this disease process, as well as clinical response to therapy, investigators have failed to offer a clear consensus regarding management and outcome issues.[69]

PNEUMATOCELE

Pneumatoceles are defined as thin-walled, air-filled, intraparenchymal pulmonary cysts and typically occur in association with underlying bacterial pneumonia. Although the formation of pneumatoceles is relatively infrequent and has been associated with a variety of underlying bacterial organisms, recent reports demonstrated that a majority are the result of staphylococcal pneumonia.[70,71] Other pathogens that have been identified as being associated with pneumatocele formation include *Streptococcus, H. influenzae, Kelbsiella, E. coli.* and *Pseudomonas.* In addition, pneumatoceles have been seen in cases of pulmonary tuberculosis and measles.[72]

Pathogenesis

Although the exact pathologic mechanisms responsible for the formation of pneumatoceles are uncertain, the development of a severe inflammatory reaction and subsequent destruction of the alveolar and interstitial architecture have been attributed to the release of bacterial exotoxins. The resulting air leak(s) occasionally culminates in a phenomenon whereby continued accumulation within the thin-walled defect results in the formation of a tension pneumatocele. The development of a tension pneumatocele may potentially compress adjacent structures or rupture into the free pleural space, resulting in a tension pneumothorax. Additional complications associated with pneumatoceles include the establishment of secondary infections, empyema, and bronchopleural fistulas.[73]

Clinical Presentation and Diagnosis

The clinical presentation and symptoms seen in children with an identified pneumatocele are usually indistinguishable from those encountered in the case of bacterial pneumonia without associated pneumatoceles. The diagnosis of pneumatoceles is typically made by chest radiograph and/or CT scan, In addition, they have occasionally been confused with simple pulmonary cysts and congenital diaphragmatic hernias. Serial examination and the overall clinical course often help to differentiate pneumatoceles from other pathologic abnormalities.

Therapy

The majority of pneumatoeceles appear to involute over time, requiring no specific therapy other than supportive care and appropriate antibiotic coverage. In the case of a rapidly enlarging and/or tension pneumatocele, resulting in respiratory compromise, urgent decompression may be required. In addition to closed-tube thoracostomy or cystostomy, recent reports describe using percutaneous catheter-drainage techniques, in combination with fluoroscopy and US, as an effective means of decompression in such clinical scenarios.[74,75] Open drainage with decortication and oversewing of the cyst wall is rarely necessary.

Outcomes

The majority of pneumatoceles decrease in size and resolve over a period of several weeks to months, assuming that the underlying infectious cause is adequately treated. In uncomplicated cases, no residual pulmonary compromise or radiologic sequelae are likely.

REFERENCES

1. Byington C, Spencer L, Johnson T, et al: An epidemiological investigation of sustained high rate of pediatric parapneumonic empyema: Risk factors and microbiological associations. Clin Infect Dis 34:434–440, 2002.
2. Adeyemo A, Adejuyibe O, Taiwo O, et al: Pleural empyema in infants and children: Analysis of 298 cases. J Natl Med Assoc 76:799–805, 1984.
3. Chonmaitree T, Powell K: Parapneumonic pleural effusion and empyema in children: Review of a 19-year experience, 1962-1980. Clin Pediatr 22:414–419, 1983.
4. Freij B, Kusmiesz H, Nelson J, et al: Parapneumonic effusions and empyema in hospitalized children: A retrospective review of 227 cases. Pediatr Infect Dis 3:578–591, 1984.
5. Jess P, Brynitz S, Mollar A: Mortality in thoracic empyema. Scand J Thorac Cardiovasc Surg 18:85–87, 1984.
6. Meier A, Smith B, Raghavan A, et al: Rational treatment of empyema in children. Arch Surg 16315:907–912, 2000.
7. American Thoracic Society. Management of non-tuberculous empyema. Am Rev Respir Dis 85:935, 1962.
8. Bartlett J, Gorbach S, Thadepalli H, et al: Bacteriology of empyema. Lancet 1:338, 1974.
9. Foglia R, Randolf J. Current indications for decortication in the treatment of empyema in children. J Pediatr Surg 22:28, 1987.
10. Gustafson R, Murray G, Warden M, et al: Role of lung decortication in symptomatic empyema in children. Ann Thorac Surg 49:940, 1990.
11. Hoff S, Neblett W, Heller R, et al: Postpneumonic empyema in childhood: Selecting appropriate therapy. J Pediatr Surg 24:659, 1989.
12. McLaughlin F, Goldman D, Rosenbaum D, et al: Empyema in children: Clinical course and long-term follow-up. Pediatrics 73:587, 1984.
13. Goeman A, Kipur N, Toppare M, et al: Conservative treatment of empyema in children. Respiration 60:182, 1993.
14. Lewis KT, Bukstein SA. Parapneumonic empyema in children: Diagnosis and management. Am Fam Physician 46:1443, 1992.
15. Kosloske AM, Cartwright KC: The controversial role of decortication in the management of children with empyema. J Thorac Cardiovasc Surg 96:166, 1988.
16. Hoff S, Neblett WW, Edwards KM: Parapneumonic empyema in children: Decortication hastens recovery in patients with severe pleural infections. Pediatr Infect Dis J 168:6, 1990.
17. Kern J, Rodgers B: Thoracosopy in the management of empyema in children. J Pediatr Surg 28:1128, 1993.
18. Wait M, Sharma S, Hohn J, et al: A randomized trial of empyema therapy. Chest 111:1548–1552, 1997.
19. Laennec RTH: De l'auscultation mediate on traite du diagnostic des maladies des poumons et du Coeur, fonde, principalement sur ce noveau moyer d'exploration. Paris, Brosson et Claude, 1819.
20. Reid LM: Reduction in bronchial subdivision in bronchiectasis. Thorax 5:233–247, 1950.
21. McGuinnea G, Naidich DP: CT of airways disease and bronchiectasis. Radiol Clin North Am 40:1–19, 2002.
22. Agasthian T, Deschamps C, Trastek VF, et al: Surgical management of bronchiectasis. Ann Thorac Surg 62:976–980, 1996.
23. Angrill J, Agusti C, De Celis R, et al: Bronchial inflammation and colonization in patients with clinically stable bronchiectasis. Am J Respir Crit Care Med 164:1628–1632, 2001.
24. Kumar NA, Nguyen B, Maki D: Bronchiectasis: Current clinical and imaging concepts. Semin Roentgenol 36:41–50, 2001.
25. Smevik B: Complementary investigations in bronchiectasis in children. Monaldi Arch Chest Dis 55:420–426, 2000.
26. Verghese A, Al-Samman M, Nabhan D, et al: Bacterial bronchitis and bronchiectasis in human immunodeficiency virus infection. Arch Intern Med 154:2086–2091, 1994.
27. Ashour M, Al-Kattan, K, Rafay MA, et al: Current surgical therapy for bronchiectasis. World J Surg 23:1096–1104, 1999.
28. Kutlay H, Canglr AK, Ennon S, et al: Surgical treatment in bronchiectasis: Analysis of 166 patients. Eur J Cardiothorac Surg 21:634–637, 2002.
29. Kosloske AM, Ball WS, Butler C, et al: Drainage of pediatric lung abscess by cough, catheter or complete resection. J Pediatr Surg 21:7;596–600, 1986.
30. Mark PH, Turner JAP: Lung abscess in childhood. Thorax 23:216–220, 1968.
31. Brook I: Lung abscess and pleural empyema in children. Adv Pediatr Infect Dis 8:159–176, 1993.
32. Mansharamani N, Koziel H: Chronic lung sepsis: Lung abscess, bronchiectasis and empyema. Curr Opin Pulmon Med 9:181–185, 2003.
33. Kirkland I: Chylothorax in infancy and childhood. Arch Dis Child 40:186–191, 1965.
34. Watson WJ, Munson DP, Christensen MW: Bilateral fetal chylothorax: Results of unilateral in-utero therapy. Am J Perinatol 13:115–117, 1996.
35. Chernick V, Reed MH: Pneumothorax and chylothorax in the neonatal period. J Pediatr 76:625–632, 1970.
36. Allen EM, Van Heeckeren DW, Spector ML, et al: Management of nutritional and infectious complications of postoperative chylothorax in children. J Pediatr Surg 26:1169, 1991.
37. Bond SJ, Guzzetta PC, Synder ML, et al: Management of pediatric postoperative chylothorax. Ann Thoracic Surg 56:469, 1993.
38. Ferguson MK. Thoracoscopy for empyema, bronchopleural fistula, and chylothorax. Ann Thorac Surg 56:644, 1993.
39. Luca R, Bini R Chessa M, et al: The effectiveness of octreotide in the treatment of postoperative chylothorax. Eur J Pediatr 161:149–150, 2002
40. Buettiker V, Hug M, Burger R: Somatostatin: A new therapeutic option for the treatment of chylothorax. Intens Care Med 27:1083–1086, 2001.
41. Au M, Weber TR, Flemmin RE: Successful use of octreotide in a case of neonatal chylothorax. J Pediatr Surg 38:1106–1107, 2003.
42. Goto M, Kawamata K, Masanao K, et al: Treatment of chylothorax in a premature infant using somatostatin. J Perinatol 23:563–564, 2003.
43. Valentine VG, Raffin TA: The management of chylothorax. Chest 102:56, 1992.
44. Graham DD, McGahren ED, Tribble CG, et al: Use of video-assisted thoracic surgery in the treatment of chylothorax. Ann Thorac Surg 57:1507–1511, 1994.
45. Buchan K, Amir-Reza H, Ritchie A. Thoracoscopic thoracic duct ligation for traumatic chylothorax. Ann Thorac Surg 72:1366–1367, 2001.
46. Fahimi H, Casselman F, Mariani M, et al: Current management of postoperative chylothorax. Ann Thorac Surg 71:448–451, 2001.
47. Wolff AB. Silen ML. Kokoska ER, et al: Treatment of refractory chylothorax with externalized pleuroperitoneal shunts in children. Ann Thorac Surg 68:1053–1057, 1999.

48. Raviglione MC, Snider DE Jr, Kochi A: Global epidemiology of tuberculosis: Morbidity and mortality of a worldwide epidemic. JAMA 273:220–226, 1995.

49. Kim WS, Moon WK, Kim IO, et al: Pulmonary tuberculosis in children: Evaluation with CT. Am J Roentgenol 168: 1005–1009, 1997.

50. Kim HY, Song KS, Good JM, et al: Thoracic sequelae and complications of tuberculosis. Radiographics 21:839–858, 2001.

51. Weber HC, Beyers N, Gie RP, et al: The clinical and radiological features of tuberculosis in adolescents. Ann Trop Paediatr 20:5–10, 2000.

52. Ip MSM, Yuen KY, Woo PCY, et al: Risk factors for pulmonary tuberculosis in bone marrow transplant recipients. Am J Respir Crit Care Med 158:1173–1177, 1998.

53. Oursler KK, Moore RD, Bishai WR, et al: Survival of patients with pulmonary tuberculosis: Clinical and molecular epidemiologic factors. Clin Infect Dis 34:752–759, 2002.

54. Efferen LS, Hyman CL: Tuberculosis reemerges: The captain remains aboard. Curr Opin Pulmon Med 2:236–245, 1996.

55. Hewitson JP, Oppell UOV: Role of thoracic surgery for childhood tuberculosis. World J Surg 21:468–474, 1997.

56. Papagiannopoulos KA, Linegar AG, Harris DG, et al: Surgical management of airway obstruction in primary tuberculosis in children. Ann Thorac Surg 68:1182–1186, 1999.

57. Perelman MI, Strelzov VP: Surgery for pulmonary tuberculosis. World J Surg 21:457–467, 1997.

58. Pomerantz BJ, Cleveland JC, Olson HK, et al: Pulmonary resection for multi-drug resistant tuberculosis. J Thorac Cardiovasc Surg 12:448–453, 2001.

59. Goldman M, Johnson P, Sarosi G: Fungal pneumonia; the endemic mycoses. Clin Chest Med 20:1–18, 1999.

60. Wheat J: Histoplasmosis: Experience during outbreaks in Indianapolis and review of the literature. Medicine 76:339–354, 1997.

61. Wheat J: Histoplasmosis. Infect Dis Clin North Am 2:841–859, 1998.

62. Turner-Warwick M: Interstitial lung disease. Semin Respir Med 6:1–102, 1984.

63. Fan L, Langston C: Chronic interstitial lung disease in children. Pediatr Pulmonol 16:184–196, 1993.

64. Bokulic RE, Hilman BC: Interstitial lung disease in children. Pediatr Clin North Am 41:543–567, 1994.

65. Kobayashi H, Gabazza EC, Taguchi O, et al: Protein C anticoagulant system in patients with interstitial lung disease. Am J Respir Crit Care Med 157L:1850–1854, 1998.

66. Howenstine M, Eigen H: Current concepts on interstitial lung disease in children. Curr Opin Pediatr 11:200–209, 1999.

67. Xaubet A, Agusti C, Luburich P: Pulmonary function tests and CT scan in the management of idiopathic pulmonary fibrosis. Am J Respir Crit Care Med 158:431–436, 1998.

68. Fan L, Lum Lung M, Wagener J: The diagnostic value of bronchoalveolar lavage in immunocompetent children with chronic diffuse pulmonary infiltrates. Pediatr Pulmonol. 23:8–13, 1997.

69. Reynolds H: Diagnostic and management strategies for diffuse interstitial lung disease. Chest 113:192–202, 1998.

70. Quigley MJ, Fraser RS. Pulmonary pneumatocele: Pathology and pathogenesis. Am J Roentgenol 150:1275–1277, 1988.

71. Oviawe O, Ogundipe O: Pneumatoceles associated with pneumonia: Incidence and clinical course in Nigerian children. Trop Geogr Med 37:264–269, 1985.

72. Glustein JZ, Kaplan M: *Enterobacter cloacae* causing pneumatocele in a neonate. Acta Pediatr 83:990–991, 1994.

73. Zuhdi MK, Bradley JS, Spear RM, et al: Fatal air embolism as a complication of staphylococcal pneumonia with pneumatoceles. Pediatr Infect Dis J 14:811–812, 1995.

74. Zuhdi MK, Spear R, Worthen M, et al: Percutaneous catheter drainage of tension pneumatocele, secondarily infected pneumatocele and lung abscess in children. Crit Care Med 42:330–333, 1996.

75. Kogutt M, Lutrell C, Pulau F, et al: Decompression of pneumatocele in a neonate by percutaneous catheter placement. Pediatr Radiol 29:488–489, 1999.

CHAPTER 23

Congenital Diaphragmatic Hernia and Eventration

Robert M. Arensman, MD, Daniel A. Bambini, MD, and Bill Chiu, MD

Congenital diaphragmatic hernia (CDH) is one of the most challenging neonatal diagnoses faced by pediatric surgeons. From the time of its first anatomic description more than 300 years ago, CDH has carried a high mortality rate. This mortality is directly related to the severity of lung hypoplasia induced by events during critical stages of fetal lung development. The increased diagnostic capabilities and tremendous advances in the care of critically ill neonates with respiratory disease have lowered the mortality rate to less than 20% in some series, yet CDH still has an overall mortality of 30% to 60% at most centers.

Although surgery continues to play a primary role in CDH, most recent advances in the care of these neonates have been nonsurgical. Early surgical intervention, once believed to be critical to survival,[1] has been replaced by a delayed surgical approach.[2-8] The repair of the diaphragmatic defect is deferred until pulmonary hypertension and persistent fetal circulation have subsided. The improved survival of the delayed surgical approach has been modest, leading many to pursue other strategies and innovative therapies, including extracorporeal membrane oxygenation (ECMO) and fetal intervention.

The treatment of CDH depends on the time of diagnosis, the clinical presentation, and institutional expertise. Perhaps no other disease encountered by pediatric surgeons has as many therapeutic and management options as does CDH. Current therapeutic approaches emphasize preoperative stabilization using ventilation strategies that avoid barotrauma and iatrogenic pulmonary injury. These new techniques have improved survival, yet the optimal management strategy for neonates with CDH remains unknown. The treatment of CDH will continue to evolve as our understanding of the disease increases.

ANATOMY OF THE DIAPHRAGM AND DIAPHRAGMATIC DEFECTS

The diaphragm is a dome-shaped musculotendinous structure that separates the thoracic and abdominal cavities. It is composed of fibrous and muscular parts.

The fibrous central tendon is the largest single component of the diaphragm and accounts for approximately one third of the total diaphragmatic surface area. Crural fibers pass around the aorta and esophagus to insert at the posterior central tendon and define the apertures for the aorta and esophagus. The anatomic pattern of the crural fibers surrounding the esophageal hiatus can be highly variable.

Congenital and acquired diaphragmatic defects commonly occur at three areas of the diaphragm (Fig. 23-1). The posterolateral diaphragmatic hernia, commonly called the Bochdalek hernia, accounts for 85% to 90% of diaphragmatic defects first seen in the neonatal period. The most commonly accepted hypothesis regarding the origin of the posterolateral defect is that it results from failed closure of the embryonic pleuroperitoneal canal. More recent embryologic studies indicate that the diaphragmatic defect appears early in gestation when the canals are still present and occurs due to malformation of the primordial diaphragm or pleuroperitoneal fold.[9] The size of the defect can range from a small slit to the complete absence of the entire hemidiaphragm (agenesis). A hernia sac is present in approximately 10% to 20% of cases. Eighty percent to 90% of posterolateral diaphragmatic defects occur on the left side.

Retrosternal hernia, usually referred to as Morgagni's hernia, accounts for 2% to 6% of congenital diaphragmatic defects. The defect is located in the anterior diaphragm immediately posterior to the xiphoid process of the sternum. It usually occurs on the right. Diaphragmatic hernias also can develop at the esophageal hiatus, but this is the least common site of congenital diaphragmatic defects.

EMBRYOLOGY OF THE DIAPHRAGM AND CONGENITAL DIAPHRAGMATIC HERNIA

The diaphragm is formed by several fused embryonic components, including the septum transversum, pleuroperitoneal membranes, esophageal mesentery, and body

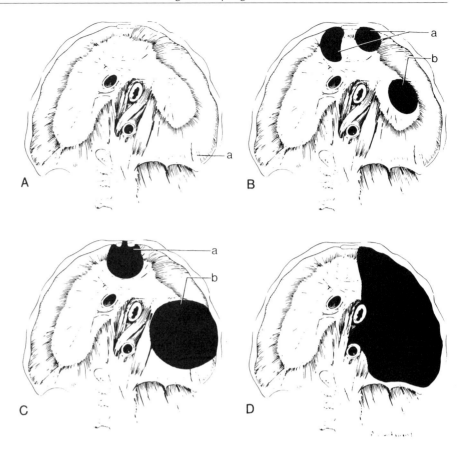

FIGURE 23-1. The inferior surface of the diaphragm and common locations of congenital diaphragmatic hernia. *A,* The normal diaphragm and the site (a) of the lumbosacral triangle, a potential area of weakness between diaphragmatic muscle fibers originating from the 12th rib and those originating from the lateral arcuate ligament. *B,* Retrosternal hernia (a) produced by failure of the sternal and costal contributions of the diaphragm to fuse at the site where the internal mammary artery traverses the diaphragm. Small posterolateral hernia (b) produced by failed closure of the pleuroperitoneal canal during embryologic development. *C,* Diaphragmatic defect and cleft sternum (a) associated with the pentalogy of Cantrell, which results from embryologic failure in the development of the septum transversum. Large posterolateral defect (b) with only a thin rim of posterior diaphragm. *D,* Agenesis of the left hemidiaphragm with absence of the left diaphragmatic crura.

wall mesoderm. The septum transversum separates the pericardial and the peritoneal cavities as it fuses dorsally with the mesodermal tissue surrounding the foregut. As this occurs, the pleuroperitoneal canals remain in continuity, connecting the pleural space and peritoneal cavity (Fig. 23-2). Closure of the pleuroperitoneal canals by the pleuroperitoneal membranes completes the formation of the primitive fetal diaphragm, separating the abdominal cavity from the paired pleural cavities. The mechanism by which this occurs is not completely understood. Nonetheless, the communication through the pleuroperitoneal canals is obliterated by week 8 of gestation. CDH has usually been attributed to a defective formation of the pleuroperitoneal membrane, perhaps as a consequence of abnormal development of the posthepatic mesenchymal plate.[10,11] Recent experimental evidence indicates that the muscular defect in CDH occurs before the time of canal closure and results from abnormal formation of the primordial diaphragm or pleuroperitoneal fold.[12] Visceral herniation through the diaphragmatic defect into the chest occurs as the intestines return to the peritoneal cavity beginning at week 10 of gestation.

LUNG DEVELOPMENT AND PULMONARY HYPOPLASIA IN CDH

Lung development is traditionally divided into four overlapping stages. The pseudoglandular stage begins with the formation of the lung bud at week 5 of gestation and lasts into week 17. During this period, the major bronchi and terminal bronchi are formed. The majority of respiratory bronchioles, alveolar ducts, and pulmonary vessels develop during the canalicular stage between weeks 16 and 25. The terminal sac period begins near week 24 and continues until birth. Alveoli begin to develop during the alveolar stage, which begins in late fetal life and continues into childhood. Although the etiology of CDH in humans remains unknown, experimental and clinical evidence suggests that pulmonary development in CDH is disrupted early in gestation. The resulting pulmonary hypoplasia and lung immaturity are the critical factors that determine the severity of illness and overall prognosis in CDH.

Visceral herniation through a diaphragmatic defect has traditionally been thought to impair lung growth by direct compression. In this context, pulmonary hypoplasia in CDH occurs as a result of in utero lung compression, which impedes both bronchial and pulmonary vascular development in the fetal lung. Recent experimental evidence suggests that the lung hypoplasia in CDH originates early in embryogenesis *before* visceral herniation has occurred.[13-15] Conceptually, a primary lung defect could lead to malformation of the fetal diaphragm, although this theory remains unproven. Pulmonary hypoplasia may be mediated by alterations in pulmonary growth factors or other mechanisms. The etiology of a primary defect in CDH lung development remains unknown, as does its relation to the diaphragmatic defect.

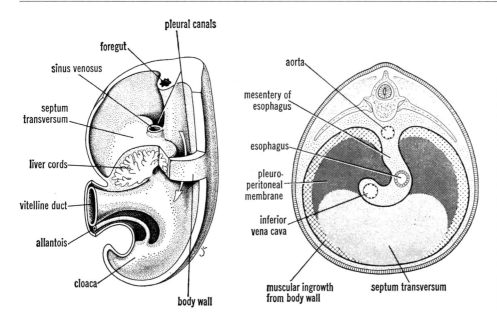

FIGURE 23-2. The embryologic relation of the developing diaphragm and pleuroperitoneal canal. The septum transversum fuses posteriorly with the mediastinal mesenchyme. The pleuroperitoneal canals (*white arrow*) allow free communication between the pleural and peritoneal cavities. Closure of these canals is completed as the pleuroperitoneal membranes develop. The four embryologic components of the developing diaphragm are shown in cross section. (From Skandalakis LJ, Colborn GL, Skandalakis JE: In Nyhus LM, Baker RJ, Fischer JE [eds]: Mastery of Surgery, 3rd ed. Boston, Little, Brown, 1996.)

Pulmonary hypoplasia in CDH is characterized by a decrease in pulmonary mass and reductions in the number of bronchial divisions, respiratory bronchioles, and alveoli. Abnormalities of septal formation within the terminal saccules and alveolar units of the lung limit gas exchange at the air-capillary interface.[16] At birth, alveoli are immature and have thickened intra-alveolar septae with increased glycogen content. Experimental models of CDH demonstrate biochemical immaturity with decreased levels of disaturated phosphatidylcholine, total lung DNA, and total lung protein.[17] Relative surfactant deficiency also may be present,[18,19] contributing to the functional immaturity of the CDH lung. The pulmonary vasculature also is hypoplastic, and the walls of the pulmonary arterioles are abnormally thickened, demonstrating increased muscularization.

The lung opposite the diaphragmatic defect also demonstrates structural abnormalities of pulmonary hypoplasia. Contralateral pulmonary hypoplasia is most severe if the visceral mass causes mediastinal shift and contralateral lung compression, yet contralateral pulmonary hypoplasia occurs even in the absence of mediastinal shift, which further suggests that mechanisms other than extrinsic compression contribute to pulmonary hypoplasia in CDH.

CONGENITAL DIAPHRAGMATIC HERNIA

Incidence and Epidemiology

Congenital diaphragmatic hernia is a relatively common anomaly that is identified in 1 of every 2000 to 5000 live births. More than 1000 babies born in the United States are affected each year.[20] Female infants are affected twice as often as males. The etiology of CDH is not known, but genetic factors may play a role because familial cases have been reported.[21,22] In familial cases, the inheritance

pattern is likely multifactorial. However, one epidemiologic study of 40 families with multiple siblings affected with CDH suggested an autosomal recessive pattern of inheritance.[23] The vast majority of cases occur sporadically, with no familial link identified. The association of CDH with other genetic abnormalities and anomalies strongly suggests an underlying genetic etiology.

Pathophysiology

Several interactive and complex mechanisms are responsible for the clinical findings and pathophysiology observed in neonates with CDH. Local and systemic factors combine to varying degrees to produce a severe, self-perpetuating cycle of hypoxia, hypercarbia, and acidosis. The severity of clinical manifestations and the survival are determined largely by the severity of pulmonary hypoplasia in each patient. Therapeutic interventions should be designed to interrupt and reverse this process.

The lungs in newborns with CDH are hypoplastic, functionally immature, and have limited capacity for gas exchange. Several vessel abnormalities contribute to the increased reactivity and increased pulmonary vascular resistance observed in infants with CDH. These vasculature abnormalities include increased muscularization of pulmonary arterioles, reduced branching of pulmonary vessels, and decreased overall cross-sectional area of the vascular bed. These vascular abnormalities contribute to sustained pulmonary hypertension in CDH, which can be severe and often is refractory to treatment.

Persistent pulmonary hypertension of the neonate (PPHN) and persistent fetal circulation (PFC) are common in neonates with CDH. A combination of factors, including hypoxia, acidosis, hypercarbia, and hypothermia, contribute to pulmonary hypertension. This results in a continued pattern of fetal circulation with right-to-left shunting through the ductus arteriosus and foramen ovale. Hypoxia caused by shunting further aggravates and perpetuates PPHN and PFC, which are risk factors for treatment failure and overall poor prognosis. Vasoactive peptides, including endothelin 1, angiotensins, thromboxanes, and prostanoids, also may contribute to the pulmonary hypertension observed in neonates with CDH.[24-27]

Associated Anomalies

Although the severity of pulmonary hypoplasia and of pulmonary vascular abnormality are the primary factors that determine survival in CDH, the contribution of associated congenital anomalies to mortality must not be underestimated. The survival advantage of infants with isolated diaphragmatic defects is significantly better than that in those with additional extradiaphragmatic malformations.[28] Ninety-five percent of stillborn neonates with CDH have major associated anomalies,[29] of which most are central nervous system defects. More than 60% of newborns with CDH who do not survive resuscitation or preoperative stabilization have associated malformations, whereas only 8% of those surviving to operation have additional anomalies.[30] Approximately 70% of infants with prenatal diagnosis of CDH have associated malformations, and 20% have chromosomal abnormalities. In contrast, the incidence of associated anomalies identified in infants with postnatally diagnosed CDH is 30% to 35%.[28]

Cardiac anomalies account for 63% of the anomalies identified.[31] The cardiac anomalies often exacerbate pulmonary hypertension, right-to-left shunting, and hemodynamic instability. The most common cardiac defects identified in neonates with CDH are heart hypoplasia, atrial septal defects, and ventricular septal defects. Other outflow tract anomalies (tetralogy of Fallot, persistent truncus, double-outlet right ventricle, coarctation) also are reported.[32] Live-born infants with both CDH and congenital heart disease are 3 times more likely to die than are those without associated heart disease.[33] Additional anomalies with CDH include pulmonary sequestration, renal and genital anomalies, neural tube defects, and chromosomal abnormalities.

Genetic abnormalities associated with CDH include both anomalies of chromosome number (Turner's syndrome; trisomies 13, 18, 21, 22, and 23) and conditions with specific chromosomal aberrations (i.e., 15q24-q26 deletions[34]). A gene distal to the 15q21 locus may be important for normal development of the diaphragm.[34,35] Congenital diaphragmatic hernia also occurs as a clinical manifestation of other genetic syndromes (i.e., Fryn's,[36,37] Brachman-de Lange,[38,39] Pallister-Killian[40]). Chromosomal anomalies associated with CDH confer a much poorer prognosis. If antenatal diagnosis of CDH is made by fetal ultrasonography (US), amniocentesis with karyotype and chromosomal analysis is warranted.

Diagnosis and Treatment

Prenatal Diagnosis

The diagnosis of CDH is made with prenatal US in approximately 50% to 60% of cases.[41] Improvements in US technology allow early diagnosis, usually between 16 and 24 weeks of gestation. At tertiary referral centers, up to 93% of neonates with CDH may be diagnosed with prenatal US.[42] Diagnosis early in the pregnancy optimizes prenatal and postnatal care of both mother and fetus and provides time for perinatal counseling, consideration of fetal intervention, or pregnancy termination.

The typical US findings in the fetus with CDH may include an echogenic chest mass, bowel loops within the chest, polyhydramnios, absent or intrathoracic gastric bubble, mediastinal shift to the contralateral side, intrathoracic liver, and fetal hydrops.[43] These sonographic features of a congenital diaphragmatic hernia are not always present at the time of the initial evaluation and may evolve over time.[44] Although suggested to be prognostic indicators of survival, none of these features can absolutely and consistently identify a fetus with a poor prognosis for survival. Antenatal diagnosis of CDH in the absence of other associated anomalies does not alter the severity of illness or survival.[45-47] In most cases, a prenatal diagnosis of CDH does not require a change in obstetric management. Although no strong evidence indicates that prenatal diagnosis should alter decisions regarding the timing or method of delivery, survival in neonates with CDH that require ECMO is better in those born near term.[48]

Clinical Presentation

Respiratory distress is the common postnatal presentation of CDH in the newborn. Respiratory distress may develop immediately after birth in association with low Apgar scores or within 24 to 48 hours after an initial period of relative stability and minimal clinical signs. Neonates that become symptomatic within 6 hours of birth are at high risk for morbidity and mortality. Initial signs include tachypnea, grunting respirations, chest retractions, pallor, cyanosis, and clinical signs of shunting and persistent fetal circulation. Physical examination often reveals a scaphoid abdomen and an increased anteroposterior chest diameter. If mediastinal shift is present, the point of maximal cardiac impulse is displaced away from the side of the diaphragmatic lesion. Bowel sounds may be auscultated within the affected hemithorax, but breath sounds are decreased bilaterally from diminished tidal volume. Breath sounds are less audible on the affected side.

The diagnosis is confirmed by chest radiography (Fig. 23-3*A, B*) performed during resuscitation. The radiographic findings of left-sided CDH include the presence of air and fluid-filled loops of bowel within the left hemithorax, with mediastinal shift to the right. Often minimal gas is noted within the abdomen, and the gastric bubble may be visualized within the left chest. Right-sided lesions are harder to appreciate and appear as lobar consolidation, fluid within the chest, or diaphragmatic eventration. The findings on plain film radiography in CDH can mimic those of congenital cystic adenomatoid malformations of the lung (Fig. 23-4). The differential diagnosis also includes cystic teratoma, pulmonary sequestration, bronchogenic cyst, neurogenic tumors, and primary lung sarcoma.

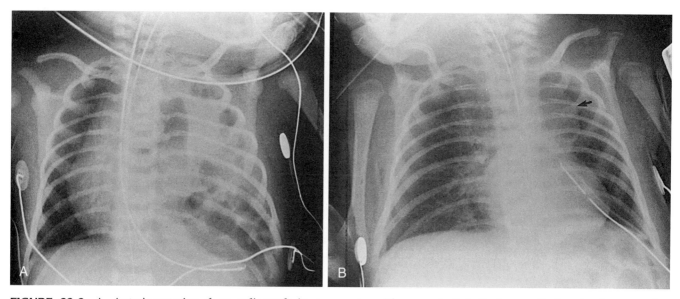

FIGURE 23-3. *A,* Anterioposterior chest radiograph in a neonate with a congenital diaphragmatic hernia demonstrating air-filled loops of bowel within the left chest. The heart and mediastinum are shifted to the right, and the hypoplastic left lung can be seen medially. *B,* Postoperative radiograph demonstrating hyperexpansion of the right lung with shift of the mediastinum to the left. The edge of severely hypoplastic left lung is again easily visualized (*arrow*).

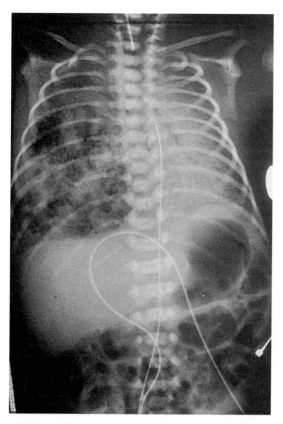

FIGURE 23-4. Anterioposterior chest radiograph in a neonate with a congenital cystic adenomatoid malformation (CCAM) of the right lung. The air-filled densities in the right chest closely resemble those that would result from bowel herniation into the chest. A normal bowel gas pattern within the abdomen helps to distinguish CCAM from congenital diaphragmatic hernia.

As many as 10 % of patients with CDH are discovered beyond the neonatal period. Most are seen initially with acute gastrointestinal symptoms. Occasionally CDH is an incidental finding in an otherwise asymptomatic patient.[49-52] In general, late-presenting CDH has an excellent prognosis because the associated lung hypoplasia and pulmonary hypertension are mild or absent. Gastric decompression can be lifesaving in an older child with severe respiratory and cardiopulmonary distress from massive distention of the intrathoracic stomach.[53] CDH results in abnormal intestinal rotation and fixation. As a result, children with unsuspected CDH may be first seen beyond the neonatal period with intestinal obstruction, volvulus, or bowel ischemia and necrosis.

Resuscitation and Stabilization

Neonates with CDH and severe respiratory distress require aggressive resuscitation. Initial interventions include endotracheal intubation, neuromuscular blockade, and positive-pressure ventilation. Mask ventilation is avoided to prevent insufflation of the stomach and small bowel with air. High airway pressures (peak inspiratory pressure [PIP] >25) should be avoided to prevent iatrogenic barotrauma. The goal of positive-pressure ventilation should be to keep the PIP less than 25 cm H_2O pressure while maintaining the preductal arterial saturation (Sao_2) above 85 %. Moderate hypercarbia ($Paco_2$, 45 to 60) is acceptable as long as the pH can be maintained above 7.3.

A nasogastric tube is inserted and placed to suction to decompress the stomach and minimize bowel distention, which can compromise cardiac and pulmonary function. Arterial and central venous lines are routinely placed for blood sampling and accurate pressure monitoring.

A right radial arterial line is preferred for monitoring preductal PaO_2, which reflects cerebral oxygenation. A urinary catheter is generally indicated to monitor closely the urine output, which reflects the adequacy of fluid resuscitation. Hypervolemia or hypovolemia should be avoided. Appropriate fluid and electrolyte management is important to ameliorate acidosis. Bicarbonate is indicated to treat metabolic acidosis (pH, <7.3) but may increase hypercarbia.

Echocardiography is performed early to identify associated cardiac anomalies and evaluate the degree of pulmonary hypertension. Although PPHN in CDH is usually apparent as a gradient between preductal and postductal arterial saturation, echocardiographic findings determine the severity of pulmonary hypertension and ductal shunting. The echocardiographic signs of pulmonary hypertension include poor contractility of the right ventricle, flattening of the interventricular septum, enlarged right heart chambers, tricuspid valve regurgitation, and right-to-left or bidirectional shunting at the ductus arteriosus. Echocardiography also provides an estimate of right ventricular pressure, which may be useful to guide therapy.

Ductal shunting can be problematic but is not necessarily harmful as long as preductal oxygenation is adequate (SaO_2, >85%) and postductal oxygen delivery is sufficient to meet tissue and organ demands. The target preductal and postductal partial pressures of oxygen (PO_2) should be at least 60 mm Hg and 40 mm Hg, respectively. Maintaining postductal PO_2 above 40 mm Hg prevents visceral and peripheral ischemia, which can cause metabolic acidosis and further worsening of pulmonary hypertension. Factors that increase pulmonary vascular resistance and precipitate PPHN (i.e., hypoxia, acidosis, hyperthermia) are avoided and quickly corrected when identified. If ductal shunting is severe or right ventricular pressure is elevated, inhaled nitric oxide (NO) may be useful. However, infants with pulmonary hypertension and CDH are less responsive to NO than are neonates with other causes of PPHN, and clinical trials have failed to demonstrate that NO is beneficial in CDH.[54] Nonetheless, NO is commonly used to treat PPHN in infants with CDH, and it may reduce right ventricular pressure and improve oxygenation. Routine use of high-dose dopamine or dobutamine is not recommended to treat PPHN in CDH. However, left ventricular dysfunction and systemic hypotension are indications for prompt administration of inotropic agents that augment left ventricular output and increase systemic pressure, minimizing right-to-left ductal shunting.

Mechanical Ventilation

The goals of ventilator therapy are to maintain adequate oxygenation while using ventilation techniques that avoid injury to the hypoplastic and immature lungs. Ventilator-induced lung injury may be largely responsible for the instability of newborns with CDH and the major contributor to mortality.[55] Initial mechanical ventilation using a fraction of inspired oxygen (FiO_2) of 1.0 is commonly required to maintain adequate oxygen delivery.

The goal of oxygen therapy is to maintain a preductal saturation of 85% or better. Reductions in FiO_2 should be made very gradually to prevent precipitation of PPHN.

Initiation of conventional ventilator management includes pressure-limited ventilation rates of 30 to 60 breaths per minute at peak inspiratory pressures of 25 cm H_2O or less to minimize barotrauma.[56,57] Spontaneous ventilation with a minimal set respiratory rate is preferred, and neuromuscular blockade is avoided. By using this strategy to avoid ventilator-induced lung injury, several groups have now achieved survival rates approaching 90%.[57–59] Hyperventilation as a ventilation strategy to induce alkalosis and decrease ductal shunting has been abandoned at most centers. Reducing lung injury with permissive hypercapnea reduces mortality in infants with CDH.[8,57,58,60] In infants with CDH, PCO_2 values in the range of 45 to 60 mm Hg are well tolerated as long as compensated acidosis exists.

The role of high-frequency oscillation (HFOV) in the ventilatory management of CDH continues to evolve. HFOV has demonstrated little or no benefit when used as a high-pressure lung recruitment ventilation strategy.[61,62] The CDH lung is likely nonrecruitable, and high mean airway pressures cause lung damage. Previously HFOV was used as a rescue mode and reserved for neonates that continued to have hypoxia and hypercarbia refractory to conventional ventilation techniques.[63,64] Many groups are now using HFOV as a primary ventilation strategy and a means to avoid barotrauma.[60,65,66] HFOV permits ventilation at lower mean airway pressures, which should be maintained at no greater than 14 to 16 cm H_2O.[65] Several groups have reported improved survival with HFOV and delayed operation.[56,60,65–67] Early use of HFOV is recommended to limit lung injury when the PIP exceeds 25 cm H_2O pressure with conventional ventilation.[56] The amplitude (peak-to-peak pressure) is adjusted in the range of 35 to 45 cm H_2O to achieve a PCO_2 of 40 to 55 mm Hg.

Nitric Oxide

Inhaled NO, a potent and selective pulmonary vasodilator, is used for the management of severe PPHN. NO stimulates soluble guanylate cyclase within vascular endothelium to produce cyclic guanosine monophosphate, a smooth-muscle relaxant. NO at doses less than 20 ppm improves systemic oxygenation and decreases the need for ECMO in neonates with respiratory failure secondary to PPHN. NO improves postductal oxygenation, reverses ductal shunting, reduces pulmonary pressures, and improves ventilation-to-perfusion matching within the lung.[64,68–71] Although NO is commonly used to treat PPHN in CDH, the benefit of this therapy is unproven. Randomized trials of the use of NO in neonates with PPHN and CDH have shown that survival was not improved, and the need for ECMO was not reduced[54,72,73] Nonrandomized studies indicated that NO is beneficial to treat PPHN in newborns with CDH,[68,74–76] but the clinical response is often inconsistent. NO failure may be related to the severity of pulmonary hypoplasia and its associated pulmonary vascular abnormalities. The response of infants with CDH to NO is unpredictable and variable but typically occurs at inhalation doses less than 20 ppm. NO should be weaned gradually as tolerated to prevent toxicity. Some neonates with CDH experience rebound pulmonary hypertension if inhaled NO is weaned abruptly.[64] Dipyridamole, a phosphodiesterase inhibitor, can augment the response to NO in newborns with CDH[77,78] and may be useful to weaning from inhaled NO therapy.[79] Recent studies suggest that NO plays a role in cell proliferation. Inhaled NO selectively modulates the pulmonary artery proliferative response that is associated with lung injury.[80] In this regard, NO may prove to be useful in CDH to attenuate or prevent the adverse pulmonary effects of ventilator-induced lung injury.

Surfactant

The lungs in newborns with CDH are immature and may have abnormalities in surfactant production and function. Experimental[81-83] and clinical[18,19,84] evidence suggest that infants with CDH are surfactant deficient and that replacement therapy might be beneficial. Surfactant phospholipids and apoprotein SP-A are decreased in animal models of CDH. Immunohistochemistry studies in an animal model demonstrated that surfactant is distributed within intercellular granules in CDH lung rather than being uniformly distributed on the alveolar surface, as is observed in the normal lung.[85] Experimentally, exogenous surfactant administration improves pulmonary blood flow, reduces pulmonary vascular resistance, and decreases ductal shunting.[86] In addition, surfactant replacement may improve gas exchange[82] and enhance NO delivery.[81] Although some authors have questioned the presence of surfactant deficiency in human CDH,[87] reasonable evidence exists that the lungs in infants with CDH are relatively surfactant deficient,[18,19] and exogenous surfactant therapy has been used. However, reports have been confined to small series or case reports,[88,89] and no controlled clinical trials have demonstrated exogenous surfactant to be beneficial in CDH. Despite a lack of proven efficacy, exogenous surfactant therapy is commonly used in infants with CDH at some centers.[90,91] The role of surfactant therapy in CDH has yet to be clearly defined. Its benefit to infants with CDH remains unproved and therefore should be used with caution.

Extracorporeal Membrane Oxygenation

ECMO is the most powerful and invasive tool for reversal of neonatal respiratory failure. It is also an expensive, labor-intensive technology associated with substantial morbidity and risk of long-term sequelae. ECMO has been used in the management of neonatal CDH since it was first reported in the late 1970s.[92] Since those early years, many reports have been published suggesting that ECMO improves survival in CDH. Currently, CDH accounts for one fourth of all neonates with severe respiratory failure treated with ECMO.[93] Overall, approximately 50% of neonates with CDH are treated with ECMO.[48,94] Before the current era of gentle ventilation

and delayed surgery, the use of ECMO in newborns with CDH increased survival by 15% to 20% over historic controls in centers reporting high mortality rates.[95-97] Currently, most centers use ECMO to stabilize infants before surgical repair of the diaphragm. Although the results of ECMO in CDH are heavily dependent on selection criteria, the overall survival rate for neonates with CDH that receive ECMO is approximately 50% to 60%.[94] Without ECMO, the predicted mortality risk for this group of critically ill neonates exceeds 80%.

ECMO, where available, is considered for almost all infants with CDH that cannot be managed with conventional therapy, provided they have no other major lethal anomalies. ECMO rescue is used in neonates with CDH and potentially reversible pulmonary hypertension. Some centers withhold ECMO for infants with severe pulmonary hypoplasia and inability to achieve a preductal SaO_2 of greater than 85% after initial resuscitation,[56,57] which may reflect inadequate lung parenchyma. In the past, some have advocated that candidates for ECMO should have at least one preductal PO_2 of at least 80 to 100 mm Hg,[98] but many survivors have been reported who have not fulfilled this criterion. Currently, no absolute predictors of lethal pulmonary hypoplasia are known in CDH, and it is not possible to predict survival with complete accuracy.

In general, selection criteria for ECMO are based on the prediction of greater than 80% to 90% mortality with maximal conventional therapy. In the past, many predictors of survival have been proposed, including PCO_2, Bohn's criteria,[99,100] best preductal or postductal PO_2, oxygenation index, and others. Although each was applied successfully at individual institutions, none was universally applicable or accepted at other neonatal centers, where management strategies and patient populations are often quite variable. In this current era of gentle ventilation and delayed operation, these earlier predictors of survival are no longer valid. Recently a study of more than 1000 neonates with CDH identified birth weight and the 5-minute Apgar score to be the best predictors of postnatal outcome,[101] which may be useful to determine which infants are candidates for ECMO. Currently, selection criteria for ECMO in CDH are institution dependent and continue to evolve as new therapies and ventilation strategies are introduced and applied.[102]

If ECMO criteria are met, extracorporeal support is considered for infants in whom signs of inadequate oxygen delivery, progressive metabolic acidosis, or organ failure develop, despite maximal medical therapy. Failure of conventional therapy may be manifested by declining preductal oxygen saturation and/or the appearance of clinical signs of barotrauma (i.e., interstitial subcutaneous emphysema, pneumothorax or pneumopericardium, persistent air leaks, and high mean airway pressures). ECMO is instituted before extreme ventilator pressures are required to prevent or minimize ventilator-induced lung injury. ECMO is considered for infants that decompensate with severe pulmonary hypertension, right-to-left shunting, and severe preductal hypoxemia. If the preductal saturation falls below 80% to 85% and is refractory to standard resuscitation and ventilatory manipulations (i.e., HFOV, FiO_2 100%, NO), ECMO should be promptly instituted. In general, ECMO is indicated when the preductal PaO_2 cannot be maintained greater than 50 mm Hg or the serum pH cannot be maintained greater than 7.15 within 1 to 2 hours despite maximal therapy. Most often the decision to proceed with ECMO is based on the infant's clinical course, rather than specific measured or calculated criteria.

Candidates for ECMO should have a birth weight that equals or exceeds 2 kg. ECMO is contraindicated in neonates with intracranial hemorrhage greater than grade I because systemic anticoagulation with heparin is required. Cranial US is performed before initiation of ECMO and is repeated daily to assess for intracranial bleeding during the first 5 days of bypass. Neonates of less than 35 weeks of gestation are at highest risk for intracranial hemorrhage. Extension of intracranial hemorrhage requires removal from ECMO.

ECMO was initially used in CDH as a rescue therapy after diaphragmatic repair.[92] In the past, more than half of newborns with CDH treated with conventional mechanical ventilation and immediate surgical repair required postoperative ECMO.[103] Delaying the repair of CDH in newborns improves survival and decreases the use of extracorporeal support.[60,104] Recent reported series from centers that have promoted gentle ventilation techniques and a delayed surgical approach indicate that ECMO was required in only 6% to 19% of neonates with CDH.[56,57]

The optimal time for surgical repair of the diaphragm after initiation of ECMO is controversial. Repair while on ECMO is reported to have a high rate of hemorrhagic complications,[105,106] but refinements in surgical technique and the use of antifibrinolytic agents has decreased these bleeding complications.[107,108] Bleeding complications also may be reduced with early repair on ECMO if performed before the development of significant edema or coagulopathy.[109] Some surgeons recommend repair after resolution of pulmonary hypertension and at the point when ECMO is ready to be discontinued.[57,110] The advantage of this approach is that ECMO can easily be reinstituted if recurrent pulmonary hypertension and respiratory failure develop postoperatively.[111] Many pediatric surgeons prefer that the patient be weaned back to conventional ventilation and decannulated before repair of CDH. Surgical repair is usually performed within 2 to 3 days after decannulation, and recurrent pulmonary hypertension is rare. Although uncommon, recurrent pulmonary hypertension after surgical repair of the diaphragm may require a second course of ECMO. Nitric oxide has been used successfully to avoid an additional course of ECMO.[74] Survival in infants requiring a second ECMO run is approximately 50%.[112]

The average duration of an ECMO course in CDH is 9 to 10 days, and a course extending beyond 2 weeks is no longer unusual.[93] Venoarterial (VA) ECMO is the mode of extracorporeal support most often chosen in CDH (86%), yet venovenous (VV) and VA ECMO are associated with similar rates of survival.[113] VV ECMO may be preferable to VA ECMO, which is associated with more neurologic complications (i.e., seizures, cerebral infarction).

Conversion from VV to VA ECMO does not appear to affect survival adversely. Failure to wean from ECMO is believed to indicate lethal pulmonary hypoplasia; support may be withdrawn, and operative repair of the diaphragm is not performed.[114] Overall survival in neonates with CDH who receive ECMO is approximately 53% to 56%.[94,115] Survival in newborns with CDH managed with delayed repair and selective preoperative stabilization with ECMO can be as high as 78% to 92%.[57,60,91,104] Infants with CDH that are born near term and require ECMO have improved survival, shorter ECMO duration, and shorter length of hospitalization than do those born before term.[48] Despite recent studies confirming that ECMO improves survival in critically ill neonates with CDH,[94] the benefit of ECMO in CDH continues to be challenged.[116,117] Some authors have reported no survival advantage with ECMO in CDH.[118,119] In infants treated with ECMO, the incidence of neurologic morbidity and chronic lung disease is higher in CDH infants than in those with other causes of PPHN.[120,121] Several centers have reported CDH survival rates of 80% to 85% *without* the use of ECMO.[122,123] As newer ventilation and therapeutic options are introduced and applied, the need for ECMO may continue to decrease.

Surgical Considerations and Postoperative Management

The timing of surgical repair of the diaphragm in CDH remains controversial. Although many centers have adopted a delayed surgical approach, this practice had not been universally accepted or applied. Surgical repair does not improve gas exchange and decreases thoracic wall and pulmonary compliance.[124] A decrease in lung compliance in a neonate with CDH with pulmonary hypoplasia and PPHN is undesirable and may cause rapid clinical deterioration. Delayed repair allows postnatal transition from fetal circulation and allows time for pulmonary vascular remodeling. Delay may produce a more stable infant more capable of tolerating the decrease in lung compliance caused by surgical repair. Delayed repair does not result in deterioration in respiratory status; in addition, it may decrease the need for ECMO and improve overall survival without increasing morbidity.[7,8,57] Despite the recent shift toward delayed operative intervention, the optimal timing of surgical repair has not been clearly demonstrated,[125] and some centers continue to favor early surgical intervention and report improved survival with this approach.[126] For individual patients, the decision about timing of repair is based on clinical or echocardiographic findings of decreased pulmonary vascular resistance and decreased pulmonary hypertension. Practically, the surgical procedure is usually performed 1 to 2 days after resolution of clinical signs of ductal shunting (i.e., differential between pre- and postductal O_2 saturation) as long as satisfactory ventilation is maintained at low ventilator pressures (PIP, <25) and low inspired oxygen requirements. When HFOV is used preoperatively, repair is usually delayed until the infant can be transitioned back to conventional pressure-limited ventilation.

Surgical repair of a CDH should be performed efficiently and expeditiously to minimize operative stress. Although both laparoscopic and thoracoscopic repairs are feasible,[127,128] these minimally invasive techniques may not be well tolerated in fragile neonates with CDH. Minimally invasive techniques are more suitable to infants and children when the diagnosis is made outside the newborn period. A transabdominal approach is the most commonly used approach to repair diaphragmatic defects in newborns. The abdomen is entered through an incision placed below the costal margin. This approach allows easy reduction of the viscera and excellent visualization of the diaphragmatic defect (Fig. 23-5). Bowel, liver, and spleen are carefully reduced from the thoracic cavity. A true hernia sac may be present in 10% to 20% of cases and should be excised. The thoracic and abdominal cavities are inspected for the presence of an associated pulmonary sequestration. Once the limits and extent of the diaphragmatic defect are precisely defined, the diaphragm is repaired.

Small defects are closed primarily with 2-0 or 3-0 permanent sutures with or without pledgets. Larger defects can be closed primarily but may produce a flattened diaphragm, poor respiratory excursion, and distortion of the thorax. In this situation, the large defect should be closed with a prosthetic patch. Polytetrafluoroethylene (1 mm thick) is a suitable material for patch closure. The patch is tailored slightly larger than the diaphragmatic defect to restore a concave shape to the reconstructed diaphragm. Restoring the "dome" shape of the diaphragm helps to expand the abdominal capacity and limits overexpansion of the ipsilateral lung. Tension-free closure of the defect in this manner also prevents constriction of the thoracic cage and limits the adverse effects of closure on pulmonary compliance. With very large defects, no apparent or easily recognizable posterior rim of diaphragm may be seen. Sutures into the abdominal wall, into the ribs, or encircling the ribs are needed to secure the prosthesis in

these cases. Recently, a bioprosthetic patch made from small intestinal submucosa has been introduced, which may be useful to reinforce or repair large diaphragmatic defects. Although unproven, bioprosthetic materials offer a theoretical advantage of better tissue ingrowth and graft incorporation than polytetrafluoroethylene, which is associated with a high rate of suture line disruption and reherniation.[113] The diaphragmatic repair is inspected for hemostasis, and fibrin sealants are often applied to the suture line in anticoagulated infants repaired while on ECMO.[129]

Tube thoracostomy is not mandatory and is probably not indicated.[8,57] The lungs will gradually enlarge, displacing fluid and air absorbed from the pleural space. Tube thoracostomy is rarely necessary unless a postoperative chylothorax develops[130] or pleural fluid accumulates, causing mediastinal shift or a contralateral pneumothorax. For surgeons who prefer thoracostomy, a chest tube is positioned and brought out through a low intercostal space before closure of the diaphragm. The chest tube can be used to adjust intrathoracic pressures and control mediastinal shift. It is connected to water seal rather than put to vacuum in the postoperative period. If air is removed from the pleural space by suction, the mediastinum will shift, allowing overdistention of the contralateral lung. Overexpansion may be a contributing factor in postoperative contralateral pneumothorax.[131] Chest tubes should be removed early to avoid infectious complications.

After completion of the diaphragmatic repair, the abdominal wall is stretched to increase the capacity of the abdominal cavity. The abdominal wall fascia is closed unless closure restricts ventilation, in which case, only skin closure is performed. The resulting abdominal wall hernia can be repaired at a later date. An alternative method is to repair the fascial defect with polyglactic acid (Vicryl) mesh, allowing the wound to heal by secondary intention. This technique frequently avoids a secondary ventral hernia repair.

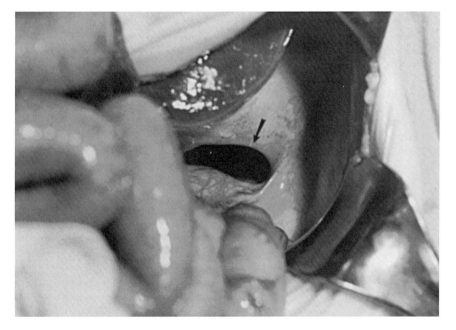

FIGURE 23-5. A small posterolateral diaphragmatic hernia (*arrow*) approached through a subcostal incision. The transabdominal approach allows easy reduction of the viscera and excellent visualization of the defect.

Postoperative ventilator management continues as before diaphragmatic repair, with continued emphasis on avoiding ventilator-induced lung injury. Surgical repair of the diaphragm decreases chest compliance initially and may adversely affect peak and mean inspiratory pressures. Surgical stress can precipitate intense pulmonary vasoconstriction and recurrence of pulmonary hypertension and persistent fetal circulation. If respiratory failure ensues and cannot be controlled with any of the previously discussed ventilation and cardiopulmonary management techniques, ECMO should be instituted. The therapeutic goal of postoperative ventilation is to minimize barotrauma. An FiO_2 of 1.0 may be required to maintain adequate oxygenation perioperatively. Rapid decreases in FiO_2 must be avoided because reductions of only 0.1 have been seen to trigger pulmonary vasospasm and recurrent pulmonary hypertension. Inhaled NO may be useful in the postoperative period to treat pulmonary hypertension[74,132] and avoid ECMO.

Several nonpulmonary complications can occur in these neonates during the postoperative period.[133] These include hemorrhage, chylothorax, and adhesive intestinal obstruction. Other long-term complications associated with CDH are gastroesophageal reflux, scoliosis, and pectus deformities. Recurrent diaphragmatic hernia occurs most frequently after prosthetic patch closure.[134]

Outcomes in Congenital Diaphragmatic Hernia

Survival

It is difficult to quantify the results of therapy and treatment of CDH owing to the tremendous variation in the strategies and techniques used to support these critically ill patients. A few points of variation between and often within institutions include differences in severity of illness, ventilation strategies, ventilator type (conventional versus HFOV), availability and selection criteria of ECMO, and variable use of other pharmacologic agents (i.e., NO, surfactant). As newer and more innovative approaches to managing CDH become available, comparisons of mortality and outcomes between institutions may become even more difficult. Recently, multi-institutional data from more than 1000 neonates with CDH were used to develop a method to stratify infants into low-, intermediate-, and high-risk categories based on birth weight and 5-minute Apgar score.[101] Risk stratification correlated closely with actual survival and may be useful to allow better comparison of outcomes data from different institutions.

Survival statistics in CDH are very institution dependent. A review of CDH outcomes from patients treated in the early 1990s indicated an overall survival rate of 60%, yet the individual institution survival rates varied from 25% to 83%.[20] Despite recent improvements in survival reported by several centers, overall survival is still only about 64%.[101] Prenatal diagnosis of CDH is associated with an increased mortality, but in the absence of other major anomalies, survival is probably not affected.[45] Nonetheless, approximately 30% of fetuses with CDH will be stillborn. Of those fetuses surviving to delivery, up to 30% to 50% will die before transfer to a neonatal center. If stillbirths and infants with CDH that die before transfer to referral centers are included, overall survival from CDH is only 40% to 60%.[46,135,136] CDH accounts for approximately 4% to 10% of neonatal deaths that are caused by congenital anomalies.[20] Prematurity and low birth weight are associated with a significantly increased risk of perinatal mortality from CDH.[137]

Three factors that have dramatically affected survival in CDH have been the introduction of ECMO, the adaptation of less barotraumatic methods of ventilation (including permissive hypercapnia), and delaying surgical repair of the diaphragm. The effect of ECMO on survival has been previously discussed. ECMO has generally been believed to improve overall survival by 15% to 20% at institutions using this technique. Many modern centers that have adapted strategies of delayed repair and gentle ventilation techniques are now reporting survival rates approaching 80% to 90% in infants with CDH without other major congenital anomalies.[8,56-58,60] The improved survival observed at these institutions also occurred with decreased morbidity and decreased use of ECMO. As more centers adapt management strategies that avoid iatrogenic barotrauma, the high overall mortality of CDH is expected to decrease.

Sequelae of CDH

The *pulmonary function* of survivors with CDH is favorable. Most CDH survivors are healthy and enjoy normal lives free of respiratory problems, but long-term pulmonary consequences of CDH are dependent on the severity of pulmonary hypoplasia at birth and the degree of lung injury. Infants that experience uneventful preoperative and postoperative courses will generally have normal lung function. For those children who require substantial support and intervention, ventilatory impairment and thoracic deformities are demonstrated in approximately 50%, despite minimal or no pulmonary symptoms. Pulmonary function tests are normal in 50% to 70% of survivors, and the remainder have findings suggesting some degree of restrictive, obstructive, or combined respiratory impairment.[138-141] Approximately one fourth of survivors tested beyond age 5 years demonstrate findings of obstructive airway disease.[141]

Functional residual capacity is reduced in the newborn after repair of CDH, but functional lung volumes may be normal over the long term. Increased bronchial reactivity seen in approximately one third of survivors is more common in those patients seen within 6 hours of birth with severe pulmonary hypoplasia and large diaphragmatic defects.[140] Pulmonary ventilation and perfusion deficiencies are more common on the side of the diaphragmatic defect,[139,140] but diffusing capacity is typically normal. The volume of the ipsilateral lung increases with time, but this increase may be secondary to emphysematous changes.[142] Air trapping within the hypoplastic lung may appear as hyperlucent areas on chest radiography. One-fourth of neonates with CDH are oxygen dependent at age 1 month, but this decreases to less than 2% at 1 year.[143]

One-third of CDH patients may have clinical and radiographic evidence of *bronchopulmonary dysplasia*,[144] which is more common in those infants managed with prolonged mechanical ventilation and O_2 supplementation. Lung function in survivors of CDH improves with age,[141,145] and alveolar multiplication continues from birth until age 7 or 8 years. Even though the hypoplastic lung may grow to be functionally normal, structurally it remains abnormal, and the number of bronchiolar and pulmonary arterial divisions is relatively fixed. It is important to note that all long-term pulmonary studies are based on survivors managed with conventional strategies (i.e., high ventilation pressures) that were associated with high mortality rates. As survival rates continue to improve with the addition of newer therapies (i.e., ECMO, NO, HFOV, permissive hypercapnia), survivors with more severe lung hypoplasia can be expected, and their long-term pulmonary sequelae may be more significant. Pulmonary problems continue to be a major source of morbidity for survivors of CDH in the first 2 years of life, even with the use of gentle ventilation techniques.[141]

Gastroesophageal reflux is a common finding in patients with CDH. The incidence of gastroesophageal reflux after successful repair of CDH is reported to exceed 50% in many series.[146–150] ECMO-treated survivors may be at greatest risk.[145,151] The gastroesophageal reflux observed in patients with CDH is part of a generalized foregut dysmotility[152,153] that also may include esophageal ectasia and delayed gastric emptying. Esophageal ectasia and dysmotility may be the result of kinking or relative obstruction at the gastroesophageal junction that is caused when the stomach translocates into the chest.[154] Large diaphragmatic defects may compromise the esophageal hiatus of the diaphragm, thereby destroying its contribution to the lower esophageal sphincter mechanism and predisposing to reflux. Management of gastroesophageal reflux and upper gastrointestinal dysmotility in patients with CDH is not different from the usual medical therapy, including prokinetic agents, H_2 antagonists, and proton pump inhibitors. Antireflux procedures are not usually necessary,[153] but surgical treatment has been required in 10% to 20% of cases.[146,149,155,156]

Intestinal obstruction is a fairly common event after CDH repair and occurs in up to 20% of patients monitored over the long term.[133,157] Small bowel obstruction may be caused by adhesions, midgut volvulus,[158] or recurrent herniation with incarceration.

Recurrent diaphragmatic hernia is common with prosthetic patch repair of large diaphragmatic defects. Overall, it occurs in approximately 5% to 20% of patients.[151,158] Prosthetic patch repair of the diaphragm results in recurrent hernia in 40% to 50% of patients within 3 years.[134] Patients requiring ECMO may be at highest risk for recurrent herniation when a prosthetic patch is used to reconstruct the diaphragm,[159] particularly if the repair is performed while on bypass.

Growth retardation and *failure to thrive* are common in survivors of CDH.[145] Poor growth affects nearly 20% of CDH survivors in the first years of life and may be caused by inadequate oral intake related to gastrointestinal dysmotility, gastroesophageal reflux, or an associated oral aversion.[143] In addition, caloric requirements may be higher because of an increased work of breathing and tachypnea.[160] In CDH survivors, more than 50% will be below the 25th percentile for weight in the first year of life, despite adequate oral intake.[156] Weight differences improve with time and may be normal for age by age 2 years.[151,153] CDH infants requiring ECMO are at greatest risk for failure to thrive. Gastrostomy may be required in up to one third of survivors.[156]

Survivors of CDH are at risk for *neurodevelopmental problems* including major motor disabilities[147] and developmental delays in both motor and verbal skills.[158] Neurocognitive deficits also are common in survivors of CDH.[121] It is difficult to separate the developmental delays that are caused by the disease process itself from those that may be caused by specific therapeutic interventions. Hyperventilation[161,162] and ECMO are both associated with potential adverse neurologic sequelae. Hyperventilation and alkalinization, although no longer recommended for treatment of pulmonary hypertension or CDH, can dramatically reduce cerebral blood flow, which is sensitive to acute changes of arterial P_{CO_2} and pH.[163] Acute hyperventilation to reduce P_{CO_2} from 40 mm Hg down to 20 mm Hg can reduce cerebral perfusion by up to 50%.[163] Alkalosis reduces oxygen delivery to all body tissues by increasing hemoglobin-oxygen affinity. Consequently, hyperventilation further reduces cerebral oxygen delivery in neonates already compromised by perinatal asphyxia, hypoxemia, and cardiovascular instability. ECMO increases the risks for cerebral palsy, sensorineural hearing loss, speech and verbal skill developmental delay, vision loss, and seizure disorder.[164] The incidence of neurologic abnormalities is greater than 50% in CDH survivors that required ECMO.[120,121,145] The hearing loss after ECMO therapy is often delayed in onset and is progressive. Significant hearing loss is detected in 4% to 28% of ECMO survivors[158,165]; serial follow-up hearing examinations are mandatory.

Novel Therapies for CDH

Fetal Intervention

Prenatal diagnosis has led to innovative fetal intervention for the fetus with CDH and prenatal features that impart a poor prognosis and high postnatal mortality. Fetal intervention is appealing as a potential method to prevent severe pulmonary hypoplasia. Selection of appropriate candidates for fetal intervention has been limited by a lack of absolute indicators of poor prognosis and improving survival (80% to 90%) in infants managed at centers using innovative mechanical ventilation techniques.[56,57,60] Only fetuses with the most severe pulmonary hypoplasia should be considered potential candidates for fetal intervention.

In centers offering fetal surgical therapy, the fetal lung-to-head ratio (LHR), as measured by US at 24 to 26 weeks of gestation, has evolved as the best predictor of severity and basis for prenatal surgical intervention. A fetal LHR of less than 1.0 is considered an indicator of poor outcome at some centers. A prospective evaluation of the LHR and survival indicated that no fetus with CDH and LHR less than 1.0 survived with postnatal therapy; all patients with LHR greater than 1.4 survived.[166] Liver herniation into the chest also is a predictor of poor prognosis for fetuses with left CDH,[167] particularly when a low LHR also is identified. Fetuses with CDH and *without* liver herniation have a favorable prognosis, even with a low LHR, and should be treated postnatally.[168,169]

Prenatal intervention is a risk to both the fetus and the mother and is justifiable only if improvements in survival or morbidity can be clearly demonstrated. All interventions must be measured against the significantly improved survival recently achieved in centers using innovative mechanical ventilation techniques. Many centers are reporting almost 90% survival with reduced use of ECMO in neonates with CDH. It is still impossible to predict accurately which fetuses will or will not survive the gestational or neonatal period.

In Utero Repair of Congenital Diaphragmatic Hernia

The rationale for in utero repair of CDH was initially based on experimental demonstration that reduction of herniated viscera in the fetus prevents lung hypoplasia and restores lung growth. The first clinical experience with in utero repair of CDH was reported in 1990.[170] Successful repair and outcome is possible in fetuses without hepatic herniation,[168] but these fetuses have good prognosis for survival with conventional postnatal therapy.[56,57] In utero CDH repair does not improve survival in fetuses without liver herniation.[168] Hepatic herniation into the chest is not correctable by in utero repair because reduction of the liver causes acute obstruction of the umbilical vein and fetal death.[167,171] Although the techniques for successful open in utero repair have been refined, currently no indication exists for in utero repair of CDH.

Tracheal Occlusion

The dynamics of fetal lung fluid have a dramatic effect on lung growth and maturity. Oligohydramnios and other conditions associated with a deficiency of fetal lung fluid cause pulmonary hypoplasia. Tracheal occlusion in utero can prevent pulmonary hypoplasia and can increase lung growth in these circumstances. Fetal tracheal ligation in experimental models of CDH accelerates lung growth, improves lung compliance, reduces herniated viscera, and improves oxygenation and ventilation after birth.[172-175] Although tracheal ligation reverses pulmonary hypoplasia, the numbers of type II pneumocytes and surfactant production are dramatically reduced at term.[176-178] Antenatal steroids and temporary occlusion may counter the effects of tracheal occlusion on type II pneumocyte function.[179,180] The timing of prenatal tracheal occlusion also may be critical to subsequent pulmonary development and function.[181]

Fetal tracheal occlusion has been successfully performed in human fetuses with CDH with both open hysterotomy and endoscopic techniques.[182-185] In prenatally diagnosed CDH with low LHR (<1.4), fetoscopic tracheal occlusion offers improved survival over that with open fetal diaphragmatic repair. Although many technical problems of fetal intervention have been solved,[167] it remains a highly experimental procedure with significant risk for complications.[182,186] Despite reversal of pulmonary hypoplasia, survival has been limited in humans.[182-184] Although theoretically promising, further experimental and clinical investigations are required before in utero tracheal occlusion becomes a recommended therapy for CDH. Currently this procedure is performed at only a few centers and only in a select group of fetuses with CDH and dismal prognosis (early diagnosis, liver herniation, LHR <1.0) with postnatal therapy.

Prenatal Glucocorticoids

The hypoplastic lungs of infants with CDH are functionally immature at birth. In addition to being relatively surfactant deficient, experimental models of CDH demonstrate several markers of biochemical immaturity including decreased levels of total lung DNA, total lung protein, and disaturated phosphatidylcholine.[17] Antenatal administration of glucocorticoids in animal models of CDH have resulted in beneficial effects including acceleration in surfactant protein synthesis and release, increases in lung volume and compliance, reduction in alveolar septal thickness, and improvements in antioxidant defense mechanisms.[187,188-192] Antenatal glucocorticoids also increase DNA synthesis and total lung protein production.[193] Although administration of antenatal glucocorticoids induces lung maturation in animal models of CDH, only limited clinical information is available regarding the use prenatal glucocorticoids in human CDH, and the benefits of such therapy are unproven. In addition, serious short-term and long-term effects may be associated with prenatal glucocorticoid therapy,[194-196] and the significance of these adverse effects in fetuses with CDH is unknown.

Prenatal steroids are routinely used to enhance lung development in premature infants and should be administered for at least 24 to 48 hours for all fetuses between 24 and 34 weeks of gestation that are at risk for preterm delivery.[197,198] Antenatal hormonal therapy is widely used to induce lung maturation in fetuses at risk of premature delivery and successfully reduces the incidence of respiratory distress syndrome. Success with preterm infants has led some to use antenatal steroids in fetuses with CDH to enhance pulmonary growth development. Reports of the use of glucocorticoids in human CDH have been limited to case reports and small anecdotal series. In one study, maternal betamethasone was administered starting at 24 to 26 weeks in 3 fetuses with CDH and features indicating a poor postnatal prognosis (early diagnosis, liver herniation, LHR <1)[199]; all three neonates survived. Despite encouraging case series reports, randomized controlled clinical trials will be required to determine whether prenatal steroids improve outcomes in fetuses with CDH.

Liquid Ventilation

Liquid ventilation is an experimental therapy that has been used in adults, children, and neonates with severe respiratory failure.[200] Partial liquid ventilation (PLV) increased functional residual capacity and improved gas exchange by enhancing recruitment of atelectatic lung regions, improving ventilation/perfusion matching, and clearing peripheral airways and alveoli by lavage. Lung compliance is improved by an effective reduction in alveolar surface tension.[201] In addition, PLV enhances pulmonary surfactant production, decreases inflammation, and reduces histologic evidence of lung injury.[202,203] During PLV, the lungs are filled with a volume of perfluorocarbon approximately equal to functional residual capacity, and ventilation is performed by using a time-cycled, pressure-controlled technique.[204] Excellent oxygenation is achieved with PLV at lower PIPs, resulting in less barotrauma.[200,201,205] PLV in combination with positive end-expiratory pressure also may protect against ventilator-induced lung injury.[206,207]

PLV has been successfully used to improve survival in infants with severe respiratory distress syndrome that were not predicted to survive.[208] Subsequently, PLV has been safely administered to high-risk newborns with CDH and severe respiratory failure on VA ECMO to improve gas exchange and pulmonary compliance.[204,209] Despite improvements in lung function, PLV has not improved survival in infants with CDH. The benefit of PLV in the treatment of neonates with CDH remains unproven.

Lung Transplantation in Congenital Diaphragmatic Hernia

Lobar lung transplantation has been successfully used as a rescue therapy in CDH.[210] In this case report, the neonate was initially stabilized with ECMO, followed by delayed repair of the diaphragm with a prosthetic patch while on ECMO. Although the neonate was successfully decannulated from ECMO, lung transplantation became necessary as a result of progressive pulmonary failure. Despite this single report, the role of lung transplantation and ECMO as a bridge to transplantation in cases of CDH with lethal pulmonary hypoplasia is not known.

Retrosternal Hernia

Retrosternal hernia occurs in two forms. The foramen of Morgagni's hernia, or parasternal hernia, is the more common of the two and represents only 2% to 6% of congenital diaphragmatic defects.[131,211] This diaphragmatic defect results from failure of the sternal and crural portions of the diaphragm to fuse at the site where the superior epigastric (internal mammary) artery traverses the diaphragm. Morgagni's hernias may be unilateral or bilateral, but occur unilaterally on the right side in approximately 90% of cases. Bilateral parasternal hernias occur in 7% of cases.[211,212] Retrosternal hernias will often appear as a midline defect at laparotomy (Fig. 23-6). A well-defined hernia sac is usually present. Morgagni's hernias are often found in association with other congenital anomalies. Trisomy 21 is present in up to 35% of children with parasternal hernias.[213,214] Congenital heart defects also are commonly reported.[215,216]

The majority of Morgagni's hernias are asymptomatic and are diagnosed from chest radiographs obtained in

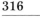

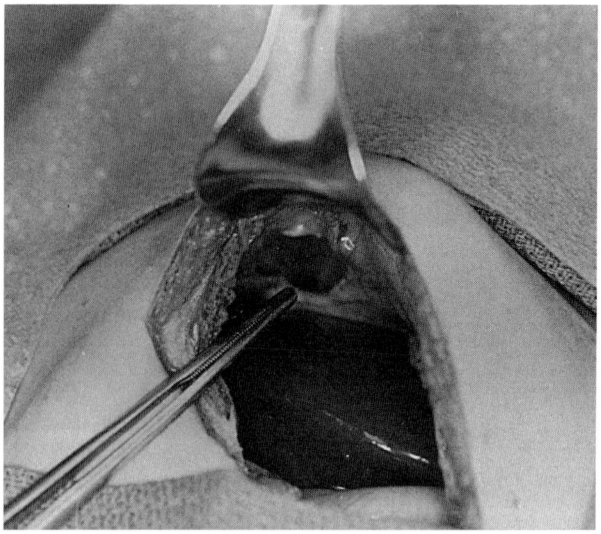

FIGURE 23-6. Retrosternal hernia viewed through a transabdominal incision. The bowel has been reduced, and the defect is seen immediately posterior to the xiphoid process.

older children or adults being evaluated for unrelated pulmonary symptoms. Children are more often symptomatic than adults with this lesion, initially seen with recurrent respiratory infection, coughing, vomiting, or epigastric discomfort.[211] Gastrointestinal symptoms may be intermittent, but intestinal obstruction,[217] ischemic bowel with necrosis,[218] and acute gastric volvulus[219,220] are possible. Cardiac tamponade is a rare presentation of this type of hernia.[221] Herniated viscera may include the transverse colon, omentum, liver, small bowel, stomach, or spleen.

Chest radiography in the neonate with a Morgagni's hernia often demonstrates a well-defined air/fluid-filled structure immediately behind the sternum (Fig. 23-7A, B). A lateral chest radiograph localizes this finding to the retrosternal space. Contrast studies obtained for evaluation of gastrointestinal symptoms will demonstrate small bowel, colon, and occasionally stomach within the thoracic cavity. Morgagni's hernias are at risk for incarceration and strangulation and should be repaired soon after the diagnosis is made. The hernia is typically repaired via a transabdominal approach, although laparoscopic repair is feasible as well.[222–224]

The less common form of retrosternal hernia occurs as a component of Cantrell's pentalogy.[225] The pentalogy of Cantrell includes a constellation of congenital defects: omphalocele; inferior sternal cleft; severe cardiac defects, including thoracoabdominal ectopia cordis; anterior diaphragmatic hernia; and a diaphragmatic pericardial defect.[226,227] The cardiac defect is the most important factor influencing morbidity and mortality. This rare congenital anomaly results from an embryologic failure in the development of the septum transversum. Repair of this complex anomaly requires correction of cardiac defects plus diaphragmatic and abdominal wall closure. Prosthetic material is often required to repair the large diaphragmatic defect.

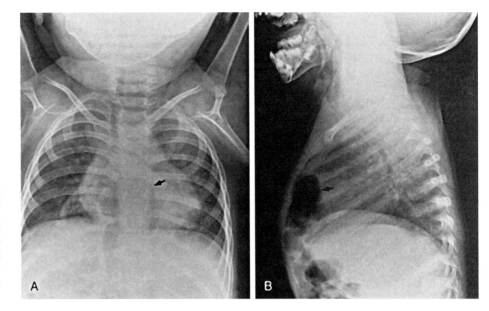

FIGURE 23-7. *A,* Chest radiograph in a neonate with a retrosternal hernia. Anteroposterior film demonstrates air-filled loops of bowel above the diaphragm and posterior to the sternum *(arrow)*. *B,* Lateral projection confirming the retrosternal position of the herniated viscera *(arrow)*.

EVENTRATION OF THE DIAPHRAGM

Eventration is an abnormal elevation of diaphragm. The affected hemidiaphragm moves paradoxically during inspiration and expiration,[228,229] which adversely affects pulmonary mechanics and function. The congenital form results from incomplete development of the muscular portion or central tendon of the diaphragm. It occurs most commonly on the left side, but bilateral diaphragmatic eventration has been reported.[230-232] Large eventrations can potentially interfere with prenatal and postnatal lung development. In cases in which the diaphragm exists as only a thin membrane, the distinction from CDH with a hernia sac is arbitrary.[103] Like CDH, congenital eventration may result in pulmonary hypoplasia, but pulmonary hypertension and persistent fetal circulation are uncommon. Eventration can occur in association with other congenital anomalies, including pulmonary sequestration, congenital heart disease, tracheomalacia, cerebral agenesis, and trisomic chromosomal abnormalities.[233,234]

Eventration in the neonate may be difficult to distinguish from diaphragmatic paralysis. Traction injury to the nerve roots of the phrenic nerve during traumatic delivery results in paralysis, sometimes with brachial plexus palsy. Iatrogenic phrenic nerve injury complicating a cardiac surgical procedure or mediastinal tumor resection is the most common cause of diaphragmatic paralysis in older infants and children. Phrenic nerve injury also can occur during surgical procedures in the neck. Inflammatory or neoplastic processes adjacent to the phrenic nerve also can cause paralysis of the diaphragm.

Although newborns with diaphragmatic eventration can be asymptomatic, most will have respiratory distress, tachypnea, and pallor. Respiratory distress results from alveolar hypoventilation and paradoxical movement of the diaphragm. During inspiration, the affected hemidiaphragm rises, and the mediastinum shifts toward the opposite side. Lung expansion becomes impaired bilaterally. Neonates with eventration often suck poorly. They tire easily during feedings and subsequently fail to gain weight. Additional clinical signs of eventration include ipsilateral dullness to percussion and unilateral or bilateral diminished breath sounds. The maximal cardiac impulse is shifted away from the side of the lesion.

Chest radiography typically demonstrates an elevated hemidiaphragm (Fig. 23-8). The diagnosis can be confirmed by fluoroscopy or US, showing paradoxical motion

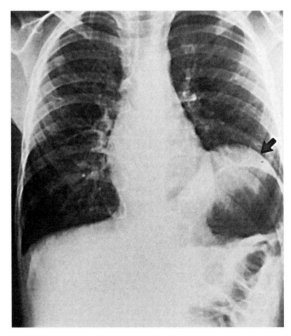

FIGURE 23-8. Anteroposterior chest radiograph demonstrates a large diaphragmatic eventration *(arrow)*. The abdominal viscera remain beneath an intact but attenuated left hemidiaphragm.

of the diaphragm and mediastinal shift with inspiration and expiration. The diagnosis of eventration or paralysis may be obscured in neonates and infants who are intubated and receiving positive pressure ventilation. A dysfunctional diaphragm may be a cause for inability to wean from mechanical ventilation. Older infants and children may have recurrent pneumonia or gastrointestinal symptoms, including intermittent vomiting, postprandial pain, dyspepsia, or gastric volvulus. Gastrointestinal complaints are more common with left-sided lesions. Computed tomography or other additional studies may be necessary to distinguish eventration from tumors, bronchogenic cysts, pulmonary sequestration or consolidation, or pleural effusions.

Initial treatment of infants with eventration includes upright positioning, supplemental oxygen, and nutritional support. Mechanical ventilation is not always necessary, but often is required to maintain adequate oxygenation and gas exchange. The indications for surgical intervention include respiratory distress requiring continued ventilatory support, recurrent pulmonary infections, and failure to thrive. Newborns with congenital eventration should undergo plication early and do not benefit from conservative management.[131,234] Small eventrations that are clinically asymptomatic may not require surgical intervention.

The surgical treatment of a symptomatic eventration is simple plication of the diaphragm.[131,229,234-236] Plication improves respiratory mechanics by increasing both tidal volume and maximal breathing capacity. The plicated diaphragm becomes immobilized to reduce its paradoxical movement and the associated contralateral shift of the mediastinum. In cases of paralysis caused by birth injury or postoperative phrenic nerve palsy, spontaneous recovery is possible; continuous positive pressure ventilation may be all that is required. Plication is indicated in patients who cannot be weaned from positive pressure ventilation after 2 to 3 weeks.[234,235,237,238] Plication does not prevent return of diaphragmatic function.[235,239] Iatrogenic phrenic nerve transection will result in permanent paralysis of the hemidiaphragm, and prophylactic plication is recommended.[131,235,240] Phrenic nerve repair has been successfully performed in older infants and children.[241,242]

Plication of the diaphragm can be performed from either the transthoracic or transabdominal approach. On the right side, a seventh intercostal space thoracotomy provides the best exposure. A left-sided eventration can easily be repaired through a left subcostal incision. Bilateral eventrations are approached through a transverse upper abdominal incision. Several rows of sutures are placed to imbricate and flatten the diaphragm. Sutures are placed carefully to avoid branches of the phrenic nerve and to obtain generous bites of tissue. Resection of the diaphragm is not necessary or indicated.

The perioperative morbidity and mortality of diaphragmatic plication are low and are mostly related to complications of prolonged mechanical ventilation.[234] In infants without major anomalies or other complicating factors, early plication results in immediate improvement in pulmonary mechanics, and long-term respiratory function is excellent.[233,235,239]

REFERENCES

1. Gross R: Congenital hernia of the diaphragm. In Gross R (ed): The Surgery of Infancy and Childhood: Its Principles and Techniques, 1st ed. Philadelphia, WB Saunders, 1953, pp 428–444.
2. Cartlidge PH, Mann NP, Kapila L: Preoperative stabilisation in congenital diaphragmatic hernia. Arch Dis Child. 61:1226–1228, 1986.
3. Langer JC, Filler RM, Bohn DJ, et al: Timing of surgery for congenital diaphragmatic hernia: is emergency operation necessary? J Pediatr Surg 23:731–734, 1988.
4. Charlton AJ, Bruce J, Davenport M: Timing of surgery in congenital diaphragmatic hernia: Low mortality after pre-operative stabilisation [comment]. Anaesthesia 46:820–823, 1991.
5. Coughlin JP, Drucker DE, Cullen ML, et al: Delayed repair of congenital diaphragmatic hernia. Am Surg 59:90–93, 1993.
6. Wilson JM, Lund DP, Lillehei CW, et al: Delayed repair and preoperative ECMO does not improve survival in high-risk congenital diaphragmatic hernia. J Pediatr Surg 27:368–375, 1992.
7. Breaux CW Jr, Rouse TM, Cain WS, et al: Improvement in survival of patients with congenital diaphragmatic hernia utilizing a strategy of delayed repair after medical and/or extracorporeal membrane oxygenation stabilization. J Pediatr Surg 26:333–338, 1991.
8. Wung JT, Sahni R, Moffitt ST, et al: Congenital diaphragmatic hernia: survival treated with very delayed surgery, spontaneous respiration, and no chest tube. J Pediatr Surg 30:406–409, 1995.
9. Greer JJ, Cote D, Allan DW, et al: Structure of the primordial diaphragm and defects associated with nitrofen-induced CDH. J Appl Physiol 89:2123–2129, 2000.
10. Iritani I: Experimental study on embryogenesis of congenital diaphragmatic hernia. Anat Embryol 169:133–139, 1984.
11. Kluth D, Keijzer R, Hertl M, et al: Embryology of congenital diaphragmatic hernia. Semin Pediatr Surg 5:224–233, 1996.
12. Greer JJ, Allan DW, Babiuk RP, et al: Recent advances in understanding the pathogenesis of nitrofen-induced congenital diaphragmatic hernia. Pediatr Pulmonol 29:394–399, 2000.
13. Jesudason EC, Connell MG, Fernig DG, et al: Early lung malformations in congenital diaphragmatic hernia. J Pediatr Surg 35:124–128, 2000.
14. Jesudason EC: Challenging embryological theories on congenital diaphragmatic hernia: Future therapeutic implications for paediatric surgery. Ann R Coll Surg Engl 84:252–259, 2002.
15. Leinwand MJ, Tefft JD, Zhao J, et al: Nitrofen inhibition of pulmonary growth and development occurs in the early embryonic mouse. J Pediatr Surg 37:1263–1268, 2002.
16. Dibbins AW: Congenital diaphragmatic hernia: Hypoplastic lung and pulmonary vasoconstriction. Clin Perinatol 5:93–104, 1978.
17. Suen HC, Catlin EA, Ryan DP, et al: Biochemical immaturity of lungs in congenital diaphragmatic hernia. J Pediatr Surg 28:471–477, 1993.
18. Lotze A, Knight GR, Anderson KD, et al: Surfactant (beractant) therapy for infants with congenital diaphragmatic hernia on ECMO: Evidence of persistent surfactant deficiency. J Pediatr Surg 29:407–412, 1994.
19. Moya FR, Thomas VL, Romaguera J, et al: Fetal lung maturation in congenital diaphragmatic hernia. Am J Obstet Gynecol 173:1401–1405, 1995.
20. Langham MR Jr, Kays DW, Ledbetter DJ, et al: Congenital diaphragmatic hernia: Epidemiology and outcome. Clin Perinatol 23:671–688, 1996.
21. Frey P, Glanzmann R, Nars P, et al: Familial congenital diaphragmatic defect: Transmission from father to daughter. J Pediatr Surg 26:1396–1398, 1991.
22. Kufeji DI, Crabbe DC: Familial bilateral congenital diaphragmatic hernia. Pediatr Surg Int 15:58–60, 1999.
23. Hitch DC, Carson JA, Smith EI, et al: Familial congenital diaphragmatic hernia is an autosomal recessive variant. J Pediatr Surg 24:860–864, 1989.
24. Kobayashi H, Puri P: Plasma endothelin levels in congenital diaphragmatic hernia. J Pediatr Surg 29:1258–1261, 1994.
25. Bos AP, Sluiter W, Tenbrinck R, et al: Angiotensin-converting enzyme activity is increased in lungs of rats with pulmonary hypoplasia and congenital diaphragmatic hernia. Exp Lung Res 21:41–50, 1995.

26. Ford WD, James MJ, Walsh JA: Congenital diaphragmatic hernia: Association between pulmonary vascular resistance and plasma thromboxane concentrations. Arch Dis Child 59:143–146, 1984.
27. Bos AP, Tibboel D, Hazebroek FW, et al: Congenital diaphragmatic hernia: Impact of prostanoids in the perioperative period. Arch Dis Child 65:994–995, 1990.
28. Bollmann R, Kalache K, Mau H, et al: Associated malformations and chromosomal defects in congenital diaphragmatic hernia. Fetal Diagn Ther 10:52–59, 1995.
29. Butler N, Claireaux A: Congenital diaphragmatic hernia as a cause of perinatal mortality. Lancet 1:659–663, 1962.
30. Sweed Y, Puri P: Congenital diaphragmatic hernia: Influence of associated malformations on survival. Arch Dis Child 69:68–70, 1993.
31. Fauza DO, Wilson JM: Congenital diaphragmatic hernia and associated anomalies: Their incidence, identification, and impact on prognosis. J Pediatr Surg 29:1113–1117, 1994.
32. Migliazza L, Otten C, Xia H, et al: Cardiovascular malformations in congenital diaphragmatic hernia: Human and experimental studies. J Pediatr Surg 34:1352–1358, 1999.
33. Cohen MS, Rychik J, Bush DM, et al: Influence of congenital heart disease on survival in children with congenital diaphragmatic hernia. J Pediatr 141:25–30, 2002.
34. Schlembach D, Zenker M, Trautmann U, et al: Deletion 15q24-26 in prenatally detected diaphragmatic hernia: Increasing evidence of a candidate region for diaphragmatic development. Prenat Diagn 21:289–292, 2001.
35. Aviram-Goldring A, Daniely M, Frydman M, et al: Congenital diaphragmatic hernia in a family segregating a reciprocal translocation t(5;15)(p15.3;q24). Am J Med Genet 90:120–122, 2000.
36. Langer JC, Winthrop AL, Whelan D: Fryns syndrome: A rare familial cause of congenital diaphragmatic hernia. J Pediatr Surg. 29:1266–1267, 1994.
37. Neville HL, Jaksic T, Wilson JM, et al: Fryns syndrome in children with congenital diaphragmatic hernia. J Pediatr Surg 37:1685–1687, 2002.
38. Cunniff C, Curry CJ, Carey JC, et al: Congenital diaphragmatic hernia in the Brachmann-de Lange syndrome. Am J Med Genet 47:1018–1021, 1993.
39. Marino T, Wheeler PG, Simpson LL, et al: Fetal diaphragmatic hernia and upper limb anomalies suggest Brachmann-de Lange syndrome. Prenat Diagn 22:144–147, 2002.
40. McLeod DR, Wesselman LR, Hoar DI: Pallister-Killian syndrome: Additional manifestations of cleft palate and sacral appendage. J Med Genet 28:541–543, 1991.
41. Garne E, Haeusler M, Barisic I, et al: Congenital diaphragmatic hernia: Evaluation of prenatal diagnosis in 20 European regions. Ultrasound Obstet Gynecol 19:329–333, 2002.
42. Benjamin DR, Juul S, Siebert JR: Congenital posterolateral diaphragmatic hernia: Associated malformations. J Pediatr Surg 23:899–903, 1988.
43. Wilcox DT, Irish MS, Holm BA, et al: Prenatal diagnosis of congenital diaphragmatic hernia with predictors of mortality. Clin Perinatol 23:701–709, 1996.
44. Vettraino IM, Lee W, Comstock CH: The evolving appearance of a congenital diaphragmatic hernia. J Ultrasound Med 21:85–89, 2002.
45. Wilson JM, Fauza DO, Lund DP, et al: Antenatal diagnosis of isolated congenital diaphragmatic hernia is not an indicator of outcome. J Pediatr Surg 29:815–819, 1994.
46. Steinhorn RH, Kriesmer PJ, Green TP, et al: Congenital diaphragmatic hernia in Minnesota: Impact of antenatal diagnosis on survival. Arch Pediatr Adolesc Med 148:626–631, 1994.
47. Clark RH, Hardin WD Jr, Hirschl RB, et al: Current surgical management of congenital diaphragmatic hernia: A report from the Congenital Diaphragmatic Hernia Study Group. J Pediatr Surg 33:1004–1009, 1998.
48. Stevens TP, Chess PR, McConnochie KM, et al: Survival in early- and late-term infants with congenital diaphragmatic hernia treated with extracorporeal membrane oxygenation. Pediatrics 110:590–596, 2002.
49. Berman L, Stringer D, Ein SH, et al: The late-presenting pediatric Bochdalek hernia: A 20-year review. J Pediatr Surg. 23:735–739, 1988.
50. Wiseman NE, MacPherson RI: "Acquired" congenital diaphragmatic hernia. J Pediatr Surg 12:657–665, 1977.
51. Newman BM, Afshani E, Karp MP, et al: Presentation of congenital diaphragmatic hernia past the neonatal period. Arch Surg 121:813–816, 1986.
52. Weber TR, Tracy T Jr, Bailey PV, et al: Congenital diaphragmatic hernia beyond infancy. Am J Surg 162:643–646, 1991.
53. Paut O, Mely L, Viard L, et al: Acute presentation of congenital diaphragmatic hernia past the neonatal period: A life threatening emergency. Can J Anaesth 43:621–625, 1996.
54. The Neonatal Inhaled Nitric Oxide Study Group (NINOS): Inhaled nitric oxide and hypoxic respiratory failure in infants with congenital diaphragmatic hernia. Pediatrics 99:838–845, 1997.
55. Sakurai Y, Azarow K, Cutz E, et al: Pulmonary barotrauma in congenital diaphragmatic hernia: A clinicopathological correlation. J Pediatr Surg 34:1813–1817, 1999.
56. Bohn D: Congenital diaphragmatic hernia. Am J Respir Crit Care Med 166:911–915, 2002.
57. Boloker J, Bateman DA, Wung JT, et al: Congenital diaphragmatic hernia in 120 infants treated consecutively with permissive hypercapnea/spontaneous respiration/elective repair. J Pediatr Surg 37:357–366, 2002.
58. Kays DW, Langham MR Jr, Ledbetter DJ, et al: Detrimental effects of standard medical therapy in congenital diaphragmatic hernia. Ann Surg 230:340–351, 1999.
59. Langham MR Jr, Kays DW, Beierle EA, et al: Twenty years of progress in congenital diaphragmatic hernia at the University of Florida. Am Surg 69:45–52, 2003.
60. Frenckner B, Ehren H, Granholm T, et al: Improved results in patients who have congenital diaphragmatic hernia using preoperative stabilization, extracorporeal membrane oxygenation, and delayed surgery. J Pediatr Surg 32:1185–1189, 1997.
61. Paranka MS, Clark RH, Yoder BA, et al: Predictors of failure of high-frequency oscillatory ventilation in term infants with severe respiratory failure. Pediatrics 95:400–404, 1995.
62. Azarow K, Messineo A, Pearl R, et al: Congenital diaphragmatic hernia: A tale of two cities: The Toronto experience. J Pediatr Surg 32:395–400, 1997.
63. Hirschl RB: Innovative therapies in the management of newborns with congenital diaphragmatic hernia. Semin Pediatr Surg 5:256–265, 1996.
64. Bohn DJ, Pearl R, Irish MS, et al: Postnatal management of congenital diaphragmatic hernia. Clin Perinatol 23:843–872, 1996.
65. Reyes C, Chang LK, Waffarn F, et al: Delayed repair of congenital diaphragmatic hernia with early high-frequency oscillatory ventilation during preoperative stabilization. J Pediatr Surg 33:1010–1016, 1998.
66. Desfrere L, Jarreau PH, Dommergues M, et al: Impact of delayed repair and elective high-frequency oscillatory ventilation on survival of antenatally diagnosed congenital diaphragmatic hernia: First application of these strategies in the more "severe" subgroup of antenatally diagnosed newborns. Intens Care Med 26:934–941, 2000.
67. Cacciari A, Ruggeri G, Mordenti M, et al: High-frequency oscillatory ventilation versus conventional mechanical ventilation in congenital diaphragmatic hernia. Eur J Pediatr Surg 11:3–7, 2001.
68. Finer NN, Etches PC, Kamstra B, et al: Inhaled nitric oxide in infants referred for extracorporeal membrane oxygenation: dose response. J Pediatr 124:302–308, 1994.
69. Kinsella JP, Abman SH: Inhalational nitric oxide therapy for persistent pulmonary hypertension of the newborn. Pediatrics 91:997–998, 1993.
70. Roberts JD, Polaner DM, Lang P, et al: Inhaled nitric oxide in persistent pulmonary hypertension of the newborn. Lancet 340:818–819, 1992.
71. Kinsella JP, Ivy DD, Abman SH: Inhaled nitric oxide improves gas exchange and lowers pulmonary vascular resistance in severe experimental hyaline membrane disease. Pediatr Res 36:402–408, 1994.
72. Finer NN, Barrington KJ: Nitric oxide in respiratory failure in the newborn infant. Semin Perinatol 21:426–440, 1997.
73. Kinsella JP, Truog WE, Walsh WF, et al: Randomized, multicenter trial of inhaled nitric oxide and high-frequency oscillatory ventilation in severe, persistent pulmonary hypertension of the newborn. J Pediatr 131:55–62, 1997.

74. Dillon PW, Cilley RE, Hudome SM, et al: Nitric oxide reversal of recurrent pulmonary hypertension and respiratory failure in an infant with CDH after successful ECMO therapy. J Pediatr Surg 30:743–744, 1995.

75. Frostell CG, Lonnqvist PA, Sonesson SE, et al: Near fatal pulmonary hypertension after surgical repair of congenital diaphragmatic hernia: Successful use of inhaled nitric oxide. Anaesthesia. 48:679–683, 1993.

76. Henneberg SW, Jepsen S, Andersen PK, et al: Inhalation of nitric oxide as a treatment of pulmonary hypertension in congenital diaphragmatic hernia. J Pediatr Surg 30:853–855, 1995.

77. Thebaud B, Saizou C, Farnoux C, et al: Dypiridamole, a cGMP phosphodiesterase inhibitor, transiently improves the response to inhaled nitric oxide in two newborns with congenital diaphragmatic hernia. Intens Care Med 25:300–303, 1999.

78. Kinsella JP, Torielli F, Ziegler JW, et al: Dipyridamole augmentation of response to nitric oxide. Lancet 346:647–648, 1995.

79. Buysse C, Fonteyne C, Dessy H, et al: The use of dipyridamole to wean from inhaled nitric oxide in congenital diaphragmatic hernia. J Pediatr Surg 36:1864–1865, 2001.

80. Roberts JD Jr, Zapol WM: Inhaled nitric oxide. Semin Perinatol 24:55–58, 2000.

81. Karamanoukian HL, Glick PL, Wilcox DT, et al: Pathophysiology of congenital diaphragmatic hernia, VIII: Inhaled nitric oxide requires exogenous surfactant therapy in the lamb model of congenital diaphragmatic hernia. J Pediatr Surg 30:1–4, 1995.

82. Wilcox DT, Glick PL, Karamanoukian H, et al: Pathophysiology of congenital diaphragmatic hernia, V: Effect of exogenous surfactant therapy on gas exchange and lung mechanics in the lamb congenital diaphragmatic hernia model. J Pediatr 124:289–293, 1994.

83. Mysore MR, Margraf LR, Jaramillo MA, et al: Surfactant protein A is decreased in a rat model of congenital diaphragmatic hernia. Am J Respir Crit Care Med 157:654–657, 1998.

84. Valls-i-Soler A, Alfonso LF, Arnaiz A, et al: Pulmonary surfactant dysfunction in congenital diaphragmatic hernia: Experimental and clinical findings. Biol Neonate 69:318–326, 1996.

85. Utsuki T, Hashizume K, Iwamori M: Impaired spreading of surfactant phospholipids in the lungs of newborn rats with pulmonary hypoplasia as a model of congenital diaphragmatic hernia induced by nitrofen. Biochim Biophys Acta 1531:90–98, 2001.

86. O'Toole SJ, Karamanoukian HL, Morin FC III, et al: Surfactant decreases pulmonary vascular resistance and increases pulmonary blood flow in the fetal lamb model of congenital diaphragmatic hernia. J Pediatr Surg 31:507–511, 1996.

87. Sullivan KM, Hawgood S, Flake AW, et al: Amniotic fluid phospholipid analysis in the fetus with congenital diaphragmatic hernia. J Pediatr Surg 29:1020–1024, 1994.

88. Glick PL, Leach CL, Besner GE, et al: Pathophysiology of congenital diaphragmatic hernia, III: Exogenous surfactant therapy for the high-risk neonate with CDH. J Pediatr Surg 27:866–869, 1992.

89. Bae CW, Jang CK, Chung SJ, et al: Exogenous pulmonary surfactant replacement therapy in a neonate with pulmonary hypoplasia accompanying congenital diaphragmatic hernia: A case report. J Korean Med Sci 11:265–270, 1996.

90. Somaschini M, Locatelli G, Salvoni L, et al: Impact of new treatments for respiratory failure on outcome of infants with congenital diaphragmatic hernia. Eur J Pediatr 158:780–784, 1999.

91. Finer NN, Tierney A, Etches PC, et al: Congenital diaphragmatic hernia: Developing a protocolized approach. J Pediatr Surg 33:1331–1337, 1998.

92. German JC, Gazzaniga AB, Amlie R, et al: Management of pulmonary insufficiency in diaphragmatic hernia using extracorporeal circulation with a membrane oxygenator (ECMO). J Pediatr Surg 12:905–912, 1977.

93. Roy BJ, Rycus P, Conrad SA, et al: The changing demographics of neonatal extracorporeal membrane oxygenation patients reported to the Extracorporeal Life Support Organization (ELSO) Registry. Pediatrics 106:1334–1338, 2000.

94. The Congenital Diaphragmatic Hernia Study Group: Does extracorporeal membrane oxygenation improve survival in neonates with congenital diaphragmatic hernia? J Pediatr Surg 34:720–725, 1999.

95. Heiss K, Manning P, Oldham KT, et al: Reversal of mortality for congenital diaphragmatic hernia with ECMO. Ann Surg 209:225–230, 1989.

96. Sawyer SF, Falterman KW, Goldsmith JP, et al: Improving survival in the treatment of congenital diaphragmatic hernia. Ann Thorac Surg 41:75–78, 1986.

97. Weber TR, Connors RH, Pennington DG, et al: Neonatal diaphragmatic hernia: An improving outlook with extracorporeal membrane oxygenation. Arch Surg 122:615–618, 1987.

98. vd Staak FH, Thiesbrummel A, de Haan AF, et al: Do we use the right entry criteria for extracorporeal membrane oxygenation in congenital diaphragmatic hernia? J Pediatr Surg 28:1003–1005, 1993.

99. Bohn DJ, James I, Filler RM, et al: The relationship between $PaCO_2$ and ventilation parameters in predicting survival in congenital diaphragmatic hernia. J Pediatr Surg 19:666–671, 1984.

100. Bohn D, Tamura M, Perrin D, et al: Ventilatory predictors of pulmonary hypoplasia in congenital diaphragmatic hernia, confirmed by morphologic assessment. J Pediatr 111:423–431, 1987.

101. The Congenital Diaphragmatic Study Group: Estimating disease severity of congenital diaphragmatic hernia in the first 5 minutes of life. J Pediatr Surg 36:141–145, 2001.

102. Wilson JM, Bower LK, Thompson JE, et al: ECMO in evolution: The impact of changing patient demographics and alternative therapies on ECMO. J Pediatr Surg 31:1116–1122, 1996.

103. De Lorimier AA: Diaphragmatic hernia. In Ashcraft KW, Holder TM (eds): Pediatric Surgery, 2nd ed. Philadelphia, WB Saunders, 1993, pp 204–217.

104. Reickert CA, Hirschl RB, Schumacher R, et al: Effect of very delayed repair of congenital diaphragmatic hernia on survival and extracorporeal life support use. Surgery 120:766–773, 1996.

105. Lally KP, Paranka MS, Roden J, et al: Congenital diaphragmatic hernia: Stabilization and repair on ECMO. Ann Surg 216:569–573, 1992.

106. Vazquez WD, Cheu HW: Hemorrhagic complications and repair of congenital diaphragmatic hernias: Does timing of the repair make a difference? Data from the Extracorporeal Life Support Organization. J Pediatr Surg 29:1002–1006, 1994.

107. Wilson JM, Bower LK, Lund DP: Evolution of the technique of congenital diaphragmatic hernia repair on ECMO. J Pediatr Surg 29:1109–1112, 1994.

108. van der Staak FH, de Haan AF, Geven WB, et al: Surgical repair of congenital diaphragmatic hernia during extracorporeal membrane oxygenation: Hemorrhagic complications and the effect of tranexamic acid. J Pediatr Surg 32:594–599, 1997.

109. Lally KP: Extracorporeal membrane oxygenation in patients with congenital diaphragmatic hernia. Sem Pediatr Surg 5:249–255, 1996.

110. Adolph V, Flageole H, Perreault T, et al: Repair of congenital diaphragmatic hernia after weaning from extracorporeal membrane oxygenation. J Pediatr Surg 30:349–352, 1995.

111. Sigalet DL, Tierney A, Adolph V, et al: Timing of repair of congenital diaphragmatic hernia requiring extracorporeal membrane oxygenation support. J Pediatr Surg 30:1183–1187, 1995.

112. Lally KP, Breaux CW Jr: A second course of extracorporeal membrane oxygenation in the neonate: Is there a benefit? Surgery 117:175–178, 1995.

113. Dimmitt RA, Moss RL, Rhine WD, et al: Venoarterial versus venovenous extracorporeal membrane oxygenation in congenital diaphragmatic hernia: The Extracorporeal Life Support Organization Registry, 1990–1999. J Pediatr Surg 36:1199–1204, 2001.

114. Atkinson JB, Kitagawa H: Extracorporeal membrane oxygenation and the management of congenital diaphragmatic hernia. Pediatr Surg Int 8:200–203, 1993.

115. Beresford MW, Shaw NJ: Outcome of congenital diaphragmatic hernia. Pediatr Pulmonol 30:249–256, 2000.

116. Schoeman L, Pierro A, Macrae D, et al: Late death after extracorporeal membrane oxygenation for congenital diaphragmatic hernia. J Pediatr Surg 34:357–359, 1999.

117. Elbourne D, Field D, Mugford M: Extracorporeal membrane oxygenation for severe respiratory failure in newborn infants: Cochrane review. Cochrane Database Syst Rev 1:CD001340, 2002.

118. Keshen TH, Gursoy M, Shew SB, et al: Does extracorporeal membrane oxygenation benefit neonates with congenital diaphragmatic hernia? Application of a predictive equation. J Pediatr Surg 32:818–822, 1997.

119. O'Rourke PP, Lillehei CW, Crone RK, et al: The effect of extra-corporeal membrane oxygenation on the survival of neonates with high-risk congenital diaphragmatic hernia: 45 cases from a single institution. J Pediatr Surg 26:147–152, 1991.

120. McGahren ED, Mallik K, Rodgers BM: Neurological outcome is diminished in survivors of congenital diaphragmatic hernia requiring extracorporeal membrane oxygenation. J Pediatr Surg 32:1216–1220, 1997.

121. Stolar CJ, Crisafi MA, Driscoll YT: Neurocognitive outcome for neonates treated with extracorporeal membrane oxygenation: Are infants with congenital diaphragmatic hernia different? J Pediatr Surg 30:366–372, 1995.

122. Pusic AL, Giacomantonio M, Pippus K, et al: Survival in neonatal congenital hernia without extracorporeal membrane oxygenation support. J Pediatr Surg 30:1188–1190, 1995.

123. Al-Shanafey S, Giacomantonio M, Henteleff H: Congenital diaphragmatic hernia: Experience without extracorporeal membrane oxygenation. Pediatr Surg Int 18:28–31, 2002.

124. Sakai H, Tamura M, Hosokawa Y, et al: Effect of surgical repair on respiratory mechanics in congenital diaphragmatic hernia. J Pediatr 111:432–438, 1987.

125. Moyer V, Moya F, Tibboel R, et al: Late versus early surgical correction for congenital diaphragmatic hernia in newborn infants. Cochrane Database Syst Rev 3:CD001695, 2002.

126. Okuyama H, Kubota A, Oue T, et al: Inhaled nitric oxide with early surgery improves the outcome of antenatally diagnosed congenital diaphragmatic hernia. J Pediatr Surg 37:1188–1190, 2002.

127. Krishna A, Zargar N: Laparoscopic repair of a congenital diaphragmatic hernia. Pediatr Surg Int 18:491–493, 2002.

128. Taskin M, Zengin K, Unal E, et al: Laparoscopic repair of congenital diaphragmatic hernias. Surg Endosc 16:869, 2002.

129. Cullen ML: Congenital diaphragmatic hernia: operative considerations. Semin Pediatr Surg 5:243–248, 1996.

130. Cheah FC, Noraida MH, Boo NY, et al: Chylothorax after repair of congenital diaphragmatic hernia: A case report. Singapore Med J 41:548–549, 2000.

131. Reynolds M: Diaphragmatic anomalies. In Raffensperger JG (ed): Swenson's Pediatric Surgery, 5th ed. East Norwalk, Conn, Appleton & Lange, 1990, pp 721–735.

132. Iocono JA, Cilley RE, Mauger DT, et al: Postnatal pulmonary hypertension after repair of congenital diaphragmatic hernia: Predicting risk and outcome. J Pediatr Surg 34:349–353, 1999.

133. Lund DP, Mitchell J, Kharasch V, et al: Congenital diaphragmatic hernia: The hidden morbidity. J Pediatr Surg. 29:258–262, 1994.

134. Moss RL, Chen CM, Harrison MR: Prosthetic patch durability in congenital diaphragmatic hernia: A long-term follow-up study. J Pediatr Surg 36:152–154, 2001.

135. Torfs CP, Curry CJ, Bateson TF, et al: A population-based study of congenital diaphragmatic hernia. Teratology 46:555–565, 1992.

136. Wenstrom KD, Weiner CP, Hanson JW: A five-year statewide experience with congenital diaphragmatic hernia. Am J Obstet Gynecol 165:838–842, 1991.

137. Puri P: Congenital diaphragmatic hernia. Curr Probl Surg 31:787–846, 1994.

138. Reid IS, Hutcherson RJ: Long-term follow-up of patients with congenital diaphragmatic hernia. J Pediatr Surg 11:939–942, 1976.

139. Falconer AR, Brown RA, Helms P, et al: Pulmonary sequelae in survivors of congenital diaphragmatic hernia. Thorax 45:126–129, 1990.

140. Vanamo K, Rintala R, Sovijarvi A, et al: Long-term pulmonary sequelae in survivors of congenital diaphragmatic defects. J Pediatr Surg 31:1096–1100, 1996.

141. Muratore CS, Kharasch V, Lund DP, et al: Pulmonary morbidity in 100 survivors of congenital diaphragmatic hernia monitored in a multidisciplinary clinic. J Pediatr Surg 36:133–140, 2001.

142. Nagaya M, Akatsuka H, Kato J, et al: Development in lung function of the affected side after repair of congenital diaphragmatic hernia. J Pediatr Surg 31:349–356, 1996.

143. Jaillard SM, Pierrat V, Dubois A, et al: Outcome at 2 years of infants with congenital diaphragmatic hernia: A population-based study. Ann Thorac Surg 75:250–256, 2003.

144. Ijsselstijn H, Tibboel D, Hop WJ, et al: Long-term pulmonary sequelae in children with congenital diaphragmatic hernia. Am J Respir Crit Care Med 155:174–180, 1997.

145. D'Agostino JA, Bernbaum JC, Gerdes M, et al: Outcome for infants with congenital diaphragmatic hernia requiring extracorporeal membrane oxygenation: The first year. J Pediatr Surg 30:10–15, 1995.

146. Nagaya M, Akatsuka H, Kato J: Gastroesophageal reflux occurring after repair of congenital diaphragmatic hernia. J Pediatr Surg 29:1447–1451, 1994.

147. Davenport M, Rivlin E, D'Souza SW, et al: Delayed surgery for congenital diaphragmatic hernia: Neurodevelopmental outcome in later childhood. Arch Dis Child. 67:1353–1356, 1992.

148. Fasching G, Huber A, Uray E, et al: Gastroesophageal reflux and diaphragmatic motility after repair of congenital diaphragmatic hernia. Eur J Pediatr Surg 10:360–364, 2000.

149. Kieffer J, Sapin E, Berg A, et al: Gastroesophageal reflux after repair of congenital diaphragmatic hernia. J Pediatr Surg 30:1330–1333, 1995.

150. Kamiyama M, Kawahara H, Okuyama H, et al: Gastroesophageal reflux after repair of congenital diaphragmatic hernia. J Pediatr Surg 37:1681–1684, 2002.

151. Van Meurs KP, Robbins ST, Reed VL, et al: Congenital diaphragmatic hernia: Long-term outcome in neonates treated with extracorporeal membrane oxygenation. J Pediatr 122:893–899, 1993.

152. Stolar CJ, Berdon WE, Dillon PW, et al: Esophageal dilatation and reflux in neonates supported by ECMO after diaphragmatic hernia repair. AJR Am J Roentgenol 151:135–137, 1988.

153. Stolar CJ, Levy JP, Dillon PW, et al: Anatomic and functional abnormalities of the esophagus in infants surviving congenital diaphragmatic hernia. Am J Surg 159:204–207, 1990.

154. Stolar CJ: What do survivors of congenital diaphragmatic hernia look like when they grow up? Sem Pediatr Surg 5:275–279, 1996.

155. Koot VC, Bergmeijer JH, Bos AP, et al: Incidence and management of gastroesophageal reflux after repair of congenital diaphragmatic hernia. J Pediatr Surg 28:48–52, 1993.

156. Muratore CS, Utter S, Jaksic T, et al: Nutritional morbidity in survivors of congenital diaphragmatic hernia. J Pediatr Surg 36:1171–1176, 2001.

157. Vanamo K, Rintala RJ, Lindahl H, et al: Long-term gastrointestinal morbidity in patients with congenital diaphragmatic defects. J Pediatr Surg 31:551–554, 1996.

158. Nobuhara KK, Lund DP, Mitchell J, et al: Long-term outlook for survivors of congenital diaphragmatic hernia. Clin Perinatol 23:873–887, 1996.

159. Atkinson JB, Poon MW: ECMO and the management of congenital diaphragmatic hernia with large diaphragmatic defects requiring a prosthetic patch. J Pediatr Surg 27:754–756, 1992.

160. Naik S, Greenough A, Zhang YX, et al: Prediction of morbidity during infancy after repair of congenital diaphragmatic hernia. J Pediatr Surg 31:1651–1654, 1996.

161. Bifano EM, Pfannenstiel A: Duration of hyperventilation and outcome in infants with persistent pulmonary hypertension. Pediatrics 81:657–661, 1988.

162. Marron MJ, Crisafi MA, Driscoll JM Jr, et al: Hearing and neurodevelopmental outcome in survivors of persistent pulmonary hypertension of the newborn. Pediatrics 90:392–396, 1992.

163. Brett C, Dekle M, Leonard CH, et al: Developmental follow-up of hyperventilated neonates: Preliminary observations. Pediatrics 68:588–591, 1981.

164. Schumacher RE, Palmer TW, Roloff DW, et al: Follow-up of infants treated with extracorporeal membrane oxygenation for newborn respiratory failure. Pediatrics 87:451–457, 1991.

165. Glass P, Miller M, Short B: Morbidity for survivors of extracorporeal membrane oxygenation: Neurodevelopmental outcome at 1 year of age. Pediatrics 83:72–78, 1989.

166. Lipshutz GS, Albanese CT, Feldstein VA, et al: Prospective analysis of lung-to-head ratio predicts survival for patients with prenatally diagnosed congenital diaphragmatic hernia. J Pediatr Surg 32:1634–1636, 1997.

167. Mychaliska GB, Bullard KM, Harrison MR: In utero management of congenital diaphragmatic hernia. Clin Perinatol 23:823–841, 1996.

168. Harrison MR, Adzick NS, Bullard KM, et al: Correction of congenital diaphragmatic hernia in utero, VII: A prospective trial. J Pediatr Surg 32:1637–1642, 1997.

169. Sbragia L, Paek BW, Filly RA, et al: Congenital diaphragmatic hernia without herniation of the liver: Does the lung-to-head ratio predict survival? J Ultrasound Med 19:845–848, 2000.

170. Harrison MR, Langer JC, Adzick NS, et al: Correction of congenital diaphragmatic hernia in utero, V: Initial clinical experience. J Pediatr Surg 25:47–56, 1990.

171. Harrison MR, Adzick NS, Flake AW, et al: Correction of congenital diaphragmatic hernia in utero, VI: Hard-earned lessons. J Pediatr Surg 28:1411–1418, 1993.

172. DiFiore JW, Fauza DO, Slavin R, et al: Experimental fetal tracheal ligation and congenital diaphragmatic hernia: A pulmonary vascular morphometric analysis. J Pediatr Surg 30:917–924, 1995.

173. Ford W, Cool J, Parsons D, et al: Congenital diaphragmatic hernia: Lung compliance after antenatal tracheal obstruction or surgical correction of the defect. Pediatr Surg Int 11:524–529, 1996.

174. O'Toole SJ, Karamanoukian HL, Irish MS, et al: Tracheal ligation: the dark side of in utero congenital diaphragmatic hernia treatment. J Pediatr Surg 32:407–410, 1997.

175. Hedrick MH, Estes JM, Sullivan KM, et al: Plug the lung until it grows (PLUG): A new method to treat congenital diaphragmatic hernia in utero. J Pediatr Surg 29:612–617, 1994.

176. O'Toole SJ, Sharma A, Karamanoukian HL, et al: Tracheal ligation does not correct the surfactant deficiency associated with congenital diaphragmatic hernia. J Pediatr Surg 31:546–550, 1996.

177. Piedboeuf B, Laberge JM, Ghitulescu G, et al: Deleterious effect of tracheal obstruction on type II pneumocytes in fetal sheep. Pediatr Res 41:473–479, 1997.

178. Flageole H, Evrard VA, Piedboeuf B, et al: The plug-unplug sequence: An important step to achieve type II pneumocyte maturation in the fetal lamb model. J Pediatr Surg 33:299–303, 1998.

179. Luks FI, Wild YK, Piasecki GJ, et al: Short-term tracheal occlusion corrects pulmonary vascular anomalies in the fetal lamb with diaphragmatic hernia. Surgery 128:266–272, 2000.

180. Kay S, Laberge JM, Flageole H, et al: Use of antenatal steroids to counteract the negative effects of tracheal occlusion in the fetal lamb model. Pediatr Res 50:495–501, 2001.

181. Wu J, Ge X, Verbeken EK, et al: Pulmonary effects of in utero tracheal occlusion are dependent on gestational age in a rabbit model of diaphragmatic hernia. J Pediatr Surg 37:11–17, 2002.

182. Harrison MR, Adzick NS, Flake AW, et al: Correction of congenital diaphragmatic hernia in utero, VIII: Response of the hypoplastic lung to tracheal occlusion. J Pediatr Surg 31:1339–1348, 1996.

183. Flake AW: Fetal surgery for congenital diaphragmatic hernia. Semin Pediatr Surg 5:266–274, 1996.

184. VanderWall KJ, Skarsgard ED, Filly RA, et al: Fetendo-clip: A fetal endoscopic tracheal clip procedure in a human fetus. J Pediatr Surg 32:970–972, 1997.

185. Harrison MR, Mychaliska GB, Albanese CT, et al: Correction of congenital diaphragmatic hernia in utero, IX: Fetuses with poor prognosis (liver herniation and low lung-to-head ratio) can be saved by fetoscopic temporary tracheal occlusion. J Pediatr Surg 33:1017–1023, 1998.

186. Graf JL, Gibbs DL, Adzick NS, et al: Fetal hydrops after in utero tracheal occlusion. J Pediatr Surg 32:214–216, 1997.

187. Losty PD, Suen HC, Manganaro TF, et al: Prenatal hormonal therapy improves pulmonary compliance in the nitrofen-induced CDH rat model. J Pediatr Surg 30:420–426, 1995.

188. Losty PD, Pacheco BA, Manganaro TF, et al: Prenatal hormonal therapy improves pulmonary morphology in rats with congenital diaphragmatic hernia. J Surg Res 65:42–52, 1996.

189. Suen HC, Bloch KD, Donahoe PK: Antenatal glucocorticoid corrects pulmonary immaturity in experimentally induced congenital diaphragmatic hernia in rats. Pediatr Res 35:523–529, 1994.

190. Schnitzer JJ, Hedrick HL, Pacheco BA, et al: Prenatal glucocorticoid therapy reverses pulmonary immaturity in congenital diaphragmatic hernia in fetal sheep. Ann Surg 224:430–439, 1996.

191. Ijsselstijn H, Pacheco BA, Albert A, et al: Prenatal hormones alter antioxidant enzymes and lung histology in rats with congenital diaphragmatic hernia. Am J Physiol 272:L1059–L1065, 1997.

192. Guarino N, Oue T, Shima H, et al: Antenatal dexamethasone enhances surfactant protein synthesis in the hypoplastic lung of nitrofen-induced diaphragmatic hernia in rats. J Pediatr Surg 35:1468–1473, 2000.

193. Oue T, Shima H, Guarino N, et al: Antenatal dexamethasone administration increases fetal lung DNA synthesis and RNA and protein content in nitrofen-induced congenital diaphragmatic hernia in rats. Pediatr Res 48:789–793, 2000.

194. Smith GN, Kingdom JC, Penning DH, et al: Antenatal corticosteroids: Is more better? Lancet 355:251–252, 2000.

195. Kay HH, Bird IM, Coe CL, et al: Antenatal steroid treatment and adverse fetal effects: What is the evidence? J Soc Gynecol Invest 7:269–278, 2000.

196. Van Tuyl M, Hosgor M, Tibboel D: Tracheal ligation and corticosteroids in congenital diaphragmatic hernia: For better for worse? Pediatr Res 50:441–444, 2001.

197. Crowley PA: Antenatal corticosteroid therapy: A meta-analysis of the randomized trials, 1972 to 1994. Am J Obstet Gynecol 173:322–335, 1995.

198. NIH Consensus Development Panel on the Effect of Corticosteroids for Fetal Maturation on Perinatal Outcomes: Effect of corticosteroids for fetal maturation on perinatal outcomes. JAMA 273:413–418, 1995.

199. Ford WD, Kirby CP, Wilkinson CS, et al: Antenatal betamethasone and favourable outcomes in fetuses with "poor prognosis" diaphragmatic hernia. Pediatr Surg Int 18:244–246, 2002.

200. Hirschl RB, Pranikoff T, Gauger P, et al: Liquid ventilation in adults, children, and full-term neonates. Lancet 346:1201–1202, 1995.

201. Major D, Cadenas M, Cloutier R, et al: Combined gas ventilation and perfluorochemical tracheal instillation as an alternative treatment for lethal congenital diaphragmatic hernia in lambs. J Pediatr Surg 30:1178–1182, 1995.

202. Steinhorn DM, Leach CL, Fuhrman BP: Partial liquid ventilation enhances surfactant phospholipid production. Crit Care Med 24:1252–1256, 1996.

203. Varani J, Hirschl RB, Dame M, et al: Perfluorocarbon protects lung epithelial cells from neutrophil-mediated injury in an in vitro model of liquid ventilation therapy. Shock 6:339–344, 1996.

204. Pranikoff T, Gauger PG, Hirschl RB: Partial liquid ventilation in newborn patients with congenital diaphragmatic hernia. J Pediatr Surg 31:613–618, 1996.

205. Fuhrman BP, Paczan PR, DeFrancisis M: Perfluorocarbon-associated gas exchange. Crit Care Med 19:712–722, 1991.

206. Reickert CA, Rich PB, Crotti S, et al: Partial liquid ventilation and positive end-expiratory pressure reduce ventilator-induced lung injury. Crit Care Med 30:182–188, 2002.

207. Lewis DA, Colton D, Johnson K, et al: Prevention of ventilator-induced lung injury with partial liquid ventilation. J Pediatr Surg 36:1333–1336, 2001.

208. Leach CL, Greenspan JS, Rubenstein SD, et al: Partial liquid ventilation with perflubron in premature infants with severe respiratory distress syndrome. N Engl J Med 335:761–767, 1996.

209. Greenspan JS, Fox WW, Rubenstein SD, et al: Partial liquid ventilation in critically ill infants receiving extracorporeal life support: Philadelphia Liquid Ventilation Consortium. Pediatrics 99:E2, 1997.

210. Van Meurs KP, Rhine WD, Benitz WE, et al: Lobar lung transplantation as a treatment for congenital diaphragmatic hernia. J Pediatr Surg 29:1557–1560, 1994.

211. Sarihan H, Imamoglu M, Abes M, et al: Pediatric Morgagni hernia: Report of two cases. J Cardiovasc Surg 37:195–197, 1996.

212. Herman TE, Siegel MJ: Bilateral congenital Morgagni hernias. J Perinatol 21:343–344, 2001.

213. Kubiak R, Platen C, Schmid E, et al: Delayed appearance of bilateral Morgagni herniae in a child with Down's syndrome. Pediatr Surg Int 13:600–601, 1998.

214. Parmar RC, Tullu MS, Bavdekar SB, et al: Morgagni hernia with Down syndrome: A rare association: Case report and review of literature. J Postgrad Med 47:188–190, 2001.

215. Pokorny WJ, McGill CW, Harberg FJ: Morgagni hernias during infancy: Presentation and associated anomalies. J Pediatr Surg 19:394–397, 1984.
216. Berman L, Stringer D, Ein SH, et al: The late-presenting pediatric Morgagni hernia: A benign condition. J Pediatr Surg 24:970–972, 1989.
217. Kimmelstiel FM, Holgersen LO, Hilfer C: Retrosternal (Morgagni) hernia with small bowel obstruction secondary to a Richter's incarceration. J Pediatr Surg 22:998–1000, 1987.
218. Ozden C, Pektas O, Baskin D: Retrosternal hernia (Morgagni) with colonic perforation due to incarceration. Pediatr Surg Int 5:274–275, 1990.
219. Estevao-Costa J, Soares-Oliveira M, et al: Acute gastric volvulus secondary to a Morgagni hernia. Pediatr Surg Int 16:107–108, 2000.
220. Cybulsky I, Himal HS: Gastric volvulus within the foramen of Morgagni. Can Med Assoc J 133:209–210, 1985.
221. de Fonseca JM, Davies MR, Bolton KD: Congenital hydropericardium associated with the herniation of part of the liver into the pericardial sac. J Pediatr Surg 22:851–853, 1987.
222. Lima M, Domini M, Libri M, et al: Laparoscopic repair of Morgagni-Larrey hernia in a child. J Pediatr Surg 35:1266–1268, 2000.
223. Ponsky TA, Lukish JR, Nobuhara K, et al: Laparoscopy is useful in the diagnosis and management of foramen of Morgagni hernia in children. Surg Laparosc Endosc Percutan Tech 12:375–377, 2002.
224. Lee KF, Chung DP, Leong HT: Laparoscopic repair of Morgagni's hernia with percutaneous placement of suture. J Laparoendosc Adv Surg Tech A 12:65–68, 2002.
225. Cantrell J, Haller J, Ravitch M: A syndrome of congenital defects involving the abdominal wall, sternum, diaphragm, pericardium and heart. Surg Gynecol Obstet 107:602–614, 1958.
226. Shamberger RC: Chest wall deformities. In Shields T (ed): General Thoracic Surgery, 4th ed. Baltimore, Williams & Wilkins, 1994, pp 529–557.
227. Herman TE, Siegel MJ: Special imaging casebook: Pentalogy of Cantrell. J Perinatol 21:147–149, 2001.
228. Symbas PN, Hatcher CR Jr, Waldo W: Diaphragmatic eventration in infancy and childhood. Ann Thorac Surg 24:113–119, 1977.
229. Wayne ER, Campbell JB, Burrington JD, et al: Eventration of the diaphragm. J Pediatr Surg 9:643–651, 1974.
230. Elberg JJ, Brok KE, Pedersen SA, et al: Congenital bilateral eventration of the diaphragm in a pair of male twins. J Pediatr Surg 24:1140–1141, 1989.
231. Wayne ER, Burrington JD, Myers DN, et al: Letter: Bilateral eventration of the diaphragm in a neonate with congenital cytomegalic inclusion disease. J Pediatr 83:164–165, 1973.
232. Shimotake T, Jikihara R, Yanagihara J, et al: Successful management of bilateral congenital eventration of the diaphragm. Pediatr Surg Int 10:173–174, 1995.
233. Sarihan H, Cay A, Akyazici R, et al: Congenital diaphragmatic eventration: Treatment and postoperative evaluation. J Cardiovasc Surg 37:173–176, 1996.
234. Smith CD, Sade RM, Crawford FA, et al: Diaphragmatic paralysis and eventration in infants. J Thorac Cardiovasc Surg 91:490–497, 1986.
235. Haller JA, Jr, Pickard LR, Tepas JJ, et al: Management of diaphragmatic paralysis in infants with special emphasis on selection of patients for operative plication. J Pediatr Surg 14:779–785, 1979.
236. Kizilcan F, Tanyel FC, Hicsonmez A, et al: The long-term results of diaphragmatic plication. J Pediatr Surg 28:42–44, 1993.
237. Mickell JJ, Oh KS, Siewers RD, et al: Clinical implications of postoperative unilateral phrenic nerve paralysis. J Thorac Cardiovasc Surg 76:297–304, 1978.
238. Langer JC, Filler RM, Coles J, et al: Plication of the diaphragm for infants and young children with phrenic nerve palsy. J Pediatr Surg 23:749–751, 1988.
239. Stone KS, Brown JW, Canal DF, et al: Long-term fate of the diaphragm surgically plicated during infancy and early childhood. Ann Thorac Surg 44:62–65, 1987.
240. Shoemaker R, Palmer G, Brown JW, et al: Aggressive treatment of acquired phrenic nerve paralysis in infants and small children. Ann Thorac Surg 32:250–259, 1981.
241. Brouillette RT, Hahn YS, Noah ZL, et al: Successful reinnervation of the diaphragm after phrenic nerve transection. J Pediatr Surg 21:63–65, 1986.
242. Merav AD, Attai LA, Condit DD: Successful repair of a transected phrenic nerve with restoration of diaphragmatic function. Chest 84:642–644, 1983.

CHAPTER 24

Mediastinal Tumors

David L. Sigalet, MD, PhD, FRCSC, FACS, and
Osama A. Bawazir, MD, FRCSI, FRCS(Ed), FRCSC, FRCS(Glas)

INCIDENCE

Thoracic masses arising from the mediastinum are a common diagnostic dilemma in the pediatric age group. These represent a wide spectrum of pathologies from congenital cysts to unusual varieties of solid and cystic malignant tumors. The patients frequently are seen initially with respiratory symptoms that can rapidly progress to obstructive emergencies because of the strategic location of the involved region and the small caliber of the airway in children. The reported incidence of malignant mediastinal tumors in children varies from 40% to as high as 72%.[1] Thus the risk of malignancy, the location of the tumors, and the potential for airway compromise make these an important aspect of pediatric surgical practice.

With the advent of antenatal ultrasonography (US), increasing numbers of thoracic masses are being detected and monitored. Thus roughly 40% of tumors will occur in infants and children younger than 2 years, and then another peak occurs in the teenage years.[2] Survival rates have improved in all age groups, and even patients with large aggressive lymphomas have a 70% to 80% survival.[3] This improvement in survival rates is predicated on accurate therapy, which often requires tissue for biopsy.[4,5]

EMBRYOLOGY

The foregut is first recognizable as an epithelium-lined tube late in the third postconceptual week, by which time the tracheal bud also is visible. Separation of the esophagus and trachea occurs over the next 2-week period by a process of cephalocaudal growth of both structures; during this interval, proliferation of foregut epithelium almost completely obliterates the esophageal lumen before subsequent tubularization. It is presumed that incomplete recanalization after the epithelial proliferative phase results in foregut duplication cysts.[6]

The thymus develops as a paired primordial structure from the ventral third pharyngeal pouch. During the seventh week, these structures elongate caudally and ventromedially to their normal position anterior to the aortic arch. Before completing descent, the thymic primordia contain a thymopharyngeal duct, which is obliterated after complete descent. The failure of this duct to obliterate may result in congenital cysts of the thymus.[6]

The embryologic development of teratomas is reviewed in Chapter 68. Mediastinal germ cell tumors and seminomas may arise from misplacement of primordial germ cells in midline locations during embryonic development or may be related to progenitors from the thymus.[7,8]

CLASSIFICATION BY REGION

Mediastinal masses are classically divided according to their site of origin: anterior mediastinum, middle mediastinum (visceral), and posterior or paravertebral mediastinum (Fig. 24-1). The anterior mediastinum is bounded by the posterior surface of the sternum; the thoracic inlet; and the anterior surface of great vessels, heart, and pericardium. This area contains the thymus and anterior surfaces of the vascular structures, as well as a few anterior lymph nodes and the rare ectopic thyroid or parathyroid. The middle mediastinum contains the heart, great vessels, trachea, and bronchi and extends to the anterior border of the vertebrae, including the esophagus, the vagus and phrenic nerves, and the descending thoracic aorta. The posterior mediastinum, or paravertebral sulcus, is bounded anteriorly by the anterior surface of the vertebral bodies. Although it is not classically a part of the mediastinum, this area is included because of the predominance of neurogenic tumors in this region.[1,3,9,10]

A thorough knowledge of the normal structures in these three areas is a prerequisite for the pediatric surgeon operating on these lesions. Lymph nodes, although arising principally in the middle mediastinum, also are present as pathologic lesions anteriorly and posteriorly. Cystic hygroma (lymphangioma) and other vascular masses are not confined to any specific mediastinal region.

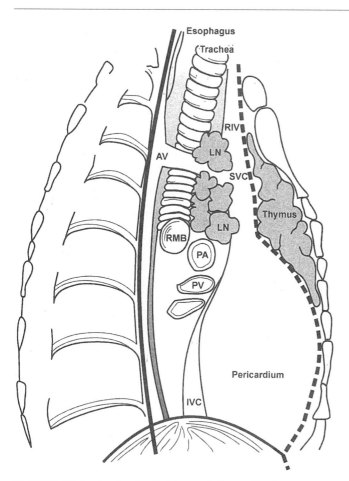

FIGURE 24-1. Anatomic divisions of the mediastinum: anterior compartment extends from the sternum to the *dotted line* anterior to the pericardium. Middle mediastinum extends posteriorly to the anterior board of the vertebrae.

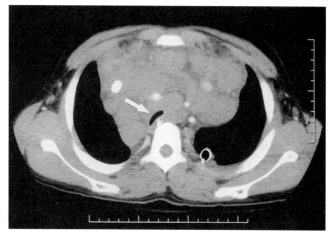

FIGURE 24-2. Computed tomography scan of a 14-year-old boy with rapidly progressive dyspnea. With attempted biopsy of a peripheral node had complete airway collapse. Note the significant airway compression. Biopsy showed non-Hodgkin's lymphoma, follow-up at 1 year showed complete regression.

CLINICAL PRESENTATION AND DIAGNOSIS

Dyspnea, noisy breathing, or a history of shortness of breath on exertion may indicate incipient airway compression. In younger children, the more classic symptoms of airway obstruction, such as shortness of breath when lying flat, may be difficult to elicit and instead may manifest as restlessness or apparent irritability, which on careful questioning can then be related to postural dyspnea. Systemic symptoms such as weight loss, night sweats, and general malaise also should be reviewed in the history. Careful physical examination should be done, focusing on the airway, including attention to signs of superior vena caval obstruction, such as plethora of the facies, venous distention, or other signs of head and neck masses, such as fullness and swelling in the supraclavicular and cervical areas.

Recognition may first occur during antenatal US. These fetuses are usually followed up closely, with intervention based on signs of progressive hydrops, cardiac failure, or mediastinal shift.[11,24,25] Such masses frequently regress. If they are asymptomatic, it is recommended that they be followed up until the infant is age 2 to 3 years, when they can be inspected thorascopically.

The chest radiograph, done in two views, should be the first diagnostic study performed in an older child first seen with a mediastinal mass. Once discovered, axial and spiral computed tomography (CT) scans with intravenous contrast are the most commonly used imaging modalities for delineation of the mass.[12] CT typically provides high-definition images of the nature of the mass and any associated airway or vascular obstruction. Airway compromise greater than 50% mandates further airway evaluation, as noted later (Fig. 24-2).[13–15] Magnetic resonance imaging (MRI) is an important diagnostic modality; however, the more lengthy examination time and need for sedation in younger patients make this study unsuitable for children with significant airway compromise.[16] In the patient with a posterior mediastinal mass who would not be likely to have airway compromise, MRI is the ideal imaging study because tumor extension into the spinal canal will be clearly defined. In some cases, a contrast esophagogram can useful to reveal deviation or compression of the esophageal lumen. Duplication cysts may contain gastric mucosa, which can be detected with technetium-99m pertechnetate scintigraphy.[2]

AIRWAY EVALUATION

Children with anterior mediastinal masses in particular are at risk for airway compromise, which may become life threatening on induction of general anesthesia (see Fig. 24-2). In most such cases, an extrathoracic approach to the diagnosis can be used (e.g., cervical or supraclavicular lymph nodes or pleural effusions from which positive cytology can be obtained) that obviates the use of general anesthesia or mediastinal invasion. Many malignancies can be diagnosed with bone marrow aspirate. However, if an extrathoracic biopsy site is not available, then a decision must made regarding the site and method of obtaining tissue. Needle biopsy of some mediastinal lesions is possible, but getting adequate tissue is often a problem, especially in Hodgkin's disease.[5,17] Pulmonary-function studies also may be helpful in evaluating the degree of obstructive and restrictive pulmonary deficits. Caution is the key, and preoperative discussion between the surgeon, anesthesiologist, and oncologist is necessary to evaluate and tailor definitive diagnostic procedures appropriately to each patient. It is critical that the surgeon and anesthesiologist be aware of the potentially disastrous airway obstruction that can occur in patients who are even minimally symptomatic as a result of a mediastinal mass. Symptomatic airway obstruction can be relieved with a short course of steroids or limited-field radiation therapy, which allows thoracoscopic biopsy or the use of the Chamberlain procedure to obtain nonirradiated tissue for definitive diagnosis.[13,17,18,26,27] Frequently, a thorough search for extrathoracic tumor sites provides adequate data for diagnosis and direction of therapy.

ANTERIOR AND SUPERIOR MEDIASTINUM

The anterior and superior mediastinums contain the thymus, great vessels, and a network of lymphatic structures as well as connective and adipose tissue. Lymphomas are the most common tumors (45% to 55% of all mediastinal masses), followed by teratomas, germ cell tumors, cystic hygromas, and thymic lesions.[1,2]

Malignant diseases such as lymphoma (see Fig. 24-2) generally are seen in the older child (mean age of Hodgkin's is 14 years, and non-Hodgkin's is 9 years) and are often associated with systemic symptoms, with adenopathy elsewhere, and frequently are associated with airway compromise.

The normal thymus may be mistaken for a pathologic mass on chest radiograph in the younger patient. The normal thymus is not a source of respiratory symptoms. It is often difficult to separate the physiologic enlargement of the infant's thymus from other anterior mediastinal masses. A 5-day course of prednisone (2 mg/kg/day) causes enough shrinkage of the normal thymus to provide an important diagnostic tool. Persistence of the mass mandates CT scanning in preparation for surgical biopsy. A lymphoma can diminish in size with steroid therapy as well, but lymphoma in children younger than 24 months is exceedingly rare.

Thymic cysts, although rare, are usually an incidental finding on chest radiographs but can become infected or hemorrhagic and produce symptoms by mass effect. These cysts, generally filled with cholesterol crystals and are sometimes noted to have a characteristic, and diagnostic, appearance on US. They can usually be resected thorascopically without major difficulty (Fig. 24-3).

Thymic tumors also can occur, including a variety of lymphomas, which may arise from the thymus proper or the surrounding lymphatic tissue. More rarely, tumors of the thymic parenchyma occur and include both benign

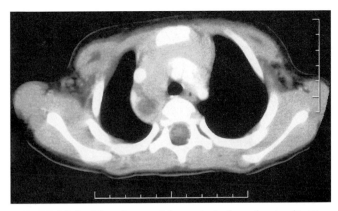

FIGURE 24-3. Thymic cyst rising anteriorly and extending to the posterior mediastinum.

and malignant cell types. The benign tumors such as thymic lipomas are slow growing and can reach a large size before presentation (Fig. 24-4).

Teratomas account for 20% of mediastinal masses in children. The mediastinum is the second most common site of teratomas in the pediatric population.[7,8] Most mediastinal teratomas originate anteriorly. Depending on their size and specific location, they may be in either hemithorax, in the middle or posterior mediastinum, in the pericardium or heart, or within lung parenchyma.

α-Fetoprotein is an effective serum tumor marker, and levels are well documented for the normal newborn; carcinoembryonic antigen and human chorionic gonadotropin are markers in some tumors and should be measured preoperatively.

Mediastinal teratomas are found, as is any other mass lesion, by incidental discovery or by symptoms of compression of contiguous structures. Respiratory symptoms are more frequent in younger patients. A teratoma may appear as a chest wall tumor and may even erode through the skin. Calcification within the mass is highly suggestive of the diagnosis of teratoma (Fig. 24-5).[22] Although it may not be seen on routine radiographs, calcification is

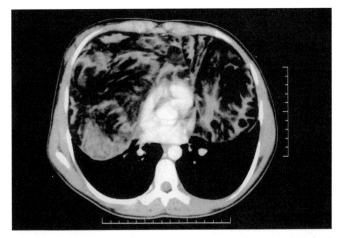

FIGURE 24-4. Extensive thymolipoma with very gradual progression of airway compression. Patient was first seen with exercise dyspnea only. Note the low-density fat signals with "alien" appearance.

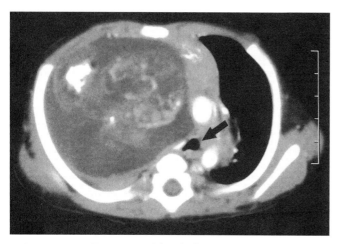

FIGURE 24-5. Teratoma with calcification within the tumor.

easily recognized on CT scan or US. These two studies help to differentiate solid from cystic lesions.

A strong association is found with Klinefelter's syndrome, and in these cases, choriocarcinoma in the teratoma can lead to precocious puberty.[27-29] Histiocytosis also has been reported with mediastinal teratoma, both with and without Klinefelter's syndrome.[29-32]

Surgical removal is indicated. Most mediastinal teratomas are cystic with one germ cell layer predominating. Ectoderm is the more common cell layer seen. The blood supply is usually singular and well defined. No gender predominance occurs, but the malignant lesions are almost exclusively found in male patients. After the age of 15 years, mediastinal teratomas have a high incidence of malignant behavior.[27]

Cystic hygromas are common mediastinal abnormalities found in children. They may result from a failure of connection of lymphatic collecting channels within their drainage systems. Hygromas most commonly occur in the neck, usually in the posterior cervical triangle, and can sometimes be extremely large and invasive, creating problems because of their size and encroachment on vital structures (Fig. 24-6). As many as 3% of patients with

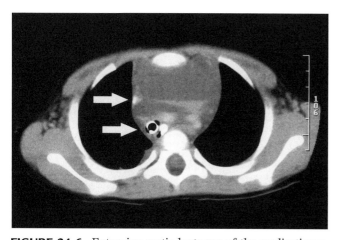

FIGURE 24-6. Extensive cystic hygroma of the mediastinum. Note bleeding in mid tumor, which caused acute airway obstruction posteriorly.

cervical cystic hygromas have extension into the superior portion of the mediastinum. Hygromas may involve all areas of the mediastinum and can extend, on rare occasions, to the diaphragm.

CT is indicated in any child whose chest radiograph suggests mediastinal extension of a cervical hygroma. Mediastinal cystic hygroma can sometimes produce chylothorax, pericardial effusion, and chylopericardium, as well as respiratory distress from airway compression. Excision is the treatment of choice, although alternatives may be found if that approach is impractical.[19] Observation has no place in the treatment of the mediastinal extension of cystic hygroma.[23] However, aggressive surgical treatment must be tempered by the benign nature of the disease, and every safeguard must be taken to prevent damage to vital structures such as the phrenic nerve.

Myasthenia Gravis

Myasthenia gravis is a disorder of the neuromuscular system seen clinically as pathologic weakness and muscle fatigue with exercise. Only 10% of patients with myasthenia gravis are children. The pathogenesis of this neuromuscular disorder is the thymus, which produces acetylcholine receptor antibodies that block the normal binding of acetylcholine at receptor sites. These antibodies also accelerate acetylcholine degradation at the end plate. Thymic antigen-specific T-helper cells also are believed to induce increased acetylcholine-receptor antibody production by lymphocytes in the peripheral circulation.

Myasthenia gravis has been described throughout the pediatric age range, although 75% of such children are older than 10 years. The symptoms of myasthenia gravis can be seen in infants born to mothers with myasthenia gravis because of transplacental passage of acetylcholine receptor antibodies. These symptoms last only for a short period, and the child fully recovers. A type of myasthenia gravis appears in infants in which the mother is not affected. These newborn patients initially have generalized weakness, but later they show only extraocular muscle symptoms of the disease, which are usually managed effectively with anticholinergic medications. Neither of these neonatal forms of myasthenia gravis benefits from thymectomy.[24]

Juvenile myasthenia gravis affects girls 4 times more often than boys. The role of median sternotomy and thymectomy is clear in acquired cases. A better outcome is seen when thymectomy is done early in the course of the disease. Preparation for surgical thymectomy includes stabilization with anticholinesterase medications, with plasmapheresis being used in refractory cases. Early thymectomy after diagnosis is believed to allow persistent symptoms to be more easily controlled. The goal of thymectomy is the reduction of drug therapy and its side effects.

Operative Technique

Median sternotomy is a preferred approach to the resection of anterior[33] mediastinal masses, whereas an anterior mediastinal window (Chamberlain procedure) is appropriate for biopsy and can be done under local anesthetic if required for airway considerations.[26]

In a median sternotomy, the cartilaginous nature of the sternum up to the age of 1 year allows it to be split with heavy Mayo scissors. In the older child up until to age 2 years, the sternum can be divided with heavier meniscus scissors, and thereafter, the electric saw is appropriate. In cases with possible superior vena cava (SVC) syndrome or airway compression, it is prudent bluntly to dissect free the deep fascial lining of the sternum, by using gauze dissector, and open the sternum in a stepwise fashion, to avoid injury to the underlying vessels.

Recent advances in minimally invasive surgery, especially thoracoscopy, have led to an evolution of new techniques for children. Thoracoscopy is a safe and effective method in experienced hands; however, a limiting factor is the size of the instruments in the small infant chest. Thus in children with asymptomatic lesions, we recommend watchful observation to the age of 2 to 4 years. This then allows the use of intrathoracic stapling devices and other such assists.[18,20]

TUMORS OF THE MIDDLE MEDIASTINUM

Middle mediastinal masses in children younger than 2 years are most often remnants of the embryonic foregut.

Esophageal duplication cysts are usually found arising within the esophageal wall near the carina. They share the muscular layer with the esophagus and often have a respiratory epithelial lining with occasional rudiments of cartilage. They may produce esophageal obstruction or erosion with bleeding.

Bronchogenic cysts are lined by respiratory epithelium and contain thick mucoid material secreted by this epithelium; many are not in close contact with the airway, and only rarely does this anomaly communicate with the airway.

Both esophageal duplications and bronchogenic cysts are most often identified in the asymptomatic patient in whom a chest radiograph has been obtained for other reasons. Either may produce obstructive respiratory symptoms, depending on the location of the cyst and its size. Infants are more likely to be seen with significant respiratory compromise for the reasons already stated. Atelectasis and hyperinflation from air trapping related to compression or deviation of the affected airway can lead to an incorrect diagnosis of congenital lobar emphysema, chronic aspiration, cystic fibrosis, or congenital cystic adenomatoid malformation. Occasionally cysts produce symptoms as a result of their strategic location, but they are too small to detect by routine chest radiograph. CT with intravenous contrast usually identifies the problem and can sometimes allow the surgeon to forego endoscopic evaluation, unless foreign body remains high in the differential diagnosis.

Treatment for either of these lesions consists of complete excision if possible. In the case of the esophageal duplication, which shares a common wall with the esophagus, the mucosal lining can be removed from the cyst to avoid major disruption of the esophageal lumen. Some esophageal lesions contain cartilage and are so obstructive that they must be excised, with esophageal anastomosis.

Enteric duplication cysts that originate below the pylorus can appear as a mass in the middle mediastinum.[21] They may be associated with lumbar vertebral anomalies and may, therefore, be differentiated from neurenteric cysts.[20] These duplications frequently contain ectopic gastric mucosa, in which case scintigraphy can be helpful in preoperative evaluation. These middle mediastinal gastrointestinal duplications, which communicate through the diaphragm or the esophageal hiatus, take their origin from the duodenum or proximal jejunum and have been labeled *thoracoabdominal duplications*.[16] If the ectopic tissue contains gastric mucosa, it may ulcerate and cause perforation with empyema in the right hemithorax. These duplications are not inherently fixed to any mediastinal structures, but their removal involves entry into both the chest and abdomen.

Pericardial cysts are benign, thin-walled, fluid-containing cysts lined with mesothelium. CT provides a sufficiently characteristic appearance to allow accurate diagnosis. If the diagnosis is uncertain or the cyst is large, these can be excised or unroofed thoracoscopically.

TUMORS OF THE POSTERIOR MEDIASTINUM

Masses in the posterior mediastinum and paravertebral sulcus are most commonly ganglioneuromas or neuroblastomas, which usually arise from the sympathetic ganglia.[22] This is the principal reason for the more favorable survival rate in children younger than 2 years who have a mediastinal tumor. Approximately 20% of all children with ganglioneuroma and neuroblastoma have a thoracic primary tumor. The mediastinal lesion may be seen with paraplegia related to tumor extension through intravertebral foramen, as dumbbell or hourglass lesions cause extradural compression of the spinal cord.[34,35]

In spite of their large size, they have an excellent prognosis, especially for stage I and II patients (Fig. 24-7). In patients with neurologic symptoms (including paraplegia), MRI should be acquired promptly, and an urgent

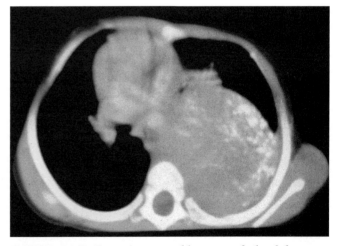

FIGURE 24-7. Extensive neuroblastoma of the left upper chest. Tumors resected intact, the child is disease free at 5 years without any requirement for chemotherapy.

laminotomy performed to excise extradural tumor and relieve cord compression before attempting intrathoracic resection of the tumor. If extradural tumor is present but the patient is asymptomatic, chemotherapy may be substituted for laminotomy or laminectomy.[36,37] See Chapter 66 for a detailed discussion of neural crest tumors.

Anterior thoracic meningocele is an extremely rare lesion. These tumors are associated with severe vertebral abnormalities. They are progressive in both size and symptoms, initially seen with weakness that progresses to paraplegia. Because it is a progressive lesion, operative correction is warranted. MRI and possibly myelography are deemed the best means for evaluating these lesions.

Neurenteric cysts are very rare cystic masses found in the posterior mediastinum. They connect the central nervous system and the gastrointestinal tract and are thought to develop very early in embryonic life as a result of failure of separation of the notochord and the foregut. These lesions usually have well-differentiated muscular layers with intestinal mucosal lining, most frequently gastric. As with anterior thoracic meningocele, the diagnosis should be considered when a posterior mediastinal cystic mass is identified adjacent to spinal anomaly. Technetium-99m pertechnetate scintigraphy may confirm ectopic gastric mucosa. MRI is the diagnostic study of choice because the communication with the intraspinal mass can be seen without the need for intraspinal contrast. The gastric mucosa in these lesions produces acid that causes inflammation and bleeding. Persistent ulceration can lead to central nervous system infection and fistulization into the spinal canal, which can be devastating.[20]

REFERENCES

1. Grosfeld JL, Skinner MA, Rescorla FJ, et al: Mediastinal tumors in children: Experience with 196 cases. Ann Surg Oncol 1:121–127, 1994.
2. Simpson I, Campbell PE: Mediastinal masses in childhood: A review from a pediatric pathologist's point of view. Prog Pediatr Surg 27:92–126, 1991.
3. Diehl V, Franklin J, Pfreundschuh M, et al: Standard and increased-dose BEACOPP chemotherapy compared with COPP-ABVD for advanced Hodgkin's disease. N Engl J Med 348:2386–2395, 2003.
4. Lehmann LE, Anupindi S, Harris NL. Case 18-2003: A 15-year-old girl with pain in the left leg and back, pruritus, and thoracic lymphadenopathy. N Engl J Med 348:2443–2451, 2003.
5. Chhieng DC, Cangiarella JF, Symmans WF, et al: Fine-needle aspiration cytology of Hodgkin disease: A study of 89 cases with emphasis on false-negative cases. Cancer 93:52–59, 2001.
6. Skandalakis JE, Gray SW, Ricketts R: The esophagus. In Skadalakis JE, Gray SW (eds): Embryology for Surgeons. Philadelphia, WB Saunders, 1994, pp 65–112.
7. Friedmann AM, Oliva E, Zietman AL, et al: Case 9-2003: An 18-year-old man with back and leg pain and a nondiagnostic biopsy specimen. N Engl J Med 348:1150–1158, 2003.
8. Moran CA, Suster S, Przygodzki RM, et al: Primary germ cell tumors of the mediastinum, II: Mediastinal seminomas: A clinicopathologic and immunohistochemical study of 120 cases. Cancer 80:691–698, 1997.
9. Pokorny WJ, Sherman JO: Mediastinal masses in infants and children. J Thorac Cardiovasc Surg 68:869–875, 1974.
10. Azarow KS, Pearl RH, Surcher R, et al: Primary mediastinal masses: A comparison of adult and pediatric populations. J Thorac Cardiovasc Surg 106:67–72, 1993.
11. Adzick NS: Fetal thoracic lesions. Semin Pediatr Surg 2:103–108, 1993.
12. Meza MP, Benson M, Slovis TJ: Imaging of mediastinal masses in children. Radiol Clin North Am 31:583–604, 1993.
13. Robie DK, Gursoy MH, Pkorny WJ: Mediastinal tumors: Airway obstruction and management. Semin Pediatr Surg 3:259–266, 1994.
14. King DR, Patrick LE, Ginn-Pease ME, et al: Pulmonary function is compromised in children with mediastinal lymphoma. J Pediatr Surg 32:292–299, 1997.
15. Shamberger RC, Holzman RS, Griscom NT, et al: CT quantitation of tracheal cross-sectional area as a guide to the surgical and anesthetic management of children with anterior mediastinal masses. J Pediatr Surg 26:138–142, 1991.
16. Siegel MJ, Nadel SN, Glazer HS, et al: Mediastinal lesions in children: Comparison of CT and MRI. Radiology 160:241–244, 1986.
17. Lange B, O'Neil JA, D'Angio G, et al: Oncologic emergencies. In Pizzo PA, Poplack DG (eds): Principles and Practice of Pediatric Oncology, 2nd ed. Philadelphia, JB Lippincott, 1993, p 953.
18. Rodgers BM: Thoracoscopic procedures in children. Semin Pediatr Surg 2:182–189, 1993.
19. Curley SA, Ablin DS, Kosloske AM: Giant cystic hygroma of the posterior mediastinum. J Pediatr Surg 24:398–400, 1989.
20. Kolski H, Vajsar J, Kim PC: Thorascopic thymectomy in juvenile myasthenia gravis. J Pediatr Surg 35:768–770, 2000.
21. Alrabeeah A, Gillis DA, Giacomantonio M, et al: Neurenteric cysts: A spectrum. J Pediatr Surg 23:752–754, 1988.
22. Saenz NC, Schnitzer JJ, Eraklis AE, et al: Posterior mediastinal masses. J Pediatr Surg 28:172–176, 1993.
23. Haberle B, Hero B, Berthold F, et al: Characteristics and outcome of thoracic neuroblastoma. Eur J Pediatr Surg 12:145–150, 2002.
24. Kuller JA, Laifer SH, Martin JG, et al: Unusual presentations of fetal teratoma. J Perinatal 11:294, 1991.
25. Meizner I, Levy A: A survey of non-cardiac fetal intrathoracic malformations diagnosed by ultrasound. Arch Gynecol Obstet 255:31, 1994.
26. Shamberger RC: Preanesthetic evaluation of children with anterior mediastinal mass. Semin Pediatr Surg 8:61–68, 1999.
27. Dehner LP: Gonadal and extragonadal germ cell neoplasms: Teratomas in childhood. In Finegold M (ed.): Pathology of Neoplasia in Children and Adolescents. Philadelphia, WB Saunders, 1986, pp 282–312.
28. Derencourt AN, Castro-Magana M, Jones KL: Mediastinal teratoma and precocious puberty in a boy with mosaic Klinefelter syndrome. Am J Med Genet 55:38–42, 1995.
29. Chaussain JL, Lemerle J, Roger M, et al: Klinefelter syndrome, tumor, and sexual precocity. J Pediatr 97:607–609, 1980.
30. Rowe MI, O'Neil JA, Grosfeld JL, et al: Teratomas and germ cell tumors. In Rowe MI, O'Neill JA, Grosfeld JL, et al. (eds.): Essentials of Pediatric Surgery. St. Louis, CV Mosby, 1995, pp 296–305.
31. Beasley SW, Tiedemann K, Howat A, et al: Precocious puberty associated with malignant thoracic teratoma and malignant histiocytosis in a child with Klinefelter's syndrome. Med Pediatr Oncol 15:277–280, 1987.
32. Sasou S, Nakamura SI, Habano W, et al: True malignant histiocytosis developed during chemotherapy for mediastinal immature teratoma. Hum Pathol 27:1099–1103, 1996.
33. Lakhoo K, Boyle M, Drake DP: Mediastinal teratomas: Review of 15 pediatric cases. J Pediatr Surg 28:1161–1164, 1993.
34. Grosfeld JL: Neuroblastoma: A 1990 overview. Pediatr Surg Int 6:9, 1991.
35. King D, Goodman J, Hawk T, et al: Dumbbell neuroblastoma in children. Arch Surg 110:888, 1975.
36. Molofsky WJ, Chutorian AM: Non-surgical treatment of intraspinal neuroblastoma. Neurology 31:1170, 1981.
37. Young DG: Thoracic neuroblastoma/ganglioneuroma. J Pediatr Surg 18:37, 1983.

The Esophagus

Keith W. Ashcraft, MD

EMBRYOLOGY

The embryonic foregut gives rise to the esophagus and trachea. Separation of these structures begins in the area of the carina with the appearance of bronchial buds. Lateral grooves can be seen in embryos; these deepen progressively to divide the airway from the esophagus up to the level of the pharynx. Most of the development of the separate trachea and esophagus occurs, however, by the process of elongation of the two structures.[1] Because of the relatively complicated way in which the esophagus and trachea divide, lesions such as esophageal atresia (Chapter 26) and tracheal atresia (Chapter 20) may occur. Because the trachea normally contains cartilage, occasional malformations that involve the esophagus contain cartilage remnants. Cystic lesions in the wall of the esophagus may be entirely esophageal duplication cysts or bronchogenic cysts, which contain either respiratory mucosa or cartilage in their walls.

The muscular wall of the esophagus comprises an inner circular muscle and an outer longitudinal muscle. It has no serosal covering. The cranial one third of the esophagus is striated muscle and under voluntary control, whereas the distal two thirds of the esophagus is composed of smooth muscle and is under autonomic control. The squamous mucosa of the esophagus is studded with its own intrinsic mucus glands that, in the presence of an acute obstruction, produce copious quantities of phlegm.

For purposes of surgical considerations, the esophagus can be divided into cervical, thoracic, and abdominal portions. The cervical portion is intimately attached to the larynx. The posterior esophagus is thinnest immediately below the cricopharyngeus muscle and is at particular risk of penetrating injury or the formation of Zenker's diverticulum. This portion of the esophagus receives its blood supply from thyrocervical vessels.

The thoracic portion of the esophagus is laterally indented by the aortic arch; it may be severely compressed by vascular ring malformations. This part of the esophagus is intimately related to the aorta and to the pericardium; therefore these adjacent structures are subject to erosion injuries from a foreign body or to damage from caustic injury. The midportion of the esophagus has a lateral or dorsal segmental blood supply. Overzealous surgical mobilization of this part of the esophagus can produce vascular insufficiency, which can adversely affect healing of an anastomosis.

The abdominal part of the esophagus is the portion that is involved with the lower esophageal sphincter (LES) mechanism (see Chapter 28). Its blood supply is generous and comes from phrenic branches and gastric vessels. Lacerations of the mucosa from forceful vomiting (Boerhaave's syndrome) and the development of varicosities from portal venous obstruction are both a potential source of major blood loss. A more detailed embryologic and anatomic discussion of the esophagus is available.[2]

CHEMICAL ESOPHAGEAL INJURIES

The natural curiosity of children and their tendency to taste everything, coupled with the availability of certain chemicals around the house, create the setting for corrosive esophageal injury. Alkaline chemicals are much more likely to produce esophageal injury than are acid chemicals. Commercially available drain cleaners, homemade lye solutions for the same purpose, and strong dishwasher detergents are the agents that most often produce liquefaction necrosis of the esophagus.[3] Concentrated alkali solutions are slick and, when put into the mouth, slip easily into the esophagus. Liquid caustic products are contrasted in their potential for injury with dry caustic products, which tend to stick to the oral mucosa and to produce intense pain, salivation, and dilution. Often dry caustics are spit out before they are swallowed.

In the presence of a suspected liquid caustic ingestion, esophageal damage is possible with little evidence of oral injury. Contact of the caustic agent with the esophageal mucosa produces intense spasm, which in turn exposes the entire circumference of the esophagus to the caustic agent. Liquefaction necrosis results. If the caustic dose is sufficient, the mucosa, submucosa, and muscular walls of the esophagus may be destroyed by continued liquefaction, until dilution alters the caustic agent to a harmless pH. The marked elevation of pH at various sites around the mediastinum, as measured by a surface electrode, has been demonstrated in the cat with an intact esophagus and an opened thorax. Because of the pattern of pH changes, this is probably more a diffusion phenomenon than a vascular dispersion. The extent of the injury both within the esophagus and into the mediastinum is probably related to the dose of hydroxyl ion.

The areas of natural closing of the esophagus are the regions of the cricopharyngeus muscle, the vicinity of the aortic arch, and the LES. In these locations, a small amount of caustic may produce a circumferential burn. Often, however, mucosal injury is extensive throughout the midportion of the esophagus as well.

Acid ingestion is much less injurious to the esophagus than is alkali ingestion, unless the acid is exceedingly potent. Acid injuries more often affect the antrum of the stomach, where mucosal necrosis and mural inflammation are produced, and antral stenosis results. Reports of antral injury due to alkali ingestion have recently been published. In some cases, extensive antral and/or pyloric strictures have resulted in cases in which recognizable esophageal injury has been absent.[4]

The sequela of caustic ingestion in the esophagus is cicatrix in the wall of the esophagus (Fig. 25-1). The depth of the burn probably indicates the amount of scar formation that will develop and the ultimate outcome of therapy. Mucosal erythema alone is usually without serious sequelae. Although published studies to date are not able to differentiate clearly full-thickness esophageal injury from superficial (and inconsequential) injury, esophageal motility appears to be a method of determining the prognosis of alkali or acid ingestion.[6] Circumferential mucosal slough usually indicates caustic injury to the muscularis, and at best, an irregular stricture will result. Similarly, full-thickness injury with continuing destruction of mediastinal structures by hydroxyl ions can lead to mediastinitis and, occasionally, to perforation of the esophagus into the contiguous structures, the most disastrous and dramatic result of which is the perforated aorta[6] (Fig. 25-2).

Immediate Therapy

Unfortunately, injury to the esophagus is almost instantaneous. Unless the dose is overwhelming, the alkali that passes into the stomach is neutralized by gastric acid, preventing further injury. It has been speculated that those patients with antral and pyloric injury from alkali ingestion may have been achlorhydric. For many years, the first-aid measure promulgated for toddlers who ingested lye was to induce vomiting, a process that allows the caustic agent a second chance to produce an injury. Unfortunately, any diluent or neutralizing agent must be given in such large quantities that vomiting is likely to be induced. The administration of acetic acid to neutralize the alkali is certainly emetic. Therefore first aid is of little or no value and may even cause further injury to the esophageal mucosa.[3]

The child is usually brought to the emergency department with a history of ingestion of lye. Its chemical

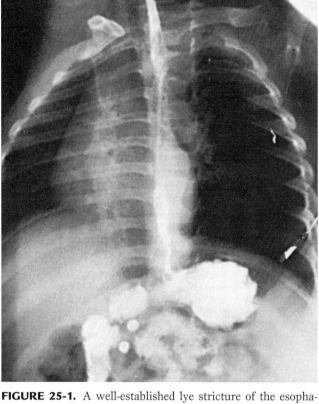

FIGURE 25-1. A well-established lye stricture of the esophagus is shown, with the most intense scarring from about the level of the aortic knob to the distal thoracic esophagus. The small amount of barium that passes makes it impossible to assess whether the stomach has been injured or whether the distal esophagus also is scarred from this lye injury. Both of these factors are important in the assessment and ultimate treatment of an extensive caustic stricture.

identification is of value, because certain agents that are common in the household, such as bleach, usually do not require endoscopy or further follow-up. An instance of gastric injury due to the ingestion of bleach has been cited, although the concentration of the agent was not reported.[4] Ingestion of sodium hydroxide or potassium hydroxide, either in solution or powdered, or powdered detergents calls for endoscopic evaluation. The status of the oral mucosa is of little or no prognostic value in determining the presence of esophageal injury. Endoscopy, usually performed within 24 hours, reveals whether the esophagus has been injured. Linear injuries to the esophagus are of less clinical significance because, unless the burn is circumferential, the remaining unburned esophagus expands to compensate for the lateral scar. General supportive care with intravenous fluids should be given in the immediate postinjury period before endoscopy or other studies are undertaken.

The use of technetium 99m–labeled sucralfate has been shown to demonstrate mucosal injury immediately after caustic ingestion. Although this technique does not have a direct correlation with the depth of injury to the esophageal wall, it has been found to be 100% accurate in excluding mucosal injury.[7]

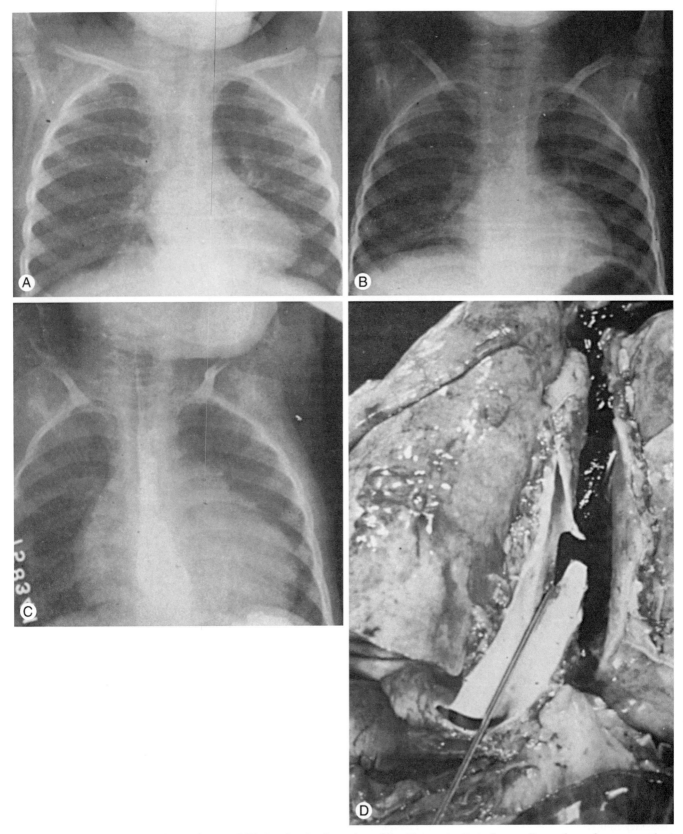

FIGURE 25-2. *A,* A chest radiograph on a child shortly after ingestion of liquid caustic. *B,* A chest radiograph on the same patient 4 days later shows a more globular appearance to the pericardium, indicating pericardial effusion. *C,* The same child 2 weeks after injury has some irregularity of the esophageal mucosa on barium study. More alarmingly, a large globular cardiac silhouette exists. *D,* The patient exsanguinated a short time after the previous radiograph. Autopsy showed a massive hole eroded into the aorta.

Rigid esophagoscopy is my choice for evaluation of the esophagus. A circumferential lesion is all that must be demonstrated. The length of the injury is not really important at this time. Passage of an endoscope beyond the area of circumferential injury may even carry a risk of esophageal disruption.

For a long time, antibiotics were thought to prevent mediastinitis, and systemic steroids were thought to prevent the ultimate formation of esophageal stricture. It is difficult to assess the depth of injury and grade the burns as first, second, or third degree, as is done with skin burns.[8] Undoubtedly, the depth of the burn is related to the eventual scar formation, which has made the assessment of steroid therapy in the healing phase difficult. The genesis of steroid treatment stems from an experimental study of standard caustic burn injuries of the esophagus in cats.[9] Treatment consisted of nothing, bougienage alone, steroids alone, antibiotics alone, or steroids and antibiotics. Animals treated with a combination of steroids and antibiotics lost less weight, and fewer died by inanition, but the therapy did not prevent the development of strictures.

A companion clinical study included 69 patients who had endoscopically demonstrated esophageal burns and who were treated with steroids and antibiotics.[10] Eight (12%) of these patients developed strictures that responded to prolonged dilation. None required esophageal replacement. By contrast, eight patients referred from other hospitals for esophageal replacement or prolonged dilatations had not been treated urgently with steroids and antibiotics. The strong impression was that the steroid/antibiotic therapy reduced the incidence of esophageal stricture but did not completely eliminate it. On the basis of these studies, steroid therapy was universally adopted, with the belief that if the steroids were administered only during the healing phase, the treatment might be beneficial. As has been subsequently shown, little else was available. Further data have suggested that, in spite of steroids and antibiotics, esophageal strictures are probably going to develop.[11] A controlled trial of steroids in children with corrosive injury of the esophagus has suggested that absolutely no statistically demonstrable benefit exists from the administration of corticosteroids in children with lye-ingestion injuries.[12]

Emergency Therapy for Massive Ingestion

If the history suggests a massive ingestion of concentrated alkali[13] in a child[14] or a suicidal ingestion of concentrated alkali in an adult or older child, immediate esophagectomy and possible gastrectomy should be considered. Whether this approach will prevent an aortoesophageal fistula that may result from continued alkali injury to mediastinal structures is not known, but some of my own experimental data and some of the clinical data available from the treatment of adults suggest that it does.[15,16] In accidental caustic ingestion in childhood, one of the standard approaches is to place a gastrostomy for feeding and sometimes to aid in prolonged dilation therapy. With massive caustic ingestion, the upper abdomen might be explored to assess the gastric wall, particularly its dependent portion, for evidence of caustic injury. If the caustic material ingested has been concentrated enough or voluminous enough to reach the stomach and produce a gastric wall injury, then the esophagus will be assumed to have been totally destroyed, and it should be removed. The recent data showing that antral and pyloric injuries from both acid and alkali may be extensive *even in the absence of recognizable esophageal injury* require that either technetium 99m–labeled sucralfate or endoscopy be used to determine the presence of severe esophageal injury before esophagectomy.[7] If the stomach does not appear to be seriously injured, a gastrostomy alone can be established, and the esophageal injury treated in the usual manner.[17]

Subacute Therapy for Caustic Injury

The most common approach to the subacute treatment of corrosive burns is observation to determine whether a stricture will develop. Most often it does.

Stenting during the healing phase has been reported to be of value both experimentally[14] and clinically, involving both children[19-22] and adults. This technique was proposed in the early 1970s and has lately gained some proponents but has not achieved widespread acceptance.

Esophageal Stricture Therapy

The long-term result of most serious caustic injuries is esophageal stenosis. The treatment is discussed later.

FOREIGN-BODY ESOPHAGEAL INJURY

The most commonly ingested foreign body that can produce injury to the esophagus is the coin. Most ingested coins pass harmlessly through the gastrointestinal (GI) tract in children, many probably unbeknownst to parents. Foreign bodies and their extraction from the esophagus are discussed in Chapter 11, but the long-term sequelae of an impacted foreign body in the esophagus, producing esophageal injury, are discussed herein.

The attitude of primary care physicians and even emergency department physicians toward the ingestion of coins is varied, extending from adamant neglect[23] to immediate action of ordering plain radiographs and contrast studies.[24] Depending on the size of the child and the size of the coin, the chances of its lodging in the esophagus are variable. If the coin is sufficiently small to pass through the cricopharyngeal area, the area of the aortic knob, and the distal esophagus into the stomach, problems are unlikely at the other narrowed or angulated portions of the GI tract (the pylorus, the ligament of Treitz, and the ileocecal valve). Given the history of coin ingestion, a chest radiograph, including the upper abdomen, should probably be done.[25] In one study, 52 consecutive children who had swallowed coins underwent radiographic examination. Those who had symptoms underwent removal of the coins. Of 30 children who had coins in the esophagus, 9 (30%) were asymptomatic.[26]

In the 3 patients whose coin had not progressed to the stomach within 24 hours, the coin was removed. In another almost simultaneous study in the same city, only a fraction of the patients whose parents called the emergency department to report a child's coin ingestion complied with the advice to get a radiograph; 20% of those children had coins in the esophagus. Most of the patients who had coins in the esophagus were symptomatic, with stridor or drooling.[27]

The consequences of an unrecognized esophageal foreign body, even one as smooth as a coin, can sometimes be disastrous.[28-30] Although some advise pushing the coin into the stomach,[31] most suggest using the Foley catheter technique to extract smooth esophageal foreign bodies.[32-34]

Esophageal injury is much more likely from sharper foreign bodies, including the detachable pop-top used on aluminum drink cans.[35,36] Because these objects are often nearly radiolucent, diagnosis comes with the late onset of esophageal obstructive symptoms.

Tracheoesophageal fistula (TEF) occasionally occurs as a result of an ingested foreign body.[37] I have had one such case. A child ingested an approximately 13-mm square plastic lattice from a badminton shuttlecock, which eroded from the esophagus into the trachea (Fig. 25-3A and B).

Of much more concern is the ingestion of the disc batteries that are used to power calculators, watches, and other small electronic gadgets.[38,39] These batteries may produce esophageal damage by one or all of three mechanisms: (1) pressure necrosis, (2) alkali or chemical injury from extravasation of the electrolytic agent, and (3) electrical current from a battery that is not exhausted. Some believe that dead batteries produce less injury.[40] Two instances of fatal erosion of disc batteries into the aorta have been reported.[41,42] These two reports were among the first reports of disc-battery ingestion.

Although some suggest that only batteries in the 22-mm or larger size range are dangerous, the potential for injury depends on the size of the esophagus and the ability of the battery to pass into the stomach.[38] Additionally, batteries that remain in the stomach for as little as 2 hours have produced mucosal staining and erosion. Whether this injury would have led to a gastric perforation cannot be determined. Batteries placed experimentally in normal saline quickly produce a pH of up to 12. Batteries in the esophagus for periods of days have produced extensive tracheoesophageal erosion.[39] This type of injury is reminiscent of that from a caustic agent because after removal of the foreign body and presumed interruption of the pathology, progressive injury has continued in several instances.[43,44]

Removal of the batteries from the esophagus can be accomplished with a Foley catheter[45] or with a magnetic device under radiographic control.[46] Removal from the stomach and even the upper portion of the small intestine also can be done with the magnetic device or with gastrotomy.[39]

Once the battery has passed through the pylorus, it probably will not cause further damage; however, one battery produced a perforation in a Meckel's diverticulum on about the third day after its ingestion.[47]

TEF or esophageal perforation resulting from foreign-body injuries to the esophagus and trachea should be

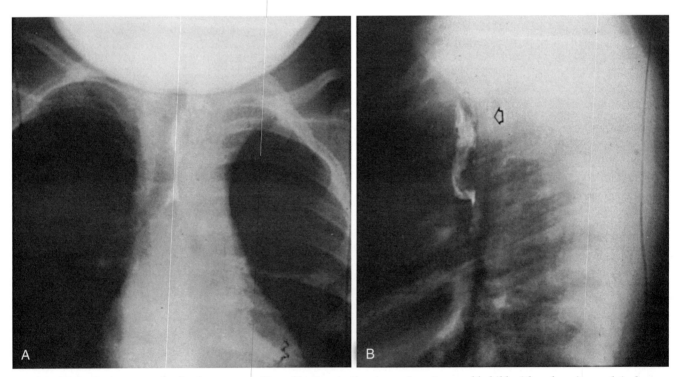

FIGURE 25-3. *A,* A communication between swallowed barium in the airway in a 4-year-old child with a chronic cough is demonstrated. *B,* A lateral radiograph on the same patient demonstrates a small lattice-like foreign body in the esophagus, which has eroded into the trachea. A piece of badminton shuttlecock had been ingested approximately 4 months before discovery of the acquired tracheoesophageal fistula.

managed individually. The battery lesions that have produced a fistula between the trachea and the esophagus are rarely as simple to treat as they might appear to be. The extent of ultimate tissue destruction is usually more troublesome than is the erosion from simple pressure necrosis.

Iatrogenic esophageal injury may occur in the intact esophagus in the newborn[48,49] and may be confused with unusual forms of esophageal atresia and TEF malformations. Mishaps of suctioning and intubation also may be responsible for esophageal perforation. Immediate surgical drainage can be carried out in many of these instances,[50] but the late diagnosis and exceedingly benign course in some would suggest that antibiotic coverage and nondrainage are satisfactory in selected cases.[51]

Spontaneous perforation of the esophagus was reported in a newborn with no history of any sort of instrumentation.[52]

Other forms of iatrogenic injury include perforations of the esophagus with an instrument, such as can occur during pneumatic dilation of achalasia by using a balloon dilator capable of achieving a 108F size.[53] Under the circumstance, the esophageal injury is not surprising. My esophageal perforation experience includes bougienage of the esophagus in a patient undergoing treatment for a lye stricture (Fig. 25-4) and repeated balloon dilation in one patient for distal peptic stricture of the esophagus. Balloon dilation is less dangerous unless unreasonable sizes are used.[54] These extravasations drained spontaneously into the lumen of the esophagus, as evidenced by follow-up radiographs, which showed prompt clearing of extravasated contrast material. Such evidence of internal drainage, coupled with a benign clinical course, obviates the need for aggressive surgical drainage.[55]

The standard treatment, however, must remain surgical drainage for any sort of perforation of the esophagus. The signs of perforation include pain and fever. A chest radiograph rarely reveals mediastinal air early after a perforation. Up to 10% of patients may have a false-negative contrast study in the presence of perforation.[56,57] Depending on the underlying disease process in the esophagus, primary closure may be accomplished, or drainage alone may be done.[55,58–61] Radical resection probably should be used for the unusual situation in which the healing potential of the esophagus is questionable.[62]

Barotrauma to the esophagus usually occurs in children who bite into high-pressure devices. It can produce severe esophageal injury.[63,64] Boerhaave's syndrome, caused by forceful vomiting, may produce an esophagopleural fistula, most commonly on the left side.[62] Primary repair and drainage should be used if the fistula is noted early.

Each esophageal perforation deserves individualized management with broad-spectrum antibiotic coverage, adequate drainage if indicated, and perhaps repair.[61] Repair may include mobilization of surrounding tissue to support the esophageal or tracheal wall. Many patients in whom esophageal injuries occur have underlying esophageal pathology, which necessitates instrumentation. These factors complicate the treatment of esophageal perforation and, undoubtedly, play a role in the selection of therapy for the perforation.

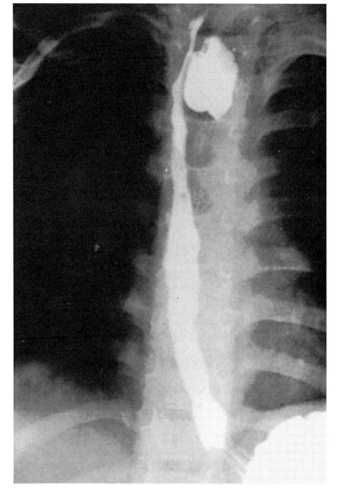

FIGURE 25-4. The cervical or high thoracic perforation of the esophagus is demonstrated after dilation of caustic stricture of the esophagus. A follow-up radiograph several hours later shows complete return of the extravasated barium to the esophagus; therefore further drainage was not undertaken. The patient eventually required esophageal replacement because of the stricture, not because of the perforation.

CONGENITAL ESOPHAGEAL STENOSIS

Congenital esophageal stenosis (CSE) is a lesion that is difficult to define, because early peptic strictures that have developed in children younger than 18 months have sometimes been included in this diagnosis. The presently accepted forms of CSE are three: (1) those with cartilage components or tracheobronchial remnants (TBRs), (2) those with fibromuscular thickening (FM), and those with membranous webs (MWs). They are often symptomatic from birth or early infancy, in retrospect, but are often not diagnosed until months or years later when nutritional failure results from the esophageal obstruction.[65]

The mainstay of diagnosis is the barium contrast esophagram, although recently endoesophageal ultrasonography (US) has been used to define further the TBR from the FM types of stenoses.[66,67] Esophageal dilation by using bougienage or balloon dilators is almost always the first line of therapy, although the accuracy of US to diagnose the TBR type of stenosis has been leading to immediate resection of these lesions. Most CSE lesions are located in the distal esophagus.[68,69] I have seen one of these lesions and, in addition, an unusual cervical esophageal stricture that contained a large cartilaginous plaque in its posterior wall. A recent report of two cases of congenital upper esophageal stenosis did not contain cartilage: one was resected, and one, dilated.[70]

CSE associated with esophageal atresia and tracheoesophageal fistula (EA/TEF) anomalies is being reported more and more frequently. Usually of the TBR type, the CSE lesion is discovered some months after successful repair of the more easily recognized EA/TEF lesion. In our experience with more than 400 patients who had EA/TEF, we have not seen a single associated CSE. CSE also is reported to be associated with Down syndrome, intestinal atresia, and anorectal malformations.

FUNCTIONAL ESOPHAGEAL DISORDERS

Diffuse Esophageal Spasm

Diffuse esophageal spasm is an uncommon condition that is also known as primary disordered motor activity.[71] The original description of this lesion is very complete.[72] Spastic pain usually occurs in the esophagus, accompanied by dysphagia. Since its early description, the pathology of diffuse esophageal spasm has been delineated as being circular muscle hypertrophy, primarily in the lower two thirds of the esophagus. The etiology is unknown.

I have had only two pediatric patients with this lesion (Fig. 25-5). One did not undergo myotomy and, when last seen, had continued intolerance of foods that were not pureed. The other patient had a distal esophageal myotomy and Thal fundoplication with limited symptomatic improvement. The intrathoracic esophageal muscle would have been split during a second procedure, if necessary. Most of the reported adult patients who have undergone long myotomy have responded favorably.

Scleroderma

Scleroderma is an uncommon collagen disorder in children. The distal two thirds of the esophagus, which is smooth muscle, loses its normal peristalsis in the patient with scleroderma. Gastroesophageal reflux is almost universally present. Esophagitis, progressing to peptic stricture of the esophagus, occurs quite commonly in scleroderma.[72] Fundoplication has resulted in clinical improvement in many patients, although the underlying systemic illness and the disordered peristalsis remain unchanged. I have seen no pediatric patients with sclerodermal involvement of the esophagus. A scleroderma-like disorder of esophageal motility and lax LES pressure was recently described in the breast-fed children of mothers who had silicone breast implants. No evidence was presented as to cause and effect.[73,74]

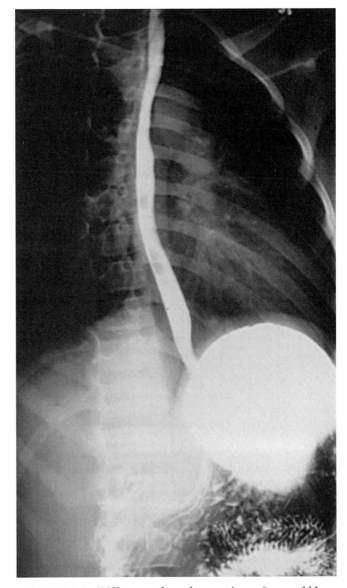

FIGURE 25-5. Diffuse esophageal spasm in an 8-year-old boy. He did not have gastroesophageal reflux nor did he respond well to repeated esophageal dilations. At last contact, he could take only soups and pureed foods.

Esophageal Diverticulum

Diverticula of the esophagus are exceedingly rare in children. In the absence of diffuse esophageal spasm, they are rare even in adults. One child was reported with Ehlers-Danlos syndrome, in whom diverticula in the esophagus, stomach, colon, and urinary bladder were noted.[75]

ESOPHAGEAL ACHALASIA

The etiology of achalasia is unknown. Histopathology in 24 muscle specimens from the distal esophagus revealed the complete absence of neural plexus in 2 patients and of ganglion cells in 10. However, ganglion cells were normal in 7 patients. These findings may be the result of ischemia or inflammation from esophagitis. In 5 patients, chronic inflammatory changes were present in the ganglion cells. Smooth muscle fibers appeared normal on light microscopy.[76] The patients were all children whose symptoms had their onset from age 5 days to 15 years. Achalasia, however, is primarily a disease of older people whose symptoms do not begin until adulthood. A congenital etiology is therefore unlikely. Teleologically, gastroesophageal reflux may certainly produce a spastic reaction in the lower end of the esophagus, which ultimately leads to a clinical picture resembling achalasia. Achalasia may occur in a familial pattern. In such situations, pyloric stenosis has been noted,[77] in which the initial symptoms are those of gastroesophageal reflux. A frequent cause of a delayed diagnosis of achalasia is confusion with symptoms of gastroesophageal reflux.[78]

I have one patient who was first seen in precisely this manner. He underwent fundoplication and was unable to swallow. Although he had an anterior fundoplication, the wrap was taken down. Continued obstruction led to the radiographic diagnosis of achalasia. An esophagomyotomy was done with a repeated anterior fundoplication. The patient has since required pyloroplasty for what appeared, at age 5 years, to be pyloric stenosis.

By the time a patient undergoes diagnostic studies, the barium examination of the distal esophagus usually shows a large proximal esophagus with ineffectual peristalsis, a bird-beak deformity of the distal esophagus, and little contrast material passing into the stomach (Fig. 25-6). This radiographic picture is diagnostic of achalasia. In the child, manometrics are not necessary to confirm the diagnosis.

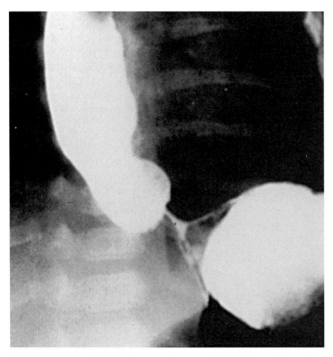

FIGURE 25-6. Achalasia in a 3-year-old child treated with a Heller myotomy and Thal fundoplication with an excellent result.

The diagnosis of achalasia may be made with barium study. In adults, it is more precisely confirmed by manometric determinations. Manometry shows that effective peristalsis is absent in the body of the esophagus, with little or no relaxation of the LES.[78,79]

Monitoring of the pH in the distal esophagus may reveal the presence of gastroesophageal reflux. This study has not been done frequently in the evaluation of achalasia.

Therapy for achalasia is surgical. A calcium channel blocker (nifedipine) was shown to reduce the LES pressure in children with demonstrated achalasia, but its effect was transient. Most likely, therefore, this treatment would not be a viable lifetime approach to the management of achalasia.[80]

Much of the literature dealing with achalasia pertains to surgery in adult patients. Comparisons of the results and the problems indicate that the management of achalasia is not much different in adults from that in children.[81] Bougienage or balloon dilation sometimes produces good symptomatic relief, but in adults, perforation rates are up to 12%.[82] Although 50% of patients were asymptomatic 4 years after dilation, 30% had symptomatic gastroesophageal reflux, and 20% had dysphagia. In the discussion of this article, it was pointed out that any operation that has a recognized 20% to 50% failure rate with a bad long-term outlook probably should not be accepted as reasonable therapy.[83] In a study of pneumatic dilation in both children and adults, the group least responsive to this form of therapy were the patients younger than 20 years. Successful balloon dilation resulted in symptomatic gastroesophageal reflux in a significant number of pediatric patients as well.[84]

The standard accepted surgical treatment for achalasia is the esophageal myotomy proposed by Heller 80 years ago. Thoracic surgeons usually use a thoracic approach, and general surgeons use an abdominal approach. The basic premise is to incise both the longitudinal and circular muscle layers of the esophagus down to the submucosa, much as is done in pyloromyotomy. In young adults, the myotomy extends 5 to 10 cm above the gastroesophageal junction, a length that should be proportionally shortened in children. An international compilation of 175 pediatric patients with achalasia demonstrated that only 54% had surgical repair through the abdomen and that 75% of those had a concomitant fundoplication when this approach was used. Better resolution of symptoms was reported with the abdominal Heller myotomy/fundoplication combination than with thoracic myotomy with or without fundoplication.[85]

My approach has been to perform a distal esophageal myotomy extending 2.5 to 5 cm up the esophagus and to cover the myotomy with an anterior fundoplication to prevent gastroesophageal reflux. Because myotomy alone has been complicated by symptomatic reflux, the question of the proper choice of operations for achalasia has been addressed.[86] In 19 patients who had undergone esophagomyotomy alone, esophagomyotomy plus a Nissen fundoplication, or a Nissen fundoplication alone, obstruction caused by the fundoplication was found in one third and gastroesophageal reflux in one third.

The remainder had inadequate esophagomyotomy. In previously untreated patients, these investigators used a combination of esophagomyotomy and Belsey fundoplication. In those patients who were followed up, 88% had a very good result documented by history, pH, and manometric studies. These investigators concluded that anterior fundoplication and esophagomyotomy were the treatments of choice for achalasia in adults. Others contend that the properly done esophagomyotomy that does not extend to the stomach is a perfectly satisfactory operation for achalasia, but that if the myotomy is extended to the stomach, a hemiwrap fundoplication is preferable to a complete wrap.[87] Many surgeons believe, as I do, that esophagomyotomy coupled with anterior fundoplication is the ideal procedure for achalasia.[76,88-91]

In one series of 21 children, however, only 5 were reported to have had fundoplications. All of these were Nissen fundoplications with good results.[81] Another study of Nissen fundoplication in children, however, stated that 50% of children who undergo esophagomyotomy for achalasia will need a fundoplication and that the Thal fundoplication is preferable.[92] In my personal experience, 26 patients have had esophagomyotomy coupled with anterior fundoplication. All had excellent long-term results.

As in many lesions today, minimally invasive techniques are in vogue. Reports of laparoscopic Heller myotomy coupled with a Dor fundoplication have shown better results than thoracoscopic Heller myotomy alone.[93,94]

ESOPHAGEAL STRICTURES

As a practical consideration, esophageal strictures in children do not involve malignancies. The etiologies of benign esophageal strictures in childhood include reflux esophagitis, corrosive ingestion, and anastomotic scarring. Anastomotic and corrosive strictures may be aggravated by the presence of gastroesophageal reflux. In many instances, therefore, the treatment program requires not only relief of the obstruction but also prevention of its recurrence by correction of the gastroesophageal reflux. Anastomotic strictures are discrete and short, whereas those strictures caused by ingested corrosives are irregular and may be long. Peptic esophageal strictures are usually located in the lower one third and may be short, but nonetheless are difficult to manage.

Esophageal stenosis has been a problem for many years, and the history of its treatment with bougienage is a fascinating one.[95] Dilation to disrupt the circular scar may be more lasting when coupled with the local injection of triamcinolone to reduce the re-formation of collagen linkage.[96-99]

The current techniques of dilation include the use of an indwelling string in the esophagus by which means Tucker's dilators can be passed in a retrograde manner via gastrostomy.[100] Hurst's mercury-filled bougies, filiforms and followers, wire-guided Savary dilators, and, most recently, balloon dilators[100] also can be used. Comparisons between the tangential dilations by bougie and the radial dilations by balloon have been made. The techniques

appear to be comparable, in terms of both complications and long-term outlook.[101,102] Radial dilation with balloons is the method that I prefer.[103]

The use of the Glidewire/Berenstein Catheter system usually applied to vascular procedures has been demonstrated to be of great value in apparently impenetrable esophageal and bronchial strictures. The procedure appears to be simple, safe, and very effective.[104]

Any method of dilation carries a risk of septicemia, including the formation of brain abscess.[105] In one series, four of nine patients had *Staphylococcus aureus* in postoperative blood cultures. The investigators recommended that appropriate antibiotic coverage should be provided for patients undergoing esophageal dilation. The threat of perforation exists regardless of the method of dilation.

In addition to the anastomotic strictures that occur after the repair of esophageal atresia, strictures can occur at either end of an interposed colon. Although in some instances, dilation of these stenoses is effective, many times, because of acid reflux, the stricture will not be resolved by dilation alone. Dilation of a proximal esophagocolonic stricture was reported to have resulted in the healing of a cervical fistula[106]; however, in my experience, these fistulas most often require revision or surgical resection to allow healing.

Peptic Strictures

Peptic stenosis of the distal esophagus has been managed successfully with dilation and nonoperative treatment of the reflux esophagitis. Most surgeons treating this combination of lesions use dilation coupled with fundoplication to prevent further reflux.[73,107-109] When given the choice between fundoplication and repeated dilation or a primary esophageal substitution procedure, fundoplication appears to provide better results and fewer long-term complications[110] (Fig. 25-7).

Rarely, a patient with epidermolysis is initially seen with esophageal stricture. These patients require esophageal substitution, because the underlying disease process does not allow dilation of the esophagus without complete disruption of the mucosa.[111,112]

Corrosive Strictures

Corrosive strictures can be successfully dilated. One study in children showed that adjunctive steroid injection into the scar made dilation treatment more lasting.[97] The problem with this approach to corrosive strictures is that if the esophagus continues to be used as a conduit for food, during the course of years, squamous cell carcinoma may develop at the site of injury. More than 130 patients are reported to have had squamous cell carcinoma develop at the site of corrosive injury. The usual scenario is that in a child in whom a stricture has developed, treated with bougienage for a number of years, progressive dysphagia develops 20 to 40 years after the ingestion. Investigation reveals squamous cell carcinoma at the site of the major burn injury, usually at the level of the aortic arch.[113-118] In one series of

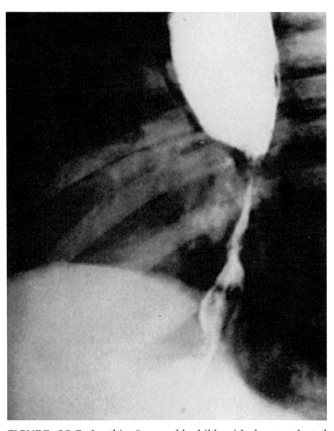

FIGURE 25-7. In this 8-year-old child with long-neglected reflux, a wide proximal esophagus, a tight esophageal stricture, and obvious gastric rugae about the level of the diaphragm are shown. A patient with these problems can be treated with fundoplication and dilation of the esophagus or distal esophageal replacement. The treatment depends on the ease with which dilation can be accomplished and the mobility of the esophagus. Often the technique cannot be assessed until the time of operation. Therefore provisions should be made for carrying out a hiatus hernia repair and fundoplication or a distal esophageal replacement with one technique or another.

63 patients, 24 were considered surgical candidates. Only 20 underwent resection, and 5 died. Of the 15 survivors, 5 were alive at 5 years. Of the radiation-treated patients, a 10% 5-year survival rate and a 5% 7-year survival rate were found. Compared with those of other patients who have carcinoma of the esophagus, the lesions in this group of patients are more resectable. The patients have a better prognosis, probably because dysphagia is apparent earlier because the esophagus is less distensible. The cicatrix in the esophageal wall also may prevent early local spread of the tumor.[118]

In my extensive literature search and in the experience of others, not a single case of carcinoma occurred in a defunctioned esophagus after lye injury.[119]

Given these concerns, the esophagus scarred by corrosives should not be relied on as a conduit for food for the remainder of the patient's life. A substitution with its attendant difficulties is probably better than leaving the esophagus in use. Whether the defunctioned esophagus should be removed at the time of substitution

remains unanswered. I have seen mucoceles develop in the residual esophagus when no way was available for the esophageal secretions to drain into the stomach, a condition that required esophagectomy.

ESOPHAGEAL REPLACEMENT

I have four principles of esophageal replacement:

1. The esophagus is the best conduit, provided that it functions near normally and has no malignant potential, as does a lye stricture or Barrett's esophagus.
2. A straight tract is best, avoiding as many twists and turns as possible, because esophagoscopy and dilations are frequently required. Almost all conduits function as passive tubes rather than by means of intrinsic peristaltic activity.
3. The prevention of reflux into any conduit is important; an interposition procedure that incorporates the distal normal esophagus with its gastroesophageal junction is best. This provides the opportunity for a low-resistance, anterior fundoplication.
4. Tenacity is exceedingly important. Anastomotic dilations should not be necessary except during the healing phase. Strictures should be revised surgically. Complex interpositions that do not function well can and should be rearranged to provide the straightest, lowest-resistance food conduit possible.

Colon Interposition

The use of the right colon as an esophageal substitute has been most popular in the United States[120] (Figs. 25-8 and 25-9). Substitution using the left colon has been more commonly done in England[121,122] and was recently described as the superior procedure in Egypt.[123] The colon segment may be placed in an antiperistaltic manner[120] or in an isoperistaltic manner.[121] Some surgeons prefer intrathoracic retrohilar placement of transverse or left colon without regard to the peristaltic orientation of the colon segment.[124–128]

In a comparison study of 80 colon replacements in 79 children, 70% were placed behind the hilum in an isoperistaltic manner, and 30% were placed retrosternally. Most esophageal atresia patients with a stump of distal esophagus have had the stump incorporated into the interposition. The incidence of proximal anastomotic leak was 31%, with a proximal anastomotic stricture developing in 15% of the retrohilar left colon anastomoses and in 41% of the retrosternal colon interpositions. Additionally, 60% of patients with substernal colon interposition had reflux. Only 18% of those with the retrohilar type had this problem. Five of 12 patients having substernal colon interposition required treatment of ulcers in the interposition. The investigators concluded that the retrohilar left colon interposition is preferable.[129] The function of any interposition is more satisfactory in the retrohilar position, according to some, because it is less tortuous.[129,130]

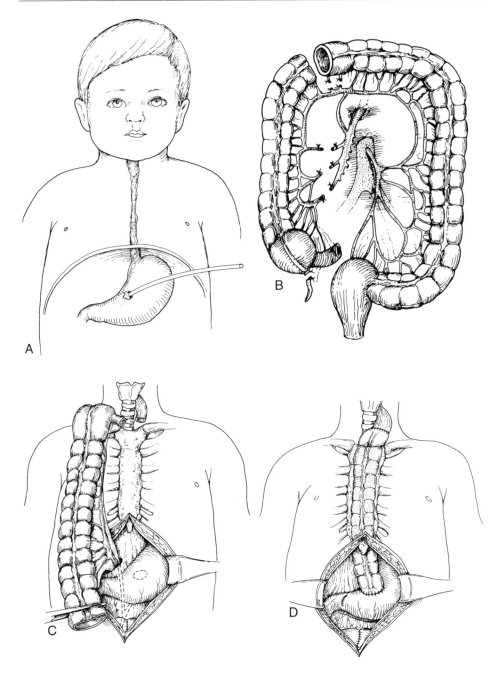

FIGURE 25-8. *A,* For any esophageal lesion in which a substitution procedure may be anticipated, the gastrostomy should be placed on the lesser curve at about the level of the incisura, so that a right or left colon or gastric tube interposition may be carried out without compromising the blood supply. *B,* The right colon and terminal ileum are isolated, based on blood supply from the arcades and from the middle colic artery. *C,* The colon on its pedicle is brought up through the lesser omentum and positioned substernally in an isoperistaltic fashion. *D,* Most frequently, excision of the terminal ileum and cecum is accomplished. Careful tailoring of the distal end allows a straight conduit to be anastomosed to the antrum. Pyloroplasty may or may not be added to the procedure. The incidence of significant gastrocolic reflux is reduced by a drainage procedure.

A recent reported series of 850 esophageal replacement procedures from one institution described 30 years' experience. Gastric pull-up procedures were done in 75 cases, retrosternal colon interpositions in 550 cases, and retrohilar colon interpositions in 225 cases. The latter procedure has evolved as the preferred procedure because it provides the most direct route and has a very low incidence of complications. Even including the last 250 cases of substernal colon interpositions, the authors report a 10% cervical anastomotic leak rate, half of whom developed anastomotic strictures and a 1% mortality rate. In only 0.6% of patients did graft stenosis develop in follow-up. These remarkable statistics perhaps reflect the value of experience rather than the intrinsic value of one procedure over another.[123]

In a much smaller series of 20 colon interpositions, the functional result seemed to be similar in the retrosternal compared with the intrathoracic group, but strictures requiring resection occurred only in the retrosternal interposition group.[131] More intraoperative ischemic complications of colon interposition have occurred with the right colon placed in the substernal position compared with the transverse or left colon placed behind the pulmonary hilum.[122] Perhaps this occurs because as many as 70% of patients have a right colon that lacks a marginal artery necessary to nourish the colon transplant.[132] Ischemia also may result from the angulation necessary for the substernal placement of the interposition.

Although one investigator reported only a 2% incidence of proximal esophageal/colonic anastomotic leak,[121] most

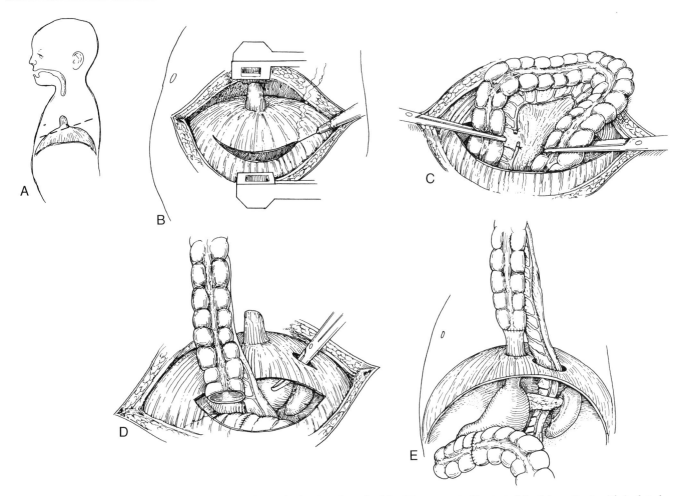

FIGURE 25-9. The left colon or transverse colon substitution described by Waterston is illustrated in this patient with isolated esophageal atresia. However, it works equally well for other lesions requiring esophageal replacement. *A,* A standard postero-lateral left thoracotomy at about the sixth intercostal space. *B,* Incision of the diaphragm peripherally. *C,* A section of colon is isolated and its vascular pedicle is developed, usually based on the left colic artery. It may be necessary to base it on the middle colic artery, in which case, this interposed colon is placed in an antiperistaltic manner. *D,* The colon and its vascular pedicle are delivered behind the spleen and pancreas and through a separate posterior opening in the diaphragm, so that the abdominal viscera do not stretch or otherwise obstruct the blood supply to this colon segment. *E,* The distal anastomosis may be made to the remnant of distal esophagus or to the posterior aspect of the stomach.

others reported an incidence of this complication of approximately 30% to 33%.[130,133,134] Esophagocolonic leak is probably caused by technical errors or minor degrees of ischemia, but stricture formation is almost undoubtedly caused by ischemia. Repeated dilation is not often successful. Therefore most anastomotic strictures that persist more than 6 months after the interposition procedure are ultimately going to need surgical revision. Both the management of esophageal leak and the surgical management of esophageal stricture are less difficult if the anastomosis is made in the neck. The proximal anastomosis is often at this level because of the cephalad extent of lye injury, if that is the cause of the replacement, or because of the shortened proximal pouch with isolated esophageal atresia when a cervical esophagostomy has been done.

I have had experience with one girl who had a colon interposition at age 3 years for caustic stricture. She did reasonably well in spite of repeated upper anastomotic strictures until age 18 years, when a fistula developed from the conduit to the skin. The original anastomosis had been between the cervical esophagus and the terminal ileum. To treat the late esophagocutaneous fistula success-fully, I split the sternum and incised the tenia to allow lengthening of the colon segment so that the terminal ileum and cecum could be discarded. Anastomosis between the esophagus and the ascending colon was then carried out. Since that procedure, she has been without symptoms. This method of elongation of the substernal colon segment was originally described by the excision of the tenia.[135] Multiple incisions of tenia, however, are more feasible and as effective.[136]

Reflux into the colon segment is less a problem when the normal distal esophagus has been used as the implantation site for the distal colonic anastomosis. Left colon placement with anastomosis of the colon to the stomach, done low on the posterior gastric wall, is reputed to prevent reflux.[137] In my experience, it does not. Although

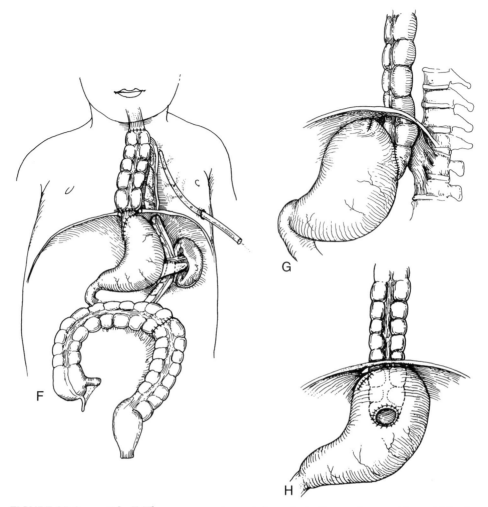

FIGURE 25-9, cont'd. *F,* The upper anastomosis is made to the esophagus either within the mediastinum or within the neck. Adequate drainage of the pleura is necessary to prevent empyema. A fundoplication after the method of Thal also may be added to this procedure, if the distal esophagus is used. This technique reduces the amount of reflux that can interfere with the healing or that can produce ulcers in the colon. *G,* A lateral view of an alternative method of cologastrostomy with Waterston's procedure. *H,* The segment of colon is shown within the abdominal cavity, which will possibly reduce the incidence of gastrocolic reflux. In my experience, reflux is not reduced.

it has anecdotally been reputed that an intra-abdominal segment of colon of 10-cm length effectively prevents reflux, cine and manometric studies show this not to be true.[138]

Construction of a submucosal tunnel has sometimes been effective in prevention of gastrocolonic reflux,[139] as has an antireflux nipple.[140] Although the creation of a Nissen fundoplication around an anterior cologastrostomy worked well in experimental animals, it has not become a common means of preventing gastrocolonic reflux in humans. Its experimental proponent suggests that colon-to-distal-esophageal anastomosis is the best method of prevention of gastrocolonic reflux.[124,141] Experience with 48 patients having a substernal, ileocolic interposition has been reported, in which the ileocecal valve served as a very effective antireflux mechanism when the cecum remains within the abdomen.[142] Leaving the ileocecal valve in the upper mediastinum as an

antireflux mechanism has been proposed,[143] but in my experience, this has not been effective.

The response of the distal colon–gastric anastomosis to acid has been studied, with the conclusion that the alkaline secretions of the colon tend to neutralize the acid or propel it back into the stomach before it can cause problems.[144] Clinically, such a fortuitous acid/alkali balance may occur, but it would be unreliable at best. Distal colonic ulcers have resulted from reflux of gastric acid. Most of these occurred in patients who did not undergo either pyloroplasty or pyloromyotomy to promote gastric drainage. Gastric drainage should be a part of any procedure that calls for a cologastric anastomosis.

Motor-activity analysis of interposed colon (as well as other esophageal-substitution conduits) has shown that the colon has a very satisfactory response to a bolus of food, although organized peristalsis is not seen.[145] Many older studies demonstrated that no matter whether the colon was placed in an isoperistaltic or antiperistaltic manner, its propulsive efforts soon were lost, and it came to serve primarily as a passive conduit for food.[128–130,138] No discernible difference regarding the ability to swallow was noted in a series of 60 patients, two thirds of whom had antiperistaltic interpositions of colon. Reflux from the stomach into the distal colon segment was common in this group of patients. Complications were infrequent, possibly because of pyloroplasty.[146] Similar findings were reported in another series of 84 patients undergoing both isoperistaltic and antiperistaltic colon interpositions.[147]

A functional assessment of interposed colon with isotope-labeled milk showed that patients who were clinically well had conduit emptying of less than 45 minutes without reflux. Those who were clinically troubled had delayed emptying of the conduit, gastrocolonic reflux, or both. The function of the colon segment may be satisfactorily assessed in this way.[148]

Late complications of colon interposition include redundancy of the colon segment, which led to one instance of obstructive volvulus of the colon.[149] Ulceration of the interposed colon can penetrate into the pericardium. In my experience, a penetrating ulcer in a substernal colon interposition has produced sternal osteomyelitis, which was troublesome to treat[150] (Fig. 25-10).

Another consideration in the selection of an interposition route is the possibility of subsequent acquired heart disease, necessitating sternotomy. In those patients in whom the substernal colon interposition has been used, this approach to the heart is difficult. Similarly, the previous use of a median sternotomy to repair the heart often necessitates an alternative route for an interposition.[151]

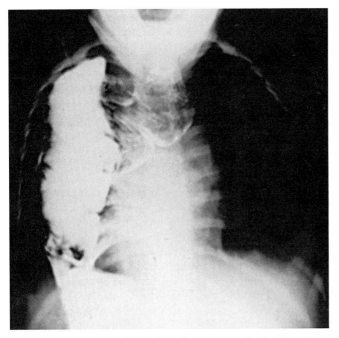

FIGURE 25-10. The elongation of a substernal colon is a difficult problem to manage at times, requiring careful tailoring of the distal end of the interposed colon without disrupting the blood supply to the upper portion.

Timing of Colon Interposition

In those patients in whom esophageal atresia exists without distal TEF and in whom attempts at stretching are not considered, the colon can be interposed in the newborn period. Most pediatric surgeons, however, create a cervical esophageal fistula, place a gastrostomy, and carry out interposition at some time after the patient is age 6 months. Some electively delay this procedure until age 12 to 18 months. Both approaches have theoretical and practical advantages. Most reported experience has been with the later procedure. However, if the patient has been without oral intake for many months, once an esophageal substitution has been made, he or she may not want to eat. Therefore sham feedings by mouth should accompany gastrostomy feedings so that the patient associates a full stomach with swallowing. In patients who have experienced failed attempts at stretching, failed anastomosis of the esophagus because of long-gap esophageal atresia with fistula, or caustic injuries, the operative procedure necessarily takes place long after the newborn period.

Passive or active drainage must accompany any esophageal anastomosis, whether in the neck or in the chest.

My personal preference for esophageal substitution by using colon is the retrohilar left or transverse colon segment placed with its vascular pedicle behind the pancreas. The distal anastomosis, whenever possible, is created by using the distal stump of esophagus. In most of these patients, I also create an anterior fundoplication to enhance the LES and to prevent gastroesophageal/colonic reflux. If this option is not available, rather than accept a cologastric anastomosis, I prefer a gastric tube interposition placed through the esophageal hiatus with anastomosis to the upper mediastinal or cervical esophagus. In these cases, the distal esophagus stump is resected, and an antireflux valve is created after the method of Toupet (see later text).

Gastric Tube Esophageal Replacement

Gastric tube replacement of the esophagus became a practicality in children in the early 1970s.[152,153] The reported experience with gastric tube esophagoplasty is much smaller than that with colon interposition, perhaps because the number of patients needing esophageal substitution has diminished in the developed world (Fig. 25-11). Awareness of caustic material hazards and changes in the chemical formulation of prepared drain cleaners have resulted in fewer serious ingestion injuries. Homemade lye solutions remain deadly.

Gastric tubes have become popular because they can be constructed rapidly with a stapling device. These tubes can be constructed from the antrum up or from the fundus down and can be constructed so that there is enough gastric tube to reach the neck.[153,154] Gastric tubes can be placed substernally or behind either pulmonary hilum. In a comparison study, the functional results of gastric tubes were similar whether they were placed transthoracically or substernally; however, in my experience, the substernal placement of the gastric tube has

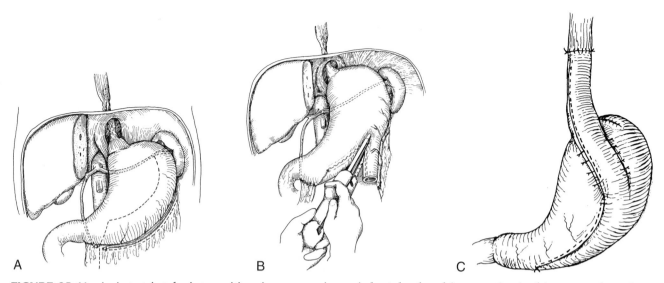

FIGURE 25-11. *A,* A gastric-tube interposition, in my experience, is best developed in an antiperistaltic manner by using a greater-curve gastric tube. Inspection of the blood supply is important before the development of a gastric tube is begun. *B,* The tube is developed with the use of the gastrointestinal anastomosis stapling device. Iatrogenic narrowing of this tube should be avoided. A large-bore red rubber catheter can prevent this unfortunate complication. Twisting of the greater curvature, which may result in a disparity between the contributions of the posterior gastric wall and the anterior gastric wall, should also be avoided. The short gastric vessels rarely must be divided for the creation of a satisfactory tube length. *C,* To be anastomosed to a remnant of esophagus in the mediastinum or in the neck, the gastric tube may be positioned in the anterior mediastinum substernally or through the esophageal hiatus. A posterior partial wrap, as illustrated, effectively prevents reflux of gastric content up into the gastric tube and reduces the likelihood of ulceration or anastomotic stricture.

resulted in necrosis in several patients and in an intractable stricture in one. The long-term results of gastric tube interposition are comparable to those of the colon interposition, and the gastric tube is simpler to construct.[153]

The gastric tube may involve peptic ulcer problems as well, both within the tube and at the junction of the gastric tube with the proximal esophagus. The ulcerations may be aggravated by stasis; therefore some authors recommend that a pyloroplasty be done in all patients undergoing gastric tube esophageal substitutions.[153] Reflux has not been a problem if at least 6 cm of gastric tube is located within the abdomen.

My preference for a gastric tube is to place it, if at all possible, behind the hilum of the lung through the esophageal hiatus and to create a posterior (Toupet) fundoplication, as illustrated in Figure 25-11. The function of such a fundoplication has been good, although in one patient, it became obstructive (Fig. 25-12). I do not routinely do pyloroplasty or pyloromyotomy. I believe that the long-term course of patients having gastric tube interposition has been much more trouble free than has the course of patients having colon interposition.

In my experience, gastric tube esophagoplasty is limited to older patients because of the percentage of stomach that must be used to create a satisfactory tube, which limits this technique in very small children.[154,155]

Gastric Interposition

Mobilization of the stomach and its repositioning into the mediastinum were strictly avoided in growing children because it was believed that the patient's growth pattern would not be normal. At the Hospital for Sick Children at Great Ormond Street, London, this technique became the interposition of choice in 1981, both for infants with esophageal atresia and for older patients with caustic injury or failed repair of esophageal atresia malformations.[156] Its use in 34 patients was reported from that institution in 1987. In total, 23 patients were younger than 12 months at the time of esophagogastrostomy. Sixteen patients had the stomach moved up into the mediastinum, and 18 had the stomach placed in a transthoracic, retrohilar position. A pyloromyotomy was done in 13, and a pyloroplasty in 20. Of the 31 survivors, 14 had uncomplicated recoveries, and 17 had one or more postoperative complication. Many of these complications were related to the fact that the patients did not know how to feed before the interposition. In one child, a leak developed in the jejunostomy feeding tube and required reexploration. A jejunostomy apparently was universally used during the healing phase in these patients. Most important, only 6 of 23 children followed up for at least a year postoperatively remained below the 30th percentile for height and weight. The others grew in a normal fashion. This experience was updated in 1995 to include a total of 83 patients. The combined mortality was 7.2%, with a 12% incidence each of an anastomotic leak and stricture. A satisfactory nutritional outcome was reported in 89%.[157,158]

A comparison of 112 Waterston retrohilar, left colon interpositions done at this same institution between 1952 and 1981 revealed that the mortality was approximately

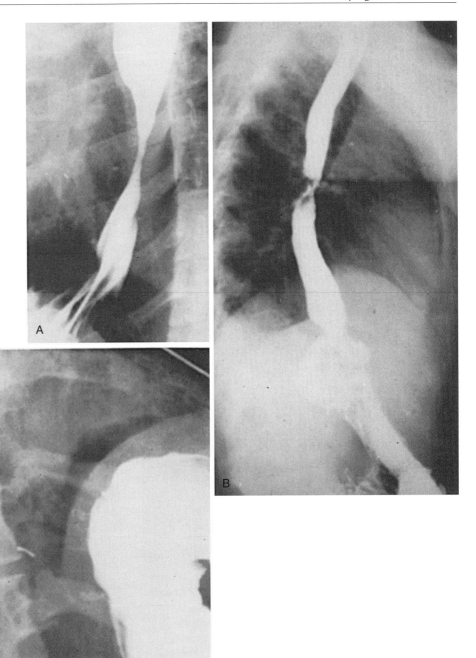

FIGURE 25-12. *A,* A mid and distal esophageal stricture caused by caustic ingestion many years before. Shortening of the esophagus with rugal folds above the diaphragm is obvious. *B,* The lateral barium study in the early postoperative period shows the gastric tube with some anastomotic edema in the portion of the midesophagus. The gastric tube has been placed through the esophageal hiatus into the posterior mediastinum. *C,* The complete absence of reflux in this interposed gastric tube can be seen with this late follow-up study. This result is probably due to the fundoplication, as illustrated in Figure 25-11.

the same but the incidence of graft failure, cervical anastomotic leak, and cervical anastomotic stricture was reduced in the gastric interposition patients, and quality of life was much improved.

I have used this interposition in four patients. One had experienced a failed colon interposition and a failed gastric tube. He underwent a successful esophagogastrostomy placed through the right chest posterior to the hilum (Fig. 25-13). He has done well. Another was a 1-year-old who had his upper atretic esophagus brought out on the neck and who had no recognizable distal esophageal stump. He has been slow to eat and to maintain his nutrition. The third patient had an ulcer-destroyed substernal right colon interposition removed, delivering her stomach in the substernal position up to the cervical esophagus. After 2 years of postprandial distress and extreme inanition, the stomach was re-placed in the abdomen, and the left colon interposed as a retrohilar, right-sided esophageal substitute. The fourth patient had a gastric pull-up at the age of 15 years because of a very dysfunctional distal esophageal segment with Barrett's changes. He had not responded to fundoplication performed at age 4 years. No collateral blood supply existed from the left to the right gastroepiploic arteries, which precluded using a reversed gastric tube.

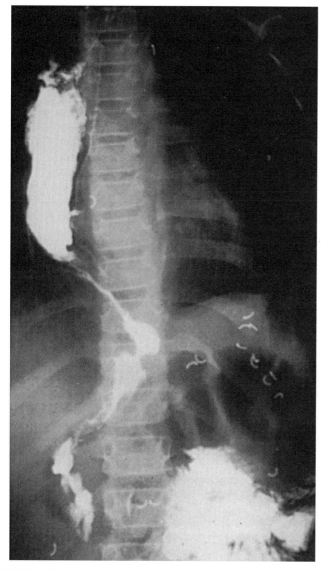

FIGURE 25-13. A patient who underwent an esophagogastrostomy after unsuccessful colon interposition and failed gastric tube. The patient also underwent a pyloroplasty at the time of the esophagogastrostomy.

Jejunal Substitution

The jejunum as an esophageal substitute has been much more common in adults than in children. Of 19 pediatric patients reported to have a segmental jejunal interposition placed into the midesophagus through the right chest, 12 were available for long-term follow-up: in 1, a stricture developed, and in 1, an elongation of the interposed jejunum developed. The surgeons preserved the distal esophagus for anastomosis whenever possible. The technique to harvest a 10- to 12-cm segment of jejunum required sacrifice of about 40 cm of jejunum, however. Some of the patients had nutritional problems, perhaps because of the loss of this much small intestine.[159]

The major use for jejunum has been as a free graft with microvascular anastomosis in the cervical position for adults with carcinoma. Extensive use of this procedure in 101 patients was reported with satisfactory results.[160] This procedure obviously would not be applicable to the pediatric population. I have done only one jejunal interposition between the cervical esophagus and stomach. Its early result was satisfactory. The patient was then lost to follow-up.

Complications of Esophageal Substitution

Substitution of the esophagus carries with it a certain number of predictable complications; the most serious one is vascular insufficiency with necrosis of the interposition. This complication is most commonly seen when using the colon, as mentioned earlier, and is recognized at the time of interposition as a blue, pulseless graft. Adjustment of the colon graft to relieve tension or twisting of the pedicle may be effective in improving the blood supply. Intraoperative hypotension may result in the colon graft taking on the appearance of vascular insufficiency. If the geometry of the graft and the patient's blood pressure are both satisfactory, the graft must be abandoned, because hoping that its vascularity will improve after interposition is usually in vain.

Interposition of a well-vascularized graft is sometimes followed several days later by fever, increased leukocytosis, and drainage from the proximal anastomosis. A contrast study may demonstrate that the mucosal pattern of the interposed segment is not normal. The interposition must be inspected and removed if necrotic. In this instance, a cervical esophagostomy should be established and a different form of substitution planned. Many investigators have reported using the left colon after failure of the right colon. I am inclined not to sacrifice that much colon and would probably resort to either gastric tube or esophagogastrostomy under the circumstances.

Proximal strictures between the esophagus and the interposition usually are the result of insufficient blood supply to the interposition. Anastomosis to a scarred esophagus also results in stricture. After a reasonable healing period, persistent strictures should be revised surgically rather than dilated repeatedly.

Ulceration in either gastric tube or interposed colon is probably the result of reflux and stasis, which may be caused by kinks or turns in the interposition or by delayed gastric emptying. The latter can be a complication of vagal injury either from the original caustic ingestion or from the surgical attempts at previous esophageal reconstruction. Whether a pyloroplasty or a drainage procedure is necessary in all interpositions is a matter of opinion. Certainly, the elimination of "sink-trap" kinks in the interposition is important to prevent ulceration. Revision of the lower end of the interposed colon to eliminate redundancy must be done with great care to prevent damage to the vascular pedicle and loss of the entire graft.

One of my patients had repeated upper anastomotic strictures because of gastrocolic reflux into a substernal colon interposition placed for esophageal atresia without fistula. I detached both ends of the colon segment through a right thoracotomy and laparotomy, delivered it back into the abdominal cavity, brought it up behind the hilum of the right lung, reanastomosed it to the upper mediastinal esophagus, shortened it, anastomosed the distal end to the distal stump of the esophagus, and performed an anterior fundoplication. An excellent outcome resulted. Such extensive revision is not often necessary but may, on occasion, turn an unsatisfactory result completely around.[162]

Colon-patch esophagoplasty for stricture of the esophagus is appropriate in certain situations,[161,162] as is myotomy and strictureplasty.[163] Alloderm patches for relief of strictures have been proposed and, in an experimental study in the normal dog esophagus, appear to be a promising, simple technique with readily available material.[164]

VASCULAR RING

The vascular malformations that involve the aortic arch and its major branches are known as vascular rings. In this chapter, only those malformations that potentially obstruct the esophagus are discussed. The complete ring, also known as the double aortic arch, is included, as are the incomplete rings, the most common of which is the aberrant subclavian vessel crossing behind the esophagus and the transverse aortic arch that crosses behind the esophagus to descend on the side opposite the ascending aorta. The incomplete rings are often associated with a ligamentum or ductus arteriosus, which limits the space available for trachea and esophagus. The incomplete rings are an unusual cause of dysphagia but are commonly seen on barium esophagram. The other much more serious vascular ring malformation is known as the pulmonary artery sling and is often related to tracheal malformation but rarely produces any esophageal symptoms.

The symptom of vascular ring is dysphagia for the most part. Dysphagia lusoria was the name attached to the symptom, attributed to an aberrant right subclavian artery, which passes behind the esophagus as it courses toward the right axilla. In fact, an aberrant right subclavian artery rarely produces dysphagia.

Because the obstruction of the esophagus is partial, the symptoms that result from vascular rings depend on how voraciously the child is eating and whether the ingested food is solid or liquid. Often these lesions are not discovered until the child is eating table food.[165]

Diagnosis

The diagnosis is established almost exclusively by barium study of the esophagus done for evaluation of dysphagia.[166] The typical radiographic picture of a double aortic arch is that of an offset in the linear axis of the esophagus. It is characteristic of the double aortic arch (Fig. 25-14) and is contrasted with the indentation without offset in the axis, as in the case of aberrant right subclavian artery (Fig. 25-15). Although echocardiography,[167] digital subtraction angiography,[168] or magnetic resonance imaging[169,170] may confirm the diagnosis, they are rarely necessary for either diagnostic or therapeutic decisions.

Surgical Treatment

The normal embryologic formation of the aortic arch requires resorption of the dorsal fourth right arch with remolding of the right subclavian and common carotid into an innominate artery arising as the first vessel off the arch. The double arch results when the resorptive process does not occur properly. If both arches persist,

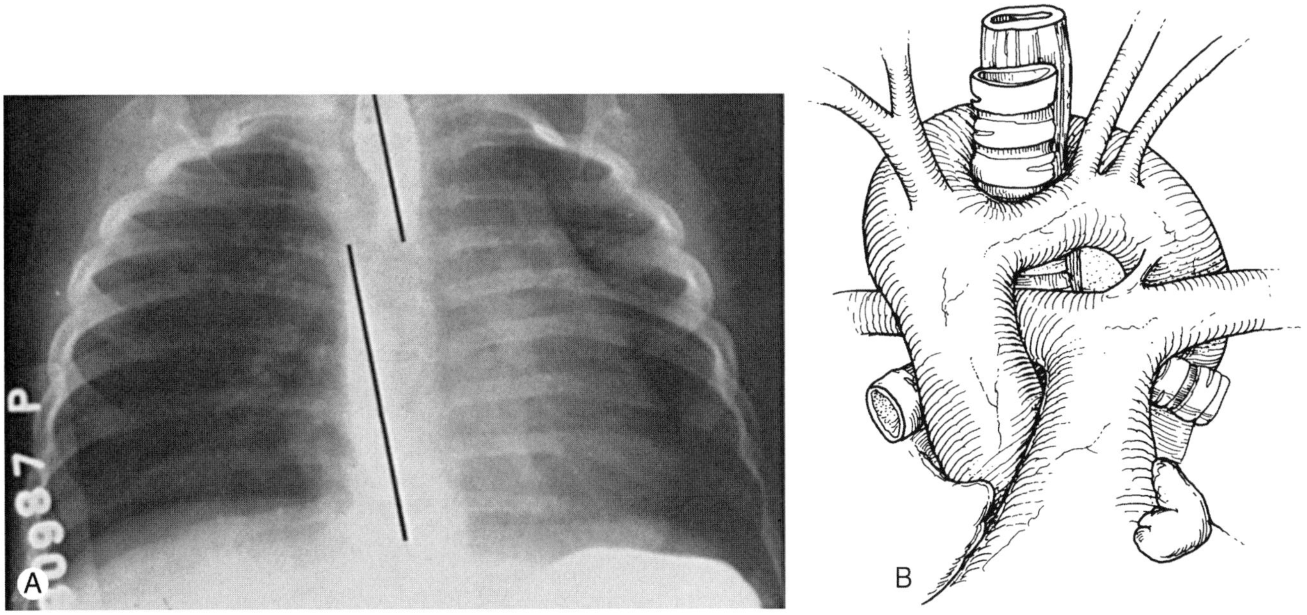

FIGURE 25-14. *A,* A double aortic arch demonstrated by barium esophagram. The axes of the proximal and distal portions of the esophagus are offset by the presence of a complete vascular ring. *B,* The double arch as drawn is usually narrowest on the left branch and is best approached for division through a left thoracotomy.

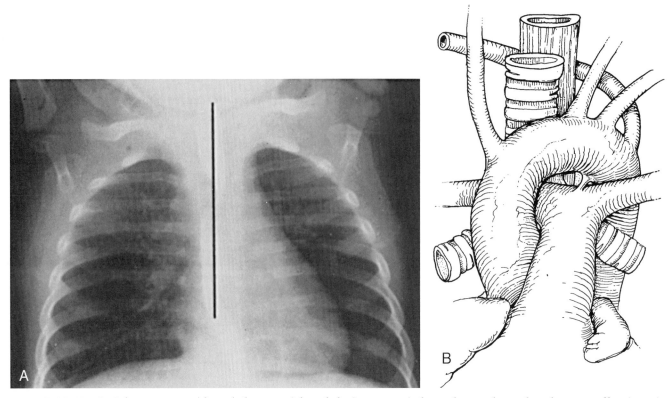

FIGURE 25-15. *A,* A longer postesophageal aberrant right subclavian artery indents the esophagus but does not offset its axis. *B,* The aberrant right subclavian artery is best divided by the left thoracotomy approach.

the right is almost always the larger of the two, with varying degrees of stenosis or even fibrosis of the left arch, forming the anterior portion of the ring. The right arch courses behind the esophagus to descend on the left. The left arch compresses the trachea and esophagus to produce the symptoms. The surgical approach to division of the vascular ring is best done through the left thorax, dividing the left arch at its narrowest point, which is either posterior to the origin of the left subclavian artery or between the ascending aorta and the origin of the left common carotid artery.[171] The ligamentum arteriosum should be divided as well to relieve the esophageal obstruction effectively. Dissection of the vessels off the trachea anteriorly and the esophagus posteriorly is usually all that is necessary to allow the trachea and the esophagus to escape the constriction and relieve the symptoms.

Although some surgeons detach the retroesophageal aberrant right subclavian artery and reimplant it on the aortic arch, most simply divide this vessel and allow the distal portion to retract across the mediastinum from behind the esophagus.[172] Thus symptoms are relieved. Therefore this anomaly can best be treated through a left thoracotomy as well. Other vascular or cardiac malformations are usually not associated with vascular ring. Any form of suspension of the vessels is usually not necessary after the division of the ring. Less invasive procedures have been applied to this, as to many other lesions within the chest.[173]

REFERENCES

1. Williams AK, Quan QB, Beasley SW: Three-dimensional imaging clarifies the process of tracheoesophageal separation in the rat. J Pediatr Surg 38:173–177, 2003.
2. Amoury RA: Structure and function of the esophagus in infancy and early childhood. In Ashcraft KW, Holder TM (eds): Pediatric Esophageal Surgery. Orlando, Grune & Stratton, pp 1–28, 1986.
3. Leape LL, Ashcraft KW, Scarpelli DG, et al: Hazard to health: Liquid lye. N Engl J Med 284:578–581, 1971.
4. Tekant G, Eroglu E, Erdogan E, et al: Corrosive injury-induced gastric outlet obstruction: A changing spectrum of agents and treatment. J Pediatr Surg 36:1004–1007, 2001.
5. Genc A, Mutaf O: Esophageal motility changes in acute and late periods of caustic esophageal burns and their relation to prognosis in children. J Pediatr Surg 37:1526–1528, 2002.
6. Ashcraft KW, Padula RT: Effect of dilute corrosives on the esophagus. Pediatrics 53:226–232, 1974.
7. Millar AJW, Numanoglu A, Mann M, et al: Detection of caustic oesophageal injury with technetium 99m-labelled sucralfate. J Pediatr Surg 36:262–265, 2001.
8. Webb WR, Koutras P, Ecker RR, et al: An evaluation of steroids and antibiotics in caustic burns of the esophagus. Ann Thorac Surg 9:95–102, 1970.
9. Haller JA, Bachman BA: Comparative effect of current therapy on experimental caustic burns of the esophagus. Pediatrics 34:236–245, 1964.
10. Haller JA, Andrews HG, White JJ, et al: Pathophysiology and management of acute corrosive burns of the esophagus: Results of treatment in 285 children. J Pediatr Surg 6:578–584, 1971.
11. Moazam F, Talbert JL, Miller D, et al: Caustic ingestion and its sequelae in children. South Med J 80:187–190, 1987.
12. Anderson KD, Rouse TM, Randolph JG: Controlled trial of corticosteroids in children with corrosive injury of the esophagus. N Engl J Med 323:637–640, 1990.

13. Edmonson MB: Caustic alkali ingestions by farm children. Pediatrics 79:413–416, 1987.
14. Shaw AN, Garvey J, Miller B: Lye burn requiring total gastrectomy and colon substitution for esophagus and stomach in a two-year-old boy. Surgery 65:837–844, 1969.
15. Estrera A, Taylor W, Mills LJ, et al: Corrosive burns of the esophagus and stomach: A recommendation for an aggressive surgical approach. Ann Thorac Surg 41:276–283, 1986.
16. Gago O, Ritter FN, Martel W, et al: Aggressive surgical treatment for caustic injury of the esophagus and stomach. Ann Thorac Surg 13:243–250, 1972.
17. Ashcraft KW: Correspondence. Ann Thorac Surg 14:221, 1972.
18. Reyes HM, Lin CY, Schlunk FF, et al: Experimental treatment of corrosive esophageal burns. J Pediatr Surg 9:317–327, 1974.
19. Reyes HM, Hill LJ: Modification of the experimental stent technique for esophageal burns. J Surg Res 20:65–70, 1976.
20. Hill LJ, Norberg HP, Smith MD, et al: Clinical technique and success of the esophageal stent to prevent corrosive strictures. J Pediatr Surg 11:443–450, 1976.
21. Wijburg FA, Heymans HSA, Urbanus NAM: Caustic esophageal lesions in childhood: Prevention of stricture formation. J Pediatr Surg 24:171–173, 1989.
22. Mills LJ, Estrera AS, Platt MR: Avoidance of esophageal stricture following severe caustic burns by the use of an intraluminal stent. Ann Thorac Surg 28:60–65, 1979.
23. Joseph PR: The pediatric forum. Management of coin ingestion. Am J Dis Child 144:449, 1990.
24. Smith PC, Swischuk LE, Fagan CJ: An elusive and often unsuspected cause of stridor or pneumonia (the esophageal foreign body). Am J Radiol Ther Nucl Med 122:80–89, 1974.
25. Foster DL: The pediatric forum: Pediatric coin ingestion. Am J Dis Child 144:450–451, 1990.
26. Schunk JE, Corneli H, Bolte R: Pediatric coin ingestions. Am J Dis Child 143:546–548, 1989.
27. Caravati EM, Bennett DL, McElwee NE: Pediatric coin ingestion: A prospective study on the utility of routine roentgenograms. Am J Dis Child 143:549–551, 1989.
28. Fernandes ET, Hollabaugh RS, Boulden T: Mediastinal mass and radiolucent esophageal foreign body. J Pediatr Surg 24:1135–1136, 1989.
29. Beal SM: Sudden infant death associated with an oesophageal problem. Med J Aust 2:91, 1979.
30. Woods I, Swan PK: Tracheal occlusion following oesophageal foreign body removal. Anaesth Intens Care 17:356–358, 1989.
31. Bonadio WA, Jona JZ, Glicklich M, et al: Esophageal bougienage technique for coin ingestion in children. J Pediatr Surg 23:917–918, 1988.
32. Bigler FC: The use of a Foley catheter for removal of blunt foreign bodies from the esophagus. J Thorac Cardiovasc Surg 51:759–760, 1966.
33. Campbell JB, Foley CL: A safe alternative to endoscopic removal of blunt esophageal foreign bodies. Arch Otolaryngol 109:323–325, 1983.
34. Campbell JB, Condon VR: Catheter removal of blunt esophageal foreign bodies in children. Pediatr Radiol 19:361–365, 1989.
35. Burrington JD: Aluminum "pop tops": A hazard to child health. JAMA 235:2614–2617, 1976.
36. Spitz J, Hirsig J: Prolonged foreign body impaction in the oesophagus. Arch Dis Child 57:551–553, 1982.
37. Takano H, Okada A, Monden Y, et al: Unusual case of acquired benign tracheoesophageal fistula caused by an esophageal foreign body. J Thorac Cardiovasc Surg 99:755–756, 1990.
38. Litovitz TL: Button battery ingestions: A review of 56 cases. JAMA 249:2495–2500, 1983.
39. Votteler TP, Nash JC, Rutledge JC: The hazard of ingested alkaline disk batteries in children. JAMA 249:2504–2506, 1983.
40. Sigalet D, Lees G: Tracheoesophageal injury secondary to disc battery ingestion. J Pediatr Surg 23:996–998, 1988.
41. Maves MD, Carithers JS, Birck HG: Esophageal burns secondary to disc battery ingestion. Ann Otol Rhinol Laryngol 93:364–369, 1984.
42. Shabino DL, Feinberg AN: Esophageal perforation secondary to alkaline battery ingestion. J Am Coll Emerg Physicians 8:360–362, 1979.
43. Vaishnav A, Spitz L: Alkaline battery-induced tracheooesophageal fistula. Br J Surg 76:1045, 1989.
44. Blatnik DS, Toohill RJ, Lehman RH: Fatal complication from an alkaline battery foreign body in the esophagus. Ann Otol 86:611–615, 1977.
45. Rumack BH, Rumack CM: Disk battery ingestion. JAMA 249:2509–2511, 1983.
46. Volle E, Beyer P, Kaufmann JH: Therapeutic approach to ingested button-type batteries: Magnetic removal of ingested button-type batteries. Pediatr Radiol 19:114–118, 1989.
47. Willis GA, Ho WC: Perforation of Meckel's diverticulum by an alkaline hearing battery. Can Med Assoc J 126:497–498, 1982.
48. Wells SD, Leonidas JC, Conkle D, et al: Traumatic prevertebral pharyngoesophageal pseudodiverticulum in the newborn infant. J Pediatr Surg 9:217–222, 1974.
49. Cohen RC, Myers NA: Traumatic oesophageal pseudodiverticulum. J Pediatr Aust 23:125–127, 1987.
50. Nagaraj HS, Mullen P, Groff DB: Iatrogenic perforation of the esophagus in premature infants. Surgery 86:583–589, 1979.
51. Grosfeld JL: Discussion: Iatrogenic perforation of the esophagus in premature infants. Surgery 86:588–599, 1979.
52. Tolstedt GE, Tudor RB: Esophagopleural fistula in a newborn infant. Arch Surg 97:780–781, 1968.
53. Adams H, Roberts GM, Smith PM: Oesophageal tears during pneumatic balloon dilatation for the treatment of achalasia. Clin Radiol 40:53–57, 1989.
54. Panieri E, Millar AJW, Rode H, et al: Iatrogenic esophageal perforation in children: Patterns of injury, presentation, management, and outcome. J Pediatr Surg 31:890–895, 1996.
55. Bolooki H, Attar S, Hankins JR, et al: Esophageal perforation: A therapeutic challenge. Ann Thorac Surg 50:50, 1990.
56. DeMeester TR: Perforation of the esophagus. Ann Thorac Surg 42:231–232, 1986.
57. Bladergroen MR, Lowe JE, Postlethwait RW: Diagnosis and recommended management of esophageal perforation and rupture. Ann Thorac Surg 42:235–239, 1986.
58. Ajalat GM, Mulder DG: Esophageal perforations. Arch Surg 119:1318–1320, 1984.
59. Cohn HE, Hubbard A, Patton G: Management of esophageal injuries. Ann Thorac Surg 48:309–314, 1989.
60. Michel L, Grillo HC, Malt RA: Esophageal perforation. Ann Thorac Surg 33:203–210, 1982.
61. Martinez L, Rivas S, Hernandez F, et al: Aggressive conservative treatment of esophageal perforations in children. J Pediatr Surg 38:685–689, 2003.
62. Hendren WH, Henderson BM: Immediate esophagectomy for instrumental perforation of the thoracic esophagus. Ann Surg 168:997–1002, 1968.
63. Conlan AA, Wessels A, Hammond CA, et al: Pharyngoesophageal barotrauma in children: A report of six cases. J Thorac Cardiovasc Surg 88:452–456, 1984.
64. Inculet R, Clark C, Girvan D: Boerhaave's syndrome and children: A rare and unexpected combination. J Pediatr Surg 31:1300–1301, 1996.
65. Amae S, Nio M, Kamiyama T, et al: Clinical characteristics and management of congenital esophageal stenosis: A report on 14 cases. J Pediatr Surg 38:565–570, 2003.
66. Kouchi K, Yoshida H, Matsunaga T, et al: Endosonographic evaluation in two children with esophageal stenosis. J Pediatr Surg 37:934–936, 2002.
67. Usui N, Kamata S, Kawahara H, et al: Usefulness of endoscopic ultrasonography in the diagnosis of congenital esophageal stenosis. J Pediatr Surg 37:1744–1746, 2002.
68. Scherer LR, Grosfeld JL: Congenital esophageal stenosis, esophageal duplication, neurenteric cyst and esophageal diverticulum. In Ashcraft KW, Holder TM (eds): Pediatric Esophageal Surgery. Orlando, Grune & Stratton, 1986, pp 53–71.
69. Domini R, Appignani A, Ceccarelli PL, et al: Congenital esophageal stenosis due to ectopic cartilaginous tissue: A case report. Ital J Pediatr Surg Sci 2:87–89, 1988.
70. Grabowski ST, Andrews DA: Upper esophageal stenosis: Two case reports. J Pediatr Surg 31:1438–1439, 1996.
71. Henderson RD, Davidson JW: Primary disordered motor activity of the esophagus (diffuse spasm). Ann Thorac Surg 18:327–336, 1974.

72. Moersch HJ, Camp JD: Diffuse spasm of the lower part of the esophagus. Ann Otorhinolaryngol 43:1165–1173, 1934.

73. Henderson RD, Henderson RF, Marryatt GV: Surgical management of 100 consecutive esophageal strictures. J Thorac Cardiovasc Surg 99:1–7, 1990.

74. Levine JJ, Ilowite NT: Scleroderma-like esophageal disease in children breast-fed by mothers with silicone breast implants. JAMA 271:213–216, 1994.

75. Toyohara T, Koneka T, Araki H, et al: Giant epiphrenic diverticulum in a boy with Ehlers-Danlos syndrome. Pediatr Radiol 19:437, 1989.

76. Nihoul-Fekete C, Bawab F, Lortat-Jacob S, et al: Achalasia of the esophagus in childhood: Surgical treatment in 35 cases with special reference to familial cases and glucocorticoid deficiency association. J Pediatr Surg 24:1060–1063, 1989.

77. Tryhus MR, Davis M, Griffith JK, et al: Familial achalasia in two siblings: Significance of possible hereditary role. J Pediatr Surg 24:292–295, 1989.

78. Rosenzweig S, Traube M: The diagnosis and misdiagnosis of achalasia. J Clin Gastroenterol 11:147–153, 1989.

79. Shoenut P, Trenholm BG, Micflikier AB, et al: Reflux patterns in patients with achalasia without operation. Ann Thorac Surg 45:303–305, 1988.

80. Smith H, Buick R, Booth I, et al: Letters to the editor. J Pediatr Gastroenterol 7:146, 1988.

81. Vane DW, Cosby K, West K, et al: Late results following esophagomyotomy in children with achalasia. J Pediatr Surg 23:515–519, 1988.

82. Sauer L, Pellegrini CA, Way LW: The treatment of achalasia. Arch Surg 124:929–932, 1989.

83. Richardson JD: Discussion. In Sauer L, Pellegrini CA, Way LW: The treatment of achalasia. Arch Surg 124:932, 1989.

84. Ponce J, Garrigues V, Pertejo V, et al: Individual prediction of response to pneumatic dilation in patients with achalasia. Dig Dis Sci 41:2135–2141, 1996.

85. Myers N, Jolley SG, Taylor R: Achalasia of the cardia in children: A worldwide survey. J Pediatr Surg 29:1375–1379, 1994.

86. Little AG, Soriano A, Ferguson MK, et al: Surgical treatment of achalasia: Results with esophagomyotomy and Belsey repair. Ann Thorac Surg 45:489–494, 1988.

87. Ellis FH: Treatment of achalasia: A continuing controversy. Ann Thorac Surg 45:473, 1988.

88. Jekler J, Lhotka J: Modified Heller procedure to prevent postoperative reflux esophagitis in patients with achalasia. Am J Surg 113:251–254, 1967.

89. Skinner DB: Myotomy and achalasia. Ann Thorac Surg 37:183–184, 1984.

90. Murray GF, Battaglini JW, Keagy BA, et al: Selective application of fundoplication in achalasia. Ann Thorac Surg 37:185–188, 1984.

91. Pai GP, Ellison RG, Rubin JW, et al: Two decades of experience with modified Heller's myotomy for achalasia. Ann Thorac Surg 38:201–206, 1984.

92. Fonkalsrud E: Discussion. In Vane DW, Cosby K, West K, et al: Late results following esophagomyotomy in children with achalasia. J Pediatr Surg 23:519, 1988.

93. Rothenberg SS, Partrick DA, Bealer JF, et al: Evaluation of minimally invasive approaches to achalasia in children. J Pediatr Surg 36:808–810, 2001.

94. Patti MG, Albanese CT, Holcomb GW III, et al: Laparoscopic Heller myotomy and Dor fundoplication for esophageal achalasia in children. J Pediatr Surg 36:1248–1251, 2001.

95. Bolstad DS: The management of strictures of the esophagus. Ann Otolaryngol 75:1019–1028, 1966.

96. Ashcraft KW, Holder TH: The experimental treatment of esophageal strictures by intralesional steroid injections. J Thorac Cardiovasc Surg 58:685–691, 1969.

97. Gandhi RP, Cooper A, Barlow BA: Successful management of esophageal strictures without resection or replacement. J Pediatr Surg 24:745–750, 1989.

98. Holder TH, Ashcraft KW, Leape L: The treatment of patients with esophageal strictures by local steroid injections. J Pediatr Surg 4:646–653, 1969.

99. Zein NN, Greseth JM, Perrault J: Endoscopic intralesional steroid injections in the management of refractory esophageal strictures. Gastrointest Endosc 41:596–598, 1995.

100. Fonkalsrud EW: Initial esophageal dilatation in infants with benign esophageal stricture. Surgery 59:883–885, 1966.

101. Tytgat Guido NJ: Dilation therapy of benign esophageal stenoses. World J Surg 13:142–148, 1989.

102. Shemesh E, Czerniak A: Comparison between Savary-Gilliard and balloon dilatation of benign esophageal strictures. World J Surg 14:518–522, 1990.

103. Yeming W, Somme S, Chenren, et al: Balloon catheter dilatation in children with congenital and acquired esophageal anomalies. J Pediatr Surg 37:398–402, 2002.

104. Gilchrist BF, Scriven R, Sanchez J, et al: The application of vascular technology to esophageal and airway strictures. J Pediatr Surg 37:47–49, 2002.

105. Golladay ES, Tepas JJ III, Pickard LR, et al: Bacteremia after esophageal dilation: A clinical and experimental study. Ann Thorac Surg 30:19–23, 1980.

106. Musher DR, Boyd A: Esophagocolonic stricture with proximal fistulae treated by balloon dilation. Am J Gastroenterol 83:445–447, 1988.

107. Little AG, Naunheim KS, Ferguson MK, et al: Surgical management of esophageal strictures. Ann Thorac Surg 45:144–147, 1988.

108. Paulson DL: Benign stricture of the esophagus secondary to gastroesophageal reflux. Ann Surg 165:765–778, 1967.

109. Ohhama U, Tsunoda A, Nishi T, et al: Surgical treatment of reflux stricture of the esophagus. J Pediatr Surg 25:758–761, 1990.

110. Isolauri J, Nordback I, Markkula H: Surgery for reflux stricture of the oesophagus. Ann Chir Gynaecol 78:120–123, 1989.

111. Fonkalsrud EW, Ament ME: Surgical management of esophageal stricture due to recessive dystrophic epidermolysis bullosa. J Pediatr Surg 12:221–226, 1977.

112. Demirogullari B, Sonmez K, Turkyilmaz Z, et al: Colon interposition for esophageal stenosis in a patient with epidermolysis bullosa. J Pediatr Surg 36:1861–1863, 2001.

113. Imre J, Kopp M: Arguments against long-term conservative treatment of oesophageal strictures due to corrosive burns. Thorax 27:594–598, 1972.

114. Kiviranta UK: Corrosion carcinoma of the esophagus: 381 cases of corrosion and nine cases of corrosion carcinoma. Acta Otolaryngol (Stockh) 42:89–95, 1952.

115. Alvarez AF, Colbert JG: Lye stricture of the esophagus complicated by carcinoma. Can J Surg 6:470–476, 1963.

116. Bigger IA, Vinson PP: Carcinoma secondary to burn of the esophagus from ingestion of lye. Surgery 28:887–889, 1950.

117. Bigelow NH: Carcinoma of the esophagus developing at the site of lye stricture. Cancer 6:1159–1164, 1953.

118. Appelqvist P, Salmo M: Lye corrosion carcinoma of the esophagus. Cancer 43:2655–2658, 1980.

119. Mansour KA, Hansen HA, Hersh T, et al: Colon interposition for advanced nonmalignant esophageal stricture: Experience with 40 patients. Ann Thorac Surg 32:584–592, 1981.

120. Gross RE, Firestone FN: Colonic reconstruction of the esophagus in infants and children. Surgery 61:955–964, 1967.

121. Belsey R, Clagett OT: Reconstruction of the esophagus with the left colon. J Thorac Cardiovasc Surg 49:33–54, 1965.

122. Kelly JP, Shackelford GD, Roper CL: Esophageal replacement with colon in children: Functional results and long-term growth. Ann Thorac Surg 36:634–644, 1983.

123. Hamza AF, Abdelhay S, Sherif H, et al: Caustic esophageal strictures in children: 30 years' experience. J Pediatr Surg 38:828–833, 2003.

124. Waterston DJ: Replacement of oesophagus with colon in childhood. In Rob C, Smith R (eds): Operative Surgery, Vol. 2 (2nd ed). London, Butterworth, 1968, pp 367–374.

125. German JC, Waterston DJ: Colon interposition for the replacement of the esophagus in children. J Pediatr Surg 11:227–234, 1976.

126. Azar H, Chrispin AR, Waterston DJ: Esophageal replacement with transverse colon in infants and children. J Pediatr Surg 6:3–9, 1971.

127. Ahmad SA, Sylvester KG, Hebra A, et al: Esophageal replacement using the colon: Is it a good choice? J Pediatr Surg 31:1026–1031, 1996.

128. Choi RS, Lillehei CW, Lund DP, et al: Esophageal replacement in children who have caustic pharyngoesophageal strictures. J Pediatr Surg 32:1083–1088, 1997.

129. Mitchell IM, Goh DW, Roberts KD, et al: Colon interposition in children. Br J Surg 76:681–686, 1989.

130. Wu M, Chiu N, Lin M, et al: Functional evaluation of esophageal substitutes. Chin Med J (Engl) 58:223–229, 1996.

131. Lindahl H, Louhimo I, Virkola K: Colon interposition or gastric tube? Follow-up study of colon-esophagus and gastric tube-esophagus patients. J Pediatr Surg 18:58–63, 1983.

132. Huang MH, Sung CY, Hsu HK, et al: Reconstruction of the esophagus with the left colon. Ann Thorac Surg 48:660–664, 1989.

133. Stone MM, Mahour GH, Weitzman JJ, et al: Esophageal replacement with colon interposition in children. Ann Surg 203:346–351, 1986.

134. West KW, Vane DW, Grosfeld JL: Esophageal replacement in children: Experience with thirty-one cases. Surgery 100:751–757, 1986.

135. Najafi H, Beattie E: Excision of teniae coli for repair of esophagocolic stricture following colon transplant: Case report. Ann Surg 162:1097–1099, 1965.

136. Lynn H: Simple method of elongating a colonic segment for esophageal replacement. J Pediatr Surg 8:391–393, 1973.

137. Belsey R: Discussion: Esophageal replacement with colon in children: Functional results and long-term growth. Ann Thorac Surg 36:641–642, 1983.

138. Sieber AM, Sieber WK: Colon transplants as esophageal replacement: Cineradiographic and manometric evaluation in children. Ann Surg 168:116–122, 1968.

139. Guzzetta PC, Randolph JG: Antireflux cologastric anastomosis following colonic interposition for esophageal replacement. J Pediatr Surg 21:1137–1138, 1986.

140. Larsson S, Lycke G, Radberg G: Replacement of the esophagus by a segment of colon provided with an antireflux valve. Ann Thorac Surg 48:677–682, 1989.

141. Butterfield WC, Massi J: Gastric reflux in colon interpositions: A method of treatment. J Thorac Cardiovasc Surg 64:229–234, 1972.

142. Raffensperger JG, Luck SR, Reynolds M, et al: Intestinal bypass of the esophagus. J Pediatr Surg 31:38–47, 1996.

143. Touloukian RJ, Tellides G: Retrosternal ileocolic esophageal replacement in children revisited. J Thorac Cardiovasc Surg 107:1067–1072, 1994.

144. Jones EL, Skinner DB, Demeester TR, et al: Response of the interposed human colonic segment to an acid challenge. Ann Surg 177:75–78, 1973.

145. Moreno-Osset E, Tomas-Ridocci M, Paris F, et al: Motor activity of esophageal substitute (stomach, jejunal, and colon segments). Ann Thorac Surg 41:515–519, 1986.

146. Isolauri J: Colonic interposition for benign esophageal disease: Long-term clinical and endoscopic results. Am J Surg 155:498–502, 1988.

147. Neville WE, Najem AZ: Colon replacement of the esophagus for congenital and benign disease. Ann Thorac Surg 36:626–633, 1983.

148. Sutton R, Sutton DM, Ackery DM, et al: Functional assessment of colonic interposition with Tc99m-labeled milk. J Pediatr Surg 24:874–881, 1989.

149. Sterling RP, Kuykendall C, Carmichael MJ, et al: Unusual sequelae of colon interposition for esophageal reconstruction: Late obstruction requiring reoperation. Ann Thorac Surg 38:292–295, 1984.

150. Pantelides ML, Fitzgerald MD: Left ventriculo-colic fistula: A late complication of colonic interposition for the oesophagus. Postgrad Med J 64:710–712, 1988.

151. Choh JH, Balderman SC, Bingham D, et al: Parasternal intrapleural colon interposition: An alternative pathway for the colon graft. Ann Thorac Surg 31:474–477, 1981.

152. Anderson KD, Randolph JG: The gastric tube for esophageal replacement in children. J Thorac Cardiovasc Surg 66:333–342, 1973.

153. Cohen DH, Middleton AW, Fletcher J: Gastric tube esophagoplasty. J Pediatr Surg 9:451–460, 1974.

154. Gavrilu D: The replacement of the oesophagus by a gastric tube. In Jamieson GG (ed): Surgery of the Oesophagus. Edinburgh, Churchill Livingstone, 1988.

155. Pedersen JC, Klein RL, Andrews DA: Gastric tube as the primary procedure for pure esophageal atresia. J Pediatr Surg 31:1233–1235, 1996.

156. Spitz L, Kiely E, Sparnon T: Gastric transposition for esophageal replacement in children. Ann Surg 206:69–73, 1987.

157. Spitz L: Esophageal atresia: Past, present, and future. J Pediatr Surg 31:19–25, 1996.

158. Ravelli AM, Spitz L, Milla PJ: Gastric emptying in children with gastric transposition. J Pediatr Gastroenterol Nutr 19:403–409, 1994.

159. Saeki M, Tsuchida Y, Ogata T, et al: Long-term results of jejunal replacement of the esophagus. J Pediatr Surg 23:483–489, 1988.

160. Coleman JJ, Tan KC, Searles JM, et al: Jejunal free autograft: Analysis of complications and their resolution. Plast Reconstr Surg 84:589–595, 1989.

161. Othersen HB, Parker EF, Smith CD: The surgical management of esophageal stricture in children. Ann Surg 207:590–597, 1988.

162. Kennedy AP, Cameron BH, McGill CW: Colon patch esophagoplasty for caustic esophageal stricture. J Pediatr Surg 30:1242–1245, 1995.

163. Anderson KD, Acosta JM, Meyer MS, et al: Application of the principles of myotomy and strictureplasty for treatment of esophageal strictures. J Pediatr Surg 37:403–406, 2002.

164. Sigalet DL, Lagerge JM, DiLorenzo M, et al: Aortoesophageal fistula: Congenital and acquired causes. J Pediatr Surg 29:1212–1214, 1994.

165. Isch JA, Engum, SA, Ruble CA, et al: Patch esophagoplasty using AlloDerm as a tissue scaffold. J Pediatr Surg 36:266–268, 2001.

166. Bonnard A, Auber F, Fourcade L, et al: Vascular ring abnormalities: A retrospective study of 62 cases. J Pediatr Surg 38:539–543, 2003.

167. Murdison KA, Andrews BA, Chin AJ: Ultrasonographic display of complex vascular rings. J Am Coll Cardiol 15:1645–1653, 1990.

168. Cherin MM, Pond GD, Bjelland JC, et al: Evaluation of double aortic arch and aortic coarctation by intravenous digital subtraction angiography. J Cardiovasc Surg 28:581–584, 1987.

169. Kastler B, Livolsi A, Germain P, et al: Magnetic resonance imaging in congenital heart disease of newborns: Preliminary results in 23 patients. Eur J Radiol 10:109–117, 1990.

170. van Son JAM, Julsrud PR, Hagler DJ, et al: Imaging strategies for vascular rings. Soc Thorac Surg 57:604–610, 1994.

171. Backer CL, Ilbawi MN, Idriss FS, et al: Vascular anomalies causing tracheoesophageal compression: Review of experience in children. J Thorac Cardiovasc Surg 97:725–731, 1989.

172. Roberts CS, Othersen HB, Sade RM, et al: Tracheoesophageal compression from aortic arch anomalies: Analysis of 30 operatively treated children. J Pediatr Surg 29:334–338, 1994.

173. Burke RP, Rosenfield HM, Wernovsky G, et al: Video-assisted thoracoscopic ring division in infants and children. J Am Coll Cardiol 25:943–947, 1995.

Esophageal Atresia and Tracheoesophageal Malformations

Lewis Spitz, PhD FRCS

The surgical correction of esophageal atresia is regarded as the epitome of neonatal surgical expertise. In 1950, Willis Potts wrote, "To anastomose the ends of an infant's esophagus, the surgeon must be as delicate and precise as a skilled watchmaker. No other operation offers a greater opportunity for pure technical artistry."[1] The evolution from a congenital abnormality incompatible with life to a condition with a survival rate of well over 90 % is remarkable. This transition has taken place over a period of only 60 years.

HISTORY[2,3]

The first recorded case of esophageal atresia was in 1670 by Durston,[4] who found a blind-ending upper esophagus in one of a pair of female thoracopagus conjoined twins. Credit, however, must be given to Thomas Gibson,[5] who, in 1697, documented the first classic description of esophageal atresia with distal fistula. He wrote as follows:

About November 1696, I was sent for to an infant that could not swallow. The child seem'd very desirous of food, and took what was offer'd it in a spoon with greediness; but when it went to swallow it, it was liked to be choaked, and what should have gone down returned by the mouth and nose, and it fell into a struggling convulsive sort of fit upon it.

Subsequent postmortem examination confirmed the diagnosis.

The next recorded case was almost 150 years later by Thomas Hill in 1840,[6] who "was called, in the night, to visit Dr. Webster's family." The newborn infant "made no effort to swallow but immediately convulsed ... and the drink which had been given returned by mouth and nose, mixed with bloody mucus." He recommended that "gently stimulating the rectum would remove the difficulty"; however, when an attempt was made to do so, there was "no vestige of an anus." By the next day, the "anxious parents, desiring that something might be done,"

he attempted to open into the rectum with an "incision about one inch long half way between the scrotum and coccygis." Hill was the first to document an associated anomaly with esophageal atresia and perhaps was the first to attempt to perform a posterior sagittal anorectoplasty.

Various single case reports followed, culminating in a thesis compiled by Harold Hirschsprung who, in 1862,[7] found a total of 10 recorded cases in the literature to which he added 4 personal cases. All 14 cases were esophageal atresia with distal tracheoesophageal fistula, and in one of the patients, a cartilaginous remnant was found in the distal esophagus.

Thomas Holmes[8] was the first to suggest the possibility of operative treatment in 1869, but he added, "the attempt ought not, I think, be made." By 1884, the number of reported cases had increased to 63. In 1888, Charles Steele[9] was the first to operate on an infant with esophageal atresia. After consultation one evening, he advised that "by day light the stomach should be opened and the oesophagus explored." If "a membrane could be made out across a continuous channel, that it should be perforated in order to give a hope of life." In the event, through a gastrotomy, the gap was found to be 1½ inches, and therefore no procedure was performed. In 1898, Hoffman performed the first gastrostomy.

In 1902, F. J. Steward[10] is reported to have operated on an infant with esophageal atresia at Great Ormond Street Hospital, London. The infant survived for 14 days, but no further details are available.

The different morphologic parts of the esophagus were noted by Keith in 1910,[11] the upper part being derived from the pharynx and having striated muscle fibers, whereas the lower part contains nonstriated muscle fibers derived from the primitive esophagus. These facts may be relevant when recommending elective paralysis to promote anastomotic healing after repair of esophageal atresia.

In 1913, Richter[12] proposed an operative plan consisting of ligation of the tracheoesophageal fistula and anastomosis of the two ends of the esophagus. Unfortunately, he did not encounter a suitable case in which to attempt the repair.

Lanman[13] was the first to perform an extrapleural repair in 1936. His patient lived for only 3 hours, and in 1940, he reported his experience with 30 operative cases, all of whom died. He stated that "with greater experience, improved technique and good luck," success would soon be reported.

The early successes with esophageal atresia are well documented, with Leven[14] and Ladd[15] in 1939 reporting the first survivors after staged repair, and Cameron Haight,[16] the first successful primary anastomosis in 1941. Haight reported on 15 cases of esophageal atresia, of whom 9 underwent thoracic exploration with 1 success. This infant girl was 12 days old on admission and had been transported over a distance of 500 miles to Ann Arbor, Michigan. The operation took place the day after admission and proceeded via a left thoracic extrapleural approach. The fistula was ligated and divided and an end-to-end anastomosis performed. Leakage at the site of the anastomosis occurred, and a gastrostomy was fashioned, which was used for feeding for 20 days. A subsequent anastomotic stricture required a single dilatation 17 months after the pioneering operation.

Thereafter improvement in survival was spectacular. Waterston and colleagues[17] reported a survival rate of 57.6% in 113 infants treated between 1951 and 1959. By the mid-1980s, mortality had fallen to less than 15% and, in some centers, success rates greater than 90% were being reported.

EMBRYOLOGY

Although the mechanisms that underlie tracheo-esophageal malformations are still a matter of debate, the development of reproducible animal models of these anomalies has allowed detailed analyses of the various stages of faulty organogenesis. By contrasting these stages with normal development, it has been possible to identify key developmental processes that may be disturbed during embryogenesis.

The mechanisms of normal tracheoesophageal development have not been clarified beyond doubt. It is generally accepted that the respiratory primordium appears as a ventral evagination on the floor of the postpharyngeal foregut at the beginning of the fourth week of gestation and that the primitive lung buds are located at the caudal end of this evagination.[18] During a period of rapid growth, the ventrally placed trachea becomes separated from the dorsally placed esophagus. According to one theory, the trachea becomes a separate organ as a result of rapid longitudinal growth of the respiratory primordium away from the foregut.[19,20] The alternative theory is that the trachea initially grows as part of an undivided foregut and then becomes a separate structure as a result of a separation process that starts at the level of the lung buds and proceeds in a cranial direction.[21,22] This process is associated with a precise temporospatial pattern of expression of the key developmental gene *Sonic hedgehog* (*Shh*) and members of its signaling cascade. A precise ventral-to-dorsal switch in foregut *Shh* expression is itself propagated cranially, ahead of

tracheoesophageal separation.[23] Furthermore, the separating foregut epithelium is marked by increased numbers of cells undergoing programmed cell death (apoptosis).[24] It is not clear how patterns of gene expression are translated into cell death.

Theories of abnormal organogenesis reflect the theories of normal development and are based largely on evidence from the doxorubicin (Adriamycin) rat model of esophageal atresia (EA) and tracheoesophageal fistula (TEF) and a more recently described mouse model.[19,23,25–32] Most studies suggest that the primary defect is the persistence of an undivided foregut, as a result of either failure of tracheal growth[23,27] or failure of the already specified trachea to separate physically from the esophagus.[32] According to both theories, the atresia of the proximal esophagus is not part of the primary malformation but rather a result of rearrangement of the proximal foregut. The failed-separation theory would link the embryology of EA/TEF to that of laryngotracheo-esophageal cleft, a much rarer form of tracheoesophageal malformations. An alternative theory suggests that atresia of the proximal esophagus is the primary event and that the malformation results secondarily from the establishment of continuity between the trachea and the stomach/distal esophagus (TEF).[29,30] The origin of the TEF also is in question. The failed-separation theory suggests it is gastrointestinal in origin, as it is essentially a continuation of the dorsal foregut, whereas the primary atresia theory suggests that it is respiratory, as it grows from the trachea to connect to the stomach. Both arguments are supported by rather conflicting expression data of the respiratory marker *Nkx2.1*.[31,32]

The development of genetic models of tracheo-esophageal malformations has provided an insight into the molecular mechanisms that underlie these defects. In the mouse, loss-of-function mutations of *Shh* and other members of its signaling pathway (*Gli2, Gli3, and Foxf1*) lead to tracheoesophageal malformations including EA/TEF.[33–35] In the case of the *Shh* mutant, failure of tracheoesophageal separation is the underlying abnormality. Interestingly, failure of tracheoesophageal separation in the Adriamycin models is associated with disturbance of the temporospatial pattern of *Shh* expression.[23,28]

INCIDENCE AND ETIOLOGY

Esophageal atresia is a relatively common congenital malformation occurring in about one in 2500 to 3000 live births. The etiology of the malformation is likely to be multifactorial and remains unknown. The overwhelming majority of cases of esophageal atresia are sporadic/nonsyndromic, although a small number within this nonfamilial group are associated with chromosomal abnormalities. Familial/syndromic cases of esophageal atresia are extremely rare, representing less than 1% of the total.

In the case of sporadic/nonsyndromic esophageal/tracheoesophageal atresia, the likely cause is an insult that occurs during the narrow gestational window of tracheoesophageal organogenesis. This is the basis of the

Adriamycin animal models and also is illustrated in the reported cases of human esophageal/tracheo-esophageal atresia that are associated with maternal intake of chemotherapeutic agents such as the thioamide methimazole.[36] The nature of the insult in the vast majority of sporadic cases remains ill defined and may be a nonspecific event such as a threatened abortion. Twin pregnancy also may disturb organogenesis, as EA is 2 to 3 times more common in twins.[37] Genetic susceptibility also could be involved, as illustrated by the few reported cases of nonsyndromic EA/TEF occurring in multiple members of the same family.[38–40] The overall risk of nonsyndromic EA/TEF in a sibling of an affected child is about 1%.

The presence of associated malformations in other organ systems could provide clues as to the possible etiology of EA/TEF. Such malformations are present in about 50% of cases of EA/TEF and can occur in distinct patterns.[41] These are described as nonrandom associations rather than syndromes because the presence of anomalies in one system makes it more likely that defects exist in another. One of the best-described nonrandom associations is the VACTERL association which consists of *v*ertebral, *a*norectal, *c*ardiac, *t*racheo-*e*sophageal, *r*enal, and *l*imb abnormalities. The pattern of these nonrandom associations is likely to be dictated by the timing of a possible insult that affects multiple morphogenetic events. In the rat model, doxorubicin exposure affects a number of systems, broadly consistent with the VACTERL association.[42] The insult could act by transiently disturbing a specific developmental signaling pathway. In the mouse, loss-of-function mutations for genes of the *Shh* pathway lead to a spectrum of anomalies that is very similar to those of VACTERL, implicating the pathway in the embryogenesis of the malformations.[43] In the human, the evidence is less conclusive, with the *Shh* mutation leading to holoprosencephaly, a malformation not associated with EA/TEF.[44] TEF and other features of VACTERL have, however, been described in patients with a mutation for *GL13*.[45]

Chromosomal abnormalities such as trisomy (18 and 21)[46] and deletions (22q11 and 17q22q23.3)[47,48] are known to be associated with EA/TEF and have been reported in up to 6% of patients who have associated malformations in other systems.[49] The presence of many of the features of the nonrandom associations described earlier in cases of chromosomal deletions (e.g., 22q11) has led to the study of all chromosomal aberrations in search of a genetic region that is likely to be involved in EA/TEF susceptibility. No such region has been identified to be linked to chromosomal abnormalities.[50]

Familial/syndromic EA/TEF is very rare. A well-studied example is Feingold syndrome (oculodigitoesophagoduodenal syndrome), which is a rare autosomal dominant disorder that includes esophageal atresia.[51,52] Studies of affected families have localized the defect to chromosome 2 (2p23-p24) and have shown that haploinsufficiency of a gene or genes in that region is associated with syndromic EA/TEF.[53] Further characterization of the genes involved could contribute to the study of the molecular basis of EA/TEF.

CLASSIFICATION

Various classification systems have been used to describe the anatomic types of EA. The original classification was devised by Vogt in 1929[54] and is still used today in certain countries. Ladd (1944)[19] and Gross (1953)[55] modified the classification, whereas Lambrecht and Kluth (1976)[56] published an extensive *Atlas of Esophageal Atresia*, which comprised 10 major types, each with numerous subtypes, based on the original Vogt classification. It is more valuable and understandable to describe the anatomic anomaly rather than to assign a label that may not be instantly recognizable to a large proportion of the specialty.

- Esophageal atresia with distal tracheoesophageal fistula (EA/TEF) (86%, Vogt IIIb, Gross C) (Fig. 26-1). This is the most common variety, in which the proximal esophagus, with a dilated, thickened muscular wall, ends blindly in the superior mediastinum at about the level of the third or fourth thoracic vertebra. The distal esophagus, which is thinner and narrower, enters the posterior wall of the trachea at the carina or, more commonly, 1 to 2 cm above the carina. The distance between the blind proximal esophagus and the distal TEF varies from overlapping to a wide gap that presents a challenge in the repair of the anomaly. Very rarely, the distal fistula may be occluded or obliterated, leading to the initial impression of an isolated atresia (Kluth type 14b[7,8]).
- Isolated EA without TEF (7%, Vogt II, Gross A) (Fig. 26-2). The proximal and distal esophagus end blindly without any connection to the trachea. The proximal esophageal segment is dilated and thick-walled and usually ends in the posterior mediastinum near the second thoracic vertebra. The distal esophagus is short and ends a variable distance above the diaphragm. The distance between the two ends will determine whether a primary repair is feasible (rarely) or a delayed primary anastomosis or esophageal replacement should be performed. It is important to exclude a proximal TEF in these cases.
- TEF without EA (isolated TEF) (4%, Gross E) (Fig. 26-3). A fistulous connection between an anatomically intact esophagus and trachea. The fistulous tract may be very narrow or may be 3 to 5 mm in diameter. An isolated TEF is commonly located in the lower cervical region. They are usually single, but two and even three fistulas have been described.
- EA with proximal TEF (2%, Vogt IIIa, and Gross B) (Fig. 26-4). This rare anomaly must be distinguished from the isolated variety. The fistula is not at the distal end of the upper pouch but is usually located 1 to 2 cm proximal on the anterior wall of the esophagus.
- EA with proximal and distal TEFs (<1%, Vogt IIIc, Gross D) (Fig. 26-5). In many of these infants, the anomaly was diagnosed and managed as a case of proximal atresia and distal fistula. As a result of recurrent respiratory infections, investigations will

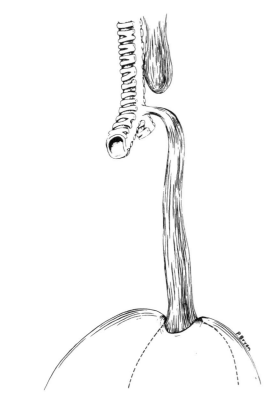

FIGURE 26-1. Esophageal atresia with distal tracheo-esophageal fistula.

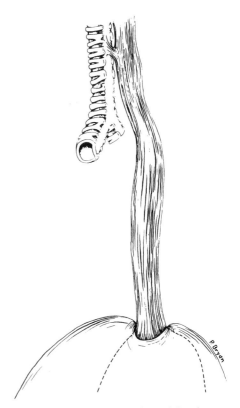

FIGURE 26-3. H-type tracheoesophageal fistula.

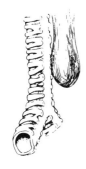

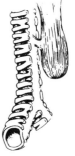

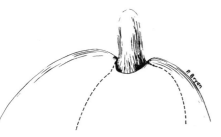

FIGURE 26-2. Pure esophageal atresia (without a tracheo-esophageal fistula).

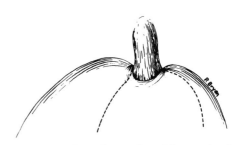

FIGURE 26-4. Esophageal atresia with proximal tracheo-esophageal fistula.

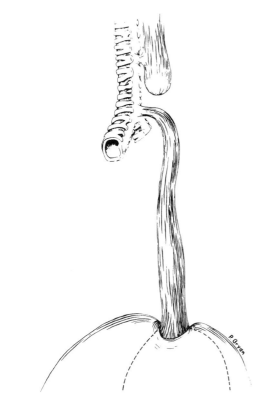

FIGURE 26-5. Esophageal atresia with proximal and distal tracheoesophageal fistulas. Note that the proximal fistula usually enters the trachea 1 to 2 cm above the blind-ending upper pouch.

reveal a TEF in the upper esophageal segment. These have often been misdiagnosed as a recurrent fistula but are located above the original, more distal fistula site. With the increasing use of preoperative endoscopy (bronchoscopy and/or esophagoscopy), recognition of the "double" fistula occurs, and complete repair performed at the initial procedure. If the proximal fistula is not diagnosed preoperatively, the diagnosis may be suspected by a large anesthetic gas leak occurring from the upper pouch while the anastomosis is being performed.

PATHOPHYSIOLOGY

The motility of the esophagus is always affected in EA. The disordered peristalsis more commonly involves the distal esophageal segment and is present even in isolated TEF without atresia. It remains to be determined whether the motility disorder is primarily due to abnormal innervation of the esophagus, as shown by the abnormality in neuropeptide distribution in the doxorubicin-induced EA in rats[57-60] and in preoperative manometric studies,[61] or secondary to vagal nerve damage occurring during the surgical repair.[61-63] Manometric studies carried out on patients with repaired EA show abnormal peristalsis in the mid and lower esophagus in the majority of cases. The resting pressure in the whole esophagus is significantly higher than that in normal patients. Closing pressure of the lower esophageal sphincter is reduced in EA.

The trachea also is abnormal in EA. The abnormality consists of an absolute deficiency of tracheal cartilage and an increase in the length of the transverse muscle in the posterior tracheal wall.[64] When severe, these abnormalities result in tracheomalacia, with collapse of the trachea during expiration, resulting in a slit-like tracheal lumen in an isolated, 1- to 2-cm segment at or around the fistula site.

DIAGNOSIS

The diagnosis of EA may be suspected prenatally by the finding of a small or absent fetal stomach bubble on ultrasonography (US) performed after the 18th week of gestation. Overall the sensitivity of prenatal US is 42%, but the combination of polyhydramnios with an absent stomach bubble increases the positive predictive value to 56%.[65] Polyhydramnios alone is an unreliable indication of EA. Available methods of improving the prenatal diagnostic rate include US examination of the fetal neck to reveal the blind-ending upper pouch[66] and magnetic resonance imaging.[67]

The newborn infant of a mother with polyhydramnios should have a nasogastric tube passed soon after delivery to exclude EA. Infants with EA are unable to swallow saliva and are noted to have "excessive" salivation, requiring repeated suctioning. At this stage, and certainly before the first feeding, a stiff wide-bore (10 to 12F) catheter should be passed through the mouth into the esophagus. In the child with EA, the catheter will not pass beyond 9 to 10 cm from the lower alveolar ridge. A plain roentgenogram of the chest and abdomen will show the tip of the catheter arrested in the superior mediastinum (T2 to 4), whereas gas in the gastrointestinal tract signifies the presence of a distal TEF (Fig. 26-6). The rigidity of the catheter is important because a fine-bore catheter may curl in the upper pouch, giving the false impression of an intact esophagus[68] (Fig. 26-7). Rarely a fine catheter may pass into the trachea and then descend into the distal esophagus through the fistula. The radiograph also may reveal additional anomalies such as the "double bubble" appearance of duodenal atresia or vertebral or rib abnormalities.

ASSOCIATED ANOMALIES

More than 50% of infants with EA have one or more additional anomalies.[69-72] The systems affected are as follows:

Cardiovascular	29%
Anorectal anomalies	14%
Genitourinary	14%
Gastrointestinal	13%
Vertebral/skeletal	10%
Respiratory	6%
Genetic	4%
Other	11%

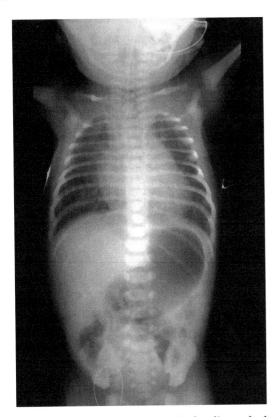

FIGURE 26-6. Plain chest and abdominal radiograph showing esophageal atresia with distal tracheoesophageal fistula. A firm 10F radio-opaque catheter has been passed; the tip of the catheter has reached the bottom of the proximal pouch. Air in the stomach, duodenum, and small intestine is indicative of a distal tracheoesophageal fistula.

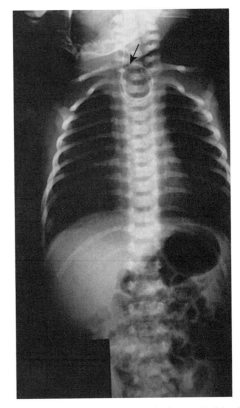

FIGURE 26-7. A fine-bore feeding tube has coiled in the upper esophageal pouch.

An increased incidence of associated anomalies occurs in pure atresia (65%), and a lower incidence, in H-type fistula (10%).

The VATER association, first described in 1973,[73] consists of a combination of anomalies including vertebral, anorectal, tracheoesophageal, and renal or radial abnormalities. This association was later expanded as the VACTERL association to include cardiac and limb defects.[74]

Other associations that may include EA are the CHARGE association (coloboma, heart defects, atresia choanae, retarded growth and development, genital hypoplasia, and ear deformities), Potter's syndrome (renal agenesis, pulmonary hypoplasia, typical dysmorphic facies), and Schisis association (omphalocele, cleft lip and/or palate, genital hypoplasia).[75] In a series of 61 patients with CHARGE association, 10 had EA + TEF. All had major cardiac defects, and 7 had major skeletal anomalies. Most of these infants had complicated postoperative courses, and 7 of the 10 died.[76] Genetic defects associated with EA include trisomy 21 and 18, and 13q deletion. Of the cardiac anomalies, the most common are ventricular septal defect and tetralogy of Fallot. Major cardiac malformations are among the main causes of mortality in infants with EA.[72,77]

The vertebral anomalies in EA are confined mainly to the thoracic region and are responsible for later development of scoliosis. The claim that the possession of 13 ribs is associated with long-gap atresia has not been substantiated.[78] Of the gastrointestinal anomalies, the most frequently encountered are duodenal atresia and malrotation, and, in addition, there is an increased incidence of pyloric stenosis found. Miscellaneous anomalies include cleft lip and palate, omphalocele, lung abnormalities, choanal atresia, and hypospadias.

MANAGEMENT

Preoperative

Once the diagnosis of esophageal atresia has been established, the infant will need to be transferred from the place of birth to a pediatric surgical center. A suction catheter, preferably of the 10F double-lumen sump type, is placed in the upper esophageal pouch to remove secretions and prevent aspiration from occurring during transfer. The infant is placed on its side in the portable incubator while the usual vital signs are monitored. Vascular access should be provided as a precautionary measure, but intravenous fluid administration is not usually necessary if the infant's condition has been diagnosed within a short period after birth and transfer is carried out within the first day of life.

The preterm infant with respiratory distress requires special attention. Clearly endotracheal intubation and mechanical ventilation are needed. In addition, the added risk of gastric overdistention due to decreased pulmonary compliance and the easy passage of respiratory gases through the distal fistula into the stomach requires monitoring. This sequence of events can be minimized by positioning the end of the endotracheal tube distal to the TEF and by applying gentle low-pressure ventilation techniques.

On arrival at the neonatal surgical center, the diagnosis of EA must be confirmed.

All infants with EA should have an echocardiogram (ECHO) before operative repair. The ECHO will define any structural anomaly of the heart or great blood vessels and occasionally may define a right-sided aortic arch that occurs in up to 2.5% of cases.[79–81] When that is suspected, a magnetic resonance imaging study is the method of choice for accurate confirmation of the diagnosis of the right aortic arch, which, in turn, will determine the approach for the operative repair. In many patients with tetralogy of Fallot, the aortic arch will be on the right side. The infant with a cyanotic congenital cardiac anomaly will need to undergo a shunting procedure before correction of the EA.[82] For example, in complicated tetralogy of Fallot, a Blalock-Taussig systemic-to-pulmonary artery shunt will alleviate the cyanotic attacks and permit safe repair of the EA a day or two later. Some associated congenital heart defects will produce congestive cardiac failure that will require medical management before repair of the esophageal anomaly.

Risk Categorization

In 1962, David Waterston[17] proposed a classification of infants born with EA into three groups "with different chances of survival." The classification is based on birth weight, associated anomalies, and pneumonia:

Group A	More than 5½ lb birth weight and well
Group B	1. Birth weight 4 to 5½ lb and well
	2. Higher birthweight, moderate pneumonia, and congenital anomaly
Group C	1. Birth weight less than 4 lb
	2. Higher birth weight, severe pneumonia, and severe congenital anomaly

This classification was applied to 113 cases treated at Great Ormond Street Hospital from 1951 to 1959. Of 38 infants in group A, 36 (95%) survived; of 43 in group B, 29 (68%) survived; whereas only 2 (6%) of the 32 in group C survived. During the subsequent 40 years, a steady improvement in the overall survival rate has occurred because of early diagnosis and prompt referral, improvements in preoperative care and diagnosis and treatment of associated anomalies, advances in anesthetic techniques, and sophisticated neonatal intensive care. Applying the Waterston classification to a series of 357 infants with EA treated at Great Ormond Street from 1980 to 1992, the results were as follows: group A, 153 (99%) of 154 survived; 72 (95%) of 76 in group B survived; and 101 (71%) of 142 in group C survived. It became obvious that a new risk-classification system, more relevant to the modern era, was needed. The new risk classification concerned birth weight and associated cardiac malformations that were previously identified as being responsible for most of the mortality.

Our revised classification[83] for survival in esophageal atresia is

Group I	Birth weight more than 1500 g *with no* major cardiac anomaly
Group II	Birth weight less than 1500 g *or* major cardiac anomaly
Group III	Birth weight less than 1500 g *PLUS* major cardiac anomaly

Major cardiac anomaly was defined as either cyanotic congenital heart disease that required palliative or corrective surgery or noncyanotic heart anomaly that required medical or surgical treatment for cardiac failure. With the new risk-classification scheme, survival was 97% in group I, 59% for group II, and 22% for group III. Two recent studies confirmed the value of this new risk classification in assessing the prognosis of infants born with EA.[84,85] A study from Montreal identified only preoperative ventilator dependence and severe associated anomalies as having prognostic significance.[86]

Selection for Nontreatment

Parents of infants with Potter's syndrome (bilateral renal agenesis) and trisomy 18, which is fatal in the first year of life in more than 90% of affected infants, should be offered the option of no treatment, allowing the infant to die. Similarly, infants with totally uncorrectable major cardiac defects or with grade IV intraventricular hemorrhage should be considered for nonoperative management as well.

Emergency Ligation of the Distal Tracheoesophageal Fistula

Generally, the operative correction of an EA is *not* regarded as an emergency procedure. The one compelling exception is the preterm infant with severe respiratory distress syndrome requiring high-pressure ventilatory support. The problem is that a majority of the respiratory gases escape through the distal fistula into the stomach, where overdistention further impedes respiratory activity. The stomach may rupture, causing a tension pneumoperitoneum, which, in turn, renders ventilatory support even more difficult (Figs. 26-8, 26-9, and 26-10).[87,88]

The traditional method of dealing with this sequence of events was to perform an emergency gastrostomy.[89,90] Unfortunately, most of these infants died, because the only problem this procedure solved was the potential gastric rupture. Attempts to alleviate the problem of inadequate ventilation, including positioning of the endotracheal tube tip distal to the fistula,[91,92] sometimes failed because of the proximity of the fistula to the carina. Others advocated blocking the fistula by using a partially inflated Fogarty catheter passed into the fistula at bronchoscopy.[93] These infants are usually preterm and in critical condition. The smallest-caliber bronchoscope will not permit ventilation with simultaneous manipulation of a Fogarty catheter into the fistula.

Since 1984, we have advocated emergency transpleural ligation of the TEF as the procedure of choice in the

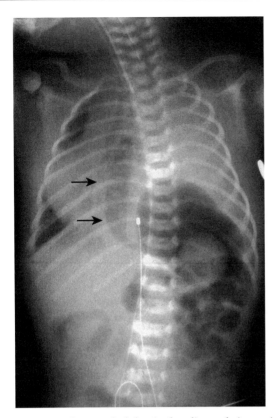

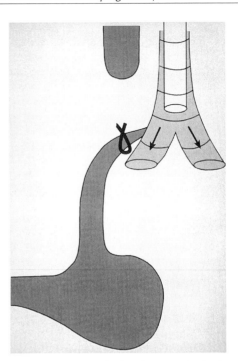

FIGURE 26-10. Ligation of the fistula in continuity in an infant with esophageal atresia and distal tracheoesophageal fistula and severe respiratory distress. Ventilatory gases are now directed toward the lungs only.

FIGURE 26-8. Chest and abdominal radiograph in an infant with esophageal atresia, distal fistula, and severe respiratory distress. The distal esophagus is very distended with air, and the stomach is dilated.

infants with this dilemma.[94–96] Occasionally a dramatic improvement in respiratory status is sufficient to allow primary repair of the EA at the time. In the majority of cases, ligation of the fistula improves the respiratory status, and the repair of the esophageal anomaly is undertaken 8 to 10 days later. A risk of recurrent fistulization exists after in-continuity ligation if a prolonged delay in repair occurs.

Operative Approach

The operation is performed under general endotracheal anesthesia with dependable vascular access. Gentle ventilatory pressure is used to prevent excess gastric distention (see Chapter 27 for a description of the thoracoscopic approach).

1. *Intraoperative endoscopy:* Preliminary bronchoscopy is carried out by many surgeons to define the site of entry of the distal TEF, as well as to assess the degree of tracheomalacia.[97,98] The fistula may enter the trachea at the level of the carina, and this may indicate a wide-gap atresia, or it may enter at the cervical level, in which case, a high thoracotomy would be an advantage. Others have relied on esophagoscopy to define the length of the upper esophagus and to exclude an upper pouch fistula, which occurs more commonly in isolated EA.
2. *Position:* The infant is placed on his or her side of the aortic arch with the arm extended above the head to lie over the ear.

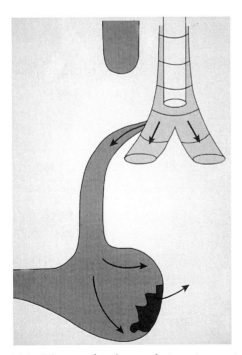

FIGURE 26-9. Diagram showing respiratory gases entering the distal esophagus via the tracheoesophageal fistula, causing gastric distention and eventually rupture of the greater curvature of the stomach. The gastric rupture results in a tension pneumoperitoneum, which adversely affects ventilation and oxygenation.

3. *Incision:* A curved incision approximately 5 to 6 cm long is made 1 cm below the scapula. The muscle of the chest wall may be either split or divided with electrocautery. In the latter case, the division of the serratus muscles should be as low as possible to preserve the long thoracic nerve. The chest is opened through the fourth or fifth intercostal space by dividing the intercostal muscles or by entry through the bed of the resected rib.

4. *Extrapleural approach:* This technique has the advantage of protecting the pleural space in the event of an anastomotic leak. Commencing posteriorly, the pleura is gently freed from endothoracic fascia by using blunt dissection. The dissection proceeds posteriorly, dissecting the pleura off the vertebral bodies, allowing access to the mediastinum. The extrapleural approach is slightly more time consuming but has theoretical advantages over the transpleural approach and is used by many surgeons.

5. *Exposure of the esophageal segments:* The azygos vein is the first structure encountered in the mediastinum (Fig. 26-11). The azygos vein is gently mobilized and divided between ligatures to expose the esophagus. The distal esophagus usually lies adjacent to the azygos vein and is identified by the vagus nerve coursing over its lateral aspect. The distal esophagus can be seen to distend with each inspiration, but it is advisable to compress the lumen of the distal esophagus gently while the anesthetist applies increased respiratory pressure. This maneuver ensures that the structure being compressed is not the right main bronchus. The blind upper esophageal pouch is identified high up in the mediastinum, aided by the anesthetist applying pressure on an oro- or nasoesophageal tube.

6. *Repair of the anomaly:* The distal esophagus is mobilized circumferentially just distal to the TEF, and a soft rubber sling is placed around it (Fig. 26-12). Traction on this sling will reduce the air leak into the distal esophagus. A marking seromuscular suture is placed in the lateral wall of the distal esophagus to maintain orientation. The distal esophagus is dissected to the level of the fistula, where the upper and lower extent of the fistula is marked with 5-0 polypropylene traction sutures. The fistula is divided so that its closure will not compromise the tracheal lumen. The tracheal side of the fistula is closed with interrupted 5-0 permanent sutures to achieve an airtight closure. The tracheal closure should be tested by instilling warm saline over the suture line while the anesthesiologist applies up to 30 cm of airway pressure.

Attention is turned to the tip of the proximal esophageal pouch, where a figure-of-eight traction suture is placed to aid in its mobilization. The proximal esophagus should be mobilized as much as necessary to produce a tension-free anastomosis. Laterally and posteriorly, the mobilization is usually accomplished by blunt dissection, but medially, fibrous adhesions to the trachea require sharp dissection. It is important to remain close to the

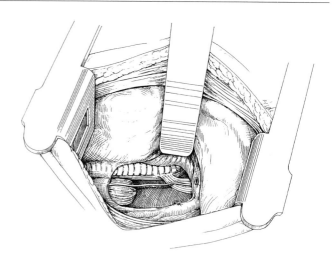

FIGURE 26-11. Extrapleural approach to esophageal atresia with tracheoesophageal fistula. The dissection follows the curve of the ribs to the mediastinum. The azygos vein is reflected anteriorly with the pleura after dividing the two highest intercostal veins as they enter the azygos. The vagus nerve is identified as it runs along the right side of both the proximal and distal esophageal segments. (From Holder TM, Manning PB: Esophageal atresia and tracheoesophageal fistula. Surg Rounds 14:492–502, 1991.)

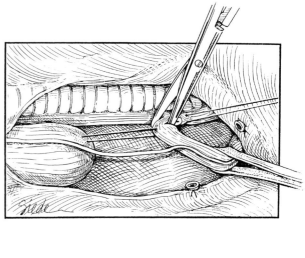

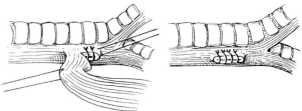

FIGURE 26-12. The distal esophagus is identified, looped, and carefully dissected up to its junction with the trachea, meticulously sparing the segmental vessels from the aorta. Traction sutures may be placed for gentle handling of the segments. The fistula is divided close to the trachea without narrowing its lumen. The tracheal end of the tracheoesophageal fistula is closed with continuous or interrupted sutures. Adjacent tissue, if available, is tacked over the closure. (From Holder TM, Manning PB: Esophageal atresia and tracheoesophageal fistula. Surg Rounds 14:492–502, 1991.)

esophageal wall and to avoid entering the membranous trachea during the mobilization. The end of the upper pouch is now opened to expose the mucosal surface.

The anastomosis between the proximal and distal esophagus should be end-to-end and fashioned with interrupted, full-thickness fine sutures (5-0 or 6-0) of either permanent or absorbable material. It is important to include the mucosa of the esophageal wall with each suture. The posterior half of the anastomosis is completed first, with sutures knotted on the mucosal surface (Fig. 26-13). If a wide gap appears, the distal esophagus can be mobilized safely well down toward the diaphragm. When tension exists on the anastomosis, all the posterior sutures should be placed before tying so that the manipulation required to place sutures does not produce unnecessary stress on the anastomosis. The sutures are then tied sequentially while the assistant supports the esophageal ends. It is almost always possible to anastomose the esophagus when a distal fistula is present. The anterior half of the anastomosis is completed with interrupted full-thickness sutures tied on the outside of the esophagus. Just before the final closure, a transanastomotic, fine-caliber nasogastric feeding tube may be passed. This provides gastric decompression and allows early feeding to take place directly into the stomach.

7. *Methods to overcome a wide gap:* Various maneuvers have been proposed to overcome a wide gap, but, in our experience, a very tense anastomosis can be achieved safely if the infant is paralyzed and ventilated postoperatively for 5 days. Very often the anastomosis will heal without leakage. Others have proposed tubularization of an upper pouch flap, circular myotomy of the upper pouch, or delayed primary anastomosis 6 to 12 weeks later.

8. *The thoracotomy incision* is now closed. If the procedure has been extrapleural and a technically satisfactory anastomosis has been performed, we prefer not to leave a drainage catheter.

Management of Isolated Esophageal Atresia

The sine qua non of isolated EA is the "gasless abdomen" (Fig. 26-14). A remote possibility exists that an occluded distal fistula will be found.[68,99] We believe that preoperative bronchoscopy should always be performed in the case of suspected isolated atresia. Evidence of either a proximal or distal fistula may be identified. The overall incidence of upper pouch fistula in EA is around 2.5%, but, in isolated EA, this occurrence is 3 to 4 times more likely.[80] In a series of 170 EA/TEF patients, 13 (7.7%) had a proximal fistula. This is much higher than generally reported.[100]

Once the existence of either a proximal or distal fistula is excluded, the next step is to perform a feeding gastrostomy and to estimate the extent of the gap between the proximal and distal esophagus. The stomach in isolated atresia is often very small and may accommodate only the

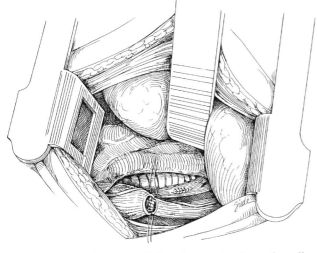

FIGURE 26-13. After mobilizing the proximal pouch well up into the thoracic inlet, the distal tip is incised, and a meticulous mucosal-to-mucosal anastomosis accomplished with a single layer of interrupted silk or long-lasting absorbable sutures. The mucosa of the proximal segment may retract and be missed if not sought for with each suture. A absorbable silicone (Silastic) stent may be left to bridge the anastomosis. A 10F neonatal chest tube is left in the retropleural space as a drain. (From Holder TM, Manning PB: Esophageal atresia and tracheoesophageal fistula. Surg Rounds 14:492–502, 1991.)

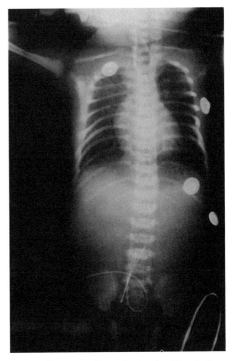

FIGURE 26-14. Pure esophageal atresia. No air is seen in the stomach or bowel. This radiographic picture also is seen in infants with esophageal atresia and a proximal tracheoesophageal fistula and in infants with a distal fistula that is plugged with mucus or is "ligamentous."

gastrostomy tube. It may not be possible to bring the stomach up to the peritoneal surface. To avoid tension and risk of necrosis of the stomach, it is preferable to leave the stomach in its native position and to allow the gastrostomy tube to traverse the peritoneal cavity. Intraoperative estimation of the gap between the esophageal ends can be done by introducing radio-opaque contrast into the stomach and distal esophagus while gently occluding the pylorus, or it may be possible to pass a metal sound through the gastrostomy site into the distal esophagus. With a radio-opaque catheter in the proximal esophagus, it is possible to measure, in terms of vertebral body heights, the gap between the two ends. A number of surgical options are possible (Table 26-1).[101-129] When the gap is less than two vertebrae, an attempt at immediate primary anastomosis should be made under extreme tension. For a gap of three to six vertebrae, delayed primary repair should be planned. Over a period of 10 to 12 weeks, while we maintain suction to the upper pouch and feed by gastrostomy, the gap gradually narrows. Regular monitoring of the gap by using metal sounds in the distal esophagus is undertaken only after the gastrostomy is matured enough to withstand removal of the tube and manipulation of the bougie. When the two esophageal ends can be approximated or overlapped, delayed primary anastomosis is undertaken (Fig. 27-15). The procedure is exactly as for regular EA/TEF but, to facilitate identification of the distal esophageal pouch, it is advantageous to have a sound or catheter in place before opening the chest (Fig. 27-16).[130,131]

When the gap between the two ends is greater than six vertebrae, the options are to proceed as described earlier and attempt delayed primary repair, or to perform a cervical esophagostomy and plan esophageal replacement at a later date. Reports have been made of successful repair

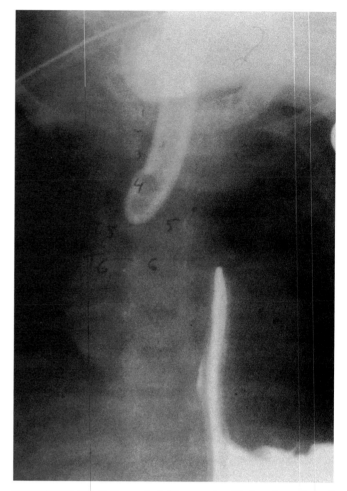

FIGURE 26-15. Before scheduling repair of isolated esophageal atresia, it is helpful to gauge the distance between the two esophageal segments with a red rubber catheter in the upper pouch and a smaller one in the lower esophagus (which was introduced through the gastrostomy). The gap in this patient was 1 to 1.5 vertebral bodies.

by using graduated tension on the esophageal ends over a period of 6 to 10 days.[132-134]

Postoperative Management

If the esophageal anastomosis has been performed under tension, the infant is electively paralyzed and mechanically ventilated for 5 postoperative days. In our experience with this regimen, no major disruptions occurred and only a few minor leaks healed spontaneously. The incidence of significant gastroesophageal reflux (GER) and the subsequent need for an antireflux procedure is much higher after anastomosis under tension.[134] In all other instances, regular pharyngeal toilet is necessary for the first few postoperative days. The suction catheter should be clearly marked to prevent the tube being passed to the depth of the anastomosis and causing damage. Transanastomotic nasogastric feeds may be commenced on the second or third postoperative day. When the infant is swallowing saliva, oral feeds may be started.

TABLE 26-1
OPERATIVE MANEUVERS IN LONG-GAP ESOPHAGEAL ATRESIA

I At the Initial Procedure
1. Anastomosis under tension[101-103]
2. Tension-relieving procedures[104-107]
3. Flap technique[108,109]
4. Suture fistula[110-112]

II Delayed Primary Anastomosis
1. With bougienage: proximal,[113,114] proximal and distal,[115] magnetic[116]
2. Without bougienage[117]
3. Esophageal lengthening techniques (e.g., flap,[108,109] myotomy,[118,119] gastric division[120])

III Transmediastinal "Thread"
1. With and without "olives"[110,121]
2. Kato technique[122]

IV Esophageal Replacement
1. Colonic interposition[123,124]
2. Gastric tube[125,126]
3. Jejunum[127]
4. Gastric transposition[128,129]

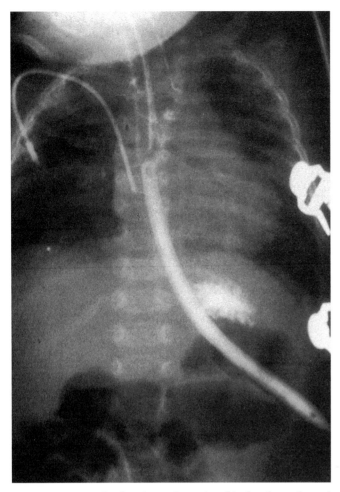

FIGURE 26-16. At the time of repair of isolated esophageal atresia, it is helpful to insert a red rubber catheter through the gastrostomy and into the lower esophagus. This maneuver greatly facilitates identification of the collapsed distal esophagus. (Reprinted with permission from Holcomb GW III: Identification of the distal esophageal segment during delayed repair of esophageal atresia and tracheoesophageal fistula. Surg Gynecol Obstet 174:323–324, 1992.)

Others have elected not to pass transanastomotic tubes and to feed the infant per mouth as early as the second postoperative day.[135]

We do not regularly perform a follow-up contrast study, but, if there is any doubt as to the integrity of the anastomosis, a water-soluble contrast study is carried out.

Complications

The early complications are anastomotic leak, anastomotic stricture and recurrent TEF. The late complications are GER, tracheomalacia, and esophageal dysmotility.

Anastomotic leaks occur in 15% to 20% of patients, but only one-third of these have a major disruption.[136] Major leaks occur in the early postoperative period (< 48 hours) and present with life-threatening

tension pneumothorax.[137,138] Emergency treatment consists of tube thoracostomy. Suction is applied to the intercostal drain while awaiting healing or stricture of the anastomosis. Immediate reoperation may be elected, with the intention of repairing the anastomosis. If the tissues do not appear to be amenable to reclosure, the creation of a cervical esophagostomy from the upper pouch and suture closure of the distal esophagus can be performed. Esophageal replacement is then accomplished at the appropriate age.

Minor leaks are often detected on the "routine" contrast study performed on the postoperative day 5 to 7.[139] Minor leaks, by definition, drain spontaneously into the lumen of the esophagus and do not require insertion or continuation of intercostal drainage.[140]

Anastomotic strictures[139,141,142] develop in 30% to 40% of cases, most of which will respond to one or two dilatations. Risk factors that have been implicated in stricture formation include anastomotic tension,[143] anastomotic leakage, and GER.[141] With meticulous handling of the esophageal ends, preservation of the blood supply, along with careful inclusion of mucosa in each and every suture of the anastomosis, strictures can be kept to a minimum.

Endoscopic dilatation of the stricture can be accomplished either with rigid esophagoscopy and semirigid bougies or with balloon dilatation introduced either at fluoroscopy or during flexible endoscopy. In either event, the balloon is carefully positioned with the stricture at its center, and contrast is gradually instilled under pressure until the "waisting" of the stricture is abolished. At the end of the procedure, a contrast esophagram should be done to ensure the integrity of the esophagus and to establish the effectiveness of the dilatation.[144,145]

Only rarely is it necessary to resort to resection of an intractable anastomotic stricture.

Recurrent Tracheoesophageal Fistula

The incidence of recurrent TEF is reported to be between 5% and 14%.[146–152] A recurrent fistula should be suspected if the infant manifests respiratory symptoms (coughing during feeds, apneic or cyanotic episodes) or has recurrent respiratory infections after "successful" repair of the EA. Urgent investigations must be undertaken to establish or exclude a recurrent fistula.

The diagnosis may be suspected on the plain chest radiograph that shows an air esophagogram. Routine contrast esophagogram has a low yield, and the most useful investigation is a video-esophagogram with the patient in the prone position. The study is begun with the catheter in the stomach, and it is slowly withdrawn as water-soluble contrast is slowly instilled (Fig. 26-17).

Bronchoscopic examination will reveal the recurrent fistula at the site of the original TEF. It is essential to pass a fine ureteral catheter across the fistula into the esophagus and to confirm the catheter to be in the esophageal lumen at esophagoscopy.[153] The passage of a catheter across the fistula also is an essential preliminary step in the operative correction of the recurrent fistula. At operation, it is useful to surround the esophagus above and

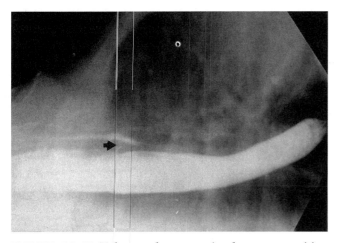

FIGURE 26-17. Tube esophagogram in the prone position showing water-soluble contrast filling the esophagus and a fine trickle of contrast (*arrow*) passing anteriorly through the recurrent tracheoesophageal fistula into the trachea.

below the site of the fistula and to insert stay sutures near the fistula before it is divided. The defects resulting from division of the recurrent fistula are closed with nonabsorbable, interrupted full-thickness sutures. If available, mediastinal pleura or a pericardial flap is interposed between the two suture lines.

Other approaches to recurrent fistula include laser ablation[154] or endoscopic application of fibrin sealant,[155,156] but the recurrence rate after these procedures is unacceptably high.[157,158]

Gastroesophageal Reflux

Significant GER occurs in 40% of infants after repair of EA, about half of whom will require surgical management.[142,159–162] GER is more common after anastomosis under tension,[163,164] after gastrostomy,[165,166] and after delayed primary repair.[140,167,168] It has been implicated in the pathogenesis of anastomotic stricture. However, reflux can still occur after an uncomplicated, tension-free anastomosis in which the distal esophagus has remained virtually undisturbed. Incompetence of the lower esophageal sphincter mechanism may be due to a primary neuromuscular disturbance inherent in the development of the EA or to technical factors involved in the repair. Tension may result in shortening of the intra-abdominal esophagus and/or abolishment of the angle of His.

Symptoms of GER may resemble those of recurrent fistula with acute or chronic respiratory problems but also may include recurrent vomiting and stricture formation. The diagnosis can be established on contrast swallow, pH monitoring, and endoscopy with biopsy of the distal esophagus. Stricture formation at the anastomosis, which is resistant to repeated dilatations, often resolves spontaneously once the GER is corrected.

Antireflux medication including gastric acid suppression is only successful in about half the cases.

Surgical treatment is problematic given the inherent dysmotility present in the distal esophagus. The fundoplication to treat the GER may in itself produce a functional obstruction at the gastroesophageal junction. The failure rate of fundoplication carried out in the first three months of life is excessively high.[159,161,162,169,170] With regard to the nature of the wrap, there are advocates for partial wrap[161] as well as for a short, floppy wrap complete wrap.

Tracheomalacia

Tracheomalacia may be defined as a structural and functional weakness of the tracheal cartilage, resulting in partial or episodic complete respiratory obstruction.[171] The structural abnormality consists of softened cartilage in the tracheal rings and an increase in the length of the transverse muscle.[64] The result is that the airway collapses during expiration, producing expiratory stridor that varies through a spectrum from a hoarse barking type of cough to acute life-threatening episodes of cyanosis or apnea.[172] The incidence of tracheomalacia is about 10% of infants, half of whom will require surgical correction. The area of collapse seen at bronchoscopy is usually restricted to the trachea at the level of the entry of the distal TEF, but it can be more extensive (Fig. 26-18). It usually is seen within the first few months of life and generally coincides with a period of rapid weight gain. The diagnosis is made at bronchoscopy or video-bronchography.

If the respiratory obstruction is severe enough to present with acute life-threatening events, treatment must be carried out promptly, and certainly before the infant leaves the hospital.[173,174] The definitive treatment consists of aortopexy, in which the ascending and arch of the aorta

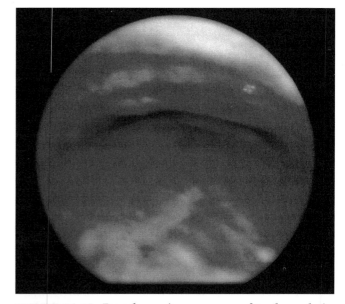

FIGURE 26-18. Bronchoscopic appearance of tracheomalacia, showing a slit-like lumen to the distal trachea.

are elevated anteriorly toward the sternum. Through a left anterolateral thoracotomy or a median sternotomy, the arch of the aorta is exposed, after excision of the lateral lobe of the thymus. Three sutures of nonabsorbable material are passed through the pericardial reflection at the aorta and the adventitia of the aortic arch and then through the sternum or the inner sternal periostium. The sutures are left untied until all three are in position, and then, as the assistant depresses the sternum, all the sutures are tied. On release of the sternum, the aortic arch is pulled forward, bringing with it the anterior wall of the trachea. The maneuver also allows space for the trachea to expand.[175,176] The result is usually dramatic, with immediate resolution of the obstruction to the air passages.[177] Tracheopexy through a cervical approach has been advocated as achieving similar success rates.[178]

Dysmotility

Children born with any of the forms of EA and TEF have dysmotility with abnormal coordination of contractions demonstrable on contrast studies of the esophagus.[179,180] The intrinsic innervation of the distal esophagus has been shown to be abnormal in the fetal rat model and affects both excitatory (SP-labeled) and inhibitory (VIP-labeled) intramural nerves.[57] The dysmotility is a major factor in the long-term swallowing problems encountered in these children. The patients are advised to take fluids liberally with meals and to avoid foods that exacerbate the problems—especially doughy white bread and cakes. Dysphagia was found in 65% of patients in all age groups in a series of 334 patients, but symptom severity decreased significantly with age. These children tend to be of normal height but subnormal weight.[181,182]

Respiratory Function

During infancy and for the first 3 years of life, patients with EA have increased frequency and duration of respiratory infections. The respiratory problems tend to lessen with time. The tendency to respiratory infections has variously been attributed to esophageal dysmotility and/or GER with recurrent aspiration or to a primary respiratory abnormality.[183] Squamous metaplasia has been found in the trachea or bronchi in 80% of infants dying in the postoperative period.[184] These findings suggested that the presence of nonciliated squamous epithelium could seriously impair the airway-clearing mechanisms and contribute to repeated attacks of bronchitis. Respiratory-function tests performed in infants soon after repair of the EA have shown abnormal patterns of air flow and also increased airway resistance.[185,186]

Congenital esophageal stenosis due to tracheo-bronchial remnants in the distal esophagus in an infant with EA is a rare but well-documented phenomenon[187,188] (see also Chapter 25). It can occur, less commonly, without associated atresia.[189,190] It is thought to arise as a result of defective separation of the trachea from the esophagus. It may be recognized at the time of the initial repair of the EA when passage of a catheter into the stomach is impeded. Alternatively, symptoms develop quite early,

with dysphagia and regurgitation of solid food. Contrast radiography shows a short well-defined narrowing in the distal esophagus, which must be differentiated from a reflux stricture. Balloon dilatation confirms the short defined narrowing, which fails to distend on inflation of the balloon.[191] Endoscopy reveals normal mucosa to the site of the stenosis that resists attempts at dilation. Treatment consists of resection and end-to-end anastomosis. A useful step at the time of operation is to pass a flexible gastroscope to the level of the stenosis to highlight the precise level of resection, as the stenosis is frequently ill defined from the external surface.

LARYNGEAL AND LARYNGOTRACHEOESOPHAGEAL CLEFT

Posterior laryngeal clefts result from failure of the posterior cricoid lamina to fuse and, in the more extensive laryngotracheoesophageal clefts, incomplete development of the tracheoesophageal septum also is found. A classification has been devised that relates well to symptoms and treatment.[192] A type I cleft may extend down to the level of the vocal cords; a type II cleft extends below the vocal cords into the cricoid; a type III cleft extends down into the cervical trachea; and the rare type IV cleft extends into the thoracic trachea and may even reach the carina (Fig. 26-19). Approximately 25% of patients with a laryngeal cleft will also have a separate TEF, but conversely, the incidence of laryngeal cleft in patients with a TEF is low. Abnormalities of the tracheal ring structure in cleft patients may result in associated tracheomalacia, which can add to the difficulties of management.

The majority of laryngeal cleft patients have other associated congenital abnormalities, of which TEF is the most common. Included in these other anomalies are GER, tracheobronchomalacia, congenital heart disease, dextrocardia, and situs inversus. Laryngeal clefts are characteristic of two syndromes. The Opitz-Frias syndrome (G syndrome) includes hypertelorism, cleft lip and palate, laryngeal cleft, and hypospadias. Pallister-Hall syndrome consists of congenital hypothalamic hamartoblastoma, hypopituitarism, imperforate anus, and postaxial polydactyly, and may include a laryngeal cleft.

Clinical Features

Symptoms are more severe the longer the cleft. Type I clefts are initially seen with cyanotic attacks with feeding and recurrent chest infections. Stridor (similar to that of laryngomalacia) may be a feature, secondary to prolapse of the cleft edges into the airway. The differential diagnosis for infants with these symptoms includes GER, neuromuscular incoordination of deglutition, vocal cord paralysis, elevated intracranial pressure, and TEF. Type II and III clefts produce dramatic aspiration with recurrent pneumonia, sometimes with stridor and an abnormal cry. Type IV clefts cause severe aspiration, cyanosis, and incipient cardiorespiratory failure.

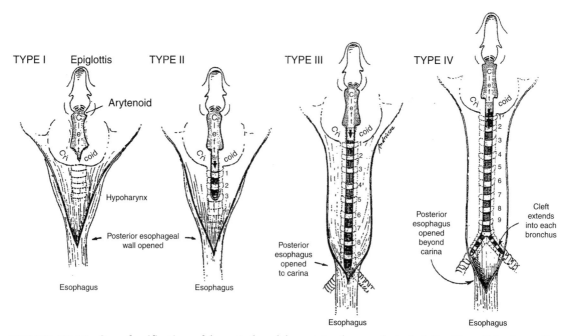

FIGURE 26-19. One classification of laryngeal and laryngotracheoesophageal clefts. Type I is above the cricoid, type II extends through the cricoid, type III extends well down the trachea toward the carina, and type IV extends out one or both main-stem bronchi. (From Ryan DP, Muehrcke DD, Doody DP, et al: Laryngotracheoesophageal cleft [type IV]: Management and repair of lesions beyond the carina. J Pediatr Surg 26:962–970, 1991.)

Investigation

Investigation of the child with aspiration and stridor requires careful microlaryngoscopy and bronchoscopy, and no other diagnostic method can replace it. Suspension microlaryngoscopy allows the use of two probes to part the arytenoids. Without this maneuver, the diagnosis may be missed, as redundant mucosa tends to prolapse into the defect and obscure it. A plain chest radiograph may show changes secondary to recurrent aspiration pneumonitis. A lateral neck radiograph may demonstrate vaguely increased laryngeal soft tissue, and a nasogastric feeding tube may be seen protruding anteriorly into the airway. Video-fluoroscopic contrast-swallow studies may not differentiate laryngeal incompetence from neuromuscular incoordination. A very high index of suspicion is required.

Treatment

The approach to treatment depends entirely on the length of the cleft. A short type I cleft with no aspiration requires no treatment. Minimal aspiration may be managed by thickening the feeds. Significant aspiration requires endoscopic repair of the cleft in two layers, by using a nasogastric feeding tube until the anastomosis has healed. A very short type II cleft also may be repaired endoscopically, albeit with difficulty, by using a nasogastric tube. However, a long type II or a type III cleft must be approached anteriorly through an extended laryngofissure. A postoperative tracheostomy and a gastrostomy are required (usually combined with fundoplication to control reflux reliably). These children take many months to

learn to swallow after successful cleft repair, and long-term gastrostomy feeding is necessary. Surgical repair of the defect is undertaken in three layers in an effort to optimize healing: the two mucosal layers are reinforced by an interposition graft of tibial periosteum or temporalis fascia. The type IV cleft presents an altogether more difficult surgical challenge. Because of the length of the cleft, a tracheostomy is not helpful in stabilizing the airway, and the convexity of the tube would tend to erode through the posterior tracheal suture line. The repair of this difficult lesion must be undertaken by using a single-stage technique with extubation taking place 7 to 10 days after surgical separation. Short type IV clefts may be managed with an anterior approach through a cervical incision, if necessary pulling the trachea up into the neck to reach the lower end of the cleft. Longer type IV clefts are best repaired by using a median sternotomy on cardiopulmonary bypass, although use of a lateral cervical approach in combination with a thoracotomy has been described. Postoperatively, tracheomalacia may prevent extubation, in which case a tracheostomy may be needed once the cleft has healed soundly.

Results

The mortality remains significant, 14% overall,[193] increasing to 66% for type IV laryngotracheoesophageal clefts and up to 100% for full-length clefts ending at the carina.[194] A large part of the mortality is from causes unrelated to the cleft, and notable morbidity is produced by other associated congenital abnormalities and sometimes by delay in reaching the correct diagnosis. Management should be in a major pediatric center where a multidisciplinary team is available with neonatal and pediatric intensive care facilities.

REFERENCES

1. Potts WJ, quoted by Cloud DT: Anastomotic technique in esophageal atresia. J Pediatr Surg 3:561–564, 1968.
2. Myers NA: Oesophageal atresia: The epitome of modern surgery. Ann R Coll Surg Engl 54:277–287, 1974.
3. Ashcraft KW, Holder TM: The story of esophageal atresia and tracheoesophageal fistula. Surgery 65:332–340, 1969.
4. Durston W: A narrative of a monstrous birth in Plymouth, October 22: Together with the anatomic observations taken thereupon by William Durston, Doctor of Physick, and communication to Dr. Tim Clerk. Philos Trans R Soc 5:2096–2098, 1670–1671.
5. Gibson T: The Anatomy of Humane Bodies Epitomized (5th ed). London, Awnsham and Churchill, 1697.
6. Hill TP: Congenital malformation. Boston Med Surg J 21:320–321, 1840.
7. Hirschsprung H: congenital occlusion of the oesophagus. Br Foreign Medico-chir Rev 30:437–442, 1962.
8. Holmes T: Cattive conformazioni nel collo. In Chiusura Congenita dell'Esofagao (2nd ed.), 1869.
9. Steele C: Case of deficient oesophagus. Lancet 2:764, 1888.
10. Steward FJ, quoted by Thomas W. On congenital occlusion of the oesophagus. Lancet 1:361–362, 1904.
11. Keith A: Constrictions and occlusion of the alimentary tract of congenital or obscure origin. Br Med J 1:301–305, 1910.
12. Richter HM: Congenital atresia of the oesophagus: An operation designed for its cure. Surg Gynecol Obstet 17:397–402, 1913.
13. Lanman TH: Congenital atresia of the esophagus. Arch Surg 41:1060–1083, 1940.
14. Levin NL: Congenital atresia of the esophagus with tracheo-esophageal fistula. J Thorac Cardiovasc Surg 10:648–657, 1941.
15. Ladd WE: The surgical treatment of esophageal atresia and tracheoesophageal fistulas. N Engl J Med 230:625–637, 1944.
16. Haight C, Towsley HA: Congenital atresia of the esophagus with tracheoesophageal fistula: Extrapleural ligation of fistula and end-to-end anastomosis of esophageal segments. Surg Gynecol Obstet 76:672–688, 1943.
17. Waterston DJ, Bonham Carter RE, Aberdeen E: Oesophageal atresia, tracheo-oesophageal: A study of survival in 218 infants. Lancet 1:819–822, 1962.
18. Ten Have-Opbroek AAW: The development of the lung in mammals: An analysis of concepts and findings. Am J Anat 162:201–219, 1981.
19. Merei J, Hasthorpe S, Farmer P, et al: Relationship between esophageal atresia and tracheoesophageal fistula and vertebral anomalies in mammalian embryos. J Pediatr Surg 33:58–63, 1998.
20. O'Rahilly R, Muller F: Respiratory and alimentary relations in staged human embryos: New embryological data and congenital anomalies. Ann Otol Rhinol Laryngol 93:421–429, 1984.
21. Qi BQ, Beasley SW: Stages of normal tracheo-bronchial development in rat embryos: Resolution of a controversy. Dev Growth Differ 42:145–153, 2000.
22. Gray SW, Skandalakis JE: The oesophagus. In Gray SW, Skandalakis JE (eds): Embryology for Surgeons, 1st ed. Philadelphia, Saunders, 1972, pp 63–99.
23. Ioannides AS, Henderson DJ, Spitz L, et al: Role of Sonic Hedgehog in the development of the trachea and esophagus. J Pediatr Surg 38:29–36, 2003.
24. Zhou B, Hutson JM, Farmer PJ, et al: Apoptosis in tracheo-esophageal embryogenesis in rat embryos with or without Adriamycin treatment. J Pediatr Surg 34:872–875, 1999.
25. Diez-Pardo JA, Baoquan Q, Navarro C, et al: A new rodent experimental model of esophageal atresia and tracheoesophageal fistula: Preliminary report. J Pediatr Surg 31:498–502, 1996.
26. Possogel AK, Diez-Pardo JA, Morales C, et al: Embryology of esophageal atresia in the Adriamycin rat model. J Pediatr Surg 33:606–612, 1998.
27. Merei JM, Farmer P, Hasthorpe S, et al: Timing and embryology of esophageal atresia and tracheo-esophageal fistula. Anat Rec 249:240–248, 1997.

28. Orford J, Manglick P, Cass DT, et al: Mechanisms for the development of esophageal atresia. J Pediatr Surg 36:985–994, 2001.
29. Crisera CA, Connelly PR, Marmureanu AR, et al: Esophageal atresia with tracheoesophageal fistula: Suggested mechanism in faulty organogenesis. J Pediatr Surg 34:204–208, 1999.
30. Crisera CA, Maldonado TS, Longaker MT, et al: Defective fibroblast growth factor signalling allows for nonbranching growth of the respiratory-derived fistula tract in esophageal atresia with tracheoesophageal fistula. J Pediatr Surg 35:1421–1425, 2000.
31. Crisera CA, Connelly PR, Marmureanu AR, et al: TTF-1 and HNF-3beta in the developing tracheo-oesophageal fistula: Further evidence for the respiratory origin of the distal esophagus. J Pediatr Surg 34:1322–1326, 1999.
32. Ioannides AS, Chowdhry B, Henderson D, et al: Dorsoventral patterning of the foregut in esophageal atresia: Evidence from a new mouse model. J Pediatr Surg 37:185–191, 2002.
33. Litingtung Y, Lei L, Westphal H, et al: Sonic hedgehog is essential for foregut development. Nat Genet 20:58–61, 1998.
34. Motoyama J, Liu J, Mo R, et al: Essential function of Gli2 and Gli3 in the formation of lung, trachea and oesophagus. Nat Genet 20:54–57, 1998.
35. Mahlapuu M, Enerback S, Carlsson P: Haploinsufficiency of the forkhead gene Foxf1, a target for sonic hedgehog signalling, causes lung and foregut malformations. Development 128:2398–2406, 2001.
36. Clementi M, Di Gianantonio E, Pelo E, et al: Methimozole embryopathy: Delineation of the phenotype. Am J Med Genet 83:43–46, 1999.
37. Orford J, Glasson M, Beasley S, et al: Oesophageal atresia in twin. Pediatr Surg Int 16:541–545, 2000.
38. Kashuk JL, Litty JR: Esophageal atresia in father and son. J Pediatr Surg 18:621–622, 1983.
39. Lipson AH, Berry AB: Oesophageal atresia in father and daughter. Aust Pediatr J 20:329, 1984.
40. Van Staey M, De Bie S, Matton MT, et al: Familial congenital oesophageal atresia: Personal case report and review of the literature. Hum Genet 66:260–266, 1984.
41. Chittmittrapap S, Spitz L, Kiely EM, et al: Oesophageal atresia and associated anomalies. Arch Dis Child 93:364–368, 1989.
42. Beasley SW, Diez Pardo J, Qi BG, et al: The contribution of the Adriamycin-induced rat model of the VATER association to our understanding of congenital abnormalities and their embryogenesis. Pediatr Surg Int 16:465–472, 2000.
43. Kim PC, Mo R, Hui CC: Murine models of VACTERL syndrome: Role of sonic hedgehog signalling pathway. J Pediatr Surg 36:381–384, 2001.
44. Roessler E, Belloni E, Gaudenz K, et al: Mutations in the human Sonic Hedgehog gene cause holoprosencephaly. Nat Genet 14:357–360, 1996.
45. Kang S, Graham JM Jr, Olney AH, et al: GK13 frameshift mutations cause autosomal dominant Pallister Hall syndrome. Nat Genet 15:266–268, 1997.
46. Beasley SW, Allen M, Myers N: The effects of Down's syndrome and other chromosomal abnormalities on survival and management in esophageal atresia. Pediatr Surg Int 12:550–551, 1997.
47. Digilio MC, Marino B, Bagalon P, et al: Microdeletion 22q11 and oesophageal atresia. J Med Genet 36:137–139, 1999.
48. Marsh AJ, Wellesley D, Burge D, et al: Interstitial deletion of chromosome 17 [del(17) (q22q23.3)] confirms a link with oesophageal atresia. J Med Genet 37:701–704, 2000.
49. Brunner HG, Winter RM: Autosomal dominant inheritance of abnormalities of the hands and feet with short palpebral features, variable microcephaly with learning disability, and oesophageal/duodenal atresia. J Med Genet 28:389–394, 1991.
50. Brewer C, Holloway S, Zawalnyski P, et al: A chromosomal deletion map of human malformations. Am J Hum Genet 63:1153–1159, 1998.
51. Courtens W, Levi S, Verbelen F, et al: Feingold syndrome: Report of a new family and review. Am J Med Genet 73:55–60, 1997.
52. Feingold M, Hall BD, Lacassie Y, et al: Syndrome of microcephaly, facial and hand abnormalities, tracheo-esophageal fistula, duodenal atresia, and developmental delay. Am J Med Genet 69:245–249, 1997.
53. Celli J, van Beusekom E, Hennekam RC, et al: Familial syndromic esophageal atresia maps to 2p23-p24. Am J Hum Genet 66:436–444, 2000.

54. Vogt EC: Congenital esophageal atresia. AJR Am J Roentgenol 22:463–465, 1929.
55. Gross RE: The Surgery of Infancy and Childhood. Philadelphia, WB Saunders, 1953.
56. Lambrecht W, Kluth D: Esophageal atresia: A new anatomic variant with gasless abdomen. J Pediatr Surg 29:564–565, 1994.
57. Qi BQ, Uemura S, Farmer P, et al: Intrinsic innervation of the oesophagus in fetal rats with oesophageal atresia. Pediatr Surg Int 15:2–7, 1986.
58. Cheng W, Bishop AE, Spitz L, et al: Abnormal enteric nerve morphology in atretic esophagus of fetal rats with Adriamycin-induced esophageal atresia. Pediatr Surg Int 15:8–10, 1999.
59. Qi BQ, Merei J, Farmer P, et al: The vagus and recurrent laryngeal nerves in the rodent experimental model of esophageal atresia. Ann Thoracic Surg 32:1580–1586, 1997.
60. Cheng W, Bishop AE, Spitz L, et al: Abnormality of neuropeptides and neural markers in the esophagus of fetal rats with an Adriamycin-induced esophageal atresia. J Pediatr Surg 32:1420–1423, 1997.
61. Shono T, Suita S, Arima T, et al: Motility function of the esophagus before primary anastomosis in esophageal atresia. J Pediatr Surg 28:673–676, 1993.
62. Duranceau A, Fisher SR, Flye M, et al: Motor function of the esophagus after repair of esophageal atresia and tracheoesophageal fistula. Surgery 82:116–123, 1977.
63. Dutta HK, Grove VP, Dwivedi SN, et al: Manometric evaluation of postoperative patients of esophageal atresia and tracheo-esophageal fistula. Eur J Pediatr Surg 11:371–376, 2001.
64. Wailoo MP, Emery JL: The trachea in children with tracheo-oesophageal fistula. Histopathology 3:329–338, 1979.
65. Stringer MD, McKenna KM, Goldstein RB, et al: Prenatal diagnosis of esophageal atresia. J Pediatr Surg 30:1258–1263, 1995.
66. Shulman A, Mazkereth R, Zalel Y, et al: Prenatal identification of esophageal atresia: The role of ultrasonography for evaluation of functional anatomy. Prenat Diagn 22:669–674, 2002.
67. Langer JC, Hussain H, Khan A, et al: Prenatal diagnosis of esophageal atresia using sonography and magnetic resonance imaging. J Pediatr Surg 36:804–807, 2001.
68. Filston HC, Shorter NA: Esophageal atresia and tracheoesophageal malformations. In Ashcraft KW, Murphy JP, Sharp RJ, et al (eds): Pediatric Surgery, 3rd ed. Philadelphia, WB Saunders, 2000, pp 348–369.
69. Holder TM, Ashcraft KW, Sharp RJ, et al: Care of infants with esophageal atresia, tracheoesophageal fistula, and associated anomalies. J Thorac Cardiovasc Surg 94:828–835, 1987.
70. Ein SH, Shandling D, Esson D, et al: Esophageal atresia with distal tracheoesophageal fistula: Associated anomalies and prognosis in the 1980s. J Pediatr Surg 24:1055–1059, 1989.
71. German JC, Mahour GH, Woolley MM: Esophageal atresia and associated anomalies. J Pediatr Surg 11:299–306, 1976.
72. Chittmittrapap S, Spitz L, Kiely EM, et al: Oesophageal atresia and associated anomalies. Arch Dis Child 64:364–368, 1989.
73. Quan L, Smith DW: The VATER association: Vertebral defects: Anal atresia: T-E fistula with esophageal atresia: Radial and Renal dysplasia: A spectrum of associated defects. J Pediatr 82:104–107, 1973.
74. Jones KL: Smith's Recognizable Patterns of Human Malformation, 5th ed. Philadelphia, WB Saunders, 1997.
75. Cseizel A: SCHISIS-association. Am J Med Genet 10:25–35, 1981.
76. Kutiyanawala M, Wyse RKH, Frereton RJ, et al: Charge and esophageal atresia. J Pediatr Surg 27:558–560, 1992.
77. Greenwood RD, Rosenthal A: Cardiovascular malformations associated with tracheoesophageal fistula and esophageal atresia. Pediatrics 57:87–90, 1976.
78. Kulkarni B, Rad RS, Oak S, et al: 13 pairs of ribs: A predictor of long gap atresia in tracheoesophageal fistula. J Pediatr Surg 32:1453–1454, 1997.
79. Bowkett B, Beasley SW, Myers NA: The frequency, significance, and management of a right aortic arch in association with esophageal atresia. Pediatr Surg Int 15:28–31, 1999.
80. Babu R, Pierro A, Spitz L, et al: The management of esophageal atresia in neonates with right-sided aortic arch. J Pediatr Surg 35:56–58, 2000.
81. Harrison MR, Hanson BA, Mahour GH, et al: The significance of right aortic arch in repair of esophageal atresia and tracheo-esophageal fistula. J Pediatr Surg 12:861–869, 1977.
82. Mee RBB, Beasley SW, Auldis AW, et al: Influence of congenital heart disease on management of oesophageal atresia. Pediatr Surg Int 7:90–93, 1992.
83. Spitz L, Kiely EM, Morecroft JA, et al: At risk groups in esophageal atresia for the 1990s. J Pediatr Surg 29:723–725, 1994.
84. Okada A, Usui N, Inoue M, et al: Esophageal atresia in Osaka: A review of 39 years' experience. J Pediatr Surg 32:1570–1574, 1997.
85. Driver CP, Shankar KR, Jones MO, et al: Phenotypic presentation and outcome of esophageal atresia in the era of the Spitz classification. J Pediatr Surg 36:1419–1421, 2001.
86. Poenaru D, Laberge J-M, Neilson IR, et al: A new prognostic classification for esophageal atresia. Surgery 113:426–432, 1993.
87. Holcomb GW III: Survival after gastrointestinal perforation from esophageal atresia and tracheoesophageal fistula. J Pediatr Surg 28:1532–1535, 1993.
88. Maoate K, Myers NA, Beasley SW: Gastric perforation in infants with oesophageal atresia and distal tracheo-oesophageal fistula. Pediatr Surg Int 15:24–27, 1999.
89. Templeton JM, Templeton JL, Schnaufer L, et al: Management of esophageal atresia and tracheo-esophageal fistula in the neonate with severe respiratory distress syndrome. J Pediatr Surg 20:394–397, 1985.
90. Jones TB, Kirchner SG, Lee FA, et al: Stomach rupture associated with atresia, tracheo-esophageal fistula and ventilatory assistance. AJR Am J Roentgenol 134:675–677, 1980.
91. Calverley RK, Johnston AE: The anaesthetic management of tracheo-oesophageal fistula: A review of 10 years' experience. Can Anaesth Soc J 1119:270–282, 1972.
92. Salem MR, Wong AY, Lin YH: Prevention of gastric distension during anesthesia for newborns with tracheo-esophageal fistulas. Anesthesiology 38:82–83, 1973.
93. Filston HC, Chitwood WR, Schkolne B, et al: The Fogarty balloon catheter as an aid to management of the infant with esophageal atresia and tracheo-esophageal fistula complicated by severe RDS or pneumonia. J Pediatr Surg 17:149–151, 1982.
94. Holmes SJK, Kiely EM, Spitz L: Tracheo-esophageal fistula and the respiratory distress syndrome. Pediatr Surg Int 2:16–18, 1987.
95. Malone PS, Kiely EM, Brain AJ, et al: Tracheo-esophageal fistula and pre-operative mechanical ventilation: A dangerous combination. Aust NZ J Surg 60:525–527, 1990.
96. Beasley SW, Myers NA, Auldist AW: Management of the premature infant with esophageal atresia and hyaline membrane disease. J Pediatr Surg 27:23–25, 1992.
97. Filston HC, Rankin JS, Grimm JK: Esophageal atresia: Prognostic factors and contribution of preoperative telescopic endoscopy. Ann Surg 199:532–537, 1984.
98. Kosloske AM, Jewell PF, Cartwright KC: Crucial bronchoscopic findings in esophageal atresia and tracheoesophageal fistula. J Pediatr Surg 23:466–470, 1988.
99. Goh DW, Brereton RJ, Spitz L: Esophageal atresia with obstructed tracheoesophageal fistula and gasless abdomen. J Pediatr Surg 26:160–162, 1991.
100. Dudgeon DL, Morrison CW, Woolley MM: Congenital proximal tracheoesophageal fistula. J Pediatr Surg 7:614–619, 1992.
101. Hagberg S, Rubenson A, Sillen U, et al: Management of long-gap esophagus: Experience with end-to-end anastomosis under maximal tension. Prog Pediatr Surg 19:88–92, 1986.
102. MacKinley GA, Burtles R: Oesophageal atresia: Paralysis and ventilation in management of long gap. Pediatr Surg Int 2:10–12, 1987.
103. Spitz L, Kiely E, Brereton RJ, et al: Management of esophageal atresia. World J Surg 17:296–300, 1993.
104. Lividitis A: Esophageal atresia: a method of overbridging large segment gaps. Z Kinderchir 13:298–306, 1973.
105. Eraklis AJ, Rosello PJ, Ballantine TVN: Circular esophagomyotomy of upper pouch in primary repair of long-segment esophageal atresia. J Pediatr Surg 11:709–712, 1976.
106. Vizas D, Ein SH, Simpson JS: The value of circular myotomy for esophageal atresia. J Pediatr Surg 13:357–359, 1978.
107. Hoffman DG, Moazam F: Transcervical myotomy for wide-gap esophageal atresia. J Pediatr Surg 19:680–682, 1984.
108. Gough MH: Esophageal atresia: Use of an anterior flap in the difficult anastomosis. J Pediatr Surg 15:310–311, 1980.

109. Davenport M, Bianchi A: Early experience with oesophageal flap oesophagoplasty for repair of oesophageal atresia. Pediatr Surg Int 5:332–335, 1990.

110. Rehbein F, Schweder N: Reconstruction of the esophagus without colon transplantation in cases of atresia. J Pediatr Surg 6:746–752, 1971.

111. Shafer AD, David TE: Suture fistula as a means of connecting upper and lower segments in esophageal atresia. J Pediatr Surg 9:669–673, 1974.

112. Schullinger NJ, Vinocur CD, Santulli TV: The suture fistula technique in the repair of selected cases of esophageal atresia. J Pediatr Surg 17:234–236, 1982.

113. Howard R, Myers NA: Esophageal atresia: A technique for elongating the upper pouch. Surgery 58:725–739, 1965.

114. Mahour GH, Woolley MM, Gwinn JL: Elongation of the upper pouch and delayed anatomic reconstruction in esophageal atresia. J Pediatr Surg 9:373–383, 1974.

115. Hays DM, Woolley MM, Snyder WH: Changing techniques in the management of esophageal atresia. Arch Surg 92:611–616, 1966.

116. Hendren WH, Hale JR: Electromagnetic bougienage to lengthen esophageal segments in congenital esophageal atresia. N Engl J Med 293:428–432, 1975.

117. Puri P, Blake N, O'Donnell B, et al: Delayed primary anastomosis following spontaneous growth of esophageal segments in esophageal atresia. J Pediatr Surg, 16:180–183, 1981.

118. Rossello PJ, Lebron H, Roman Franco AA: The technique of myotomy in esophageal reconstruction: An experimental study. J Pediatr Surg 15:430–432, 1980.

119. Kimura K, Nishijima E, Tsugawa C, et al: A new approach for the salvage of unsuccessful esophageal atresia repair: A spiral myotomy and delayed definitive operation. J Pediatr Surg 22:981–983, 1987.

120. Scharli AF: Esophageal reconstruction in very long atresias by elongation of the lesser curvature. Pediatr Surg Int 7:101–105, 1992.

121. Okmian F, Boss D, Ekelund L: An endoscopic technique for Rehbein's silver-olive method. Z Kinderchir 16:212–215, 1975.

122. Kato T, Hollmann G, Hopner F, et al: Ein neues Instrument zur Fadenleghung ohne Thorakotomie in ausgewählten Fällen von Osophagusatresie. Z Kinderchir 6:206–214, 1980.

123. Waterston D: Colonic replacement of esophagus (intrathoracic). Surg Clin North Am 44:1441, 1964.

124. Freeman NV, Cass DT: Colon interposition: A modification of the Waterston technique using the normal oesophageal route. J Pediatr Surg 17:17–21, 1982.

125. Heimlich HJ: Elective replacement of the oesophagus. Br J Surg 53:913, 1966.

126. Anderson KD, Randolph JG: The gastric tube for esophageal replacement in infants and children. J Thor Cardiovasc Surg 66:333, 1973.

127. Ring WS, Varco RL., L'Heureux PR, et al: Esophageal replacement with jejunum in children: An 18 to 33-year follow-up. J Thorac Cardiovasc Surg 83:918, 1982.

128. Spitz L: Gastric transposition via the mediastinal route for infants with long-gap esophageal atresia. J Pediatr Surg 19:149–154, 1984.

129. Spitz L: Gastric transposition for esophageal substitution in children. J Pediatr Surg 27:252–259, 1992.

130. Boyle EM Jr, Irwin ED, Foker JE: Primary repair of ultra-long gap esophageal atresia: Results without a lengthening procedure. Ann Thorac Surg 57:576–579, 1994.

131. Holcomb GW III: Identification of the distal esophageal segment during delayed repair of esophageal atresia and tracheoesophageal fistula. Surg Gynecol Obstet 174:323–324, 1992.

132. Foker JE, Linden BC, Boyle EM Jr, et al: Development of a true primary repair for the full spectrum of esophageal atresia. Ann Surg 226:533–543, 1997.

133. Al-Qahtani AR, Yazbeck S, Rosen NG, et al: Lengthening technique for long gap esophageal atresia and early anastomosis. J Pediatr Surg 38:737–739, 2003.

134. Spitz L, Kiely E, Brereton RJ, et al: Management of oesophageal atresia. World J Surg 17:296–300, 1993.

135. Patel SB, Ade-Ajayi N, Kiely EM: Oesophageal atresia: A simplified approach to early management. Pediatr Surg Int 18:87–89, 2002.

136. Chittmittrapap S, Spitz L, Kiely EM, et al: Anastomotic leakage following surgery for esophageal atresia. J Pediatr Surg 27:29–32, 1992.

137. Holder RM, Ashcraft KW: Developments in the care of patients with esophageal atresia and tracheoesophageal fistula. Surg Clin North Am 61:1051–1061, 1981.

138. Martin LW, Alexander F: Esophageal atresia. Surg Clin North Am 65:1099–1113, 1985.

139. Lundertse-Verloop K, Tibboel D, Hazebrock FWJ et al: Postoperative morbidity in patients with esophageal atresia. Pediatr Surg Int 2:2–5, 1987.

140. Sillen U, Hagberg S, Rubeson A, et al: Management of esophageal atresia: Review of 16 years' experience. J Pediatr Surg 23:805–809, 1988.

141. Chittmittrapap S, Spitz L, Kiely EM, et al: Anastomotic stricture following repair of esophageal atresia. J Pediatr Surg 25:508–511, 1990.

142. Holder TM, Ashcraft KW, Sharp RJ et al: Care of infants with esophageal atresia, tracheoesophageal fistula and associated anomalies. Thorac Cardiovasc Surg 94:828–835, 1087.

143. Jolly SG, Johnston DG, Roberts CC, et al: Patterns of gastro-esophageal reflux in children following repair of esophageal atresia and distal tracheoesophageal fistula. J Pediatr Surg 15:857–862, 1980.

144. Tam PKH, Sprigg A, Cudmore RE, et al: Endoscopy-guided balloon dilatation of esophageal strictures and anastomotic strictures after esophageal replacement in children. J Pediatr Surg 26:1101–1103, 1991.

145. Allmendinger N, Hallisey MJ, Markowitz SK, et al: Balloon dilatation of esophageal strictures in children. J Pediatr Surg 31:334–336, 1996.

146. Ghandour KE, Spitz L, Brereton RJ et al: Recurrent tracheo-oesophageal fistula: experience with 24 patients. J Paediatr Child Health 26:89–91, 1990.

147. Verloop K, Leendertse P, Tibboel D, et al: Post-operative morbidity in patients with oesophageal atresia. Paediatr Surg Int 2:2–5, 1987.

148. Hicks LM, Mansfield PB: Oesophageal atresia and tracheo-oesophageal fistula: Review of thirteen years' experience. J Thorac Cardiovasc Surg 81:358–363, 1981.

149. Bishop PJ, Klein MD, Philipart AI, et al: Transpleural repair of esophageal atresia without a primary gastrostomy: 240 patients treated between 1951 and 1983. J Pediatr Surg 20:823–824, 1985.

150. Beardmore HE, Pietsch JB, Stokes KB: Esophageal atresia with tracheo-esophageal fistula. J Pediatr Surg 13:677–681, 1978.

151. Touloukian RJ: Long-term results following repair of esophageal atresia by end-to-side anastomosis and ligation of the tracheo-esophageal fistula. J Pediatr Surg 16:983–988, 1981.

152. Ein SH, Stringer DA, Stephans CA, et al: Recurrent tracheo-esophageal fistulas: Seventeen-year review. J Pediatr Surg 18:436–441, 1983.

153. Filston HC, Rankin JC, Kirks DR: The diagnosis of primary and recurrent tracheo-esophageal fistulas: Value of selective catheterization. J Pediatr Surg 17:144–148, 1982.

154. Bhatnagar V, Lal R, Sriniwas M, et al: Endoscopic treatment of tracheoesophageal fistula using electrocautery and the Nd:YAG laser. J Pediatr Surg 34:464–467, 1999.

155. Willets IE, Dudley NE, Tam PK: Endoscopic treatment of recurrent tracheo-oesophageal fistulae: Long-term results. Pediatr Surg Int 13:256–258, 1998.

156. Hoelzer DJ, Luft JD: Successful long-term endoscopic closure of a recurrent tracheoesophageal fistula with fibrin glue in a child. Int J Pediatr Otorhinolaryngol 25:48:259–263, 1999.

157. Rangecroft L, Bush GH, Lister J, Irving IM: Endoscopic diathermy: Obliteration of recurrent tracheo-esophageal fistulae. J Pediatr Surg 19:41–43, 1943.

158. Izzidien Al-Samarrai AY, Jessen K, Haque K: Endoscopic obliteration of a recurrent tracheo-esophageal fistula. J Pediatr Surg 232:993, 1987.

159. Curci MR, Dibbins AW: Problems associated with a Nissen fundoplication following tracheoesophageal fistula and esophageal atresia repair. Arch Surg 123:618–620, 1988.

160. Parker AF, Christie DL, Cahill JL, et al: Incidence and significance of gastroesophageal reflux following repair of esophageal atresia and tracheoesophageal fistula and the need for antireflux procedures. J Pediatr Surg 14:5–8, 1979.

161. Snyder CL, Ramachandran V, Kennedy AP, et al: Efficacy of partial wrap fundoplication for gastroesophageal reflux after repair of esophageal atresia. J Pediatr Surg 32:1089–1092, 1997.
162. Wheatley MJ, Coran AG, Wesley JR: Efficacy of the Nissen fundoplication in the management of gastroesophageal reflux following esophageal atresia repair. J Pediatr Surg 28:53–55, 1993.
163. Guo W, Fonkalsrud EW, Swaniker F, et al: Relationship of esophageal anastomotic tension to the development of gastroesophageal reflux. J Pediatr Surg 32:1337–1340, 1997.
164. Spitz L: Esophageal atresia: Past, present, and future. J Pediatr Surg, 31:19–25, 1996.
165. Kiely E, Spitz L: Is routine gastrostomy necessary in the management of oesophageal atresia? Pediatr Surg Int 2:13–15, 1987.
166. Black TL, Fernandez Et, Ellis DG, et al: The effect of tube gastrostomy on gastroesophageal reflux in patients with esophageal atresia. J Pediatr Surg 26:168–170, 1991.
167. Peiretti R, Shandling B, Stephens CA: Resistant esophageal stenosis associated with reflux after repair of esophageal atresia. J Pediatr Surg 9:355–357, 1994.
168. Myers NA, Beasley SW, Audlist AW: Secondary esophageal surgery following repair of esophageal atresia with distal tracheoesophageal fistula. J Pediatr Surg 25:773–777, 1960.
169. Kubiak R, Spitz L, Kiely EM: Effectiveness of fundoplication in early infancy. J Pediatr Surg 34:295–299, 1999.
170. Lindahl H, Rintala R, Louhimo I, et al: Failure of the Nissen fundoplication to control gastroesophageal reflux in esophageal atresia patients: Evaluation of lower esophageal sphincter function in infants and children following esophageal surgery. J Pediatr Surg 24:985–987, 1989.
171. Spitz L: Tracheomalacia. Surg Child Int 3:160–162, 1999.
172. Benjamin B, Cohen D, Glasson M: Tracheomalacia in association with congenital tracheoesophageal fistula. Surgery 79:504–508, 1978.
173. Filler RM, Messineo A, Vinograd I: Severe tracheomalacia associated with esophageal atresia: Results of surgical treatment. J Pediatr Surg 27:1136–1141, 1992.
174. Messineo A, Filler RM: Tracheomalacia. Semin Pediatr Surg 3:253–258, 1993.
175. Kiely EM: Aortopexy: In Spitz L, Coran AG (eds): Rob & Smith's Operative Surgery: Paediatric Surgery, 5th ed. London, Chapman & Hall Medical, 1995, pp 132–135.
176. Kiely EM, Spitz L, Brereton R: Management of tracheomalacia by aortopexy. Pediatr Surg Int 2:13–15, 1978.
177. Corbally MT, Spitz L, Kiely EM, et al: Aortopexy for tracheomalacia in oesophageal anomalies. Eur J Pediatr Surg 3:264–266, 1993.
178. Vaishnav A, MacKinnon AE: New cervical approach for tracheopexy. Br J Surg 73:441–442, 1986.
179. Biller JA, Allen JL, Schuster SR, et al: Long-term evaluation of esophageal and pulmonary function in patients with repaired esophageal atresia and tracheoesophageal fistula. Dig Dis Sci 32:985–990, 1978.
180. Duranceau A, Fisher SR, Flye M, et al: Motor function of the esophagus after repair of esophageal atresia and tracheoesophageal fistula. Surgery 82:116–123, 1977.
181. Chetcuti P, Phelan PD: Gastrointestinal morbidity and growth after repair of oesophageal atresia and tracheo-oesophageal fistula. Arch Dis Child 68:163–166, 1993.
182. Puntis JW, Ritson DG, Holden CE, et al: Growth and feeding problems after repair of oesophageal atresia. Arch Dis Child. 65:84–88, 1990.
183. Delius RE, Wheatley MJ, Coran AG: Etiology and management of respiratory complications after repair of esophageal atresia with tracheoesophageal fistula. Surgery 112:527–532, 1992.
184. Emery JL, Haddadin AJ: Squamous epithelium in the respiratory tract of children with tracheo-oesophageal fistula. Arch Dis Child 41:236–242, 1971.
185. Beardsmore CS, MacFadyen UM, Johnstone MS, et al: Clinical findings and respiratory function in infants following repair of oesophageal atresia and tracheo-oesophageal fistula. Eur Respir J 7:1039–1047, 1994.
186. Agrawal L, Beardsmore CS, MacFadyen UM: Respiratory function in childhood following repair of oesophageal atresia and tracheoesophageal fistula. Arch Dis Child 81:404–408, 1999.
187. Spitz L: Congenital oesophageal stenosis distal to associated oesophageal atresia. J Pediatr Surg 8:973–974, 1973.
188. Yeung CK, Spitz L, Brereton RJ, et al: Congenital esophageal stenosis due to tracheobronchial remnants: A rare but important association with esophageal atresia. J Pediatr Surg 27:852–855, 1992.
189. Amae S, Nio M, Kamiyama T, et al: Clinical characteristics and management of congenital esophageal stenosis: A report on 14 cases. J Pediatr Surg 38:565–570, 2003.
190. Liu YX, Xue F: Congenital oesophageal stenosis due to tracheobronchial cartilage. Int J Pediatr Otolaryngol 14:95–100, 1987.
191. Shorter NA, Mooney DP, Vaccaro TJ, et al: Hydrostatic balloon dilatation of congenital esophageal stenosis associated with esophageal atresia. J Pediatr Surg 35:1742–1745, 2000.
192. Benajamin B, Inglis A: Minor congenital laryngeal clefts: Diagnosis and classification. Ann Otol Rhinol Laryngol 98:417–420, 1989.
193. Evans KL, Courtney-Harris R, Bailey CM, et al: Management of posterior laryngeal and laryngotracheoesophageal clefts. Arch Otolaryngol Head Neck Surg 121:1380–1385, 1995.
194. Shehab ZP, Bailey CM: Type IV laryngotracheoesophageal clefts: Recent 5 year experience at Great Ormond Street Hospital for Children. Inter J Pediatr Otorhinolaryngol 60:1–9, 2002.

CHAPTER 27

Thoracoscopy in Infants and Children

Steven Rothenberg, MD

Thoracoscopy is a technique that has been described since the early 1900s, but has undergone an exponential increase in utilization over the last decade. Jacobeus[1] first reported this technique in 1910 and described inserting a cystoscope through a rigid cannula into the pleural space to lyse adhesions and collapse the lung as treatment for tuberculosis. He later reported a large experience in more than 100 patients. During the next 70 years, thoracoscopy was used sparingly, primarily in Europe, for biopsy of pleural-based tumors and limited thoracic explorations in adults, but widespread utilization was minimal.[2,3]

In the 1970s and 1980s, the first significant experience in children was reported.[4,5] Equipment modified for pediatric patients was used for biopsy of various intrathoracic lesions and for limited pleural debridement in cases of empyema.[6] Even though an increasing recognition existed of the morbidity associated with a standard thoracotomy, especially in small infants and children, little acceptance or adoption of this minimal-access approach occurred.[7] It was not until the early 1990s, with the dramatic evolution in technology associated with laparoscopic surgery in adults, that more advanced diagnostic and therapeutic procedures were performed in children.[8] The development of high-resolution, microchip, and now digital cameras, smaller instrumentation, and better optics has enabled pediatric surgeons to perform even the most complicated thoracic procedure by using an endoscopic approach.[9]

The recent advances in endoscopic surgical technology have dramatically altered the approach to intrathoracic lesions in the pediatric patient. Most operations can now be performed by using a thoracoscopic approach. Whereas a thoracoscopic approach will not always result in a significant decrease in hospitalization, it may result in a significant decrease in the overall morbidity for the patient. Thoracoscopic surgery has clearly shown significant benefits over standard open thoracotomy in many cases, and, with continued improvement and miniaturization of the equipment, the procedures that can be performed and the advantages to the patient should continue to grow.

INDICATIONS

Currently, a wide variety of indications are recognized for thoracoscopic procedures in children (Table 27-1), and this number continues to expand with advances and refinements in technology and technique. Thoracoscopy is being used extensively for lung biopsy and pulmonary wedge resection in cases of interstitial lung disease (ILD) and metastatic lesions.[10,11] More extensive pulmonary resections including segmentectomy and lobectomy also have been performed for infectious reasons, cavitary lesions, bullous disease, sequestrations, lobar emphysema, congenital adenomatoid malformations, and neoplasms.[12–15] Thoracoscopy also is advantageous in the evaluation and treatment of mediastinal masses.[16] It provides excellent access and visualization for biopsy and resection of mediastinal structures such as lymph nodes, thymic and thyroid lesions, cystic hygromas, foregut duplications, ganglioneuromas, and neuroblastomas.[17–19] Other advanced intrathoracic procedures, such as decortication for empyema, ligation of patent ductus arteriosus (PDA), repair of hiatal hernia and congenital diaphragmatic defects, esophageal myotomy for achalasia, thoracic sympathectomy for hyperhydrosis, anterior spinal fusion for severe scoliosis, and, most recently, primary repair of esophageal atresia with fistula have been described in children.[20–28]

PREOPERATIVE WORKUP

The preoperative evaluation varies considerably, depending on the procedure to be performed. Most intrathoracic lesions require routine chest radiographs as well as a computerized tomographic (CT) or magnetic resonance imaging (MRI) scan. A thin-cut, high-resolution CT scan is especially helpful in evaluating patients with ILD, as it can identify the most affected areas and help determine the site of biopsy (Fig. 27-1), as the external appearance of the lung is usually not helpful. CT-guided needle localization also can be used to direct biopsies for focal

TABLE 27-1	
INDICATIONS FOR THORACOSCOPIC PROCEDURES IN CHILDREN	
Lung biopsy	PDA ligation
Lobectomy	Thoracic duct ligation
Sequestration resection	Esophageal atresia repair
Cyst excision	TEF repair
Decortication	Aortopexy
Foregut duplication resection	Mediastinal mass excision
Esophageal myotomy	Thymectomy
Anterior spine fusion	Sympathectomy
Diaphragmatic hernia/plication	Pericardial window

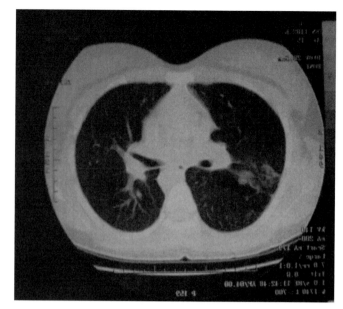

FIGURE 27-1. Computed tomography scan of patient with interstitial lung disease. The areas of greatest involvement can be identified for biopsy.

lesions, which may be deep in the parenchyma and therefore not visible on the surface of the lung. This localization is usually performed just before the thoracoscopy, with the radiologist marking the visceral pleura overlying the lesion with a small blood patch or dye (Fig. 27-2). On occasion, a wire may be placed, as in breast biopsies, but it may become dislodged during collapse of the lung at the time of surgery. As intraoperative ultrasonography (US) imaging advances, this may provide a more sensitive means for the surgeon to detect lesions deep to the surface of the lung and compensate for the lack of tactile sensation. Unfortunately, in its current state, this technology is still unreliable.[29] An MRI scan may be more useful in evaluating vascular lesions or masses that may arise from or encroach on the spinal canal, or in the case of vascular rings. These studies can be extremely important in determining how the patient is positioned at the time of operation and the initial port placement.

Another major consideration for the successful completion of most thoracoscopic procedures is whether the patient will tolerate single-lung ventilation, thus allowing collapse of the ipsilateral lung to ensure adequate visualization and room for manipulation. Unfortunately, no specific preoperative test will yield this answer. However, most patients, even those who are ventilator dependent, can tolerate short periods of single-lung ventilation. This should allow adequate time to perform most diagnostic procedures such as lung biopsy. In cases in which single-lung ventilation cannot be tolerated, other techniques may be used and are discussed next.

PREOPERATIVE PREPARATION

Anesthetic Considerations

Whereas single-lung ventilation is achieved relatively easily in adult patients by using a double-lumen endotracheal tube, this technique is more difficult in the infant or small child. The smallest available double-lumen endotracheal tube is 28F, which is usually too large for a patient weighing less than 30 kg. Another option is a bronchial blocker. This device contains an occluding balloon attached to a stylet on the side of the endotracheal tube. After main-stem intubation, this stylet is advanced into the bronchus to be occluded, and the

balloon is inflated. Unfortunately, size is again a limiting factor, as the smallest bronchial blocker currently available is a 6F tube.

For the majority of cases in infants and small children, selective main-stem intubation of the contralateral bronchus with a standard uncuffed endotracheal tube is effective. This can usually be accomplished blindly without the aide of a bronchoscope, simply by manipulating the head and neck. It also is important to use an endotracheal tube one half to one size smaller than would be selected for standard intubation, or the tube may not pass into the main-stem bronchus, especially on the left side. At times this technique will not lead to total collapse of the lung, as some overflow ventilation may occur because the endotracheal tube is not totally occlusive. This problem is overcome by the routine use of a low-flow (1 L/min), low-pressure (4 mm Hg) CO_2 insufflation during the procedure to help keep the lung compressed. If adequate visualization is still not achieved, then the pressure and flow can be gradually increased until adequate lung collapse is achieved. Pressures of 10 to 12 torr can be tolerated without significant respiratory or hemodynamic consequences in most cases. This technique requires the use of a valved cannula rather than a nonvalved port. It also can be used on patients who cannot tolerate single-lung ventilation. By using small tidal volumes, lower peak inflating pressures, and a higher respiratory rate, enough lung collapse usually can be achieved to allow adequate exploration and biopsy. In neonates with esophageal atresia and fistula or other congenital malformations, CO_2 alone can be used to deflate the lung. Once the lung is collapsed, it will remain compressed until the anesthesiologist makes an effort to re-expand it. The low surface tension of the collapsed alveoli in the newborn keeps the lung collapsed without excessive insufflation pressure.

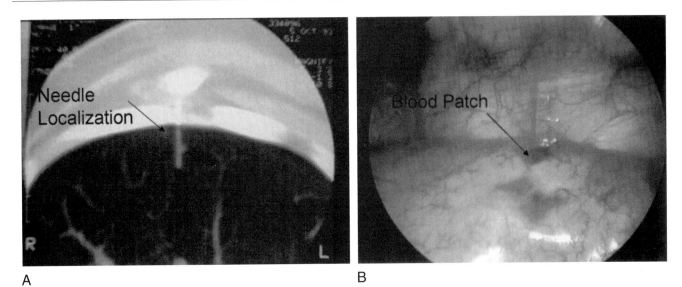

FIGURE 27-2. Needle localization of presumed metastatic lesion under computed tomographic guidance (*A*). Small blood patch visible on pleural surface marking the underlying nodule (*B*).

This insufflation technique also is useful if bilateral procedures are being performed, such as in the case of sympathectomy.[30] A slight tension pneumothorax gives adequate exposure to visualize the sympathetic chain without the need for manipulating the endotracheal tube. Whatever method is chosen, it is imperative that the anesthesiologist and surgeon have a clear plan and good communication to prevent problems with hypoxia and excessive hypercapnia.[31]

Patient Positioning

Patient positioning depends on the site of the lesion and the type of procedure. Most open thoracic operations are performed with the patient in a lateral decubitus position. Thoracoscopic procedures should be performed with the patient in a position that allows the greatest access to the target area with the aid of gravity to keep the uninvolved lung or other tissues out of the field of view.

For routine lung biopsies or lung resections, the patient is placed in a standard lateral decubitus position (Fig. 27-3). This position allows excellent visualization and access to all surfaces of the lung. Moreover, it is the most beneficial setup for decortications, pleurodesis, and other procedures for which the surgeon may need access to the entire pleural or lung surface. For anterior mediastinal masses, the patient should be placed supine with the affected side elevated 20 degrees to 30 degrees (see Fig. 27-3). This affords excellent visualization of the entire anterior mediastinum while allowing gravity to retract the lung posteriorly without the need for retractors. The surgical ports may then be placed between the anterior and midaxillary lines, giving clear access to the anterior mediastinum. This patient position should be used for thymectomy, aortopexy, and biopsy or resection of anterior tumors or lymph nodes. For posterior mediastinal masses, foregut duplications, esophageal

atresia, and operations on the esophageal hiatus, the patient should be placed in a modified prone position with the affected side elevated slightly (see Fig. 27-3). The patient can then be placed in the Trendelenburg or reverse Trendelenburg position, as needed, to help keep the lung out of the viewing field.

Once the patient is appropriately positioned and draped, the viewing monitors can be positioned. For most thoracoscopic procedures, it is advantageous to have one monitor on either side of the table. The monitors should be placed between the patient's shoulders and hips, depending on the site of the lesion. The principle is to keep the surgeon in line with the camera/telescope, the pathology, and the monitor. This allows the surgeon to work in the most efficient and ergonomic way. In some procedures such as decortication, the field of dissection may constantly change. In such cases, the monitors should be placed at the patient's shoulder level and moved as necessary.

The majority of operations can be performed with a surgeon and one assistant/camera holder. The surgeon should stand on the side of the table opposite the target area, so that he or she can work in line with the camera. For most thoracic procedures, such as biopsy or wedge resection, it is best to have the assistant/camera holder on the same side of the table as the surgeon so that he or she is not working paradoxically to the surgeon. This concept is even more important when the field of dissection is localized primarily to one region. Operations such as biopsy of a mediastinal mass, esophageal atresia repair, or more complicated lung resections are quite complex, and it is imperative that both the surgeon and the assistant are working in line with the field of view to allow efficient movements. In cases such as decortication, in which the field of view and dissection are constantly changing and the majority of movements are relatively gross, having the surgeon and assistant on opposite sides of the table is appropriate and may actually expedite the procedure.

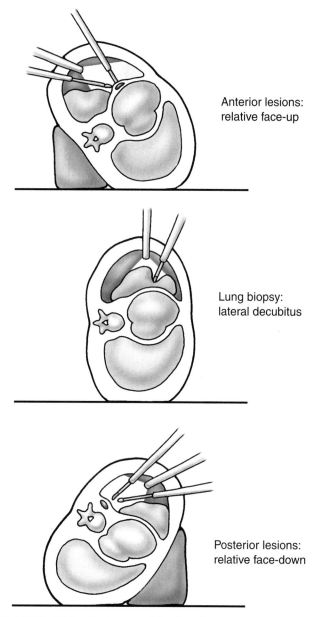

Anterior lesions:
relative face-up

Lung biopsy:
lateral decubitus

Posterior lesions:
relative face-down

FIGURE 27-3. Patient positioning for the thoracoscopic approach to mediastinal and pulmonary lesions in children is important. The relative positions of the three cannulas also are illustrated for these lesions.

Cannula Placement

The placement of the cannulas varies widely with the procedure being performed and the site of the lesion. Thoughtful positioning of the cannulas is more important than that in laparoscopic surgery because the chest wall is rigid, and therefore the mobility of the instruments will be somewhat restricted as compared with the pliable abdominal wall. The most commonly performed operations such as lung biopsy or decortication may require wide access to many areas in the thoracic cavity, and therefore the ports are positioned to facilitate this need. This may, however, result in some degree of paradoxical movements during portions of the procedure. Other operations are directed toward a very restricted

area, and the ports are placed to allow the best visualization and access to this specific spot. In general, the camera/telescope port should be situated slightly above and between the working ports to allow the surgeon to look down on the field of view, much as in open surgery. This also will minimize instrument dueling, which can be a significant problem, especially in smaller infants.

For lung biopsy, the camera port is usually in the midaxillary line at the fifth or sixth interspace, and the other cannulas should usually be placed between the fourth and eighth intercostal spaces. If an endoscopic stapler is used, it requires a 12-mm port and therefore should be placed in the lowest interspace possible, especially in smaller children, as these lower interspaces are wider and better able to accommodate the larger port. If the lesion is anterior, the stapler port should be placed closer to the posterior axillary line and vice versa. This positioning will allow the greatest amount of space between the chest wall and the lesion, as the working head of the stapler requires at least 45 to 50 mm of space. The third or grasping port is placed closer to the lesion and provides traction on the lesion during biopsy. This arrangement allows the surgeon, camera, and primary working port to be in line with the area from which the biopsy is to be taken. The midaxillary camera/telescope port should be placed first to allow modification of the other two ports once an initial survey of the chest cavity has been completed. A triangular arrangement of the cannulas also has been described because it allows rotation of the telescope and instruments between the three ports, giving excellent access to all areas. Especially in children, the number of large ports should be limited. Therefore careful planning should be directed to port placement to limit the numbers and sizes of ports needed. Generally the port placement can be tentatively planned based on preoperative imaging studies and then modified once the initial cannula is introduced.

Instrumentation

The equipment used for thoracoscopy is similar to that used for laparoscopy. In general, 5-mm and 3-mm instrumentation is adequate, and therefore 5-mm and smaller cannulas can be used. In most cases, valved trocars are used for the reasons previously discussed. Basic equipment should include 5-mm 0-degree and 30-degree or 45-degree telescopes. If procedures are being performed in small children and infants, it also is helpful to have shorter telescopes as well. A high-resolution digital camera and high-power light source also are extremely important for adequate visualization, especially when using smaller telescopes, which transmit less light. Basic instrumentation should include curved dissecting scissors, curved dissectors, atraumatic clamps, a fan retractor, a suction/irrigator, and needle holders. Disposable instrumentation that should be available includes hemostatic clips, pre-tied ligatures, and an endoscopic linear stapler. The endoscopic stapler is quite advantageous for performing wedge resections of the lung, but its current size requires placement of a 12-mm port, precluding its use in patients weighing less than 10 kg because of the limited size of the

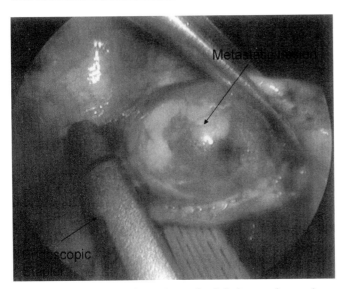

FIGURE 27-4. The endoscopic stapler is being used to excise a presumed metastatic lesion.

thoracic cavity (Fig. 27-4). A number of other energy sources are available for hemostasis and tissue ligation/ division. These include monopolar and bipolar cautery, ultrasonic coagulating shears, and the Ligasure (U.S. Surgical Corp., Norwalk, CT), all of which can be helpful in difficult dissections. It also is advantageous to have one of the various tissue glues available for sealing lung and pleural surfaces.

EMPYEMA

Empyema is the most common intrathoracic problem encountered by pediatric surgeons and has traditionally been treated with antibiotics and some form of chest drainage, including pleurocentesis, tube thoracostomy, minithoracotomy, and formal thoracotomy. Aggressive intervention has often been delayed because of the perceived morbidity associated with surgical intervention. This delay has often led to days, weeks, or even months of antibiotics and pulmonary compromise, as these infections were allowed to persist without adequate surgical drainage. Thoracoscopic debridement offers an opportunity to provide early intervention to diminish the morbidity and recovery time associated with an empyema while limiting the surgical trauma.[32,33] It is rare that thoracoscopic decortication is not an appropriate first step (Fig. 27-5). However, these patients are often septic, with compromised pulmonary and cardiovascular status. The patient's condition should be optimized with fluid resuscitation, aggressive pulmonary care, and antibiotics. In many cases, it is helpful to obtain a preoperative CT scan or US. This information will help to decide if thoracoscopy is appropriate by documenting the amount of loculated fluid, inflammatory peel, and any evidence of parenchymal injury (Fig. 27-6). Although it is unusual to have significant blood loss during the procedure, the patient should be typed and crossed for a unit of blood as a precaution. Many of these patients are anemic, and

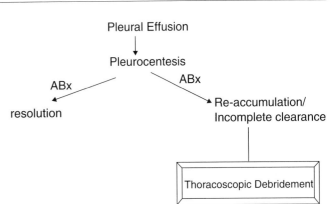

FIGURE 27-5. Algorithm for treatment of pleural effusions and empyema in children.

preoperative transfusion may be necessary to help prepare the child for the operation.

The procedure is performed under general anesthesia with endotracheal intubation. Single-lung isolation with either a double-lumen endotracheal tube or main-stem intubation of the contralateral side is preferred but not mandatory. Single-lung isolation may help to prevent cross contamination of the contralateral airways during manipulation of the affected side. It also may aid in maintaining an adequate working space by preventing reinflation of the trapped lung as the inflammatory peel is removed. However, even without single-lung ventilation, CO_2 insufflation usually is adequate to maintain lung collapse until attempts are made to actively re-expand the lung with positive pressure. Therefore the patient's respiratory status should not be compromised further, and excessive time should not be expended by trying to obtain single-lung isolation.

The procedure is best performed with the patient in a formal lateral decubitus position, which allows the greatest access to the entire pleural cavity. The patient is

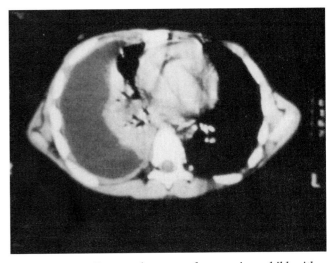

FIGURE 27-6. Computed tomography scan in a child with a large right empyema. The large pleural peel and consolidated lung are easily identified.

supported on a bean-bag or towel rolls. As with all procedures performed in a lateral decubitus position, it is important to place an axillary roll and sufficient padding at all pressure points. Adhesive tape or a strap can be used to support the patient's hips. Patients with severe pulmonary compromise may not tolerate having the ventilated lung restricted by being in a dependant position. In these cases, a modified supine position can be used, with the affected side elevated 25 degrees to 30 degrees.

For this operation, the surgeon and the assistant are positioned on each side of the patient, which allows visualization of the entire pleural cavity. Moreover, the surgeon and assistant are able to manipulate the camera and instruments from both sides, depending on which side is most favorable to approach a specific area. The scrub nurse may be positioned toward the feet on whichever side is convenient. Monitors should be situated on both sides at approximately the level of the shoulders. Port placement can be somewhat variable, depending on the size of the patient and the area of the chest cavity most involved. In general, the procedure can be performed with just two ports. These are placed in the anterior and posterior axillary lines at the fifth or sixth interspace. If necessary, a third port can be positioned as needed to reach an area not readily accessible by the other two or if retraction is helpful. If the patient is large enough, one of the cannulas should be 10 mm in diameter to facilitate removal of the inflammatory peel. However, it is important to remember that the larger the port size, the more limited the range of motion will be at that site because of the rigid rib cage.

With two or three ports, mobilization of the fibrous peel can start in a systematic method under direct vision. The larger (10-mm) port should be placed at the site where the pleural space is most inflamed. A blunt grasper is used to grasp some of the peel, and a sweeping motion is used to strip as much peel as possible off the visceral and parietal pleura (Fig. 27-7). The tissue can almost be removed in strips. If the peel is less fibrous, much of it

may be able to be broken up and removed with the suction catheter. Work should proceed in a clockwise fashion to ensure that all areas are addressed. When an area becomes difficult to reach, the telescope and grasper are exchanged, usually allowing a better view and exposure to the area. If the surgeon is working out of the smaller port and the peel cannot be easily brought out through the port, it can simply be mobilized and left in the pleural cavity and then removed through the larger cannula when convenient.

The monitors also may require repositioning to keep the surgeon in line with the camera and the target area. Because the field of dissection is constantly changing, it is acceptable for the surgeon, at times, to be operating out of a partial paradox, as the stripping of the peel does not require fine motor movements. Once the majority of the peel is removed and all loculations lysed, the chest cavity is irrigated with copious amounts of saline with or without antibiotics.

A single chest tube is placed through the anterior port site and directed posteriorly so that it lies in a dependent position. If an adequate debridement was performed, it is rare to need two drainage tubes. The incisions are closed in layers with absorbable suture. If the patient is stable, it is usually possible to extubate him or her at the end of the procedure. The limited surgical trauma allows aggressive postoperative physiotherapy. Having the patient spontaneously breathe and cough should aid in keeping the lung expanded and the airway clear.

The desired goal of the procedure is to remove the majority of infected fluid and tissue, break down all loculations, free and re-expand the trapped lung, and establish adequate drainage. It is not necessary to remove every piece of the peel. The time of the procedure should be minimized to avoid a prolonged anesthetic. If adequate drainage and lung re-expansion is achieved, then the residual infected peel will be reabsorbed, as long as the patient's clinical picture improves.

Some surgeons have advocated the preoperative instillation of urokinase or other agents through a chest tube to dissolve the inflammatory peel or, in some cases, during or after the surgery.[34,35] Although a role may be found for this adjuvant therapy, its efficacy is yet to be determined. In many cases, the child would still need a general anesthetic for the chest tube and urokinase insertion, and it seems unlikely that this technique will surpass debridement under direct visualization.

LUNG LESIONS

Lung biopsy is one of the most commonly performed thoracoscopic procedures. Under general anesthesia, contralateral single-lung ventilation is obtained, as previously described. The patient is then placed in a lateral decubitus position. The chest wall is first pierced with a Veress needle followed by low-flow (1 L/min), low-pressure (4 mm Hg) insufflation to help further collapse the lung. Valved ports are used to help maintain the slight tension pneumothorax. In general, three cannulas are usually sufficient. The first port is always placed in the

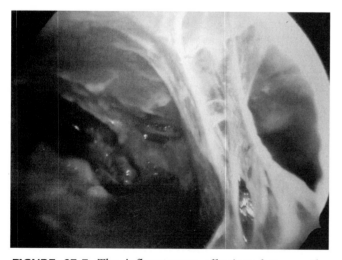

FIGURE 27-7. The inflammatory adhesions between the visceral and parietal pleural surfaces are seen in this endoscopic view.

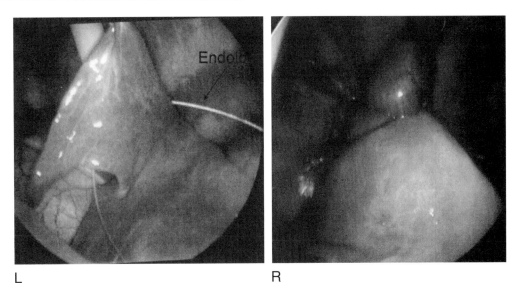

L   R

FIGURE 27-8. An endo-loop is being applied to a tongue of lung tissue for lung biopsy in a small child (*left*). A second endo-loop is being snared down to provide an air- and water-tight seal (*right*).

fifth or sixth intercostal space at the midaxillary line for the initial survey and also because injury to the lung, diaphragm, or other structures is unlikely to occur at this level. After the initial survey, the other two ports are introduced. In small children, 3- or 5-mm ports are used. In children near 10 kg or larger, a single 12-mm port is needed for introduction of the endoscopic stapler. If a biopsy is being taken from the ventral surface of the lung, the telescope should be placed through the midaxillary cannula, the grasper through the anterior port, and the stapler through the inferior and posterior site. For biopsies on the posterior surface of the lung, the position of the telescope and grasper are reversed. In smaller patients whose chest cavity cannot accommodate the stapler, endo-loops can be used to encircle and ligate sections of lung. Two endo-loops are placed at the base of the specimen, and the tissue is sharply excised distal to the ligatures (Fig. 27-8). This technique provides a hemostatic and air-tight seal equivalent to that obtained with the stapler. Specimens of 2 to 3 cm can be obtained in this manner and are adequate for diagnosis. Biopsies can easily be obtained from all five lobes by using this technique.

For biopsy of metastatic lesions, port placement is altered, depending on the site of the lesion. Although the majority of nodules are peripheral, lesions smaller than 1 cm in diameter or deep in the parenchyma of the lung may not be readily visible on the pleural surface. In these cases, preoperative CT-guided localization, as previously described (see Fig. 27-2), should be considered. At the time of operation with the lung collapsed, the marked area can easily be identified. If the lesion itself is not visible, then the area underlying the blood patch can be excised. A frozen section should be obtained to ensure that the lesion is included with the specimen. Ongoing improvements in endoscopic US probes may eventually make this the preferred technique for localization.

Resection of bullae or infectious cavitary lesions can be accomplished by using similar techniques (Fig. 27-9). The minimal morbidity associated with thoracoscopy has shifted the algorithm for treatment, and earlier surgical intervention is often being requested (Fig. 27-10). In the case of bullous disease with a spontaneous pneumothorax, it is usually advisable to combine the bullectomy with localized pleurodesis or pleurectomy. This can easily be accomplished by abrading the parietal pleura (usually the apex) with an endoscopic instrument or a small sponge placed through one of the port sites. In recurrent or severe cases, a formal pleurectomy may be

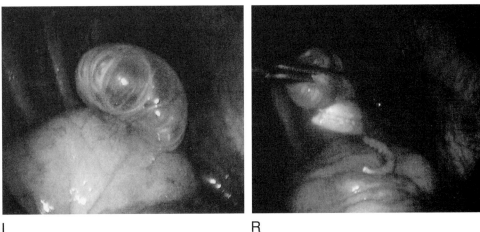

L   R

FIGURE 27-9. An apical bleb is seen in a patient with a spontaneous pneumothorax (*left*). The stapler is being used to resect the bleb (*right*).

Pneumothorax

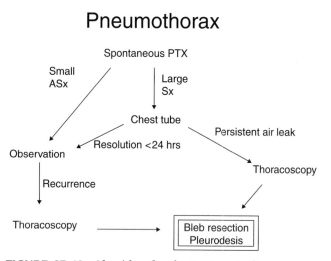

FIGURE 27-10. Algorithm for the treatment of spontaneous pneumothorax in children (Sx, symptomatic; ASx, asymptomatic).

indicated. Some surgeons prefer to use a chemical or talc pleurodesis, and these agents can all be instilled through the endoscopic ports, but, in general, this extensive pleurodesis is not necessary. Chemical pleurodesis is generally needed only in cases of malignant effusions.

Any potentially malignant or infectious lesion that is too big to fit through the cannula sleeve should be placed in an endoscopic specimen bag to prevent possible intrathoracic seeding.[36] Once the procedure is completed, a small chest tube or drain is placed through one of the port sites, and the collapsed lung is ventilated. In most cases, especially with adequate hemostasis and no effusion present, the chest tube can be removed before extubation in the operating room if no evidence of an air leak is present. This early removal avoids the considerable discomfort associated with the chest tube in the postoperative period. A chest radiograph is obtained in the recovery room, and if the lung is fully expanded, no further films are needed.

THORACOSCOPIC LOBECTOMY

The initial experience with minimally invasive lobectomy required a video-assisted approach. This technique combined the use of two to three ports and standard laparoscopic instruments with a minithoracotomy, through which standard thoracic instruments and staplers could be easily introduced.[14] These operations were technically demanding and often arduous but did spare the patient the morbidity of a formal thoracotomy. The minithoracotomy was placed in the midaxillary line, and a total muscle-sparing technique was used. With improvement in endoscopic staplers as well as energy sources that can seal both pulmonary vessels and lung parenchyma, the need for the minithoracotomy has been eliminated. These procedures can now be accomplished completely thoracoscopically through 3-, 5-, 10-, and 12-mm ports in a safe and efficacious manner.[15]

Sealing devices such as the Ligasure allow the surgeon to seal the main pulmonary vessels in smaller patients without the need for suture ligation, clips, or staples. It also seals lung tissue, preventing both bleeding and air leak. In larger patients, the articulating endoscopic stapler can be used to complete the interlobar fissure as well as ligate and divide the main pulmonary vessels and bronchi. These technical advances allow the surgeon to perform the lobectomy endoscopically. However, the surgeon's view is limited to a two-dimensional plane, and it is difficult to manipulate the lobe to look at both the anterior and posterior surfaces for a three-dimensional perspective. Therefore it is critical for the surgeon to have a good understanding of the anatomic spatial relations between the vessels, parenchyma, and bronchi, as these structures may not be visible and cannot be palpated.

The operation is performed with the patient in a lateral decubitus position, and the surgeon works from the anterior-to-posterior direction. In general, the pulmonary arterial branches are taken before the vein to minimize lung congestion, which can make the lobe even more difficult to manipulate (Fig. 27-11). Lower lobectomies are generally easier than upper ones, as dissection can proceed along the major fissure, and any vessel or bronchus crossing it is considered an end vessel and can be ligated. Upper lobectomies are much more difficult, as dissection must proceed along the main pulmonary artery, sacrificing each segmental branch to the upper lobe as it is encountered, with care taken not to injure the main trunk. Once the lobectomy is completed, the inferior port site is enlarged slightly, and the lung is removed in a piecemeal fashion if necessary. A chest tube is left overnight but can usually be removed on the first postoperative day.

ESOPHAGEAL AND POSTERIOR MEDIASTINAL LESIONS

During resection of extrapulmonary lesions such as mediastinal masses or esophageal lesions, the patient

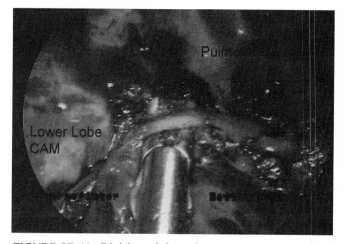

FIGURE 27-11. Division of the pulmonary artery as it transverses the major fissure during excision of a right lower lobe cystic adenomatoid malformation.

should be positioned to allow gravity to retract the lung from the field of view. This is usually accomplished by positioning the patient in a modified supine or full-prone position as already described (see Fig. 27-3). In regard to port placement, the goal is to position the telescope so that direct visualization of the area is achieved. The working ports are then situated so that the surgeon is working in line with the camera. The cannulas should not be placed too close together, as the instruments and telescope will end up dueling, making the dissection much more difficult. If possible, the telescope should be positioned superior to the working ports to avoid this problem. A 30-degree telescope allows the surgeon to look down on the instruments, much as in open surgery, and is extremely helpful when the working space is limited.

When working in the posterior mediastinum or on the esophagus, it is useful to have a flexible gastroscope, bougie, or nasogastric tube in the esophagus during the dissection. This helps to identify the esophagus by illumination or by palpation with the thoracoscopic instruments. It may also be useful for identifying any iatrogenic injuries to the esophagus. This is especially true when performing a thoracoscopic esophagomyotomy for achalasia. Having the esophagoscope in the esophagus during the myotomy not only helps identify the esophagus and check for mucosal perforations, but this internal visualization also helps to assure that the myotomy has been extended far enough distally. This visualization should help prevent an incomplete myotomy. The myotomy can be performed by using a number of different instruments, but most surgeons find a hook cautery or sharp dissection works extremely well. Care must be taken not to cause thermal injury to the mucosal lining when using these energy devices. With the hook cautery, the surgeon pulls the circular muscles away from the underlying submucosa, and the muscle is cauterized. The only question surrounding the use of a thoracoscopic approach for myotomy is whether it is appropriate to perform the myotomy without the addition of a partial fundoplication to prevent postoperative gastroesophageal reflux (GER). Most authors now believe that a significant risk of severe GER is involved after myotomy and therefore recommend performing a partial wrap with the myotomy. These two operations are more easily achieved by using a laparoscopic approach.

The same thoracoscopic exposure can be used to approach the esophageal hiatus in patients with a hiatal or paraesophageal hernia. This is especially useful in patients who have undergone a previous abdominal fundoplication and whose wrap is intact but has herniated into the mediastinum. By using thoracoscopy, the surgeon is able to approach the hiatus without having to dissect a previously operated-on field and avoids the need to take down the fundoplication wrap for adequate exposure. Both the right and left diaphragmatic crus can be exposed from the left chest, and an excellent hiatal repair can be achieved.

Other esophageal procedures that have been successfully performed and reported include resection of alimentary tract duplications, esophageal diverticula, and esophageal-wall tumors. Foregut duplications are relatively common entities that are easily approached thoracoscopically (Fig. 27-12). Once identified, the lesion is circumferentially separated from the overlying pleura. This can be accomplished either with sharp dissection, as the plane is usually avascular or by using any number of different energy sources. Generally a well-defined stalk is at the base of the duplication, although the majority do not have a luminal connection with the esophagus. They can be dissected off the muscular wall of the esophagus without entering the esophageal lumen. If a connection is present, this can be sutured or, in larger patients, an endoscopic stapler can be used to divide and seal the tract.

Bronchogenic cysts are approached similarly with dissection of the cyst down to its common wall with either the membranous trachea or bronchus. However, in these cases, the common wall often cannot be separated without causing injury or perforation of the airway. Therefore it is usually better to leave that small common portion of the back wall of the cyst intact and either excise or ablate the retained mucosal lining.

Most recently, successful repair of esophageal atresia and tracheoesophageal fistula has been successfully performed.[37-39] This operation is performed with the patient in a modified prone position with the right side slightly

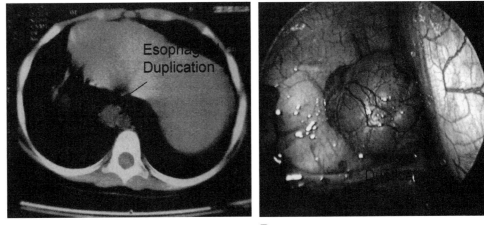

FIGURE 27-12. A foregut duplication cyst is seen on a computed tomography scan (*left*) and at thoracoscopy (*right*).

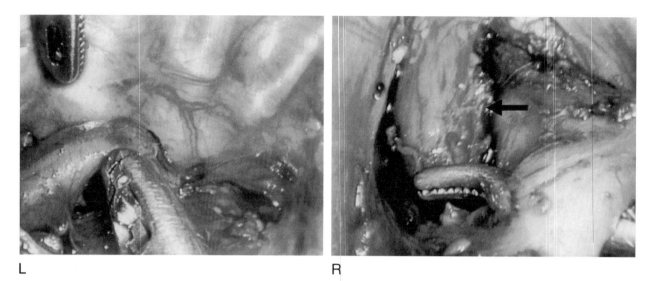

L   R

FIGURE 27-13. The distal esophagus is being mobilized near its insertion into the membranous fistula (*left*). The angled telescope is rotated to visualize the back side of the tracheoesophageal fistula (*right*). The distended proximal esophagus also is seen (*arrow*).

elevated. A three-port technique with the telescope in the posterior axillary line and the working ports in the midaxillary line allows excellent exposure. In general, CO_2 insufflation alone is adequate to collapse the right lung, and time should not be spent trying to obtain single-lung isolation. The principles of the thoracoscopic operation are similar to those of the open procedures. The first step is division of the azygous vein, which provides a good landmark for the level of the fistula. The lower esophageal segment is identified and dissected proximal to its insertion into the membranous trachea (Fig. 27-13). This is actually visualized much better than through a thoracotomy because the telescope is at a right angle to the fistula and provides a significantly magnified view. A 5-mm surgical clip or suture is used to ligate the fistula at its insertion into the trachea. The upper esophageal

pouch is then identified by asking the anesthesiologist to provide downward pressure on the oroesophageal catheter. The upper pouch is dissected free into the thoracic inlet to ensure adequate mobilization. The distal tip of the upper pouch is resected, and an end-to-end anastomosis is performed. The posterior portion of the anastomosis is performed first with a series of interrupted simple sutures, with the knots lying intraluminally. This is accomplished with 4-0 or 5-0 silk or polydioxanone suture, with the initial stitches tied extracorporeally because of the limited space. Once the back row is secured, the esophageal tube is advanced through the anastomosis into the stomach, and the anterior anastomosis is completed (Fig. 27-14). A chest tube or drain is inserted through the lower port site and advanced to a point adjacent to the anastomosis.

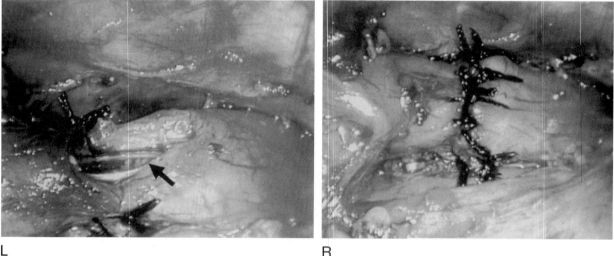

L   R

FIGURE 27-14. The posterior row of the esophageal anastomosis has been accomplished, and a small feeding catheter (*arrow*) is advanced through the anastomosis into the stomach (*left*). The completed anastomosis is seen on the right.

ANTERIOR MEDIASTINAL PROCEDURES

The entire anterior mediastinum can be easily visualized thoracoscopically and allows access to anterior mediastinal, paratracheal, and hilar masses. This is an excellent technique for lymph node biopsy and can avoid a more invasive anterior minithoracotomy or a more limited and potentially dangerous mediastinal exploration in which access and visualization is limited. These biopsies can usually be performed with three 3-mm or 5-mm cannulas. The patient is placed in a modified supine position, and the ports are placed between the third and fifth interspace and between the anterior and midaxillary line. The mass can usually be easily visualized, and resection or biopsy can be obtained without difficulty. Care should be taken in all anterior mediastinal procedures to avoid injury to the phrenic nerve, which is usually easily seen. Teratomas and mediastinal thyroid tumors also can be excised with this approach. On occasion, a minithoracotomy may be necessary to remove the specimen.

Thymectomy for myasthenia gravis also is well suited to the thoracoscopic approach. The thymus can be approached from either the right or left chest, depending on the surgeon's preference. The ports are placed in a position similar to that for other anterior mediastinal masses. The ipsilateral inferior horn is dissected first, taking care to avoid the phrenic nerve. Dissection is carried cephalad to the isthmus, and then the upper pole is mobilized. Usually a posterior thymic vessel drains into the innominate vein. Once this is sealed and divided, the contralateral horns are easily retracted to the surgeon's side and fully mobilized under direct vision.

In all these cases, the specimens can be removed through a slightly enlarged cannula site, usually in the midaxillary line.

PATENT DUCTUS ARTERIOSUS LIGATION

Closure of a persistent patent ductus arteriosus (PDA) has routinely been performed through a standard posterolateral thoracotomy with either suture ligation or vascular-clip closure of the ductus. Over the last decade, an increasing experience with intravascular occlusive devices such as coils and plugs has developed, but these techniques are often limited by the size of the patient and the diameter of the PDA.[40] Thoracoscopic closure offers an alternative to these two nonoperative techniques and affords many of the same benefits seen in other thoracoscopic procedures.

The procedure is performed with the patient in a modified prone position, with the left side elevated approximately 30 degrees. Two 3-mm ports and one 5-mm port are used to perform the operation. A right main-stem intubation is obtained, and the collapsed left lung is retracted anteriorly by gravity, exposing the ductus. The pleura overlying the ductus is dissected, starting in the middle, and it is then retracted medially. This exposes the ductus as well as mobilizes the vagus nerve out of the field of dissection. The endoscope allows excellent visualization of the ductus and the recurrent laryngeal nerve, which should help prevent injury to this structure. A 5-mm endoscopic clip can then be safely applied to the ductus, thereby occluding flow. In some cases, it is necessary to use a larger clip or to perform a suture ligation. In these cases, the 5-mm port is removed, and a standard hemo-clip can be placed through a widened cannula incision. To date, excellent results have been obtained with this technique with minimal morbidity and a significant decrease in recovery and hospitalization.

ANTERIOR SPINAL PROCEDURES

The treatment for severe scoliosis and kyphosis in children often involves extensive surgical procedures with significant associated pain and morbidity. These procedures are usually a joint effort between the pediatric access surgeon and the pediatric spine surgeon and consist of an anterior thoracotomy with release, diskectomy and fusion, followed by posterior correction and fixation with rods. Many of these children already have severe pulmonary compromise, and these procedures can lead to severe morbidity and even death. Application of thoracoscopic techniques has allowed these patients to avoid a painful thoracotomy, resulting in a decrease in postoperative pulmonary complications.

The patient is placed in a modified lateral decubitus position, tilted slightly prone, to aid in keeping the lung out of the visual field. The anterior release can usually be performed through four or five incisions, which are each 5 to 10 mm in length. Port placement depends on the number and levels of the disks to be removed. In general, the initial port is situated near the apex of the spinal deformity near the midaxillary line. The disk spaces are then evaluated, and the other ports introduced. All ports are kept in the midaxillary line so that the telescope and instruments can be interchanged as the surgeon moves up and down along the spine.

The first step is exposure of the disk spaces by incising and then clearing the overlying pleura at each level. The segmental vessels can be either preserved or ligated and divided, depending on the preference of the spine surgeon. The spine surgeon performs the diskectomy by using modified spine instrumentation and packs the disk space with allograft or other bone graft to enhance fusion. The disk spaces from T2 to T12 can be reached in this manner. The diaphragm can be locally mobilized to give access to the first and second lumbar vertebrae if needed.

A single chest tube is placed through one of the lower port sites, and the other cannula incisions closed. The operative time for this technique is now comparable to that of the open approach, and the postoperative recovery seems improved. Some centers have even started performing anterior instrumentation, but the experience is now limited to a very small number of programs. Other spinal procedures including vertebral body biopsies and hemivertebrectomy also can be accomplished in a similar fashion.

POSTOPERATIVE CARE

The postoperative care in the majority of patients undergoing a thoracoscopic operation is straightforward. Most patients after biopsy or limited resection can be admitted directly to the surgical floor with limited monitoring (i.e., a pulse oximeter for 6 to 12 hours) and are generally observed for 23 hours. If a chest tube is inserted, it can usually be removed on the first postoperative day. Pain management is usually not a significant problem. Local anesthetic is injected at each port site before insertion of the port, and one or two doses of intravenous narcotic are usually adequate in the immediate postoperative period. By that evening or the following morning, most patients are comfortable on oral codeine or acetaminophen. It is very important, especially in patients with compromised lung function, to initiate early and aggressive pulmonary toilet. The significant decrease in postoperative pain associated with the thoracoscopic approach results in much less splinting and allows for more effective deep breathing. This has resulted in a reduction in postoperative pneumonia and other pulmonary complications.

REFERENCES

1. Jacobeus HC: The practical importance of thoracoscopy in surgery of the chest. Surg Gynecol Obstet 4:289–296,1921.
2. Bloomberg HE: Thoracoscopy in perspective. Surg Gynecol Obstet 147:433–443, 1978.
3. Page RD, Jeffrey RR, Donnelly RJ: Thoracoscopy: A review of 121 consecutive surgical procedures. Ann Thorac Surg 48:66–68, 1989.
4. Rodgers BM, Moazam F, Talbert JL: Thoracoscopy in children. Ann Surg 189:176–180, 1979.
5. Ryckman FC, Rodgers BM: Thoracoscopy in the management of empyema in children. J Pediatr Surg 17:521–524, 1982.
6. Kern JA, Rodgers BM: Thoracoscopy in the management of empyema in children. J Pediatr Surg 28:1128–1132, 1993.
7. Rothenberg SS, Pokorny WJ: Experience with a total muscle sparing approach for thoracotomies in neonates, infants and children. J Pediatr Surg 27:1157–1160, 1992.
8. Rodgers BM: Pediatric thoracoscopy. Where have we come, what have we learned? Ann Thorac Surg 56:705–707, 1993.
9. Rothenberg SS: Thoracoscopy in infants and children. Semin Pediatr Surg 3:277–288, 1994.
10. Rothenberg SS, Wagener JS, Chang JHT, et al: The safety and efficacy of thoracoscopic lung biopsy for diagnosis and treatment in infants and children. J Pediatr Surg 31:100–104, 1996.
11. Smith JJ, Rothenberg SS, Brooks M, et al. Thoracoscopic surgery in childhood cancer. J Pediatr Hematol Oncol 24:429–435, 2002.
12. Hazelrigg SR: Thoracoscopic management of pulmonary blebs and bullae. Semin Thorac Cardiovasc Surg 5:327–331, 1993.
13. McKenna RJ: Lobectomy by video-assisted thoracic surgery with mediastinal node sampling. J Thorac Cardiovasc Surg 107:879–882, 1994.
14. Walker WS: Video assisted thoracic surgery: Pulmonary lobectomy. Semin Laparosc Surg 3:233–244, 1996.
15. Rothenberg SS: Experience with thoracoscopic lobectomy in infants and children. J Pediatr Surg 38:102–104, 2003.
16. Mack MJ: Thoracoscopy and its role in mediastinal disease and sympathectomy. Semin Thorac Cardiovasc Surg 5:332–336, 1993.
17. Partrick DA, Rothenberg SS: Thoracoscopic resection of mediastinal masses in infants and children: An evolution of technique and results. J Pediatr Surg 36:1165–1167, 2001.
18. Kogut KA, Bufo AJ, Rothenberg SS: Thoracoscopic thymectomy for myasthenia gravis in children. J Pediatr Surg 35:1576–1577, 2000.
19. Holcomb GW III: Indications for minimally invasive surgery in pediatric oncology. J Laparoendosc Adv Surg Tech B 6:299–304, 2001.
20. Laborde F, Noirhomme P, Karam J, et al: A new video assisted technique for the interruption of patent ductus arteriosus in infants and children. J Thorac Cardiovasc Surg 105:278–280, 1993.
21. Rothenberg SS, Chang JHT, Towes WH, et al: Thoracoscopic closure of patent ductus arteriosus: A less traumatic and more cost effective technique. J Pediatr Surg 30:1057–1060, 1995.
22. Rothenberg SS: Thoracoscopic closure of patent ductus arteriosus in infants and children. J Pediatr Endosurg Innovative Tech 5:109–112, 2001.
23. Sartorelli KH, Rothenberg SS, Karrer FM, et al: Thoracoscopic repair of hiatal hernia following fundoplication: A new approach to an old problem. J Laparoendosc Surg 6:S91–S93, 1996.
24. Pellegrini C, Wetter A, Patti M, et al: Thoracoscopic esophagomyotomy: Initial experience with a new approach for the treatment of achalasia. Ann Surg 216:291–299, 1992.
25. Rothenberg SS, Partrick DA, Bealer JF, at al: Evaluation of minimally invasive approaches to achalasia in children. J Pediatr Surg 36:808–810, 2001.
26. Mack MJ, Regan JJ, McAfee PC, et al: Video assisted thoracic surgery for the anterior approach to the thoracic spine. Ann Thorac Surg 54:142–144, 1995.
27. Rothenberg SS, Erickson M, Eilert R, et al: Thoracoscopic anterior spinal procedures in children. J Pediatr Surg. 33:1168–1171, 1998.
28. Rothenberg SS: Thoracoscopic repair of tracheo-esophageal fistula and esophageal atresia in newborns. J Pediatr Surg 37:869–872, 2002.
29. Waldenhausen JH, Tapper D, Sawin RS: Minimally invasive surgery and clinical decision making for pediatric malignancy. Surg Endosc 14:250–253, 2000.
30. Cohen Z, Shinar D, Levi I, et al: Thoracoscopic upper sympathectomy for primary hyperhydrosis in children and adolescents. J Pediatr Surg 30:471–473, 1995.
31. Tobias JD. Anesthesia for minimally invasive surgery in children. Best Pract Res Clin Anaesthesiol 16:115–116, 2002.
32. Rothenberg SS, Chang JHT: Thoracoscopic decortication in infants and children. Surg Endosc II:93–94, 1997.
33. Merry CM, Bufo AJ, Shah RS, et al. Early definitive intervention by thoracoscopy in pediatric empyema. J Pediatr Surg 9:178–181, 1999.
34. Rosen H, Nadkarni V, Theroux M, et al: Intrapleural streptokinase as adjunctive treatment for persistent empyema in pediatric patients. Chest 103:1190–1193, 1993.
35. Cochran JB, Techlenburg FW, Turner RB: Management of empyema. Pediatr Crit Care Med 4:122–123, 2003.
36. Sartorelli KH, Patrick D, Meagher DP: Port-site recurrence after thoracoscopic resection of pulmonary metastasis owing to osteogenic sarcoma. J Pediatr Surg 31:1443–1444, 1996.
37. Lobe TE, Rothenberg SS, Waldschmidt J, et al: Thoracoscopic repair of esophageal atresia in an infant: A surgical first. J Pediatr Endosurg Innovative Tech 3:141–143, 1999.
38. Rothenberg SS: Thoracoscopic repair of tracheoesophageal fistula in a newborn. J Pediatr Endosurg Innovative Tech 4:289–294, 2000.
39. Bax NM, Van der Zee DC: Feasibility of thoracoscopic repair of esophageal atresia with distal fistula. J Pediatr Surg 37:192–196, 2002.
40. Gray DT, Fyler DC, Walker AM, et al: Clinical outcomes and cost of the transcatheter as compared with the surgical closure of patent ductus arteriosus. N Engl J Med 329:1517–1523, 1993.

CHAPTER 28

Gastroesophageal Reflux

Jose Boix-Ochoa, MD, and Keith W. Ashcraft, MD

Gastroesophageal reflux (GER) is defined as a return of gastric contents into the esophagus. It is common for infants to have recurrent problems with "spitting up" or "vomiting" during the first year of life. The severity of the condition varies from an occasional burp to persistent emesis. Evaluation of most of these infants reveals no definable anatomic, metabolic, infectious, or neurologic etiology.

Because vomiting is so common as to be almost universal and is also socially acceptable in early infancy, the symptom is generally ignored, and most babies give up the disgusting and messy habit within a few months. Accordingly, GER should cause concern only when associated with additional problems such as abnormal persistence, growth retardation, and respiratory symptoms. The spectrum of clinical symptoms in pathologic GER disease (GERD) is wide, and complications are at times severe. Appropriate diagnostic studies and therapeutic steps should follow recognition of possible pathologic vomiting.

The natural history of untreated GER in children reveals that symptoms of GER almost invariably begin within the first 6 weeks of life. Sixty to sixty-five percent of such infants are essentially free of symptoms and in good health by age 2 years without treatment. Also untreated, the remainder have persistent and significant symptoms until at least age 4 years. In about 4% of the total group, esophageal strictures will develop, and 5% of the total group will die, usually of inanition or pulmonary infection.[1]

Since the late 1960s, GER has increasingly been recognized as a condition that frequently affects children with potentially serious consequences. Until the 1990s, medical treatment was relatively ineffective, and in all likelihood, most of those babies and children who did become asymptomatic did so because of the natural course of the disease. A number of effective and safe antireflux surgical procedures were developed during these years, and by adapting one or more of these techniques, pediatric surgeons were soon performing large numbers of such operations. [2–4] Antireflux procedures continue to rank second or third in frequency of major operations performed by pediatric surgeons, generally to

good effect. Long-term results in several large series are excellent, and complications are relatively few.[5–7] However, significant complications and failures do occur, and long-term results, although generally good, are by no means perfect.

Recently two major advances in management are changing the therapeutic scenario in GERD. Of most importance, the proton-pump inhibitors have revolutionized medical treatment. These drugs cure esophagitis with an effectiveness that is truly amazing in comparison with antacids, histamine-receptor antagonists, and motility-enhancing drugs. Second, antireflux operations are being performed laparoscopically in increasing numbers. Although not a fundamental change in concept, this technique shows considerable promise in terms of reducing both short-term postoperative morbidity and long-term complications such as intestinal obstruction.

In addition to these therapeutic advances, basic investigations have focused on the pathophysiologic mechanisms of reflux itself. Much information has come from studies of lower esophageal pressure profiles in normal human beings and in patients with reflux esophagitis.[8,9] Wide variations have been found in basal lower esophageal sphincter (LES) pressure that bear little relation to reflux, refuting the widely held concept of a direct relation between a low basal LES and reflux. Instead, reflux has been demonstrated to occur most often during periods of inappropriate, complete LES relaxation. These relaxations were transient (termed TLESR) and inappropriate in the sense that they were not secondary to esophageal peristalsis initiated by pharyngeal swallowing. Confirmation of these findings has led to the proposition that such inappropriate LES relaxations are the *primary* mechanism leading to reflux. Additional research with similar technical approaches has expanded our knowledge of normal and abnormal esophageal peristalsis, the role of the diaphragm in prevention of reflux, and the unsolved question of delayed gastric emptying (DGE) as important factors in this knotty puzzle. Our understanding of the multiple and complex factors controlling the esophagogastric junction has increased remarkably in the last decade but remains far from complete.

ANATOMY AND GENETICS

Various attempts to define esophageal segments have been reported. We believe that division into cervical, upper, middle and lower thoracic, and abdominal segments is adequate. With respect to GERD, the lower thoracic and abdominal segments are the most important, because the antireflux mechanism, which prevents return of gastric material into the esophagus, depends on their anatomy and physiology. The anatomic state of this area, the gastroesophageal junction, results from the complex but coordinated development of the esophagus, diaphragm, and stomach, together with the autonomic nerve innervation and the blood supply of these viscera.[11] Failure of development and maturation of the gastroesophageal junction results in structural defects and functional abnormalities that can lead to GER.

Lately, attention has focused on the possibility that GER may have a genetic basis. A specific locus associated with pediatric GER has been identified on chromosome 13. The identification of the molecular mechanisms underlying familial pediatric GERD will have important consequences, both for our understanding of the pathophysiology of this common and costly disorder and for our ability to target treatments more accurately at those mechanisms.[12–14]

HISTORY

The recognition that observed lesions in the esophagus were a result of reflux of gastric contents required about a century.[5,16–18] In 1935, Winkelstein[19] described in detail for the first time the gastroesophageal reflux syndrome. In 1947, Neuhauser and Berenberg[20] brought the disease entity of GER to the attention of pediatricians. They coined the term *achalasia* to describe a lax gastoesophageal sphincter mechanism. They outlined the clinical findings in children and suggested positional therapy for reflux. Roviralta,[1,21] in 1950, developed the concept of the "phrenicopyloric" syndrome and offered a basis for conservative treatment. The landmark work of Ivo Carré[20,22] (who termed the lesion *partial thoracic stomach* as the anatomic etiology of GERD) described the natural history of the disease and also demonstrated the salutary therapeutic effects of gravity on infants maintained mostly in the upright position.

Because little other than positional therapy existed for GERD at that time, various operative procedures were developed in the decade from 1957 until the late 1960s. The procedures described by Lortat-Jacob,[23] Hill,[24,25] Belsey,[26,27] Nissen and Rosetti,[28] and Thal[3] have contributed most importantly to the surgical procedures used today.

Refinements in diagnostic procedures and, consequently, in understanding the pathophysiology of GERD have continued from the 1960s to the present. Recently, esophageal manometry, esophagoscopy and esophageal biopsy, "esophageal clearance" and immunologic defense of the esophageal mucosa, acidity tests, 24-hour pH esophageal monitoring, scintiscan, alterations in gastroduodenal motility, duodenogastric reflux, and factors that influence the peptic activity of the gastric content on the esophageal mucosa have been the subjects of most of the publications relating to GERD.

The development of very effective pharmaceutical agents continues to be an important part of the developing story of GERD both in adults and children.

GER is perhaps one of the aspects of pediatric surgery that has advanced most over the last few years and generated the most interest, because of its frequency, variety of pathologic manifestations, and associated complications. For many years, the syndrome of GERD was termed *hiatus hernia,* a term used to describe an anatomic anomaly that may or may not be accompanied by reflux. That term has been abandoned for the more appropriate description of the pathophysiology, *gastroesophageal reflux* or GER, which implies the incompetence of the antireflux barrier to be the etiology of the disease.

PATHOPHYSIOLOGY

The pathophysiology of GERD involves acid/pepsin in the refluxate being in direct contact with the esophageal epithelium. Some acid/pepsin reflux is normal. A combination of defects in the antireflux barrier and luminal clearance mechanisms for acid/pepsin must be present to overwhelm an intact epithelium, or defects must exist within the epithelium that enable normal acid contact times to become damaging to the epithelium.

Three major tiers of defense serve to limit the degree of GER and to minimize the risk of reflux-induced injury to the esophagus. The first line of defense is the "antireflux barrier," consisting of the LES, the diaphragmatic pinchcock, and the angle of His. This barrier serves to limit the frequency and volume of refluxed gastric contents. When this first line of defenses fails, the second, "esophageal clearance," assumes greater importance to limit the duration of contact between luminal contents and esophageal epithelium. Gravity and esophageal peristalsis serve to remove volume from the esophageal lumen, whereas salivary and esophageal secretions (the latter from esophageal submucosal glands) serve to neutralize acid. The third line of defense, "tissue or esophageal mucosal resistance," comes into play when esophageal clearance is defective or not operative (e.g., motility disorders, sleep). These mechanisms are discussed.

The Antireflux Barrier

The Lower Esophageal Sphincter

In 1956, as a result of the development of esophageal manometry, a high-pressure zone (HPZ) near the esophagogastric junction was described. A sphincter muscle in the lower esophagus was proposed as the mechanism for maintaining this pressure.[29] Unfortunately, no such anatomic structure exists. Meticulous dissections of the esophagus have revealed an oblique gastroesophageal ring caused by a meager increase in muscle mass.[30] This asymmetrical muscle thickening cannot reasonably be called a sphincter. Nonetheless, a well-defined HPZ does exist in the lower esophagus and is referred to as the LES.

Patients who have had surgical removal of the distal esophagus (esophagogastrectomy) have, in manometric studies, an HPZ at the thoracoabdominal junction that relaxes on swallowing and increases with an increase in intraabdominal pressure.[31]

Esophageal peristalsis normally begins in the pharynx, progressing down the esophagus and producing, at the appropriate time, relaxation of the LES. This relaxation is brief, but it results in effective and rapid passage of ingested food and liquid from the pharynx to the stomach. Presumably, afferent and efferent vagal neural pathways controlled by brainstem nuclei mediate this sequence of events.[32]

The presence of a segment of intraabdominal esophagus is vital to the antireflux barrier[33,34] and is the key to the whole LES system.[35-38] The greater the length of the intraabdominal esophagus, the more effective the LES becomes.[39-42] When intraabdominal pressure increases, the esophagus responds as a soft tube and collapses. The diameter of the esophagus is, at most, one-fifth that of the stomach. Hence, according to Laplace's law, when the intraabdominal pressure on the esophagus is sufficient to enable it to act as a closing valve, the pressure on the stomach will increase only by one-fifth or less.

All effective surgical procedures depend on the establishment of a sufficient segment (> 2 cm) of intraabdominal esophagus.[33] In newborns and older infants, we have demonstrated that the intraabdominal segment (the pars abdominalis) is the cornerstone of the antireflux barrier.[43] Although demonstrably lacking in the neonatal period, by age 45 days, the pars abdominalis increases in relation to the total length of the LES and therefore exerts the maximal antireflux effect at beyond this age.

To understand the minimal anatomic conditions and physiological pressures necessary to ensure an antireflux barrier, we revisited our data from 6000 manometric studies and 2000 24-hour pH-monitoring studies. By using our Biomedical Statistic Studies Department to analyze all the data obtained in normal subjects and patients with GERD, we determined that a competent gastroesophageal junction depends on:

1. A gastroesophageal gradient of 2 mm of mercury, once the LES pressure has reached 6 mm, and
2. An overall LES length of 2 cm or more.

An intraabdominal pressure between 6 and 8 cm H_2O is necessary to maintain the competence of the LES, compressing the intraabdominal esophagus and sealing the gastroesophageal junction. Loss of intraabdominal pressure (omphalocele, gastroschisis, muscular weakness) can result in GER. However, increased intraabdominal pressure does not produce reflux if the positive esophageal gradient is maintained.[44,45]

Pinchcock Action

The esophagus passes through the diaphragm at the hiatus, a sling-shaped orifice formed by the right crus of the diaphragm. The crural diaphragm constitutes the external mechanism of the LES.[46,47] The anatomic disposition of this diaphragmatic sling pulls the esophagus to the right and downward, narrowing its lumen during deep inspiration.[48-52] As the esophagus passes through the hiatus, it is surrounded by the phrenoesophageal membrane, a fibroelastic ligament arising from the subdiaphragmatic fascia as a continuation of the transversalis fascia lining the abdomen. The insertion of the phrenoesophageal membrane[53-55] marks the level at which the esophagus changes from an intrathoracic to an intraabdominal structure.[56-59] This pinchcock action of the diaphragm can easily be observed during endoscopy[60] and functions to increase the LES pressures through the combination of elongation of the pars abdominalis and diaphragmatic pressure.[55,59,61-65]

Thus essentially two sphincter mechanisms are found at the GE junction: the LES and the diaphragmatic pinchcock. The two mechanisms are necessary because the pressure gradient between the esophagus and the stomach is constantly changing. Because this gradient is the driving force behind the prevention of GER, the esophagogastric junction pressure must constantly adapt to counteract these changes. This adaptive response is mediated through interaction of the LES and the crural diaphragm.[52]

Angle of His

The angle of His is that angle formed by the juncture of the esophagus with the stomach. In children with an abdominal esophagus of normal length, the angle of His is acute. This acute angle creates a double antireflux effect. When the patient attempts to vomit, more gastric contents strike the fundus than escape through the esophagus. Pressure of the contents striking the fundus narrows the angle and compresses the esophagus. However, if the angle is obtuse (e.g., as occurs from a short esophagus, hiatus hernia, or esophageal atresia), the upper stomach is converted into a funnel, and the fluids are directed into the esophagus. We have experimentally demonstrated this phenomenon in dogs.[61] The concept of the angle of His must be kept in mind when considering the most appropriate surgical technique to correct reflux in children.[66]

Mucosal Rosette

In the presence of a normal angle of His, a convoluted fold of mucosa with a rosette-like configuration is seen at the GE junction. With increases in intragastric pressure or with negative pressure in the thoracic esophagus, these mucosal folds squeeze together and act as an additional weak antireflux valve.[54,67]

Delayed Gastric Emptying (DGE)

Gastric retention and dilatation creates a distracting force producing an increase in the tension of the gastric wall directed toward the esophagus. This reduces LES length until the sphincter opens. The damaging effect of increased diameter could be reversed only by increasing the sphincter length, but gastric distention logically shortens the overall length of the intraabdominal segment, taking away the patient's last chance against reflux.[9,45]

A lot of attention and an equal amount of controversy have centered on the role of DGE in GER. In a study of the patterns of reflux, patients who had reflux in the upright position tended to have their reflux episodes within 2 hours after a meal.[68] A radionuclide gastric-emptying study in one of these patients showed significant DGE. The authors thought that pylorospasm might account for this delay, which, combined with active gastric contractions, could increase intragastric pressure above distal esophageal pressure and result in reflux. A follow-up on this observation studied patients with symptoms suggestive of GER.[69] Gastric emptying was normal in those with reflux but without esophagitis and in the controls, but those with esophagitis had significant DGE. The researchers also found that reflux episodes in those with esophagitis were significantly more numerous than in those without it.

Radionuclides in the study of gastric emptying have shown DGE in more than 40% of patients with GER.[70] Gastric emptying in patients with reflux was studied before and after fundoplication.[71] With both liquid and solid meals, gastric emptying was significantly more rapid 6 months after fundoplication than preoperatively.

Studies using isotope in water have shown DGE in children with GER,[72] but other studies using apple juice as the vehicle found no significant differences in gastric emptying between patients with and without reflux.[73] In a separate study, investigators focused on the relation of gastric emptying to retching symptoms that occurred after antireflux surgery.[74] This proved to be a complex issue. Twelve of 66 postoperative patients studied had persistent retching, and 6 of the 12 also had dumping. Those with postoperative retching and dumping had increased effective gastric emptying; those with postoperative retching alone had DGE. Of those with preoperative DGE, postoperative retching developed in only 13%. With normal preoperative gastric emptying, postoperative retching is unlikely.

Experience with a large group of children treated surgically for GER has led some to advocate pyloroplasty in conjunction with fundoplication when preoperative DGE is found.[5] In a review of 420 children treated surgically, the conclusion was that reflux and DGE were often a part of a more generalized intestinal motor disorder. Some 50% of children with symptoms of reflux also have DGE, and this percentage is much higher in those with severe mental impairment. In this report, 60 of the last 275 children who had a fundoplication also had a pyloroplasty. No leaks and no anastomotic obstructions were found in those who had pyloroplasty added and, of particular importance, no instances of persistent dumping. Again, the high risk of DGE with refluxing children who have serious mental retardation is emphasized.[75]

Another study of gastric emptying in 99 children with GER revealed 28 with DGE.[76] Of the patients with DGE, 75% were neurologically impaired (NI). Some reported findings in NI children with GER are totally at variance to this report.[77] Forty such patients with DGE had either fundoplication and pyloroplasty or fundoplication alone.

No differences between the two groups were found in incidence of recurrent symptoms, readmissions, or reoperations. Those with added pyloroplasty had significantly more postoperative complications. Another group of NI children with reflux who underwent fundoplications were studied for gastric emptying preoperatively and were divided into those with DGE and those without DGE. No postoperative differences in feeding tolerance, complications, or recurrent symptoms were noted; understandably, the authors of this report thought that pyloroplasty added no benefit for these children. Another retrospective study in refluxing children with neurologic disorders confirmed that pyloroplasty was of little benefit.[78]

Because no way is known to predict which patients with normal preoperative gastric emptying would show DGE postoperatively and because the large majority of those with preoperative DGE demonstrate normal gastric emptying afterward, a gastric-drainage operation at the time of the antireflux procedure is not thought to be warranted.[79]

Clearly, this issue remains unsettled. It is our opinion, because an antireflux operation often results in more rapid gastric emptying and because many children with DGE revert to normal gastric-emptying patterns after antireflux procedures, perhaps it is reasonable to delay a decision to perform a gastric-drainage procedure until after the antireflux procedure.

GERD: When the Barrier Breaks

Recognition of TLESR, rather than low basal LES, as the primary mechanism of reflux clearly is a major step in our understanding of this disease. In TLESR, the decrease in pressure is abrupt and profound and lasts, on average, considerably longer than the normal LES pressure decreases associated with swallowing. Furthermore, and of significance, TLESR is not associated with a peristaltic wave effective in esophageal clearance; the esophageal mucosa is exposed to the noxious effects of acid gastric contents for relatively long periods (Fig. 28-1). Nonetheless, the previously described parts of the antireflux barrier remain essential to the prevention of reflux, whatever the exact causative mechanism of the reflux episodes may be. Hence therapy, medical or surgical, must continue to address and correct, whenever possible, the deficiencies in the antireflux barrier mechanism.

Once the gastric juice gains access to the esophageal mucosa, the resultant damage depends on the balance between the erosive factors and the defense mechanisms.

Erosive Factors

Four components of gastric juice theoretically can damage the esophageal epithelium. These are: (1) hydrochloric acid (HCl), (2) pepsin, (3) bile salts (conjugated and unconjugated), and (4) pancreatic enzymes (trypsin, lipase). In the typical circumstance, however, when the gastric pH is acid, the major injurious factors are HCl and the acid-activated proteolytic enzyme, pepsin.[80] Unconjugated bile salts and pancreatic enzymes are ineffective at acid pH because the acidity renders them either insoluble

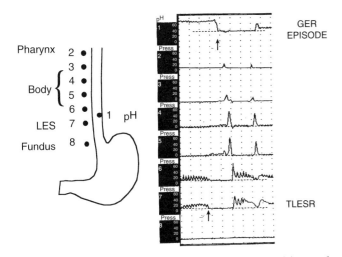

FIGURE 28-1. Abrupt LES relaxation not preceded by swallowing and resulting in a decline in esophageal pH in transient lower esophageal sphincter relaxation (TLESR). GER, Gastroesophageal reflux; LES, lower esophageal sphincter. (Manometric trace courtesy of Prof. S. Cucchiara, University of Naples.)

or inactive.[81,82] Although acid/pepsin are crucial for the generation of the symptoms and signs of GERD, the rates of gastric acid and pepsin secretion in patients with GERD remain similar to those of healthy subjects. This similarity indicates that fundamentally GERD is not a disease of excess acid/pepsin but instead is a disease resulting from the breakdown of one or more elements of the esophageal defense system.

The number and concentration of hydrogen ions obviously are intimately related to the volume and acidity of gastric secretion. We have demonstrated[83,84] that children with GER and elevated maximal acid output (MAO) are at high risk of being symptomatic. However, in spite of the symptomatology, recent studies in adults fail to show a direct correlation between esophageal mucosal damage and gastric hypersecretion. Clearly further investigation in this area is required.

Defensive Factors

Luminal acid clearance mechanisms and tissue resistance represent the hallmarks of esophageal defense.

Although not directly involved with the antireflux barrier, prompt and efficient *clearing of the esophagus* by normal peristalsis is necessary to avoid GERD. The sophistication and reliability of esophageal manometry have increased greatly with miniaturization of the manometric assemblies.[85] We now know that essentially normal esophageal peristalsis occurs in healthy preterm and term babies. These patterns were found in premature newborns as young as 33 weeks of postconceptual age.[86] Pharyngeal swallowing produced esophageal contractions 95% of the time, and of these, 70% were peristaltic and propulsive. In both infants and children, peristaltic waves ranged from 2 to 6 seconds in all age groups.[87,88] In newborns and infants (age 14 days to 11 months) with mild regurgitation and normal growth, peristaltic waves

after swallowing were comparable with those of nonregurgitating infants in terms of duration, pressure, and progression. A study of infants with significant reflux, however, shows a different picture. Thirty-four infants were evaluated for possible GER. Peristalsis was normal in those with vomiting but who were otherwise healthy. In those with failure to thrive or recurrent pulmonary disease (GERD), the amplitude of the peristaltic waves was significantly reduced, and the frequency of nonperistaltic contractions was significantly increased.

Those patients with severe esophageal mucosal disease (esophagitis, stricture, Barrett's esophagus) showed impaired esophageal peristalsis that increased with the severity of the mucosal injury. Rarely was impairment of esophageal peristalsis found in the patients who had GER but normal esophageal mucosa. The histology of resected esophageal specimens that were removed owing to stricture or Barrett's esophagus revealed both increased submucosal collagen and replacement of muscularis propria by collagen, in comparison with specimens examined at autopsy from patients without esophageal disease.

One study was interpreted to show that the impaired peristalsis with defective clearance is a result of injury to the esophageal wall. Patients with reflux esophagitis were compared with normal patients without reflux and with patients with reflux without mucosal inflammation.[89] The amplitude of peristaltic waves was lower in the esophagitis patients, and the degree of lowering increased with the severity of the esophagitis.

A comparable study of esophageal peristalsis was done in 27 infants with reflux, age 3 to 20 months, dividing the patients into those with esophagitis and those without.[90] Those with esophagitis had significantly lower amplitude of esophageal peristalsis than did those with reflux alone, and nonspecific motor defects were more frequent in the first group. Most of the reflux episodes in both groups resulted from TLESR, and this phenomenon was more frequent in those with esophagitis.

Whether the impairment of motor function of the esophagus is a primary element of the disease or is secondary to acid reflux is not absolutely clear, but the available evidence weighs in favor of its being a secondary phenomenon.

Although clearance mechanisms minimize contact between acid and epithelium, the cumulative acid contact time even in healthy subjects is significant, estimated to be 1 to 2 hours per day. This observation emphasizes the importance of the third tier of esophageal defense against reflux injury, *tissue resistance*. Tissue resistance is not a single factor but a group of dynamic mucosal structures and functions that interact to minimize damage during contact of epithelium with noxious luminal contents. For discussion purposes, tissue resistance can be broken down into three areas: pre-epithelial, epithelial, and postepithelial defense.[91,92] Traditional dogma holds that GER is a condition primarily resulting from defects in the antireflux barrier. A strong case can be made, however, for GERD, at least in part, being due to impairment in tissue resistance.[93]

The *pre-epithelial* defense in the esophagus is the least well-developed mechanism, with neither a well-defined mucus layer nor the capacity of surface cells to secrete bicarbonate into the unstirred water layer. The *epithelial* defense in the esophagus consists of structural and functional components. Structural components include the cell membranes and intercellular functional complex. These protect by limiting the rate of HCl diffusion into and between the cells. The functional components of tissue resistance include the ability of esophageal epithelial cells to buffer and transport acid. The *postepithelial* defense in the esophagus is provided principally by the blood supply. Blood flow delivers oxygen, nutrients, and bicarbonate and removes H^+ and CO_2. These functions provide protection by maintaining the normal tissue acid/base balance.

As a result of esophagitis, an increase occurs in the regional blood flow, increasing the local tissue content of prostaglandin E_2. Prostaglandin increases the permeability of the mucosa to acid, which enhances inflammation.

Esophagitis leads to irritation, dysfunction, and inflammation of the local vagal nerve endings, producing pylorospasm.[94] Pylorospasm-induced DGE promotes further GER. Effective treatment depends on measures to disrupt this vicious cycle. Esophageal strictures[95] and Barrett's esophagus are the worst complications of esophagitis.[96] In Barrett's esophagus, columnar epithelium replaces the eroded squamous epithelium in the lower esophagus.[97-99] Although it is a rare complication in children, the possibility of progression to adenocarcinoma makes early diagnosis and treatment of GERD clearly important.[100-104]

CLINICAL MANIFESTATIONS

Regurgitation is, by far, the most common symptom of GER in infancy. A distinctive type of regurgitation begins early in infancy, usually within the first week of life. The regurgitation usually is effortless and occurs with burping or when the infant is returned to his or her crib after feeding. The vomitus does not contain blood or bile. This type of vomiting, termed *chalasia,* is benign, self-limited, and rarely requires more than the simplest of treatment.[20] Occasionally, however, the regurgitation or vomiting is forceful or even projectile, so that other causes, such as pyloric stenosis, must be considered. Most babies with such vomiting grow normally, and other complications do not develop. Vomiting of this character may be considered physiologic and requires little in terms of either diagnosis or treatment.

Still, in a considerable number of vomiting infants, significant problems develop (Table 28-1). Some *fail to thrive* and become malnourished because of the loss of caloric intake. Others refuse feedings, perhaps because swallowing is painful owing to esophagitis.[105] *Irritability* is another symptom, which, like refusal to eat, may be secondary to esophagitis and its associated discomfort. *Respiratory symptoms* are particularly important in babies with GER and range from coughing, wheezing, or stridor secondary to aspiration to acute life-threatening respiratory events such as apnea and *near-miss sudden infant death syndrome* (SIDS).[106,107] Because many respiratory symptoms in infants obviously arise from other sources, primarily the

TABLE 28-1
SYMPTOMS OF GASTROESOPHAGEAL REFLUX IN CHILDREN
Vomiting
Rumination
Failure to thrive
Esophageal manifestations
Anemia, hematemesis
Chest pain, heartburn
Dysphagia
Stricture
Respiratory manifestations
Aspiration pneumonia
Laryngospasm, hoarseness
Reactive airway disease
Chronic cough
Choking, otitis, sinusitis
Apnea
Neurologic problems
Infantile irritability
Seizure-like events
Sandifer's syndrome
Respiratory
Obstruction: foreign body, cyst, tumor
Bronchial hyperreactivity caused by allergens
Infection, inflammation, cystic fibrosis
Neurobehavioral
Seizure-like spells
Vestibular disorders
Reaction to drugs
Nonspecific irritability

lungs, the causal relation between such symptoms and GER should be established as firmly as possible before surgical treatment.[108,109] Gross aspiration of gastric contents obviously can produce pneumonia, but this mechanism is rare with GER. Microaspiration with acidification of the trachea is more common, leading to laryngospasm or bronchospasm. Spasm of the larynx and bronchi also may be caused by gastric acid stimulation of vagal afferents in the esophageal wall. Esophagitis probably enhances this mechanism.[106,108]

The effects of GER on premature infants with respiratory problems have been studied.[110] Most of these infants were intubated for varying periods owing to respiratory distress syndrome or bronchopulmonary dysplasia. In the former group, GER was responsible for deteriorating pulmonary status requiring intubation. In the latter, deterioration of pulmonary status plus failure to thrive and anorexia led to the diagnosis of GER. All improved with correction of the GER.[111]

Children, in contrast to infants, less frequently regurgitate, and the symptoms of *esophagitis* predominate, as with adults. Heartburn, or substernal pain, is common. The pain is increased with ingestion of acid juices and relieved by ingestion of antacids. Pain or dysphagia may occur on swallowing. Esophagitis may progress to an obstructing stricture in addition to pain.

Although *Barrett's esophagus* does not produce specific symptoms, the condition is serious owing to the potential complications of stricture, ulcer, and adenocarcinoma. More than half of the children who have Barrett's metaplasia have associated strictures.[112,113] Neither the response to adequate treatment of GERD nor the risk of carcinoma in these children is as yet clearly defined. These children are obviously at high risk, and vigorous treatment to control or eradicate the reflux plus long-term surveillance are imperative.

The child with *Sandifer's syndrome* moves his or her head, neck, and sometimes, upper trunk into strange and contorted positions. Torticollis without spasm of the neck muscles is common. The neck may be extended or twisted. The movements may be more striking with eating but cease with sleep. This syndrome, although rare, is associated with esophagitis.[114] Owing to dystonia and bizarre posturing of the head, neck, and back, some children may be misdiagnosed as having a neurologic or even a psychiatric disturbance. The posturing disappears with appropriate management of the reflux.[115]

Diagnosis of Gastroesophageal Reflux Disease

Diagnostic procedures other than clinical evaluation should be used when the results will strongly influence treatment or will identify complications.[116,117] For the infant with frequent regurgitation but who is thriving and is otherwise well, none is needed.

Radiologic Examination

When the diagnosis of obstruction is considered or when GERD is evident, a barium study of the esophagus, stomach, and duodenum is appropriate. In expert hands, the diagnosis of reflux itself is made with a high degree of accuracy. A skilled, experienced radiologist is essential. Associated abnormalities are relatively uncommon, but conditions such as hiatus hernia, pyloric obstruction, malrotation, or some other anatomic lesion responsible for vomiting can occasionally be clearly identified.[118] *The barium study provides important anatomic information not available by other tests.* However, the study is rarely useful for quantitation of the reflux. The radiologist also can evaluate the esophagus with respect to possible structural or mucosal irregularities. Esophageal peristalsis also may be usefully evaluated, together with an estimation of the efficiency of esophageal clearance. Owing to the inert nature of the barium meal, the study does not permit a critical evaluation of gastric emptying.

Scintigraphy

This technique, by using a technetium isotope, has a number of advantages. Reflux is accurately demonstrated. The study can be prolonged for perhaps an hour until the isotope has left the stomach, thus permitting images to be taken while the infant is quiet and undisturbed. It can be used with meals or formulas that neutralize gastric acidity, an advantage over pH monitoring in this circumstance. Some measure of esophageal clearance is possible. Evaluation of aspiration by detection of the isotope in the lungs would be a major contribution from the technique,

but, unfortunately, its sensitivity for this purpose is low.[119,120] The technique is of use in measuring gastric emptying.

24-Hour Esophageal Monitoring

This technique was developed in the early 1970s for use in adults,[121] but it was soon adapted for children.[122] A pH electrode of appropriate size is positioned transnasally at the junction of the middle and lower thirds of the esophagus (usually 2.5 to 3 cm above the LES). The pH is continuously measured and recorded either on a strip chart or by a computerized pH recorder. A pH of 4.0 or less denotes reflux of acid gastric contents. The frequency and duration of reflux episodes are recorded. The number of such episodes longer than 5 minutes, the longest episode, and the percentage of time with pH less than 4.0 also are determined. Finally, with the help of a parent or nurse, the relation of reflux to a variety of activities is noted: sleep, body position, eating, and symptoms such as fussiness or coughing. Normal values have been determined, and a number of patterns of reflux have been demonstrated.[123,124] In the past, the study usually was performed in the hospital, but many are now being done quite satisfactorily at home.[125] The test is the most reliable study available for finding occult episodes of reflux and for correlating reflux and symptoms.[126] The percentage of time the pH is less than 4.0 (reflux index) is clinically useful as well as quantification of GER with a sensitivity and specificity of 94% or more.[123]

The 24-hour pH-monitoring study is indicated in the following specific circumstances:

1. Infants who have respiratory symptoms (apnea, near-miss SIDS)
2. Infants who are irritable, intractably crying, and anorectic
3. Children who have reactive airway disease (asthma) or unexplained or recurrent pneumonia
4. Children who are unresponsive to medical measures and in whom the role of GER in their symptoms is uncertain

The study also should be done in those children who again become symptomatic after fundoplication. Conversely, the study generally is not useful or necessary for infants with uncomplicated regurgitation, children with esophagitis already found by endoscopy and biopsy, and children with dysphagia or heartburn thought to be caused by GER. Three patterns of reflux have been described in symptomatic infants, as determined by extended esophageal pH monitoring[123]: continuous, discontinuous, and mixed. Those infants with the discontinuous type rarely required a surgical antireflux operation, whereas approximately half of those with the other two types did. One should keep in mind that medical treatment at the time of this study was much less effective than that in the late 1990s. Nonetheless, this study indicates that pH monitoring can be useful in sorting out infants with GER who may or may not require an antireflux procedure.[124,125] Incidentally, all of the infants in this study, including normal controls, refluxed frequently in the first 2 hours after feeding of apple juice for this study.

Newer Diagnostic Studies

We have always assumed that retrograde flow of acid/pepsin material from the stomach into the esophagus was the basic pathologic event of reflux disease. It is becoming clear that the situation is not this straightforward. Attempts to correlate symptoms other than spitting and vomiting to pH-probe–detected reflux episodes have been particularly problematic. For example, in babies with spells of choking or colicky crying, a close association between pH-probe–detected acid reflux and these symptoms cannot routinely be demonstrated. Some spells coincide with reflux episodes, but many do not. Similar questions can be raised when looking at pH-probe data on the relation between acid reflux episodes and apnea/bradycardia spells of premature infants or between wheezing, cough, dental erosion, sleep disturbance, and all the other myriad symptoms attributed to reflux.

By using one old diagnostic technique and one new, some of the disparities between pH-probe observations and "events" may be better understood. This is based on the recent observations that some reflux of "new" acid into the lower esophagus occurs while the intraesophageal pH is less than 4 after a traditional acid-reflux episode. This is called "acid rereflux" and will be missed by using only pH-monitoring techniques.[127] Acid rereflux is most likely to occur in patients with severe esophagitis, postprandially and in the recumbent posture. It is thought to be a common cause of prolonged acid contact. Detecting acid rereflux provides a better estimation of the incompetence of the antireflux barrier than do traditional pH-probe evaluations.

Two methods may be used to evaluate acid rereflux. The first is scintigraphy, which directly measures radiolabeled liquid gastric contents flowing into the esophagus, independent of the pH of the refluxate or the esophageal lumen. The second is multichannel intraluminal impedance (MII), a method that recognizes the flow of gastric contents into the esophagus by detecting decreases in impedance from high (the esophagus) to low (the stomach) values across electrode pairs placed throughout the esophagus and into the stomach. MII also can distinguish liquid from gas refluxate.[128–130]

Recent studies using MII suggest that measuring acid reflux may not be the best method of evaluating GERD.[131] These studies indicate that the pH probe does not simultaneously detect the majority of reflux events as defined by impedance monitoring, presumably because the rereflux boluses are not acid.

Endoscopy and Biopsy

Suspicion of esophagitis is the prime indication for this diagnostic procedure. Irritability and anorexia in infants and heartburn or upper abdominal pain in children raise this suspicion. Dysphagia is another indication. The study is of particular value in NI children with vomiting, growth failure, and other confusing symptoms. The endoscopist may be unable to discern esophagitis on gross inspection.[132,133] One study recorded abnormal mucosa in only 52% of children with documented reflux.

When the study did show inflammation, however, the finding was 100% specific, and in none of the nonrefluxing patients was mucosal inflammation found. Owing to the lack of sensitivity of esophagoscopy alone, mucosal biopsies are essential. Biopsies and microscopic diagnoses are both highly specific and sensitive (95%) in the diagnosis of esophagitis.[134–136] The histologic criteria for esophagitis on biopsy examination are well established. Intraepithelial inflammatory cells, eosinophils particularly, plus morphometric measures of basal cell–layer thickness and papillary height are highly specific for esophagitis. Clearly, the biopsy diagnosis of esophagitis is a most important finding because it demands prompt and vigorous treatment.

Esophagoscopy shows other esophageal abnormalities as well, particularly ulcer, stricture, and Barrett's esophagus. All three are serious complications of long-standing reflux and often coexist. Combining 35 patients from three separate studies on Barrett's esophagus in children, 16 strictures were identified.[137,138] The endoscopist often does not recognize the characteristic pink/red velvety appearance of Barrett's esophagus, emphasizing the importance of biopsies. The typical gross appearance of Barrett's esophagus at endoscopy occurs in only a minority of patients; the diagnosis rests on histologic biopsy examinations.[134] Three types of metaplastic columnar epithelium may be identified: cardiac, fundic, and intestinal. Some correlation appears between the type of columnar epithelium found and the potential for dysplasia or carcinoma.[139]

In addition to esophagitis and its complications, esophagoscopy also may show isolated patches of gastric epithelium, perhaps of congenital origin, in the proximal esophagus. Postoperative complications of repaired esophageal atresia, such as stricture or recurrent fistula, may be visualized.

Manometry

Manometry is responsible for much of our knowledge concerning GER. Maturation of the LES in early infancy was first demonstrated by this technique, only to be disputed later with the advent of more sophisticated micromanometric assemblies.[85,86] The crucial importance of TLESR to reflux changed our entire concept of the cause of GER. The technique demonstrates normal and abnormal patterns of esophageal peristalsis and clearance. Pharyngeal swallowing has been shown to be the primary factor in clearing refluxed gastric fluid in the esophagus by a study using esophageal pH monitoring in conjunction with manometry. Development of smaller and more sophisticated pressure transducers and recording devices has permitted 24-hour esophageal-motility monitoring on an ambulatory basis. With this method, deterioration of esophageal motility has been shown to parallel increasing degrees of esophagitis secondary to reflux in adults, and its use will surely be extended to children.[140]

A considerable potential for manometry exists in evaluating children with GER, but at the moment, it has limited clinical roles. It cannot directly detect reflux or injury to esophageal mucosa. It does have a role in the child with a repaired esophageal atresia in whom reflux develops.[141] The lower esophagus in such a child characteristically has poor and disorganized peristalsis, and such impairment is a major factor in determining treatment. Actually the most promising device that needs further development is the Sphinctometer, a solid-state "sleeve-like system" that has been reported to record LES pressure in the ambulatory setting. The major advantage of this system is that it does not require any water infusion; therefore it is convenient for prolonged LES pressure recording in the ambulatory setting.[142] However, only a handful of studies have been reported with this system, and it is not clear whether it can record TLESR, the major mechanism of GER in normal subjects and patients with GERD. Further improvement in sphinctometer technology is needed before it can be recommended for routine clinical use.

TREATMENT OF GASTROESOPHAGEAL REFLUX DISEASE

Once GERD has been diagnosed, the question is, which treatment should be applied, medical or surgical?[4] The decision should be selected for the individual, depending on age, anatomic information, severity, and social environment, which will affect compliance with a treatment regimen. In the majority of cases, nonoperative treatment is the therapy of choice.

Position and Feeding

Nonoperative therapy for GERD in children has been based on postural changes for many years. Alteration in the size and consistency of feedings also has been a longstanding adjunct to positional therapy. It is extremely important to assess accurately the caloric needs of the individual child so that reducing volumes of each feeding does not result in caloric deprivation. It also is important that, when adding cereal to thicken feedings, too many calories are not provided so that the child becomes overnourished. Not every infant will respond in the same manner to thickened feeds, as demonstrated by pH studies after feeding milk with cereal and milk alone.[143,144] Postural and dietary modifications alone will result in clinical improvement in the vast majority of infants with GERD.[145,146] We have obtained approximately 90% good results in 3000 patients of younger than 1 year, with a follow-up of more than 25 years in some cases.

In older children, dietary alterations include a diet low in fat, and the elimination of chocolate, coffee, tea, carbonated drinks, and spicy foods. If symptoms persist despite these dietary alterations, sodium alginate (Gaviscon) has been shown to reduce the frequency of GER as well as esophageal mucosal acid exposure.[147]

The seated semiupright position (approximately 45 degrees) for an infant with reflux has been recommended since 1956. In the 1960s, Carré[20,22] showed that 60% of children with GER treated in this way improved by the age of weaning, and an additional 30% improved

by age 4 years.[1] Other studies confirmed the effectiveness of this approach,[20,22] and in Europe, positional therapy in the chalasia chair remained the therapy of choice for many years. However, it is possible that the improvement found in the symptoms was simply due to the natural evolution of the illness, because a series of articles published between 1976 and 1983 showed by means of pH monitoring that the semiupright position worsened GER in some adults[68] and children.[146]

The European Society of Gastroenterology and Nutrition (ESPGAN) then recommended positioning babies in semielevated prone position until the flat prone position was found to be an independent risk factor for SIDS.[148] Today, the ESPGAN still recommends the 30-degree head-up, prone position, but only as the third step after thickening of feedings and the administration of prokinetic agents (e.g., cisapride) have failed in improving symptoms.

In our experience, a program of semiseated position (30 to 45 degrees), 24 hours a day and thickened and frequent small feedings to avoid overfilling the stomach, gives satisfactory results in 80% to 90% of babies younger than 14 months. Once instituted, this regimen should be continued for at least 6 months.

Failure of postural therapy may be related to social problems, chronic infections, or impaired gastric clearance. In older patients, postural treatment is impractical because of the virtual impossibility of maintaining the desired semisitting posture for sleep. Close attention to the details of postural therapy by the family members is most important to its success.[148]

Pharmacologic Therapy

If symptoms persist despite a well-monitored program of postural therapy and dietary modifications, pharmacologic measures should be added. Medical therapy includes the administration of one or more drugs that increase esophageal peristalsis, increase LES pressure, increase gastric emptying, or lessen gastric acid production.

Prokinetic Agents

A prokinetic drug (bethanecol, metaclopramide, domperidone, cisapride) is ordinarily tried first. The drug most commonly used today is cisapride (0.2 to 0.3 mg/kg dose). Although it has not been proven to diminish the frequency of TLESR, it increases the basal pressure of the sphincter, improves esophageal clearance, and accelerates gastric emptying; all are beneficial effects in the treatment of pathologic reflux. Because cisapride is generally free from significant side effects, its use has been recommended by some on the basis of a clinical diagnosis alone.[149]

Recent concerns about safety of cisapride have prompted a critical analysis of all reported adverse events and have resulted in the following conclusions and recommendations[150]: Cisapride should be administered only to patients in whom the use of prokinetic agents is justified according to current medical knowledge. If cisapride is given to pediatric patients who can be considered healthy except for their gastrointestinal motility disorder, and the maximum dose does not exceed 0.8 mg/kg per day in three to four administrations of 0.2 mg/kg (not exceeding 40 mg/day), no special safety procedures regarding potential cardiac adverse events are recommended. However, in patients who are known to be or are suspected of being at increased risk for drug-associated increases in QT interval, great care must be taken with the administration of cisapride. Such patients include those

1. With a previous history of cardiac dysrhythmias,
2. Receiving drugs known to inhibit the metabolism of cisapride and/or adversely effect ventricular repolarization,
3. With immaturity and or disease causing reduced cytochrome P450 3A4 activity, or
4. With electrolyte disturbances. In such patients, electrocardiography (ECG) monitoring to quantitate the QT interval should be used before initiation of therapy and after 3 days of treatment to ascertain whether a cisapride-induced cardiac adverse effect is present.[151]

Acid Alteration

Measures to reduce gastric acidity should be given to patients with complicated reflux, especially with esophagitis.[152] Alteration in gastric acid may be accomplished by neutralization with antacids, competition with histamine H_2–receptor antagonists or by proton-pump inhibitors. Histamine H_2–receptor antagonists or antacids are being used less and less today, although the latter seems particularly useful in controlling heartburn. H_2-receptor antagonists may have a beneficial effect for patients whose respiratory symptoms are suspected of being caused by microaspirations.

The proton-pump inhibitor, omeprazole, has been demonstrated to reduce gastric acid production to zero.[153-155] It is a very powerful drug that affects gastric acid production for 72 hours after cessation of administration. A prospective study determined that, within the therapeutic dose range (0.7 to 3.3 mg/kg/day), omeprazole was both efficacious and safe for children. To date, problems due to hypergastrinemia observed in the gastric mucosa of children with long-term treatment with the drug ($\leq$4 years) are benign (fundic polyps, expansion of the parietal cells, and pseudohypertrophy of individual parietal cells).[156,157] PPIs inhibit the final step of gastric acid secretion by blocking proton production.

Experience with these drugs in children is more limited than that in adults; however, some reports indicate that they can be used in very resistant esophagitis and in special situations, such as in lieu of surgical procedures for GERD in NI individuals. An initial dosage of 0.7 mg/kg/day has been suggested, with subsequent adjustment by repeated prolonged intraluminal esophagogastric pH determinations.[153]

A recent study showed that omeprazole is highly effective in even grade IV esophagitis.[154] A dosage of 0.7 mg/kg/day healed 45% of patients, and 1.4 mg/kg/day healed another 30%. On a bodyweight basis, the dosages

required in children are generally higher than those in adults. For children unable to swallow the whole capsule, it is suggested to open the capsule and give the granular contents in a weakly acidic vehicle such as orange juice, yoghurt, or cranberry juice. The granules are stable in acid but are degraded in a neutral or alkaline pH. New proton-pump inhibitor (PPI) medications (lansoprazole, rabeprazole, pantoprazole, esomeprazole), promise to offer better medical therapeutic possibilities.[158-161]

Recently it was demonstrated that in normal subjects, the γ-aminobutyric acid (GABA)$_B$ agonist, baclofen, significantly reduces GER by inhibition of transient LES relaxations.[162] These findings suggest that GABA$_B$ agonists may be useful as therapeutic agents for the management of reflux in patients with GERD, acting centrally on the pattern generator in the brainstem to inhibit the triggering of TLESR.[163-167] This drug appears to offer great potential as the major inhibitory neurotransmitter within the central nervous system controlling the rate of TLESR, the key mechanism underlying most episodes of GER.

Compared with other available agents, baclofen is available as an oral agent and does not have adverse effects on basal LES pressure or acid clearance. Side effects are common, however, and include drowsiness, nausea, and the lowering of the threshold for seizures. It is hoped that new compounds with more specific and better-targeted action will be developed in the future.[168]

Surgical Treatment of Gastroesophageal Reflux Disease

The pediatric surgeon must bring to any discussion of "definitive" therapy the question of whether medications are simply delaying the final treatment; an operation that may offer a better quality of life. Certainly antireflux surgery may provide a more permanent and less expensive solution to refractory GERD in children. Although PPIs appear to be well tolerated for short-term use (3 to 7 months), studies to assess long-term safety are needed, because the significance of elevated gastrin levels in children is unknown. Patient compliance and drug expense over many years are certainly considerations in selecting definitive therapy.

GERD is a disease that can be mitigated by the reduction of gastric acid production. Successful therapy with nonoperative means does not mean that the natural history of the GER can be ignored. Clearly adults with GERD must continue medications or have recurrence of symptoms. Very likely those adults who have GERD had GER as children and represent those who did not spontaneously achieve lasting relief. In the authors' experience of treating pediatric GERD for 3 decades, we expected a successful operation to "last" indefinitely. In those patients who have recurrence of symptoms, we have almost always demonstrated breakdown of the fundoplication. In the instances in which we have personally followed up asymptomatic patients for a decade or two, the few patients in whom we could justify repeat upper gastrointestinal radiologic studies and/or extended pH monitoring, the fundoplications were intact, many having had the operation within the first year of life.

When conservative treatment fails, however, or age, type of anatomic anomaly, severity, respiratory complications, or social environment make it necessary, surgery is the next step, and one that should be effected without delay.

Short- and long-term results and low complication rates of fundoplication make this a safe therapeutic method with very few risks.[169] Results of surveys among parents show that 97% of them were satisfied with the postoperative results in their children, in contrast to surveys of patient satisfaction in adults, in whom symptoms persist in 27% to 54% of patients.[170–174]

Two different concepts govern the most commonly used operative procedures. Many surgeons subscribe to the complete wrap of the fundus around the newly established intraabdominal esophageal segment, as typified by the Nissen fundoplication. Recent research in adults suggests that this "mechanical mechanism" has a functional counterpart in the form of inhibition of triggering of transient LES relaxations in addition to effectively making a 360-degree angle of His, where intragastric pressure prevents complete relaxation of the LES. The alternative surgical aim is to correct the abnormal anatomy while permitting the normal physiologic antireflux mechanisms to remain effective. The Thal[3] and the Boix-Ochoa[62,175] partial-wrap fundoplications are examples. The essentials of these operations, which differ only slightly, are the provision of a sufficiently long intraabdominal esophagus, fixation of the intraabdominal esophagus by the 180-degree wrap and restoration of the normal angle of His (Fig. 28-2). Both the Thal and the Boix-Ochoa techniques allow a physiologic degree of GER, avoid the "gas-bloat" problem, and even permit vomiting. The reader may sense that these procedures are our personal preferences. Results of using either surgical approach are excellent, at least in neurologically normal (NN) children, although the Nissen procedure is followed by a higher incidence of complications (Fig. 28-3).[176–178]

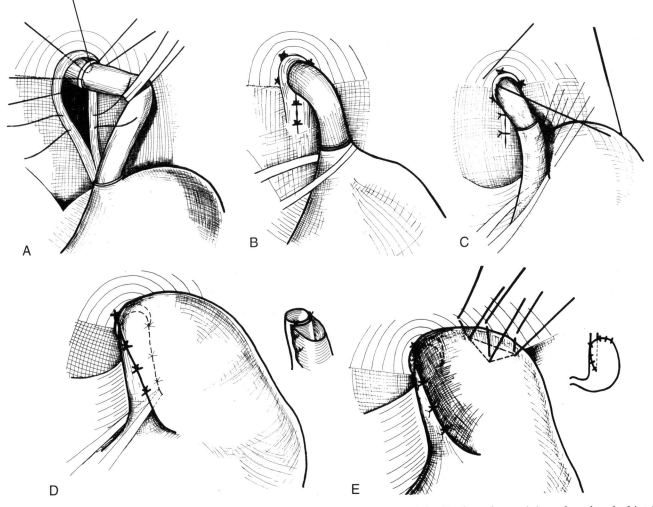

FIGURE 28-2. Boix-Ochoa technique. *A* and *B*, After exposure and mobilization of the distal esophagus, it is anchored to the hiatal crura to ensure as long an intraabdominal segment of esophagus as possible. The posterior pillars are closed. *C*, Restoration of the angle of His by a suture from the fundus to the right crura. *D*, The anterior plication is constructed by placing sutures between the gastric fundus and the intraabdominal esophagus. *E*, Three sutures, which suspend the fundus superiorly, are placed between the fundus and the undersurface of the left diaphragm.

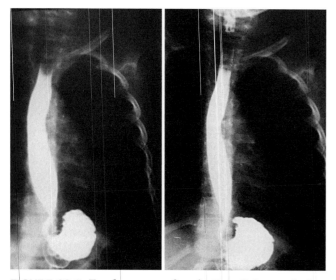

FIGURE 28-3. Esophagogram after the Boix-Ochoa antireflux procedure.

The most widely used procedure is the Nissen.[2] The reasons for this choice on the part of the majority of surgeons is not entirely clear because the creation of a satisfactory Nissen fundoplication requires great care. Because the newly created antireflux mechanism is often too competent, concomitant gastrostomy is recommended by some authorities to act as a vent for postoperative wrap protection, for gastric venting if the "gas bloat" occurs, and for postoperative feeding.[179,180]

The Nissen fundoplication has been used much more frequently than any other operation. The lower esophagus is mobilized so that an adequate intraabdominal length is assured. A cuff of stomach is thus created by passing the fundus from left to right behind the esophagus; usually requiring division of at least some of the short gastric vessels. The right and left margins of the wrap are sutured together anteriorly, including the anterior esophageal wall in the two or three sutures. The superior margin of the wrap is fixed to the hiatus with a few additional sutures. The wrap should be relatively short (depending on the age of the child) and constructed loosely (floppy) around a large intraesophageal bougie placed during the operation. The wrap transmits intragastric pressure to the lower esophagus, raises the LES pressure, and acts as an effective one-way valve. A gastrostomy is almost routinely added in NI children. Early postoperative complications are uncommon.[181,182] Small bowel obstruction has been reported in 4% to 9% in the first 2 years after operation.[183-185] Most of these resulted from intraabdominal adhesions after the open Nissen procedure. A more significant problem is failure of the wrap, occurring in from 4% to 12% in the larger series.[183-188] These failures usually resulted from disruption of the wrap or herniation of the wrap upward through the hiatus. Reoperation on those with a failed wrap was successful on a long-term basis in about 75% to 80%, and overall long-term good results are reported at about 90%.

In the Thal and Boix-Ochoa procedures, the lower esophagus is similarly mobilized, and the crura approximated posterior to the esophagus to reestablish a hiatus of "normal" size. The hiatus closure, described as a "limiting" stitch, also is used to affix the esophagus posteriorly to the hiatus, aiding in the maintenance of the intraabdominal esophageal segment. Early experience in which this step was omitted resulted in an unacceptable rate of recurrent hiatus hernia. A partial, 180-degree anterior fundal wrap is then constructed, plicating the available upper fundus to the easily accessible anterior esophageal wall. The procedure does not require division of short gastric vessels, is technically simpler than a Nissen procedure, and has a shorter operating time. The Boix-Ochoa procedure differs from the Thal in that the remaining fundus is fixed by interrupted sutures to the underside of the left hemidiaphragm to ensure the angle of His. The incidence of postoperative intestinal obstruction is low (<1%), probably due to the authors' use of the transverse upper abdominal incision with minimal exposure of the intestine.[189] In a series of 1150 patients who had Thal's fundoplication at one institution, disruption of the fundoplication and recurrent GER occurred in only 2%, and with recurrent hiatus hernia, in another 2%. A distinct advantage of a lesser wrap is the very low incidence of gas-bloat syndrome, so that a gastrostomy is done only when the patient's underlying condition requires prolonged tube feeding. These children are able to burp or even, when necessary, vomit. Overall good results exceed 90%. In both of the authors' experience, the number of NI children was low, whereas in most other large series of Nissen fundoplications, the incidence of NI children is often 50% or higher. The partial-wrap procedures seem to be more attractive to the parents of NN children with GERD because the complication rates are lower than reported with Nissen fundoplications, and parental satisfaction was extremely high.

Another partial-wrap method is the Toupet procedure, also developed to minimize the gas-bloat problem. In this operation, a partial, 270-degree wrap is positioned posterior to the esophagus. The preliminary steps of the technique are identical to those of the previous two procedures. The Toupet procedure can be performed through an upper abdominal transverse incision, so that exposure of the intestine is largely avoided. After the crura have been approximated to restore the size of the hiatus to normal, the gastric fundus is passed posterior to the esophagus. Division of some of the short gastric vessels is often necessary. The posterior aspect of the wrap is sutured to the right crura. The margins of the wrap on either side are then sutured to the right and left margins of the esophagus, leaving the anterior esophageal wall free. Experience with this operation in 112 patients revealed that 30% were NI.[190] The early postoperative course was generally described as benign, but in 2, intestinal obstruction developed. On late follow-up evaluation, the outcome was excellent in 90%. Six reoperations were necessary because of recurrent GER. Dysphagia was a temporary problem in 6, and gas bloat was not a problem.

In 1991, the feasibility of performing Nissen fundoplication in 12 adults by using a laparoscopic approach was demonstrated.[191] In rapid succession, additional reports appeared confirming the practicability and safety of this technique in adults. To show how the pendulum has swung in some quarters vis-à-vis medical treatment, a recent report proposed laparoscopic fundoplication as a reasonable alternative to omeprazole.[192] Laparoscopic approaches to fundoplication in children are being reported with increasing frequency and have served only to increase the relative percentage of Nissen fundoplications for pediatric GERD. Technically, the laparoscopic Nissen is much easier to perform that either the Thal or the Boix-Ochoa. Reports of endoscopic antireflux operations performed on children document both feasibility and satisfactory short-term results.[193,194] One group's experience not only detailed the learning curve but also described a rapid decrease in the percentage of cases in which conversion to an open operation was required, from 30% after the first 20 cases to a cumulative rate of 7.5% after 160 cases.[195] A similar decline in complication rate also was noted, falling from an early 12% rate to a final cumulative rate of 7.4%. Some proponents of laparoscopic partial-wrap fundoplications maintain that the establishment of a more physiologic LES is worth the extra effort involved.[196]

The larger question is not which operation, but rather, when. Until the mid-1990s, the indications for surgery were reasonably easy to define. The results of nonoperative therapy for the severe or potentially dangerous complications of reflux were generally unsatisfactory; thus failure of medical management was common in those children at the highest risk of significant morbidity or even death. As a consequence of omeprazole and the appearance of other new drugs that have enhanced medical treatment, the most appropriate therapy for children with severe GERD is evolving, and our present indications for surgery are changing.

Postoperative Complications

As has been found in most other studies of fundoplication operations, the complications occurred significantly more often in the NI than in the NN. The early complications after laparoscopic Nissen were 41% in NI patients versus 17% in NN patients. The late complications occurred in 13% of NI patients and none of NN patients. The authors conclude that the laparoscopic technique is superior to the open method in the performance of Nissen antireflux procedures.

The results of the combined experience with antireflux operations from seven large pediatric surgical departments are encouraging.[169] In total, 7467 children were included. Significant clinical improvement was recorded in 94% of NN children and in 84.6% of the NI group. Major postoperative complications were recorded in an average of 4.2% of the NN patients and in 12.8% of the NI patients. Postoperative deaths (within 1 month of operation) were found in 0.07% of the NN patients and in 0.8% of the NI patients. Reoperation was necessary, on average, in 3.6% of the NN and 11.8% of the NI groups. These data show the significant differences between NN and NI children, but more important, they emphasize the satisfactory overall outcome in both groups. The unique problems of the NI children with GER, feeding problems, or both are addressed in more depth in a later section on GER and neurologic impairment. In the previously cited study, only minor variations occurred in the overall results or complication and reoperation rates, irrespective of the type of antireflux procedure used.

Critics of this large, combined study take issue with some of the data and conclusions.[197] They point to the relatively high morbidity of antireflux procedures in high-risk children such as those who are NI and those who had previous repairs of esophageal atresia. The excellent short-term results with omeprazole in these high-risk groups make the medication a viable alternative. At the least, drug therapy may provide a considerable amount of relief and permit postponement of the decision for or against operation for a considerable time.

It is probably true that no one technique will be the best for all patients, and the antireflux operation should be tailored to the child's situation. One has to be very cautious in interpreting the results published, because the groups are different in the percentages of composition.[198,199] If the results of the Boix-Ochoa procedure appear too good in comparison with other publications, the key is that we are dealing with a patient population group in which only 7% of the patients are NI, in contrast with other groups. The NI patient is the most difficult to deal with and has more complications. A recent report stated, "In our experience, the Boix-Ochoa antireflux procedure should be the procedure of choice in the surgical treatment of G.E.R. in otherwise normal children, while the Nissen fundoplication is preferable in neurologically impaired children and in patients with G.E.R. following esophageal atresia repair."[200]

GASTROESOPHAGEAL REFLUX DISEASE AND NEUROLOGIC IMPAIRMENT

The most difficult clinical problem in the field of GER is the overall management of the severely NI child with persistent vomiting. To begin, such vomiting is common, much more so than with normal children; 15% of institutionalized, severely retarded children had recurrent vomiting, with a frequency of at least eight episodes per month.[201] Three-fourths of the vomiting children were shown to have GER. Although a few prior reports pointed out the occurrence of reflux or hiatus hernia in such children, this study strongly enforced the magnitude of the problem and paved the way for many studies and therapies designed to ameliorate it.

Earlier, such vomiting was largely thought to be psychogenic in origin or simply part of the primary neurologic disease, and little effort was made to investigate the cause critically. Perhaps for this reason, although the vomiting often began early in infancy, diagnosis was usually made relatively late. In those for whom a surgical antireflux procedure was eventually done, the average age at operation was considerably older than for normal children.

At least half of normal children have their operations in infancy, whereas retarded children's representative average and mean ages at operation were 7.5 and 5.9 years, respectively.[202,203]

A number of manifestations or complications of the primary neurologic disease are common. This may both delay the diagnosis of and predispose the child to the development of GER. Vomiting, already mentioned, is the most common of these complications, and its misinterpretation is a major factor in delay of diagnosis. Difficulty in feeding or even refusal of feedings is a frequent problem in these children, a problem not uncommon with GER as well. The vast majority of the NI children are nonverbal; communication and proper identification of symptoms may be exceedingly difficult. A similar proportion also are nonambulatory; therefore gravity as an aid to esophageal propulsion is not helpful. Increased intraabdominal pressure also probably plays a role. Scoliosis, spastic quadriplegia, and seizures all are problems in many of these children, and all result in periodic elevations of intraabdominal pressure, enough to overcome the normal antireflux barrier and allow chronic reflux. Severe growth retardation also is common in these children, a complication shared with some normal children with reflux and obviously accentuated in the NI children in whom reflux develops.

Complications of GER itself are generally more advanced in NI children than in the NN group. Esophagitis is the most prominent of these. Esophagoscopy has been used as a major diagnostic tool in many reported studies, and esophagitis has been a common finding (66% to 100%).[204,205] Esophageal stricture, as expected, is frequently identified.[206] Barrett's esophagus, a condition associated with both esophagitis and stricture, also has been found much more commonly in NI than in NN individuals. In one study of institutionalized adults, 26% had Barrett's esophagus changes on esophagoscopy and biopsy.[207] Another study in children and young adults found a strikingly higher incidence in the mentally retarded group as compared with the NN group.[208] Respiratory problems, particularly repeated episodes of pneumonia, are common and almost always require hospitalization. Various investigators have documented these problems in from 35% to 85% of the patients.[202-206] One group of investigators found that 18% of the children had a history of apneic episodes before surgery.[209] Obviously, many of these complications, both of the neurologic disease and of GER, are interrelated, and a careful, methodical evaluation is essential when planning appropriate management. Equally obvious, most of these children have a serious and advanced degree of reflux disease.

Diagnostic studies in this group of children are basically the same as in the NN group, but a few modifications are in order. The radiologist, while performing the barium upper gastrointestinal series, must pay particular attention to the possibility of orotracheal aspiration. This is relatively common and must be appreciated before any surgical operation. An antireflux procedure may not be helpful if oropharyngeal aspiration is significant, and, indeed, the problem of aspiration might be worsened.

Abnormal esophageal motility is relatively common, perhaps secondary to esophagitis. Hiatus hernia is more often found in NI patients than in the NN group, 51% in one study.[210] Extended esophageal pH monitoring can be accomplished as a standard method, but in some, the probe is poorly tolerated and may be pulled out repeatedly. Endoscopy with biopsy is helpful, as noted previously, because the incidence of esophagitis, stricture, Barrett's esophagus, and hiatus hernia is relatively high.[208]

Enteral Feeding

The provision of adequate nutrition in NI children is often the primary goal. Enteral feedings via a nasogastric tube generally were considered impractical, except as a short-term method in infants with malnutrition secondary to GER. In one study, 12 infants (11 NN) were treated with continuous infusion of formula through a small-caliber nasogastric feeding tube for 11 to 13 days. Of the 12 infants, 8 had a favorable early response with adequate weight gain and cessation of vomiting. Ten were followed up for 3 to 12 months, 5 of whom continued to grow normally and did not require fundoplication.[1] In this small series, the solitary NI patient did not respond.[211]

Gastrostomy is the most common long-term solution for enteral feeding. The procedure can be done by a standard Stamm gastrostomy or by the percutaneous endoscopic gastrostomy (PEG) method.[212] The Stamm gastrostomy can be done via a laparotomy or laparoscopically. PEG is a quick and simple technique and has been widely adopted, although it has some unique complications of its own. In a substantial number of children without prior clinical evidence of GER, reflux develops after a gastrostomy, irrespective of whether the procedure is a Stamm or a PEG.[213-216] In about two-thirds of children who have normal studies before gastrostomy, GER develops postoperatively, and about half eventually become symptomatic.[217] Why gastrostomy causes GER remains undetermined; widening the angle of His by pulling down the fundus during the procedure is one possible explanation. Owing to the high incidence of reflux after gastrostomy, routine antireflux operations have been recommended and practiced in a number of pediatric surgical centers. Many, however, believe that all patients referred for feeding gastrostomy should be evaluated for GER and that only those with significant clinical reflux should have a concomitant antireflux procedure. For those in whom clinical reflux develops postoperatively, the antireflux procedure may be done at that time.[218] Fundoplication *after* gastrostomy is a much more difficult procedure than is fundoplication *with* gastrostomy.

One should realize that an antireflux operation is not necessarily mandatory in the NI child with reflux whose primary problem is nutrition. Converting bolus gastrostomy feedings to continuous feedings can dramatically resolve vomiting and result in excellent weight gain and markedly diminished pulmonary complications.[219] Another option in NI children who need a feeding gastrostomy and who have minimal to moderate reflux is to place the gastrostomy tube on the lesser curvature, thus fixing the stomach to the posterior right rectus fascia, as in a Boerema anterior gastropexy. This modification was reported in nine NI children, only two of whom had moderate GER preoperatively. All did well without clinical symptoms of GER and with marked nutritional improvement. Postoperative barium studies in eight did not show reflux.[220]

Still another approach in these children is to use a jejunostomy. By one technique, a percutaneous gastrostomy is established under fluoroscopic control while a small plastic tube is threaded through the gastrostomy tube and guided into the jejunum. Comparison of this technique with a Nissen fundoplication showed a strikingly lower incidence of complications in the former.[221] Obviously, this same principle could be achieved by passing the jejunal tube through a preexisting gastrostomy. One annoying problem in such methods is occasional displacement of the feeding jejunal tube upward into the stomach and the necessity for its replacement under fluoroscopic control. This technique does not directly treat the GER, and medical management must be continued. A final method along these same lines is a Roux-en-Y jejunostomy for feeding. A gastrostomy for decompression is done at the same time if one is not already in place.[222] This procedure obviously is more complex, but the results in a small series have been excellent in terms of improved nutritional status and dramatic decrease in GER symptoms.

Antireflux Surgery in Neurologic Impairment

Surgical measures to correct reflux have been the standard treatment since the 1970s in both NI and NN children, owing to the generally poor response to medical therapy, including upright positioning, thickening of feedings, and drugs such as H_2-receptor antagonists and prokinetic agents. The exact percentage of NI children without demonstrable GER who receive an antireflux procedure in conjunction with a feeding gastrostomy is difficult to determine, but in one series, the indication for the antireflux operation was prophylactic in 30%.[223]

All of the various antireflux surgical procedures have been used in NI children. The Nissen has been most often used, as with NN children, but the Thal operation also has been used almost exclusively in some series.[224,225] The most vexing problem with these children is the high rate of both postoperative complications and deaths within the perioperative period as compared with NN children undergoing the same procedures. One series noted an early complication rate of 11% and a late complication rate of 26%.[226] All but one of the early complications were small bowel obstructions; more than half of the later complications were wrap herniations or wrap failure. NN children from this same institution had one-third the number of early complications and less than half the rate of late complications. Reoperation for late complications was required in 19%. The Nissen fundoplication was used in about 80% of the NI children, and Thal fundoplications in the remainder. Another series reported on 35 profoundly disabled children who had antireflux procedures, almost all of which were

Nissen fundoplications.[223] Perioperative complications, which were nonfatal, developed in 17%, and three additional complications were responsible for death. Late complications included bowel obstruction requiring laparotomy (3 patients) and recurrent GER (7 patients). A second antireflux operation was performed in 6 patients. The results of the anterior gastropexy of Boerema in 50 NI children were similar: 25 early and 9 late complications, 17 reoperations, and 2 deaths related to the operation.[227] A still larger series reported distressingly high complication rates after Nissen fundoplications in 193 patients.[228] Both of the authors reporting on fundoplication questioned the advisability of continuing with operations that were designed to improve the quality of life in these children but that were plagued with numerous problems.

Experience with the Thal operation suggests a more optimistic picture, with an 8% failure rate and an 11% complication rate.[224] The complication rate is about the same as with the NN children, but the failure rate in the NN is only 2%. In a series of Thal procedures in 141 NI children, recurrent GER or recurrent hiatus hernia required reoperation in 10%.[225] Only 6% required a later pyloroplasty due to DGE for symptoms of gagging and retching.

It is more than apparent that antireflux operations in NI children carry a considerably higher risk than in otherwise normal children. The reasons for the high incidence of wrap failure have not been clarified. Certainly, those with severe growth failure may have impaired wound healing. Chronic or periodic increased intraabdominal pressure from retching, recumbency, and seizures may be important causative factors. Because the Thal procedure permits belching and vomiting, less strain against this partial wrap may occur than against a complete wrap; thus a partial wrap may be the preferable option. These disquieting results are cause for serious consideration as to the best therapy available for these children. However, in all the series cited, most of the children were much improved, and parents and other caregivers expressed a high degree of satisfaction with the outcome. In a study that examined this important issue, feeding indices were improved, and the child's comfort and quality of life were perceived to be significantly better.[229] Furthermore, the level of frustration in caring for the child was less, and the quality of life for the parents as well as for the child was improved.

ESOPHAGEAL ATRESIA AND GASTROESOPHAGEAL REFLUX DISEASE

GER after repair of esophageal atresia malformations is common. The frequency is difficult to establish precisely, but significant reflux occurs in at least 50% of these babies.[230–233] In cases of isolated esophageal atresia (no tracheoesophageal fistula [TEF]), the incidence of GER after primary repair was 100% in a series of nine infants.[234]

The cause of the GER has been assumed by many to be secondary to the repair of the esophageal atresia itself. Tension on the anastomosis with upward displacement of the lower esophageal segment may shorten the intra-abdominal esophagus and widen the angle of His. Dissection of the TEF and the lower esophageal segment may damage the vagal innervation, or scarring secondary to the dissection may have the same effect. A study of 25 such children revealed that excessive tension at the anastomosis was the only factor studied that was associated with an increased incidence of GER.[232] However, most investigators in the field now believe that the cause is a primary, probably congenital, defect in the motor function of the distal esophagus.[235–238] Esophageal dysmotility, aperistalsis, nonprogressive contractions with low amplitude, and disorganized contractions all have been observed.

The long-term follow-up study of 22 adolescents or young adults who had repair of esophageal atresia and distal TEF as newborns examined some of these problems.[239] The technique used was a combination of 24-hour esophageal manometry and pH monitoring on an ambulatory basis. Half had a pattern of long nocturnal episodes of reflux with very slow clearance. All had markedly diminished esophageal contractibility, disorganized propulsive activity, and absence of acid-clearing capacity. Propulsion of ingested fluids and solids as well as clearance of refluxed fluids was accomplished largely by gravity. GER was noted in more than half of these patients, so that it is clear that the reflux noted early in life in these children persists indefinitely.

The clinical manifestations of reflux are similar in many ways to those of otherwise normal children with GER. Respiratory symptoms, such as recurrent pneumonia, are common, and life-threatening episodes of apnea or cyanosis may occur.[233,240] Failure to thrive due to recurrent vomiting, dysphagia, and esophagitis is often a problem. The esophageal anastomosis may become tight, and the stricture often does not respond to dilation, presumably because of the frequent reflux of acid fluid. Esophagitis is particularly common (Fig. 28-4).

Conventional medical treatment is effective in about half of the children. This includes upright positioning, thickening of the feedings, H_2 blockers, and prokinetic drugs such as cisapride. Owing to dysphagia, supplemental gastrostomy feedings may be necessary. Infusion gastrostomy feedings are probably more effective than bolus feedings because less vomiting results. Omeprazole has not been reported as treatment for these infants to date, but it surely is being tried and may be helpful because esophagitis and persistent strictures are common.

When medical measures are not effective and complications such as failure to thrive, apneic spells, recurrent pneumonia, or anastomotic strictures persist, some form of antireflux surgical procedure is necessary. Many reports document excellent results. Fifteen infants with tight anastomotic strictures failing to respond to repeated dilations were reported.[241] The cause was thought to be frequent episodes of reflux, and all were managed with an antireflux operation. The stenoses were cured in all. Another group of children was reported to have excellent but slightly less spectacular relief of stricture, vomiting, pneumonia, and dysphagia.[242] Nissen fundoplications were performed in all nine with no major complications and with relief of their reflux symptoms in all. Respiratory problems were markedly diminished, and the strictures were successfully managed.

However, surgical treatment of reflux in this group of children has been, by no means, uniformly successful. The experience with fundoplications used in 14 children with GER after repair of esophageal atresia and TEF was reported to be distressing.[230] After fundoplication, half

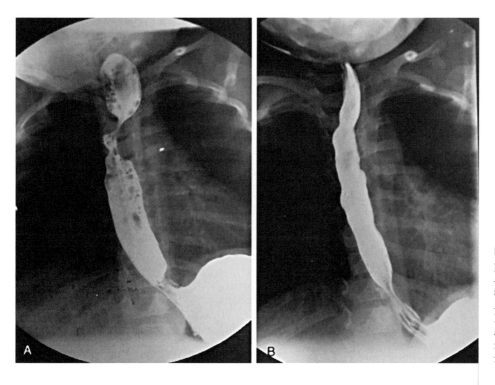

FIGURE 28-4. Esophagogram of a patient with esophageal atresia. *A,* Stenosis of the suture line and small hiatus hernia with reflux. *B,* Patient treated with cisapride, H_2-antagonists, and bougie dilations, and ultimately the pH monitoring reverted to normal values. Antireflux surgery was not necessary.

had dysphagia requiring gastrostomy supplementation, and in 5 of the 7, the dysphagia persisted beyond 1 year. All had competent fundoplications on follow-up study, but all also had absent esophageal peristalsis below the anastomosis. Another report relates similar problems with Nissen fundoplications in this scenario.[231] The investigators thought that the dysphagia was secondary to the inability of the defective distal esophageal motility to overcome the increased resistance of the fundoplication.

What appeared to be excellent short-term results proved to be poor long-term results with fundoplications in another report.[234]

In other reports, the problems are not so severe. Reoperation was required in 18% of those children with a Nissen fundoplication and in 15% of patients who had a Thal fundoplication after esophageal atresia/TEF repair.[243,244] Reoperation rates, of course, do indicate failure but do not necessarily reflect the total incidence of morbidity after antireflux surgery.

Obviously, a clear consensus has not been reached concerning the children who have successfully overcome the original problem of esophageal atresia only to develop GER. Some of the early problems of GER are life threatening or are responsible for growth failure, recurrent pneumonia, and severe esophagitis with resistant anastomotic strictures. Medical treatment alone often does not prove effective, yet antireflux surgery is beset with significant drawbacks.

ESOPHAGEAL STRICTURE AND BARRETT'S ESOPHAGUS

The treatment of esophageal stricture secondary to esophagitis has changed little in the past 30 years.[245] Esophagoscopy is essential initially to demonstrate the type and extent of the lesion and the possibility of dilatation. Dilatations are then initiated. If the stricture is particularly tight or long, a gastrostomy will be necessary, not only for alimentation but also for the placement of an indwelling string to permit retrograde dilatations. Even with improvement from dilatations, some form of antireflux operation is necessary; and dilatations may have to be continued postoperatively for some time.[246] All but the most recalcitrant strictures respond to a regimen of repeated dilatations coupled with an effective antireflux procedure.

Rarely the stricture is limited to a short segment, which allows for resection and anastomosis. If the stricture is long and unyielding, esophageal replacement occasionally may be required, either by gastric tube or by colon replacement. Better knowledge of the consequences of GER and its pathophysiology, earlier diagnosis, and effective therapy account for the fact that strictures from reflux esophagitis are now seen less frequently than in past decades. Why strictures develop in some patients but not in others remains an unanswered question. The answer may well be found in variability of the mucosal defense mechanisms and the noxiousness of the refluxate.

In recent years, our group has been treating the severe strictures with "autoexpanding" prothesis, with excellent results, lower morbidity, longer time between dilatations,

family and child satisfaction, and a high percentage of success.[247,248]

A large number of reports confirm the effectiveness of omeprazole in the treatment of esophagitis in children.[95,248–250] Perhaps the drug will eventually have a role as an adjunct in managing reflux strictures, but no reports on this use have appeared. Although its effectiveness in esophagitis is apparent, its success in truly advanced esophagitis is not so impressive; less than half of grade 4 esophagitis healed with omeprazole. Recurrence seems to be inevitable when the drug is stopped.

Barrett's esophagus is a complication of esophagitis and is often accompanied by stricture.[251,252] Although it is usually regarded as quite uncommon in childhood, the incidence has been reported at 4% and 14% of children with GER in two series. In another report, Barrett's esophagus was found in 25% of the children with reflux strictures. In adults, progressive increase in the incidence and severity of dysplasia in the columnar epithelium has been documented on repeated endoscopic and biopsy observations over a period of years.[253]

The progressive increase in the incidence and severity of dysplasia, together with the development of carcinoma, make Barrett's esophagus most worrisome. Two cases of carcinoma arising in Barrett's esophagus in children were reported from one institution.[254] One patient was age 11 years, and the other, age 14 years at diagnosis of the malignancy. A report exists of an esophageal adenocarcinoma located adjacent to the esophagogastric junction in a 20-year-old woman who had repair of esophageal atresia and TEF as a newborn.[255] She was managed with an extensive resection with restoration of continuity by a colon-segment interposition. The specimen did not show Barrett's epithelium, but certainly a reasonable possibility exists that Barrett's esophagus was present at one time but was obliterated by the tumor.

How best to handle the child with reflux and Barrett's esophagus is obviously a major problem. One child, age 12 years, was treated with antireflux operation with an excellent clinical result.[256] Two years later, on both gross endoscopic examination and histologic review, distinct evidence of regression was found, with replacement of the columnar epithelium by squamous epithelium, and this regression continued over a further 3-year period. In another case, complete regression followed antireflux surgery.[257]

Generally, however, Barrett's esophagus in childhood does not regress after antireflux surgery. Prolonged follow-up evaluation with endoscopy and biopsy are recommended if dysplastic changes are to be found, and carcinoma can either be prevented or found at an early stage.[258] The use of endoscopic laser ablation of the epithelium was recently reported.[259] Prophylactic esophagectomy[260] or mucosectomy[261] has been proposed for severe dysplasia.

REFERENCES

1. Carré IJ: The natural history of the partial thoracic stomach in children. Arch Dis Child 34:344–353, 1959.
2. Nissen R: Gastropexy and fundoplication in surgical treatment of hiatal hernia. Am J Dig Dis 6:954–961, 1961.

3. Thal AP: A unified approach to surgical problems of the esophagogastric junction. Ann Surg 168:542–549, 1968.

4. Boix-Ochoa J: The physiologic approach to the management of gastric esophageal reflux. J Pediatr Surg 21:1032–1039, 1986.

5. Fonkalsrud EW, Foglia RP, Ament ME, et al: Operative treatment for the gastroesophageal syndrome in children. J Pediatr Surg 24:525–529, 1989.

6. Ashcraft K: Gastroesophageal reflux. In Ashcraft KW, Holder TM (eds): Pediatric Surgery, 2nd ed. Philadelphia, WB Saunders, 1993, pp 270–287.

7. Tunell WP, Smith EI, Carson JA: Gastroesophageal reflux in childhood: The dilemma of surgical success. Ann Surg 197:560–565, 1983.

8. Dent J, Dodds WJ, Friedman RH, et al: Mechanism of gastroesophageal reflux in recumbent asymptomatic human subjects. J Clin Invest 65:256–267, 1980.

9. Dodds WJ, Dent J, Hogan WJ, et al: Mechanisms of gastroesophageal reflux in patients with reflux esophagitis. N Engl J Med 307:1547–1552, 1982.

10. Winter HS: Disorders of the oesophagus. In Avery ME, Taeusch HV (eds): Schaffer's Diseases of the Newborn. Philadelphia, WB Saunders, 1984, pp 234–331.

11. Kilgore SP, Ormsby A, Gramlich T, et al: The gastric cardia: Fact or fiction? Am J Gastroenterol 95:921–925, 2000.

12. Hu FZ, Preston RA, Post JC, et al: Mapping of a gene for severe pediatric gastroesophageal reflux to chromosome 13q14. JAMA 284:325–334, 2000.

13. Hu FZ, Post JC, Johnson S, et al: Refined localization of a gene for pediatric gastroesophageal reflux makes HTR2A an unlikely candidate gene. Hum Genet 107:519–525, 2000.

14. Orenstein SR, Shalaby TM, Pfuetzer RH, et al: Autosomal dominant infant GERD: Exclusion of a 13q14 locus in 6 well-characterized families suggest genetic heterogeneity [abstract]. Gastroenterology 120(suppl):A211, 2001.

15. Bright R: Account of a remarkable misplacement of the stomach. Guys Hosp Rep 1:598, 1836.

16. Billard P: Maladie des Enfants Nouveau-Nés. París, 1828.

17. Allison PR, Johnston AS, Royce GB: Short esophagus with simple peptic ulceration. J Thorac Cardiovasc Surg 12:432, 1943.

18. Tileston W: Peptic ulcer of the esophagus. Am J Med Sci 132:240, 1906.

19. Winkelstein A: Peptic esophagitis: A new clinical entity. JAMA 104:906, 1935.

20. Carré IJ: Postural treatment of children with a partial thoracic stomach (hiatus hernia) in children. Arch Dis Child 35:569, 1960.

21. Roviralta E.: El Lactante Vomitador. Barcelona, Jane Ed, 1950.

22. Holloway RH: The antireflux barrier and mechanisms of gastroesophageal reflux. Baillieres Clin Gastroenterol 14–15: 681–699, 2000.

23. Lortat-Jacob JL: Le traitement chirurgical des maladies du reflux gastroesophagienne. Presse Med 65:457, 1957.

24. Hill LD: An effective operation for hiatal hernia: An eight-year appraisal. Ann Surg 166:681, 1967.

25. Hill LD: Surgery and gastroesophageal reflux. Gastroenterology 63:183, 1972 pp. nos.

26. Belsey R: Surgery of the diaphragm. In Brown JM (ed): Surgery of Children. Baltimore, Williams & Wilkins, 1963, p 762.

27. Belsey R: Gastroesophageal Reflux and Hiatal Hernia. Boston, Little, Brown, 1972.

28. Nissen R, Rossetti M: Die Behandlung von hiatushernie und reflux-oesophagitis mit gastropexie und fundoplicatio. Stuttgart, Georg Thieme Verlag, 1959.

29. Fyke FE, Code CF, Schlegel JF: The gastroesophageal sphincter in healthy human beings. Gastroenterologia 86:135–150, 1956.

30. Liebermann-Meffert D, Allgower M, Schmid P, et al: Muscular equivalent of the lower esophageal sphincter. Gastroenterology 76:31–38, 1979.

31. Klein WA, Parkman HP, Dempsey DT, et al: Sphincterlike thoracoabdominal high-pressure zone after esophagogastrectomy. Gastroenterology 105:1362–1369, 1993.

32. Mittal RK, Balaban DH: The esophagogastric junction. N Engl J Med 336:924–932, 1997.

33. Bonavina L, Evander A, DeMeester TR: Length of the distal esophageal sphincter and competency of the cardia. Am J Surg 15:25, 1986.

34. O'Sullivan GC, DeMeester TR, Joelsson BE: Interaction of lower esophageal sphincter pressure and length of sphincter in the abdomen as determinants of gastroesophageal competence. Am J Surg 143:40, 1982.

35. Fyke FE, Code CF, Schlegel JF: The gastroesophageal sphincter in healthy human beings. Gastroenterologia 86:135, 1956.

36. Boix-Ochoa J: Gastroesophageal reflux. In Welch K, Randolph JG, Ravitch MM, (eds): Pediatric Surgery. St. Louis, Mosby-Year Book, 1986.

37. O'Sullivan GC, DeMeester TR, Joelsson BE, et al: Interaction of lower esophageal sphincter pressure and length of sphincter in the abdomen as determinants of gastroesophageal competence. Am J Surg 143:40–47, 1982.

38. DeMeester TR, Wernly JA, Bryant GH, et al: Clinical and in vitro analysis of determinants of gastroesophageal competence. Am J Surg 137:39–46, 1979.

39. Winans CS, Harris LD: Quantitation of lower esophageal sphincter competence. Gastroenterology 52:773–778, 1967.

40. Johnson HD: The Antireflux Mechanism in the Cardia and Hiatus. Springfield, Ill, Charles C Thomas, 1968.

41. Wernly MD, DeMeester TR, Bryant GH: Intraabdominal pressure and manometric data of the distal esophageal sphincter, their relationship to gastroesophageal reflux. Arch Surg 115:534, 1980.

42. Thor KB, Hill LD, Mercer DD, et al: Reappraisal of the flap valve mechanism in the gastroesophageal junction. Acta Chir Scand 153:25–28, 1987.

43. Boix-Ochoa J, Canals J: Maturation of the lower esophagus. J. Pediatr Surg 11:749, 1976.

44. Dent J, Dodds WJ, Hogan WJ, et al: Factors that influence induction of gastroesophageal reflux in normal human subjects. Dig Dis Sci 33:270–275, 1988.

45. Dent J, Holloway RH, Toouli J, et al: Mechanisms of lower oesophageal sphincter incompetence in patients with symptomatic gastrooesophageal reflux. Gut 29:1020–1028, 1988.

46. Mittal RK, Sivri B, Schirmer BD, et al: Effect of crural myotomy on the incidence and mechanism for gastroesophageal reflux in cats. Gastroenterology 105:740–747, 1993.

47. Altorki NK, Skinner DB: Pathophysiology of gastroesophageal reflux. Am J Med 86:685–689, 1989.

48. Cotton BR, Smith G: The lower oesophageal sphincter and anaesthesia. Br J Anaesth 56:37–46,1984.

49. Dent J: Recent views on the pathogenesis of gastro-esophageal reflux disease. Ballieres Clin Gastroenterol 1:727–745, 1987.

50. Bombeck CT, Dillard DH, Nyhus LM: Muscular anatomy of the gastroesophageal junction and role of phrenoesophageal competence. Ann Surg 164:643, 1966.

51. Mann CV, Greenwood RK, Ellis FH: The esophagogastric junction. Surg Gynecol Obstet 104:853, 1964.

52. Vantrappen G, Texter EC, Barborka CJ, et al: The closing mechanism at the gastroesophageal junction. Am J Med 28:564, 1960.

53. Orenstein SR: Gastroesophageal reflux. Curr Probl Pediatr 21:193–241, 1991.

54. Altschuler SM, Boyle JT, Nixon TE, et al: Simultaneous reflex inhibition of lower esophageal sphincter and crural diaphragm in cats. Am J Physiol 249:586–591, 1985.

55. Boyle JT, Altschuler SM, Nixon TE, et al: Role of the diaphragm in the genesis of lower esophageal sphincter pressure in the cat. Gastroenterology 88:723–730, 1985.

56. Dev NB, Boyle JT: Phasic contraction of the diaphragm during respiration impedes its role in the gastroesophageal antireflux barrier. Gastroenterology 96:120, 1989.

57. Mittal RK, Rochester DF, McCallum RW: Effect of the diaphragmatic contraction on lower oesophageal sphincter pressure in man. Gut 28:1564–1568, 1987.

58. Mittal RK, Rochester DF, McCallum RW: Sphincteric action of the diaphragm during a relaxed lower esophageal sphincter in humans. Am J Physiol 256:139–144, 1989.

59. Mittal RK, Rochester DF, McCallum RW: Electrical and mechanical activity in the human lower esophageal sphincter during diaphragm contraction. J Clin Invest 81:1182–1189, 1988.

60. Biancani P, Zabinski MP, Behar J: Pressure, tension, and force of closure of the human lower esophageal sphincter and esophagus. J Clin Invest 56:476–483, 1975.

61. Bardaji C, Boix-Ochoa J: Contribution of the His angle to the gastroesophageal antireflux mechanism. Pediatr Surg Int 1:172, 1986.

62. Boix-Ochoa J, Casasa JM, Gil-Vernet JM: Une chirurgie physiologique pour les anomalies du secteur cardiohiatal. Chir Pediatr 24:117, 1983.

63. Johnson HD: The Antireflux Mechanism in the Cardia and Hiatus. Springfield, Ill, Charles C Thomas, 1968, pp 57–59.

64. Pettersson GB, Bombech CT, Nyhus LM: The lower esophageal sphincter: Mechanisms of opening and closure. Surgery 88:307, 1980.

65. Delattre JF, Palot JP, Ducasse A, et al: The crura of the diaphragmatic passage. Anat Clin 7:271–283, 1985.

66. Sloan S, Rademaker AW, Kahrilas PJ: Determinants of gastroesophageal junction incompetence: Hiatal hernia, lower esophageal sphincter, or both? Ann Intern Med 117:977–982, 1992.

67. Roussos C, Macklem PT: The respiratory muscles. N Engl J Med 307:786–797, 1982.

68. DeMeester TR, Johnson LF, Joseph GJ, et al: Patterns of gastroesophageal reflux in health and disease. Ann Surg 184:459–470, 1976.

69. Little AG, DeMeester TR, Rezai-Zadeh K, et al: Abnormal gastric emptying in patients with gastroesophageal reflux. Surg Forum 28:347–348, 1977.

70. Horowitz M, Cook DJ, Collins PJ, et al: The application of techniques using radionuclides to the study of gastric emptying. Surg Gynecol Obstet 155:737–744, 1982.

71. Maddern GJ, Jamieson GG: Fundoplication enhances gastric emptying. Ann Surg 201:296–299, 1985.

72. Euler AR, Byrne WJ: Gastric emptying times of water in infants and children: Comparison of those with and without gastroesophageal reflux. J Pediatr Gastroenterol Nutr 2:595–598, 1983.

73. Jolley SG, Leonard JC, Tunell WP: Gastric emptying in children with gastroesophageal reflux, I: An estimate of effective gastric emptying. J Pediatr Surg 22:923–926, 1987.

74. Jolley SG, Tunell WP, Leonard JC, et al: Gastric emptying in children with gastroesophageal reflux, II: The relationship to retching symptoms following antireflux surgery. J Pediatr Surg 22:927–930, 1987.

75. Fonkalsrud EW, Ament ME: Gastroesophageal reflux in childhood. Curr Probl Surg 33:10–70, 1996.

76. Papaila JG, Wilmot D, Grosfeld JL, et al: Increased incidence of delayed gastric emptying in children with gastroesophageal reflux. Arch Surg 124:933–936, 1989.

77. Maxson RT, Harp S, Jackson RJ, et al: Delayed gastric emptying in neurologically impaired children with gastroesophageal reflux: The role of pyloroplasty. J Pediatr Surg 29:726–729, 1994.

78. Campbell JR, Gilchrist BF, Harrison MW: Pyloroplasty in association with Nissen fundoplication in children with neurologic disorders. J Pediatr Surg 24:375–377, 1989.

79. Brown RA, Wynchank S, Rode H, et al: Is a gastric drainage procedure necessary at the time of antireflux surgery? J Pediatr Gastroenterol Nutr 25:377–380, 1997.

80. Tobey NA, Hosseimi S, Caymaz-Bor C, et al: The role of pepsin in acid injury to esophageal epithelium. Am J Gastroenterol 96:3062–3070, 2001.

81. Littlemoe K, Johnson LF, Harmon JW: Alkaline esophagitis: A comparison of the ability of components of gastroduodenal contents to injure the rabbit esophagus.Gastroenterology 85:62–68, 1983.

82. Salo JA, Lehto VP, Kivilaakso E: Morphologic alterations in experimental esophagitis: Light microscopic and scanning and transmission electron microscopic study. Dig Dis Sci 28:440–448, 1983.

83. Casasa JM, Boix-Ochoa J: Surgical or conservative treatment in hiatal hernia in children: A new decisive parameter. Surgery 82:573–576, 1977.

84. Boix-Ochoa J: Diagnosis and management of gastroesophageal reflux in children. Surg Ann 13:123–136, 1981.

85. Omari TI, Dent J: Assessment of oesophageal motor function in children and neonates. J Jpn Soc Pediatr Surg 33:25–30, 1997.

86. Omari T, Miki K, Fraser R, et al: Esophageal body and lower esophageal sphincter function in healthy premature infants. Gastroenterology 109:1757–1764, 1995.

87. Gryboski JD, Thayer WR Jr, Spiro HM: Esophageal motility in infants and children. Pediatrics 31:382–395, 1983.

88. Hillemeier AC, Grill BB, McCallum R, et al: Esophageal and gastric motor abnormalities in gastroesophageal reflux during infancy. Gastroenterology 84:741–746, 1983.

89. Kahrilas PJ, Dodds WJ, Hogan WJ, et al: Esophageal peristaltic dysfunction in peptic esophagitis. Gastroenterology 91:897–904, 1986.

90. Cucchiara S, Staiano A, DiLorenzo G, et al: Pathophysiology of gastroesophageal reflux and distal esophageal motility in children with gastroesophageal reflux disease. J Pediatr Gastroenterol Nutr 7:830–836, 1988.

91. Orlando RC: Pathophysiology of gastroesophageal reflux disease, esophageal epithelial resistance. In Astell DO, Richter JE (eds): The Esophagus, 3rd ed. Philadelphia, Lippincott Williams & Wilkins, 1999, pp 409–420.

92. Orlando RC: Pathophysiology of gastroesophageal reflux disease, offensive factors and tissue resistance. In Orlando RC (ed): Gastroesophageal Reflux Disease. New York, Marcel Dekker, 2000, pp 165–192.

93. Orlando RC: Pathogenesis of gastroesophageal reflux disease. Gastroenterol Clin North Am 31:S35–S44, 2002.

94. Black DD, Haggit RC, Orenstein SR, et al: Esophagitis in infants: Morphometric histological diagnosis and correlation with measures of gastroesophageal reflux. Gastroenterology 98:1408–1414, 1990.

95. Boix-Ochoa J, Rehbein F: Esophageal stenosis due to reflux esophagitis. Arch Dis Child 40:197, 1965.

96. Cheu HW, Grosfeld JL, Heifetz SA, et al: Persistence of Barrett's esophagus in children after antireflux surgery: Influence on follow-up care. J Pediatr Surg 27:260–266, 1992.

97. Barrett NR: The lower esophagus lined by columnar epithelium. Surgery 41:881–894, 1957.

98. Berardi RS, Devaiah KA: Barrett's esophagus. Surg Gynecol Obstet 156:521–538, 1983.

99. Bozymski EM, Herlihi KJ, Orlando RC: Barrett's esophagus. Ann Intern Med 97:103–107, 1982.

100. Brand DL, Ylvisaker JT, Gelfand M, et al: Regression of columnar esophageal (Barrett's) epithelium after anti-reflux surgery. N Engl J Med 302:844–848, 1980.

101. Cameron AJ, Otto BJ, Payne WS: The incidence of adenocarcinoma in columnar-lined (Barrett's) esophagus. N Engl J Med 313:857–859, 1985.

102. Dahms BB, Rothstein FC: Barrett's esophagus in children: A consequence of chronic gastroesophageal reflux. Gastroenterology 86:318–323, 1984.

103. Hoeffel JC, Nihoul-Fekete C, Schmidt M: Esophageal adenocarcinoma after gastroesophageal reflux in children. J Pediatr 115:259–261, 1989.

104. Spechler SJ, Robbins AH, Bloomfield H, et al: Adenocarcinoma and Barrett's esophagus: An overrated risk? Gastroenterology 87:927–933, 1984.

105. Hyman PE. Gastroesophageal reflux: One reason why baby won't eat. J Pediatr 125(suppl):S103–S109, 1994.

106. del Rosario JF, Orenstein SR: Evaluation and management of gastroesophageal reflux and pulmonary disease. Curr Opin Pediatr 8:209–215, 1996.

107. Jolley SG, Halpern LM, Tunell WP, et al: The risk of sudden infant death from gastroesophageal reflux. J Pediatr Surg 26:691–696, 1991.

108. Jolley SG, Herbst JJ, Johnson DG, et al: Esophageal pH monitoring during sleep identifies children with respiratory symptoms from gastroesophageal reflux. Gastroenterology 80:1501–1506, 1981.

109. Andze GO, Brandt ML, St. Vil D, et al: Diagnosis and treatment of gastroesophageal reflux in 500 children with respiratory symptoms: The value of pH monitoring. J Pediatr Surg 26:295–300, 1991.

110. Hrabovsky EE, Mullett MD: Gastroesophageal reflux and the premature infant. J Pediatr Surg 21:583–587, 1986.

111. Orenstein SA: An overview of reflux-associated disorders in infants: Apnea, laryngospasm, and aspiration. Am J Med 111:60S–63S, 2001.

112. Hassall E, Weinstein WM, Ament ME: Barrett's esophagus in childhood. Gastroenterology 89:1331–1337, 1985.

113. Otherson HB Jr, Ocampo RJ, Parker EF, et al: Barrett's esophagus in children. Ann Surg 217:676–681, 1993.

114. Mandel H, Tirosh E, Berant M: Sandifer syndrome reconsidered. Acta Paediatr Scand 78:797–799, 1989.

115. Bray PF, Herbst JJ, Johnson DG, et al: Childhood gastroesophageal reflux: Neurologic and psychiatric syndromes mimicked. JAMA 237:1342–1345, 1977.

116. Kahrillas PJ: Diagnosis of symptomatic gastroesophageal reflux disease. Am J Gastroenterology 98:S15–S23, 2003.

117. Fas R, Tolugas G: Functional heartburn: The stimulus, the pain, and the brain. Gut 51:885–892, 2002.

118. Al-Khaxari Hanaa A, Sinan TS, Seymour H: Diagnosis of gastro-oesophageal reflux in children: Comparison between oesophageal pH and barium examinations. Pediatr Radiol 32:765, 2002.

119. Fawcett HD, Hayden CK, Adams JC, et al: How useful is gastro-sophageal reflux scintigraphy in suspected childhood aspiration? Pediatr Radiol 18:311–313, 1988.

120. Berdon WE, Mellins RB, Levy J: On the following paper by Fawcet HD, Hayden CK, Adams JC and Swischuk LE: How useful is gastroesophageal reflux scintigraphy in suspected childhood aspiration? Pediatr Radiol 18:309–310, 1988.

121. Johnson LF, DeMeester TR: Twenty-four hour pH monitoring of the distal esophagus: A quantitative measure of gastroesophageal reflux. Am J Gastroenterol 62:325–332, 1974.

122. Hill JL, Pelligrini CA, Burrington JD, et al: Technique and experience with 24-hour esophageal pH monitoring in children. J Pediatr Surg 12:877–887, 1977.

123. Jolley SG, Herbst JJ, Johnson DG, et al: Patterns of postcibal gastroesophageal reflux in symptomatic infants. Am J Surg 138:946–950, 1979.

124. Colletti RB, Christie DL, Orenstein SR: Indications for pediatric esophageal pH monitoring. J Pediatr Gastroenterol Nutr 21:253–262, 1995.

125. Jamieson JR, Stein HJ, DeMeester TR, et al: Ambulatory 24-hour esophageal pH monitoring: Normal values, optimal thresholds, specificity, sensitivity, and reproducibility. Amer J Gastroenterol 87:1102–1111, 1992.

126. Boix-Ochoa J, Lafuente JM, Gil-Vernet JM: Twenty-four hour esophageal pH monitoring in gastroesophageal reflux. J Pediatr Surg 15:74–78, 1980.

127. Shay SS, Johnson LF, Richter JE: Acid Rereflux. Dig Dis Sci 48:1–9, 2003.

128. Wenzl TC, Moroder C, Trachterna M, et al: Esophageal pH monitoring and impedance measurement: A comparison of two diagnostic tests for gastroesophageal reflux. J Pediatr Gastroenterol Nutr 34:519–523, 2002.

129. Vela MF, Camacho-Lobato L. Srinivasan R, et al: Simultaneous intraesophageal impedance and pH measurement of acid and nonacid gastroesophageal reflux: Effect of omeprazole. Gastroenterology 120:1599–1606, 2001.

130. Sifrim D, Holloway RH, Silny J, et al: Acid, nonacid and gas reflux in patients with gastroesophageal reflux disease during 24-hr ambulatory pH-impedance recordings. Gastroenterology 120:1588–1598, 2001.

131. Kahrilas P: Will impedance testing rewrite the book on GERD? Gastroenterology 120:1862–1864, 2001.

132. Biller JA, Winter HS, Grand RJ, et al: Are endoscopic changes predictive of histologic esophagitis in children? J Pediatr Surg 103:215–218, 1983.

133. Meyers WF, Roberts CC, Johnson DG, et al: Value of tests for evaluation of gastroesophageal reflux in children. J Pediatr Surg 20:515–520, 1985.

134. Black DD, Haggitt RC, Orenstein SR, et al: Esophagitis in infants. Gastroenterology 98:1408–1414, 1990.

135. Orenstein SR: Gastroesophageal reflux. In Wyllie R, Hyams JS (eds): Pediatric Gastrointestinal Disease. Philadelphia, WB Saunders, 1993, pp 337–369.

136. Glassman M, George D, Grill B: Gastroesophageal reflux in children. Gastroenterol Clin North Am 24:71–98, 1995.

137. Dahms BB, Rothstein FC: Barrett's esophagus in children: A consequence of chronic gastroesophageal reflux. Gastroenterology 86:318–323, 1984.

138. Cooper JE, Spitz L, Wilkins BM: Barrett's esophagus in children: A histologic and histochemical study in 11 cases. J Pediatr Surg 22:191–196, 1987.

139. Hameeteman W, Tytgat GNJ, Houthoff JH, et al: Barrett's esophagus: Development of dysplasia and adenocarcinoma. Gastroenterology 96:1249–1256, 1989.

140. Stein HJ, DeMeester TR: Indications, technique, and clinical use of ambulatory 24-hour esophageal motility monitoring in a surgical practice. Ann Surg 217:128–137, 1993.

141. Shepard R, Fenn S, Seiber WK: Evaluation of esophageal function in postoperative esophageal atresia and tracheoesophageal fistula. Surgery 59:608–617, 1966.

142. Pehlivanov N, Jianmin L, Tania A, et al: Lower esophageal sphincter monitoring with sphinctometer: in vitro and in vivo studies. Am J Physiol 277:G577–G1999, 2002.

143. Bailey DJ, Andreas JM, Danek GD, et al: Lack of efficacy of thickened feedings as treatment for gastroesophageal reflux. Pediatrics 110:187–189, 1987.

144. Salvia G, De Vizia B, Manguso F, et al: Effect of intragastric volume and osmolality on mechanisms of gastroesophageal reflux in children with gastroesophageal reflux disease. Am J Gastroenterol 96:1725–1732, 2001.

145. Katz PO: Treatment of gastroesophageal reflux disease: use of algorithms to aid in management. Am J Gastroenterol 94:3–10, 1999.

146. Orenstein SR, Whitington PF, Orestein DM: The infant seat as a treatment for gastroesophageal reflux. N Engl J Med 309:760–763, 1983.

147. Buts JP, Barudi C, Otte JB: Double-blind controlled study on the efficacy of sodium alginate (Gaviscon) in reducing gastroesophageal reflux assessed by 24h continuous pH monitoring in infants and children. Eur J Paediatr 146:156–158, 1987.

148. Ponsonby AL, Dwyer T, Gibbons LE, et al: Factors potentiating the risk of sudden infant death syndrome associated with the prone position. N Engl J Med 329:377–382, 1993.

149. Vandenplas Y, Belli DC, Benatar A, et al: The role of cisapride in the treatment of pediatric gastroesophageal reflux. J Pediatr Gastroenterol Nutr 28:528–528, 1999.

150. Levy J, Hayes C, Kern J, et al: Does cisapride influence cardiac rhythm? Results of a United States multicenter, double-blind, placebo-controlled pediatric study. J Pediatr Gastroenterol Nutr 32:458–463, 2001.

151. Benatar A, Feenstra A, Decraene T, et al: Effects of cisapride on corrected QT interval, heart rate, and rhythm in infants undergoing polysomnography. Pediatrics 106:E85, 2000.

152. Dimand RJ: Use of H2-receptor antagonists in children. Ann Pharmacother (suppl) 24:42–46, 1990.

153. Zimmermann AE, Walters JK, Katoma BG, et al: A review of omeprazole use in the treatment of acid-related disorders in children. Clin Ther 2385:660–679, 2001.

154. International Pediatric Omeprazole Study Group: Omeprazole for treatment of chronic erosive esophagitis in children: A multi study efficacy, safety, tolerability and dose requirements. J Pediatr 137:800–807, 2000.

155. International Pediatric Omeprazole Pharmacokinetic Group: Pharmacokinetics of orally administered omeprazole in children. Am J Gastroenterol 95:3101–3106, 2000.

156. Israel DM, Hassal E, Dimmich JE: Gastric polyps in children receiving omeprazole. Gastroenterology 108:A110, 1995.

157. Hassall E, Dimmick JE, Israel DM: Parietal cell hyperplasia in children receiving omeprazole. Gastroenterology 108:A121, 1995.

158. Role of drugs therapy in the treatment of gastro-oesophageal reflux disorder in children. Paediatr Drugs 2:263–272, 2000.

159. Scaillon M, Cadranel S: Safety data required for proton-pump inhibitor use in children. J. Pediatr Gastroenterol Nutr 35:113–118, 2002.

160. Castell DO, Kahrillas PJ, Richter JE: Esomeprazole (40 mg) compared with lansoprazole (30 mg) in the treatment of erosive esophagitis. Am J. Gastroenterol 97:575–586, 2002.

161. Frazzoni M, De Micheli E, Grisendi A, et al: Effective intra-oesophageal acid suppression in patients with gastro-oesophageal reflux disease: Lansoprazole vs. Pantoprazole. Aliment Pharmacol Ther 17:235–241, 2003.

162. Lidums I, Lehmann A, Checklin A, et al: Control of transient lower esophageal sphincter relaxations and reflux by the GABAß agonist baclofen in normal subjects. Gastroenterology 118:7–13, 2000.

163. Brooks PA, Glaum SR, Miler RJ, et al: The actions of baclofen on neurones and synaptic transmission in the nucleus tractus solitarii of the rat in vitro. J Physiol (Lond) 457:115–129, 1992.

164. Bolser DC, De Gennaro FC, O'Reilly, et al: Peripheral and central sites of action of GABAß agonists to inhibit the cough reflex in the cat and guinea pig. Br J Pharmacol 113: 1344–1348, 1994.
165. Page AJ, Blackshaw LA: Baclofen inhibits responses to graded mechanical stimuli of gastro-oesophageal vagal afferents in vitro. Gastroenterology 116:A1057, 1999.
166. Blackshaw LA, Grundy D, Scratcherd T: Vagal afferent discharge from gastric mechanoreceptors during contraction and relaxation of the ferret corpus. J Auton Nerv Syst 18:19–24, 1987.
167. Vela MF, Tutuian R, Katz PO, Castell DO: Baclofen decreases acid and non-acid post-prandial gastro-oesophageal reflux measured by combined multichannel intraluminal impedance and pH. Aliment Pharmacol Ther 17:243–251, 2003.
168. Richter JE: Novel medical therapies for gastroesophageal reflux disease beyond proton-pump inhibitors. Gastroenterol Clin North Am 31:S111–S116, 2002.
169. Fonkalsrud EW, Ashcraft KW, Coran AG, et al: Surgical treatment of gastroesophageal children: A combined hospital study of 7467 patients. Pediatrics 101:419–422, 1998.
170. Harnsberger JK, Corey JJ, Johnson DJ, et al: Long-term follow-up of surgery for gastroesophageal reflux in infants and children. J Pediatr Surg 102–508, 1983.
171. Kazerooni NL, Vancamp J, Hirschl RB, et al: Fundoplication in 160 children under 2 years of age. J Pediatr Surg 29:677–681, 1994.
172. Jolley SG, Tunell WP, Hoelzer DJ, et al: Intraoperative esophageal manometry and early postoperative esophageal pH monitoring in children. J Pediatr Surg 24:336–340, 1989.
173. Spitz L, Coran A: Operative Surgery-Pediatric Surgery. 5th ed. Chaptman and Hall Medical. 265–285.
174. Weber TR: Toupet fundoplication for gastroesophageal reflux in childhood. Arch Surg 134:717–720, 1999, discussion 720–721.
175. Boix-Ochoa J: The physiologic approach to the management of gastro esophageal reflux. J Pediatr Surg 21:1032–1039, 1986.
176. Hassall E: Wrap session: Is the Nissen slipping? Am J Gastroenterol 90:1212–1220, 1995.
177. Dedinsky GK, Vane DW, Black CT, et al: Complications and reoperation after Nissen fundoplication in childhood. Am J Surg 153:177–183, 1987.
178. Taylor LA, Weiner T, Lacey SR, et al: Chronic lung disease is the leading risk factor correlating with the failure (wrap disruption) of antireflux procedures in children. J Pediatr Surg 29:161–166, 1994.
179. Bustorff-Silva J, Fonkalsrud EW, Peres CA, et al: Gastric emptying procedures decrease the risk of postoperative recurrent reflux in children with delayed gastric emptying. J Pediatr Surg 34:79–82, 1999.
180. Fonkalsrud EW, Foglia RP, Ament ME, et al: Operative treatment for the gastroesophageal reflux syndrome in children. J Pediatr Surg 24:525–529, 1989.
181. Leape LL, Ramenofsky ML: Surgical treatment of gastroesophageal reflux in children. Am J Dis Child 134:935–938, 1980.
182. St. Cyr JA, Ferrara TB, Thompson TR, et al: Nissen fundoplication for gastroesophageal reflux in infants. J Thorac Cardiovasc Surg 92:661–666, 1986.
183. Turnage RH, Oldham KT, Coran AG, et al: Late results of fundoplication for gastroesophageal reflux in infants and children. Surgery 105:457–464, 1989.
184. Jolley SG, Tunell WP, Hoelzer DJ, et al: Postoperative small bowel obstruction in infants and children: A problem following Nissen fundoplication. J Pediatr Surg 21:407–409, 1986.
185. Dedinsky GK, Vane DW, Black CT, et al: Complications and reoperation after Nissen fundoplication in childhood. Am J Surg 153:177–183, 1987.
186. Caniano DA, Ginn-Pease ME, King DR: The failed antireflux procedure: Analysis of risk factors and morbidity. J Pediatr Surg 25:1022–1026, 1990.
187. Price MR, Janik JS, Wayne ER, et al: Modified Nissen fundoplication for reduction of fundoplication failure. J Pediatr Surg 32:324–327, 1997.
188. Wheatley MJ, Coran AG, Wesley JR, et al: Redo fundoplication in infants and children with recurrent gastroesophageal reflux. J Pediatr Surg 26:758–761, 1991.
189. Lelli JL, Ashcraft KW: Gastroesophageal reflux. Semin Thorac Cardiovasc Surg 6:240–246, 1994.
190. Bensoussian AL, Yazbeck S, Carceller-Blanchard A: Results and complications of Toupet partial posterior wrap: 10 years' experience. J Pediatr Surg 29:1215–1217, 1994.
191. Dallemagne B, Weerts JM, Jehaes C, et al: Laparoscopic Nissen fundoplication: Preliminary report. Surg Laparosc Endosc 1:138–142, 1991.
192. Anvari M, Allen C, Borm A: Laparoscopic Nissen fundoplication is a satisfactory alternative to long-term omeprazole therapy. Br J Surg 82:938–942, 1995.
193. Lobe TE, Schropp KP, Lunsford K: Laparoscopic Nissen fundoplication in childhood. J Pediatr Surg 28:358–361, 1993.
194. Georgeson KE: Laparoscopic gastrostomy and fundoplication. Pediatr Ann 22:675–677, 1993.
195. Meehan JJ, Georgeson KE: The learning curve associated with laparoscopic antireflux surgery in infants and children. J Pediatr Surg 32:426–429, 1997.
196. Ref for Lap Thals.
197. Hassall E: Antireflux surgery in children: Time for a harder look. Pediatrics 101:467–468, 1998.
198. Dela Vecchia LK, Grosfeld JL, West KW, et al: Reoperation after Nissen fundoplication in children with gastroesophageal reflux: Experience with 130 patients. Ann Surg 226:315–323, 1997.
199. Caniano DA, Ginn-Pease ME, King DR: The failed antireflux procedure: Analysis of risk factors and morbidity. J Pediatr Surg 25:1022–1026, 1990.
200. Cohen Z, et al: Nissen fundoplication and Boix-Ochoa antireflux procedure: Comparison between two surgical techniques in the treatment of gastroesophageal reflux in children. Eur J Pediatr Surg 9:289–293, 1999.
201. Sondheimer JM, Morris BA: Gastroesophageal reflux among severely retarded children. J Pediatr 94:710–714, 1979.
202. Spitz L: Surgical treatment of gastroesophageal reflux in severely mentally retarded children. J R Soc Med 75:525–529, 1982.
203. Vane DW, Harmel RP Jr, King DR, et al: The effectiveness of Nissen fundoplication in neurologically impaired children with gastroesophageal reflux. Surgery 98:662–666, 1985.
204. Bohmer CJM, Niezen-de Boer MC, Klinkenberg-Knol EC, et al: Gastroesophageal reflux disease in intellectually disabled individuals: Leads for diagnosis and the effect of omeprazole. Am J Gastroenterol 92:1475–1479, 1997.
205. Byrne WJ, Campbell M, Ashcraft E, et al: A diagnostic approach to vomiting in severely retarded patients. Amer J Dis Child 137:259–262, 1983.
206. Wilkinson JD, Dudgeon DL, Sondheimer JM: A comparison of medical and surgical treatment of gastroesophageal reflux in severely retarded children. J Pediatr Surg 99:202–205, 1981.
207. Roberts IM, Curtis RL, Madara JL: Gastroesophageal reflux and Barrett's esophagus in developmentally disabled patients. Am J Gastroenterol 81:519–523, 1986.
208. Snyder JD, Goldman H: Barrett's esophagus in children and adults: Frequent association with mental retardation. Dig Dis Sci 35:1185–1189, 1990.
209. Spitz L, Roth K, Kiely EM, et al: Operation for gastroesophageal reflux associated with severe mental retardation. Arch Dis Child 68:347–351, 1993.
210. Cameron BH, Cochran WJ, McGill CW: The uncut Collis-Nissen fundoplication: Results for 79 consecutively treated high-risk children. J Pediatr Surg 32:887–891, 1997.
211. Ferry GD, Selby M, Pietro TJ: Clinical response to short-term nasogastric feeding in infants with gastroesophageal reflux and growth failure. J Pediatr Gastroenterol Nutr 2:57–61, 1983.
212. Gauderer MWL: Percutaneous endoscopic gastrostomy: A 10 year experience with 220 children. J Pediatr Surg 26:288–294, 1991.
213. Wesley JR, Coran AG, Sarahan TM, et al: The need for evaluation of gastroesophageal reflux in brain-damaged children referred for feeding gastrostomy. J Pediatr Surg 16:866–871, 1981.
214. Mollitt DL, Golladay S, Seibert JJ: Symptomatic gastroesophageal reflux following gastrostomy in neurologically impaired patients. Pediatrics 75:1124–1126, 1985.
215. Grunow JE, Al-Hafidh A, Tunell WP: Gastroesophageal reflux following percutaneous endoscopic gastrostomy in children. J Pediatr Surg 24:42–45, 1989.

216. Jolley SG, Smith EI, Tunell WP: Protective antireflux operation with feeding gastrostomy. Ann Surg 201:736–740, 1985.

217. Langer JC, Wesson DE, Ein SH, et al: Feeding gastrostomy in neurologically impaired children: Is an antireflux procedure necessary? J Pediatr Gastroenterol Nutr 7:837–841, 1988.

218. Isch JA, Rescorla FJ, Scherer T III, et al: The development of gastroesophageal reflux after percutaneous endoscopic gastrostomy. J Pediatr Surg 32:321–323, 1997.

219. Berezin S, Schwarz SM, Halata MS, et al: Gastroesophageal reflux secondary to gastrostomy tube placement. Amer J Dis Child 140:699–701, 1986.

220. Stringel G: Gastrostomy with antireflux properties. J Pediatr Surg 25:1019–1021, 1990.

221. Albanese CT, Towbin RB, Ulman I, et al: Percutaneous gastrojejunostomy versus Nissen fundoplication for enteral feeding of the neurologically impaired child with gastroesophageal reflux. J Pediatr Surg 123:371–375, 1993.

222. DeCou JM, Shorter NA, Karl SR: Feeding Roux-en-Y jejunostomy in the management of severely neurologically impaired children. J Pediatr Surg 28:1276–1280, 1993.

223. Smith CD, Otherson HB Jr, Gogan NJ, et al: Nissen fundoplication in children with profound neurologic disability. High risks and unmet goals. Ann Surg 215:654–659, 1992.

224. Tuggle DW, Tunell WP, Hoelzer DJ, et al: The efficacy of Thal fundoplication in the treatment of gastroesophageal reflux: The influence of central nervous system impairment. J Pediatr Surg 23:638–640, 1988.

225. Ramachandran V, Ashcraft KW, Sharp RJ, et al: Thal fundoplication in neurologically impaired children. J Pediatr Surg 31:819–822, 1996.

226. Pearl RH, Robie DK, Ein SH, et al: Complications of gastroesophageal antireflux surgery in neurologically impaired versus neurologically normal children. J Pediatr Surg 25:1169–1173, 1990.

227. Borgstein ES, Heij HA, Beugelaar JD, et al: Risks and benefits of antireflux operations in neurologically impaired children. Eur J Pediatr 153:248–251, 1994.

228. Martinez DA, Ginn-Pease ME, Caniano DA: Sequellae of antireflux surgery in profoundly disabled children. J Pediatr Surg 27:267–273, 1992.

229. O'Neill JK, O'Neill PJ, Goth-Owens T, et al: Care-giver evaluation of anti-gastroesophageal reflux procedures in neurologically impaired children: What is the real-life outcome? J Pediatr Surg 31:375–380, 1996.

230. Curci MR, Dibbins AW: Problems associated with a Nissen fundoplication following tracheoesophageal fistula and esophageal atresia repair. Arch Surg 123:618–620, 1988.

231. Wheatley MJ, Coran AG, Wesley JR: Efficacy of the Nissen fundoplication in the management of gastroesophageal reflux following esophageal atresia repair. J Pediatr Surg 28:53–55, 1993.

232. Jolley SG, Johnson DG, Roberts CC, et al: Patterns of gastroesophageal reflux in children following repair of esophageal atresia and distal tracheoesophageal fistula. J Pediatr Surg 15:857–862, 1980.

233. Engum SA, Grosfeld JL, West KW, et al: Analysis of morbidity and mortality in 227 cases of esophageal atresia and/or tracheoesophageal fistula over two decades. Arch Surg 130:502–509, 1995.

234. Lindahl H, Rintala R: Long-term complications in cases of isolated esophageal atresia treated with esophageal anastomosis. J Pediatr Surg 30:1222–1223, 1995.

235. Orringer MB, Kirsh MM, Sloan H: Long-term esophageal function following repair of esophageal atresia. Ann Surg 186:436–443, 1977.

236. Duranceau A, Fisher SR, Flye MW, et al: Motor function of the esophagus after repair of esophageal atresia and tracheoesophageal fistula. Surgery 82:116–123, 1977.

237. Romeo G, Zuccarello B, Proietto F, et al: Disorders of the esophageal motor activity in atresia of the esophagus. J Pediatr Surg 22:120–124, 1987.

238. Shono T, Suita S, Arima T, et al: Motility function of the esophagus before primary anastomosis in esophageal atresia. J Pediatr Surg 28:673–676, 1993.

239. Tovar JA, Diez Pardo JA, Murcia J, et al: Ambulatory 24-hour manometric and pH metric evidence of permanent impairment of clearance capacity in patients with esophageal atresia. J Pediatr Surg 30:1224–1231, 1995.

240. Parker AF, Christie DL, Cahill JL: Incidence and significance of gastroesophageal reflux following repair of esophageal atresia and tracheoesophageal fistula and the need for antireflux procedures. J Pediatr Surg 14:5–8, 1979.

241. Pieretti R, Shandling B, Stephens CA: Resistant esophageal stenosis associated with reflux after repair of esophageal atresia: A therapeutic approach. J Pediatr Surg 9:355–357, 1974.

242. Fonkalsrud EW: Gastroesophageal fundoplication for reflux following repair of esophageal atresia: Experience with nine patients. Arch Surg 114:48–51, 1979.

243. Lindahl H, Rintala R, Louhimo I: Failure of the Nissen fundoplication to control gastroesophageal reflux in esophageal atresia patients. J Pediatr Surg 24:985–987, 1989.

244. Snyder CL, Ramachandran V, Kennedy AP, et al: Efficacy of partial wrap fundoplication for gastroesophageal reflux after repair of esophageal atresia. J Pediatr Surg 32:1089–1092, 1997.

245. O'Neill JA, Betts J, Ziegler MM, et al: Surgical management of reflux strictures of the esophagus in childhood. Ann Surg 196:453, 1982.

246. Broto J, Asensio M, et al: Conservative treatment of caustic esophageal injuries in children: 20 years of experience. Pediatr Surg Int 15:323–325, 1999.

247. Broto J, Asensio M, Gil Vernet JM: Results of a new technique in the treatment of severe esophageal stenosis in children: Poliflex stents. J Pediatr Gastroenterol, 2003, in press.

248. Hetzel DJ, Dent J, Reed WD, et al: Healing and relapse of severe peptic esophagitis after treatment with omeprazole. Gastroenterology 95:903–912, 1988.

249. Kato S, Ebina K, Fujii K, et al: Effect of omeprazole in the treatment of refractory acid-related diseases in childhood: Endoscopic healing and 24-hour intragastric acidity. J Pediatr Surg 128:415–421, 1996.

250. DeGiacomo C, Bawa P, Franceshi M, et al: Omeprazole for severe reflux esophagitis in children. J Pediatr Gastroenterol Nutr 24:528–532, 1997.

251. Fitzgerald RC: Significance of acid exposure in Barrett's esophagus. Am J Gastroenterol 98:699–700, 2003.

252. Boyce HW: Barrett's esophagus: endoscopic findings and what to biopsy. J Clin Gastroenterol 36:S6–S18, 2003.

253. Robert ME: Defining dysplasia in Barrett's esophagus. J Clin Gastroenterol 36:S19–S25, 2003.

254. Hoeffel JC, Nihoul-Fekete C, Schmitt M: Esophageal adenocarcinoma after gastroesophageal reflux in children. J Pediatr Surg 115:259–261, 1989.

255. Adzick NS, Fisher JH, Winter HS, et al: Esophageal adenocarcinoma 20 years after esophageal atresia repair. J Pediatr Surg 24:741–744, 1989.

256. Hassall E, Weinstein WM: Partial regression of childhood Barrett's esophagus after fundoplication. Am J Gastroenterol 87:1506–1512, 1992.

257. Nibali SC, Barresi G, Tuccari G, et al: Barrett's esophagus in an infant: A long standing history with final postsurgical regression. J Pediatr Gastroenterol Nutr 7:602–607, 1988.

258. Cheu HW, Grosfeld JL, Heifetz SA, et al: Persistence of Barrett's esophagus in children after antireflux surgery: Influence on follow-up care. J Pediatr Surg 27:260–266, 1992.

259. Salo JA, Salminen JT, Kiviluoto TA, et al: Treatment of Barrett's esophagus by endoscopic laser ablation and antireflux surgery. Ann Surg 227:40–44, 1998.

260. Heitmiller RF: Prophilactic esophagectomy in Barrett's esophagus with high-grade dysplasia. Langenbecks Arch Surg 388:83, 2003.

261. Fitzgerald RC: Ablative mucosectomy is the procedure of choice to prevent Barrett's cancer. Gut 52:16–17, 2003.

CHAPTER 29

Lesions of the Stomach

Brain F. Gilchrist, MD, FACS, and Marc S. Lessin, MD

The stomach of a child is the seat of a plethora of disturbances, diseases, and disabilities. Because of advances in endoscopic diagnosis and treatment, our ability to remedy these afflictions is better and less invasive than it was in the past. However, the lesions discussed in the following pages have remained essentially the same for countless years.

EMBRYOLOGY AND ANATOMY

The stomach as a distinct entity is discernible at the 10-mm embryonic stage. The dorsal aspect of the developing stomach elongates more rapidly than the ventral, a fact that produces the greater curvature and the rotation of the stomach on its longitudinal axis.

It is the transposition of the ventrum and the dorsum that leads to the stomach's unique relation with the vagus nerve branches. The rotation that occurs early in development brings the originally right-sided surface dorsally, and the left, ventrally. Thus the right vagus nerve is distributed mainly to the dorsum of the stomach, and the left vagus supplies mainly the ventral surface.

Ultimately the stomach develops and continues to enlarge after birth. Its mean capacity varies with age, being 30 mL at birth, increasing gradually to 1000 mL at puberty, and finally reaching 1500 mL in adults. The stomach is subject to many maladies and pathologies during infancy and childhood, the first of which has its etiology in the embryologic development of the gastric attachments, gastric volvulus.

GASTRIC VOLVULUS

Gastric volvulus, although rare, has been known for more than 3 centuries.[1,2] Chronic gastric volvulus is far greater in frequency, but the acute form is far more serious. The usual cause of both forms is a constellation of laxities: laxity of the gastrophrenic ligaments, the esophageal hiatus, the vasa brevia, and the gastrocolic ligaments.

Gastric volvulus also can occur when these ligamentous entities are absent.

Gastric volvulus most often is initially seen with symptoms of foregut obstruction. However, if vascular compromise is present, systemic and local signs of ischemia will be noted. One should also keep in mind that a mass might be felt in the epigastrium because of volvulus-induced pyloric obstruction.

Classification of gastric volvulus is done along geometric lines. Organoaxial volvulus is a twist along the stomach's long axis. Mesenterioaxial volvulus is a twist along the horizontal line of axis (i.e., from the greater to the lesser curvatures of the stomach) (Fig. 29-1). The torsion in either plane may be total or incomplete.

Plain roentgenograms of the abdomen may reveal gastric dilatation. A contrast study may demonstrate a high-grade obstruction of the gastroesophageal junction (Fig. 29-2).

Detorsion is an emergency surgical procedure if gastric necrosis is to be avoided. Emergency intraoperative decompression of the stomach can be done with needle or trocar. One caveat, however, is to close the puncture wound before reduction of the torsion, as the site may later be inaccessible. Gastrostomy or anterior gastropexy is then performed. Gastric perforations, which may have occurred, must be debrided and closed or used as the site of a gastrostomy. Recurrence of gastric volvulus has been reported but should be rare, if fixation has been adequate.

GASTRIC PERFORATION IN THE NEWBORN

Gastric perforation in a newborn is remarkable for a number of reasons. The massive pneumoperitoneum that results is startling. Traumatic perforation of a newborn's stomach can be the result of bag-mask ventilation, a misplaced endotracheal tube, or perforation from insertion of a rigid nasogastric tube. Perforation of a newborn's stomach also can occur because of ischemia associated with birth asphyxia, maternal use of cocaine, volvulus, and necrotizing entercolitis totalis. However, some cases

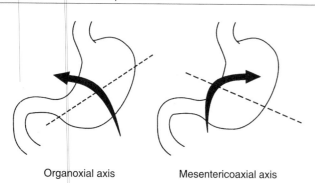

Organoxial axis   Mesentericoaxial axis

FIGURE 29-1. Schematic representation of the two types of gastric volvulus with their lines of rotation.

of spontaneous perforation are not easily explicable. Some have invoked an intrinsic deficiency in the musculature of the newborn's stomach wall,[3] but to date, no all-encompassing answer to the riddle of spontaneous perforation is known.

The surgical strategy in all of these cases, irrespective of the etiology, is to maintain as much stomach as possible. Operative management revolves around the size of the perforation and what can be done to establish closure safely. Although massive gastric resections and subsequent Hunt-Lawrence pouch formation have been necessary in cases in which maternal opiate use was apparent, the usual situation necessitates a two-layer closure of a rent along the

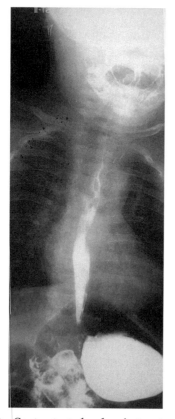

FIGURE 29-2. Contrast study showing organ axial gastric volvulus. Air outlines the greater curvature of the stomach to be against the diaphragm.

greater curvature. Mortality from these cases is predicated on the underlying condition of the child.

FOREIGN BODIES AND BEZOARS

The presence of a foreign body in a child's stomach is a cause of great concern, apprehension, and misinformation. Almost all foreign bodies that find their way into the stomach will pass without problem. However, the rules followed by most pediatric surgeons are that objects that linger in the stomach for 30 days or more, objects that are sharp on both ends, and batteries of any type must be removed either endoscopically or surgically.[4]

Bezoars also are problematic for children, as they commonly cause gastric outlet obstruction. A bezoar is an accumulation of indigestible material A bezoar can be derived from vegetable matter (phytobezoar), undigested milk products (lactobezoar), hair, or other fibers (tricobezoar).[5] A bezoar, regardless its type, ultimately becomes problematic when it reaches a critical mass, forms a cast in the contour of the stomach, and obstructs the outflow tract (Fig. 29-3*A* and *B*).

Upper abdominal distention is seen when the bezoar has reached obstructive proportions. Many pediatric surgeons will opt for immediate operative intervention regardless the type of bezoar. It is thought that attempting to digest phytobezoars partially with papain or cellulase is time consuming and often futile. Some, however, would attempt to fragment a fibrous bezoar endoscopically and remove it piecemeal via an endoscope. A lactobezoar may be amenable to nasogastric decompression and saline washout via the tube.[6]

CHILDHOOD OBESITY

Morbid obesity in children is discussed in detail in Chapter 78. It is apparent in the United States that childhood obesity is an insidiously developing national epidemic.[7] An obese child very often becomes an obese adult and suffers through all stages of life. Obesity leads to diabetes, hypertension, joint diseases, and vascular and cardiopulmonary pathology.[8] Once the obesity has reached morbid dimensions, diets and behavior modifications rarely are effective.[9] The need for early and safe intervention is obvious. The development of minimally invasive, reversible operations is both appealing and logical for the pediatric population.[10]

Some centers have developed a program to address pediatric morbid obesity. Multispecialty involvement in the evaluation of each child seen for possible bariatric intervention is essential. Our morbid obesity team includes members of the University departments of Ethics and Philosophy, so that issues such as informed consent and compliance are examined in a reasoned and appropriate manner. A diverse group with differing perspectives must determine patient selection, quality assurance, and surgical suitability. The role of pediatric surgeons in the surgical treatment of morbid obesity is just beginning to be defined.[11]

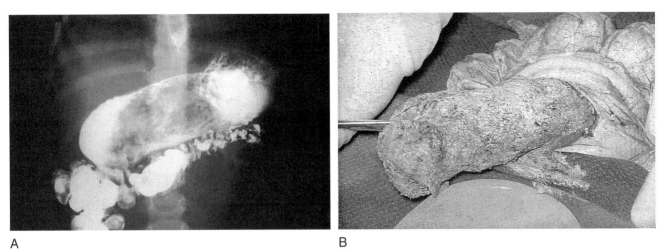

A   B

FIGURE 29-3. *A*, Contrast radiograph of tricobezoar in stomach. *B*, Gastrostomy with removal of barium-stained tricobezoar.

Without doubt, institutional resources, commitment, and expertise to manage the many psychosocial issues that are associated with morbid obesity must be well examined and developed. Preoperative, operative, and postoperative issues are equally important. Research into pediatric morbid obesity and the result of surgical intervention on the physiology of obese children is expanding.[12]

PYLORIC STENOSIS

Pyloric stenosis (PS) is the most common surgical cause of vomiting in infancy. It was first described as a disease by the famous pathologist, Hirschsprung,[13] in 1888, who named the entity as congenital hypertrophic pyloric stenosis. The first report of successful treatment was in 1898, with a gastrojejunostomy. Surgical mortality was high until Borgwardt and Ramstedt[14] in 1912 described the extramucosal muscle-splitting operation that remains essentially the same today.

Incidence

The incidence of pyloric stenosis has been increasing from approximately 1:900 live births reported in 1957[15] to 1:150 reported in 1988.[16] PS is rare in African-American and Asian children, occurring more commonly in the white population.[17] Male infants are affected 4 times more frequently than are girls. The commonly held historic predisposition for PS in first-born male infants has been disputed.[18] A hereditary disposition to PS has been noted, with approximately 1 in 20 male offspring and 1 in 50 female offspring from an affected male parent.[19] The incidence of PS in a male offspring of an affected mother is approximately 15%.[20] PS has an increased incidence in babies with intestinal malrotation, obstructive uropathy, and esophageal atresia.

Pathophysiology

The pyloric musculature in PS demonstrates hypertrophy without hyperplasia.[19] The thickened pyloric muscle protrudes distally into the duodenal lumen, producing a reflection of duodenal mucosa that is subject to injury at the time of the pyloromyotomy. Extending the pyloromyotomy distal to the pyloric vein can result in entry into the duodenal lumen.

Although several etiologies for this condition have been hypothesized, the true etiology is not known. Congenital redundancy of the pyloric mucosa has been implicated.[19] Milk curds passing through the channel narrowed by redundant pyloric mucosa may result in edema, leading to further obstruction.[21] Other theories implicate abnormalities of local enteric innervation and diminished levels of nitric oxide synthase.[22,23] Exposure to erythromycin either prenatally or up to the first 2 weeks of life has been associated with a significant increase in PS.[24] If PS is not treated surgically, it will eventually resolve. In Europe, PS in the past was treated with frequent small-volume, low-curd feedings, such as dextrose water or breast milk. The pyloric hypertrophy would eventually resolve. However, this takes several months and is associated with significant morbidity. The Japanese have used atropine successfully for treatment, although it requires intravenous administration and is associated with a significant failure rate.[25] Neither of these nonoperative techniques has gained acceptance in the United States.

Clinical Presentation

The typical age at presentation is 2 to 8 weeks. In previously premature infants, which account for 10% of cases, it typically occurs when the child reaches 42 to 50 weeks of postconceptual age.[26] Only 4% of cases occur beyond age 3 months.[27] The child has postprandial, forceful, nonbilious vomiting, commonly referred to as "projectile." Rarely the emesis may be bloody from gastritis or esophageal trauma. The infant typically is hungry after vomiting, eager to eat, only to vomit once again. Often multiple formula changes have been attempted before the diagnosis. Less vomiting occurs with low-curd feedings such as breast milk, or dextrose with water. The progression, if not recognized, will lead to weight loss, often below birth weight. Today with increased awareness among pediatricians and family practitioners, more than 90% are initially seen without serious dehydration or electrolyte disturbance.[28]

In addition to pylorospasm, the differential diagnosis includes viral enteritis and gastroesophageal reflux.

Diagnosis

Today, more than two-thirds of patients will have the suspicion of pyloric stenosis confirmed with ultrasonography (US). Almost 100% of patients have imaging before surgical repair, in contradistinction to traditional diagnosis on the basis of physical examination.[28,29] The abdomen is scaphoid, particularly after recent emesis. Occasionally, gastric peristaltic waves can be seen through the abdominal wall. The hypertrophic pylorus can be palpated in the right upper quadrant by an experienced diagnostician in more than 90% of cases. This is best accomplished by emptying the stomach with an orogastric tube and then giving the baby a dextrose/water solution or pacifier during the examination. Palpation of the hypertrophied pylorus, which has the feel of an olive, confirms the diagnosis, and no further imaging is necessary. An impression of a hypertrophied pylorus can be given by palpation of the caudate lobe of the liver, the right kidney, the vertebrae, or an orogastric tube in the distal stomach. US has almost exclusively replaced the upper gastrointestinal contrast study as the confirmatory study. A sonogram shows a thickened pylorus wall in excess of 3 mm, a length in excess of 15 mm, along with a classic appearance of the narrowed pyloric channel and redundant thickened mucosa[30,31] (Fig. 29-4A). US has a sensitivity of 97% and a specificity of 100%.[32] Pylorospasm may initially be mistaken for PS, but the experienced ultrasonographer will recognize periods of relaxation and make the correct diagnosis. Pylorospasm has been hypothesized to be an early stage of PS, but this has not been proven. If US is not diagnostic, an upper gastrointestinal series may be obtained. Positive studies will show a narrow pyloric channel, the so-called "string sign," and the "shoulder sign," which is caused by the impression of the pylorus into the stomach (see Fig. 29-4B).

Preoperative Preparation

Although it is rare that infants have severe electrolyte disturbances, the serum electrolytes should always be determined. The most common abnormality is hyponatremic, hypochloremic, hypokalemic metabolic alkalosis with paradoxical aciduria. The loss of gastric secretion secondary to protracted vomiting will result in dehydration. As a result, through aldosterone-stimulated absorption, potassium is excreted in the urine in an attempt to conserve sodium. As potassium depletion worsens, sodium resorption across the renal tubule is then achieved in exchange for a hydrogen ion, thereby creating paradoxical aciduria.[33] Mild electrolyte disturbances can be corrected preoperatively with 0.45% normal saline with 5% dextrose. Severe disturbances require correction with 0.9% normal saline bolus of 10 to 20 mL/kg, followed by administration of 0.9% normal saline in 5% dextrose solution. Potassium can be added if necessary when urine output is established. Fluid should be administered at a rate 25% to 50% above maintenance. Although preoperative nasogastric tube placement

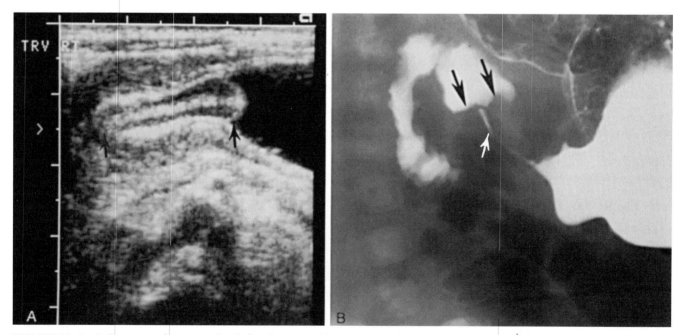

FIGURE 29-4. *A,* Sonogram demonstrating infant hypertrophic stenosis with an elongated pylorus (note the distance between the *arrows*) and a thickened pyloric wall with increased total diameter. *B,* Classic appearance of infant hypertrophic pyloric stenosis with a barium contrast study. Note the gastric distention, narrowed pyloric channel (*small arrow*), and a fornix or "shoulder effects" of bulging hypertrophic muscle at the distal duodenal end of the pylorus (*large arrows*). (Courtesy of G. W. Taylor, MD.)

is somewhat controversial, most will stop vomiting with cessation of feeds. Most pediatric surgeons do not place a gastric decompression tube preoperatively, as it is believed to exacerbate the loss of gastric secretions. The procedure is not an emergency. Common sense requires the correction of electrolyte disturbances before operative correction of the obstruction, with a particular goal of reducing the serum bicarbonate to less than 30 mEq/dL because of potential myocardial dysfunction and respiratory depression when it is elevated above this level.[34]

Occasionally children with PS will have jaundice due to a transient impairment of glucuronyl transferase activity. This is self-limited once postoperative feeding is initiated.[35]

Operative Management

Infants undergoing pyloromyotomy are assumed to have a full stomach. Evacuation of the stomach in the operating room is indicated. Most pediatric anesthesiologists prefer awake intubation to protect against aspiration.

Preoperative antibiotics are controversial, and data supporting their use with the standard right upper quadrant incision are scant.[36] They may be of benefit when performing the operation through the umbilical skin fold.[37]

The basic operation has remained the same since described by Ramstedt nearly 100 years ago. Several incisions have been described to expose the pylorus and perform the extramucosal pyloromyotomy. Classically, the operation has been approached through a right upper quadrant muscle-splitting approach. A transverse incision is made midway between the umbilicus and the xiphoid. The anterior and posterior rectus sheaths can be divided transversely or longitudinally. The omentum is delivered through the incision by placing a moist sponge and then withdrawing it. Traction on the omentum delivers the transverse colon and stomach. The stomach proximal to the pylorus is delivered, and the pyloric "tumor" is gently rocked until it is delivered through the incision. The serosa is incised from 1 to 2 mm proximal to the pyloric vein or the obvious color change between pylorus and duodenum (Fig. 29-5*A–C*). The superficial incision is extended proximally onto the stomach 1.5 cm beyond the proximal portion of the hypertrophied muscle. The outer longitudinal and inner circular muscle fibers are split with the blunt end of the scalpel handle until the mucosa pouts through the muscular defect. The back side of a curved hemostat or a special pyloric spreader designed for the operation can be used to complete the separation of the thickened muscle. Extreme care must be used

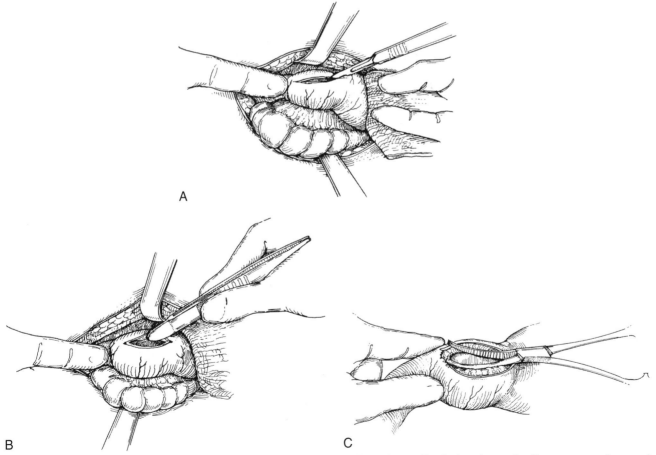

A

B

C

FIGURE 29-5. *A,* The serosa over the hypertrophied pylorus is incised from the small pyloric vein proximally onto normal stomach. *B,* The blunt end of the scalpel is used to divide most of the hypertrophied muscle. *C,* A blunt spreader completes the pyloromyotomy. (From Ashcraft KW, et al: Atlas of Pediatric Surgery, 1994.)

in dividing the last few muscle fibers on the duodenal end of the incision, as this can result in entry into the duodenum where the duodenal mucosa has been folded back over the hypertrophied pyloric muscle. The adequacy of the pyloromyotomy is demonstrated with the index finger so that both sides move independently. Gentle "milking" of the duodenum, observing for the presence of bile or gas, will demonstrate a perforation of the mucosa. If the lumen has been entered on either end of the incision, it can be repaired with a fine absorbable suture without reapproximating the muscle or closing the pyloromyotomy. Alternatively, and particularly for a central laceration of the mucosa, the pyloromyotomy should be closed, the pylorus rotated 180 degrees, and a new pyloromyotomy performed on the opposite side. In this case, a nasogastric decompression is necessary for 24 hours after the procedure, and the initiation of feeding is delayed. Mild bleeding may occur from the pyloromyotomy incision due to venous congestion that will resolve with return of the pylorus to the peritoneal cavity. Arterial bleeding from the muscular edge can be sutured or cauterized.

Two alternative approaches have recently become popular: a supraumbilical transverse skin-fold incision and laparoscopic pyloromyotomy. These approaches appear to be equally effective and result in better long-term cosmesis. The complication rates may be higher, although this may be related to the learning curve.[37,38]

Postoperative Management

Postoperative nasogastric decompression is not necessary unless the mucosa has been entered and repaired. Postoperative pain management seldom requires narcotic medication. Infants are particularly prone to apnea, and these medications have a long half-life in the infant. Acetaminophen is usually all that is necessary. Several feeding schedules have been advocated after surgery. Traditional structured feeding regimens as opposed to more rapid initiation and advancing feeding schedules are probably unnecessary.[39] Feedings are begun 4 to 6 hours after operation, normally with low-volume balanced electrolyte or dextrose solution initially, and rapidly advanced to full feeds of formula over the next 12- to 24-hour period. If the patient vomits, which is common after this procedure, the same volume feed that caused the emesis can be repeated. The patient is usually discharged the day after operation.

Postoperative complications include wound infection and dehiscence in about 1%.[40,41] Persistent vomiting beyond 48 hours, thought to be due to gastric atony, occurs in about 3%. Unrecognized perforation during pyloromyotomy is a serious but rare problem demanding immediate reoperation. Incomplete pyloromyotomy may occur but is difficult to distinguish from gastroesophageal reflux. Unfortunately, imaging studies done postoperatively are difficult to interpret and usually not helpful. If complete gastric-outlet obstruction is present on a contrast study, repeated pyloromyotomy is necessary.

After a surgical pyloromyotomy, the pyloric muscle subsides to a normal size, and when viewed during subsequent operations, is usually visible only as a fine line over the pylorus at the site of the myotomy.

PEPTIC ULCER DISEASE

Peptic ulcer disease in children and adolescents is rare. The original classification of ulcers, which is still used today, was described in 1963.[42] Ulcers have been classified as primary when no etiologic factors are apparent and secondary when they result from disorders elsewhere in the body. The presence of *Helicobacter pylori* infection is an important etiologic factor now recognized in primary ulceration. Similar etiologic factors noted in adults have been noted in children, including hyperacidity with duodenal ulcers and type O blood. A familial predisposition[43] may be related to bacterial transmission. Environmental factors have been implicated, such as cigarette smoking, alcohol use, caffeine, anti-inflammatory medications, corticosteroids, and stress.[44]

Primary ulcer disease is seen in the absence of underlying illness. The ulcers are usually duodenal or prepyloric and are uncommon in neonates and small children. A strong relation exists between *H. pylori* infection and duodenal ulcers, and to a lesser extent, gastric ulcers. Appropriate testing for *H. pylori* should be carried out in any patient with duodenal or gastric ulcers.[45] The rate of *H. pylori* infection is 10% to 80% in different parts of the world, with the highest prevalence in underdeveloped countries. Worldwide, 50% of children are infected by age 10 years. This infection is spread through oral-to-oral contact or fecal-to-oral contamination, as well as by contamination of the water supply in the Third World. In addition to association with peptic ulcer disease, *H. pylori* has been associated with gastric adenocarcinoma and mucosa-associated lymphoid tumor (MALToma).[46] The diagnosis is established by endoscopy with biopsy submitted for urease testing. The standard testing for eradication of *H. pylori* is urea breath testing. Eradication therapy is indicated in the symptomatic patient in the face of positive testing for *H. pylori*. The evidence does not support therapy for abdominal pain or non–ulcer-related dyspepsia. The treatment is a proton-pump inhibitor, amoxicillin, and either metronidazole or clarithromycin for 10 to 14 days.[47]

Secondary ulcers are usually associated with stress, systemic illness, or medications. The most commonly implicated medications are corticosteroids and nonsteroidal anti-inflammatory medications.[48] Zollinger-Ellison syndrome and Crohn's disease can result in secondary gastric ulceration.[49,50] Stress ulcers are usually multiple and associated with gastritis. They are believed to be associated with disruption of the protective mucosal barrier complicated by hyperacidity. Cushing's ulcers are associated with traumatic head injury and occur equally in the stomach and duodenum.[51] Curling's ulcers are associated with serious burn injuries and are more common in the duodenum.[52]

Peptic ulcer disease may initially appear with pain, obvious bleeding, occult blood in the stool, or vomiting. A thorough history should be taken for common etiologic causes, including particularly a medication history. Endoscopic evaluation in children is usually indicated, whereas a presumptive diagnosis in adults can be treated without endoscopic verification. A biopsy should be performed of gastric ulcers to rule out rare tumors. Ulcers in unusual locations, such as the stomach, distal duodenum, and jejunum, should raise suspicion of gastrin-secreting tumors.[53] The diagnosis is confirmed by an elevated serum gastrin determination.

Surgical intervention is rarely indicated. Significant hemorrhage or perforation may warrant surgical repair or control[54] (Fig. 29-6). In a child, surgical intervention is generally considered after transfusion of half of the blood volume. Control of the bleeding usually requires only oversewing of the ulcer. A vagotomy is seldom indicated, considering the availability of the newer acid-suppressing medications.

GASTROPARESIS

Gastroparesis is defined as delayed gastric emptying in the absence of an anatomic obstruction. Symptoms include nausea, vomiting, abdominal distention, and epigastric pain. Infants may have irritability and failure to thrive. Delayed gastric emptying often occurs in association with gastroesophageal reflux.[55] The condition is often drug induced and may be associated with narcotic medications and tricyclic antidepressants.[56] Postviral gastroparesis can be an acute, self-limiting condition, or it may be chronic. Antroduodenal motility studies demonstrate postprandial antral hypomotility. Nuclear medicine studies with a tagged meal will demonstrate a 50% retention of the tracer beyond 60 to 90 minutes, adjusted for the age of the patient.

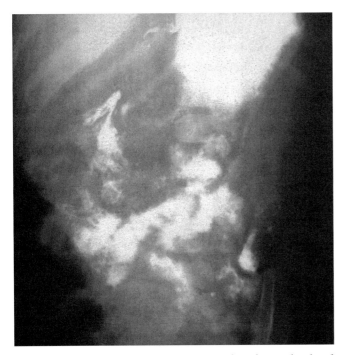

FIGURE 29-6. Contrast demonstration of perforate duodenal ulcer in a 1-year-old child. The extravasated barium has created a "7" sign on the underside of the liver.

Gastroparesis commonly occurs in conjunction with diffuse motility dysfunction of the gastrointestinal tract. Children with intestinal pseudoobstruction, cerebral palsy, and muscular dystrophy often have symptoms of delayed gastric emptying.[57,58] Some have advocated performing gastric-emptying studies on all neurologically delayed children before fundoplication, and if abnormal, performing a concomitant pyloroplasty.[59,60]

Dietary modification can be invoked to treat mild delays in gastric emptying. Medications such as metoclopramide (a dopamine antagonist) and erythromycin (a motilin agonist) have been used with some success. Because gastroparesis is usually self-limited, surgical intervention is seldom necessary. A nasojejunal tube can be placed as a temporizing measure. In chronic conditions lasting several months, it may be necessary to perform a pyloromyotomy or pyloroplasty, most often in conjunction with placement of a gastrostomy. Occasionally when gastric retention is severe, a gastrostomy tube can be placed for decompression, and a jejunal tube, for feeding.

MICROGASTRIA

The cause of hypoplasia of the stomach is a lack of fetal rotation. This lack of rotation arrests the differentiation of the stomach into its component parts of fundus cardia, antrum and pyloric channel. The gastroesophageal junction is thus incompetent, and the esophagus assumes the storage function in the foregut.[61] Malrotation, nonrotation, esophageal atresia without tracheoesophageal fistula, and other anomalies may be present. Vomiting from birth is the principal clinical presentation.

GASTRIC DUPLICATIONS

Gastric duplications account for fewer than 4% of all gastrointestinal tract duplications. The majority are located along the greater curvature, are cystic in nature, and are not in continuity with the lumen of the stomach.[62] Duplications elsewhere in the gastrointestinal tract with heterotopic gastric mucosa are not considered true gastric duplications. Approximately half are discovered in the neonatal period and are seen with vomiting, poor feeding, and an epigastric mass.[63] Duplications in the region of the pylorus can mimic PS.[64] US will show a cystic mass. Nuclear medicine technetium scanning will show uptake if gastric mucosa is in the duplication. Communication with the pancreatic duct and recurrent pancreatitis have been reported.[65] Extralobar bronchopulmonary sequestrations may attach to the gastroesophageal junction and be associated with a gastric duplication.[66,67] When continuity exists with the stomach lumen, the patient may have hematemesis or melena.

The treatment of a gastric duplication is excision. Most will not communicate directly with the stomach lumen. When communication exists, a two-layer closure of the defect is all that is necessary. When a duplication involves the entire greater curvature, mucosal stripping through multiple incisions in the duplication can be performed. Excision is curative.

GASTRIC POLYPS

Gastric polyps are a rare entity in children. Gastric polyps, particularly in the fundus, are associated with the polyposis syndromes. More than 50% of patients with familial polyposis coli syndrome will develop gastric polyps, most often in adulthood. Polyps associated with familial adenomatous polyposis have malignant potential and should be removed.[68] Most solitary polyps are hyperplastic/inflammatory, with no malignant potential.[69] An association has been reported with omeprazole therapy for gastroesophageal reflux. These do not appear to have malignant potential.[70] Polyps can occasionally result in gastric-outlet obstruction or bleeding. Removal can be accomplished endoscopically or, if necessary, through a gastrotomy. Asymptomatic, incidentally discovered gastric polyps need not be removed unless they are encountered in conjunction with familial adenomatous polyposis, Peutz-Jeghers syndrome, or diffuse juvenile polyposis.

FOVEOLAR HYPERPLASIA

Idiopathic foveolar hyperplasia is a rare condition in infants, seen as a gastric-outlet obstruction. It may mimic pyloric stenosis and has been associated with the development of PS.[71,72] Infants receiving prostaglandin therapy to maintain patency of the ductus arteriosus are at risk. The effects appear to be dose related and usually resolve when the prostaglandin is discontinued.[73]

GASTROSTOMY

Gastrostomy provides direct access to the stomach for feeding, decompression, or administration of medication. It is often used in children with neurologic impairment and is done frequently in conjunction with fundoplication. The insertion of a gastrostomy changes the anatomic position of the stomach by displacing the organ anteriorly and inferiorly, resulting in widening of cardioesophageal angle of His.[74] This has been implicated in both causation of de novo reflux and worsening of preexisting reflux.[75] Children with significant clinical reflux should undergo fundoplication at the time of gastrostomy tube placement. Gastrostomy tube placement should be in the anterior gastric wall slightly medial to the greater curvature of the stomach. Some have advocated placement along the lesser curvature to lessen the effects of reflux.[76] Antral tube placement has been associated with worsening reflux.[77] Additionally, placement near the pylorus can result in gastric-outlet obstruction and preclude the use of bolus feedings, which would enter directly into the duodenum. Several techniques for gastrostomy tube placement with a variety of devices are available. Open techniques have been used less

frequently with the advent of laparoscopic and percutaneous endoscopic techniques.

Open gastrostomy is placed through a small upper midline or left upper quadrant incision. A double purse-string suture is placed in the desired location of the anterior wall of the stomach. A gastrostomy tube with an end balloon or a silicone (Silastic) mushroom catheter is brought through the abdominal wall in the left upper quadrant and introduced into the stomach through a gastrotomy made in the center of the previously placed purse-string sutures. The balloon is inflated, the purse-strings secured, and the stomach is sutured to the peritoneum at four points circumferentially around the tube (Fig. 29-7A–C). Alternatively, a low-profile gastrostomy device can be placed primarily.

Percutaneous endoscopic gastrostomy (PEG) has been popularized by pediatric gastroenterologists. The relative contraindications to a PEG procedure are coagulopathy, massive abdominal distention, ascites, and suspected adhesions from previous abdominal surgery. The procedure requires an endoscopist, a gastroscope with a working channel, and an assistant working on the abdominal wall. A guide wire, passed into the stomach through the abdominal wall, is retrieved by the endoscopist and delivered through the esophagus and the mouth. A gastrostomy tube with a rigid flange on the end is secured to the wire. The wire is pulled back through the abdominal wall, with the gastrostomy tube trailing along. The flange within the stomach approximates the serosa of the stomach to the abdominal wall peritoneum. The fibrous union formed between stomach and abdominal wall allows safe removal of the gastrostomy in about 3 months, with replacement by a low-profile device. This requires a second endoscopy to remove the flange, although an alternative is to cut the tube close to the abdominal wall and let the flange pass per rectum.

Complications of this technique include skin necrosis under the bolster used to fix the tube to the abdominal wall, tube dislodgement, and misplacement of the tube transfixing an adjacent viscus, such as the transverse colon or small intestine.[78,79] Inadvertent placement of PEG tubes include placement on the posterior wall of the stomach, placement too near the pylorus, and placement too high on the greater curvature. Accurate positioning of the tube along the stomach requires experience. Failure to position the tube properly along the greater curvature can make subsequent fundoplication, if necessary, difficult, without repositioning the gastrostomy. In an effort to obviate these mishaps, laparoscopy through the umbilicus has been used to visualize the intraperitoneal component of the gastrostomy tube placement.[80]

An alternative method of PEG exists. T-fasteners deployed through hollow needles can be placed through the abdominal wall into the stomach at several points. A guide wire passed through a needle in the center of the T-fasteners is followed by progressive dilators until a breakaway sheath can be placed that will admit a 14F gastrostomy button or tube.[81] The suture attached to the T-fasteners is then secured over a bolster or around the button on the skin surface to hold the stomach against the abdominal wall. It is important to remove these sutures in 1 week to avoid pressure necrosis. Primary

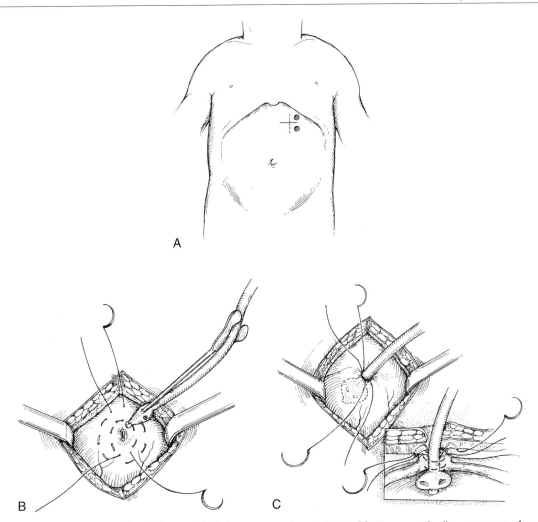

FIGURE 29-7. *A,* Gastrostomy incision is located in left upper quadrant. *B,* Double "purse-string" sutures are placed before the insertion of the depressor gastrostomy catheter. *C,* Tying of the purse-string sutures creates a serosal tunnel. (From Ashcraft KW, et al: Atlas of Pediatric Surgery, 1994.)

button placement has been described as placing two large transfixion sutures (U-stitches) through the full thickness of the abdominal wall, incorporating the stomach under laparoscopic vision and using the needle/guide wire/dilator system to place the button. The sutures are then secured around the low-profile device so that it does not become dislodged. The sutures are removed in 3 days.[82]

Laparoscopic gastrostomy tube placement is performed by placing a lens through an umbilical port. A second port is placed in the left upper quadrant at a site specified before establishment of the pneumoperitoneum for the gastrostomy tube. The stomach is grasped and pulled through the trocar site and secured to the peritoneum. A purse-string is placed around the stomach, and a gastrotomy is made. An inflatable balloon tube is placed in the stomach during visualization with the laparoscope. The purse-string is secured, and the tube is secured to the skin. This can be converted to a low-profile button in approximately 4 weeks without further anesthesia.

Gastrostomy tube placement is often associated with problems. Most are minor and self-limited, such as leakage, granulation tissue, and infection at the site. More serious complications include perforations of the esophagus or stomach, bleeding from gastric erosions, and tube dislodgement. Tube dislodgement is particularly problematic in the early postoperative period when there is not a well-formed tract. Attempting to replace a gastrostomy tube before the stomach has become adherent to the abdominal wall can result in gastric leakage or infusion of formula into the peritoneal cavity. All gastrostomy tubes replaced in the period up to 3 months after initial placement should have their position confirmed by a contrast radiographic study.

Gastrostomy tracts will often close spontaneously with removal or dislodgement of the tube. Tubes that have been out for as little as 1 to 2 hours can be difficult to replace and may require dilation of the tract. Caretakers should be instructed regarding tube replacement or insertion of a temporary catheter into a well-established tract, pending definitive gastrostomy tube replacement.

When the gastrostomy is no longer needed, the tube can simply be removed. Most of the time, the tract will close spontaneously within the first 24 hours. Tracts that do not close will require surgical closure.

REFERENCES

1. Berti A: Singolare attortigliamento dell' esofago col duodeno sequito da rapida morte. Gass Med Ital 9:139, 1866.
2. DeLorimier AA, Penn L: Acute volvulus of the stomach, emphasizing management hazards. AJR Am J Roentgenol 77:627, 1957.
3. Izraeli S, Freud E, et al: Neonatal intestinal perforation due to congenital defects in the intestinal muscularis. Eur J Pediatr 151:300–303, 1992.
4. Schwartz GF, Polsky HS: Ingested foreign bodies of the gastrointestinal tract. Am Surg 51:173, 1985,
5. Bennett P, Herman S: Curious curd. Lancet 1:1430, 1975.
6. Yoss BS: Human milk lactobezoars. J Pediatr 1984;105:819.
7. Stephen AM, Wald NJ: Trends in individual consumption of dietary fat in the United States, 1920-1984. Am J Clin Nutr 52:457–469, 1990.
8. Harris TB, Ballard-Barbasch R, Madans J, et al: Overweight, weight loss and risk of coronary heart disease in older woman. The NHANES-I Follow up study. Am J Epidemiol 137:1318–1327, 1993.
9. Henry RR, Gumbiner B: Benefits and limitations of very low calorie diet therapy in obese NIDDM. Diabetes Care 14: 802-823, 1991.
10. O'Brien PE, Brown WA, Smith, A, et al: Prospective study of a laparoscopically placed, adjustable gastric band in the treatment of morbid obesity. Br J Surg 85:113–118, 1999.
11. Fielding GA, Rhodes M, Nathanson, LK: Laparoscopic gastric banding for morbid obesity. Surg Endosc 13:550–554, 1999.
12. Hsu GLK, Benotti PN, Dwyer J, et al: Nonsurgical factors that influence the outcome of bariatric surgery: Psychosom Med 60:338–346, 1998.
13. Hirschsprung H: Falle von angeborener pylorus stenose. Jb Kinderheilk 27:61, 1888.
14. Borgwardt G, Ramstedt C: An appreciation. Z Kinderchir 41:195–200, 1986.
15. Laron Z, Horne LM: The incidence of infantile pyloric stenosis. Am J Dis Child 94:151, 1957.
16. Jed MB, Melton J, Griffin MR, et al: Factors associated with infantile hypertrophic pyloric stenosis. Am J Dis Child 142:334–337, 1988.
17. Klein A, Cremin BJ: Racial significance in pyloric stenosis. S Afr Med J 44:1130–1134, 1970.
18. Hugenard JR, Staples GE: Incidence of congenital hypertrophic pyloric stenosis within sibships. J Pediatr 81:45–49, 1972.
19. Rowe et al. (eds.).Essentials of Pediatric Surgery. Mosby, 1995, pp 481–485.
20. Carter CO, Evans KA: Inheritance of congenital hypertrophic pyloric stenosis. J Med Genet 6:233–254, 1969.
21. Lynn H: The mechanism of pyloric stenosis and its relationship to preoperative preparation. Arch Surg 81:453, 1960.
22. Langer JC, Berezin I, Daniel EE: Hypertrophic pyloric stenosis: Ultrastructural abnormalities of enteric nerves and interstitial cells of Cajal. J Pediatr Surg 30:1535–1543, 1995.
23. Vanderwinden JM, Pierre M, Schiffman SN, et al: Nitric oxide synthase activity in infantile hypertrophic pyloric stenosis. N Engl J Med 327:511–515, 1992.
24. Cooper WO, Griffin MR, Arbogast P, et al: Very early exposure to erythromycin and infantile hpertrophic pyloric stenosis. Arch Pediatr Adolesc Med 156:647–650, 2002.
25. Nagita A, Yamaguchi J, Amemoto K: Management and ultrasonographic appearance of infantile hypertrophic pyloric stenosis with intravenous atropine sulfate. J Pediatr Gastroenterol Nutr 23:172–177, 1996.
26. Tack ED et al: Pyloric stenosis in the sick premature infant: Clinical and radiologic findings. Am J Dis Child 142:68, 1988.
27. Zhang AL, Cass DT, Dubois RS, et al: Infantile hypertrophic stenosis: A clinical review from a general hospital. J Pediatr Child Health 29:372–378, 1993.
28. Chen EA, Luks FI, Gilchrist BF, et al: Pyloric stenosis in the age of ultrasonography: Fading skills, better patients? J Pediatr Surg 31:829–830, 1996.
29. Papdakis K, Chen EA, Luks FI, et al: The changing presentation of pyloric stenosis. Am J Emerg Med 17:67–69, 1999.
30. Keller H, Waldermann D, Greiner P: Comparison of preoperative sonography with intraoperative findings in congenital hypertrophic pyloric stenosis. J Pediatr Surg 22:950, 1987.
31. Lamki N, Athey PA, Round ME, et al: Hypertrophic pyloric stenosis in the neonate—diagnosis criteria revisited. Can Assoc Radiol J 44:21, 1993.
32. Godbole P, Sprigg A, Dickson JA, et al: Ultrasound compared with clinical examination in infantile hypertrophic pyloric stenosis. Arch Dis Child 75:335–337, 1996.
33. Goh DW, Hall SK, Gornall P, et al: Plasma chloride and alkalaemia in pyloric stenosis. Br J Surg 77:922–923, 1990.
34. Steven IM, Allen TH, Sweeny DB: Congenital hypertrophic pyloric stenosis: the anesthetist's view. Anaesth Intens Care 1:544–546, 1073.
35. Woolley MM, Felsher BF, Asch MJ, et al: Jaundice, hypertrophic pyloric stenosis, and hepatic glucoronyl transferase. J Pediatr Surg 9:359–363, 1974.
36. Nour S, MacKinnon AE, Dickson JAS, et al: Antibiotic prophylaxis for infantile pyloromyotomy. J R Coll Surg Edinb 41:178–180, 1996.
37. Leinwand MJ, Shaul DB, Anderson KD: The umbilical fold approach to pyloromyotomy: Is it a safe alternative to the right upper-quadrant approach? J Am Coll Surg189:362–367, 1999.
38. Harmon CM, Barnhart DC, Georgeson KE, et al: Comparison of the incidence of complications in open and laparoscopic pyloromyotomy: A concurrent single institution series, presentation (abstract) at 34th Annual meeting American Pediatric Surgical Assn, Ft. Lauderdale, FL, 2003.
39. Puapong D, Kahng D, Ko A, et al: Ad libitum feeding: safely improving the cost-effectiveness of pyloromyotomy. J Pediatr Surg 37:1667–1668, 2002.
40. Bell MJ: Infantile pyloric stenosis: Experience with three hundred and five cases at the Louisville Children's Hospital. Surgery 64:983–989, 1968.
41. Gibbs MK, vanHeerden JA, Lynn HB: congenital hypertrophic pyloric stenosis: Surgical experience. Mayo Clin Proc 50:312–316, 1975.
42. Schuster SR, Gross RE: Peptic ulcer disease in childhood. Am J Surg 105:324, 1963.
43. Blodgett MD, Morris N, Lurie HJ: children with peptic ulcers and their families. J Pediatr 62:280, 1963.
44. Mezoff AG, Balistreri WF: Peptic ulcer disease in children Pediatr Rev 16:257, 1995.
45. Dohil R, Hassall E, Jevon G, et al: Gastritis and gastropathy of childhood. J Pediatr Gastroenterol Nutr 29:378–394, 1999.
46. Huang J-Q, Sridhars CY, Hunt RH: Meta-analysis of the relationship between Helicobacter pylori seropositivity and gastric cancer. Gastroenterology 115:642–648, 1998.
47. Gold BD, Colletti RB, Abbott M, et al: Helicobacter pylori infection in children: Recommendations for diagnosis and treatment. J Pediatr Gastroenterol Nutr 31:490–497, 2000.
48. Mulberg AE, Linz C, Verhave M: Identification of nonsteroidal antiinflammatory drug-induced gastroduodenal injury in children with juvenile rheumatoid arthritis. J Pediatr 122:647, 1993.
49. Hirschowitz BI: Zollinger -Ellison syndrome: pathogenesis, diagnosis and management. Am J Gastroenterol 92(suppl 4):445–485, 1996.
50. Moonka D, Lichtenstein GR, Levine MS, et al: Giant gastric ulcers: an unusual manifestation of Crohn's disease. Am J Gastroenterol 88:297–299, 1993.
51. Kumar D, Spitz L: Peptic ulceration in children. Surg Gynecol Obstet 159:63, 1984.
52. Williams JW, Pannell WP, Sherman RT: Curling's ulcer in children. J Trauma 16:639, 1976.
53. Rosenlund ML: The Zollinger-Ellison syndrome in children: A reveiw. Pediatrics 141:894, 1967.
54. Curci MR, Little K, Sieber WK, et al: Peptic ulcer disease in childhood reexamined. J Pediatr Surg 11:329–335, 1976.
55. Cucchiara S, Salvia G, Borrelli O, et al: Gastric electrical dysrhythmias and delayed gastric emptying in gastroesophageal reflux disease. Am J Gastroenterol 92:1103–1108, 1997.
56. Nimmo WS: Drugs, diseases and altered gastric emptying, Clin Pharmacokinet 1:189–203, 1976.
57. Hyman PE: chronic intestinal pseudo-obstruction in childhood: progress indiagnosis and management. Scand J Gastroenterol 213:39–46, 1995.

58. Staiano A, Carraziari E, Andreotti MR, et al: Upper gastrointestinal tract motility in children with progressive muscular dystrophy. J Pediatr 121:720–724, 1992.

59. Bustorff-Silva J, Fonkalsrud EW, Perez CA, et al: Gastric emptying procedures decrease the risk of postoperative recurrent reflux in children with delayed gastric emptying. J Pediatr Surg 34:79–82, 1999.

60. Maxson RT, Harp S, Jackson RJ, et al: Delayed gastric emptying in neurologically impaired children with gastroesophageal reflux: The role of pyloroplasty. J Pediatr Surg 29:726–729, 1994.

61. Blank E, Chisholm AJ: Congenital microgastria: A case report with a 26 year follow-up. Pediatrics 51:1037–1045, 1973.

62. Kremer RM, Kepoff RB, Izant RJ: Duplications of the stomach. J Pediatr Surg 5:360, 1070.

63. Cooper S, Abrams RS, Carbaugh RA: Pyloric duplications: Review and case study. Am Surg 61:1092–1094, 1995.

64. Patel MP, Meisheri IV, Waingankar VS, et al: Duplication cyst of the pylorus: A rare cause of gastric outlet obstruction in the newborn. J Postgrad Med 43:43–45, 1997.

65. Hoffman M, et al: Gastric duplication cyst communicating with aberrant pancreatic duct: A rare cause of recurrent acute pancreatitis. Surgery 101:369, 1987.

66. Spanos C, Lessin M, Brisson P, et al: Thoracoabdominal extralobar sequestration with an unusual combination of congenital anomalies in a neonate. Surg Rounds 22:654–656, 1999.

67. Saggess A, Carbonara A, Russo R, et al: Intra-abdominal extra lobar pulmonary sequestration communicating with gastric duplication: A case report. Eur J Pediatr Surg 12:426–428, 2002.

68. Marcello PW, Asbun HJ, Veidenheimer MC, et al: Gastroduodenal polyps in familial adenomatous polyposis. Surg Endosc 1:418–421, 1995.

69. Attard TM, Yardley JH, Cuffari C: Gastric polyps in pediatrics: An 18-year hospital based analysis. 97:298–301, 2002.

70. Pashankar DS, Israel DM: Gastric polyps and nodules in children receiving long-term omeprazole therapy. J Pediatr Gastroenterol Nutr 35:658–662, 2002.

71. Holland AJ, Freeman JK, Le Quesne GW, et al: Idiopathic focal foveolar hyperplasia in infants. Pediatr Surg Int 12:497–500, 1997.

72. Callahan MJ, McCauley RG, Patel H, et al: The development of hypertrophic pyloric stenosis in a patient with prostaglandin-induced foveolar hyperplasia. Pediatr Radiol 29:748–751, 1999.

73. Pelad N, Dagan O, Babyn P, et al: Gastric outlet obstruction induced by prostaglandin therapy in neonates. N Engl J Med 327:505–510, 1992.

74. Jolley SG, Tunnell WP, Hoelzer J, et al: Lower esophageal pressure changes with tube gastrostomy: A causative factor of gastroesophageal reflux in children? J Pediatr Surg 21:624–627, 1986.

75. Berzein S, Schwartz SM, Halata MS, et al: Gastroesophageal reflux secondary to gastrostomy tube placement. Am J Dis Child 140:699–701, 1986.

76. Seekri IK, Rescorla FJ, Canal DF, et al: Lesser curvature gastrostomy reduces the incidence of postoperative gastroesophageal reflux. J Pediatr Surg 26:982–986, 1991.

77. Razeghi S, Behrens R: Influence of percutaneous endoscopic gastrostomy on gastroesophageal reflux: A prospective study in 68 children. J Pediatr Gastroenterol Nutr 27-3-, 2002.

78. Boey CCM, Goh K-L, Sithasanan N, et al: Jejunal perforation complication PEG insertion in a child. Gastrointest Endosc 55:607–608, 2002.

79. Dwivedi AJ, Chahin F, Patel J, et al: Cologastric and colocutaneous fistulae: Unusual complications of percutaneous endoscopic gastrostomy. Surg Rounds 11:654–656, 2000.

80. Stringel G, Geller ER, Lowenheim MS: Laparoscopic-assisted percutaneous endoscopic gastrostomy. J Pediatr Surg 30:1209–1210, 1995.

81. Tomicic JT, Luks FI, Shalon L: Laparoscopic gastrostomy in infants and children. Eur J Pediatr Surg 12:107–110, 2002.

82. Sampson LK, Georgeson KE, Winters DC: Laparoscopic gastrostomy as an adjunctive procedure to laparoscopic fundoplication in children. Surg Endosc 10:1106–1110, 1996.

Intestinal Atresia and Stenosis

Alastair J. W. Millar, MBChB, FRCS, FRCS(Edin), Heinz Rode,
MBChB, MMed(Surg), FRCS(Edin), and Sidney Cywes,
MMed(Surg), FRCS, FRCS(Edin)

Congenital defects in continuity of the intestine are morphologically divided into either stenosis or atresia and constitute one of the most common causes of neonatal intestinal obstruction.[1-5]

Pyloric atresia is rare and familial, and it has a well-documented association with epidermolysis bullosa.

Congenital duodenal atresia occurs once in approximately 2500 live births, is associated with Down syndrome, and is more frequent in populations with a high rate of consanguinity.[6] Although first described in the 18th century, it was not until the first decade of the 20th century that the surgical treatment began with gastrojejunostomy.[7,8] At present, duodenoduodenostomy, with or without tapering duodenoplasty, has become standard.[8-12]

Most jejunoileal atresias or stenoses result from intrauterine ischemia, although familial cases with multiple atresias have been described.[13] The incidence of jejunoileal atresia is approximately 1 in 1000 live births.[4,14-18] The first successful surgical repair of an intestinal atresia was in 1911.[19] Until the mid-1950s, the prognosis was very poor, largely due to late presentation and dysmotility of the proximal dilated atretic portion of bowel, leading to chronic obstruction, blind-loop syndrome, and inanition. Louw, focusing on the ischemic etiology, reported marked improvement in outcome with back resection of the dilated portion and primary anastomosis.[40] Nixon[20] emphasized the poor prograde peristalsis of the dilated segment, and Benson advocated back resection and primary anastomosis, and these factors, along with advances in neonatal care, made the treatment of intestinal atresia an extraordinary achievement. Only those few with severe congenital abnormalities or very short bowel will not have a good prognosis.[21]

PYLORIC ATRESIA

Pyloric atresia is a rare autosomal genetic defect,[22,23] in which the pyloric lumen is completely obliterated by either a diaphragm or a solid core of tissue, or a complete absence of the pylorus with loss of bowel continuity is noted. Nonbilious vomiting and upper abdominal distention result. Abdominal radiograph shows a single gas bubble or air/fluid level and no distal air in the gastrointestinal (GI) tract (Fig. 30-1). The differential diagnosis includes high duodenal atresia and malrotation with volvulus of the midgut. Gastric perforation may lead to peritonitis and toxemia.[24]

Surgical excision for membranous atresia or a side-to-side gastroduodenostomy successfully restores continuity. Gastrojejunostomy should be avoided. Long-term outcome is excellent except for those with epidermolysis bullosa.[25] We treated two cases that were sporadic and not associated with epidermolysis. Both had a solid core of tissue and were cured with side-to-side gastroduodenostomy.

DUODENAL ATRESIA AND STENOSIS

Etiology

Duodenal atresia and stenosis are most commonly believed to be caused by a failure of recanalization, although others contest this theory.[26-29] During the third week of embryonic development, the second part of the duodenum gives off biliary and pancreatic buds that lead to the formation of the hepatobiliary system and pancreas. Simultaneously, the duodenum passes through a solid phase, with its lumen being reestablished by coalescence of vacuoles between weeks 8 and 10. An embryologic insult during this period may lead to intrinsic webs, atresia, and stenoses.

Occasionally the atresia is associated with pancreatic tissue that may surround the duodenum. This phenomenon is probably a failure of duodenal development rather than a true annular pancreas.[10,30] The distal biliary tree is often abnormal and may open proximal or distal to the atresia.[31,32] Biliary atresia, agenesis of the gallbladder, and stenosis of the common bile duct have been reported

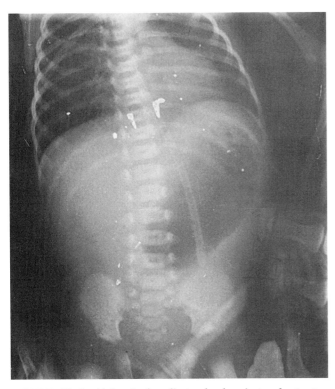

FIGURE 30-1. Abdominal radiograph showing a large gas-filled stomach with no distal air, typical of pyloric obstruction.

to occur in association with duodenal atresia and particularly with double atresias, a rare occurrence having a distinct familial incidence.[5,33–36]

Classification

Stenosis, or incomplete obstruction, may be due to a diaphragm or web with a small opening. A thin web that has ballooned distally is referred to as a *windsock*.[37,38] *Atresia*, or complete obstruction, may be seen with duodenal muscular continuity or with a gap that is usually filled in with pancreatic tissue (Fig. 30-2).

Prematurity, growth retardation, and coexistent malformations are common. Almost 50% of duodenal atresias are associated with some other anomaly (e.g., cardiac, genitourinary, anorectal, or, occasionally, esophageal atresia), and up to 40% have trisomy 21.[39–41]

Pathology

Although the site of obstruction is usually classified as preampullary or postampullary, the majority are postampullary. Depending on the degree of obstruction, the proximal duodenum and stomach dilate to several times their normal size. The pylorus is distended and hypertrophic. The bowel distal to the obstruction is collapsed, and in cases of complete atresia, thin walled. Because the obstruction is high, it is decompressed proximally in utero, and perforation is rare.[42] Associated polyhydramnios is recorded in up to one half of cases, with premature

delivery in one third.[5] Growth retardation also is common, which may imply that the fetus has been deprived of the nutritional contribution of swallowed amniotic fluid.

Diagnosis

Polyhydramnios results from high intestinal obstruction because the reabsorption of amniotic fluid is disturbed. The dilated stomach and proximal duodenum may be seen on antenatal ultrasonography (US), as may associated cardiac abnormalities. Most cases of duodenal atresia are detected between months 7 and 8 of intrauterine life, but a normal US of the fetus with polyhydramnios at that time does not absolutely exclude duodenal obstruction.[43]

The vomiting of clear or bile-stained fluid usually starts within hours of birth. Distention or abnormal stooling may or may not be present. Aspiration via a nasogastric tube of more than 20 mL of gastric contents in a newborn suggests intestinal obstruction; the normal aspirate is less than 5 mL.[44] The diagnosis of an incomplete obstruction (stenosis or web) may be delayed until well beyond the neonatal period.[45] Because most duodenal obstructions occur distal to the ampulla, the vomitus is bile stained in more than two thirds. Occasionally, blood-stained vomitus results from gastritis. Abdominal distention may not be evident, owing to vomiting. Delayed diagnosis may result in dehydration, hyponatremia, and hypochloremia. Jaundice, if present, is rarely obstructive and is more likely due to prematurity and dehydration.

An upright abdominal radiograph using instilled air, if necessary, as contrast, is sufficient to confirm the diagnosis (Fig. 30-3). Intestinal gas beyond the duodenum indicates incomplete obstruction. A contrast meal is then required to exclude malrotation and volvulus (Fig. 30-4) Rarely, the biliary tree is air filled, and a variety of pancreatic and biliary anomalies have been demonstrated[44] (Fig. 30-5). It has not been our practice to perform a contrast enema before operative treatment because colonic atresia is rarely seen, and an enema is an inexact method of determining malrotation.[46]

Management

Once the diagnosis has been established, gastric decompression and correction of fluid and electrolyte disturbances are begun. Other associated anomalies should be excluded by appropriate investigation with radiography, US, and echocardiography. Urgent surgery is indicated if malrotation and volvulus remain as possible diagnoses. Only after the baby has been resuscitated is operative correction performed.

A supraumbilical transverse abdominal incision is preferred. The duodenal obstruction is exposed by mobilizing the ascending and transverse colon to the left and by identifying any associated malrotation, which occurs in approximately 30% of these patients.[5] The pancreas may appear to be annular in nature. Occasionally, an anterior portal vein may be identified. The duodenum and jejunum distal to a complete obstruction are collapsed and thin walled compared with the hypertrophied and

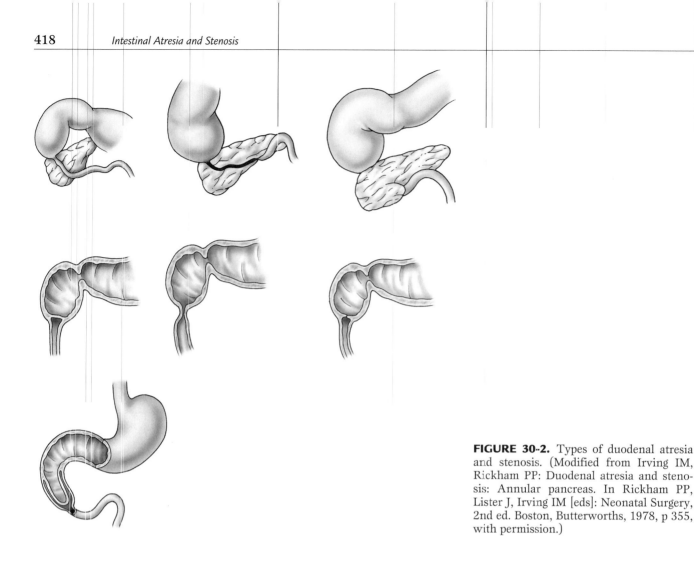

FIGURE 30-2. Types of duodenal atresia and stenosis. (Modified from Irving IM, Rickham PP: Duodenal atresia and stenosis: Annular pancreas. In Rickham PP, Lister J, Irving IM [eds]: Neonatal Surgery, 2nd ed. Boston, Butterworths, 1978, p 355, with permission.)

dilated proximal obstructed duodenum. A sufficient length of duodenum distal to the atresia is mobilized. The operation preferred by most is a diamond-shaped or side-to-side duodenoduodenostomy, by using a transverse incision at the inferior aspect of the proximal blind-ending bulbous part and a longitudinal incision on the distal bowel[47] (Fig. 30-6). Muscular continuity of the duodenal wall suggests a windsock deformity or diaphragm that calls for extra vigilance in the operative correction, as dilated and collapsed bowel, both distal to the windsock duodenal membranes, have been anastomosed in error.[37,48]

Although duodenotomy and web excision have been advocated, a potential exists for bile duct injury with this approach, which seems to have no functional advantage over duodenoduodenostomy.[32,38,39,48] In some cases, a tapering duodenoplasty is performed, excising a wedge of the anterolateral aspect of the second part of the duodenum[12,49]; this is most simply done by using a GI anastomosis stapling device. One must be careful not to narrow the duodenum or injure the ampulla of Vater.[11] Ladd's procedure should be performed when needed. Postoperative nasogastric decompression instead of gastrostomy has been shown to decrease hospitalization from a mean of 20 days to 8 days.[50] Survival rates are in excess of 90%;

mortality, in most cases, is due to an associated cardiac anomaly or chromosomal disorder.[39,42]

Early postoperative complications may be associated with anastomotic leak and local sepsis. Surgical injury to the bile duct has resulted in "acquired atresia."[35] Long-term complications include alkaline reflux and peptic ulceration or duodenal stasis with blind-loop syndrome, recurrent abdominal pain, and diarrhea.[51–53] Gallstones also have been observed after duodenal atresia repair.[54] Protracted follow-up is mandatory.

Patient Review

Over the 44-year period of 1959 to 2003, 187 infants and children with duodenal atresia or stenosis were treated at the Red Cross Children's Hospital in Cape Town. The 115 treated between 1977 and 2003 have been analyzed in detail. Of these 115 patients, maternal polyhydramnios was noted in 12.5% with stenosis and in 65% with atresia. The obstruction was due to stenosis in 22, multiple stenosis in 1, duodenal membrane in 20, single atresia in 73, and multiple atresias in 2. Thirty-eight (32%) had Down syndrome, 19 had congenital heart disease, and 8 had esophageal and anorectal anomalies (Fig. 30-7). More than 50% of those with stenosis or fenestrated

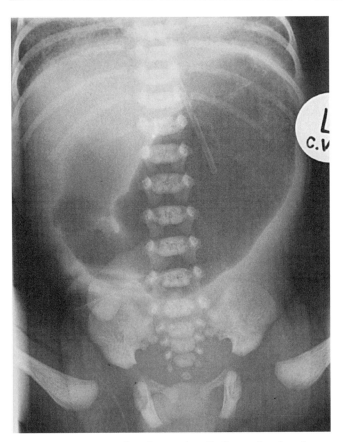

FIGURE 30-3. Duodenal atresia. Radiograph showing a dilated gas-filled stomach and duodenum, with a gasless distal abdomen indicating complete obstruction.

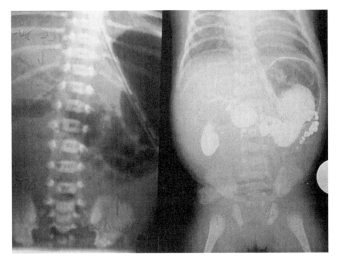

FIGURE 30-4. Duodenal atresia with biliary air and contrast meal outlining bile ducts. Radiograph (*A*) patient with duodenal atresia. Note the gas outlining bile ducts. *B,* A contrast meal in the same patient with contrast filling the dilated intrahepatic bile ducts.

membranes were first seen late (5 weeks to 14 years). Prematurity was much more frequent with atresia (43%) as compared with incomplete obstructions (23%). Only 6 patients were recorded as having a bile duct insertion proximal *and* distal to the obstruction. The 3 patients with multiple membranes were siblings and had associated immunodeficiency.[36] Neither duodenoplasty nor web excision was attempted. Gastrostomy was routinely used until 1992, when a prospective study demonstrated that time to full oral feeding was 15 days with gastrostomy

patients and only 8 days in the group without gastrostomy. Ladd's procedure was performed only if the mesentery was unfixed and the residual pedicle was narrow, thus predisposing the patient to volvulus. No episodes of midgut volvulus in association with duodenal atresia have been recorded in our experience.[46] In this series, only 2 patients required reoperation, which was done at age 6 years, for chronic abdominal pain and residual megaduodenum. Tapering duodenoplasty resolved their symptoms.

JEJUNOILEAL ATRESIA AND STENOSIS

Etiology

Although several mechanisms have been postulated to explain the intestinal atresia malformations,[27,28,55,56] the most favored theory is that of a localized intrauterine

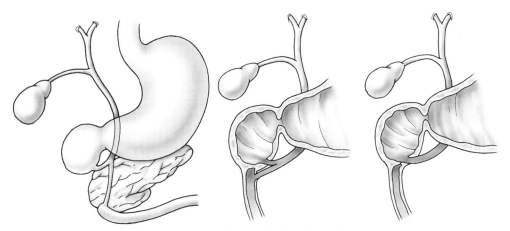

FIGURE 30-5. Types of biliary abnormalities in duodenal atresia.

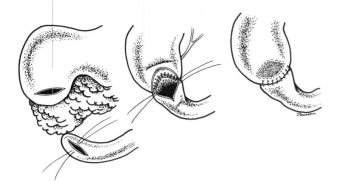

FIGURE 30-6. Duodenoduodenostomy.

vascular accident with ischemic necrosis of the sterile bowel and subsequent resorption of the affected segment or segments[13,40] (Fig. 30-8). This theory was based on results of an investigation of 79 children with intestinal atresia treated at The Hospital for Sick Children in London.[4]

Mesenteric vascular insults, such as ligation of a loop of intestine to simulate the effect of the volvulus, intussusception, and interference with segmental blood supply, were created in fetal dogs, leading to different degrees and patterns of intraluminal obstruction, exactly reproducing the spectrum of stenosis and atresia found in people.[13,14]

It was clearly demonstrated that devitalized segments of bowel were rapidly absorbed, the proximal and distal bowel separated from the devascularized segment and sealed to form rounded blind ends, and adhesions in the vicinity of the pathologic process disappeared unless a perforation led to meconium peritonitis. The interval between producing the ischemic insult and the birth of the experimental animals was too short to establish the histopathology of the event. Sequential histologic studies of this process in fetal rabbits showed rapid liquefaction, absorption, and resolution of necrotic tissue after vascular occlusion. Subsequently, these experimental findings were observed in several different animal models.[57–60]

These findings, together with clinical evidence of presence of bile, lanugo hair, and squamous epithelial cells from swallowed amniotic fluid distal to an atresia, support this hypothesis.[40,59,61,62] In addition, evidence of intrauterine fetal intussusception, midgut volvulus, thromboembolic

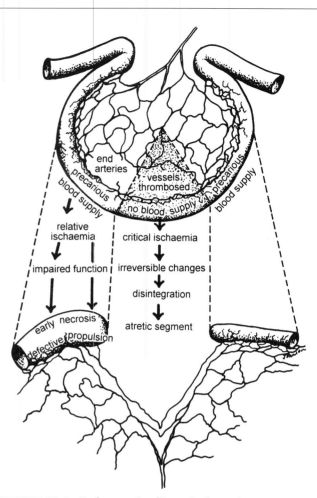

FIGURE 30-8. Pathogenesis of intestinal atresia.

occlusions, transmesenteric internal hernias, and incarceration or snaring of bowel in an omphalocele or gastroschisis has been noted in the fetus and newborn and has led to wide acceptance of this hypothesis.[1,3,15,59,62–67] In our series, the GI anomalies associated with jejunoileal atresia were mostly of such a nature as to predispose to strangulation of the fetal bowel. Anomalous fixation of the intestinal mesentery was reported in 45% of infants born with jejunoileal atresia and multiple occlusions.[4] Evidence of a

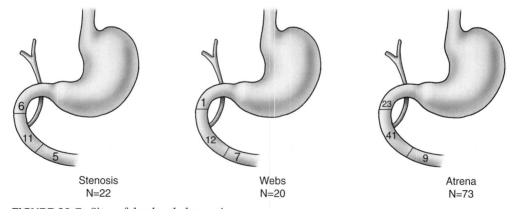

Stenosis
N=22

Webs
N=20

Atrena
N=73

FIGURE 30-7. Sites of duodenal obstruction.

"vascular accident" was present in 118 (41%) of the 292 neonates with jejunoileal atresia in our series. Malrotation or volvulus was detected in 91, exomphalos in 5, gastroschisis in 3, meconium ileus in 5, meconium peritonitis in 7, Hirschsprung's disease with proximal atresia in 5, and internal hernia in 1 neonate. Intrauterine intussusception with postnatal evidence of the intussusception and proximal atresia was seen in 2 patients and generally is responsible for 0.6% to 1.3% of atresias. The site of atresia with this etiology is usually at the ileocecal level.[68] The low prevalence of associated abnormalities is in keeping with the pattern observed in developing countries.[1]

Evidence of bowel infarction was present in 42% of 449 cases of jejunoileal atresia in a collated series.[69] The localized nature of the vascular accident occurring late in fetal life would explain the low incidence (<10%) of coexisting abnormalities of the extra-abdominal organs.[14,69] In rare instances, jejunoileal atresia has been found to be associated with esophageal, gastric, duodenal, colonic, and rectal atresias, as well as biliary atresia, meningomyelocele, and Hirschsprung's disease.[14,15,69-72] Methylene blue, used for amniocentesis in twin pregnancies, has been implicated in causing small bowel atresia.[73]

The anomaly is usually not genetically determined, although affected monozygotic twins and siblings have been described, all having multiple webs.[74] A syndrome of hereditary multiple gastrointestinal atresias has been described with an increased incidence in areas with a high incidence of consanguineous families and is possibly transmitted by autosomal-recessive inheritance.[74-78] No correlation is found between jejunoileal atresia and parental age or maternal disease. Although chromosomal abnormalities are relatively common in duodenal atresia, they are seen in fewer than 1% of more distal atresias.[2,69]

One in three infants is significantly premature and often weighs less than is appropriate for gestational age.[69] Amniotic fluid may contribute to fetal growth, especially in the last week of gestation. Despite this, the intrauterine growth pattern is generally not very different from that in other infants.

Pathology

The morphologic classification of jejunoileal atresia into three types has been of significant prognostic and therapeutic value.[40,56,79] Modification has retained the original classification but added a special category of type III(b) (apple peel or Christmas tree appearance) and considered multiple atresias as type IV.[17] This emphasized the importance of associated loss in intestinal length, abnormal

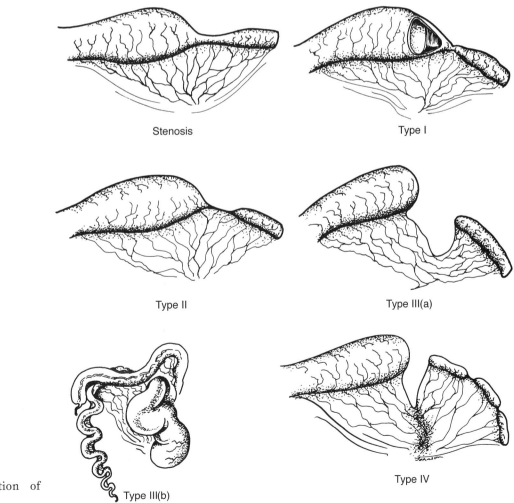

Stenosis

Type I

Type II

Type III(a)

Type III(b)

Type IV

FIGURE 30-9. Classification of small bowel atresia.

collateral intestinal blood supply, and concomitant atresias or stenoses[80] (Fig. 30-9). The most proximal atresia determines whether it is classified as jejunal or ileal atresia. Although a single atresia is most common, multiple atretic segments may be encountered in 6% to 21% of cases.[2,3,69]

Stenosis

Stenosis is defined as a localized narrowing of the intestinal lumen without disruption of continuity or defect in the mesentery. At the stenotic site, a short, narrow, somewhat rigid segment with a minute lumen is found where the muscularis is often irregular and the submucosa thickened. Stenosis may also take the form of a type I atresia with a fenestrated web. The small intestine is of normal length.

Atresia Type I

In *atresia type I,* the obstruction is caused by a membrane or web formed by mucosa and submucosa. The proximal dilated bowel and distal collapsed bowel are in continuity without a mesenteric defect. Increased intraluminal pressure in the proximal bowel can produce bulging of the web into the distal intestine, creating a conical transition zone, the windsock effect. The bowel length is not foreshortened.

Atresia Type II

In *atresia type II* (blind ends joined by a fibrous cord), the proximal bowel terminates in a bulbous blind end, which is connected to the collapsed distal bowel by a short fibrous cord along the edge of an intact mesentery. The proximal bowel is always dilated and hypertrophied for several centimeters and may become cyanosed as a result of ischemia from increased intraluminal pressure. The distal collapsed bowel commences as a blind end, which sometimes assumes a bulbous appearance, owing to the remains of an intussusception. The total small bowel length is usually normal.

Atresia Type III(a)

In *atresia type III(a)* (disconnected blind ends), the atresia ends blindly both proximally and distally, as in type II, but the fibrous connecting cord is absent, and a V-shaped mesenteric defect of varying size is seen (see Fig. 30-9). The dilated and blind-ending portion of proximal bowel is often aperistaltic and more frequently may undergo torsion or become overdistended, with necrosis and perforation as a secondary event.[4] The total length of the bowel is subnormal and variable, owing to intrauterine resorption of the compromised bowel. Cystic fibrosis is commonly associated with this variety.[81]

Atresia Type III(b)

Atresia type III(b) (apple-peel,[59] Christmas tree,[82] or Maypole deformity[18]) consists of a proximal jejunal atresia near the ligament of Treitz, absence of the superior mesenteric artery beyond the origin of the middle colic branch and of the dorsal mesentery, significant loss of intestinal length, and a large mesenteric defect. The distal small bowel lies free in the abdomen and assumes a helix configuration around a single perfusing vessel arising from the ileocolic or right colic arcades (Fig. 30-10). Occasionally, further type I or type II atresias are found in the bowel closest to the distal blind end. Vascularity of the distal bowel is often impaired. This type of atresia has been found in families with a pattern suggestive of an autosomal recessive mode of inheritance. It also has been encountered in siblings with identical lesions and in twins.[18,72,74,75,83,84]

The occurrence of conventional intestinal atresia in other affected siblings, the association of multiple atresias (15%), and the discordance in a set of apparently monozygotic twins may point to more complex genetic transmission with an overall recurrence rate of 18%.[72,85–87] Babies with this anomaly are often premature (70%), have malrotation (54%), and may have short gut syndrome (74%) with increased morbidity (63%) and mortality (54%).[69,72] The deformity is most likely the consequence of a proximal superior mesenteric arterial occlusion with extensive infarction of the proximal segment of the midgut on a basis of a thrombus or embolus, or of a strangulating obstruction owing to a midgut volvulus.[40,72,82,88] A primary failure of development of the distal superior mesenteric artery also has been suggested as an etiologic factor, although this is unlikely because meconium is found in the bowel distal to the atresia, which indicates that the atresia was acquired after bile secretion began, which occurs around week 12 of intrauterine life.[89]

Atresia Type IV

In *atresia type IV,* multiple-segment atresias of a combination of types I to III are present, often having the morphologic appearance of a string of sausages. A familial incidence is noted, with prematurity, a grossly shortened

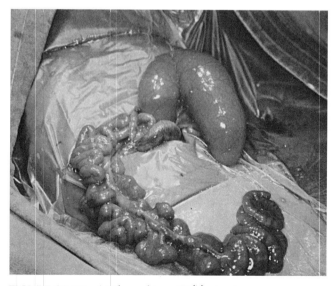

FIGURE 30-10. Apple-peel type III(b) atresia.

bowel length, and an increased mortality.[74,83] Up to 25 separate atresias have been encountered, usually with sparing at the terminal ileum.[90] Concomitant bile duct dilation also has been described.[91] A rare autosomal recessive pattern of transmission has been documented in several neonates with multiple atresias from the stomach to the rectum. Seven babies were reported from four related French Canadian families in Quebec.[76,79]

Multiple atresias also could be the consequence of multiple ischemia infarcts, an intrauterine inflammatory process, or a malformation of the GI tract occurring during early embryonic life.[79,92] Pathologic findings in the familial cases would support the concept that a developmental process early in intrauterine life, and affecting the whole GI tract, may be responsible, and not an ischemic or inflammatory process.[93,94]

Based on the wide distribution of these atresias and the presence of multiple lumina, each surrounded by muscularis mucosa, the atresia may represent an example in which the solid state of epithelial proliferation took place throughout the intestine with incomplete recanalization. The recognition of familial polyatresia may be helpful in genetic counseling. Embolization of thromboplastin-rich material from a dead monozygotic fetal twin to the living one through placental vascular anastomoses also could account for single or multiple intestinal atresias.[95,96] Multiple areas of intestinal atresias also have been seen in association with severe immunodeficiency.[36]

Among the 292 patients in our series were 31 (11%) stenoses and 261 (89.3%) atresias. The incidence of the various types of atresias is shown in Table 30-1. These findings are similar to those of surveys done in 1969 and 1971, except that a much higher incidence of jejunal atresias is found in our series.[69]

Pathophysiology

The ischemic insult not only causes the morphologic abnormalities but also adversely influences the structure and subsequent function of the remaining proximal and distal bowel.[4,13,18,20,40,97–99] The blind-ended proximal bowel is dilated and hypertrophied with histologically normal villi, but it is without effective peristaltic activity. A deficiency of mucosal enzymes and muscular adenosine triphosphatase also is found.[18,100] At the level of the atresia, the ganglia of the enteric nervous system are atrophic and hypocellular with minimal acetylcholinesterase activity. These changes are most likely the result of local ischemia, although obstruction per se can elicit the same but less severe morphologic and functional abnormalities.[100]

The histologic and histochemical abnormalities progressively normalize proximally, although up to 20 cm cephalad to the atretic segment, muscular hyperplasia and hypertrophy with concomitant hyperplasia of ganglia may still be observed.[97,98,100] The discrepancy in diameter between the lumen of the proximal and distal bowel may vary from 2 to 20 times depending on the completeness of the obstruction and its distance from the stomach.[101] These abnormalities of the proximal atretic segment may be the reason for lack of prograde movement of intraluminal contents, in addition to decreased secretion and absorptive capabilities if this segment is retained when bowel continuity is restored.[40,62,102] The changes can be so extensive that a state of decompensation is reached, with no effective prograde movement of contents.

Canine experiments have shown that progressive obstruction of the proximal bowel results in diminished intraluminal pressure and circumferential contractions, which fail to achieve prograde movement of contents during active peristaltic activity.[20,103] In addition, the viability of the bulbous atretic segment may be at risk, with further compromise from the excessive distention, which can lead to ischemia and perforation (9.7% to 20%) and allow the transmural migration of bacteria. Histologic studies of the distal bowel have demonstrated hypertrophied, tortuous, and intertwined villi, often obliterating the tiny lumen of the distal segment.[104] The apparent hypertrophy could, however, result from mucosal crowding within the unused distal lumen rather than from true villous enlargement.[105] The distal small bowel is unused and potentially normal in length and function, as is the unused microcolon, although diminished contractile activity has been demonstrated.[106]

Experimental studies showing that intestinal atresia resulted from ischemic necrosis of intestine would imply precarious blood supply to the proximally dilated loop of bowel,[13,21,40] and postmortem injection of barium sulfate into mesenteric vessels has confirmed this suspicion.[89]

It was, however, postulated that the intestine is not ischemic at birth and becomes so only on swallowing air, with subsequent distention and increased intraluminal pressure or with secondary torsion.[20] The excellent results obtained with tapering procedures without resection of the bulbous portion would support the contention that the blood and nerve supply to the bowel adjacent to the atresia is adequate.[20,107] However, the insult may have interfered with mucosal and neural function. Defective peristalsis is commonly noticed in this area, and no doubt resection of the dilated bulbous proximal end produced better results. The proximal end of the distal atretic bowel has been subjected to a similar insult and requires resection at the time of surgical correction of the atresia.[40]

Insufficient bowel length (as a result of the primary insult), excessive removal of residual bowel, or ischemic insult to the remaining bowel, as well as postoperative

TABLE 30-1			
JEJUNOILEAL ATRESIA AND STENOSIS: RED CROSS CHILDREN'S HOSPITAL EXPERIENCE, 1959 TO 2003			
Type	Jejunum	Ileum	Total (%)
Stenosis	19	12	31 (11)
Type I	53	15	68 (23)
Type II	18	12	30 (10)
Type III(a)	24	23	47 (16)
Type III(b)	55	—	55 (19)
Type IV	47	14	61 (21)
Total	**216**	**76**	**292**

N = 292 patients.

complications or the inappropriate use of hyperosmolar feeds or medication can lead to a short-gut syndrome with long-term sequelae for growth and development. The brown bowel syndrome also has been identified and is most likely the result of malabsorption of fat-soluble vitamins (vitamin E), resulting in lipofuscinosis of the GI tract.[108]

Clinical Manifestations

Prompt recognition of intestinal atresia is essential for adequate management to be instituted.[1,3,4,14,61,69,70] The differentiation among atresia, intrinsic bowel obstruction, and extrinsic obstruction owing to midgut volvulus or internal hernia is the most important consideration, requiring immediate diagnostic studies. In recent years, US has contributed substantially to the prenatal diagnosis of jejunoileal atresia and has improved the management of the mother and her unborn baby.[109] This is especially so in pregnancies complicated by third-trimester polyhydramnios associated with small bowel atresia, volvulus, and meconium peritonitis.[3,69] Polyhydramnios, however, may not be present early in gestation or with distal obstruction. A family history may help identify hereditary forms. A modified dominant mode of inheritance has been suggested in atresias occurring in two aunts and two nephews who were siblings.[76,85]

Type III(b) atresia also has a familial tendency, based on anomalies of intestinal rotation or fixation. A 3.4% incidence of anomalies in siblings has been reported in a large survey of children with jejunoileal atresias.[69] Familial combined duodenal and jejunoileal atresia is uncommon.[110] Bile staining and increased bile acid concentration in the amniotic fluid may indicate the presence of intestinal obstruction distal to the ampulla of Vater.[111]

In babies with atresia or stenosis, bilious vomiting usually develops on the first day of life, but in 20% of children, it may be delayed for 2 to 3 days.[1,2,4,14] The higher the obstruction, the earlier and more forceful the vomiting.[70] Dehydration, fever, unconjugated hyperbilirubinemia, and aspiration pneumonia occur with delay in diagnosis.

Abdominal distention is more pronounced with distal small bowel obstruction. Sixty percent to 70% of these babies fail to pass meconium on the first day of life.[3,4] Although the meconium may appear normal, it is more common to find gray plugs of mucus passed via the rectum.[61] Tenderness, rigidity, edema, and erythema of the abdominal wall are signs of bowel ischemia or peritonitis.[14] Occasionally, if ischemic distal bowel is present in type III(b) atresia, altered blood may be passed through the rectum.

Intestinal stenosis is more likely to create diagnostic difficulty. Intermittent partial obstruction or malabsorption may subside without treatment.[62,70,112] Investigations may initially be normal. These babies usually fail to thrive, and complete intestinal obstruction ultimately develops, which requires exploration.

The diagnosis of jejunoileal atresia is by radiographic examination of the abdomen with only swallowed air as contrast.[112,113] Swallowed air reaches the proximal bowel by 1 hour and the distal small bowel by 3 hours in a normal vigorous infant in whom its passage is blocked, but this pattern may be delayed in premature or sick infants with poor sucking.[114]

Jejunal atresia patients have a few gas-filled and fluid-filled loops of small bowel, but the remainder of the abdomen is gasless (Fig. 30-11). Air/fluid levels may be scanty or absent and may become evident only after decompression via a nasogastric tube (Fig. 30-12). Fewer air/fluid levels are evident, with a typical ground-glass appearance of inspissated meconium when the atresia is associated with cystic fibrosis. A limited-contrast meal may be useful if intestinal stenosis is suspected.

Distal ileal atresia may be difficult to differentiate from colonic atresia because haustral markings are rarely seen in neonates. A contrast enema shows the large bowel distal to the obstruction; the bowel typically has an unused appearance. The rare colonic atresia that we have seen with jejunoileal atresia and malrotation of the colon may be discovered on this study.[14,46,113,115] Omission of a diagnostic barium enema with reliance on the intraoperative injection of saline to confirm distal bowel patency may fail to identify an associated colonic or rectal atresia.[116,117] Rotational abnormalities and volvulus were observed in 36% of our patients. If the atresia occurred late in intrauterine life, the bowel distal to the atresia may have a more normal caliber. Occasionally, air and meconium can accumulate proximal to an atresia, mimicking the radiologic appearance of meconium ileus. Total colonic aganglionosis may be difficult to differentiate from atresia.[113]

Ten percent of babies with atresia have meconium peritonitis.[3,69,112] The perforation usually occurs proximal to the obstruction in the bulbous blind end. The radiologic appearance of a meconium pseudocyst containing a large air/fluid level is related to the late intrauterine perforation of bowel and can easily be identified on radiographs. Intraluminal calcification of meconium or intramural dystrophic calcification in the form of diffuse punctate or rounded aggregations has been reported with intestinal stenosis or atresia.[118] Meconium calcification in patients with hereditary multiple GI atresia produces a "string of pearls," which is pathognomonic of this condition.[76,94]

The clinical and radiologic picture of jejunoileal stenosis is determined by the level and degree of stenosis, and the diagnosis may be delayed for years.[69,70] Morphologic and functional changes in the proximal obstructed intestine vary depending on the degree of obstruction (Fig. 30-13).

Differential Diagnosis

Diseases that are initially seen with symptoms and signs mimicking jejunoileal atresia include colonic atresia, midgut volvulus, meconium ileus, duplication cysts, internal hernia, ileus due to sepsis, birth trauma, maternal medications, prematurity, and hypothyroidism.[3,14,15,70,119] Special investigations, including upper-GI contrast studies, contrast enema, rectal biopsy, and a delta F508 gene deletion assay or a sweat test to rule out associated cystic fibrosis, may be needed.[15,81]

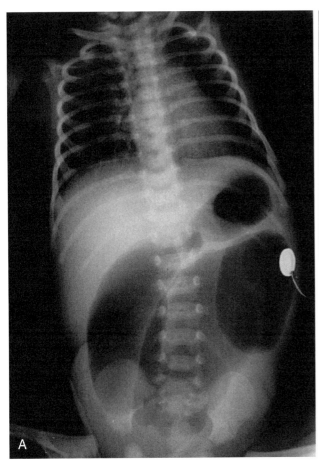

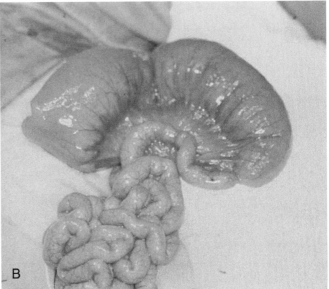

FIGURE 30-11. Jejunal atresia. *A,* Abdominal radiograph. *B,* Operative photograph.

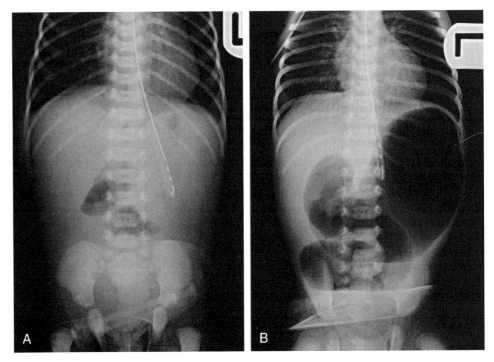

FIGURE 30-12. Abdominal radiograph *(A)* before and *(B)* after injection of air.

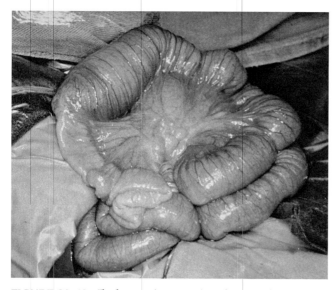

FIGURE 30-13. Ileal stenosis: operative photograph.

Management

Delay in diagnosis may lead to impairment of viability (50%), frank necrosis and perforation (10% to 20%) of the bulbous proximal end, fluid and electrolyte abnormalities, and increased incidence of sepsis.[4,61,70]

Electrolyte and volume resuscitation is started. Nasogastric or orogastric tube decompression may improve diaphragmatic excursion and prevent vomiting and aspiration.

Surgical Considerations

The operative procedure depends on the pathologic findings. Resection of the proximal dilated and hypertrophied bowel with primary end-to-end (end-to-back) anastomosis with or without tapering of the proximal bowel is most common[3,4,13,14,21,40,48,59,61,62] (Fig. 30-14).

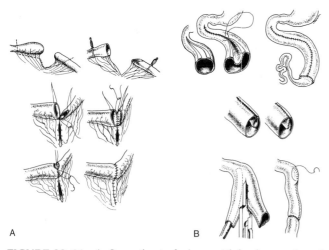

A   B

FIGURE 30-14. *A,* Operative technique with back resection of proximal bowel and end-to-end anastomosis. *B,* Tapering techniques, antimedsenteric seromuscular strip resection and inversion placation, mication, and tapering, respectively.

As recently as 1952, the surgical mortality was 80% to 90%.[14,70] The present survival rate is approximately 90%.[4,14,21] Understanding that the proximal dilated and hypertrophied bowel was dysfunctional, improvement of anastomotic technique and suture material, and development of total parenteral nutritional (TPN) support are the primary reasons for the greatly improved survival in the years that have followed. Appropriate management of the short-bowel syndrome should lead to further improvements.

Operative Considerations

A transverse supraumbilical incision provides access to the abdominal contents. Intraperitoneal fluid should be sent for Gram stain and culture. In uncomplicated cases, the bowel can easily be delivered into the wound by gentle pressure on the wound edges. Any perforation is identified and sutured before further exploration, and the abdominal cavity is irrigated with warm saline until all macroscopic debris has been removed. Division of vascularized adhesions may be required.[15] All of the bowel should be exteriorized and carefully inspected to determine the site and type of obstruction and to exclude other atresias or stenoses, malrotation, or meconium ileus. Malrotation should be corrected by derotation and division of Ladd's bands.

The length of the bowel estimated to be functional should be carefully measured along the antimesenteric border, because this is of prognostic significance and may determine the method of reconstruction. The patency of the bowel distal to the anastomotic site must be verified by injecting saline into the distal bowel and observing free flow into the cecum. If colonic patency has not been established preoperatively, patency of the colon must be confirmed by injection of saline either directly or via a prepositioned transrectal catheter.

If the total usable bowel length is adequate (> 80 cm + ileocecal valve), the bulbous hypertrophied bowel proximal to the atresia is resected to approximately normal bowel diameter.[4,40] In high jejunal atresia, the resection may extend into the second portion of the duodenum, with derotation of the duodendum and mobilization of the colon to the left side. The blood supply to the cut ends of the intestine must be carefully preserved.

A short segment (4 to 5 cm) of the distal atretic bowel is removed obliquely so that the mesenteric side is the longest. An incision along the antimesenteric border to create a "fish mouth" may be needed to equalize the openings for anastomosis.[18,21,40]

A one-layer modification of the end-to-back anastomosis using 5-0 or 6-0 monofilament absorbable sutures is preferred.[2,4] Alternatively, an extramucosal anastomosis can be performed. Once the anastomosis has been completed, the suture line is tested for leaks, and reinforcing sutures are placed as required. The mesenteric defect is repaired, taking great care not to kink the anastomosis.[18] It may be difficult at this time to close the mesenteric defect without distorting or kinking the anastomotic site. The preserved mesentery of the resected proximal bowel can be used as a vascularized flap to close any residual defects.[120]

A similar technique is used for stenosis and intraluminal membranes. Procedures such as simple transverse enteroplasties, excision of membranes, and bypassing techniques are not recommended primarily because they fail to remove the abnormal segments of bowel, which may produce blind-loop syndromes. The end-to-side ileo–ascending colonic anastomosis for low ileal atresia is also obsolete.[21] Neither decompression gastrostomy[121,122] nor transanastomotic stents are recommended.[123] Our practice is to place a nasogastric tube for decompression and to rely on short-term TPN with early introduction of graduated enteral feeding.

At completion of the operation, the bowel is carefully returned into the abdomen to avoid kinking or volvulus of the bowel.

Prognostic Factors

The normal small bowel length in term neonates is approximately 250 cm, and in preterm infants, is 160 to 240 cm.[21] Previous estimates that small bowel length of 100 cm or more is necessary to sustain oral intake and survival may no longer be applicable, owing to the advent of TPN, special enteral diets, and pharmacologic management of short-gut syndrome.[21] Nevertheless, the preservation of as much bowel length as possible at the risk of creating a poorly functioning anastomosis has little merit.[4,69,107,124] In one series, an average of 15 cm (SD, 13.4) of intestine proximal and 5 cm (SD, 6.5) distal to the atresia was resected, with a mean of 101 cm (SD, 57) of functional intestine remaining.[112]

If proximal resection is not possible, tapering or plication of the dilated bowel is indicated.[48,103,107,122,125,126] Tapering enteroplasty as proximal as the second midpart of the duodenum, if necessary, is accomplished by resecting an antimesenteric strip of the dilated proximal bowel, with either suture or staple closure to ensure adequate lumen size.[126] Particularly with type III atresias, during performance of a tapering duodenojejunoplasty, the duodenum is derotated, and the cecum moved to the left to avoid kinking at the anastamosis.[127] The tapering can safely be done over a length of 35 cm.[126] The tapered bowel may be primarily anastomosed to the distal bowel or may be exteriorized as a stoma, if necessary.

Plication or infolding along the antimesenteric border is preferred by some surgeons because it conserves mucosal surface area and may facilitate the return of bowel function.[125] Plication also reduces the risk of leak from the antimesenteric suture line. More than one half of the bowel circumference may be folded into the lumen over an extended length without causing obstruction. Breakdown of the plication suture line results in a functional obstruction.[48] The plication is less likely to be disrupted if a longitudinal antimesenteric seromuscular strip is resected before plication.[128,129]

From 1978, when tapering was introduced into our practice, to 2003, 186 infants were treated with proximal resection and end-to-end anastomosis. Sixty-five (35%) had some proximal resection along with antimesenteric excision and tapering or inversion plication. These were done predominantly to conserve bowel length in type

III(b) atresia patients or to reduce disparity in anastomotic size. Tapering also was used to correct a failed inversion plication procedure and as a secondary procedure to improve function in a persistently dilated nonfunctioning megaduodenum. Tapering was successful in all 65 children, although 1 required further proximal tapering. No anastomotic leaks were encountered. Inversion plication was performed in 7 patients, of whom 4 required revision, owing to breakdown of the plication with persistent dysfunction. Dysfunction is manifested by persistent vomiting. Contrast studies revealed a partially obstructed anastomosis with ineffective prograde movement in the dilated bowel. We have not seen this problem when a seromuscular excision strip was added to the inversion plication procedure (9 patients; see Fig. 30-14).

Primary anastomosis may be contraindicated in cases of peritonitis, volvulus with vascular compromise, meconium ileus, and type III(b) atresia.[17,101] Under these circumstances, exteriorization of both ends has been recommended. However, we do not favor the use of initial surgical stomas because it may increase the incidence of systemic sepsis and the mortality rate.[14,59,61,112,130–133] The proximal bowel often remains dilated in spite of exteriorization, and fluid and electrolyte losses may be severe. None of the babies in our series required bowel exteriorization. Primary anastomosis has been shown to be effective, with no anastomosis-related mortality.[134]

Atresia encountered in gastroschisis may be single or multiple and may be located in either the small or the large bowel.[63,135] Rarely is the bowel suitable for primary anastomosis. Exteriorization is an option if the proximal bowel has perforated or is minimally dilated.[17,63,115] Identification of the atresia may be extremely difficult, and the safest course is to reduce the eviscerated bowel, with the atresia left undisturbed. Primary closure of the abdominal wall or silo reduction is done. Resolution of the bowel edema then occurs, allowing safe delayed resection and anastomosis 14 to 21 days later.[63,136]

Although isolated type I atresias are best dealt with by primary resection and end-to-end anastomosis,[21,69] multiple diaphragms have been successfully perforated and dilated with bougies passed along the entire length of small intestine.

In surgery for type III(b) atresia, restricting bands along the free edge of the distal coiled and narrow mesentery should be divided to ensure maximal vascular flow. The potential for kinking the precarious single marginal artery and vein also requires careful return of the bowel into the abdominal cavity.[82] The proximal dilated bowel should be partly resected with tapering, and limited resection of the distal bowel end may be required for questionable viability.[86,137]

Bowel-length conservation methods, such as multiple anastomoses for multiple atresias, may result in increased morbidity.[21,61,138] An intraluminal absorbable silicone (Silastic) catheter stent can facilitate the completion of multiple primary anastomoses and serve, simultaneously, as a conduit for radiologic evidence of anastomotic integrity, luminal patency, and enteral feeding.[139] Multiple atresias, which are present in as many as 18% of patients, are often localized; therefore resection of the bowel segment with several atresias and one anastomosis may be preferable.[138]

There is no place for a bowel-lengthening procedure at the initial operation, but this procedure may ultimately obviate the need for prolonged TPN.[140]

Postoperative Care

Parenteral nutrition should begin as soon as a stable postoperative state has been reached and continued until total enteral nutrition (TEN) is established.

Paradoxically, the more proximal the atresia, the longer the period of postoperative intestinal dysfunction, necessitating nasogastric decompression. In general terms, oral intake is commenced only when the baby is alert, sucks well, has clear gastric aspirate of less than 5 mL/hour, has a soft flat abdomen, and is passing flatus or feces. Delay in function beyond 14 days may be an indication for a contrast upper GI study.[102]

Abdominal distention, vomiting, evidence of peritonitis, and a pneumoperitoneum present more than 24 hours after operation suggest an anastomotic leak, and immediate re-exploration should be performed. The leaking anastomosis may be resected and reanastomosed, or it may be exteriorized.[15] It is important to reconfirm patency of the distal bowel.

A Silastic transanastomotic tube (TAT) passed via the lumen of a gastrostomy tube or transnasally allows for the early introduction of enteral feeding. TAT feeding is started 24 hours after surgery with 1 mL iso-osmolar solution once every 4 hours and increased as tolerated. Continuous infusion of a polymeric formula should be instituted as soon as intestinal motility has returned.[62,101,102,141,142]

Improvements in quality and delivery of TPN have reduced the urgency and necessity of early TAT or oral feeding, although the judicious intraluminal deposition of expressed breast milk or iso-osmolar formula stimulates reactive hyperplasia in the residual intestinal mucosa and should enhance intestinal adaptation. Adaptation begins almost immediately after resection and continues for more than a year.[102,143] Our experience with the gastrostomy/transanastomotic tube (GT/TAT) system revealed that TEN feedings were established at 17 days and full oral intake at an average of 25 days (14 to 44 days). With nasogastric decompression, with or without a transnasal TAT, full oral intake was established at an average of 20 days (16 to 23 days). Three major problems were encountered with TAT: migration of the tube into the stomach, tube blockage, and small-bowel perforation. The effect of early enteral feeding on the induction of gut hormones on bowel growth, secretions, and motility on intermediate metabolism and, ultimately, on bowel adaptation is relatively unknown.[144–146]

Adequate oral nutrition should consist of a complete infant formula with approximately 62% carbohydrate, 18% fat, and 12% protein. Intraluminal fat is the most potent stimulus for intestinal mucosal growth, and as little as 20% of the total daily caloric requirements in the form of long-chain triglycerides is sufficient to maintain the structure and function of the small bowel.[143] The unique role of glutamine in stimulating mucosal cell growth and metabolism has not been fully determined. Caloric intake should not be less than 120 cal/kg/day. As tolerance develops, the patient's oral intake is gradually increased.

Transient GI dysfunction is frequently observed in infants with jejunal and ileal atresia and is multifactorial in etiology.[3,4,62,102] Lactose intolerance, malabsorption owing to stasis with bacterial overgrowth, intestinal hurry, and diarrhea may be significant in children with short-bowel syndrome after surgery for multiple atresias, surgery for the apple-peel anomaly, and loss of the ileocecal valve. These infants require a gradual transition period for the eventual goal of TEN to be reached. Regular monitoring for clinical signs and biochemical evidence of intestinal overload or intolerance is required. Disaccharide and even monosaccharide intolerance, indicative of gross intestinal brush-border malfunction, should be assessed by regular biochemical evaluation of stool samples.[102] Warning signs are water-loss stools, increasing stool frequency, hematochezia, fecal-reducing substances, a decreasing stool pH, an increase in gastric residual volume, and increasing breath hydrogen excretion levels.[102] Unintentional injury to the fragile mucosa can be caused by sugars, high-osmolality feeds, oral medications, and intestinal bacterial and viral infections. Pharmacologic control of altered GI function may hasten adaptation. Loperamide hydrochloride decreases intestinal peristaltic activity, and cholestyramine is effective in binding bile salts.[147] Cholestyramine should not be given unless water-loss stools are evident. Vitamin B_{12} and folic acid should be given regularly to the patient without a terminal ileum to prevent megaloblastic anemia.

Results

Before 1952, our mortality rate for small bowel atresia was 90%, decreasing to 28% between 1952 and 1955.[4,40] A change in the surgical procedure from primary anastomosis without resection to liberal resection of the blind ends and primary end-to-end anastomosis significantly improved the survival to 78% over the next 3 years.[40] During the 44-year period 1959 to 2003, 292 patients with jejunoileal atresia and stenosis were admitted to our pediatric surgical service; 30 have died, giving an overall mortality rate of 10.3% (Table 30-2). The highest mortality was encountered in type III atresia (16.5%) Eight neonates were moribund on admission, with infarction of the proximal bowel owing to volvulus of the bulbous end and established peritonitis—one type I, one type II, two type III(a), two type III(b), and two type IV—reemphasizing the need for prompt surgical management. Eight neonates died of infection related to pneumonia or peritonitis, 2 from an anastomotic leak owing to unrecognized colonic atresia. This experience and 3 deaths that have been reported due to undiagnosed colonic atresia in infants treated for jejunoileal atresia[116] have prompted us to insist on a contrast enema before repair of a jejunoileal atresia. Support was withdrawn from 3 patients with less than 10 cm residual small bowel. One neonate died

TABLE 30-2
MORTALITY RELATED TO TYPE OF ATRESIA

Type	Patients	Mortality	(%)
Stenosis	31	0	(0)
Type I	68	4	(6)
Type II	30	3	(10)
Type III(a)	47	8	(17)
Type III(b)	55	9	(16)
Type IV	61	6	(10)
Total	**292**	**30**	

Overall mortality, 10.3%.

18 hours after birth of hemorrhagic disease. Seven died in the early phase because of short-bowel syndrome, line sepsis, and liver failure. The final neonate died of peritonitis after jejunal perforation from a transanastomotic tube. Other researchers report that mortality also is influenced by prematurity, associated disease processes or congenital abnormalities, malrotation, postoperative volvulus and bowel infarction, and anastomotic dysfunction or leak.[14,15,17,18,21,69,112,148] Owing to the small size and delicate blood supply of the distal bowel in type III(b) atresia, anastomotic leaks (15%), stricture formation (15%), and gangrene of the proximal end of the distal segment (7%) have been reported in a collected review.[72] Delay in presentation, coupled with inadequate medical facilities and nutritional support, accounted for a mortality rate of 52% in children with jejunoileal atresia in one series from a developing country.[1] A collective review of mortality from 1950 to 2002 is depicted in Table 30-3.

Short-gut syndrome after surgical correction of jejunoileal atresia may be due to extensive intrauterine bowel loss, overzealous resection, operative ischemic injury to the bowel, or postoperative complications. Short-bowel syndrome is defined as residual jejunoileal length of less than 75 cm with permanent malabsorption.[149] Although many factors influence survival, long-term survival is possible in infants with an 11- to 15-cm jejunoileum and an intact ileocecal valve or with 25- to 40-cm small bowel length without an ileocecal valve.[149,150]

TABLE 30-3
JEJUNOILEAL ATRESIA AND STENOSIS: IMPROVEMENT IN SURVIVAL

Authors	Years of Study	N	Survival (%)
Evans[14]	1950	1498	9.3
Gross[61]	1940–1952	71	51
Benson et al.[21]	1945–1959	38	55
De Lorimer[69]	1957–1966	587	65
Nixon and Tawes[18]	1956–1967	62	62
Louw[119]	1959–1967	33	94
Martin and Zerella[79]	1957–1975	59	64
Cywes et al.[2]	1959–1978	84	88
Danismend et al.[133]	1967–1981	101	77
Smith and Glasson[112]	1961–1986	84	61
Vecchia et al.	1972–1997	128	84
Cywes et al.	1959–2003	292	90

A survival rate of 46% to 69% can be anticipated in most infants with less than 25 cm of jejunoileum.[149-151] Careful and accurate measurement of the total residual bowel length (small bowel plus colon) is imperative to determine the infant's potential for adaptation.

The following factors must be considered in determining the final functional status of the bowel. Rapid jejunoileal growth occurs during the later stages of gestation from the mean of 115 cm at 19 to 27 gestational weeks to 250 cm at 35 to 40 weeks.[152] Postnatal growth in intestinal length can further facilitate intestinal adaptation.[151] The small intestine (digestion and assimilation areas) continues to grow and elongate most rapidly during infancy until total body length reaches about 60 cm. Thereafter, intestinal growth slows and remains constant once 100 to 140 cm of total body length has been reached.[153] These findings emphasize the importance of maintaining overall somatic growth in these children during the period of type I intestinal adaptation until full oral intake can be achieved.[143] The dilated bowel proximal to the atresia is stretched, leading to overestimation of its functional capabilities, in contradistinction to the collapsed unused distal bowel, where the functional length is up to twice the measured length. Bowel length also may be underestimated in infants with gastroschisis.[136] Of critical importance is an intact ileocecal valve, which allows accelerated intestinal adaptation with shorter residual jejunoileal length.[142,151] The residual bowel becomes dilated, and both villus height and crypt depth increase, resulting in an increase in the absorption surface area per unit length of bowel and enhanced absorption. The adaptive response to jejunal loss is more marked than that for ileal resection, and with loss of the ileocecal valve, infants are more susceptible to rapid bowel transit, malabsorption, diarrhea, and increased bacterial proliferation in the small bowel.[143] Early introduction of intraluminal feeding facilitates and hastens the period of intestinal adaptation, thereby reducing the dependency on TPN as the sole provider of adequate nutrition for growth and development.[143,145,150,151]

Infants with short-bowel syndrome are divided into four main functional groups: uncorrectable intestinal insufficiency, adequate bowel function for survival, adequate alimentary function for growth and development, and normal alimentary function with a degree of intestinal reserve.[2] Long-term outlook for most of these children is optimistic, although TPN-associated complications are frequent and sometimes fatal.[141,151] Several surgical procedures have been described to improve short-bowel syndrome, including interposition of colonic segments, reversal of bowel segments, and methods to increase mucosal surface area. Most are obsolete, except for bowel-lengthening procedures. An isoperistaltic bowel-lengthening procedure has proved successful for the short-term and intermediate-term intestinal function.[140,154-156] Intestinal transplantation is indicated when permanent dependency on TPN is expected.[157] Although intestinal transplantation in the tacrolimus immunosuppression era is feasible, morbidity and mortality remain daunting, mainly because of the ongoing immunogenicity of transplanted bowel and the increased level of immunosuppression required to achieve graft acceptance. Improved survival may come with advances in immunosuppressive therapy.[158] One-year graft and patient survival in the best centers are greater than 50%, both with small bowel alone and with small bowel with other visceral grafts.[157]

The 42 patients with short-bowel syndrome in our series had an average small bowel length of 39 cm, 6 without an ileocecal valve. Five early deaths were due to extremely short bowel: 9 cm, 10 cm, 12 cm, 17 cm, and 22 cm. Two other early deaths were due to sepsis and liver failure in patients with residual bowel, ranging from 26 cm to 50 cm. Four late deaths occurred: 2 months, 7 1/2 months, 11 months, and 2 1/2 years after the initial operation, all related to complications of TPN. Thus the lack of sufficient residual bowel was responsible for considerable morbidity or a miserable quality of life in the other patients. In most instances, maximal intestinal adaptation occurred within 6 to 12 months but was delayed for 18 months in 2 patients. Of the 31 survivors, 15 have developed normally, whereas 16 had delayed milestones and were below the third percentile for weight.

Colonic Atresia

Atresia of the colon is a rare form of intestinal atresia and composes from 1.8% to 15% of all intestinal atresias and stenoses.[115,116] Atresias can occur at any level, but type III lesions to the right of the splenic flexure and type I lesions distal to the vascular watershed predominate.[115] Complicated colonic atresia with partial or complete absence of the hindgut is frequently associated with major anterior abdominal wall and genitourinary defects (i.e., vesicointestinal fissure and extrophy of the bladder) and in ischiopagus-conjoined twins.[159] Concomitant small bowel atresia, Hirschsprung's disease, and gastroschisis are not infrequently associated with colonic atresia. The atresia is most likely due to mesenteric vascular impairment or intrauterine volvulus.[13,71,160]

Prenatal diagnosis can be suspected on US in the presence of bowel obstruction and if the diameter of the colon is larger than expected for gestational age.[161]

These infants are usually term and have rapidly progressing findings of distal intestinal obstruction. Delay in diagnosis can lead to ischemia and proximal bowel perforation.

Abdominal radiographs confirm distal bowel obstruction, often with a disproportionately large loop corresponding to the ectatic and dilated proximal colonic segment.[162] This dilation can be so massive that it mimics a pneumoperitoneum (Fig. 30-15A). A contrast enema confirms colonic atresia, showing a small-diameter colon that terminates adjacent to the obstructed colonic segment (Fig. 30-16A and B).

The surgical approach depends on the clinical status of the patient, the level of atresia, the status of the bowel proximal to the atresia, any associated small intestinal

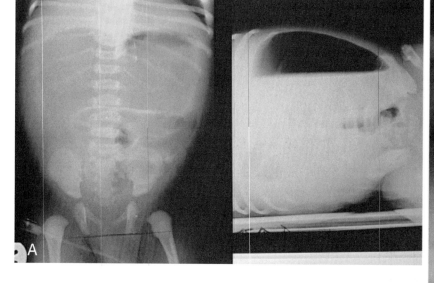
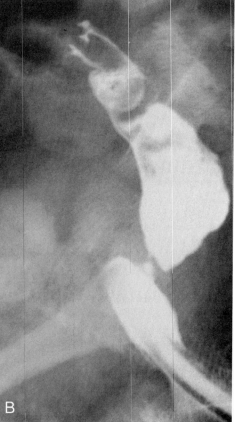

FIGURE 30-15. *A,* Abdominal radiograph of colonic atresia showing huge air-filled proximal colon mimicking a pneumoperitoneum. *B,* Right colonic atresia with rectal stenosis.

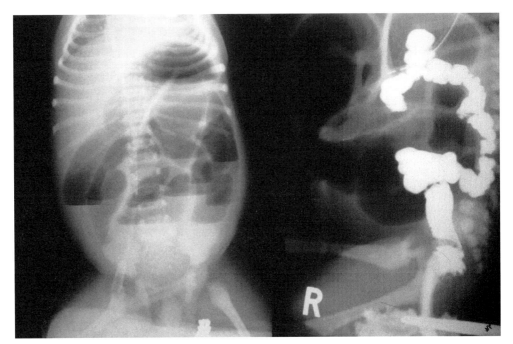

FIGURE 30-16. Abdominal radiograph showing distal bowel obstruction and barium enema confirming type I transverse colonic atresia.

atresia, the patency of the bowel distal to the atresia, and complications. It is important to ensure patency of the entire colon, because multiple atresias and stenosis can occur, and to exclude Hirschsprung's disease.[71,163] A staged surgical approach is generally preferred, with initial resection of the dilated colon, colostomy, and distal mucous fistulas. Primary resection and anastomosis have a higher incidence of complications, usually owing to undiagnosed distal pathology.[164,165]

Prognosis is usually excellent but depends on residual small bowel length, concomitant small bowel pathology, and associated anomalies.

Patient Material

We have treated 12 patients with colonic atresia, excluding those with complete vesicointestinal malformations and conjoined twins. Of the 7 girls and 5 boys, 11 were term: An ultrasonic antenatal diagnosis was made in three cases. Seven were type III(a); 4, type I; and 1, type II. Two atresias were in the right colon, five involved the transverse colon (see Fig. 30-16A and B), and five were more distal. One of the infants with atresia of the right colon had two further stenoses in the rectosigmoid colon (see Fig. 30-15B). Four patients had associated small bowel atresia, of whom 3 had extensive loss of more proximal bowel, which led to short-bowel syndrome in two. Four had malrotation, 1 had gastroschisis, and 1 had distal colon Hirschsprung's disease. One had neuronal intestinal dysplasia distally. In this patient, an anastomotic leak required a Hartman's procedure and colostomy formation with subsequent closure. Four had primary resection and anastomosis, and 3 had associated small bowel atresias. In one of these patients, the colonic

atresia was missed because no preoperative contrast enema had been done. Anastomotic disruption resulted in death of sepsis. In another infant with a primary anastomosis, postoperative functional bowel obstruction developed, and Hirschsprung's disease of the distal colon was confirmed. Colostomy and later pull-through was required. Eight had colostomy and delayed anastomosis. One of these was well for 7 months, but protein-losing enteropathy developed and was extensively investigated. Despite essentially normal contrast studies, it was only at laparotomy that a chronic 360-degree midgut volvulus was found with a completely unfixed mesentery and gross venous and lymphatic congestion. Ladd's procedure was curative.

REFERENCES

1. Adeyemi D: Neonatal intestinal obstruction in a developing tropical country: Patterns, problems, and prognosis. J Trop Pediatr 35:66, 1989.
2. Cywes S, Davies MRQ, Rode H: Congenital jejuno-ileal atresia and stenosis. S Afr Med J 57:630, 1980.
3. Grosfeld JL: Jejunoileal atresia and stenosis, section 3: The small intestine. In Ravitch MM, Welch KJ, Benson CD, et al (eds): Pediatric Surgery. Chicago, Year Book Medical, 1986, p 838.
4. Louw JH: Congenital intestinal atresia and severe stenosis in the newborn. S Afr J Sci 3:109, 1952.
5. Irving IM, Rickham PP: Duodenal atresia and stenosis: Annular pancreas. In Rickham PP, Lister J, Irving IM (eds): Neonatal Surgery, 2nd ed. Boston, Butterworths, 1978, p 355.
6. Al-Salem A, Khwaja S, Grant C, et al: Congenital intrinsic duodenal obstruction: Problems in the diagnosis and management. J Pediatr Surg 24:1247, 1989.
7. Calder J: Two examples of children born with preternatural conformation of the guts. Med Essay (Edinb) 1:203, 1733. Cited by: Kelly PM. Br J Surg 29:245, 1941.
8. Madsen CM: Duodenal atresia: 60 years of follow-up [case report]. Prog Pediatr Surg 10:61, 1977.

9. Ernst NP: A case of congenital atresia of the duodenum treated successfully by operation. BMJ 1:644, 1916.
10. Jackson JM: Annular pancreas and duodenal obstruction in the neonate: A review. Arch Surg 87:37, 1963.
11. Bowen J, Dickson A, Bruce J: Reconstruction for duodenal atresia: Tapered or non-tapered duodenoplasty. J Pediatr Surg 11:474, 1996.
12. Adzick NS, Harrison MR, de Lorimier AA: Tapering duodenoplasty for megaduodenum associated with duodenal atresia. J Pediatr Surg 21:311, 1986.
13. Louw JH, Barnard CN: Congenital intestinal atresia: Observations on its origin. Lancet 2:1065, 1955.
14. Evans CH: Atresias of the gastrointestinal tract. Int Abstr Surg 92:1, 1951.
15. Hays DM: Intestinal atresia and stenosis. In Ravitch M (ed): Current Problems in Surgery. Chicago, Year Book Medical, 1969, p 3.
16. World Health Organization: Congenital Malformations [bulletin]. WHO 34:38, 1966.
17. Grosfeld JL, Ballantine TVN, Shoemaker R: Operative management of intestinal atresia and stenosis based on pathologic findings. J Pediatr Surg 14:368, 1979.
18. Nixon HH, Tawes R: Etiology and treatment of small intestinal atresia: Analysis of a series of 127 jejunoileal atresias and comparison with 62 duodenal atresias. Surgery 69:41, 1971.
19. Fockens P: Operativ geheilter Fall von kongenitaler Dunndarmatresie. Zentralbl Chir 38:532, 1911.
20. Nixon HH: An experimental study of the propulsion in isolated small intestine, and applications to surgery in the newborn. Ann R Coll Surg Engl 27:105, 1960.
21. Benson CD, Lloyd JR, Smith JD: Resection and primary anastomosis in the management of stenosis and atresia of the jejunum and ileum. Pediatrics 26:265, 1960.
22. Bar-Moar JA, Nissan S, Nero P: Pyloric atresia, a hereditary congenital anomaly with autosomal recessive transmission. J Med Genet 9:70, 1972.
23. Bronsther B, Nadear MR, Abrams MW: Congenital pyloric atresia: A report of three cases and a review of the literature. Surgery 69:1, 130, 1971.
24. Burnett HA, Halpert B: Perforation of stomach of newborn infants with pyloric atresia. Arch Pathol 44:318, 1947.
25. Hayashi AH, Galliani CA, Gillis DA: Congenital pyloric atresia and junctional epidermolysis bullosa: A report of long-term survival and a review of the literature. J Pediatr Surg 11:1341, 1991.
26. Tandler J: Zur Entwicklungsgeschichte des Menschlichen Duodenums im frühen Embryonal Stadiem. Gegenbaurs Morphol Jahrb 29:187, 1900.
27. Boyden EA, Cope JG, Bill AH: Anatomy and embryology of congenital intrinsic obstruction of the duodenum. Am J Surg 114:139, 1967.
28. Lynn HB, Espinas EE: Intestinal atresia: An attempt to relate location to embryologic processes. Arch Surg 79:357, 1959.
29. Movtosouris C: The "solid stage" and congenital intestinal atresia. J Pediatr Surg 1:446, 1966.
30. Elliot GB, Kliman R, Elliot KA: Pancreatic annulus: A sign or a cause of duodenal obstruction? Can J Surg 11:357, 1968.
31. Gourevitch A: Duodenal atresia in the newborn. Ann R Coll Surg Engl 48:141, 1971.
32. Jona JZ: Duodenal anomalies and the ampulla of Vater. Surg Gynecol Obstet 143:565, 1976.
33. Brereton RJ, Cudmore RE, Bouton JM: Double atresia of the duodenum. Z Kinderchir 31:60, 1980.
34. Coughlin JP, Rector RE, Klein MD: Agenesis of the gallbladder in duodenal atresia: Two case reports. J Pediatr Surg 27:1304, 1992.
35. Davenport M, Saxena R, Howard E: Acquired biliary atresia. J Pediatr Surg 31:1721, 1996.
36. Moore SW, de Jongh G, Buic P, et al: Immune deficiency in familial duodenal atresia. J Pediatr Surg 31:1733, 1996.
37. Bill AH, Pope WM: Congenital duodenal diaphragm. Surgery 35:482, 1954.
38. Rowe M, Buckner D, Clatworthy HW: Windsock web of the duodenum. Am J Surg 116:444, 1968.
39. Grosfeld JL, Rescoria FJ: Duodenal atresia and stenosis: Reassessment of treatment and outcome based on antenatal diagnosis, pathologic variance, and long-term follow-up. World J Surg 17:301, 1993.
40. Louw JH: Congenital intestinal atresia and stenosis in the newborn: Observations on its pathogenesis and treatment. Ann R Coll Surg Engl 25:209, 1959.
41. Bodian M, White LLR, Carter CO, et al: Congenital duodenal obstruction and mongolism. BMJ 1:77, 1952.
42. Fonkalsrud EW, de Lorimier AA, Hays DM: Congenital atresia and stenosis of the duodenum: A review compiled from the members of the Surgical Section of the American Academy of Pediatrics. Pediatrics 43:79, 1969.
43. Hancock BJ, Wiseman NE: Congenital duodenal obstruction: The impact of an antenatal diagnosis. J Pediatr Surg 24:1027, 1989.
44. Britton JR, Britton HL: Gastric aspirate volume at birth as an indicator of congenital intestinal obstruction. Acta Paediatr 85:945, 1995.
45. Brown RA, Millar AJW, Linegar A, et al: Fenestrated duodenal membranes: An analysis of symptoms, signs, diagnosis, and treatment. J Pediatr Surg 29:429, 1994.
46. Millar AJW, Rode H, Brown RA, et al: The deadly vomit: Malrotation and midgut volvulus: A review of 137 cases. Pediatr Surg Int 2:172, 1987.
47. Kimura L, Tsugawa C, Ogawa K, et al: Diamond-shaped anastomosis for congenital duodenal obstruction. Arch Surg 112:1262, 1977.
48. Richardson WR, Martin LW: Pitfalls in the management of the incomplete duodenal diaphragm. J Pediatr Surg 4:303, 1969.
49. de Lorimier AA, Harrison MR: Intestinal plication in the treatment of atresia. J Pediatr Surg 18:734, 1983.
50. Waever E, Nielson OH, Arnbjornsson E, et al: Operative management of duodenal atresia. Pediatr Surg Int 10:322, 1995.
51. Kokkonen ML, Kalima T, Jaaskelainen J: Duodenal atresia: Late follow-up. J Pediatr Surg 23:216, 1988.
52. Ein SH, Shandling B: The late nonfunctioning duodenal atresia repair. J Pediatr Surg 21:798, 1986.
53. Spigland N, Yazbeck S: Complications associated with surgical treatment of congenital intrinsic duodenal obstruction. J Pediatr Surg 25:1127, 1990.
54. Tchirkow G, Highman LM, Shafer AD: Cholelithiasis and cholecystitis in children after repair of congenital duodenal anomalies. Arch Surg 115:85, 1980.
55. Harris J, Kallen B, Robert E: Descriptive epidemiology of alimentary tract atresia. Teratology 52:15, 1995.
56. Bland-Sutton J: Imperforated ileum. Am J Med Sci 18:457, 1889.
57. Abrams JS: Experimental intestinal atresia. Surgery 64:185, 1968.
58. Koga Y, Hayashida Y, Ikeda K, et al: Intestinal atresia in fetal dogs produced by localized ligation of mesenteric vessels. J Pediatr Surg 10:949, 1975.
59. Santulli TV, Blanc WA: Congenital atresia of the intestine: Pathogenesis and treatment. Ann Surg 154:939, 1961.
60. Tibboel D, van der Kamp AWM, Molenaar JC: An experimental study of the effect of an intestinal perforation at various developmental stages. Z Kinderchir 37:62, 1982.
61. Gross RE: Congenital atresia of the intestine and colon. In Gross RE (ed): The Surgery of Infancy and Childhood. Philadelphia, WB Saunders, 1953, p 150.
62. Nixon HH: Intestinal obstruction in the newborn. Arch Dis Child 30:13, 1955.
63. Amoury RA, Ashcraft KW, Holder TM: Gastroschisis complicated by intestinal atresia. Surgery 82:373, 1977.
64. Grosfeld JL, Clatworthy HW Jr: The nature of ileal atresia due to intrauterine intussusception. Arch Surg 100:714, 1970.
65. Murphy DA: Internal hernias in infancy and childhood. Surgery 55:311, 1964.
66. Spriggs NI: Congenital intestinal occlusion. Guys Hosp Rep 66:143, 1912.
67. Vassy LE, Boles ET: Iatrogenic ileal atresia secondary to clamping of an occult omphalocoele. J Pediatr Surg 10:797, 1975.
68. Todani T, Tavuchi K, Tanaka S, et al: Intestinal atresia due to intrauterine intussusception: Analysis of 24 cases in Japan. J Pediatr Surg 10:445, 1975.
69. de Lorimier AA, Fonkalsrud EW, Hays DM: Congenital atresia and stenosis of the jejunum and ileum. Surgery 65:819, 1969.
70. Lister J, Rickham PP: Intestinal atresia and stenosis, excluding the duodenum. In Rickham PP, Lister J, Irving IM (eds): Neonatal Surgery. London, Butterworths, 1978, p 381.

71. Moore SW, Rode H, Millar AJW, et al: Intestinal atresia and Hirschsprung's disease. Pediatr Surg Int 5:182, 1990.
72. Seashore JH, Collins FS, Markowitz RI, et al: Familial apple peel jejunal atresia: Surgical, genetic, and radiographic aspects. Pediatrics 80:540, 1987.
73. Nicolini U, Monni G: Intestinal obstruction in babies exposed in utero to methylene blue. Lancet 336:1258, 1990.
74. Mishalany HG, Der Kaloustian VM: Familial multiple-level intestinal atresias: Report of two siblings. J Pediatr 79:124, 1971.
75. Mishalany HG, Najjar FB: Familial jejunal atresia: Three cases in one family. J Pediatr 73:753, 1968.
76. Guttman FM, Braun P, Garance PH, et al: Multiple atresias and a new syndrome of hereditary multiple atresias involving the gastrointestinal tract from stomach to rectum. J Pediatr Surg 8:633, 1973.
77. Gakukamble DB, Adrian ABM, Al-Gadi Musa: Atresias of the gastrointestinal tract in an inbred previously unstudied population. Pediatr Surg Int 18:40, 2002.
78. Lambrecht W, Kluth D: Hereditary multiple atresias of the gastrointestinal tract: Report of a case and review of the literature. J Pediatr Surg 33:794, 1998.
79. Martin LW, Zerella JT: Jejunoileal atresia: A proposed classification. J Pediatr Surg 11:399, 1976.
80. Davies MRQ, Louw JH, Cywes S, et al: The classification of congenital intestinal atresias [letter]. J Pediatr Surg 17:224, 1982.
81. Blanck C, Okmian L, Robbe H: Mucoviscidosis and intestinal atresia: A study of four cases in the same family. Acta Paediatr Scand 54:557, 1965.
82. Weitzman JJ, Vanderhoof RS: Jejunal atresia with agenesis of the dorsal mesentery with "Christmas tree" deformity of the small intestine. Am J Surg 111:443, 1966.
83. Blyth H, Dickson JAS: Apple peel syndrome: Congenital intestinal atresia. J Med Genet 6:275, 1969.
84. Olson LM, Flom LS, Kierney CMP, et al: Identical twins with malrotation and type IV jejunal atresia. J Pediatr Surg 22:1015, 1987.
85. Rickham PP, Karplus M: Familial and hereditary intestinal atresia. Helv Paediatr Acta 26:561, 1971.
86. Zerella JT, Martin LW: Jejunal atresia with absent mesentery and a helical ileum. Surgery 80:550, 1976.
87. Smith MB, Smith L, Wells JW, et al: Concurrent jejunal atresia with "apple peel" deformity in premature twins. Pediatr Surg Int 6:425, 1991.
88. Dickson JAS: Apple peel small bowel: An uncommon variant of duodenal and jejunal atresia. J Pediatr Surg 5:595, 1970.
89. Jimenez FA, Reiner L: Arteriographic findings in congenital abnormalities of the mesentery and intestine. Surg Gynecol Obstet 113:346, 1961.
90. Rittenhouse EA, Beckwith JB, Chappel JS, et al: Multiple septa of the small bowel: Description of an unusual case, with review of the literature and consideration of etiology. Surgery 71:371, 1972.
91. McHugh K, Daneman A: Multiple gastrointestinal atresias: Sonography of associated biliary abnormalities. Pediatr Radiol 21:355, 1991.
92. Tsujimoto K, Sherman FE, Ravitch MM: Experimental intestinal atresia in the rabbit fetus: Sequential pathological studies. Johns Hopkins Med J 131:287, 1972.
93. Arnal-Monreal F, Pombo F, Capdevila-Puerta A: Multiple hereditary gastrointestinal atresias: Study of a family. Acta Paediatr Scand 72:773, 1983.
94. Puri P, Guiney EJ, Carroll R: Multiple gastrointestinal atresias in three consecutive siblings: Observations on pathogenesis. J Pediatr Surg 20:22, 1985.
95. Benirschke K: Twin placenta in perinatal mortality. N Y State J Med 61:1499, 1961.
96. Braun F, Ferrier S, Berclaz J, et al: Multiple intestinal atresias and encephalomalacia in the survivor after in-utero death of a monozygous co-twin. Pediatr Surg Int 2:249, 1987.
97. Cloutier R: Intestinal smooth muscle response to chronic obstruction: Possible applications in jejunoileal atresia. J Pediatr Surg 10:3, 1975.
98. Tepas JJ, Wyllie RG, Shermeta DW, et al: Comparison of histochemical studies of intestinal atresia in the human newborn and fetal lamb. J Pediatr Surg 14:376, 1979.
99. Baglaj SM, Czernik J, Koryszko J, Kuropka P: Natural history of experimental intestinal atresia: Morphologic and ultrasound study. J Pediatr Surg 36:9;1428, 2001.
100. Pickard LR, Santoro S, Wyllie RG, et al: Histochemical studies of experimental fetal intestinal obstruction. J Pediatr Surg 16:256, 1981.
101. Touloukian RJ: Intestinal atresia. Clin Perinatol 5:3, 1978.
102. Haller JA, Tepas JJ, Pickard LR, et al: Intestinal atresia: Current concepts of pathogenesis, pathophysiology, and operative management. Am Surg 49:385, 1983.
103. de Lorimier AA, Norman DA, Gooding CA, et al: A model for the cinefluoroscopic and manometric study of chronic intestinal obstruction. J Pediatr Surg 8:785, 1973.
104. Touloukian RJ, Wright HK: Intrauterine villus hypertrophy with jejunoileal atresia. J Pediatr Surg 8:779, 1973.
105. Tovar JA, Sunol M, de Torre LB, et al: Mucosal morphology in experimental intestinal atresia: Studies in the chick embryo. J Pediatr Surg 26:184, 1991.
106. Doolin EJ, Ormsbee HS, Hill JL: Motility abnormalities in intestinal atresia. J Pediatr Surg 22:320, 1987.
107. Thomas CG: Jejunoplasty for the correction of jejunal atresia. Surg Gynecol Obstet 129:545, 1969.
108. Ward HC, Leake J, Millar PJ, et al: Brown bowel syndrome: A late complication of intestinal atresia. J Pediatr Surg 27:1593, 1992.
109. Lee TG, Warren BH: Antenatal ultrasonic demonstration of fetal bowel. Radiology 124:471, 1977.
110. Gross E, Aarmon Y, Abu-Dalu K, et al: Familial combined duodenal and jejunal atresia. J Pediatr Surg 31:1573,1996.
111. Deleze G, Sidiropoulus D, Paumgartner G: Determination of bile acid concentration in human amniotic fluid for prenatal diagnosis of intestinal obstruction. Pediatrics 59:647,1977.
112. Smith GHH, Glasson M: Intestinal atresia: Factors affecting survival. Aust N Z J Surg 59:151, 1989.
113. Cremin BJ, Cywes S, Louw JH: Small intestine. In Cremin BJ, Cywes S, Louw JH (eds): Radiological Diagnosis of Digestive Tract Disorders in the Newborn: A Guide to Radiologists, Surgeons, and Paediatricians. London, Butterworths, 1973, pp 62–89.
114. Wasch MG, Marck A: The radiographic appearance of the gastrointestinal tract during the first day of life. J Pediatr 32:479, 1948.
115. Boles ET Jr, Vassy LE, Ralston M: Atresia of the colon. J Pediatr Surg 11:69, 1976.
116. Benson CD, Lofti MW, Brough AJ: Congenital atresia and stenosis of the colon. J Pediatr Surg 3:253, 1968.
117. Jackman S, Brereton RJ: A lesson in intestinal atresias. J Pediatr Surg 23:852, 1988.
118. Aharon M, Kleinhaus U, Lightig C: Neonatal intramural intestinal calcifications associated with bowel atresia. AJR Am J Roentgenol 130:999, 1986.
119. Louw JH: Resection and end-to-end anastomosis in the management of atresia and stenosis of the small bowel. Surgery 62:940, 1967.
120. Malcynski JT, Shorter NA, Mooney DP: The proximal mesenteric flap: A method for closing large mesenteric defects in jejunal atresia. J Pediatr Surg 29:1607, 1994.
121. Holder TM, Gross RE: Temporary gastrostomy in pediatric surgery: Experience with 187 cases. Pediatrics 26:36, 1960.
122. Howard ER, Othersen HB: Proximal jejunoplasty in the treatment of jejunoileal atresia. J Pediatr Surg 8:685, 1973.
123. Ehrenpreis TH, Sandblom PN: Duodenal atresia and stenosis. Acta Paediatr Scand 39:109, 1949.
124. Louw JH: Congenital atresia and stenosis of the small intestine: The case for resection and primary end-to-end anastomosis. S Afr J Surg 4:57, 1966.
125. Ramanujan TM: Functional capability of blind small bowel loops after intestinal remodelling techniques. Aust N Z J Surg 54:145, 1984.
126. Kimura K, Perdzynski W, Soper RT: Elliptical seromuscular resection for tapering the proximal dilated bowel in duodenal or jejunal atresia. J Pediatr Surg 31:1405, 1996.
127. Kling K, Applebaum H, Dunn J, et al: A novel technique for correction of intestinal atresia at the ligament of Treitz. J Pediatr Surg 35:353, 2000.

128. Weber TR, Vane DW, Grosfeld JL: Tapering enteroplasty in infants with bowel atresia and short gut. Arch Surg 117:684, 1982.
129. Kizilkan F, Tanyel FC, Hicsonmez A, et al: Modified plication technique for the treatment of intestinal atresia. Pediatr Surg Int 6:233, 1991.
130. Bishop HC, Koop CE: Management of meconium ileus, resection, roux-en-Y anastomosis, and ileostomy irrigation with pancreatic enzymes. Ann Surg 145:410, 1957.
131. Rehbein F, Halsband H: A double-tube technique for the treatment of meconium ileus and small bowel atresia. J Pediatr Surg 3:723, 1968.
132. Swenson O: End-to-end aseptic intestinal anastomosis in infants and children. Surgery 36:192, 1954.
133. Danismend EN, Frank JD, Brown ST: Morbidity and mortality in small bowel atresia: Jejuno-ileal atresia. Z Kinderchir 42:17, 1987.
134. Turncock RR, Brereton RJ, Spitz L, et al: Primary anastomosis in apple-peel bowel syndrome. J Pediatr Surg 26:718, 1991.
135. Shah R, Woolley MM: Gastroschisis and intestinal atresia. J Pediatr Surg 26:788, 1991.
136. van Hoorn WA, Hazebroek FWJ, Molenaar JC: Gastroschisis associated with atresia: A plea for delay in resection. Z Kinderchir 40:368, 1985.
137. Waldhausen JHT, Sawin RS: Improved long-term outcome for patients with jejunoileal apple peel atresia. J Pediatr Surg 32:1307, 1997.
138. El Shafie M, Rickham PP: Multiple intestinal atresias. J Pediatr Surg 5:655, 1970.
139. Chaet MS, Warner BW, Sheldon CA: Management of multiple jejunoileal atresias with an intraluminal Silastic stent. J Pediatr Surg 29:1604, 1982.
140. Bianchi A: Intestinal loop lengthening: A technique for increasing small intestinal length. J Pediatr Surg 15:145, 1980.
141. Thompson JS, Pinch LW, Vanderhof JA, et al: Experience with intestinal lengthening for the short bowel syndrome. J Pediatr Surg 26:721, 1991.
142. Schwartz MZ, Maeda K: Short bowel syndrome in infants and children. Pediatr Clin North Am 32:1265, 1985.
143. Dowling RH: Small bowel adaptation and its regulation. Scand J Gastroenterol 17:53, 1982.
144. Bristol JB, Williamson RCN: Mechanisms of intestinal adaptation. Pediatr Surg Int 3:233, 1988.
145. Lentze MJ: Nutritional aspects of the short bowel syndrome. Pediatr Surg Int 3:312, 1988.
146. Gleeson MH, Bloom SR, Polak JM, et al: Endocrine tumour in kidney affecting small bowel structure, motility, and absorptive function. Gut 12:773, 1971.
147. Remmington M, Malagelada JR, Zinsmeister A, et al: Abnormalities in gastrointestinal motor activity in patients with short bowel: Effect of a synthetic opiate. Gastroenterology 85:629, 1983.
148. Louw JH, Cywes S, Davies MRQ, et al: Congenital jejuno-ileal atresia: Observations on its pathogenesis and treatment. Z Kinderchir 33:3, 1981.
149. Wilmore DW: Factors correlating with a successful outcome following extensive intestinal resection in newborn infants. J Pediatr 80:88, 1972.
150. Dorney SFA, Ament ME, Berquist WE, et al: Improved survival in very short small-bowel of infancy with use of long-term parenteral nutrition. J Pediatr 107:521, 1985.
151. Caniano DA, Starr J, Ginn-Pease ME: Extensive short-bowel syndrome in neonates: Outcome in the 1980s. Surgery 105:119, 1989.
152. Touloukian RJ, Smith GJ: Normal intestinal length in preterm infants. J Pediatr Surg 18:720, 1983.
153. Siebert JR: Small-intestine length in infants and children. Am J Dis Child 134:593, 1980.
154. Weber TR, Powel MA: Early improvement on intestinal function after isoperistaltic bowel lengthening. J Pediatr Surg 31:61, 1996.
155. Kimura K, Soper RT: A new bowel elongating technique for the short-bowel syndrome using the isolated bowel segment Iowa models. J Pediatr Surg 28:792, 1993.
156. Chahine AA, Ricketts RR: A modification of the Bianchi intestinal lengthening procedure with a single anastomosis. J Pediatr Surg 33:1292, 1998.
157. Goulet O, Jan D, Brousse N, et al: Intestinal transplantation. J Pediatr Gastroenterol Nutr 25:1, 1997.
158. Rowe PM: Signalling an end to transplant rejection? Lancet 350:1526, 1997.
159. Cywes S, Millar AJW, Rode H, et al: Conjoined twins: The Cape Town experience. Pediatr Surg Int 12:234, 1997.
160. Erskine JM: Colonic stenosis in the newborn: The possible thromboembolic etiology of intestinal stenosis and atresia. J Pediatr Surg 5:321, 1970.
161. Anderson N, Malpas T, Robertson R: Prenatal diagnosis of colon atresia. Pediatr Radiol 23:63, 1993.
162. Winters WD, Weinberger E, Hatch EI: Atresia of the colon in neonates: Radiograph findings. AJR Am J Roentgenol 159:1273, 1992.
163. Williams MD, Burrington JD: Hirschsprung's disease complicating colon atresia. J Pediatr Surg 28:637, 1993.
164. Kim PCW, Superina RA, Ein S: Colonic atresia combined with Hirschsprung's disease: A diagnostic and therapeutic challenge. J Pediatr Surg 30:1216, 1995.
165. Pohlson EC, Hatch EI, Glick PL, et al: Individualized management of colonic atresia. Am J Surg 155:690, 1988.

CHAPTER 31

Malrotation

John J. Aiken, MD, and Keith T. Oldham, MD

Malrotation describes a spectrum of anatomic abnormalities of incomplete rotation and fixation of the intestine during fetal development. Disorders of intestinal rotation and fixation are of paramount importance in pediatric practice because they most commonly are seen initially in infancy and childhood as midgut volvulus with the potential for ischemic infarction of the intestine from the duodenum to the mid-transverse colon. The normal development of the human intestine involves two processes: complete rotation of the midgut and subsequent fixation of the colon and mesentery.[1] This concept of the normal embryology of the human intestine is based on the studies of Mall[2] and Frazer and Robbins.[3] In 1923, Dott[4] published the classic article on this subject, correlating the embryology of abnormalities of rotation and fixation with clinical cases and their surgical aspects. The surgical management of malrotation of the intestines was first described by William Ladd in 1932.[5] Ladd originally described 10 cases of malrotation with volvulus and their surgical treatment by counterclockwise detorsion. Ladd's subsequent article[6] in 1936 focused on liberation of the duodenum from constricting peritoneal bands in the right upper quadrant as a key component of the surgical management of malrotation of the intestines. The fundamentals of modern surgical management of malrotation remain unchanged from these original descriptions. An understanding of the embryology of the intestine is essential in the recognition and appropriate surgical management of these conditions.

Embryology

The primitive intestinal tract is first recognized at approximately 4 weeks of gestation as a roughly linear tube from the stomach to the rectum and, at this point, subdivides into foregut, midgut, and hindgut.[1] Ventrally the midgut is connected to the yolk sac via the omphalomesenteric duct, and this connection explains the close relation of the midgut to the umbilicus in the embryo. During the next few weeks, growth of the developing midgut is faster than the growth of the body. To accommodate this period of rapid growth, the midgut normally herniates out of the peritoneal cavity into the umbilical cord at about week 5 of development in the human fetus and returns to the abdominal cavity at about week 10 of gestation. Simultaneous with return of the intestine to the abdominal cavity, the intestines undergo a process of rotation and fixation, culminating in the final position of the small intestine and colon in the term infant. The axis for rotation of the primary midgut loop is the superior mesenteric artery (SMA). The two components of the midgut, duodenojejunal (cranial segment) and cecocolic (caudal segment), rotate separately but in parallel. The duodenum returns to the abdominal cavity first and begins rotation from right to left (counterclockwise) and beneath the SMA. The colon follows and is directed to the left upper quadrant and begins its rotation from left to right ventral to the SMA. Normal rotation of both the duodenojejunal limb and the cecal limb of the midgut is critical to the formation of the normal broad mesenteric base for the SMA and proper fixation of the mesentery to the posterior body wall. Interruption, reversal, or arrest of this complex process at any stage results in a rotational anomaly and may place the patient at risk for intestinal obstruction or volvulus. The unifying theme for the many possible anatomic abnormalities is a narrow SMA pedicle and lack of fixation of the midgut mesentery. This anatomic derangement allows axial rotation of the midgut around the SMA, resulting in midgut volvulus. For descriptive purposes, normal intestinal rotation and fixation may be divided into three stages: (1) herniation, (2) return to the abdomen, and (3) fixation. The key components of each stage are described according to the way in which they affect the two ends of the intestinal tract, that is, the proximal duodenojejunal loop and the distal cecocolic loop and the simultaneous rotation of these two components around the SMA.

As the midgut begins the phase of rapid growth and elongation during week 4 of gestation, it herniates into the base of the umbilical cord (Fig. 31-1A to C). The midgut will become the intestinal tract from the distal duodenum to the mid-transverse colon supplied by the SMA. The SMA is the axis of the herniation and divides the midgut into cranial (prearterial, duodenojejunal) and

435

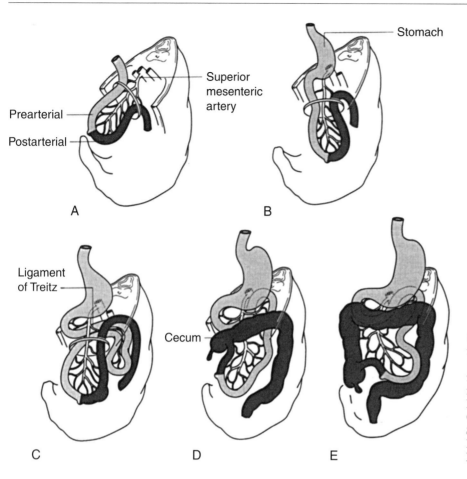

FIGURE 31-1. Normal midgut rotation is shown beginning in gestational week 5 (*A*), through completion of the process in week 12 (*E*) (see text). (Adapted from Oldham KT: Pediatric abdomen. In Greenfield LJ, Mulholland M, Oldham KT, et al. [eds]: Surgery: Scientific Principles and Practice. Philadelphia, Lippincott-Raven, 1997. Illustrations by Holly R. Fischer.)

caudal (postarterial, cecocolic) segments. The rate of growth of the duodenojejunal segment is greater than that of the cecocolic segment during this first stage. As the midgut herniates and continues to grow outside the body, the duodenojejunal segment is pushed inferiorly by the developing liver and left umbilical vein and begins to rotate around the SMA. Starting above the SMA, the duodenojejunal segment first rotates 90 degrees to the right (counterclockwise), resulting in a horizontally oriented midgut and placing the duodenojejunal junction to the right of the SMA. As development proceeds, the duodenojejunal segment undergoes an additional 90-degree rotation such that at the end of this first stage (herniation), the duodenojejunal junction has rotated counterclockwise 180 degrees and lies directly posterior to the SMA. Rotation of the cecocolic segment of the midgut during the first stage directly parallels rotation of the duodenojejunal segment. The ileocecal junction begins immediately inferior to the SMA, and as the duodenojejunal segment undergoes its first 90-degree rotation to the right of the SMA, the ileocecal junction rotates 90 degrees to the left of the SMA (counterclockwise) (see Fig. 31-1*D*). Just before returning to the abdomen, the ileocecal junction rotates another 90 degrees so it also has rotated 180 degrees, and at this point, lies directly ventral to the SMA.

The second phase is return of the midgut loops into the abdominal cavity. The developing intestine begins its return to the abdominal cavity during gestational week 10, and return is completed by week 11. The duodenojejunal limb returns first to the abdomen and, in this process, completes an additional 90-degree rotation around the SMA. The final result is a 270-degree counterclockwise rotation around the SMA. This completed rotation of the duodenojejunal limb yields the normal adult anatomic relations with the stomach above or anterior to the artery: the second portion of the duodenum to the right of the artery; the third portion of the duodenum beneath the artery; and the distal duodenum and proximal jejunum to the left of the artery. The distal segment (fourth portion of the duodenum and proximal jejunum) becomes fixed posteriorly to the body wall at the ligament of Treitz.

As the cecocolic limb returns to the abdomen, it also undergoes an additional 90-degree rotation, thus completing a 270-degree counterclockwise rotation around the SMA. This brings the cecocolic limb to the right, with the transverse colon overcrossing the root of the mesentery. After rotation is complete, the cecum descends to its final position in the right iliac fossa to the right of the SMA (see Fig. 31-1).

The final step in the normal midgut-positioning process is fixation of the intestine to the posterior abdominal wall. The process of fixation begins after week 12 of gestation and continues until after birth. Proper fixation is not possible unless normal rotation of the midgut has occurred. Normal points of fixation include the cecum in the right iliac fossa and the duodenojejunal junction in the left upper quadrant at the ligament of Treitz to the left of the aorta and anterior to the left renal vein (Fig. 31-2). Once the duodenojejunal junction and the cecum become fixed in their appropriate locations, the midgut mesentery becomes adherent to the posterior abdominal wall. The resulting oblique fixation of the intestinal mesentery from the ligament of Treitz to the cecum is broad based and normally not at risk for volvulus. In contrast, when rotation and fixation are interrupted, the cecum typically is just to the left of midline in the upper abdomen, and the duodenojejunal limb lies just to the right of midline; fixation of the mesentery is absent. Because of the narrow mesenteric vascular pedicle and absent fixation, the midgut is at risk of volvulus, resulting in obstruction and potentially intestinal ischemia and necrosis. In addition, normal fixation of the bowel includes peritoneal bands that form to anchor the ascending and descending colon in the right and left paracolic gutters, respectively. If the cecum and right colon do not fully rotate to the right side of the peritoneal cavity, these peritoneal bands (Ladd's bands) cross the duodenum in their course to the abnormally located cecum and can cause duodenal obstruction from external compression.

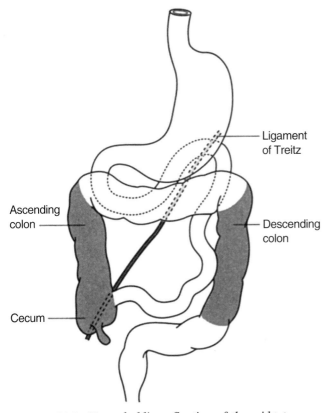

FIGURE 31-2. Normal oblique fixation of the midgut mesentery extends from the ligament of Treitz to the cecum in the right iliac fossa. The *shaded* portions of the ascending and descending colon are fixed in the retroperitoneum as well. (Adapted from Oldham KT: Pediatric abdomen. In Greenfield LJ, Mulholland M, Oldham KT, et al. [eds]: Surgery: Scientific Principles and Practice. Philadelphia, Lippincott-Raven, 1997. Illustrations by Holly R. Fischer.)

Incidence

The true incidence of malrotation of the midgut is unknown because the spectrum of anatomic forms of malrotation includes minor derangements that predictably are asymptomatic and therefore undiagnosed. In addition, even *complete* malrotation can remain asymptomatic. The incidence of malrotation leading to clinical disease has been reported to occur with a frequency of 1 in 6000 live births.[7] Complete nonrotation, whereby the entire small bowel is located on the right side of the abdomen, and the colon, on the left, has been reported in 0.5% of autopsies[8] and as an asymptomatic and incidental finding in 0.2% of contrast studies of the gastrointestinal (GI) tract at any age.[9] The concept of malrotation as an asymptomatic finding on an intestinal contrast study is a controversial one, as most patients are being evaluated for abdominal complaints, but the symptoms and the rotational abnormality may be unrelated. A relatively common scenario is for patients to be demonstrated to have a rotational abnormality, typically malrotation without volvulus, by a GI contrast study performed in evaluation for chronic nonspecific abdominal complaints such as recurring abdominal pain or constipation. In children younger than 1 year, malrotation is more common in boys than in girls.[10]

Associated Anomalies

Malrotation may occur as an isolated abnormality or in conjunction with other developmental abnormalities. Nonrotation or incomplete rotation is always a component of congenital diaphragmatic hernia (CDH) and abdominal wall defects: omphalocele and gastroschisis. Other congenital anomalies are reported to occur in 30% to 62% of patients with malrotation and most often are related to the GI tract.[11] As many as 50% of patients with duodenal atresia and one third of those with jejunoileal atresia have associated malrotation.[12] The presumed etiology of jejunoileal atresia in this setting is in utero volvulus with interruption of the mesenteric blood supply, resulting in an atresia. Other anomalies that may be

TABLE 31-1
ASSOCIATED ANOMALIES

Anomaly*	%
Intestinal atresia	5–26
Imperforate anus	0–9
Cardiac anomalies	7–13
Duodenal web	1–2
Meckel's diverticulum	1–4
Hernia	0–7
Trisomy 21/mental retardation	3–10
Rare: esophageal atresia, biliary atresia, mesenteric cyst, craniosynostosis, Hirschsprung's disease, cystic duplication of stomach	

*Patients with malrotation have the approximate incidence of the anomaly indicated.`

found in association with malrotation are summarized in Table 31- 1.[13-16] In addition, pyloric stenosis[17] and abnormalities of the gallbladder and extrahepatic biliary tree[18] have been described in association with malrotation. Familial occurrence of malrotation has been reported,[19] and the association with craniofacial and limb abnormalities[20] has raised the suggestion of a common genetic link.[21] Intrinsic duodenal obstruction from a luminal web or stenosis has been reported to occur in 8 % to 12 % of infants with rotational anomalies,[22] and therefore, eliminating this possibility is an important technical obligation either at or before the time of operative intervention.

CLASSIFICATION OF MALROTATION

Interruption or arrest of the precise sequence of intestinal rotation and fixation can occur at any point, and therefore the term *malrotation* encompasses a spectrum of anatomic abnormalities. For convenience, rotational anomalies are classified by separate consideration of the rotations of the duodenojejunal limb and the cecocolic limb of the midgut. The most important aspect of abnormalities of rotation and fixation is the degree to which the specific derangement results in a narrow SMA vascular pedicle at risk for volvulus or an abnormally positioned duodenum at risk of obstruction from kinking or peritoneal bands. In clinical practice, the most common abnormalities encountered are complete nonrotation of the midgut and incomplete rotation of the midgut. These are described together because the distinction between the two is arbitrary and often clinically indistinguishable in their appearance in the abdominal cavity. Several intermediate or mixed forms also are relatively common and are described. More rare are mesocolic hernias and other abnormalities. Not all rotational abnormalities will lead to clinical symptoms or be at risk of volvulus. An understanding of the most common forms of rotational and fixation anomalies should aid in their recognition and proper surgical management.

Nonrotation and Incomplete Rotation

Nonrotation is the most frequently encountered rotational anomaly and occurs when *both* the duodenojejunal limb and the cecocolic limb fail to undergo rotation around the SMA on their return to the abdomen. Normally, the duodenum rotates 270 degrees posterior to the SMA so that the duodenojejunal junction (ligament of Treitz) is to the left of midline and at the level of the gastric antrum. In cases of nonrotation, the rotation is either absent or arrested before exceeding 90 degrees (Fig. 31-3). The duodenojejunal junction is on the right side of the spine. Incomplete rotation is characterized by arrest of the normal rotational process at or near 180 degrees. The result in both cases for the duodenojejunal limb is a duodenum that is typically truncated, anterior, and often has a spiral or corkscrew configuration, all to the right of the midline. Nonrotation or incomplete rotation of the cecal limb leaves the colon in the left abdomen, typically with the cecum at or near the midline (Fig. 31-4). The colon and the duodenum in the upper

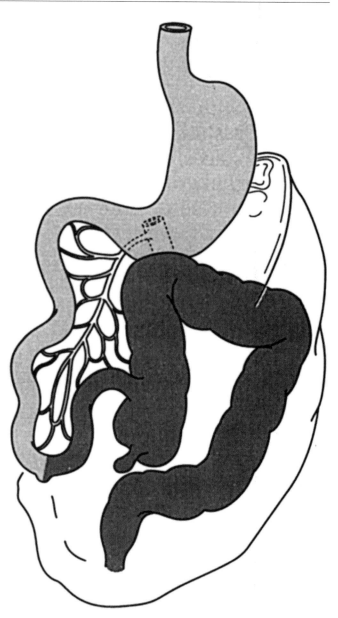

FIGURE 31-3. Nonrotation. The prearterial midgut (*lightly shaded*) resides on the patient's right and the postarterial segment (*darkly shaded*) is on the left. Neither segment of the midgut has undergone rotation in this illustration. (Adapted from Oldham KT: Pediatric abdomen. In Greenfield LJ, Mulholland M, Oldham KT, et al. [eds]: Surgery: Scientific Principles and Practice. Philadelphia, Lippincott-Raven, 1997.)

abdomen are often fused near the midline with a narrow mesentery through which courses the SMA. The adhesions connecting the duodenum and the colon result in a fold to the mesentery, and separation of these structures is an integral component of the complete surgical correction of malrotation, discussed later. Fixation of the bowel is absent. These conditions predispose the patient to midgut volvulus, which can severely or completely obstruct the blood supply to the bowel involved, with potential ischemic necrosis of the midgut. The normal anatomic arrangement, with the ligament of Treitz in the left upper quadrant and the cecum in the right lower quadrant, provides a broad-based mesentery, and along

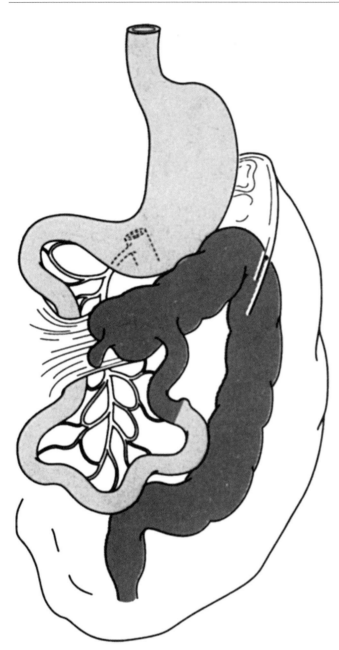

FIGURE 31-4. Incomplete rotation. The prearterial midgut segment (*lightly shaded*) has failed to undergo 270-degree rotation and resides largely to the patient's right. The postarterial segment has rotated to reside anterior to the duodenum. Note that (Ladd's) bands fixing the cecum to the posterior body may compress and obstruct the duodenum.

with proper fixation of the bowel, a low risk of volvulus occurs. In addition to volvulus, nonrotation and incomplete rotation can result in duodenal obstruction from kinking of the duodenum in its abnormal position and course or from external compression from Ladd's bands as they cross to the abnormally positioned cecum.

Mixed Rotational Abnormalities

Mixed rotational abnormalities are a less common and highly variable group of anomalies in which the rotational process is arrested or disrupted with reference to *either* the

duodenojejunal or cecocolic midgut limb. The spectrum of possible anatomic abnormalities ranges from variations with little clinical consequence, such as an incompletely descended cecum, to configurations associated with a narrow SMA vascular pedicle and absent fixation of the bowel, at risk for midgut volvulus. It is important for the surgeon to be familiar with these mixed rotational anomalies so that when they are encountered, they are properly recognized and managed.

The most commonly encountered mixed rotational anomaly is nonrotation of the duodenojejunal limb followed by normal rotation and fixation of the cecocolic limb. In this setting, the duodenojejunal junction and the cecocolic limb are separated satisfactorily to maintain a broad base to the mesentery, such that the risk of midgut volvulus is low; however, the duodenum occupies an anterior position, and duodenal obstruction may occur because of its abnormal position and course or from peritoneal bands from the colon. A rare rotational anomaly has been termed *reverse rotation*.[23] This abnormality involves some degree of midgut rotation in a clockwise direction around the SMA. Reverse rotation of the duodenojejunal limb results in the duodenum lying anterior to the SMA rather than in its usual posterior position. If the cecocolic limb also undergoes reverse rotation, the mid-transverse colon lies posterior to the SMA and creates the potential for obstruction of the transverse colon. If, conversely, the cecocolic limb rotates normally, a right mesenteric pouch (or paraduodenal hernia) is produced. The hernia sac is produced by the mesentery of the right colon as it rotates from the left upper quadrant to the right lower quadrant, passing anterior to the SMA and covering over the duodenojejunal limb of the intestine.

Incomplete rotation of the duodenojejunal limb occurs if the duodenojejunal limb fails to complete its normal 270-degree counterclockwise rotation posterior to the SMA. This aberration is encountered relatively commonly in clinical practice as cases in which the duodenojejunal junction is demonstrated on contrast study inferior and to the right of its normal left upper quadrant location. The risk of midgut volvulus in this setting varies, depending on the rotation of the cecocolic limb and the precise position of the ligament of Treitz.

Nonrotation of the cecocolic limb may be seen with normal rotation or rotational abnormalities of the duodenojejunal limb. Any time nonrotation of the cecocolic limb occurs, generally absent fixation of the intestine is found, and there is a risk of midgut volvulus similar to complete nonrotation of both limbs. Nonrotation of the cecocolic limb also is associated with aberrant peritoneal bands (Ladd's bands) that may cause partial duodenal obstruction by external compression, depending on the position of the duodenum. The more the duodenum lies anteriorly (fails to rotate posteriorly), the greater the risk of this form of obstruction. Incomplete fixation of the cecum also may predispose the patient to cecal volvulus.

Mesocolic Paraduodenal Hernias

Mesocolic (paraduodenal) hernias are a rare but surgically important group of malformations that result from failure of fixation of either the right or left mesocolon to the posterior body wall in the normal fashion (see Fig. 31-2). These are referred to with a variety of names, including paraduodenal hernia. The resulting spaces offer the potential for sequestration and entrapment of the small intestine between the mesocolon and posterior body wall on either the right or left side.

A right-sided mesocolic hernia is associated with non-rotation of the duodenojejunal limb. The major portion of the small bowel remains to the right of the SMA. If the cecocolic limb rotates in a normal counterclockwise manner, as fixation of the posterolateral peritoneum takes place, the small intestine is trapped in a sac that is the mesentery of the right side of the colon.[24] The ileocolic, right colic, and middle colic vessels lie within the anterior wall of the sac.

A left mesocolic hernia is produced when, during embryonic development, the unsupported area of the descending mesocolon between the inferior mesenteric vein and the posterior parietal attachment is invaginated by the small intestine as it migrates to the left superior portion of the abdominal cavity. The inferior mesenteric artery and vein and their branches are an integral part of the hernia sac.[24] As with any hernia, both right and left mesocolic hernias imply a potential risk for obstruction, incarceration, and strangulation of the small bowel. Their surgical correction is discussed later.

Clinical Manifestations

Malrotation can manifest clinically in many ways, including midgut volvulus, partial duodenal obstruction, and chronic abdominal complaints. The onset of symptoms can be acute, intermittent, or recurrent, and the manner of presentation tends to be age dependent (Table 31-2).[13] The classic and most common presentation is the acute onset of bilious emesis in a previously healthy infant in

the neonatal period. A subacute presentation may occur when malrotation causes partial or intermittent duodenal obstruction from kinking of the duodenum or Ladd's bands but without midgut volvulus. Malrotation also may be seen as chronic nonspecific abdominal symptoms or as an incidental finding in an otherwise asymptomatic patient. Less common manifestations of malrotation usually seen in older patients include chronic abdominal pain, chronic pancreatitis, weight loss, failure to thrive, early satiety, or intermittent diarrhea or blood per rectum.[10,13] Malrotation can be clinically silent until adulthood and then become symptomatic, and in some patients with malrotation, symptoms will never develop. The following is a discussion of the more common presentations.

Volvulus

The classic presentation of malrotation is a previously healthy newborn infant in the first few weeks to months of life with the acute onset of bilious emesis due to midgut volvulus. Fifty percent to 75% of patients with malrotation who become symptomatic do so in the first month of life, and approximately 90% of clinical symptoms occur in children younger than 1 year.[25] Midgut volvulus is a true surgical emergency, because delay in operative correction is associated with a high risk of intestinal necrosis and possible short bowel or death. Bilious emesis is a cardinal manifestation of neonatal intestinal obstruction, and this presentation in any child younger than 1 year should be considered malrotation with midgut volvulus until proven otherwise. Although other conditions may cause bilious emesis in a newborn, if the diagnosis is malrotation with volvulus, the intestine is typically strangulated, and any time delay in diagnosis and management is potentially devastating. Once clinical signs of intestinal compromise appear, the process has reached life-threatening severity, and the outcome may be poor. Physical findings in infants with volvulus are variable but typically include gastric and duodenal distention secondary to duodenal obstruction. The infant typically is irritable and may rapidly demonstrate signs and symptoms of dehydration due to vomiting and third spacing of fluid into the bowel and abdominal cavity. As the volume loss and intestinal ischemia progress, the infant can become lethargic and display signs and symptoms of septic shock, including abdominal wall erythema, peritonitis, hypotension, respiratory failure, systemic acidosis, thrombocytopenia, and either leukocytosis or leukopenia. Hematemesis, melena, or both also may result from intestinal mucosal ischemia. It is important to note that early in the disease process, particularly if the mesenteric and intestinal obstruction is only partial, physical examination findings, plain abdominal radiographs, and laboratory studies may all appear remarkably normal. It is incumbent on the clinician to evaluate rapidly all infants and children with bilious emesis for possible malrotation, and this can be done definitively only by upper GI contrast study. Furthermore, based on presentation and physical examination, a child younger than 1 year who has bilious emesis may undergo laparotomy without an upper GI study in the interest of time.

TABLE 31-2

CLINICAL PRESENTATION OF PATIENTS WITH MALROTATION RELATED TO AGE

Symptom/Sign	Age <2 mo %	Age <2 mo Duration*	Age >2 mo %	Age >2 mo Duration
Vomiting				
Bilious	71	2	49	19
Nonbilious	25	10	49	213
Diarrhea	23	5	14	64
Abdominal pain	0	—	31	241
Constipation	6	4	23	76
Anorexia or nausea	11	14	14	35
Irritability	11	5	9	7
Apnea (intermittent)	11	2	6	75
Lethargy	9	1	9	1
Failure to thrive	6	12	23	112
Blood in stool	17	4	17	2
Fever	9	2	23	2

*Average duration of symptom (days).
Adapted from Powell D, Othersen HB, Smith CD: Malrotation of the intestines in children: The effect of age on presentation and therapy. J Pediatr Surg 24:777-780, 1989.

Potentially, a delay in diagnosis of only a few hours may lead to extensive bowel loss and the predictable morbidity and mortality.[14]

Midgut volvulus also may be incomplete or intermittent. This is clearly a less common mode of presentation. Typically, patients are older and have chronic nonspecific symptoms of abdominal pain, intermittent episodes of emesis (which may be nonbilious), early satiety, weight loss, failure to thrive, or malabsorption and diarrhea.[10,13] With partial volvulus, the resultant mesenteric venous and lymphatic obstruction may cause chylous ascites or impair nutrient absorption and produce protein loss into the gut lumen. Melena or guiac-positive stools may result from mucosal ischemia as a result of arterial insufficiency.

Duodenal Obstruction

Duodenal obstruction is common with malrotation, and several etiologies exist, including kinking of the abnormally positioned and tortuous duodenum, duodenal obstruction from narrowing of the lumen due to torsion from volvulus, extrinsic obstruction from Ladd's peritoneal bands in the right upper quadrant crossing the duodenum as they extend to the cecum, and occasionally intrinsic duodenal obstruction from atresia or stenosis. The duodenal obstruction may be partial or intermittent. Patients with malrotation seen clinically because of duodenal obstruction typically demonstrate the classic signs and symptoms of high intestinal obstruction: bilious emesis, abdominal pain, or both. Occasionally the emesis may be nonbilious if the degree of obstruction is mild or the point of obstruction is preampullary. Physical findings are similar to those in patients with volvulus, and abdominal distention secondary to gastric and proximal duodenal obstruction are typical. Patients are at risk for dehydration and may demonstrate hypochloremic, hypokalemic metabolic alkalosis early in the course of illness, secondary to vomiting. Later in the course of illness, the intravascular volume may become so depleted as to result in poor perfusion and metabolic acidosis. Plain abdominal radiographs are again variable and may demonstrate findings suggestive of proximal intestinal obstruction (dilated proximal intestine and stomach with little distal gas) or may be nonspecific and unremarkable.

Intermittent or Chronic Abdominal Pain/Nonspecific Abdominal Complaints

Malrotation may be the cause of chronic abdominal pain or chronic nonspecific abdominal symptoms in rare patients. Typically these patients are older, and symptoms are the result of intermittent volvulus or intermittent partial duodenal obstruction. The symptoms are likely due to distention of the bowel, resulting in colicky abdominal pain and vomiting. Additional symptoms may include early satiety, failure to thrive, weight loss, or intermittent diarrhea. Chronic or intermittent abdominal symptoms also may result from partial or intermittent occlusion of the mesenteric venous and lymphatic systems, causing edema of the bowel wall, mesentery, and mesenteric

lymph nodes. Chronic arterial insufficiency caused by a partial volvulus may result in diarrhea, chronic pain, worsening pain after meals (intestinal angina), or melena as a result of intestinal mucosal ischemia.

Asymptomatic Patient

Malrotation may be demonstrated during contrast studies for nonspecific abdominal complaints or discovered as an incidental finding during operation for unrelated reasons. A relatively common scenario is the older child discovered to have malrotation on upper gastrointestinal barium study in evaluation for chronic abdominal pain or constipation. It is difficult to determine in this group of patients whether the symptoms that prompted evaluation are related to the malrotation or whether the malrotation is truly an incidental finding. Although midgut volvulus leading to vascular insufficiency of the midgut is uncommon in older children or adults, any patient with malrotation is at some risk for volvulus and acute vascular compromise of the bowel. Because the consequences of midgut volvulus (need for emergency surgery, short-gut syndrome, or death) are potentially so devastating, and operative correction is generally accomplished with minimal morbidity, all patients who are identified to have rotation anomalies should undergo operative correction. The low risk of volvulus in these patients allows the surgical procedure to be scheduled electively. If their symptoms persist after correction of the malrotation, further workup can be performed.

Diagnosis

For newborn infants or children with bilious emesis, the immediate consideration is for the possibility of intestinal obstruction, and the imaging evaluation begins with plain abdominal radiographs; anteroposterior flat plate, and either upright or lateral decubitus view, depending on the age of the child. The plain radiographic findings of malrotation/midgut volvulus are of several general patterns. The most consistent radiographic findings of malrotation with volvulus are those of proximal bowel obstruction: a distended stomach (gastric air bubble) and proximal duodenum with a paucity of air in the distal small bowel.[26] These findings are the consequence of the duodenal obstruction, and a "double-bubble" sign may be present. Although the classic double-bubble sign on plain radiograph is pathognomonic for duodenal atresia, diminished but discernible distal small bowel air is typical of malrotation. For this reason, in cases of suspected duodenal atresia or stenosis, the finding of any discernible gas beyond the duodenum raises the possibility of malrotation with volvulus and mandates an expeditious upper GI contrast study to avoid the potential disastrous consequences of any delay in diagnosis. In addition, normal or nonspecific abdominal radiographs in an infant with bilious emesis do not exclude the diagnosis of malrotation. Patients with malrotation also may have plain radiographs demonstrating high-grade small bowel obstruction with multiple dilated loops of bowel with air/fluid levels. Because the mechanical obstruction of malrotation and volvulus is characteristically more proximal, this radiographic finding or abdominal tenderness or peritonitis on physical examination is suggestive of intestinal strangulation. In patients with plain radiograph findings of high-grade or complete bowel obstruction or a classic presentation and worrisome findings on physical examination, no further radiographic evaluation is needed. Aggressive fluid resuscitation and electrolyte correction should be performed, followed by emergency operative exploration.

In stable patients without peritonitis, an upper GI contrast study is the standard examination for the definitive diagnosis of malrotation (Fig. 31-6A). The study is performed in the fluoroscopy suite by using either barium or water-soluble contrast by a trained radiologist. These patients should have a nasogastric tube in place because of their presentation with bilious emesis, and the contrast agent is instilled through the tube. Fundamental supportive-care measures include efforts to keep the patient warm, running intravenous fluids, and precautions to avoid aspiration. Typically, malrotation with volvulus produces a high-grade or complete obstruction

in the second or third portion of the duodenum and has the appearance of a "bird's beak" on the upper GI contrast study (Fig. 31-5).[26] If only partial obstruction of the duodenum is present, a spiral or corkscrew (coiled-spring) appearance of the duodenum and proximal small bowel is the classic appearance. The diagnosis of duodenal atresia is generally made on plain films with the classic double-bubble sign. The findings on upper GI series in cases of duodenal atresia include: complete proximal duodenal obstruction, a smoother duodenal contour, without the coiled-spring or bird's beak appearance, and without external compression on the duodenum typically seen with malrotation. Duodenal stenosis with incomplete obstruction, particularly if located in a more distal location, may be indistinguishable from malrotation radiographically, even with intraluminal contrast. Uncertainty requires immediate operative exploration because the outcome with midgut volvulus is time dependent. Furthermore, radiographic differentiation of malrotation with and without midgut volvulus may be unreliable; therefore it is potentially hazardous to defer operative exploration owing to the radiographic expectation that volvulus has not occurred.

In patients with malrotation but without volvulus, the diagnosis of malrotation is made based on the position of the duodenojejunal junction (ligament of Treitz) (see Fig. 31-6A). The normal position of the duodenojejunal junction is to the left of the spine at the level of the gastric antrum, fixed tightly to the posterior body wall. In patients with malrotation, the duodenojejunal junction is typically found on the right side of the spine, inferior to the duodenal bulb, and more anterior than expected. The lateral view is very useful in assessing the anterior and posterior relations of the duodenojejunal junction. Dilated, fluid-filled loops of bowel not evident on plain radiographs can displace the duodenojejunal junction

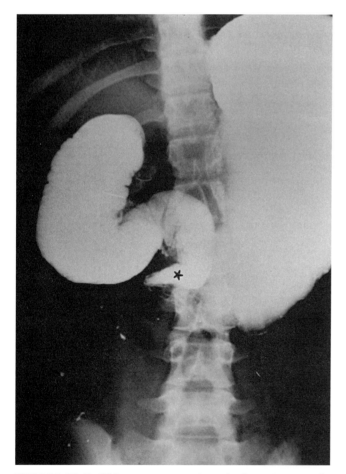

FIGURE 31-5. This upper gastrointestinal contrast study shows malrotation with volvulus. The "beak" is illustrated by the asterisk. Note the malposition of the distal duodenum as well. (From Oldham KT: Pediatric abdomen. In Greenfield LJ, Mulholland M, Oldham KT, et al. [eds]: Surgery: Scientific Principles and Practice. Philadelphia, Lippincott-Raven, 1997.)

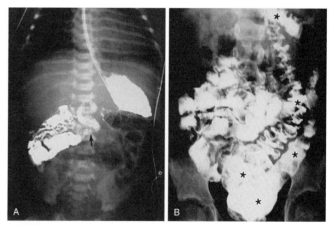

FIGURE 31-6. *A,* This upper gastrointestinal contrast series in a patient with malrotation without volvulus illustrates typical malposition of the duodenal-jejunal juncture (*arrow*). This corresponds to the ligament of Treitz and is located more caudad, right, and anterior than normal. *B,* This radiograph again illustrates malrotation. The small bowel is to the right of midline, and the colon and cecum (*asterisks*) are to the left. (Adapted from Oldham KT: Pediatric abdomen. In Greenfield LJ, Mulholland M, Oldham KT, et al. [eds]: Surgery: Scientific Principles and Practice. Philadelphia, Lippincott-Raven, 1997.)

inferiorly and thus mimic malrotation. If an upper GI study is performed and results in the diagnosis of malrotation, significant duodenal dilation should alert the surgeon to the possibility of intrinsic duodenal obstruction to ensure that this possibility is further evaluated during the corrective operation. This can be done in several ways, including passage of a nasogastric or orogastric tube beyond the stomach and through the proximal jejunum; use of a Fogarty embolectomy catheter or Foley catheter, which is passed from the mouth or nose into the distal duodenum and then withdrawn after inflating the balloon a small amount; or creation of an anterior gastrotomy to perform these same techniques. If the upper GI contrast study is not diagnostic, further evaluation by using a contrast enema to determine the position of the cecum may be helpful. Other findings on upper GI contrast study in malrotation include all loops of the proximal jejunum on the right side of the abdomen. Interpretation of an upper GI tract contrast series in this situation is somewhat subjective and operator dependent. For maximal value, the study requires an experienced pediatric radiologist, a high-quality fluoroscopic study in the radiology suite, and direct involvement of the surgeon.

The contrast enema is often the primary study helpful in evaluating children with more general concerns of neonatal intestinal obstruction, but it is less reliable with regard to malrotation because the position of the cecum and the colon are highly variable and may even appear to be normal.[27] The finding of a high right-sided or left-sided cecum is suggestive of malrotation, but is also reported in about 15% of normal infants without malrotation. With malrotation, the small bowel typically resides in the right abdomen, and the colon and the cecum are often on the left (see Fig. 31-6B). Finally, and most important, duodenal obstruction caused by malrotation may occur in the presence of a normally positioned cecum. With these limitations in mind, the findings of malrotation by contrast enema include the entire colon within the left abdomen (as seen in complete nonrotation), and an abnormally short ascending colon with the cecum positioned above the right iliac wing.

Other imaging studies that demonstrate axial relations such as US or computed tomography may periodically demonstrate evidence of malrotation.[28] US is frequently used to evaluate infants with emesis for the possibility of pyloric stenosis and may demonstrate findings suggestive of volvulus. The typical finding here is reversal in the relation of the SMA to the superior mesenteric vein (SMV). Normally, the SMV is positioned to the right of the SMA. If the SMV lies in an aberrant location, either anterior or to the left of the SMA, malrotation may be present. If present, this finding is noteworthy but not sufficiently reliable to establish the diagnosis of malrotation with volvulus.[29] Likewise, studies have shown that a normal SMA/SMV relation does not always exclude malrotation. Although attractive as a diagnostic tool because it is noninvasive and generally can be quickly performed, its lack of sensitivity and specificity limit its helpfulness. Its role may be confined to suggesting the need for further evaluation in a vomiting child referred for US, in whom pyloric stenosis has been ruled out.

Treatment

Infants and children with acute presentation of midgut volvulus or complete bowel obstruction require urgent operative correction. The immediate resuscitation of the acutely ill child in this setting includes administration of intravenous fluids, placing a nasogastric tube and Foley catheter, typing and cross-matching blood, and giving broad-spectrum antibiotics. These resuscitative measures should all be conducted concurrent with diagnostic imaging, as indicated, so that a diagnosis of malrotation is followed immediately by laparotomy. Time is critical, as a delay of a few hours may determine whether ischemic intestine remains viable and therefore salvageable. If the midgut is not salvageable at laparotomy, the survival rate is approximately 50% and has historically been achieved only with permanent or long-term parenteral hyperalimentation.[30] More recently, intestinal transplantation (with or without liver transplantation) has become an alternative, but without question, these complex approaches are to be avoided if possible.[31] In cases of classic presentation of a previously healthy newborn with the acute onset of bilious emesis associated with signs and symptoms of compromised intestine, such as abdominal-wall erythema, bloody stool, or tenderness on physical examination, laparotomy may proceed without confirmatory contrast studies. No reason exists to delay surgical exploration when the clinical diagnosis is malrotation with possible midgut volvulus.

In the patient in whom malrotation has been radiographically established but without volvulus, several factors affect the urgency of operative correction. In the symptomatic patient, laparotomy and operative correction should proceed as early as possible because contrast studies are not completely reliable in determining whether volvulus has occurred. In the asymptomatic patient, the urgency of operative correction is lessened, but it must be noted that acute vascular insufficiency of the midgut may occur at any age, and this possibility dictates the approach to malrotation at any age. In the case of a young child, especially younger than 1 year, operative correction should proceed electively at the earliest possibility, because this age group is at the highest risk for volvulus with vascular insufficiency. The management of the older asymptomatic patient with malrotation is more controversial. Often the diagnosis of malrotation in the older patient is made during the evaluation of nonspecific symptoms such as chronic abdominal pain or constipation. It is difficult to be certain whether the symptoms that prompted the imaging study are being caused by the malrotation. In addition, some patients have mixed rotational abnormalities in which the resultant anatomic derangement seems minimal. No reliable imaging technique can determine whether the breadth of the SMA vascular pedicle places a particular patient at risk for volvulus. Some authors have recommended laparoscopy to assess the width of the mesenteric fixation and possible laparoscopic correction, if necessary, but this technique is not now widely practiced.[32,33] Older children with intermittent symptoms over a prolonged period are at lower risk for a volvulus developing within a few days after diagnosis. Because the potential consequences of malrotation with volvulus are so devastating and the corrective procedure is associated with a low morbidity, an electively scheduled operative correction seems the most reasonable approach in this setting.

Regardless of age, incidental rotational abnormalities discovered at laparotomy should be evaluated and corrected when encountered, because in this circumstance, it is generally straightforward and adds no additional morbidity.

One additional dilemma is the circumstance of midgut rotational abnormalities associated with congenital heart disease in the heterotaxia syndromes.[34] In this circumstance, careful observation of the asymptomatic patient and deferral of the Ladd's procedure until the cardiac physiology is surgically stabilized appears to be appropriate.

Operative Technique

The operative management of malrotation and midgut volvulus has not changed since the original description by William Ladd and involves six principles. Entry into the abdomen can be accomplished via a variety of incisions, but in the infant, generally a transverse right upper quadrant incision is used. Key elements of the procedure are illustrated in Figure 31-7 and are summarized in the following paragraphs.

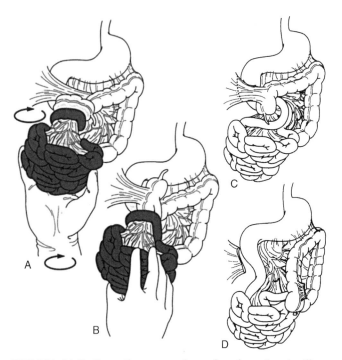

FIGURE 31-7. Operative correction of malrotation is illustrated. Counterclockwise detorsion is shown in (*A*) and (*B*). The division of Ladd's cecal bands and broadening of the superior mesenteric artery mesentery are shown in (*C*) and (*D*). Note the final cecal position on the left and the incidental appendectomy. (Adapted from Oldham KT: Pediatric abdomen. In Greenfield LJ, Mulholland M, Oldham KT, et al. [eds]: Surgery: Scientific Principles and Practice. Philadelphia, Lippincott-Raven, 1997. Illustrations by Holly R. Fischer.)

After abdominal entry and rapid exploration, complete evisceration of the intestine and mesentery is performed. Complete evisceration of the entire bowel permits complete assessment of the mesentery for the presence or absence of volvulus, as well as other abnormalities or causes of obstruction. If malrotation with volvulus is present, the surgeon often encounters chylous ascites as a result of the lymphatic obstruction induced by the volvulus. Peritoneal cultures may be sent if any concern exists that the fluid is contaminated. Alternatively, if the fluid is turbid or purulent, it may reflect bacterial contamination from ischemic or necrotic bowel.

If no volvulus is encountered, the subsequent steps for correction of the malrotation are undertaken (see later). If present, midgut volvulus is relieved by rotating the affected small intestine opposite to the direction of torsion, generally in a counterclockwise direction. It is helpful to remember the phrase "turning back the hands of time" when looking down on the twisted bowel. The degree of torsion is variable but may involve one or more complete twists of the mesentery requiring reduction (Fig. 31-8*A*). After untwisting, the intestine may appear congested, edematous, and some areas may appear necrotic. A period of intraoperative warming and observation is often necessary, and placement of warm lap pads and observation for a period often improves the appearance of the intestine where the vascular integrity has been compromised. If areas of the bowel do not recover and are obviously necrotic, resection is performed, generally with creation of one or more stomas. Primary anastomosis may be appropriate if the resected margins are completely viable to avoid further loss of intestinal length at the time of stoma takedown or to avoid the associated fluid and electrolyte problems predictable with a proximal stoma. The guiding principle at this point should be preservation of bowel length. Marginal or questionable segments of bowel should be left in place, and a second-look procedure performed within 24 to 36 hours. The difficult situation in which all of the midgut appears nonviable may call for a second-look procedure in 24 to 36 hours, before proceeding with an extensive resection. If the entire midgut is necrotic, options include resection with one or more stomas and plan for central line placement for parenteral nutrition and eventual stoma closure and gastrostomy tube placement. If an extended length of intestine must be resected, consideration should be given to placement of a gastrostomy tube to provide options for maximizing enteral nutrition. This may be especially helpful in patients struggling to get off parenteral nutrition. Alternatively, when the entire midgut is necrotic, closure without resection and palliative care may be an appropriate approach after discussion with the family.

Division of Ladd Bands

Ladd's bands (see Fig. 31-7*C*) are peritoneal bands extending from the posterior abdominal wall to the cecum. In cases of malrotation, the cecum typically resides in the right abdomen, and thus these bands can cause external compression and obstruction of the

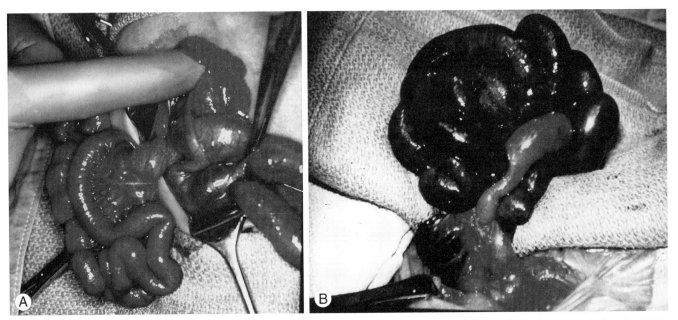

FIGURE 31-8. Operative photographs in two infants with malrotation and midgut volvulus. *A,* The midgut here is clearly viable, although the uncorrected superior mesenteric artery vascular pedicle is less than a fingerbreadth. A Ladd's procedure as shown in Figure 31-7 is definitive therapy. *B,* The midgut here is clearly infarcted and presents a much more difficult set of decisions (see text).

duodenum as they pass anteriorly and laterally across the duodenum. The bands should be divided completely on both the lateral and medial aspects of the duodenum. A generous Kocher maneuver is performed, and all bands are divided to the level of the portal triad superiorly and to the duodenojejunal junction inferiorly. The medial bands to be divided lie between the duodenum and the ascending colon. During this portion of the procedure, the duodenum must be checked for any mechanical kinking caused by adhesions and for the possibility of intrinsic duodenal obstruction. Kinking and adhesions can cause a corkscrew configuration of the duodenum and should be corrected by careful inspection from the pylorus to the proximal jejunum and division of all adhesions. A helpful maneuver is to pass a nasogastric tube from the mouth to the distal duodenum. This is made technically easier in this situation by the generous Kocher maneuver. This ensures that no kinking of the duodenum is present and checks for any associated intrinsic duodenal obstruction. Alternatively, a Foley catheter or a Fogarty embolectomy catheter may be used. The surgeon directs the catheter into the distal duodenum, inflates the balloon, and then withdraws the catheter into the stomach. This maneuver also can be performed by using a gastrotomy, although this is typically not necessary.

Widening of the Mesenteric Base

The base of the mesentery (see Fig. 31-7*D*) normally extends from the ligament of Treitz in the left upper quadrant to the cecum in the right lower quadrant. The base of the mesentery in patients with malrotation is formed by the SMA running through the space between the duodenum and ascending colon. The division of

Ladd's bands from the right lateral abdominal wall to the ascending colon exposes the duodenum and relieves any external compression, but the right colon is still attached to the duodenum. Division of the coloduodenal bands allows the mesentery to unfold, widens the mesenteric base to a broad-based attachment, moves the duodenum and small bowel clearly right of midline, and moves the cecum and right colon left of midline. With further sharp and blunt dissection to separate these structures, the mesenteric base opens widely, and the tendency to volvulize is lessened. The peritoneal bands and adhesions between duodenum, cecum, and the leaves of the mesentery around the SMA are divided. With regard to the SMA pedicle, it is important to carry the dissection and division of the bands down to the SMA and SMV themselves. Much of the mesenteric broadening results in the final portion of this dissection; therefore this should be done completely, proceeding down to the pancreas and the SMVs. Clearly, injury to these structures must be meticulously avoided. Properly opened, the mesenteric pedicle is at low risk for recurrent volvulus. Postoperatively, small bowel obstruction is reported in 10% of patients or fewer, generally as a result of simple adhesion formation. Some authors have advocated pexy of the cecum and duodenum to maintain their position, but this has not been demonstrated to have long-term benefit and is not generally recommended.

Incidental Appendectomy

Appendectomy is considered standard because the malposition of the cecum and the attached appendix in the left abdomen can make acute appendicitis a difficult diagnosis to make if it were to develop in the future. Because the appendix is typically normal at the time of a Ladd's procedure, the appendectomy can be done by using an inversion technique, if preferred, to avoid entry into the GI tract. At the conclusion of the procedure, the intestine is replaced into the abdomen without mesenteric torsion, generally, the small intestine on the right side, and the cecum and colon on the left. Efforts to secure the mesentery surgically by cecal or duodenal attachment to the posterior body wall have been abandoned for lack of supportive data.

Repair of Mesocolic Hernias

Mesocolic hernias appear more complex, largely because they are rarer and thus unfamiliar. A right mesocolic hernia is corrected simply by dividing the lateral peritoneal attachments of the cecum and right colon to the posterior body wall, and the colon is reflected to the left, thus eliminating this potential retrocolic space. This allows the small bowel to reside in the right abdomen and the cecum and colon to occupy the left. In addition, the SMA pedicle should be broadened as much as possible by using the aforementioned techniques. It is tempting to open the sac, but this should be avoided because the right, middle, and left colic vessels are part of the anterior wall of the sac and at risk of injury. In addition, it is not possible to reduce the hernia completely. Left mesocolic hernias are more involved technically; the elements of the procedure are to mobilize the inferior mesenteric vein on the right side of the sac, reduce the small bowel from the hernia sac, and close the neck of the mesocolic sac to eliminate the potential space. Again, the small bowel comes to lie on the right and the colon on the left when this is done. This group of anomalies is more variable, and treatment must necessarily be individualized. An alternative is simply to enlarge the mesocolic space by mobilizing the left colon and opening the neck of the sac sufficiently so that no opportunity is afforded for strangulation. The final position of the intestine has no physiologic relevance; to eliminate the opportunity for entrapment, obstruction, or volvulus is important.

Results

Contemporary results after surgical correction of malrotation are generally excellent, with normal life expectancy in the absence of compromised bowel at the time of the initial procedure. In modern practice, the mortality rate for the operative correction of malrotation ranges from 3% to 9% and is increased in patients with intestinal necrosis, prematurity, and the presence of other abnormalities.[11] Advances in pediatric surgical intensive care, including enteral and parenteral nutritional support, have decreased morbidity and mortality even in cases complicated by intestinal necrosis or associated abnormalities.

Complications associated with malrotation include recurrent volvulus, intestinal dysmotility and prolonged ileus, adhesive bowel obstruction, and short-gut syndrome. Recurrent volvulus is a rare complication with a reported incidence of none to 10% in most series.[14,35] GI-motility disturbances are common after operative correction for malrotation and may be related to postoperative adhesions or ischemic injury to the intestines. The most serious complication of malrotation is short-gut syndrome. Malrotation with midgut volvulus accounted for 18% of all children with short-gut syndrome in the pediatric population in one report.[36] Early diagnosis and urgent operative intervention remain the critical factors to minimizing morbidity and mortality.

REFERENCES

1. Gray SW, Skandalakis J E: Embryology for Surgeons. Philadelphia, Saunders, 1972, pp129–141
2. Mall FP: Develpoment of the human intestine and its position in the adult. Johns Hopkins Hosp Bull 9:197–208, 1898.
3. Frazer TE, Robbins RF: On the factors concerned in causing rotation of the intestine in man. J Anat Physiol 50:74–110, 1915.
4. Dott NM: Anomalies of intestinal rotation: Their embryology and surgical aspects, with the report of five cases. Br J Surg 11:251–286, 1923.
5. Ladd WE: Congenital obstruction of the duodenum in children. N Engl J Med 206:277–283, 1932.
6. Ladd WE: Surgical diseases of the alimentary tract in infants. N Engl J Med 215:705, 1936.
7. Byrne WJ: Disorders of the intestine and pancreas. In Taeusch WH, Ballard RA, Avery ME, (eds): Disease of the Newborn. Philadelphia, WB Saunders, 1991, pp 685–693.
8. Skandalakis JE, Gray SW, Ricketts R, et al: The small intestines. In Skandalakis JE, Gray SW, (eds): Embryology for Surgeons, 2nd ed. Baltimore, Williams & Wilkins, 1994, pp 184.
9. Kantor JL: Anomalies of the colon: Their roentgen diagnosis and clinical significance: Resume of 10 years study. Radiology 23:651–662, 1934.
10. Spigland N, Brandt ML, Yazbeck S: Malrotation presenting beyond the neonatal period. J Pediatr Surg 25:1139–1142, 1990.
11. Warner BW: Malrotation. In Oldham KT, Colambani PM, Foglia RP (eds): Surgery of Infants and Children: Scientific Principles and Practice. Philadelphia, Lippincott-Raven, 1997, pp 1229–1240.
12. Smith IE: Malrotation of the intestine. In: Welch KJ, Randolph JG, Ravich MR, et al. (eds): Pediatric Surgery, 4th ed. Chicago, Year Book Medical Publishers, 1986, pp 882–895.
13. Powell D, Otterson HB, Smith CD: Malrotation of the intestines in children: The effect of age on presentation and therapy. J Pediatr Surg 24:777–780, 1989.
14. Stewart DR, Colodny AL, Daggett WC: Malrotation of the bowel in infants and children: A 15 year review. Surgery 79:716–720, 1976.
15. Filston HC, Kirks DR: Malrotation: The ubiquitous anomaly. J Pediatr Surg 16:614–620, 1981.
16. Yanez R, Spitz L: Intestinal malrotation presenting outside the neonatal period. Arch Dis Child 61:682–685, 1986.
17. Croitoru D, Neilson I, Guttman FM: Pyloric stenosis associated with malrotation. J Pediatr Surg 1991;26:1276–1278.
18. Campbell KA, Sitzmann JV, Cameron JL: Biliary tract anomalies associated with intestinal malrotation in the adult. Surgery 113:312–317, 1993.
19. Smith SL. Familial midgut volvulus. Surgery 72:420–426, 1972.
20. Barone CM, Marion R, Shanske A, et al: Craniofacial, limb, and abdominal anomalies in a distinct syndrome: Relation to the spectrum of Pfeiffer syndrome type 3. Am J Med Genet 45:745–750, 1993.
21. Stalker HJ, Chitayat D: Familial intestinal malrotation with midgut volvulus and facial anomalies: A disorder involving a gene controlling the normal gut rotation? Am J Med Genet 44:46–47, 1992.
22. Firor H, Steiger E: Morbidity of rotational abnormalities of the gut beyond infancy. Clev Clin Q 50:303–309, 1983.
23. Wang C, Welch CE: Anomalies of intestinal rotation in adolescents and adults. Surgery 54:839–855, 1963.
24. Willwerth BM, Zollinger RM, Izant RJ: Congenital mesocolic (paraduodenal) hernia: Embryologic basis of repair. Am J Surg 128:358–361, 1974.

25. Gross RE: Malrotation of the intestine and colon. In Gross RE, (ed): The Surgery of Infancy and Childhood. Philadelphia, WB Saunders, 1953, p 192.

26. Kirks DR, Caron KH: Gastrointestinal tract. In Kirks DR (ed): Practical Pediatric Imaging, 2nd ed. Philadelphia, JB Lippincott, 1991, p 710.

27. Slovis TL, Klein MD, Watts FB: Incomplete rotation of the intestine with a normal cecal position. Surgery 87:325–330, 1980.

28. Weinberger E, Winters WD, Liddell RM, et al: Sonographic diagnosis of intestinal malrotation in infants: Importance of the relative positions of the superior mesenteric vein and artery. Am J Radiol 159:825–828, 1992.

29. Zerin JM, DiPietro MA. Superior mesenteric vascular anatomy at US in patients with surgically proved malrotation of the midgut. Radiology 183:693–694, 1992.

30. Seashore JH, Toloukian RJ: Midgut volvulus. Arch Pediatr Adolesc Med 148:43–46, 1994.

31. Reyes J, Bueno J, Kocoshis S, et al: Current status of intestinal transplantation in children. J Pediatr Surg 33:243–254, 1998.

32. Gross E, Chen MK, Lobe TE: Laparoscopic evaluation and treatment of intestinal malrotation in infants. Surg Endosc 10:936–937, 1996.

33. Frantzides CJ, Cziperle DJ, Spergel K, et al: Laparoscopic Ladd and cecopexy in the treatment of malrotation beyond the neonatal period. Surg Laparosc Endosc 6:73–75, 1996.

34. Chang J, Brueckner M, Touloukian RJ: Intestinal rotation and fixation abnormalities in heterotaxia: Early detection and management. J Pediatr Surg 28:1281–1285, 1993.

35. Stauffer UG, Hermann P. Comparison of late results in patients with corrected intestinal malrotation with and without fixation of the mesentery. J Pediatr Surg 15:9, 1980.

36. Warner BW, Ziegler MM. Management of the short bowel syndrome in the pediatric population. Pediatr Clin North Am 40:1335, 1993.

Meconium Disease

Michael G. Caty, MD, Michael S. Irish, MD, and Daniel Little, MD

Neonatal intestinal obstruction (NIO) is one of the most common admitting diagnoses to the neonatal intensive care unit, accounting for as many as one third of all admissions.[1] Failure to pass meconium within the first 24 to 48 hours of life, feeding intolerance, abdominal distention, and bilious emesis are hallmarks of NIO and evoke a differential diagnosis of obstruction based on anatomic, metabolic, and functional considerations. Strictly speaking, the term *meconium disease* refers to meconium ileus (MI) and meconium plug syndrome (MPS). These conditions are considered separately from functional or anatomic causes of neonatal intestinal obstruction such as Hirschsprung's disease, intestinal atresia, and anorectal malformations.

MECONIUM ILEUS

MI is a misnomer. The true connotation of the term *meconium ileus* is intestinal obstruction due to inspissated meconium within the terminal ileum. This results from abnormal composition of fetal meconium due to cystic fibrosis.

MI is one of the most common causes of intestinal obstruction in the newborn, accounting for 9% to 33% of neonatal intestinal obstructions.[2] It is characterized by extremely viscid, protein-rich, inspissated meconium causing obstruction of the distal ileum. It is the earliest clinical manifestation of cystic fibrosis (CF), occurring in approximately 16% of patients with CF.[3] MI may be an early indication of a more severe phenotype of cystic fibrosis. This has been suggested by significantly lower pulmonary function found in children with a history of MI compared with age- and gender-matched children who did not have MI.[4]

Because of abnormalities of exocrine mucous secretion, the meconium in MI differs from normal meconium in that it has less water content (meconium ileus, 65%; normal, 75%), lower sucrase and lactase levels, increased albumin, and decreased pancreatic enzymes.[5,6]

Therefore more viscous intestinal mucus results in thick, dehydrated meconium that obstructs the intestine.[7]

CYSTIC FIBROSIS

Incidence

CF is an autosomal recessive disease with a heterozygote frequency estimated to be 1 in 29 in the white population, affecting approximately 30,000 children and young adults in the United States. With an incidence of 1 in 3000 live births, approximately 1200 infants with CF are born each year in the United States. The disease is less common in nonwhite populations. The incidence in African-American births is 1 in 15,000 but is much lower in native Africans. Incidences for other populations are 1 in 31,000 in Asian-American births, 1 in 10,500 live Native American Aleut (Eskimo) births, and 1 in 13,500 in Hispanic-white births.

Genetics

In 1989, the CF locus was localized through linkage analysis to the long arm of human chromosome 7, band q31.[8,9] The disease results from mutations in the gene coding for a cell membrane protein termed the *cystic fibrosis transmembrane (conductance) regulator* (CFTR).[10,11] This protein has been found to be an adenosine 3',5'-cyclic adenosine monophosphate (cAMP)-induced chloride channel, which also regulates the flow of other ions across the apical surface of epithelial cells. The alteration in CFTR results in an abnormal electrolyte content in the environment external to the apical surface of epithelial membranes. This leads to desiccation and reduced clearance of secretions from tubular structures lined by affected epithelia.

The most common mutation of the *CFTR* gene, the ΔF508 mutation, is a 3–base pair deletion, which results in the removal of a phenylalanine residue at amino acid position 508 of the *CFTR*. More than 1000 CFTR mutations have been reported to the CF Genetic Consortium.

Gastrointestinal Pathophysiology

Clinically, CF is characterized by the triad of chronic obstruction and infection of the respiratory tract, insufficiency of the exocrine pancreas, and elevated sweat chloride levels.[12] Other clinical variants, such as adult men with bilateral absence of the vas deferens but who have little other clinical involvement, were recently described.[13-15] Secondary manifestations and complications of CF are discussed later.

Pancreas

In 1905, the association of inspissated meconium in a newborn with pathologic changes in the pancreas was first described.[16] In 1936, the term *cystic fibrosis* was first used to describe the combination of pancreatic insufficiency and chronic pulmonary disease in childhood.[17] Two years later, the coexistence of MI and CF was described, and the histologic lesions in the pancreas were noted to be identical in both conditions.[18]

Development of both the pancreas and intestinal tract in fetuses with CF is abnormal. In patients with CF, abnormal pancreatic secretions obstruct the duct system, leading to autodigestion of the acinar cells, fatty replacement, and ultimately fibrosis. Beginning in utero, this process occurs variably over time. Pancreatic insufficiency is prevalent in young infants with CF and has a significant impact on growth and nutrition.[19]

Early investigation suggested that pancreatic insufficiency played a central role in the pathogenesis of MI.[20] This is supported by the fact that two thirds of infants found to have CF by neonatal screening are pancreatic insufficient at birth.[21] However, approximately 10% of patients with CF are pancreatic sufficient and will tend to have a milder course.[22] This suggests that pancreatic insufficiency is not the sole cause of abnormal meconium in MI.[22,23] The lack of concordance between MI and severity of pancreatic disease suggests that intraluminal intestinal factors also contribute to the development of MI.

Intestine

Inspissation of meconium, caused by abnormal intestinal mucus, was first suggested in 1946.[24] Chemical analysis of inspissated meconium from infants with MI was carried out as early as 1952.[25] In 1953, the abnormally viscid nature of meconium in MI was first attributed to the secretion of abnormal mucus by the intestines of patients with CF.[26] Meconium in patients with CF has a higher protein and lower carbohydrate concentration than does that of controls.[20,27]

Abnormal intestinal motility also may contribute to the development of MI. Some patients with CF have been found to have prolonged small intestinal transit times.[28,29] Non-CF diseases associated with abnormal gut motility, such as Hirschsprung's disease and chronic intestinal pseudo-obstruction, have been associated with MI-like disease, suggesting that decreased peristalsis may play some role in the development of MI.[30-32] One can speculate that the CFTR ion-channel defect leads to dehydration of intraluminal contents.[33]

PRENATAL DIAGNOSIS AND SCREENING

In consideration of the diagnosis of MI, the risk of CF in the fetus must be considered. Antenatal diagnosis of MI can be made in two different groups: a *high-risk* group and a *low-risk* group. In the low-risk group, the diagnosis is suspected when the sonographic appearances of MI are found on routine prenatal ultrasound (US) examination. All pregnancies subsequent to the birth of a CF-affected child are considered at high risk, and parents of a child with CF are considered to be obligate carriers of a CF mutation.

Pediatric surgeons are often consulted to evaluate fetuses with suspected bowel obstruction. MI must be considered in the differential diagnosis, particularly in the high-risk fetus. An algorithm may be used in the decision making and the management of the fetus suspected of having MI[34-36] (Fig. 32-1). The obvious advantage of prenatal diagnosis is that it allows the clinician to prepare for the medical and psychological needs of the parents, fetus, and newborn before, during, and after delivery. In a pregnancy in which CF is suspected, sonographic examinations are performed on a monthly basis until delivery. This evaluation allows the early detection of potential complications as they occur and prepares the clinicians for special or urgent medical or surgical needs on delivery.

Sonographic Evaluation

Sonographic characteristics associated with MI include a hyperechoic, intra-abdominal mass of inspissated meconium, dilated bowel, and nonvisualization of the gallbladder. Normal fetal meconium, when visualized in the second and third trimesters, is usually hypoechoic or isoechoic compared with adjacent abdominal structures[37-42] (Fig. 32-2). The sensitivity of intra-abdominal echogenic masses in the detection of MI/CF is reported to be only between 30% and 70%. Using echogenicity as a sonographic marker of meconium ileus is problematic because it is a subjective assessment, and a lengthy associated differential diagnosis exists. In addition to MI,[37-40,43,44] hyperechoic bowel has been reported with Down syndrome,[45,46] intrauterine growth retardation,[37,39,40,45-47] prematurity,[48] in utero cytomegalovirus (CMV) infection,[49] intestinal atresia, abruptio placenta, and fetal death.[47] The usefulness of hyperechoic fetal bowel is related to gestational age at detection, ascites, calcification, volume of amniotic fluid, and the presence of other fetal anomalies.[42] Furthermore, the prenatal diagnosis of MI by using the sonographic feature of hyperechoic bowel must take into account the a priori

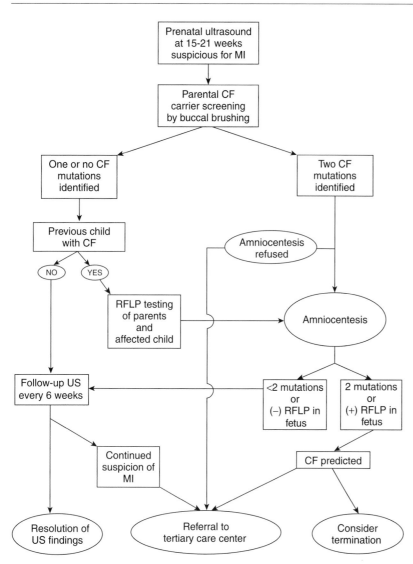

FIGURE 32-1. Suggested algorithm for antenatal management of suspected meconium ileus and cystic fibrosis. (Reprinted from Irish MS, Ragi JM, Karamanoukian H, et al: Prenatal diagnosis of the fetus with cystic fibrosis and meconium ileus. Pediatr Surg Int 12:434–436, 1997.)

risk of the parents. The positive predictive value of hyperechoic masses in a high-risk fetus is estimated to be 52%, whereas in the low-risk fetus, the estimate is only 6.4%.[37]

Although reviews of pregnancies with a 1 in 4 risk of CF show a 25% to 60% association between hyperechoic bowel and CF,[44,48] this association is less prevalent in the general population. In a review of 12,776 fetal US studies performed after 14 weeks of gestation, hyperechoic bowel was noted in only 30 (0.2%) fetuses.[37] CFs was found in 13.3% of these. It is crucial to note that hyperechoic bowel has been found to be a normal variant in both the second and third trimesters.[41,42,50]

The finding of dilated bowel on prenatal US, in association with CF, has been reported less frequently than that of hyperechoic bowel. In MI, bowel dilation is caused by obstruction by meconium, but mimics findings in midgut volvulus, congenital bands, intestinal atresia, intestinal duplication, internal hernia, MPS, and Hirschsprung's disease.[51] The correlation of dilated fetal bowel with MI suggests that dilated fetal bowel warrants

parental testing for CF and continued sonographic surveillance of the fetus.

Inability to visualize the gallbladder on fetal US also has been associated with CF.[52] Combined with other sonographic features, nonvisualization of the gallbladder can be useful in the prenatal detection of the disease. However, caution should be exercised in the interpretation of an absent gallbladder, as the differential diagnosis also includes biliary atresia, omphalocele, and diaphragmatic hernia.

The sonographic characteristics of fetal bowel obstruction are neither sensitive nor specific for MI. Again, the interpretation of sonographic findings must include consideration of the risk of the fetus of having CF. Certainly findings suggesting MI in the high-risk fetus indicate a high probability of CF.[52] In the low-risk fetus, suggestive US findings warrant consideration of prenatal screening by DNA testing or, at the very least, serial follow-up examinations.

The utility of prenatal screening for CF in fetuses with intestinal obstruction was recently examined by

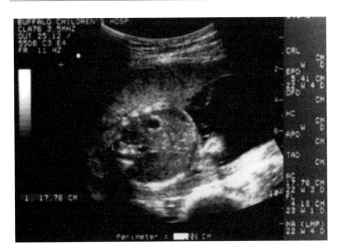

FIGURE 32-2. Sonogram a 22-week gestation demonstrating a 2 × 3 cm intraluminal (distal ileum) mass consistent with meconium inspissation (meconium ileus). (Reprinted from Irish MS, Ragi JM, Karamanoukian H, et al: Prenatal diagnosis of the fetus with cystic fibrosis and meconium ileus. Pediatr Surg Int 12:434–436, 1997.)

prospectively reviewing patients with MI, MPS, meconium peritonitis, jejunoileal atresia, and volvulus. Prenatal US signs were correlated with postnatal findings of CF and type of bowel obstruction. Immunoreactive trypsin measurement, genetic studies, and sweat tests were performed to confirm or rule out CF. Of the 80 patients reviewed, 30 (37.5%) had a prenatal diagnosis of an intestinal anomaly. The overall incidence of CF with a prenatal diagnosis of an intestinal anomaly was 13% or 333 times the estimated risk of CF in the general population. A hyperechoic pattern with dilated bowel was associated with higher specificity for CF (100%), followed by hyperechoic bowel with ascites (75%). These authors suggest that prenatal screening for CF is indicated in all pregnancies with US patterns of specific intestinal disorders, and all neonates with any type of NIO should be screened for CF.[53] Neonatal screening also has been noted to lead to better preservation of lung function in the long term, to prevent severe malnutrition, and to improve long-term growth in CF patients.[54]

MI is categorized as either *simple* or *complicated*. In either form, thickened meconium begins to form in utero and, as it obstructs the midileum, proximal dilatation, bowel wall thickening, and congestion occur. In *complicated* MI, volvulus, atresia, necrosis, perforation, meconium peritonitis, and pseudocyst formation may occur.

CLINICAL PRESENTATION IN NEWBORNS

Simple Meconium Ileus

Newborns with uncomplicated MI appear healthy immediately after birth. The bowel obstruction in the patient with MI is clinically similar to many types of neonatal small bowel obstruction. Therefore the clinician should simultaneously consider and evaluate for malrotation, small intestinal atresia, colonic atresia, and MPS. The history, physical examination, and contrast enema can help make these distinctions.

Failure to pass meconium leads to progressive abdominal distention and bilious vomiting. Dilated loops of bowel become visible on examination and have a doughy character that indents on palpation.[55] The rectum and anus are often narrow, a finding that may be misinterpreted as anal stenosis.[56]

Complicated Meconium Ileus

Fifty percent of patients with MI have complications: volvulus, intestinal necrosis, bowel perforation, intestinal atresia, or meconium peritonitis.[57-60] The incidence of CF in neonates with meconium peritonitis is reported to be 15% to 40%.

Complicated MI may appear dramatically and immediately after birth. In others, symptoms will develop within 24 hours of birth. As a result of in utero perforation or bowel compromise, signs of peritonitis including distention, tenderness, and abdominal wall edema, and clinical evidence of sepsis may be present on the initial neonatal examination. Abdominal distention can be so severe as to cause immediate respiratory distress. A palpable mass suggests pseudocyst formation, which results from in utero bowel perforation.[55,56] Often the neonate is *in extremis* and needs urgent resuscitation and surgical exploration.

Historically, segmental volvulus was reported in larger series to be the most common complication of MI.[57,58] A twist of the bowel, without vascular compromise, is not necessarily a serious condition, yet interruption of mesenteric blood flow will lead to segmental necrosis and produce an intestinal atresia with an associated mesenteric defect. Atretic segments are common in MI, and the affected bowel may appear viable, showing no evidence of previous perforation or gangrene.

Four types of meconium peritonitis have been recognized, including adhesive meconium peritonitis, giant cystic meconium peritonitis, meconium ascites, and infected meconium peritonitis.[61] In addition to MI, other causes of in utero bowel perforation also must be considered (atresia, stenosis, colonic disorders, imperforate anus) in this clinical setting.

Each form of meconium peritonitis shares a common etiology, bowel perforation. The differences in clinical presentation are secondary to the timing of perforation and whether the perforation seals spontaneously. The site of perforation has usually closed by birth. Mortality is increased in cases in which the perforation remains patent.[62]

Initially, meconium peritonitis is a nonbacterial, chemical and foreign-body peritonitis occurring during intrauterine or early neonatal life as a result of a connection between the bowel and peritoneal cavity.[63] As meconium escapes the obstructed bowel, a sterile chemical peritonitis ensues. After delivery, however, bacterial superinfection can occur after colonization of the gastrointestinal tract.

RADIOGRAPHIC FEATURES

Uncomplicated MI is characterized by a pattern of unevenly dilated loops of bowel on abdominal radiograph with variable presence of air-fluid levels.[59,64,65] As air mixes with the tenacious meconium, bubbles of gas may be seen. This *soap-bubble* appearance depends on the viscosity of the meconium and is not a constant feature[59,64] (Fig. 32-3). Although each of these features alone is not diagnostic of MI, collectively, and with a family history of CF, they strongly suggest the diagnosis.[66]

If uncomplicated MI is clinically and radiographically suspected, a contrast enema with barium may establish the diagnosis, but it should be followed by a therapeutic water-soluble enema. To avoid two agents, we advocate water-soluble contrast for both diagnosis and treatment (see Nonoperative Management later). In MI, contrast instillation is monitored fluoroscopically and will demonstrate a colon of small caliber, described as the *microcolon of disuse* (Fig. 32-4), often containing small *rabbit pellets* of inspissated mucus (Fig. 32-5).

Radiographic findings in complicated MI vary according to the complication. Prenatal US findings include ascites, intra-abdominal cystic masses, dilated bowel, and calcification.[67] Neonatal radiographic findings may include air-fluid levels, free air, intra-abdominal calcifications, or a combination of these. Air-fluid levels may be minimally present or absent, misleading the clinician to make an incorrect diagnosis of uncomplicated MI.

Speckled calcifications on abdominal plain films are highly suggestive of intrauterine intestinal perforation and meconium peritonitis. A pseudocyst is suggested by the radiographic findings of obstruction and a large dense mass with a rim of calcification. These calcium deposits will be linear, coursing the parietal peritoneum and serosal surface of the visceral organs.[68]

Interestingly, one third of cases of complicated MI have no radiologic findings suggesting a complication of MI.[69] It is important to remember that in utero perforation (CF or non-CF related) can lead to meconium peritonitis or meconium pseudocyst formation; therefore in these situations, only intraoperative inspection may differentiate CF- from non-CF–related meconium peritonitis or meconium pseudocyst formation. Water-soluble enemas are contraindicated in patients with complicated MI.

NONOPERATIVE MANAGEMENT

After birth, both simple and complicated MI should initially be managed as a newborn intestinal obstruction. Resuscitative measures include mechanical respiratory support, if necessary, and intravenous hydration. Gastric decompression to prevent progressive abdominal distention, aspiration, and pulmonary compromise is important. The administration of vitamin K to correct any coagulopathy and empirical antibiotic coverage complete the initial management. When MI is suspected or diagnosed, immediate pediatric surgical evaluation should be obtained.

The majority of newborns with MI can be managed nonoperatively with hyperosmolar water-soluble enemas. Acknowledged criteria for proceeding with this therapy require that (1) the infant show signs of uncomplicated MI with no clinical or radiologic evidence of complicating factors, such as volvulus, gangrene, perforation, peritonitis, or atresia of the small bowel; (2) an initial diagnostic contrast enema must exclude other causes of neonatal distal intestinal obstruction; (3) the infant should be well prepared for the enema, with adequate fluid and electrolyte replacement and correction of hypothermia; (4) the enema must be done under fluoroscopic control; (5) intravenous antibiotics should be administered; and (6) close surgical supervision, from the initial evaluation and throughout the hospital course, is imperative.[69]

Gastrografin (Bristol-Meyers Squibb, Princeton, NJ) is meglumine diatrizoate, a hyperosmolar, water-soluble, radiopaque solution containing 0.1% polysorbate 80 (Tween 80) and 37% organically bound iodine. The osmolarity of the solution is 1900 mOsm/L (roughly 6 times the osmolarity of serum). On instillation, fluid is

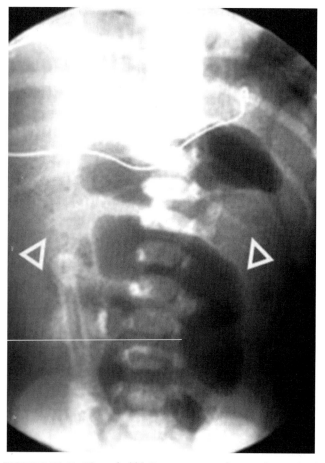

FIGURE 32-3. "Soap bubble" appearance of meconium mixed with water-soluble contrast material. (Reprinted from Irish MS, Gollin Y, Borowitz DS, et al: Meconium ileus: Antenatal diagnosis and perinatal care. Fetal Matern Med Rev 8:79–83, 1996.)

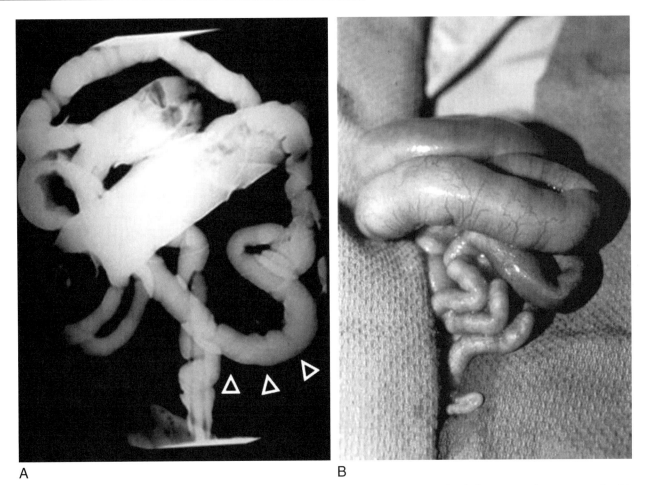

FIGURE 32-4. "Microcolon of disuse" (*arrow*) as seen on contrast enema radiography (*A*). At operation, compared with dilated ileum (*B*). (Reprinted from Irish MS, Gollin Y, Borowitz DS, et al: Meconium ileus: Antenatal diagnosis and perinatal care. Fetal Matern Med Rev 8:79–83, 1996.)

drawn into the intestinal lumen, hydrating and softening the meconium mass. Both transient osmotic diarrhea and diuresis follow. Thus adequate resuscitation and hydration in anticipation of these fluid losses is important.

Under fluoroscopic control, a 25% to 50% solution of Gastrografin is infused slowly at low hydrostatic pressure through a catheter inserted into the rectum. To minimize the risk of rectal perforation, balloon inflation is avoided. On completion, the catheter is withdrawn, and an abdominal radiograph is obtained to exclude perforation. The infant is then returned to the neonatal care unit for intensive monitoring and fluid resuscitation. Warm saline enemas containing 1% N-acetylcysteine may be given to help complete the evacuation.[55] Usually rapid passage of semiliquid meconium continues in the ensuing 24 to 48 hours. Radiographs should be taken in 8 to 12 hours, or as clinically indicated, to confirm evacuation of the obstruction and to exclude late perforation. In the nonoperative management of MI, if evacuation is incomplete, or if the first attempt at Gastrografin evacuation does not reflux contrast into dilated bowel, a second enema may be necessary. Serial Gastrografin enemas can be repeated at 6- to 24-hour intervals if necessary. However, if progressive distention, signs of

peritonitis, or clinical deterioration occurs, surgical exploration is indicated.

After successful evacuation and resuscitation, 5 mL of a 10% N-acetylcysteine solution may be administered every 6 hours through a nasogastric tube to liquefy upper gastrointestinal secretions. Feedings, with supplemental pancreatic enzymes for those infants confirmed with CF, may be initiated when signs of obstruction have subsided.[70] The success rate of patients with uncomplicated MI, treated with Gastrografin enemas, ranges between 63% and 83%.[71]

Several potential complications exist with the use of hyperosmolar enemas in treating MI. The risk of rectal perforation can be avoided with careful placement of the catheter under fluoroscopic guidance and avoidance of inflating balloon-tipped catheters. A 23% perforation rate has been demonstrated in patients in whom inflated balloon catheters were used.[72] Early perforation, occurring during the administration of the enema, is usually readily apparent under fluoroscopy. The risk of perforation increases with repeated enemas.[73] Late perforation, occurring between 12 and 48 hours after the enema, can occur. Potential causes for late perforation include severe bowel distention by fluid osmotically drawn into the

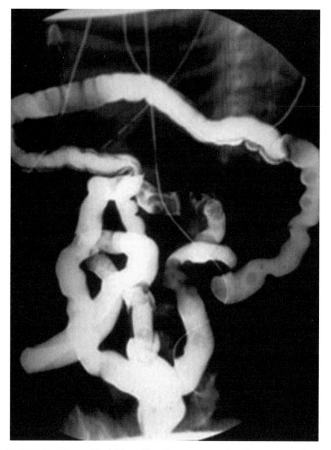

FIGURE 32-5. "Rabbit-pellets" are seen in the microcolon. (Reprinted from Irish MS, Gollin Y, Borowitz DS, et al: Meconium ileus: Antenatal diagnosis and perinatal care. Fetal Matern Med Rev 8:79–83, 1996.)

intestine or direct injury to the bowel mucosa by the contrast medium.[73] The former appears to be the etiology in experimental models.[74,75] Delayed perforation associated with extensive bowel necrosis has been reported.[76,77] The pathogenesis of intestinal perforation associated with necrotizing enterocolitis is believed to be the ischemia produced by intestinal distention.[76] Hypovolemic shock is a risk with delivery of hypertonic enemas. Ischemia caused by overdistention is worsened by hypoperfusion caused by hypovolemia due to inadequate fluid resuscitation. Adequate fluid resuscitation (150 mL/kg/day, minimum) with anticipation of fluid losses due to osmotic diarrhea and diuresis is essential. The addition of 1% N-acetylcysteine to the enema solution will aid in dissolution of the inspissated meconium. Slow infusion, carefully monitored under fluoroscopy, is recommended.[76]

OPERATIVE MANAGEMENT

The indications for operative management of *simple MI* are inadequate meconium evacuation or a complication of the contrast enema, such as perforation. Failure of

nonoperative treatment with Gastrografin enemas may result from the technical inability to advance the column of Gastrografin into the ileum to a sufficient distance. Failure also may result from an unsuspected, associated intestinal atresia. If the Gastrografin enema fails to promote passage of meconium within 24 to 48 hours, an operative approach is indicated.

Before the widespread acceptance of hyperosmolar enemas, several operative strategies predominated as initial therapy.[36] Many of these therapies involved the use of proximal and distal stomas. This allowed the decompression of the dilated intestine and provided access for intestinal irrigation.

In 1948, the first successful surgical management of five infants with MI with intraoperative disimpaction of meconium with saline via a tube enterostomy was reported.[78] A similar technique was reported in 1989, in which an appendectomy was performed and a cecostomy catheter was introduced through the appendiceal stump for insertion of irrigant and evacuation of impacted meconium.[79] Over the years, a number of surgical approaches in the treatment of uncomplicated MI have been proposed.[55,60,79–83] Success rates with each of these methods have been variable. The approach to each infant should be individualized, with the goal of operative management being relief of obstruction with preservation of maximal intestinal length.

Several techniques have involved placing indwelling intestinal tubes for the purpose of postoperative bowel irrigation, decompression, feeding, or a combination of these. These have involved tube enterostomies, with and without resection, and T-tubes. Irrigations are begun in the early postoperative period, and after the successful clearance of meconium, the tubes are removed, and the entercutaneous fistula is allowed to close spontaneously.[82,84]

Other, older operative approaches revolved around resection, anastomosis, and enterostomy, through which postoperative irrigations can be delivered. The Mikulicz double-barreled enterostomy has three distinct advantages. First, because complete evacuation of inspissated meconium is not necessary, operative and anesthetic times are reduced. Second, an intra-abdominal anastomosis is avoided, preventing the risk of anastomotic leakage. Third, the bowel can be opened after complete closure of the abdominal wound, thereby reducing the risk of intraperitoneal contamination. After operation, solubilizing agents can be administered through both the proximal and distal limbs of the stoma, as well as per rectum or via nasogastric tube.[66,81] As classically described, a crushing clamp may be applied to the two intestinal limbs to create continuity for distal flow of intestinal fluids. Disadvantages of this and other procedures with resection and stoma(s) are potential postoperative fluid losses through high-volume stomas, bowel shortening by resection, and the need for a second procedure to re-establish intestinal continuity.

A distal chimney enterostomy (Bishop-Koop) involves resection of the segment of ileum containing the mass of meconium. The distal ileum is brought out as an irrigating and decompressive ileosotomy. An anastomosis is created between the end of the proximal segment and the side of the distal segment of bowel just within the abdominal cavity.[80] This technique allows normal gastrointestinal transit while providing a means for managing distal obstruction through the ileostomy, should it occur. The advantage to this arrangement of the small bowel is that, in the absence of distal obstruction, the intestinal contents will continue "downstream," and the stoma output is usually not a problem. A similar procedure (Santulli) involves creating a proximal enterostomy with creation of an anastomosis between the side of the proximal ileum and the end of the distal limb just inside the abdominal wall.[60,85] With this arrangement, proximal irrigation and decompression are enhanced. Moreover, it is not necessary to evacuate the proximal small bowel at the time of operation. Like the distal chimney enterostomy, catheter access to the distal limb can be achieved through the stoma, thus providing means of irrigating the distal bowel. The apparent disadvantage with this technique is the presence of a high-output stoma with the risk of dehydration. Care must be taken to replenish fluids, electrolytes, and nutrients in the face of high stoma output. Reinstillation of stoma output from the proximal to the distal limb is often performed via an indwelling catheter.[60,66]

Resection with primary anastomosis was first described in 1962.[83] Anastomotic leakage complicated early attempts with this approach. Improved results have been more recently reported.[86,87] Successful application of resection with primary anastomosis depends on adequate resection of compromised bowel, complete proximal and distal evacuation of meconium, and preservation of adequate blood supply to the anastomosis.

With any of the operative techniques, manual evacuation of the inspissated meconium is aided by intraoperative instillation of Gastrografin. Gastrografin can be passed prograde through a nasogastric tube, retrograde through the appendiceal stump, or directly into the meconium through an enterotomy. The dissolved meconium can be milked into the colon. Often the tenacious meconium must be removed directly through an enterotomy. The surgeon must take care to avoid spilling the meconium in the peritoneal cavity when using this strategy. Once the meconium is cleared, the enterotomy or appendiceal stump can be closed. In some situations, a T-tube can be left in the enterotomy to allow postoperative irrigation with Gastrografin, saline, or *N*-acetylcysteine.[88]

An operative approach is always indicated in cases of *complicated MI*. Optimal management includes early recognition, debridement of necrotic material, pseudocyst resection, diverting stoma(s), antibiotics, and meticulous postoperative care.[89] Creation of an ostomy is the fastest and safest course, alleviating concern over bowel discrepancy, anastomotic breakdown, and return of bowel activity. Whereas meconium peritonitis is best managed in this fashion, both segmental volvulus and intestinal atresia in stable patients without peritoneal contamination may be managed with resection, irrigation of the bowel to remove inspissated contents, and end-to-end or end-oblique anastomosis, depending on the relative size of the intestinal segments to be joined.

Initial postoperative management involves ongoing resuscitation. Maintenance fluids and replacement of insensible fluids, as well has gastrointestinal losses (nasogastric suction and ileostomy), must be carefully monitored. Instillation of *N*-acetylcysteine via a nasogastric tube or through an ileostomy will help solubilize residual meconium. In the patient with fetal or neonatal bowel obstruction, CF must be suspected, and diagnostic tests should be performed as soon as possible. Stomas created should be closed as soon as possible (4 to 6 weeks) to help avoid prolonged problems with fluid, electrolyte, and nutritional losses.

NUTRITIONAL MANAGEMENT IN THE POSTOPERATIVE PERIOD

With relief of the obstruction and resumption of bowel function, infants with uncomplicated MI and CF may be given breast milk or routine infant formula, along with supplemental pancreatic enzymes and vitamins.[90,91] Caution must be used when prescribing enteric enzyme medication to patients with MI or CF. Treatment failures and complications such as fibrosing colonopathy from excessive enzyme doses[90] and distal intestinal obstruction syndrome (DIOS)[32] from inadequate enzyme therapy or generic substitutions for proprietary medications have been reported.[92-94] Those who have a complicated surgical course will require either continuous enteral drip feedings or total parenteral nutrition (TPN). The use of a predigested infant formula is recommended initially for enterally fed infants. Prestenotic dilation of the small bowel caused by the obstructing meconium theoretically may lead to mucosal damage, which could contribute to poor peristalsis or malabsorption. In patients with complicated MI, or in those who have had sizeable loss of intestine, continuous feeding with predigested, diluted formula is suggested. If this is well tolerated, the concentration of the formula should be increased before increasing the volume, all the while observing for signs of feeding intolerance (i.e., abdominal distention, gastric residual, heme-positive stools, and/or increasing emesis). Once enteral feedings are begun, pancreatic enzymes must be given (even with predigested formula), starting at 2,000–4,000 lipase units per 120 mL of full-strength formula. Capsules containing enteric-coated microspheres can be opened and the contents mixed with formula or applesauce in older infants. These microcapsules should not be crushed, as this will expose the enzymes to the acid of the stomach, and they will be destroyed. Uncrushed pancreatic enzymes should be given even with medium-chain triglyceride (MCT) formulas.[95]

Infants with MI are at increased risk for cholestasis, particularly if they are receiving TPN. Alkaline phosphatase, alanine aminotransferase (ALT), aspartate aminotransferase (AST), and bilirubin should be monitored weekly. The fluid and nutritional status of infants who have had significant bowel resection (more than one third) may be difficult to manage. In addition, the presence of an ileostomy may lead to excessive fluid and sodium losses, so it is preferable to close an enterostomy as soon as possible. In the interim, if access to the distal, defunctionalized bowel is feasible, drip feeds of glutamine-enriched formula or instillation of the effluent from the proximal stoma may be carefully fed into the distal ileum to enhance intestinal growth and help prevent bacterial translocation.

Gastric acid hypersecretion is seen in patients who have short-bowel syndrome. An acidic intestinal environment inactivates pancreatic enzymes and prevents dissolution of enteric-coated microcapsules. H_2-blocking agents may be used as an adjunct to pancreatic enzyme therapy in patients who have had significant bowel resections. Patients with excessive sweat and intestinal sodium losses need compensation for total body sodium deficit. Urine sodium should be measured in infants with an enterostomy, especially when failure to grow is noted, even if serum sodium levels are normal. Those with urine sodium less than 10 mEq/L will need sodium (and possibly bicarbonate) supplementation.[96]

PULMONARY MANAGEMENT

Although clinical pulmonary complications of CF do not usually develop early, mucus plugging and atelectasis can be seen. Prophylactic pulmonary care with chest physiotherapy is initiated immediately postoperatively. The head-down position should not be used, as this increases the risk of gastroesophageal reflux (GER) and aspiration. Infants should receive nebulized albuterol (2.5 mg) twice a day, followed by chest physiotherapy. Prophylactic antibiotics are not necessary. If antibiotic therapy is needed, it should be based on sensitivities directed by respiratory tract cultures.

PROGNOSIS

The prognosis for infants with MI was uniformly poor despite surgical treatment before the mid-1900s. Early series showed mortality rates of 50% to 67%.[57,80,81,97] Improved survival in infants with MI can be attributed to many factors. With advances in prenatal diagnosis, neonatal intensive care, nutrition, nonoperative management, improvements in operative management and continued understanding of the pathophysiology and treatment of the complications of cystic fibrosis, the prognosis for infants with both complicated and simple MI has improved dramatically.[98,99] Survival rates of 85% to 100% have been reported in uncomplicated MI[66] and up to 85% in complicated cases.[97] Long-term follow-up of CF patients shows pulmonary function at age 13 years to be no different between those born with MI and those without MI.[98] Conversely, comparison of the nutritional status of a similar population of patients with CF suggests that those with MI have long-term nutritional complications[100] as well as other problems.

MECONIUM PLUG SYNDROME

The meconium plug syndrome (MPS) was first described in 1956.[101] The term "plugged-up babies" was coined, and it was hypothesized that either colonic motility or the character of the meconium was altered, which prevented normal passage and evacuation of the colon in the newborn period. Under normal conditions, the leading 2 cm of neonatal meconium is firm in texture, forming a whitish cap. Most newborns pass this cap of meconium prenatally, during, or shortly after delivery. One in 500 newborns will have a longer, more tenacious obstructive plug. Failure to pass this results in MPS, another cause of newborn colonic obstruction.[101]

Pathologic causes of MPS include CF, small left colon syndrome, and Hirschsprung's disease.[102–104] Less common causes include congenital hypothyroidism, maternal narcotic addiction, and neuronal intestinal dysplasia.

The presentation of MPS is similar to that of MI. Signs include failure to pass meconium, bilious vomiting, and abdominal distention with an obstructive pattern on plain abdominal radiographs. Often the meconium plug may become dislodged after digital stimulation of the anus and rectum. Fortunately, colon function is generally preserved and returns to normal after passage of the mass. Ultimately, most of these infants are found to be healthy. The remaining affected newborns require a contrast enema, which may be therapeutic as well as diagnostic. After resolution, a sweat test should be performed to exclude CF, and a thyroid-stimulating hormone (TSH) level should be checked. All patients with slow passage of meconium require close observation of their stool pattern. If bowel dysfunction persists, a rectal biopsy should be performed to evaluate for Hirschsprung's disease.[55,102]

COMPLICATIONS OF MECONIUM ILEUS AND CYSTIC FIBROSIS

Gastroesophageal Reflux Disease

GER occurs with increased prevalence in patients with CF. Pathological reflux with endoscopic and histologic esophagitis is present in more than 50% of CF patients. It is clear that early diagnosis and treatment of this condition is of prime importance if the complications of pathologic reflux are to be avoided. Uncontrolled GER also may aggravate the respiratory status of the CF patient.

Biliary Tract Disease

The most common hepatic complications of cystic fibrosis are steatosis, fibrosis, biliary cirrhosis, atretic gallbladder, cholelithiasis, sclerosing cholangitis, and biliary dyskinesia. Although more common in older patients with CF, intrahepatic cholestasis can be seen in neonates. Prolonged cholestatic liver disease in CF patients may lead to cirrhosis, portal hypertension and, ultimately, to liver failure and death or to liver transplantation.

Inspissated bile syndrome producing cholestasis secondary to plugging of macroscopically normal bile ducts also can occur. In advanced cases in neonates with profound intrahepatic cholestasis, this process can be associated with a marked decrease in ductal diameter, varying from hypoplasia to atresia, and is suggested by prolonged jaundice unresponsive to choleretics, nondilated bile ducts and gallbladder on US, absent biliary excretion on nuclear scan, and characteristic liver biopsy. Severely atrophic or atretic extrahepatic bile ducts may be best managed with reconstruction.[105–107]

Distal Intestinal Obstruction Syndrome

DIOS (formerly called MI equivalent) is a recurrent partial or complete intestinal obstruction unique to patients with CF.[108] Most cases occur in adolescents and adults, but all age groups can be affected, with an overall incidence of approximately 15%.[109–113] DIOS describes a broad range of chronic clinical manifestations stemming from partial to complete bowel obstruction secondary to abnormally viscid mucofeculent material in the distal ileum and right colon.

The etiology of DIOS is unclear, but these patients are more likely to have a history of steatorrhea from pancreatic exocrine insufficiency despite adequate enzyme therapy. A number of aspects peculiar to gastrointestinal function of the CF patient may help to explain this syndrome. In addition to inherently slow intestinal motility, other contributing factors may include thickening of chyme secondary to presence of undigested protein and fat,[114] precipitation of undigested protein and bile acids in duodenal fluid with a reduced pH,[114–116] lower water content of pancreatic and duodenal secretions, hyperviscosity of mucus resulting from abnormal ion and water transport,[115,116] abnormal regulation of mucin secretion,[117] and altered biochemical properties of CF mucus glycoprotein.[114–117] Precipitating factors include sudden withdrawal of, or noncompliance with, adequate enzyme supplementation, immobilization, dehydration, and respiratory tract infections. However, in the majority of cases, no identifiable cause will be found.

Opinions remain varied on the incidence of DIOS. Most reports claim that this condition occurs in up to 15% of CF patients, particularly in those with associated pancreatic insufficiency with malabsorption and severe pulmonary limitations.[103,118–121] The lowest incidence is reported at 5.4 cases per 1000 patient years.[122] Others have noted a higher incidence up to 37%.[123–125] Children with normal fat absorption are rarely affected.

Historic features of DIOS are crampy abdominal pain, often localized to the right lower quadrant, and a decreased frequency of defecation. Other patients may complain of an insidious, debilitating abdominal pain. Physical examination in uncomplicated DIOS usually reveals abdominal distention and a tender mass in the right lower quadrant, with no evidence of peritonitis. Typically, no fecal impaction is seen on rectal examination, and the stool is heme negative. Varying degrees of obstruction will develop, from partial obstruction, which is most common, to complete obstruction with vomiting, abdominal distention, and obstipation.

Supine and erect abdominal radiographic studies are the most helpful initial investigation when any bowel obstruction is suspected. In the presence of DIOS, these will show distended small bowel with scattered air-fluid levels and a granular, bubbly pattern of intestinal gas representing the mixing of air and inspissated meconium in the right lower quadrant. The suspected inspissated material in the right colon and distal ileum can be demonstrated with a water-soluble contrast enema. This study may be therapeutic as well as diagnostic and, in addition, will exclude the presence of an intussusception that also may occur in CF patients.

Other potential causes of abdominal pain and intestinal obstruction in CF patients also must be considered. These include small bowel obstruction due to adhesions from previous abdominal procedures, intussusception, and appendicitis, which occurs in 1.5% to 2% of patients with CF. Because abdominal pain is a common complaint of patients with CF, and as they often undergo prolonged treatment with antibiotics and steroids, the classical clinical signs and symptoms of appendicitis are often masked, and the diagnosis missed. As a result, a high incidence of perforation is seen with its attendant morbidity in this patient group. Despite the blunting of clinical signs, the patient may still have fever and leukocytosis. Depending on the location of the appendix, a contrast enema may show an inflammatory deformity of the cecum with a mass. An abdominal US or, if necessary, a computed tomography (CT) scan will show free fluid or an abscess collection in the region of the cecum. In such cases, appendectomy is indicated. If the diagnosis is still unclear, the surgeon may opt to do a laparoscopic investigation and then proceed, depending on the findings.

In the absence of small bowel obstruction due to adhesions, intussusception, or appendiceal disease, the initial attempt at management of DIOS is to relieve the distal bowel obstruction nonoperatively. After adequate rehydration and cleansing enemas, a balanced polyethylene glycol–electrolyte solution, such as GoLytely or Colyte, can be given orally or by nasogastric tube. The dose is 20–40 mL/kg/hr, with a maximum of 1200 mL/hr. Alternatively, ingestion of a nonabsorbable intestinal lavage solution such as Gastrografin may produce the most striking improvement in DIOS.[126] A single oral dose of Gastrografin is successful in the majority of patients. Careful attention to fluid resuscitation is vital. Oral administration of Gastrografin should be withheld in cases in which dehydration, obstruction, or peritoneal signs suggest an acute abdomen. Younger patients will usually require insertion of a nasogastric tube, whereas older children may be able to ingest sufficient volumes of lavage solution to relieve the impacted material.

Successful treatment is judged by the passage of stool, resolution of symptoms, and the disappearance of a previously palpable right lower quadrant abdominal mass. Sequential plain abdominal radiographs will help to document the resolution of DIOS, but if symptoms persist, the differential diagnosis already outlined should be reconsidered. Some authors have recommended prophylaxis for DIOS with use of scheduled laxatives and high dietary roughage.[103,118]

When complete obstruction or evidence of peritonitis is noted, surgical intervention is necessary, and all oral or rectal therapies are contraindicated. A nasogastric tube should be introduced for decompression, and adequate resuscitative measures initiated. At laparotomy the bowel wall will feel thickened and filled with tenacious material. It can be decompressed and irrigated with Gastrografin usually via a small catheter placed through the appendiceal stump as previously described for uncomplicated MI. It also is possible to leave an irrigating device such as a T-tube in situ to irrigate the bowel postoperatively.

Fibrosing Colonopathy

Fibrosing colonopathy is a newly described entity in children with CF.[90,91,110,127–129] Findings at laparotomy include colonic strictures with histopathologic changes of postischemic ulcer scarring, mucosal and submucosal fibrosis, and destruction of the muscularis mucosa. In some patients, a change from conventional enteric-coated pancreatic enzymes to high-strength products 12 to 15 months before presentation has been described. In the largest case-control study reported, the absolute dose of pancreatic enzymes, rather than the type of enzyme, was the strongest predictor of fibrosing colonopathy.

The diagnosis of fibrosing colonopathy should be considered in CF patients who have been exposed to high doses of pancreatic enzymes and who have symptoms of abdominal pain, distention, chylous ascites, change in bowel habit, or failure to thrive. Continued diarrhea also may be a prominent feature, which unfortunately may prompt the family to increase supplemental enzymes further. On occasion, the diarrhea may be bloody. A barium enema may reveal mucosal irregularity, loss of haustral markings with a foreshortened colon, and varying degrees of stricture formation. In some cases, the whole colon has been involved. Colonoscopy may show an erythematous mucosa and areas of narrowing,[59] from which it is advisable to take multiple biopsies.

Initial management should include reduction of enzyme dosage to the recommended levels of 500 to 2500 lipase units/kg per meal. This should be accompanied with adequate nutritional supplementation, which may be enteral elemental feeding or even TPN for a time. Those patients who show signs of unrelenting failure to thrive, obstruction, uncontrollable diarrhea, or chylous ascites will need surgical intervention.

When an operation is planned electively for patients with intractable symptoms, a gentle preoperative bowel preparation can be given. The aim of surgical intervention is to resect the affected bowel and perform a primary anastomosis. Unfortunately, this is not possible in the event of pancolonic or rectal involvement, and as a result, the patient may require an ileostomy or colostomy. It also is not clear if this condition completely resolves with a reduction in enzyme dosage and surgical resection. Therefore the patients requiring operation also require regular follow-up for any signs of deterioration or recurrence.

REFERENCES

1. Lister J: Intestinal obstruction: General considerations. In Lister J, Irving IM (eds): Neonatal Surgery. London, Butterworth, 1990, pp 421–423.
2. DeLorimier AA, Fonkalsrud EW, Hays DM: Congenital atresia and stenosis of the jejunum and ileum. Surgery 65:819–827, 1969.
3. FitzSimmons SC: The changing epidemiology of cystic fibrosis. J Pediatr 122:1–9, 1993.
4. Evans AK, Fitzgerald DA, McKay KO: The impact of meconium ileus on the clinical course of children with cystic fibrosis. Eur Respir J 18:784–789, 2001.
5. Antonowicz I, Lebenthal E, Schwachman H: Disaccharidase activities in small intestinal mucosa in patients with cystic fibrosis. J Pediatr 92:214–219, 1978.
6. Schwachman H, Antionowicz I: Studies on meconium. In Lebenthal E (ed): Textbook of Gastroenterology and Nutrition in Infancy. New York, Raven Press, 1981, pp 83–93.
7. Eggermont E, De Boeck K: Small-intestinal abnormalities in cystic fibrosis patients. Eur J Pediatr Surg 150:824–828, 1991.
8. Rommens JM, Iannuzzi MC, Kerem B, et al: Identification of the cystic fibrosis gene: Chromosome walking and jumping. Science 245:1059–1065, 1989.
9. Kerem B, Rommens JM, Buchanan JA, et al: Identification of the cystic fibrosis gene: Genetic analysis. Science 245:1073–1080, 1989.
10. Welsh MJ, Anderson MP, Rich DP, et al: Cystic fibrosis transmembrane conductance regulator: A chloride channel with novel regulation. Neuron 8:821–829, 1992.
11. Riordan JR, Rommens JM, Kerem B, et al: Identification of the cystic fibrosis gene: Cloning and characterization of complementary DNA [published erratum appears in Science 29:1437, 1989]. Science 245:1066–1073, 1989.
12. Boat T, Welsh M, Beaudet A: Cystic Fibrosis. In: Scriver C, Beaudet A, Sly W, et al (eds): The Metabolic Basis of Inherited Disease. New York, McGraw-Hill, 1989, pp 2649–2680.
13. Dohle GR, Veeze HJ, Overbeek SE, et al: The complex relationships between cystic fibrosis and congenital bilateral absence of the vas deferens: Clinical, electrophysiological and genetic data. Hum Reprod 14:371–374, 1999.
14. Jarvi K, McCallum S, Zielenski J, et al: Heterogeneity of reproductive tract abnormalities in men with absence of the vas deferens: Role of cystic fibrosis transmembrane conductance regulator gene mutations. Fertil Steril 70:724–728, 1998.
15. Shin D, Gilbert F, Goldstein M, et al: Congenital absence of the vas deferens: Incomplete penetrance of cystic fibrosis gene mutations. J Urol 158:1794–1799, 1997.
16. Landsteiner K: Darmverschluss durch eingedicktes Meconium: Pankreatitis. Zentralbl Allg Pathol 16:903–907, 1905.
17. Fanconi G, Uehlinger E, Knauer C: Das Coeliakiesyndrom bei angeborener zystischer pancreasfibromatose und bronchiektasien. Wien Med Wochenschr 27:753–756, 1936.
18. Anderson D: Cystic fibrosis of the pancreas and its relationship to celiac disease. Am J Dis Child 56:344–399, 1938.
19. Bronstein MN, Sokol RJ, Abman SH, et al: Pancreatic insufficiency, growth, and nutrition in infants identified by newborn screening as having cystic fibrosis. J Pediatr 120:533–540, 1992.
20. Green M, Clarke J, Shwachman H: Studies in cystic fibrosis of the pancreas: Protein pattern in meconium ileus. Pediatrics 21:635, 1958.
21. Foulkes AG, Harris A: Localization of expression of the cystic fibrosis gene in human pancreatic development. Pancreas 8:3–6, 1993.
22. Kerem E, Corey M, Kerem BS, et al: The relation between genotype and phenotype in cystic fibrosis: Analysis of the most common mutation (delta F508). N Engl J Med 323:1517–1522, 1990.
23. Farber S: The relation of pancreatic achylia to meconium ileus. J Pediatr 24:387–392, 1944.
24. Glanzmann E: Dysporia entero-bronco-pancreatica congenita familiaris. Ann Paediatr 166:289, 1946.
25. Buchanan D, Rapoport S: Chemical comparison of normal meconium and meconium from patients with meconium ileus. Pediatrics 9:304–310, 1952.
26. Bodian M (ed): Fibrocystic Disease of the Pancreas: Congenital Disorder of Mucus Production: Mucosis. New York, Grune & Stratton, 1953.

27. Stephan U, Busch EW, Kollberg H, et al: Cystic fibrosis detection by means of a test-strip. Pediatrics 55:35–38, 1975.

28. Bali A, Stableforth DE, Asquith P: Prolonged small-intestinal transit time in cystic fibrosis. Br Med J Clin Res Ed 287:1011–1013, 1983.

29. Dalzell AM, Freestone NS, Billington D, et al: Small intestinal permeability and orocaecal transit time in cystic fibrosis. Arch Dis Child 65:585–588, 1990.

30. Toyosaka A, Tomimoto Y, Nose K, et al: Immaturity of the myenteric plexus is the aetiology of meconium ileus without mucoviscidosis: A histopathologic study. Clin Auton Res 4:175–184, 1994.

31. Emery JL: Colonic retention syndrome (megacolon) associated with immaturity of intestinal intramural plexus. Proc R Soc Med 66:222–223, 1973.

32. Wilcox DT, Borowitz DS, Stovroff MC, et al: Chronic intestinal pseudo-obstruction with meconium ileus at onset. J Pediatr 123:751–752, 1993.

33. Emery J: Laboratory observations of the viscidity of meconium. Arch Dis Child 29:34, 1954.

34. Irish MS, Gollin Y, Borowitz DS, et al: Meconium ileus: Antenatal diagnosis and perinatal care. Fetal Matern Med Rev 8:79–83, 1996.

35. Irish MS, Ragi JM, Karamanoukian H, et al: Prenatal diagnosis of the fetus with cystic fibrosis and meconium ileus. Pediatr Surg Int 12:434–436, 1997.

36. Irish M, Borowitz DS, Glick PL: Meconium ileus. In Ziegler MM, Azizkhan RG, Gauderer MWL, et al (eds): Operative Pediatric Surgery. Stamford, Conn: Appleton & Lange, 2003, pp 597–607.

37. Dicke JM, Crane JP: Sonographically detected hyperechoic fetal bowel: Significance and implications for pregnancy management. Obstet Gynecol 80:778–782, 1992.

38. Denholm TA, Crow HC, Edwards WH, et al: Prenatal sonographic appearance of meconium ileus in twins. Am J Roentgenol 143:371–372, 1984.

39. Caspi B, Elchalal U, Lancet M, et al: Prenatal diagnosis of cystic fibrosis: Ultrasonographic appearance of meconium ileus in the fetus. Prenat Diagn 8:379–382, 1988.

40. Benacerraf BR, Chaudhury AK: Echogenic fetal bowel in the third trimester associated with meconium ileus secondary to cystic fibrosis: A case report. J Reprod Med 34:299–300, 1989.

41. Fakhry J, Reiser M, Shapiro LR, et al: Increased echogenicity in the lower fetal abdomen: A common normal variant in the second trimester. J Ultrasound Med 5:489–492, 1986.

42. Lince DM, Pretorius DH, Manco-Johnson ML, et al: The clinical significance of increased echogenicity in the fetal abdomen. Am J Roentgenol 145:683–686, 1985.

43. Goldstein RB, Filly RA, Callen PW: Sonographic diagnosis of meconium ileus in utero. J Ultrasound Med 6:663–666, 1987.

44. Boue A, Muller F, Nezelof C, et al: Prenatal diagnosis in 200 pregnancies with a 1-in-4 risk of cystic fibrosis. Hum Genet 74:288–297, 1986.

45. Bromley B, Doubilet P, Frigoletto FD Jr, et al: Is fetal hyperechoic bowel on second-trimester sonogram an indication for amniocentesis? Obstet Gynecol 83:647–651, 1994.

46. Nyberg DA, Resta RG, Luthy DA, et al: Prenatal sonographic findings of Down syndrome: Review of 94 cases. Obstet Gynecol 76:370–377, 1990.

47. Gollin Y, Shaffer W, Gollin G, et al: Increased abdominal echogenicity in utero: A marker for intestinal obstruction. Am J Obstet Gynecol 168:349–355, 1993.

48. Bahado-Singh R, Morotti R, Copel JA, et al: Hyperechoic fetal bowel: The perinatal consequences. Prenat Diagn 14:981–987, 1994.

49. Forouzan I: Fetal abdominal echogenic mass: An early sign of intrauterine cytomegalovirus infection. Obstet Gynecol 80:535–537, 1992.

50. Paulson EK, Hertzberg BS: Hyperechoic meconium in the third trimester fetus: An uncommon normal variant. J Ultrasound Med 10:677–680, 1991.

51. De Backer AI, De Schepper AM, Deprettere A, et al: Radiographic manifestations of intestinal obstruction in the newborn. JBR-BTR 82:159–166, 1999.

52. Duchatel F, Muller F, Oury JF, et al: Prenatal diagnosis of cystic fibrosis: Ultrasonography of the gallbladder at 17-19 weeks of gestation. Fetal Diagn Ther 8:28–36, 1993.

53. Casaccia G, Trucchi A, Nahom A, et al: The impact of cystic fibrosis on neonatal intestinal obstruction: The need for prenatal/neonatal screening. Pediatr Surg Int 19:75–78, 2003.

54. Farrell PM, Kosorok MR, Rock MJ, et al: Early diagnosis of cystic fibrosis through neonatal screening prevents severe malnutrition and improves long-term growth: Wisconsin Cystic Fibrosis Neonatal Screening Study Group. Pediatrics 107:1–13, 2001.

55. Andrassy R, Nirgiotis J: Meconium disease of infancy: Meconium ileus, meconium plug syndrome, and meconium peritonitis. In: Holder T, Ashcraft K (eds): Pediatric Surgery. Philadelphia, WB Saunders, 1990, pp 331–340.

56. Lloyd D: Meconium ileus. In Welch K, Randolph J, Ravitch M, et al (eds): Pediatric Surgery, 4th ed. Chicago, Year Book Medical Publishers, 1986, pp 849–858.

57. Donnison AB, Shwachman H, Gross RE: A review of 164 children with meconium ileus seen at the Children's Hospital Medical Center, Boston. Pediatrics 37:833–850, 1966.

58. Holsclaw DS, Eckstein JB, Nixon HH: Meconium ileus: 20 year review of 109 cases: AMA. Med J Dis Child 109:101–113, 1965.

59. Leonidas JC, Berdon WE, Baker DH, et al: Meconium ileus and its complications: A reappraisal of plain film roentgen diagnostic criteria. AJR Am J Roentgenol Radium Ther Nucl Med 108:598–609, 1970.

60. Santulli T, Blanc W: Congenital atresia of the intestine: Pathogenesis and treatment. Ann Surg 154:939–948, 1961.

61. Martin LW: Meconium peritonitis. In Ravitch MM, Welch KJ, Benson CD, et al (eds): Pediatric Surgery. Chicago, Year Book Medical Publishers, 1979, pp 952–955.

62. Speck CR, Moore TC, Stout FE: Antenatal roentgen diagnosis of meconium peritonitis. Am J Radiol 88:566–570, 1962.

63. Bendel WL, Michel MLJ: Meconium peritonitis: Review of the literature and report of a case with survival after surgery. Surgery 34:321–333, 1953.

64. Herson RE: Meconium ileus. Radiology 68:568–571, 1957.

65. White H: Meconium ileus: A new Roentgen sign. Radiology 66:567–571, 1956.

66. Ziegler MM: Meconium ileus. Curr Probl Surg 3:731–777, 1994.

67. Dirkes K, Crombleholme TM, Craigo SD, et al: The natural history of meconium peritonitis diagnosed in utero. J Pediatr Surg 30:979–982, 1995.

68. Foster MA, Nyberg DA, Mahony BS, et al: Meconium peritonitis: Prenatal sonographic findings and their clinical significance. Radiology 165:661–665, 1987.

69. Noblett HR: Treatment of uncomplicated meconium ileus by Gastrografin enema: A preliminary report. J Pediatr Surg 4:190–197, 1969.

70. Noblett H: Meconium ileus: In Ravtch M, Welch K, Benson C, et al (eds): Pediatric Surgery, 3rd ed. Chicago, Year Book Medical Publishers, 1979, pp 943–951.

71. Rowe MI, Furst AJ, Altman DH, et al: The neonatal response to Gastrografin enema. Pediatrics 48:29–35, 1971.

72. Ein S, Shandling B, Reilly B, et al: Bowel perforation with nonoperative treatment of meconium ileus. J Pediatr Surg 22:146–147, 1987.

73. Rowe MI, Seagram G, Weinberger M: Gastrografin-induced hypertonicity: The pathogenesis of a neonatal hazard. Am J Surg 125:185–188, 1973.

74. Lutzger LG, Factor SM: Effects of some water-soluble contrast media on the colonic mucosa. Radiology 118:545–548, 1976.

75. Wood BP, Katzberg RW, Ryan DH, et al: Diatrizoate enemas: Facts and fallacies of colonic toxicity. Radiology 126:441–444, 1978.

76. Leonidas JC, Burry VF, Fellows RA, et al: Possible adverse effect of methylglucamine diatrizoate compounds on the bowel of newborn infants with meconium ileus. Radiology 121:693–696, 1976.

77. Grantmyre EB, Butler GJ, Gillis DA: Necrotizing enterocolitis after Renografin-76 treatment of meconium ileus. Am J Roentgenol 136:990–991, 1981.

78. Hiatt R, Wilson P: Therapy of meconium ileus: report of 8 cases with review of the literature. Surg Gynecol Obstet 87:317–327, 1948.

79. Fitzgerald R, Conlon K: Use of the appendix stump in the treatment of meconium ileus. J Pediatr Surg 24:899–900, 1989.

80. Bishop H, Koop C: Management of meconium ileus: Resection, Roux-en-Y anastomosis and ileostomy irrigation with pancreatic enzymes. Ann Surg 145:410–414, 1957.

81. Gross R: The Surgery of Infants and Childhood. Philadelphia, WB Saunders, 1953.

82. Harberg FJ, Senekjian EK, Pokorny WJ: Treatment of uncomplicated meconium ileus via T-tube ileostomy. J Pediatr Surg 16:61–63, 1981.

83. Swenson O: Pediatric Surgery, 2nd ed. New York, Appleton-Century-Crofts, 1962.

84. O'Neill JAJ, Grosfeld JL, Boles ET Jr, et al: Surgical treatment of meconium ileus. Am J Surg 119:99–105, 1970.

85. Santulli T: Meconium ileus. In Holder T, Ashcraft K (eds): Pediatric Surgery. Philadelphia, WB Saunders, 1980, pp 356–373.

86. Mabogunje OA, Wang CI, Mahour H: Improved survival of neonates with meconium ileus. Arch Surg 117:37–40, 1982.

87. Chappell JS: Management of meconium ileus by resection and end-to-end anastomosis. S Afr Med J 52:1093–1094, 1977.

88. Steiner Z, Mogilner J, Siplovich L, et al: T-tubes in the management of meconium ileus. Pediatr Surg Int 12:140–141, 1997.

89. Careskey JM, Grosfeld JL, Weber TR, et al: Giant cystic meconium peritonitis (GCMP): Improved management based on clinical and laboratory observations. J Pediatr Surg 15:484–489, 1982.

90. FitzSimmons SC, Burkhart GA, Borowitz D, et al: High-dose pancreatic-enzyme supplements and fibrosing colonopathy in children with cystic fibrosis. N Engl J Med 336:1283–1289, 1997.

91. Borowitz DS, Grand RJ, Durie PR: Use of pancreatic enzyme supplements for patients with cystic fibrosis in the context of fibrosing colonopathy: Consensus Committee. J Pediatr 127:681–684, 1995.

92. Hendeles L: Use bioequivalency rating to select generics [letter]. Am Pharm NS29:6, 1989.

93. Hendeles L, Dorf A, Stecenko A, et al: Treatment failure after substitution of generic pancrelipase capsules: Correlation with in vitro lipase activity [see comments]. JAMA 263:2459–2461, 1990.

94. Irish MS, Glick PL, Borowitz DS, et al: An asfaliogenic complication arising from profit-motivated decision-making [letter]. Pediatrics 99:503–504, 1997.

95. Durie PR, Newth CJ, Forstner GG, et al: Malabsorption of medium-chain triglycerides in infants with cystic fibrosis: Correction with pancreatic enzyme supplement. J Pediatr 96:862–864, 1980.

96. Bower TR, Pringle KC, Soper RT: Sodium deficit causing decreased weight gain and metabolic acidosis in infants with ileostomy. J Pediatr Surg 23:567–572, 1988.

97. Rescorla FJ, Grosfeld JL, West KJ, et al: Changing patterns of treatment and survival in neonates with meconium ileus. Arch Surg 124:837–840, 1989.

98. Kerem E, Corey M, Kerem B, et al: Clinical and genetic comparisons of patients with cystic fibrosis, with or without meconium ileus. J Pediatr 114:767–773, 1989.

99. McPartlin JF, Dickson JA, Swain VA: Meconium ileus: Immediate and long-term survival. Arch Dis Child 47:207–210, 1972.

100. Lai HC, Kosorok MR, Laxova A, et al: Nutritional status of patients with cystic fibrosis with meconium ileus: A comparison with patients without meconium ileus and diagnosed early through neonatal screening. Pediatrics 105:53–61, 2000.

101. Clatworthy H, Howard W, Lloyd J: The meconium plug syndrome. Surgery 39:131–142, 1956.

102. Flake AW, Ryckman FC: Meconium plug syndrome. In Fanaroff AA, Martin RJ (eds): Neonatal-Perinatal Medicine, Disease of the Fetus and Infant, 5th ed. St. Louis, Mosby-Year Book, 1992, pp 1054–1055.

103. Rosenstein BJ, Langbaum TS: Incidence of meconium abnormalities in newborn infants with cystic fibrosis. Am J Dis Child 134:72–73, 1980.

104. Stewart DR, Mixon GW, Johnson DG, et al: Neonatal small left colon syndrome. Ann Surg 186:741–795, 1977.

105. Shapira R, Hadzic N, Francavilla R, et al: Retrospective review of cystic fibrosis presenting as infantile liver disease. Arch Dis Child 81:125–128, 1999.

106. Greenholz SK, Krishnadasan B, Marr C, et al: Biliary obstruction in infants with cystic fibrosis requiring Kasai portoenterostomy. J Pediatr Surg 32:175–180, 1997.

107. Oppenheimer EH, Esterly JR: Hepatic changes in young infants with cystic fibrosis: Possible relation to focal biliary cirrhosis. J Pediatr 86:683–689, 1975.

108. Rasor R, Stevenson C: Cystic fibrosis of the pancreas: A case history. Rocky Mt Med J 38:218, 1941.

109. Agrons GA, Corse WR, Markowitz RI, et al: Gastrointestinal manifestations of cystic fibrosis: Radiologic-pathologic correlation. Radiographics 16:871–893, 1996.

110. Eggermont E: Gastrointestinal manifestations in cystic fibrosis. Eur J Gastroenterol Hepatol 8:731–738, 1996.

111. Hamosh A, Fitz-Simmons SC, Macek M Jr, et al: Comparison of the clinical manifestations of cystic fibrosis in black and white patients. J Pediatr 132:255–259, 1998.

112. Fuchs JR, Langer JC: Long-term outcome after neonatal meconium obstruction. Pediatrics 101:E7, 1998.

113. Wilschanski M, Rivlin J, Cohen S, et al: Clinical and genetic risk factors for cystic fibrosis-related liver disease. Pediatrics 103:52–57, 1999.

114. Zentler-Munro PL: Progress report: Cystic fibrosis: A gastroenterological cornucopia. Gut 28:1531–1547, 1987.

115. Marino CR, Gorelick FS: Scientific advances in cystic fibrosis. Gastroenterology 103:681–693, 1992.

116. Kopelman H, Corey M, Gaskin K, et al: Impaired chloride secretion, as well as bicarbonate secretion, underlies the fluid secretory defect in the cystic fibrosis pancreas. Gastroenterology 95:349–355, 1988.

117. McPherson MA, Dormer RL, Bradbury NA, et al: Defective beta-adrenergic secretory responses in submandibular acinar cells from cystic fibrosis patients. Lancet 2:1007–1008, 1986.

118. Hanly JG, Ritzgerald MX: Meconium ileus equivalent in older patients with cystic fibrosis. Br Med J 286:1411–1413, 1983.

119. Dalzell AM, Heaf DP, Carty H: Pathology mimicking distal intestinal obstruction syndrome in cystic fibrosis. Arch Dis Child 65:540–541, 1990.

120. Matseshe JW, Go VLW, Dimagno E: Meconium ileus equivalent complicating cystic fibrosis in post-neonatal children and young adults. Gastroenterology 72:732–736, 1972.

121. Park RW: Gastrointestinal manifestation of cystic fibrosis: A review. Gastroenterology 81:1143–1161, 1981.

122. Anderson HO, Hjelt K, Waever E, et al: The age related incidence of meconium ileus equivalent in a cystic fibrosis population: The impact of high energy intake. J Pediatr Gastroenterol Nutr 11:356–360, 1990.

123. Hodson ME, Norman AP, Batten JC: Cystic Fibrosis. London: Bailliere Tindall, 1983.

124. Lloyd-Still J (ed): Textbook of Cystic Fibrosis. Boston: John Wright, PSG, 1983.

125. O'Halloran SM, Gilbert J, McKendrick OM, et al: Gastrografin in acute meconium ileus equivalent. Arch Dis Child 61:1128–1130, 1986.

126. Cleghorn GJ, Forstner GG, Stringer DA, et al: Treatment of distal intestinal obstruction syndrome in cystic fibrosis with a balanced intestinal lavage solution. Lancet 1:8–11, 1986.

127. Lloyd-Still JD, Beno DW, Kimura RM: Cystic fibrosis colonopathy. Curr Gastroenterol Rep 1:231–237, 1999.

128. Serban DE, Florescu P, Miu N: Fibrosing colonopathy revealing cystic fibrosis in a neonate before any pancreatic enzyme supplementation. J Pediatr Gastroenterol Nutr 35:356–359, 2002.

129. Dialer I, Hundt C, Bertele-Harms RM, et al: Sonographic evaluation of bowel wall thickness in patients with cystic fibrosis. J Clin Gastroenterol 37:55–60, 2003.

Necrotizing Enterocolitis

Shawn D. St. Peter, MD, and Daniel J. Ostlie, MD

EPIDEMIOLOGY

Necrotizing enterocolitis (NEC) is the most common gastrointestinal (GI) emergency in newborns. Its incidence is estimated to be about 3 per 1000 live births, and 30 per 1000 in low-birth-weight neonates. NEC occurs in about 5% of all infants admitted to the neonatal intensive care units.[1-4] Although it can occur in term infants, NEC is predominantly a disease of prematurity, with preterm infants representing 90% of cases of NEC.[3,4] Recent data from the National Institute of Child Health and Human Development Neonatal Research Network demonstrated a 7% incidence of NEC in all newborns less than 1500 g.[2] The estimated incidence of NEC among healthy term infants is about 0.05 per 1000 live births.[5] Its incidence in urban communities is 1.5 times higher than that in rural areas. Similarly, the overall incidence of NEC for blacks is significantly greater than that for non-Hispanic whites, and this difference remains significant after controlling for birth weight.[6]

The incidence of NEC has remained relatively stable over the past two decades, with a slight recent decline.[2,7,8] Although improvements in neonatal care have reduced the incidence of NEC, the susceptible population is increasing, as more very premature infants survive.

The social and financial impact of NEC is immense. Data compiled from a single center in the United States from 1992 to 1994 found that total hospital charges for infants with surgically treated NEC averaged $186,200 in excess of those for controls, and $73,700 more for infants with medically managed NEC.[9] The additional hospital charges for NEC in this series were $6.5 million per year or $216,666 per survivor. These data provide a potent financial stimulus for research to curb the incidence and impact of this disease.

CLINICAL PRESENTATION

NEC is a manifestation of multiple pathologic events, and the diagnosis depends on the overall clinical picture, as opposed to an individual finding or abnormal test. This clinical picture is best described by outlining the combination of physiologic signs, physical findings, and radiographic abnormalities.

Physiologic Signs

Physiologic abnormalities begin with mild temperature instability, apnea, bradycardia, and lethargy. Disease progression is marked by the development of acidosis and thrombocytopenia, followed by neutropenia, disseminated intravascular coagulation (DIC), sepsis syndrome, and cardiovascular collapse.

Neonates manifesting NEC within the first 7 days of life, which are typically of a greater gestational age, have been shown to have a higher incidence of thrombocytopenia, leucopenia, and apnea.[10]

Physical Signs

Ileus is recognized by feeding intolerance, increased residual gastric volume, mild abdominal distention, and possibly bilious emesis and is the earliest physical sign of NEC. GI mucosal deterioration leads to occult blood in the stools that may progress to obvious bleeding per rectum. Abdominal distention and tenderness progress from localized to generalized peritonitis. Advanced physical signs include discoloration of the anterior abdominal wall, with ecchymotic changes of the skin and occasionally a palpable abdominal mass in the right lower quadrant (Fig. 33-1).

Because the early physiologic signs of NEC are nonspecific and common in the neonatal intensive care unit (NICU), the physical findings of NEC are usually necessary to draw attention to the diagnosis. The most common findings that initiate clinical concern are abdominal distention and blood in the stool.[3]

It has been suggested that in the presence of ascites, fluid samples should be obtained. Exudative fluid and a positive Gram stain imply gangrenous bowel and may warrant surgical intervention.[11,12]

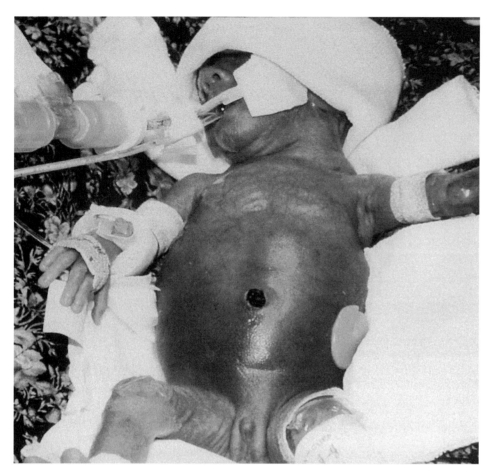

FIGURE 33-1. An infant with necrotizing enterocolitis is shown. Notice the abdominal wall ecchymosis extending from the suprapubic region to above the umbilicus and laterally to the flanks.

Radiographic Signs

Early in the disease process, plain radiographs of the abdomen may be normal or demonstrate mild ileus with intestinal dilation. As the disease progresses, intestinal dilation worsens, and pneumatosis intestinalis develops (Fig. 33-2). It is important to note that pneumatosis intestinalis does not necessarily equate with necrosis of the gut.[13]

Further progression results in the appearance of portal venous air (Fig. 33-3), ascites and finally pneumoperitoneum (Fig. 33-4), indicating intestinal perforation. Pneumatosis and portal venous air are pathognomonic of NEC, but their absence does not exclude the diagnosis. The specificity of both pneumatosis and portal venous air for the presence of NEC are approximately 100%, but the sensitivity is only about 44% for pneumatosis and 19% for portal venous air.[14]

In premature infants with ambiguous signs and clinical findings, a contrast enema may help exclude the diagnosis of NEC,[15] but the risk is that the infant with NEC may be made worse by the study.

Staging

The classification system used by most authors when reporting clinical data is presented in Table 33-1. This classification is a tool that provides consistency in terminology with regard to the severity and progression of NEC in infants.

Pathology

The most common pathologic changes identified in resected intestinal specimens affected with NEC are coagulation or ischemic necrosis of the gut.[16–18] In about 50% of cases, necrosis involves both large and small intestine.[19] Perforation usually occurs on the antimesenteric border at the junction between normal and devitalized bowel but may occur within the necrotic segments.[18,19] Regions of viable bowel are often interspersed with the nonviable bowel, and intramural hemorrhage may be confused with necrosis.[19,20]

PATHOGENESIS

NEC has no single predisposing risk factor, pathogen, or pathologic process defined as causative. As clinically described, NEC is the visible end point of tissue injury. Several factors may initiate the disease process, whereas the response of the host will define the course and outcome. The factors thought to promote the initiation of NEC do not address the pathways of tissue injury after the process has been set into motion. The factors of disease initiation and the mechanism of disease progression will be considered separately.

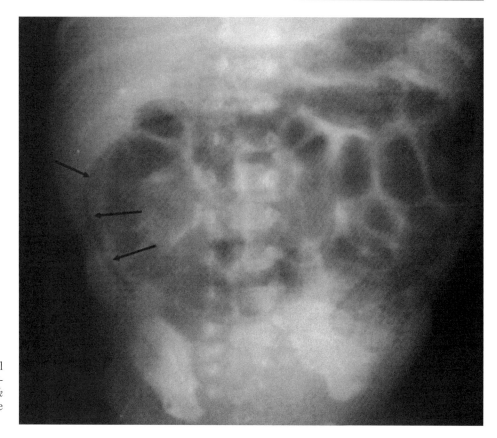

FIGURE 33-2. An abdominal plain radiograph is shown depicting pneumatosis intestinalis (*black arrows*) in the wall of the intestine in the right lower quadrant.

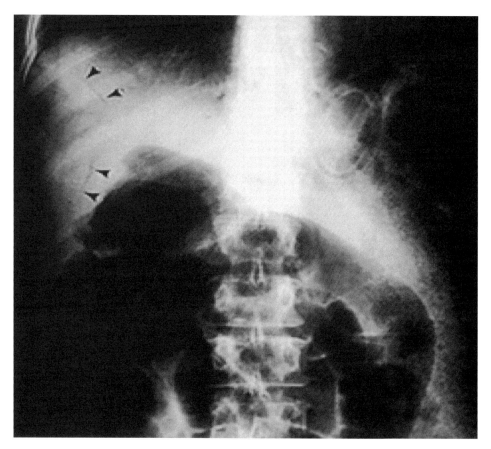

FIGURE 33-3. Portal venous gas is seen (*black arrowheads*) in this plain abdominal radiograph of an infant with necrotizing enterocolitis.

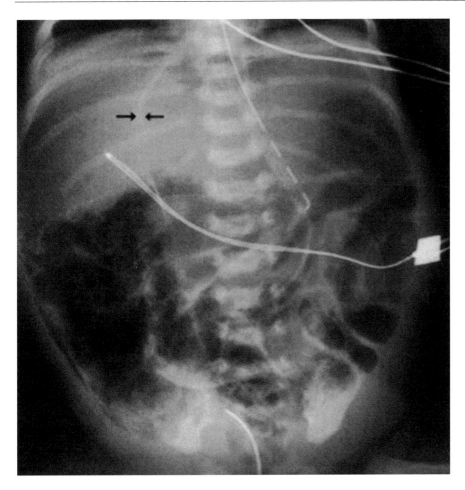

FIGURE 33-4. An abdominal radiograph of an infant with necrotizing enterocolitis and massive pneumoperitoneum. The falciform ligament is clearly identified (between the *black arrows*) as a result of the pneumoperitoneum.

Initiation of Disease

Although background clinical variables of infants stricken with NEC are somewhat inhomogeneous, the suspected factors contributing to the initiation of NEC include enteral feeding, intestinal ischemia, and enteric microorganisms (Fig. 33-5). Studies in the rat model have shown that exposing animals to asphyxia, formula feeding, and bacteria results in very high NEC rates with correspondingly high mortality.[21] Interestingly, in this model, asphyxia was clearly the most significant instigating factor. Formula feeding was much less important, and bacterial colonization was not a significant determinant. However, the relative impact of each of these variables has not been clinically defined for NEC in humans.

TABLE 33-1			
MODIFIED BELL'S CLASSIFICATION OF NEC			
	Stage 1	Stage 2	Stage 3
Physiologic signs	Temperature instability, apnea, bradycardia, lethargy ⟶	Metabolic acidosis, thrombocytopenia ⟶	Neutropenia, DIC, sepsis syndrome, cardiovascular collapse
Physical signs	Feeding intolerance, increased residuals, mild abdominal distension, and bilious emesis ⟶	Bloody stools, moderate abdominal tenderness/distention, mild discoloration, palpable mass ⟶	Diffuse pertonitis, severe abdominal tenderness, distention and discoloration, palpable right lower quadrant mass
Radiographic signs	Mild ileus ⟶	Moderate to severe ileus, fixed loops of bowel, pneumatosis intestinalis ⟶	Pneumoperitoneum, portal venous gas

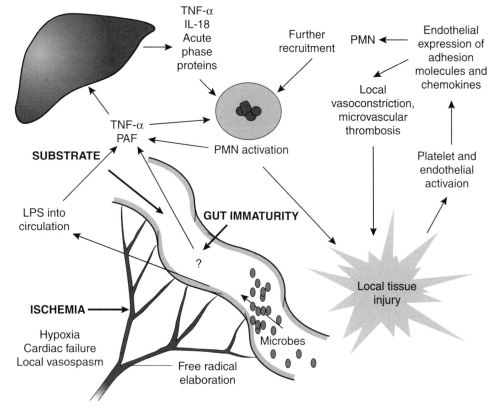

FIGURE 33-5. Enteral feeds (substrate) introduced to an immunologically and physiologically immature gut produce a maladaptive interaction in some neonates for reasons that have yet to be defined. Ischemia likely promotes, exacerbates, and may even produce the events leading to gut injury. Microbes can opportunistically facilitate a worsening condition under such circumstances. Inflammatory mediators released from the gut activate polymorphonuclear neutrophils (PMNs) and stimulate hepatic elaboration of stress factors and more inflammatory mediators. PMNs initiate tissue injury and facilitate systemic response, as outlined in Figure 33–6.

Ischemia

Ischemia has long been implicated as a causative factor in the development of NEC. Whereas local intestinal ischemia is almost certainly responsible for the necrotic lesions occurring in NEC, the precise role of ischemia within the cascade of events culminating in NEC remains unclear. Further, the mechanisms accounting for local ischemia remain to be elucidated. Angiotensin-mediated pathways have been proposed as a theoretical participant in local vasoconstriction, and it has been shown that intestinal vasculature is rich in angiotensin receptors.[22,23] In experimental models of shock, ischemic colitis secondary to mesenteric vasoconstriction is not ameliorated by adrenergic blockade, but it is by inhibition of angiotensin-converting enzyme (ACE).[24]

Microorganisms

Support exists for enteric pathogens as contributing factors to the NEC syndrome. First, the disease develops after oral feeding and bacterial colonization has begun. Second, in animal models, the entire NEC syndrome cannot be replicated in the presence of a sterile GI tract.[25] Bacterial endotoxin, lipopolysaccharide (LPS), has been shown in experimental models to act through, and/or with, the release of inflammatory mediators to cause intestinal necrosis and a clinical syndrome similar to NEC.[26,27] Enteric pathogens are not exclusively causative, considering that a wide range of organisms,

including gram-positive, gram-negative and anaerobic bacteria, and even viruses, have been cultured from both stool and blood of NEC patients.[28–32] Further, microorganisms recovered from NEC patients have been found to mirror those of the typical fecal flora within the neonatal ICU.[33] Analysis of these trends has revealed no significant correlation between the disease and either the age of the infant or the intestinal site of disease.[31] Similarly, analysis of duodenal microflora has demonstrated no association between strain pattern and NEC.[34] It is more plausible that pathogens in the abnormal intestinal environment of NEC infants become opportunistic participants in the disease process, taking advantage of the physiologically attenuated host.

Enteral Feeding

Enteral feeding has been considered an etiology of NEC from the beginning of its recognition as a clinical entity, with more than 90% of cases occurring after the initiation of feeds.[35–38] Depending on the type and volume of enteral nutrition, changes occur within the gut, including: the initial introduction of organisms, alterations of the spectrum of flora, type and amount of byproducts of microbial life, and oxygen demand.[39,40] Of course, these changes occur in the intestine of all neonates after feeding, and therefore they do not explain the development of NEC, which occurs in relatively few. The understanding of the complex interplay between luminal stimuli and host response is currently being elucidated.[41–43]

Understanding the defects in the elaborate immunologic armamentarium of the intestine may lead to understanding the causations of NEC.

Progression of Disease

Once the chain of clinical and biologic events has initiated NEC, defense mechanisms begin to proliferate through molecular communication and culminate in the destruction of tissue through the inflammatory pathways and tissue responses to ischemia and reperfusion.

Mediators of Tissue Injury

On initiation of the pathologic process of NEC, cellular communication through inflammatory mediator molecules results in a multitude of events, culminating in the end-organ damage seen in NEC patients. Understanding these steps may clarify and help to ameliorate the effects of the disease. As knowledge of the molecular basis of systemic stress response continues to evolve, two inflammatory mediators have received considerable attention: tumor necrosis factor α (TNF-α) and platelet-activating factor (PAF), which have been shown in multiple animal studies to result in ischemic bowel necrosis similar to NEC.[22,44–46,48]

Tumor Necrosis Factor-α

TNF-α is a mediator of ischemia-induced injury, and NEC infants have been shown to have elevated circulating levels of TNF-α.[49] Specifically, TNF-α acts through neutrophils to produce local organ damage during ischemia.[50] In addition, the release of TNF-α after injury plays a role in distant organ dysfunction.[51,52] Further, undefined mechanisms of tissue toxicity by TNF-α are not coupled with neutrophil activity.[53] Neutralization of TNF-α has been shown to decrease hepatocellular damage after ischemia.[53] TNF-α neutralization may serve as "molecule-targeted" therapy for NEC.

Platelet Activating Factor

The role of PAF has been more clearly defined than most of the pathways involved in NEC. PAF induces TNF-α expression and activates diverse inflammatory gene transcription through the nuclear factor κB (NF-κB). NF-κB is a potent cornerstone in the pathogenesis of inflammation. Activation of this ubiquitous transcription factor results in gene expression of cytokines, chemokines, growth factors, immunoreceptors, and cell adhesion molecules, which have been demonstrated to participate in tissue injury in ischemia models.[35–38,53,54,56] In animal NEC models, intestinal NF-κB activation has been shown to result in increased mucosal permeability, promoting endotoxemia, culminating in intestinal necrosis.[22]

The evidence for PAF and TNF-α participation offers little insight into precipitating events that lead to the proliferation of these inflammatory molecules or why they occur in premature infants to produce the syndrome of NEC. However, PAF levels in both serum and stool have been shown to increase after enteral feedings.[57,58] Specific to the timing of NEC susceptibility, PAF-degrading enzyme acetylhydrolase (PAF-AH) demonstrates low activity in newborns, reaching normal adult values at about age 6 weeks.[59] In animal models, PAF-AH can prevent bowel necrosis induced by PAF,[60] providing a scientific basis for the clinical observation that breast milk (which possesses PAF-AH activity) decreases the risk of NEC when compared with formula (which lacks PAF-AH activity).[61] PAF, similar to TNF-α or other inflammatory mediators, is certainly not the cause of NEC. However, it plays a large enough role in the mechanisms leading to tissue injury that therapy targeting this molecule may curtail the clinical consequences of the disease.

Nitric Oxide

Although their precise role deserves further clarification, nitric oxide (NO) pathways are likely important mediators in the development of intestinal damage and systemic manifestations of NEC. Evidence suggests that NO produced by enterocytes in the intestinal wall of infants with NEC precipitates apoptosis of enterocytes in apical villi via peroxynitrite formation.[62] Within the liver, nitric oxide appears to mediate hepatic injury during severe systemic illness (shock and sepsis),[63–65] and hepatic NO synthesis has been shown to be increased during NEC.[66,67]

Liver-Gut Axis

The liver appears to play an integral role in the final clinical picture of NEC. The liver is the initial filter for all substances originating from the intestine (via the portal vein), including by-products of ischemia, debris from necrosis, and inflammatory mediators. Intestinal ischemia, or at least circulatory disturbance, is thought to be an important contributing factor to the development of NEC,[68–72] and inflammatory-mediated hepatic dysfunction after ischemia-reperfusion injury to the gut, as in NEC, has been well documented.[63,73–75]

Kupffer cells are reticuloendothelial macrophages located exclusively in the liver. They represent 80% to 90% of the body's resident macrophages, with an enormous potential for releasing inflammatory mediators.[76] Emerging evidence suggests that within the liver-gut interactions, Kupffer cells and their elaboration of communication molecules in the inflammatory pathways are important in the development of NEC. In a rat model of NEC, Kupffer cell activation with subsequent upregulation of interleukin (IL)-18 and TNF-α has been demonstrated to correlate with the degree of ileal injury.[66] Interestingly, the same study found no significant difference between NEC animals and controls in the levels of IL-1α, IL-1β, IL-6, and IL-12, all of which are proinflammatory cytokines. Of these, IL-1 and IL-6 are thought to be significant contributing molecules in the pathways of systemic inflammatory response syndrome (SIRS).[21,77,78] Although sepsis appears to be a contributing factor for the development of NEC, this evidence provides a molecular basis for uncoupling these two processes, as they appear to be the result of at least partially independent inflammatory profiles.

Effectors of Tissue Injury

Inflammatory mediators do not cause the majority of tissue injury directly, but rather stimulate terminal events that engender injury. The product of inflammatory injury is ultimately the effect of interweaving mechanisms including changes in microcirculation, free radical formation, and stimulation of immune-mediated injury (see Fig. 33-5).

Among circulating leukocytes, polymorphonuclear neutrophils (PMNs) possess an enormous capacity for cytodestruction through free radical release and are a central cellular component of ischemia-reperfusion injury.[79,80] Activated PMNs also elaborate proteolytic enzymes causing direct tissue injury and inflammatory mediators that cause microvascular alteration, increased vascular permeability, complement and leukocyte activation, and leukocyte migration, all leading to subsequent tissue injury (Fig. 33-6).[81–83] Data from neutrophil inactivation studies have implicated PMNs as the dominant cells in the late phase of injury in ischemia models.[84] PAF and TNF-α initiate PMN proliferation and vascular changes leading to local PMN accumulation.[85–88] The orchestration of deleterious events that follow PMN activation is schematically outlined in Figure 33-6.

Local vasoconstriction, microvascular thrombus, hemodynamic instability, and other undefined mechanisms contribute to local ischemia leading to free radical production. In the absence of oxygen, accumulating products of adenosine triphosphate (ATP) breakdown provide a substrate for a "respiratory burst" of oxygen free radical release on the reintroduction of oxygen, leading to lipid peroxidation and cellular destruction.[89] These reactive oxygen species, including those involved in PAF-mediated pathways, are known to be important in the terminal events during NEC development.[90,91]

CLINICAL RISK FACTORS

Preterm Infants

The risk of a newborn's having NEC is most significantly related to the degree of prematurity, and its incidence is inversely related to gestational age.[2,7,8,92–96,97,98] The age-specific attack rate of NEC declines sharply after 35 weeks of gestational age.[9] Similarly, the incidence and severity of NEC are higher in neonates with smaller birth weight,[7,97–99] with very low birth weight infants in whom NEC develops being more likely to require operative intervention.[99–101]

Congenital heart disease is associated with NEC development in infants, regardless of gestational age. Within the population of infants with congenital heart disease, specific variables found to be associated with the development of NEC include hypoplastic left heart syndrome, truncus arteriosus, and episodes of poor systemic perfusion during shock.[102]

Umbilical artery catheterization has previously been implicated as an etiologic agent of NEC.[103] The suggestion that umbilical artery catheters cause a decrease in mesenteric blood flow led to the recommendation that cautious consideration should be given to their use in hemodynamically unstable neonates or in those with GI disease.[104] However, data from a prospective, randomized trial demonstrate that premature infants in stable

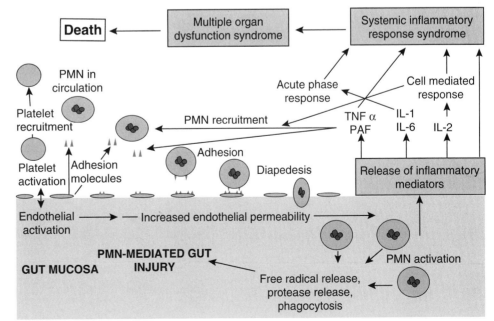

FIGURE 33-6. Activated endothelial cells in turn activate platelets and a signal for polymorphonuclear netrophils (PMNs) by the release of adhesion molecules and chemokines. PMNs localized to the activated areas of endothelium migrate through the endothelium because of increased endothelial permeability (diapedesis). Once out of circulation, the PMNs can cause local tissue injury through several mechanisms and stimulate the systemic response.

condition who receive enteral feedings with an umbilical artery catheter in place have no increase in feeding complications compared with those who receive enteral feedings 24 hours after catheter removal.[105] In addition, the position of the catheter tip and the location of the perfusion hole have not been shown to make a difference in the rate of NEC; however, high position and end-hole catheters are recommended to decrease the rate of other catheter-related complications.[106–108]

Polycythemia requiring exchange transfusion has been implicated as a risk factor for the development of NEC.[109] However, subsequent analysis of exchange-transfusion patients does not support the procedure as an independent risk factor.[110] Data from small clinical series and animal models suggest that hemolytic disease, particularly polycythemia, is a risk factor for developing NEC, independent of exchange transfusion.[111,112] Oxygen delivery may suffer because of increased viscosity associated with polycythemia. An inverse linear correlation has been identified between blood pH at birth and hematocrit measured 2 hours after delivery in preterm patients with polycythemia.[113] Although polycythemia as a risk factor is theoretically sound with decreased oxygen delivery, impaired microvascular rheology, and possible promotion of microvascular thrombosis, the additional risk from this diagnosis appears to be small.[114] Further, polycythemia may be a parallel, rather than preceding, event, as it shares predisposing risk factors with NEC such as perinatal asphyxia and intrauterine hypoxia.[115]

Several drugs have been implicated in the development of NEC. Exposure to maternal cocaine use by preterm neonates smaller than 1500 g results in earlier presentation and more severe disease than that in a nonexposed equivalent cohort. The significance of this single variable and its impact on overall incidence remain unknown.[116] Enteral theophylline, especially in very low birthweight infants, has been suggested as a predisposing factor to GI disturbances and NEC.[117,118] However, evaluation of all patients treated with theophylline, either oral or intravenous, compared with those without theophylline exposure, has failed to validate this.[119] Antenatally, theophylline administered to high-risk mothers does appear subsequently to increase the risk of NEC in premature infants.[120]

Finally, general physiologic compromise, including lower 1- and 5-minute Apgar scores, prolonged hypotension, persistent respiratory distress, and septicemia, has been shown to increase significantly the incidence of NEC.[8,121–124] Additionally, hypothermia appears to increase significantly the risk of NEC in a dependent fashion, relative to the degree of prematurity.[125]

Term Infants

In preterm infants, maturity of the gut mucosa is clearly a dominant variable in the development of NEC. However, the development of NEC in term infants requires an alternative explanation. The etiology of NEC in term infants should be viewed as a different disease process from that occurring in the premature neonates.[4,10,126–128] As an example, NEC presentation in term infants occurs earlier as gestational age increases.[4,10,16,99,126,129–132]

Other risk factors implicated in the development of NEC in the term population include prolonged rupture of membranes, chorioamnionitis, Apgar score less than 7 at 1 and 5 minutes, respiratory difficulties, congenital heart disease, hypoglycemia, exchange transfusions, and infection.[3,129,133,134] Evidence suggests that in term infants, maternal status has a less important role in NEC susceptibility. Specifically, maternal variables shown to have no impact on the incidence of NEC in term infants include pre-eclampsia, maternal diabetes, drug abuse (including cocaine), fever during labor, magnesium sulfate treatment, or meconium-stained amniotic fluid.[129]

Indicators of Disease and Prognosis

Monitoring plasma levels of PAF may have clinical utility in the NEC-susceptible population. Investigation of neonates at risk for NEC demonstrated that PAF levels increased as the severity of NEC increased, and subsequently decreased with NEC resolution.[135] In this study, a PAF level of 10.2 ng/mL, used to define NEC, had a positive predictive value of 100%.

Several other molecules may have a role in predicting severity of NEC. Concentrations of both IL-8 and IL-10 are significantly higher during the first 24 hours of illness in infants with stage III NEC compared with those in infants with less severe disease (stages I and II). Similarly, IL-1–receptor antagonist, a counterinflammatory cytokine, was found to be significantly more elevated at diagnosis in patients who subsequently progressed to more severe disease. A concentration of more than 130,000 pg/mL has been shown to have sensitivity and specificity for predicting stage III NEC of 100% and 92%, respectively. Serum concentrations of IL-10 follow a similar pattern, with a level of more than 250 pg/mL having a sensitivity of 100% and specificity of 90% in identifying stage III NEC.[136]

Thrombocytopenia defined as a platelet count less than 100×10^4/mL, or a precipitate decline in the platelet count, has been associated with poor prognosis. However, platelet counts alone have not been demonstrated to predict accurately the extent of the disease or survival rate.[137]

Glutamine and arginine, amino acids essential to intestinal integrity, have been demonstrated to be significantly lower in infants with NEC 7 days before its onset.[138] These amino acids may serve as a potential means of detecting neonates at higher risk, and hence their replacement could possibly represent an avenue of prevention. Similarly, plasma arginine concentration is known to be decreased at the time of NEC diagnosis in premature infants.[139] In a randomized, double-blinded, placebo-controlled study to evaluate the role of oral supplementation with L-arginine, it was shown that oral supplementation reduced the incidence of all stages of NEC.[140]

The activation of the Thomsen-Friedenreich cryptantigen (TCA) portends a risk of hemolysis after transfusion of blood products: 22% of the NEC patients investigated at a single center demonstrated the presence of TCA, suggesting an association between TCA and advanced NEC. Screening of neonates with advanced NEC for TCA may be prudent to identify those at risk of hematologic complications requiring low-titer anti-T fresh frozen plasma and washed platelets.[141]

Technologic advances, including GI tonometry or duplex ultrasonography (US), may improve our ability to detect and deter NEC. GI tonometry provides the ability to measure intramucosal pH continuously and has been used to monitor for intestinal ischemia. It may hold promise for early detection of NEC in susceptible patients.[142] Studies using duplex-pulsed Doppler US to determine blood-flow velocities in the celiac axis and superior mesenteric artery of neonates demonstrated that neonates at risk of developing NEC have abnormal gut blood-flow velocities.[143] Similarly, antenatal Doppler velocimetry of the umbilical artery and the fetal superior mesenteric artery in identified high-risk pregnancies may be used to predict the patient likely to have NEC and maybe an increased risk of mortality in the early neonatal period.[144-147]

Prevention

Breast milk has long been recognized for its protective effects in reducing the incidence of NEC.[61,148] Maternal milk contains a variety of immunomodulators that help explain this phenomenon, including PAF-AH, the degradative enzyme of PAF.[149,150] When maternal breast milk is not available, a meta-analysis found that feeding with donor human milk significantly reduced the relative risk of NEC.[151]

Standardized feeding regimens within the neonatal intensive care unit have been shown to improve early detection of feeding intolerance that reduced the incidence of advanced-stage disease[152] and the overall incidence of NEC. This declination is independent of birth weight, prenatal steroid exposure, breast milk, day of life of first feed, and the number of days to reach full feeds.[153] Whereas it appears that homogeneous feeding schedules in newborns improve institutional care of premature infants, the rate of feeding advancement has not been shown to alter the incidence of clinically significant NEC cases.[154]

Clinical data suggest that the incidence of NEC is significantly reduced after prenatal steroid treatment, and although postnatal steroid treatment does not decrease the incidence as effectively as prenatal therapy, it may improve clinical outcomes.[155] At present, further clinical evidence is needed to support the use of steroids in these patients.

One of the postulated mechanisms of steroid-induced NEC protection is the enhanced release of PAF-AH. Increasing serum levels of PAF-AH by medications, recombinant enzyme supplementation, or targeted cell-receptor stimulation may allow the progress of disease to be tempered.[156,157] Experimental models of PAF-receptor antagonists (WEB 2170 and WEB 2086) have been used to reduce the incidence and severity of NEC.[45,158]

Experimental animal models are presently available to allow the study of therapies to protect against the development of NEC. Dietary supplementation of anti-inflammatory omega-3 fatty acids has been shown to suppress intestinal inflammatory mediators, causing a subsequent reduction in hypoxia-induced bowel necrosis.[159] Polyunsaturated fatty acids, the metabolites of omega-3 and omega-6 fatty acids, also have been shown to be protective in a neonatal rat model of NEC.[161] In a murine model, dietary supplementation with L-arginine and L-carnitine significantly decreased lipid peroxidation, thereby ameliorating the histologic evidence of ischemia-reperfusion intestinal injury.[161] Experimental intestinal immunomodulation has shown some potential for attenuating the development of NEC.

Clearly a better understanding of the developmental aspects of GI function in health and disease will lead to further advances in prevention of NEC.[162]

TREATMENT

Initial/Medical Management

Once NEC is suspected, enteral feedings are withheld. If abdominal distention is present, a nasogastric tube should be placed on low continuous suction with intravenous replacement of measured losses. Precise fluid management is important to optimize intestinal perfusion. Parenteral nutrition should be initiated.

Aggressive monitoring with frequent clinical and radiographic assessment is recommended. Supine AP abdominal radiographs should be performed every 6 to 8 hours during the initial phase to establish disease progression evident by worsening pneumatosis (see Fig. 33-2), portal venous gas (see Fig. 33-3), or pneumoperitoneum (see Fig. 33-4). The necessity for surgical intervention is usually evident within 24 hours. If this level of illness is not reached, conservative management should be continued, during which enteral feedings are generally withheld for 10 to 14 days after radiographic evidence of disease has abated.

Broad-spectrum antibiotic coverage should be started in anticipation of bacterial translocation, leading to bacteremia and subsequent septicemia. Ampicillin, gentamicin, and clindamycin are a common regimen of antimicrobial treatment.[163] However, cultures of isolates from the peritoneal fluid of NEC patients have been shown to be resistant to this regimen,[164] underscoring the importance of obtaining cultures and following sensitivity profiles. It also is valuable to consider the institutional microbial resistance patterns in selecting an antibiotic regimen. Alternative antimicrobial regimens have not been extensively studied, but comparative investigation with traditional triple-antibiotic coverage with matched controls has shown that cefotaxime and vancomycin reduce the risk of culture-positive peritonitis and thrombocytopenia that lead to decreased mortality.[165] Given that continual evolution of microbial resistance is inevitable,[166,167] it may not be possible to delineate any optimal antimicrobial treatment in NEC patients.[163]

Of note, magnesium and copper deficiency have been implicated as a cause of compromised host defense and oxidative injury.[168] Therefore mineral measurement and replacement should be incorporated into NEC management.

Surgical Management

The presence of pneumoperitoneum is considered an absolute indication for surgical intervention. Relative indications include the presence of a fixed, dilated loop of bowel on serial radiographs, portal venous gas, a palpable abdominal mass, abdominal wall erythema, positive peritoneal fluid cultures, or progressive illness despite maximal medical measures (e.g., worsening thrombocytopenia, acidosis, or cardiovascular collapse).

The risk of operation is considerable. However, in an appropriate setting, operative intervention under general anesthesia is well tolerated, even in very low birth weight infants.[169] A multicenter review found that the incidence of complications after operations for NEC was high, but similar in very low birth weight (<1000 g) infants compared with infants heavier than 1000 g.[170] The risk of hypothermia in the neonatal population has led many surgeons to operate in the NICU directly under an infant radiant-warmer system to reduce the detrimental effects of transport to the operating room, which have been associated with deterioration of multiple physiologic parameters.[171] Regardless of operative setting, once the need for surgical intervention has been established the parents should be appropriately counseled that multiple operations are likely, and complications are to be expected.[172]

Focal Disease

At laparotomy, surgical decision making is based on the extent of disease encountered. In focal disease with isolated perforation, limited resection with proximal enterostomy is most common. Primary anastomosis has been advocated as an alternative.[173-177] Advocates of primary anastomosis make note of the high morbidity of enterostomy in neonates.[176] It has been reported that length of hospital stay, time to full feeds, and length of ventilator requirements are all shorter in patients treated with primary anastomosis.[177] Conversely, proponents of enterostomy have brought attention to the fact that most stomal complications are amenable to repair without major operations and that early stomal closure can be performed after NEC abates, even in infants weighing less than 2000 g.[163,178,179] The experience of a single center that selected primary anastomosis for focal perforation as the procedure of choice found higher mortality rates that led to the abandonment of this procedure in favor of proximal enterostomy.[180] The results of this series emphasize that primary anastomosis is probably not applicable to most focal NEC perforations. The consequences of anastomotic dehiscence after a primary anastomosis are a far greater hazard to the neonate than are stomal complications.

Diffuse Disease

Understandably, extent of involvement at laparotomy directly correlates with mortality.[181,182] Extensive intestinal involvement with NEC not only increases mortality but also places survivors at higher risk of long-term sequellae such as more frequent bowel movements, fecal incontinence, short bowel syndrome, dependence on parenteral nutrition, and progressive liver failure.[160,183-186] Therefore it is a surgical priority to minimize the amount of bowel resection when extensive involvement is encountered at laparotomy, and most surgical techniques for panintestinal NEC involvement are founded on this goal.

Peritoneal Drainage

Over the past two decades, peritoneal drainage to facilitate stabilization and delay or avert the need for laparotomy has become recognized as sometimes the preferable technique in the management of severe NEC.[187-196] Peritoneal drainage is performed at the bedside with local anesthesia via percutaneous placement of one or two drains into the peritoneal cavity, usually in the right lower quadrant (Fig. 33-7) Peritoneal drainage has been shown to provide immediate clinical improvement and, in some cases, afford definitive treatment.[190,195,196] However, most patients treated with drainage will still require laparotomy, leading some authors to consider drainage a measure of resuscitation for the critically ill.[193,197,198] Comparative studies have shown mortality rates for initial laparotomy versus percutaneous drainage to be comparable.[199] Meta-analysis of the available data has failed to demonstrate that one approach is superior.[200] On the basis of these data, critics of peritoneal drainage argue that assessing the extent of disease and removing necrotic bowel at initial laparotomy can hasten recovery and subsequent discharge, while simultaneously allowing informed surgical decision making and parental counseling.[199] Multiple logistic regression analysis of comorbid variables in a comparative study between initial operation versus drainage identified that the total number of comorbidities predicts outcome. independent of the initial treatment modality.[201] Therefore individualized care with evaluation of all patient factors that affect survival is likely more valuable than applying a single treatment strategy for all patients. Primary peritoneal drainage can be considered a useful adjunct in resuscitating critically ill NEC infants, particularly very small premature infants, but may not serve as an alternative to laparotomy, which is usually necessary after clinical stabilization.[163,188,193,198]

Operative Strategy

Although several procedures have been described to negotiate the tenuous circumstance of extensive intestinal necrosis, all modern techniques adhere to the principle of maximal bowel preservation. Therefore aggressive resection to clearly viable bowel is not advocated as primary therapy. Similarly, multiple stoma formation compromises final enteric length secondary to trimming at the time of takedown and is not advocated.

Minimal resection of only obvious nonviable intestine with proximal stoma formation and a second look within 36 hours can facilitate survival of critically ill NEC patients while maintaining as much intestinal length as

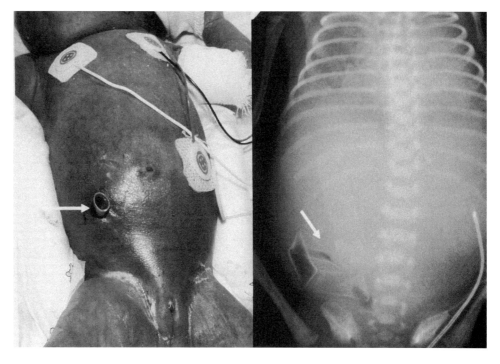

FIGURE 33-7. A micropremature infant with necrotizing enterocolitis and perforation is shown with her corresponding abdominal radiograph. A percutaneous drain (*white arrows*) has been placed in the right lower quadrant for drainage of the intestinal perforation. Note that the drain is placed at a position below the level of the umbilicus to avoid injury to the lower edge of the right lobe of the liver.

possible.[202] Similarly, some authors propose no resection at the time of exploration if extensive disease is encountered, but rather simply perform proximal enterostomy.[163,203,204] This technique commits the patient to re-exploration, but does allow more accurate demarcation of viable bowel to maximize bowel length by preventing the resection of reversible regions.

Another approach to avoid the loss of intestinal length associated with stomal closure has been termed the "clip and drop-back" technique. This technique involves resection of only obvious nonviable segments, with the placement of occlusive surgical clips on the ends of remaining bowel. The abdomen is closed, leaving behind blind-ended segments of intestine. Re-exploration with delayed anastomosis is performed in 48 to 72 hours. This approach has been used with success in severely ill infants with extensive necrosis, bowel perforation, and peritonitis; however, its use has not been widely applied.[205] An alternative procedure has been described in which a feeding tube is placed through the lumen of the viable intestinal segments without anastomosis of the intestinal segments.[206] In one case, a diverting jejunostomy and a mucous fistula were made, with the tube used to orient the defunctionalized intervening intestinal segments. In another patient, the remaining intestine was left in continuity, with the feeding tube brought into the jejunum proximal to the first area of resection and out distally through the tip of the appendix. In both cases, a subsequent contrast study showed autoanastomosis of the intestinal segments.

After an infant has survived the initial intervention, it is not uncommon for intestinal obstructive symptoms to develop. Stricture formation is a common postintervention complication and likely develops secondary to ischemic injury to the intestine. The most common location for stricture formation after NEC is colonic, followed by distal ileal and jejunal. Laparotomy with resection and primary anastomosis is usually required in this setting; however, occasionally, stricturoplasty may be used.

Because of the complexity of the surgical dilemma created by multisegmental or extensive disease, it is not useful to propose a definitive algorithm for surgical treatment in this setting. No well-documented prospective comparative trials exist to separate the relative benefits of the aforementioned surgical techniques. It is therefore prudent for the practicing pediatric surgeon to be cognizant of the presently described procedures to broaden the armamentarium of treatment for this condition, depending on the operative findings and clinical scenario.

Survivor Outcomes

If a neonate survives the initial disease, the chance of long-term survival after NEC is approximately 90%.[207] Unfortunately, most NEC infants invest much of their biologic resources combating the severe physiologic stress during a vital period of growth and development. Therefore children surviving NEC should not be expected to demonstrate normal development after infancy. In particular, neurosensory development outcome is adversely affected by NEC.[207–209] Very low birth weight infants with NEC have been shown to have a significantly higher rate of severe psychomotor retardation when compared with equal-weight premature infants without NEC.[207,208] The risk of neurodevelopmental delay appears to increase with severity of NEC.[210] Those requiring surgical treatment display a higher rate of impairment compared with those managed nonoperatively.[207,209] The most recent data from prospective studies estimate the rate of severe psychomotor retardation in very low birth weight infants with NEC as high as 55% at age 20 months.[208,209] Among extremely low birth weight infants (<800 g) with or without NEC, a higher incidence of neurosensory impairment among affected boys compared with girls has been identified, although no plausible reason for this difference has been forwarded.[211-213]

Although premature children trail the growth curves of term infants, recent data suggest that premature infants with NEC may not display somatic growth retardation compared with matched-control premature infants without NEC.[208] These data should not distract from the point that long-term growth is substantially disturbed in most NEC patients. Approximately 50% of this cohort will follow a course of physical maturity below the 5th percentile in both height and weight on standard growth tables, and of the remainder, most will be under the 25th percentile.[184,214,215]

The documented attenuation in objective neurosensory development in the NEC cohort is detected by fine neurologic testing at a young age (2 years).[207-209] However, a recent survey of gross subjective function in older survivors of NEC revealed more encouraging results.[185] At a mean follow-up age of 7.5 years, 83% were enrolled in school full-time. All children ate by mouth, and nearly all were toilet trained. Expectedly, all were less than the 50th percentile for height and weight. Although the follow-up in this series incorporated only 61% of their total NEC survivors during the investigation time frame, the majority of respondents had survived stage 3 disease.

REFERENCES

1. Pokorny WJ, Garcia-Prats JA, Barry YN: Necrotizing enterocolitis: Incidence, operative care, and outcome. J Pediatr Surg 21:1149–1154, 1986.
2. Lemons JA, Bauer CR, Oh W, et al: Very low birth weight outcomes of the National Institute of Child Health and Human Development Neonatal Research Network, January 1995 through December 1996: NICHD Neonatal Research Network. Pediatrics 107:E1, 2001.
3. Kliegman RM, Fanaroff AA: Neonatal necrotizing enterocolitis: A nine-year experience. Am J Dis Child 135:603–607,1981.
4. Wiswell TE, Robertson CF, Jones T, et al: Necrotizing enterocolitis in full-term infants: A case control study. Am J Dis Child 142:532–535, 1988.
5. Bolisetty S, Lui K, Oei J, Wojtulewicz J: A regional study of underlying congenital diseases in term neonates with necrotizing enterocolitis. Acta Paediatr 89:1226–1230, 2000.
6. Llanos AR, Moss ME, Pinzon MC, et al: Epidemiology of neonatal necrotising enterocolitis: A population-based study. Paediatr Perinat Epidemiol 16:342–349, 2002.
7. Uauy RD, Fanaroff AA, Korones SB, et al: Necrotizing enterocolitis in very low birth weight infants: Biodemographic and clinical correlates: National Institute of Child Health and Human Development Neonatal Research Network. J Pediatr 119:630–638, 1991.
8. Ryder RW, Shelton JD, Guinan ME: Necrotizing enterocolitis: A prospective multicenter investigation. Am J Epidemiol 112:113–123, 1980.
9. Bisquera JA, Cooper TR, Berseth CL: Impact of necrotizing enterocolitis on length of stay and hospital charges in very low birth weight infants. Pediatrics 109:423–428, 2002.
10. Yaseen H, Khawaja, Okasha I, et al: Necrotizing enterocolitis in term and near term neonates: Presentation and outcome. Neonatal Intens Care 9:17–23, 1996.
11. Kosloske AM, Goldthorn J: Paracentesis as an aid to the diagnosis of intestinal gangrene. Arch Surg 117:571–573, 1982.
12. Kosloske AM, Lilly JR: Paracentesis and lavage for diagnosis of intestinal gangrene in neonatal necrotizing enterocolitis. J Pediatr Surg 13:315–320, 1978.
13. St Peter SD, Abbas MA, Kelly KA: The spectrum of pneumatosis intestinalis. Arch Surg 138:68–75, 2003.
14. Tam AL, Camberos A, Applebaum H: Surgical decision making in necrotizing enterocolitis and focal intestinal perforation: Predictive value of radiologic findings. J Pediatr Surg 37:1688–1691, 2002.
15. Uken P, Smith W, Franken EA, et al: Use of the barium enema in the diagnosis of necrotizing enterocolitis. Pediatr Radiol 18:24–27, 1988.
16. Polin RA, Pollack PF, Barlow B, et al: Necrotizing enterocolitis in term infants. J Pediatr 89:460–462, 1976.
17. DeSa DJ. The spectrum of ischemic bowel disease in the newborn. Perspect Pediatr Pathol 3:273–309, 1976.
18. Ballance WA, Dahms BB, Shenker N, et al: Pathology of neonatal necrotizing enterocolitis: A ten-year experience. J Pediatr 117:S6–S13, 1980.
19. Amoury RA: Necrotizing enterocolitis: A continuing problem in the neonate. World J Surg 17:363–373, 1993.
20. Kliegman RM, Hack M, Jones P, et al: Epidemiologic study of necrotizing enterocolitis among low-birth-weight infants: Absence of identifiable risk factors. J Pediatr 100:440–444, 1982.
21. Chen J, Zhou YP, Rong XZ: An experimental study on systemic inflammatory response syndrome induced by subeschar tissue fluid. Burns 26:149–155, 2000.
22. Hsueh W, Caplan MS, Qu XW, et al: Neonatal necrotizing enterocolitis: Clinical considerations and pathogenetic concepts. Pediatr Dev Pathol 6:6–23, 1993.
23. Sechi LA, Valentin JP, Griffin CA, et al: Autoradiographic characterization of angiotensin II receptor subtypes in rat intestine. Am J Physiol 265:G21–G27, 1993.
24. Bailey RW, Bulkley GB, Hamilton SR, et al: Protection of the small intestine from nonocclusive mesenteric ischemic injury due to cardiogenic shock. Am J Surg 153:108–116, 1987.
25. Musemeche CA, Kosloske AM, Bartow SA, et al: Comparative effects of ischemia, bacteria, and substrate on the pathogenesis of intestinal necrosis. J Pediatr Surg 21:536–538, 1986.
26. Hsueh W, Gonzalez-Crussi F, Arroyave JL: Platelet-activating factor: An endogenous mediator for bowel necrosis in endotoxemia. FASEB J 1:403–405, 1987.
27. Gonzalez-Crussi F, Hsueh W: Experimental model of ischemic bowel necrosis: The role of platelet-activating factor and endotoxin. Am J Pathol 112:127–135, 1983.
28. Kliegman RM, Fanaroff AA, Izant R, et al: *Clostridia* as pathogens in neonatal necrotizing enterocolitis. J Pediatr 95:287–289, 1979.
29. Mollitt DL, Tepas JJ III, Talbert JL: The microbiology of neonatal peritonitis. Arch Surg 123:176–179, 1988.
30. Rotbart HA, Nelson WL, Glode MP, et al. Neonatal rotavirus-associated necrotizing enterocolitis: Case control study and prospective surveillance during an outbreak. J Pediatr 112:87–93, 1988.
31. Mollitt DL, String DL, Tepas JJ III, et al: Does patient age or intestinal pathology influence the bacteria found in cases of necrotizing enterocolitis? South Med J 84:879–882, 1991.
32. Alfa MJ, Robson D, Davi M, et al: An outbreak of necrotizing enterocolitis associated with a novel *Clostridium* species in a neonatal intensive care unit. Clin Infect Dis 1;35(suppl 1):S101–S105, 2002.
33. Peter CS, Feuerhahn M, Bohnhorst B, et al. Necrotising enterocolitis: Is there a relationship to specific pathogens? Eur J Pediatr 158:67–70, 1999.
34. Hoy CM, Wood CM, Hawkey PM, et al: Duodenal microflora in very-low-birth-weight neonates and relation to necrotizing enterocolitis. J Clin Microbiol 38:4539–4547, 2000.
35. Read MA, Whitley MZ, Gupta S, et al. Tumor necrosis factor alpha-induced E-selectin expression is activated by the nuclear factor-kappaB and c-JUN N-terminal kinase/p38 mitogen-activated protein kinase pathways. J Biol Chem 272:2753–2761, 1997.
36. Collins T, Read MA, Neish AS, et al: Transcriptional regulation of endothelial cell adhesion molecules: NF-kappa B and cytokine-inducible enhancers. FASEB J 9:899–909, 1995.
37. Read MA, Whitley MZ, Williams AJ, et al: NF-kappa B and I kappa B alpha: An inducible regulatory system in endothelial activation. J Exp Med 179:503–512, 1994.

38. Shu HB, Agranoff AB, Nabel EG, et al: Differential regulation of vascular cell adhesion molecule 1 gene expression by specific NF-kappa B subunits in endothelial and epithelial cells. Mol Cell Biol 13:6283–6289, 1993.

39. Mannick E, Udall JN Jr: Neonatal gastrointestinal mucosal immunity. Clin Perinatol 23:287–304, 1996.

40. Udall JN Jr: Gastrointestinal host defense and necrotizing enterocolitis. J Pediatr 117:S33–S43, 1990.

41. Simmons CP, Clare S, Dougan G: Understanding mucosal responsiveness: Lessons from enteric bacterial pathogens. Semin Immunol 13:201–209, 2001.

42. Neutra MR: Current concepts in mucosal immunity: V Role of M cells in transepithelial transport of antigens and pathogens to the mucosal immune system. Am J Physiol 274:G785–G791, 1998.

43. Smith TJ, Weis JH: Mucosal T cells and mast cells share common adhesion receptors. Immunol Today 17:60–63, 1996.

44. Ewer AK: Role of platelet-activating factor in the pathophysiology of necrotizing enterocolitis. Acta Paediatr Suppl 91:2–5, 2002.

45. Caplan MS, Hedlund E, Adler L, et al: The platelet-activating factor receptor antagonist WEB 2170 prevents neonatal necrotizing enterocolitis in rats. J Pediatr Gastroenterol Nutr 24:296–301, 1997.

46. Caplan MS, Sun XM, Hsueh W: Hypoxia causes ischemic bowel necrosis in rats: The role of platelet-activating factor (PAF-acether). Gastroenterology 99:979–986, 1990.

47. Zhang C, Hsueh W, Caplan MS, et al: Platelet activating factor-induced shock and intestinal necrosis in the rat: Role of endogenous platelet-activating factor and effect of saline infusion. Crit Care Med 19:1067–1072, 1991.

48. Hsueh W, Caplan MS, Sun X, et al: Platelet-activating factor, tumor necrosis factor, hypoxia and necrotizing enterocolitis. Acta Paediatr Suppl 396:11–17, 1994.

49. Caplan MS, Hsueh W: Necrotizing enterocolitis: Role of platelet activating factor, endotoxin, and tumor necrosis factor. J Pediatr 117:S47–S51, 1990.

50. Colletti LM, Remick DG, Burtch GD, et al: Role of tumor necrosis factor-alpha in the pathophysiologic alterations after hepatic ischemia/reperfusion injury in the rat. J Clin Invest 85:1936–1943, 1990.

51. Colletti LM, Kunkel SL, Walz A, et al: The role of cytokine networks in the local liver injury following hepatic ischemia/reperfusion in the rat. Hepatology 23:506–514, 1996.

52. Remick DG, Colletti LM, Scales WA, et al: Cytokines and extrahepatic sequelae of ischemia-reperfusion injury to the liver. Ann N Y Acad Sci 723:271–283, 1994.

53. Colletti LM, Remick DG, Burtch GD, et al: Role of tumor necrosis factor-alpha in the pathophysiologic alterations after hepatic ischemia/reperfusion injury in the rat. J Clin Invest 85:1936–1943, 1990.

54. Shimizu H, Mitomo K, Watanabe T, et al: Involvement of a NF-kappa B-like transcription factor in the activation of the interleukin-6 gene by inflammatory lymphokines. Mol Cell Biol 10:561–568, 1990.

55. Scheinman RI, Cogswell PC, Lofquist AK, et al: Role of transcriptional activation of I kappa B alpha in mediation of immunosuppression by glucocorticoids. Science 270:283–286, 1995.

56. Baldwin AS: The NF-kappa B and the I kappa B proteins: New discoveries and insights. Annu Rev Immunol 14:649–681, 1996.

57. Amer MD, Caplan MS: Neonatal necrotizing enterocolitis increases platelet activating factor levels in the stool of newborn infants. Clin Res 42:372A, 1994.

58. MacKendrick W, Hill N, Hsueh W, et al: Increase in plasma platelet-activating factor levels in enterally fed preterm infants. Biol Neonate 64:89–95, 1993.

59. Caplan M, Hsueh W, Kelly A, et al: Serum PAF acetylhydrolase increases during neonatal maturation. Prostaglandins 39:705–714, 1990.

60. Furukawa M, Lee EL, Johnston JM: Platelet-activating factor-induced ischemic bowel necrosis: The effect of platelet-activating factor acetylhydrolase. Pediatr Res 34:237–241, 1993.

61. Lucas A, Cole TJ: Breast milk and neonatal necrotising enterocolitis. Lancet 336:1519–1523, 1990.

62. Ford H, Watkins S, Reblock K, Rowe M: The role of inflammatory cytokines and nitric oxide in the pathogenesis of necrotizing enterocolitis. J Pediatr Surg 32:275–282, 1997.

63. Wang JH, Redmond HP, Wu QD, et al: Nitric oxide mediates hepatocyte injury. Am J Physiol 275:G1117–G1126, 1998.

64. Menezes JM, Hierholzer C, Watkins SC, et al: The modulation of hepatic injury and heat shock expression by inhibition of inducible nitric oxide synthase after hemorrhagic shock. Shock 17:13–18, 2002.

65. Menezes J, Hierholzer C, Watkins SC, et al: A novel nitric oxide scavenger decreases liver injury and improves survival after hemorrhagic shock. Am J Physiol 277:G144–G151, 1999.

66. Halpern MD, Holubec H, Dominguez JA, et al: Hepatic inflammatory mediators contribute to intestinal damage in necrotizing enterocolitis. Am J Physiol Gastrointest Liver Physiol 284:G695–G702, 2003.

67. Pfeiffer S, Lass A, Schmidt K, Mayer B. Protein tyrosine nitration in cytokine-activated murine macrophages: Involvement of a peroxidase/nitrite pathway rather than peroxynitrite. J Biol Chem 276:34051–34058, 2001.

68. Caplan MS, Hedlund E, Adler L, et al: Role of asphyxia and feeding in a neonatal rat model of necrotizing enterocolitis. Pediatr Pathol 14:1017–1028, 1994.

69. Sibbons PD, Spitz L, van Velzen D: Necrotizing enterocolitis induced by local circulatory interruption in the ileum of neonatal piglets. Pediatr Pathol 12:1–14, 1992.

70. Nowicki PT, Nankervis CA: The role of the circulation in the pathogenesis of necrotizing enterocolitis. Clin Perinatol 21:219–234, 1994.

71. Crissinger KD: Regulation of hemodynamics and oxygenation in developing intestine: Insight into the pathogenesis of necrotizing enterocolitis. Acta Paediatr Suppl 396:8–10, 1994.

72. Reber KM, Nankervis CA, Nowicki PT: Newborn intestinal circulation: Physiology and pathophysiology. Clin Perinatol 29:23–39, 2002.

73. Horie Y, Wolf R, Chervenak RP, et al: T-lymphocytes contribute to hepatic leukostasis and hypoxic stress induced by gut ischemia-reperfusion. Microcirculation 6:267–280, 1999.

74. Mori N, Horie Y, Nimura Y, et al: Hepatic microvascular responses to ischemia-reperfusion in low-density lipoprotein receptor knockout mice. Am J Physiol Gastrointest Liver Physiol 279:G1257–G1264, 2000.

75. Wang JH, Redmond HP, Watson RW, et al: Role of lipopolysaccharide and tumor necrosis factor-alpha in induction of hepatocyte necrosis. Am J Physiol 269:G297–G304, 1995.

76. Arii S, Imamura M: Physiological role of sinusoidal endothelial cells and Kupffer cells and their implication in the pathogenesis of liver injury. J Hepatobiliary Pancreat Surg 7:40–48, 2000.

77. Sander A, Armbruster W, Sander B, et al: Hemofiltration increases IL-6 clearance in early systemic inflammatory response syndrome but does not alter IL-6 and TNF alpha plasma concentrations. Intens Care Med 23:878–884, 1997.

78. Taniguchi T, Koido Y, Aiboshi J, et al: Change in the ratio of interleukin-6 to interleukin-10 predicts a poor outcome in patients with systemic inflammatory response syndrome. Crit Care Med 27:1262–1264, 1999.

79. Suzuki S, Toledo-Pereyra LH, Rodriguez F, Lopez F: Role of Kupffer cells in neutrophil activation and infiltration following total hepatic ischemia and reperfusion. Circ Shock 42:204–209, 1994.

80. Suzuki S, Toledo-Pereyra LH, Rodriguez FJ: Role of neutrophils during the first 24 hours after liver ischemia and reperfusion injury. Transplant Proc 26:3695–3700, 1994.

81. Flick MR, Perel A, Staub NC: Leukocytes are required for increased lung microvascular permeability after microembolization in sheep. Circ Res 48:344–351, 1981.

82. Weiss SJ, Curnutte JT, Regiani S: Neutrophil-mediated solubilization of the subendothelial matrix: Oxidative and nonoxidative mechanisms of proteolysis used by normal and chronic granulomatous disease phagocytes. J Immunol 136:636–641, 1986.

83. Baird BR, Cheronis JC, Sandhaus RA, et al: O₂ metabolites and neutrophil elastase synergistically cause edematous injury in isolated rat lungs. J Appl Physiol 61:2224–2229, 1986.

84. Jaeschke H, Farhood A, Smith CW: Neutrophils contribute to ischemia/reperfusion injury in rat liver in vivo. FASEB J 4:3355–3359, 1990.

85. Sun XM, Qu XW, Huang W, et al: Role of leukocyte beta 2-integrin in PAF-induced shock and intestinal injury. Am J Physiol 270:G184–G190, 1996.

86. Sun X, Rozenfeld RA, Qu X, et al: P-selectin-deficient mice are protected from PAF-induced shock, intestinal injury, and lethality. Am J Physiol 273:G56–G61, 1997.

87. Tedder TF, Steeber DA, Chen A, Engel P: The selectins: Vascular adhesion molecules. FASEB J 9:866–873, 1995.

88. Kubes P, Suzuki M, Granger DN: Modulation of PAF-induced leukocyte adherence and increased microvascular permeability. Am J Physiol 259:G859–G864, 1990.

89. St Peter SD, Moss AA, Mulligan DC: Effects of tacrolimus on ischemia-reperfusion injury. Liver Transplant 9:105–116, 2003.

90. Cueva JP, Hsueh W: Role of oxygen derived free radicals in platelet activating factor induced bowel necrosis. Gut 29:1207–1212, 1988.

91. Qu XW, Rozenfeld RA, Huang W, et al: The role of xanthine oxidase in platelet activating factor induced intestinal injury in the rat. Gut 44:203–211, 1999.

92. Kanto WP Jr, Wilson R, Breart GL, et al. Perinatal events and necrotizing enterocolitis in premature infants. Am J Dis Child 141:167–169, 1987.

93. Wilson R, Kanto WP Jr, McCarthy BJ, et al: Epidemiologic characteristics of necrotizing enterocolitis: A population-based study. Am J Epidemiol 114:880–887, 1981.

94. Wilson R, Kanto WP Jr, McCarthy BJ, et al: Age at onset of necrotizing enterocolitis: An epidemiologic analysis. Pediatr Res 16:82–85, 1982.

95. De Curtis M, Paone C, Vetrano G, et al: A case control study of necrotizing enterocolitis occurring over 8 years in a neonatal intensive care unit. Eur J Pediatr 146:398–400, 1987.

96. Yu VY, Joseph R, Bajuk B, et al: Perinatal risk factors for necrotizing enterocolitis. Arch Dis Child 59:430–434, 1984.

97. Stoll BJ, Kanto WP Jr, Glass RI, et al: Epidemiology of necrotizing enterocolitis: A case control study. J Pediatr 96:447–451, 1980.

98. Covert RF, Neu J, Elliott MJ, et al: Factors associated with age of onset of necrotizing enterocolitis. Am J Perinatol 6:455–460, 1989.

99. Snyder CL, Gittes GK, Murphy JP, et al: Survival after necrotizing enterocolitis in infants weighing less than 1000 g: 25 years' experience at a single institution. J Pediatr Surg 32:434–437, 1997.

100. Rowe MI, Reblock KK, Kurkchubasche AG, Healey PJ: Necrotizing enterocolitis in the extremely low birth weight infant. J Pediatr Surg 29:987–990; discussion 990–991, 1994.

101. Fasching G, Hollwarth ME, Schmidt B, Mayr J: Surgical strategies in very-low-birthweight neonates with necrotizing enterocolitis. Acta Paediatr Suppl 396:62–64, 1994.

102. McElhinney D, Hedrick H, Bush D, et al: Necrotizing enterocolitis in neonates with congenital heart disease: Risk factors and outcomes. Pediatrics 106:1080–1087, 2000.

103. Bunton GL, Durbin GM, McIntosh N, et al: Necrotizing enterocolitis: Controlled study of 3 years' experience in a neonatal intensive care unit. Arch Dis Child 52:772–777, 1977.

104. Rand T, Weninger M, Kohlhauser C, et al: Effects of umbilical arterial catheterization on mesenteric hemodynamics. Pediatr Radiol 26:435–438, 1996.

105. Davey AM, Wagner CL, Cox C, Kendig JW: Feeding premature infants while low umbilical artery catheters are in place: A prospective, randomized trial. J Pediatr 124:795–799, 1994.

106. Kempley ST, Bennett S, Loftus BG, et al: Randomized trial of umbilical arterial catheter position: clinical outcome. Acta Paediatr 82:173–176, 1993.

107. Barrington KJ: Umbilical artery catheters in the newborn: Effects of position of the catheter tip. Cochrane Database Syst Rev CD000505, 2000.

108. Barrington KJ: Umbilical artery catheters in the newborn: Effects of catheter design (end vs side hole). Cochrane Database Syst Rev 2:CD000508, 2000 Review.

109. Black VD, Rumack CM, Lubchenco LO, Koops BL: Gastrointestinal injury in polycythemic term infants. Pediatrics 76:225–231, 1985.

110. Hein HA, Lathrop SS: Partial exchange transfusion in term, polycythemic neonates: Absence of association with severe gastrointestinal injury. Pediatrics 80:75–78, 1987.

111. Roig JC, Burchfield DJ: Term neonates with hemolytic disease of the newborn and necrotizing enterocolitis: A report of two cases. J Perinatol 14:201–203, 1994.

112. LeBlanc MH, D'Cruz C, Pate K: Necrotizing enterocolitis can be caused by polycythemic hyperviscosity in the newborn dog. J Pediatr 105:804–809, 1984.

113. Carmi D, Wolach B, Dolfin T, Merlob P: Polycythemia of the preterm and full-term newborn infant: Relationship between hematocrit and gestational age, total blood solutes, reticulocyte count, and blood pH. Biol Neonate 61:173–178, 1992.

114. Wiswell TE, Cornish JD, Northam RS: Neonatal polycythemia: Frequency of clinical manifestations and other associated findings. Pediatrics 78:26–30, 1986.

115. Werner EJ: Neonatal polycythemia and hyperviscosity. Clin Perinatol 22:693–710, 1995.

116. Lopez SL, Taeusch HW, Findlay RD, Walther FJ: Time of onset of necrotizing enterocolitis in newborn infants with known prenatal cocaine exposure. Clin Pediatr (Phila) 34:424–429, 1995.

117. Hufnal-Miller CA, Blackmon L, Baumgart S, Pereira GR: Necrotizing enterocolitis in the first 24 hours of life. Pediatrics 73:476–480, 1984.

118. Grosfeld JL, Dalsing MC, Hull M, Weber TR: Neonatal apnea, xanthines, and necrotizing enterocolitis. J Pediatr Surg 18:80–84, 1983.

119. Davis JM, Abbasi S, Spitzer AR, Johnson L: Role of theophylline in pathogenesis of necrotizing enterocolitis. J Pediatr 109:344–347, 1986.

120. Zanardo V, Trevisanuto D, Cagdas S, et al: Prenatal theophylline and necrotizing enterocolitis in premature newborn infants. Pediatr Med Chir 19:153–156, 1997.

121. Santulli TV, Schullinger JN, Heird WC, et al: Acute necrotizing enterocolitis in infancy: A review of 64 cases. Pediatrics 55:376–387, 1975.

122. Frantz ID III, L'heureux P, Engel RR, Hunt CE: Necrotizing enterocolitis. J Pediatr 86:259–263, 1975.

123. Milner ME, de la Monte SM, Moore GW, Hutchins GM: Risk factors for developing and dying from necrotizing enterocolitis. J Pediatr Gastroenterol Nutr 5:359–364, 1986.

124. Mufti P, Bhutta ZA: Necrotizing enterocolitis in infants weighing less than 2000 g. J Pak Med Assoc 42:37–39, 1992.

125. Buch NA, Ahmad SM, Ali SW, Hassan HM: An epidemiological study of neonatal necrotizing enterocolitis. Saudi Med J 22:231–237, 2001.

126. Bolisetty S, Lui K, Oei J, et al: A regional study of underlying congenital diseases in term neonates with necrotizing enterocolitis. Acta Paediatr 89:1226–1230, 2000.

127. Bolisetty S, Lui K: Necrotizing enterocolitis in full-term neonates. J Paediatr Child Health. 37:413–414, 2001.

128. Yaseen H, Kamaledin K, Al Umran K, et al: Epidemiology and outcome of "early-onset" vs "late-onset" necrotizing enterocolitis. Indian J Pediatr 69:481–484, 2002.

129. Martinez-Tallo E, Claure N, Bancalari E: Necrotizing enterocolitis in full-term infants: Risk factors. Biol Neonate 71:292–298, 1997.

130. Andrews D, Sawin R, Ledbetter D, et al: Necrotizing enterocolitis in term neonates. Am J Surg 159:507–509, .

131. Wilson R, Del Prtillo M, Schmidt E, et al: Risk factors for necrotizing enterocolitis in infants weighing more than 2,000 grams at birth: A case-control study. Am J Dis Child 71:19–22, 1983.

132. Thilo EH, Lazarte RA, Hernandez JA: Necrotizing enterocolitis in the first 24 hours of life. Pediatrics 73:476–480, 1984.

133. Koloske AM: Pathogenesis and prevention of necrotizing enterocolitis: A hypothesis based on personal observation and review of the literature. Pediatrics 74:1086–1092, 1984.

134. Koloske AM, Ulrich JA: A bacteriologic basis for presentations of necrotizing enterocolitis. J Pediatr Surg 15:558–564, 1980.

135. Rabinowitz SS, Dzakpasu P, Piecuch S, et al: Platelet-activating factor in infants at risk for necrotizing enterocolitis. J Pediatr 138:81–86, 2001.

136. Edelson MB, Bagwell CE, Rozycki HJ: Platelet-activating factor in infants at risk for necrotizing enterocolitis. J Pediatr 138:81–86, 2001.

137. Ververidis M, Kiely EM, Spitz L, et al: The clinical significance of thrombocytopenia in neonates with necrotizing enterocolitis. J Pediatr Surg 36:799–803, 2001.

138. Becker RM, Wu G, Galanko JA, et al: Reduced serum amino acid concentrations in infants with necrotizing enterocolitis. J Pediatr 137:785–793, 2000.

139. Zamora SA, Amin HJ, McMillan DD, et al: Plasma L-arginine concentrations in premature infants with necrotizing enterocolitis. J Pediatr 131:226–232, 1997.

140. Amin HJ, Zamora SA, McMillan DD, et al: Arginine supplementation prevents necrotizing enterocolitis in the premature infant. J Pediatr 140:425–431, 2002.

141. Hall N, Ong EG, Ade-Ajayi N, et al: T cryptantigen activation is associated with advanced necrotizing enterocolitis. J Pediatr Surg 37:791–793, 2002.

142. Hatherill M, Tibby SM, Denver L, et al: Early detection of necrotizing enterocolitis by gastrointestinal tonometry. Acta Paediatr 87:344–345, 1998.

143. Coombs RC, Morgan ME, Durbin GM, et al: Abnormal gut blood flow velocities in neonates at risk of necrotising enterocolitis. J Pediatr Gastroenterol Nutr 15:13–19, 1992.

144. Bhatt AB, Tank PD, Barmade KB, Damania KR: Abnormal Doppler flow velocimetry in the growth restricted foetus as a predictor for necrotising enterocolitis. J Postgrad Med 48:182–185, 2002.

145. Soregaroli M, Bonera R, Danti L, et al: Prognostic role of umbilical artery Doppler velocimetry in growth-restricted fetuses. J Matern Fetal Neonatal Med 11:199–203, 2002.

146. Korszun P, Dubiel M, Breborowicz G, et al: Fetal superior mesenteric artery blood flow velocimetry in normal and high-risk pregnancy. J Perinat Med 30:235–241, 2002.

147. Robel-Tillig E, Vogtmann C, Bennek J: Prenatal hemodynamic disturbances: Pathophysiological background of intestinal motility disturbances in small for gestational age infants. Eur J Pediatr Surg 12:175–179, 2002.

148. Kosloske AM: Breast milk decreases the risk of neonatal necrotizing enterocolitis. Adv Nutr Res 10:123–137, 2001.

149. Caplan MS, Amer M, Jilling T: The role of human milk in necrotizing enterocolitis. Adv Exp Med Biol 2002;503:83–90.

150. Kelleher SL, Lonnerdal B: Immunological activities associated with milk. Adv Nutr Res 10:39–65, 2001.

151. Premji S, Chessell L: Continuous nasogastric milk feeding versus intermittent bolus milk feeding for premature infants less than 1500 grams. Cochrane Database Syst Rev :CD001819, 2003.

152. Patole SK, Kadalraja R, Tuladhar R, et al: Benefits of a standardised feeding regimen during a clinical trial in preterm neonates. Int J Clin Pract 54:429–431, 2000.

153. Kamitsuka MD, Horton MK, Williams MA: The incidence of necrotizing enterocolitis after introducing standardized feeding schedules for infants between 1250 and 2500 grams and less than 35 weeks of gestation. Pediatrics 105:379–384, 2000.

154. Rayyis SF, Ambalavanan N, Wright L, Carlo WA: Randomized trial of "slow" versus "fast" feed advancements on the incidence of necrotizing enterocolitis in very low birth weight infants. J Pediatr 134:293–297, 1999.

155. Halac E, Halac J, Begue EF, et al: Prenatal and postnatal corticosteroid therapy to prevent neonatal necrotizing enterocolitis: A controlled trial. J Pediatr 117:132–138, 1990.

156. Narahara H, Nishioka Y, Johnston JM: Secretion of platelet-activating factor acetylhydrolase by human decidual macrophages. J Clin Endocrinol Metab 77:1258–1262, 1993.

157. Caplan MS, Lickerman M, Adler L, et al: The role of recombinant platelet-activating factor acetylhydrolase in a neonatal rat model of necrotizing enterocolitis. Pediatr Res 42:779–783, 1997.

158. de Boissieu D, Canarelli JP, Cordonnier C, et al: Effect of BN 50727 on pathological findings and tissue platelet activating factor levels during ileal ischemia in newborn piglets. J Pediatr Surg 31:1675–1679, 1996.

159. Akisu M, Baka M, Coker I, et al: Effect of dietary n-3 fatty acids on hypoxia-induced necrotizing enterocolitis in young mice: N-3 fatty acids alter platelet-activating factor and leukotriene B4 production in the intestine. Biol Neonate 74:31–38, 1998.

160. Caplan MS, Russell T, Xiao Y, et al: Effect of polyunsaturated fatty acid (PUFA) supplementation on intestinal inflammation and necrotizing enterocolitis (NEC) in a neonatal rat model. Pediatr Res 49:647–652, 2001.

161. Akisu M, Ozmen D, Baka M, et al: Protective effect of dietary supplementation with L-arginine and L-carnitine on hypoxia/reoxygenation-induced necrotizing enterocolitis in young mice. Biol Neonate 81:260–265, 2002.

162. Kliegman RM, Walker WA, Yolken RH: Necrotizing enterocolitis: research agenda for a disease of unknown etiology and pathogenesis. Pediatr Res 34:701–708, 1993.

163. Nadler EP, Upperman JS, Ford HR: Controversies in the management of necrotizing enterocolitis. Surg Infect (Larchmt) 2:113–119; discussion 119–120, 2001.

164. Chan KL, Saing H, Yung RW, et al: A study of pre-antibiotic bacteriology in 125 patients with necrotizing enterocolitis. Acta Paediatr Suppl 396:45–48, 1994.

165. Scheifele DW, Ginter GL, Olsen E, et al: Comparison of two antibiotic regimens for neonatal necrotizing enterocolitis. J Antimicrob Chemother 20:421–429, 1987.

166. Musoke RN, Revathi G: Emergence of multidrug-resistant gram-negative organisms in a neonatal unit and the therapeutic implications. J Trop Pediatr 46:86–91, 2000.

167. Toltzis P, Blumer JL: Antibiotic-resistant gram-negative bacteria in the critical care setting. Pediatr Clin North Am 42:687–702, 1995.

168. Caddell JL: A review of evidence for a role of magnesium and possibly copper deficiency in necrotizing enterocolitis. Magnes Res 9:55–66, 1996.

169. Anveden-Hertzberg L, Gauderer MW: Surgery is safe in very low birthweight infants with necrotizing enterocolitis. Acta Paediatr 89:242–245, 2000.

170. Horwitz JR, Lally KP, Cheu HW, et al: Complications after surgical intervention for necrotizing enterocolitis: A multicenter review. J Pediatr Surg 30:994–998, 1995.

171. Frawley G, Bayley G, Chondros P: Laparotomy for necrotizing enterocolitis: Intensive care nursery compared with operating theatre. J Paediatr Child Health 35:291–295, 1999.

172. Chwals WJ, Blakely ML, Cheng A, et al: Surgery-associated complications in necrotizing enterocolitis: A multi-institutional study. J Pediatr Surg 36:1722–1724, 2001.

173. Fasoli L, Turi RA, Spitz L, et al: Necrotizing enterocolitis: Extent of disease and surgical treatment. J Pediatr Surg 34:1096–1099, 1999.

174. Ade-Ajayi N, Kiely E, Drake D, et al: Resection and primary anastomosis in necrotizing enterocolitis. J R Soc Med 89:385–388, 1996.

175. Parigi GB, Bragheri R, Minniti S, Verga G: Surgical treatment of necrotizing enterocolitis: When? How? Acta Paediatr Suppl 396:58–61, 1994.

176. O'Connor A, Sawin RS: High morbidity of enterostomy and its closure in premature infants with necrotizing enterocolitis. Arch Surg 133:875–880, 1998.

177. Griffiths DM, Forbes DA, Pemberton PJ, Penn IA: Primary anastomosis for necrotising enterocolitis: A 12-year experience. J Pediatr Surg 24:515–518, 1989.

178. Gertler JP, Seashore JH, Touloukian RJ: Early ileostomy closure in necrotizing enterocolitis. J Pediatr Surg 22:140–143, 1987.

179. Weber TR, Tracy TF Jr, Silen ML, Powell MA: Enterostomy and its closure in newborns. Arch Surg 130:534–537, 1995.

180. Cooper A, Ross AJ III, O'Neill JA Jr, Schnaufer L: Resection with primary anastomosis for necrotizing enterocolitis: A contrasting view. J Pediatr Surg 23:64–68, 1988.

181. de Souza JC, da Motta UI, Ketzer CR: Prognostic factors of mortality in newborns with necrotizing enterocolitis submitted to exploratory laparotomy. J Pediatr Surg 36:482–486, 2001.

182. Voss M, Moore SW, van der Merwe I, Pieper C: Fulminating necrotising enterocolitis: Outcome and prognostic factors. Pediatr Surg Int 13:576–580, 1998.

183. Kliegman RM, Fanaroff AA: Necrotizing enterocolitis. N Engl J Med 310:1093–1103, 1984.

184. Ladd AP, Rescorla FJ, West KW, et al: Long-term follow-up after bowel resection for necrotizing enterocolitis: Factors affecting outcome. J Pediatr Surg 33:967–972, 1998.

185. Stanford A, Upperman JS, Boyle P, et al: Long-term follow-up of patients with necrotizing enterocolitis. J Pediatr Surg 37:1048–1050, 2002.

186. Ricketts RR: Surgical treatment of necrotizing enterocolitis and the short bowel syndrome. Clin Perinatol 21:365–387, 1994.

187. Demestre X, Ginovart G, Figueras-Aloy J, et al: Peritoneal drainage as primary management in necrotizing enterocolitis: A prospective study. J Pediatr Surg 37:1534–1539, 2002.

188. Ahmed T, Ein S, Moore A: The role of peritoneal drains in treatment of perforated necrotizing enterocolitis: Recommendations from recent experience. J Pediatr Surg 33:1468–1470, 1998.

189. Cass DL, Brandt ML, Patel DL, et al: Peritoneal drainage as definitive treatment for neonates with isolated intestinal perforation. J Pediatr Surg 35:1531–1536, 2000.

190. Rovin JD, Rodgers BM, Burns RC, McGahren ED: The role of peritoneal drainage for intestinal perforation in infants with and without necrotizing enterocolitis. J Pediatr Surg 34:143–147, 1999.

191. Morgan LJ, Shochat SJ, Hartman GE: Peritoneal drainage as primary management of perforated NEC in the very low birth weight infant. J Pediatr Surg 29:310–314, 1994.

192. Azarow KS, Ein SH, Shandling B, et al: Laparotomy or drain for perforated necrotizing enterocolitis: Who gets what and why? Pediatr Surg Int 12:137–139, 1997.

193. Wang YH, Su BH, Wu SF, et al: Clinical analysis of necrotizing enterocolitis with intestinal perforation in premature infants. Acta Paediatr Taiwan 43:199–203, .

194. Badowicz B, Latawiec-Mazurkiewicz I: Necrotising enterocolitis (NEC): Methods of treatment and outcome: A comparative analysis of Scottish (Glasgow) and Polish (Western Pomerania) cases. Eur J Pediatr Surg 10:177–181, 2000.

195. Ein SH, Shandling B, Wesson D, Filler RM: A 13-year experience with peritoneal drainage under local anesthesia for necrotizing enterocolitis perforation. J Pediatr Surg 25:1034–1036, 1990.

196. Lessin MS, Luks FI, Wesselhoeft CW Jr, et al: Peritoneal drainage as definitive treatment for intestinal perforation in infants with extremely low birth weight (<750 g). J Pediatr Surg 33:370–372, 1998.

197. Noble HG, Driessnack M: Bedside peritoneal drainage in very low birth weight infants. Am J Surg 181:416–419, 2001.

198. Cheu HW, Sukarochana K, Lloyd DA: Peritoneal drainage for necrotizing enterocolitis. J Pediatr Surg 23:557–561, 1988.

199. Camberos A, Patel K, Applebaum H: Laparotomy in very small premature infants with necrotizing enterocolitis or focal intestinal perforation: postoperative outcome. J Pediatr Surg 37:1692–1695, 2002.

200. Moss RL, Dimmitt RA, Henry MC, et al: A meta-analysis of peritoneal drainage versus laparotomy for perforated necrotizing enterocolitis. J Pediatr Surg 36:1210–1213, 2000.

201. Ehrlich PF, Sato TT, Short BL, Hartman GE: Outcome of perforated necrotizing enterocolitis in the very low birth weight neonate may be independent of the type of surgical treatment. Am Surg 67:752–726, 2001.

202. Weber TR, Lewis JE: The role of second-look laparotomy in necrotizing enterocolitis. J Pediatr Surg 21:323–325, 1986.

203. Sugarman ID, Kiely EM: Is there a role for high jejunostomy in the management of severe necrotising enterocolitis? Pediatr Surg Int 17:122–124, 2001.

204. Luzzatto C, Previtera C, Boscolo R, et al: Necrotizing enterocolitis: Late surgical results after enterostomy without resection. Eur J Pediatr Surg 6:92–94, 1996.

205. Vaughan WG, Grosfeld JL, West K, et al: Avoidance of stomas and delayed anastomosis for bowel necrosis: The "clip and drop-back" technique. J Pediatr Surg 31:542–545, 1996.

206. Lessin MS, Schwartz DL, Wesselhoeft CW Jr: Multiple spontaneous small bowel anastomosis in premature infants with multisegmental necrotizing enterocolitis. J Pediatr Surg 35:170–172, 2000.

207. Tobiansky R, Lui K, Roberts S, Veddovi M: Neurodevelopmental outcome in very low birthweight infants with necrotizing enterocolitis requiring surgery. J Paediatr Child Health 31:233–236, 1995.

208. Sonntag J, Grimmer I, Scholz T, et al: Growth and neurodevelopmental outcome of very low birthweight infants with necrotizing enterocolitis. Acta Paediatr 89:528–532, 2000.

209. Chacko J, Ford WD, Haslam R: Growth and neurodevelopmental outcome in extremely-low-birth-weight infants after laparotomy. Pediatr Surg Int 15:496–499, 1999.

210. Walsh MC, Kliegman RM, Hack M: Severity of necrotizing enterocolitis: Influence on outcome at 2 years of age. Pediatrics 84:808–814, 1989.

211. Hirata T, Epcar JT, Walsh A, et al: G. Survival and outcome of infants 501 to 750 gm: A six-year experience. J Pediatr 102:741–748, 1983.

212. Brothwood M, Wolke D, Gamsu H, et al: Prognosis of the very low birthweight baby in relation to gender. Arch Dis Child 61:559–564, 1986.

213. La Pine TR, Jackson JC, Bennett FC: Outcome of infants weighing less than 800 grams at birth: 15 years' experience. Pediatrics 96:479–483, 1995.

214. Whiteman L, Wuethrich M, Egan E: Infants who survive necrotizing enterocolitis. Matern Child Nurs J 14:123–133, .

215. Cikrit D, West KW, Schreiner R, Grosfeld JL: Long-term follow-up after surgical management of necrotizing enterocolitis: Sixty-three cases. J Pediatr Surg 21:533–535, 1986.

CHAPTER 34

Hirschsprung's Disease

Alexander Holschneider, MD, PhD, and Benno M. Ure, MD, PhD

INCIDENCE

One in 5000 newborns is initially seen with Hirschsprung's disease (HD),[1] and 70% to 80% are boys. HD is observed in all races but is less common in blacks. Siblings and offspring of familial cases have an increased risk of being afflicted. The reported incidence in these children varies from 1.5% to 17.6%[2,3] which is 130 times higher for boys and 360 times higher for girls than that in the general population.[4] HD is more likely to be transmitted by a mother with aganglionosis than by a father. As many as 12.5% of the siblings of patients with total aganglionosis of the colon (Zuelzer-Wilson syndrome) will have the same disease.[5] Associated anomalies are present in 25% of familial cases, compared with 10% in nonfamilial HD cases. One report[6] describes four families with 22 affected siblings, most of them having long-segment aganglionosis. The overall incidence of neurocristopathies, including all inborn errors of the enteric nervous system (ENS) is not known. Familial cases of intestinal neuronal dysplasia (IND) are described, but the incidence of this condition or other neuronal intestinal malformations has not been reported.[7]

GENETIC FACTORS

Although Harald Hirschsprung[8] gave the first detailed description of congenital megacolon in 1888 and more than 500 articles have been published to elucidate the pathophysiology, the etiology of the disease is still unknown. In recent years, increasing attention has been focused on genetic defects.

Human beings are not the only species to have aganglionosis. Aganglionosis has been observed in mice, rats, horses, cows, dogs, and cats. The first description of aganglionosis in mice was published in 1957.[9] The first genetic transmission in a human being was reported in 1992.[10] The spotted lethal (sl) rat model has two subgroups: one with total colonic aganglionosis, and the second, less numerous group, in which ganglion cells extend to the proximal half of the colon.[11,12] The lethal spotted (ls) mice have approximately 2 mm of aganglionosis.[13] whereas another strain showed a deficiency of ganglion cells over approximately 10 mm. Studies in which a linkage of genes and gene "knockouts" were analyzed revealed that the RET knockout gene deleted on chromosome 10 was responsible for human HD.[14]

Early genetic studies of familial occurrence of nonsyndromic HD in humans[15] resulted in a multigenetic model to explain the nonmendelian inheritance pattern. The average risk of recurrence in siblings of 3% to 4%, reaching 17% in certain families, was 200-fold higher than the risk in the general population. The higher proportion of affected siblings in female patients is thought to be the result of a greater contribution of genetic factors in female patients.[16] It is not understood why familial incidence is lower for short HD than for long HD. In a recent study, Bolk Gabriel et al.[17] investigated 49 families with short HD, with a total of 106 affected individuals all with nonsyndromic HD. The authors undertook a genome-wide linkage scan covering more than 92% of the human genome. The main gene conferring susceptibility was confirmed to be RET in 17 of 43 linked families. The failure to identify coding-region mutations in some of the RET-linked families suggested the existence of mutations in regulatory regions.

We know that the migration of neural crest–derived intestinal ganglion cells involves genes in three different signaling pathways.[18–21] These genes include the RET-receptor tyrosine kinase pathway with genes encoding the RET receptor and its ligands, the glial cell line–derived neurotrophic factor (GDNF), the endothelin type B–receptor pathway with the EDNR receptor and its ligand, endothelin-3 (EDN3), and the SOX10-mediated transcription (Table 34-1). Mutations in these eight partially independent genes are associated with HD. The mutations are not fully penetrant. Dominant mutations in RET have been found in about 50% of familial patients with HD and in about 15% to 35% of isolated cases. The EDNRB mutations are recessive, with a penetrance of 30% to 80% (14b). Table 34-1 shows the genes implicated in the etiology of HD (see Table 34-1).

TABLE 34-1

GENES IMPLICATED IN THE ETIOLOGY OF HIRSCHSPRUNG'S DISEASE

Gene	Location	Main Effect	Penetrance
RET	10q11.2	Dominant, loss-of-function	50%–72%
GDNF	5p13.1	Dominant/recessive	Unknown
EDNRB	13q22	Recessive	30%–85%
EDN3	20q13	Recessive	Unknown
SOX10	22q13	Dominant/recessive	>80%
ECE1	1p36	Dominant/recessive	Unknown
NTN	19p13	Unknown	Unknown
SIP1	2q22	Sporadic	Unknown

Most effects seem to be interdependent, and mutant alleles usually do not segregate in a mendelian pattern.
According to Passarge E: Genetic heterogenicity and recurrence risk of congenital intestinal aganglionosis. Birth Defects Orig Artic Ser VIII:63, 1972.

However, the high frequency of sporadic HD cases, the varying expressivity in different members of an affected family, and the sex-independent differences in the extent of aganglionosis confirm the multifactorial genesis of the condition. It has not been clarified whether the genetic defects result in neural crest cell deficiency, in migration problems of the ganglion cells, or in a peripheral microenvironment deficiency. Therefore the link between genetic defects and pathophysiology remains to be elucidated.

PATHOPHYSIOLOGY

The basic pathophysiology in HD is a lack of propagation of propulsive waves and an abnormal or absent relaxation of the internal anal sphincter due to aganglionosis, hypoganglionosis, or dysganglionosis of the bowel. However, innervation abnormalities in HD and allied cristopathies are qualitative, not quantitative.

Peristaltic Reflex

Peristalsis consists of a reflex relaxation below and a contraction of the circular muscle layer above an intraluminal bolus (Fig. 34-1). In addition, the longitudinal muscle layer contracts simultaneously over the bowel content, which leads to aboral propagation. The neural reflex circuit is generated by distention of the bowel and spontaneous depolarization of pacemaker cells in the smooth muscle layers. The electrical impulses are carried by cholinergic neurons to interneurons situated in the submucous and myenteric plexus. The interneurons are of nonadrenergic, noncholinergic (NANC) origin, but they depend on adenosine triphosphate, vasoactive intestinal peptide (VIP), and nitric oxide (NO) directly inhibiting the smooth muscle cells. The ganglia of the intramural plexus contain four to six ganglion cells and are modulated by cholinergic and adrenergic influences running to the ganglia and blood vessels (adrenergic fibers) via extramural neural pathways. Adrenaline modulates the acetylcholine release at cholinergic

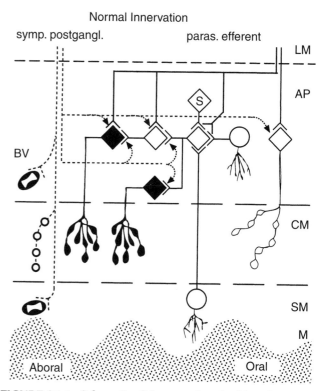

Normal Innervation

FIGURE 34-1. Schematic of the normal peristaltic reflex, showing the intramural plexus and the postganglionic adrenergic and preganglionic cholinergic axons entering the bowel. The sensory neurons are indicated by *circles*. The impulses from the mechanoreceptor cells are transmitted via interneurons (*white squares*) over cholinergic synapses to the nonadrenergic inhibitory neurons (*dark squares*). The finely drawn neuron with *white circles* in its terminal axons represents a postganglionic axon. The neuron labeled S symbolizes a pacemaker neuron with spontaneous activity. Stimulation of the nonadrenergic inhibitory neurons leads to a neurogenically produced relaxation beyond the bolus. Above the bolus, a myogenically produced contraction of the circular muscle occurs (rebound excitation). The sympathetic system acts as a modulator of the acetylcholine release at the cholinergic synapses. AP, Auerbach's plexus; BV, blood vessel; CM, circular muscle; LM, longitudinal muscle; M, mucosa; S, pacemaker neuron with spontaneous activity; SM, submucosa.

synapses. In addition to these nerve fibers and the submucous and myenteric plexus, the interstitial cells of Cajal seem to play an important regulatory role in human gut muscle function.[22]

NO has recently been recognized as a neurotransmitter that mediates relaxation of the smooth muscles of the gastrointestinal tract. It is identical to reduced nicotinamide adenine nucleotide phosphate (NADPH)-diaphorase, which can therefore be used as a diagnostic marker for HD. Other than NO-containing inhibitory neurons, various other peptidergic neurons storing VIP, substance P, enkephalin, neurokinin A, histidine, isoleucin, gastrin-releasing peptide, and many others are involved in the peristaltic reflex. They are absent or abnormal in HD and allied disorders. Currently, the absence of NO-producing neurons is thought to be the cause of the failure of the aganglionic bowel to relax.

The Internal Anal Sphincter

The internal anal sphincter is influenced by four neuronal mechanisms:

α-Adrenergic excitatory stimuli, which travel in the hypogastric nerves and maintain the sphincter tone via α-excitatory receptors

β-Adrenergic inhibitory receptors relaxing the smooth muscle

Cholinergic neurons, whose influence on the sphincter is not yet adequately known

Nonadrenergic and noncholinergic neurons leading to internal sphincter relaxation by the mediation of NO, VIP, and other peptidergic neurons[23]

The relaxation phase of the peristaltic reflex below a fecal bolus is similar to the internal sphincter relaxation, which opens the anal channel at the beginning of defecation. Evidence of this most caudal peristaltic reflex can therefore be considered a proof of normal neurotransmission down to the end of the gastrointestinal tract and thus exclude HD. Bowel dysfunction in HD is the result of a complex malformation of the intrinsic nerve system of the bowel, which includes the absence of cholinergic ganglia, NANC interneurons, different peptidergic nerve fibers, and probably connective tissue structures of the bowel wall (Fig. 34-2). Cholinergic axons from the sacral parasympathetic plexus proliferate into the bowel wall and act directly with the smooth muscle cells, producing unopposed contraction. The acetylcholine released at the nerve endings is inactivated by a similar amount of acetylcholinesterase (AChE). Therefore the staining for AChE provides a very useful diagnostic tool for HD. However, misleading results occur in 10% of cases with AChE-stained biopsies. The frequency of misleading information was highest in long-segment HD.[24] The aganglionic segment remains in permanent contraction, unable to relax because of the lack of NANC interneurons and NO, but it is elastic and able to produce some uncoordinated motility. This may allow some degree of fecal transport and could be the reason HD is sometimes diagnosed later in life. This also applies to patients with hypoganglionosis and IND who show markedly reduced neural cell adhesion molecules and NAPD-diaphorase activity.[25] Conversely, the adrenergic axons (which synapse directly on the excitatory α-receptors of the smooth muscle cells) are normal. The internal anal sphincter therefore remains permanently unable to relax.

Hypoganglionosis

Proximal to the aganglionic segment of HD is generally a zone of hypoganglionosis. Hypoganglionosis also can represent an isolated disease entity. Hypoganglionosis is defined as the state in which the number of ganglion cells is reduced by a factor of 10, and the density of the nerve fibers, by a factor of 5.[26-28] AChE-positive fibers are rarely seen. The number of nerve cells in the myenteric plexus is 50% of that of normal innervated colon, and the distances between the ganglia are doubled. The mean area of the ganglia is 3 times smaller than that in controls. However, isolated hypoganglionosis and hypoganglionosis associated with HD or IND do not differ histochemically. Hypoganglionosis sometimes involves only a short length of colon and occasionally may involve the whole bowel. As a consequence, a few ganglion cells found on microscopy of frozen-section biopsies taken during an operation do not prove normal bowel innervation or guarantee normal bowel motility. In hypoganglionosis, internal sphincter relaxation is often missing or rudimentary.[29]

Immaturity of Ganglion Cells

Immature ganglion cells with monopolar small dentrites can be identified with lactate dehydrogenase (LDH) staining. Nerve cells in the immature ganglia have not developed a dehydrogenase-containing cytoplasm. Therefore a differentiation between Schwann cells and nerve cells cannot be made. The maturity of ganglion cells is most reliably determined by using the succinyldehydrogenase (SDH) reaction, which tests for this specific mitochondrial enzyme. Enzyme activity is low during the first weeks of life. Maturation of ganglion cells, as determined by the SDH reaction, demonstrates that full maturity requires 2 to 4 years. Immaturity may be seen with IND or hypoganglionosis, and the condition may eventually cause bowel obstruction.[28] The association of hypoganglionosis and immaturity is called hypogenesis.[30,31]

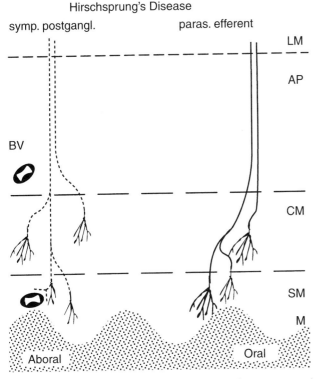

Hirschsprung's Disease

FIGURE 34-2. Schematic of intramural neurons in Hirschsprung's disease, showing the absence of ganglion cells and interneurons and the increased adrenergic and cholinergic influence on the smooth muscle cells. AP, Auerbach's plexus; BV, blood vessel; CM, circular muscle; LM, longitudinal muscle; M, mucosa; SM, submucosa.

Intestinal Neuronal Dysplasia

HD represents an abnormality of neural crest cell migration. Therefore it is not surprising that in addition to aganglionosis and hypoganglionosis, incomplete maturation of the enteric nerve plexus or dysganglionosis can occur.[32] In 1971, IND was first described as either a separate obstructive disease or as one that could coexist with classic HD.[33] IND type A (which is characterized by a malformation of the adrenergic nerve supply to the blood vessels) was distinguished from IND type B, in which the submucous plexus is involved.

The diagnosis of IND type B was based mainly on the occurrence of giant ganglia, containing on average 7 to 10, and occasionally up to 16 LDH-positive ganglion cells (Fig. 34-3). These large ganglia represent only 60% of all ganglia seen in a given case and are usually not observed in the distal rectum.[34] Moreover, the morphology of the nerve cell groups and nerve cell fibers is abnormal. They form budlike cell formations and pearl string–like nerve fibers. Often the muscularis mucosa and sometimes the lamina propria mucosa contain heterotopic nerve cells or ganglia. The AChE activity is increased in the nerve fibers of the lamina propria but mostly normalizes at age 9 to 18 months. One authority believes that 40 serial sections must be investigated with LDH reaction to establish the diagnosis reliably. Of these sections, 30% to 55% do not contain ganglia in the submucosa. Of the remainder, one in four will contain giant ganglia. At least four giant ganglia must be identified.[27] The diagnosis of IND is difficult, and these criteria generally are not accepted.[35] In children older than 4 years, IND is often associated with hypoganglionosis, hypogenesis, and heterotopia of the myenteric plexus. A recent study was performed by sending each biopsy under an anonymous code to three pediatric pathologists, who followed the criteria established by Meier-Ruge and colleagues.[36] An excellent consensus was found in the diagnosis of HD, but none in the diagnosis of IND.[37,38] It may be that this misjudgment was due to interobserver variation, differences in experience with the diagnosis, and differences in histochemical parameters for IND used. We have concluded from our studies on children with imperforate anus that IND also could be an expression of neuromuscular hypertrophy proximal to a congenital intestinal obstruction.[39]

IND type A is characterized by a lack or immaturity of the adrenergic innervation of the myenteric plexus, arterial vessels, and mucosa (Fig. 34-4). It is very rare and observed in less than 2% of all neuronal intestinal malformations.[40,41]

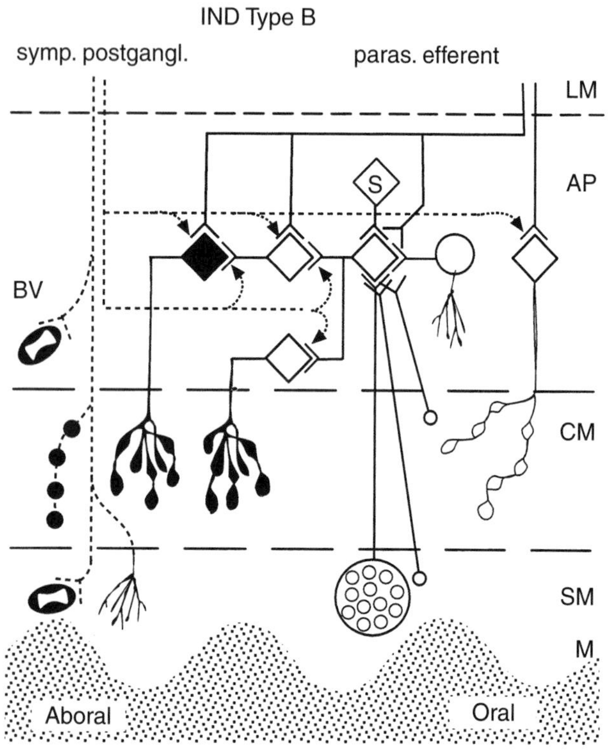

FIGURE 34-3. Schematic of bowel innervation in intestinal neuronal dysplasia type B. Note the increased size of ganglia, increased number of ganglion cells, increased density of ganglions, and heterotopic ganglion cells in the muscularis mucosae and lamina propria mucosae. AP, Auerbach's plexus; BV, blood vessel; CM, circular muscle; LM, longitudinal muscle; M, mucosa; S, pacemaker neuron with spontaneous activity; SM, submucosa.

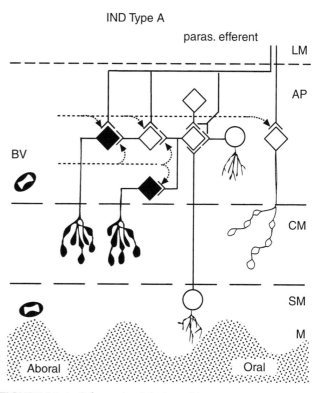

FIGURE 34-4. Schematic of the bowel innervation in intestinal neuronal dysplasia type A: aplasia or hypoplasia of the sympathetic innervation of the myenteric plexus and the arterial vessels. AP, Auerbach's plexus; BV, blood vessel; CM, circular muscle; LM, longitudinal muscle; M, mucosa; SM, submucosa.

Desmosis of the Colon

Desmosis of the colon recently was described as a cause of heterotopia of ganglion cells. The disease is characterized by a defect or a partial lack of the connective tissue net of the muscular wall of the intestine, leading to impairment of propulsive gut activity.[42]

Acquired Ganglion Cell Damage

Acquired aganglionosis and hypoganglionosis may be nonvascular or vascular in origin. Nonvascular causes for acquired aganglionosis include *Trypanosoma cruzi* infection (Chagas' disease), vitamin B$_1$ deficiencies, and chronic infections such as tuberculosis. Ischemic ganglion cell damage is caused by an inadequate blood supply in a pull-through segment, tension on both the arterial and venous blood supply during a pull-through procedure, or damage to the mesenteric vessels. Five cases were analyzed, with 11 additional cases from the literature.[43] In all children, a pull-through procedure according to Swenson, Duhamel, or Soave had been performed. We know of one case of acquired hypoganglionosis.[44]

Associated Malformations

Associated abnormalities are present in 11% to 30% of the children with HD.[2] However, when HD patients were routinely screened by a clinical geneticist, the number with associated anomalies increased to 48%. In our recent series of 203 patients, the familial pattern was observed in 11%,[41] with 35% having associated malformations. The most common disorders were of the urogenital tract (11%), cardiovascular system (6%), and gastrointestinal system (6%), with 8% having various other malformations such as cataract, coloboma, cleft palate, and extremity or cerebral defects. Prematurity is reported in as many as 10% of the children with HD.

Down Syndrome

Three percent of HD patients are reported to have Down syndrome, which is 4 times the incidence in the population as a whole.[45] In our series, 6% of the patients with HD had Down syndrome.[41] Constipation in Down syndrome patients also may be caused by hypothyroidism, hypotonia, or mental retardation. Therefore difficulties in the differential diagnosis of constipation in patients with Down syndrome result in a high incidence of enterocolitis. In addition to trisomy 21, other chromosomal anomalies are associated with HD, such as deletion of chromosomes 2, 10, and 13, and partial trisomies 11 and 22.

Waardenburg's and Other Syndromes

The sympathetic ganglia of the gastrointestinal tract originate from neuroectodermal cells. These neural crest cells, especially those of the somites 4 and 5, migrate from the neural tube to the gut and contribute to the ENS. The neural crest caudal to somite 3 is primarily responsible for ENS formation in the colon. Studies indicate that ENS precursors might migrate along a ventrolateral pathway, whereas cells from the rhombencephalic neural crest down to the caudal boundary of somite 3 migrate predominantly via dorsolateral pathways to the pharyngeal arches.[46] Some evidence also exists of different migration pathways between the anterior and posterior vagal neural crest. While migrating to their final position in the gut, the neural crest cells receive signals from the enteric microenvironment, which indicate when and where to stop migration and to form ganglia. One of these factors might be laminin, an extracellular matrix molecule normally present in the basal laminae of the mucosal and serosal epithelium and of the smooth muscle cells of the gut. The neural crest cells acquire a receptor for laminin while migrating to the gut. The interaction of laminin and its receptor may determine the destination of neural crest cells, but the factors that interfere with ganglion cell formation are unknown.

Waardenburg's syndrome is characterized by pigmentation anomalies caused by the fact that neural crest cells almost all form melanocytes. The syndrome is associated with inner ear deafness combined with facial abnormalities. Shah-Waardenburg's syndrome, the association of Waardenburg's syndrome with HD, is probably dependent on *SOX10* gene mutation.[47] The mode of inheritance of Waardenburg's syndrome has been proposed as autosomal dominant.[34]

In addition to Shah-Waardenburg's syndrome, several other specific pedigrees and phenotypes have been reported. HD with microcephaly, mental retardation, and facial dysmorphisms (hypertelorism, megalocornea, dense eyebrows, and anteverted ears) represents a syndrome that was eventually correlated with *EDNRB* Ser 305 Asn-variant.[48] HD with congenital central hypoventilation syndrome (Haddad's syndrome)[49] probably is correlated with incomplete penetrance of *GDNF* and *RET* mutations, as observed in HD and *EDN3* gene mutation in congenital hypoventilation syndrome, "Ondine's curse." Twenty-seven percent of 161 cases with Ondine's syndrome in the literature were associated with HD.[50-52] Multiple endocrine neoplasia type II (MEN-II) is an association of medullary thyroid carcinoma, pheochromocytoma, multiple mucosal neuromas, characteristic phenotype, and, occasionally, HD. The association of pheochromocytoma, medullary thyroid carcinoma, hyperparathyroidism, and Cushing's disease is called Sipple's syndrome.[53] The association of medullary thyroid carcinoma, pheochromocytoma, and multiple ganglioneuromas is designated MEN-IIA, and the combination without parathyroid disease but with severe constipation due to multiple intestinal ganglioneuromas or aganglionosis, MEN-IIB syndrome.[54] The genetic defect for these familial syndromes is not yet known.

Associated Anomalies of the Intestine

Congenital atresia of the small or large intestine, meconium ileus, and imperforate anus are sometimes associated with HD, hypoganglionosis, or IND. In 1994, we reported on 19 HD patients with small bowel atresia.[39]

Five also had hypoganglionosis, and 2, IND. In a recent study, just more than half of 52 patients with anorectal malformations had ENS disorders: 9 had aganglionosis in the rectal pouch specimens, 11 had hypoganglionosis, 4 had IND type B, and 3 had dysganglionosis.[55] Only in 2 (4%) patients were the innervation patterns of the fistula or rectal pouch found to be normal. Another report of 30 children with intestinal atresia who had associated HD emphasizes the association.[56]

Other Associated Anomalies

Associated urogenital anomalies have been reported with a frequency of 23%.[1] In our series, the incidence was 11%.[41] However, it became evident that voiding problems frequently occur in patients with an enlarged rectum, which compresses the bladder neck, with subsequent bladder neck obstruction and megacystis. Bladder function in these patients may mimic that of patients with spinal lesions, and it might be difficult to wean these patients from the urinary catheter in the postoperative period.

The incidence of cardiac abnormalities in HD has been reported to range from 2% to 8%, compared with 0.5% to 1% in the normal population.[45] This pertains not only to patients with Down syndrome, who frequently have associated endocardial cushion defects. A 12% incidence of associated eye abnormalities, including microphthalmia and anophthalmia, also is found.[45] We have seen a child with total intestinal HD, who also had glaucoma affecting both eyes.

CLINICAL PRESENTATION

Most children with HD have intestinal obstruction or severe constipation during the neonatal period. The cardinal symptoms are failure of passage of meconium within the first 24 hours of life, abdominal distention, and vomiting. The severity of these symptoms and the degree of constipation vary considerably between patients and in individual cases. Therefore some infants have complete intestinal obstruction, whereas others have relatively few symptoms in the first weeks or months of life. They may later have persistent constipation, particularly in response to changes in feeding, such as weaning from the breast to cow's milk or weaning onto solids. Patients in whom HD is diagnosed later in life have a long history of constipation, severe abdominal distention with a dilated drumlike belly, multiple fecal masses, and, often, enterocolitis. In some, growth impairment may occur. In these children, fecal retention and meteorism lead to secondary symptoms such as anorexia and cachexia with subsequent hypoproteinemia and anemia.

Rectal examination, a rectal tube, thermometer, or washouts may induce explosive discharge of fluid stool and gas suggestive of enterocolitis. This may lead to a remission of symptoms for a short time, and then abdominal distention recurs. On rectal examination, the anal sphincter is hypertonic, and the rectum is typically empty.

Diarrhea is common and was found in as many as one third of the children whose HD was diagnosed before age 3 months.[57] It may also be considered to be a symptom of enterocolitis, which is the most serious complication of aganglionosis. However, HD-associated enterocolitis has not been clearly defined. Whereas some authors consider diarrhea alone a mild form of enterocolitis,[53,54] others confine enterocolitis to instances with mucosal ulceration and sepsis.[58,60,61]

Enterocolitis is reported to occur in 12% to 58% of patients with HD.[59,62-65] Various hypotheses have been postulated to explain its occurrence. Fecal stasis has been suggested to result in mucosal ischemia with bacterial invasion and translocation. Furthermore, alterations in mucin components and mucosal defense mechanisms,[66-68] alterations in intestinal neuroendocrine cell populations,[69] an increased prostaglandin E_1 activity,[70] and infection with *Clostridium difficile*[71] or rotavirus[72] have been suggested to cause the condition. The pathogenesis of HD-associated enterocolitis remains unclear, and patients may have persistent symptoms even after diversion of the fecal stream by colostomy.[67,73,74]

Enterocolitis in its most severe form may lead to life-threatening toxic megacolon. It is characterized by fever, bile-stained vomiting, explosive diarrhea, abdominal distention, dehydration, and shock.[57,59] Ulceration and ischemic necrosis of the mucosa above the aganglionic segment may lead to sepsis, pneumatosis, and perforation. Therefore the possibility of underlying HD should be considered in all children with necrotizing enterocolitis. Spontaneous perforation has been reported in as many as 3% of the patients with HD.[59,75] A strong correlation exists between the length of the aganglionic bowel and the incidence of perforation.

DIAGNOSIS

HD is suspected on the basis of history and clinical findings. The diagnosis is established with radiologic examination, anorectal manometry, and histochemical analysis of biopsy specimens.

Radiologic Diagnosis

The diagnosis may be suspected when supine and erect plain abdominal radiographs show air/fluid levels in the colon. In children with suspected HD, a contrast enema is routinely applied. Newborns should not have digital examination or rectal washouts before contrast enema, as these procedures may result in a false-negative diagnosis. In particular, in patients with suspected meconium ileus or meconium plug syndrome, a water-soluble contrast medium should always be preferred to barium to reduce the obstruction. The classic finding is that of a normal-caliber rectum or narrow distal segment, a funnel-shaped dilation at the level of the transition zone, and a marked dilation of the proximal colon. In questionable cases, retention of contrast medium in the colon for more than 24 hours may be helpful in establishing the diagnosis (Fig. 34-5).

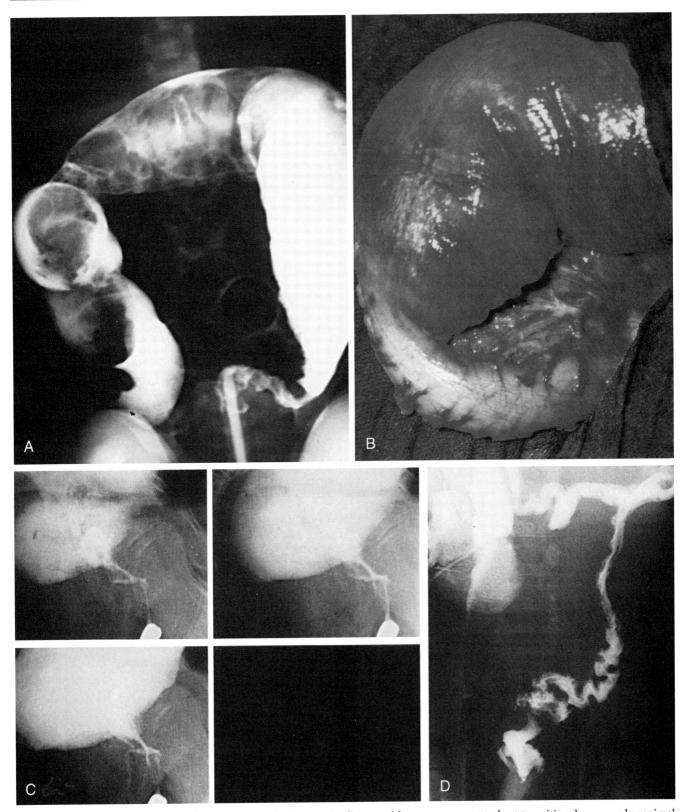

FIGURE 34-5. *A,* Classic radiographic finding of Hirschsprung's disease with narrow segment, short transitional zone, and proximal dilation. *B,* Intraoperative picture. *C,* Defecography showing ultrashort Hirschsprung's disease. *D,* Long-segment Hirschsprung's disease (Zuelzer–Wilson syndrome).

Contrast enema examination has been reported to be inconclusive in 10% of children with confirmed HD and in 29% of cases with HD-associated IND type B.[41] In children with total aganglionosis, the colon is not significantly narrowed, and reflux into the distended ileum may be diagnostic.[76] Children with enterocolitis may show thickening of the bowel wall with mucosal irregularity and grossly distended bowel loops on plain films. In these cases, a characteristic transitional zone may not be present because of inflammatory impairment of muscular function in the normally innervated colon.

The assessment of the intestinal transit time by using radiopaque markers offers an opportunity to identify the level of an eventual impairment of transport. The transit time is always prolonged in classic aganglionosis, and determining the most distal point reached by transport markers may help in identifying the level of resection. In addition, the clinical impact of associated intestinal neuronal malformations such as IND type B or hypoganglionosis can be determined.[77] No one method of evaluation of intestinal transport is generally accepted. One study used three different forms of markers given on 3 consecutive days with an abdominal radiograph on day 4.[78] Others rely on radiographs on days 5 or 7.[79] We give 20 markers simultaneously, repeating the abdominal radiograph every 24 hours for 3 days (Fig. 34-6).

The technique also can be used in children with an enterostoma before a pull-through procedure to measure the transport from the distal stoma to the anus.

Anorectal Electromanometry

The diagnostic accuracy of anorectal manometry for HD has been reported to be as high as 85%.[41,80–82] Normally, distention of the rectum by using a balloon results in relaxation of the internal sphincter. In HD, the pressure profile of the anal canal and lower rectum in conjunction with the distending stimulus shows characteristic changes that also occasionally are found in other intestinal malformations. In children with aganglionosis, multisegmental rhythmic contractions or waves were pathognomonic (Fig. 34-7). On distention of a balloon in the rectum, no rectal or anal inhibitory response is noted. The anorectal pressure profile is sometimes elevated. Patients with hypoganglionosis or IND also may have a missing or rudimentary response.[41] However, anorectal manometry can be misleading in newborns. We believe that the normal rectosphincteric reflex is complete by day 12 of life.[83] This reflex has not been identified in children younger than 39 weeks in gestational age or in those weighing less than 2.7 kg. With these caveats, anorectal manometry is an excellent screening tool for HD and allied disorders.

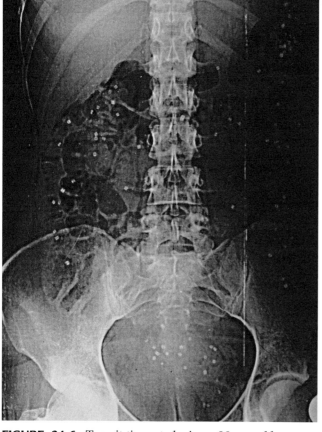

FIGURE 34-6. Transit-time study in a 36-year-old woman with intestinal neuronal dysplasia 11 days after ingestion of barium pellets.

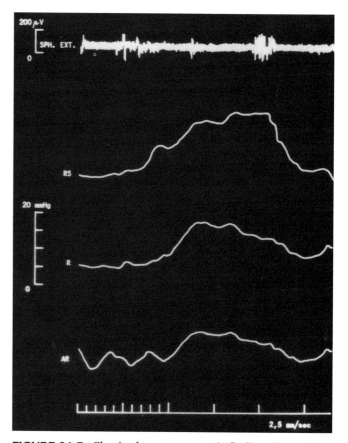

FIGURE 34-7. Classic electromanometric findings in a patient with Hirschsprung's disease: no internal sphincter relaxations but multisegmental mass contractions.

Rectal Biopsy

HD is diagnosed with examination of rectal biopsy specimens. Since the introduction of suction biopsy techniques,[84] the procedure has become less traumatic and can be performed without anesthesia. Suction biopsy specimens are taken at 2 cm, 3 cm, 5 cm, and, if possible, higher up above the dentate line. They also may be taken proximal and distal to a proposed stoma. However, the optimal size of a biopsy is approximately 3.5 mm in diameter, to include submucosa. Perforation and bleeding due to suction biopsies have been reported in newborns. Ganglion cells in the newborn can be immature and not clearly visible without special staining techniques (LDH, SDH reaction). Small suction biopsies are not always representative for the whole involved segment. Aganglionosis may therefore be overdiagnosed at birth, leading to unnecessary resections if the definitive procedure is performed in the newborn period. Hypoganglionosis may be missed when the biopsies contain only submucous plexus. In children with suspected hypoganglionosis or heterotopia of the myenteric plexus, full-thickness biopsies are recommended (Figs. 34-8 and 34-9).

DIFFERENTIAL DIAGNOSIS

In the newborn infant, it may be clinically difficult to differentiate between meconium plug syndrome, small left colon syndrome, HD, and allied ENS disorders. In addition, neonatal sepsis and brain injury may result in a delayed passage of meconium. However, newborns and infants with symptoms of an ileus or enterocolitis should always be suspected to have HD or one of the allied disorders. In these patients, a contrast enema, histochemical examination of suction biopsies, and perhaps manometry will establish the diagnosis of aganglionosis.

Various other conditions may cause chronic constipation and intestinal obstruction in infants and children. These include inadequate dietary habits, psychological disorders, hypomotility caused by medication, and metabolic or endocrine conditions such as uremia or

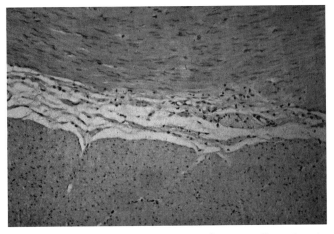

FIGURE 34-8. Histologic examination (hematoxylin and eosin staining): aganglionosis of the myenteric plexus.

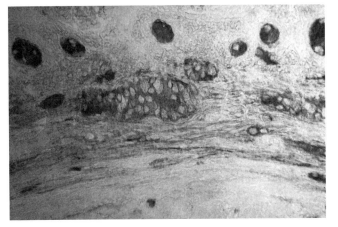

FIGURE 34-9. Histochemical examination: giant and heterotopic ganglion cells in the submucous plexus of a patient with intestinal neuronal dysplasia.

hypothyroidism. Other conditions that may produce constipation include disorders of the intrinsic enteric nerves (diabetes or dysautonomia), central nervous system diseases, and smooth muscle dysfunction. Intestinal smooth muscle disorders include hollow visceral myopathy syndrome and other myopathic disorders. Abnormalities of contractile proteins and connective tissue disorders such as scleroderma or dermatomyositis also may lead to persistent constipation.

Megacystis/microcolon/intestinal hypoperistalsis syndrome, a rare cause of chronic intestinal obstruction in the newborn, is generally fatal. Degenerative changes in the smooth muscle cells with an abundant amount of connective tissue may be the cause of the disease, but the etiology remains unclear.[85] Not more than 70 cases have been described.[86] Abdominal distention is caused by lax abdominal musculature and a distended bladder. Characteristically incomplete intestinal rotation and microcolon with decreased peristalsis are found. Barium enema demonstration of a microcolon and ultrasonographic or intravenous urographic evidence of hydronephrosis and megacystis help to differentiate the condition from HD.

MANAGEMENT

The ENS is the brain of the intestine. Similar to the brain, it functions automatically to some degree, even when some neural mechanisms are deficient. Therefore affected newborns may be admitted with intestinal obstruction, whereas others are first seen later in childhood or adulthood with chronic constipation. Once symptomatic, most patients require decompression as the first step of management.

Decompression

Decompression in the obstructed newborn is performed by introducing a nasogastric tube and by repeated emptying of the rectum with rectal tubes and irrigations. After the diagnosis is established by radiologic, electromano-metric, and histochemical techniques, an appropriate stoma is established if necessary. Occasionally patients can be managed satisfactorily over longer periods with irrigations or other conservative means to ensure daily evacuation.

Colostomy

Our preference in the newborn who is obstructed by HD is to establish an enterostomy. We believe that the definitive procedures can be performed more satisfactorily outside the newborn period. In our opinion, enterostomy can be avoided only in children who are older than 3 to 5 months when the diagnosis is established.

Before performing a colostomy, a bowel washout is mandatory. Antibiotics are given intravenously 30 minutes before the operation. A urethral catheter is introduced to achieve bladder decompression during the operation and to provide postoperative drainage. We usually create a "loop" colostomy or ileostomy with a skin bridge beneath. Care should be taken not to narrow the proximal stoma, which might create a partial obstruction. Prolapse of the bowel, the second most frequent complication, can be avoided by suturing the afferent and efferent segments of the bowel loop together within the abdomen. The stoma is preferably constructed by using the right transverse colonic flexure, to be left in place during the definitive resection. It will be closed 2 weeks later. When near-total or total colectomy is necessary, the procedure is protected by an ileostomy.

A leveling end colostomy with frozen-section confirmation of the level of ganglion cells is an alternative management technique. In this case, the aganglionic distal bowel is closed as a Hartmann pouch. The pull-through is not protected by a colostomy.

DEFINITIVE PROCEDURES

Swenson and Bill[87] performed the first resection of an aganglionic segment in 1948. Since then, three other basic techniques have been developed (Fig. 34-10).

Swenson's Technique

The patient is positioned to provide simultaneous surgical access to the abdomen and perineum. Seromuscular or full-thickness biopsies are taken to establish the proximal extent of aganglionosis by rapid staining techniques. The proximal colon and mesentery are dissected to achieve a sufficient length for reconstruction without compromising the blood supply.

The peritoneal reflection at the rectosigmoid is then incised, both ureters and vas deferens are identified, and the deep pelvic dissection commenced. The dissection is performed close to the rectal wall to protect the pelvic autonomic nervous system. Division of the rectosigmoid is accomplished by a stapling device at a convenient level. A long, curved clamp is then inserted through the anus to grasp the rectosigmoid stump and

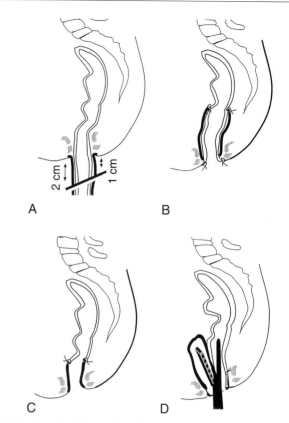

FIGURE 34-10. Schematic of principles of pull-through and anastomotic techniques according to Swenson (*A*), Soave (*B*), Rehbein (*C*), and Duhamel (*D*).

invert it. The mucocutaneous line should be clearly visible. An oblique incision is made through the anterior half of the prolapsed rectum, and a clamp is inserted into the pelvis to grasp and pull through the proximal ganglionated segment through the anus. The proximal bowel wall is now divided, and an extra-anal anastomosis is performed with interrupted absorbable sutures approximating first the muscular coats and then the mucosal layers. Finally, the anastomosis is permitted to recede into the pelvis (see Fig. 34-10*A*).

Duhamel-Grob Procedure

The principles of this procedure are preservation of the internal anal sphincter; opening of the retrorectal space only, followed by retrorectal pull-through of the ganglionic part of the colon; and elimination of the colorectal septum. The rectum is divided and closed just above the peritoneal reflection. Resection of the aganglionic colon is then performed. The retrorectal space is developed bluntly down to the pelvic floor. In the original Duhamel procedure,[88,89] a long, curved forceps fitted with a small sponge is pushed into this space to evert the posterior rectal wall through the anus. The posterior half of the rectum is incised just above the dentate line. Grob[90] incised the posterior wall 1.5 to 2.5 cm above the mucocutaneous junction. The sponge can then be grasped by another curved clamp, which is pushed in a retrograde manner into the pelvis. The colon then can easily be pulled through the endoanal incision. At a level where ganglion cells have been demonstrated, the colon is transected and anastomosed to the cut edge of the rectum, creating an end-to-side colorectal anastomosis. The ultimate side-to-side anastomosis of the anterior aganglionic rectum and posterior ganglionated colon is created either by crushing the septum or by use of a long stapling device. Today, the rectocolic anastomosis is most often performed with a stapling device.[91] This technique must avoid the creation of an anterior blind rectal pouch, which will lead to retention of feces and obstruction (see Fig. 34-10*D*).

Anterior Resection According to Rehbein

Rehbein's technique differs from Swenson's procedure, in that the anastomosis is a low, anterior colorectal anastomosis. The pelvirectal dissection is completed, leaving the aganglionic terminal 2 to 3 cm of the rectum in infants and 4 to 5 cm in older children. Vigorous sphincter dilation with Hegar's bougies is performed intraoperatively up to one size over the size of the stapling instrument chosen for anastomosis. We perform this bougienage under direct vision to avoid bowel rupture. Dilation of the internal anal sphincter is extremely important and must be repeated in later years because the internal anal sphincter remains aganglionic (sphincter achalasia). However, deep dissection of the upper and middle rectum decreases the resting internal anal sphincter tone.

The anastomosis may be performed by using a circular end-to-end anastomosis (EEA) stapling instrument introduced through the anus[92] or by direct suture deep in the pelvis. In these cases, the anastomosis is constructed by using interrupted 4-0 absorbable sutures. An extraperitoneal drain is placed, the peritoneum is closed above the anastomosis, and a transanastomotic drain is inserted through the anus. The drain can be removed after 10 to 12 days when a contrast enema shows a healed anastomosis. Gentle dilation of the anus with Hegar dilators is then commenced. The size of the dilators is gradually increased with time until the fifth finger can easily pass the anastomosis (see Fig. 34-10*C*).

Endorectal Pull-Through

The use of extramucosal dissection of the rectosigmoid was proposed[93,94] for the treatment of high imperforate anus and was later used by Soave[95] in HD cases to avoid primary anastomosis. The first steps of the procedure are similar to the techniques described previously. After opening of the peritoneal reflection, the rectum is dissected over at least an additional 2 cm extraperitoneally. Procaine hydrochloride in saline solution (0.5%) is injected between the mucosal and muscular layers of the upper rectum to facilitate the dissection. The rectal muscle is incised, and the mucosal tube is freed distally. The mucosal dissection is continued to the level of the dentate line. The progress of the dissection may be assessed by having an assistant's finger introduced into the anus. The mucosa is incised circumferentially at about 1 cm above the dentate line. Soave's procedure requires more

mobilization of the colon than does Rehbein's technique. The mucosal sleeve is grasped and used as a tractor to pull the colon through to the established level of ganglion cells. This pull-through may be done by attaching the mucosa to a catheter introduced transanally or by using a ring forceps. The abdominal part of the operation is completed by suturing the proximal free end of the aganglionic rectal cuff to the seromuscular layer of the pulled-through colon. The perineal stage is completed by anchoring the serosa of the colon to the everted anal canal mucosa. A Penrose drain is placed extraperitoneally between the rectal muscle sleeve and then pulled through colon.

After 10 days, when the serosa of the ganglionic colon is adherent to the rectal muscle sleeve, the protruding colon stump is amputated, and a mucosa-to-mucosa anastomosis is done (see Fig. 34-10*B*).

Boley's procedure uses the same endorectal technique but is completed at one sitting with a primary two-layer anastomosis at the pectinate line.[96] Others have added a posterior rectal myotomy and a partial sphincterectomy to avoid anorectal dysfunction, which could result from anal sphincter achalasia.[97,98] However, sphincteromyectomy increases the risk of fecal incontinence. Boley's procedure has become the more popular in neonates.

Laparoscopic Pull-Through Techniques

Advancements in minimally invasive surgery and instrumentation have resulted in pull-through procedures being performed with laparoscopic techniques. The postulated advantages are minimal postoperative pain, more rapid return of bowel function, shorter postoperative recovery, and improved cosmetic appearance. However, the advantages of laparoscopic pull-through techniques have not yet been assessed by randomized trials comparing laparoscopy with the open technique.

Most surgeons who treat HD endoscopically have used a modified Swenson's pull-through technique,[99-101] but the Duhamel method and the Soave technique have been performed laparoscopically as well. The reported techniques were used both for primary pull-through and in patients with diverting enterostomy. Laparoscopic Swenson's pull-through is performed by using three 5-mm trocars and standard laparoscopic instruments. The mesentery is mobilized laparoscopically up to the level of the inferior mesenteric artery, which may be divided in patients with a high transition zone. Dissection close to the bowel wall results in minimal bleeding. Laparoscopic pelvic dissection is extended circumferentially to the level of the prostate or cervix and the coccyx. After some transanal submucosal dissection, the smooth muscle fibers of the rectal sleeve are transected, and the colon is pulled through. The colon is transected and sutured to the everted rectal wall.[100]

The laparoscopic Duhamel procedure is performed via four trocars.[102] After laparoscopic mobilization of the colon, the rectum is divided at the peritoneal level by using a stapler. The colon is pulled through an incision made through the posterior rectal wall, and a side-to-side anastomosis is performed as usual. Two or more applications of the stapling device inserted through the anus may be necessary.[103,104]

Operative times required for the laparoscopic Swenson procedure have been reported to be similar to those for the open technique.[99,100] The duration of the Duhamel procedure was somewhat longer.[102,105] Most children were discharged from the hospital between postoperative days 2 and 7, which is shorter than the duration of hospital stay with the conventional open technique. The reported rate of complications was not higher with laparoscopy. However, the experience with the technique remains limited to special centers, and the number of patients who have undergone the procedure to date is extremely small. Laparoscopic therapy of HD is a promising technique, particularly with refinements in instrumentation.

Laparoscopic Soave was used, too, and is now the procedure of choice in the modification of de la Torre-Monragoú and Ortega Salgados[106] technique of transanal endorectal pull-through. This operation is frequently performed as a primary procedure without colostomy.

Primary Pull-Through

Primary pull-through in the newborn was introduced mostly by surgeons who prefer Boley's procedure.[107–109] They postulate that endorectal dissection is more difficult to perform in older children than in infants because of tenacious adhesions in the submucous plane caused by chronic proctitis and daily enemas. During the first 3 months of life and especially in the newborn, the rectum shows less inflammation, and the dissection between the submucous layer and muscular cylinder is easy to perform. Primary endorectal pull-through usually does not require a protective colostomy, except in patients with enterocolitis. However, the dissection of the last 1 to 2 cm just above the pectinate line is difficult in the newborn, and the mucosal cylinder is very easily damaged.

A reliable histologic and histochemical diagnosis is difficult to establish in the newborn. Adequate suction biopsies taken above the peritoneal reflection can be dangerous in newborns, and perforations have been reported in that age group. At birth, ganglion cells may be immature, and the cytoplasm may not be visualized by hematoxylin and eosin staining. Because ganglia may not mature for months or years, primary pull-through procedures may lead to excessive or inadequate resection in some newborns. The reported results of primary pull-through are not better than those of staged treatment. In a reported series of 24 patients, 1 died, bowel volvulus developed in 1, 9 (39%) had recurrent enterocolitis, and 12 (42%) were constipated.[110]

Transanal Endorectal Pull-Through

Primary transanal rectosigmoidectomy has been growing in popularity with acceptable early results in the recent years.[106,111–117] After full anal dilatation and preparation of the anorectal cavity with povidine-iodine, the rectal mucosa is incised circumferentially 1 to 1.5 cm above the dentate line, as described by Boley.[96] With blunt dissection, a submucosal space is developed and extended 6 to

7 cm. After we pull on the mucosa, the denuded rectum protrudes out of the anus and begins to form a muscular sleeve. The rectal muscle is now completely incised to reach the perirectal tissue. This can be done with laparoscopic help to avoid damage to intrapelvic structures such as the ureters. Perirectal tissue and smooth muscle fibers of the rectum are dissected to liberate the muscle sleeve, which can now return to its original position. A posterior myotomy of the sleeve completes this step of the operation. The rectum can now easily be pulled down, and the mesenteric vessels divided. If the colon is completely freed, the transitional zone can be observed macroscopically. Full-thickness biopsy specimens are examined to assure normoganglionosis. Finally, the aganglionic and hypoganglionic transitory segment is removed and a Boley-type anastomosis of the pulled-through colon and the rectal mucosa is established.

The results are so far very encouraging, but late results have not yet been published. The technique seems to be the treatment of choice for typical HD cases with aganglionosis at the level of the rectosigmoid. Whether it is best performed as a primary procedure in the newborn and with or without protective colostomy is not yet clear.

TREATMENT OF TOTAL COLONIC AGANGLIONOSIS

For the treatment of total colon aganglionosis, Martin[118,119] introduced a long side-to-side anastomosis between the normal ileum and aganglionic descending colon and the rectum—essentially an extension of the Duhamel side-to-side anastomosis. Theoretically, the long aganglionic rectosigmoid segment should allow resorption of fluid and electrolytes, and recent experience has borne this out.[120] The operation should be performed at age 1 year, when the performing of the rectal and pelvic anastomosis is easier. A stapler is applied twice or more to create a long side-to-side anastomosis between the aganglionic rectum and the ganglionated terminal ileum.

Unfortunately, Martin's modification of Duhamel's procedure has not completely eliminated complications such as frequent and liquid stools, excoriated perineum, enterocolitis, and nighttime incontinence, which occur in as many as 60% of the patients.[121] Therefore we prefer the Rehbein deep anterior resection in patients with total colonic aganglionosis.[122] The persistent rectal achalasia increases transit time and the resorption capability of the ileum without increasing the frequency of enterocolitis. We use a protective ileostomy to protect the anastomosis during the healing phase. Improved bowel resorptive function has been reported by establishment of a right colon onlay patch.[123,124]

POSTOPERATIVE CARE

Some patients experience normal bowel function shortly after the operation. However, in more extended resections, frequent and liquid stools cause excoriation of the perineum. In these patients, loperamide may reduce the frequency of defecation, and kaolin-pectin suspension may help to solidify the stools. In some children, allergic diarrhea develops after they consume milk products, food preservatives, nuts, strawberries, or other substances. In patients without an ileocecal valve or with a short remnant colon, cholestyramine is helpful to bind bile salts, which should be absorbed in the terminal ileum. Special diets are often necessary to improve stool consistency (e.g., bananas, carrots, blueberries) or to treat constipation (e.g., rhubarb, prune juice, bran).

COMPLICATIONS

The predominant problems after Swenson's and Duhamel's procedures are fecal incontinence and persistent constipation. The major complication after Rehbein's technique is anastomotic leakage, with subsequent stricture formation. Soave's and Boley's operations are complicated by bowel retraction, cuff abscesses, and rectal stenosis caused by the aganglionic rectal muscle cuff. However, all these methods achieve an excellent result in more than 90% of the children.[125]

Early Complications

Complications that become manifest within the first 4 weeks after operation are usually the result of technical errors or infection.[126] In an international study of 439 patients with HD from 16 different pediatric surgical centers, anastomotic leaks were observed in 7%, anastomotic strictures in 15%, and wound infections in 11% of the children.[125] The pulled-through colon retracted in 3% of the children who had Swenson's procedure and in 7% who underwent Soave's technique. Rehbein's technique showed a leak in 2.8% of 176 cases.

The most frequent early complications after Swenson's and Duhamel's procedures were anastomotic leaks. A survey of the surgical section of the American Academy of Pediatrics (AAP),[127] which included more than 5000 procedures performed by 181 surgeons, revealed anastomotic leaks in 11% after Swenson's procedure and 2.4% after Duhamel's procedure. One-fourth of the children with anastomotic disruption after Swenson's technique required a second pull-through, and 11% ultimately had a permanent colostomy. A collected series of 1628 procedures for HD in Japan revealed that anastomotic leaks occurred in 8% after rectosigmoidectomy (Swenson or Rehbein), 7% after Duhamel's procedure, 1% after Soave's endorectal pull-through, and 7% after a Boley procedure.[63] The data from Children's Memorial Hospital in Chicago, which include Swenson's personal experience, revealed anastomotic leaks in 5.6% of 880 patients.[75] In a smaller experience with the Duhamel procedure from another institution, only 1 of 185 patients experienced a leak.[128] Fecal fistulas resulted from a leak in 6% of cases using the Swenson procedure, 3% of those using a Duhamel pull-through, and 1% of those using Soave's procedure.

Factors known to increase the risk of anastomotic leak are tension on the anastomosis, ischemia of the rectal cuff or distal colonic segment, incomplete anastomotic suture, and inadequate stapling. Anastomotic leaks always result in anastomotic stricture. Obstruction distal to the anastomosis increases the risk of disruption, so we advise a transanastomotic tube for the first 10 postoperative days. In case of any anastomotic leakage, an immediate enterostomy should performed. Almost all leaks heal spontaneously within 4 to 5 months.

Cuff abscess and retraction of the pull-through segment are most serious complications after Soave's and Boley's operations. Contamination of the cuff, incomplete removal of the mucosa, hemorrhage, or insufficient drainage may lead to formation of a cuff abscess or mucocele in as many as 5% of the patients. The lower anal channel should be meticulously inspected with a speculum during the operation to prevent leaving islands of mucosa. Creating an anastomosis without any tension but with good blood supply and interrupted full-thickness sutures may help to prevent this complication.

Disturbances of micturition occur more frequently in children who undergo surgery later in life. It is sometimes difficult to wean patients from the urinary catheter placed for the short postoperative period. Dribbling, incomplete urinary control, bladder atony, and ureteric obstruction all have been reported in children after pull-through operations.[129] Voiding dysfunction occurred mostly after Swenson's technique (12%) and Duhamel's technique (4%). The condition does not result from a malformation of the autonomic nerve supply to the bladder. Nerve fibers are most probably damaged during the operative procedure or by compression from the enlarged rectum before the operation.

Wound infections or intra-abdominal adhesions occur at a rate comparable to those for other major abdominal operations. No early mortality rate is seen for classic HD in the present day. However, for total colonic aganglionosis, the AAP Surgical Section survey conducted in the 1970s reported a mortality of 18%.[127] Current results have improved.

Late Complications

Chronic constipation, enterocolitis, and encopresis are the most relevant long-term problems. They are found more frequently during the first postoperative months and decrease within the following years. We found that 33% of the children with HD had constipation shortly after the operation, but only 9% reported persistent constipation after an average of 5 years.[73] The frequency of enterocolitis and of encopresis decreased with the passage of time.

Chronic constipation occurs mostly because of anal sphincter achalasia, incomplete resection, stricture formation, and fecaloma. Persistent constipation was reported in 6% of the patients after Swenson's procedure,[130] in 10% after Duhamel's technique,[131] and in 7% after Rehbein's resection.[132]

Anal sphincter achalasia is a frequent postoperative phenomenon. In our series,[125] 32% of patients underwent repeated sphincter dilation, and 13% required sphincteromyectomy. After Rehbein's technique, sphincter dilations are part of the follow-up plan, and bougienage is performed for weeks or months until the anastomosis can no longer be detected by rectal palpation. In Swenson's technique, Duhamel's technique, and some modifications of Soave's technique, internal sphincter myectomy is part of the original procedure. We found the anorectal resting pressure profile to be increased in only 8% of the children after 5 years, with no significant difference between the operative procedures used. Internal sphincter relaxations that had not been observed before treatment were present in 10% of the children at follow-up.

Incomplete resection cannot be avoided regardless of technique. Proximal to an aganglionic segment, hypoganglionosis is always found, and often, IND.[133] The extent of these associated malformations varies considerably in individual patients. Short-segment aganglionosis can be associated with long-segment hypoganglionosis and vice versa. Rapid staining techniques such as hematoxylin and eosin do not allow the reliable diagnosis of either hypoganglionosis or IND.[134] One analysis of 4873 patients with HD from the literature revealed recurrent constipation in 9%.[135] In our opinion, these patients continue to have constipation and/or attacks of enterocolitis due to insufficient resection of segments with hypoganglionosis or IND proximal to the aganglionosis. A second resection may be required when repeated sphincter dilations fail. We recently reported that reoperation was necessary in 5% of 81 children.[41] Reoperation was necessary in 20 of 215 children in another study; 9 underwent sphincteromyectomy, and 11 required a repeated pull-through.[136]

Enterocolitis was reported in the Surgical Section survey to occur in 16% of the children undergoing rectosigmoidectomy (Swenson or Rehbein), in 6% undergoing Duhamel's pull-through, in 15% undergoing the Soave technique, and in 2% undergoing the Boley procedure.[127] After Rehbein's procedure, enterocolitis was diagnosed in 10%.[41] In our international study, enterocolitis was identified in 4% of the patients after rectosigmoidectomy, in 6% after anterior resection, in 13% after endorectal pull-through without anastomosis, and in 5% after retrorectal pull-through.[108] A literature review found an overall incidence of 8% in 5919 patients.[135] In 1628 Japanese patients, enterocolitis occurred in 34% after Swenson's procedure, in 14% after Duhamel's procedure, in 20% after Soave's procedure, and in 12% following Boley's operation.[63] According to published reports, the incidence of enterocolitis after repair of HD has not changed during recent years.[137]

Strictures result from anastomotic leaks, a narrow rectal muscle cuff around a pulled-through colon, or damage to the blood supply of the cuff or colon. Strictures occurred in 7% of patients having a retrorectal pull-through and 9% of patients having an endorectal pull-through.[137]

Fecal incontinence (soiling, encopresis) does not occur after Rehbein's technique[135] but occurred in 12% of the cases after Swenson's procedures, in 7% after Duhamel's technique, and in 3% following Soave's procedure. Two of 81 of our patients had encopresis; both had sphincteromyectomies performed elsewhere.[41] Incontinence was noted in 9% of the children after Swenson's procedure but in only 3% after Duhamel's technique in the Japanese study.[63] Soiling was noted in 22 of 63 children after Duhamel's operation,[136] in 8% after Swenson's,[130] and in 3% after Soave's[138]; however, in this study, soiling occurred in only 1% after Boley's operation. Long-segment disease is associated with a higher incidence of incontinence and soiling, which occur particularly during nighttime. Fecaloma is a complication unique to Duhamel's technique. One study reported that in 17.5% of the patients, fecal impaction and overflow incontinence developed.[125]

Long-term voiding dysfunction is rare and is observed in mostly older children with long-lasting chronic constipation and an enlarged rectum. In these patients, a large atonic bladder develops, sometimes with enlargement of the ureters and pelvis of the kidney as a result of compression of the bladder neck. The condition is mostly reversible within months after definitive repair. In a urodynamic study on 68 patients with HD, we found a spontaneous improvement of urinary incontinence from 22% to 6% within 10 years of follow-up.[139] Three children had occasional enuresis, and one girl with mental retardation remained incontinent. Sexual dysfunction has been reported in 9% of the patients after Duhamel's procedure and in 10% after Swenson's operation.[138] The authors found dyspareunia in female patients and primary infertility, poor erections, low sperm counts, and psychosexual problems in male patients.

The late mortality compiled from published data[135] ranged from 2% after Soave's procedure to 5% after Swenson's technique and involved mostly patients with long-segment aganglionosis. Similar results were reported by the Surgical Section of the AAP,[127] with a mortality ranging from 1% for Boley's technique to 3% for Soave's two-stage procedure.

ULTRASHORT-SEGMENT DISEASE

Ultrashort-segment HD is not rare. However, data on the incidence vary considerably because the term *ultrashort* is not clearly defined. One study estimated the incidence of ultrashort HD at 11% to 14% in relation to all aganglioses.[140] Another group reported on 10 children with ultrashort-segment disease of 106 children with chronic constipation.[141] In a group of patients diagnosed with HD, short-segment disease was found in 2.6% of patients.[23] The gender ratio was estimated to be five male patients to one female.

The postulated length of the ultrashort segment varied from 2 cm[142] to 10 cm.[143] In our opinion, the term should be restricted to the lowermost 2 to 4 cm of the anal channel above the mucocutaneous line, which means that the aganglionic segment comprises the lower half of the rectum from the dentate line upward to the third sacral vertebra. Shorter distances restricted to the internal anal sphincter are referred to as *neurogenic anal sphincter achalasia*. Preterm newborns were found to have a

2-mm "physiologic" aganglionic zone in the myenteric plexus and an aganglionic zone of 5 mm of the submucous plexus.[144] The length of this normal zone increased with age of the baby. In contrast, another anatomic study found few ganglion cells in the internal anal sphincter, with decreasing numbers as more distal sections were studied.[145] No clear definition exists of ultrashort-segment aganglionosis or of anal sphincter achalasia, and considerable individual variation in the ganglion cell distribution in the most distal intestinal tract may be found.

The pathophysiology and symptoms of this form of the malformation are similar to those of classic aganglionosis. Agenesis of NO fibers and increased AChE activity in the lamina propria mucosae and submucous plexus (but not in the myenteric plexus) are the most important pathophysiologic parameters.[119,146,147] The limited extent of the disease allows treatment with extended sphincteromyotomy. The procedures can be performed from inside the anus,[148] or from a posterior sagittal approach.[149] An ultrashort aganglionic segment can be associated with an extensive zone of hypoganglionosis, leading to persistent severe chronic constipation after sphincteromyotomy.

INTERNAL ANAL SPHINCTER ACHALASIA

Internal anal sphincter achalasia (IASA) is defined as the inability of the internal anal sphincter to relax. IASA may be an isolated disease of the ENS, or it may be an acquired condition of psychological (functional) origin with normal innervation patterns. However, it also may be part of HD or allied disorders (neurogenic anal sphincter achalasia).[23,25] The inability of the sphincter to relax can be shown by electromanometry and defecography. The findings are similar to the pathognomonic signs for HD. In hypoganglionosis, IND, and ganglion cell immaturity, the relaxation reflex may be absent, rudimentary, or normal.[41]

On rectal digital examination, the sphincter is hypertonic, but the rectum is impacted with stool just above the anal ring. Confirmation of the diagnosis requires biopsies taken at the mucocutaneous junction and a few centimeters above. Anal sphincter dilation under general anesthesia may be sufficient to treat the condition. In cases with persistent constipation, sphincteromyectomy is indicated. Functional (or psychogenic or acquired) IASA is found in 95% of the cases with chronic constipation. An α receptor–blocking medication (phenoxybenzamine) in addition to psychological treatment may be helpful[150] (see also Chapter 36).

INTESTINAL NEURONAL DYSPLASIA AND ALLIED DISORDERS

The diagnosis of intestinal neuronal malformations has become popularized after Meier-Ruge and other investigators classified IND, hypoganglionosis, and other dysganglionoses.[33,37,151,152] These malformations were found proximal to the aganglionic segment in HD,[41,65,153-155] and in patients with various clinical presentations such as chronic constipation,[41,153,156] intestinal pseudo-obstruction,[157] neurofibromatosis,[158] mucoviscidosis,[41,159] MEN-IIb,[157] anorectal malformations,[39,55] and small bowel atresia.[39] Numerous studies have dealt with the sequelae of these malformations, but the causal relation between specific histologic findings and clinical symptoms remains somewhat controversial.

Intestinal Neuronal Dysplasia Type A

IND type A is characterized by the paucity of sympathetic fibers and dysplasia of the submucous plexus. Clinical parasympathetic overactivity results in spasticity and ulceration of the colon.[160] The condition is extremely rare. Its dramatic clinical course is characterized by bloody stools combined with ileus.[40,160,161] Unanimous agreement is found that children with IND type A should undergo rectosigmoidectomy or even more extended resection of the colon.[160,161]

Intestinal Neuronal Dysplasia Type B

IND type B may be associated with a great variability of symptoms. Constipation was reported in 53% of children; more significant obstruction in 20%; colitis in 12%; and bloody stools, diarrhea, or vomiting, in fewer than 10%.[162] Other associated symptoms were encopresis, enuresis, or behavioral problems.[154] It remains unclear why some children have a dramatic clinical course such as meconium peritonitis, volvulus, or intussusception.[29,163]

Multiple treatment plans have been suggested, including laxatives and enemas, total parenteral nutrition, sphincteromyotomy, colostomy, and partial or total resection with or without leaving IND-affected bowel in place. The results have been discordant because of the wide variations in histochemical involvement and severity of symptoms. In our experience, 25% of the patients require surgical treatment including bowel resection, temporary enterostomy, and sphincteromyotomy.[41] Another surgeon found constipation to be so severe that bowel resection was required in five of nine patients, three of whom died.[151] Posterior sphincteromyotomy was reported to be necessary in 59% of patients in one series, with a cure rate of 90% within 3 months.[161] No bowel was resected in this series. The concept of "temporary" colostomy in patients with severe symptoms is supported by a study that identified a normalization of biopsy findings after 5 years.[164] It has been postulated that in patients with IND type B, normal colon motility often spontaneously develops with increasing age,[40,160,161] but the clinical course after closure of the enterostomy has been investigated in only small series.[153,165] However, medical treatment with laxatives and enemas remains the method of first choice in children without disabling obstruction,[32,41,161,164] and this may be expected to be successful in 75% of the patients.

HYPOGANGLIONOSIS

The analysis of the intramural plexus is essential to establish the diagnosis of hypoganglionosis.[27,28,166] The diagnosis is often missed in patients who undergo suction biopsies. Full-thickness biopsies show a reduced number of myenteric ganglia, low AChE activity in the lamina propria, and hypertrophy of the muscularis mucosae and circular muscle. Only small series of patients with hypoganglionosis of the myenteric plexus have been investigated so far. The symptoms were always severe, and constipation did not improve with time. Seven of nine children in one series[29] and 11 of 12 patients in another required resection.[167]

OTHER NEURONAL INTESTINAL MALFORMATIONS

Isolated heterotopia of the myenteric plexus is extremely rare. The heterotopic neurons of the myenteric plexus in the circular and longitudinal muscles contain practically no plexus in the space between the two layers of muscle.[35] This results in severe symptoms, mostly requiring bowel resection.[29,40] The clinical significance of other intestinal malformations remains controversial. Heterotopia of the submucous plexus in the muscularis mucosa is extremely common and seems to be a normal variant.[40] It rarely requires surgical therapy in form of sphincteromyotomy. This also accounts for patients with ganglion-cell hypogenesis, immature ganglion cells, or dysganglionosis.[32,40,161,168]

ASSOCIATION OF HIRSCHSPRUNG'S DISEASE AND OTHER INTESTINAL NEURONAL MALFORMATIONS

Abnormal innervation patterns may be expected in the colon proximal to an aganglionic segment in nearly all children with HD.[168] The reported incidence of associated IND type B is 20% to 75%.[41,153-155,161,162,169] Hypoganglionosis proximal to the aganglionic segment was seen in 63%, and heterotopic nerve cells of the myenteric plexus, in 20% of patients with HD.[29] It has been postulated that the acute onset of obstruction in patients with IND-associated aganglionosis indicates an additive effect of both lesions. As many as 73% of patients in whom aganglionosis was combined with IND type B had ileus, as compared with 32% with isolated aganglionosis.[142,153,154]

IND type B may be the cause of persistent constipation or obstructive symptoms after resection for HD. Nine of 16 children investigated for persistent obstructive symptoms had IND type B in one study.[129] Ten children who had enterocolitis, soiling, or constipation after resection for HD were found to have associated IND type B.[155] In another series, six of seven children underwent repeated resection, because they also had IND type B.[29] As a consequence, it has been postulated that children who have HD with associated IND type B should undergo a more extended resection at the initial operation.[32] Reports of HD associated with other intestinal malformations are rare, and the clinical significance of these findings remains unclear. We reported 15 HD patients with associated heterotopia of the myenteric plexus who did not have significantly more frequent postoperative symptoms compared with patients with classic aganglionosis.[170]

REFERENCES

1. Ehrenpreis TH: Hirschsprung's Disease. Chicago, Year Book Medical Publishers, 1970.
2. Kaiser G, Bettex M: Clinical generalities. In Holschneider AM (ed): Hirschsprung's Disease. Stuttgart, Thieme Stratton, 1982, pp 43–53.
3. Russel MB, Russel CA, Niebuhr E: Familial occurrence of Hirschsprung's disease. Clin Genet 45:231, 1994.
4. Passarge E: Genetic heterogenicity and recurrence risk of congenital intestinal aganglionosis. In Birth Defects. Original article series VIII, No 2, 63. Baltimore, Williams & Wilkins, 1972, pp 116–122.
5. Engum SA, Petrites M, Rescorla FJ, et al: Familial Hirschsprung's disease: 20 cases in 12 kindreds. J Pediatr Surg 28:1286, 1993.
6. Schiller M, Levy P, Shawa RA, et al: Familial Hirschsprung's disease: A report of 22 affected siblings in four families. J Pediatr Surg 25:322, 1990.
7. Moore SW, Kaschul ROC, Cywes S: Familial and genetic aspects of neuronal intestinal dysplasia and Hirschsprung's disease. Pediatr Surg Int 8:406, 1993.
8. Hirschsprung H: Stuhlträgheit Neugeborener infolge Dilatation und Hypertrophie des Colons. Jahresber Kinderheilkd 27:1, 1888.
9. Derrick EH, St. George-Brambauer BM: Megacolon in mice. J Bacteriol Pathol 73:569, 1957.
10. Martuciello G, Bjocchi M, Dodero P, et al: Total colonic aganglionosis associated with interstitial deletion of the long arm of chromosome 10. J Pediatr Surg 7:308, 1992.
11. Ikadai H, Fujita H, Agematsu Y, et al: Observation of congenital aganglionosis rat (Hirschsprung's disease rat) and its genetic analysis. Congen Anom 19:31, 1979.
12. Ikadai H, Suzufi K, Fujita H, et al: Animal models of human disease: Hirschsprung's disease. Comp Pathol Bull 13:3, 1981.
13. Lane PW, Liu HM: Association of megacolon with two recessive spotting genes in the mouse. J Hered 57:181, 1966.
14. Cass D: Animal models of aganglionosis. In Holschneider AM, Puri P (eds): Hirschsprung's Disease and Allied Disorders. London, Harwood Academic Publishers, 2000, pp 59–68.
15. Passarge E: Genetics of Hirschsprung's disease. N Engl J Med 276:138–143, 1967.
16. Passarge E: Dissecting Hirschsprung's disease. Nat Genet 31:11–12, 2002.
17. Bolk Gabriel S, et al: Segregation at three loci explains familial and population risk in Hirschsprung disease. Nat Genet 31:89–93, 2002.
18. Lyonnet S, et al: A gene for Hirschsprung disease maps to the proximal long arm of chromosome 10. Nat Genet 4:346–350, 1993.
19. Angrist M, et al: A gene for Hirschsprung disease (megacolon) in the pericentromeric region of human chromosome 10. Nat Genet 4:351–356, 1993.
20. Wakamatsu N: Mutations in SIP1, encoding Smad interacting protein-1, cause a form of Hirschsprung disease. Nat Genet 27:369–370, 2001.
21. Hofstra RM: RET and GDNF gene scanning in Hirschsprung patients using two dual denaturing gel systems. Hum Mutat 15:418–429, 2000.
22. Christensen J: Normal colonic motor function and relevant structure. In Holschneider AM, Puri P (eds): Hirschsprung's Disease and Allied Disorders. London, Harwood Academic Publishers, 2000, pp 89–108.
23. Holschneider AM: Anal sphincter achalasia and ultrashort Hirschsprung's disease. In Holschneider AM, Puri P (eds): Hirschsprung's Disease and Allied Disorders. London, Harwood Academic Publishers 2000.

24. Athow AC, Filipe MI, Drake DP: Problems and advantages of acetylcholinesterase histochemistry of rectal suction biopsies in the diagnosis of Hirschsprung's disease. J Pediatr Surg 25:520, 1990.

25. Kobayashi H, Hirakawa H, Puri P: Abnormal internal anal sphincter innervation in patients with Hirschsprung's disease and allied disorders. J Pediatr Surg 31:794, 1996.

26. Meier-Ruge W: New aspects in the pathophysiology of the hypoganglionic megacolon. Verh Dtsch Ges Pathol 53:237, 1969.

27. Meier-Ruge W: The histologic diagnosis and differential diagnosis of Hirschsprung's disease. In Holschneider AM, Puri P (eds): Hirschsprung's Disease and Allied Disorders. London, Harwood Academic Publishers, 2000, pp 252–264.

28. Meier-Ruge W, Brunner LA, Engert J, et al: A correlative morphometric and clinical investigation of hypoganglionosis of the colon. Eur J Pediatr Surg 2:67, 1999.

29. Ure BM, Holschneider AM, Schulten D, et al: Clinical impact of intestinal neuronal malformations: A prospective study in 141 patients. Pediatr Surg Int 12:377, 1997.

30. Ikeda K, Goto S, Nagasaki A, et al: Hypogenesis of intestinal ganglion cells: A rare cause of intestinal obstruction simulating aganglionosis. Z Kinderchir 43:52, 1988.

31. Munakata K, Okabe I, Morita K: Histologic studies of rectocolic aganglionosis and allied diseases. J Pediatr Surg 13:67, 1978.

32. Holschneider AM, Meier-Ruge W, Ure BM: Hirschsprung's disease and allied disorders: A review. Eur J Pediatr Surg 4:260, 1994.

33. Meier-Ruge W: Über ein Krankheitsbild mit Hirschsprung's symptomatik. Verh Dtsch Ges Pathol 55:506, 1971.

34. Badner JA, Chakravati A: Waardenburg syndrome and Hirschsprung's disease: Evidence for pleiotropic effects of a single dominant gene. Am J Med Genet 35:100, 1990.

35. Kobayashi H, Hirakawa H, Puri P: What are the diagnostic criteria for intestinal neuronal dysplasia? Pediatr Surg Int 10:459, 1995.

36. Meier-Ruge WA, Brönnimann PB, Gambazzi F, et al: Histopathological criteria for intestinal neuronal dysplasia of the submucous plexus (type B). Virchows Arch 426:549, 1995.

37. Borchard F, Meier-Ruge W, Wiebecke B, et al: Innervationsstörungen des Dickdarms-Klassifikation und Diagnostik. Pathologe 12:171, 1991.

38. Koletzko S, Jesch I, Faus-Kebetaler T, et al: Rectal biopsy for diagnosis of intestinal neuronal dysplasia in children: A prospective multicentre study on interobserver variation and clinical outcome. Gut 44:853, 1999.

39. Holschneider AM, Pfrommer W, Gerrescheim B: Results in the treatment of anorectal malformations with special regard to the histology of the rectal pouch. Eur J Pediatr Surg 4:303, 1994.

40. Meier-Ruge W: Epidemiology of congenital innervation defects of the distal colon. Virchows Arch Pathol Anat 420:171, 1992.

41. Ure BM, Holschneider AM, Meier-Ruge W: Neuronal intestinal malformations: A retro- and prospective study on 203 patients. Eur J Pediatr Surg 4:279, 1994.

42. Meier-Ruge W: Desmosis of the colon: A working hypothesis of primary chronic constipation. Eur J Pediatr Surg 8:299–303, 1998.

43. West KW, Grosfeld JL, Rescorla FJ, et al: Acquired aganglionosis: A rare occurrence following pull-through procedures for Hirschsprung's disease. J Pediatr Surg 25:104, 1990.

44. Dajani OM, Slim MS, Mansour A: Acquired hypoganglionosis after endorectal pullthrough procedure: A case report. Z Kinderchir 41:248, 1986.

45. Brown RA, Cywes S: Disorders and congenital malformations associated with Hirschsprung's disease. In Holschneider AM, Puri P (eds): Hirschsprung's Disease and Allied Disorders. London, Harwood Academic Publishers, 2000, pp 137–146.

46. Meyers SHC: The development of the enteric nerve system. In Holschneider AM, Puri P (eds): Hirschsprung's Disease and Allied Disorders. London, Harwood Academic Publishers, 2000, pp 9–18.

47. Pingault V, Bondurand N, Kuhlbrodt K, et al: *SOX 10* mutations in patients with Waardenburg-Hirschsprung disease. Paper presented at The Third International Meeting: Hirschsprung's Disease and Related Neurocristopathies, Feb 5–8, 1998, Evian, France.

48. Brooks AS, Breubing MH, Meijers C: Spectrum of phenotypes associated with Hirschsprung's disease: An evaluation of 239 patients from a single institution. Paper presented at The Third International Meeting: Hirschsprung's Disease and Related Neurocristopathies, Feb 5–8, 1998, Evian, France.

49. Hahhad GG, Mazza NM, Defendini R, et al: Congenital failure of automatic control of ventilation, gastrointestinal motility and heart rate. Medicine (Baltimore) 57:517, 1978.

50. Elhalaby E, Coran A: Hirschsprung's disease associated with Ondine's course: Report of three cases and review of the literature. J Pediatr Surg 29:530, 1994.

51. Gaultier CI, Trang-Pham H, Dauger S, et al: Congenital central hypoventilation syndrome phenotypes. Paper presented at The Third International Meeting: Hirschsprung's Disease and Related Neurocristopathies, Feb 5–8, 1998, Evian, France.

52. Nakahara S, Yokomori K, Tamura K, et al: Hirschsprung's disease with Ondine's course: A special subgroup? J Pediatr Surg 30:1481, 1995.

53. Steiner AL, Goodman AD, Powers SR: Study of a kindred with pheochromocytoma, medullary thyroid carcinoma, hyperparathyroidism and Cushing disease: Multiple endocrine neoplasia type II. Medicine (Baltimore) 47:371, 1968.

54. Khan AH, Desjardins JG, Youssef S, et al: Gastrointestinal manifestations of Sipple syndrome in children. J Pediatr Surg 22:719, 1987.

55. Holschneider AM, Ure BM, Pfrommer W, et al: Innervation patterns of the rectal pouch and fistula in anorectal malformations: A preliminary report. J Pediatr Surg 31:357, 1996.

56. Akgur FM, Tanyel FC, Buyukpamukcu N, et al: Colonic atresia and Hirschsprung's association shows further evidence for migration of enteric neurons. J Pediatr Surg 28:635, 1993.

57. Puri P, Wester T: Enterocolitis complicating Hirschsprung's disease. In Holschneider AM, Puri P (eds): Hirschsprung's Disease and Allied Disorders. London, Harwood Academic Publishers, 2000, pp 296–300.

58. Bill AH, Chapman ND: The enterocolitis of Hirschsprung's disease: Its natural history and treatment. Am J Surg 103:70–74, 1962.

59. Elhalaby EA, Coran AG, Blane CE, et al: Enterocolitis associated with Hirschsprung's disease: A clinical-radiological characterization on 168 patients. J Pediatr Surg 30:76, 1995.

60. Harrison MW, Deitz DE, Campbel JR, et al: Diagnosis and management of Hirschsprung's disease: A 25-year perspective. Am J Surg 152:49, 1986.

61. Sieber WK: Hirschsprung's disease. In Welch KJ, Randolph JG, Ravitch MM, et al (eds): Pediatric Surgery, 4th Ed. Chicago, Yearbook Medical Publishers, 1986, p 995.

62. Carneiro PMR, Brereton RJ, Drake DP, et al: Enterocolitis in Hirschsprung's disease. Pediatr Surg Int 7:356, 1992.

63. Ikeda K, Goto S: Diagnosis and treatment of Hirschsprung's disease in Japan: Analysis of 1628 patients. J Pediatr Surg 199:400, 1984.

64. Shanbhouge LKR, Bianchi A: Experience with primary Swenson resection and pullthrough for neonatal Hirschsprung's disease. Pediatr Surg Int 5:446, 1990.

65. Surana R, Quinn FMJ, Puri P: Evaluation of risk factors in the development of enterocolitis complicating Hirschsprung's disease. Pediatr Surg Int 9:234, 1994.

66. Akahary S, Sahwy E, Kandil W, et al: A histochemical study of the mucosubstances of the colon in cases of Hirschsprung's disease with and without enterocolitis. J Pediatr Surg 24:1272, 1989.

67. Fujimoto T, Puri P: Persistence of enterocolitis following diversion of faecal stream in Hirschsprung's disease. A study of mucosal defense mechanisms. Pediatr Surg Int 3:141, 1988.

68. Wilson-Storey D, Scobie WG: Impaired gastrointestinal mucosal defense in Hirschsprung's disease: A clue to the pathogenesis of enterocolitis. J Pediatr Surg 24:462, 1989.

69. Soeda J, O'Brian DS, Puri P: Regional reduction in intestinal neuroendocrine cell populations in enterocolitis complicating Hirschsprung's disease. J Pediatr Surg 28:1063, 1993.

70. Lloyd-Stil JD, Demers LM: Hirschsprung's enterocolitis, prostaglandins, and response to cholestyramine. J Pediatr Surg 13:417, 1978.

71. Thomas DFM, Fernie DS, Bayston R, et al: Enterocolitis in Hirschsprung's disease: A controlled study of the etiologic role of *Clostridium difficile*. J Pediatr Surg 21:22, 1986.

72. Wilson-Storey D, Scobie WG, McGenity KG: Microbiological studies of the enterocolites of Hirschsprung's disease. Arch Dis Child 65:1338, 1990.

73. Lifschitz CH, Bloss R: Persistence of colitis in Hirschsprung's disease. J Pediatr Gastroenterol Nutr 4:291, 1985.

74. Teitelbaum DH, Caniano DA, Qualman SJ: The pathophysiology of Hirschsprung's associated enterocolitis: Its importance and histologic correlates. J Pediatr Surg 24:1271, 1989.

75. Sherman JO, Snyder ME, Weitzman JJ, et al: A 40-year multinational retrospective study of 880 Swenson procedures. J Pediatr Surg 24:833, 1989.

76. Blake NA: Radiological diagnosis of Hirschsprung disease and allied disorders. In Holschneider AN, Puri P (eds): Hirschsprung's Disease and Allied Disorders. London, Harwood Academic Publishers, 2000, pp 273–279.

77. Ure BM, Holschneider AM, Schulten D, et al: Intestinal transit time in children with intestinal neuronal malformations mimicking Hirschsprung's disease. Eur J Pediatr Surg 2:91, 1999.

78. Benningha MA, Büllar HA, Staalman CR, et al: Defecation disorders in children, colonic transit time versus the Barr-score. Eur J Pediatr 154:1277, 1995.

79. Papadopoulou A, Clayden GS, Booth IW: The clinical value of solid marker transit studies in childhood constipation and soiling. Eur J Pediatr 153:560, 1994.

80. Holschneider AM: Clinical and electromanometrical investigations of postoperative continence in Hirschsprung's disease. Z Kinderchir 29:39, 1980.

81. Holschneider AM: Elektromanometrie des Enddarms: Diagnostik und Therapie der Inkontinenz und der chronischen Obstipation. 2. Munich, Urban & Schwarzenberg, 1983.

82. Holschneider AM: Functional diagnosis of Hirschsprung's disease and allied disorders. In Holschneider AM, Puri P (eds): Hirschsprung's Disease and Allied Disorders. London, Harwood Academic Publishers, 2000, pp 230–251.

83. Holschneider AM, Kellner E, Streibl P, et al: The development of anorectal continence and its significance in the diagnosis of Hirschsprung's disease. J Pediatr Surg 11:151, 1976.

84. Noblett HR: A rectal suction biopsy tube for use in the diagnosis of Hirschsprung's disease. J Pediatr Surg 4:406, 1969.

85. Puri P, Lake BD, Gorman F, et al: Megacystis-microcolon-intestinal hypoperistalsis syndrome: A visceral myopathy. J Pediatr Surg 18:64, 1983.

86. Puri P: Megacystis-microcolon-intestinal hypoperistalsis syndrome. In Holschneider AM, Puri P (eds): Hirschsprung's Disease and Allied Disorders. London, Harwood Academic Publishers, 2000, pp 185–196.

87. Swenson O, Bill AH: Resection of rectum and rectosigmoid with preservation of sphincter for benign spastic lesions producing megacolon. Surgery 24:212, 1948.

88. Duhamel B: Une nouvelle operation pour le megacolon congenital: L'abaissement retrorectal et transanal du colon et son application possible au traitement de quelques autres malformations. Press Med 64:2249, 1956.

89. Duhamel B: Retrorectal and transanal pullthrough procedure for the treatment of Hirschsprung's disease. Dis Colon Rectum 7:455, 1964.

90. Grob M: Intestinal obstruction in the newborn infant. Arch Dis Child 35:40, 1960.

91. Steichen FM, Spigland NA, Nunez D: The modified Duhamel operation for Hirschsprung's disease performed entirely with mechanical sutures. J Pediatr Surg 22:436, 1987.

92. Holschneider AM, Söylet Y: Die anteriore Resektion nach Rehbein in der Behandlung des Megacolon congenitum Hirschsprung: Hand oder Stapler Anastomose. Eine vergeichende Studie. Z Kinderchir 44:216, 1989.

93. Romualdi P: Eine neue Operationstechnik fur die Behandlung einiger Rectum-Missbildunger. Langenbecks Arch Dtsch Z Chir 279:37, 1960.

94. Rehbein F: Intraabdominelle Resektion oder Rektosigmoidektomie bei der Hirschsprung'schen Krankheit. Chirurg 29:366, 1964.

95. Soave F: A new original technique for treatment of Hirschsprung's disease. Surgery 56:1007, 1964.

96. Boley SJ: New modification of the surgical treatment of Hirschsprung's disease. Surgery 56:1015, 1964.

97. Marks RM: Endorectal split sleeve pull-through procedure for Hirschsprung's disease. Surg Gynecol Obstet 136:627, 1973.

98. Kasai M, Suzuki H, Watanabe K: Rectal myotomy with colectomy: A new radical operation for Hirschsprung's disease. J Pediatr Surg 6:36, 1971.

99. Curran TJ, Raffensperger JG: Laparoscopic Swenson's pull-through: A comparison with the open procedure. J Pediatr Surg 31:1155, 1995.

100. Georgeson KE, Fuenfer MM, Hardin WD: Primary laparoscopic pull-through for Hirschsprung's disease in infants and children. J Pediatr Surg 30:1017, 1995.

101. Hoffmann K, Schier F, Waldschmidt J: Laparoscopic Swenson's procedure in children. Eur J Pediatr Surg 6:15, 1996.

102. Bax NMA, van der Zee DC: Laparoscopic removal of aganglionic bowel using the Duhamel-Martin method in five consecutive infants. Pediatr Surg Int 10:116, 1995.

103. van der Zee DC, Bax KN: One-stage Duhamel-Martin procedure for Hirschsprung's disease: A 5-year follow-up study. J. Pediatr Surg 35:1434–1436, 2000.

104. de Laguasie P, Berrebi D, Geib G, et al: Laparoscopic Duhamel procedure: Management of 30 cases. Surg Endosc 13:972–974, 1999.

105. Smith BM, Lobe TE, Steiner RB: Laparoscopic Duhamel pullthrough procedure for Hirschsprung's disease in childhood. J Laparoendosc Surg 4:273–266, 1994.

106. De la Torre-Mondragon L, Ortega-Salgado JA: Transanal endorectal pull-through for Hirschsprung's disease. J Pediatr Surg 33:1283–1286, 1998.

107. Carcassone M, Morisson-Lacombe G, LeTourneau JW: Primary corrective operation without decompression in infants less than three months of age with Hirschsprung's disease. J Pediatr Surg 17:241, 1982.

108. Cilley RE, Slatter MB, Hirschl RB, et al: Definitive treatment of Hirschsprung's disease in the newborn with a one-stage procedure. Surgery 115:551, 1994.

109. So HB, Schwartz DL, Becker JM, et al: Endorectal pull-through without preliminary colostomy in neonates with Hirschsprung's disease. J Pediatr Surg 15:470, 1980.

110. Teitelbaum DH, Drongowski RA, Chamberlain JN, et al: Long-term stooling patterns in infants undergoing primary endorectal pull-through for Hirschsprung's disease. J Pediatr Surg 32:1049, 1997.

111. Langer JC, Minkes RK, Mazziotti MV, et al: Transanal one stage Soave procedure for infants with Hirschsprung's disease. J Pediatr Surg 34:148–152, 1999.

112. Langer JC, Seifert M, Minkes RK: One stage Soave pull-through for Hirschsprung's disease: A comparison of the transanal and open approaches. J Pediatr Surg 35:820–822, 2000.

113. Albanese CT, Jennings RW, Smith B, et al: Perineal one stage pull-through for Hirschsprung's disease. J Pediatr Surg 34:377–380, 1999.

114. Shankar KR, Losty PD, Turnoch RR: Transanal endorectal coloanal surgery for Hirschsprung's disease: Experience in two centers. J Pediatr Surg 35:1209–1213, 2000.

115. Gao Y, Li G, Zhang X, et al: Primary transanal rectosigmoidectomy for Hirschsprung's disease: Preliminary results in the initial 33 cases. J Pediatr Surg 36:1816–1819, 2002.

116. Rintala RJ: Transanal coloanal pull-through with a short muscular cuff for classic Hirschsprung's disease. Eur J Pediatr Surg 13:181–186, 2003.

117. Hahhidi A: Transanal endorectal pull-through for Hirschsprung's disease: A comparison with open technique. Eur J Pediatr Surg 13:176–180, 2003.

118. Martin LW: Surgical management of Hirschsprung's disease involving the small intestine. Arch Surg 97:183, 1968.

119. Martin LW: Surgical management of total colonic aganglionosis. Am Surg 176:343, 1972.

120. Heath AL, Spitz L, Milla PJ: The absorptive function of colonic aganglionic intestine: Are the Duhamel and Martin procedures rational? J Pediatr Surg 20:34, 1985.

121. Ein SH, Shandling B: Long Duhamel procedure. In Holschneider AM, Puri P (eds): Hirschsprung's Disease and Allied Disorders, 2nd ed. London, Harwood Academic Publishers, 1999.

122. Dübbers M, Holschneider AM, Meier-Ruge W: Results of total and subtotal resections in children. Eur J Pedriatr Surg 13:195–200, 2003.

123. Emslie J, Krishnamoorthy M, Allebaum H: Long-term follow up of patients treated with ileoendorectal pull-through and right colon onlay patch form total colonic aganglionosis. J Pediatr Surg 32:1542, 1997.

124. Suita S, Taguchi T, Kamimura T, et al: Total colonic aganglionosis with or without small bowel involvement: A changing profile. J Pediatr Surg 32;1537, 1997.

125. Holschneider AM: Clinical and electromanometric studies of postoperative continence in Hirschsprung's disease: Relationship to the surgical procedures. In Holschneider AM (ed): Hirschsprung's Disease. Stuttgart, Thieme Stratton, 1982, pp 221–241.

126. Holschneider AM: Complication after surgical treatment of Hirschsprung's disease. In Heberer G (ed): Anglo-German Coloproctology Meeting, 1981. Berlin, Springer, 1981, pp 112–124.

127. Kleinhaus S, Boley SJ, Sheran M, et al: Hirschsprung's disease: A survey of the members of the surgical section of the American Academy of Pediatrics. J Pediatr Surg 14:588, 1979.

128. Rescorla FJ, Morrison AM, Engles D, et al: Hirschsprung's disease: Evaluation of mortality and long-term function in 260 cases. Arch Surg 127:934, 1992.

129. Moore SW, Millar AJ, Cywes S: Long-term clinical, manometric, and histological evaluation of obstructive symptoms in the postoperative Hirschsprung's patient. J Pediatr Surg 29:106, 1994.

130. Liem NT, Hau BD, Thu NX: The long-term follow up result of Swenson's operation in the treatment of Hirschsprung's disease in Vietnamese children. Eur J Pediatr Surg 14:110, 1993.

131. Heij HA, de Vries X, Bremer I, et al: Long-term anorectal function after Duhamel operation for Hirschsprung's disease. J Pediatr Surg 30:430, 1995.

132. Wester T, Hoehner J, Olsen L: Rehbein's anterior resection in Hirschsprung's disease, using a circular stapler. Eur J Pediatr Surg 5:358, 1995.

133. Schulten D, Holschneider AM, Meier-Ruge W: Proximal segment histology of resected bowel in Hirschsprung's disease predicts postoperative bowel function. Eur J Pediatr Surg 10:378–381, 2000.

134. Kobayashi H, Wang Y, Hirakawa H, et al: Intraoperative evaluation of extent of aganglionosis by a rapid acetylcholinesterase histochemical technique. J Pediatr Surg 30:248, 1995.

135. Joppich I: Late complications of Hirschsprung's disease. In Holschneider AM (ed): Hirschsprung's Disease. Stuttgart, Hippokrates, 1982, pp 25–26.

136. Banani SA, Forootan HR, Kumar PV: Intestinal neuronal dysplasia as a cause of surgical failure in Hirschsprung's disease: A new modality for surgical management. J Pediatr Surg 31:572, 1996.

137. Snyder CL, Ashcraft KW: Late complications of Hirschsprung's disease. In Holschneider AM, Puri P (eds): Hirschsprung's Disease and Allied Disorders. London, Harwood Academic Publishers, 2000, pp 431–440.

138. Moore SW, Albertyn R, Cywes S: Clinical outcome and long-term quality of life after surgical correction of Hirschsprung's disease. J Pediatr Surg 31:1496–1502, 1996.

139. Holschneider AM, Kraeft H, Scholtissek CH: Urodynamic investigations of bladder disturbances in imperforate anus and Hirschsprung's disease. Z Kinderchir 35:64, 1982.

140. Meier-Ruge W, Schärli AF: The epidemiology and enzyme histotopochemical characterization of ultrashort-segment Hirschsprung's disease. Pediatr Surg Int 1:37, 1986.

141. Clayden GS, Lawson JON: Investigation and management of long-standing chronic constipation in childhood. Arch Dis Child 51:918, 1976.

142. Bettex M: Megakolon. In Zenker R, Deucher F, Schink W (eds): Chirurgie der Gegenwart, vol. 7. München, Urban & Schwarzenberg, 1976, pp 89–97.

143. Nissan S, Bar-Moar JA: Further experience in the diagnosis and surgical treatment of short-segment Hirschsprung's disease and idiopathic megacolon. J Pediatr Surg 6:738, 1971.

144. Aldrige RT, Campbell PE: Ganglion cell distribution in the normal rectum and anal canal: A basis for the diagnosis of Hirschsprung's disease by anorectal biopsy. J Pediatr Surg 3:475, 1968.

145. Müntefering H, Welskop J, Fadda B, et al: Enzymhistotopochemische Befunde bei der neurogenen Achalasie des M. Sphincter ani internus. Verh Dtsch Ges Pathol 70:622, 1986.

146. Meier-Ruge W: Der ultrakurze M. Hirschsprung: Ein bioptisch zuverlässig objectivierbares Krankheitsbild. Z Kinderchir 40:146–150, 1985.

147. Puri P: Hirschsprung's disease: Clinical and experimental observations. World J Surg 17:374, 1993.

148. Bentley JFR: Some new observations on megacolon in infancy and childhood with special reference to the management of megasigmoid and megarectum. Dis Colon Rectum 7:462, 1964.

149. Lynn HB: Rectal myectomy for aganglionic megacolon. Mayo Clin Proc 41:289, 1966.

150. Holschneider AM, Kraeft H: Die Wirkung von Alpha-Blockern auf den Muskulus sphincter ani internus. Z Kinderchir 30:152, 1980.

151. Munakata K, Morita K, Okabe I, et al: Clinical and histologic studies of neuronal intestinal dysplasia. J Pediatr Surg 20:231, 1985.

152. Puri P, Fujimoto T: Diagnosis of allied functional bowel disorders using monoclonal antibodies and electron microscopy. J Pediatr Surg 23:546, 1988.

153. Briner J, Oswald HW, Hirsig J, et al: Neuronal intestinal dysplasia: Clinical and histochemical findings and its association with Hirschsprung's disease. Z Kinderchir 41:282, 1986.

154. Fadda B, Pistor G, Meier-Ruge W, et al: Symptoms, diagnosis, and therapy of neuronal intestinal dysplasia masked by Hirschsprung's disease. Pediatr Surg Int 2:76, 1987.

155. Kobayashi H, Hirakawa H, Surana R, et al: Intestinal neuronal dysplasia is a possible cause of persistent bowel symptoms after pull-through operation for Hirschsprung's disease. J Pediatr Surg 30:253, 1995.

156. Koletzko S, Ballauff A, Hadzilelimovic F, et al: Is histological diagnosis of neuronal intestinal dysplasia related to clinical and manometric findings in constipated children? Results of a pilot study. J Pediatr Gastroenterol Nutr 17:59, 1993.

157. Navarro J, Sonsino E, Boige N, et al: Visceral neuropathies responsible for chronic intestinal pseudo-obstruction syndrome in pediatric practice: Analysis of 26 cases. J Pediatr Gastroenterol Nutr 11:179, 1990.

158. Saul RA, Sturner RA, Burger PC: Hyperplasia of the myenteric plexus: Its association with early infantile megacolon and neurofibromatosis. Am J Dis Child 136:852, 1982.

159. Wildhaber J, Seelentag WKF, Spiegel R, et al: Cystic fibrosis associated with neuronal intestinal dysplasia type B: A case report. J Pediatr Surg 31:951, 1996.

160. Fadda B, Maier WA, Meier-Ruge W, et al: Neuronal intestinal Dysplasie: Eine kritische 10-Jahres-Analyse klinischer und bioptischer Diagnostik. Z Kinderchir 38:305, 1983.

161. Schärli AF: Neuronal intestinal dysplasia. Pediatr Surg Int 7:2, 1992.

162. Csury L, Pena A: Intestinal neuronal dysplasia. Pediatr Surg Int 10:441, 1995.

163. Sacher P, Briner J, Stauffer UG: Unusual cases of neuronal intestinal dysplasia. Pediatr Surg Int 6:225, 1991.

164. Simpser E, Kahn E, Kenigsberg K, et al: Neuronal intestinal dysplasia: Quantitative diagnostic criteria and clinical management. J Pediatr Gastroenterol Nutr 12:61, 1991.

165. Rintala R, Rapola J, Louhimo I: Neuronal intestinal dysplasia. Progr Pediatr Surg 24:186, 1989.

166. Meier-Ruge W, Schärli AF, Stoss F: How to improve histopathological results in the biopsy diagnosis of gut dysganglionosis. Pediatr Surg Int 10:454, 1995.

167. Munakata K, Okabe I, Morita K: Hypoganglionosis. Pediatr Surg Int 7:8, 1992.

168. Ure BM, Holschneider AM: Treatment of intestinal neuronal malformations mimicking Hirschsprung's disease. In Holschneider AM, Puri P (eds): Hirschsprung's Disease and Allied Disorders. London, Harwood Academic Publishers, 2000, pp 375–388.

169. Hanimann B, Inderbitzin D, Briner J, et al: Clinical relevance of Hirschsprung-associated neuronal intestinal dysplasia (HANID). Eur J Pediatr Surg 2:147, 1992.

170. Schulten D, Holschneider AM, Meier-Ruge W: Proximal segment histology of resected bowel in Hirschsprung's disease predicts postoperative bowel function. Eur J Pediatr Surg 10:378–381, 2000.

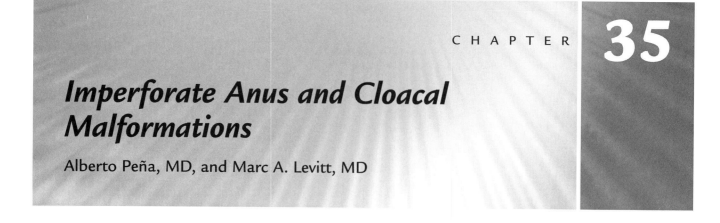

CHAPTER **35**

Imperforate Anus and Cloacal Malformations

Alberto Peña, MD, and Marc A. Levitt, MD

HISTORY

"Imperforate anus" has been a well-known condition since antiquity.[1-3] For many centuries, physicians, as well as individuals who practiced medicine, tried to help these children by creating an orifice in the perineum. Many of these children survived, most likely because they had a type of defect that is now recognized as "low." Those with a "high defect" did not survive that kind of treatment. Amussat, in 1835, was the first to suture the rectal wall to the skin edges, which could be considered the first actual anoplasty.[2] During the first 60 years of the 20th century, most surgeons performed a perineal anoplasty without a colostomy for the so-called "low malformations." A colostomy performed during the newborn period was followed by an abdominal perineal pull-through operation for the treatment of "high malformations." The decision to create the colostomy was based mainly on the radiologic information obtained by the "invertogram."[4] During the era of the abdominoperineal pull-through operation, the specific recommendation was to pull the bowel as close to the sacrum as possible to avoid trauma to the genitourinary (GU) tract. Stephens[5] made a significant contribution to the field by performing the first objective anatomic studies of human specimens. In 1953, Stephens proposed an initial sacral approach followed by an abdominoperineal operation, when necessary. The purpose of the sacral stage of the procedure was to preserve the puborectalis sling, considered a key factor in maintaining fecal continence.[5] Since then, different surgical techniques have been proposed by others.[6-9] All those techniques have as a common denominator: the protection and use of the puborectalis sling.

The posterosagittal approach for the treatment of imperforate anus was performed first in September of 1980, and its description was published in 1982.[10,11]

This approach allowed direct exposure of this important anatomic area. The unique opportunity arose to correlate the external appearance of the perineum with the operative findings and, subsequently, with the clinical results. Significant implications emerged in terms of terminology and classification.

Incidence, Types of Defects, and Terminology

Imperforate anus occurs in one of every 4000 to 5000 newborns.[12-14] The estimated risk for a couple having a second child with an anorectal malformation is approximately 1%.[15-17] The frequency of this defect is slightly higher in boys than in girls. The most frequent defect in male patients is imperforate anus, with a rectourethral fistula.[18] The most frequent defect in female patients is rectovestibular fistula.[18] Imperforate anus without a fistula is a rather unusual defect; it occurs in about 5% of the entire group of malformations.[18] Persistent cloaca was, in the past, considered an unusual defect[19]; instead, a high incidence of rectovaginal fistula was reported in the literature.[19] In retrospect, it seems that the presence of the cloaca is a much more common defect in female patients.[20] Moreover, a persistent cloaca is the third most common defect in female patients after perineal fistulas and vestibular fistulas. Rectovaginal fistula is an almost nonexistent defect, present in fewer than 1% of all cases.[20,21] Probably most patients with a persistent cloaca were erroneously thought to have a rectovaginal fistula. Many of those patients underwent surgical procedures, and the rectal component of the malformation was repaired, but the patients were left with a persistent urogenital (UG) sinus.[20] Recent evidence[20] also shows that most rectovestibular fistulas were erroneously called "rectovaginal fistula." Recto–bladder neck fistula in male patients is the only real supralevator malformation and fortunately occurs in only about 10% of all male patients.[18] It is the only defect in male patients that requires an abdominal approach (either laparotomy or laparoscopy), in addition to the posterior sagittal approach because it is the only malformation in male patients in which the rectum is unreachable through the posterior sagittal incision.

Anorectal malformations represent a wide spectrum of defects. The terms *low, intermediate,* and *high* are arbitrary and not useful in therapeutic or prognostic terms. Within the group of anorectal malformations traditionally referred to as high, defects are included with different therapeutic and prognostic implications. For instance, rectoprostatic fistula and recto–bladder neck fistula were both considered high, yet the first can be repaired with a posterior sagittal approach alone, and the second requires, in addition, an abdominal approach. Furthermore, the prognosis for each type is completely different. Therefore a more therapeutic and prognostically oriented classification is depicted in Table 35-1.

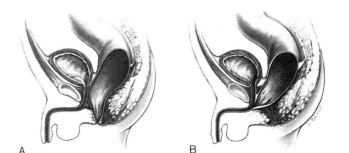

FIGURE 35-1. Spectrum of defects in male patients. *A,* Perineal fistula. *B,* Rectourethrobulbar fistula. (From Peña A: Atlas of Surgical Management of Anorectal Malformations. New York, Springer-Verlag, 1990, p 26.)

MALE DEFECTS

Rectoperineal Fistulas

Rectoperineal fistula is what traditionally was known as a low defect. The rectum is located within most of the sphincter mechanism. Only the lowest part of the rectum is anteriorly mislocated (Fig. 35-1*A*). Sometimes the fistula does not open into the perineum but rather follows a subepithelial midline tract, opening somewhere along the midline perineal raphe, scrotum, or even at the base of the penis. The diagnosis is established by perineal inspection. No further investigations are required.

Most of the time, the anal fistula opening is abnormally narrow (stenosis). The terms *covered anus, anal membrane,* and *anteriorly mislocated anus,* as well as *bucket-handle malformations,* refer to different external manifestations of perineal fistulas.

Rectourethral Fistulas

Imperforate anus with rectourethral fistula is the most frequent defect in male patients.[18] The fistula may be located at the posterior part of the urethra (bulbar urethra; see Fig. 35-1*B*) or higher (Fig. 35-2*A*).

Immediately above the fistula site, the rectum and urethra share a common wall. This important anatomic fact has significant technical and surgical implications. The rectum is usually distended and surrounded laterally and posteriorly by the levator muscle. Between the rectum and the perineal skin, a portion of striated voluntary muscle called the muscle complex is present. The contraction of these muscle fibers elevates the skin of the anal dimple. At the level of the skin, a group of voluntary muscle fibers, called parasagittal fibers, are located on both sides of the midline. Lower urethral (bulbar) fistulas are usually associated with good-quality muscles, a well-developed sacrum, a prominent midline groove, and a prominent anal dimple. Higher urethral (prostatic) fistulas are more frequently associated with poor-quality muscles, an abnormally developed sacrum and a flat perineum, with a poor midline groove, and a hardly visible anal dimple. However, exceptions to these rules exist. Occasionally, the infant passes meconium through the urethra, which is an unequivocal sign of rectourinary fistula.

TABLE 35-1
CLASSIFICATION

Males
Cutaneous (perineal fistula)
Recto-urethral fistula
   Bulbar
   Prostatic
Recto–bladder neck fistula
Imperforate anus without fistula
Rectal atresia

Females
Cutaneous (perineal fistula)
Vestibular fistula
Imperforate anus without fistula
Rectal atresia
Cloaca
Complex malformations

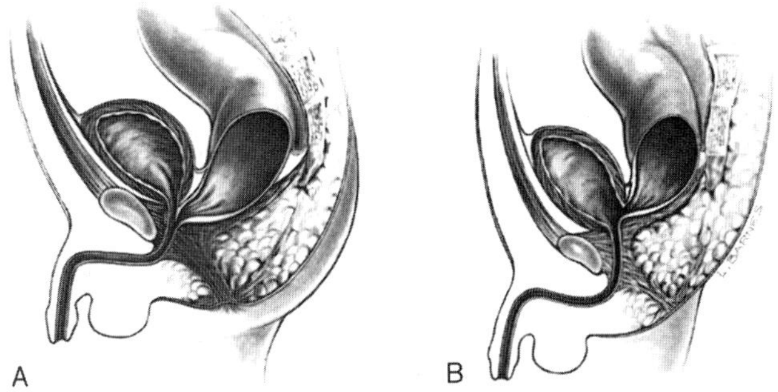

FIGURE 35-2. Spectrum of defects in male patients. *A,* Rectourethroprostatic fistula. *B,* Recto–bladder neck fistula. (From Peña A: Atlas of Surgical Management of Anorectal Malformations. New York, Springer-Verlag, 1990, p 26.)

Rectovesical Fistulas

In this defect, the rectum opens at the bladder neck (Fig. 35-2*B*). The patient has a poor prognosis because the levator muscle, muscle complex, and external sphincter frequently are poorly developed. The sacrum is often deformed, and the entire pelvis seems to be underdeveloped. The perineum is often flat, with evidence of poor muscle development. About 10 % of male imperforate anus cases are in this category.[18]

Imperforate Anus without Fistula

Interestingly, most patients with this unusual defect have a well-developed sacrum and good muscles. The rectum ends approximately 2 cm from the perineal skin. The patient usually has a good prognosis in terms of bowel function.[18] Even when the patient does not have a communication between rectum and urethra, these two structures are separated only by a thin, common wall, which is an important anatomic detail with technical implications. About half of the patients with no fistula also have Down syndrome, and more than 90 % of the patients with Down syndrome and imperforate anus have this specific defect, hinting at a chromosomal link.[22] The fact that these patients have Down syndrome does not seem to interfere with the good prognosis in terms of bowel control.[22]

Rectal Atresia

In this extremely unusual defect in male patients, the lumen of the rectum may be totally (atresia) or partially (stenosis) interrupted. The upper pouch is represented by a dilated rectum, whereas the lower portion is represented by a small anal canal that is in the normal location and measures approximately 1 to 2 cm deep. These two structures may be separated by a thin membrane or by a dense portion of fibrous tissue. These defects occur in approximately 1 % of the entire group of malformations.[18] Patients with this defect have all the necessary elements to be continent and have an excellent functional prognosis. Because they have a well-developed anal canal, they have normal sensation in the anorectum. They also have an almost normal voluntary sphincter.

FEMALE DEFECTS

Rectoperineal Fistulas

From the therapeutic and prognostic points of view, this common defect is equivalent to the perineal fistula described in the male patients.[18] The rectum is well located within the sphincter mechanism, except for its lower portion, which is anteriorly located. Rectum and vagina are well separated (Fig. 35-3*A*).

Rectovestibular Fistulas

Patients with rectovestibular fistulas are frequently erroneously diagnosed as having rectovaginal fistula. The rectovestibular fistula is by far the most commonly seen

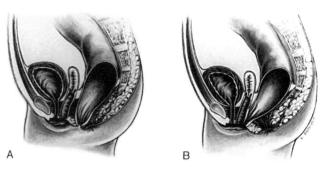

FIGURE 35-3. Spectrum of defects in female patients. *A,* Perineal fistula. *B,* Vestibular fistula. (From Peña A: Atlas of Surgical Management of Anorectal Malformations. New York, Springer-Verlag, 1990, p 50.)

defect in girls. It has an excellent functional prognosis. The precise diagnosis is a clinical one; a meticulous inspection of the newborn genitalia is needed for the diagnosis. The clinician will observe a normal urethral meatus and normal vagina, with a third hole in the vestibule, which is the rectovestibular fistula (Fig. 35-3*B*). About 10 % of these patients have two hemivaginas.

A number of pediatric surgeons repair this defect without a protective colostomy. This is a well-recognized trend in the management of anorectal malformations.[23,24] The advantage of this approach consists in avoiding the potential morbidity of a colostomy and reducing the number of operations from three (colostomy, repair, and colostomy closure) to one. Many patients do very well with a single neonatal primary operation without a protective colostomy. However, a perineal infection followed by dehiscence of the anal anastomoses and recurrence of the fistula provokes severe fibrosis that may interfere with the sphincteric mechanism. In such a case, the patient may have lost the best opportunity for an optimal functional result, because secondary operations do not render the same good prognosis as do successful primary operations.[18] Thus a protective colostomy is still the safest way to avoid these complications. The decision related to establishing a colostomy or operating primarily in these cases must be taken individually by the surgeon, taking into consideration his or her experience and the clinical conditions of the patient. At our institution, patients who are born with this kind of malformation without serious associated defects are operated on primarily as newborns without a colostomy.

The term *vaginal fistula* is frequently erroneously used in dealing with the patients who actually have a vestibular fistula or a cloaca. A real vaginal fistula occurs in fewer than 1 % of all cases,[20,21] and therefore is not considered as part of the proposed classification.

Imperforate Anus without Fistula

This defect in female patients carries the same therapeutic and prognostic implications as those described for male patients.

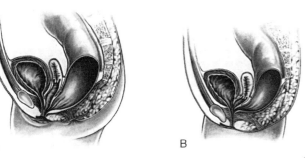

FIGURE 35-4. Spectrum of cloacae. *A*, Most common type of cloaca. *B*, Long common channel. (From Peña A: Atlas of Surgical Management of Anorectal Malformations. New York, Springer-Verlag, 1990, p 60.)

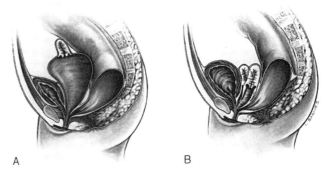

FIGURE 35-6. *A*, Associated hydrocolpos. *B*, Double vagina and double uterus. (From Peña A: Atlas of Surgical Management of Anorectal Malformations. New York, Springer-Verlag, 1990, p 61.)

PERSISTENT CLOACA

This group of defects represents the extreme in the spectrum of complexity of female malformations. A cloaca is defined as a defect in which the rectum, vagina, and urinary tract meet and fuse, creating a single common channel (Figs. 35-4 to 35-6).

The diagnosis of persistent cloaca is a clinical one. This defect should be suspected in a girl born with imperforate anus and small-looking genitalia. Careful separation of the labia discloses a single perineal orifice. The length of the common channel varies from 1 to 7 cm, which has technical and prognostic implications. Common channels longer than 3 cm usually are associated with complex defects (Fig. 35-4*B*) where the mobilization of the vagina is difficult. Therefore in these patients with a long common channel, some form of vaginal replacement is often used during the definitive repair. A common channel of less than 3 cm usually means that the defect can be repaired with a posterior sagittal operation without opening the abdomen (Fig. 35-4*B*). Sometimes the rectum opens high into the dome of the vagina (Fig. 35-5*A*). Therefore a laparotomy must be part of the procedure to mobilize the bowel. Frequently the vagina is abnormally distended and full of secretions (hydrocolpos) (Fig. 35-6*A*). The distended vagina compresses the trigone and interferes with the drainage of the ureters, and the malformation therefore is frequently associated with megaureters.

The dilated vagina also can become infected, which is called pyocolpos, and may lead to perforation and peritonitis. Conversely, such a large vagina may represent a technical advantage for the repair, because having more vaginal tissue will facilitate its reconstruction. A frequent finding in cloacal malformations is the presence of different degrees of vaginal and uterine septation or duplication (Fig. 35-6*B*). The rectum usually opens in between the vaginas. Some of these patients also may have cervical atresia. During puberty, they are unable to drain menstrual blood through the vagina. These patients accumulate menstrual blood into the peritoneal cavity and have at times required emergency operation.[25] Low cloacal malformations (< 3 cm) (Figs. 35-4*A* and 35-5*B*) are usually associated with a well-developed sacrum, a normal-appearing perineum, and adequate muscles and nerves. Therefore a good functional prognosis is expected.

Complex Malformations

Unusual and bizarre anatomic arrangements can be seen in this group. Each case represents a unique challenge to the surgeon, with a different prognosis and therapeutic implications. No general guidelines can be drawn for the management of these patients. Each case must be individualized.

ASSOCIATED DEFECTS

Sacrum and Spine

Sacral deformities seem to be the most frequently associated defect. One or several sacral vertebrae may be missing. One missing vertebra does not seem to have important prognostic implications.[18] However, more than two absent sacral vertebrae represent a poor prognostic sign in terms of bowel continence and, sometimes, urinary control. A hemisacrum is usually associated with a presacral mass and poor bowel control. Other sacral abnormalities, such as spinal hemivertebra, have a negative implication for bowel control.

A sacral ratio has been developed to make a more objective evaluation of the sacrum (Fig. 35-7). This sacral

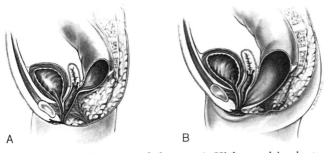

FIGURE 35-5. Spectrum of cloacae. *A*, High rectal implantation into the vagina. *B*, Short common channel. (From Peña A: Atlas of Surgical Management of Anorectal Malformations. New York, Springer-Verlag, 1990, p 61.)

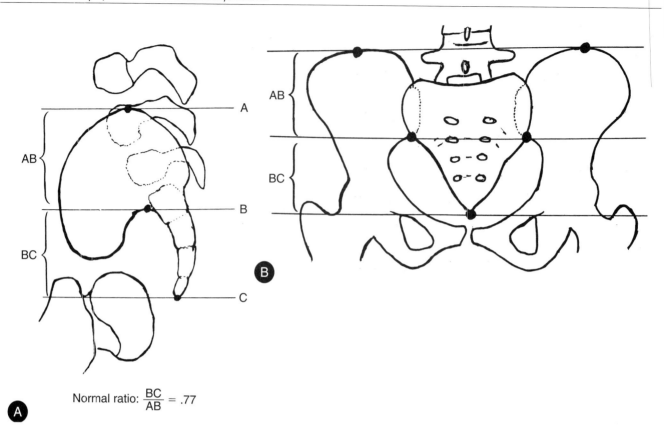

FIGURE 35-7. Sacral ratios. *A,* Anteroposterior view. *B,* Lateral view.

ratio in normal children is 0.77. Children with anorectal malformation have different degrees of sacral hypodevelopment, and therefore the sacral ratio varies from 0.0 to 1.0. We have never seen a patient develop good bowel control with a sacral ratio of less than 0.3.[18]

Emphasis has been placed on the diagnosis and treatment of tethered cord, which is a defect frequently associated with anorectal malformations.[26,27] It has been assumed that presence of tethered cord is associated with poor functional prognosis in these children. A review of our own series showed that 25% of patients with anorectal malformations have a tethered cord.[28] It is true that most of these children have a poor prognosis. However, the presence of tethered cord by itself coincides with the presence of very high defects, a very abnormal sacrum, or myelodysplasia. Therefore it is very difficult to know whether the tethered cord itself is responsible for the bad prognosis. We could not find evidence that the operation to release the tethered cord changed the functional prognosis of the patient.

Genitourinary Defects

The frequency of associated GU defects varies from 20% to 54%.[29-39] The accuracy and thoroughness of the urologic evaluation may account for the reported variation.

In our series, 48% of patients (55% girls and 44% boys) had associated GU anomalies.[35] These figures may not reflect the real incidence of GU defects in a broad population, because ours is a referral center, where we see a high proportion of complex malformations not representative of the entire spectrum of defects.

The higher the malformation, the more frequent are associated urologic abnormalities. The patients with persistent cloaca or rectovesical fistulas have a 90% chance of having an associated GU abnormality.[35] Conversely, children with low defects (perineal fistulas) have less than a 10% chance of an associated urologic defect. Hydronephrosis, urosepsis, and metabolic acidosis from poor renal function represent the main source of morbidity and mortality in newborns with anorectal malformations. Thus a thorough urologic investigation is mandatory in cases of high defects. These studies represent a higher priority than the colostomy itself. The urologic evaluation also is mandatory, although not as urgent in cases of rectovestibular and rectourethral fistulas. In cases of low defects, the urologic evaluation can be postponed and performed on an elective basis. The urologic evaluation in every child with imperforate anus must include an ultrasonographic (US) study of the kidneys and the entire abdomen to rule out the presence of hydronephrosis or any other urologic obstructive process. This study is particularly vital in patients with cloaca to rule out the presence of hydrocolpos. If this study is abnormal, further urologic evaluation is necessary.

INITIAL APPROACH

Figure 35-8 shows the decision-making algorithm for the initial management of male patients. During the last few years, the tendency by the pediatric surgical community worldwide has been to operate on patients with anorectal malformations primarily without a protective colostomy. We promote this trend but also alert all to the potential negative consequences of doing these operations without the necessary experience.

When one is called to see a newborn boy with an anorectal malformation, a thorough perineal inspection must be performed. This usually gives us the most important clues about the type of malformation that the patient has. It is important not to make a decision about colostomy or primary operation before age 24 hours. The reason for this is that it requires a significant intraluminal pressure for the meconium to be forced through a fistula orifice. The passing of meconium through a fistula will be the most valuable sign of the location of the fistula in these babies. If meconium is seen on the perineum, that is an evidence of a perineal fistula. If meconium is in the urine, that makes the diagnosis of a rectourinary fistula. Radiologic evaluations do not show the real anatomy before 24 hours, because the rectum is collapsed, and it takes a significant amount of intraluminal pressure to overcome the muscle tone of the sphincters that surround the lower part of the rectum. Therefore radiologic evaluations done before 24 hours most likely will suggest the presence of a "very high rectum," giving a false diagnosis. During the first 24 hours, the baby should receive intravenous fluids and antibiotics, and the clinician should use those hours to rule out the presence of associated defects that potentially may represent a risk for the baby's life: cardiac malformations, esophageal atresia, and urinary defects. An echocardiogram can be performed to look for cardiac anomalies, and the continuity of the esophagus may easily be demonstrated. A radiograph of the lumbar spine and the sacrum are essential, as well as a spinal US to rule out the presence of tethered cord. US of the abdomen will rule out the presence of hydronephrosis. If the baby has signs of a perineal fistula, we recommend the performance of an anoplasty without a protective colostomy during the first 48 hours of life.

If, after 24 hours, no meconium is seen on the perineum, we recommend performing a cross-table lateral plain roentgenogram with the baby in the prone position. If air in the rectum is seen located below the coccyx and the baby is in good condition with no significant associated defects, one may consider performing a posterior sagittal operation without a protective colostomy. A more conservative alternative could be to perform the posterior sagittal repair and a protective colostomy in the same stage.

Conversely, if the rectal gas does not extend beyond the coccyx, the patient has meconium in the urine, an abnormal sacrum is present, and particularly in the presence of a flat bottom, we strongly recommend the performance of a colostomy. We would elect to perform the anorectoplasty 4 weeks later, provided the baby is gaining weight normally.

After recovery from the colostomy, the patient is discharged from the hospital.

Performing the definitive repair at age 1 month has important advantages for the patient, including less time with an abdominal stoma, less size discrepancy between proximal and distal bowel at the time of colostomy closure, simpler anal dilation, and no recognizable psychological sequela from painful perineal maneuvers.

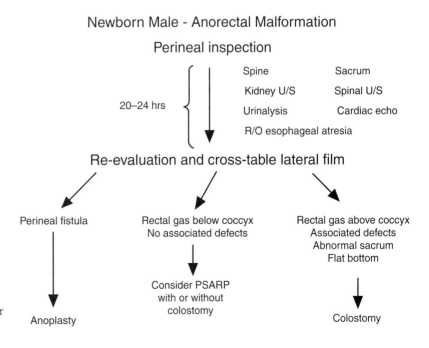

FIGURE 35-8. Decision-making algorithm for male newborns with anorectal malformations.

In addition, placing the rectum in the correct location early in life may be an advantage in terms of the potential for acquired local sensation.[40]

All these potential advantages of an early operation must be weighed against the possible disadvantages of an inexperienced surgeon who is not familiar with the minute anatomic structures of the pelvis of a young infant.

A temptation to repair these defects without a protective colostomy, always exists.[23,24] Repair without colostomy limits the anatomic information that may be very helpful to the surgeon. The worst complications we have seen involved patients operated on without a colostomy and a distal colostogram. Proceeding with the posterior sagittal approach looking for the rectum has resulted in a spectrum of different serious injuries including damage to the urethra, complete division of the urethra, pull-through of the urethra, pull-through of the bladder, injury of the ureters, and division of the vas deferens or seminal vesicles.[41]

Figure 35-9 shows a decision-making algorithm for the initial management of female patients. Again, in female babies, the perineal inspection is the most important step in diagnosis and decision making. The first 24 hours also should be used to rule out important serious, potentially lethal associated defects, as previously described. The perineal inspection may disclose the presence of a single perineal orifice, establishing the diagnosis of a persistent cloaca. A persistent cloaca carries a high risk of an associated urologic defect. The patient needs a complete urologic evaluation including a pelvic US to look for hydrocolpos.

These girls require a colostomy. It is important to perform the divided sigmoid colostomy in such a manner as to leave enough redundant, distal rectosigmoid to allow a pull-through. During the establishment of the colostomy, it is mandatory to drain the hydrocolpos when present. If the hydrocolpos is not large enough to be brought to the abdominal wall above the bladder, it can be drained with an indwelling catheter. Because a significant number of these patients have two hemivaginas, the surgeon must be certain that both are drained. Occasionally, a vaginovaginostomy will have to be created to drain both vaginas with one catheter. At times, the hydrocolpos is of such size that it may produce respiratory distress. The giant vaginas may be drained by creating a tubeless vaginostomy. Many persistent cloaca patients are unable to empty their bladders completely, either because of the narrow common channel or because of an inherent neurologic defect in the bladder musculature. In such circumstances, the baby may require a vesicostomy or a suprapubic cystotomy. Endoscopic examination of the cloaca is recommended to delineate the anatomy.

The perineal inspection may show the presence of a rectoperineal fistula. In these patients, we recommend performing a primary anoplasty without a colostomy. Occasionally, if the baby has severe associated defects or

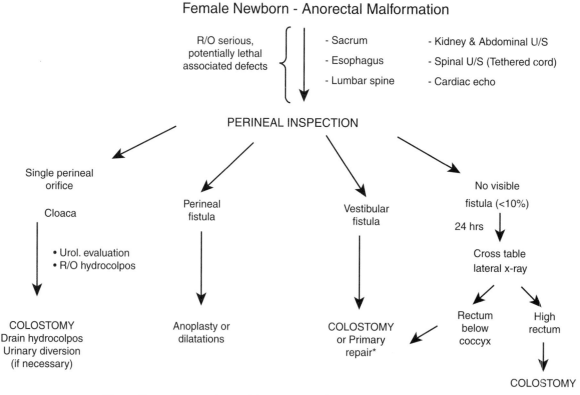

FIGURE 35-9. Decision-making algorithm for female newborns with anorectal malformations.

is ill, the surgeon may elect to dilate the fistula or to do a simple "cut back" to facilitate the emptying of the colon while concomitant issues are addressed.

The presence of a vestibular fistula is the most common finding in female patients. Most surgeons also repair this malformation during the neonatal period without a protective colostomy. Although these operations have been successful many times, they represent the most common source of operative complications in these female patients. To decide to repair this malformation primarily or to establish a protective colostomy is a personal decision that should be based on the experience of the particular surgeon. Colostomy is still the most effective way to protect these patients from the complications associated with the presence of feces in a recently operated on field. Alternatively, the surgeon could perform the rectal repair and also establish a colostomy during the same operation.

When newborn patients with a vestibular fistula are repaired primarily at our institution, we keep the patient 5 days with nothing by mouth, receiving parenteral nutrition. Conversely, when the patient has a primary repair of a vestibular fistula or perineal fistula without colostomy later in life, we are very strict about a preoperative bowel irrigation 24 hours in advance to be sure that the intestine is completely clean. During the operation, we insert a central venous line and keep the patient 7 days receiving parenteral nutrition with nothing by mouth. With this regimen, no infections have occurred in these patients.

In fewer than 10% of the girls, no visible fistula exists with no evidence of meconium after 24 hours of observation. This small group of patients require a cross-table lateral, prone radiographic study. This situation in female patients is extremely unusual. If the radiograph shows gas in the rectum approximating the skin, it means that the patient likely has a very narrow perineal fistula. Conversely, if the distal extent of the rectal gas is located about 1 to 2 cm above the skin, it is most likely the patient has an imperforate anus with no fistula. If the patient is in good condition, one can perform a primary operation without a colostomy, depending again on the surgeon's experience. Many of these patients with no fistula also have Down syndrome. In the event that associated conditions make the rectal repair unfeasible in the newborn period, a colostomy should be done. Those patients can be repaired later in life.

COLOSTOMY

A divided descending colostomy is ideal for the management of anorectal malformations. The completely diverting colostomy provides bowel decompression as well as protection for the final repair of the malformation. In addition, this colostomy permits the performance of the distal colostogram, which is the most accurate diagnostic study to determine the detailed anatomy of these defects.[42]

The descending or upper sigmoid colostomy has definite advantages over a right or transverse colostomy.[43] It is important to have a relatively short segment of defunctionalized distal colon. In some patients, atrophy of the

bowel distal to a more proximal colostomy occurs with development of a microcolon, preventing either retrograde or prograde drainage of the rectosigmoid. Megarectosigmoid may result. Mechanical cleansing of the distal colon before the definitive repair is much less difficult when the colostomy is located in the descending portion of the colon. In the case of a large rectourethral fistula, the patient frequently voids into the colon, and a more distal colostomy allows urine to escape through the distal stoma without significant absorption. With a more proximal colostomy, the urine is absorbed in the colon, increasing the incidence of metabolic acidosis. A loop colostomy permits the passage of stool from the proximal stoma into the distal bowel, which may lead to urinary tract infection or distal rectal pouch dilation and fecal impaction or both. Prolonged distention of the rectal pouch may produce an irreversible hypomotility disorder, leading to severe constipation later in life. An analysis of our experience demonstrated that the problem of colostomy prolapse is more frequent in loop colostomies.[43] A colostomy established in the mid to lower rectosigmoid may interfere with the mobilization of the rectum during the pull-through. This is the most common iatrogenic error we have seen in these patients.

SURGICAL TECHNIQUES

In the past, many surgical techniques to repair anorectal malformations have been described. These included endorectal dissection,[6,8,9] anterior perineal approach to a rectourethral fistula,[44] and many different types of anoplasties.[45] It seems that most pediatric surgeons now use the posterior sagittal approach to repair these malformations, with or without laparotomy or laparoscopy. The debate recently has been centered more on the possibility of performing these operations primarily without a colostomy or with a protective colostomy.

Posterior Sagittal Approach

The patient is placed in the prone position with the pelvis elevated. The use of an electrical stimulator to elicit muscle contraction during the operation is recommended. This contraction serves as a guide to make the incision in the midline, leaving equal amount of muscle on both sides. The length of the incision varies with the type of defect and can be extended to achieve the exposure necessary to allow a satisfactory repair. Thus a perineal fistula requires a minimal posterior sagittal incision (2 cm), whereas higher defects may require a full posterior sagittal incision that usually runs from the middle portion of the sacrum toward the base of the scrotum in the male patient or to the single perineal orifice in cases of a persistent cloaca. The incision includes the skin, subcutaneous tissue, parasagittal fibers, muscle complex, and levator muscles. In simple defects (perineal and vestibular), the incision includes the parasagittal fibers and the muscle complex, but it is not usually necessary to open the levator muscle. Once the sphincter mechanism has been divided, the next most important step of the operation is the separation of the rectum from the UG structures, the most delicate part of the procedure. Magnification and meticulous dissection are necessary to prevent serious injury during this part of the operation.[41]

About 90% of defects in boys can be repaired via the posterior sagittal approach without opening the abdomen and without laparoscopy.[18] Each case has individual anatomic variants that mandate technical modifications. An example is the size discrepancy frequently seen between an ectatic rectum and the space available for pull-through. If the discrepancy is significant, the surgeon must tailor the rectum to fit. In the last 20 years, rectal dilation is less commonly seen, and therefore tailoring is less frequently required. We attribute this to the fact that the patients are receiving more effective colostomies and are referred for definitive repair earlier in life.

If a colostomy has been done, the posterior sagittal approach should never be attempted without a technically adequate high-pressure distal colostogram to determine the exact position of the rectum and the fistula.[42] Attempting the repair without this important information significantly increases the risk of potential damage to the seminal vesicles, prostate, urethra, and bladder innervation.[41]

REPAIR OF SPECIFIC DEFECTS IN BOYS

Perineal Fistula

The operation in these babies is performed in prone position with the pelvis elevated. Multiple 6-0 silk traction sutures are placed in the fistula orifice. An incision is created dividing the entire sphincter mechanism located posterior to the fistula. The incision usually measures about 2 cm in length. The sphincter is divided, and the posterior rectal wall is identified by its characteristic whitish appearance. This plane is easy to find. The dissection of the rectum continues laterally, following that specific plane. The last part of the dissection consists in separating the anterior rectal wall from its intimate relation with the urethra. The most common and serious complication in these relatively simple operations involves injuring the urethra. The patient must have a Foley catheter. The best way to avoid urethral injury is to be aware continuously of the fact that the common wall has no plane of dissection and that the surgeon must create two walls out of one.

Rectourethral Fistula

A Foley catheter is inserted through the urethra. About 20% of the time, this catheter goes into the rectum rather than into the bladder. Under these circumstances, the surgeon may attempt bladder catheterization, again by using a catheter guide, or relocate the catheter into the bladder under direct visualization during the operation.

The incision is performed as previously described (Fig. 35-10); the parasagittal fibers, muscle complex, and levator muscle fibers are completely divided. Sometimes the coccyx can be split in the midline with a cautery,

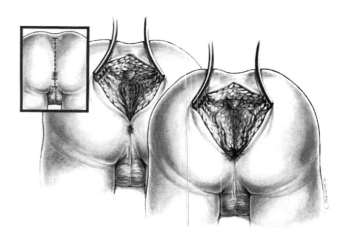

FIGURE 35-10. Posterior sagittal incision. Separation of parasagittal fibers and exposure of the muscle complex.

particularly in those cases of rectoprostatic fistula in which the surgeon requires more exposure in the upper part of the incision. The higher the malformation, the deeper the levator muscle. When the entire sphincter mechanism has been divided, the surgeon expects to find the rectum. It is at this point in the operation that the importance of a good high-pressure distal colostogram cannot be overstated. If the radiologic image showed the presence of a bulbar urethral fistula, the surgeon can be sure that the rectum is going to be found just below the levator, with little risk of inadvertent injury to the urinary tract. In this situation, the rectum actually bulges through the incision when the sphincter mechanism is divided. (Fig. 35-11) Mobilization of the rectum is rather minimal, because only a short gap exists between the rectum and the perineum.

Conversely, if the preoperative distal colostogram shows a rectoprostatic fistula, the surgeon must be particularly careful because the rectum joins the urinary tract much higher. The initial search for the rectum should be near the coccyx. Looking for the rectum lower than that risks injury

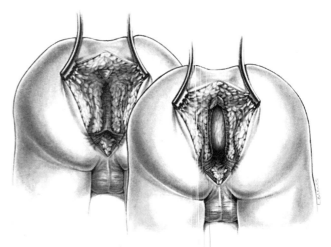

FIGURE 35-11. Dividing muscle complex and levator muscle. Rectum is exposed.

into the bulbar urethra. If the colostogram disclosed the presence of a recto–bladder neck fistula, the posterior sagittal approach is not appropriate as a means of identifying the distal bowel. The rectum is identified and separated from the urinary bladder by the abdominal approach.

In all of the cases in which the rectal fistula is at the bulbar level or higher, silk traction sutures are placed in the posterior rectal wall on both sides, and the rectum is opened in the midline. The incision is extended distally, exactly in the midline, down to the fistula site. Additional silk traction sutures are placed on the edges of the opened posterior rectal wall. When the fistula site is visualized, a last silk suture is placed in the fistula orifice.

The anterior rectal wall above the fistula is part of a common wall, with no natural plane of separation between the urinary tract and the rectum. The plane of separation must be created in that common wall. For this, multiple 6-0 silk traction sutures are placed in the rectal mucosa immediately above the fistula site. The rectal mucosa is then separated from the urethra for approximately 5 to 10 mm above the fistula site (Fig. 35-12*A–C*). This dissection obviously may be the source of serious complications during this repair. If the surgeon has little experience in these dissections, he must be particularly careful. We recommend creating a lateral plane of dissection on either side of the rectum to help with the delineation of the rectal wall from the urethra and prostate. The rectum is covered by a thin fascia that contains fat vessels and nerves that must be preserved on the back side of the bladder. This tissue should be completely stripped from the rectum to be sure that one is working as close as possible to the rectal wall. This is the only way to prevent denervation of the bladder or injury to the vas deferens. Once the rectum is fully separated from the deep structures of the urinary tract, circumferential perirectal dissection is performed to gain enough rectal length to reach the perineum.

In cases of rectoprostatic fistula, the perirectal dissection is considerably more difficult. During this dissection, uniform traction is applied on the multiple silk traction sutures that were originally placed on the rectal edges and also on the mucosa above the fistula. Uniform traction creates and demonstrates the rectal wall and allows the identification

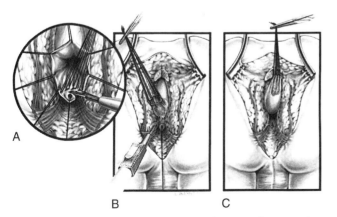

FIGURE 35-12. *A* and *B,* Separation of rectum from urethra. *C,* Rectum is completely separated.

of fibrous bands and vessels that hold the rectum in the pelvis. These bands must be carefully separated from the rectal wall by using cautery, because they contain vessels that tend to retract into the pelvis once divided. The rectum should be dissected as close as possible to the rectal wall without injuring the rectal wall itself.

At the completion of the dissection in prostatic fistula cases, we have sacrificed many of the extrinsic vessels that supply the rectum, but the rectum should be quite viable provided we preserve the intramural blood supply. Although one would think that denervation of the rectum would provoke a motility disorder, leading to severe constipation, this has not been our experience. Patients with lower defects are bothered by more severe postoperative constipation than are patients with higher defects.[18] We do not have an explanation for this.

The circumferential dissection of the rectum must continue until enough length has been gained to allow a rectoperineal anastomosis without tension. At this point, the size of the rectum can be evaluated and compared with the available space. If necessary, the rectum can be tapered, removing part of the posterior wall. In such cases, the rectal wall is reconstructed with two layers of interrupted long-lasting absorbable sutures. The anterior rectal wall is frequently damaged to some degree as a consequence of the mucosal separation between rectum and urethra. To reinforce this wall, both smooth muscle layers can be approximated with interrupted 5-0 long-lasting absorbable sutures. The urethral fistula is sutured with the same material. The rectal tapering should never be performed anteriorly, as this would leave a rectal suture line adjacent to the urethral fistula repair and may lead to a recurrent fistula.

The limits of the anal sphincter mechanism are electrically determined and marked with temporary silk sutures at the skin level. Sometimes those limits are obvious in patients with good sphincter mechanism, even without electrical stimulation. The limits of the sphincter are identified where the muscle complex crosses the parasagittal fibers that run perpendicular and lateral to the muscle complex and parallel to the posterior sagittal incision. The perineal body is reconstructed, bringing together the anterior limits of the external sphincter previously marked with the temporary silk sutures. The rectum must be placed in front of the levator and within the limits of the muscle complex (Fig. 35-13*A,B*). Long-lasting 5-absorbable sutures are placed on the posterior edge of the levator muscle.

The posterior limit of the muscle complex also must be reapproximated behind the rectum. These sutures must include part of the rectal wall as fixation to prevent rectal prolapse (Fig. 35-13*B*). An anoplasty is performed with 16 interrupted long-lasting absorbable sutures (Fig. 35-14*A,B*). The wound is closed with a subcuticular 5-0 absorbable monofilament. Before this, the ischiorectal fossa and the subcutaneous tissue are reapproximated with the same suture material. The Foley catheter inserted before the beginning of the operation remains in place for 5 to 10 days. The patient receives broad-spectrum antibiotics for 24 hours. These patients can be fed after recovery from anesthesia because of the diverting colostomy.

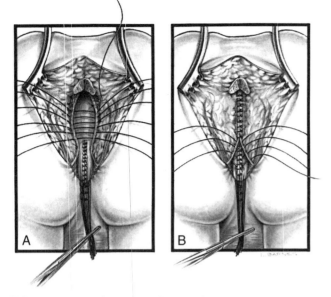

FIGURE 35-13. *A,* Rectum is passed in from of the levator muscle. *B,* Muscle complex sutures anchor the rectum.

Recently some surgeons have been repairing rectourethral fistulas laparoscopically.[46] The preliminary experience shows that these procedures are feasible. We are not convinced that a laparoscopic approach for a rectourethral fistula is necessarily less invasive than the posterior sagittal approach.

Recto–Bladder Neck Fistulas

For this repair, a total body preparation is performed. The entire lower part of the patient's body is included in the sterile field. The initial incision is posterior sagittal. All the muscle structures are divided in the midline. After creating the tunnel through the muscle complex through which the rectum will eventually be pulled, this wound is closed, leaving a rubber tube in the tract to be retrieved from the abdominal dissection. The size of the tube should be chosen to represent the space available for the pull-through. The patient is then placed in the lithotomy position so that the surgeon can work simultaneously in the abdomen and in the perineum. At this point,

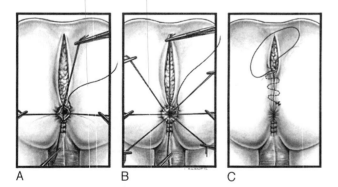

FIGURE 35-14. *A* and *B,* Anoplasty. *C,* Skin suture.

laparoscopy represents an excellent minimally invasive alternative to a laparotomy.

In the patient with a bladder neck fistula, the rectum connects to the bladder neck, approximately 2 cm below the peritoneal reflection. The higher the malformation, the shorter the common wall between the rectum and the urinary tract. This means that the rectum joins with the urinary tract a nearly a right angle, with little common wall. This anatomic fact makes separation of the rectum from the bladder much easier. The laparoscopic approach provides an excellent view of the peritoneal reflection, the ureters, and the vas deferens, which must be kept under direct view to prevent injury to them.

We recommend dividing the peritoneum around the distal rectum to create a plane of dissection to be followed distally. The rectum rapidly narrows as it communicates with the bladder neck, at which point it is divided, and bladder side is sutured. The rectum is now fully separated from the urinary tract. The vessels that supply the distal rectum are divided with electrocautery or between ligatures until we have enough estimated length to pull the rectum comfortably down to the perineum. At this point, the rubber tube that was left through the muscle complex and sphincter from below is located in the retroperitoneum (Fig. 35-15*A,B*). The tube is removed and replaced from the perineum with a long narrow hemostat used to grasp the traction sutures on the rectal side of the fistula. Traction on the rectum from below will demonstrate further lines of tension that must be divided to allow the rectum to reach the perineum.

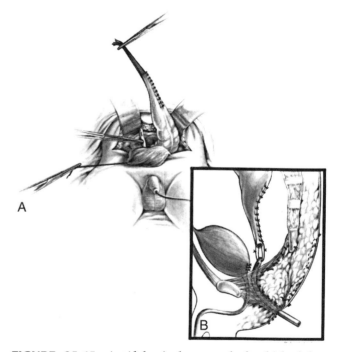

FIGURE 35-15. *A,* Abdominal approach for high defects (recto–bladder neck fistula). Rectum has been separated from the bladder neck. The presacral rubber tube is identified. *B,* Rectum is anchored to the rubber tube to guide the pull-through.

One limitation of laparoscopy is that tapering of the rectum, if necessary, is not easy. Tapering is much more efficiently done with the abdomen open.

Imperforate Anus without Fistula

In these cases, the blind end of the rectum is usually located at the level of the bulbar urethra and is easily reachable from the posterior sagittal approach. The rectum must be carefully separated from the urethra, because both structures have a common wall, even though no fistula is present. The rest of the repair must be performed as described for the rectourethral fistula defect.

Rectal Atresia and Stenosis

The approach to these malformations also is posterior sagittal. The upper rectal pouch is opened, as well as the little distal anal canal. An end-to-end anastomosis is performed under direct visualization, followed by a meticulous reconstruction of the muscle mechanism posterior to the rectum.

FEMALE PATIENTS

Rectoperineal Fistulas

This defect is repaired in the same way as described for male patients. The difference in these cases is that the rectum is not usually intimately attached to the vagina, and therefore the chances of a vaginal injury are remote.

Vestibular Fistulas

The complexity of this defect is frequently underestimated. Multiple 5-0 silk traction sutures are placed at the mucocutaneous junction of the fistula. The incision used to repair this defect is shorter than the one used to repair the male rectourethral fistula. The incision continues down to the fistula and around the fistula into the vestibule. Once the entire sphincter mechanism has been divided, one identifies the posterior rectal wall by its characteristic whitish appearance. The fascia that surrounds the rectum must be removed to be sure that one is dissecting as close as possible to the rectal wall. The dissection is aided by working from each side of the rectum as well as from below, while applying traction on the multiple silk traction sutures. One must keep in mind that a long common wall exists between the vagina and the rectum and that two walls must be created out of one by using a very meticulous, delicate technique. The dissection continues cephalad until the rectal and vaginal walls are fully separated (Fig. 35-16*A*). If the rectum and the vagina are not completely separated, a tense anoplasty anastomosis predisposes the patient to dehiscence and retraction.

Once the dissection has been completed, the perineal body is repaired (Fig. 35-16*B*). The anterior edge of the muscle complex is reapproximated, as previously described. The muscle complex must be reconstructed

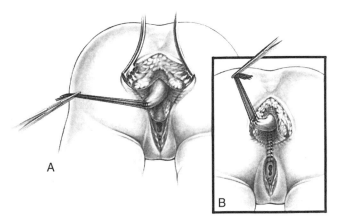

FIGURE 35-16. Repair of rectovestibular fistula. *A*, Rectum is completely separated from vagina. *B*, Perineal body is repaired.

posterior to the rectum. The sutures must include the posterior edge of the muscle complex and the posterior rectal wall to avoid rectal prolapse (Fig. 35-17*A*). The anoplasty is performed as previously described (Fig. 35-17*B*).

CLOACA

Before undertaking the repair of these defects, the surgeon should perform an endoscopic study of the cloaca malformation, with the specific purpose of determining the approximate length of the common channel. Our experience of more than 342 patients allows us to define two well-characterized groups of patients with cloaca.[47] These two groups represent different technical challenges and must be recognized preoperatively. The first is represented by patients that are born with a common channel shorter than 3 cm. Fortunately, these patients represent more than 60% of the entire group of persistent cloaca patients. The great majority of these patients can be repaired with a posterior sagittal approach only, without a laparotomy. We believe that the operation indicated to repair this variant is a reproducible one that can be done by most pediatric surgeons.

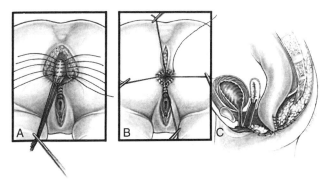

FIGURE 35-17. Repair of vestibular fistula. *A*, Muscle complex sutures anchor the rectum. *B*, Anoplasty. *C*, Operation is finished.

The second group is represented by patients with a long common channel; these usually need a laparotomy. In this group of patients, decision-making processes benefit from a large experience and special training in urology. We believe, therefore, that it is in the best interest of the patients that they be referred to centers with special dedication to the repair of complex cloacal malformations.

Cloacas with Common Channel Shorter than 3 Centimeters

The incision extends from the middle portion of the sacrum down to the single perineal orifice (Fig. 35-18A). All the sphincter mechanism is divided in the midline. The first structure that the surgeon will find after the division of the sphincter mechanism is the rectum (Fig. 35-18B). However, because of the special complexity of these malformations, the surgeon must be prepared to find bizarre anatomic arrangements of the rectum and vagina. The rectum is opened in the midline (Fig. 35-18C), and silk traction sutures are placed along the edges of the posterior rectal wall. The incision is extended distally to the perineum through the entire common channel. The common channel is thus exposed, which allows us to measure and confirm the length of the common channel under direct vision. The next step of this procedure consists in separating the rectum from the vagina (Fig. 35-19). This is performed in the same way as described during the repair of the rectovestibular fistula. The rectum and vagina share the same common wall described earlier.

Once the rectum has been completely separated from the vagina, we perform what we call total UG mobilization.[48] In the past, we used to separate the vagina from the urinary tract, which was a technically challenging, not very reproducible maneuver with a significant morbidity. The total UG mobilization consists of bringing both vagina and urethra to the perineum as a unit, without separating them. After the rectum has been dissected

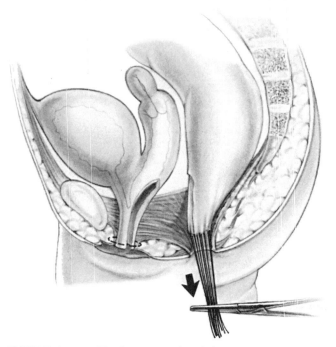

FIGURE 35-19. Total urogenital mobilization. Rectum separated from vagina. (From Peña A: Total urogenital mobilization: An easier way to repair cloacas. J Pediatr Surg 32:263–268, 1997.)

away from the cloaca, multiple silk traction sutures are placed in the edges of the vagina and the common channel, to apply uniform traction on the UG sinus as it is mobilized. Another series of fine traction sutures is placed across the UG sinus approximately 5 mm proximal to the clitoris (Fig. 35-20). The UG sinus is transected between the last row of silk stitches and the clitoris. The anterior part of the UG sinus is dissected from the pubic symphysis, taking advantage of the fact that a natural plane exists between it and the pubis. This dissection is usually easy and relatively bloodless. At the upper edge of the pubis, we find the fibrous, avascular suspensory ligaments that give support to vagina and bladder. While we apply traction to the multiple UG sinus sutures, the suspensory ligaments are divided, which immediately provides 2 to 3 cm of additional mobilization of the UG sinus. Lateral and posterior dissection of the UG sinus will provide an addition of 0.5 to 1.0 cm of length (Fig. 35-21). Both the urethral meatus and the vaginal introitus are anastomosed to the perineum in the appropriate positions. Approximately 60% of all persistent cloaca malformations can be very satisfactorily repaired with this technique. This maneuver has the additional advantage of preserving excellent blood supply to both urethra and vagina, while placing the urethral opening in a visible location to facilitate intermittent catheterization when necessary (Fig. 35-22). It also provides a smooth urethra that can be easily catheterized. What used to be the common distal UG channel is divided in the midline and used to create labia for the patient. The vaginal edges are mobilized to reach the skin

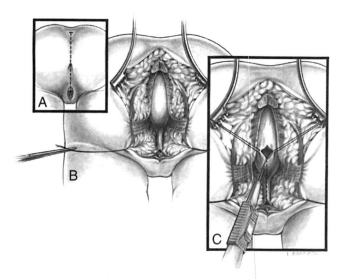

FIGURE 35-18. Cloaca repair. *A*, Incision. *B*, Rectum and common channel are exposed. *C*, Rectal opening.

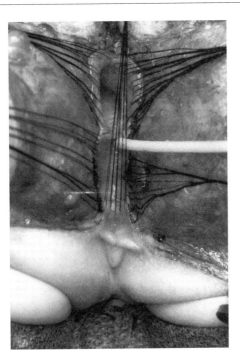

FIGURE 35-20. Total urogenital mobilization. Stitches placed on the edges of the sinus and across, near the clitoris.

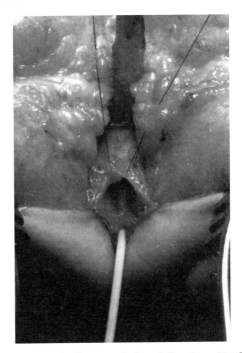

FIGURE 35-22. Total urogenital mobilization. Urethra and vagina sutured in their new positions.

to create a surprisingly natural-looking introitus. The limits of the rectal sphincter are electrically determined, and the perineal body is reconstructed, bringing together the anterior limit of the sphincter. The rectum is placed within the limits of the sphincter, as described earlier (Fig. 35-23). The patients can eat the same day, and the pain is usually controlled easily. The patients are discharged 48 hours after the surgical procedure.

Cloacas with a Common Channel Longer than 3 Centimeters

When the endoscopy shows that the patient has a long common channel, the surgeon must be prepared to face a very significant technical challenge. We would emphasize again that no substitute for experience exists when treating these difficult patients.

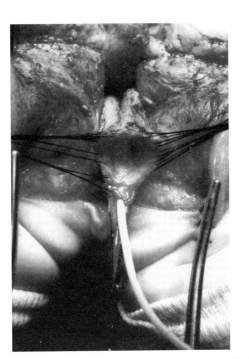

FIGURE 35-21. Total urogenital mobilization. Urogenital sinus fully mobilized.

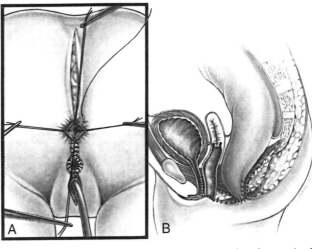

FIGURE 35-23. *A,* Urethra and vagina are already repaired. Anaplasty. *B,* Operation is completed. (From Peña A: Atlas of Surgical Management of Anorectal Malformations. New York, Springer-Verlag, 1990, p 69.)

In the presence of a long common channel, the patient should be prepped so that the entire lower body is accessible, because it is likely that the patient will require a laparotomy after the initial exploration by the posterior sagittal approach. As before, the rectum is separated from the vagina and urethra, and the length of the common channel of the UG sinus is determined. The presence of a common channel of more than 5 cm means that total UG mobilization from below will not be enough to repair the malformation, and it is advisable to leave the common channel intact for use as a urethra. This will eventually be used for intermittent catheterization. In that situation, the vagina is separated from the urinary tract from below, by placing traction sutures to aid in creating the plane of dissection. This is a very delicate, meticulous, and tedious maneuver. With this dissection, one can gain a separation of the vagina from the urinary tract for approximately 2 cm. The posterior wall of the previous common channel is closed with interrupted sutures of absorbable material. The rest of the separation must be completed through the abdomen.

A midline laparotomy is recommended. The bladder is opened in the midline, and feeding tubes are placed into the ureters for identification to protect them. Both the ureters run through the large common wall between the vagina and the bladder. The stents provide easy identification of the ureters during this difficult dissection.

The surgeon must be familiar with techniques of ureteral reimplantations, because frequently the ureters will require reimplantation after the separation of the bladder and vagina is complete. We also confirm the patency of the müllerian structures by injecting saline through a no. 3 feeding tube inserted through the fimbria of the fallopian tubes. If one of the tubes is not patent, we recommend its excision, along with its hemiuterus if the system is bifid. The ovary and its blood supply are preserved.

When both müllerian structures are atretic, we recommend leaving both in place, informing the parents, and monitoring the patient for a long period so that we may help with further decisions when she reaches puberty, at which time techniques may be available to address this cause of infertility.

With the abdomen open, surgical decisions must be based on the specific anatomic findings. In the presence of a single vagina of normal size, the surgeon must separate a vagina from the urinary tract, being sure to preserve its blood supply that comes from the uterine vessels. It is brought to the perineum, and the introitus is constructed. When the vagina is found to be too short, the patient requires some form of vaginal replacement, which can be constructed with the rectum, colon, or small bowel.

Vaginal Switch Maneuver

Some girls with persistent cloaca malformations are born with hydrocolpos, two hemivaginas and two uteri. The hemivaginas are very large, and the two uteri are widely separated, the distance between the uteri being longer than the length of both the hemivaginas. In those cases, it is ideal to perform a maneuver called a "vaginal switch."

One of the uteri and its fallopian tube are resected (Fig. 35-24), preserving the ovary with its blood supply.

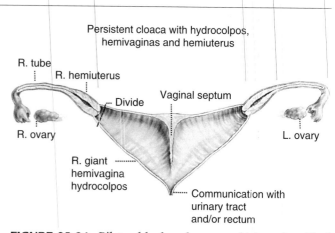

FIGURE 35-24. Bilateral hydrocolpos, very high vagina. Ideal anatomy to be repaired with vaginal switch maneuver. (From Kiely EM, Peña A: Anorectal malformations. In O'Neil JA, Rowe MI, Grosfeld JL, et al [eds]: Pediatric Surgery. St. Louis, Mosby-Yearbook, 1998, p. 1442.)

The blood supply of the ipsilateral hemivagina must be sacrificed, but most of the time, collateral vessels from the opposite vagina will support both. The vaginal septum is resected, creating a single long vagina. The cut end of the ipsilateral vagina is turned down to the perineum (Fig. 35-25). This is an excellent procedure to use to construct a viable and very functional vagina.

Vaginal Augmentation or Replacement or Both

A short vagina can be augmented or totally absent vagina constructed from a bowel segment in case of a very high or absent vagina. The choices are rectum, colon, or small bowel.

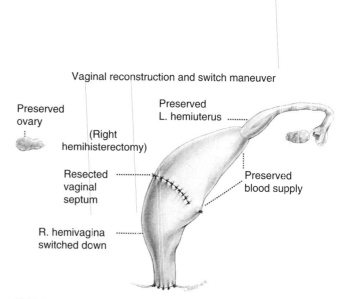

FIGURE 35-25. Vaginal switch maneuver. (From Kiely EM, Peña A: Anorectal malformations. In O'Neil JA, Rowe MI, Grosfeld JL, et al [eds]: Pediatric Surgery. St. Louis, Mosby-Yearbook, 1998, p. 1442.)

1. The vagina can be constructed from the rectum when the patient has a megarectum that can be divided longitudinally, preserving the mesenteric blood supply (Fig. 35-26*A,B*). This is feasible only in patients that have a megarectum large enough to allow the formation of an adequate-sized rectum. The blood supply of the rectum will be provided transmurally from branches of the inferior mesenteric vessels.

2. Vaginal replacement with colon. The colon is an ideal substitute for the vagina. At times the location of the colostomy interferes with this type of reconstruction. When available, the sigmoid colon is preferable. One must take the most mobile portion of the colon to use a piece that has a long mesentery. When the patient has internal genitalia or a little cuff of vagina or cervix, the upper part of the bowel used for replacement must be sutured to the vaginal cuff. When the patient has no vagina and no uterus, the neovagina is closed at its upper end and is used only for sexual purposes but obviously not for reproduction (Fig. 35-27).

3. Small bowel. If a colon segment is not available, then the most mobile portion of the small bowel is used for vaginal reconstruction. The most mobile portion of the small bowel is located approximately 15 cm proximal to the ileocecal valve (Fig. 35-28*A*). We believe that it is the best portion of the small bowel to be used for vaginal replacement. A portion of this ileum is isolated and pulled down, preserving its blood supply (Fig. 35-28*B* and *C*).

The most difficult type of cloacal malformation consists of those in which two little hemi vaginas attach to the bladder neck or the trigone of the bladder. In these cases, the rectum also opens in the trigone (Fig. 35-29). The separation of these structures is done via the abdomen. Unfortunately, when that separation is completed, the patient is frequently left with a nonfunctional bladder neck. The surgical decision then must be between an attempt to reconstruct the bladder neck or to close it permanently. In the first situation, most patients will need to rely on intermittent catheterization to empty the bladder. If permanent closure of the bladder neck is elected, a vesicostomy is created, delaying a continent diversion procedure until the patient is 3 to 4 years old. In this type of malformation, vaginal replacement should be done by using one of the substitutes previously described.

We have abandoned using skin flaps or vaginal flaps because we found that the maneuvers described here provide better results.

Postoperative Management and Colostomy Closure

Postoperatively, the patients generally have a smooth course. Pain is not a complaint, except for those who have undergone a laparotomy. In the simple cloacal repair, the Foley catheter remains in place for 8 to 14 days. In very complex malformations, for example, in cases with a bladder neck reconstruction, we prefer to leave a

TECHNIQUE FOR VAGINAL REPLACEMENT USING RECTUM

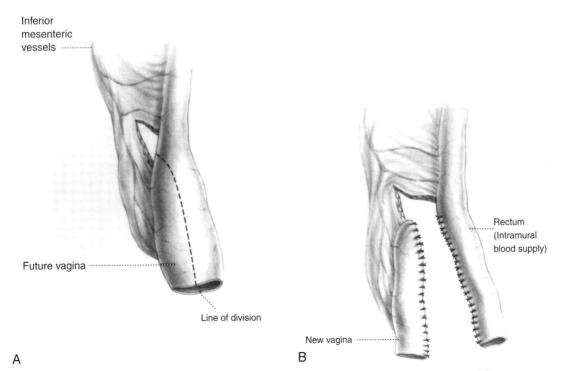

Inferior mesenteric vessels

Future vagina

Line of division

Rectum (Intramural blood supply)

New vagina

A

B

FIGURE 35-26. A, Vaginal replacement with rectum. Planning the neovagina. B, Neovagina separated from rectum.

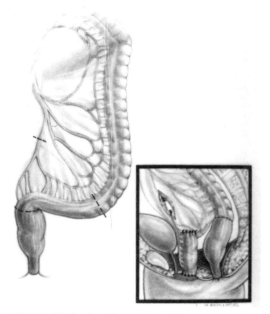

FIGURE 35-27. Vaginal replacement with sigmoid colon.

suprapubic tube. In patients in whom the bladder neck was surgically obliterated, we establish a vesicostomy. Male patients with rectourethral fistulas are kept on Foley catheter drainage for 7 days. If the catheter should become dislodged, the patients often can void without any problem and do not require replacement of the catheter.

Intravenous antibiotics are administered for 48 hours. Antibiotic ointment is applied to the perineal suture lines for 8 to 10 days. Most patients go home 2 days after a posterior sagittal repair and 3 to 4 days after a laparotomy.

Two weeks after the repair, anal dilatations are started. A dilator that fits snugly into the anus should be used. This procedure is done twice daily by the parents. Every week, the size of the dilator is increased, until the rectum reaches the desired size, which depends on the patient's age (Table 35-2). Once this desired size is reached, the colostomy may be closed. The frequency of dilatation may be reduced once the parents feel that the dilator goes in easily with no resistance. After that, our dilatation schedule is as follows.

At least once a day for 1 month
Ever third day for 1 month
Twice a week for 1 month
Once a week for 1 month
Once a month for 3 months

Severe strictures have occurred in cases when the dilation program was not carried out as prescribed or when the blood supply of the distal rectum was insufficient.

At the time of colostomy closure and especially in the patients who had a persistent cloaca, we perform an endoscopy to be sure that the repair is intact. After the colostomy is closed, the patient may have multiple bowel movements, and perineal excoriation may develop. A constipating diet may be helpful in the treatment of this problem. After several weeks, the number of bowel movements decreases, and most patients will begin to experience constipation. After 6 months, a more regular bowel-movement pattern develops. A patient, who has one to three bowel movements per day, remains clean in between bowel movements and shows evidence of a feeling or pushing during bowel movements, has a good bowel-movement pattern, usually has a good prognosis. This type of patient is trainable. A patient with multiple bowel movements or one who is passing stool constantly without showing any signs of sensation or pushing usually has a poor functional prognosis.

We usually keep the cloaca patients on Foley catheter drainage for 2 to 3 weeks. In our series, about 20% of the patients with a common channel shorter than 3 cm require long-term intermittent catheterization to empty the bladder. Patients with common channels longer than 3 cm will require intermittent catheterization 70% to 80% of the time. Therefore we leave the Foley catheter until the perineal wounds are healed sufficiently to allow catheterization. If the urethral meatus is not clearly visible, we prefer to keep the Foley catheter in place. Once we are able to see the urethral orifice, then we remove the Foley catheter in the clinic and observe the baby to see if she is capable of spontaneous voiding and emptying the bladder. If she cannot pass urine, then we can teach the mother at that time the techniques of intermittent catheterization. In cases of a very long common channel, we prefer to leave a suprapubic tube. One month after repair, we perform a suprapubic cystogram and begin clamping the tube. We measure the residual urine, which is an indicator of bladder function. The suprapubic tube remains in place until we have evidence of good bladder function or the mother learns to catheterize the bladder per urethra when indicated.

FUNCTIONAL DISORDERS AFTER REPAIR OF ANORECTAL MALFORMATIONS

Most patients who have undergone repair of an anorectal malformation will experience some degree of a functional defecating disorder, and all have from some degree of abnormality in their fecal continence mechanism.

Fecal continence depends on three main factors.

1. *Voluntary muscle structures.* These structures are represented by the levator muscle, muscle complex, and external sphincter. Normally they are used only for brief periods, when the fecal mass reaches the anorectal area, propelled by the involuntary peristaltic contraction of the rectosigmoid, only minutes before defecation. These voluntary muscle structures are used only occasionally during the rest of the day and night. Patients with anorectal malformations have abnormal voluntary striated muscles with variable degrees of underdevelopment.

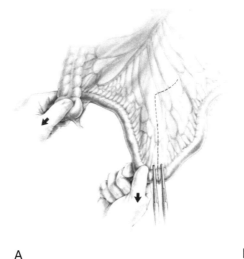

A

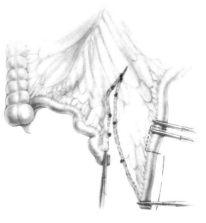

B

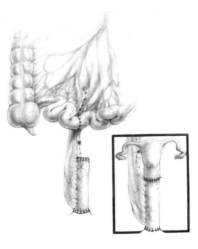

C

FIGURE 35-28. *A,* Vaginal replacement with small bowel, using that portion with the longest mesentery. *B,* Pulling the small bowel down. *C,* Operation completed.

Voluntary muscles can be used only when the patient feels that it is necessary to use them. For that sensation, the patient needs information that can be derived only from an intact sensory mechanism, a mechanism that many patients with anorectal malformations lack.

2. *Sensation.* Exquisite sensation in normal individuals resides in the anal canal. Except for patients with rectal atresia, most patients with anorectal malformations are born without an anal canal; therefore sensation either does not exist or is rudimentary. Evidence exists that distention of the rectum is felt in many of these patients, provided the rectum has been located accurately within the muscle structures. This sensation seems to be a consequence of stretching the voluntary muscle (proprioception). The most important clinical implication of this is that liquid stool or soft fecal material may not be felt by the patient with anorectal malformations, as the rectum is not distended. Thus to achieve some degree of sensation

and bowel control, the patient must have the capacity to form solid stool.

3. *Bowel motility.* Perhaps the most important and largely underestimated factor in fecal continence is bowel motility. In a normal individual, the rectosigmoid remains quiet for variable periods (1 to several days), depending on individual defecation habits. During that time, anorectal sensation and the voluntary muscle structures are almost not necessary because the stool remains in the rectosigmoid if it is solid.

The peristaltic contraction of the rectosigmoid that occurs before defecation is normally felt by the patient. Voluntarily, the normal individual will relax the striated muscles, which allows the rectal contents to migrate down into the highly sensitive area of the anal canal. There, accurate information is provided concerning the consistency and quality of the stool. The voluntary muscles may be used to push the rectal contents back up into the

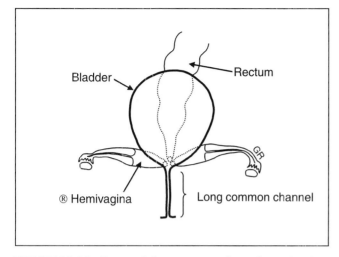

FIGURE 35-29. Extremely long common channel. Hemivaginas and rectum connected to bladder neck.

rectosigmoid and to hold them if desired, until the appropriate time for evacuation. At the time of defecation, the voluntary muscle structures relax, allowing the fecal mass to pass into and through the anorectum.

The main factor that initiates the emptying of the rectosigmoid is a massive involuntary peristaltic contraction helped sometimes by a Valsalva maneuver. Most patients with anorectal malformation have a serious disturbance of this sophisticated bowel motility mechanism. Patients who have undergone a posterior sagittal anorectoplasty or any other type of sacroperineal approach, in which the most distal part of the bowel was preserved, show evidence of an overefficient bowel reservoir (megarectum). The main clinical manifestation of megarectum is constipation, which seems to be more severe in patients with lower defects. Vestibular fistula patients, in particular, are more prone to this problem. We believe that a loop colostomy is sometimes associated with a fecal impaction in the blind rectal pouch, before repair that leads to severe postrepair constipation. The enormously dilated rectosigmoid with normal ganglion cells behaves like a myopathic type of hypomotility disorder. The patients

TABLE 35-2

SIZE OF DILATOR ACCORDING TO AGE

Age	Hegar Dilator (No.)
1–4 mo	12
4–12 mo	13
8–12 mo	14
1–3 yr	15
3–12 yr	16
>12 yr	17

with overflow fecal incontinence based on rectosigmoid constipation are manageable with enemas.

Those patients treated with techniques in which the most distal part of the bowel was resected (endorectal dissection)[6,9] clinically behave as individuals without a rectal reservoir. This is a situation equivalent to a perineal colostomy. Depending on the amount of colon resected, the patient may have loose stools. In these cases, medical management consisting of enemas plus a constipating diet and medications to slow the colonic motility is indicated.

Evaluation of Results

Each defect described here has a different prognosis. When evaluating clinical results, the error of oversimplification should be avoided. Classifications such as "high," "intermediate," and "low," or even "high" and "low," do not accurately correlate with the results that we have obtained, because the so called high and intermediate defects frequently include individual malformations with different prognoses. The patients with low defects usually have excellent results, except when technical errors have been made.

Table 35-3 shows the results obtained in our series. The patients with a sacral ratio of less than 0.3 and a flat perineum have fecal incontinence regardless of the type of malformation or the quality of the repair.

Because persistent cloaca represents another spectrum of defects, they must be subclassified on the basis of potential for bowel and urinary control. The length of the common channel seems to be the most important prognostic factor.

Complications

In our series of 1640 patients, 7 patients experienced wound infection in the immediate postoperative period. Three of these patients had a loop colostomy, which was not completely diverting. Fortunately, the infections affected only the skin and subcutaneous tissue, and all healed secondarily, without functional sequelae. Anal strictures may be the consequence of lack of discipline in following the protocol of dilatations. When trying to prevent discomfort for the patient, some surgeons dilate the anus once a week, frequently under anesthesia. This serious error can eventually create a severe, intractable fibrous stricture. Patients who underwent tapering did not have more constipation compared with those who did not. Constipation was the most common functional disorder observed in patients who underwent posterior sagittal anorectoplasty (see Table 35-3). Patients with the best prognosis have the highest incidence of constipation. Patients with very poor prognosis, such as bladder-neck fistula, have a low incidence of constipation and a high rate of incontinence. The analysis of our series indicates that the constipation seems to be related directly to the degree of preoperative rectal ectasia. Colostomies that do not allow cleaning and irrigation of the distal colon lead to megarectum.

TABLE 35-3									
GLOBAL FUNCTIONAL RESULTS									
	Voluntary Bowel Movement		Soiling		Totally Continent		Constipated	
	Pts.	%	Pts.	%	Pts.	%	Pts.	%
Perineal fistula	39/39	100	3/43	20.9	35/39	89.7	30/53	56.6
Rectal atresia or stenosis	8/8	100	2/8	25	6/8	75	4/8	50
Vestibular fistula	89/97	92	36/100	36	63/89	70.8	61/100	61
Imperforate anus without fistula	30/35	86	18/37	48.6	18/30	60	22/40	55
Bulbar-urethral fistula	68/83	82	48/89	53.9	34/68	50	52/81	64.2
Prostatic fistula	52/71	73	67/87	77.1	16/52	30.8	42/93	45.2
Cloaca: short common channel	50/70	71	50/79	63.3	25/50	50	34/85	40
Cloaca: long common channel	18/41	44	34/39	87.2	5/18	27.8	17/45	34.8
Vaginal fistula	3/4	75	4/5	80	1/3	33.3	1/5	20
Bladderneck fistula	8/29	28	39/43	90.7	1/8	12.5	7/45	15.6

Severe anorectal strictures occurred in three of our patients as a result of devascularization of the rectum during the rectal mobilization. Dilations were more difficult than usual. One patient required a secondary operation. Tapering was not responsible for a stricture in any of the patients.

Urethrovaginal fistula has been the most common and feared complication in cases of persistent cloaca before the introduction of the total UG mobilization maneuver.[48] In cases in which vaginal mobilization and separation from the neourethra resulted in opposing suture lines, 90-degree rotation of the vagina failed to decrease the incidence of a postoperative fistula. In four patients, complete fibrosis of the vagina developed secondary to an excessive dissection in an attempt to mobilize a high vagina. Additionally, in two of the vaginal-switch patients, acquired atresia of the pulled-through vagina developed.

Transient femoral nerve palsy was observed in three adolescent patients, a consequence of excessive pressure in the groin during the operation. This problem can be avoided by adequate cushioning of the patient's groin area.

During a secondary operation, a recurrent rectourethral fistula that closed spontaneously developed in one patient. This patient had a severe pelvic inflammatory process secondary to a retained foreign body from a previous operation.

Many of our patients were referred because of severe complications after a failed repair of an anorectal malformation. A review of 572 of those patients[41] revealed that significant urologic injuries were the most common complications in male patients. Failure to obtain a good distal colostogram to delineate the anatomy precisely was the most important source of these complications.

Neurogenic bladder in male patients as a result of the anorectal malformation itself must be extremely unusual, because it happens only in patients with a very abnormal sacrum (Table 35-4). Otherwise, it reflects poor surgical technique with denervation of the bladder and bladder neck during the repair.[41]

Most persistent cloaca patients have a flaccid, smooth, large bladder that does not empty completely. We do not see the "Christmas tree" cystographic image of the typical neurogenic bladder seen in patients with a myelodysplasia. Fortunately, most of the patients with a persistent cloaca have a competent bladder neck. The combination of a competent bladder neck with a flaccid bladder make these patients ideal candidates for intermittent catheterization, which keeps them completely dry. Two exceptions to this rule are found; one is represented by patients that have a very long common channel, wherein the hemivaginas are attached to the bladder neck. After even the most careful separation of these structures, the patient is left with no bladder neck or a very damaged bladder neck. The second group is represented by a small number of patients that are born with separated pubic bones. These patients have a congenital absence of the bladder neck and will eventually require continent urinary diversion.

MEDICAL MANAGEMENT FOR FECAL INCONTINENCE

For those patients with bowel dysfunction, a program of bowel management should be implemented. We believe that all patients with anorectal malformations, regardless

TABLE 35-4		
URINARY INCONTINENCE		
	Pts.	%
Rectal atresia or stenosis	0/8	0
Perineal fistula	0/38	0
Bulbar-urethral fistula	2/85	2.4
Imperforate anus without fistula	1/37	2.7
Prostatic fistula	7/85	8.2
Bladderneck fistula	7/38	18.4
Cloaca: short common channel	5/18	27.8
Vaginal fistula	1/5	20
Cloaca: long common channel	37/48	77.1

of the complexity of the defect, can be kept completely dry of urine and clean of stool. The patients with more favorable lesions achieve bowel and urinary control with simple intervention. The more difficult patients achieve continence of urine and stool because we implement a more complicated program to keep them dry and clean.

With the rational administration of bowel irrigations, diet, and drugs, most patients, including those with severe fecal incontinence, are able to remain clean for 24 hours.[49] In our experience, only those patients with severe diarrhea secondary to an absent or a short colon have been candidates for a permanent colostomy.

Patients with fecal incontinence are evaluated and classified into those with constipation, and those with increased motility will tend to have diarrhea.

In the first group, bowel irrigations must be aggressive. A rubber tube is usually introduced high into the sigmoid to clean the bowel. This program succeeds because the decreased bowel motility allows them to remain clean for 24 hours after an effective irrigation. No laxatives or diets are given as part of this protocol. The second group, or those patients with increased bowel motility due to loss of the rectal reservoir, require a constipating diet, medication to decrease the bowel motility, and a program of colonic irrigations to promote defecation at a appropriate time.[49]

We adjust this treatment by trial and error over a period of 1 week, and 95% of the patients remain clean and have an acceptable social life. Bowel management is started when the patient has to go to school, and all his or her classmates are already wearing regular underwear. Most patients and parents are very happy with the implementation of this program.[49] However, when the patient reaches the age of 7 to 12 years or sometimes younger, he or she usually needs more independence. At that point, the creation of a continent appendicostomy (Malone procedure) is recommended.[50,51] This operation creates a communication between the abdominal wall and the cecum through the appendix of the patient, creating a valve mechanism that allows the catheterization of the cecum for enema administration, but prevents leakage of stool. This allows the patient to administer his or her own enema while sitting on the toilet. The operation consists of plicating the cecum around the native appendix of the patient and exteriorizing the tip of the appendix in the deepest part of the umbilicus to make it inconspicuous. A significant number of patients do not have an appendix. In such cases, we tubularize a flap of the cecum, plicate the cecum around it, and create a stoma at the umbilicus. Most patients who have had this operation express a great deal of satisfaction.

REFERENCES

1. Aegineta P: On the imperforate anus. In Adams F (translator): The Seven Books (book 6). London, Sydenham Society, 1844, pp 405–406.
2. Amussat JZ: Gustiure d'une operation d'anus artifical practique avec success par un nouveau procede. Gaz Med Paris 3:735–758, 1835.
3. Roux de Brignoles JN: De l'imperforation de l'anus chez les nouveaux-nex-Rapport et discussion sur l'operation a tenter dans ces cas. Gaz Med Paris 2:411–412, 1834.
4. Wangensteen OH, Rice CO: Imperforate anus: A method of determining the surgical approach. Ann Surg 92:77–81, 1930.
5. Stephens FD: Imperforate rectum: A new surgical technique. Med J Aust 1:202–206, 1953.
6. Kiesewetter WB: Imperforate anus, II: The rationale and technique of sacroabdominoperineal operation. J Pediatr Surg 2:106–117, 1967.
7. Louw JH, Cywes S, Cremin BJ: The management of anorectal agenesis. S Afr J Surg 9:21–30, 1971.
8. Rehbein F: Imperforate anus: Experiences with abdominoperineal and abdominosacroperineal pull-through procedures. J Pediatr Surg 2:99–105, 1967.
9. Soave F: Surgery of the rectal anomalies with preservation of the relationship between the colonic muscular sleeve and puborectal muscle, J Pediatr Surg 4:705–712, 1969.
10. deVries P, Peña A: Posterior sagittal anorectoplasty. J Pediatr Surg 17:638–643, 1982.
11. Peña A, deVries P: Posterior sagittal anorectoplasty: Important technical considerations and new applications. J Pediatr Surg 17:796–881, 1982.
12. Brenner EC: Congenital defects of the anus and rectum. Surg Gynecol Obstet 20:579–588, 1915.
13. Santulli TV: Treatment of imperforate anus and associated fistulas. Surg Gynecol Obstet, 95:601–614, 1952.
14. Trusler GA, Wilkinson RH: Imperforate anus: A review of 147 cases. Can J Surg 5:169–177, 1962.
15. Anderson RC, Read SC: The likelihood of recurrence of congenital malformations. Lancet 74:175–176, 1954.
16. Cozzi F, Wilinson AW: Familial incidence of congenital malformations. Lancet 74:175–176, 1954.
17. Murken JD, Albert A: Genetic counseling in cases of anal and rectal atresia. Progr Pediatr Surg 9:115–118, 1976.
18. Peña A: Posterior sagittal anorectoplasty: Results in the management of 322 cases of anorectal malformations. Pediatr Surg Int 3:94–104, 1988.
19. Stephens FD, Smith ED: Incidence, frequency of types, etiology. In Stephens FD, Smith ED, Paul NW (eds): Anorectal Malformations in Children. Chicago, Year Book Medical, 1971, pp 160–171.
20. Rosen NG, Hong AR, Soffer SZ, et al: Recto-vaginal fistula: A common diagnostic error with significant consequences in female patients with anorectal malformations. J Pediatr Surg 37:961–965, 2002.
21. Bill AH, Hall DG, Johnson RJ: Position of rectal fistula in relation to the hymen in 46 girls with imperforate anus. J Pediatr Surg 10:361–365, 1975.
22. Torres P, Levitt MA, Tovilla JM, et al: Anorectal malformations and Down's syndrome. J Pediatr Surg 33:2–5, 1998.
23. Goon HK: Repair of anorectal anomalies in the neonatal period. Pediatr Surg Int 5:246–249, 1990.
24. Moore TC: Advantages of performing the sagittal anoplasty operation for imperforate anus at birth. J Pediatr Surg 25:276–277, 1990.
25. Levitt MA, Stein DM, Peña A: Gynecological concerns in the treatment of teenagers with cloaca. J Pediatr Surg 33:88–193, 1998.
26. Karrer FM, Flannery AM, Nelson MD Jr, et al: Anorectal malformations: Evaluation of associated spinal dysraphic syndromes. J Pediatr Surg 23:45–48, 1988.
27. Davidoff AM, Thompson CV, Grimm JK, et al: Occult spinal dysraphism in patients with anal agenesis. J Pediatr Surg 26:1001–1005, 1991.
28. Levitt MA, Patel M, Rodriguez G, et al: The tethered spinal cord in patients with anorectal malformations. J Pediatr Surg 32:362–468, 1997.
29. Belman BA, King LR: Urinary tract abnormalities associated with imperforate anus. J Urol 108:823–824, 1972.
30. Hoekstra WJ, Scholtmeijer RJ, Molenar JC, et al: Urogenital tract abnormalities associated with congenital anorectal anomalies. J Urol 130:962–963, 1983.
31. Munn R, Schillinger JF: Urologic abnormalities found with imperforate anus. Urology 21:260–264, 1983.
32. Parrott TS: Urologic implications of anorectal malformations. Urol Clin North Am 12:13–21, 1985.
33. Wiener ES, Kiesewetter WB: Urologic abnormalities associated with imperforate anus. J Pediatr Surg 8:151–157, 1973.
34. William DI, Grant J: Urological complications of imperforate anus. Br J Urol 41:660–665, 1969.

35. Rich MA, Brock WA, Peña A: Spectrum of genitourinary malformations in patients with imperforate anus. Pediatr Surg Int 3:110–113, 1988.
36. Stephens FD, Smith ED: Incidence, frequency of types, etiology. In Stephens FD, Smith ED (eds): Anorectal Malformations in Children. Chicago, Year Book Medical, 1971, pp 289–292.
37. Spence HM: Anomalies and complications of the urogenital tract associated with congenital imperforate anus. J Urol 71:453–463, 1954.
38. Smith ED: Urinary anomalies and complications in imperforate anus and rectum. J Pediatr Surg 3:337–342, 1968.
39. Carcassonne M, Monfort G, Isman H: Les problemes urologiques des malformations ano-rectales. Arch Franc Pediatr 28:723–739, 1971.
40. Freeman NV, Burge DM, Soar JS, et al: Anal evoked potentials. Z Rinderchir 31:22–30, 1980.
41. Hong AR, Rosen N, Acuña MF, et al: Urological injuries associated with the repair of anorectal malformations in male patients. J Pediatr Surg 37:339–344, 2002.
42. Gross GW, Wolfson PJ, Peña A: Augmented-pressure colostogram in imperforate anus with fistula. Pediatr Radiol 21:560–563, 1991.
43. Wilkins S, Peña A: The role of colostomy in the management of anorectal malformations. Pediatr Surg Int 3:105–109, 1988.
44. Mollard P, Soucy P, Luis D, Meunier P: Preservation of infralevator structures in imperforate anus repair. J Pediatr Surg 24:1023–1026, 1989.
45. Nixon JJ: Nixon anoplasty. In Stephens FD, Smith ED (eds): Anorectal Malformations in Children: Update 1988. New York, Alan R. Liss, 1988, pp 378–381.
46. Georgeson KE, Inge TH, Albanese CT: Laparoscopically assisted anorectal pull through for high imperforate anus: A new technique. J Pediatr Surg 35:927–931, 2000.
47. Peña A, Levitt MA, Hong AR, Midulla PS: Surgical management of cloacal malformations: A review of 339 patients. J Pediatr Surg 39:470–479, 2004.
48. Peña A: Total urogenital mobilization-an easier way to repair cloacas. J Pediatr Surg 32:263–268, 1997.
49. Peña A, Guardino K, Tovilla JM, et al: Bowel management for fecal incontinence in patients with anorectal malformations. J Pediatr Surg 33:133–137, 1998.
50. Malone PS, Ransley PG, Kiely EM: Preliminary report: The anterograde continence enema. Lancet 336:1217–1218, 1990.
51. Levitt MA, Soffer SZ, Peña A: Continent appendicostomy in the bowel management of fecal incontinent children. J Pediatr Surg 320:1630–1633, 1997.

Anorectal Continence and Management of Constipation

Gerard Weinberg, MD, and Scott J. Boley, MD

Of the many benign disorders afflicting children, abnormal defecation often has the most disruptive effect on the family. Although enormous progress has been made in the diagnosis and management of infections and metabolic diseases, children with functional constipation remain a source of continuing frustration to themselves, their parents, and their physicians. Normal anorectal function, so frequently taken for granted, is a complex balance of three interrelated functions: (1) the transport of fecal contents from the colon into the rectum (i.e., colonic motility); (2) the intermittent, rather than continuous, evacuation of stool from the rectum (i.e., defecation); and (3) the total retention of intestinal contents between acts of defecation (i.e., continence). Social continence is the ability not only to evacuate stool intermittently but also to do so only at socially appropriate times. Any alterations in the physiologic or anatomic mechanisms controlling any one of these functions can produce abnormalities that affect the others.

ANATOMY

Important anatomic structures involved in defecation and continence include both those with primarily a sensory role and those with primarily a motor role. The primary muscles are the internal anal sphincter (IAS), the external anal sphincter (EAS), and the puborectalis muscle; the other levator ani muscles play less important roles. The two major sites of sensation are the tension receptors in the rectal wall, especially in the adjacent puborectalis muscles, and the nerve endings in the anal mucosa, which are sensitive to pain, touch, and temperature.

The smooth-muscle IAS lies one third below the dentate line and two thirds above it. The striated-muscle EAS lies outside of and surrounds the IAS. The puborectalis muscle forms a sling posteriorly around the rectum. It is contiguous with the deep portion of the EAS (Fig. 36-1). These two striated muscles are supplied by the pudendal nerve. Often acting as a unit, they are sometimes referred to as the *striated muscle complex*.[1]

Internal Anal Sphincter

The IAS is a smooth muscle in a tonic state of contraction. It provides at least 85% of the resting anal canal pressure.[2] The EAS and the puborectalis muscle provide the remainder. The tonic contraction of the IAS is primarily an intrinsic property of the smooth muscle itself, but it may be supplemented by intrinsic neural input. The IAS may be capable of slightly increased contraction, but the major change in its resting tone is relaxation in response to rectal distention. This inhibitory reflex is an intrinsic neural reflex (Fig. 36-2).[3]

The sensory receptors of the anal canal are limited to the mucosa just superior to the dentate line. In the more proximal rectum, no sensory receptors are present. Thus the determination of whether fluid, solid stool, or gas is being passed occurs in the distal anal canal. To facilitate this discrimination, the proximal IAS relaxes, which allows the material to pass to the distal canal. The material is identified by the sensory receptors and either contained or released as appropriate.

The innervation of the smooth-muscle portion of the sphincter is complex and not completely elucidated. Sympathetic innervation is supplied by both lumbar splanchnic nerves from the lumbar spinal cord and by hypogastric nerves from the inferior mesenteric ganglion. Parasympathetic innervation comes via the pelvic nerves from the sacral spinal cord.[4]

The sympathetic motor effect is primarily excitatory, but an inhibitory component may be present. α-Adrenergic stimulation is excitatory, but β-adrenergic stimulation is inhibitory. The parasympathetic nerves cause relaxation. However, cholinergic agonists actually cause excitation, whereas the cholinergic antagonist atropine produces either excitation or inhibition, depending on the experimental model.[5] Thus excitatory innervation appears to be dual, both cholinergic and adrenergic. Both adrenergic and nonadrenergic inhibitory innervations also may be present.[6]

Intrinsic innervation of the internal sphincter is the primary system for producing relaxation in response to rectal distention. This relaxation response occurs even in

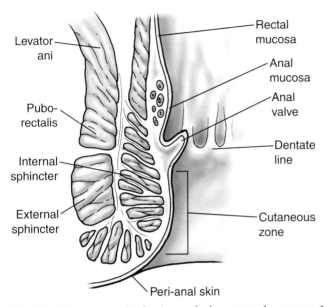

FIGURE 36-1. A sagittal view of the normal anorectal anatomy demonstrates the location of the internal and external anal sphincters and the puborectalis and levator ani muscles.

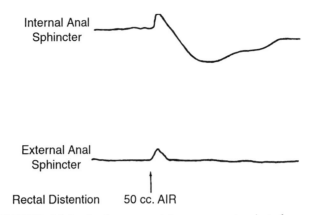

Rectal Distention   50 cc. AIR

FIGURE 36-2. Anal manometric pressure tracing demonstrates normal relaxation of the internal anal sphincter in response to a 50-cc bolus of air into a balloon positioned in the rectum. The increased intra-anal pressure caused by the expanding balloon is reflected in the momentary pressure elevation in the external anal sphincter pressure tracing.

the presence of spinal anesthesia. The nerves involved lie in the intramural plexuses and the myenteric and submucosal ganglia. They are nonadrenergic and noncholinergic in nature.[7] Evidence suggests vasoactive intestinal polypeptide as the possible inhibitory neurotransmitter, but additional neurotransmitters may be involved.[8]

External Anal Sphincter

The EAS muscle is a striated muscle and, hence, capable of phasic contraction. Like the IAS, the EAS may have some tonic contraction.[9] Unlike the IAS, the tonic contraction of the EAS depends exclusively on efferent nervous input. The phasic contractions are both voluntary and involuntary. The external sphincter muscle provides part of the resting tone of the sphincter complex. Depending on the situation, increased contraction of the

external sphincter muscle can aid either in resisting defecation or in emptying the distal anal canal.[10]

With rectal distention, the EAS contracts reflexively: the "inflation reflex" (see Fig. 36-2), which is an extrinsic arc. The puborectalis muscle also contracts reflexively with rectal distention. The two muscles work together to enhance continence during rectal distention. After defecation, the EAS and puborectalis muscle reflexively contract, the "deflation reflex." This process empties the last part of the rectal canal.

The nervous innervation of the EAS comes exclusively from the sacral cord via the pudendal nerves. Pudendal nerve injury paralyzes the EAS.

The internal and external sphincters work together in response to rectal distention. The external sphincter contracts reflexively via extrinsic reflex pathways, whereas the internal sphincter relaxes reflexively via intrinsic reflex pathways. Spinal anesthesia blocks the external contraction, but the internal sphincter relaxation is unaffected.

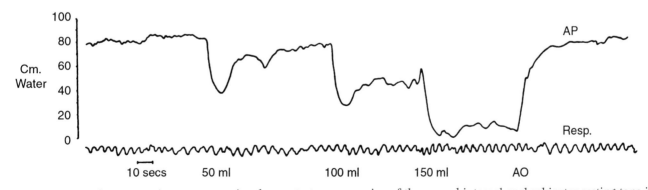

FIGURE 36-3. Anal manometric pressure tracing demonstrates suppression of the normal internal anal sphincter resting tone in response to increasing inflation of an intrarectal balloon. At each 50-cc increment, the anal canal pressure returns to a level below preinsufflation, until the inhibition reflex of the internal anal sphincter is totally suppressed at 150 cc. When the air in the balloon is fully withdrawn, the anal canal pressure returns to normal. AO, air out; AP, anal pressure. (From Lane RHS, Parks, AG: Function of the anal sphincters following the colo-anal anastomosis. Br J Surg 64:599, 1977.)

The reflexive contraction of the external sphincter with rectal distention is one of the primary mechanisms of continence. To defecate, this resistance is overcome through (1) voluntarily increasing intraperitoneal and rectal pressure, or (2) under normal circumstances, increasing rectal distention, which produces reflex total inhibition of the EAS and puborectalis muscles when a maximal tolerable volume is reached (Fig. 36-3).

Puborectalis Muscle

The puborectalis muscle is the most anterior and deepest of the levator ani muscles. It forms a sling behind the rectum. The puborectalis muscle is not attached posteriorly; hence with contraction, it pulls anteriorly, forming the anorectal angle (Fig. 36-4). The other levator ani muscles are attached posteriorly; hence they contract in a vertical plane, forming a funnel but not altering the anorectal angle. If the puborectalis muscle function is lost, incontinence almost always results, regardless of the state of contraction of the internal and external anal sphincters.

The anorectal angle is normally present when any individual is erect. The puborectalis muscle is relatively relaxed during recumbency and is not needed to preserve continence. With resumption of the erect state, tonic activity of the puborectalis muscle is increased markedly, the anorectal angle is reestablished, and gross continence is maintained.

The puborectalis muscle must remain in a state of tonic contraction, a feat previously considered to be limited to smooth muscle. The puborectalis muscle is capable of both voluntary and involuntary phasic contractions that reinforce the tonic state. The muscle has two distinct types of fibers that can be differentiated biochemically, histologically, and anatomically. These fibers even develop at different stages of maturation.[11] The small "red" myocytes contain a larger amount of myoglobin and maintain the tonic state of the sphincter, whereas the "white" cells contract the sphincter to maintain continence, even in the face of sudden increases in either intrarectal or intra-abdominal pressure.

The persistent tonic state depends on a proprioceptive reflex mechanism. The sensory receptors lie within the puborectalis and levator ani muscles, with the ganglia in the lumbosacral spine. The involuntary phasic contractions are produced by a reflex arc from the puborectalis sensory receptors to the lumbosacral spinal cord and back. Transection of the cord superior to the lumbosacral region does not affect these involuntary phasic contractions. Voluntary contractions depend on cortical centers. They are abolished with cord transection.

The combination of normally functioning internal and external sphincters and the puborectalis muscle produce both gross and fine continence. Gross continence, or the ability to withhold periodically large volumes of solid or liquid feces, is a function primarily of the intact anorectal angle produced by the actions of puborectalis muscle. Fine continence, or the control of small volumes of often semi-soft feces, is primarily controlled by the sphincter muscles. The critical site of fine continence is the distal 2 cm of the anal canal, that portion below the puborectalis muscle.

PHYSIOLOGY

The nerves and muscles work to produce normal colonic motility and controlled defecation. Colonic motility produces slow transit to facilitate fluid absorption and mass movement to facilitate defecation. Three types of colonic activity exist: (1) localized segmental contractions, which produce slow forward movement of feces; (2) peristaltic contractions, which produce retrograde and slow forward movement; and (3) mass contractions, which empty long segments of the colon in a prograde fashion. The mass movements are not the peristaltic movements typical of the more proximal gastrointestinal tract. Rather they are contractions of long segments of colon preceded by aboral waves of relaxation, so-called descending inhibition, which empty long segments of the colon.[12]

The process of defecation can be divided into five stages (Fig. 36-5):

1. *Stage one.* The rectal ampulla begins to fill with stool, which produces a transient reflex contraction of the external sphincter and puborectalis muscles and a relaxation of the internal sphincter. This activity can occur even before any conscious awareness of rectal distention occurs.
2. *Stage two.* The second stage occurs when the ampulla is approximately one-fourth full, which is the threshold for the awareness of stool in the rectum. At this point, a slight urge to defecate occurs, but voluntary inhibition of defecation can be prolonged. The EAS

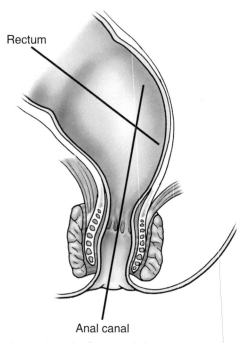

Rectum

Anal canal

FIGURE 36-4. A sagittal view of the normal anal canal and rectum, which demonstrates the anorectal angle. (Modified from Pemberton JH, Kelly KA: Achieving enteric continence: Principles and applications. Mayo Clin Proc 61:586-599, 1986.)

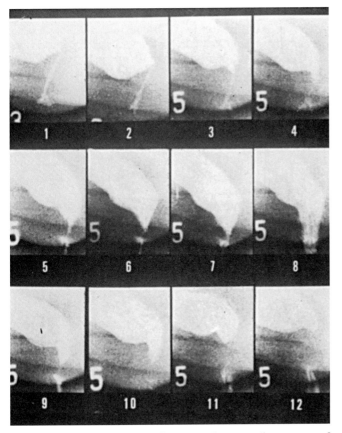

FIGURE 36-5. Defecogram illustrates the normal sequence of changes in the anorectum during defecation. (Modified from Kerremans R: Radiocinematographic examination of the rectum and the anal canal in cases of rectal constipation: A radiocinematographic and physical explanation of dyschezia. Acta Gastroenterol Belg 31:561–570, 1968.)

and puborectalis muscles are voluntarily contracted to reinforce the tonic reflex contractions. The rectum stretches, which decreases the pressure and eliminates the urge to defecate.

3. *Stage three.* The volume and the pressure in the rectum increase as more stool is pushed into it. As the urge to defecate increases in intensity, the reflex relaxation of the IAS becomes greater in degree and longer in duration. The reflex suppression of tonic contraction of the EAS and puborectalis muscles begins. If time and place are appropriate, the person has gone to the toilet and is ready to allow the urge to be satisfied.

4. *Stage four.* This stage involves defecation. Voluntary defecation is begun in response to the irresistible urge to defecate. Tonic activity in the IAS, the EAS, and the puborectalis muscles is totally inhibited, and phasic activity in the striated muscle is suppressed voluntarily. The anorectal angle straightens, and the levator ani muscles fall, which leaves the rectal contents free to pass through the anal canal. Evacuation is abetted by voluntary straining and increased intra-abdominal pressure.

5. *Stage five.* The emptying of the rectal vault initiates a reflex contraction of the striated muscle: the deflation reflex. This reflex serves to empty the anal canal and initiates the return of tonic activity to the striated muscles and to the internal sphincter. The anorectal angle is reestablished, and the components of continence are again operative.

PATHOPHYSIOLOGY

Constipation can be viewed as a failure of the ability to undertake and complete the defecatory process satisfactorily. The inability may result from (1) a failure of any of the five stages of defecation, (2) a more proximal defect of small intestinal, colonic, or generalized motility, or (3) abnormal stool in the presence of a normal motility and defecation pattern.

Although constipation among children has been the most common disorder of anorectal function and has been recognized for thousands of years, its definition remains a source of disagreement among physicians. Defecation patterns vary widely among normal children. A pattern that worries one child's mother may be of no concern to another. Several bowel movements a day or only one every 5 to 7 days may be normal in children older than 1 year. Nonetheless, constipation should be considered to be present when two or more of the following occur for an extended period: (1) fewer than three bowel movements per week, (2) excessive straining and pain accompanying 25% or more of bowel movements, and (3) passage of hard or pellet-like stools with at least 25% of bowel movements.

During the first year of life, lack of a bowel movement at least every other day warrants an evaluation. In the neonatal period, any delay of passage of meconium should raise a suspicion of underlying pathologic condition and should result in vigorous investigative efforts. Although only distressed fetuses pass meconium in utero, 94% to 98% of term and 76% of preterm normal babies have bowel movements during the first 24 hours; 100% of term and 98.8% of preterm normal babies pass meconium within the first 48 hours.[13]

The problem resulting in constipation may be of major or minor importance. The causes vary in frequency by age but, in any case, can be subdivided into one of five general categories: (1) changes in stool character, (2) structural problems, (3) extrinsic disorders of nerves or muscles, (4) intrinsic motility disorders, and (5) functional constipation.

Abnormal Stool Character

Abnormal stool character may result from inappropriate diet. Underfeeding or insufficiency of fluid or sugar may reduce fecal bulk or produce excessively viscid or hard stools. Cystic fibrosis with its pancreatic exocrine function disturbances may cause a similar problem, as may any upper intestinal disorder that limits adequate intake, such as pyloric stenosis.

Local Structural Abnormalities

Local structural abnormalities of the anorectum, including anorectal stenosis, may present actual physical barriers to normal evacuation. Even minor abnormalities, such as an anteriorly placed ectopic anus, can produce severe constipation. Those structural abnormalities may be associated with absence of the normal defecatory reflexes, so that even structural corrections do not alleviate constipation.

Another commonly seen problem in infants and children that may lead to disorders of defecation are perirectal abscesses. These usually result from infection in the anal glands that enter the anus in crypts at the level of the anal valves. The pain resulting from the infection causes rectal spasm, inhibiting normal defecation. Anal fissures are painful and can cause voluntary stool withholding and result in constipation. Hard and very bulky stools may aggravate the fissure and can turn an acute problem into a chronic one. Similarly, tumors that compress or narrow the rectum interfere with normal defecation.[14]

Extrinsic Neurologic or Muscular Abnormalities

Extrinsic neurologic or muscular abnormalities interfere with anal sensation. When the patient cannot sense a full rectum, incontinence may result from the reflex suppression of the EAS and puborectalis muscle. With the loss of the urge to defecate, constipation may lead to dilation of the rectum. Impairment of the rectal and anal reflexes, changes in sphincter tone, and neurogenic bladder often accompany neurologic defects. Constipation or incontinence also may occur. More general muscular weakness may diminish the increase in intra-abdominal pressure from the diaphragm and abdominal muscles, inhibiting defecation and producing constipation. The disorders that can cause this condition include meningomyelocele, cerebral palsy, polio, or polyneuritis.

Intrinsic Motility Abnormalities

Intrinsic motility abnormalities may be caused by (1) generalized causes of abnormal motility; (2) local intramural neuromuscular derangements; (3) metabolic and endocrine disturbances, including hypercalcemia, hyperkalemia, hyperparathyroidism, and abnormal thyroid function; and (4) pharmacologic agents, including phenothiazines and opiates, which may slow intestinal motility at any age. This list includes drugs taken by the mother in the prenatal period. Motility abnormalities may be seen in premature infants in the absence of organic pathology, especially in those with respiratory distress, sepsis, or deranged electrolytes.

The local intramural defects run a spectrum from neurologic immaturity through classic Hirschsprung's disease to ultrashort-segment aganglionosis. The most common of these causes is Hirschsprung's disease (see Chapter 34). Another entity that has been described and whose mechanism is more clearly understood is neuronal intestinal dysplasia, also known as intestinal *hyperganglionosis*. The condition is characterized by the increased number and size of ganglia in the submucosal and myenteric plexuses in conjunction with hypoplasia or aplasia of the sympathetic innervation of the myenteric plexus.[15] This disorder shares many clinical characteristics more commonly seen with Hirschsprung's disease, and several patients have been reported as having both conditions.[16] Bowel activity is irregular and uncoordinated, resulting in ineffectual evacuation of stool. In addition, the internal sphincter is often spastic. Special nerve stains have been used to elucidate the various abnormalities that cause this condition.

Rare conditions that can affect the innervation of the anorectum include Chagas' disease and neurofibromatosis. These disorders produce constipation either by ineffective propulsive activity or by failure of the IAS to relax in response to rectal distention.

Functional Constipation

Functional constipation is the most common form of constipation in children. However, it almost certainly represents the combining of multiple causes under one rubric.

The classic concept of functional constipation is the conscious or subconscious suppression by the child of the urge to defecate. Eventually, the rectum dilates and remains dilated. Higher intrarectal pressures become necessary to initiate the normal defecation response. The stool volume necessary to initiate the defecation reflex is too large and often too hard to pass easily. Diminution in the sensitivity of rectal stretch receptors also occurs, which can affect the intrinsic internal sphincter relaxation response but usually does not. Rather, the conscious sensation of the urge to defecate becomes suppressed.

This discordance between the volume that produces reflex relaxation and that which causes conscious sensation has been studied. In children with a marked discrepancy between reflex relaxation and conscious sensation, encopresis often occurs. In children with a lesser discrepancy, a lower incidence of encopresis occurs. In children with no discrepancy, encopresis is rare.[17]

Loss of the urge to defecate is not the only abnormality in those with "functional constipation." Hypertonia of the puborectalis muscle has been observed, with failure to relax and straighten the anorectal angle. Not surprisingly, the child so affected also has constipation. In one study of the inhibiting reflex in children considered to have functional constipation, some had failure of internal sphincter relaxation, similar to that in Hirschsprung's disease; some had relaxation of the IAS, but it was minimal; others had hypertonia of the IAS with a paradoxical hyperrelaxation when the rectum was distended.[18]

The multitude of problems that have been designated *functional constipation* is equaled by the number of different psychogenic problems implicated as underlying causes. Repeated use of enemas or suppositories during infancy, disturbances in parent/child relationships, early or strict toilet training, and neurodevelopmental disorders all have been cited as causes.

DIAGNOSIS

When constipation is one manifestation of a generalized disorder, its cause is usually apparent. Similarly, simple physical inspection usually allows the recognition of anorectal malformations, muscular disorders, or extrinsic neurologic defects when they are responsible for the constipation.

The major diagnostic difficulties lie in differentiating between functional constipation and intrinsic motility disorders. Features of Hirschsprung's disease that distinguish it from functional constipation include onset in infancy, absence of fecal soiling, rarity of abdominal pain, empty rectal ampulla, and commonly, malnutrition.

The clinical presentation is not always so classic, and no one feature is pathognomonic. Especially when Hirschsprung's disease involves only a short segment, symptoms may not be seen until later in life. The finding of impacted stool in the rectum, and even fecal soiling in some patients, is not uncommon. In addition, some of the diseases described as intrinsic motility disorders are impossible to differentiate clinically from Hirschsprung's disease. Thus other diagnostic modalities are necessary. The three most important of these are radiologic studies, anorectal manometry, and tissue biopsy.

In a child with Hirschsprung's disease, barium enema examination usually demonstrates a normal-sized or contracted aganglionic rectum with a transitional zone that leads to the dilated ganglionic colon. In the newborn, failure to evacuate barium within 24 hours of instillation may be the most pertinent finding. With short-segment aganglionosis, the barium enema may appear similar to functional constipation, with a markedly dilated rectum down to the anus.

Anorectal manometry is performed with either pressure transducers or perfused catheters. In a normal child, distention of the rectum with 10 to 30 cc of air results in reflex contraction and then relaxation of the internal sphincter, accompanied by contraction of the external sphincter. With functional constipation, a reduced sensation of rectal distention is present because of the

markedly dilated rectum. Greater volumes of air are needed to create an urge to defecate. Nevertheless, normal internal sphincter relaxation does occur with these greater volumes, and relaxation may occur even at normal volumes of air. The latter may account for the uncontrolled passage of liquid around an impaction.

In children with Hirschsprung's disease, the internal sphincter fails to relax on rectal distention. Contraction may occur. With manometry, it is less difficult to exclude Hirschsprung's disease than to confirm its presence. Absence of internal sphincter relaxation may result from technical problems. Lack of relaxation may be found in young neonates and premature babies with normal colons, especially in those with respiratory distress syndrome, sepsis, or electrolyte disturbances (Fig. 36-6).

Anorectal manometry can be used in conjunction with electromyography in the evaluation of problems of defecation and continence from anorectal malformations and neurologic disorders. Tissue for study can be obtained by punch or suction biopsy without anesthesia or by surgical excision of a full-thickness section of rectal wall with anesthesia. Specimens obtained with punch or suction techniques contain only mucosa and a portion of submucosa. About 50 to 100 sections must be examined for ganglion cells by an experienced pathologist. Full-thickness sections, which are less difficult to interpret, include Auerbach's plexus.

The identification of increased acetylcholinesterase activity in superficial suction biopsies is an accurate means for diagnosing Hirschsprung's disease. This test has obviated the need for full-thickness biopsies in many cases.

TREATMENT

The treatment of most of the causes of constipation is straightforward. Metabolic and endocrine disturbances are corrected, anatomic obstructions are surgically removed, and responsible drugs are eliminated. The treatment of the two common causes of constipation, Hirschsprung's disease and functional constipation, is

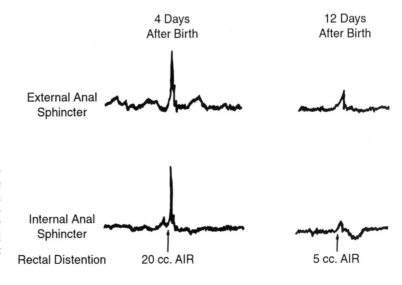

FIGURE 36-6. Anorectal manometric pressure tracings from a patient at age 4 days demonstrate the absence of a normal internal sphincter relaxation in response to z transient 20-cc bolus of air into a balloon placed in the rectum. At a subsequent study done at age 12 days, normal relaxation of the internal anal sphincter is present in response to a transient 5-cc bolus of air.

more complex. The management of Hirschsprung's disease is discussed in detail in Chapter 34.

Treatment of functional constipation should be approached in a systematic way. The rectum is emptied, and stool reaccumulation, prevented. The rectum is allowed to return to its original size. The child experiences the urge to defecate when the rectum is only mildly distended by stool entering it. The initial removal of the fecal mass can usually be aided by the administration of 5 to 10 tablespoons of mineral oil or a hypertonic phosphate enema (e.g., Fleet enema). Repeated administration may be necessary. Sufficient amounts of mineral oil should be given to cause two to four loose bowel movements each day. The dose should be titrated against the child's response: several tablespoons or more each day are commonly needed. In several instances, we have given 24 tablespoons per day of mineral oil for refractory cases. The anal discharge of oil usually indicates seepage around a still-retained fecal mass, in which case, the dose should be increased. To make the mineral oil more palatable and to increase compliance with the regimen, the oil may be refrigerated or flavored with fruit juice. The mineral oil may be taken all at once or divided into two daily portions. Administration of mineral oil may have to be continued for several months. It should be discontinued gradually. The regimen is sufficient in many cases of simple constipation. Osmotic agents also have been successfully used for long-term therapy in children with severe refractory constipation. PEG (polyethylene glycol 350), a chemically inert polymer that does not contain any absorbable salt, can be used for long-term therapy at a dose of 0.3 g/kg/day. The side effects were minimal, and the children drank the agent with minimal resistance.[19]

If the child is old enough (usually older than 3 years), regular toilet training is started by having the patient sit on the toilet at the same time each day for 10 to 20 minutes, usually shortly after a major meal, to take advantage of the gastrocolic reflex. If the child's legs do not reach the floor, a small stool should be provided so that pressure can be applied to help move the bowels.

In other cases, careful exploration of family events and emotional factors that lead to the fecal retention is needed to help the family resolve parent/child conflicts and to establish sympathetic, but firm, guidelines for dealing with the patient and the patient's problems. Psychiatric referral may be helpful in some severely disturbed families. Treatment of constipation in mentally retarded children usually is unsatisfactory.

About half of all children with functional constipation contract the EAS, the puborectalis, and pelvic floor muscles during defecation attempts instead of relaxing them. Because these structures are voluntary striated muscles, they should be amenable to control and modulation by the use of biofeedback techniques.[20]

The rectum is emptied and allowed to return to a more normal size before biofeedback training is begun. A balloon, which is connected to pressure transducers, is inserted into the rectum, and the pressure tracings are displayed on a monitor. The balloon is inflated, and the child is shown the pressure tracing that he or she generated in response to the rectal distention. The child is then urged to mimic defecation while the intrarectal pressures are monitored. In many of these children, the external sphincter contracts, generating a high-pressure tracing. The child is then shown a normal tracing of external sphincter relaxation during defecation. The child is then encouraged to mimic the normal tracing. Additional biofeedback reinforcement can be accomplished by adding a variety of audio and visual stimuli to the pressure apparatus. Most important, the child should be encouraged and rewarded when progress is made toward a normal response. This process takes time, patience, and good rapport between the child and coach. As a final step in the process, the rectal balloon is removed, and the child then practices voluntary external sphincter relaxation on command. Most children need about five sessions at weekly intervals to achieve a satisfactory response. Biofeedback training has proven useful in children with abnormal defecation dynamics. Most of these children can learn a more normal pattern of muscle relaxation and then go on to achieve normal defecation.[21]

Anorectal myectomy or vigorous anal dilation by using anesthesia has been successful in some patients who failed to respond to all of the aforementioned measures. In this procedure, a strip of rectal muscular wall, starting just below the dentate line and extending upward to the level of the puborectalis muscle, is removed. The lowest portion of the internal sphincter is not divided.[22]

Considerable interest has been demonstrated in even more aggressive surgical management of some particularly difficult to treat constipated youngsters. A recent report of patients treated with sigmoid resections has demonstrated some encouraging results; this approach, however, has not met with wide acceptance.[23] Another surgical approach to aid in the management of constipation is the antegrade enema through a continent appendicostomy or button cecostomy. These surgical options make the administration of enemas less traumatic and have the advantage of cleaning out the entire colon, leaving the child soilage free for more hours.[24,25]

ANTERIORLY DISPLACED ANUS

A controversial entity, which several investigators claim is a major cause of constipation, is the anteriorly displaced anus, or anterior ectopic anus. The controversy concerning this entity arises from the different definitions of the abnormality, the real relation between the anatomic abnormality and constipation, the operation to be performed, and the incidence of the entity.[26]

In 1958, a variant of the spectrum of anomalies carried under the overall term *imperforate anus* was termed an *anteriorly placed rectal opening in the perineum*, or *ectopic anus*.[27] In 30 patients, all of the openings were in the perineum anterior to the normal anal position and the external sphincter. Some 20 years later, in two independent series, anterior anus and anterior ectopic anus were reported as a frequently unrecognized cause of constipation. One report, although not specifically stating so, appears to describe an anterior anal opening within the external sphincters.[28] The other report specifically describes an apparently normal sphincter except for its anterior ectopia.[29] In 1984, another report described a structural abnormality in seven children with anterior perineal anus: the absence of a portion of the triple loop system of EASs.[30]

General agreement exists that anal openings anterior to the external sphincters can produce constipation, which is relieved by operation. Most pediatric surgeons remain skeptical, however, about the importance and even the identification of anteriorly displaced anal openings within the external sphincters. One group of workers made the diagnosis of anal ectopia solely by inspection, describing an anus that is well forward of the normal location, midway between the vaginal fourchette and the tip of the coccyx. In another report, the eccentric placement of the anal opening was emphasized. Indeed, in 20% of the patients, the anus did not appear to be anteriorly displaced. An anal-position index has been described based on examination of 200 newborn infants, which can be used to identify anterior displacement of the anus.[31] An abnormal index is not an indication for operation, however.

Despite specifically looking for these abnormalities in a large number of constipated children, we have not found a clearly identified anteriorly displaced anus or an eccentrically placed anus to be common. Palpation of a posterior shelf or cul-de-sac behind the sphincter is the other physical finding associated with this entity. This finding is similar to the shelf that is present in the patient with the anterior ectopic anus as originally described.[27] In the few patients we have operated on for anterior ectopic anus, the shelf was the most impressive finding.

A prominent posterior shelf found on barium enema has been described as indicative of this entity.[32] However, the presentations are no different from those we have seen in other children and adolescents with chronic constipation. The abnormally prominent shelf is due to a hypertrophied puborectalis muscle and is much improved within weeks of vigorous dilation of the puborectalis by using anesthesia.

The operations performed for anterior ectopic anus include transplantation of the anus (a simple cut-back procedure) and posterior advancement of a mucosal flap with and without posterior sphincterotomy. We have found a simple cut-back, including the sphincter, to be effective and the simplest procedure, but care must be taken not to include the puborectalis muscle accidentally.

Anteriorly displaced anus clearly occurs, but infrequently in our experience. It is sometimes associated with chronic constipation. Some children are helped by an operation. We share the viewpoint of most pediatric surgeons, however, that this entity is an uncommon cause of chronic constipation and that children should be operated on only after a trial of medical management and careful evaluation.

REFERENCES

1. Swenson O, Bill AH: Resection of the rectum and rectosigmoid with preservation of the sphincter. Surgery 24:212–220, 1948.
2. Culver PS, Rattan S: Genesis of anal canal pressures in the opossum. Am J Physiol 251:765–771, 1986.
3. Schuster MM, Hentrix TR, Mendeloff AI: The internal and sphincter response: Manometric studies on its normal physiology, neural pathways and alteration in bowel disorders. J Clin Invest 42:196–207, 1963.
4. Aldridge RT, Campbell PE: Ganglion cell distribution in the normal rectum and anal canal. J Pediatr Surg 3:475–496, 1968.
5. Bitar Kid, Makhlow GM: Purinergic receptors on isolated smooth muscle cells. Gastroenterology 82:1018–1027, 1982.
6. Garrett JR, Howard ER, Jones W: The internal anal sphincter in the cat: A study of nervous mechanisms affecting tone and reflex activity. J Physiol 243:153–166, 1974.
7. Frenckner B, Ihre T: Influence of autonomic nerves on the internal anal sphincter in man. Gut 17:306–312, 1976.
8. Nurko S, Rattan S: Role of vasoactive intestinal polypeptide in the internal anal sphincter relaxation in the opossum. J Clin Invest 81:1146–1153, 1988.
9. Christensen J: Motility of the colon. In Johnson LR (ed): Physiology of the Gastrointestinal Tract, 2nd ed. New York, Raven Press, 1987, pp 445–467.
10. Monges H, Salducci J, Nardi B, et al: Electrical activity of internal anal sphincter. In Christensen J (ed): Gastrointestinal Motility. New York, Raven Press, 1980, pp 495–502.
11. Holschneider AM: The problem of anorectal continence. Prog Pediatr Surg 9:85–97, 1976.
12. Ritchie JA: Mass peristalsis in the human colon after contact with oxyphenisation. Gut 13:211–219, 1972.
13. Clark DA: Times of first void and first stool in 500 newborns. Pediatrics 60:457–459, 1977.
14. Loening-Baucke VA: Factors responsible for persistence of childhood constipation. J Pediatr Gastroenterol Nutr 6:915–922, 1987.
15. Munakata K, Morita K, Okabe I, et al: Clinical and histologic studies in neuronal intestinal dysplasia. J Pediatr Surg 20:231–235, 1985.
16. Fadda B, Pistor G, Meier-Ruge W, et al: Symptoms, diagnosis, and therapy of neuronal intestinal dysplasia masked by Hirschsprung's disease. Pediatr Surg Int 2:76–80, 1987.
17. Martelli H, Devroede G, Arhan P, et al: Mechanisms of idiopathic constipation: Outlet obstruction. Gastroenterology 75:623–631, 1978.
18. Meunier P, Louis D, Jaubert de Beaujeu M: Physiologic investigation of primary chronic constipation in children: Comparison with the barium enema study. Gastroenterology 87:1351–1357, 1984.
19. Minor ML, Gleghorn EE: A new polyethylene glycol-based, small volume medication for constipation/encopresis in children. J Pediatr Gastroenterol Nutr 31:S34, 2000.
20. Loening-Baucke VA: Modulation of abnormal defecation dynamics by biofeedback treatment in chronically constipated children with encopresis. J Pediatr 116:214–222, 1990.
21. Benninga MA, Buller HA, Taminiau JA: Biofeedback training in constipation. Arch Dis Child 68:126–129, 1993.
22. Pena A, Levitt MA: Colonic inertia disorders in pediatrics. Curr Probl Surg 39:666–730, 2002.
23. Youssef NN, Barksdale E Jr, Griffiths JM, et al: Management of intractable constipation with antegrade enemas in neurologically intact children. J Pediatr Gastroenterol Nutr 34:402–405, 2002.
24. Pinho M, Yoshioka K, Keighley MRB: Long-term results of anorectal myectomy for chronic constipation. Br J Surg 76:1163–1164, 1989.
25. Ottolenghi A, Sulpasso M, Bianchi S, et al: Ectopic anus in childhood. Eur J Pediatr Surg 4:145–150, 1994.

26. Lee SL, DuBois JJ, Montes-Garces RG, Inglis K, et al: Surgical management of chronic unremitting constipation and fecal incontinence associated with megarectum: A preliminary report. J Pediatr Surg 37:76–79, 2002.
27. Bill AH Jr, Johnson RJ, Foster RA: Anteriorly placed rectal opening in the perineum, "ectopic anus": A report of 30 cases. Ann Surg 147:173–179, 1958.
28. Hendren WH: Constipation caused by anterior location of the anus and its surgical correction. J Pediatr Surg 13:505–511, 1978.
29. Leape LL, Ramenofsky ML: Anterior ectopic anus: A common cause of constipation in children. J Pediatr Surg 13:627–630, 1978.
30. Upadhyaya P: Mid-anal sphincteric malformation, cause of constipation in anterior perianal anus. J Pediatr Surg 19:183–186, 1984.
31. Bar-Maor JA, Eitan A: Determination of the normal position of the anus. J Pediatr Gastroenterol Nutr 6:559–561, 1987.
32. Reisner SH, Sivan Y, Nitzan M, et al: Determination of anterior displacement of the anus in newborn infants and children. Pediatrics 73:216–217, 1984.

CHAPTER 37

Acquired Anorectal Disorders

Keith W. Ashcraft, MD

PERIANAL AND PERIRECTAL ABSCESSES

Perianal or perirectal abscesses develop primarily in infants. The abscess usually appears as a tender mass lateral to the anal opening. A history of stool abnormalities is not often noted in these children, either before development of the abscess or during its maturation. In my experience, approximately an equal incidence of perirectal abscess is found in male and female infants. Virtually all these patients are seen first when they are younger than 12 months. However, other reports suggest that perianal abscesses are much more common in male children and are frequent in children older than 2 years.[1]

Sitz baths (or their equivalent for the infant) are prescribed if the abscess does not appear to be fluctuant and in need of immediate drainage. Approximately one third of abscesses thus treated resolve without recurrence. Approximately two thirds require surgical drainage or drain spontaneously. Surgical drainage can be done in the infant without anesthesia or with a topical anesthetic ointment. In the child who is older than 1 year, the procedure usually must be done by using general anesthetic, with curettage and packing of the abscess cavity. Approximately 40% to 50% of perianal abscesses progress to fistula in ano.[2]

It is unusual to find ischiorectal abscesses in children unless associated with chronic inflammatory bowel diseases.

FISTULA IN ANO

Fistula in ano appears predominantly in male patients.[3] The child is usually seen first after two or more flare-ups of a perianal abscess that either continues to drain or to form a small pustule that ruptures, only to form again.[4] The fistula is commonly located lateral to the anus rather than in the midline. Occasionally, two fistulas occur simultaneously in one child. In several patients, fistulas have occurred in a serial fashion.

An intriguing theory has been suggested that fistula in ano results from infection in abnormally deep crypts that are under the influence of androgens.[1,3] Fistula in ano almost never follows a perianal abscess in female children.[5] The levels of circulating sex hormones have been found to be normal in adult male and female patients with idiopathic fistula in ano.[6]

The preferred surgical procedure for fistula in ano is cryptectomy or fistulectomy (rather than fistulotomy), removing the entire crypt with its granulation tissue. Hydrogen peroxide has been used as a means of identifying the associated crypt intraoperatively.[7] It has been postulated that in addition to the fistulotomy or fistulectomy, multiple cryptotomy should be carried out to prevent serial fistulization. I have had no experience with this technique, nor have I sought to confirm the presence of abnormal crypts. The wound is left open, which provides some distress on the part of the parents but little discomfort on the part of the child. I have not seen difficulties with healing in any of these patients, nor have I seen a recurrence of the same fistula with this approach. Suture closure has been reported to result in satisfactory healing without infection.[1]

FISSURE IN ANO

Fissure in ano develops in toddlers whose diet changes from liquid to solid and whose stool consistency changes from soft to firm. A period of constipation often precedes a hard, bulky stool that results in a posterior midline anal tear. The discomfort associated with a fissure in ano often leads to further constipation, which, in turn, aggravates the fissure with each stool and prevents healing. Fissure in ano is usually seen in the toddler who is capable of repressing the urge to defecate because of anticipated pain. The diagnosis is made through the history of blood streaking on the stool, the child's crying during bowel movements, and the recognition of a split in the skin of the anus.

Excision is rarely necessary. I prefer to manage these patients with sitz baths and with milk of magnesia used as a stool softener. Any other form of stool softening that is effective works as well.

A fissure in ano in an older child or a teenager very often is associated with chronic inflammatory bowel disease, usually Crohn's disease (see Chapter 41).[8] The diagnosis of Crohn's disease may follow by some months the demonstration of a fissure in ano, but if the clinician is persistent, the inflammatory changes of Crohn's disease can ultimately be detected. Some of the perianal manifestations of Crohn's disease can be very destructive.[9] Treatment of Crohn's disease concomitant with surgical treatment of the anal manifestations usually results in healing of the fissure or fistula.[10,11] Rectourethroperineal fistula also may result from Crohn's disease and may require complex procedures for correction.[12,13]

HEMORRHOIDS

Hemorrhoids are uncommon in the pediatric population unless associated with portal hypertension. Formerly, extrahepatic portal vein thrombosis was the primary cause of portal hypertension, but currently the most common etiology is cystic fibrosis (CF). Rarely is it necessary to perform surgical procedures on these hemorrhoids. Symptomatic local therapy reduces the likelihood of bleeding and pruritus. Careful local hygiene is an important aspect of this treatment. Perianal skin tags can be managed with good hygiene, but if the skin tag is enlarging in a smaller child, excision is reasonable. Skin tag is rarely an indication of other disease, although it may result from a healed fissure.

Surgical treatment of hemorrhoids should be conservative. Sphincter preservation is paramount. According to Bornemeier, "The sphincter [ani] apparently can differentiate between solid, fluid, and gas. It apparently can tell when its owner has his pants on or off. No other muscle in the body is such a protector of the dignity of man, yet so ready to come to his relief. A muscle like this is worth protecting."[14]

Thrombosed hemorrhoids resulting from prolonged extrusion require incision and evacuation of clot. Little treatment exists for bleeding hemorrhoids other than to reduce portal hypertension. Cryptitis, which produces sphincter spasm and results in venous engorgement, may be successfully treated with local measures or with multiple cryptotomy.

RECTAL PROLAPSE

Rectal prolapse is relatively common in young children and usually occurs as a result of a diarrheal illness, constipation, wasting illness, or malnutrition.[15,16] Prolapse is probably a herniation of the rectum, in most cases through a dilated levator mechanism.[17] Straining at stool and long periods of sitting on the toilet, because of protracted diarrhea or constipation, allows stretching of the pelvic diaphragm, the suspensory vessels, and other less well-defined suspensory structures of the rectum, resulting in prolapse.[15,18] Sometimes what appears to be rectal prolapse is an intussusception of the sigmoid colon.[19,20]

In these cases, an intact rectal suspension system exists, but a dilated levator mechanism produced by straining at stool, coupled with a redundant sigmoid colon, allows prolapse.[18] The pelvic diaphragm is a muscular structure. If the prolapse is prevented from recurring, the muscle fibers shorten, and the situation may be self-limiting. Improvement in nutrition also may result in a spontaneous resolution of rectal prolapse.

The diagnosis is usually made by the parent, who sees the rosette of rectum or sigmoid when the child complains of discomfort at the anus. Bleeding is occasionally noted as the primary symptom. Rarely is rectal prolapse in children the source of significant disability. One unusual case of a pig-bite was reported in a 2-year-old Indian child.[21] The prolapse either reduces spontaneously, as the child gets off the toilet, or the parent pushes it back in. Many 3-year-old children very quickly learn to reduce their own prolapse. It generally does not recur until the next episode at stool. It is uncommon for the child to be able to produce the prolapse in the examining room. Occasionally the prolapse can be demonstrated during a brief session on the toilet. Most often, the prolapse is not seen during examination because the patient does not relax the anus and strain sufficiently. The typical prolapse is a rosette of mucosa, sometimes slightly longer posteriorly than anteriorly (Fig. 37-1). One should be able to slip a finger alongside the prolapse and feel the sulcus 1 to 2 cm up inside the anus. A deeper sulcus suggests sigmoid intussusception rather than rectal prolapse. It is often difficult to differentiate the two clinically, even in the face of rectal examination at the time of prolapse or radiologic studies obtained to clarify the situation.[20]

If the child continues straining at stool once the pelvic diaphragm and rectal sphincters have been stretched,

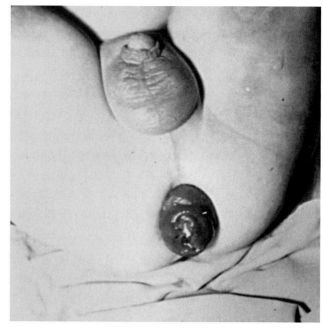

FIGURE 37-1. Rectal prolapse occurring in a child who had severe burns on his legs. Despite its being reduced repeatedly for several weeks, this prolapse continued to occur several times daily and required surgical correction.

little chance exists that the prolapse will correct itself. A change in bowel habits that eliminates the persistent urge to defecate, which seems to be common in many of these children, may allow the pelvic musculature to resume its normal tone. The stretched suspensory mechanism of the rectum then has a chance to shrink, and the process may spontaneously resolve.

Diagnostic Studies

At least in the United States, it is probably worthwhile to investigate the patient with rectal prolapse for the possibility of CF. In personal experience with 47 patients with rectal prolapse who underwent operative treatment, only two had CF. One was a known CF patient, and the other's condition was discovered by a screening sweat test while the child was being evaluated for rectal prolapse.

Barium enema studies are rarely of diagnostic benefit, because at the time of the barium enema, the prolapse is reduced, and the relations may not appear to be abnormal at all. In several patients, my colleagues and I have demonstrated, by an intra-abdominal injection of water-soluble contrast material, a deep sulcus of the pelvic peritoneum that extended downward, forming a "hernia sac" between the bladder and the rectum in male patients or the vagina and the rectum in female patients (Fig. 37-2). Although this herniogram may help distinguish a sigmoid intussusception from a true rectal prolapse, we have not often used it because it is an extremely uncomfortable procedure.

Treatment

The nonoperative treatment of rectal prolapse consists of attempts to alter the stool disorder that led to the prolapse. One of the early authorities advised against allowing the child to use the toilet or potty until the problem was resolved, suggesting that the child defecate in a squatting position on a newspaper.[15,22] Eliminating the cause of intractable diarrhea or chronic constipation seems to be the most practical approach, but success depends on recognition of the cause. Enzymatic therapy for CF is an example of nonoperative therapy.[23]

Surgical therapy has taken a number of forms. In Europe, the Middle East, and Asia, perianal cerclage has been used frequently, because it can be done as an outpatient procedure. It tightens the anal outlet and prevents prolapse from recurring while the musculature of the pelvis reestablishes its more normal relations.[24] The fact that the cerclage procedure is commonly used bespeaks its effectiveness, although erosion of the anus may occur from a wire or other suture being placed too tightly. Local infection is occasionally reported.[25]

Sclerotherapy with 30% saline, 5% phenol, or 25% glucose injected into the retrorectal space produces an inflammatory response and scar that theoretically prevents the rectum from sliding downward.[26-28] Whatever the injection material, it sometimes must be repeated and must always be done by using general anesthesia in the child, owing to the associated discomfort. I do not recommend injection therapy.

Various sorts of cauterization therapy have been used for rectal prolapse, including quadrant cauterization, reduction, and taping of the buttocks.[15] Endorectal cauterization or mucosal stripping as an alternative to suspension and plication procedures may be effective by allowing restoration of the suspensory apparatus.[29] Little reason exists to believe that rectal prolapse is due to mucosal overabundance.

An open sclerosing procedure, in which the retrorectal space is developed and packed with gauze, is done through an incision posterior to the anus but anterior to the coccyx. The gauze packing is removed gradually over a 10-day period. The packing produces enough inflammatory response that the rectum remains suspended. The major proponent of this operation has suggested that, when the sphincter mechanism is grossly stretched, a "plastic operation" may be needed to maintain the rectal suspension.[15]

Transanal suture fixation of the rectum (as described in 1909) has recently been used in a group of children with good success.[30] Its benefit probably derives from prevention of recurrent prolapse, while inflammation produced by the mattress suture, which extends from the rectal lumen to the skin, produces adhesions. An extensive plication or reefing of the posterior rectal wall via coccygectomy incision has recently been reported to have good results, but the potential for fistula formation from the multiple suture "bites" makes this a worrisome technique.[31]

My colleagues and I approach this lesion as if it were a true hernia. Through a natal cleft incision, we remove the coccyx, narrow the muscular hiatus, and suspend the rectum from the cut edge of the sacrum so that it cannot slide downward (Fig. 37-3).[32,33] This maneuver immediately reestablishes the suspensory mechanism and narrows the hiatus, which are the ultimate therapeutic outcomes of all the nonoperative and operative methods of treatment. We have used this technique in 53 patients over a 23-year period, with 50 of them being available for follow-up from periods of 2 months to 10 years.[21]

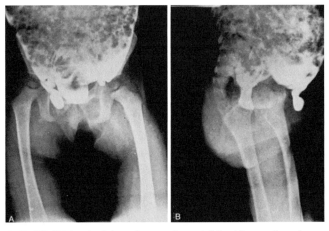

FIGURE 37-2. *A,* A herniogram in a child with rectal prolapse shows the overlapping sacs filled with contrast material. The right inguinal hernia sac is seen just medial to the hip joint, and the rectal prolapse extension of the peritoneum is located in the midline. *B,* A lateral view of the posterior prolapse sac and the anterior hernia sac.

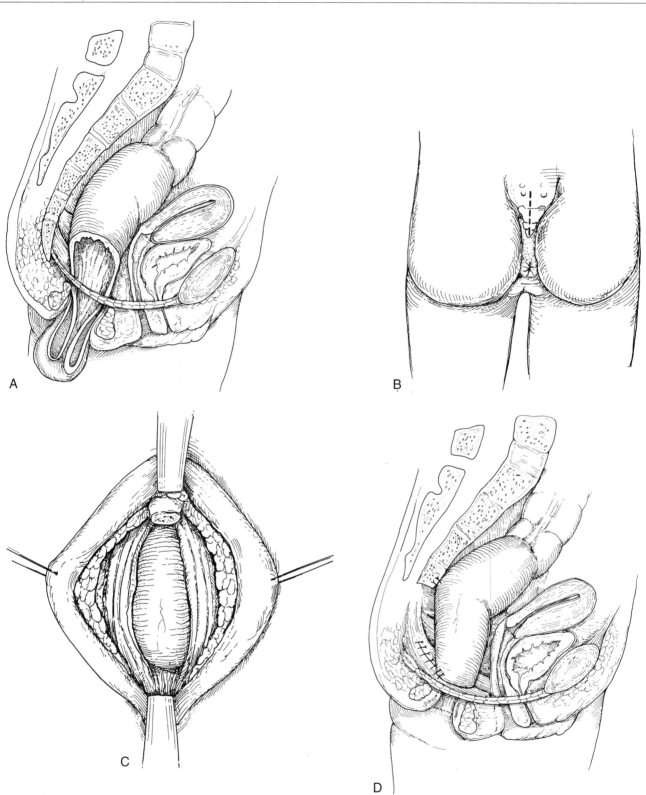

FIGURE 37-3. *A,* A cut-away sagittal view to illustrate the failure of the rectal suspensory mechanism to hold the rectum within the pelvis. *B,* The posterior sagittal incision for the suspension. *C,* The coccyx has been removed, and the posterior rectal wall exposed. *D,* The pelvic diaphragm is closed posterior to the reduced rectum. The rectum is sutured laterally to the pelvic diaphragm. The rectum is further suspended from the cut edge of the sacrum. (*A* and *D* redrawn from Ashcraft KW, Amoury RA, Holder TM: Levator repair and posterior suspension for rectal prolapse. J Pediatr Surg 12:241–245, 1977; *B* and *C,* from Ashcraft KW: Atlas of Pediatric Surgery. Philadelphia, WB Saunders, 1994, p 217.)

Of these patients, 40 had excellent initial results. Three patients had mild mucosal prolapse that gradually spontaneously resolved, and one had transanal trimming of the mucosa 1 month after the posterior suspension. Four patients had recurrent "prolapse," which proved to be intussusception of the sigmoid colon. One of these required transanal resection and anastomosis.[34,35] One case resolved spontaneously, and two other patients underwent transabdominal sigmoid resections. In one patient, a preoperative barium study was interpreted as normal, only later to show findings consistent with an intussusception. One case of caudal dysgenesis was a total failure.

This operation can be performed quite satisfactorily as an outpatient procedure. Modifications of the posterior sagittal approach have been reported and seem to have considerable merit.[19,25]

RECTAL TRAUMA

Rectal trauma in pediatric patients generally occurs by one of two mechanisms. The first is an accidental impalement injury. For example, one child jumped out of a boat to put on water skis and was impaled by a hidden tree branch beneath the water. The branch entered and penetrated the anus and penetrated through the bladder into the peritoneum. Another example is that of a 12-year-old boy who was riding a bicycle that did not have a seat; he had a laceration of the anus from the bicycle post when he had a collision. Bicycle crossbar injuries or "monkey-bar" injuries to the perineum rarely cause anal trauma. In female patients, straddle injuries most often affect the introitus. In male patients, they affect the urethra as a crushing type of injury.

The second and most common rectal trauma is a result of sexual abuse. Digital or penile penetration of the anorectum or other instrumentation may be seen immediately with bleeding or bruising. The most common clinical presentation is that of a chronic stellate laceration of the anus with lymphedema (Fig. 37-4). Perianal condylomata are a common occurrence in cases of sexual abuse involving the anus.

History

The patient with an accidental injury to the anus usually is seen immediately after the accident occurs. An accurate and consistent history of the mechanism of injury is needed. Evidence of sexual abuse is strengthened with a more chronic type of injury, an inconsistent history of the mechanism of injury, or no satisfactory explanation of how the condylomata came to occur. Careful questioning may reveal that a male member of the immediate family has penile condylomata. However, as many as 25% of males who carry human papillomavirus in the urethra have no external evidence of the virus.[36]

As with other forms of sexual abuse involving genital penetration in female patients or manipulation in male patients, difficulty is often encountered in obtaining an adequate history from the victim owing to fear, threats of

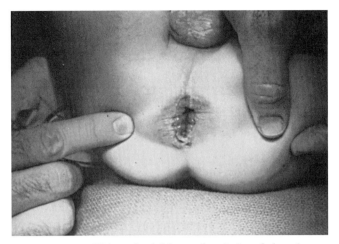

FIGURE 37-4. This male child was the victim of chronic sexual abuse and shows the typical stellate lacerations of the anal mucosal skin with exudate.

retaliation, or guilt. Unexplained injuries to the rectum must be considered a manifestation of sexual abuse and must be investigated through the appropriate social service authorities.[37]

Examinations

The child who has an acute traumatic rectal injury is often difficult to examine adequately owing to the associated discomfort. Penetration of a foreign object by impalement may require voiding cystourethrography followed by rectal examination and sigmoidoscopy under a general anesthetic.

The child who is sexually abused and who has either condylomata or lacerations of a more chronic nature can often be examined while awake. Making the diagnosis does not often require radiographic examination.

Treatment

Treatment of penetrating rectal injuries often requires a diverting colostomy.[38] Extensive perianal lacerations are repaired at the same time to reapproximate the sphincter muscle mechanism as much as possible. Closure of the colostomy is performed once satisfactory healing is demonstrated. Some rectal injuries may be repaired primarily without fecal diversion, but the risk of a bad result producing fecal incontinence hardly seems justified.[39]

Treatment of sexual abuse lesions involves interruption of the abuse pattern, which may require removal of the child from the home environment. The anal lesions usually heal much more quickly than the psychological trauma that has occurred with the sexual abuse. In the sexual abuse victim who may have an acute laceration extending up the rectal wall, it is rarely necessary to do a diverting colostomy, because these lacerations are not often full thickness. In two patients, however, sexual abuse resulted in laceration of the pelvic peritoneum; the resulting peritonitis caused the death of one of those patients.

REFERENCES

1. Fitzgerald RJ, Harding B, Ryan W: Fistula-in-ano in childhood: A congenital etiology. J Pediatr Surg 20:80–81, 1985.
2. Poenaru D, Yazbeck S: Anal fistula in infants: Etiology, features, management. J Pediatr Surg 28:1194–1195, 1993.
3. Shafer AD, McGlone TP, Flanagan RA: Abnormal crypts of Morgagni: The cause of perianal abscess and fistula-in-ano. J Pediatr Surg 22:203–204, 1987.
4. Ross ST: Fistula in ano. Surg Clin North Am 68:1417–1426, 1988.
5. Al-Salem AH, Laing W, Talwalker V: Fistula-in-ano in infancy and childhood. J Pediatr Surg 29:436–438, 1944.
6. Lunniss PJ, Jenkins PJ, Besser GM, et al: Gender differences in incidence of idiopathic fistula-in-ano are not explained by circulating sex hormones. Int J Colorect Dis 10:25–28, 1995.
7. Glen DL: Use of hydrogen peroxide to identify internal opening of anal fistula and perianal abscess. Aust N Z J Surg 56:433–435, 1986.
8. Sweeney L, Ritchie JK, Nichols RJ: Anal fissure in Crohn's disease. Br J Surg 75:57, 1988.
9. Markowitz J, Grancher K, Rosa J, et al: Highly destructive perianal disease in children with Crohn's disease. J Pediatr Gastroenterol Nutr 21:149–153, 1995.
10. Levien D, Surrell J, Mazier WP: Surgical treatment of anorectal fistula in patients with Crohn's disease. Surg Gynecol Obstet 169:133–136, 1989.
11. Bayer I, Gordon PH: Selected operative management of fistula-in-ano in Crohn's disease. Dis Colon Rectum 37:760–765, 1994.
12. Fazio VW, Jones IT, Jagelman DG, et al.: Rectourethral fistulas in Crohn's disease. Surg Gynecol Obstet 164:148–150, 1987.
13. Stamler JS, Bauer JJ, Janowitz HD: Rectourethroperineal fistula in Crohn's disease. Am J Gastroenterol 80:111–112, 1985.
14. Bornemeier WC: Sphincter protecting hemorrhoidectomy. Am J Proctol 11:48–52, 1960.
15. Lockhart-Mummery JP: Surgical procedures in general practice: Rectal prolapse. BMJ 1:345–347, 1939.
16. Severijnen R, Festen C, Van Der Staak F, et al: Rectal prolapse in children. Neth J Surg 41:149–151, 1989.
17. Moschcowitz AV: The pathogenesis, anatomy and care of prolapse of the rectum. Surg Gynecol Obstet 15:7, 1912.
18. Nigro ND: Restoration of the levator sling in the treatment of rectal procidentia. Dis Colon Rectum 1:123–127, 1958.
19. Pai GK, Pai PK: A case of congenital colonic stenosis presenting as rectal prolapse. J Pediatr Surg 25:699–700, 1990.
20. Theuerkauf FJ, Beahrs OH, Jill JR: Rectal prolapse: Causation and surgical treatment. Ann Surg 171:819–835, 1970.
21. Gangopadhyay AN, Gupta DK, Dhulkotia A, et al: Pig bite of prolapsed rectum in a child. J Pediatr Surg 37:657–658, 2002.
22. Kopel FB: Gastrointestinal manifestations of cystic fibrosis. Gastroenterology 62:483–491, 1972.
23. Shwachman H, Redmond A, Khaw K-T: Studies in cystic fibrosis: Report of 130 patients diagnosed under 3 months of age over a 20-year period. Pediatrics 46:335–343, 1970.
24. Sempsky WT, Rosenstein BJ: The cause of rectal prolapse in children. Am J Dis Child 142:338–339, 1988.
25. Pearl RH, Ein SH, Churchill B: Posterior sagittal anorectoplasty for pediatric recurrent rectal prolapse. J Pediatr Surg 24:1100–1102, 1989.
26. Kay NRM, Zachary RB: The treatment of rectal prolapse in children with injections of 30 per cent saline solutions. J Pediatr Surg 5:334–337, 1970.
27. Wyllie GG: The injection treatment of rectal prolapse. J Pediatr Surg 14:62–64, 1979.
28. Chan WK, Kay SM, Laberge JM, et al: Injection sclerotherapy in the treatment of rectal prolapse in infants and children. J Pediatr Surg 33:255–258, 1998.
29. Groff D, Nagaraj H: Rectal prolapse in infants and children. Am J Surg 160:531–532, 1990.
30. Schepens MA, Verhelst AA: Reappraisal of Ekehorn's rectopexy in the management of rectal prolapse in children. J Pediatr Surg 28:1494–1497, 1993.
31. Tsugawa C, Matsumoto Y, Nishijima E, et al: Posterior plication of the rectum for rectal prolapse in children. J Pediatr Surg 30:692–693, 1995.
32. Ashcraft KW, Amoury RA, Holder TM: Levator repair and posterior suspension for rectal prolapse. J Pediatr Surg 12:241–245, 1977.
33. Ashcraft KW, Garred JL, Holder TM: Rectal prolapse: 17 year experience with the posterior repair and suspension. J Pediatr Surg 25:992–995, 1990.
34. Altemeier WA, Culbertson WR, Schowengerdt C, et al: Nineteen years' experience with the one-stage perineal repair of rectal prolapse. Ann Surg 173:993–1006, 1971.
35. Chwals W, Brennan L, Weitzman J, et al: Transanal mucosal sleeve resection for the treatment of rectal prolapse in children. J Pediatr Surg 25:715–718, 1990.
36. Rosemberg SK, Husain M, Herman GE, et al: Sexually transmitted papillomaviral infection in the male: VI. Simultaneous urethral cytology-ViraPap testing of male consorts of women with genital human papillomaviral infection. Urology 36:38–41, 1990.
37. Finkel MA: Anogenital trauma in sexually abused children. Pediatrics 84:317–322, 1989.
38. Trunkey D, Hays RJ, Shired GT: Management of rectal trauma. J Trauma 13:411–415, 1973.
39. Levine JH, Longo WE, Pruitt C, et al: Management of selected rectal injuries by primary repair. Am J Surg 172:575–579, 1996.

Intussusception

Mary E. Fallat, MD

Intussusception is a frequent cause of bowel obstruction in infants and toddlers. It was first described by Paul Barbette[1] of Amsterdam in 1674. Jonathan Hutchinson[2] reported the first successful operation for intussusception in a 2-year-old child in 1873. In 1876, Harald Hirschsprung[3] described a systematic approach to hydrostatic reduction. In the United States, Ravitch[4] popularized the use of barium enema reduction for this problem. His 1959 monograph reviewing all aspects of intussusception remains a classic.

PRIMARY IDIOPATHIC INTUSSUSCEPTION

Pathogenesis

Intussusception is the telescoping of one portion of the intestine into another. An intussusception is customarily described by the proximal portion of intestine (intussusceptum) first and the distal portion of intestine (intussuscipiens) last. More than 80% of intussusceptions are ileocolic. The ileoileal, cecocolic, colocolic, and jejunojejunal varieties occur with increasing rarity.[5] An intussusception may have an identifiable lesion that serves as a lead point, drawing the proximal bowel into the distal bowel by peristaltic activity. In almost every patient examined at operation, marked hypertrophy of the lymphoid tissue of the ileal wall is encountered at the leading edge of the intussusceptum.[5] Intussusception occurs frequently in the wake of an upper respiratory infection or an episode of gastroenteritis, providing an etiology for hypertrophy of Peyer's patches. Adenoviruses, and to a much lesser extent rotavirus, have been implicated in up to 50% of cases.[5,6] These swollen Peyer's patches protrude into the lumen of the intestine and are the likely cause of the initial invagination.

The incidence of a definite anatomic lead point ranges from 2% to 12% in reported series.[7] These include Meckel's diverticulum, the appendix, polyps, carcinoid tumors, submucosal hemorrhage resulting from Henoch-Schönlein purpura, non-Hodgkin's lymphoma, foreign bodies, ectopic pancreas or gastric mucosa, and intestinal duplication. The most common pathologic lead point is a Meckel's diverticulum. The incidence of anatomic lead points increases in proportion to age.[8] Small-bowel intussusceptions related to gastrojejunostomy tubes also have been described.[9]

As the mesentery of the proximal bowel is drawn into the distal bowel, it is compressed, which results in venous obstruction and edema of the bowel wall. If reduction of the intussusception does not occur, arterial insufficiency and bowel wall necrosis follow. Although spontaneous reduction undoubtedly occurs, the natural history of an intussusception is to progress to a fatal outcome as a result of sepsis unless the condition is recognized and appropriately treated. For many reasons, the morbidity and mortality rates have decreased dramatically at children's hospitals in North America since the mid-1940s.[7]

SECONDARY INTUSSUSCEPTION

Patients with cystic fibrosis are prone to intussusception, and reduction may be required on multiple occasions. It is probable that inspissated secretions and thick fecal matter in the intestinal lumen act as a lead point to produce repeated intussusception in this disease. These conditions are seen in children at an average age of 9 to 12 years.[5]

INCIDENCE

Idiopathic intussusception can occur at any age; however, the greatest incidence occurs in infants between ages 5 and 9 months. More than half of all cases occur within the first year of life, and only 10% to 25% of cases occur after age 2 years.[5,10] The condition has been described in premature infants and has been postulated as the cause of small bowel atresia in some cases.[11]

Most patients are well-nourished, healthy infants. Approximately two-thirds are boys.[5] It seems reasonable to be more suspicious of intussusception during peaks of respiratory infection and epidemics of gastroenteritis.

CLINICAL PRESENTATION

Intussusception produces cramping abdominal pain, which begins acutely with signs of severe discomfort in an infant who has previously been comfortable. The child may stiffen and pull the legs up to the abdomen. Hyperextension, writhing, and breath holding may be followed by vomiting. The attack often ceases as suddenly as it started. Between attacks, the child may appear comfortable or may fall asleep. After some time, the child becomes lethargic between episodes of pain. Vomiting at some stage is almost universal, consisting of undigested food initially and later becoming bilious. Small or normal bowel movements may result initially from the straining as the colon evacuates distal to the obstruction. Later in the course, the stools may be tinged with blood. Still later in the progression of the bowel ischemia, dark red mucoid clots or "currant jelly" stools are passed.

PHYSICAL EXAMINATION

The child's vital signs are usually normal early in the course of the disease. During episodes of pain, hyperperistaltic rushes may be audible.

Between episodes of cramping, the right lower abdominal quadrant may appear flat or empty. This finding is due to progression of the cecum and ileocecal portion of the intussusception into the right or transverse colon. During the relaxed interval between pains, a mass may be delineated almost anywhere in the abdomen. The mass is often curved because it is tethered by the blood vessels and mesentery on one side. On rectal examination, blood-stained mucus or blood may be encountered. The longer the duration of symptoms, the more likely the probability of identifying gross or occult blood. Palpation of the intussuscepted mass on bimanual examination is possible. Actual contact with the rectal examining finger is rare.

If the obstructive process has been prolonged, dehydration and bacteremia ensue, leading to tachycardia and fever. Occasionally, the child is first seen in hypovolemic or septic shock.

Prolapse of the intussusceptum through the anus is a grave sign, particularly when the intussusceptum is blue/black. Certainly rectal protrusion of an ileal lead point is an indication of extensive telescoping and severe compromise of blood supply and ischemic damage to the gut. Such a patient undoubtedly exhibits signs of systemic illness. The greatest danger in a case of prolapse of the intussusceptum is that the examiner will misdiagnose the condition and reduce what is thought to be merely a small rectal prolapse. To avoid such a tragedy, a lubricated tongue blade should be passed up along the side of the protruding mass before reduction is attempted. Prolapse of a colocolic intussusception may easily be mistaken for simple rectal prolapse. If the blade can be inserted more than a centimeter or two into the anus alongside of the mass, the diagnosis of intussusception should be considered. Rectal prolapse, while producing discomfort, should not be accompanied by vomiting or signs of sepsis.

DIAGNOSTIC STUDIES

In about half of cases, the diagnosis of intussusception can be suspected on plain abdominal radiographs (Fig. 38-1). Suggestive radiographic abnormalities on a plain film include an abdominal mass, abnormal distribution of gas and fecal contents, sparse large bowel gas, and air/fluid levels in the presence of bowel obstruction.[12] These signs are not diagnostic, however, and controversy exists over whether the limited accuracy warrants this study.[13]

Ultrasonography

Ultrasonographic (US) examination of the abdomen is now used in many medical centers to evaluate a child with a possible intussusception.[13,14] The sonographic pattern of intussusception was first reported in 1977.[15] Since then, numerous studies have described the characteristic findings of a "target" lesion and a "pseudokidney" sign. The target lesion is seen on transverse section and consists of two rings of low echogenicity separated by a hyperechoic ring. The pseudokidney sign is seen on longitudinal section and appears as superimposed hypoechoic and hyperechoic layers (Fig. 38-2). This pattern represents the edematous walls of the intussusception.

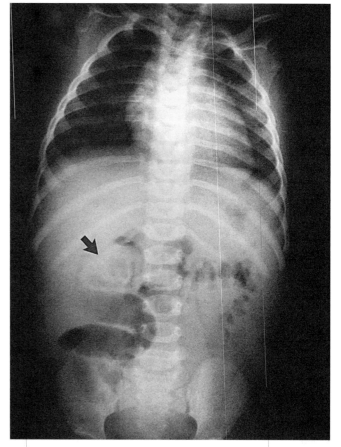

FIGURE 38-1. Abdominal radiograph showing dilated loops of small bowel in the right lower quadrant and a soft tissue mass density in the vicinity of the transverse colon near the hepatic flexure (*arrow*).

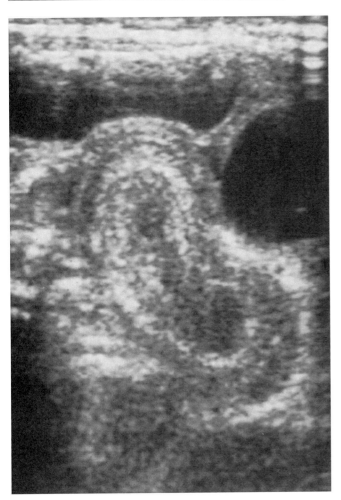

FIGURE 38-2. Sonogram showing the "pseudokidney" sign seen with intussusception on longitudinal section.

Successful reduction results in a smaller "donut," with an echogenic rim representing edema of the terminal ileum and ileocecal valve.

A virtue of screening US is that it is highly accurate in experienced hands and decreases the number of unnecessary contrast enemas, thus reducing exposure to ionizing radiation.[13] Methods used to reduce the intussusception after diagnosis include using a sonographically guided 10% meglumine ioxitamalate enema in balanced salt solution to reduce it, or using sonographically guided pneumatic pressure.[16,17] The use of US-guided reduction has a lower success rate in cases in which entrapped fluid is present or the intussusception is located in the left abdomen.[16] If a child has classic clinical findings with colic, an abdominal mass or currant jelly stools or both, and no clinical evidence is noted of peritonitis, a contrast enema for diagnosis and reduction represents safer practice.[12]

Computed Tomography

Intussusception has been described on computed tomography (CT) imaging as an intraluminal mass with a characteristic layered appearance or fat or both within the mass or in continuity with adjacent mesenteric fat (Fig. 38-3).

Transient small-bowel intussusception has been noted on both CT and US, and the majority of these are not clinically significant.[18] These intussusceptions are usually short-segment with no recognizable lead point. Intervention should be dictated by clinical findings in symptomatic patients.[19]

NONOPERATIVE MANAGEMENT

Once the diagnosis of intussusception is considered, a nasogastric tube may be needed to decompress the stomach. Intravenous fluid resuscitation is begun. A complete blood count and serum electrolytes are obtained. A pneumatic or contrast enema is still the mainstay of diagnosis and the first line of reduction treatment in many centers. Few complications are expected, as long as certain guidelines are followed.

Pneumatic or hydrostatic enema reduction should be attempted only under controlled conditions. Evidence of peritonitis, perforation, advancing sepsis, and possible gangrenous bowel precludes pneumatic or hydrostatic enema reduction. This should be the surgeon's decision. The longer the history of symptoms, the greater the possibility that enema reduction will not be successful and the more dangerous it may be.

Hydrostatic Reduction

One of the first studies evaluating the technique of intussusception reduction by using hydrostatic pressure was published in 1926.[20] These reductions were not fluoroscopically controlled with contrast agent but were performed under anesthesia by using saline solution. Fundamentals of this method of management were incorporated into the present technique of hydrostatic reduction. A lubricated straight catheter or Foley catheter is inserted into the rectum and held in place by firmly taping the buttocks together; balloon occlusion of the anus is avoided by most radiologists. The child is restrained. The contrast material is allowed to run into the rectum from a height of 3 ft above the patient. Filling of the bowel is observed fluoroscopically. Constant hydrostatic pressure is continued as long as reduction is occurring. In the absence of progress, the contrast material is allowed to drain. This procedure can be repeated a second or third time.

Typically, reduction of the ileum back to the area of the ileocecal valve is simple. Usually, a delay occurs at that point, until a free flow of contrast into the distal small bowel is seen.

The nonoperative enema technique of intussusception reduction has several obvious advantages over operative reduction, including decreased morbidity, cost, and length of hospital stay. A successful reduction is dependent on free reflux of contrast into the distal small bowel (Fig. 38-4). Hydrostatic reduction with barium under fluoroscopic guidance was the standard method until the mid-1980s.[13] Water-soluble isotonic contrast is a more ideal alternative for hydrostatic reduction, owing to the risk of barium extravasation with perforation.

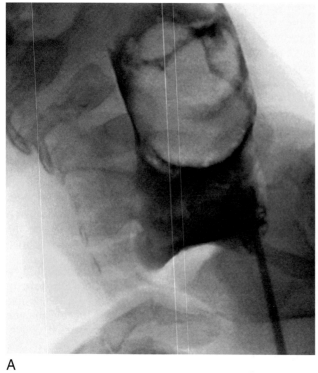

A

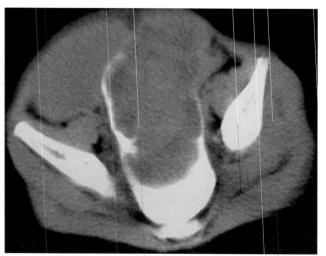

B

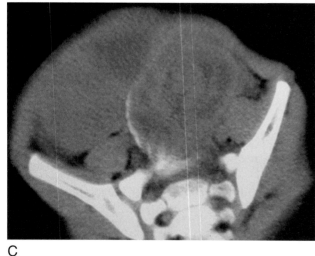

C

FIGURE 38-3. Concurrent contrast enema and pelvic computed tomography image of an intussusception. *A,* Contrast study showing intussusception low in pelvis. *B,* Computed tomography image of intussusception. *C,* Computed tomography image of the "layered" intussuscepted mass.

Pneumatic Reduction

Air reduction of intussusception was described in 1897 by Holt.[21] Adoption of the air enema or pneumatic technique has become more widespread since the late 1980s, owing to the higher rates of successful reduction reported in large international series.[10] The procedure is fluoroscopically monitored as air is insufflated into the rectum. The maximum safe air pressure is 80 mm Hg for younger infants and 110 to 120 mm Hg for older infants. Advocates of the air enema believe that the method is quicker, safer, less messy, and decreases the exposure time to radiation. Accurate pressure measurements are possible, and reduction rates are higher than with hydrostatic

techniques (Fig. 38-5).[22] Potential drawbacks of using pneumatic reduction include the possibility of development of a tension pneumoperitoneum, poor visualization of lead points, and relatively poor visualization of the intussusception and reduction process, resulting in false-positive reductions (Fig. 38-6).[22-24]

Attempts at hydrostatic or pneumatic reduction are continued *as long as progress is evident.* Many knowledgeable physicians think that if the patient's general condition permits, two or three attempts at reduction should be done before abandoning the procedure.

Success rates of reduction by using hydrostatic techniques reported between 1980 and 1991 were found to be

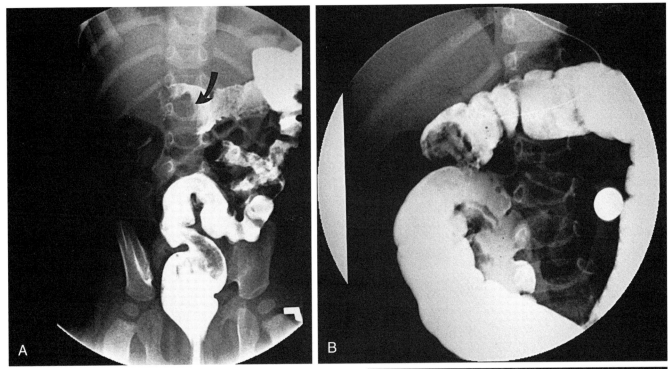

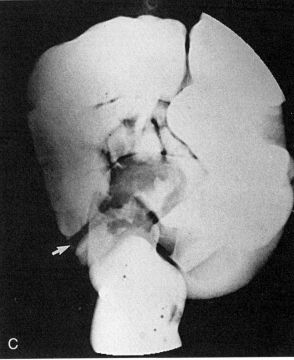

FIGURE 38-4. Fluoroscopic examination using isotonic contrast for hydrostatic reduction of intussusception. *A,* Intussusception (*arrow*) seen in midtransverse colon. *B,* Reduction has occurred to hepatic flexure. *C,* Complete reduction with reflux of contrast into terminal ileum. Note edematous ileocecal valve (*arrow*).

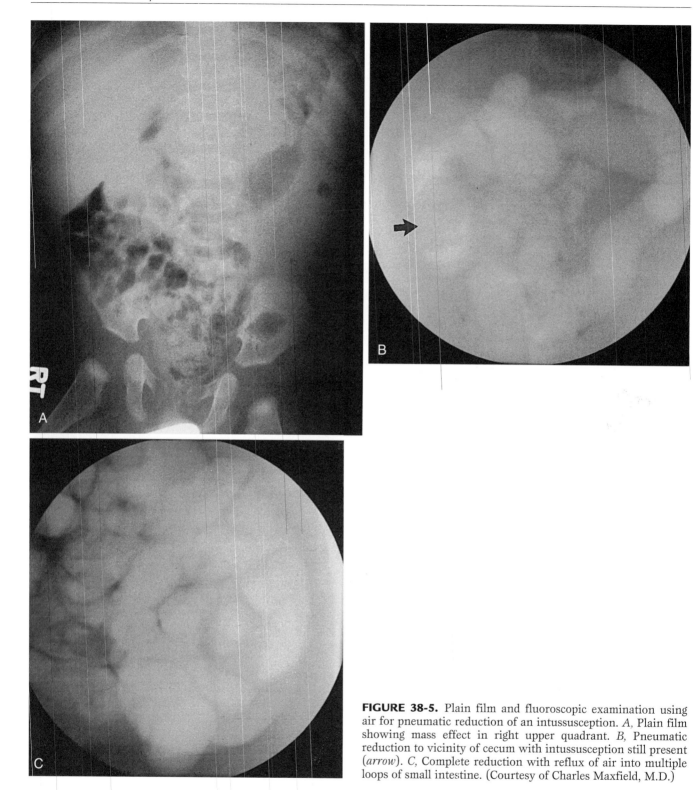

FIGURE 38-5. Plain film and fluoroscopic examination using air for pneumatic reduction of an intussusception. *A,* Plain film showing mass effect in right upper quadrant. *B,* Pneumatic reduction to vicinity of cecum with intussusception still present (*arrow*). *C,* Complete reduction with reflux of air into multiple loops of small intestine. (Courtesy of Charles Maxfield, M.D.)

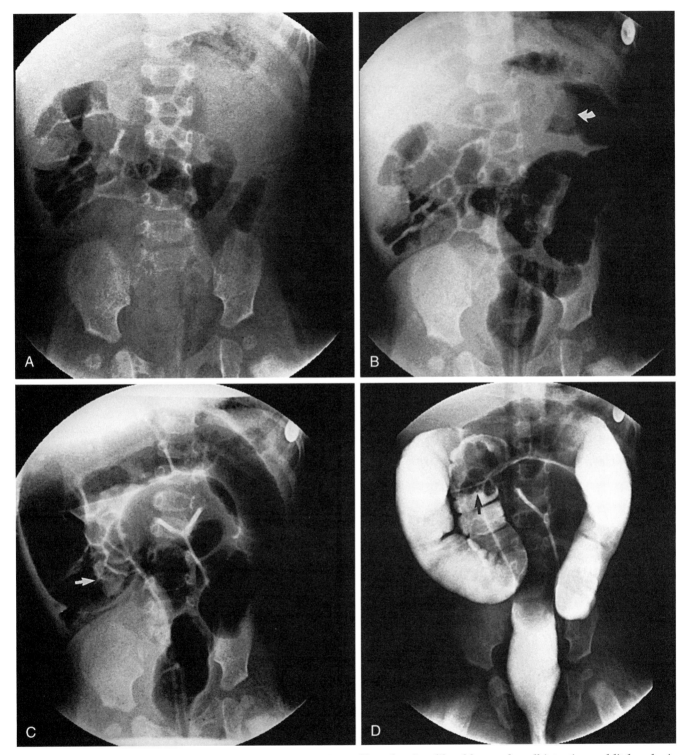

FIGURE 38-6. Incomplete reduction of intussusception. *A,* Scout films showing dilated loops of small intestine and little colonic gas. *B,* Pneumatic reduction to transverse colon showing intussusceptum (*arrow*). *C,* Further reduction with persistent intussusception (*arrow*). *D,* Attempted reduction with isotonic contrast, showing cecum in right upper quadrant. This child had an upper gastrointestinal series, which was normal, to rule out malrotation, followed by operative reduction.

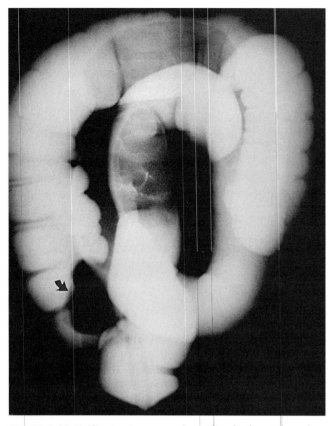

FIGURE 38-7. Contrast enema view after hydrostatic reduction of an intussusception to the ileocecal junction. A persistent filling defect (*arrow*) is present without free reflux into the terminal ileum.

50% to 78% compared with 75% to 94% with pneumatic reduction between 1986 and 1991.[5] A second trial of hydrostatic or air reduction may be undertaken within a few hours if the child does not have signs of an intra-abdominal catastrophy and the symptoms seem relieved, but the original reduction failed to show reflux into the terminal ileum (Fig. 38-7).[10,25]

A colon perforation rate of 0.16% to 2.8% during gas enema reductions is published.[22,24] Excessive pressure may disrupt the compromised bowel wall, or reduction may unmask an existing occult perforation.

After successful reduction under fluoroscopic monitoring, the patient should be observed for several hours on intravenous fluids with nothing being given by mouth.[26] The family should be advised of the possibility of recurrence, which exists regardless of whether the intussusception is reduced by enema or by operation.

OPERATIVE TREATMENT

Laparotomy is required in children with signs of shock or peritonitis and in those who have incomplete hydrostatic pressure or pneumatic reduction. Preoperative preparation includes gastric decompression, intravenous fluid resuscitation, and the administration of prophylactic antibiotics.

Successful enema reduction of an intussusception does not completely exclude a lead point that might result

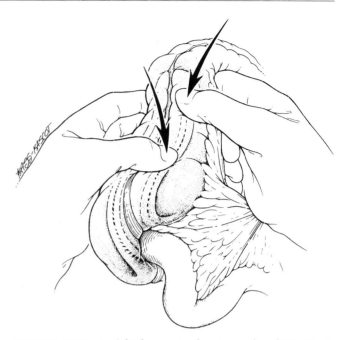

FIGURE 38-8. A right lower quadrant muscle-splitting incision allows delivery of the intussusception into the wound. Gentle and continuous massage from distal to proximal usually results in reduction of an intussusception.

in recurrence or that might otherwise be hazardous to the patient. Some studies suggest that the incidence of a lead point increases with age.[8] A residual intraluminal filling defect after enema reduction with terminal ileal reflux is an indication for laparotomy.[27]

A right lower abdominal muscle-splitting incision is usually satisfactory for exposure. The involved bowel can almost always be readily reduced to this area, even when the intussusceptum has progressed to the rectosigmoid. The option of extension of the incision is available.

Gentle manipulation of the bowel is needed, pushing (rather than pulling) the lead point of the intussusceptum back toward its normal position (Fig. 38-8). When resistance to reduction reaches the point of serosal tearing, the surgeon must decide whether further attempts at reduction are likely to be fruitful or might result in intestinal rupture and contamination. As hydrostatic reduction has become more efficient, fewer patients are requiring operation, but the incidence of resection at operation has increased.[6]

Even when reduction is complete, the viability of the bowel may be questionable. In such cases, the application of warm saline packs may improve the circulation and relieve doubt about the necessity of resection. When serious vascular impairment has developed, resection is usually the safest course (Fig. 38-9).

Once operative reduction has been achieved, examination for a pathologic lead point must be performed, and appropriate measures must be taken (Fig. 38-10A and B). The most concerning cases are those in which the patient is older than 2 years. An appendectomy is usually performed because the location of the healed scar suggests that an appendectomy has been performed.

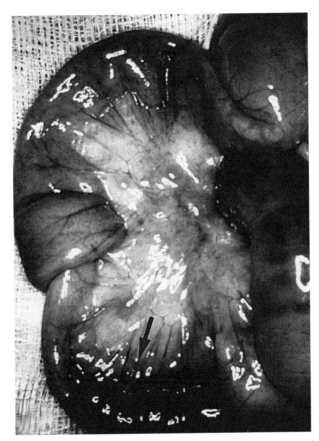

FIGURE 38-9. Operative view of an incompletely reduced intussusception. The intestine in the lower half of the photograph has been reduced, and the bowel wall is ecchymotic, with at least one area of questionable viability (*arrow*).

RECURRENT INTUSSUSCEPTION

Recurrent intussusception has been described in 2% to 20% of cases, with about one-third occurring within 1 day and the majority within 6 months of the initial episode.[27-29] Recurrences usually have no defined lead point, and they are less likely to occur after surgical reduction or resection. Multiple recurrences can occur in the same patient. Success rates with enema reduction after one recurrence are comparable to those with the first episode and are better if the child did not previously require operative reduction. Patients tend to be seen earlier with recurrent intussusception, and they have fewer symptoms. Irritability and discomfort may be the only clues during the early state of a recurrence.

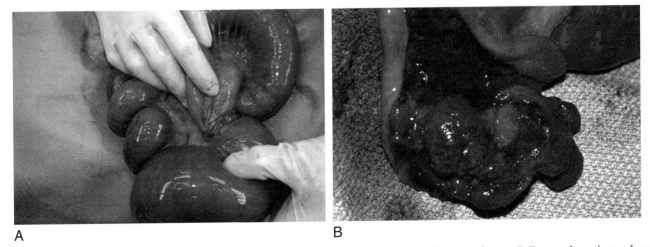

A   B

FIGURE 38-10. *A*, Operative view of an intussuscepted mass in a child with Peutz-Jeghers syndrome. *B*, Resected specimen shows a large jejunal polyp that was a lead point for the intussusception.

An overriding concern in recurrent intussusception is occult malignancy, although multiple recurrences are not a contraindication to attempted radiologic reduction.[27] Unfortunately, the clinical findings or pattern of recurrence do not predict the presence of a pathologic lead point. A careful imaging search is mandatory, and US has been recommended as the imaging study of choice.[27,30] Indications for operation include (1) irreducible recurrence, (2) clinical evidence to suggest a pathologic lead point, (3) documentation of a pathologic lead point by an imaging procedure, or (4) persistence of clinical symptoms after the completion of the enema.[27]

POSTOPERATIVE INTUSSUSCEPTION

Intussusception occurs after operations done for a variety of conditions. Thoracic as well as abdominal operations have been followed by latent intussusception. Because ileus and adhesive obstruction more frequently come to mind as a cause for intestinal obstruction, these intussusceptions may not be diagnosed preoperatively, although US has proved to be a successful diagnostic modality.[31] Most postoperative intussusceptions occur within a month of the initial procedure, and an interval of about 10 days between initial operation and development of symptoms is average.[32] Most postoperative intussusceptions are ileoileal and respond to operative reduction without resection.[31,32]

REFERENCES

1. Barbette P: Oeuvres Chirugiques et Anatomiques. Geneva, Francois Miege, 1674, p 522.
2. Hutchinson J: A successful case of abdominal section for intussusception. Proc R Med Chir Soc 7:195–198, 1873.
3. Hirschsprung H: Et Tilfaelde af suakut Tarminvagination. Hospitals-Tidende 3:321–327, 1876.
4. Ravitch MM: Intussusception in Infants and Children. Springfield, Ill, Charles C Thomas, 1959.
5. Stringer MD, Pablot SM, Brereton RJ: Paediatric intussusception. Br J Surg 79:867–876, 1992.
6. Montgomery EA, Popek EJ: Intussusception, adenovirus, and children: A brief reaffirmation. Hum Pathol 25:169–174, 1994.
7. Meier DE, Coln CE, Rescorla FJ, et al: Intussusception in children: International perspective. World J Surg 20:1035–1040, 1996.
8. Blakelock RT, Beasley SW: The clinical implications of non-idiopathic intussusception. Pediatr Surg Int 14:163–167, 1998.
9. Hughes UM, Connolly BL, Chait PG, et al: Further report of small-bowel intussusceptions related to gastrojejunostomy tubes. Pediatr Radiol 30:614–617, 2000.
10. Guo J, Ma X, Zhou Q: Results of air pressure enema reduction of intussusception: 6,396 cases in 13 years. J Pediatr Surg 21:1201–1203, 1986.
11. Mooney DP, Steinthorsson G, Shorter NA: Perinatal intussusception in premature infants. J Pediatr Surg 31:695–697, 1996.
12. Smith DS, Bonadio WA, Losek JD, et al: The role of abdominal x-rays in the diagnosis and management of intussusception. Pediatr Emerg Care 8:325–327, 1992.
13. Daneman A, Navarro O: Intussusception, Part 1: A review of diagnostic approaches. Pediatr Radiol 33:79–85, 2003.
14. Henrikson S, Blane CE, Koujok K: The effect of screening sonography on the positive rate of enemas for intussusception. Pediatr Radiol 33:190–193, 2003.
15. Burke LF, Clarke E: Ileocolic intussusception: A case report. J Clin Ultrasound 5:346–347, 1977.
16. Crystal P, Hertzanu Y, Farber B, et al: Sonographically guided hydrostatic reduction of intussusception in children. J Clin Ultrasound 30:343–348, 2002.
17. Gu L, Zhu H, Wang S: Sonographic guidance of air enema for intussusception reduction in children. Pediatr Radiol 30:339–342, 2000.
18. Strouse PJ, DiPietro MA, Saez F: Transient small-bowel intussusception in children on CT. Pediatr Radiol 33:316–320, 2003.
19. Kornecki A, Daneman A, Navarro O, et al: Spontaneous reduction of intussusception: Clinical spectrum, management and outcome. Pediatr Radiol 30:58–63, 2000.
20. Hipsley P: Intussusception and its treatment by hydrostatic pressure: Based on an analysis of 100 consecutive cases so treated. Med J Aust 2:201–206, 1926.
21. Holt LE: The Diseases of Infancy and Childhood: For the Use of Students and Practitioners of Medicine. New York, Appleton, 1897, pp 378–388.
22. Kirks DR: Air intussusception reduction: "The winds of change." Pediatr Radiol 25:89–91, 1995.
23. Peh WCG, Khong PL, Chan KL, et al: Sonographically guided hydrostatic reduction of childhood intussusception using Hartmann's solution. AJR Am J Roentgenol 167:1237–1241, 1996.
24. Maoate K, Beasley SW: Perforation during gas reduction of intussusception. Pediatr Surg Int 14:168–170, 1998.
25. Sandler AD, Ein SH, Connolly B: Unsuccessful air-enema reduction of intussusception: Is a second attempt worthwhile? Pediatr Surg Int 15:214–216, 1999.
26. LeMasne A, Lortat-Jacob S, Sayegh N, et al: Intussusception in infants and children: Feasibility of ambulatory management. Eur J Pediatr 158:707–710, 1999.
27. Daneman A, Alton DJ, Lobo E, et al: Patterns of recurrence of intussusception in children: A 17-year review. Pediatr Radiol 28:913–919, 1998.
28. Champoux AN, Del Beccaro MA, Nazar-Stewart V: Recurrent intussusception. Arch Pediatr Adolesc Med 148:474–478, 1994.
29. Fecteau A, Flageole H, Nguyen LT, et al: Recurrent intussusception: Safe use of hydrostatic enema. J Pediatr Surg 31:859–861, 1996.
30. Navarro O, Dugougeat F, Kornecki A, et al: The impact of imaging in the management of intussusception owing to pathologic lead points in children. Pediatr Radiol 30:594–603, 2000.
31. Linke F, Eble F, Berger S: Postoperative intussusception in childhood. Pediatr Surg Int 14:175–177, 1998.
32. Holcomb GW, Ross AJ, O'Neill JA: Postoperative intussusception: Increasing frequency or increasing awareness? South Med J 84:1334–1339, 1991.

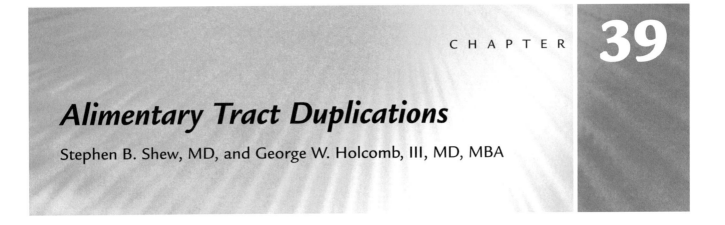

CHAPTER 39

Alimentary Tract Duplications

Stephen B. Shew, MD, and George W. Holcomb, III, MD, MBA

Alimentary tract duplications are rare congenital anomalies that can occur in any portion of the gastrointestinal tract from the mouth to the anus. Duplications may initially be seen with symptoms of bleeding or obstruction, or they may be asymptomatic and discovered only incidentally. The majority of duplications are diagnosed by age 2 years, with an increasing number being diagnosed by prenatal ultrasonography. The surgical goal is to remove the duplication to eliminate symptoms and prevent recurrence. Duplications are benign conditions, but the risk of peptic ulceration due to the presence of ectopic gastric mucosa and the rare malignant transformation within the duplication remain secondary therapeutic concerns. Duplications frequently share a common vasculature with the native alimentary tract, and simple resection is generally required. The management of extensive thoracoabdominal or long intra-abdominal duplications can be challenging; however, radical resections are rarely in the patient's best interest. The prognosis after surgical treatment is generally favorable but is predicated on the severity of the presenting illness and the morbidity and mortality of associated congenital anomalies.

HISTORY

Calder[1] is credited with the first published report in 1733 describing an infant with a duodenal duplication. One hundred fifty years later, Reginald Fitz[2] was the first to apply the term *duplication* to describe what he thought was a remnant of the omphalomesenteric duct. Subsequently, a variety of terms were used to designate the origin or location of these anomalies, including "enterogenous cyst" and "ileum duplex." However, William Ladd[3] was the first to coin the phrase *duplication of the alimentary tract* in 1937 to describe a pattern of these anomalies found in a case series of 10 patients. He noted that all the anomalies had three specific findings in common, independent of their location: a well-developed coat of smooth muscle, an epithelial lining from the alimentary tract, and an attachment to some part of the alimentary tract. Later, Gross et al.[4] supported and adopted this term to help simplify the classification of these diversely located anomalies.

EMBRYOLOGY

Alimentary tract duplications can first be seen at any age, and they occur with an incidence of 1 in 4500 births.[5] Duplications are thought to arise from disturbances in the embryonic development of the alimentary tract and hence are considered to be congenital malformations. No genetic predisposition is known. Duplications can be found in association with anomalies of the vertebrae, spinal cord, and genitourinary tract in 30% to 50% of the patients.[4,6] Infrequently, these lesions also may be associated with intestinal atresia and malrotation.[7]

Several theories have been proposed regarding the etiology of these anomalies. One early theory postulated that duplications were the result of a persistent embryonic diverticulum during the formation of the alimentary tract.[8] Several decades later, these anomalies were suggested to be the result of aberrant recanalization of the lumen of the alimentary tract.[9] Still later, a theory of partial twinning was espoused to rationalize the association between tubular duplications of the colon and duplications of the genitourinary systems, with similar anomalies found in conjoined twins.[10,11] Others theorized that local environmental factors such as hypoxia played a large role in the development of duplications.[12] An extension of this postulate suggested that spared viable areas within ischemic segments of intestine secondary to in utero vascular occlusive events lead to duplications as part of a spectrum of intestinal atresias.[13] The "split notochord" theory was developed to explain the association between spinal anomalies and enteric duplications from a series of five patients.[14] Despite further evidence for notochord involvement in the etiology of various foregut and hindgut malformations with spinal anomalies,[15,16] the exact mechanism for the formation of alimentary tract duplications remains elusive. Although most of these speculations are supported by clinical observations made from subsets of patients with duplications, no single theory is able to explain adequately the variety of alimentary tract duplications and all of the possible associated anomalies.

CLINICAL PRESENTATION AND DIAGNOSIS

Alimentary tract duplications do not have a classic presentation. Although duplications of the stomach are more frequently found in female patients, alimentary tract duplications as a whole do not exhibit a gender preponderance.[4,7,17,18] More than 75% of patients are younger than 2 years when they become symptomatic.[7] However, duplications may be seen at the extremes of age, from the fetus to the geriatric patient.[19,20] Symptoms can be vague or attributed to other more common etiologies that can make the diagnosis difficult. In general, symptoms are related to the shape, size, location, and type of mucosa in the duplication. Most alimentary tract duplications are cystic, whereas the minority are tubular (Fig. 39-1). Because these lesions do not communicate with the native bowel, a colorless mucoid fluid will generally be found within the duplication. Large duplications can compress adjacent organs, whereas smaller ones may create a lead point for intussusception and intestinal obstruction. In the majority of reported series, the jejunum and ileum are the most common sites for duplications (Table 39-1). Histologically, most duplications are lined by the indigenous mucosa specific to the location of the lesion. Ectopic tissue

is present in 30% of all duplications,[4] and the prevalence will vary depending on its location along the alimentary tract (Table 39-2). The most common ectopic tissue is gastric mucosa, followed by pancreatic exocrine and endocrine tissue.[21] However, any type of intestinal epithelium can be found in an ectopic location. Frequently, ectopic gastric mucosa will cause peptic ulceration, leading to hemorrhage and perforation (Fig. 39-2). The type of mucosal lining will determine the nature of the intraluminal contents. Although some reports of duplications containing malignant cells have been seen in adults, duplications found in infancy and childhood are considered benign.[22] Because many duplications are asymptomatic, it is not unusual for them to be discovered incidentally on imaging studies or at surgical exploration.

Diagnosis of Suspected Duplications

A variety of imaging studies are useful for diagnosis. Plain radiographs may demonstrate a posterior mediastinal mass, suggestive of an esophageal duplication. Contrast studies may be useful for demonstrating duplications with an extrinsic mass effect or by demonstrating communication to the native gastrointestinal tract. Computerized tomography (CT) scans can be particularly useful in delineating a soft tissue mass in the thoracic and abdominal cavities. An enhancing rim of tissue around a fluid-filled cyst can be diagnostic of an alimentary tract duplication. Moreover, ultrasonography (US) may be particularly efficacious in diagnosing gastrointestinal duplications by demonstrating hyperechoic mucosa surrounded by hypoechoic muscular layers and the presence

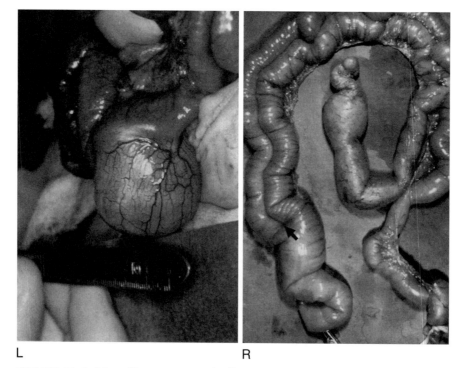

L   R

FIGURE 39-1. Most alimentary tract duplications are cystic in nature *(left)*. On the right is a tubular duplication. Note that the native bowel is bifurcated *(arrow)* into the tubular duplication and native intestine.

TABLE 39-1

ALIMENTARY TRACT DUPLICATIONS BY LOCATION

Authors	Institution	#D (pt)	Oral	Esophagus	Thoraco-abdominal	Stomach	Duodenum	Jejunum/ileum	Colon	Rectum	Other
Gross, 1952	Children's, Boston	68 (67)	1	13	3	2	4	32	10	3	0
Basu, 1960	A. H. Children's, Liverpool	33 (28)	0	7	0	1	3	16	4	2	0
Grosfeld, 1970	Children's, Columbus	23 (23)	0	4	2	1	0	9	7	0	0
Favara, 1971	Children's, Denver	39 (37)	1	6	0	3	4	20	4	0	1
Bower, 1977	Children's, Pittsburgh	78 (64)	0	15	1	6	6	34	12	2	2
Hocking, 1981	RHSC, Glasgow	60 (53)	-	8	2	8	1	32	4	5	0
Ildstad, 1988	Children's, Cincinnati	20 (17)	0	6	0	1	0	5	8	0	0
Bissler, 1988	Children's, Akron	11 (11)	0	1	0	1	2	4	2	1	0
Holcomb,1989	Children's, Philadelphia	101 (96)	0	21	3	8	2	47	15	5	0
Pinter, 1992	Hungary	30 (28)	-	6	2	4	3	9	3	3	0
Bajpai, 1994	IIMS, New Delhi, India	15 (14)	0	8	1	0	1	1	3	1	0
Stringer, 1995	Hosp Sick Child, London	77 (72)	2	15	6	10	3	21	10	6	4
Iyer, 1995	Children's, Los Angeles	29 (27)	2	0	0	3	1	9	8	6	0
Yang, 1996	NTUH, Taipei, China	20 (17)	0	2	0	1	0	14	3	0	0
Karnak, 2000	Ankara, Turkey	42 (38)	1	7	2	1	3	17	9	2	0
Puligandla, 2003	Montreal Children's	73 (73)	-	-	0	6	7	51	5	4	0
Totals		**719 (665)**	**7 (1%)**	**119 (17%)**	**22 (3%)**	**56 (8%)**	**40 (6%)**	**321 (45%)**	**107 (15%)**	**34 (6%)**	**7 (1%)**

TABLE 39-2

ECTOPIC GASTRIC MUCOSA BY LOCATION

Authors	Esophageal	Small Bowel	Colorectal
Gross, 1952	7/16	8/36	0/10
Favara, 1971	3/6	6/24	0/4
Bower, 1977	7/16	5/40	0/14
Hocking, 1981	5/10	21/33	2/9
Ildstad, 1988	2/6	5/13	0/8
Holcomb, 1989	8/24	12/49	1/20
Bajpai, 1994	9/9	2/2	1/4
Stringer, 1995	9/21	7/24	0/16
Puligandla, 2003	-	30/58	3/9
	50/108 (46%)	**96/279 (34%)**	**7/94 (7%)**

of intraluminal debris[23] (Fig. 39-3). With the increased use of prenatal US, a greater number of alimentary tract duplications are being discovered in utero.[24] Because a high percentage of duplications contain ectopic gastric mucosa, technetium-99 scintigraphy may be helpful in the diagnostic evaluation.[25,26] A CT-myelogram or magnetic resonance imaging (MRI) study can delineate a neuroenteric communication between the spinal column and an alimentary tract duplication.[27–29]

Classification and Treatment by Location

The variety of presentations and surgical management of duplications are better understood if these anomalies are categorized based on their location along the alimentary tract. A compilation of the major case series of alimentary tract duplications published in the past 50 years is seen in Table 39-1. In total, 719 duplications in 665 children

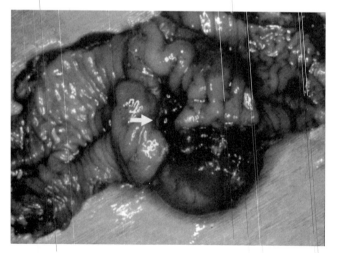

FIGURE 39-2. Most intestinal bleeding from duplications is caused by tubular duplications with communication to the intestine. However, in this photograph, the bleeding was due to mucosal ulceration (*solid arrow*) secondary to an adjacent cystic duplication. (From Holcomb GW III, Gheissari A, O'Neill JA, et al: Surgical management of alimentary tract duplications. Ann Surg 209:167–174, 1989.)

collected from 16 institutional reports show the location and relative frequency of alimentary tract duplications.[4,6,7,13,17,27,30–39] Approximately 8% of patients had a duplication at more than one site.

Oropharyngeal Duplications

Oropharyngeal duplications are rare, encompassing less than 1% of all alimentary tract duplications. They are usually asymptomatic cysts found in the floor of the oral cavity in infants. These oral duplication cysts frequently contain ectopic gastric or colonic mucosa. When present, an oral duplication can be approached through the mouth, and the oral mucosa reapproximated after resection of the cyst.[40]

Esophageal Duplications

One fifth of all alimentary tract duplications originate from the esophagus. Duplications may occur along the length of the esophagus. Although esophageal duplications have been reported in the cervical region, the vast majority are located on the right side adjacent to the thoracic esophagus. Although they may be asymptomatic, esophageal duplications in infants usually are first seen with dyspnea or chronic stridor secondary to tracheal compression. Obstructing cervical esophageal duplications may require tracheostomy before definitive resection.[13] With esophageal deviation and compression, patients also may have dysphagia, more common in older children. Most esophageal duplications are cystic and do not share a common muscular wall with the native esophagus, nor do they have a communication with the esophageal lumen. Approximately one half of esophageal duplications contain ectopic gastric mucosa. Compared with other alimentary tract duplications, esophageal duplications more frequently contain gastric mucosa (see Table 39-2). Therefore patients with esophageal duplications have a propensity to have occult anemia or even hematemesis.

Esophageal duplications will often be demonstrated as a soft tissue mass in the posterior mediastinum on plain chest radiograph and as an extrinsic compressive mass on an esophagram. Because some of the mediastinal duplications may extend below the diaphragm, further characterization of the mass by chest and abdominal CT scan or MRI is indicated (Fig. 39-4). Abdominal US may be useful as a screening tool to assess intra-abdominal extension of the duplication or the presence of an additional abdominal duplication. Neuroenteric communication to the spine or extension of the duplication into the abdominal cavity (i.e., thoracoabdominal duplication) will alter the surgical management, as a more extensive dissection will be necessary. Vertebral and spinal cord anomalies have been found in up to 20% of esophageal duplications and may necessitate multidisciplinary involvement.[6] Otherwise, treatment is excision of the duplication when found. Most often, this is accomplished through a right thoracotomy. However, because of the benign nature of the duplication and the increasing experience with video-assisted thoracoscopic surgery, thoracoscopic resection is

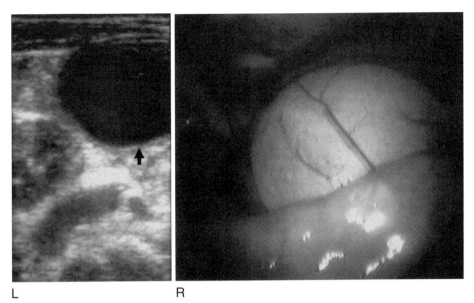

FIGURE 39-3. Ultrasound is a frequent imaging modality for diagnosing abdominal duplications. *Left,* A sonogram showing a cystic mass (*arrow*) in an infant with symptoms of intestinal obstruction. *Right,* A laparoscopic view of this same patient showing a cystic duplication of the ileum.

becoming the preferred approach for uncomplicated esophageal duplications in many institutions.[41,42]

Thoracoabdominal Duplications

Infrequently, esophageal duplications may extend into the abdominal cavity through the diaphragmatic hiatus. These are uncommon (3% of all duplications) and are known as thoracoabdominal duplications. They may extend a variable distance distally along the gastrointestinal tract, most commonly to the jejunum.[6,7] As with isolated esophageal duplications, thoracoabdominal duplications may be asymptomatic. Likewise, symptomatic thoracoabdominal duplications usually are seen with dyspnea or dysphagia. An even higher association with vertebral

anomalies may occur in thoracoabdominal compared with isolated esophageal duplications (Fig. 39-5).[6] Therefore it is important to exclude neuroenteric communication. CT scan and MRI are the imaging modalities of choice for this purpose. The current treatment is a one-stage combined thoracoabdominal approach for resection.

Gastric Duplications

Gastric duplications encompass approximately 8% of all alimentary tract duplications and usually become symptomatic in early childhood. Unlike other alimentary tract duplications, duplications of the stomach occur more commonly in girls than in boys.[11] Symptomatic gastric

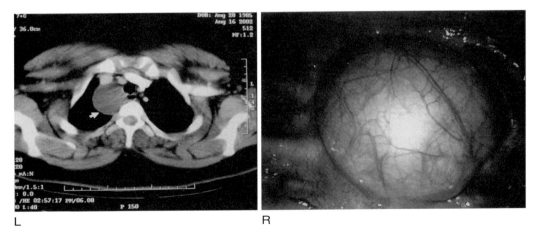

FIGURE 39-4. This 16-year-old was found to have a posterior mediastinal mass on a chest radiograph. *Left,* a computed tomography scan showed the duplication (*arrow*) to be adjacent to the trachea and the esophagus. *Right,* A view of the duplication as seen at thoracoscopy.

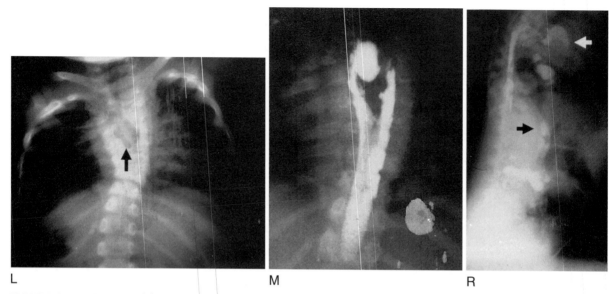

L   M   R

FIGURE 39-5. A 3-year-old was found to have a right paravertebral mass. *Left,* A large anterior defect in the vertebral bodies of the upper thoracic spine (*arrow*). *Middle,* A myelogram that shows the filling defect caused by a neuroenteric cyst. *Right,* The contrast from the myelogram is seen in the neuroenteric cyst (*upper arrow*) with extension subdiaphragmatically (*lower arrow*) into the distal small intestine. (From Holcomb GW III, Gheissari A, O'Neill JA, et al: Surgical management of alimentary tract duplications. Ann Surg 209:167–174, 1989.)

duplications may initially be seen with nonbilious emesis, hematemesis, or vague abdominal pain. On physical examination, a tender, epigastric mass may be appreciated. Gastric duplications are usually cystic and occur mostly along the greater curvature of the stomach (Fig. 39-6). Infrequently, they may be along the lesser curvature or in association with the pylorus. When intraluminal communication exists between the duplication and the native stomach, peptic ulceration with hemorrhage and perforation may occur.

The diagnostic evaluation usually proceeds along the direction of the presenting symptoms. However, CT scan with oral contrast or abdominal US may be the most sensitive means for evaluating these lesions. Gastric duplications may be confused with pancreatic pseudocysts on imaging studies, and caution is warranted as treatment differs. Asymptomatic gastric duplications should be excised to prevent gastrointestinal bleeding. Usually, complete excision can be accomplished without entering the gastric lumen. However, limited partial gastrectomy may be required for large or complex lesions. Carcinoma has been reported in an adult with a gastric duplication.[22]

Duodenal Duplications

Analogous to gastric duplications, duodenal duplications are uncommon and are seen in a similar fashion during early childhood. Emesis due to partial obstruction or gastrointestinal bleeding from ulceration due to ectopic gastric mucosa may be the presenting features. As most duodenal duplications are cystic and are located on the mesenteric side of the first or second portion of the duodenum, bilious emesis, jaundice, and the development of

pancreatitis are possible.[13] Thus the diagnosis may be easily confused with a choledochal cyst.

Abdominal CT scan and US are the preferred imaging studies for duodenal duplications. Particularly on US, motility of the cyst wall in question may assist in the diagnosis. The treatment of duodenal duplications is complicated by their tenuous location. If possible, simple excision is preferred as long as the blood supply to the native duodenum can be preserved. If no ectopic gastric mucosa is identified on frozen section, the preferred operation may be a roux-en Y cystjejunostomy to protect the vasculature of the duodenum and biliary system.[43] If the duplication is large and contains gastric mucosa, duodenal resection may be necessary to eliminate effectively the potential of future gastrointestinal hemorrhage in some cases.

Small Bowel Duplications

Small bowel duplications account for almost one half of all duplications. They can be tubular or cystic, with the majority being cystic (see Fig. 39-3). Tubular duplications can vary in length from a few centimeters to the entire length of bowel (Fig. 39-7). Duplications may be separate, attached with a separate muscular wall, or share a wall with the native intestine. They are found on the mesenteric side of the bowel and share a common blood supply. The most common site is in the distal ileum.

Small bowel duplications are frequently discovered in early childhood secondary to emesis, melena, hematochezia, or the presence of an abdominal mass and tenderness. They can lead to intestinal obstruction secondary to volvulus, can create a lead point for intussusception, or can cause

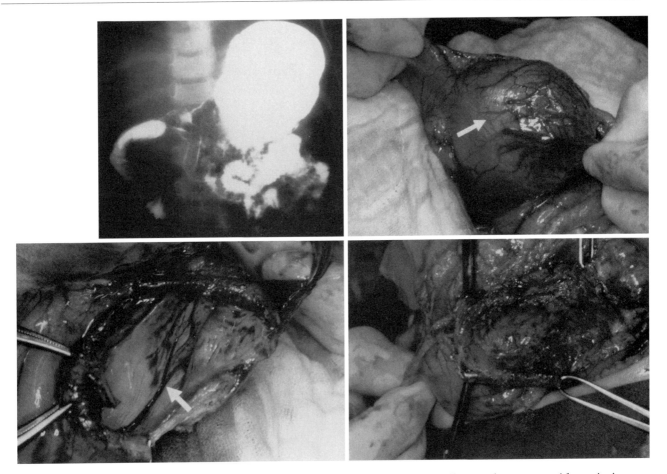

FIGURE 39-6. This patient had nonbilious emesis and was found to have a mass effect on the antrum with extrinsic compression of the second portion of the duodenum on a contrast study (*top left*). *Upper right,* A gastric duplication was found emanating from the inferior aspect of the greater curvature (*arrow*) of the gastric antrum at operation. It was thought best to marsupialize the duplication, as a significant partial gastrectomy would be required to remove this lesion completely. *Lower left,* The duplication has been marsupialized, and the mucosa of the duplication lying on the common wall with the stomach is seen (*arrow*). *Lower right,* The mucosa has been stripped, leaving intact the common wall between the duplication and the gastric antrum. (From Holcomb GW III, Gheissari A, O'Neill JA, et al: Surgical management of alimentary tract duplications. Ann Surg 209:167–174, 1989.)

peritonitis secondary to perforation. US is the usual imaging study for evaluating these lesions. Ectopic gastric mucosa is present in 80% of the tubular but in only 20% of the cystic small bowel duplications.[39] The ectopic gastric mucosa may be the source of peptic ulceration leading to hemorrhage, causing the duplication to be mistaken for a bleeding Meckel's diverticulum on a technetium scan. Contrast small bowel follow-through studies and CT scans are probably less helpful in distinguishing the etiology of an abdominal mass. The use of laparoscopy for diagnostic purposes as well as possible limited resection has been recently advocated[39,44] (see Fig. 39-3). This approach may be preferable to open exploration for uncertain diagnoses that may be amenable to more conservative measures or for laparoscopic resection.

The surgical management of small bowel duplications varies depending on the location and nature of the lesion. Segmental small bowel resection and primary reanastomosis of native bowel is the usual surgical approach. Infrequently, a cystic duplication can be enucleated without sacrificing the enteric blood supply. Management of long tubular duplications is more complicated, as the blood supply is intimately associated with that of the native bowel. Therefore preservation of bowel length may be compromised with resection of long tubular duplications. As a novel approach to prevent the risk of peptic ulceration, a technique has been described in which the mucosa of the duplication is stripped in stepwise fashion by using multiple duplication enterotomies to excise the ectopic gastric mucosa.[45] With this technique, the muscular layers of the duplication are left in situ, which should not lead to further complications. Another novel approach is to anastomose the tubular small bowel duplication containing gastric mucosa to the stomach, which will allow drainage of the acid produced by the duplication into the stomach and yet preserve native bowel length.[46]

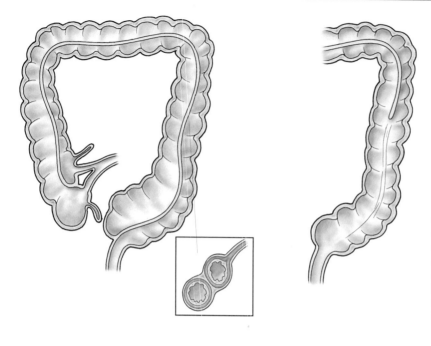

FIGURE 39-7. Ileal and colonic tubular duplications vary in length and complexity. *Left,* The terminal ileum is seen to bifurcate into native colon and duplicated colon, which is medial to the native colon. The duplicated colon ends blindly in the upper rectum. *Right,* The duplicated colon communicates with the native colon and forms a common descending colon.

Colonic Duplications

Colonic duplications account for approximately 15% of all duplications. Most occur in the cecum and are cystic in shape. However, some are tubular and vary in length and complexity. Unlike many other types of duplications, colonic duplications rarely contain ectopic gastric mucosa, and patients less frequently are initially seen with symptoms of bleeding. Colonic duplications are usually found on the antimesenteric aspect of the bowel. Patients with colonic duplications are prone to develop a large bowel obstruction secondary to compression, volvulus, or intussusception. A higher than usual number of associated anomalies occur in children with tubular colonic duplications. Complete colorectal duplication may be associated with doubling anomalies of other pelvic organs (e.g., bladder, uterus, vagina, and anus), which gave rise to the partial twinning theory of embryogenesis for duplications.[47]

Tubular colonic duplications are seen in such a variety of ways, that it has been stated that no two are similar.[48] Compared with cystic duplications, tubular colonic duplications often have one or more communications with the native bowel lumen. To categorize the assortment of anatomic variations, a classification system of colonic duplications has been suggested.[49] Colonic duplications were placed into one of two general classes. Type I duplications were those limited to the alimentary tract, whereas type II were those duplications associated with genital or urinary tract duplications.

Imaging studies can be helpful in establishing the diagnosis in the presence of nonemergency symptoms. Unfortunately, plain radiographs will demonstrate only nonspecific findings such as partial intestinal obstruction. However, the abnormal radiographs usually lead to further diagnostic evaluation with contrast studies, US, or CT scans based on symptoms. A contrast enema may be useful in demonstrating a duplication and its communication to the native bowel, if present, whereas CT scans and US are more sensitive but less specific in establishing the diagnosis. However, colonic duplications are sometimes discovered at surgical exploration regardless of prior imaging studies.

The treatment of colonic duplications is individualized according to the symptoms and location of the lesion. Cystic colonic duplications occasionally can be enucleated from the colon but more commonly require resection and anastomosis. The surgical approach to tubular duplications is more complex. For symptomatic duplications, surgical resection is the goal when feasible. However, the majority of long and complex colonic duplications are not entirely resectable, as lengthy resection of the native colon would be required. Therefore it is acceptable to resort to conservative management with stool softeners in asymptomatic cases in which a distal communication to the native colon or rectum is demonstrated. Although rare, carcinoma has been reported in adults with undiagnosed cystic and tubular duplications.[22,50,51] However, none has been reported when the duplication has a distal communication to the native bowel. Unlike small bowel duplications, in which a risk of peptic ulceration exists from ectopic gastric mucosa, it is not often necessary to excise the mucosa of a colonic duplication. If a distal communication between the duplication and colon or rectum is not present, one can be created with either an end-to-side or side-to-side anastomosis to the colon or rectum to relieve the obstruction. A fistulous tract to the uterus or bladder should be resected.

Rectal Duplications

Rectal duplications account for approximately 6% of all duplications and are commonly found in the presacral

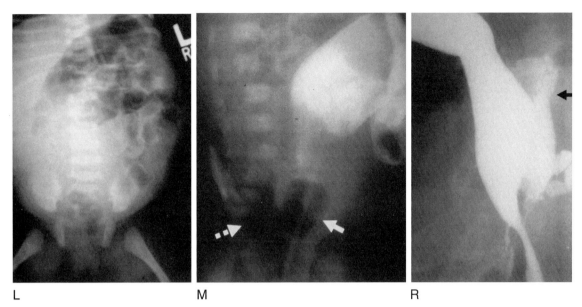

L   M   R

FIGURE 39-8. This newborn had abdominal distention and evidence of a pelvic mass (*left*). On rectal examination, a mass was palpable posterior to the rectum. *Middle,* A contrast study in which an 8 Foley catheter was introduced into the rectum, and the balloon was inflated with air (*solid arrow*). Posterior to the rectum and compressing it is a rectal duplication with air (*dotted arrow*), indicating communication to the gastrointestinal tract. A colostomy was initially performed because of the rectal obstruction. *Right,* A barium enema performed at age 6 months in this patient. On this lateral radiograph, filling of the posterior rectal mass is seen (*arrow*). (From Holcomb GW III, Gheissari A, O'Neill JA, et al: Surgical management of alimentary tract duplications. Ann Surg 209:167–174, 1989.)

region, posterior to the native rectum (Fig. 39-8). A fistulous communication to the perineum may lead to the development of a perirectal abscess. As a consequence of the posterior rectal obstruction, chronic constipation also is a prominent symptom of rectal duplications. As expected, a posterior rectal mass may be appreciated on digital rectal examination. The differential diagnosis of a presacral mass would include a rectal duplication, teratoma, and anterior meningocele. Treatment options for rectal duplications include marsupialization through a transanal approach, division of the septum between the duplication and rectum, or complete excision of the noncommunicating duplication through a posterior sagittal approach. An initial colostomy may be necessary as well.

REFERENCES

1. Calder JL: Two examples of children born with preternatural conformation of the guts. Med Essays Obers 1:203–206, 1733.
2. Fitz RH: Persistent omphalo-mesenteric remains: Their importance in the causation of intestinal duplication, cyst formation, and obstruction. Am J Med Sci 88:30–57, 1884.
3. Ladd WE: Duplications of the alimentary tract. South Med J 30: 363–371, 1937.
4. Gross RE, Holcomb GW, Farber S: Duplications of the alimentary tract. Pediatrics 9:449–467, 1952.
5. Schalamon J, Schleef J, Hollworth ME: Experience with gastrointestinal duplications in childhood. Langenbeck's Arch Surg 385:402–405, 2000.
6. Stringer MD, Spitz L, Abel R, et al: Management of alimentary tract duplication in children. Br J Surg 82:74–78, 1995.
7. Holcomb GW III, Gheissari A, O'Neill JA, et al: Surgical management of alimentary tract duplications. Ann Surg 209:167–174, 1989.
8. Lewis FT, Thyng FW. Regular occurrence of intestinal diverticula in embryos of pig, rabbit, and man. Am J Anat 7:505–519, 1908.
9. Bremer JL: Diverticula and duplications of the intestinal tract. Arch Pathol 38:132–140, 1944.
10. Smith ED: Duplication of the anus and genitourinary tract. Surgery 66:909–921, 1969.
11. Lewis PL, Holder T, Feldman M: Duplication of the stomach: Report of a case and review of the English literature. Arch Surg 82:634–640, 1961.
12. Mellish RWP, Koop CE: Clinical manifestations of duplication of the bowel. Pediatrics 27:397–407, 1961.
13. Favara BE, Franciosi RA, Akers DR: Enteric duplications: Thirty-seven cases: A vascular theory of pathogenesis. Am J Dis Child 122:501–506, 1971.
14. Bentley JFR, Smith JR: Developmental posterior enteric remnants and spinal malformations: The split notochord syndrome. Arch Dis Child 35:76–86, 1960.
15. Qi BQ, Beasley SW, Williams AK: Evidence of a common pathogenesis for foregut duplications and esophageal atresia with tracheo-esophageal fistula. Anat Rec 264:93–100, 2001.
16. Qi BQ, Beasley SW, Frizelle FA: Evidence that the notochord may be pivotal in the development of sacral and anorectal malformations. J Pediatr Surg 38:1310–1316, 2003.
17. Grosfeld JL, O'Neill JA, Clatworthy HW: Enteric duplications in infancy and childhood: An 18 year review. Ann Surg 172:83–90, 1970.
18. Wieczorek RL, Seidman I, Ranson JH, et al: Congenital duplications of the stomach: Case report and review of the English literature. Am J Gastroenterol 79:597–602, 1984.
19. Martinez-Ferro M, Milner R, Voto L, et al: Intrathoracic alimentary tract duplication cysts treated in utero by thoracoamniotic shunting. Fetal Diagn Ther 13:343–347, 1998.
20. Mair WS, Abbott CR: Perforation of ileal duplication in old age. Br Med J 11:621, 1976.
21. Qazi FM, Geisinger KR, Nelson JB, et al: Symptomatic congenital gastroenteric duplication cyst of the esophagus containing exocrine and endocrine pancreatic tissues. Am J Gastroenterol 85:65–67, 1990.

22. Orr MM, Edwards AJ: Neoplastic change in duplications of the alimentary tract. Br J Surg 62:269, 1975.

23. Kangerloo H, Sample F, Hansen G, et al: Ultrasonic evaluation of abdominal gastrointestinal tract duplication in children. Radiology 131:191–194, 1979.

24. Markert DJ, Grumbach K, Haney PJ: Thoracoabdominal duplication cyst: Prenatal and postnatal imaging. J Ultrasound Med 15: 333–336, 1996.

25. Lecouffe P, Spyckerelle C, Venel H, et al: Use of pertechnetate 99m Tc abdominal scanning in localizing an ileal duplication cyst: Case report and review of the literature. Eur J Nucl Med 19:65–67, 1992.

26. Macpherson RI: Gastrointestinal tract duplications: Clinical, pathologic, etiologic, and radiologic considerations. Radiographics 13:1063–1080, 1993.

27. Bajpai M, Mathur M: Duplications of the alimentary tract: clues to the missing links. J Pediatr Surg 29:1361–1365, 1994.

28. Azzies G, Beasley S: Diagnosis and treatment of foregut duplications. Semin Pediatr Surg 38:768–770, 2003.

29. Haddon MJ, Bowen A: Bronchopulmonary and neuroenteric forms of foregut anomalies: Imaging for diagnosis and management. Radiol Clin North Am 29:241–254, 1991.

30. Basu R, Forshall I, Rickham PP: Duplications of the alimentary tract. Br J Surg 47:477, 1960.

31. Bower RJ, Sieber WK, Kiesewetter WB: Alimentary tract duplications in children. Ann Surg 188:669–674, 1977.

32. Hocking M, Young DG: Duplications of the alimentary tract. Br J Surg 68:92–96, 1981.

33. Ildstad ST, Tollerud DJ, Weiss RG, et al: Duplications of the alimentary tract. Ann Surg 208:184–189, 1988.

34. Bissler JJ, Klein RL: Alimentary tract duplications in children: Case and literature review. Clin Pediatr 27:152–157, 1988.

35. Pinter AB, Schubert W, Szemledy F, et al: Alimentary tract duplications in infants and children. Eur J Pediatr Surg 2:8–12, 1992.

36. Iyer CP, Mahour GH: Duplications of the alimentary tract in infants and children. J Pediatr Surg 30:1267–1270, 1995.

37. Yang MC, Duh YC, Lai HC, et al: Alimentary tract duplications. J Formos Med Assoc 95:406–409, 1996.

38. Karnak I, Ocal T, Senocak ME, et al: Alimentary tract duplications in children: Report of 26 years experience. Turk J Pediatr 42: 118–125, 2000.

39. Puligandla PS, Nguyen LT, St-Vil D, et al: Gastrointestinal duplications. J Pediatr Surg 38:740–744, 2003.

40. Chen MK, Gross E, Lobe TE: Perinatal management of enteric duplication cysts of the tongue. Am J Perinatol 14:161–163, 1997.

41. Merry C, Spurbeck W, Lobe TE: Resection of foregut-derived duplications by minimal-access surgery. J Pediatr Surg Int 15: 224–226, 1999.

42. Michel JL, Revillon Y, Montupet P, et al: Thoracoscopic treatment of mediastinal cysts in children. J Pediatr Surg 33:1745–1748, 1998.

43. Leenders EL, Osman MZ, Sukarochana K: Treatment of duodenal duplication with international review. Am Surg 36:368, 1970.

44. Danzer E, Schier F, Gorsler C: Laparoscopic management of ovarian cysts in infants, children, and adolescents. Pediatr Endosurg Innov Technol 5:349–353, 2001.

45. Wrenn EL Jr: Tubular duplication of the small intestine. Surgery 52:494–498, 1962.

46. Jewett TC Jr, Walker AB, Cooney DR: A long term follow-up on a duplication of the entire small intestine treated by gastroduplication. J Pediatr Surg 18:185–188, 1983.

47. Smith ED, Stephens FD: Duplication and vesicointestinal fissure. Birth Defects Orig Artic Ser 24:551, 1988.

48. Yousefzadeh DK: Tubular colonic duplication: Review of 1876-1981 literature. Pediatr Radiol 13:65, 1983.

49. Kottra JJ, Dodds WJ: Duplication of the large bowel. Am J Roentgenol 113:310, 1971.

50. Crowley LV, Page HG: Adenocarcinoma arising in presacral enterogenous cyst. Arch Pathol 69:64, 1960.

51. Tammery HJ, Testra RE: Carcinoma arising in a duplicated colon. Cancer 20:478, 1967.

CHAPTER 40

Meckel's Diverticulum

Kurt P. Schropp, MD

The most common congenital malformation of the small intestine, a diverticulum named after the German anatomist Johann Meckel, is a vitelline duct anomaly. In utero, the vitelline (omphalomesenteric) duct forms the connection between the fetal gut and yolk sac. The duct usually involutes during the fifth to sixth week of gestation. When the portion of the vitelline duct that is on the antimesenteric border of the ileum fails to regress, it forms a true diverticulum. Its persistence may be present in a number of anatomic variations and may be asymptomatic or the cause of a number of complications.

Although this malformation has been known for many years, recently some significant improvements have occurred in the diagnosis and treatment of Meckel's diverticulum (MD). Still, controversies remain, such as the best method of diagnosing a bleeding diverticulum and the proper treatment of an incidentally discovered, asymptomatic malformation.

INCIDENCE

Because the majority of patients that have an MD are asymptomatic, its true incidence is unknown. Most studies quote the incidence to be around 2% of the general population, with an increased percentage in patients with certain congenital anomalies of the umbilicus (patent omphalomesenteric duct, omphalocele), alimentary tract, central nervous system, and the cardiovascular system.[1] Overall, about 4% of patients with an MD become symptomatic, meaning that about 8/10000 people will manifest complications.[2] The male-to-female complication rate ratio is about 3:1, and 50% to 60% of all cases of symptomatic MD are discovered in the first 2 years of life.[3] Only about 15% of children first seen with a symptomatic MD are older than 4 years.[4]

Heterotopic tissue is the cause of most of the complications, consisting mostly of gastric tissue but less commonly of pancreatic, jejunal, or colonic tissue.[3] Symptomatic MDs have a 10-fold increased incidence of heterotopic tissue, but it is estimated that only 50% to 60% of patients with ectopic tissue become symptomatic.[5]

PATHOPHYSIOLOGY

A wide spectrum of omphalomesenteric abnormalities may be present, depending on the degree of involution of the vitelline duct[6] (Fig. 40-1). The classic description is that the MD is about 2 feet from the ileocecal valve, 2 cm in diameter, 2 inches in length, and is not attached to the abdominal wall. As previously stated, most of the complications with this abnormality are related to ectopic tissue, usually gastric mucosa, causing a bleeding ulcer. Occasionally, gastric or pancreatic tissue can act as a lead point for an intussusception, resulting in a bowel obstruction. Intestinal obstruction also may be caused by an MD that is attached to the umbilicus by a fibrous cord. This may lead to a volvulus around the cord and may be difficult to diagnose because the patient usually will not have undergone any previous abdominal operations, and adhesive bowel obstruction is not high on the differential diagnosis. Similarly, a persistent vitelline artery, which is an end artery from the superior mesenteric artery, may cause obstruction and/or volvulus. Often this will cause a fibrous band from the base of the mesentery across the ileum and onto the diverticulum.

Because of the association of *Helicobacter pylori* and gastroduodenal ulceration, it had been suggested that the gastritis and ulceration/bleeding of MDs may be due to colonization with *H. pylori*. Eradicating the *H. pylori* potentially would decrease the bleeding associated with ectopic gastric tissue. Recently, though, studies have shown a very low colonization rate with *H. pylori* in children with MD.[7,8]

Besides anatomic considerations and ectopic gastric mucosa, other tissues may lead to pathologic findings with MD. In a recent report in an asymptomatic MD in a patient with Beckwith-Wiedemann syndrome, nesidioblastosis was found in ectopic pancreatic tissue.[9]

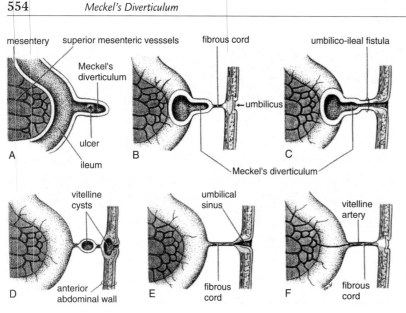

FIGURE 40-1. Drawing illustrating Meckel's diverticuli and other remnants of the yolk sac. (From Moore KL: The Developing Human. Philadelphia, WB Saunders, 1988.)

Moreover, being composed mostly of small bowel mucosa, the MD also may contain a wide variety of tumors such as carcinoid, leiomyoma, angioma, and neurofibroma, which are often found incidentally, but may be the cause of serious complications.

CLINICAL PRESENTATION

The clinical presentation in symptomatic patients with MD is quite varied and dependent on the configuration of the MD and whether it has ectopic tissue. The three main forms of presentation are hemorrhage, 40% to 60%; obstruction, 25%; and diverticulitis, 10% to 20%.[3] The classic presentation of a child with a bleeding MD is a preschool patient with painless rectal bleeding. This may consist of dark, tarry stools in small amounts or red, gross blood if bleeding is heavy. The hemorrhage is episodic and usually ceases without treatment. Rarely will a child need immediate operation to control the bleeding. Sometimes the hemorrhage is insidious and not appreciated by the family. A young child with hemoglobin-positive stools and a chronic iron deficiency anemia must be investigated for a bleeding MD. The hemorrhage is often at the junction of the gastric and ileal mucosa, but can be on the mesenteric border of the ileum, away from the MD, especially with short, wide-based diverticulae.

Patients seen with obstruction secondary to an intussusception usually have classic signs and symptoms of an idiopathic intussusception, including crampy abdominal pain, progressing to bilious vomiting and obstipation. They will often have currant-jelly stools. Patients with artery/band obstruction also demonstrate bilious vomiting and abdominal distention, but be in extremis if volvulus and ischemia develop. As mentioned earlier, the intussusception or obstruction is often diagnosed preoperatively, but MD as the cause often is not.

Patients with diverticulitis often have symptoms that resemble appendicitis. Periumbilical pain is usually the first presenting symptom. They usually do not have the same amount and intensity of nausea and vomiting as do children with appendicitis. Moreover, their point of maximal tenderness may migrate across the abdomen as the child moves. Many of these children have been previously hospitalized with similar symptoms but did not undergo exploration because the diagnosis of diverticulitis was not entertained. About the same percentage of patients with diverticulitis will appear with perforation, as do those with appendicitis.

Finally, MD may be seen in a number of less common, unusual manners. A Littre's hernia is an inguinal hernia with an incarcerated MD. It also can be incarcerated in a spigelian hernia,[10] be a cause of intra-abdominal hemorrhage,[11] or be a cystic mass.[12] It has been diagnosed in a child age 4 hours.[13] It is extremely rare to have MD diagnosed by prenatal ultrasound.

DIAGNOSIS

The diagnosis of a symptomatic MD is dependent on the anatomic configuration of the MD and its presentation, signs, and symptoms. Routine history and physical examination are probably the most important diagnostic methods. For example, patients with lower gastrointestinal bleeding need a complete description of the quality and frequency of the bloody stools. A nasogastric tube should be placed to help exclude gastric bleeding as the cause. Rectal examination, and occasionally lower endoscopy, is useful in identifying other causes of lower gastrointestinal bleeding, such as polyps and rectal tears. Radiologic examination also may be helpful in diagnosing the complications of MD, such as obstruction caused by an MD that has formed an intussusception, or intestinal inflammation caused by Meckel's diverticulitis. Of the three most common presentations, though, a hemorrhaging diverticulum is probably most often diagnosed preoperatively by radiographic procedures.

Technetium-99m pertechnetate scintigraphy abdominal scanning has become commonly used to help detect ectopic gastric tissue in an MD. Unfortunately, ectopic gastric mucosa also may be found in intestinal duplications and in the small bowel separate from an MD. Technetium-99m pertechnetate is secreted by the tubular gland cells of gastric mucosa. Therefore any MD with ectopic gastric mucosa potentially may be diagnosed with scintigraphy. Unlike many other invasive and noninvasive tests for bleeding, an active hemorrhage is not a prerequisite for a positive diagnosis.

The study itself is fairly easily performed. If possible, the child should fast for 3 to 4 hours before the scan. Optimally, no barium studies should be performed in the preceding 24 hours, nor should enemas or laxatives be given. After the injection of the Tc-99m, the only focal accumulation of tracer should be in the urinary tract or the stomach. A positive study is characterized by a focal tracer uptake that appears simultaneous with the stomach and increases in intensity over time[14] (Fig. 40-2). A number of causes of false-positive results may be found, including intussusception, inflammation of the bowel, intestinal duplication, an abnormal urinary collecting system, a hemangioma, or an arteriovenous malformation. False-negative scans are probably even more problematic. They may result from having only a small amount of gastric mucosa, residual barium from a previous study, or an MD that is low in the pelvis and obscured by the bladder.

Controversy exists as to the utility of pharmacologic enhancement of the uptake of the isotope to increase the accuracy of scintigraphy. The most commonly used medications for this purpose are pentagastrin and H$_2$ blockers. Pentagastrin enhancement works by stimulating acid production by parietal cells. H$_2$-blocker enhancement works by decreasing the washout of pertechnetate from the gastric glands, enhancing the visualization of the scan. Because no conclusive evidence exists that pharmacologic enhancement clearly increases accuracy, many use the drugs only when a study is inconclusive (not clearly positive or negative).

Even though the presence of ectopic gastric mucosa in a patient with a bleeding MD approaches 100%, the accuracy of Tc-99m scanning does not. The specificity of scintigraphy is probably adequate at 95% or higher, but the sensitivity is significantly worse at around 60%. Therefore a negative scan result does not necessarily exclude a bleeding MD. A number of authors advocate laparotomy, or more recently, laparoscopy, to exclude MD as the cause of bleeding[15] with a negative scintigram but a high clinical suspicion of a bleeding MD. Some authors have touted the utility of angiography for bleeding MD if high suspicion exists of a bleeding MD in the presence of a negative scintigram.[16] One difficulty with angiography, besides being very invasive, is that the ulcer must be actively bleeding for the study to be diagnostic.

A new, noninvasive diagnostic technique that may aid in the diagnosis of a bleeding MD is wireless capsule endoscopy. With this study, the patient swallows a capsule, and numerous pictures of the intestine are taken. Occasionally, patients who have had many other diagnostic procedures will undergo a capsule endoscopy that is positive.[17]

The patient with a nonhemorrhaging MD will have a low incidence of heterotopic gastric mucosa. In this setting, scintigraphy will not be useful. Patients with obstruction secondary to an intussuscepted MD can often be diagnosed with air enema. On occasion, the air enema will reduce the ileocolic portion of the intussusception, and an unrecognized ileoileal component will remain. This component often will not be reducible with the enema, and if it does reduce, it will often recur. Ultrasonography remains fairly reliable in skilled hands to diagnose the intussusception. It also may demonstrate an inflamed MD (Fig. 40-3). Sometimes a combination of ultrasonography, computerized tomography, and contrast enema may aid in the diagnosis of complicated, scintigraphy-negative MD.[18]

TREATMENT

The treatment of symptomatic MD begins with adequate resuscitation. If the patient initially is seen with hemorrhage, adequate resuscitation to an appropriate

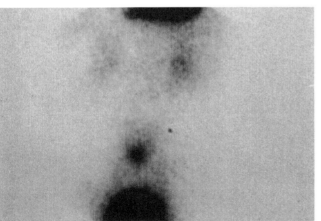

FIGURE 40-2. Technetium-99m pertechnetate scan of a patient with Meckel's diverticulum. Note the blush above the bladder. (Courtesy of Kyo Lee, MD)

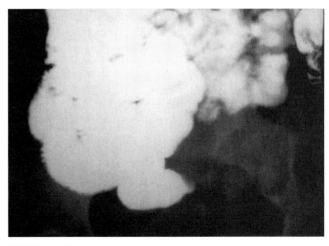

FIGURE 40-3. Contrast small bowel enema depicting a Meckel's diverticulum in the pelvis. Note the protrusion of gastric mucosa into the lumen. (Courtesy of Kyo Lee, MD)

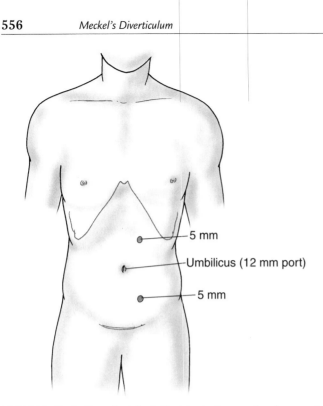

5 mm

Umbilicus (12 mm port)

5 mm

FIGURE 40-4. Drawing depicting typical cannula placement for an elective Meckel's diverticulectomy.

hemoglobin level should be accomplished before operation. In the last decade, laparoscopy has become the standard of care for elective diverticulectomy for bleeding MD. Multiple techniques have been described. A typical procedure may include the umbilical placement of a cannula large enough for introduction of the endoscopic stapler (12 mm) with two additional small cannulae for grasping instrumentation. Typical placement for these smaller cannulae will be in the left upper and left lower abdominal quadrants, similar to port placement for laparoscopic appendectomy (Fig. 40-4). Once the cecum is located, the ileocecal valve is identified and the small bowel can then be easily inspected in a retrograde fashion until the MD is located. Once it is found, the decision must be made whether it is safe merely to staple transversely across the base of the MD or to perform a partial ileal resection.

Most authors suggest that it is important to resect the ulcer, if present, caused by the gastric secretions. Because most narrow-based MDs have the gastric tissue at the tip, the ulcer is usually in the MD itself. A simple diverticulectomy by stapling transversely across the base would be appropriate in this setting. After removal from the abdomen in an endoscopic bag, the diverticulum should be opened to ensure that the ulcer is resected. Conversely, some believe that resection of the ulcer is not necessary as long as all the gastric mucosa has been removed. If the diverticulum is wide based, then an increased chance exists the ectopic mucosa could be anywhere in the diverticulum, and therefore an ileal resection should probably be performed. This can be accomplished intracorporeally by stapling across the ileum on either side of the diverticulum and then performing a stapled

intracorporeal anastomosis. Because this procedure is often needed in infants and small children, adequate working space for endoscopic stapling is limited. Thus many surgeons may feel more comfortable extending the umbilical incision to exteriorize the two ileal segments and perform an extracorporeal anastomosis. Whichever method is used to remove the diverticulum, an incidental appendectomy is appropriate if no compelling reasons are found for its being left in situ. The presence of scars on the abdomen will lead subsequent examiners to assume that the appendix has been removed.

Because the other presentations often are found unexpectedly at operation, the feasibility of resection is determined on a case-by-case basis. For example, if an intussuscepted MD can be reduced, it may or may not be wise to staple across the base of the MD, depending on the thickness of the base, the appearance of the intussusceptum itself, its ease of removal, and any damage that occurred because of the intussusception.

Postoperatively, if the procedure is performed laparoscopically with simple diverticulectomy, the child may be fed almost immediately. If an ileal resection is needed, it is best to wait until bowel function returns before feeding is resumed.

CONTROVERSIES

The major controversy is whether to resect an incidentally discovered MD at operation. In adults, some evidence exists that more morbidity occurs with resection than does risk that a complication will be found in the future from the diverticulum.[19] Others argue that, because it is difficult to predict who will become symptomatic and because of the low incidence of surgical morbidity, no contraindication to removal exists.[20] If palpable gastric mucosa is noted in the tip and simple excision is feasible, it seems reasonable that the MD should be removed. In young children, because of a life-long potential for complications and the low morbidity with resection, an incidentally encountered MD probably should be resected.

REFERENCES

1. Simms MH, Corkery JJ: Meckel's diverticulum: Its association with congenital malformation and the significance of atypical morphology. Br J Surg 67:216–219, 1980.
2. Soltero MJ, Bill AH: The natural history of Meckel's diverticulum and its relation to incidental removal: A study of 202 cases of diseased Meckel's diverticulum found in King County, Washington, over a fifteen-year period. Am J Surg 132:168–173, 1976.
3. Kempe CH, Silver HK, O'Brien D, et al: Current Pediatric Diagnosis and Treatment. Los Altos, Calif, Lange Medical Publications, 1980.
4. Vane DW, West KW, Grosfeld JL: Vitelline duct anomalies: Experience with 217 childhood cases. Arch Surg 122:542–547, 1987.
5. Kapischke M, Bley K, Delz E: Meckel's diverticulum: A disease associated with a colored clinical picture. Surg Endosc 17:U7–U14, Feb 2003.
6. Moore KL: The Developing Human. Philadelphia, WB Saunders, 1988.
7. Finn LS, Christie DL: *Helicobacter pylori* and Meckel's diverticula. J Pediatr Gastroenterol Nutr 32:150–155, 2001.

8. Ergun O, Celik A, Akarca US, et al: Does colonization of *elicobacter pylori* in the heterotopic gastric mucosa play a role in bleeding of Meckel's diverticulum? J Pediatr Surg 37:1540–1542, 2002.

9. Schier F, Sauerbrey A, Kosmehl H: A Meckel's diverticulum containing pancreatic tissue and nesidioblastosis in a patient with Beckwith-Wiedemann syndrome. Pediatr Surg Int 16:124–127, 2000.

10. Dixon E, Heine JA: Incarcerated Meckel's diverticulum in a spigelian hernia. Am J Surg 180:126, 2000.

11. Jelene F, Strlic M, Gvardijancic D: Meckel's diverticulum perforation with intraabdominal hemorrhage. J Pediatr Surg 37:E18, 2002.

12. Oguzkurt P, Arda S, Kayaselcuk F, et al: Cystic Meckel's diverticulum: A rare cause of cystic pelvic mass presenting with urinary symptoms. J Pediatr Surg 36:1855–1858, 2001.

13. Sy ED, Shan YS, Tsai HM, et al: Meckel's diverticulum associated with ileal volvulus in a neonate. Pediatr Surg Int 18:529–531, 2002.

14. Emamian SA, Shalaby-rana E, Majd M: The spectrum of heterotopic gastric mucosa in children detected by Tc-99m pertechnetate scintigraphy. Clin Nucl Med 26:529–535, 2001.

15. Swaniker F, Soldes O, Hirschl RB: The utility of technetium 99m pertechnetate scintigraphy in the evaluation of patients with Meckel's diverticulum. J Pediatr Surg 34:760–764, 1999.

16. Huang MC, Huang FC, Cheng YF, et al: The value of angiography in diagnosis of Meckel's diverticulum: Case report. Changgeng Yi Xue Za Zhi 23:716–719, 2000.

17. Mylonaki M, MacLean D, Fritscher-Ravens A, et al: Wireless capsule endoscopic detection of Meckel's diverticulum after nondiagnostic surgery. Endoscopy 34:1018–1020, 2002.

18. Daneman A, Lobo E, Alton DJ, et al: The value of sonography, CT and air enema for detection of complicated Meckel diverticulum in children with nonspecific clinical presentation. Pediatr Radiol 28:928–932, 1998.

19. Peoples JB, Lichtenberger EJ, Dunn MM: Incidental diverticulectomy in adults. Surgery 118:649–652, 1995.

20. Arnold JF, Pellicane JV: Meckel's diverticulum: A ten-year experience. Am Surg 63:354–355, 1997.

CHAPTER 41

Inflammatory Bowel Disease and Intestinal Cancer

Edmund Y. Yang, MD, PhD, Sidney Johnson, MD, and Moritz M. Ziegler, MD

The inflammatory bowel diseases (IBDs) represent a spectrum of disorders that are characterized principally by an immune response directed at the intestine. The two primary disorders are Crohn's disease (CD) and ulcerative colitis (UC). Although etiologic similarities may exist between these two disorders, clinical differences distinguish them from one another. CD usually is an insidious disease that causes full-thickness injury anywhere in the gastrointestinal tract. In contrast, UC often is initially more acute, with the disease limited to the colonic mucosa. UC begins in the rectum and extends proximally. About 15% of patients with IBD have a disorder that is difficult to diagnose as either CD or UC. These patients are classified as having indeterminate colitis.

ULCERATIVE COLITIS

Incidence and Etiology

Although several reports suggest that the incidence of IBD is increasing,[1] when examined separately, any increases have been limited to CD.[2,3] The overall incidence of UC (1.5 to 2.0 cases per 10^5 children) has not shown any recent, consistent increase. These trends point toward environmental factors as a primary influence in the etiology of IBD, especially for CD. A higher incidence of IBD is found in industrialized countries, and immigration to industrialized countries has been associated with an increasing incidence of disease.[4,5] The environmental exposure is thought to occur early in life.[6]

Genetic factors are clearly important as well. A family history of disease is a very strong risk factor for IBD, with an odds ratio of 5:6.[7] Genetic predisposition is seen clinically in the increased prevalence of IBD among descendents of Ashkenazi Jews in the United States.[4] Patients with the *HLA-DR2* allele are more likely to have UC.[8] Animal models of UC provide a unifying hypothesis for the clinical and epidemiologic findings. Knockout mice deficient in either interleukin (IL)-10[9] or IL-2[10] demonstrate forms of colitis that are dependent on environmental germ exposure. When these animals are raised in germ-free environments, colitis is absent or attenuated. Further studies are required to determine whether similar mechanisms exist in human UC.

Diagnosis of Ulcerative Colitis in Childhood

UC is usually diagnosed during the pediatric age period between 5 and 16 years.[11] About 80% to 90% of patients are 9 years or older when symptoms develop, and boys and girls are equally affected.[12] Generally, children do worse clinically than do adults. A greater likelihood of pan-colonic involvement (about 50%), a greater likelihood of proximal extension of initially localized disease, and a greater need for colectomy exist.[12,13] Early diagnosis in infancy does not necessarily portend a poor prognosis. Newer modes of medical management have decreased the rate of colectomy for UC. The rate of total colectomy for children was 49% during the period between 1955 and 1965, whereas it was 26% between 1965 and 1974.[14]

The diagnosis of IBD should be suspected in any child with unexplained gastrointestinal symptoms. UC is often difficult to diagnose because of the diverse array of symptoms with which children are first seen (Table 41-1) and the multitude of organ systems that can be affected (Table 41-2). Most patients have either abdominal pain or diarrhea, although in retrospect, extraintestinal symptoms are often present for months or years.[15] About 10% of patients have a fulminant form of colitis, manifested as severe abdominal pain, rectal bleeding, fever, hypoalbuminemia, and anemia. In these patients, abdominal radiographs may demonstrate signs of toxic megacolon. These patients require hospitalization, bowel rest, and an intense trial of medical therapy.

The investigation should address the presenting symptoms and exclude extraintestinal manifestations (see Table 41-2). Developmental, psychological, and nutritional status should be documented, and laboratory

TABLE 41-1

PRESENTING SYMPTOMS AT THE TIME OF DIAGNOSIS OF ULCERATIVE COLITIS

Presenting Symptom	UC Children Affected (%)
Abdominal pain	76
Rectal bleeding	41
Bloody diarrhea	38
Diarrhea	38
Vomiting	14
Weight loss	27
Anemia	5
Extraintestinal symptom	5

Data from 105 children with UC. From Barton JR, Ferguson A: Clinical features morbidity, and mortality of Scottish children with inflammatory bowel disease. Q J Med 75: 423–439, 1990.

studies may be helpful for determining whether coexisting primary sclerosing cholangitis or renal disease is present. Enteric infection should be excluded by analysis for *Clostridium difficile, Escherichia coli,* and stool for culture, ova and parasites, especially in those patients with fulminant colitis.

As opposed to CD, radiographic studies have a lesser role in diagnosing UC. Ultimately, the diagnosis rests on colonoscopic demonstration of friable, erythematous mucosa with ulceration and pseudopolyp formation that begins in the rectum and extends proximally in a continuous manner. Biopsies should be taken. Histopathologically, the diseased intestine demonstrates a spectrum of findings from chronic inflammation of the lamina propria and goblet cell dropout to mucosal ulceration with crypt abscesses.[16] In fulminant colitis, the lamina propria is thinned. Moreover, complete mucosal ulceration is seen along with submucosal fibrosis, inflammation, and hyperemia.

Medical Management of Ulcerative Colitis

A number of drugs are available for the medical management of UC (Table 41-3). The aminosalicylates are used as maintenance therapy for UC. Immunosuppressants such as corticosteroids and cyclosporine are used to control flare-ups, to induce remission, and, in the setting

TABLE 41-2

DIVERSE ARRAY OF EXTRAINTESTINAL SYMPTOMS

Extraintestinal Symptom

Weight loss
Arthralgias and arthritis
Delayed growth
Delayed sexual maturation
Malabsorption
Nutritional deficiency
Mucocutaneous lesions
Renal disease
Hepatobiliary disease
Ocular complications

TABLE 41-3

MEDICATIONS FOR CHILDREN WITH ULCERATIVE COLITIS

Medication	Dose
Aminosalicylates	
Sulfasalazine	50–75 mg/kg/day PO divided tid or qid
Mesalamine (5′ aminosalicylate)	30–50 mg/kg/day PO divided bid or tid
Mesalamine enemas	2–4 g qhs
Mesalamine suppository	0.5 g qhs
Immunosuppressants	
Prednisone	1–2 mg/kg/day
Methylprednisolone	1.0–1.5 mg/kg/day IV
Hydrocortisone enema	80 mg qhs
6-Mercaptopurine	1.0–1.5 mg/kg/day
Azathioprine	1.5–2.0 mg/kg/day IV
Cyclosporine	
Initial	2.0 mg/kg IV bid or continuous infusion
Maintenance	4–6 mg/kg PO bid

Modified from Kirschner BS: Ulcerative colitis in children. Pediatr Clin North Am 43:235–254, 1996.

of inevitable operative intervention, to decrease the acuity of inflammation and allow nutritional repletion.

Mild disease is usually controlled with oral sulfasalazine. If side effects are not tolerated, then mesalamine can be used. Disease that is localized to the rectum can be treated with mesalamine or hydrocortisone enemas. For patients with more severe disease with symptoms of abdominal cramping, tenderness, bloody diarrhea, and anemia, intravenous steroids are used to decrease inflammation quickly. Parenteral nutrition and bowel rest should be instituted if abdominal symptoms are severe. Serial abdominal radiographs are useful to exclude the development or progression of toxic megacolon. With clinical improvement, a low-residue diet can be instituted, and conversion to oral steroids and aminosalicylates can be initiated.

Cyclosporine can achieve remission in cases of steroid-refractory UC. Improvement in symptoms is usually seen within 7 to 10 days. However, relapse and the need for surgical therapy are seen in 38% to 70% of patients within 6 months after stopping cyclosporine.[17] Therefore cyclosporine merely delays the need for operation. Discontinuation of steroids or cyclosporine can be overlapped with the administration of other immunosuppressants, such as 6-mercaptopurine (6-MP) or azathioprine (AZA), to prolong the period of relapse.[18]

Indications for Surgical Therapy

As opposed to CD, operative therapy for UC is potentially curative and is indicated for both emergency and elective reasons. Overall, about 20% to 25% of children undergo a major operation within 10 years of diagnosis, and more than 50% of children have operative therapy within 20 years of diagnosis.[12,19]

Emergency operation is indicated for patients with fulminant colitis resistant to medical therapy, toxic megacolon, perforation, or severe colonic bleeding. About 10% of children with UC have fulminant colitis and require hospitalization. If clinical improvement is not seen within 3 to 4 days of medical therapy, then an operation should be considered. In a few patients, toxic megacolon develops and requires emergency surgical treatment. In only 5 of 90 children with UC did toxic megacolon develop over a 10-year period in one series.[19] The need for operation for perforation or severe colonic bleeding also is rare.

Elective indications for operation include growth failure, failure of medical management, unacceptable quality of life, and increased cancer risk. Patients with these indications represent the majority. Careful, serial documentation of growth parameters is required to assess the need for elective surgical intervention. More commonly, repeated hospitalization, complications from medications, and frustration or non-compliance with medical management are the decisive reasons for operation. A lower threshold for elective operative therapy may be justified. Aggressive medical therapy may result in patients being initially seen with more severe fulminant colitis. Consequently, these patients may have more complications, a higher incidence of emergency surgical procedures, and a higher incidence of staged colectomy before restoration of intestinal continuity.[20,21]

The risk of colon cancer in UC is a long-term complication and is related to the duration of disease. Nevertheless, this issue should be discussed during the pediatric period. Studies demonstrate that the risk of colon cancer does not begin until about 10 years after the time of diagnosis.[22] Thus colonoscopic surveillance should begin at this time. After the first decade, the risk of cancer increases 0.5% per year for the second decade and then 1% per year for the third and fourth decades.[22] After 40 years, the cancer risk increases dramatically, with cancer or dysplasia developing in approximately 20% of patients per year.[23]

Surgical Options

Subtotal Colectomy with Ileostomy

Patients with an emergency need for operation due to fulminant colitis, toxic megacolon, perforation, or bleeding should undergo subtotal colectomy with ileostomy. This operation has been performed extensively in UC patients. The primary goal is removal of the entire diseased colon while sparing the rectum, followed by recovery and eventual improvement in nutritional and immunologic status in preparation for a future second-stage ileoanal pull-through operation. This operation can be performed through a midline incision or, on occasion, laparoscopically. The colon is fully mobilized and resected. The rectum is oversewn near the peritoneal reflection, and an end ileostomy is created. Symptoms may persist from disease in the retained rectum, but the magnitude is typically markedly reduced.

This operation has several advantages. It can be done quickly for the sickest patients. The pelvis is left undissected, thus retaining the native tissue planes for future procedures, and preventing the possible complications of impotence and bleeding. Recovery from this operation is fairly rapid, and most patients do not have problems with malabsorption secondary to the ileostomy.

Subtotal Colectomy with Ileorectal Anastomosis

This is not an appropriate operation in the emergency setting because of the increased risk of anastomotic leak. Furthermore, the child is left with a significant long-term cancer risk of 13% to 20% in the retained rectum.[24,25] Thus subtotal colectomy with ileorectal anastomosis is not a recommended operation in the pediatric patient.

Restorative Proctocolectomy with Ileoanal Pull-Through

Technically, this operation involves a subtotal colectomy, rectal mucosectomy, ileal pouch construction, and ileoanal anastomosis. Patients with medically controlled disease are ideal candidates to have the ilioanal pull-through (IAPT) as a single-stage operation. Those patients that have undergone subtotal colectomy with end ileostomy and closure of the spared rectum are also candidates for restoration of intestinal continuity by endorectal mucosectomy and IAPT. Usually this is performed as a second-stage operation at least 3 months after the colectomy.

The rectal mucosectomy and ileoanal anastomosis were first described in 1947.[26] The major advance was the sphincter-preserving rectal mucosectomy. The ileal pouch was added to the operation after the success of the Koch ileostomy reservoirs, in which the frequency of bowel movements is decreased as compared with the straight ileoanal anastomosis.[27,28] Thus the operation accomplishes complete removal of all diseased mucosa while restoring intestinal continuity and provides acceptable bowel habits. Because no pelvic dissection is done near the anal sphincter complex, postoperative fecal incontinence is less common, although rectal urgency and fecal soiling may occur. Furthermore, the mucosal dissection and anastomosis can be carried down very close to the dentate line, eliminating nearly all risk of future colon carcinoma. The major disadvantages of the IAPT are primarily related to pouch dysfunction and operative complications.

The IAPT begins with a standard colon mobilization to a point about 10 cm above the dentate line. The terminal ileum is separated from the colon, the mesentery is mobilized and divided, and the ileum is checked for adequate pelvic length. The longest loop of ileum should reach the pubic symphysis. In the rare case that the ileum will not reach, then one should consider an end ileostomy as an alternative option, with closure of the rectum followed by repeated operation after steroid taper and weight loss. If adequate ileal length is available, then the pull-through procedure can proceed. The rectal mucosectomy is performed transanally. The dissection is begun just above the dentate line, and it is facilitated by submucosal injection of 1:100,000 epinephrine (Fig. 41-1). Once the mucosa has been separated to a point above the intra-abdominal dissection, the muscular wall of the

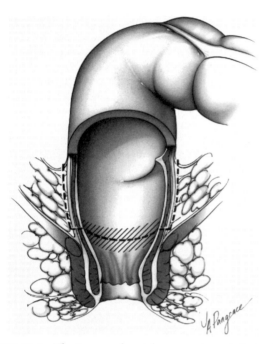

FIGURE 41-1. The transanal rectal mucosectomy is begun 1 to 2 cm above the dentate line. The ease of entry into a circumferential submucosal plane of dissection is facilitated by the injection of 1:100,000 epinephrine, which also aids in limiting the local bleeding that tends to obscure the operative field.

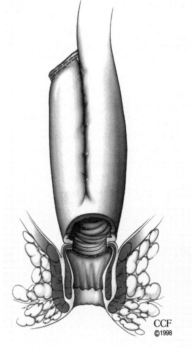

FIGURE 41-2. A J pouch reservoir is configured from distal ileum. After mucosectomy, the small bowel is pulled through the muscular sleeve of spared rectum, and the ileoanal anastomosis is completed by placement of interrupted absorbable sutures.

rectum is circumferentially transected, the mucosal sleeve and colon are removed, leaving the muscular cuff of the rectum.

A J pouch is the most commonly configured internal ileal reservoir (Fig. 41-2). Although lateral S and W pouches have been described, these constructions use more length of ileum and offer only minor improvements in postoperative bowel habits in adults.[29,30] The J pouch is simple and quick to construct. The loop of ileum is folded back on itself for a distance of 15 cm by using stay sutures. An enterotomy is made at the apex of the J pouch, and a gastrointestinal stapler is used to join the two limbs along the antimesenteric border. The pouch is brought down to the pelvis, through the muscular cuff of rectum, and a transanal hand-sewn anastomosis is made by using full-thickness, absorbable sutures.

It is our preference to create a diverting end ileostomy to protect the pouch. Pelvic drains and antibiotics are continued for 5 postoperative days, and a diet is advanced with resumption of bowel function. Routine anal dilatations are not performed. We have found that a digital examination at 2 weeks after surgery usually suffices for lysing any anastomotic adhesions. If the examination is abnormal, then intraoperative anoscopy is scheduled to examine the anastomosis. A J pouch radiographic contrast study is obtained 6 weeks after the operation. If this is normal, then biofeedback training is begun with progressively larger pouch enemas over a 6-week period. With this method, children gain biofeedback in pelvic sensation. Follow-up studies demonstrate a high resting anal pressure and a minimal rate of incontinence.[31] Usually 3 months after the IAPT, patients are ready to have an ileostomy takedown.

The question as to whether fecal diversion is required in the IAPT is unanswered in children. Although the number of patients was small, a single study in children demonstrated no significant differences in pouch-related complications or functional outcome with and without a temporary diverting ileostomy.[32] Adult studies have demonstrated no significant difference in outcome with and without diversion unless the patient is taking significant steroids (>20 mg).[33,34] The ileostomy does add significant risk of bowel obstruction, as well as the need for an additional operation.[33] However, if a patient is taking supraphysiologic doses of corticosteroids, if tension is present on the anastomosis, or if ischemia is evident in the pouch, then diversion should be used to protect the pouch and ileoanal anastomosis. In the absence of these situations, an ileostomy may not be necessary. In our protocol, diversion also affords the patient a period for biofeedback training.

Further controversy exists surrounding the use of a hand-sewn versus a stapled ileoanal anastomosis. Although adult studies have demonstrated that the stapled ileoanal anastomosis gives rise to a higher resting anal pressure and lower risk of incontinence,[35,36] the stapled anastomosis leaves a few centimeters of anal transition zone for the life of the patient. Prospective 10-year follow-up studies in adult patients demonstrated a 5% long-term risk of dysplasia and an unknown risk of carcinoma. Thus most pediatric surgeons prefer complete excision of the diseased mucosa through rectal mucosectomy followed by the hand-sewn anastomosis.

The overall results from the IAPT operation are very good. In adults, 90% of patients report an excellent quality of life, with a median of six stools daily.[37] These results were consistent over 8 years of follow-up, suggesting no deterioration in pouch function. In a comprehensive review of 20 adult series, the overall mortality was 0.5%, with a 10% rate of small bowel obstruction (SBO) and a 12% rate of operation-specific mortality.[38] SBO is a frequent early complication, occurring in 26% of adult patients.[39] As discussed, an ileostomy can add a threefold increase in the frequency of SBO.[33] Postoperative sepsis occurs in 2% to 15% of cases, usually because of pouch leak and rarely because of pouch infarction or anastomotic breakdown. The sepsis is managed with antibiotics, percutaneous drainage of any abscesses and, if necessary, fecal diversion in those patients without an ileostomy.[39,40] Pouch stricture occurs in 10% to 15% of cases.[41] The stricture is usually at the site of anastomosis and responds to serial anal dilatations. More proximal pouch strictures are probably due to ischemia and may require endoscopic dilatation or surgical revision or both.

Long-term complications are most commonly due to the J pouch and its limited ability to act as a fecal reservoir. Pouchitis occurs in 10% to 40% of adult patients.[42] The frequency of pouchitis in children may be lower and approximates 12%.[43] However, the episodes may be more severe than those in adults.[44] Patients have fever, malaise, pelvic pain, and bloody diarrhea. Although the etiology of pouchitis is multifactorial, bacterial overgrowth and stasis certainly contribute, because effective emptying decreases the rate of pouchitis.[45] Endoscopy of the pouch demonstrates inflamed mucosa, and biopsies should be performed to exclude granulomatous changes suggestive of CD. Most cases respond well to metronidazole or ciprofloxacin treatment. In severe cases, diversion may be necessary. Pouch excision should be considered a last resort for repeated, severe pouchitis.

Laparoscopic Subtotal Colectomy and Ileoanal Pull-Through

The role of laparoscopy in the treatment of UC is gaining acceptance. A number of studies in adults and children confirmed the feasibility and safety of laparoscopic procedures for UC.[46,47] The laparoscopic IAPT is really a laparoscopic-assisted approach in which the colon is mobilized and the mesentery is transected intracorporeally. A Pfannenstiel incision is then made to remove the colon, construct the J pouch, mobilize the small bowel mesentery, and complete the pull-through with the ileoanal anastomosis. The laparoscopic subtotal colectomy is performed by using a similar technique, but the colon is removed through the ileostomy site. This procedure has been performed in adults and children for the treatment of fulminant colitis.[48,49] Although the laparoscopic procedures are significantly longer than similar open operations, potential advantages include improved cosmetic appearance, shorter length of hospitalization, quicker return of bowel function, and reduced wound complications. However, these potential advantages have not been completely realized. Only two retrospective studies have demonstrated reduced length of stay,[48,50] and two retrospective studies demonstrated a quicker return of bowel function.[48,49] One study demonstrated reduced wound complications,[51] but the rate of operation-specific complications did not differ between open and laparoscopic patients. An adequate-size, randomized, prospective trial has yet to be performed. With improvements in laparoscopic technique, instrumentation, and shorter laparoscopic operating times, clinical differences may eventually emerge. One would anticipate a reduced rate of postoperative SBO in laparoscopic versus open patients. The value for the improved cosmesis resulting from a laparoscopic procedure in a child is not known.

CROHN'S DISEASE

Classically, CD is characterized by chronic, transmural inflammation of the gastrointestinal tract. The etiology is unknown. Drs. Crohn, Ginzburg, and Oppenheimer were initially credited with describing "Crohn disease" in 1932. Of historical interest to pediatric surgeons, this first description was of a young teenage patient with terminal ileal disease.[1] Further characterization of the disease as a chronic, transmural inflammation that can involve any part of the digestive tract, from the oral cavity to anal canal, continued over the next 11 years, until CD was described in 48 more children with multiple manifestations of the disease.

Although originally described as "terminal ileitis," as patient experience grew, it became apparent that the inflammatory process can affect any portion of the alimentary tract. The colonic form of CD was distinguished from UC by Brooke in 1959 and further by Lockhart-Mummery in 1960.

Although first described in children, CD is now recognized as a relatively rare condition in children. The concept of CD as a nonchildhood illness developed as diagnostic modalities increased, specifically with the wide use of endoscopic evaluation and histologic studies of biopsy materials. As a result, a steady growth of the frequency of CD has occurred since the middle of the 1980s. Today the incidence of CD in the United States is approximately 5 per 100,000 persons. Evidence exists that the worldwide incidence of CD has increased during the past several decades, although in the United States during the last 10 years, the incidence of newly diagnosed IBD has reached a plateau. CD incidence is equal in men and women and is five times more prevalent in whites than in blacks. The incidence is sharply increased in Jewish populations.

Etiology

Despite intense investigation, the exact etiology of CD remains unclear. Infectious, environmental, and immunologic links are present, but no distinct etiology has been identified. Ethnic clustering, racial predisposition, and therapeutic response to immunomodulators suggest a genetic source and immunologic predisposition. It seems most probable that unidentified environmental triggers in genetically susceptible individuals are important in the CD cycle.

Difficult to distinguish at times from UC, CD can be distinguished and characterized by using anti-neutrophil cytoplasmic antibodies (ANCAs) and anti-*Saccharomyces cerevisiae* antibodies (ASCA) antibody screening. This supports the notion that an immune basis for the disease exists, perhaps a poorly regulated immunologic response to as yet unidentified antigens. Various antigens may include bacteria, antibiotics, food antigens, and environmental sources. In the future, such antibodies and other genetic markers may be helpful in stratifying patients into different therapeutic modalities for CD.

Pathology

CD is a chronic transmural granulomatous inflammation that can involve any part of the digestive system from the oral cavity to the anal canal. Grossly, or endoscopically, small ulcers in the mucosa can produce a characteristic "cobblestone" appearance. Deep fissures can occur parallel to the long axis of the intestine. These ulcerations and fissures may penetrate completely through the muscularis and serosal layers of the bowel, leading to adhesions, sinus tracts, abscesses, or chronic fistulae. Transmural and segmental areas of inflammation are the hallmark signs of CD. The classic histology in CD shows noncaseating granulomas, but this finding occurs in as few as 30% of patients.

Although CD can affect the alimentary tract at any point, it does have a predisposition for the ileocecal region. The majority of patients will have disease in the terminal ileum. Involvement of the colon is present in 60% of patients, and 50% of those will have pancolitis. Traditional teaching is that 30% of patients have upper gastroduodenal inflammation; however, more recent reports of endoscopic surveillance in children with CD suggest this may be more prevalent. Perirectal disease is present in 20% of patients with CD and is usually associated with patient misery and a difficult clinical course.

Natural History/Prognosis

CD is recognized with increasing frequency in children. It is most commonly diagnosed among young adults, but the onset of symptoms may occur in the early teen years. Although rectal bleeding is a hallmark of UC, it is much less frequent in the patient with CD. If a patient with CD does have bleeding, it is usually associated with colonic disease. In 60% to 70% of children with CD, a diagnostic delay of more than 1 year usually occurs. In one series, more than one-third of patients with CD were first treated for a nongastrointestinal disorder before proper diagnosis. Unfortunately, children with CD tend to have a fairly chronic and protracted course. Children are most commonly affected with ileocolonic disease, and ileocolectomy is the most common operative procedure in children with CD.

Clinical Presentation/Extraintestinal Manifestations

In children with IBD, failure to thrive is an ominous sign. When found at the time of presentation, it often confirms CD as the correct diagnosis, and it may be a distinguishing point between UC and CD. Linear growth failure is a common finding in patients with early-onset CD. Many pediatric patients with CD have failure to thrive and colonic and perianal disease. Presenting symptoms include weight loss, diarrhea, abdominal pain, fever, and anorexia. At times, these extraintestinal manifestations precede the clinical diagnosis of CD.

The extraintestinal manifestations of CD are similar to those described for UC. Extraintestinal manifestations that are distinct from UC include severe failure to thrive and weight loss that is more pronounced in the child with CD. Additionally, children with CD may have clubbing of the distal digits. Other extraintestinal manifestations include skin lesions, anemia, stomatitis, uveitis, and delayed sexual maturation. Biopsy of oral lesions may reveal granulomas typical of CD.

Medical Therapy for Crohn's Disease

The medical treatment of CD has progressed dramatically over the past decade. In general, medical therapy is based on distinct classes of medications, and therapy is directed toward an individual patient response. Medical therapy can be divided into four general classes: anti-inflammatory medications, immunomodulatory or immunosuppressive therapy, nutritional therapy, and the relatively new field of "biologic therapy." Biologic therapy refers to the class of medicines directed at modulation of the body's hyperregulated inflammatory response in CD.

Nutritional Therapy

Nutritional therapy may be most useful in maintaining remission in CD while promoting linear growth. Although nutritional therapy may be useful as an adjunct, a combination of nutritional and pharmacologic approaches is optimal for all but the most mildly affected children with CD. Elemental or semielemental enteral nutrition has been advocated to induce remission. Unfortunately, relapse is common after primary nutritional therapy is discontinued. Adjunctive nutritional therapies, especially evolving biologic and probiotic agents, offer some hope for improving future treatment.

Prolonged nutritional treatment for CD usually mandates concomitant pharmacologic therapy with either 6-MP or AZA. A recent meta-analysis of multiple studies looking at nutritional therapy for CD concluded that corticosteroid therapy is more effective than enteral nutrition for inducing remission of active CD. In this meta-analysis, no significant difference in the efficacy of elemental and nonelemental diets was found for induction of remission of CD.[2]

Anti-Inflammatory Medications/Steroids

Traditional medical treatment for CD consists of aminosalicylates and corticosteroids as the cornerstone of therapy. As the severity of the intestinal manifestation of the disease increases, CD often responds best in the short term to high-dose corticosteroids. To date, no study has prospectively compared the efficacy of oral versus parenteral corticosteroids in a randomized controlled fashion. Traditionally, parenteral corticosteroids are used in more severely active CD. Recently, the oral steroid budesonide has been used in the treatment of CD. The creation of an oral formulation was directed largely at minimizing the debilitating side effects of high-dose parenteral steroid therapy. The oral preparation of budesonide possesses an approximately 90% first-pass metabolism. Consequently, budesonide has an improved toxicity profile when compared with conventional corticosteroids (e.g., prednisone and methylprednisolone). In recent prospective, randomized, double-blind clinical trials, oral budesonide was shown to be effective in the treatment of active CD.[56] Data have not been supportive of the use of oral budesonide for the maintenance of remission in CD. Budesonide has been shown to have efficacy similar to that of conventional corticosteroids, with fewer systemic side effects and less likelihood of adrenal suppression.[57]

Corticosteroids have not been shown to be beneficial for maintenance of remission in patients with CD. Today, in most cases, steroids are coupled with 6-MP or AZA to help maintain long-term remission. Multimodal therapy tends to minimize toxicity. In children with CD, particular emphasis must be placed on the growth suppression and other toxic effects of corticosteroids.

Immunomodulators

Many centers advocate the early introduction of immunosuppressives (such as AZA or 6-MP) as maintenance treatment in CD. Although arguably more toxic, methotrexate also may serve as an alternative therapy in CD. The rationale for the use of immunomodulators in CD is founded in observations implicating immunologic mechanisms in the pathogenesis of IBD. The most common immunomodulators are AZA and 6-MP. Because studies have shown that these agents are effective in inducing and maintaining remission in patients with CD, current trends favor the use of immunomodulatory agents over colectomy for children with intractable Crohn's colitis. A recent meta-analysis of randomized controlled trials looking at immunomodulatory therapy demonstrated an overall response rate of 55% for the treatment of active CD with AZA and 6-MP.[3] Consistent remission with this therapy is achieved in approximately 67% of patients.[4] One important utility of AZA and 6-MP in this setting is their steroid-sparing effect. Limited data suggest other potential benefits of these agents including the management of perianal and fistulous disease and the prevention of postoperative recurrence.

Practice trends indicate that pediatric gastroenterologists have widely accepted the use of immunomodulators in the treatment of children and adolescents with IBD. Since the early 1990s, the use of immunomodulation has been useful for treating perianal and nonperianal fistulas, for managing growth failure, for prophylaxis against postoperative recurrence, and as initial therapy.

Biologic Therapy

Recent significant advances that assist in the design of new therapies have been made in our understanding of the pathogenesis of IBD. Infliximab, a monoclonal antibody to the proinflammatory cytokine tumor necrosis factor (TNF-α) has shown significant promise in the treatment of CD. This is based on the observation that the concentration of TNF-α is increased in the gastrointestinal mucosa of patients with active CD. Neutralization of TNF with infliximab decreases the mucosal inflammatory response in many adults with CD. Although the majority of the evidence for the use of infliximab is in adult patients, more pediatric centers are now accumulating experience. The ACCENT I trial (*A Crohn's Disease Clinical Trial Evaluating Infliximab in a New Long-term Treatment Regimen*) looked specifically at benefits of treating with infliximab in adults. Overall, this trial showed three general findings. First, a clinical response at 54 weeks was achieved in 43% to 53% of patients receiving infliximab maintenance therapy compared with 17% in patients receiving placebo maintenance therapy ($P<0.001$).[5] The remission rates at 54 weeks were 28% to 38% in patients receiving infliximab maintenance therapy contrasted with 14% in the placebo group. Second, this study demonstrated the superiority of a three-dose regimen compared with a single-infusion regimen for inducing remission. Last, the ACCENT I study showed the steroid-sparing benefit of infliximab.[6] In another landmark study in adults with moderate to severe CD, a single infusion of infliximab resulted in a 50% to 81% clinical response rate (81% with a 5-mg/kg dose) and a 25% to 48% remission rate (48% remission with 5-mg/kg dose) at 4 weeks. The characteristic response to infliximab is rapid, occurring within 1 to 2 weeks after medication infusion, and the effect persists for 8 to 12 weeks.[62]

Infliximab also has been used for the treatment of two specific complications of CD: strictures and fistulas. In one adult study, complete closure of more than half of all fistulas was achieved in 62% of patients, and complete closure of all fistulas occurred in 46% of patients.[63] In contrast, it appears that once a stricture is established in CD, it generally does not respond well to therapy. The response rate of strictures to infliximab may be diminished, as it often represents end-stage inflammation. The role of infliximab in Crohn's strictures is still unclear, but it may have a role in stricture prevention rather than in treatment. Studies also indicate that treating patients with CD with infliximab does not lead to the development of intestinal strictures, as was previously speculated.[64] Importantly, treatment with infliximab may be protective against the development of late strictures. The ACCENT I study demonstrated the importance of the inflammatory component on the development of strictures, and it also showed a beneficial effect of infliximab in deterring the development of strictures. Prospectively, individuals in the ACCENT I study who received the higher aggregate amounts of infliximab were less likely to develop symptomatic intestinal strictures over time.[65] The use of infliximab is associated with rapid and remarkable short-term clinical improvement in children with CD. Unfortunately, fairly rapid return of disease activity occurs when it is discontinued.

Other new therapies have focused on modulating the neovascularity and inflammatory migration of cells in CD. Monoclonal antibodies that target the α-4 integrins or their CAM ligands (natalizumab) can ameliorate inflammation in CD. Treatment with natalizumab in reducing signs and symptoms of CD appears to be comparable to that of infliximab in early studies. Therapy with natalizumab in the future may prove to be a useful adjunct to infliximab, but more data are needed to establish clear safety, efficacy, and clinical indications.

Last, antiangiogenic agents, specifically thalidomide, have been used in patients with CD. Thalidomide also has been shown to reduce selectively the TNF-α production by inflammatory cells. The effects of thalidomide on the intestinal manifestations of CD can be marked and impressive. Although thalidomide seems to be a safe and effective treatment in pediatric patients with CD, it should probably be used as a last resort, preferably in male or prepubescent female patients.

Surgical Treatment

Multimodal medical therapy, as previously described, is the first-line treatment for CD. In general, operative intervention provides only palliative relief for patients with CD. As such, surgical intervention is largely reserved for complications of CD.

Complications of Crohn's Disease

Despite the focus on the medical management of CD, with an emphasis on prevention and maintenance therapy, the majority of patients with CD will require surgical intervention at some point during their lives. Historically, up to 70% to 80% of patients with CD have undergone some surgical intervention for the treatment of the complications of their disease. Interventions range from the surgical treatment of perianal disease to complex intra-abdominal operations. It may be that this number will decrease significantly in the future because of the recent advances in immunologic and biologic therapy.

Patient presentation tends to vary according to the underlying pathologic location of the disease focus. For instance, in patients with ileocecal disease, the majority will have intestinal obstruction. In contrast, a minority of patients with isolated colonic disease will have intestinal obstruction. The patients with isolated colonic disease tend to have intractable or even bloody diarrhea. In contrast to UC, rectal bleeding is much less frequent in patients with CD, but does happen in about 15% of patients.

In general, complications leading to surgical intervention in the CD patient population include the following: ileocolonic stricture and bowel obstruction, enterocutaneous fistula, enteroenterofistula, enterovesicle fistula, enterovaginal fistula perianal disease and fistulization, intra-abdominal and perirectal abscesses, growth retardation, medical intractability, intestinal bleeding, and rarely, free intraperitoneal perforation with sepsis.

Failure of Medical Therapy

Somewhat surprisingly, in children with CD, the most common indication for operative intervention is failure of medical management. Specifically, medical therapy commonly fails in children because of growth retardation, chronic steroid dependence, inability to participate in normal daily activities, and prolonged absence from school.[66]

Because of the inherent problems of malnutrition frequently encountered in patients with CD, many patients benefit from preoperative bowel rest. Limited evidence is based on data in adult patients that a short-term preoperative course of total parenteral nutrition may help reduce perioperative complications.

Perianal Crohn's Disease

Treatment of the perianal manifestations of CD may be one of the most frustrating and difficult aspects of the disease. Importantly, in the pediatric population, perianal fistula and abscesses may herald signs of Crohn's colitis. It is not uncommon for perianal symptoms to antedate the abdominal symptoms associated with CD by several years. Specifically, in patients with an early presentation of perianal abscess or fistula in childhood or the early teen years and in patients with recurrent perianal disease, the suspicion of CD is raised. Recurrent fistula, multiple fistulas, and perianal fistulas in atypical locations (rectovaginal, anterior fistulas) in particular should raise this suspicion.

Perianal CD can often be best managed with medical therapy. Perianal fistulas are often best treated with local wound care and metronidazole or ciprofloxacin or both. More extensive cases may require treatment with 6-MP or even infliximab. Early operation is not indicated because of the chronic nature and underlying pathology of these complications. Nonhealing fistulas are sometimes operatively removed once active infection around the fistula has resolved. Only with total failure of local wound care in the treatment of fistulas would it be prudent to consider a diverting colostomy, ileostomy, or even a possible proctectomy. Perianal disease, in the face of isolated intra-abdominal ileocolic disease, may improve after ileocolectomy.

Fistula

Perianal disease is usually a consequence of the development of rectal/cutaneous abscesses and fistulization. Many children with CD also are plagued by intra-abdominal fistulization. In a recent series from Boston Children's Hospital, 14% of children that underwent operation did so because of intra-abdominal fistula.[66]

Fistulas may be enteroenteral, enterocolonic, or enterovesical. These children are not likely to heal these fistulas with total parenteral nutrition alone.[67] Fistulas may be asymptomatic, but more commonly, they are the cause of chronic abdominal pain, vague complaints, weight loss, or pneumouria. The majority of intra-abdominal fistulas in children arise from the terminal ileum or proximal small bowel.[66]

En bloc resection of the diseased intestine and fistula with primary anastomosis is the preferred treatment of enteroenteral and enterocolic fistulas. Fistulas to the bladder also may be treated with resection and anastomosis of the diseased segment of bowel, with primary repair of the bladder.

Stricture

Because of the relatively high incidence of ileocolonic disease in the pediatric-age population, the need for operative treatment is still common in children with CD. Bowel obstruction from stricture formation secondary to terminal ileal disease is the most common presentation in the pediatric population. As outlined earlier, such strictures are the result of chronic inflammation. As a result, by the time pediatric patients are seen with obstructive symptoms, their strictures are usually well established and respond poorly to immunologic or biologic therapy. Recent trends have been directed at a minimally invasive approach to the surgical treatment for CD, including strictureplasty and laparoscopic bowel resection.

The former is designed to preserve as much bowel length as possible (Fig. 41-3).

Limited Disease

Because ileocecal disease is the most common location for CD, a common indication for operative intervention in the pediatric age group is directed to relieve partial or complete bowel obstruction or chronic pain secondary to small bowel or colonic strictures. With disease limited to the small bowel or with short-segment ileocolonic disease, resection and primary anastomosis may be the most efficient treatment. Strictureplasty also may be considered as long as the ileocecal valve is not involved.

The best operative results are seen when short-segment CD is limited to the small bowel. Patients with extensive colonic disease have mixed results. In short-segment colonic disease, treatment options include segmental resection and anastomosis, resection and diverting proximal ileostomy, subtotal colectomy with ileostomy with consideration for later ileostomy takedown, and ileoproctostomy. In one review, the patients did best with subtotal colectomy and ileostomy and reported minimal problems with disease within the rectal stump.[66]

Multicentric/Long-Segment Disease

Although the accepted standard for short-segment complicated CD has been bowel resection, recently surgeons have directed intervention toward strictureplasty in an

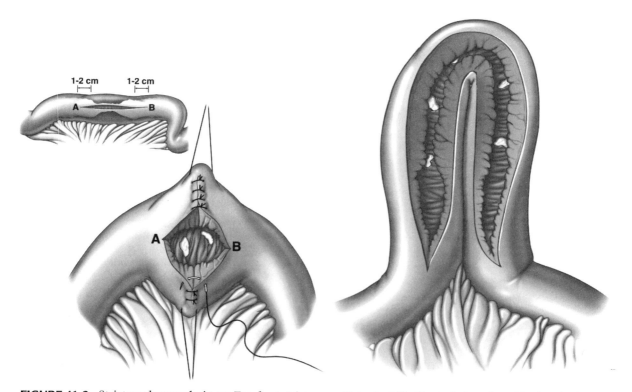

FIGURE 41-3. Strictureplasty techniques. For short strictures, a Heineke-Mikulicz technique for widening the lumen may be used (*A*). For longer strictures, a side-to-side anastomosis may be created by using the Finney technique (*B*).

attempt to preserve bowel length (see Fig. 41-3). In several reviews, strictureplasty in CD patients with extensive stricture disease has been shown to be an effective surgical option for relieving obstruction while sparing bowel length.

Some pediatric series have shown a fairly high incidence of postoperative recurrence of the manifestations of CD. High recurrence rates for CD most closely correlate with the severity of disease at the time of operation, colonic disease, and the use of preoperative 6-MP. However, the early institution of 6-MP for maintenance therapy may well prevent some resurgence of the disease. Interestingly, strictureplasty also may be associated with a lower postoperative recurrence rate. The mechanism is unclear, but some adult series indicate that postoperative bowel obstruction and recurrent stricture may be less frequent after strictureplasty. In addition, some pediatric series also support strictureplasty.[68] Moreover, in many series, the results of strictureplasty are superior to those of intestinal resection, both in regard to the incidence and timing of recurrences as well as to complications.

Laparoscopy

With the increasing use of minimally invasive surgery, laparoscopy has been recognized as a useful adjunct in the surgical diagnosis and treatment of CD. Several adult series have established the laparoscopic approach as a viable option for the surgical treatment of CD. Trends have been observed toward shorter hospital stay, decreased pain and postoperative ileus, smaller incisions, decreased cost, and fewer complications with laparoscopic resection when compared with open resection. In turn, two specific series of pediatric patients have been treated with minimally invasive techniques.[69,70] The first involved laparoscopy for diagnosis and intestinal mobilization for extracorporeal resection and anastomosis. The second series looked specifically at total intracorporeal intestinal resection and anastomosis for CD. Both pediatric series demonstrate that bowel resection for CD can be performed safely with the laparoscopic approach. Surgical outcomes were comparable with open techniques with acceptable operating time and morbidity.

No reports exist of laparoscopy-assisted strictureplasty, although an extracorporeal technique seems feasible.

INTESTINAL CANCER

Intestinal cancer is an infrequent entity in pediatric solid tumor oncology; however, an understanding of its pathophysiology is necessary for effective treatment. Such surgical therapy ranges from prophylactic intestinal resection to radical resection of the tumor and the regional lymphatics, or to palliative resection with relief of intestinal obstructive symptoms. This section reviews the heritable intestinal cancers, which include the polyposis syndromes; the primary intestinal tumors, benign and malignant, that may arise from the anatomic components of the intestinal wall; gastrointestinal lymphomas; and neuroendocrine tumors.

Heritable Intestinal and Colorectal Cancer: Intestinal Polyps and the Polyposis Syndromes

Almost 20% of colorectal cancers occur in the presence of a family history of the disease.[71] The most commonly occurring familial colorectal cancer syndrome is hereditary nonpolyposis colorectal cancer (HNPCC), first described more than 100 years ago, which may be responsible for 5% to 7% of all colorectal cancers. These high-grade more proximal colon tumors are characterized by a younger age at onset, few or solitary sessile adenomas, an improved overall survival, and an association with other cancers of the endometrium, small bowel, ureter, or renal pelvis.[71] However, because this is predominantly a disease of young adults, and because recommended surveillance screening begins at about age 25 years, this chapter does not elaborate further on this entity.

Intestinal polyps most frequently are isolated, benign, and self-limited entities, characterized either by being asymptomatic, producing intermittent bright red rectal bleeding, or by showing with signs and symptoms of intestinal obstruction, infrequently by mass effect and more likely by serving as a lead point for intussusception.

TABLE 41-4				
FEATURES OF GASTROINTESTINAL POLYPS IN CHILDREN				
Syndrome	Gene Defect	Population Frequency	GI Cancer Risk	Defining Features
Common juvenile polyps	Unknown	1:50–1:100 (1%–2% of children)	None known	Hamartoma
Juvenile polyposis	*Smad 4* (18q21.1) *PTEN* Autosomal dom.	1:100,000	Up to 50%	50–200 hamartomas; 5–50 mm diameter
Peutz-Jeghers syndrome	*LKB1* (19p13.3) Autosomal dom.	1:120,000	20%–40%	Muscle polyp core, mucocutaneous pigment
Familial adenomatous polyposis	*APC* (5q21) Autosomal dom. or spont mutation	1:5,000–1:17,000	100%	Adenomatous polyps colon and small bowel

GI, gastrointestinal.

Table 41-4 summarizes the polyp entities, the known genetic aberrations, the histology, their frequency, and the gastrointestinal cancer risk.

Juvenile Polyps

Juvenile, retention, or hamartomatous polyps are the most frequent of the intestinal polyps of childhood.[72] They occur in as many as 1% to 2% of the childhood population. They are diagnosed most often in the first decade, with a peak incidence at age 2 to 5 years and a rare occurrence at younger than 1 year. Although their genetic and developmental origin is unknown, their hamartomatous histology with fluid or mucus-filled cystic spaces suggests a developmental origin. The natural history of these large, vascular, and fleshy polyps may be that their growth exceeds their blood supply, with secondary intraluminal bleeding being a result of mucosal ulceration or autoamputation, the bleeding in the latter case being from the residual central artery. Such polyps are occasionally recovered in the stool. Therefore the gastrointestinal bleeding that forms the basis for the presenting symptoms of such polyps may be small and intermittent, at times associated with an iron-deficiency anemia, or it may be more sudden and extensive. Fortunately, in the latter case, it will typically prove to be self-limited, and it will spontaneously cease either with operative endoscopic polypectomy or after autoamputation, during which interval, patient-supportive therapy alone is typically effective.

Therapeutically, if a patient has rectal bleeding, thorough evaluation is warranted. At times the offending lesion may spontaneously prolapse through the anus, where it can be directly visualized. At other times, it can be palpated at rectal examination, extracted by the transanal route, its stalk suture ligated, and the polyp operatively amputated. Although an air-contrast barium enema radiograph or proctoscopy or both are useful screening tools, the most sensitive diagnostic tool is colonoscopy.[73] This technique also can be therapeutic, serving as the route for polypectomy. Colonoscopy has the added advantage of identifying the patient who harbors more than one juvenile polyp, even in the right or transverse colon, a likelihood that occurs in as many as 50% of children with a polyp. Pancolonoscopy in the face of a known juvenile polyp has demonstrated five or more polyps in as many as 18% of patients.

Juvenile Polyposis Syndrome

In the presence of multiple colonic juvenile polyps, typically 50 to 200 in number, that vary from 5 to 50 mm in diameter, and a strong family history, the autosomal dominant juvenile polyposis syndrome is likely. Approximately 25% of cases are secondary to an inactivating mutation of *Smad 4,* a transforming growth factor-β intracellular signaling molecule whose gene is found on chromosome 18q21.1. Rare additional kindreds with protein tyrosine phosphatase and tensin homologue (PTEN) mutations also have been described. Because juvenile polyps at times also are characterized by adenomatous change and

because in as many as 50% of patients with juvenile polyposis, gastrointestinal cancer develops, serial surveillance with polyp biopsy or polypectomy is recommended. Only in the face of dysplasia or actual malignant degeneration would a more aggressive segmental or total colon resection be warranted. Prophylactic colectomy has to date not been recommended.

When this syndrome occurs in children younger than 2 years, *infantile juvenile polyposis,* the multiple large polyps may be associated with rectal bleeding, protein-losing diarrhea with secondary malnutrition and failure to thrive, and intussusception. A more aggressive operative approach with proctocolectomy may be necessary to reverse this symptom pattern if polypectomy alone proves impractical or unsuccessful.

When *diffuse gastrointestinal juvenile polyposis* occurs, it is typically transmitted as an autosomal recessive trait. The polyps found throughout the gastrointestinal tract should be subjected to an aggressive program of polypectomy and intestinal surveillance.

Peutz-Jeghers Syndrome

This entity is defined by the association of multiple hamartomatous polyps, found typically in the jejunum but also in the duodenum as well as the stomach, with brownish-blue mucocutaneous melanin pigmentation.[72] This latter finding around the lips and oral mucosa occurs in as many as 95% of cases, although the pigmentation also has been seen on the hands, feet, perineum, and in the periorbital area. Interestingly, this pigmentation may antedate the presence of polyps by several years. The polyps are typically multiple, of variable size, and their histology is that of a smooth muscle core that takes its origin from the muscularis mucosa, surrounded by normal-appearing intestinal epithelium. This familial disease is transmitted by autosomal dominant inheritance with a variable penetrance, and approximately one third of patients are identified during childhood. The Peutz-Jeghers syndrome gene has been identified as the *LKB1* gene found on chromosome 19p13.3. It encodes for serine-threonine kinase *STKII* and acts as a tumor-suppressor gene.

Syndrome treatment is again directed at symptom relief in the child with either small bowel or ileocolic intussusception, gastrointestinal bleeding, or for the diagnosis or prevention or both of malignant degeneration that may occur in as many as 20% of patients. Enteroscopy used preoperatively to localize the extent of disease may either avoid operation altogether or at least limit the extent of resection, thus avoiding secondary short-bowel syndrome. The malignant transformation is more common for gastric and duodenal polyps, and surveillance with polypectomy is recommended. Interestingly, in addition to an apparent increased risk for gastrointestinal cancer, female patients with Peutz-Jeghers syndrome are more prone to uterine, breast, and ovarian tumors, and male patients are more prone to testicular and head and neck malignancy, an overall 18-fold increased risk for cancer when compared with the general population.[71]

Familial Adenomatous Polyposis

This inherited disease is the most common genetic polyposis syndrome occurring at a prevalence of 1:5,000 to 1:17,000.[71] The genetic abnormality in familial adenomatous polyposis (FAP) is a germline defect in the adenomatosis polyposis coli gene (*APC*), a tumor-suppressor gene that maps to chromosome 5q21. *APC* regulates β-catenin degradation, a protein whose functions include regulation of cytoskeletal organization, organization of tissue architecture, cell migration and adhesion, intracellular signaling, and gene transcription. Autosomal dominant inheritance accounts for the majority of such patients, but as many as 30% of cases are secondary to spontaneous mutations.[72] Many (>400) *APC* mutations have been found, most located in a region (domain) responsible for β-catenin degradation, and a recognized correlation exists between *APC* gene mutation location and the clinical presentation of FAP. An attenuated FAP occurs with a truncating mutation in the 5′ portion of the *APC* gene; and conversely, mutations between codons 1250 and 1464 are associated with earlier onset and a more diffuse distribution of polyps.[74]

A few adenomatous polyps typically begin their onset in the mid-teenage years, ultimately expanding to hundreds or thousands distributed throughout the colon and rectum. The earliest age at onset of an adenomatous polyp undergoing transformation to a malignant adenocarcinoma was reported before age 10 years. On the other end of the spectrum, progression to adenocarcinoma is considered inevitable by the fifth decade of life.[75] The presence of gastric and duodenal polyps significantly increases the risk of duodenal and periampullary carcinoma.

The diagnosis of FAP today is accomplished by genetic screening of the patient and first-degree relatives of peripheral blood lymphocytes in protein truncation assays. The test is considered to be negative only if an affected family member has had a positive result.[72] The appropriate time to screen children first is at approximately age 8 to 10 years. All screening, positive or negative, should be associated with appropriate genetic counseling. Once a mutant allele is confirmed, annual upper and lower endoscopy with polyp biopsy is prudent. Children who have a family member with an identified mutation but who themselves have had negative genetic testing should undergo screening endoscopy once per decade.

Multiple extraintestinal manifestations also may characterize FAP. The findings of such benign lesions as

desmoid tumors, epidermoid cysts, osteomas, congenital hypertrophy of the retinal pigment epithelium, fibromas, and lipomas may suggest FAP in at-risk patients. The eye findings are particularly sensitive. Table 41-5 summarizes these extracolonic manifestations of FAP along with its phenotypic variants, Gardner's syndrome and Turcot's syndrome.[72,74,76,77] In addition, in patients with FAP, an increased risk exists of pancreatic adenocarcinoma, cholangiocarcinoma, and thyroid carcinoma. A child born to a parent with FAP has an 850 times greater risk than the general population to develop a hepatoblastoma.

The contemporary management of FAP includes both a medical and a surgical component.[78,79] The use of nonsteroidal anti-inflammatory agents, as well as cyclooxygenase inhibitors, have been considered as a preemptive therapy to reduce the number of at-risk adenomatous polyps.[80–85] Table 41-6 summarizes these outcomes. Operatively, the definitive therapy is total proctocolectomy with restorative ileoanal endorectal pull-through, done with or without an internal reservoir, done with or without laparoscopic assist, and done in either two stages or in a single stage without a protecting proximal enterostomy.[86] Enthusiasm has been expressed for the potentially "less morbid" ileorectal anastomosis with sparing of the rectum, especially in Europe. Several prospective studies support such a strategy.[87] However, the presence of a putative cancer-harboring rectum that requires continued and frequent surveillance along with the documented persisting rectal cancer mortality has dimmed the enthusiasm for this option in the United States.

The most difficult decisions that deal with the optimal management of FAP revolve around the preferred timing for preventive colectomy and the management of duodenal adenomas. Various registry studies suggest that although isolated case reports of colorectal cancer associated with FAP occur before age 10 years, such occurrence is extremely rare. Therefore in the absence of suggestive lesions found at yearly surveillance colonoscopy and biopsy, and especially in the absence of the *APC* genetic mutation high-risk disease variants, optimal timing for proctocolectomy, rectal mucosectomy, and endorectal pull-through can be deferred to approximately age 15 years.[88] Prevention or limitation is the preferred management of the highly morbid desmoid tumors that occur in up to 12.4% of FAP patients, tumors that follow laparotomy and colectomy and that are typically resistant to conventional anticancer therapy. Risk factors for desmoids that might further delay the timing of elective

TABLE 41-5			
FEATURES OF THE VARIANTS OF FAMILIAL ADENOMATOUS POLYPOSIS			
Syndrome	Germline Mutation	Cancer Risk	Clinical Features
Familial adenomatous polyposis	*APC*	100% by age 40 yr	CHRPE, desmoid tumors, thyroid and liver cancer risk
Gardner's syndrome	*APC*	Same as FAP	Osteomas, lipomas, sebaceous cysts, dental lesions, desmoids
FAP-related Turcot syndrome	*APC*	Same as FAP	Medulloblastomas
Attenuated FAP	*APC*	70% by age 65 yr	<100 and right-sided colon and fundic polyps

CHRPE, congenital hypertrophy of retinal pigment epithelium.

TABLE 41-6

PHARMACOLOGIC MANAGEMENT OF ADENOMATOUS POLYPS

Agent	Drug Family	Outcome Data
Acetylsalicylic acid (Aspirin)	NSAID; nonselective COX inhibitor	81 mg better than 325 mg for moderate prevention
Sulindac	NSAID; nonselective COX inhibitor	150 mg and 300 mg not preventive; 300 mg reduces number/size
Celecoxib (Celebrex)	NSAID; selective COX-2 inhibitor	800 mg reduces colon and duodenal polyps

NSAID, nonsteroidal anti-inflammatory drug; COX, cyclo-oxygenase.

colectomy in FAP and that might instead encourage aggressive medical management with polyp-reducing strategies include female gender, clinical presence of osteomas, *APC* mutations beyond codon 1444, and a family history of desmoids.[89]

Management of upper gastrointestinal polyps in patients with FAP remains challenging. Routine surveillance upper endoscopy with biopsy is typically deferred until defined colonic polyps are seen in an at-risk patient. Medical management as noted earlier may reduce polyp number and size, but it will produce neither a complete nor a sustained polyp resolution. Fundic gland gastric polyps are frequently seen in patients with FAP, and as many as a third to a half of afflicted patients have evidence of dysplasia.[90] Endoscopic surveillance with polypectomy is the preferred management method. Periampullary polyps are still more challenging, and in face of dysplasia or frank neoplasia, a pancreas-sparing duodenectomy has been reported to be a safe and a long-term effective treatment.[91]

Outcomes

Debate continues over the comparison of functional outcomes in FAP patients treated with ileorectal versus ileoanal anastomosis. An advantage may occur with ileorectal anastomosis related to day and night stool frequency, soiling, flatus and feces discrimination, and the need for antidiarrheal medication. In large series of FAP adolescents, the quality-of-life scores are generally favorable for ileoanal anastomosis; and although a morbidity is associated with the procedure itself (pelvic sepsis, bleeding, small bowel obstruction), the major longer-term issues include day and night stool soiling and an increased stool frequency.[92] Use of the J pouch reservoir is a common adjunct that may improve this morbidity[93] (see Fig. 41-2). Although less commonly done, especially in adolescents, an alternative procedure would be an abdominoperineal total proctocolectomy coupled with a continent ileostomy.[94] However, in one-third of such patients, this reservoir is eventually removed because of an associated morbidity; but in the remaining two-thirds, the results are considered excellent.

A persistent and ongoing mortality from rectal cancer occurs in patients treated with subtotal colectomy and ileorectal anastomosis, despite the addition of regular surveillance and biopsy. However, total proctocolectomy, rectal mucosectomy, and ileoanal anastomosis with a small bowel reservoir does not preclude the development

of adenomatous polyps in the pulled-through small bowel.[95,96] As many as 35% of pouch reservoirs demonstrate adenomas. Over a 15-year postoperative surveillance interval, as many as 75% of pouches develop polyps.[96] Such pouch adenomas are more frequently associated with duodenal and periampullary adenomas; however, no correlation of such findings is noted with *APC* mutation analysis nor is evidence of malignant transformation found at routine surveillance. Finally, a recent report suggested a substantive reduction in female fecundity after proctocolectomy and ileal pouch/anal anastomosis, a diminution not so great as that seen after the same operation for ulcerative colitis. However, the diminished fertility is statistically more significant than that seen in the general population, than seen in FAP patients before operation, and than seen in FAP patients treated with colectomy and ileorectal anastomosis.[97] The mechanism explaining this observation remains unresolved.

NONPOLYPOSIS SMALL INTESTINAL TUMORS

The variety of potential primary small bowel tumors is indicated by the tabulation in Table 41-7. However, such tumors in aggregate remain rare entities. When they are located in the small bowel, they typically are secondary to signs and symptoms produced by their mass effect (pain, obstruction, perforation), their elaboration of endocrine chemical products (fever, flushing, diarrhea), or to acute or chronic gastrointestinal bleeding.[98]

TABLE 41-7

NONPOLYPOSIS SMALL BOWEL TUMORS

Benign	Malignant
Leiomyoma	Adenocarcinoma
Lipoma	Leiomyosarcoma
Vascular lesions	Non-Hodgkin's lymphoma
Malformations	Lymphoblastic
Hemangiomas	Undifferentiated, small cell
Lymphoid hyperplasia	Large cell
Hamartomas	
Neuroendocrine	
Carcinoid	
Neurogenic	
Gastrinomas	

The diagnostic evaluation for small bowel lesions requires a high index of suspicion in the face of chronic abdominal signs and symptoms, occult stool blood, or iron-deficiency anemia. Most often, the most sensitive diagnostic studies of the upper and lower gastrointestinal tract have relied on endoscopic evaluation, whereas examination of the small bowel has been done with enteroclysis radiography. The tumor mass effect can be evaluated with conventional extracorporeal or endoscopic ultrasound (US), computerized tomographic (CT) or magnetic resonance imaging (MRI), and the application of extended endoscopy or even diagnostic laparoscopy. The endoscopic evaluation of the small bowel in children can be facilitated by using newer smaller and longer endoscopes that permit small bowel inspection for 40 to 60 cm beyond the ligament of Treitz. Currently being applied as well as experimentally studied is the use of a released endoscopic video capsule that traverses the gastrointestinal tract and records and transmits images of the small bowel en route.

The following brief discussion elaborates greater detail on several of the important individual tumors.

Benign Small Bowel Tumors

Leiomyoma

This rare intestinal stromal tumor is most commonly found in the jejunum or ileum.[98] Such tumors can be configured as intraluminal, intramural, extraluminal, or dumbbell shaped, and this anatomy dictates the presenting symptoms of obstruction, bleeding with ulceration, a lead point for intussusception, or a mass effect. These well-differentiated smooth muscle tumors are characterized by rare or absent mitoses and the expression of α-smooth muscle actin on CD 117 (KIT). Whether diagnosed preoperatively or found incidentally, segmental resection with primary intestinal anastomosis should be curative.

Lipoma

These rare tumors typically occur more distally in the small bowel, and they rarely produce symptoms. Their fat content produces a unique imaging characteristic on both endoscopic assessment and by CT image, and if they are symptom producing, either excision or segmental resection is curative.

Vascular Lesions

The vascular lesions can be further classified into the congenital vascular malformations or the hemangiomas.[99] *Malformations* are more likely to produce symptoms of bleeding, and they rarely cause either obstruction or perforation. Their diagnosis is typically secondary to peripheral clinical findings (for example, cutaneous lesions as seen in the blue-rubber bleb nevus syndrome) or by endoscopic appearance. A variety of endoscopic or radiographic techniques, angiography, or nuclear medicine bleeding scans can localize the actual site of bleeding. The most effective therapy designed to ameliorate symptoms relates to ablation or removal of the mucosal or submucosal lesions with operative excision, segmental resection, sclerosis, laser destruction, or a staged removal. "Cure," if achievable, is dependent on the identification and removal of all present malformations.

Intestinal hemangiomas less frequently produce symptoms and typically are first seen as a part of a more systemic manifestation of hemangiomatosis that includes hepatic lesions. Such hemangiomas also are amenable to medical management with antiangiogenic therapies such as corticosteroids, interferon α, or low-dose thalidomide. If such medical therapy is unsuccessful, then devascularization by sclerosis or actual excision may be needed.

Intestinal Lymphoid Hyperplasia (Lymphoid Nodular Hyperplasia, Intestinal Nodular Hyperplasia)

In this benign condition, hyperplasia of lymph follicles in the lamina propria and submucosa, centrally umbilicated "polyps" of mucosa protrude into the lumen.[100] The etiology remains uncertain, but it may be secondary to a variety of infectious agents, allergic responses, or even an immune deficiency. Such lesions may be asymptomatic, but they also may be the cause of abdominal pain, diarrhea, gastrointestinal hemorrhage, or a lead point for intussusception. Their diagnosis is typically endoscopic or by air-contrast radiographic imaging. In this latter case, the findings may overlap with those of intestinal lymphomas. Management typically has been excision or resection for symptom-producing lesions, although more recently, interest has focused both on antihistamines and corticosteroids as effective medical therapy. Evidence exists that a child with recurrent intussusception, with suggestive lymphoid hyperplasia and no other evidence of a lead point, should first be treated with a 1- to 3-month trial of corticosteroids rather than a more radical approach that would mandate an ileocolic resection.[100]

Hamartomas

The polyp syndromes, notably Peutz-Jeghers syndrome, were previously described as an etiology of hamartomatous polyps. Hamartomas involving duodenal Brunner's glands (Brunner's gland hamartoma, brunneroma) are rare and infrequently produce symptoms of obstruction or bleeding. Because they are not premalignant lesions, treatment is limited to only those that produce symptoms.

Malignant Bowel Tumors

Malignant bowel tumors may be subdivided into the following categories: the heritable bowel cancer syndromes; the polyposis lesions; tumors secondary to nonhereditary factors; tumors associated with other chronic disease such as CD, UC, or celiac sprue; tumors secondary to immunoincompetence or chronic immunosuppression; the independent lymphomas; and metastatic disease from another nonbowel primary tumor. The following section elaborates further details on those important malignant bowel tumors of childhood not already discussed.

Adenocarcinoma

Primary carcinoma of the colon or small bowel in children, not associated with a genetic or nongenetic predisposition, is very rare.[101,102] The tumor biology is that of a highly aggressive, poorly differentiated tumor that typically has been resistant to resection plus adjuvant chemotherapy, and the outcomes are almost uniformly fatal. Primary adenocarcinoma of the small bowel is even rarer in the pediatric age group.[103,104] Such tumors are initially seen with abdominal pain, anemia, and signs of obstruction. Tumors most frequently are located in the duodenum, including adenocarcinoma of the ampulla of Vater, and they are least frequent in the ileum. Risk factors that have a negative impact on patient outcomes include positive surgical resection margins, extramural tumor venous spread, lymph node metastases, poor tumor differentiation, depth of tumor invasion, and a history of CD.

Colorectal carcinoma of childhood, although representing but 1% of all colorectal cancers, remains the most common carcinoma of the pediatric age group. Despite the hereditary nature of both polyposis and nonpolyposis-related cancers, most cases of colorectal cancer arise in children with no previous underlying abnormality.[101] The presenting signs and symptoms of pain, vomiting, constipation or diarrhea, weight loss, and either indolent or more profuse rectal bleeding are similar to those in adults. The frequent finding of right lower quadrant pain reflects the more frequent right colon location of these tumors in children.

Pediatric colorectal cancers are typically highly aggressive pathologically, and the mucinous poorly differentiated tumors account for more than half.[102] The low likelihood of diagnosis, the right-side location, and the aggressive tumor biology all contribute to a more advanced disease with transmural extension, frequent nodal involvement, and a not infrequent presence of metastases to the liver (Duke stage B, C, or D) at the time of diagnosis.

The treatment goal for even advanced-stage disease is to achieve tumor removal by en bloc resection of the primary tumor and regional lymph nodes, attaining tumor-free margins of resection with early vascular control, and with the avoidance of tumor perforation or spill. Adjuvant therapy is then typically applied in Dukes B, C, and D lesions. Disease outcomes remain significantly less favorable for children than for adults, largely secondary to the more advanced stage of disease at the time of the initial diagnosis and treatment.

Leiomyosarcoma

These rare soft tissue tumors typically are first seen early in life, and they are more common in girls. Unlike adenocarcinomas, their anatomic distribution frequency is jejunum, ileum, and duodenum, from highest to lowest frequency. Their rare occurrence also may account for the frequent delay in diagnosis and their progression to a palpable mass by the time a clinical diagnosis is made. The distinction of benign from malignant is based on evidence of invasiveness as well as on tumor pathology: size,

degree of necrosis, and cellular mitotic index.[98] In addition, the benign leiomyomas express the γ-smooth muscle isoactin gene that the leiomyosarcomas do not.

Resection with disease-free margins is needed to effect a cure and to prevent local recurrence, the latter being the most common adverse outcome. Adjuvant chemotherapy and radiation therapies offer no benefit.

Lymphoma

Lymphomas are the third most common childhood cancer behind the leukemias and brain tumors.[105] Non-Hodgkin's lymphoma (NHL) is the most common malignant primary small bowel tumor of childhood, representing one-half of the 30% to 40% of NHLs that are abdominal in location.[106] Gastrointestinal NHL—stomach, small bowel, and colon—account for as many as 20% of all NHLs, and the gastrointestinal tract is the most common extranodal site for the presentation of lymphoma. This is particularly relevant in pediatrics, in which almost all NHL cases are extranodal in origin.

Childhood NHLs can be divided into three histologic groups: lymphoblastic lymphoma, undifferentiated or small, non–cleaved cell lymphoma, and large cell lymphoma.[105] Lymphoblastic lymphomas are indistinguishable from acute lymphoblastic leukemia, and they are largely of T-cell origin. The rare large cell lymphomas may be of T-cell, B-cell, or histiocytic cell origin. Undifferentiated tumors, indistinguishable from Burkitt's lymphoma except by the degree of cellular pleiomorphism, are of B-cell origin, and they account for as many as 90% of intestinal lymphomas. NHL is very rare in the child younger than 5 years, and the disease is more prevalent in white children and in boys. Its location is most commonly in the ileum.

The etiology of NHL remains unknown. An association is found of endemic Burkitt's lymphoma with the Epstein-Barr virus, and a recognized increase in NHL occurs secondary to immunodeficiency syndromes, including human immunodeficiency virus (HIV) infection, abdominal solid organ transplantation, and after multimodal therapy for Hodgkin's disease and other solid tumors.

The staging of Burkitt's lymphoma in childhood typically is done by the Murphy system (Table 41-8). Staging for non-Burkitt's NHL is done with the St. Jude staging system (see Table 41-8).[106] NHL of the bowel most commonly is first seen with abdominal pain, signs and symptoms of obstruction, intermittent gastrointestinal bleeding, and the potential for intestinal perforation. A palpable abdominal mass may be found in the right lower quadrant. Rapid enlargement of the mass or the rapid accumulation of ascites or both is typical. A clinical picture of intussusception may precipitate sudden symptoms, and nonoperative hydrostatic or pneumatic reduction will be unsuccessful.

Operation with biopsy, especially in the face of urgent symptoms, is often the diagnostic tool used. Staging laparotomy does not play a pre-emptive role in intestinal NHL. Other diagnostic tools include cytologic analysis of ascitic fluid removed by paracentesis or bone marrow

	Murphy Classification	St. Jude Staging
TABLE 41-8 **LYMPHOMA STAGING SYSTEMS**		
I	Involvement of single nodal group or single extranodal site	A single tumor (extranodal) or single anatomic area (nodal), with the exclusion of mediastinum or abdomen
II	Involvement of more than one nodal group on same side of diaphragm or single extranodal site and adjacent lymph nodes	A single tumor (extranodal) with regional node involvement; two or more nodal areas on the same side of the diaphragm; two single (extranodal) tumors with or without regional node involvement on the same side of the diaphragm; a primary GI tumor with or without involvement of associated mesenteric nodes
III	Disseminated disease on both sides of diaphragm, extensive unresectable abdominal disease, or primary skin involvement	Two single tumors (extranodal) on opposite sides of the diaphragm; two or more nodal areas above and below the diaphragm; all primary intrathoracic tumors (mediastinal, pleural, thymic); all extensive primary intra-abdominal disease; all paraspinal or epidural tumors, regardless of other tumor sites
IV	Addition of bone marrow or central nervous system involvement	Any of the above with initial central nervous system or bone marrow involvement

GI, gastrointestinal.

biopsy when diagnosing and staging an unknown abdominal mass, the latter being positive in as many as 20% to 40% of abdominal NHL. Cerebrospinal fluid cytologic evaluation also is required. Radiographic imaging is less invasive and less specific, but it may prove useful in identifying nodal disease in association with a primary mass. Serologic evaluation also may be useful to demonstrate tumor load by measuring serum lactate hydrogenase and uric acid as well as serum phosphate and potassium. Such an analysis may prove useful in the aggressive early management of the tumor-lysis syndrome or uric acid nephropathy that may characterize patients with bulky tumors, particularly rapidly doubling Burkitt's lymphoma.

NHL is a systemic disease, and multimodal therapy is indicated. Operation is reserved for biopsy and intra-abdominal assessment, typically while treating an acute surgical emergency such as intestinal obstruction or perforation. Because multiagent postoperative chemotherapy with or without radiation therapy is the rule, extensive operation that leaves multiple anastomoses, large raw denuded surfaces, and a large incision to heal may only inappropriately delay the needed nonoperative therapy. However, in the face of localized symptomatic tumor amenable to resection, operative resection that includes tumor-free margins and the adjacent mesentery may be preferred not only to treat the emergency symptoms but also to debulk primary tumor burden. In the face of more extensive disease, biopsy only should be done, including biopsy of the apparent primary tumor but also noting, and, where safe, performing a biopsy of tumor on peritoneal surfaces, in the omentum, and on other viscera. Proper fresh handling of the tumor specimens and the nodal disease is paramount to assuring diagnostic accuracy.

Multidrug chemotherapy has been the mainstay of treatment for NHL, and the use of cyclophosphamide, doxorubicin, vincristine, and prednisone (CHOP regimen) is preferred. For higher risk Burkitt's lymphoma, additional agents include methotrexate, cytarabine, and cisplatin. In addition to this primary treatment, radiation therapy and operative resection have served as adjuvants directed at achieving local disease control.

The treatment of lymphoma in the immunocompromised transplant patient depends on the characterization of the tumor. Toxic therapy is limited in these already immunocompromised patients. After transplantation, "polyclonal premalignant lymphomas" may effectively be treated with a reversal or withdrawal of immunosuppression; in more aggressive or "monoclonal lymphoma" disease or both, aggressive chemotherapy is indicated, along with operation or radiation therapy if achievement of local control is feasible.

Outcomes from NHL may be favorable, with a greater than 90% survival in the face of local primary tumor control after operative resection and multimodal chemotherapy. In the presence of either bulk disease not amenable to resection, cure rates decrease to 60% to 90%. With bone marrow, central nervous system, or local relapse, outcomes are less favorable, with 5-year survivals being in the 25% to 30% range. Poor prognostic factors include tumor beyond the regional lymph nodes, tumor size greater than 10 cm, immunoblastic histology, presence of aneuploidy, T-lymphocyte immunoperoxidase staining, and the clinical presentation as an acute abdomen. Outcomes from the intestinal T-cell lymphomas are generally less favorable.

Neuroendocrine Tumors

Carcinoid Tumors

These rare tumors are typically described by their site of origin as foregut, midgut, or hindgut. Intestinal carcinoids typically secrete serotonin (5-hydroxytryptamine) or serotonin precursors and account for almost three-fourths of the body's carcinoid tumors.[98] The frequency of location for gastrointestinal carcinoids is the

TABLE 41-9			
CHARACTERISTICS OF CARCINOID TUMORS			
Characteristic	Foregut	Midgut	Hindgut
Distribution	Bronchi Stomach Duodenum Pancreas	Small bowel Cecum Ascending colon	Remainder of colon Rectum
Primary secreting agents	5-HTP, histamine	Serotonin	Rare
Clinical manifestations	Atypical flushing	Flushing, diarrhea	None
Metastases	Bone	Liver	Bone
Carcinoid syndrome	Atypical	Classic	Rare

HTP, hydroxytryptophan.

following: small bowel, 29%, appendix, 19%, and the rectum, 12.5%. The tumor is more frequent in African Americans and in aged adults, although it does occur in children. Table 41-9 summarizes the tumor characteristics. The tumors typically are first seen in one of three ways: they most commonly are incidental findings at laparotomy; they may be seen secondary to a mass effect with pain, intussusception, intermittent bowel obstruction, or indolent gastrointestinal bleeding; or in only 10% of cases, they appear with the symptomatic carcinoid syndrome—cramps, diarrhea, flushing, bronchospasm, and cyanosis—secondary to the elaboration of 5-hydroxytryptophan (HTP), histamine, or serotonin (see Table 41-9).

The definitive diagnosis of the carcinoid syndrome depends first on establishing the biochemical evidence: a urinary 5-hydroxyindoloacetic acid level greater than 10 mg per 24 hours. Serotonin elevation also may be documented. Rarely, imaging may be diagnostic with nuclear medicine techniques and somatostatin-receptor agents, such as octreotide, that bind to receptors expressed in more than 80% of carcinoid tumors. Operation may be required to localize, resect, and definitely diagnose the tumor.

The extent of resection is dictated by the size of the primary tumor, which further influences the potential for tumor metastases. Carcinoids larger than 2 cm in diameter are frequently associated with additional nonlocalized regional tumors, and thus extended bowel resection with en bloc lymph node removal is preferred. This implies that the application of a right hemicolectomy is preferred when an appendiceal carcinoid tumor exceeds 2 cm in diameter. In contrast, appendiceal carcinoid tumors smaller than 1 cm in diameter are best treated with appendectomy alone.

Outcomes from carcinoid tumors vary by size and site of location. Five-year survivals from appendiceal carcinoid tumors approximate 85%, and from small bowel carcinoids, 55%. Not only is the somatostatin analogue octreotide effective in decreasing the 5-hydroxyindoloacetic acid excretion, but it also may improve the symptoms of the syndrome.

Neurogenic Tumors

Neuroblastoma or ganglioneuroma or both may either occur within or encroach on the bowel lumen. In addition, selected neuroblastomas influence the gastrointestinal tract by secreting vasoactive intestinal peptide (VIP) that may produce a diarrheagenic effect that can be profound. At times somatostatin analogues may be effective in limiting, although not ameliorating, these effects, and conventional neuroblastoma tumor therapy remains the mainstay of treatment (see Chapter 66).

Gastrinomas

These gastrin-elaborating tumors are more common in the stomach, duodenum, or the pancreas, and they are not further discussed in this chapter.

REFERENCES

1. Barton JR, Gillon S, Ferguson A: Incidence of inflammatory bowel disease in Scottish children between 1968 and 1983: Marginal fall in ulcerative colitis, three-fold rise in Crohn's disease. Gut 30:618–622, 1989.
2. Souza MH, Troncon LE, Rodrigues CM, et al: Trends in the occurrence (1980-1999) and clinical features of Crohn's disease and ulcerative colitis in a university hospital in southeastern Brazil. Arq Gastroenterol 39:98–105, 2002.
3. Urne FU, Paerregaard A: [Chronic inflammatory bowel disease in children: An epidemiological study from eastern Denmark 1998-2000]. Ugeskr Laeger 164:5810–5814, 2002.
4. Roth MP, Petersen GM, McElree C, et al: Geographic origins of Jewish patients with inflammatory bowel disease. Gastroenterology 97: 900–904, 1989.
5. Probert CS, Jayanthi V, Hughes AO, et al: Prevalence and family risk of ulcerative colitis and Crohn's disease: An epidemiological study among Europeans and south Asians in Leicestershire. Gut 34:1547–1551, 1993.
6. Montgomery SM, Lambe M, Wakefield AJ, et al: Siblings and the risk of inflammatory bowel disease. Scand J Gastroenterol 37:1301–1308, 2002.
7. Gilat T, Hacohen D, Lilos P, et al: Childhood factors in ulcerative colitis and Crohn's disease: An international cooperative study. Scand J Gastroenterol 22:1009–1024, 1987.
8. Toyoda H, Wang SJ, Yang HY, et al: Distinct associations of HLA class II genes with inflammatory bowel disease. Gastroenterology 104:741–748, 1993.
9. Kuhn R, Lohler J, Rennick D, et al: Interleukin-10-deficient mice develop chronic enterocolitis. Cell 75:263–274, 1993.
10. Sadlack B, Merz H, Schorle H, et al: Ulcerative colitis-like disease in mice with a disrupted interleukin-2 gene. Cell 75:253–261, 1993.
11. Chong SK, Blackshaw AJ, Morson BC, et al: Prospective study of colitis in infancy and early childhood. J Pediatr Gastroenterol Nutr 5:352–358, 1986.
12. Ferguson A: Assessment and management of ulcerative colitis in children. Eur J Gastroenterol Hepatol 9:858–863, 1997.

13. Ament ME, Vargas JH: Medical therapy for ulcerative colitis in childhood. Semin Pediatr Surg 3:28–32, 1994.
14. Michener WM, Whelan G, Greenstreet RL, et al: Comparison of the clinical features of Crohn's disease and ulcerative colitis with onset in childhood or adolescence. Cleve Clin Q 49:13–16, 1982.
15. Hyams JS: Extraintestinal manifestations of inflammatory bowel disease in children. J Pediatr Gastroenterol Nutr 19:7–21, 1994.
16. Coulson WF: Pathological features of inflammatory bowel disease in childhood. Semin Pediatr Surg 3:8–14, 1994.
17. Lichtiger S, Present DH, Kornbluth A, et al: Cyclosporine in severe ulcerative colitis refractory to steroid therapy. N Engl J Med 330:1841–1845, 1994.
18. Ramakrishna J, Langhans N, Calenda K, et al: Combined use of cyclosporine and azathioprine or 6-mercaptopurine in pediatric inflammatory bowel disease. J Pediatr Gastroenterol Nutr 22:296–302, 1996.
19. Nicholls S, Vieira MC, Majrowski WH, et al: Linear growth after colectomy for ulcerative colitis in childhood. J Pediatr Gastroenterol Nutr 21:82–86, 1995.
20. Ferzoco SJ, Becker JM: Does aggressive medical therapy for acute ulcerative colitis result in a higher incidence of staged colectomy? Arch Surg 129:420–423; discussion 423–424, 1994.
21. Heuschen UA, Hinz U, Allemeyer EH, et al: One- or two-stage procedure for restorative proctocolectomy: Rationale for a surgical strategy in ulcerative colitis. Ann Surg 234:788–794, 2001.
22. Solomon MJ, Schnitzler M: Cancer and inflammatory bowel disease: Bias, epidemiology, surveillance, and treatment. World J Surg 22:352–358, 1998.
23. Lashner BA: Colorectal cancer in ulcerative colitis patients: Survival curves and surveillance. Cleve Clin J Med 61:272–275, 1994.
24. Baker WN, Glass RE, Ritchie JK, et al: Cancer of the rectum following colectomy and ileorectal anastomosis for ulcerative colitis. Br J Surg 65:862–868, 1978.
25. Grundfest SF, Fazio V, Weiss RA, et al: The risk of cancer following colectomy and ileorectal anastomosis for extensive mucosal ulcerative colitis. Ann Surg 193:9–14, 1981.
26. Ravitch M, Sabiston D: Anal ileostomy with preservation of the sphincter: A proposed operation in patients requiring total colectomy for benign lesions. Surg Gynecol Obstet 84:1095–1097, 1947.
27. Parks AG: Transanal technique in low rectal anastomosis. Proc R Soc Med 65:975–976, 1972.
28. Parks AG, Nicholls RJ: Proctocolectomy without ileostomy for ulcerative colitis. Br Med J 2:85–88, 1978.
29. Nasmyth DG, Williams NS, Johnston D: Comparison of the function of triplicated and duplicated pelvic ileal reservoirs after mucosal proctectomy and ileo-anal anastomosis for ulcerative colitis and adenomatous polyposis. Br J Surg 73:361–366, 1986.
30. Tuckson WB, Fazio VW: Functional comparison between double and triple ileal loop pouches. Dis Colon Rectum 34:17–21, 1991.
31. Shamberger RC, Lillehei CW, Nurko S, et al: Anorectal function in children after ileoanal pull-through. J Pediatr Surg 29:329–332; discussion 332–333, 1994.
32. Dolgin SE, Shlasko E, Gorfine S, et al: Restorative proctocolectomy in children with ulcerative colitis utilizing rectal mucosectomy with or without diverting ileostomy. J Pediatr Surg 34:837–839; discussion 839–840, 1999.
33. Gorfine SR, Gelernt IM, Bauer JJ, et al: Restorative proctocolectomy without diverting ileostomy. Dis Colon Rectum 38:188–194, 1995.
34. Tjandra JJ, Fazio VW, Milsom JW, et al: Omission of temporary diversion in restorative proctocolectomy: Is it safe? Dis Colon Rectum 36:1007–1014, 1993.
35. Remzi FH, Church JM, Bast J, et al: Mucosectomy vs. stapled ileal pouch-anal anastomosis in patients with familial adenomatous polyposis: Functional outcome and neoplasia control. Dis Colon Rectum 44:1590–1596, 2001.
36. Johnston D, Holdsworth PJ, Nasmyth DG, et al: Preservation of the entire anal canal in conservative proctocolectomy for ulcerative colitis: A pilot study comparing end-to-end ileo-anal anastomosis without mucosal resection with mucosal proctectomy and endo-anal anastomosis. Br J Surg 74:940–944, 1987.
37. Kohler LW, Pemberton JH, Hodge DO, et al: Long-term functional results and quality of life after ileal pouch-anal anastomosis and cholecystectomy. World J Surg 16:1126–1131; discussion 1131–1132, 1992.
38. Becker JM: Ileal pouch-anal anastomosis: current status and controversies. Surgery 113:599–602, 1993.
39. Blumberg D, Opelka FG, Hicks TC, et al: Restorative proctocolectomy: Ochsner Clinic experience. South Med J 94:467–471, 2001.
40. Fleshman JW, Cohen Z, McLeod RS, et al: The ileal reservoir and ileoanal anastomosis procedure: Factors affecting technical and functional outcome. Dis Colon Rectum 31:10–16, 1988.
41. Blumberg D, Beck DE: Surgery for ulcerative colitis. Gastroenterol Clin North Am 31:219–235, 2002.
42. Nicholls RJ, Banerjee AK: Pouchitis: Risk factors, etiology, and treatment. World J Surg 22:347–351, 1998.
43. Fonkalsrud EW: Surgery for pediatric ulcerative colitis. Curr Opin Pediatr 7:323–327, 1995.
44. Fonkalsrud EW: Surgical management of ulcerative colitis in childhood. Semin Pediatr Surg 3:33–38, 1994.
45. Fonkalsrud EW: Clinical and physiologic studies with restorative proctocolectomy. Langenbecks Arch Chir Suppl Kongressbd 1118–1122, 1994.
46. Ky AJ, Sonoda T, Milsom JW: One-stage laparoscopic restorative proctocolectomy: An alternative to the conventional approach? Dis Colon Rectum 45:207–210; discussion 210–211, 2002.
47. Georgeson KE: Laparoscopic-assisted total colectomy with pouch reconstruction. Semin Pediatr Surg 11:233–236, 2002.
48. Bell RL, Seymour NE: Laparoscopic treatment of fulminant ulcerative colitis. Surg Endosc 16:1778–1782, 2002.
49. Proctor ML, Langer JC, Gerstle JT, et al: Is laparoscopic subtotal colectomy better than open subtotal colectomy in children? J Pediatr Surg 37:706–708, 2002.
50. Marcello PW, Milsom JW, Wong SK, et al: Laparoscopic restorative proctocolectomy: Case-matched comparative study with open restorative proctocolectomy. Dis Colon Rectum 43:604–608, 2000.
51. Seshadri PA, Poulin EC, Schlachta CM, et al: Does a laparoscopic approach to total abdominal colectomy and proctocolectomy offer advantages? Surg Endosc 15:837–842, 2001.
52. Barton JR, Ferguson A: Clinical features, morbidity and mortality of Scottish children with inflammatory bowel disease. Q J Med 75:423–439, 1990.
53. Kirschner BS: Ulcerative colitis in children. Pediatr Clin North Am 43:235–254, 1996.
54. Crohn BB, Ginzburg L, Oppenheimer GD: Regional ileitis: A pathologic and clinical entity. JAMA 99:1323–1329, 1932.
55. Krok KL, Lichtenstein GR: Nutrition in Crohn's disease. Curr Opin Gastroenterol 19:148–153, 2003.
56. Ewe K, Bottger T, Buhr HJ, et al: Low-dose budesonide treatment for prevention of postoperative recurrence of Crohn's disease: A multicentre randomized placebo-controlled trial: German Budesonide Study Group. Eur J Gastroenterol Hepatol 11:277–282, 1999.
57. Greenberg GR, Feagan BG, Martin F, et al: Oral budesonide as maintenance treatment for Crohn's disease: A placebo-controlled, dose-ranging study: Canadian Inflammatory Bowel Disease Study Group. Gastroenterology 110:45–51, 1996.
58. Pearson DC, May GR, Fick GH, et al: Azathioprine and 6-mercaptopurine in Crohn's disease: A meta-analysis. Ann Intern Med 123:132–142, 1995.
59. Pearson DC, May GR, Fick G, et al: Azathioprine for maintaining remission of Crohn's disease. Cochrane Database Syst Rev 2000:CD000067.
60. Hanauer SB, Feagan BF, Lichtenstein GR, ACCENT I Study Group, et al: Maintenance infliximab for Crohn's disease: The ACCENT I randomized trial. Lancet 359:1541–1549, 2002.
61. Hanauer SB, Feagan BG, Lichtenstein GR, et al: Maintenance infliximab (Remicade) is safe, effective and steroid-sparing in Crohn's disease: preliminary results from the ACCENT I trial. Gastroenterology 120:A21, 2001.
62. Targan SR, Hanauer SB, van Deventer SJ, et al: A short-term study of chimeric monoclonal antibody cA2 to tumor necrosis factor alpha for Crohn's disease: Crohn's Disease cA2 Study Group. N Engl J Med 337:1029–1035, 1997.

63. Present DH, Rutgeerts P, Targan S, et al: Infliximab for the treatment of fistulas in patients with Crohn's disease. N Engl J Med 340:1398–1405, 1999.

64. Weinberg AM, Rattan S, Lewis JD, et al: Strictures and response to infliximab in Crohn's disease. Am J Gastroenterol 97:S255, 2002.

65. Lichtenstein GR, Olson A, Bao W, et al: Infliximab treatment does not result in an increased risk of intestinal strictures or obstruction in Crohn's disease patients: Accent I study results. Am J Gastroenterol 97:S254, 2002.

66. Patrel HI, Leichtner AM, Shamberger RC: Surgery for Crohn's disease in infants and children. J Pediatr Surg 32:1063–1068, 1997.

67. Block GE, Moosa AR, Simonowitz D: The operative treatment of Crohn's disease in childhood. Surg Gynecol Obstet 144:713–717, 1977.

68. Abriola GF, DeAngelis P, Dall'Oglio L, et al: Strictureplasty: An alternative approach in long segment bowel stenosis in Crohn's disease. J Pediatr Surg 38:814–818, 2003.

69. Dutta S, Rothenberg SS, Chang J, et al: Total intracorporeal laparoscopic resection of Crohn's disease. J Pediatr Surg 38:717–719, 2003.

70. Diamond IR, Langer JC: Laparoscopic-assisted versus open ileocolic resection for Crohn's disease. J Pediatr Gastroenterol Nutr 33:543–547, 2001.

71. Boardman LA: Heritable colorectal cancer syndromes: Recognition and preventive management. Gastroenterol Clin North Am 31:1107–1131, 2002.

72. Corredor J, Wambach J, Barnard J: Gastrointestinal polyps in children: Advances in molecular genetics, diagnosis, and management. J Pediatr 138:621–628, 2001.

73. Winawer SJ, Stewart ET, Zauber AG, et al: A comparison of colonoscopy and double-contrast barium enema for surveillance after polypectomy: National Polyp Study Work Group. N Engl J Med 342:1766–1772, 2000.

74. Friedl W, Caspari R, Sengteller M, et al: Can APC mutation analysis contribute to therapeutic decisions in familial adenomatous polyposis? Experience from 680 FAP families. Gut 48:515–521, 2001.

75. Church JM, McGannon E, Burke C, et al: Teenagers with familial adenomatous polyposis: What is their risk for colorectal cancer? Dis Colon Rectum 45:887–889, 2002.

76. Soravia C, Berk T, McLeod RS, et al: Desmoid disease in patients with familial adenomatous polyposis. Dis Colon Rectum 43:363–369, 2000.

77. Bertario L, Russo A, Sala P, et al: Genotype and phenotype factors as determinants of desmoid tumors in patients with familial adenomatous polyposis. Int J Cancer 95:102–107, 2001.

78. Vasen HF, van Duijvendijk P, Buskens E, et al: Decision analysis in the surgical treatment of patients with familial adenomatous polyposis: A Dutch Scandinavian collaborative study including 659 patients. Gut 49:231–235, 2001.

79. Gwyn K, Sinicrope FA: Chemoprevention of colorectal cancer. Am J Gastroenterol 97:13–21, 2002.

80. Gardiello FM, Yang VW, Hylind LM, et al: Primary chemoprevention of familial adenomatous polyposis with sulindac. N Engl J Med 346:1054–1059, 2002.

81. Steinbach G, Lynch PM, Phillips RK, et al: The effect of celecoxib, a cyclooxygenase-2 inhibitor, in familial adenomatous polyposis. N Engl J Med 342:1946–1952, 2000.

82. Giardiello FM, Hamilton SR, Krush AJ, et al: Treatment of colonic and rectal adenomas with sulindac in familial adenomatous polyposis. N Engl J Med 328:1313–1316, 1993.

83. Phillips RK, Wallace MH, Lynch PM, et al: A randomized, double blind, placebo controlled study of celecoxib, a selective cyclooxygenase-2 inhibitor, on duodenal polyposis in familial adenomatous polyposis. Gut 50:857–860, 2002.

84. Baron JA, Cole BF, Sandler RS, et al: A randomized trial of aspirin to prevent colorectal adenomas. N Engl J Med 348:891–899, 2003.

85. Khosraviani K, Weir HP, Hamilton P, et al: Effect of folate supplementation on mucosal cell proliferation in high risk patients with colon cancer. Gut 51:195–199, 2002.

86. Moslein G, Pistorius S, Saeger HD, et al: Preventive surgery for colon cancer in familial adenomatous polyposis and hereditary nonpolyposis colorectal cancer syndrome. Langenbecks Arch Surg 388:9–16, 2003.

87. van Duijvendijk P, Slors JF, Taat CW, et al: Functional outcome after colectomy and ileorectal anastomosis compared with proctocolectomy and ileal pouch-anal anastomosis in familial adenomatous polyposis. Ann Surg 230:648–654, 1999.

88. Fonkalsrud EW, Thakur A, Beanes S: Ileoanal pouch procedures in children. J Pediatr Surg 36:1689–1692, 2001.

89. Wehrle BM, Weiss SW, Yandow S, et al: Gardner-associated fibromas (GAF) in young patients: A distinct fibrous lesion that identifies unsuspected Gardner syndrome and risk for fibromatosis. Am J Surg Pathol 25:645–651, 2001.

90. Attard TM, Yardley JH, Cuffari C: Gastric polyps in pediatrics: an 18-year hospital-based analysis. Am J Gastroenterol 97:298–301, 2002.

91. Kalady MF, Clary BM, Tyler DS, et al: Pancreas-preserving duodenectomy in the management of duodenal familial adenomatous polyposis. J Gastrointest Surg 6:82–87, 2002.

92. Parc YR, Moslein G, Dozois RR, et al: Familial adenomatous polyposis: Results after ileal pouch-anal anastomosis in teenagers. Dis Colon Rectum 43:893–898, 2000.

93. Rintala RJ, Lindahl HG: Proctocolectomy and J-pouch ileo-anal anastomosis in children. J Pediatr Surg 37:66–70, 2002.

94. Litle VR, Barbour S, Schrock TR, et al: The continent ileostomy: Long-term durability and patient satisfaction. J Gastrointest Surg 3:625–632, 1999.

95. Martinez ME, Sampliner R, Marshall JR, et al: Adenoma characteristics as risk factors for recurrence of advanced adenomas. Gastroenterology 120:1077–1078, 2001.

96. Parc YR, Olschwang S, Desaint B, et al: Familial adenomatous polyposis: Prevalence of adenomas in the ileal pouch after restorative proctocolectomy. Ann Surg 233:360–364, 2001.

97. Olsen KO, Juul S, Bulow S, et al: Female fecundity before and after operation for familial adenomatous polyposis. Br J Surg 90:227–231, 2003.

98. Gill SS, Heuman DM, Mihas AA: Small intestinal neoplasms. J Clin Gastroenterol 33:267–282, 2001.

99. Fishman SJ, Burrows PE, Leichtner AM, et al: Gastrointestinal manifestations of vascular anomalies in childhood: Varied etiologies require multiple therapeutic modalities. J Pediatr Surg 33:1163–1167, 1998.

100. Shteyer E, Koplewitz BZ, Gross E, et al: Medical treatment of recurrent intussusception associated with intestinal lymphoid hyperplasia. Pediatrics 111:682–685, 2003.

101. Lynch HT, de la Chapelle A: Genetic susceptibility to nonpolyposis colo rectal cancer. J Med Genet 36:801–818, 1999.

102. Radhakrishnan CN, Bruce J: Colorectal cancers in children without any predisposing factors: A report of eight cases and review of the literature. Eur J Pediatr Surg 13:66–68, 2003.

103. Abrahams NA, Halverson A, Fazio VW, et al: Adenocarcinoma of the small bowel: A study of 37 cases with emphasis on histologic prognostic factors. Dis Colon Rectum 45:496–502, 2002.

104. Howe JR, Karnell LH, Menck HR, et al., and The American College of Surgeons Commission on Cancer and the American Cancer Society: Adenocarcinoma of the small bowel: Review of the National Cancer Data Base, 1985–1995. Cancer 86:2693–2706, 1999.

105. Shorter NA: Tumors of the small bowel. In Oldman KT, Colombani PM, Foglia RP (eds): Surgery of Infants and Children: Scientific Principles and Practice. Philadelphia, Lippincott-Raven, 1997, pp 1249–1252.

106. Koniaris LG, Drugas G, Katzman P, et al: Management of gastrointestinal lymphoma. J Am Coll Surg 197:127–141, 2003.

CHAPTER 42

Appendicitis

Stephen E. Morrow, MD, and Kurt D. Newman, MD

HISTORY

Although the symptoms of appendicitis were first recorded more than 5 hundred years ago, the disease remained a mystery until the 19th century.[1] Autopsies performed in the early 19th century suggested that cecal inflammation was responsible for the pathophysiology seen in appendicitis, and the term *typhillitis* reflected that assumption. In 1886, American pathologist Reginald Fitz[2] identified the true source of inflammation in typhillitis was in the appendix, not the cecum, and he coined the term *appendicitis*. After the introduction of anesthesia, successful appendectomies were reported in the late 19th century by Groves, Grant, Morton, Senn, and McBurney. In 1889, McBurney[3] described the point of maximal abdominal tenderness in appendicitis and recommended appendectomy as the proper treatment. Experiments by Wangensteen[4] in 1939 demonstrated that luminal obstruction initiates the inflammatory process in appendicitis. Prompt appendectomy became the standard treatment for appendicitis in the beginning of the 20th century and has remained so to the present day. Refinements in the last half-century have included the use of antibiotics, nonoperative management for selected patients with or without interval appendectomy, improved diagnostic imaging techniques, radiologic-guided percutaneous abscess drainage, and the use of laparoscopy for appendectomy.

CLINICAL FEATURES

Appendicitis is the most common cause of the acute surgical abdomen in children and adults and currently accounts for approximately one third of childhood hospitalizations for abdominal pain.[5] The lifetime risk of appendicitis is estimated to be 8.67% for boys and 6.7% for girls.[6] Appendicitis is most common in older children and adolescents, with a peak incidence between ages 12 and 18 years. A genetic predisposition appears operative in some cases, particularly in children in whom appendicitis develops before age 6 years.[7] A family history of appendicitis is obtained in 36% of patients with proven appendicitis compared with 14% of patients with right lower quadrant pain without appendicitis.[8]

Most authors believe the cause of appendicitis is luminal obstruction caused by lymphoid hyperplasia, inspissated fecal matter, an ingested foreign body, or parasites. Submucosal lymphoid follicles are few in number at birth but multiply steadily, to reach a peak number in the teen years. Appendiceal lymphoid tissue then sharply declines after age 30 years.[9] Both fecoliths and appendicitis are more frequent in developed countries with a high consumption of refined, low-fiber diets than in developing nations consuming high-fiber diets.[10] After appendiceal obstruction occurs, mucus production and bacterial proliferation raise intraluminal pressure, which in turn impairs lymphatic and venous drainage and causes tissue edema. Congestion of the organ compromises arterial inflow, and tissue ischemia, necrosis, and perforation follow thereafter. Although this sequence of events seems to occur in most cases of appendicitis, luminal obstruction is not always found on histologic examination. Bacteria such as *Yersinia, Salmonella,* and *Shigella* spp. and viruses such as mumps, coxsackie B, and adenovirus have been implicated in appendicitis.[11,12] Case reports of appendicitis after blunt abdominal trauma have been reported.[13] In children with cystic fibrosis, painful distention of the appendix may develop from abnormal mucus production without inflammation.[14] Appendicitis in neonates is rare and warrants evaluation for cystic fibrosis as well as Hirschsprung's disease.[15] Neonatal appendicitis also can be indistinguishable from focal necrotizing enterocolitis confined to the appendix.[16]

Like those of most human diseases, the diagnosis of appendicitis is best made with a careful history and physical examination. The clinician must remember that appendicitis in children often deviates from the classic description of the disease and that the differential diagnosis varies with the age of the child. Appendicitis classically begins with anorexia followed by vague periumbilical pain. However, it is not unusual for older children with appendicitis to say that they are hungry if asked. The periumbilical pain migrates after several hours to the right lower quadrant. Once localized, the pain is steady and is aggravated by movement. Nausea and vomiting classically follow the pain, but many children will vomit before the onset of pain. Diarrhea is a significant finding in perforated appendicitis but also may occur with acute, nonperforated appendicitis. It also is common in infants and toddlers[17] and may lead to the misdiagnosis of gastroenteritis. In general, however, repeated episodes of vomiting and diarrhea are more suggestive of gastroenteritis than of appendicitis, especially in older children. Ruptured appendicitis may be initially seen as a bowel obstruction, particularly in infants and young children. Fever, if present, is usually low grade in acute appendicitis; high fever accompanies appendiceal rupture. The appendix commonly, but by no means always, ruptures about 24 to 48 hours after the onset of symptoms. As appendicitis may mimic many diseases, a careful review of systems to consider alternative diagnoses is important.

Physical examination usually demonstrates percussion tenderness near McBurney's point, which he described originally as the point "one and a half to two inches from the anterior superior iliac process along a line drawn from the process to the umbilicus."[3] Other methods of eliciting peritoneal irritation often produce pain as well, depending on the degree of inflammation and location of the appendix. "Rebound" tenderness, elicited by deep palpation of the abdomen followed by abrupt removal of pressure, is very painful, has poor correlation with peritonitis and should be avoided. Children with retrocecal appendices or large, thick abdominal walls often have less tenderness on abdominal palpation. Determination of tenderness in a crying, resistant child can be difficult. The examiner often requires gentleness, patience, warm hands, and the assistance of a reassuring parent to obtain a reliable examination. In difficult cases, sedation may be necessary. Digital rectal examination is unlikely to contribute to the evaluation of appendicitis in children.[18] However, it remains important in cases of suspected pelvic abscess or ovarian pathology. Bowel sounds are usually absent when perforation has occurred or are hyperactive with gastroenteritis. High-pitched sounds and "rushes" suggest obstruction. A mass in the right lower quadrant can easily be missed if the patient has muscular guarding or rigidity. Often such masses are first palpated on the operating table after anesthesia has been induced.

Laboratory studies are not very sensitive or specific for appendicitis but may alter the clinician's suspicion of the disease. The leukocyte count is typically mildly elevated (11,000 to 16,000/mm^3) but may be normal or, rarely, even markedly elevated, even in nonperforated cases. However, a very high white cell count usually suggests perforation or another diagnosis. The urine should be free of bacteria but may have a few red or white blood cells if the inflamed appendix is adjacent to the ureter or bladder. The urine is often concentrated and contains ketones from diminished oral intake and vomiting.

Electrolytes and liver chemistries are usually normal. Several studies recently examined C-reactive protein in appendicitis and found that it usually increases in proportion to the degree of appendiceal inflammation. It becomes markedly elevated with perforation but is less reliably elevated in children than in adults.[19,20] No studies have demonstrated the superiority of C-reactive protein to the white blood cell count. Furthermore, a normal C-reactive protein and white blood cell count do not exclude appendicitis.[21] Thus C-reactive protein is not routinely measured in the diagnostic evaluation of appendicitis.[20,22]

Several reports described clinical scoring systems incorporating specific elements of the history, physical examination, and laboratory studies designed to improve diagnostic accuracy. A few authors found that such scores are remarkably accurate,[23] but others found that their sensitivity and specificity is only modest (76% to 78%),[24] thus rendering them no better than experienced clinical judgment. To date, all efforts to find clinical features or laboratory tests, either alone or in combination, that are able to diagnose appendicitis with 100% sensitivity or specificity have proven futile. However, diagnostic accuracy with clinical criteria alone can be improved in equivocal cases by repeating the physical examination and laboratory studies over a period of 12 to 24 hours. The patient's clinical course during this observation period often simplifies the decision to discharge the patient or proceed with appendectomy. Observation with repeated examination is cost-effective and often avoids radiologic imaging. Fewer than 2% of children's appendixes will perforate while under observation.[25]

Spontaneous resolution of appendicitis occasionally occurs,[26] as does relapsing or "chronic" appendicitis.[27] Perforation is most common in young children, with rates as high as 82% noted among children younger than 5 years and 100% in 1-year-olds.[28] The overall rupture rate varied from 20% to 76%, with a median of 36%, in a recent analysis of data from 30 pediatric hospitals in the United States.[29] In a study of 1366 pediatric appendectomies performed in 147 Department of Defense hospitals worldwide over a 1-year period, the perforation rate and the negative appendectomy rate were both 20%. Major complications occurred in 1.2% of cases of acute appendicitis compared with 6.4% of perforated appendicitis cases.[30] Predictably, length of hospitalization is increased from a median of 3 days in nonperforated cases to 9 days in perforated appendicitis.[28] The delayed diagnosis of appendicitis and corresponding perforation rates have been attributed by various authors to socioeconomic factors such as access to health care, insurance status, and patient-referral patterns. For example, children with perforation are much more likely to have been initially referred to a pediatrician rather than to a surgeon.[31]

RADIOLOGIC IMAGING

Delay in the diagnosis and treatment of appendicitis leads to substantial increases in morbidity, length of hospitalization, and cost. Traditionally, negative laparotomy rates of 10% to 20% were considered appropriate to keep perforation rates low. Many authors have recently criticized previously accepted negative laparotomy rates, citing the risks and expense of unnecessary surgery.[32] When properly performed and interpreted, imaging studies are generally more accurate than a surgeon's clinical diagnosis. This fact has led many primary care and emergency physicians to order imaging studies before consulting a surgeon. Interestingly, modern imaging has not improved the overall rate of negative appendectomies.[34] However, some reports from children's hospitals cite negative appendectomy rates of less than 2% with the use of diagnostic imaging[29] (Fig. 42-1).

Plain films, the oldest and simplest radiologic study, may show sentinel loops of bowel caused by a localized ileus or mild scoliosis from psoas spasm. They also demonstrate a fecolith in approximately 10% to 15% of cases of perforated appendicitis. Fecoliths are very suggestive of appendicitis when present in a patient with abdominal pain.[34] However, plain films have a very low sensitivity for appendicitis and are not recommended unless a bowel obstruction, a mass, or free peritoneal air is suspected.[35] Barium enemas were used in the past but have been supplanted by ultrasonography (US) and computerized tomography (CT).

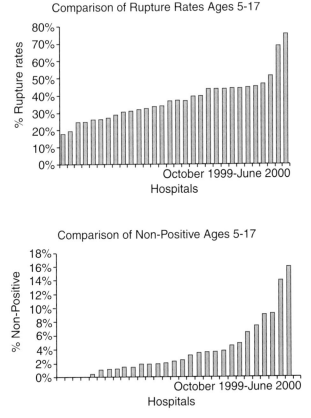

FIGURE 42-1. *A,* Ruptured appendectomy rates among 30 children's hospitals. *B,* Nonpositive appendectomy rates among the same hospitals. (From Newman K, Ponsky T, Kittle K, et al: Appendicitis 2000: Variability in practice, outcomes, and resource utilization at thirty pediatric hospitals. J Pediatr Surg 38:372–379, 2003.)

US has excellent specificity in most series (>90%) but variable sensitivity (50% to 92%), according to the skill of the technician and patient factors such as obesity, cooperation, and peritoneal irritation.[36] A normal appendix must be visualized to exclude appendicitis by US. The US criteria for appendicitis include the presence of a noncompressible tubular structure 6 mm or greater in diameter, a complex mass in the right lower quadrant, or a fecolith (Fig. 42-2). Reports from centers with skilled ultrasonographers often recommend US for all children with suspected appendicitis.[37] Other reports cite the superiority of US over surgical judgment in clinically equivocal cases.[38-40] US is recommended by many authors as the best first-line study in most children because of its low cost and freedom from both patient preparation and ionizing radiation.

CT is not operator dependent and has a higher sensitivity and specificity than US in most pediatric series (>95% for both).[41] However, CT is more expensive than US, may require contrast administration, and may call for sedation in uncooperative children. The radiation exposure from a single CT scan also subjects each child to an estimated one in a thousand lifetime mortality risk from radiation-induced malignancy.[42] Children typically have less intra-abdominal fat than do adults, which makes the identification of periappendiceal fat-stranding more difficult and thus lowers the diagnostic accuracy in some pediatric studies. For this reason, some authors recommend colonic contrast in children to improve accuracy[43] (Fig. 42-3). Others report excellent accuracy with unenhanced CT scans in children (99% vs. 91% for US).[44] Still others have found that CT offers no improvement in diagnostic accuracy for appendicitis over a standard history, physical examination, and laboratory analysis.[45,46]

The use of magnetic resonance imaging (MRI) to evaluate acute abdominal pain in children has been limited because it is more time consuming, usually requires sedation or general anesthesia, is more expensive, and is less accessible than US or CT. One study of MRI in 45 children found unenhanced T_2-weighted imaging was 100% sensitive for appendicitis.[47] MRI appears to offer the accuracy of CT without radiation exposure and could become the future imaging modality of choice for the evaluation of abdominal pain if its disadvantages can be minimized or eliminated.

Finally, radionuclide-labeled white blood cell scans have been used in some centers under unusual circumstances when other imaging modalities are inconclusive. Tagged white cell scans have a very high sensitivity but only modest specificity (97% vs. 80%).[48]

The impressive accuracy of imaging studies has led some practitioners to order them for all children with possible appendicitis to reduce the negative laparotomy rate without increasing the perforation rate. However, the accuracy of both clinical judgment and imaging studies varies significantly from one medical center to another. Imaging studies, like all medical tests, cost money, can delay treatment, and can be falsely positive or negative. The false-negative risk of an imaging study is increased when used in children with a high clinical suspicion of appendicitis, just as the false-positive risk of a study is

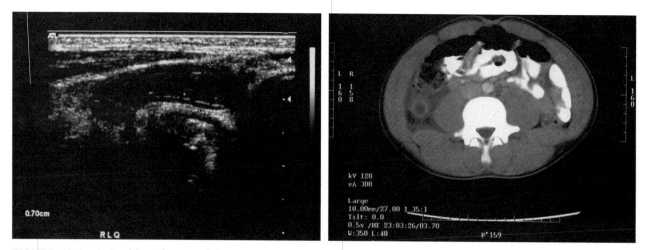

FIGURE 42-2. *A*, Positive ultrasound for acute appendicitis: a noncompressible tubular structure >6 mm in diameter. *B*, Computed tomography scan showing acute appendicitis. *Arrow,* Enlarged appendix and adjacent "fat-stranding" consistent with inflammation. (Courtesy of Dorothy Bulas, MD, Department of Radiology, Children's National Medical Center, Washington, DC.)

increased when used in children with a low clinical suspicion.[49] Thus maximal benefit of imaging is obtained when its use is limited to children with clinically equivocal presentations, yet the lack of consensus on this issue is reflected by the fact that the use of diagnostic imaging recently varied from 18% to 89% of cases of suspected appendicitis at 30 American pediatric hospitals.[29] Our general preference is to begin with US in equivocal cases of appendicitis and then follow with a CT scan if the US is inconclusive. CT is our first-line test for obese children, probable advanced appendicitis, clinically suspected alternative diagnoses, and whenever US is not readily available. This approach is both highly accurate and cost-effective.[49,50]

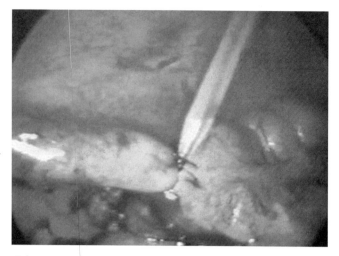

FIGURE 42-3. Intraoperative photograph of laparoscopic appendectomy for acute appendicitis. Endoloop ligature being applied to base of appendix. (Courtesy of David Powell, MD, Department of Surgery, Children's National Medical Center, Washington, DC.)

DIFFERENTIAL DIAGNOSIS

Appendicitis in children is first seen in an "atypical" fashion in approximately 50% of cases and can mimic many other diseases. Thus the diagnosis of appendicitis continues to challenge even the most astute clinician. Other inflammatory disorders such as cecal, sigmoid, or Meckel's diverticulitis; inflammatory bowel disease; cholecystitis; pancreatitis; gastroenteritis; mesenteric adenitis; pneumonia; neutropenic typhillitis; urinary tract infection; and pelvic inflammatory disease can masquerade as appendicitis. Gastroenteritis is the diagnosis most commonly made in cases of missed appendicitis.[31] Ovarian cysts, follicle rupture, and torsion are important considerations in girls. Blunt abdominal trauma may cause pain similar to that of appendicitis; indeed, some authors believe trauma can even cause appendicitis.[51] Lymphoma and tumors of the appendix (carcinoid, adenocarcinoma), large and small intestine, and ovary may simulate appendicitis as well.

TREATMENT

The treatment of appendicitis depends on both the patient's general condition and the state of the appendix. Children with appendicitis are often dehydrated and may be febrile, acidotic, and even septic. Intravenous fluids and antibiotics are always indicated preoperatively. The antibiotic regimen selected should be effective against the bacterial flora found in the appendix. Anaerobic bacteria make up most of the colonic flora and include *Bacteroides, Clostridia,* and *Peptostreptococcus* spp. Gram-negative aerobic bacteria such as *Escherichia coli, Pseudomonas aeruginosa, Enterobacter,* and *Klebsiella* spp. also are important. Gram-positive organisms are less commonly found in the colon, and the need to provide antibiotic coverage for them (primarily enterococcus) is controversial. For non-perforated appendicitis, a single agent such as cefoxitin, cefotetan, ampicillin/sulbactam, ticarcillin/clavulanate, or piperacillin/tazobactam is typically prescribed. In perforated appendicitis, most surgeons select either traditional "triple" antibiotics (ampicillin, gentamycin, and clindamycin or metronidozole) or a combination such as ceftriaxone/metronidozole or ticarcillin/clavulanate plus gentamycin. In one study, ticarcillin/clavulante plus gentamycin was superior to ampicillin/gentamycin/clindamycin in terms of decreased length of stay, duration of fever, and complications.[52] Another study found equal efficacy with piperacillin/tazobactam compared with triple antibiotics in perforated appendicitis.[53]

If the patient has early, nonperforated appendicitis, prompt appendectomy is indicated. Appendectomy has traditionally been treated as a semiemergency procedure. Recent data suggest that perforation rates and clinical morbidity are not increased if appendectomy is delayed for 12 to 24 hours.[54,55] Appendectomy is less urgent in perforated appendicitis. If peritonitis is present, most surgeons will proceed with appendectomy after preoperative fluid resuscitation and antibiotics have been initiated. Others will continue nonoperative management and avoid appendectomy completely or perform an interval appendectomy in 8 to 12 weeks if the patient returns to normal. A child who fails to improve within 24 to 72 hours needs an appendectomy. One study found nonoperative treatment fails 84% of the time if the patient has greater than 15% band forms in the differential white cell count.[56] When choosing among treatment options, the surgeon should keep in mind that some cases are difficult to categorize accurately as perforated or nonperforated preoperatively.

Interval appendectomy is controversial. Some authors do not perform this procedure, citing a low risk (approximately 14%) of recurrent appendicitis.[57] Others emphasize the high rate of pathologic findings in interval appendectomy specimens.[58,59] In a recent survey of the members of the American Pediatric Surgical Association (APSA), 86% perform interval appendectomy routinely after nonoperative management of perforated appendicitis.[60] In cases of a single, contained appendiceal abscess, percutaneous drainage under radiologic guidance is commonly performed and may be easier and safer than operative drainage. If operation is undertaken with advanced appendicitis, the surgeon may encounter an extremely inflamed appendix and cecum, with densely adherent loops of small bowel. Injury to the intestine and ureter may occur. In this situation, a safe appendectomy may be difficult. Options include drainage alone, appendectomy with extra steps taken to secure stump closure (such as ligation with inversion, stump coverage with omentum or pericolonic fat, or use of a stapling device), tube cecostomy, and even partial cecectomy or ileocecectomy with primary anastamosis.[61] Each of these techniques has advantages and disadvantages.

Culture of the peritoneal fluid during appendectomy has been shown to be of no benefit.[62,63] Standard antibiotic regimens that cover the appendiceal flora usually cover any pathogens that grow in culture, and the bacteria that are cultured may not be the clinically significant pathogens. One study demonstrated that children whose peritoneal fluid was cultured actually did somewhat worse than those whose fluid was not cultured.[63] However, cultures should be obtained in cases of tertiary peritonitis because previous antibiotics may have selected resistant organisms. Peritoneal lavage with saline or antibiotic solution has never been shown to reduce the incidence of postoperative abscess.[64] Similarly, the use of drains has not proved useful except in cases of walled-off abscess cavities.[65,66] Nevertheless, many surgeons use these adjuncts. Injection of bupivacaine into the wound has been shown to reduce postoperative pain significantly in a randomized controlled trial in children.[67]

Appendectomy has been performed through a muscle-splitting right lower quadrant incision for more than 100 years. In the past 2 decades, laparoscopic appendectomy (LA) has become increasingly popular (see Fig. 42-3). Some surgeons perform LA routinely, others use LA selectively, and still others prefer open appendectomy (OA) for all patients. Although considerable variation exists in study methods and outcome measures in published series concerning LA, pediatric studies generally conclude that LA is comparable to OA in most aspects. Postoperative pain has not been shown to be significantly reduced by LA in randomized pediatric trials. Some studies cite a decreased length of stay for LA.[68-70] These same studies, however, cite a seemingly long length of stay for OA, raising the question of bias based on traditional practice or the perception that minimally invasive procedures should automatically correlate with early hospital discharge. The cosmetic advantage of the laparoscopic approach varies with the child's body habitus. In thin children, OA can be performed with a single incision approximately 2 cm long and competes easily with multiple cannula sites in such patients. LA is more expensive,[71] may be technically challenging and take longer to perform,[68,72] and increases the risk of postoperative abscess when used in perforated appendicitis.[72,73] A review of 45 recently published trials of LA compared with OA showed that LA reduced the rate of wound infections by one half but increased the rate of intra-abdominal abscess 4 times.[74] The threshold for operation may be lowered by some clinicians who use the laparoscopic technique, as some studies note that more normal appendices are removed with the laparoscope (21% vs. 13% for OA).[33,68] This finding is significant, considering that some laparoscopic surgeons leave a normal-appearing appendix in situ, especially if another cause of the patient's symptoms is found.[74] A purported advantage of this approach is a reduced negative appendectomy rate. However, the argument against the removal of a normal appendix is the cost and complication risk to the patient, and these factors are not significantly altered by the use of diagnostic laparoscopy. The pathology report also does not always correlate with the surgeon's diagnosis. Thus leaving untouched a "normal" appendix risks leaving early but progressive appendicitis in situ or facing postoperatively the dilemma of persistent or recurrent symptoms.

Inadvertent injury to other abdominal structures seems to occur slightly more commonly with LA but is still rare. We prefer to use the laparoscopic approach in obese children, in those with suspected alternative diagnoses, in children with inconclusive radiologic studies, and in menstruating girls and use the open technique in most of the remaining children.

Postoperatively, most surgeons advocate 24 hours of antibiotic coverage in cases of acute appendicitis and advance the diet as tolerated. Most children are discharged from the hospital within 24 to 48 hours. In cases of perforated appendicitis, intravenous antibiotics are typically continued until the patient is afebrile for 24 hours and the white blood cell count has returned to normal. This approach has been validated prospectively.[75] Many children are able to complete their antibiotic therapy at home. Studies have demonstrated that home antibiotics are safe and cost-effective, with an approximate 7% readmission rate for abscess or bowel obstruction.[76] Evidence also exists that the use of oral antibiotics at home after return of enteral function, regardless of fever or leukocytosis, may be equivalent to intravenous antibiotic regimens.[77]

COMPLICATIONS

Most complications from appendicitis arise from the infectious nature of the entity. Wound infections are most common, yet are substantially less common in children than in adults. In a recent survey, 80% of American pediatric surgeons perform primary wound closure after open appendectomy, even in perforated cases.[60] Despite this practice, a wound-infection rate of just 3% to 11% is reported.[78,79] Some surgeons avoid primary wound closure in obese children, those taking steroids, and immuno-compromised children, although the literature does not support this practice.[80] In very rare cases, necrotizing fasciitis may develop, with life-threatening consequences. Excessive wound pain, high fever, tachycardia, and "dishwater" drainage are classic findings of this complication. Prompt recognition, broad-spectrum antibiotics, and aggressive debridement to healthy bleeding tissue are essential. Intra-abdominal abscess occurs in approximately 1% to 2% of children with perforated appendicitis.[81] It occasionally occurs in nonperforated cases as well. In contrast to that in adults, percutaneous drainage of postappendectomy abscesses is rarely needed in children. Intravenous or oral antibiotics or both alone lead to successful abscess resolution in more than 90% of cases.[82] Sepsis is not rare in advanced appendicitis but usually responds promptly to antibiotics, fluids, and other supportive measures. Multisystem organ failure and death still occasionally occur, particularly in neonates and immuno-compromised children. In a 1986 literature review, mortality in neonatal appendicitis was 71%, with survivors limited to neonates having an inflamed appendix within an inguinal hernia sac.[83]

Adhesive bowel obstruction occurs in approximately 5% of perforated cases. Postoperative intestinal ileus is almost universal in cases of perforated appendicitis. Gastric decompression and intravenous nutrition may be necessary while waiting for intestinal peristalsis to resume. Early adhesive postoperative bowel obstruction may be safely managed with bowel rest during the first 3 weeks after appendectomy because intestinal ischemia is highly unusual in this setting. Failure to resolve may require operative adhesiolysis. In contrast, children seen initially with a bowel obstruction due to appendicitis rarely improve without operation. The diagnosis of postoperative intussusception is typically delayed because it occurs with nausea, vomiting, and distention, all of which are common after laparotomy. Of note, one study found that 5 of 11 children with postappendectomy intussusception had undergone an inversion appendectomy.[84]

OTHER ISSUES

Children with a ventriculoperitoneal shunt may present a diagnostic challenge because spontaneous bacterial peritonitis and pseudocysts occur in these children and may masquerade as appendicitis. Radiologic imaging takes on an increased role in caring for these children. Contrary to popular assumption, ascending infection of the shunt tubing and cerebrospinal fluid rarely occurs with primary peritoneal infections such as appendicitis. Thus the shunt tubing may be left in place after appendectomy, even in cases of perforated appendicitis.[85] However, intra-abdominal infection may impair drainage of cerebrospinal fluid and necessitate shunt removal on that basis. Infected pseudocysts and the presence of cerebrospinal fluid contamination require exteriorization of the shunt. Children with cerebral palsy and spina bifida present similar diagnostic challenges. One study noted a 14% mortality in children with spina bifida and appendicitis.[86]

Differentiating appendicitis from typhillitis in neutropenic children also is challenging. Imaging studies are essential in these children. Despite careful clinical evaluation, a diagnostic error rate of 37% has been reported.[87] Incidental appendectomy during exploration for a malignant intra-abdominal tumor has been urged by some authors to prevent potentially fatal appendicitis occurring during chemotherapy-induced neutropenia.[88] In one study of 1910 children with Wilms' tumor, only 24% had incidental appendectomy during nephrectomy. No difference was found in infectious postoperative complications between those who had appendectomy and those who did not, nor was a difference in complications seen between the inversion and standard appendectomy techniques. However, in only 0.2% of children who did not have an incidental appendectomy was acute appendicitis noted during a median follow-up period of 5 years.[89]

One traditional argument for aggressive operative management in cases of suspected appendicitis was the belief that female fertility is impaired after ruptured appendicitis.[90] However, more recent studies have found that perforated appendicitis did not increase the risk of infertility.[91,92] Conclusive studies on this issue are lacking.

Recently, clinical practice guidelines for the management of appendicitis based on the best available evidence have been designed in an effort to minimize hospital stay and cost while improving patient care and outcome.[35,93]

One impetus for these guidelines has been the realization that a wide variety of management strategies exist. In a recent survey of the APSA membership, only 17% of pediatric surgeons follow a formal clinical practice guideline, whereas 24% follow an informal guideline based on a consensus within their practice group. The majority (59%) simply follow their individual preferences.[60] Other studies demonstrate that length of hospitalization and cost have both decreased under practice guidelines without increasing complications.[35,94] Additionally, length of stay, costs, and complication rates are lower when children are cared for by pediatric surgeons as compared with general surgeons.[95,96]

Surgeons are very familiar with children who have complete and prompt symptom resolution after appendectomy despite having a histologically normal appendix removed. Recent reports of "neuropathic" or "neuroimmune" appendicitis describe increased expression of neuropeptides S-100, vasoactive intestinal polypeptide (VIP), substance P, and growth-associated protein 43 (GAP-43) in histologically normal appendices removed for suspected appendicitis compared with those in incidentally removed asymptomatic controls.[97,98] Neuroimmune appendicitis may be less common in children compared with adults.[99] Other investigators propose "appendiceal colic" to explain the finding that children with recurrent episodes of right lower quadrant pain but normal imaging studies had an 88% rate of symptom relief with appendectomy.[100]

Incidental appendectomy has been debated for many years. Advocates for appendiceal preservation often cite the fact that the appendix can be used for a number of procedures such as a conduit for urinary tract and biliary tract reconstruction and for antegrade colonic enemas. However, the likelihood of using the appendix for any of these procedures in children who do not already have specific underlying conditions for which it might be useful is far less than the likelihood of future appendicitis. Other reasons for leaving the appendix in situ may be the lack of reimbursement for its removal and the potential for postoperative complications. Studies have examined the risk of future appendicitis against the risk of performing an incidental appendectomy. Analysis of demographic data seems to support the performance of incidental appendectomy for patients younger than 30 years, provided specific contraindications do not exist.[101] Contraindications to incidental appendectomy include impaired immunity, presence of surgical implants, intraoperative instability, history of abdominal radiation, and an inaccessible appendix. Concern about potential contamination has been addressed with the inversion appendectomy technique; however, this technique has been implicated in reports of intussusception[84,102] and failure of the appendix to slough, with later presentation as a cecal mass or appendicitis.[103] Careful attention to ligation of the entire appendiceal blood supply when using the inversion technique is essential for prevention of this complication. To avoid future diagnostic confusion, most pediatric surgeons perform an incidental appendectomy during a Ladd procedure for malrotation and when making a right lower quadrant incision for intussusception.

Tumors of the appendix are rare. The carcinoid tumor is by far the most common tumor of the appendix; this tumor has been found incidentally in 0.3% to 0.8% of appendices removed for symptoms.[104] Carcinoids are usually benign, located near the tip of the appendix, and appear with right lower quadrant pain. Almost all are cured by simple appendectomy. Right hemicolectomy is advised for mesenteric lymph node metastases and for tumors larger than 2 cm. Mucoceles, hyperplastic polyps, adenomas, and mucinous tumors of unknown potential also occur in the appendix. Carcinomas of the appendix have not been reported in pediatric patients.

REFERENCES

1. Meade JL: The evolution of surgery for appendicitis. Surgery 55:741, 1964.
2. Fitz RH: Perforating inflammation of the vermiform appendix, with special reference to its early diagnosis and treatment. Am J Med Sci 1:321–346, 1886.
3. McBurney C: Disease of the vermiform appendix. N Y Med 50:676–684, 1889.
4. Wangensteen OH, Dennis C: Experimental proof of obstructive origin of appendicitis. Ann Surg 110:629, 1939.
5. Wagner JM, McKinney WP, Carpenter JL: Does this patient have appendicitis? JAMA 276:1589–1594, 1996.
6. Addiss DG, Shaffer N, Fowler BS, et al: The epidemiology of appendicitis and appendectomy in the United States. Am J Epidemiol 132:910–924, 1990.
7. Brender JD, Marcuse EK, Weiss NS, et al: Is childhood appendicitis familial? Am J Dis Child 139:338–340, 1985.
8. Gauderer MW, Crane MM, Green JA, et al: Acute appendicitis in children: The importance of family history. J Pediatr Surg 36:1214–1217, 2001.
9. Anderson KD, Parry RL: Appendicitis. In O'Neill JA, Rowe MI, Grosfeld JL, et al (eds): Pediatric Surgery, 5th ed. St. Louis, Mosby-YearBook Inc., 1998, p 130.
10. Jones BA, Demetriades D, Segal I: The prevalence of appendiceal fecoliths in patients with and without appendicitis: A comparative study from Canada and South Africa. Ann Surg 202:80–82, 1985.
11. Karmali MA, Toma S, Shiemann DA, et al: Infection caused by *Yersinia enterolcolitica* serotype 0:21. J Clin Microbiol 15:596–598, 1982.
12. Arda IS, Ergin F, Varan B, et al: Acute abdomen caused by *Salmonella typhimurium* infection in children. J Pediatr Surg 36:1849–1852, 2001.
13. Hennington MH, Tinsley EA, Proctor HJ, et al: Acute appendicitis following blunt abdominal trauma. Incidence or coincidence? Ann Surg 214:61–63, 1991.
14. Coughlin JP, Gauderer MW, Stern RC, et al: The spectrum of appendiceal disease in cystic fibrosis. J Pediatr Surg 25:835–839, 1990.
15. Martin LW, Perrin EV: Neonatal perforation of the appendix in association with Hirschsprung's disease. Ann Surg 166:799, 1967.
16. Stiefel D, Stallmach T, Sacher P: Acute appendicitis in neonates: Complication or morbus sui generis? Pediatr Surg Intl 14:122–123, 1998.
17. Horwitz JR, Gursoy M, Jaksic T, et al: Importance of diarrhea as a presenting symptom of appendicitis in very young children. Am J Surg 173:80–82, 1997.
18. Dunning PG, Goldman MD: The incidence and value of rectal examination in children with suspected appendicitis. Ann R Coll Surg Engl 73:233–234, 1991.
19. Paajanen H, Mansikka A, Laato M, et al: Are serum inflammatory markers age dependent in acute appendicitis? J Am Coll Surg 184:303–308, 1997.
20. Rodríguez-Sanjuán JC, Martín-Parra JI, Seco I, et al: C-reactive protein and leukocyte count in the diagnosis of acute appendicitis in children. Dis Colon Rectum 42:1325–1329, 1999.

21. Gronroos JM: Do normal leukocyte count and C-reactive protein value exclude acute appendicitis in children? Acta Pediatr 90:649–651, 2001.

22. Jaye DL, Waites KB: Clinical applications of C-reactive protein in pediatrics. Pediatr Infect Dis J 16L:735–746, 1997.

23. Samuel M: Pediatric appendicitis score. J Pediatr Surg 37:877–881, 2002.

24. Macklin CP, Radcliffe GS, Merei JM, et al: A prospective evaluation of the modified Alvarado score for acute appendicitis in children. Ann R Coll Surg Engl 79:203–205, 1997.

25. Dolgin SE, Beck AR, Tartter PI: The risk of perforation when children with possible appendicitis are observed in the hospital. Surg Gynecol Obstet 175:320–324, 1992.

26. Heller MB, Skolnick LM: Ultrasound documentation of spontaneously resolving appendicitis. Am J Emerg Med 11:51–53, 1993.

27. Mattei P, Sola JE, Yeo CJ: Chronic and recurrent appendicitis are uncommon entities often misdiagnosed. J Am Coll Surg 178:385–389, 1994.

28. Nance ML, Adamson WT, Hedrick HL: Appendicitis in the young child: A continuing diagnostic challenge. Pediatr Emerg Care 16:160–162, 2000.

29. Newman K, Ponsky T, Kittle K, et al: Appendicitis 2000: Variability in practice, outcomes, and resource utilization at thirty pediatric hospitals. J Pediatr Surg 38:372–379, 2003.

30. Pearl RH, Hale DA, Molloy M, et al: Pediatric appendectomy. J Pediatr Surg 30:173–178, 1995.

31. Cappendijk VC, Hazebroek FW: The impact of diagnostic delay on the course of acute appendicitis. Arch Dis Child 83:64–66, 2000.

32. Flum DR, Koepsell T: The clinical and economic correlates of misdiagnosed appendicitis: Nationwide analysis. Arch Surg 137:799–804, 2002.

33. Flum DR, Morris A, Koepsell T, et al: Has misdiagnosis of appendicitis decreased over time? A population-based analysis. JAMA 286:1748–1753, 2001.

34. Buonomo C, Taylor GA, Share JC, et al. Gastrointestinal tract. In Kirks DP, Griscom NT (eds): Practical Pediatric Imaging: Diagnostic Radiology of Infants and Children, 3rd ed. Philadelphia, Lippincott-Raven, 1998, p 946.

35. Warner BW, Kulick RM, Stoops MM, et al: An evidenced-based clinical pathway for acute appendicitis decreases hospital duration and cost. J Pediatr Surg 33:1371–1375, 1998.

36. Hahn HB, Hoepner FU, Kalle, et al: Ultrasonography in suspected acute appendicitis in children: 7 years experience. Pediatr Radiol 28:147–151, 1998.

37. Rubin SZ, Martin DJ: Ultrasonography in the management of possible appendicitis in childhood. J Pediatr Surg 25:737–740, 1990.

38. Lessin MS, Chan M, Catallozzi M, et al: Selective use of ultrasonography for acute appendicitis in children. Am J Surg 177:193–196, 1999.

39. Dilley A, Wesson D, Munden M, et al: The impact of ultrasound examinations on the management of children with suspected appendicitis: A 3-year analysis. J Pediatr Surg 36:303–308, 2001.

40. Ramachandran P, Sivit CJ, Newman KD, et al: Ultrasonography as an adjunct in the diagnosis of acute appendicitis: A 4-year experience. J Pediatr Surg 31:164–167, 1996.

41. Sivit CJ, Applegate KE, Stallion A, et al: Imaging evaluation of suspected appendicitis in a pediatric population: Effectiveness of sonography versus CT. AJR Am J Roentgenol 175:977–980, 2000.

42. Brenner D, Elliston C, Hall E, et al: Estimated risks of radiation-induced fatal cancer from pediatric CT. AJR Am J Roentgenol 176:289–296, 2001.

43. Mullins ME, Kircher MF, Ryan DP, et al: Evaluation of suspected appendicitis in children using limited helical CT and colonic contrast material. AJR Am J Roentgenol 176:37–41, 2001.

44. Lowe LH, Penney MW, Stein SM, et al: Unenhanced limited CT of the abdomen in the diagnosis of appendicitis in children: Comparison with sonography. AJR Am J Roentgenol 176:31–35, 2001.

45. Stephen AE, Segev KL, Ryan DP, et al: The diagnosis of appendicitis in a pediatric population: To CT or not to CT. J Pediatr Surg 38:367–371, 2003.

46. Patrick DA, Janik JE, Janik JS, et al: Increased CT scan utilization does not improve the diagnostic accuracy of appendicitis in children. J Pediatr Surg 38:659–662, 2003.

47. Horman M, Paya K, Eibenberger K, et al: MR imaging in children with nonperforated acute appendicitis: Value of unenhanced MR imaging in sonographically selected cases. AJR Am J Roentgenol 171:467–470, 1998.

48. Yan DC, Shiau YC, Wang JJ, et al: Improving the diagnosis of acute appendicitis in children with atypical clinical findings using the technetium-99m hexamethylpropylene amine oxime-labelled white-blood-cell abdomen scan. Pediatr Radiol 32:663–666, 2002.

49. Guillerman RP, Brody AS, Kraus SJ: Evidence-based guidelines for pediatric imaging: The example of the child with possible appendicitis. Pediatr Ann 31:629–640, 2002.

50. Peña BM, Taylor GA, Fishman SJ, et al: Costs and effectiveness of ultrasonography and limited computed tomography for diagnosing appendicitis in children. Pediatrics 106:672–676, 2000.

51. Hennington MH, Tinsley EA, Proctor HJ, et al: Acute appendicitis following blunt abdominal trauma: Incidence or coincidence? Ann Surg 214:61–63, 1991.

52. Rodriguez JC, Buckner D, Schoenike S, et al: Comparison of two antibiotic regimens in the treatment of perforated appendicitis in pediatric patients. Int J Clin Pharmacol Ther 38:492–499, 2000.

53. Fishman SJ, Pelosi L, Klavon SL, et al: Perforated appendicitis: Prospective outcome analysis for 150 children. J Pediatr Surg 35:923–926, 2000.

54. Surana R, Quinn F, Puri P: Is it necessary to perform appendectomy in the middle of the night in children? Br Med J 306:1168, 1993.

55. Yardeni D, Hirschl RB, Drongowski RA, et al: Delayed versus immediate surgery in acute appendicitis: Do we need to operate during the night? J Pediatr Surg 39:464–469, 2004.

56. Kogut KA, Blakely ML, Schropp KP, et al: The association of elevated percent bands on admission with failure and complications of interval appendectomy. J Pediatr Surg 36:165–168, 2001.

57. Ein SH, Shandling B: Is interval appendectomy necessary after rupture of an appendiceal mass? J Pediatr Surg 31:849–850, 1996.

58. Gahukamble DB, Gahukamble LD: Surgical and pathological basis for interval appendectomy after resolution of appendicular mass in children. J Pediatr Surg 35:424–427, 2000.

59. Mazziotti MV, Marley EF, Winthrop AL, et al: Histopathologic analysis of interval appendectomy specimens: Support for the role of interval appendectomy. J Pediatr Surg 32:806–809, 1997.

60. Chen C, Botelho C, Cooper A, et al: Current practice patterns in the treatment of perforated appendicitis in children. J Am Coll Surg 196:212–221, 2003.

61. Lane JS, Schmit PJ, Chandler CF, et al: Ileocecectomy is definitive treatment for advanced appendicitis. Am Surg 67:117–122, 2001.

62. Bilik R, Burnweit C, Shandling B: Is abdominal cavity culture of any value in appendicitis? Am J Surg 175:267–270, 1998.

63. Kokoska ER, Silen ML, Tracy TF, et al: The impact of intraoperative culture on treatment and outcome in children with perforated appendicitis. J Pediatr Surg 34:749–753, 1999.

64. Sherman JO, Luck SR, Borger JA: Irrigation of the peritoneal cavity for appendicitis in children: A double blind study. J Pediatr Surg 11:371–374, 1976.

65. Kokoska ER, Silen ML, Tracy TF, et al: Perforated appendicitis in children: Risk factors for the development of complications. Surgery 124:619–625, 1998.

66. David IB, Buck JR, Filler RM: Rational use of antibiotics for perforated appendicitis in childhood. J Pediatr Surg 17:494–500, 1982.

67. Wright JE: Controlled trial of wound infiltration with bupivacaine for postoperative pain relief after appendectomy in children. Br J Surg 80:110–111, 1993.

68. Meguerditchian AN, Prasil P, Cloutier R, et al: Laparoscopic appendectomy in children: A favorable alternative in simple and complicated appendicitis. J Pediatr Surg 37:695–698, 2002.

69. Lintula H, Kokki H, Vanamo K: Single-blind randomized clinical trial of laparoscopic versus open appendectomy in children. Br J Surg 88:510–514, 2001.

70. Canty TG, Collins D, Losasso B, et al: Laparoscopic appendectomy for simple and perforated appendicitis in children: The procedure of choice? J Pediatr Surg 35:1582–1585, 2000.

71. Little DC, Custer MD, May BH, et al: Laparoscopic appendectomy: An unnecessary and expensive procedure in children? J Pediatr Surg 37:310–317, 2002.

72. Lintula H, Kokki H, Vanamo K, et al: Laparoscopy in children with complicated appendicitis. J Pediatr Surg 37:1317–1320, 2002.

73. Horwitz JR, Custer MD, May BH, et al: Should laparoscopic appendectomy be avoided for complicated appendicitis in children? J Pediatr Surg 32:1601–1603, 1997.

74. Eypasch E, Sauerland S, Lefering R, et al. Laparoscopic versus open appendectomy: Between evidence and common sense. Dig Surg 19:518–522, 2002.

75. Hoelzer DJ, Zabel DD, Zern JT: Determining duration of antibiotic use in children with complicated appendicitis. Pediatr Infect Dis J 18:L979–L982, 1999.

76. Bradley JS, Behrendt CE, Arrieta AC, et al: Convalescent phase outpatient parenteral anti-infective therapy for children with complicated appendicitis. Pediatr Infect Dis J 20:19–24, 2001.

77. Gollin G, Abarbanell A, Morres D: Oral antibiotics in the management of perforated appendicitis in children. Am Surg 68:1072–1074, 2002.

78. Serour F, Efrati Y, Klin B, et al: Subcuticular skin closure as a standard approach to emergency appendectomy in children: Prospective clinical trial. World J Surg 20:38–42, 1996.

79. Burnweit C, Bilik R, Shandling B: Primary closure of contaminated wounds in perforated appendicitis. J Pediatr Surg 26:1362–1365, 1991.

80. Tsang TM, Tam PK, Saing H: Delayed primary wound closure using skin tapes for advanced appendicitis in children: A prospective, controlled study. Arch Surg 127:451–453, 1992.

81. Neilson IT et al: Appendicitis in children: Current therapeutic recommendations. J Pediatr Surg 25:1113–1116, 1990.

82. Okoye BO, Rampersad B, Marantos, et al: Abscess after appendectomy in children: The role of conservative management. Br J Surg 85:1111–1113, 1998.

83. Massad M: Neonatal appendicitis: Case report and a revised review of the English literature. Z Kinderchir 41:241–243, 1986.

84. Holcomb GW III, Ross AJ, O'Neill JA: Postoperative intussusception: Increasing frequency or increasing awareness? South Med J: 84:1334–1339, 1991.

85. Pumberger W, Löbl M, Geissler W: Appendicitis in children with a ventriculoperitoneal shunt. Pediatr Neurosurg 28:21–26, 1998.

86. Worley G, Wiener JS, George TM, et al: Acute abdominal symptoms and signs in children and young adults with spina bifida: Ten years' experience. J Pediatr Surg 36:1381–1386, 2001.

87. Angel CA, Rao BN, Wrenn E, et al: Acute appendicitis in children with leukemia and other malignancies: Still a diagnostic dilemma. J Pediatr Surg 27:476–479, 1992.

88. Steinberg R, Freud E, Yaniv I, et al: A plea for incidental appendectomy in pediatric patients with malignancy. Pediatr Hematol Oncol 16:431–435, 1999.

89. Ritchey M, Haase GM, Shochat SJ, et al: Incidental appendectomy during nephrectomy for Wilms' tumor. Surg Gynecol Obstet 176:423–426, 1993.

90. Mueller BA, Daling JR, Moore DE, et al: Appendectomy and the risk of tubal infertility. N Engl J Med 315:1506–1508, 1986.

91. Puri P, McGuinness EPJ, Guiney EJ: Fertility following perforated appendicitis in girls. J Pediatr Surg 24:547–549, 1989.

92. Anderson R, Lambe M, Bergström R: Fertility patterns after appendicectomy: Historical cohort study. BMJ 318:L963–L967, 1999.

93. Johnson PA, Chavanu KE, Newman KD: Guiding practice improvements in pediatric surgery using multidisciplinary clinical pathways. Semin Pediatr Surg 11:20–24, 2002.

94. Lelli JL, Drongowski RA, Raviz S, et al: Historical changes in the postoperative treatment of appendicitis in children: Impact on medical outcome. J Pediatr Surg 35:239–244, 2000.

95. Alexander F, Magnuson D, DiFiore J, et al: Specialty versus generalist care of children with appendicitis: An outcome comparison. J Pediatr Surg 36:1510–1513, 2001.

96. Kokoska ER: Effect of pediatric surgical practice on the treatment of children with appendicitis. Pediatrics 107:1298–1301, 2001.

97. Di Sebastiano P, Fink T, di Mola FF, et al: Neuroimmune appendicitis. Lancet 354:461–466, 1999.

98. Bouchard S, Russo P, Radu A, et al. Expression of neuropeptides in normal and abnormal appendices. J Pediatr Surg 36:1222–1226, 2001.

99. Franke C, Gerharz CD, Böhner H, et al: Neurogenic appendicopathy in children. Eur J Pediatr Surg 12:28–31, 2002.

100. Gorenstin A, Serour F, Katz R, et al: Appendiceal colic in children: A true clinical entity? J Am Coll Surg 182:246–250, 1996.

101. Fisher KS, Ross DS: Guidelines for therapeutic decision in incidental appendectomy. Surg Gynecol Obstet 171:95–98, 1990.

102. Hoehneer JC, Kimura K, Soper RT: Intussusception as a complication of inversion appendectomy. Pediatr Surg Int 10:51, 1995.

103. McCarville MB, Ross MB, Rao BN, et al: Sonographic appearance of appendicitis in a neutropenic pediatric patient after inversion appendectomy. Pediatr Radiol 31:578–80, 2001.

104. Gouzi JL, Laigneau P, Delalande JP, et al: Indications for right hemicolectomy in carcinoid tumors of the appendix. Surg Gynecol Obstet 176:543–547, 1993.

Biliary Tract Disorders and Portal Hypertension

Takeshi Miyano, MD

BILIARY ATRESIA

Introduction

Biliary atresia (BA) is an obstructive condition of the bile ducts causing neonatal jaundice. The obstruction is of unknown etiology but results from a progressive obliterative process of variable extent. Biliary atresia is rare. Reliable incidence figures are available from France (1 in 19,500 live births), the U.K. and Eire (1 in 16,700 live births), Georgia in the United States, and Sweden (1 in 14,000 live births).[1-4] The highest recorded incidence is in French Polynesia.[1] No significant seasonal variation or clustering appears, and in most large series, a slight female preponderance is found.

In the late 1950s, Morio Kasai, a Japanese surgeon, reported the presence of patent microscopic biliary channels at the porta hepatis in young infants with BA. Exposing these channels by radical excision of atretic extrahepatic biliary remnants resulted in effective drainage of bile in some cases, especially if drainage was performed within 8 weeks of birth. The Kasai portoenterostomy is now accepted as the standard initial operation for BA. However, despite the great improvement in prognosis associated with the introduction of the Kasai procedure, BA remains the foremost indication for liver transplantation in infants and children.

History[2,3]

BA appears as a distinct disease entity in the Edinburgh Medical Journal in 1891, and in 1916, the concepts of "correctable" and "noncorrectable" types of disease were introduced after a comprehensive review of all reported cases.[5,6] Successful surgical treatment for the correctable type was reported for the first time in 1928 and repeated over the next three decades.[7] However, only a few long-term survivors remained, all of whom had the favorable correctable type, which represents only a minority of all BA patients.[8,9]

For the majority with "noncorrectable"-type disease, a number of procedures designed to relieve biliary obstruction, including impalement of the liver with metal tubes, incisions into the hilum with a cardiac valvulotome, and partial hepatectomy to create biliary fistulas, were developed and used.[10-12] In addition, lymphatic drainage through the thoracic duct was attempted.[13,14] Despite occasional hopeful reports, all techniques failed to provide adequate biliary decompression. Timing of surgical intervention was controversial, with some surgeons recommending that all infants with obstructive jaundice undergo early diagnostic laparotomy and cholangiography to identify those with correctable variants, whereas others[15,16] concluded that early age is a contraindication for surgical treatment. They emphasized that neonatal hepatitis could be worsened by surgical intervention and recommended that surgical procedures should be postponed until at least age 4 months. The argument for early surgical correction also was weakened by reports describing "spontaneous" cure.[17,18] Second-look surgical exploration also was recommended at one stage because of a rather mystical belief that a totally fibrotic extrahepatic ductal system might subsequently become patent.[19]

After a long, hopeless era for patients with noncorrectable-type disease, the now common hepatic portoenterostomy procedure was reported in 1959 for the surgical treatment of BA.[20] The original report was in Japanese and received little attention until it was published in English in 1968.[21] Effective bile drainage could be achieved after portoenterostomy, but early surgical repair was crucial. Bile drainage could be achieved in more than 50% of patients if surgical treatment was performed before age 2 months. Conversely, effective bile drainage was observed in only 7% if the operation was performed after age 4 months.[22] The portoenterostomy procedure gradually gained popularity in the United States during the 1970s, and in the 1990 report of the BA Registry, more than 90% of infants with BA had had the procedure.[23]

Etiology and Pathogenesis

Despite intensive interest and investigation, the cause of BA remains unknown. Two different forms are described.[24] In syndromic BA (also known as the embryonic type), associated congenital anomalies are found, such as an interrupted inferior vena cava, preduodenal portal vein, intestinal malrotation, situs inversus, cardiac defects, and polysplenia. In this variety, which accounts for about 10% to 20% of all cases, BA is likely to be due to a developmental insult occurring during differentiation of the hepatic diverticulum from the foregut of the embryo. A possible relation between syndromic BA and maternal diabetes has been reported.[25] Nonsyndromic BA (also known as the perinatal type) may have its origins later in gestation and run a different clinical course, with biliary obstruction being progressive.

No ideal animal model exists for BA, a fact that has slowed the understanding of its pathogenesis. Various etiologic mechanisms have been postulated, including intrauterine or perinatal viral infection, genetic mutation, abnormal ductal plate remodeling, vascular or metabolic insult to the developing biliary tree, pancreaticobiliary ductal malunion, and immunologically mediated inflammation. Recent observations would suggest that BA is not a single disease entity. Some infants even have pigmented stools at birth. Reovirus type 3 infection, rotavirus, cytomegalovirus, papillomavirus, and Epstein-Barr virus have all been proposed as possible etiologic agents, but conclusive evidence is lacking. Reovirus type 3 can cause an inflammatory cholangiopathy in weanling mice, but the condition is not progressive, and the animals recover.

Generally, BA is not considered to be an inherited disorder. However, genetic mutations that result in defective morphogenesis may be important in syndromic BA. Transgenic mice with a recessive deletion of the inversin gene have situs inversus and an interrupted extrahepatic biliary tree.[24,26] Mutations of the *CFC1* gene, which is involved in left-right axis determination in humans, have recently been identified in a few patients with syndromic BA.[27]

Intrahepatic bile ducts are derived from primitive hepatocytes, which form a sleeve (the ductal plate) around intrahepatic portal vein branches and associated mesenchyme in early gestation. Remodeling of the ductal plate in fetal life results in the formation of the intrahepatic biliary system. This emphasized similarities in cytokeratin immunostaining between biliary ductules in BA and normal first-trimester fetal bile ducts.[28] They suggested that nonsyndromic BA might be caused by a failure of bile duct remodeling at the hepatic hilum, with persistence of fetal bile ducts poorly supported by mesenchyme.

Several studies have investigated whether bile duct epithelial cells are susceptible to immune/inflammatory attack because of abnormal expression of human leukocyte antigen (HLA) antigens or intracellular adhesion molecules on their surface.[29,30] A greater than threefold increase in HLA-B12 antigen is found in BA patients compared with controls, particularly in those with no associated malformations and increases in haplotypes A9-B5 and A28-B35.[31] Aberrant expression of class II HLA-DR antigens on biliary epithelial cells and damaged hepatocytes in BA patients may render these tissues more susceptible to immune-mediated damage by cytotoxic T cells or locally released cytokines.[32] Increased expression of intercellular adhesion molecule-1

(ICAM-1) is noted on bile duct epithelium in patients with BA, a finding that may play a role in immune-mediated damage.[30] Strong expression of ICAM-1 also has been found on proliferating bile ductules, endothelial cells, and hepatocytes in BA,[33] and a direct relation exists between the degree of ductular expression of ICAM-1 and disease severity, suggesting that ICAM-1 might be important in the development of cirrhosis.

More recently, interest has focused on co-stimulatory molecules. Two processes are involved in the activation of T lymphocytes by antigen-presenting cells (APCs). One relates to the expression of major histocompatibility complex class II molecules, which interact directly with T-cell receptors. The other depends on the expression of B7 antigens on APCs and provides the second (co-stimulatory) signal to T lymphocytes through CD28.[34] In postoperative BA patients with good liver function, co-stimulatory antigens (B7-1, B7-2, and CD40) are expressed only on bile duct epithelial cells, whereas in patients with failing livers, these markers are found on the surfaces of Kupffer cells, dendritic cells, sinusoidal endothelial cells, and in the cytoplasm of hepatocytes.[35] This suggests that the biliary epithelium and hepatocytes in BA are susceptible to immune recognition and destruction. Agents that block or prevent co-stimulatory pathways might offer a new therapeutic approach to controlling liver damage.

None of these mechanisms is mutually exclusive. It is not clear which signs and symptoms are primary or secondary with respect to some theories. One current hypothesis is that in the etiology of nonsyndromic BA, a viral or other toxic insult to the bile duct epithelium, induces the expression of new antigens on the biliary epithelial cell surface.[36] Coupled with a genetically predetermined susceptibility mediated via histocompatibility antigens, these neoantigens are recognized by circulating T lymphocytes, resulting in a cell-mediated, immune, fibrosclerosing bile duct injury.

Classification and Histopathology

Although the term BA implies a static process with complete obstruction or absence of bile ducts, it is more a dynamic process of progressive obliteration and sclerosis of bile ducts. The areas that are affected and the degrees of fibrosis are variable and presumably reflect different sites of primary involvement by an as-yet-unknown cause.

The disease can be classified by using macroscopic appearance and cholangiography findings according to three main categories: (1) main type, (2) subtypes according to the pattern of distal bile ducts, and (3) subgroups according to the pattern of hilar hepatic radicles. Types I, II, and III are defined as atresia at the site of the common bile duct (CBD), at the site of the hepatic duct, and up to the porta hepatis, respectively. Most patients have type III. Cystic dilatation at the distal end of a patent duct is seen in some cases of type I BA (Fig. 43-1). Of the subtypes, patent distal ducts through the gallbladder to the duodenum are seen in 20%, and atretic distal ducts are seen in 62% of cases. Of the subgroups, a patent duct that can be anastomosed to the intestine at the porta hepatis is present in 5% of cases (i.e., "correctable" type).

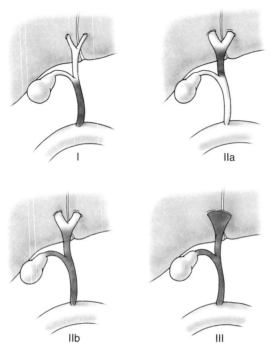

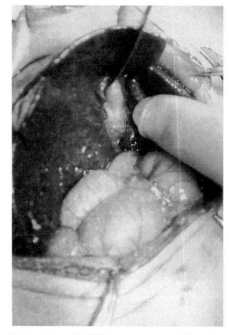

FIGURE 43-1. Morphologic classification of biliary atresia based on macroscopic and cholangiographic findings. Type I, occlusion of common bile duct; type IIa, obliteration of common hepatic duct; type IIb, obliteration of common bile duct, hepatic and cystic ducts, with cystic dilatation of ducts at the porta hepatis, and no gallbladder involvement; type III, obliteration of common, hepatic, and cystic ducts without anastomosable ducts at porta hepatic. (From Lefkowitch JH, et al: Biliary atresia. Mayo Clinic Proc 73:99, 1998.)

FIGURE 43-2. Type III biliary atresia with enlarged, firm, green liver and hypoplastic small gallbladder.

In more than 90% of cases, however, no normal ductal structures are seen at the porta hepatis (i.e., "noncorrectable" type).[37]

Early in the course of BA, the liver is enlarged, firm, and green. The gallbladder may be small and filled with white mucus, or it may be completely atretic (Fig. 43-2). Microscopically, the biliary tracts contain inflammatory and fibrous cells surrounding miniscule ducts that are probably remnants of the original embryonic duct system. The liver parenchyma is fibrotic and shows signs of cholestasis. Proliferation of biliary neoductules is seen (Fig. 43-3). This process develops into end-stage cirrhosis if good drainage cannot be achieved. These early changes are often nonspecific and may be confused with neonatal hepatitis and metabolic disease.

It is generally accepted that the pathologic changes seen in BA are panductal, affecting the intrahepatic biliary tree as well as the extrahepatic bile duct system; the intrahepatic bile ducts can be narrowed, distorted in configuration, or irregular in shape.[38–40] However, some authors believe that secondary damage occurs only to the extrahepatic biliary system as a result of obliteration of extrahepatic bile ducts during development of the liver.[41] This theory is strongly supported by the fact that outcome is better if corrective surgery is performed early. In any case, the intrahepatic biliary tree is important not

only pathologically but also clinically. The degree of damage that is present in the intrahepatic biliary system is actually responsible for much of the morbidity after hepatic portoenterostomy. Ductal proliferation includes ductal plate malformation, such as disturbance of adequate remodeling of the ductal plate and ductular metaplasia of hepatocytes.[42] Paucity or absence of intralobular bile ducts along with architectural disturbances, even in jaundice-free infants after successful hepatic portoenterostomy, has been observed by some investigators.[43] The nature and fate of intrahepatic biliary involvement is still a subject of great controversy.

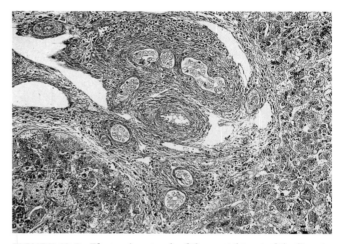

FIGURE 43-3. Photomicrograph of the portal tract of the liver in a 60-day-old infant with biliary atresia. Ductal plate malformation can be seen in the center of the portal space with portal fibrosis. Note ductal metaplasia of hepatocytes (Azan stain, × 100).

Diagnosis

The cardinal signs and symptoms of BA are jaundice, clay-colored stools, and hepatomegaly. However, meconium staining is normal in most patients, and in the neonatal period, feces are yellowish or light yellowish in more than half of patients.[44] Urine becomes dark brown. Anemia, malnutrition, and growth retardation develop gradually because of malabsorption of fat-soluble vitamins, although patients are active, and their growth appears to be normal during the first few months of life. In infancy, jaundice that persists beyond 2 weeks should no longer be considered physiologic, particularly if the elevation in bilirubin is mainly of the direct fraction. Neonatal hepatitis and interlobular biliary hypoplasia are most likely to be confused with BA, and conventional liver function tests alone are useless for establishing a definitive diagnosis of BA.

A number of diagnostic protocols have been published, but the emphasis must always be on early diagnosis (Table 43-1).[45,46] For definitive diagnosis of BA, further investigations, including special biochemical studies, tests to confirm the patency of the extrahepatic bile ducts, and needle biopsy of the liver, are often required. Several authors consider liver biopsy to be the most reliable test for establishing the diagnosis.[47,48] Serum lipoprotein-X is positive in all patients with BA, although it also is positive in 20% to 40% of patients with neonatal hepatitis. Serum bile acid levels increase in infants with cholestatic disease, but both the total bile acid level and the ratio of chenodeoxycholic acid to cholic acid have no value for differentiating BA from other cholestatic diseases.[49] Duodenal fluid aspiration is recommended as an easy, noninvasive, and rapid test, because BA can be excluded if typical yellow bilirubin-stained fluid is aspirated.[50] Hepatobiliary scintigraphy with technetium-labeled agents is widely used for differentiating BA from other cholestatic diseases. In BA, nucleotide uptake by hepatocytes is rapid, but excretion into the bowel is absent, even on the delayed image. In hepatocellular jaundice, isotope uptake is delayed owing to parenchymal disease, and excretion into the intestine may or may not be demonstrated.

Ultrasonography (US), a safe and noninvasive test, should be performed in all jaundiced infants. Hepatobiliary US will exclude other surgical causes of jaundice such as choledochal cyst and inspissated bile. In BA, the intrahepatic ducts are not dilated on US because they are affected by inflammatory processes. Various sonographic features have been targeted in the attempt to distinguish BA from other causes of conjugated hyperbilirubinemia in infants.[51-55] In BA, a small, shrunken, noncontractile gallbladder is found and increased echogenicity of the liver. The presence of other associated anomalies of the polysplenia syndrome is pathognomonic of BA.[56] Differentiation from choledochal cyst and type I BA also is rapid and simple with US.[57] Irrespective of interobserver variation, failure to visualize the CBD is not diagnostic of BA, because a patent distal CBD can be found in up to 20% of affected infants. An absent gallbladder or one with an irregular outline is suggestive of BA.[55] In some cases, a well-defined triangular area of high reflectivity is seen at the porta hepatis, corresponding to fibrotic ductal remnants (the "triangular cord" sign) (Fig. 43-4).[52,53]

Endoscopic retrograde cholangiopancreaticography (ERCP) and laparoscopy have been used for the diagnosis of BA at some institutions.

Most patients with BA can be correctly diagnosed by using an appropriate combination of the investigations listed. However, to differentiate accurately between BA, biliary hypoplasia, and severe neonatal hepatitis, surgical cholangiography may be required.

TABLE 43-1

CLINICAL FINDINGS AND EXAMINATION FOR DIAGNOSIS OF BA

Routine Examinations
   Color of stool
   Consistency of the liver
   Conventional liver function tests, including test
      for γ-glutamyl transpeptidase
   Coagulation times (PT, aPTT)

Special Examinations
Special biochemical studies
   Hepatitis A, B, C serologies
   TORCH titers
   α_1-Antitrypsin level
   Serum lipoprotein-X
   Serum bile acid
Confirmation of patency of extrahepatic bile ducts
   Duodenal fluid aspiration
   Ultrasonography
   Hepatobiliary scintigraphy
   Endoscopic retrograde cholangiopancreatography
   Near-infrared reflectance spectroscopy
Needle biopsy of the liver for histopathologic studies
Laparoscopy
Surgical cholangiography

PT, prothrombin time; aPTT, activated partial thromboplastin time; TORCH, toxoplasmosis, other viruses, rubella, cytomegalovirus, and herpes simplex virus.

Treatment

Preoperative Management

Daily doses of vitamin K are usually given for several days before operation. The bowel should be prepared with oral kanamycin. Oral feeding is discontinued 24 to 48 hours before the procedure, and glycerin enemas are given. Preoperative broad-spectrum antibiotics are administrated intravenously.

Surgical Technique

HEPATIC PORTOENTEROSTOMY. The patient is placed in the supine position on an operating table with facilities for intraoperative cholangiography. An extended right subcostal incision, dividing the muscle layers, is used to expose the inferior margin of the liver. After division of the falciform and triangular ligaments, the liver is delivered

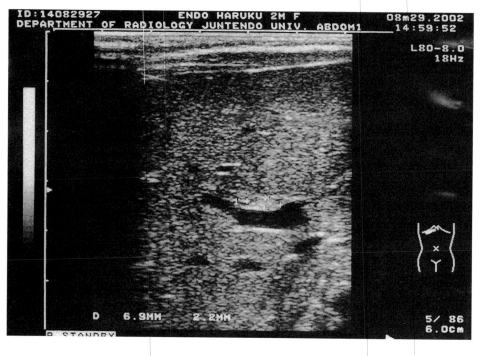
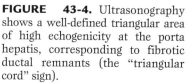

FIGURE 43-4. Ultrasonography shows a well-defined triangular area of high echogenicity at the porta hepatis, corresponding to fibrotic ductal remnants (the "triangular cord" sign).

from the abdominal cavity. This procedure provides an excellent operative field for dissection of the porta hepatis. Cholangiography is important to determine the type of BA present and can be used to differentiate BA from neonatal hepatitis (Fig. 43-5). The fundus of the gallbladder is mobilized from the liver bed, and a 4F to 6Fr feeding tube is passed into the gallbladder through a small incision. If bile is detected on aspiration of the gallbladder, a small amount of contrast material is injected. Unless the normal anatomy of the intrahepatic biliary system is observed, a hepatic portoenterostomy should be performed.[21,58] Liver biopsy is usually carried out on the right lobe, as histopathologic findings are important for predicting prognosis.[59-61] The cystic artery is ligated and divided, and the gallbladder is dissected from the liver bed.

The mobilized gallbladder is used as a guide for locating the fibrous remnant of the CBD. After the lower end of the CBD is ligated and divided at the upper border of the duodenum, the upper portion with the gallbladder is dissected upward above the bifurcation of the portal vein. The portal vein and the hepatic arteries are exposed along their whole course. For better portal dissection, the right and left hepatic arteries and the right and left portal branches are individually encircled by vessel loops (Fig. 43-6). The fine veins extending between the portal vein and the base of the portal fibrous mass are carefully ligated and divided. After the dissection reaches the rim of the right and left portal vein branches, the portal fibrous mass is transected at its border with the liver. The transection can be performed very accurately by using

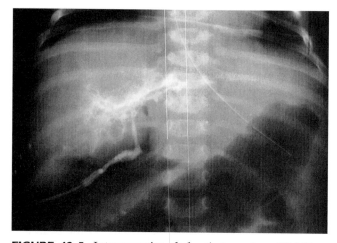

FIGURE 43-5. Intraoperative cholangiogram, type III biliary atresia. Note atretic common bile duct.

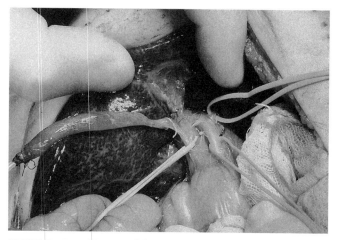

FIGURE 43-6. Type III biliary atresia. The tape is around the atretic bile duct (*A*) and hepatic artery (*B*).

scissors or a scalpel. Transection of liver parenchyma should be avoided to prevent obstruction of the remnant bile duct by scar tissue. The 5/0 absorbable sutures are usually placed in the liver surface of the posterior side of the remnant fibrous mass before transection, for use in the portoenterostomy. It is important to have enough distance between these sutures and the remnant fibrous mass. Bleeding points are controlled by packing with gauze. Diathermy electrocautery is not used because it can cause damage to the remnant bile duct (Fig. 43-7). Intraoperative histopathology of the transected portal fibrous mass is important. If openings of microscopic bile duct structures are present at the transected surface, additional transection of the portal fibrous mass should be performed. A 30- to 40-cm Roux-en-Y loop is prepared by transecting the jejunum approximately 15 to 25 cm downstream from the ligament of Treitz (Fig. 43-8). The distal end may be oversewn or left open. It is passed in a retrocolic position to the hepatic hilum. Continuity of the small bowel is established with an end-to-side enteroenterostomy. Hepatic portoenterostomy is performed in an end-to-side or end-to-end using interrupted sutures. Jejunal sutures are placed by using the 5/0 sutures that had been placed in the posterior side of the remnant fibrous mass before transection, as a guide. When all sutures are placed on the posterior margin, the jejunal loop is brought into position, and the sutures are gently tied in series. The anterior margin of the jejunum is then sutured to the surface of the liver. Adequate separation should exist between the anterior margin and the remnant fibrous mass. A small drain is placed in the foramen of Winslow through a separate stab wound in the abdominal wall. The wound is closed conventionally.

HEPATICOENTEROSTOMY. In "correctable" BA, Roux-en-Y hepaticojejunostomy is usually performed.

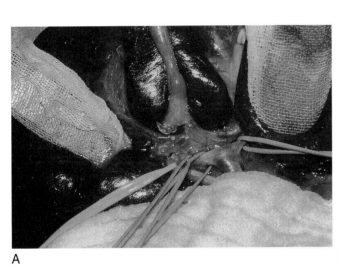

A

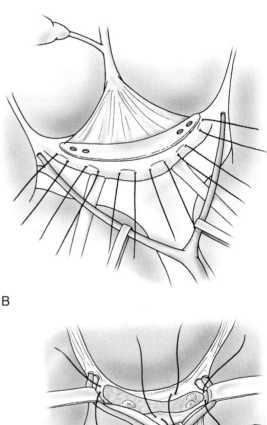

B

C

FIGURE 43-7. The portoenterostomy operation. *A,* Photograph of the initial mobilization of the gallbladder and atretic bile ducts and dissection/exposure of the porta hepatis. After the common bile duct remnants are severed from the duodenal side, the proximal end is pulled up, and the portal bile duct remnants are freed from underlying structures. The portal vein and hepatic artery are taped. Several small vessel branches between the portal vein to the fibrous remnants can be identified and should be divided between ligatures. (*A,* from Howard ER, Stringer MD, Colombani PM, et al: Surgery of the Liver, Bile Ducts, and Pancreas in Children, 2nd ed. 2002.) *B,* The portal bile duct remnants must be dissected to 5 to 6 mm proximal of the anterior branch of the right hepatic artery on the right side and to the umbilical point of the left portal vein on the left side. After completion of portal dissection, the portal bile duct remnants should be transected at the site of the line drawn. *C,* The end of the intestine is anastomosed around the transected end of the portal bile duct remnants. Sutures must not be placed into the transected surface of the bile duct remnant because minute bile ducts may be present. (*B, C,* from O'Neill JA, Rowe MI, Grosfeld JL, et al: Pediatric Surgery, 5th ed. Vol 2. 1471, 1998.)

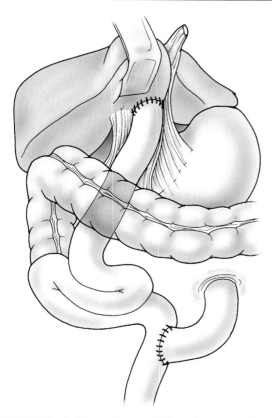

FIGURE 43-8. A 40-cm Roux-en-Y loop is prepared by transecting the jejunum ~20 to 30 cm downstream from the ligament of Treitz. The distal end is oversewn and passed in a retrocolic position to the hepatic hilum. (From Tagge DU, Tagge EP, Drongowski RA, et al: A long-term experience with biliary atresia. Ann Surg 214:591, 1991.)

Although a wide and deep portal dissection is not required, excision of the patent duct to the liver hilum is required. Any cystlike structure should be excised and must not be used for anastomosis to the intestine. Failure to remove all abnormal duct tissue results in anastomotic stricture and cholangitis.[62]

REPEATED HEPATIC PORTOENTEROSTOMY.

Pediatric surgeons have recently reached a consensus about repeated hepatic portoenterostomy.[63] Bile drainage after reoperation is significant only in patients who had good bile excretion after the initial surgical procedure.[64] Because liver transplantation is a treatment option, repeated hepatic portoenterostomy should be considered only in patients in whom good bile flow ceased suddenly.

Postoperative Management

Patients are given oxygen and intravenous fluids, and nasogastric tube drainage is used. Broad-spectrum antibiotics are continued postoperatively to prevent cholangitis. Corticosteroids also are given intravenously or orally, although the efficacy of this therapy is currently being evaluated by a randomized controlled trial in the U.K.

Both antibiotic and steroid use is largely empirical; steroids are used both for their choleretic effect and to decrease scarring at the anastomosis site.[65,66] Ursodeoxycholic acid may be useful in augmenting bile flow, but only in the presence of a patent bile duct. Fat-soluble vitamins (A, D, E, and K) and formula feeds enriched with medium-chain triglycerides also are prescribed.

Complications

CHOLANGITIS.

Cholangitis is the most frequent complication occurring after portoenterostomy and occurs most commonly in the first 2 years. Approximately 40% of infants are affected. All conduits become colonized within a month of surgery. Cholestasis is the main risk factor for cholangitis, and all BA patients have very small ducts.

Cholangitis is initially seen with fever, decreased quantity and quality of bile, elevations in serum bilirubin, and a variety of signs associated with any intercurrent infection. Nonetheless, prompt treatment is necessary because recurring attacks cause progressive liver damage. After initial blood cultures, broad-spectrum antibiotics with good gram-negative coverage are started, and favorable response is usually prompt. If stools become acholic, a pulse of steroids is useful. To decrease the risk for cholangitis, Roux-en-Y biliary reconstruction has been modified by various maneuvers including lengthening the Roux-en-Y limb from 50 to 70 cm, total diversion of the biliary conduit, intestinal valve formation, and use of a physiologic intestinal valve.[67-71] An intussusception-type intestinal valve is associated with a lower incidence of cholangitis. Stomas complicate liver transplantation, which may be required later. At this time, the antireflux intussusception valve may be the modification of choice. A gallbladder conduit is not recommended when the lumen of the patent duct is narrow or when pancreaticobiliary maljunction is demonstrated on cholangiography.

CESSATION OF BILE FLOW.

Loss of fecal bile pigment in a patient with a well-functioning portoenterostomy is a depressing scenario in the practice of pediatric surgery. Prompt reestablishment of bile flow is imperative to avoid liver damage. Parents should be encouraged to report changes in stool color or signs of cholangitis. If cessation of bile flow occurs, a pulse of steroids is usual.[65,66] Steroids both augment bile flow and reduce inflammation. If bile flow is reestablished, then steroid dosage is reduced. If bile flow is not reestablished, steroids are stopped. If the child had good bile flow previously, it is reasonable to consider reoperation. However, multiple attempts at reoperation are not useful and increase the technical difficulties for subsequent transplantation.

PORTAL HYPERTENSION.

Portal hypertension is common after portoenterostomy, even in infants with good bile flow. The basic inflammatory process affecting the extrahepatic ducts also damages the intrahepatic branches, albeit at variable rates. Continuing fibrosis has been demonstrated in some children despite successful portoenterostomy.[72] Clinical manifestations of portal hypertension include esophageal variceal hemorrhage, hypersplenism, and ascites (Fig. 43-9). Of special note is the finding that over time, susceptibility to complications of portal hypertension seems to decrease, resulting in reduced frequency and severity of variceal bleeding. This observation is difficult to explain and may be related to improvement in hepatic histology or development of spontaneous portosystemic shunts. In any case, this general observation justifies a nonsurgical approach to the management of portal hypertension, as long as hepatic function is preserved (i.e., the patient remains anicteric, with no coagulopathy and normal serum albumin level). In the presence of poor hepatic function, however, complications of portal hypertension are an indication for liver transplantation.

INTRAHEPATIC CYSTS. Biliary cysts or "lakes" may develop within the livers of long-term survivors and cause recurrent attacks of cholangitis (Fig. 43-10).[73] Prolonged antibiotic treatment and ursodeoxycholic acid may be helpful in preventing cholangitis, but unremitting infection is an indication for liver transplantation.

HEPATOPULMONARY SYNDROME. Diffuse intrapulmonary shunting may occur as a complication of chronic liver disease in children with BA, probably as a result of vasoactive compounds from the mesenteric circulation bypassing sinusoidal inactivation. The syndrome is characterized by cyanosis, dyspnea on exertion, hypoxia, and finger clubbing. It is more prevalent in children with syndromic BA. The diagnosis is confirmed by using a combination of arterial blood gas estimations with and without inspired oxygen, radionuclide lung scans with macroaggregated albumin to quantify the degree of shunting, and contrast bubble echocardiography. This complication is progressive and can usually be reversed by liver transplantation. Pulmonary hypertension is a

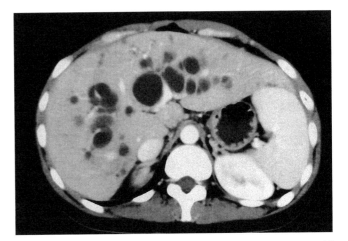

FIGURE 43-10. Computed tomography scan of a 17-year-old with biliary atresia. Multiple biliary cysts or "lakes" have developed within the liver of this long-term survivor and cause recurrent attacks of cholangitis.

rarer complication but also may develop in long-term survivors after portoenterostomy.

HEPATIC MALIGNANCY. Rarely, malignant change (hepatocellular carcinoma or cholangiocarcinoma) may complicate long-standing biliary cirrhosis after portoenterostomy.

OTHER COMPLICATIONS. Metabolic problems associated with malabsorption of fat, protein, vitamins, and trace minerals can occur postoperatively because of impairment of bile flow to the gut that may occur for many months, because of the presence of residual hepatic disease.[74,75] Weight gain after surgical correction may be retarded if hepatic dysfunction persists. Essential fatty acid deficiencies and rickets are common problems related to metabolic derangements.[76] Careful monitoring of clinical symptoms and adequate nutritional supplementation are required in the long term. Ectopic intestinal variceal bleeding and pulmonary arteriovenous fistulas are sometimes seen in long-term survivors with incomplete relief of impaired liver function.[37,46]

Results and Prognosis

Without question, the hepatic portoenterostomy has positively altered the prognosis for infants with BA. The results of surgical treatment have steadily improved during the last 30 years. However, a wide discrepancy exists in reported long-term postoperative results. One study from Japan found the postoperative outcome to be excellent, with a 10-year survival rate of more than 70% if corrective surgery was performed before age 60 days.[77] However, a nationwide survey of the surgical section of the American Academy of Pediatrics found that long-term survival was only 25%.[23] Other reported survival rates include 40% to 50% from the U.K., and 68% for a French national study on 10-year overall survival.[1,78] Results are considerably worse if the infant is older than 100 days at the time of portoenterostomy because

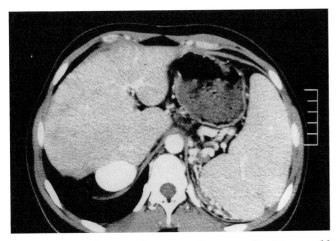

FIGURE 43-9. Computed tomography scan of a 20-year-old girl in whom severe portal hypertension developed. It shows marked atrophy of the left lobe of the liver, severe splenomegaly, and varices around the stomach.

obliterative cholangiopathy and hepatic fibrosis are more advanced.[78,79] The major determinants of satisfactory outcome after portoenterostomy are (1) age at initial operation, (2) successful achievement of postoperative bile flow, (3) presence of microscopic ductal structures at the hilum, (4) degree of parenchymal disease at diagnosis, and (5) technical factors of the anastomosis. The age at which the surgical drainage is performed is the single most widely quoted prognostic variable. Favorable outcome is expected if the procedure is performed before age 60 days.[66] Cirrhosis is present by age 3 to 4 months. Infants who show a significant decrease in serum bilirubin and have fecal signs of good bile excretion also have improved results. Serum bilirubin at 3 months after surgical correction can be used to predict long-term survival.[80] The presence of microscopic ducts at the hilum is somewhat controversial. Some authors have suggested that duct size is important, but not all agree.[81,82] Types I and II BA generally have a good prognosis if treated early. In the more typical type III BA, the presence of larger bile ductules at the porta hepatis ($>150~\mu m$ in diameter) is associated with better prognosis. The subgroup of infants with syndromic BA have worse outcomes in terms of both clearance of jaundice and overall mortality.[1,25] The latter is related to associated malformations, particularly congenital heart disease, a predisposition to developing hepatopulmonary syndrome, and possibly immune compromise from functional hyposplenism. Anecdotal evidence suggests that infants with concomitant cytomegalovirus infection fare less well after a portoenterostomy.

The importance of surgical technical experience was demonstrated by a British survey in which patients who underwent treatment at centers treating one case per year had significantly worse outcome than patients who underwent surgical treatment at centers performing more than five cases per year. The level of surgical skill and the experience with postoperative management are critical factors for optimizing outcome.[83]

Certain substances may act as prognostic factors in BA. Serum levels of interleukin (IL)-6, IL-1ra, vascular cell adhesion molecule-1 (VCAM-1), and ICAM-1 correlate with liver dysfunction in postoperative BA patients.[33,84] Immunohistochemically, a reduction in the expression of CD68 and ICAM-1 at the time of portoenterostomy is associated with better postoperative prognosis.[85] Postoperative prognosis could be better predicted after further research on such substances and would have direct impact on the timing of decision to perform liver transplantation.

Liver Transplantation

Infants whose jaundice is not cleared after portoenterostomy and those in whom complicated or end-stage chronic liver disease develops despite an initially successful portoenterostomy require liver transplantation. BA is the most common indication for liver transplantation in children, and the majority of affected children will eventually come to transplant. Most of these cases require a transplant in the first few years of life. The indications for liver transplantation in postoperative BA

patients are (1) no bile drainage at all, because major clinical deterioration will be inevitable; (2) presence of signs of developmental retardation or their sequelae if they become uncontrollable; and (3) complications/side effects being socially unacceptable.

A high hepatic artery resistance index measured on Doppler US is an ominous sign and an indication for relatively urgent transplantation. Deterioration in hepatic status may be precipitated by adolescence or pregnancy.[86] However, as many as 20% of patients undergoing portoenterostomy will remain well and reach maturity with good native liver function.

The dramatic improvement in survival after liver transplantation that has accompanied the use of cyclosporin and FK-506 immunosuppression raises the question of transplantation becoming a more conventional form of surgical treatment for BA. Donor supply is always a problem, alleviated to some extent by reduced-size liver transplantation. Favorable experience with living-related liver transplantation at Kyoto University in Japan has been widely reported.[87]

Five-year survival after liver transplantation for BA is currently 80% to 90%, and techniques such as split-liver grafting and living-related liver transplantation have minimized the risk of dying on the waiting list. The combination of Kasai portoenterostomy and liver transplantation has transformed a disease that was almost invariably fatal in the 1960s into one with an overall 5-year survival of about 90%. Furthermore, long-term studies have shown BA survivors have relatively good quality of life after portoenterostomy alone and after liver transplantation.[88,89]

Although we are aware of the debate over whether hepatic portoenterostomy or primary liver transplantation should be performed as the initial surgical procedure for BA, the consensus among pediatric surgeons all over the world is that hepatic portoenterostomy is still the most reasonable first choice. However, liver transplantation has an important role in the management of BA.

CHOLEDOCHAL CYST

Choledochal cysts, or dilatations of the CBD, were first reported by Douglas in 1852.[90] The condition is a relatively rare abnormality, with an estimated incidence in Western populations of one in 13,000 to 15,000.[91] However, this condition is far more common in the East, with rates as high as one per 1,000 having been described in Japan. The etiology remains unknown, but choledochal cysts are likely to be congenital. The pathologic features of the condition frequently include an anomalous junction of the pancreatic and CBDs (pancreaticobiliary malunion: PBMU), intrahepatic bile duct dilatation with or without downstream stenosis, and various degrees of hepatic fibrosis.

Choledochal cysts are usually classified into three groups, based on anatomy.[92] However, other forms and subgroups have been described, based on the cholangiographic findings of intrahepatic ducts or the presence of a long common duct shared by the liver and the pancreas (the so-called pancreaticobiliary malunion or PBMU).[93,94] Based on our experience, we prefer to classify choledochal cysts into groups according to presence or absence of PBMU (Fig. 43-11). The vast majority of choledochal cysts are associated with PBMU. Thus the following comments are related primarily to cystic (saccular), fusiform, and forme fruste choledochal cysts (FFCCs).

Pathogenesis

A number of theories have been proposed for the etiology of the choledochal cyst. Congenital weakness of the bile duct wall, a primary abnormality of proliferation during embryologic ductal development, and congenital obstruction have been given as possible causes.[95–97]

An obstructive factor in the early developmental stage was stressed as a causative factor. It is based on an experimental study in which cystic dilatation of the CBD was produced by ligation of the distal end of the CBD in the neonatal lamb, but not in a later stage of development.[98]

In 1969, the so called "long common channel theory" was proposed as a new concept. It was theorized that PBMU allows reflux of pancreatic enzymes into the CBD, which leads to disruption of the ductal wall. This theory is supported by the high amylase content in the fluid aspirated from a choledochal cyst. In theory, the CBD could become obstructed distally because of edema or fibrosis caused by refluxed pancreatic fluid.[99]

We support the "long common channel theory" anatomically because almost all choledochal cyst patients have PBMU, but we cannot agree with the hypothesis that the weakness of the choledochal wall is due to the reflux of pancreatic fluid. Our experimental data in puppies showed that the chemical reaction in the CBD initiated by refluxed pancreatic fluid is extremely mild.[100]

It also is generally recognized that a number of patients who have PBMU and high amylase levels in the gallbladder show no dilation of the CBD. The diagnosis of choledochal cyst may be made as early as the fifth month of gestation, at which time, the fetal pancreas does not produce functional enzymes. The exact role of the pancreatic fluid is unclear.

From research on human fetuses, it was demonstrated that the pancreaticobiliary ductal junction is located outside the duodenal wall before the eighth week of gestation and then migrates normally toward the duodenal lumen, suggesting that PBMU may persist as a result of arrest of this migration.[101]

Based on these studies, we believe that PBMU combined with congenital stenosis is the basic causative factors of the choledochal cyst rather than destruction caused by reflux of pancreatic fluid.

Clinical Presentation

Choledochal cysts can appear at any age, but more than half of patients are initially seen within the first decade of life. Clinical manifestations of choledochal cysts differ according to the age at onset.

An infant may have obstructive jaundice, acholic stools, and hepatomegaly, which resembles BA. These patients sometimes have advanced liver fibrosis. Studies will reveal a patent communication to the duodenum and well-developed intrahepatic bile duct (IHBD) tree, as shown by surgical cholangiography. Young infants may have a large upper abdominal mass without jaundice.

The presenting symptom of choledochal cysts in children after early infancy can be divided roughly into two groups: right upper quadrant mass with intermittent jaundice due to biliary obstruction, seen in patients with

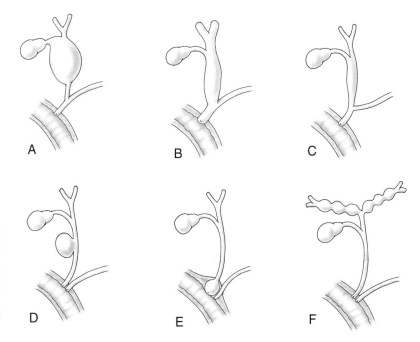

FIGURE 43-11. Classification of choledochal cysts with pancreaticobiliary malunion (PBMU). *A,* Cystic dilatation of the extrahepatic bile duct. *B,* Fusiform dilatation of the extrahepatic bile duct. *C,* Forme fruste choledochal cyst without PBMU. *D,* Cystic diverticulum of the common bile duct. *E,* Choledochocele (diverticulum of the distal common bile duct). *F,* Intrahepatic bile duct dilatation alone (Caroli's disease). (From Miyano T, Yamataka A: Choledochal cysts. Curr Opin Pediatr 9:284, 1997.)

saccular choledochal cysts, and abdominal pain due to pancreatitis, which is characteristic of the fusiform or the FFCCs.

Choledochal cysts in adolescence and adulthood that have gone undiagnosed for many years may first be seen with cholelithiasis, cirrhosis, portal hypertension, hepatic abscess, and biliary carcinoma. Surgical treatment in this group is much more difficult than that in children, and the incidence of postoperative complications is quite high, even after primary cyst excision.[102]

Pathology

The bile duct mucosa shows erosion, epithelial desquamation, and papillary hyperplasia with regenerative atypia.[103]

Dysplasia in the bile duct mucosa without carcinoma is frequently found in patients with choledochal cysts.[104] Additionally, metaplastic changes, such as mucous cells, goblet cells, and Paneth cells can be seen. Hyperplasia and metaplasia increase with age and progress to carcinoma in adult cases. These changes are seen in all types of choledochal cysts.[105]

The gallbladder mucosa in patients with PBMU shows cholecystitis, cholesterolosis, adenomyosis or adenomyomatosis, polyp including adenoma, and epithelial hyperplasia. The gallbladder mucosa in the FFCC is characterized by diffuse epithelial hyperplasia, with or without metaplasia of pyloric glands, goblet cells, and Paneth cells.

Diagnosis

For the diagnosis of choledochal cyst, it is important to detect not only dilatation of the extrahepatic bile duct, but also PBMU.

Currently abdominal US is probably the best screening method in patients who are suspected of having a choledochal cyst. In recent years, the number of patients who are diagnosed by antenatal US is increasing. US also clearly demonstrates IHBD dilatation and the state of the liver parenchyma.

ERCP can accurately visualize preoperatively the configuration of the pancreaticobiliary ductal system in fine detail. However, it is invasive and therefore unsuitable for repeated use and is contraindicated during acute pancreatitis.

Magnetic resonance cholangiopancreatography (MRCP) can provide excellent visualization of the pancreaticobiliary ducts, allowing detection of narrowing, dilatation, and filling defects with medium to high degrees of accuracy (Fig. 43-12).[106,107] MRCP is noninvasive and can be useful in delineating the pancreatic and biliary ducts proximal to an obstruction. However, in children younger than 3 years, MRCP may not visualize the pancreaticobiliary ductal system because of the small caliber.

Percutaneous transhepatic cholangiography also is valuable, especially for the patient with IHBD dilatation and severe jaundice.

Intraoperative cholangiography is unnecessary if the entire biliary system has been delineated before cyst

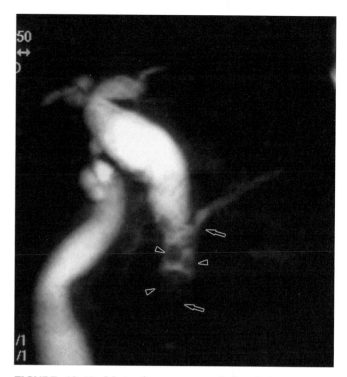

FIGURE 43-12. Magnetic resonance cholangiopancreatography in a patient with a choledochal cyst, showing fusiform dilatation of the extrahepatic bile duct, long common channel (between *arrows*), protein plugs (*arrowheads*), and pancreatic duct. (From Miyano T, Yamataka A: Choledochal cysts. Curr Opin Pediatr 9:285, 1997.)

excision, but it should be used if the pancreaticobiliary ductal system is not completely visualized.

Treatment

Cyst excision is the definitive treatment of choice for choledochal cyst because of the high morbidity and high risk of carcinoma after internal drainage, a commonly used treatment in the past. Recently, more attention has been paid to treatment of intrahepatic and intrapancreatic ductal diseases such as IHBD dilatation, focal stenosis, debris in the IHBD, and protein plugs or stones in the common channel.[108,109] The transection level of the common hepatic duct and excisional level of the intrapancreatic bile duct also are highly controversial.[108,110]

The Common Bile Duct

Usually more adhesions are found between a saccular choledochal cyst and the portal vein and hepatic artery, especially in the older children and when compared with the fusiform choledochal cyst. In the adolescent and adults, the adhesions are often very dense, and great care is required during cyst excision.

Before dissection of the cyst, we always open the anterior wall of the choledochal cyst transversely (Fig. 43-13). After opening the anterior wall of the cyst, the posterior wall of the cyst is visible directly from

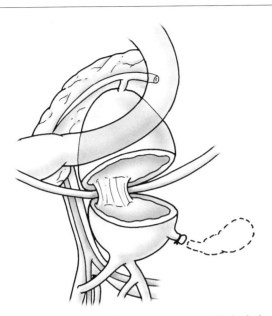

FIGURE 43-13. Schema of transaction of choledochal cyst. (From Miyano T: Congenital biliary dilatation. In Puri P (ed): Newborn Surgery. Oxford, UK, Butterworth-Heinemann, 1996, p 436.)

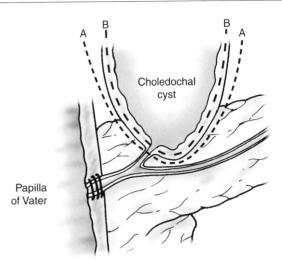

FIGURE 43-15. Operative procedure for the excision of the distal portion of choledochal cyst (*A*, full-thickness layer; *B*, mucosectomy layer). (From Miyano T: Congenital biliary dilatation. In Puri P (ed): Newborn Surgery. Oxford, UK, Butterworth-Heinemann, 1996, p 437.)

the inside, facilitating the dissection of the portal triad. If the cyst is extremely inflamed and adhesions are very dense, mucosectomy of the cyst (Figs. 43-14, 43-15) should be performed rather than attempting full-thickness dissection (see Figs. 43-13 and 43-15) to minimize the risk of injuring the portal vein and the hepatic artery.

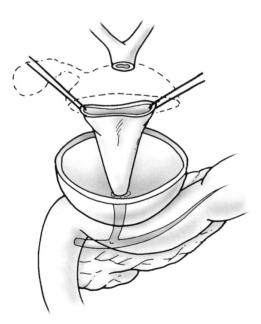

FIGURE 43-14. Schema of mucosectomy of distal portion of choledochal cyst. (From Miyano T: Congenital biliary dilatation. In Puri P (ed): Newborn Surgery. Oxford, UK, Butterworth-Heinemann, 1996, p 437.)

The Distal Common Bile Duct

To prevent postoperative pancreatitis or stone formation or both in a remnant cyst, the distal CBD should be resected as close as possible to the pancreaticobiliary ductal junction. In the saccular type, the distal CBD is sometimes so narrow that it cannot be identified. Thus in the saccular choledochal cyst, it is unlikely that a residual cyst will develop within the pancreas. In contrast, in fusiform choledochal cyst, the delineation of the diseased duct is more difficult, because the distal CBD is still wide at the pancreaticobiliary ductal junction, and the likelihood of leaving some remnant of distal CBD is high. If the distal CBD is resected along line 1 (Fig. 43-16), over time, a cyst will reform around the distal CBD left within the pancreas, leading to recurrent pancreatitis, stone formation, or malignancy in the residual cyst (Fig. 43-17). In contrast, if the distal duct is resected along line 3 (see Fig. 43-16), that is, just above the pancreaticobiliary ductal junction, cyst reformation due to residual duct within the pancreas is unlikely.[93]

Before the introduction of intraoperative endoscopy, it was difficult to excise the pancreatic portion of the fusiform-type choledochal cyst completely and safely because of risk of injury to the pancreatic duct. Endoscopy now allows safe excision of most of the fusiform choledochal cyst wall in the pancreas without damaging the pancreatic duct, and we believe that this reduces the risk of postoperative complications.

The Proximal Common Bile Duct

The common hepatic duct is transected at the level of distinct caliber change. Because any remaining proximal cyst mucosa is prone to malignant changes, care must be taken to excise it completely, especially when a large anastomosis is present (Fig. 43-18).

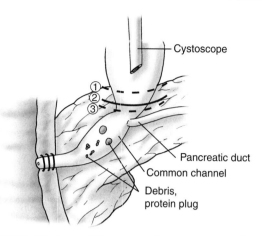

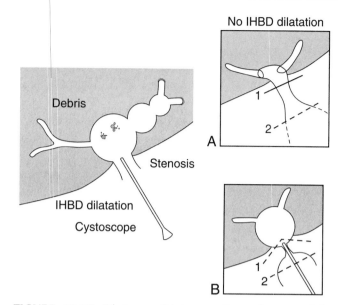

FIGURE 43-16. Diagram of intraoperative endoscopy of the bile duct distal to a cyst with debris and protein plug. After identification of the orifice of the pancreatic duct, the cyst is excised at level 1. Likelihood of leaving the residual cyst. Level 2, Adequate excision level of the cyst. Level 3, likelihood of injuring the pancreatic duct. (From Miyano T, Yamataka A, Long Li: Congenital biliary dilatation. J Pediatr Surg 9:190, 2000.)

FIGURE 43-18. Diagrams of intraoperative endoscopy of the bile duct proximal to a cyst. *A,* Ideal level of resection of the common hepatic duct is safely determined without injuring the orifices of the intrahepatic duct and without leaving any redundant common hepatic duct. *B,* Stenosis of the common hepatic duct near the hepatic hilum is safely excised, and a wide anastomosis is made. Level 1, Adequate level of resection of the common hepatic duct. Level 2, Inadequate level of resection. (From Miyano T, Yamataka A, Long Li: Dilatation of the intrahepatic duct. Semin Pediatr Surg 9: 187–195, 2000.)

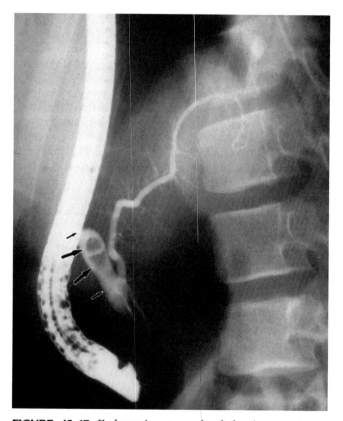

FIGURE 43-17. Endoscopic retrograde cholangiopancreatography showing stones (*arrows*) in the residual intrapancreatic terminal choledochus after excision of fusiform type choledochal cyst. (From Yamataka A, Ohshiro K, Okada Y, et al: Complications after cyst excision with hepaticoenterostomy for choledochal cyst and their surgical management in children versus adults. J Pediatr Surg 32:1099, 1997.)

Dilatation of the peripheral IHBD in patients with choledochal cysts may be associated with late complications such as recurrent cholangitis, stone formation, and anastomotic stricture. Severe dilatation of the IHBD can be managed by segmentectomy of the liver, intrahepatic cystoenterostomy, or balloon dilatation of a stenotic lesion at the time of cyst excision.[111-114] However, the incidence of the late complications appears to be low, especially in younger children, so such excessive surgical intervention may be unnecessary, except in specific cases. If IHBD dilatation persists even after definitive surgery, careful follow-up is mandatory.

Intraoperative endoscopy also is useful for examining for the presence of debris in the dilated IHBD (Fig. 43-19). Recently we found a high incidence of IHBD debris that was not detected by preoperative radiologic investigations, and some debris that had been shown in the preoperative studies was overlooked. These facts indicate that intraoperative endoscopy is necessary at the time of cyst excision. Another striking finding was that there could be debris even when the IHBD were not dilated, although this was uncommon. We believe endoscopic inspection of the IHBD should be a routine part of the operative treatment of choledochal cysts.[115]

The Anastomosis

End-to-end anastomosis of the jejunem to the upper remnant of the CBD is recommended if the ratio between the diameters of the CBD and the proximal Roux-en-Y

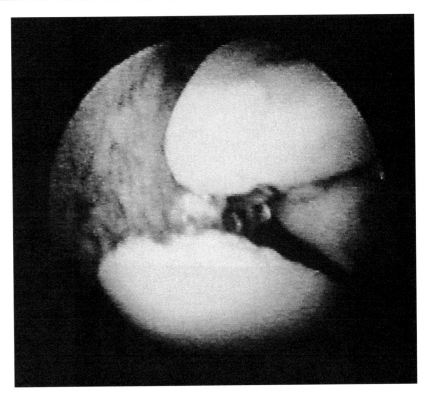

FIGURE 43-19. Massive debris in the intrahepatic bile duct observed through the pediatric cystoscope. From Shima H, Yamotaka A, Yanai T, et al: Intracorporeal electrohydraulic lithotripsy for intrahepatic bile duct stone formation after choledochal cyst excision. Pediatr Surg Int 20:70–72, 2004.

jejunum is less than or equal to 1 (common hepatic duct) to 2.5 (jejunum) (Fig. 43-20). If the biliary duct is too small, then an end-to-side anastomosis is unavoidable. The anastomosis should be created as close as possible to the closed end of the duodenal limb (see Fig. 43-20, *inset*). An end-to-side anastomosis performed far from the closed end of the proximal jejunum will allow formation of a blind pouch as the child grows (Fig. 43-21). Bile stasis in the blind pouch can lead to intrahepatic stone formation, especially if the intrahepatic ducts are dilated. We believe that using an end-to-end hepaticojejunostomy and our end-to-side jejunojejunostomy technique will help prevent both stone formation and ascending cholangitis.

Some surgeons predetermine the length of the Roux-en-Y jejunal limb without considering the size of the child, which causes the Roux-en-Y jejunal limb to be unnecessarily long, especially in infants and younger children. Redundancy of the Roux-en-Y limb is likely as the patient grows, leading to bile stasis in the limb itself, that leads, in turn, to cholangitis or stone formation. Construction of the Roux-en-Y as shown (see Fig. 43-20) should prevent redundancy of the Roux-en-Y limb. We recommend that the jejunal limb from the ligament of Treitz and the Roux-en-Y jejunal limb be approximated side to side for about 8 cm proximal to the end-to-side anastomosis to ensure the smooth flow of bile and succus entericus distally. Without performing this, the jejunojejunostomy will tend to be T-shaped, promoting reflux of jejunal contents into the Roux-en-Y limb, a situation we recently encountered in a patient who was operated on at another hospital (see Fig. 43-21).[116]

Results

A satisfactory surgical outcome with low morbidity in the short to mid term is expected in patients after cyst excision. In the long-term follow-up, many complications are reported. Careful long-term follow-up is mandatory.

In an American survey in 1981, 14 of 198 patients with choledochal cysts were reported to have died of biliary atresia, cholangitis with sepsis, hepatic failure, or carcinoma.[117] Other late and serious complications were cholangitis, obstructive jaundice, pancreatitis, stone formation, and portal hypertension. Thirty-six patients had been lost to follow-up, and only 115 patients were alive without liver disease.

In 1997 we reported 200 children who had cyst excision performed at age 15 years or younger.[102] The onset of symptoms was 5 years or younger in 175 children, and between 6 and 15 years in the remaining 25 children. The mean age of initial symptoms was 3 years. The mean age at cyst excision was 4.2 years. Primary cyst excision was performed in 176, five had cyst excision converted from internal drainage, and 19 had cyst excision converted from other biliary surgery such as percutaneous transhepatic cholangiodrainage, T-tube drainage, and cholecystectomy. Intraoperative endoscopy was used in 70 children. The mean follow-up period was 10.9 years.

Roux-en-Y hepaticojejunostomy was performed in 188 patients, 11 had standard hepaticoduodenostomy, and 1 had a jejunal interposition hepaticoduodenostomy. No operative mortality occurred. Eighteen (9%) children had 25 complications after cyst excision, including ascending cholangitis, intrapancreatic terminal CBD calculi, pancreatitis, and bowel obstruction (Table 43-2).

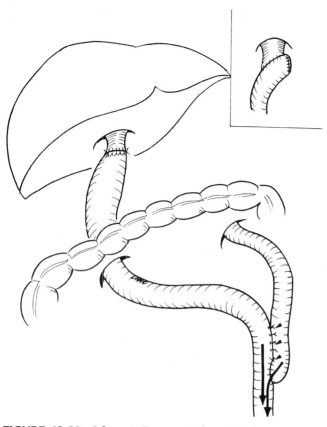

FIGURE 43-20. Adequate Roux-en-Y hepaticojejunostomy at the time of cyst excision. *Arrowheads,* Approximated native jejunum and distal Roux-en-Y limb. *Arrows,* smooth flow without reflux of small bowel contents. (From Yamataka A, Kobayashi H, Shimotakahara A, et al: Recommendations for preventing complications related to Roux-en-Y hepatico-jejunostomy performed during excision of choledochal cyst in children. J Pediatr Surg 38:1830–1832, 2003.)

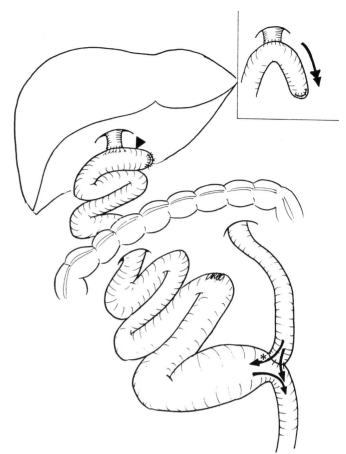

FIGURE 43-21. Inadequate Roux-en-Y (RY) hepaticojejunostomy (HJ) at the time of cyst excision. Note HJ far from the closed end of the blind pouch (*arrowhead*). *Double arrows in the inset,* Elongation of the blind pouch. *Arrow with an asterisk,* Reflux of jejunal contents into the RY limb through a T-shaped RY jejunojejunostomy. (From Yamataka A, Kobayashi H, Shimotakahara A, et al: Recommendations for preventing complications related to Roux-en-Y hepatico-jejunostomy performed during excision of choledochal cyst in children. J Pediatr Surg 38:1830–1832, 2003.)

Fifteen of the 18 children required surgical interventions such as revision of the hepaticoenterostomy, percutaneous transhepatic cholangioscopic lithotomy, excision of the residual intrapancreatic terminal CBD, endoscopic sphincterotomy, pancreaticojejunostomy, or laparotomy for bowel obstruction. Neither stone formation, anastomotic stricture, nor cholangitis was seen in the 70 children who had intraoperative endoscopy. No occurrence of malignancy was reported.

In patients who underwent cyst excision at age 5 years or younger, no major complications such as intrahepatic stones, intrapancreatic terminal CBD calculi, or stricture of the hepaticoenterostomy were seen. Thus we believe that early diagnosis followed by cyst excision and intraoperative endoscopy is extremely important to prevent postoperative complications.

Even after primary cyst excision, malignancy can arise from the intrapancreatic terminal CBD,[118] the hepaticojejunostomy anastomosis site,[119] and from the IHBD.[120] Of the 40 adult patients in our series who had cyst excision at age 16 years or older, two died of cholangiocarcinoma. One of these patients had had a primary cyst excision at age 25 years.

In the past 18 years, we have performed a total of 92 Roux-en-Y hepaticojejunostomies (70 end-to-end anastomoses and 22 end-to-side anastomoses) by using our cyst-excision technique with intraoperative endoscopy and the Roux-en-Y hepaticojejunostomy technique mentioned in the section on treatment. All patients are well after a mean follow-up period of 8.0 years (range, 9 months to 16 years) without any major complications.[116]

OTHER BILIARY TRACT DISORDERS

Biliary Hypoplasia

Biliary hypoplasia is a lesion characterized by an exceptionally small but grossly visible and radiographically patent extrahepatic biliary duct system. The diagnosis is made at the time of surgical exploration for the investigation of jaundice in infancy. Biliary hypoplasia is not a specific disease entity but a manifestation of a variety of hepatobiliary disorders: neonatal hepatitis, α_1-antitrypsin

TABLE 43-2

COMPLICATIONS AFTER CYST EXCISION IN CHILDREN VERSUS ADULTS

Incidence in 200 Children	Post-CEHE Complications	Incidence in 40 Adults
3	Ascending cholangitis	9
3	Intrahepatic bile duct stones	5
3*	Intrapancreatic terminal choledochus calculi	1
1	Pancreatic duct calculus	1
1*	Stones in the blind pouch of the end-to-side Roux-en-Y hepaticojejunostomy	0
9†	Bowel obstruction	3‡
0	Cholangiocarcinoma	2
0	Liver dysfunction	1
5	Pancreatitis	5
25 (18)	Total	27 (17)

Note. The numbers in parentheses indicate the patients who had complications after cyst excision (18 children and 17 adults had 25 and 27 complications after cyst excision, respectively).
*One patient with intrapancreatic terminal choledochus calculi also had a stone in the blind pouch of the end-to-side hepaticojejunostomy.
†Adhesions in six and intussusception in three.
‡Adhesions in all three.
From Yamataka A, Ohshiro K, Okada Y, et al: Complications after cyst excision with hepaticoenterostomy for choledochal cysts and their surgical management in children versus adults. J Pediatr Surg 32:1098, 1997, with permission.

deficiency, intrahepatic biliary atresia, Alagille's syndrome, and nonsyndromic paucity of IHBDs. Biliary hypoplasia cannot be improved by surgical maneuvers. The prognosis is highly variable, depending on the primary disease. Some die in infancy; others live to adolescence, often with jaundice, pruritus, and stunted growth; and still others recover fully.

Alagille's syndrome is a genetic defect that results in a typical constellation of features: peculiar facies with a high, prominent forehead and deep-set eyes, chronic cholestasis, posterior embryotoxon, butterfly-like vertebral arch defects, and heart disease (usually peripheral pulmonary stenosis). These patients often respond to supportive measures such as treatment with ursodeoxycholic acid and phenobarbital.[121] They often have hypercholesterolemia and may eventually require liver transplantation because of ongoing hepatic scarring and the development of hepatocellular carcinoma.

Nonsyndromic paucity of the bile ducts may be associated with liver changes similar to those seen in Alagille's syndrome but without the associated findings. Treatment is similar for both conditions.

Idiopathic Perforation of Bile Ducts: Bile Ascites

Bile ascites typically is first seen with gradually worsening abdominal distention with jaundice in a newborn infant. The disease may be associated with an episode of sepsis or ABO incompatibility; but, more typically, it is an isolated finding, probably related to duct malformation.

The almost universal site of perforation is at the junction of the cystic duct with the CBD. The diagnosis is made by hepatobiliary scan, demonstrating radioactivity in the free peritoneal cavity.

At operation, sterile bile ascites and bile staining are found. An operative cholangiogram should be performed, by using the gallbladder. The lesion is almost always self-limiting, and the perforation seals with drainage. Aggressive surgical intervention is not indicated because the small, delicate, presumably congenitally weakened bile duct may be further damaged during attempts at anastomosis.[122]

Gallbladder Disease

Gallbladder disease in children is being diagnosed with increasing frequency. This is related both to increased sensitivity of detection associated with more widespread use of routine US and to increased incidence secondary to dietary changes that occur with modernization in developing countries. Gallbladder disease also may develop in infants supported with total parenteral nutrition.

Hydrops of the Gallbladder

Acute distention of the gallbladder with edema of the gallbladder wall has been reported in association with a number of septic or shocklike states, including Kawasaki disease, severe diarrhea with dehydration, hepatitis, scarlet fever, familial Mediterranean fever, leptospirosis, and mesenteric adenitis. Hydrops is suspected if a palpable mass of the gallbladder is confirmed by US. In most cases, hydrops resolves spontaneously. If symptoms intensify, cholecystectomy may be necessary.[123]

Acalculous Cholecystitis

Hydrops and acalculous cholecystitis are probably manifestations of the same disease entity and usually arise after a patient has been resuscitated from a state of primary sepsis or shock. Presumably, asymptomatic hydrops of the gallbladder then develops, becoming secondarily infected. Patients are often intubated in an intensive care unit setting, so early manifestations of the disease are not evident: the most common presentation is one of deterioration and signs of sepsis in a previously stable patient. If it is suspected, the diagnosis can be confirmed by US, which demonstrates gallbladder distention and intraluminal echogenic debris. Hepatobiliary scans show nonfunction of the gallbladder. Treatment in mild cases can be conservative with antibiotics. However, if the patient's condition deteriorates, then cholecystectomy is indicated. In patients who are very ill, percutaneous or open cholecystostomy may be a useful temporary measure.

Hemolytic Cholelithiasis

In the past, the usual cause of gallstones in children was hemolytic disease. Hereditary spherocytosis, sickle cell anemia, and thalassemia are the most common hemolytic disorders resulting in the development of gallstones. Jaundice also may occur intermittently because of hemolysis, and therefore does not necessarily mean that common duct calculi are present. In patients with spherocytosis, US is recommended before splenectomy. Demonstration of stones dictates that simultaneous cholecystectomy should be performed. In sickle cell disease, the incidence of stones progresses from 10% to 55% as the child grows older. Cholecystectomy is currently not recommended for children with sickle cell disease, unless symptomatic, and cholecystectomy should be performed electively rather than as an emergency procedure during an hemolytic crisis.[124] Partial exchange transfusion is necessary before operation to reduce the hemoglobin S level to less than 40%. In patients with thalassemia major, the incidence of gallstones is now 2% to 3% because of hypertransfusion regimens.

Cholesterol Cholelithiasis

Cholesterol gallstones appear to occur in children and adolescents because of the same pathophysiologic disturbances that cause these stones in adults. In most North American institutions, the incidence is increasing and has come to surpass hemolytic disease as the leading cause of cholelithiasis in pediatric patients. The typical patient is a markedly obese young girl; the clinical symptoms are usually of vague abdominal pain, with minimal physical findings. The classic history of fatty food intolerance is often not present. The diagnosis is usually made by using US, and the treatment is typically laparoscopic cholecystectomy. Cholesterol stones can occur in infants on prolonged total parenteral nutrition or after ileal resection. Cholecystectomy is still the treatment of choice, although these patients typically have had multiple previous operations, and laparoscopy may not be possible.

Congenital Deformities

A variety of abnormal configurations and locations of the gallbladder, such as gallbladder agenesis, duplication, bilobation, floating gallbladder, diverticula, and ectopia, have been reported. They are usually of no real clinical relevance unless they impair gallbladder emptying. In such cases, calculi are frequent, and treatment is almost always cholecystectomy.

PORTAL HYPERTENSION

Portal hypertension in children produces some of the most uniquely challenging therapeutic problems encountered in clinical pediatric practice. Although the predictable consequences of increased pressure in the portal system (bleeding esophageal varices, hypersplenism, and ascites) are the same in adults and children, their etiology, outcome, and appropriate management are very different. As an example, the onset of bleeding esophageal varices in an adult is often a preterminal event or, at best, a grave prognostic indicator of impending clinical deterioration. In children, at least half

of all esophageal variceal bleeding occurs as an isolated, albeit life-threatening, problem in a setting of normal liver metabolism in which portal hypertension has resulted from portal vein thrombosis. Even when portal hypertension has resulted from cirrhosis, the overall outcome in children is much better than that in adults. For these reasons, palliation per se is almost never the treatment goal in children. Rather, the aim is for growth, development, and improvement in quality and length of life. Modern therapeutic management of isolated manifestations of portal hypertension should not limit any chance a child has for liver transplantation. As a result, treatment has moved increasingly away from shunting toward nonshunt management, such as esophageal variceal endosclerosis, splenic embolization, vigorous nutritional support, and diuretics.

Pathophysiology

Portal hypertension results from an increase in resistance to venous flow through the liver. The site of obstruction is categorized anatomically as being prehepatic, intrahepatic, or suprahepatic. Prehepatic causes of portal hypertension are relatively unique to the pediatric age group, hepatic parenchymal function is well maintained, and coagulopathy plays no role in abnormal bleeding. Intrahepatic and suprahepatic causes typically have associated liver dysfunction, which increases the risk for bleeding resulting from coagulopathy, increases the formation of ascites, and affects all aspects of the patient's care.

The hemodynamic effects of portal venous obstruction are complex. In experimental animals, it has been shown that, in addition to portal venous obstruction, an increase in mesenteric arterial flow is required to cause an increase in portal venous pressure.[125] The interplay of these hemodynamic changes coupled with the development of collateral vessels in the growing child makes any prediction of long-term outcome after therapy difficult and emphasizes the importance of long-term follow-up.

Prehepatic Obstruction

In the past, portal vein thrombosis was the most common cause of portal hypertension in children.[126] Now, with extended survival achieved through operative bile drainage in children with BA, intrahepatic obstruction (hepatic fibrosis) nearly equals portal vein thrombosis as a cause for portal hypertension in children.[127] Portal vein thrombosis may result from perinatal omphalitis, cannulation of the umbilical vein in the newborn period, intra-abdominal sepsis, or dehydration, but in more than half the cases, no causal event is known. In contrast to those with cirrhosis, patients with portal vein thrombosis usually have normal liver synthetic function (bilirubin, prothrombin time, albumin), but manifestations of portal hypertension (variceal hemorrhage and hypersplenism) are pronounced.

Intrahepatic Obstruction

Biliary atresia is the single most common cause of intrahepatic obstruction leading to portal hypertension in children. Even when bile drainage is achieved, histopathologic studies show that the liver is affected by hepatic fibrosis of varying degrees, even in the newborn period. Approximately one-third of patients with biliary atresia with successful bile drainage do well, have normal liver function, and continue normal growth and development. The remaining two thirds have clinical evidence of liver disease, with half requiring liver transplantation to survive, and the other half growing, but with clinical or laboratory manifestations of liver dysfunction. In the last group, postsinusoidal obstruction is the result of hepatic venous compression by regenerating nodules.

Congenital hepatic fibrosis may occur as an isolated disease of the liver characterized by hepatosplenomegaly that becomes manifest at age 1 to 2 years, or in association with multiple forms of kidney disease, the most common of which is infantile polycystic disease. The disease is defined histopathologically by the presence of linear fibrous bands within the liver that result in presinusoidal obstruction. Although hepatomegaly is present, no stigmata of chronic liver disease are seen. In the liver, the parenchyma is spared (presinusoidal obstruction), hepatocellular function is preserved, and serum bilirubin, transaminase, and alkaline phosphatase levels and prothrombin time are usually normal. Portal hypertension is the most frequent complication of congenital hepatic fibrosis.[128] Children commonly are first seen with hepatosplenomegaly and frequently have bleeding esophageal varices.

Other causes of intrahepatic portal hypertension in children include focal biliary cirrhosis, α_1-antitrypsin deficiency, chronic active hepatitis, and complications secondary to radiation or chemotherapy. The incidence of focal biliary cirrhosis with portal hypertension occurring in patients with cystic fibrosis ranges from 0.5% to 8% in children and from 5% to 20% in adolescents and young adults.[129]

Suprahepatic Obstruction

Obstruction of the hepatic veins (Budd-Chiari syndrome) is a rare cause of portal hypertension in children. This syndrome may be seen in association with coagulation disorders, use of oral contraceptives, malignant disease, autoimmune disorders, and hepatic vein webs. The course is typically insidious, with a long interval between the onset of hepatomegaly, abdominal pain, and ascites and the recognition of the syndrome. If symptoms develop urgently, it can be associated with sudden severe liver enlargement and liver damage with central lobular congestion and necrosis.

Clinical Presentations of Portal Hypertension

Variceal hemorrhage occurs most commonly from the distal esophagus. Increased portal pressure leads to dilation of the portal systemic collateral veins, the most important of which link the coronary vein to the short gastric and the submucosal plexus of the lower esophagus. As blood flow through the system increases, esophageal varices develop and can be frighteningly large.

The typical presentation is one of vomiting bright red blood, but melena also may occur. Retroperitoneal, periumbilical, and hemorrhoidal collaterals also develop, and although these can be large, they do not tend to cause significant bleeding.

After control of an acute hemorrhage, the cause for the bleeding (i.e., portal hypertension) is sought. In a patient without stigmata of liver disease, portal vein thrombosis is by far the most likely diagnosis. Physical examination typically shows an enlarged spleen and a normal-sized liver, and Doppler US is nearly 100% diagnostic. In contrast, patients with concurrent liver disease usually have signs of liver failure, and the liver is almost always firm and enlarged, with associated malnutrition, splenomegaly, ascites, and jaundice.

Occasionally, splenomegaly and hypersplenism are the first signs of portal hypertension in children. Splenic size does not correlate with the degree of venous pressure elevation, but the hematologic effects of hypersplenism do correlate with the size of the spleen. All formed blood elements may be affected. Long-standing portal hypertension can cause splenic fibrosis, which then reduces the hematologic consequences. This also makes the effects of subsequent shunting less efficacious.

Diagnosis and Treatment

Initial management of upper gastrointestinal hemorrhage is the same regardless of etiology and involves fluid-volume resuscitation, nasogastric tube placement for gastric lavage, and stabilization. Accurate monitoring of cardiovascular parameters and urine output and frequent laboratory determination of blood counts necessitate an intensive care setting. Balloon tamponade with a Sengstaken-Blakemore tube may be necessary initially to control hemorrhage, and children require tracheal intubation, sedation, and ventilation. Once the patient's condition is stabilized, endoscopic and Doppler US are used to delineate the status of the portal vein. US can accurately document portal venous thrombosis as well as cirrhosis with hepatofugal flow, and quantify arterial inflow. Liver function tests document hepatic functional status. Esophagoscopy can be performed electively to document clinical status and for therapeutic purposes.

Endoscopic varix sclerosis in children requires deep sedation and tracheal intubation. Short-term results are typically excellent in experienced hands.[130] Patients with acute hemorrhage are reinjected every 2 to 3 days until bleeding ceases. Patients who are not actively bleeding should have repeated endoscopy at 6-week intervals until all varices are obliterated. Nearly complete control of bleeding can be achieved by using this regimen. Minor complications include superficial esophageal ulceration, pleural effusion, and atelectasis. Occasionally, very serious complications of varix injection can occur, such as esophageal stricture, perforation, spinal cord paralysis, systemic venous thrombosis, and respiratory distress syndrome related to the use of excessive volumes of sclerosant.[131,132]

An alternative to sclerosants is band ligation of esophageal varices. It is just as effective for controlling bleeding[133] and has fewer systemic complications (Fig. 43-22).

Other therapy after acute esophageal bleeding is dependent on the underlying pathophysiology. Portal hypertension resulting from intraparenchymal liver disease most likely will require liver transplantation. Evaluation for transplantation is usually already under way, and variceal bleeding usually expedites assessment in these patients. Conversely, if patients are found to have good liver function with either suprahepatic or portal venous obstruction, other surgical intervention may be more appropriate. For patients who have a prehepatic

cause for portal hypertension, shunt therapy should be considered after the first bleed and is specifically indicated if repeated bleeding occurs despite sclerotherapy.[134,135] Because these patients typically have good liver function, the incidence of postshunt encephalopathy is low.[136,137] Selective splenorenal shunting also is a satisfactory option,[138] but the increased complexity of this procedure, coupled with the observations that most children at the time of shunt surgery already have hepatofugal flow in the portal vein, and loss of selectivity of the distal splenorenal shunt occurs over time, usually work against its use in pediatric patients.[139]

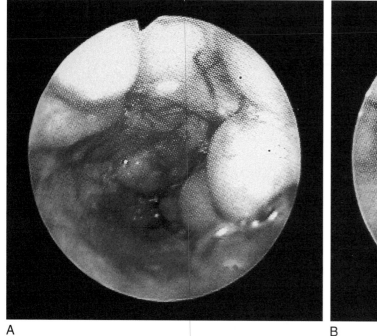

A

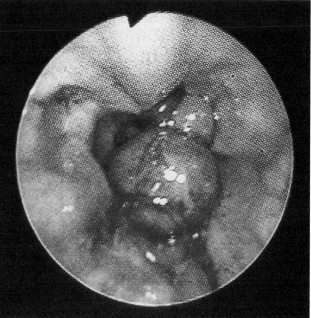

B

C

FIGURE 43-22. EVL, Endoscopic variceal ligation. *A,* Before EVL. *B,* EVL with rubber band. *C,* After EVL.

Of special consideration are those patients who bleed from varices in the stomach, small bowel, or colon. These vessels are not amenable to sclerotherapy, and thus these patients may require earlier intervention with shunt therapy. Recently, a new operative technique using direct bypass of an extrahepatic portal venous obstruction (a cavernoma) was reported.[140] In this procedure, the obstructive lesion was bypassed by interposing a venous jugular autograft between the superior mesenteric vein and the distal portion of the left portal vein. Although this procedure is restricted to those patients in whom the intrahepatic left portal branch can be confirmed to be patent by Doppler US, it can be regarded as an option.

Long-standing splenomegaly is occasionally accompanied by clinically significant hypersplenism. Because of the recognized hazard of postsplenectomy sepsis in children, embolization methods aimed at eliminating hypersplenism while conserving splenic immune function have been developed. Maddison[141] was the first to perform embolization for hypersplenism in 1973. Since that time, improvements in materials and methods have made splenic embolization the treatment of choice for hypersplenism in children. The technique usually involves injection of surgical gel (Gelfoam) particles until 60% to 80% splenic infarction has been achieved. The immediate postembolization morbidity rate is high, with fever and pain being present in all children. Ileus, pleural effusion, and atelectasis also are common. However, major complications such as splenic rupture and splenic abscess are rare, and postsplenectomy sepsis has not developed over long-term follow-up.[142]

ASCITES

Children can have severe ascites, typically associated with end-stage liver disease, and portal hypertension. Ascites may contribute to respiratory embarrassment because of elevation of the diaphragm and to malnutrition because of protein loss. Occasionally, chylous ascites may develop as a result of portal hypertension and liver disease. Long-term total parenteral nutrition and use of somatostatin analogues reduce the volume of fluid produced.[143] Conservative management consists of dietary sodium and water restriction, spironolactone, furosemide, and periodic paracentesis. In the absence of infection in the ascitic fluid, coagulopathy, and primary cardiac failure, peritoneovenous shunt procedures can return the ascitic fluid to the circulating blood volume, but this is rarely performed in the pediatric age group. Most patients with refractory ascites require liver transplantation, and therapy should be directed at preparing the patient for that procedure.

REFERENCES

1. Chardot C, Carton M, Spire-Bendelac N, et al: Prognosis of biliary atresia in the era of liver transplantation: French national study from 1986 to 1996. Hepatology 30:606–611, 1999.
2. McKiernan PJ, Baker AJ, Kelly DA: The frequency and outcome of biliary atresia in the UK and Ireland. Lancet 355:25–29, 2000.
3. Yoon PW, Bresee JS, Olney RS, et al: Epidemiology of biliary atresia: A population-based study. Pediatrics 99:376–382, 1997.
4. Fischler B, Haglund B, Hjern A: A population-based study on the incidence and possible pre- and perinatal etiologic risk factors of biliary atresia. J Pediatr 141:217–222, 2002.
5. Thomson J: On congenital obliteration of the bile ducts. Edinburgh Med J 37:523–531, 604–616, 724–735, 1891.
6. Holmes JB: Congenital obliteration of the bile ducts: Diagnosis and suggestions for treatment. Am J Dis Child 11:405–431, 1916.
7. Ladd WE: Congenital atresia and stenosis of the bile ducts. JAMA 91:1082–1085, 1928.
8. Bill AH: Biliary atresia. World J Surg 2:557–559, 1987.
9. Gross RE: The Surgery of Infancy and Children. Philadelphia, WB Saunders, 1953, pp 508–523.
10. Sterling JA: Experiences with Congenital Biliary Atresia. Springfield, Ill, Charles C Thomas, 1960, pp 3–68.
11. Potts WJ: The Surgeons and the Child. Philadelphia, WB Saunders, 1959, pp 137–143.
12. Longmire WP, Sanford MC: Intrahepatic cholangiojejunostomy with partial hepatectomy for biliary obstruction. Surgery 24:264–276, 1948.
13. Fonkalsrud EW, Kitagawa S, Longmire WP: Hepatic drainage to the jejunum for congenital biliary atresia. Am J Surg 112:188–194, 1966.
14. Williams LF, Dooling JA: Thoracic duct-esophagus anastomosis for relief of congenital biliary atresia. Surg Forum 14:189–191, 1963.
15. Swenson O, Fisher JH: Utilization of cholangiogram during exploration for biliary atresia. N Engl J Med 249:247, 1952.
16. Thaler MM, Gellis SS: Studies in neonatal hepatitis and biliary atresia, II: The effect of diagnostic laparotomy on long-term prognosis of neonatal hepatitis. Am J Dis Child 116:262–270, 1968.
17. Kanof A, Donovan EJ, Berner H: Congenital atresia of the biliary system: Delayed development of correctability. Am J Dis Child 86:780–787, 1953.
18. Kravetz LJ: Congenital biliary atresia. Surgery 47:453–467, 1960.
19. Carlson E: Salvage of the "noncorrectable" case of congenital extrahepatic biliary atresia. Arch Surg 81:893–898, 1960.
20. Kasai M, Suzuki S: A new operation for noncorrectable biliary atresia: Hepatic portoenterostomy. Shujutu 13:733–739, 1959.
21. Kasai M, Kimura S, Asakura Y, et al: Surgical treatment of biliary atresia. J Pediatr Surg 3:665–675, 1968.
22. Kasai M: Treatment of biliary atresia with special reference to hepatic portoenterostomy and its modification. Progr Pediatr Surg 6:5–52, 1974.
23. Karrer FM, Lilly JR, Stewart BA, et al: Biliary atresia registry, 1976–1989. J Pediatr Surg 25:1076–1081, 1990.
24. Perlmutter DH, Shepherd RW: Extrahepatic biliary atresia: A disease or a phenotype? Hepatology 35:1297–1304, 2002.
25. Davenport M, Savage M, Mowat AP, et al: The biliary atresia splenic malformation syndrome. Surgery 113:662–668, 1993.
26. Mazziotti MV, Willis LK, Heuckeroth RO, et al: Anomalous development of the hepatobiliary system in the *Inv* mouse. Hepatology 30:372–378, 1999.
27. Jacquemin E, Cresteil D, Raynaud N, et al: *CFC1* gene mutation and biliary atresia with polysplenia syndrome. J Pediatr Gastroenterol Nutr 34:326–327, 2002.
28. Tan CEL, Driver M, Howard ER, et al: Extrahepatic biliary atresia: A first-trimester event? Clues from light microscopy and immunohistochemistry. J Pediatr Surg 29:808–814, 1994.
29. Seidman SL, Duquesnoy RJ, Zeevi A, et al: Recognition of major histocompatibility complex antigens on cultured human biliary epithelial cells by alloreactive lymphocytes. Hepatology 13:239–246, 1991.
30. Dillon P, Belchis D, Tracy T, et al: Increased expression of intercellular adhesion molecules in biliary atresia. Am J Pathol 145:263–267, 1994.
31. Silveira TR, Salzano FM, Donaldson PT, et al: Association between HLA and extrahepatic biliary atresia. J Pediatr Gastroenterol Nutr 16:114–117, 1993.
32. Kobayashi H, Puri P, O'Brian DS, et al: Hepatic overexpression of MHC class II antigens and macrophage-associated antigen (CD68) in patients with biliary atresia of poor prognosis. J Pediatr Surg 32:590–593, 1997.
33. Kobayashi H, Horikoshi K, Li L, et al: Serum concentration of adhesion molecules in postoperative biliary atresia patients: Relationship to disease activity and cirrhosis. J Pediatr Surg 36:1297–1301, 2001.

34. Allison JP: CD28-B7 interactions in T-cell activation. Curr Opin Immunol 6:414–419, 1994.
35. Kobayashi H, Li Z, Yamataka A, et al: Role of immunologic co-stimulatory factors in the pathogenesis of biliary atresia. J Pediatr Surg 38:892–896, 2003.
36. Sokol RJ, Mack C: Etiopathogenesis of biliary atresia. Semin Liver Dis 21:517–524, 2001.
37. O'Neill JA, Rowe MI, Grosfeld JL, et al: Pediatric Surgery, 5th ed. St. Louis, Mosby-Year Book, 1998.
38. Ito T, Horisawa M, Ando H: Intrahepatic bile ducts in biliary atresia: A possible factor determining the prognosis. J Pediatr Surg 18:124–130, 1983.
39. Raweily EA, Gibson AAM, Burt AD: Abnormalities of intrahepatic bile ducts in extrahepatic biliary atresia. Histopathology 17:521–527, 1990.
40. Lilly JR, Altman RP: Hepatic portoenterostomy (the Kasai operation) for biliary atresia. Surgery 78:76–86, 1975.
41. Ohi R, Chiba T, Endo N: Morphologic studies of the liver and bile ducts in biliary atresia. Acta Paediatr Jpn 29:584–589, 1987.
42. Desmet VJ: Intrahepatic bile ducts under the lens. J Hepatol 1:545, 1987.
43. Sherlock S: The syndrome of disappearing intrahepatic bile ducts. Lancet 2:493–496, 1987.
44. Chiba T, et al: Japanese biliary atresia registry: Biliary atresia. Tokyo Icom Assoc 1991.
45. Altman RP, Levy J: Biliary atresia. Pediatr Ann 14:481–485, 1985.
46. Okazaki T, Kobayashi H, Yamataka A, et al: Long-term post surgical outcome of biliary atresia. J Pediatr Surg 34:312–315, 1998.
47. Balistreri WF: Neonatal cholestasis. J Pediatr 106:171–184, 1985.
48. Brough H, Houssin D: Conjugated hyperbilirubinemia in early infancy: A reassessment of liver biopsy. Hum Pathol 5:507–516, 1974.
49. Javitt NB, Keating JP, Grand RJ, et al: Serum bile acid patterns in neonatal hepatitis and extrahepatic biliary atresia. J Pediatr 90:736–739, 1977.
50. Faweya AG, Akinyinka OO, Sodeinde O: Duodenal intubation and aspiration test: Utility in the differential diagnosis of infantile cholestasis. J Pediatr Gastroenterol Nutr 13:290–292, 1991.
51. Azuma T, Nakamura T, Moriuchi T, et al: Preoperative ultrasonographic diagnosis of biliary atresia with reference to the presence or absence of the extrahepatic bile duct: Paper presented at the 38th Annual Congress of the Japanese Society of Pediatric Surgeons, Tokyo, Japan, June 2001.
52. Park WH, Choi SO, Lee HJ: The ultrasonographic "triangular cord" coupled with gallbladder images in the diagnostic prediction of biliary atresia from infantile intrahepatic cholestasis. J Pediatr Surg 34:1706–1710, 1999.
53. Kotb MA, Kotb A, Sheba MF, et al: Evaluation of the triangular cord sign in the diagnosis of biliary atresia. Pediatrics 108:416–420, 2001.
54. Tan Kendrick AP, Ooi BC, Tan CE: Biliary atresia: Making the diagnosis by the gallbladder ghost triad. Pediatr Radiol 33:311–315, 2003.
55. Farrant P, Meire HB, Mieli-Vergani G: Ultrasound features of the gallbladder in infants presenting with conjugated hyperbilirubinaemia. Br J Radiol 73:1154–1158, 2000.
56. Abramson SJ, Berdon WE, Altman RP, et al: Biliary atresia and noncardiac polysplenia syndrome: US and surgical consideration. Radiology 163:377–379, 1987.
57. Han BK, Babcock DS, Gelfand MM: Choledochal cyst with bile duct dilatation: Sonographic and 99mTc-IDA cholescintigraphy. AJR Am J Roentgenol 136:1075–1079, 1981.
58. Miyano T, Fujimoto T, Ohya T, et al: Current concept of the treatment of biliary atresia. World J Surg 17:332–336, 1993.
59. Kobayashi H, Horikoshi K, Yamataka A, et al: Alpha-Glutathione-S-transferase as a new sensitive marker of hepatocellular damage in biliary atresia. Pediatr Surg Int 16:302–305, 2000.
60. Kobayashi H, Horikoshi K, Yamataka A, et al: Hyaluronic acid: A specific prognostic indicator of hepatic damage in biliary atresia. J Pediatr Surg 34:1791–1794, 1999.
61. Miyano T, Suruga K, Tsuchiya H, et al: A histopathological study of the remnant of extrahepatic bile duct in so-called uncorrectable biliary atresia. J Pediatr Surg 12:19–25, 1977.
62. Kimura K, Tsugawa C, Matsumoto T, et al: The surgical management of the unusual forms of biliary atresia. J Pediatr Surg 14:653–660, 1979.
63. Freitas L, Gauthier F, Valayer J: Second operation for repair of biliary atresia. J Pediatr Surg 22:857–860, 1987.
64. Ibraham M, et al: Indication and results of reoperation for biliary atresia: Biliary atresia. Tokyo Icom Association, 1991.
65. Muraji T, Higashimoto Y: The improved outlook for biliary atresia with corticosteroid therapy. J Pediatr Surg 32:1103–1107, 1997.
66. Karrer FM, Lilly JR: Corticosteroid therapy in biliary atresia. J Pediatr Surg 20:693–695, 1985.
67. Suruga K, Miyano T, Kimura K, et al: Reoperation in the treatment of biliary atresia. J Pediatr Surg 17:1–6, 1982.
68. Sawaguchi S, et al: The treatment of congenital biliary atresia with special reference to hepatic portoenteroanastomosis. Paper presented at the Fifth annual meeting of the Pacific Association of Pediatric Surgeons, Tokyo, 1972.
69. Nakajo T, Hashizume K, Saeki M, et al: Intussusception-type antireflux valve in Roux-en-Y loop to prevent ascending cholangitis after hepatic portojejunostomy. J Pediatr Surg 25:311–314, 1990.
70. Tanaka K, Shirahase I, Utsunomiya H, et al: A valved hepatic portoduodenal intestinal conduit for biliary atresia. Ann Surg 213:230–235, 1990.
71. Endo M, Katsumata K, Yokoyama J, et al: Extended dissection of the porta hepatis and creation of an intussuscepted ileocolic conduit for biliary atresia. J Pediatr Surg 12:784–793, 1983.
72. Altman RP, Chandra R, Lilly JR: Ongoing cirrhosis after successful portoenterostomy with biliary atresia. J Pediatr Surg 10:685–691, 1975.
73. Bu LN, Chen HL, Ni YH, et al: Multiple intrahepatic biliary cysts in children with biliary atresia. J Pediatr Surg 37:1183–1187, 2002.
74. Andrews WS, Pau CM, Chase HP, et al: Fat soluble vitamin deficiency in biliary atresia. J Pediatr Surg 16:284–290, 1981.
75. Greene HL, Helinek GL, Moran R, et al: A diagnostic approach to prolonged obstructive jaundice by 24-hour collection of duodenal fluid. J Pediatr Surg 95:412–414, 1979.
76. Barkin RM, Lilly JR: Biliary atresia and the Kasai operation: Continuing care. J Pediatr Surg 96:1015–1019, 1980.
77. Kasai M, Mochizuki I, Ohkohchi N, et al: Surgical limitation for biliary atresia: Indication for liver transplantation. J Pediatr Surg 24:851–854, 1989.
78. Davenport M, Kerkar N, Mieli-Vergani G, et al: Biliary atresia: The King's College Hospital experience (1974–1995). J Pediatr Surg 32:479–485, 1997.
79. Chardot C, Carton M, Spire-Bendelac N, et al: Is the Kasai operation still indicated in children older than 3 months diagnosed with biliary atresia? J Pediatr Surg 138:224–228, 2001.
80. Ohhama Y, Shinkai M, Fujita S, et al: Early prediction of long-term survival and the timing of liver transplantation after the Kasai operation. J Pediatr Surg 35:1031–1034, 2000.
81. Chandra RS, Altman RP: Ductal remnants in extrahepatic biliary atresia: A histopathologic study with clinical correlation. J Pediatr Surg 93:196–200, 1978.
82. Tan EL, Davenport M, Driver M, et al: Does the morphology of the extrahepatic biliary remnants in biliary atresia influence survival? A review of 205 cases. J Pediatr Surg 29:1459–1464, 1994.
83. McClement JW, Howard ER, Mowat AP: Results of surgical treatment for extrahepatic biliary atresia in the United Kingdom 1980–1982. BMJ 290:345–347, 1985.
84. Kobayashi H, Yamataka A, Lane GJ, et al: Levels of circulating anti-inflammatory cytokineinterleukin-1 receptor antagonist and proinflammatory cytokines at different stages of biliary atresia. J Pediatr Surg 37:1038–1041, 2002.
85. Davenport M, Gonde C, Redkar R, et al: Immunohistochemistry of the liver and biliary tree in extrahepatic biliary atresia. J Pediatr Surg 36:1017–1025, 2001.
86. Broide E, Farrant P, Reid F, et al: Hepatic artery resistance index can predict early death in children with biliary atresia. Liver Transplant Surg 3:604–610, 1997.
87. Tanaka K, Uemoto S, Tokunaga Y, et al: Surgical techniques and innovations in living related liver transplantation. Ann Surg 217:82–91, 1993.

88. Howard ER, MacClean G, Nio M, et al: Biliary atresia: Survival patterns after portoenterostomy and comparison of a Japanese with a UK cohort of long-term survivors. J Pediatr Surg 36:892–897, 2001.

89. Bucuvalas JC, Britto M, Krug S, et al: Health-related quality of life in pediatric liver transplant recipients: A single-center study. Liver Transplant 9:62–71, 2003.

90. Douglas AH: Case of dilatation of the common bile duct. Monthly J Med Sci 14:97–99, 1852.

91. McEvoy CF, Suchy FJ: Biliary tract disease in children. Pediatr Clin North Am 43:82–83, 1996.

92. Alonso-Lej J, Rever WB, Pessagno DJ: Congenital choledochal cyst, with a report of 2, and an analysis of 94 cases. Int Abst Surg 108:1–30, 1959.

93. Todani T, Narusue M, Watanabe Y, et al: Management of congenital choledochal cyst with intrahepatic involvement. Ann Surg 187:272–280, 1977.

94. Komi N, Takehara H, Kunitomo K, et al: Does the type of anomalous arrangement of the pancreaticobiliary ducts influence the surgery and prognosis of choledochal cyst? J Pediatr Surg 6:728–731, 1992.

95. Ryckman FC, Noseworthy J: Neonatal cholestatic conditions requiring surgical reconstruction. Semin Liver Dis 7:134–154, 1987.

96. Yotsuyanagi S: Contributions to aetiology and pathology of idiopathic cystic dilatation of common bile duct, with reports of three cases: New aetiological theory. Gann 30:601, 1936.

97. Miyano T, Suruga K, Suda K: Abnormal choledocho-pancreaticoductal junction related to the etiology of infantile obstructive jaundice diseases. J Pediatr Surg 14:16–25, 1979.

98. Spitz L: Experimental production of cystic dilatation of the common bile duct in neonatal lambs. J Pediatr Surg 12:39, 1977.

99. Babbitt DP: Congenital choledochal cyst: new etiologic concepts on anomalous relationships of the common bile and pancreatic bulb. Ann Radiol 12:231–241, 1969.

100. Miyano T, Suruga K, Shimomura H, et al: Choledochopancreatic elongated common channel disorders. J Pediatr Surg 19:165, 1984.

101. Wong KC, Lister J: Human fetal development of the hepatopancreatic junction. J Pediatr Surg 16:139–145, 1981.

102. Yamataka A, Ohshiro K, Okada Y, et al: Complications after cyst excision with hepaticoenterostomy for choledochal cyst and their surgical management in children versus adults. J Pediatr Surg 32:1097–1102, 1997.

103. Suda K, Miyano T, Matsumoto Y, et al: A clinicopathological study of the carcinogenic process in patients with pancreaticobiliary maljunction. In Koyanagi Y (ed): Pancreaticobiliary Maljunction. Tokyo, Igakutosho, 2002, pp 243–252.

104. Suzuki F, Eguchi M, Mizuguchi K, et al: Histopathological studies of choledochus and gallbladder in congenital choledochal cyst: With special reference to premalignant lesion. Biliary Tract 1:69–76, 1987.

105. Shimotakahara A, Yamataka A, Kobayashi H, et al: Forme fruste choledochal cyst: Long-term follow-up with special reference to surgical technique. J Pediatr Surg 38:1833–1836, 2003.

106. Yamataka A, Kuwatsuru R, Shima H, et al: Initial experience with non-breath-hold magnetic resonance cholangiopancreatography: A new noninvasive technique for the diagnosis of the choledochal cyst in children. J Pediatr Surg 32:1560–1562, 1997.

107. Shimizu T, Suzuki R, Yamashiro Y, et al: Progressive dilatation of the main pancreatic duct using magnetic resonance cholangiopancreatography in a boy with chronic pancreatitis. J Pediatr Gastroenterol Nutr 30:102–104, 2000.

108. Miyano T, Yamataka A, Kato Y, et al: Choledochal cysts: special emphasis on the usefulness of intraoperative endoscopy. J Pediatr Surg 30:482–484, 1995.

109. Uno K, Tsuchida Y, Kawasaki H, et al: Development of intrahepatic cholelithiasis long after primary excision of choledochal cysts. J Am Coll Surg 183:583–588, 1996.

110. Ando H, Ito T, Nagaya M, et al: Pancreaticobiliary maljunction without choledochal cysts in infants and children: Clinical features and surgical therapy. J Pediatr Surg 30:1658–1662, 1995.

111. Ando H, Ito T, Kaneko K, et al: Intrahepatic bile duct stenosis causing intrahepatic calculi formation following excision of a choledochal cyst. J Am Coll Surg 183:56–60, 1996.

112. Warren KW, Kune GA, Hardy KJ, et al: Biliary duct cysts. Surg Clin North Am 88:567–577, 1968.

113. Eagle J, Salmon PA, et al: Multiple choledochal cysts. Arch Surg 88:345–349, 1964.

114. Tsuchida Y, Taniguchi F, Nakahara S, et al: Excision of a choledochal cyst and simultaneous hepatic lateral segmentectomy. Pediatr Surg Int 11:496–497, 1996.

115. Shimotakahara A, Yamataka A, Kobayashi H, et al: Massive debris in the intrahepatic bile ducts in choledochal cyst: Possible cause of postoperative stone formation. Pediatr Surg Int 20:61–69, 2004.

116. Yamataka A, Kobayashi H, Shimotakahara A, et al: Recommendations for preventing complications related to Roux-en-Y hepatico-jejunostomy performed during excision of choledochal cyst in children. J Pediatr Surg 38:1830–1832, 2003.

117. Kim SH: Choledochal cyst: Survey by the surgical section of the American Academy of Pediatrics. J Pediatr Surg 16:402–407, 1981.

118. Yoshikawa K, Yoshida K, Shirai Y, et al: A case of carcinoma arising in the intrapancreatic terminal choledochus 12 years after primary excision of a giant choledochal cyst. Am J Gastroenterol 81:378–384, 1986.

119. Yamamoto J, Shimamura Y, Ohtani I, et al: Bile duct carcinoma arising from the anastomotic site of hepaticojejunostomy after the excision of congenital biliary dilatation: A case report. Surgery 119:476–479, 1996.

120. Chaudhuri PK, Chaudhuri B, Schuler JJ, et al: Carcinoma associated with congenital cystic dilatation of bile ducts. Arch Surg 117:1349–1351, 1982.

121. Alagille D: Alagille syndrome today. Clin Invest Med 19:325–330, 1996.

122. Lilly JR, Weintraub WH, Altman RP: Spontaneous perforation of the extrahepatic bile ducts and bile peritonitis in infancy. Surgery 75:664–673, 1974.

123. Mercer S, Carpenter B: Surgical complication of Kawasaki disease. J Pediatr Surg 16:444–448, 1981.

124. Ware R, Filston HC, Schultz WH, et al: Elective cholecystectomy in children with sickle hemoglobinopathies. Ann Surg 208:17–22, 1988.

125. Witte CL, Tobin GR, Clark DS, et al: Relationship of splanchnic blood flow and portal venous resistance to elevated portal pressure in the dog. Gut 17:122, 1976.

126. Shaldon S, Sherlock S: Obstruction to the extrahepatic portal system in children. Lancet 1:63, 1962.

127. Altman RP. Krug J: Portal hypertension: American Academy of Pediatrics, Surgical Section Survey. J Pediatr Surg 17:567, 1982.

128. Alvarez F, Bernard O, Brunelle F, et al: Congenital hepatic fibrosis in children. J Pediatr 99:370–375, 1981.

129. Psacharopoulos HT, Mowat AP: The liver and biliary system. In Hodson ME, Norman AP, Bratten JC (eds): Cystic Fibrosis. London, Balliere Tindall, 1983, p 164.

130. Howard E, Stinger MD, Mowat AP: Assessment of injection sclerotherapy in the management of 152 children with oesophageal varices. Br J Surg 75:404–408, 1988.

131. Seidman E, Weber AM, Morin CL, et al: Spinal cord paralysis following sclerotherapy for esophageal varices. Hepatology 4:950–954, 1984.

132. Vallgren S, Sigurdsson GH, Moberger G, et al: Influence of intravenous injection of sclerosing agents on the respiratory function. Acta Chir Scand 154:271–276, 1998.

133. Hall RJ, Lilly JR, Stiegmann GV: Endoscopic esophageal varix ligation: Technique and preliminary results in children. J Pediatr Surg 23:1222–1223, 1988.

134. Gauthier F, De Dreuzy O, Valyer J, et al: H-type shunt with an autologous venous graft for treatment of portal hypertension in children. J Pediatr Surg 24:1041–1043, 1989.

135. Sigalet DL, Mayer S, Blanchard H: Portal venous decompression with H-type mesocaval shunt using autologous vein graft: A North American experience. J Pediatr Surg 36:91–96, 2001.

136. Alagille D, Carlier JC, Chiva M, et al: Long-term neuropsychological outcome in children undergoing portal-systemic shunts for

portal vein obstruction without liver disease. J Pediatr Gastroenterol Nutr 5:861–866, 1986.

137. Alvarez F, Bernard O, Brunelle F, et al: Portal obstruction in children, I: Clinical investigation and hemorrhage risk. J Pediatr 103:696–702, 1983.

138. Evans S, Stovroff M, Heiss K, et al: Selective distal splenorenal shunts for intractable variceal bleeding in pediatric portal hypertension. J Pediatr Surg 30:1115–1118, 1995.

139. Belghiti J, Grenier P, Novel O, et al: Long-term loss of Warren's shunt selectivity: Angiographic demonstration. Arch Surg 116:1121–1124, 1981.

140. De Goyet JV, Alberti D, Clapuyt P, et al: Direct bypassing of extrahepatic portal venous obstruction in children: A new technique for combined hepatic portal revascularization and treatment of extrahepatic portal hypertension. J Pediatr Surg 33:597–601, 1998.

141. Maddison F: Embolic therapy of hypersplenism. Invest Radiol 8:280–281, 1973.

142. Brandt CT, Rothbarth LJ, Kump DA, et al: Splenic embolization in children: Long-term efficacy. J Pediatr Surg 24:642–645, 1989.

143. Sharpiro AM, Bain VG, Sigalet DL, et al: Rapid resolution of chylous ascites after liver transplantation using somatostatin analog and total parenteral nutrition. Transplantation 61:1410–1411, 1996.

CHAPTER 44

Solid Organ Transplantation in Children

Frederick C. Ryckman, MD, Maria H. Alonso, MD, and Greg M. Tiao, MD

INTRODUCTION

The ability to undertake successful solid organ transplantation in children has led to a remarkable improvement in both survival and quality of life. Although the vast majority of solid organ transplant recipients are adults, the innovative techniques that have been developed to meet the challenges of pediatric transplantation and the unique demands of immunosuppression in infancy continue to be a forum for the advancement of transplant care. Virtually all of the pediatric population, from the newborn to the young adult, have benefited from the advancements this chapter discusses. Kidney transplant offered the initial experience and success with immunosuppression and perioperative care that formed the foundation for the development of liver transplantation. The significant challenges of limited donor availability and the constraints imposed on donor size in pediatric liver transplantation have driven the evolution of unique and innovative technical developments such as reduced-size transplantation and living donation. This experience and the need for combined liver/intestinal transplantation for children with short-gut syndromes spurred the more recent innovations in multivisceral combined liver, small bowel, and pancreas transplantation. In this chapter, we examine each of the solid organ transplant procedures including the indications, operative procedure, and postoperative complications relevant to the practicing pediatric surgeon.

LIVER TRANSPLANTATION

Few subspecialties have undergone the dramatic improvements in success and survival that have occurred in pediatric liver transplantation. In the early 1980s, survival rates of 30% limited the enthusiasm for this costly and work-intense operation.

The introduction of more effective immunosuppression along with refinements in the operative and postoperative management of infants and children improved survival rates to more than 90% in many centers specializing in pediatric transplantation. When compared with the universally fatal outcome these patients would experience without transplantation, it is not surprising that liver transplantation has been embraced as the preferred therapy for many progressive liver diseases.

With this improved survival rate has come an increasing need for transplant donor organs suitable for pediatric recipients of all ages and sizes. This wide spectrum of needs, coupled with the national shortage of transplant donor organs, has stimulated the pioneering development of surgical procedures such as reduced-size liver transplantation, "split liver" transplantation, and living donor (LD) liver transplantation. However, the excellent survival and organ availability offered by the complementary use of these transplant options cannot overshadow the need for comprehensive evaluation and selective application of liver transplantation.

The Selection Process

The primary aim of the evaluation process is to define which patients require or would benefit from orthotopic liver transplantation (OLT) and when such therapy should be undertaken. Evaluation should be directed toward the identification of (1) progressive deterioration of hepatocellular function, (2) portal hypertension and gastrointestinal (GI) bleeding, or (3) nutritional and growth failure. Referral for transplantation should occur when progressive deterioration is noted and before the development of life-threatening complications.

Indications for Transplantation

The most common clinical presentations prompting transplant evaluation in children can be classified as follows: (1) progressive primary liver disease with the expected outcome of hepatic failure, (2) stable liver disease with remarkable morbidity or known mortality, (3) hepatic-based metabolic disease, and (4) fulminant hepatic failure of known or unknown etiology. In addition, children with hepatic malignancy, particularly hepatoblastoma, whose tumors are not resectable by conventional means, but who have no unresectable metastatic disease, have been

609

identified as excellent candidates for complete liver replacement. Children with diffuse and extensive arteriovenous anomalies or benign vascular tumors leading to irreversible heart failure should also be considered for complete resection and transplantation. Rarely, patients with liver disease secondary to systemic illness such as cystic fibrosis or primary hepatic malignancy are seen as candidates for pediatric transplantation.

Table 44-1 reviews primary diagnoses leading to pediatric transplantation. These disease entities define the bimodal age distribution of pediatric transplant recipients. Infants and children in the first 2 years of life represent

TABLE 44-1

INDICATIONS FOR LIVER TRANSPLANTATION, CINCINNATI CHILDREN'S HOSPITAL MEDICAL CENTER 1986–2003

Primary Diagnosis	No. of Patients	% Total
Neonatal Cholestasis	*133*	*51.15*
Biliary atresia	114	43.8
Alagille syndrome	7	2.7
Ideopathic cholestasis	4	1.5
1° Sclerosing cholangitis	5	1.9
TPN induced	3	1.
Metabolic Disease	*44*	*17*
α_1-Antitrypsin deficiency	22	8.5
Tyrosinemia	7	2.7
Glycogen storage disease-IV	3	1
Hyperoxyluria	3	1
Wilson's disease	2	.7
Cystic fibrosis	1	.38
Hemochromatosis	2	.7
Urea cycle defects	4	1.5
Fulminant Hepatic Failure	*39*	*15*
Non-A Non-B hepatitis	32	12.3
Drug induced	4	1.5
Wilson's disease	2	.7
X-linked LPD (Duncan's syndrome)	1	.38
Hepatitis	*10*	*3.85*
Neonatal-chronic active	5	1.9
Autoimmune	5	1.9
Cirrhosis	*20*	*7.7*
Crytogenic	15	5.7
Short-gut syndrome/TPN cholestasis	5	1.9
Tumor	*9*	*3.5*
Hepatoblastoma	9	3.5
Other	*5*	*1.9*
Total Primary Transplants	*260*	
Retransplantation	*44*	*16*
Second allograft	37	14
Third allograft	4	
Primary transplant elsewhere	3(1 each, 2nd, 3rd, 4th allograft)	
Total Transplants	*304*	

TPN, total parenteral nutrition; LPD, lymphoproliferative disease.

patients with biliary atresia and, occasionally, rapidly progressive hepatic failure secondary to metabolic abnormalities such as neonatal tyrosinemia and hemochromatosis or neonatal hepatic vascular tumors. Patients with metabolic disturbances, fulminant viral hepatitis, and cirrhosis are seen for OLT as older children and adolescents.

Neonatal Cholestatic Syndromes

Biliary Atresia

Children with extrahepatic biliary atresia constitute at least 50% of the pediatric liver transplant population. Successful biliary drainage achieving an anicteric state after the Kasai portoenterostomy is the most important factor affecting preservation of liver function and long-term survival. Primary transplantation without portoenterostomy is not recommended in patients with biliary atresia unless the initial presentation is older than 120 days and the liver biopsy shows advanced cirrhosis.[1,2] We believe that the Kasai portoenterostomy should be the primary surgical intervention for all other infants with extrahepatic biliary atresia. Patients with progressive disease after a portoenterostomy should be offered early OLT. The sequential use of these two procedures optimizes overall survival and organ use.[2]

Patients with extrahepatic biliary atresia who are seen for transplantation form several cohorts. Infants with a failed portoenterostomy have recurrent bacterial cholangitis, ascites, rapidly progressive portal hypertension, malnutrition, and progressive hepatic synthetic failure. Most require OLT within the first 2 years of life. Children having a successful portoenterostomy have an improved prognosis, but this alone does not preclude the development of progressive cirrhosis with eventual portal hypertension, hypersplenism, variceal hemorrhage, and ascites formation. These patients are seen in later childhood for OLT. Individual patients with mild hepatocellular enzyme and bilirubin elevation and mild portal hypertension can be safely observed with ongoing medical therapy. Approximately 15 to 20% of all biliary atresia patients do not require OLT.[3,4]

Alagille Syndrome

Alagille syndrome (angiohepatic dysplasia) is an autosomal dominant genetic disorder manifest as bile duct paucity leading to progressive cholestasis and pruritus, xanthomas, malnutrition, and growth failure. Liver failure occurs late, if at all. Occasionally, severe growth retardation, hypercholesterolemia, and pruritus can compromise the patient's overall well-being to the point at which transplantation is valuable. Exact criteria for OLT are difficult to quantitate. Evaluation must include assessment for congenital cardiac disease and renal insufficiency, both of which are associated with this syndrome. Hepatocellular carcinoma also has been seen occasionally in these patients.[5,6]

Experience using external biliary diversion or internal ileal bypass accompanied by ursodeoxycholic acid therapy has demonstrated a significant decreased in both pruritus and complications of hypercholesterolemia.[7,8]

Both of these procedures may ameliorate the ongoing liver destruction and cirrhosis, further decreasing the need for liver transplantation. The vast improvement in growth and nutrition and the resolution of pruritus, hypercholesterolemia, and xanthoma allow quality-of-life issues to be criteria for consideration for OLT.[9-11]

Metabolic Disease

The leading indication for hepatic transplantation in older children is hepatic-based metabolic disease. In these patients, OLT not only is lifesaving but also it often accomplishes phenotypic and functional cure. A review of these diseases and their mode of presentation is given in Tables 44-2 and 44-3.

Hepatic replacement to correct the metabolic defect should be considered before other organ systems are affected and before complications that would preclude transplantation develop, such as in patients with tyrosinemia, in whom a high risk of hepatocellular carcinoma is found.[5] Although results of transplantation are excellent in the metabolic disease subgroup, replacement of the entire liver to correct single enzyme deficiencies is an inefficient but presently necessary procedure. Current research efforts may show that orthotopic partial hepatic replacement, hepatocyte transplantation, and gene therapy may better serve this patient population in the future.[12-16] Patients with primarily extrahepatic manifestations of their disease, such as cystic fibrosis, are occasionally helped by liver transplantation, although their prognosis is most often a function of their primary illness.[17]

Fulminant Hepatic Failure

Patients with fulminant hepatic failure without recognized antecedent liver disease present diagnostic and prognostic difficulties. Rapid clinical deterioration frequently makes establishment of a definitive diagnosis impossible before an urgent need exists for transplantation. Acute viral hepatitis of undefined type makes up the largest group, followed by drug toxicity and toxin exposure. Previously unrecognized metabolic disease also must be considered. The prognosis for these patients is difficult to predict, and neurologic outcome is potentially suboptimal.[15,16,18,19] When acceptable clinical and metabolic stability make liver biopsy safe, diagnostic information allowing directed treatment of the primary liver disease is helpful. The presence of ongoing coagulopathy often dictates the need for an open approach.

Use of intracranial pressure (ICP) monitoring in patients with progressive encephalopathy has allowed early recognition and treatment of increased ICP. Monitoring should be instituted for patients with advancing grade III encephalopathy and in all patients with grade IV encephalopathy. Intracranial monitoring is continued intraoperatively and for 24 to 48 hours after OLT because significant increases in ICP have been identified throughout the entire clinical course. Failure to maintain a cerebral perfusion pressure (mean blood pressure – ICP) of greater than 50 mm Hg and an ICP less than 20 mm Hg has been associated with very poor neurologic recovery.[19] Survival after transplantation is significantly decreased in patients who reach grade IV encephalopathy.

Efforts to identify and perform transplantation in children before encephalopathy develops is of utmost importance. When candidates are identified before irreversible neurologic abnormalities develop, the results of transplantation are dramatic. Hepatocyte transplantation can provide neurologic protection during organ acquisition or while awaiting spontaneous recovery.[15,16,18]

Malignancy

Transplantation for primary hepatic malignancy has historically been uncommon in children; thus experience is limited.[7] Transplantation for hepatoblastoma is recommended only for individuals with neoplasm confined to the liver and unresectable by conventional means after the initial administration of several chemotherapy courses. Individuals with isolated resectable metastatic lung disease, or children in whom a prior isolated metastasis has disappeared while undergoing preoperative chemotherapy can be considered in selected instances as well. Factors associated with a favorable prognosis include (1) absence of prior surgical resection attempts, (2) unifocal rather than multifocal involvement, (3) absence of vascular invasion, and (4) fetal histology compared with anaplastic or embryonal histology. In addition to these staging factors, a favorable response to pretransplant chemotherapy suggests a more favorable prognosis. Total hepatic and occasionally inferior vena cava (IVC) resection with transplantation and postoperative chemotherapy has led to an overall survival of 88% in our experience.[20] Recurrent disease has historically accounted for half of the postoperative mortality.[21] Despite this success, transplantation must still be viewed as salvage therapy. The primary treatment for hepatoblastoma continues to be conventional surgical resection and chemotherapy.

TABLE 44-2
TRANSPLANTATION FOR METABOLIC DISEASE IN CHILDREN

Wilson's disease
α_1-Antitrypsin deficiency
Crigler-Najjar syndrome (type I)
Tyrosinemia
Cystic fibrosis
Glycogen storage disease-IV
Branched-chain amino acid catabolism disorders
Hemophilia A
Protoporphyria
Homozygous hypercholesterolemia
Urea cycle enzyme deficiencies
Primary hyperoxaluria
Iron storage disease

Reprinted from Balistreri WF, Ohi R, Todani T, et al: Hepatobiliary, Pancreatic and Splenic Disease in Children: Medical and Surgical Management, 1997, pp 395–399.

TABLE 44-3

MODE OF PRESENTATION*

Cirrhosis	Liver Tumor	Life-Threatening Progressive Liver Disease	Failure of Secondary Organ, Normal Liver
α_1-ATD	Tyrosinemia	Urea cycle defect	Type 1 hyperoxalosis
Wilson's disease	GSD-1	Protein C deficiency	Hypercholesterolemia
Hemochromatosis	Galactosemia	Crigler-Najjar syndrome type 1	
Byler's disease	FHD	Niemann-Pick disease	
Cystic fibrosis	Hemochromatosis	Hemochromatosis	
Tyrosinemia	α_1-ATD	Tyrosinemia	
GSD-IV		BCAA	
FHD			
EPP			

*Classification of inherited metabolic disorders according to clinical modes of presentation.
α_1-ATD, α_1-antitrypsin deficiency; BCAA, branched-chain amino acid catabolism disorders; EPP, erythropoietic protoporphyria; FHD, fumaryl hydrolase deficiency; GSD, glycogen storage disease.
Reprinted from Balistreri WF, Ohi R, Todani T, et al: Hepatobiliary, Pancreatic and Splenic Disease in Children: Medical and Surgical Management, 1997, pp 395–399.

Transplantation for hepatocellular carcinoma is complicated by less successful chemotherapy options and frequent extrahepatic involvement. The reported 2-year survival rates of 20% to 30% compare unfavorably with the experience with hepatoblastoma. Most deaths are due to recurrent carcinoma within the allograft or to extrahepatic tumor involvement. When primary hepatocellular carcinoma is discovered incidentally within the cirrhotic native liver at the time of hepatectomy, the overall prognosis is unaffected by the tumor.[22]

Patients with vascular tumors represent a group with diffuse pathology who can benefit significantly from transplantation. Children with progressive, intractable congestive heart failure, even when caused by non-neoplastic arteriovenous malformations or hemangioendotheliomas, offer a unique opportunity for complete removal of the vascular malformation and correction of congestive heart failure. Transplantation in these instances, in our experience, offers significantly better long-term survival compared with embolization or hepatic artery occlusion, which can precipitate sudden and widespread hepatic necrosis. Pretransplant biopsy is essential in large or complex lesions to exclude angiosarcoma.

Contraindications

Contraindications to transplantation include (1) serology positive for human immunodeficiency virus (HIV), (2) primary unresectable extrahepatic malignancy, (3) malignancy metastatic to the liver, (4) progressive terminal nonhepatic disease, (5) uncontrolled systemic sepsis, and (6) irreversible neurologic injury.

Relative contraindications to transplantation that must be individually evaluated include (1) advanced or partially treated systemic infection, (2) advanced hepatic encephalopathy (grade IV), (3) severe psychosocial abnormalities, and (4) portal venous thrombosis extending throughout the mesenteric venous system.

Prioritization of Candidates

Candidate evaluation and selection is undertaken by a multidisciplinary team who establish candidate acceptability and medical urgency and initiate preoperative intervention and education.

Preoperative Preparation

Efforts to correct abnormalities noted during candidate evaluation decrease both the operative risk and postoperative complications. Complications of portal hypertension and malnutrition are vigorously treated. Assessment of prior viral exposure and meticulous attention to the delivery of all normal childhood immunizations, particularly the live-virus vaccines, are imperative, if time allows, before OLT. Additionally, patients receive a one-time inoculation with pneumococcal vaccine, as well as appropriate administration of hepatitis B vaccine. Preoperative assessment of specific cardiopulmonary reserve and hepatic vascular anatomy also is necessary.

Operative Treatment

Donor Options

The single factor limiting the availability of OLT is the limited supply of donor organs. The number of patients awaiting liver transplantation has increased by 11-fold since 1991. Available donor resources have not kept pace with this need. As a consequence of this donor shortage, the time to transplant (waiting time) for all pediatric age groups has increased significantly, with young children and infants most affected (Figs. 44-1 and 44-2). This severely limited supply of available donor organs has driven the advancement of many innovative liver transplant surgical procedures. The development of reduced-size liver transplantation allowed significant expansion

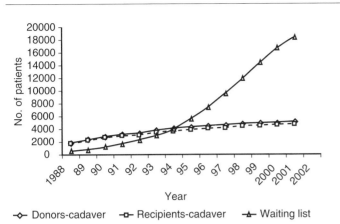

FIGURE 44-1. Number of patients on the United Network of Organ Sharing waiting list for liver transplantation compared with the number of cadaver donors and cadaver liver recipients, 1988 to 2002.

of the donor pool for infants and small children. This not only improved the availability of donor organs but also allowed access to donors with improved stability and organ function. Evolution of these operative techniques has allowed the development of both split-liver transplantation and LD transplantation.

In the hands of experienced transplant teams, these procedures all have success equivalent to that of whole organ transplantation. Furthermore, access to these many donor options has reduced the waiting list mortality rate to less than 5%. Infants and children requiring transplantation benefit greatly by having access to all of these transplant options to minimize waiting time and optimize organ use.

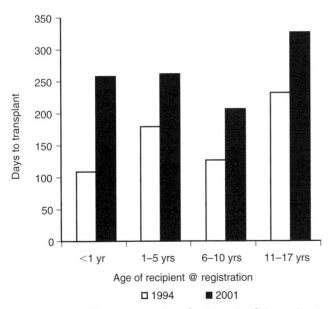

FIGURE 44-2. Time to transplant (waiting time) for pediatric liver transplant recipients subdivided by age at the time of registration. Comparison of 1994 to 2001 waiting times.

Orthotopic Transplant Techniques

Donor Factors

The success of OLT has led to an increase in transplantation that has not been matched by an increase in donor volume. This increased shortage of donor organs has led to expanded efforts to use individuals of advanced age and marginal stability.

Assessment of donor organ suitability is undertaken by evaluating clinical information, static biochemical tests, and dynamic tests of hepatocellular function. The clinical factors reviewed identify donors who are at the limits of age, have had prolonged intensive care hospitalization with potential sepsis, and have vasomotor instability requiring excessive vasoconstricting inotropic agents. Static biochemical tests identify preexisting functional abnormalities or organ trauma but do not serve as good benchmarks to differentiate among acceptable and poor donor allografts. Dynamic tests of hepatic function, which directly measure hepatocyte function, such as MEG-X (monoethylglycine-xylidide), have come closer to identifying limits for organ acceptability.[23] Donor liver biopsy is helpful in questionable cases to identify preexisting liver disease or donor liver steatosis.

Donor Liver Selection

Anatomic replacement of the native liver in the orthotopic position requires selection or surgical preparation of the donor liver to fill but not to exceed available space in the recipient. When using full-sized allografts, a donor weight range 15% to 20% above or below that of the recipient is usually appropriate, taking into consideration body habitus and factors that would increase recipient abdominal size, such as ascites and hepatosplenomegaly.

Surgical preparation of reduced-size liver allografts is based on the anatomy of the hepatic vasculature and bile ducts. Prolonged cold ischemic preservation allows the safe application of the extensive hypothermic bench surgical procedure necessary for reduction technology. The need for this preparation also limits the acceptability of "marginal donors" for these procedures because of the prolonged cold ischemic time necessary. The three primary reduced-size allografts used clinically, prepared ex vivo, are the right lobe, the left lobe, and the left lateral segment.

The right lobe graft, using segments 5 to 8, can be accommodated when the weight difference is no greater than 2:1 between the donor and the recipient. The thickness of the right lobe makes this allograft of limited usefulness in small recipients. Similar right lobe anatomic grafts from LDs have become widely used in adults. The left lobe, using segments 1 to 4, is applicable with a donor-to-recipient (D/R) disparity from 4:1 to 5:1, and a left lateral segment (segments 2 and 3) can be used with up to a 10:1 D/R weight difference. For a left or right lobe graft, the parenchymal resection follows the anatomic lobar plane through the gallbladder fossa to the vena cava.[24,25] A crush-and-tie technique is preferred to achieve good closure of vascular and biliary structures. The middle hepatic vein is retained with the graft in all left lobe and many right lobe preparations. The bile duct, portal vein, and hepatic artery are divided and ligated at the right or left confluence. The vena cava is left incorporated with the allograft in both right and left lobe preparations. Vena caval reduction by posterior caval wall resection and closure is only occasionally necessary. Resection of the inferior protruding portion of the caudate lobe is necessary during left lobe preparation to reduce the likelihood of arterial angulation, which can result in arterial thrombosis. This also facilitates shortening of the inferior vena cava to fit in a small recipient.[26]

When using left lateral segment allografts, the parenchymal dissection follows the right margin of the falciform ligament, with preservation of the left hilar structures. Direct implantation of the left hepatic vein into the combined orifice of the right and middle/left hepatic veins in the recipient vena cava is preferred; the donor vena cava is not retained with this segmental allograft.

Biliary reconstruction in all allograft types is achieved through an end-to-side choledochojejunostomy. Primary bile duct reconstruction is not used with reduced-sized allografts owing to the risk of ischemia in the common bile duct. The bile ducts are perfused by a dense arterial plexus, which travels within the common connective tissue "vasobiliary sheath."[27] Dissection should be limited to that necessary to identify the bile duct for anastomosis.

The use of LDs has increased greatly in past years, with the safety and success of this procedure now well demonstrated[28–30] (Fig. 44-3). In most pediatric cases, the left lateral segment donated from an adult is used as the graft. In situ dissection of the left lateral segment, preserving the donor vascular integrity until the parenchymal division is completed, is undertaken. At the time of harvest, the left hepatic vein is divided from the vena cava, and the left branch of the portal vein and proper hepatic artery are removed with the allograft.[31] Vascular continuity of the hepatic arterial branches to segment IV is maintained if possible. Recently, increased experience has been gained in using the right lobe as an LD allograft for larger recipients such as adolescents and adults.[28,32,33] This more extensive operation has proven to be a challenge to the donor and recipient alike, with complication and mortality rates significantly exceeding that of left lateral segmentectomy. Despite these risks, the number of right lobe LD recipients now greatly exceeds the number of children receiving LD grafts. Recent appreciation of the donor risk of this operation has moderated the early rapid rise in operative cases (see Fig. 44-3). Cryopreservation and implantation follow standard reduced-size orthotopic liver transplant (RSOLT) techniques.

One of the critical elements of LD transplantation is the proper selection of a donor, usually a parent or relative. This procedure is performed on the assumption that donor safety can be assured and that the donor's liver function is normal. Donors should be aged 21 to 55 years, have an ABO-compatible blood type, and have no acute or chronic medical condition. After a satisfactory medical and psychological examination by a physician not directly involved with the transplant program, computed tomography (CT) scanning is used to measure the volume of the potential donor segment to assure that it will meet the metabolic needs but not exceed the space available in the recipient (Table 44-4). If acceptable, arteriography is undertaken to assess the hepatic arterial anatomy, thereby excluding potential donors with multiple arteries to segments 2 and 3, and facilitating minimal hilar vascular dissection at the time of OLT.

Experience has shown that, when donors were deemed unacceptable, 90% of patients were excluded on the basis of history, examination, laboratory screening, and ABO type. Only 10% were excluded after angiography.[34] Donor safety has been excellent in all pediatric LD series.[31,35,36]

Split-liver grafting involves the preparation of two allografts from a single donor. Two similar techniques have been used to accomplish hepatic division in the donor with similar overall success. *The ex situ split* procedure divides the right lobe allograft (segments 5 to 8) from the left lateral segment allograft (segments 2 and 3) after the whole donor organ has been procured. Because this division is undertaken under vascular hypothermic conditions without hepatic perfusion, the vascular integrity of segment 4 is difficult to assess, and it is frequently discarded. Conventional techniques for implanting the respective allografts are then used.[29] The successful experience with *in situ* division of the living donor organ left lateral segment is a basis for the *in situ*

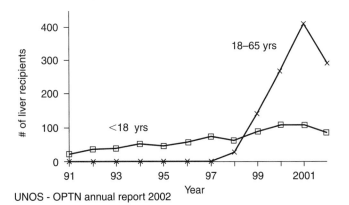

FIGURE 44-3. Number of living donor transplants per year subdivided by age of the transplant recipient, 1991–2000.

TABLE 44-4
ESTIMATION OF ALLOGRAFT SIZE FOR LIVING DONOR TRANSPLANT

Urata formula

$$ELV \ (mL) = 706.2 \times BSA \ (m^2) + 2.4$$

$$ELV \ (mL) = 2.223 \times BW \ (kg)^{0.425} \times BH \ (cm)^{0.682}$$

Revised Urata formula

$$ELV \ (mL) = 1072.8 \times BSA \ (m^2) - 345.7 \ (white \ population)^{179}$$

Graft estimate to weigh ≥ 1% body weight of recipient.
Best to weigh 2%–3% of recipient body weight.

BW, body weight; ELV, estimated liver volume; BSA, body surface area.

split procedure. Here the left lateral segment is prepared identically to a living related donor. The viability of segment 4 can be examined at the time of the division, and it is usually incorporated with the right lobe graft to increase the cellular mass of the allograft. Because this procedure adds considerably to the donor procurement time, and the necessary skill of the donor team, it is more demanding and occasionally difficult to orchestrate successfully. This technique is, however, despite these considerations, the preferred method for split-liver donor preparation.[30,32,37,38]

The obvious benefits of split-liver transplantation are best achieved when ideal donors are selected. Strict restrictions on age, vasopressor administration, predonation hepatic function, and limited donor hospitalization have been used to select optimal candidates for this donor procedure. When these donors are selected, the results from both *in situ* and *ex situ* techniques are similar, with both techniques now having patient survival for both allografts of 90% to 93% and graft survival rates of 86% to 89%.[39]

The selection of a donor segment with an appropriate parenchymal mass for adequate function is critical to success. However, the minimal mass necessary for recovery is not yet established. Any calculation must take into account loss of function after preservation damage, acute rejection, and technical problems. When the D/R weight range is within the normal 8:1 to 10:1 ratio, risk is minimal. Estimates of donor graft–to–recipient body weight ratio (GRWR) may prove to be a more accurate predictor of adequate graft volume. When the GRWR is less than 0.7%, overall allograft and patient survival suffered. In extreme cases in which small-for-size grafts are used, excessive portal flow can lead to hemorrhagic necrosis of the graft. Large-for-size allografts (GRWR > 5.0%) have a less deleterious effect.[40] A review of these donor anatomic options is shown in Figure 44-4.

Creative use of the techniques refined for reduced-size liver transplantation has allowed additional donor options in individual cases. Resection of the left lobe of the native liver followed by auxiliary partial orthotopic transplantation of a reduced-size left lateral segment allograft has been successfully undertaken for patients with metabolic disease (ornithine transcarbamylase deficiency, Crigler-Najjar syndrome) and fulminant hepatic failure.[41,42] This provides for normal hepatic synthesis and function while leaving the right lobe of the donor liver in situ. The auxiliary partial orthotopic transplantation technique also has been undertaken by using an LD for similar indications.[43] Auxiliary placement of a reduced-size allograft also has been undertaken successfully for fulminant hepatic failure in patients deemed too unstable for OLT. In these cases, recovery of the recipient native liver function can ultimately allow discontinuation of immunosuppression and atrophy of the donor allograft if it is no longer required to supplement organ function.[44,45]

The Transplant Procedure

The transplant procedure is carried out through a combined upper midline/bilateral subcostal incision. Meticulous ligation of portosystemic collaterals and vascularized adhesions is necessary to avoid slow but relentless hemorrhage. Dissection of the hepatic hilum, with provision for division of the hepatic artery and portal vein above their bifurcation, allows maximal recipient vessel length to be achieved. The bile duct, when present, is divided high in the hilum to preserve the length and vasculature of the distal duct in case it is needed for later reconstruction in older recipients. Preservation of the Roux-en-Y in biliary atresia patients who have undergone Kasai portoenterostomy simplifies later biliary reconstruction. Complete mobilization of the liver, with dissection of the suprahepatic vena cava to the diaphragm and the infrahepatic vena cava to the renal veins, completes the hepatectomy.

In children with serious vascular instability who cannot tolerate caval occlusion, and in LD transplantation, "piggyback" implantation is possible. In this procedure, the recipient vena cava is left intact, and partial caval occlusion allows end-to-side implantation of a combined donor hepatic vein patch. Access to the infrarenal aorta to implant the celiac axis of the donor liver or iliac artery vascular conduits, provided by mobilizing the right colon and duodenum, is our preference for arterial reconstruction in complex allograft recipients.

Control of hemorrhage is essential during the recipient hepatectomy, requiring meticulous surgical technique. Coagulation factor assays (V, VII, VIII, fibrinogen, platelets, prothrombin time, partial thromboplastin time) allow specific blood-product supplementation to improve clotting function. Use of venovenous bypass is reserved for recipients weighing more than 40 kg who demonstrate hemodynamic instability at the time of venous interruption. Venovenous bypass is rarely necessary in patients who weigh less than 40 kg. Early institution of venovenous bypass combined with high-dose vasopressin (0.2 to 0.6 units/min) is occasionally used in patients with marked friable retroperitoneal variceal hypertension before completing hepatic mobilization.

Removal of the diseased liver is completed after vascular isolation is achieved. Retroperitoneal hemostasis is achieved before implanting the donor liver. In standard OLT, the suprahepatic vena cava is prepared by suture ligating any large phrenic orifices and creating one caval lumen out of the hepatic vein (vena cava confluence). The donor liver is implanted by using conventional vascular techniques and monofilament suture for the vascular anastomosis. In small recipients, interrupted suture techniques, monofilament dissolving suture material, and a "growth factor" knot have all been used to allow for vessel growth. When left lateral segment reduced-size grafts are used, the left hepatic vein orifice is anastomosed directly to the anterolateral surface of the infradiaphragmatic IVC by using the combined right-middle hepatic vein orifices. The left lateral segment allograft is later fixed when necessary to the undersurface of the diaphragm to prevent torsion and venous obstruction of this anastomosis. Similar fixation is not necessary with right or left lobe allograft or with whole organ transplants.

Before completing the vena caval anastomosis in all allografts, the hyperkalemic preservation solution is flushed from the graft by using 500 to 1000 mL of hypothermic normokalemic intravenous (IV) solutions.

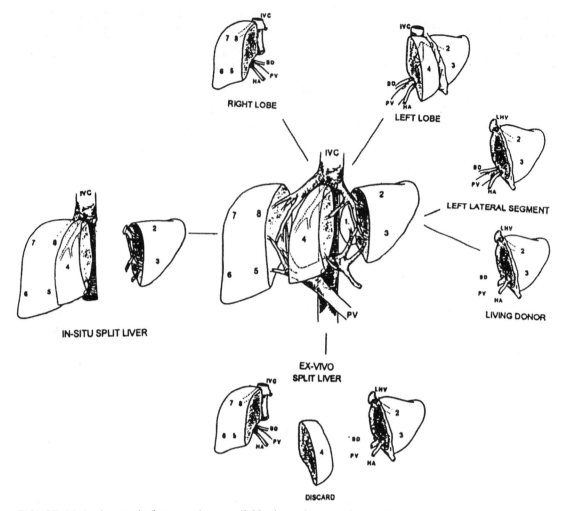

FIGURE 44-4. Anatomic donor options available through surgical reduction.

When using full-sized grafts in older patients, we prefer to complete all venous anastomoses before reconstructing the hepatic artery. In reduced-size allografts and in small recipients in whom we prefer direct aortic vascular inflow reconstruction, the hepatic arterial anastomosis is completed before reconstructing the portal vein to improve visibility of the infrarenal aorta without placing traction on the portal vein anastomosis. We prefer to complete all anastomoses during vascular isolation before organ reperfusion, although some transplant teams reperfuse after venous reconstruction is complete.

Before re-establishing circulation to the allograft, anesthetic adjustments must be made to address the large volume of blood needed to refill the liver and the presence of hypothermic solutions released at reperfusion. Inotropic support with dopamine (5 to 10 mg/kg/min) is begun. Calcium and sodium bicarbonate are administered to combat the effects of hyperkalemia from any remaining preservation solution and systemic acidosis after aortic and vena caval occlusion. Sufficient blood volume expansion, administered as packed red blood cells to increase the central venous pressure (CVP) to 15 to 20 cm H_2O and

the hematocrit to 40%, minimizes the development of hypotension on unclamping and prevents dilutional anemia. Communication between the surgical and anesthesia teams facilitates a smooth sequential reestablishment of vena caval, portal venous, and then arterial recirculation to the allograft.

Biliary reconstruction in patients with biliary atresia or in those weighing less than 25 kg is achieved through an end-to-side choledochojejunostomy by using interrupted dissolving monofilament sutures. A multifenestrated polymeric silicone (Silastic) internal biliary stent is placed before completing the anastomosis (Fig. 44-5). In most cases, the prior Roux-en-Y can be used, with a 30- to 35-cm length being preferred. Primary bile duct reconstruction without stenting is used in older patients with whole organ allografts.

When closing the abdomen, increased intra-abdominal pressure should be avoided. In many cases, avoidance of fascial closure and the use of mobilized skin flaps and running monofilament skin closure are advisable. Musculofascial abdominal closure can be completed before patient discharge.

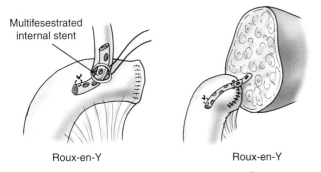

FIGURE 44-5. Bile duct reconstruction in to be Roux-en-Y with placement of an internal multifenestrated biliary stent. (Redrawn from Ryckman F: Liver Transplantation. In Ziegler MM, Azizkhan RG, Weber T [eds]: Operative Pediatric Surgery. New York, McGraw-Hill, 2003, p 1275.)

Immunosuppressive Management

Most centers use an immunosuppressive protocol based on the administration of multiple complementary medications. All use corticosteroids and cyclosporine or tacrolimus. Additional antimetabolites (azathioprine, mycophenolate) are used when more antirejection treatment is needed. Prior protocols using polyclonal or monoclonal induction therapy have been abandoned in most cases because of the extent of the immunosuppressive potency. The recent introduction of humanized monoclonal antibodies to interleukin (IL)-2 (basiliximab, daclizumab) has stimulated interest in induction immunosuppression protocols, as these agents appear to have a low risk of opportunistic infections. The role that they will play in the future is not clear at present. A sample protocol is given in Table 44-5.

Postoperative Complications

Most postoperative complications are seen as cholestasis; increasing hepatocellular enzyme levels; and variable fever, lethargy, and anorexia. This nonspecific symptom complex requires specific diagnostic evaluation before instituting treatment. Therapy directed at the specific causes of allograft dysfunction is essential; empirical therapy of presumed complications is fraught with misdiagnoses, morbidity, and mortality. A flow diagram outlining this evaluation is shown in Figure 44-6.

Primary Nonfunction

Primary nonfunction (PNF) of the hepatic allograft implies the absence of metabolic and synthetic activity after transplantation. Complete nonfunction requires immediate retransplantation before irreversible coagulopathy and cerebral edema occur. Lesser degrees of allograft dysfunction occur more frequently and can be associated with several donor, recipient, and operative factors (Table 44-6).

The status of the donor liver contributes significantly to the potential for PNF. Ischemic injury secondary to anemia, hypotension, hypoxia, or direct tissue injury is often difficult to ascertain in the history of multiple trauma victims. Donor liver steatosis also has been

TABLE 44-5			
IMMUNOSUPPRESSION PROTOCOL			
Day/Wk	Methylprednisolone (mg/kg/day)	Tacrolimus (mg/kg/day)	Tacrolimus Target Level (mg/kg/day)
Intra-Op	15	0	
1	10	0.3	
2	8	0.3	
3	6	0.3	
4	4	0.3	12–15
5	3	0.3	
6	2	0.3	
7	1	0.3	
Week 2	1	Adjust as needed	12–15
Week 3	0.9		
Week 4	0.8		
Week 5	0.7		8–12
Week 6	0.6		
Week 7	0.5		
Week 8	0.4		
Month 3	0.3		
Month 4	0.2		
Month 5	0.1		
Month 6	0.1 qod		7–10
Month 7–9	D/C		
Month 10–12	—		4–7
>1 yr	—		

D/C, discontinue.

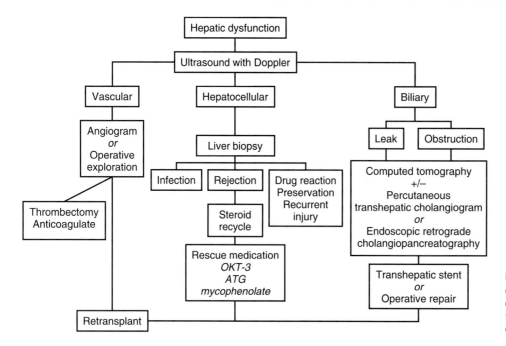

FIGURE 44-6. Schematic flow diagram for management of postoperative liver allograft dysfunction. ATG, antithymocyte globulin; OKT-3, monoclonal antibody.

recognized as a factor contributing to severe dysfunction or nonfunction in the donor liver. *Macrovesicular steatosis* on donor liver biopsy is somewhat more common in adult than in pediatric donors and, when severe, is recognized grossly by the enlarged yellow, greasy consistency of the donor liver. The risk of PNF increases as the degree of fatty infiltration increases. Microscopic findings are classified as mild if less than 30% of the hepatocytes have fatty infiltration, moderate if 30% to 60% are involved, and severe if more than 60% of the hepatocytes have fatty infiltration. Livers with severe fatty infiltration should be discarded, and donors with moderate involvement are used with some concern, with the degree of steatosis and the condition of the recipient

determining use of the allograft. *Microvesicular steatosis* is not related to PNF.[46–49,50–52]

Immediate post-transplant immunologic events, such as humoral antibody-mediated hyperacute rejection, can occur but are uncommon after OLTx. Initial reports suggested that a positive cytotoxic antibody crossmatch between the donor and recipient did not affect the viability or function of the allograft.[53] However, more recent experience with crossmatch-positive donors has demonstrated significantly decreased allograft and patient survival.[54,55]

The use of ABO-incompatible donors has been controversial. Allograft and patient survival rates in adult recipients have not been comparable to those achieved by using ABO identical or compatible donors.[56,57] However, pediatric recipients of ABO-incompatible allografts have achieved survival rates equivalent to those using ABO-compatible and ABO-identical donors, by using either cadaveric donors (CDs) or LDs.[58–60]

Documentation of functional hepatic recovery is best undertaken by evaluating the ongoing hepatic output of clotting factors (V, VII) with improvement in coagulation parameters (prothrombin time, partial thromboplastin time) and the synthesis of bile. Protocol hepatic biopsies assist in the documentation of hepatic histologic and immunologic events, but they cannot accurately predict the likelihood of recovery.

Vascular Thrombosis

Hepatic artery thrombosis (HAT) occurs in children 3 to 4 times more frequently than in adult transplant series, occurring most often within the first 30 days after transplantation. Factors influencing the development of HAT are listed in Table 44-7.

TABLE 44-6

FACTORS RELATED TO PRIMARY NONFUNCTION

Donor Factors
Preexisting disease or injury to donor, anemia, hypoxia, hypotension before organ harvest
Donor organ steatosis (>60% macrovesicular fat)

Transplant Factors
Prolonged cold ischemic storage (>12–8 hr)
Prolonged warm ischemic time at implantation
Complex vascular anastomosis requiring surgical revision
Significant size discrepancy between donor and recipient

Recipient Factors
Postreperfusion hypotension
Vascular thrombosis
Immunologic factors
ABO incompatible, positive crossmatch

TABLE 44-7

FACTORS AFFECTING VASCULAR THROMBOSIS

Donor/Recipient Age/Weight Allograft Type
Whole organ > reduced size
Living donor ≥ reduced size

Anastomotic Anatomy
Primary hepatic artery > direct aortic

Allograft Edema—Increased Vascular Resistance
Ischemic injury secondary to prolonged preservation;
    prolonged implantation
Rejection
Fluid overload

Recipient Hypotension Hypercoagulability
Administration of coagulation factors, fresh-frozen plasma
Procoagulant factor deficiencies

HAT has a variable clinical picture that may include (1) fulminant allograft failure, (2) biliary disruption or obstruction, or (3) systemic sepsis. Doppler ultrasound (US) imaging has been accurate in identifying arterial thrombosis, and it is used as the primary screening modality to assess blood flow after transplantation or whenever complications arise. Acute HAT with allograft failure most often requires immediate retransplantation. Successful thrombectomy and allograft salvage is possible if reconstruction is undertaken before allograft necrosis.[61] Biliary complications are particularly common after HAT. Ischemic biliary disruption with intraparenchymal biloma formation or anastomotic disruption is seen with cholestasis associated with systemic sepsis. The development of systemic septicemia or multifocal abscesses in sites of ischemic necrosis secondary to gram-negative enteric bacteria, *Enterococcus*, anaerobic bacteria, or fungi also can be seen. Antibiotic therapy directed toward these organisms, along with surgical drainage, is indicated when specific abscess sites are identified. Percutaneous drainage and biliary stenting may control bile leakage and infection until retransplantation is undertaken.

Late postoperative thrombosis can be asymptomatic or be seen with slowly progressive bile duct stenosis. Rarely, allograft necrosis occurs. Arterial collaterals from the Roux-en-Y limb can provide a source of revascularization of the thrombosed allograft through hilar collaterals. These collateral channels develop during the first postoperative months, making late thrombosis an often silent clinical event. Conversely, disruption of this collateral supply during operative reconstruction of the central bile ducts in patients with HAT can precipitate hepatic ischemia and parenchymal necrosis. When HAT is asymptomatic, careful follow-up alone is indicated.

Prevention of HAT requires meticulous microsurgical arterial reconstruction at the time of transplantation. Anatomic reconstruction is preferred in whole organ allografts; direct implantation of the celiac axis into the infrarenal aorta is recommended for all reduced-size liver allografts. All complex vascular reconstructions of the donor hepatic artery should be undertaken ex vivo whenever possible by using microsurgical techniques before transplantation. When vascular grafts are required, they also should be directly implanted into the infrarenal aorta.[62] No systemic anticoagulation was routinely used in our series, but aspirin (20 to 40 mg/day) is administered to all children for 100 days. Complex protocols administering both procoagulants and anticoagulants also have been very successful.[49]

Portal vein thrombosis is uncommon in whole organ allografts unless prior portosystemic shunting has altered the flow within the splanchnic vascular bed or unless severe portal vein stenosis in the recipient has impaired flow to the allograft. Preexisting portal vein thrombosis in the recipient can be overcome by thrombectomy, portal vein replacement, or extra-anatomic venous bypass. In biliary atresia recipients, preexisting portal vein hypoplasia is best corrected by anastomosis to the confluence of the splenic and superior mesenteric veins in the recipient. When inadequate portal vein length is present on the donor organ, iliac vein interposition grafts are used. Early thrombosis after transplantation requires immediate anastomotic revision and thrombectomy. Discrepancies in venous size imposed by reduced-size allografts can be modified to allow anastomotic construction.[63,64] Deficiencies of anticoagulant proteins, such as protein C and S, and antithrombin III deficiency in the recipient also must be excluded as a contributing cause for vascular thrombosis.[65] Failure to recognize portal thrombosis can lead to either allograft demise or, on a more chronic basis, significant portal hypertension with hemorrhagic sequelae or intractable ascites.

Biliary Complications

Complications related to biliary reconstruction occur in approximately 10% of pediatric liver transplant recipients. Their spectrum and treatment is determined by the status of the hepatic artery and the type of allograft used. Although whole and reduced-size allografts have an equivalent risk of biliary complications, the spectrum of complications differs.[66,67]

Primary bile duct reconstruction is the preferred biliary reconstruction in adults, but it is less commonly used in children. It has the advantage of preserving the sphincter of Oddi, decreasing the incidence of enteric reflux and subsequent cholangitis, and not requiring an intestinal anastomosis. Early experience with primary choledochocholedochostomy without a T-tube has been favorable.[68] Late complications after any type of primary ductal reconstruction include anastomotic stricture, biliary sludge formation, and recurrent cholangitis. Endoscopic dilation and internal stenting of anastomotic strictures has been successful in early postoperative cases. Roux-en-Y choledochojejunostomy is the preferred treatment for recurrent stenosis or postoperative leak.

Roux-en-Y choledochojejunostomy is the reconstruction of choice in small children and is required in all patients with biliary atresia. Recurrent cholangitis, a theoretical risk, suggests anastomotic or intrahepatic biliary stricture formation or small bowel obstruction within the

Roux or distal to the Roux-en-Y anastomosis. In the absence of these complications, cholangitis is uncommon.

Reconstruction of the bile ducts in patients with reduced-size allografts is more complex. Division of the bile duct in close proximity to the cut-surface margin of the allograft, with careful preservation of the biliary duct collateral circulation, decreases but does not eliminate ductal stricture formation secondary to ductal ischemia. In our early experience, in 14% of patients with left lobe reduced-size allografts, a short segmental stricture developed, requiring biliary anastomotic revision (Fig. 44-7). Operative revision of the biliary anastomosis and reimplantation of the bile ducts into the Roux-en-Y is necessary. Percutaneous transhepatic cholangiography is essential to define the intrahepatic ductal anatomy before operative revision, and temporary catheter decompression of the obstructed bile ducts allows treatment of cholangitis and elective reconstruction. Operative reconstruction is accompanied by transhepatic passage of exteriorized multifenestrated biliary ductal stents, which remain in place until reconstructive success is documented and late stenosis is unlikely. Dissection remote from the vasobiliary sheath in the donor has significantly decreased the incidence of this complication.

Biliary complications have been seen with an increased frequency after living donation in pediatric recipients. The left lateral segment 2 and 3 bile ducts are frequently separate at the plane of parenchymal division. The need for individual drainage of these small biliary ducts makes the development of late anastomotic stenosis more frequent. Individual segmental strictures may not lead to jaundice in the recipient but rather are identified by elevated γ-glutamyl transferase enzymes or through US surveillance. Reoperation after ductal dilatation successfully reestablishes bile drainage.

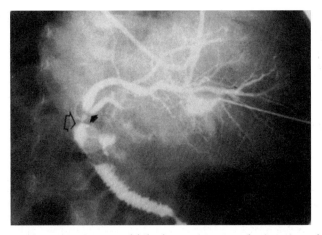

FIGURE 44-7. Segmental bile duct stricture at the junction of the left lateral and left medial segmental bile ducts in a left lobe reduced-size allograft. *Solid arrow,* bile duct stricture; *open arrow,* Roux-en-Y loop and bile duct anastomosis. (From Ryckman FC: Liver Transplantation in Children. In Suchy FJ [ed]: Liver Disease in Children. St. Louis, CV Mosby, 1994, p 941.)

Rejection

Acute Cellular Rejection

Allograft rejection is characterized by the histologic triad of endothelialitis, portal triad lymphocyte infiltration with bile duct injury, and hepatic parenchymal cell damage.[69] Allograft biopsy is essential to establish the diagnosis before treatment. The rapidity of the rejection process and its response to therapy dictate the intensity and duration of antirejection treatment.

Acute rejection occurs in approximately two thirds of patients after OLT.[70] The primary treatment of rejection is a short course of high-dose steroids. Bolus doses administered over a period of several days with a rapid taper to baseline therapy is successful in 75% to 80% of cases.[71] When refractory or recurrent rejection occurs, antilymphocyte therapy with the monoclonal antibody OKT-3 or Thymoglobulin is successful in 90% of cases.[72]

Retransplantation for refractory rejection is necessary in fulminant cases in which vascular thrombosis occurs and in cases unresponsive to treatment. In refractory cases, retransplantation should be undertaken before using multiple courses of corticosteroids or antilymphocyte agents to avoid the overwhelming risks of infection or lymphoproliferative disease. However, modern immunosuppressive treatment makes this an uncommon event.

Chronic Rejection

Uniform diagnosis and management of chronic rejection is complicated by the lack of a consistent definition or clinical course. Chronic rejection occurs in 5% to 10% of transplanted patients. Its incidence appears to be decreasing in all transplant groups, perhaps related to better overall immunosuppressive strategies. Some suggestion has been made that the use of primary Tacrolimus-based immunosuppression is a key element in this apparent decrease.[73,74] Risk factors for its development are many, and no factor predicts the outcome of treatment. The chronic rejection rate was significantly lower in recipients of LD grafts than in recipients of cadaveric grafts; African-American recipients had a significantly higher rate of chronic rejection than did white recipients; and the number of acute rejection episodes, transplantation for autoimmune disease, occurrence of post-transplantation lymphoproliferative disorder (PTLD), and cytomegalovirus (CMV) infection also were significant risk factors for chronic rejection.[75] The primary clinical manifestation is a progressive increase in biliary ductal enzymes (alkaline phosphatase, γ-glutamyl transferase) and progressive cholestasis. This course can be initially asymptomatic or often will follow an unsuccessful treatment course for acute rejection. The syndrome can occur within weeks of transplantation or later in the clinical course.

Chronic rejection can follow one of two clinical forms.[76] In the first, the injury is primarily to the biliary epithelium, and the clinical course is typically slowly progressive with preservation of synthetic function. Histologic evidence shows interlobular bile duct destruction in the absence of ischemic injury or the presence of hepatocellular necrosis. In full expression, this lesion is characterized as acute *vanishing bile duct syndrome* when severe ductopenia is seen in at least 20 portal tracts.[77,78] The eventual spontaneous resolution of up to one half of affected patients with tacrolimus therapy has led to the development of enhanced immunosuppression protocols for this patient subgroup.[76] Retransplantation is occasionally necessary but rarely an emergency.

The second subtype is characterized by the early development of progressive ischemic injury to both bile ducts and hepatocytes, leading to ductopenia and ischemic necrosis with fibrosis. The clinical picture of cholestasis is accompanied by significant synthetic dysfunction with superimposed vascular thrombosis or biliary stricture formation. The vascular endothelial injury responsible for the progressive ischemic changes is characterized by the development of subintimal foam cells or fibrointimal hypertrophy. The clinical course is relentlessly progressive and nearly always requires retransplantation. Unfortunately, recurrence of chronic rejection in the retransplanted allograft is common.[77]

The immunologic nature of this process is emphasized by the primary target role played by the biliary and vascular endothelium, the only tissues in the liver that express class II antigens. Other interdependent cofactors such as CMV infection, human leukocyte antigen (HLA) mismatching, positive B-cell cross-matching, and differing racial demographics of the donor-to-recipient combination have all failed to show consistent correlation with the development of chronic rejection.[76,77]

RENAL INSUFFICIENCY

The long-term success of liver transplantation has been related to the effective immunosuppression with calcineurin inhibitors (CIs), such as cyclosporine and tacrolimus. However, nephrotoxicity associated with their long-term use has become a major problem which affects up to 70% of all nonrenal recipients. Only with the prolonged survival that is now possible has this problem been unmasked. Renal insufficiency is seen in many ways after CI administration and liver transplantation. When this occurs during the initial post-transplant weeks, it is most often related to transient excessive blood levels and is reversible with appropriate dose correction. The role these transient elevations may play in the long-term development of renal insufficiency is yet unclear. Impaired glomerular filtration rate (GFR) seen in pediatric recipients with stable graft function represents a more serious problem. Up to 20% may have a decrease in their GFR to less than 50 mL/min/1.73 m^2, and 5% may progress to end-stage renal failure. Adult studies have shown a progressive increase in chronic renal failure from 0.9% at year 1 to 8.6% at year 13 after OLTx.[79] Similarly, end-stage renal disease (ESRD) increased from 1.6% at year 1 to 9.5% at year 13 after OLTx, yielding a total incidence of renal dysfunction of 18%. The presence of an elevated serum creatinine before OLTx, at 1 year after transplant, and the presence of hepatorenal syndrome before transplant were all identified risk factors.[79,80]

Cyclosporine and tacrolimus both appear to be similar in risk.

In our review of our children who were more than 3 years after liver transplant, we found that 32% had a GFR less than 70 mL/min/1.73 m^2.[81] The factors primarily related to lower GFR were the presence of an elevated creatinine at 1 year after transplant and the length of time after transplantation. Our data supported the concept of a continued decline in renal function after liver transplantation. Considering the long survival for children undergoing liver transplantation, the possibility of progressive asymptomatic renal insufficiency leading to severe kidney disease poses a critical challenge.

Efforts to reverse ongoing renal insufficiency by using protocols that include instituting non-nephrotoxic agents, such as mycophenolate mofetil (MMF) while decreasing the CI dose, have shown some limited success in improving GFR while protecting against unacceptable risks of acute rejection at the time of immunosuppressive drug conversion.[82] Efforts also have been undertaken to use the new class of monoclonal anti-CD25 antibodies for induction therapy coupled with MMF and steroids in an effort to avoid administration of CI during the first post-transplant week. These agents appear to afford sufficient protection against rejection to allow the successful late administration of CI. Whether these efforts will prevent the later development of renal insufficiency is yet unproven.[83] Efforts to eliminate CI administration completely have been complicated by acute or ductopenic rejection. Present efforts suggest that earlier staged reduction of CI before the development of severe GFR reduction will decrease but not eliminate this complication. Once established, chronic renal failure does not appear to resolve with CI dose adjustment. Although CI toxicity is now appreciated, the association of both hepatic and renal disease in many metabolic diseases of childhood also may contribute to the identified GFR abnormalities seen in post-transplant patients.

INFECTION

Infectious complications have become the most common source of morbidity and mortality after transplantation. Multiple-organism infection is common, as are concurrent infections by different infectious agents.

Bacterial infections occur in the immediate post-transplant period and are most often caused by gram-negative enteric organisms, *Enterococcus,* or *Staphylococcus* species. Intra-abdominal abscesses or infected collections of serum along the cut surface of the reduced-size allograft are best addressed with extraperitoneal or laparotomy drainage; percutaneous drainage has been less successful in our experience. Intrahepatic abscesses suggest hepatic artery stenosis or thrombosis, and treatment is directed by the vascular status of the allograft and associated bile duct abnormalities. Sepsis originating at sites of invasive monitoring lines can be minimized by replacing or removing all intraoperative lines soon after transplantation. Antibacterial prophylactic antibiotics are discontinued as soon as possible to prevent the development of resistant organisms.

Fungal sepsis represents a significant potential problem in the early post-transplant period. Aggressive protocols for pretransplant prophylaxis are based on the concept that fungal infections originate from organisms colonizing the GI tract of the recipient. Selective bowel decontamination was successful in eliminating pathogenic gram-negative bacteria from the GI tract in 87% of adult patients; in all cases, *Candida* was eliminated.[84,85] However, these protocols have not been practical in pediatric patients because a long waiting time exists for pediatric organs, and the taste of the antibiotics used is poorly accepted. These regimens are, however, commonly used in the preoperative preparation for combined liver/small intestinal transplantation. Fungal infection most often occurs in patients requiring multiple operative procedures and in those who have had multiple antibiotic courses. Development of fungemia or urosepsis requires retinal and cardiac investigation and a search for renal fungal involvement; antifungal therapy should be promptly undertaken. Severe fungal infection has a mortality rate greater than 80%, making early treatment essential. All patients undergoing OLT should receive antifungal prophylaxis with fluconazole.

The majority of early and severe viral infections are caused by viruses of the Herpesviridae family, including Epstein-Barr virus (EBV), CMV, and herpes simplex virus (HSV). CMV transmission dynamics are well studied and serve as a prototype for herpesvirus transmission in the transplant population. The likelihood that CMV infection will develop is influenced by the preoperative CMV status of the transplant donor and recipient.[86,87] Seronegative recipients receiving seropositive donor organs are at greatest risk, with seropositive D/R combinations at the next greatest risk. Use of various immune-based prophylactic protocols including IV immunoglobulin G (IgG) or hyperimmune anti-CMV IgG, coupled with acyclovir or ganciclovir/valganciclovir, have all achieved success in decreasing the incidence of symptomatic CMV infection, although seroconversion in naive recipients of seropositive donor organs inevitably occurs.

The clinical diagnosis of CMV infection is suggested by the development of fever, leukopenia, maculopapular rash, hepatocellular abnormalities, respiratory insufficiency, or GI hemorrhage. Hepatic biopsy or endoscopic biopsy of colonic or gastroduodenal sites allows early diagnosis with immunohistochemical recognition. Rapid blood and urine assays for CMV also can expedite diagnosis. In suspected cases, treatment should be instituted while awaiting culture or biopsy results, owing to the potential rapidity and severity of this infection in a previously naive child. The treatment of CMV has been greatly improved by the development of ganciclovir. Early treatment with IV IgG and ganciclovir is successful in most cases.

HSV syndromes, similar to those seen in nontransplant patients, require treatment with acyclovir when diagnosed.

Other viruses leading to significant post-transplant infectious complications include adenovirus hepatitis, varicella, and enterovirus-induced gastroenteritis. Recurrent viral hepatitis is an uncommon problem in pediatric transplantation, but it is commonly seen in adult patients. *Pneumocystis* infection has been nearly eliminated by the prophylactic administration of sulfamethoxazole-trimethoprim or aerosolized pentamidine.

EBV infection occurring in the perioperative period represents a significant risk to the pediatric transplant recipient.[88] It has a varying presentation including a mononucleosis-like syndrome, hepatitis-simulating rejection, extranodal lymphoproliferative infiltration with bowel perforation, peritonsillar or lymph node enlargement, or encephalopathy. In small children, its primary portal of entry is often the tonsils, making asymptomatic tonsillar hypertrophy a common initial presentation.[89] EBV infection can occur as a primary infection or after reactivation of a past primary infection. When serologic evidence of active infection exists, an acute reduction in immunosuppression is indicated. It has become clear that continuous surveillance is necessary, as the presentation is often nonspecific, and the prognosis is related to early diagnosis. Screening by determination of EBV blood viral load by quantitative polymerase chain reaction (PCR) appears to be the best present predictor of risk. However, viral loads have been identified in asymptomatic patients and patients recovering from PTLD, limiting the specificity of this test. The balance between viral load measured by quantitative PCR and specific cellular immune response, perhaps mediated by CD8 T cells specific to EBV, may explain this lack of specificity to viral load alone.[90–92]

Many pediatric transplant centers now use serially measured quantitative EBV-DNA PCR as an indication for primary immunosuppression modulation. We recommend monthly EBV-DNA PCR counts to monitor increased genomic expression. Increasing viral load levels warrant more frequent monitoring, as often as every week. In the EBV seronegative pretransplant patients, more than 40 genomes/10^5 peripheral blood leukocytes (PBLs), and more than 200 genomes/10^5 PBLs identify patients for reduction in primary immunosuppression by 25% to 100%. Institution of antiviral therapy with ganciclovir and CMV-IgG also is used in most cases, although only nonrandomized observational studies support their use. Both agents are active in vitro against linear replicating forms of the EBV, but have no activity against the circular episome in immortalized B cells. Treatment should be continued until symptoms of lymphadenopathy have resolved and viral EBV-DNA PCR has returned to baseline.[88,93] It should, however, be cautioned that PTLD can develop and progress without increases in EBV-PCR viral load.[94]

PTLD, a potentially fatal abnormal proliferation of B lymphocytes, can occur in any situation in which immunosuppression is undertaken. The importance of PTLD in pediatric liver transplantation is a result of the intensity of the immunosuppression required, its lifetime duration, and the absence of prior exposure to EBV infection in 60% to 80% of pediatric recipients. PTLD is the most common tumor in children after transplantation, representing 52% of all tumors compared with 15% in adults. About 80% occur within the first 2 years after transplantation.[90]

Multiple studies analyzing immunosuppressive therapy and the development of PTLD have shown a progressive increase in the incidence of PTLD with (1) an increase in total immunosuppressive load, (2) the EBV-naïve recipients, and (3) intensity of active viral load.[95] No single immunosuppressive agent has been directly related to PTLD, although high-dose cyclosporine, tacrolimus, polyclonal antilymphocyte sera (MALG, ALG), and monoclonal antibodies (OKT-3) have all been implicated. Immunosuppressive strategies using these agents as sequential therapy in low doses have not produced an increase in PTLD when successful induction prevents recurrent high-dose or long-duration immunotherapy for rejection. However, prolonged treatment with anti–T-cell agents and the duration, intensity, and total immunosuppressive load are the origin of the defective immunity that creates the background for neoplasia.

The second pathogenic feature influencing PTLD appears to be EBV infection. Primary or reactivation infections usually precede the recognition of PTLD. Active EBV infection, whether primary or reactivation, involves the B-lymphocyte pool, causing B-cell proliferation. A simultaneous increase in cytotoxic T-cell activity is the normal primary host mechanism preventing EBV dissemination. Loss of this natural protection as a result of the administration of T-cell–inhibitory immunotherapy allows polyclonal B-cell proliferation to progress. Polyclonal proliferation of B-lymphocytes occurs after EBV viral replication and release. These EBV proliferating cells express specific viral antigens that represent possible targets for the immune system, which explains the well-described regression of PTLD after immunosuppressive tapering. With time, transformation of a small population of cells results in a malignant monoclonal aggressive B-cell lymphoma.[91,96–98]

Most tumors seen in children are large cell lymphomas, 86% being of B-cell origin. Extranodal involvement, uncommon in primary lymphomas, is seen in 70% of PTLD cases. Extranodal sites include central nervous system, 27%; liver, 23%; lung, 22%; kidney, 21%; intestine, 20%; and spleen, 13%. Allograft involvement is common and can mimic rejection. T-cell and B-cell immunohistochemical markers of the infiltrating lymphocyte population define the B-cell infiltrate and assist in establishing an early diagnosis.

Treatment of PTLD is stratified according to the immunologic cell typing and clinical presentation.[99] Documented PTLD requires an immediate decrease in or discontinuation of immunosuppression and institution of anti-EBV therapy. We prefer to use IV ganciclovir for initial antiviral therapy owing to the high incidence of concurrent CMV infection. Acyclovir is used for long-term treatment. The development of newer antiviral alternatives such as valganciclovir may offer better long-term treatment options in the future.[100] Patients with polyclonal B-cell proliferation frequently show regression with this treatment.[88,93] If tumor cells express B-cell marker CD 20 at histology, the anti-CD 20 monoclonal antibody rituximab can be given in four weekly infusions of 375 mg/m². Although it is associated in many cases with significant reduction in tumor mass, patients have frequently experienced reversible neutropenia requiring granulocyte colony-stimulating factor (G-CSF) and hypogammaglobulinemia requiring supplementation.[101] Acute liver rejection has frequently been seen during Rituximab treatment. Patients with aggressive monoclonal malignancies have poor survival even with immunosuppressive reduction, acyclovir, and conventional chemotherapy or radiation therapy. These additional treatment modalities often precipitate the development of fatal systemic infection. Efforts to reconstitute the EBV-specific cellular immunity by using partially HLA-matched EBV-specific cytotoxic T cells may offer improved treatment outcome for advanced cases, and future development of anti-EBV vaccine may decrease the present significant risks of this unique complication of pediatric transplantation.[102,103] When treatment is successful, careful follow-up to identify recurrent disease or delayed central nervous system involvement is essential.

Retransplantation

The vast majority of retransplantation procedures in pediatric patients are done as a result of acute allograft death caused by HAT or PNF. Acute rejection, chronic rejection, and biliary complications are more uncommon causes. Many of these complications are associated with concurrent sepsis, which further complicates reoperation and compromises success. Survival after transplantation is directly related to prompt identification of appropriate patients and acquisition of a suitable organ. When retransplantation is promptly undertaken for early graft failure, patient survival rate, in our experience, is 73%. However, when retransplantation is undertaken for chronic allograft failure, often complicated by multiple organ system insufficiency, the survival rate is only 45%.[104]

Similar findings were reported by United Network of Organ Sharing (UNOS) Region I in their combined experience; patients undergoing retransplantation for acute organ failure experienced twice the overall survival rate as those undergoing retransplantation for chronic disease.[105] In addition, acute retransplantation survival was significantly influenced by the time to acquire a retransplant organ, with a greater than 3-day wait decreasing the survival rate from 52% to 20%. The overall incidence of retransplantation is 15% in our series and ranges in others' experience from 8% to 29%. This incidence is similar when primary whole organ allografts are compared with primary reduced-size allografts. Reduced-size allografts are frequently used when retransplantation is required, in view of their improved availability and their decreased incidence of allograft-threatening complications.[126,106,107] These findings emphasize the need for early identification of children requiring retransplantation and expeditious reoperation before the development of multisystem organ failure or sepsis.

Outcome After Transplantation

Although the potential complications after liver transplantation are frequent and severe, the overall results are rewarding. Improvements in organ preservation, operative management, immunosuppression, and treatment of postoperative complications have all contributed to the excellent survival rate that is seen. Factors influencing the survival of children undergoing transplantation are detailed in Table 44-8. Most successful transplant programs have reached overall 1-year survival rates of 90%, with greatly decreased risk thereafter.[108,109] Similar if not better results are associated with living donor transplantation, especially for small recipients.[110–112] Infants younger than 1 year or weighing less than 10 kg have historically had reported survival rate of 65% to 88% overall, an improvement over initial reported rates of 50% to 60% during the early era of OLTx development.[106,113,114] Survival rates in infants now equal those seen in older children.[115] Improved survival in these small recipients is consistent throughout all levels of medical urgency and results from a decrease in life-threatening and graft-threatening complications, such as HAT and PNF, in the reduced-size donor organ.

Patients with fulminant hepatic failure have an overall survival rate that is significantly lower than other diagnostic groups, with patients having metabolic disease having the highest survival rate. Prior surgical procedures, especially in patients who have undergone multiple reoperations, and the presence of multiple episodes of subacute bacterial peritonitis before OLTx influence the incidence of complications, especially bowel perforation, but do not adversely affect overall survival in most cases. However, the most important factor determining survival is the severity of the patient's illness at the time of transplantation.[26,116] When stratified for illness by PELD scores, Pediatric Risk of Mortality (PRISM) score, and the previous UNOS score, the PRISM score was the most accurate in predicting both survival and morbidity during the perioperative period.[117] Present efforts to use surgically altered allografts, such as RSOLT, LD-OLT, and split-liver OLT, have experienced similar survival rates as those for whole organ recipients (Fig. 44-8).[106,118]

The increased donor availability for small recipients achieved through the use of surgically reduced, split, or LD organs also brought about a significant decrease in waiting-list mortality. In our center, mortality rate for patients awaiting transplantation decreased from 29% to 2%, and similar results have been reported by other pediatric centers.[106,107,118] Efforts to enhance donor availability, allowing transplantation of children before they reach critical status, is essential before major improvements in postoperative survival rates can occur.

The significant success now achieved after liver transplantation cannot overshadow the need for improved management of post-transplant consequences of

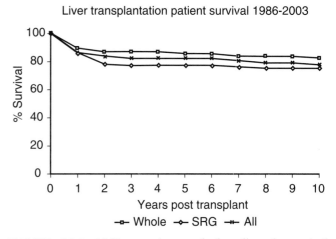

FIGURE 44-8. 10-Year patient and the allograft survival subdivided by whole and surgically reduced grafts, Cincinnati Children's Hospital Medical Center, Liver Care Center.

immunosuppression and pre-OLTx chronic disease. The most significant factors contributing to long-term failure of the allograft or patient death in our program and others are consequences of immunosuppressive medications, such as late infection, and PTLD, and chronic rejection of the allograft.[109,119–121] Our ability to address these challenges successfully will determine the life-long success of transplantation for our youngest recipients.

Follow-up

The overriding objective of hepatic transplantation in children is complete rehabilitation with improved quality of life. Factors contributing to the attainment of this goal include improved nutritional status with appropriate growth and development, as well as enhanced motor and cognitive skills, allowing social reintegration.

Nutrition and Growth

Optimal postoperative nutrition significantly facilitates recovery and rehabilitation. This initially requires providing 100 to 130 calories/kg/day in recipients weighing less than 10 kg. Hepatic synthetic function, gut absorption, and appetite all improve after successful pediatric liver transplantation.

Despite these improvements, growth disturbances do not immediately resolve.[122–124] In the first year after transplantation, very little catch-up growth occurs. During the second and third year after transplantation, patients usually show significant catch-up growth, with the potential for catch-up growth being directly correlated with the degree of preoperative growth retardation. Decreased corticosteroid administration improves this recovery, and the effect is further improved by the use of alternate-day steroids or complete steroid withdrawal in patients with stable allograft function 2 years after OLTx.[125] The "steroid-sparing" effects of new immunosuppressive agents, such as tacrolimus, could diminish this unwanted consequence of immune modulation.

TABLE 44-8
FACTORS AFFECTING TRANSPLANT SURVIVAL

Medical status at orthotopic liver transplantation
Primary diagnosis
Age and size
Comorbid conditions
   Encephalopathy
   Infection
   Multiple organ dysfunction

Neuropsychological Outcome

Although most pediatric transplant recipients are returning to normal age-appropriate activities (e.g., accomplishing normal developmental milestones, re-entering school), recent studies indicate that they may be experiencing subtle functional difficulties.[126–128] Neuropsychological function studies of children after transplantation demonstrate multiple deficits involving learning and memory, abstraction, concept formation, visual-spatial function, and motor function. The well-documented neurologic and cerebral abnormalities associated with chronic cirrhosis precede transplantation but certainly influence these results.[127,129–131]

The long-term impact that transplantation has on the psychosocial and financial health of the entire family unit also is the subject of much concern. Long-term pediatric liver transplant survivors need in-depth, multicenter longitudinal studies to clarify these issues.

Health-related quality of life (HRQOL) surveys of post-transplant families and patients demonstrate improved health and physical perception compared with their pretransplant status; however, as can be imagined, the overall impact on the family is significant. Age at transplantation, the time elapsed since transplantation, hospitalizations within the previous year, maternal education, and race were significant predictors of physical health. Age at transplantation and maternal education predicted psychosocial function. HRQOL was decreased in a population of pediatric liver transplant recipients compared with the general population and similar to that for children with chronic illness.[132] Both younger children and adolescents continue to have self-confidence and body-image concerns, and their participation in out-of-family activities and sports is often limited. Caregivers, and mothers in particular, are heavily affected by the need for care of their chronically ill children before transplant and during their recovery. Many have experienced job losses, career changes, and significant family stress. The importance in providing these caregivers with critical support and psychological help is essential for the entire family to survive and flourish after the difficult times that inevitably follow liver transplantation.

SMALL INTESTINAL TRANSPLANTATION

Introduction

Intestinal failure is a significant problem in the pediatric population. Parenteral alimentation (TPN) remains the first line of therapy of children who have a loss of GI function and is a proven, effective means of treatment; however, complications of long-term parenteral alimentation such as TPN-induced cholestatic liver disease, a paucity of access due to venous thrombosis, and recurrent catheter sepsis may preclude its long-term use. When complications of long-term TPN become life threatening, the only alternative is intestinal transplantation. Although the exact incidence of intestinal failure in children is unclear, more than two thirds of the patients who are currently on the national intestinal transplantation waiting list are in the pediatric age group.[133]

Recent developments in the use of immunosuppression and the technical aspects of surgical procedures have improved the outcome of patients who have undergone intestinal transplantation.[134,135] With the improved outcome, the role of intestinal transplantation has evolved from a heroic last effort to salvage patients who have no remaining treatment options to a standard part of the armamentarium in the management of patients with intestinal failure. As a result, in October 2000, the Centers for Medicare and Medicaid Services issued a memorandum approving federal reimbursement for intestinal transplantation for selected indications.[136] In this section of the chapter, we review the role of intestinal transplantation in patients with intestinal failure.

Indications

Intestinal failure is the inability of the native GI tract to provide nutritional autonomy. Patients with intestinal failure require TPN to maintain a normal state of nutrition, fluid and electrolyte balance, and growth and development. The cause of intestinal failure can be divided into three categories: the short bowel syndrome (SBS), the intestinal dysmotility syndromes, and the congenital epithelial mucosal disorders. The SBS, usually caused by the loss of intestinal length due to surgical resection for an intra-abdominal catastrophe, is the most common cause of intestinal failure. Disease processes necessitating surgical intervention that may result in SBS range from of necrotizing enterocolitis and gastroschisis in the newborn period to Crohn's disease and traumatic injury to the main intestinal blood supply in the older population. Midgut volvulus, another frequent cause of SBS, may occur at any age, although the majority of cases occur in infants.

The intestinal dysmotility syndromes include total intestinal aganglionosis (Hirschsprung's disease) and the constellation of disorders known as chronic idiopathic intestinal pseudo-obstruction. Congenital epithelial mucosal diseases, which, through impaired enterocyte absorption, lead to intractable diarrhea, include microvillus inclusion disease, epithelial dysplasia, and autoimmune enteritis. Although these disorders are rare, affected children face life-long difficulty with GI function and require TPN for survival.

Parenteral alimentation is the standard treatment for patients who experience acute intestinal failure. Bowel rehabilitation should be attempted, as intestinal adaptation may result in eventual enteral autonomy. Bowel-rehabilitation programs using a combination of TPN, gradual reintroduction of enteral feeds, and intestinal antimotility agents are successful in achieving enteral autonomy in some patients.[137,138] Bowel-lengthening procedures may be beneficial in selected patients.[139] Survival and complete return of GI function may be predicted when the postresection length of intestine exceeds 5% of normal for gestational age when the ileocecal valve remains, or greater than 10% of normal if the ileocecal valve has been lost.[140] Unfortunately, for a subset of patients, bowel rehabilitation will fail, and they will require life-long TPN for survival.

Although parenteral alimentation is life saving, complications of long-term TPN may eventually preclude its use. The current Medicare-approved indications for intestinal transplantation are shown in Table 44-9.[136]

Impending liver failure from TPN-induced cholestasis is associated with a significant mortality and, unless TPN can be stopped, is a strong indication for combined liver/intestinal transplantation. Recent studies have shown that the presence of hyperbilirubinemia greater than 3 mg/dL or bridging fibrosis and cirrhosis found on liver biopsy in a infant dependent on TPN is associated with a 1-year survival of less than 30%.[141] All of the remaining indications reflect patients with chronic problems from continued TPN use and are relative indicators for intestinal transplantation.

Currently, with improved outcomes after intestinal transplantation, some centers advocate early intestinal transplantation before the onset of TPN-induced complications.[134,135] These groups believe that graft and patient survival after intestinal transplantation may improve if recipients undergo transplantation before the onset of secondary organ damage, especially liver disease. Furthermore, the quality of life in patients who have undergone successful intestinal transplantation may be better than that of patients who require long-term TPN. This issue is controversial and requires further study.

Contraindications

The contraindications to intestinal transplantation are similar to those for any other solid organ transplantation. The presence of an active nonresectable malignancy, severe neurologic disabilities, or life-threatening extraintestinal illness precludes intestinal transplantation.

Operative Considerations

Currently, three forms of intestinal transplantation are in use: multivisceral, liver/small bowel composite, and small bowel alone. The type of intestinal transplant used is dictated by the needs of the individual patient. The biggest limitation to intestinal transplantation is the need for size-matched grafts. Patients with intestinal failure generally have limited abdominal domain (due in part to a lack of intestine volume), which necessitates near-identical size donors. Recent developments using reduced-size liver grafts have increased the flexibility of D/R size match,[142] but still between 40% and 50% of patients on the intestinal transplant waiting list die before undergoing transplantation because of the lack of appropriate donors.[133,143] Recipients who are cytomegalovirus naïve should not receive intestinal grafts from CMV-positive donors, as they can experience a severe potentially life-threatening CMV infection after transplantation.[144]

In all variants of intestinal transplant, the donor colon is removed during procurement, as it has been shown that colonic transplantation is associated with increased septic complications.[145] An ileostomy is created in all recipients so that surveillance endoscopy and biopsy of the small bowel mucosa can be performed to monitor the allograft for rejection. A feeding jejunostomy is usually created at the time of transplantation to allow the controlled introduction of enteral nutrition. If absent, a Stamm gastrostomy also is placed so that the gastric decompression is possible.

Multivisceral

Multivisceral transplantation entails transplantation of the stomach, duodenum, pancreas, small intestine, and if necessary, the liver. In the pediatric population, the primary indications for this form of transplantation are the intestinal dysmotility syndromes. On occasion, a giant desmoid tumor of the mesentery that infiltrates the blood vessels of all the intra-abdominal viscera may require this form of transplantation. Exenteration of the native intra-abdominal viscera is followed by transplantation of the multivisceral graft by using arterial inflow through the donor celiac and superior mesenteric arteries. Venous outflow is through the transplanted liver placed in the standard orthotopic position.

Liver/Small Bowel Composite

A liver/small bowel composite graft is a modification of the multivisceral graft in which the stomach is removed during procurement. This form of transplantation is indicated in patients with intestinal failure and impending or overt TPN-induced liver failure and is the most common type of intestinal transplant used today (Fig. 44-9). The recipient's liver and residual small intestine are removed, whereas the native stomach, duodenum, pancreas, and spleen are left intact. A portacaval shunt from the native portal vein to IVC is necessary to provide venous outflow from the recipient's foregut organs (Fig. 44-10). The donor celiac and superior mesenteric arteries remain the source of arterial inflow to the transplanted organs. The donor portal vein and biliary tree are intact, having not undergone dissection during procurement, and as a result, no portal vein or bile duct reconstruction is necessary. The pancreas is left intact to protect the peribiliary ductal vessels and to prevent the possibility of pancreatic

---

TABLE 44-9

MEDICARE-APPROVED INDICATIONS FOR INTESTINAL TRANSPLANTATION

1. Impending or overt liver failure due to TPN-induced liver injury. Liver failure defined as increased serum bilirubin or liver enzyme levels or both, splenomegaly, thrombocytopenia, gastroesophageal varices, coagulopathy, stomal bleeding, hepatic fibrosis, or cirrhosis
2. Thrombosis of two or more central veins (subclavian, jugular, or femoral)
3. The development of two or more episodes of systemic sepsis secondary to line infection that requires hospitalization or a single episode of line-related fungemia, or septic shock or acute respiratory distress syndrome or both
4. Frequent episodes of severe dehydration despite intravenous fluid supplementation in addition to TPN

TPN, total parenteral nutrition.

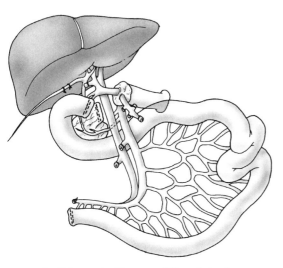

FIGURE 44-9. Schematic diagram of liver/intestine composite allograft. (From Abu-elmagd K, Reyes J, Todo S, et al: Clinical intestinal transplantation: New perspectives and immunologic considerations. J Am Coll Surg 186:512–527, 1998.)

leak from a divided surface. Venous outflow from the transplanted organs is once again provided by the donor liver placed in a standard orthotopic fashion. If the liver is too large, an ex vivo hepatic lobectomy can be performed, usually removing the right lobe of the liver (Fig. 44-11). Luminal continuity from the patient's stomach and duodenum to the newly transplanted bowel is achieved by anastomosis of the recipient's duodenum to the donor jejunum. If the recipient has any colonic remnants, a donor ileum–to–recipient colonic anastomosis is created distal to the ileostomy.

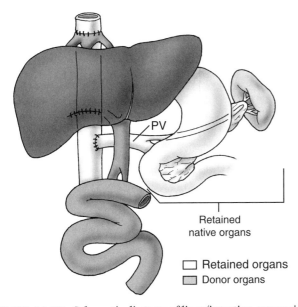

FIGURE 44-10. Schematic diagram of liver/intestine composite allograft with native portocaval shunt. (Adapted from Starzl TE, Todo S, Tzakis A, et al: The many faces of multivisceral transplantation. Surg Gynecol Obstet 172:335–344, 1991.)

Small Intestine Alone

Transplantation of the small intestine alone entails procurement of only the jejunum and ileum. During procurement, the superior mesenteric artery and vein are divided just below the third portion of the duodenum at the root of the mesentery, generating a graft of jejunum and ileum (Fig. 44-12). This type of transplant is indicated in patients with intestinal failure without other organ dysfunction. Depending on space requirements, the recipient's residual small bowel is removed. Arterial inflow is provided by anastomosis of the superior mesenteric artery to the recipient's aorta. Venous drainage of the transplanted intestines is directly into either the IVC or the native superior mesenteric vein. Initially, it was thought that venous drainage into the native portal circulation was beneficial to the liver, but recent studies suggest minimal benefit.[146] Therefore now the most common form of venous reconstruction is to perform an end-to-side anastomosis of the donor superior mesenteric vein to the native vena cava. Luminal continuity is restored by anastomosis of the recipient's proximal bowel to the transplanted jejunum. Once again, if residual colon is present, a donor ileum-to-colonic anastomosis is created downstream of the ileostomy.

POSTOPERATIVE COMPLICATIONS

Although the success rate after intestinal transplantation continues to improve, postoperative complications are common. A breakdown of intestinal integrity either at sites of anastomosis or in areas of mucosal injury from ischemia and reperfusion will necessitate re-exploration. Bowel perforation also may occur during surveillance endoscopy. Patients with a significant amount of peritoneal contamination after bowel perforation may require serial operative exploration to clear foci of intra-abdominal infection. Postoperative bleeding is frequent, especially in patients who undergo liver/small intestine composite grafts, as preexisting portal hypertension results in varices throughout the abdomen. Chylous leaks also are frequent, as lymphatic drainage may be disrupted during both the procurement and the recipient operative procedures. Most chylous leaks can be managed conservatively. Almost all patients who undergo intestinal transplantation will require re-exploration at some point in the postoperative period.

Immunosuppression/Rejection

The most significant advances in the management of an intestinal transplant recipient have occurred in the use of immunosuppression. Rejection remains the most common complication after intestinal transplantation, with virtually every patient experiencing an episode of rejection in the first 6 months after transplantation. Overwhelming rejection was one of the most frequent causes of graft loss during the initial experience with intestinal transplantation, due in part to the limited number of immunosuppressive agents available. The

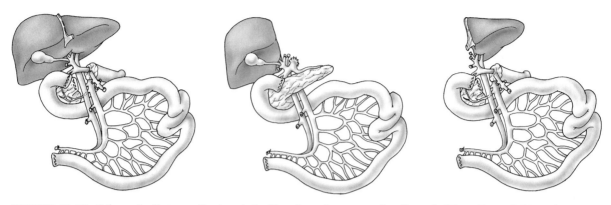

FIGURE 44-11. Schematic diagram of reduced-size liver/intestine composite allograft. (From Reyes J, Mazariegos GV, Bond GMD, et al: Pediatric intestinal transplantation: Historical notes, principles and controversies. Pediatr Transplant 2002:6:193–207.)

development of the CI tacrolimus ushered in the era of successful transplantation, but high-dose immunosuppression was necessary to prevent rejection. Infections and PTLD, side effects of high-dose immunosuppression, became frequent causes of poor outcome. The goal of current immunosuppressive regimens is to use just enough immunosuppression to prevent rejection but not in excess, such that infections and PTLD become common. The management of immunosuppression in patients who undergo intestinal transplantation remains the most challenging aspect of patient care.

Surveillance endoscopy and biopsy is initiated 5 days after transplantation to rule out rejection and is performed

at least 2 to 3 times per week for the first postoperative month. Significant progress in the definition of the histologic characteristics of small bowel rejection has been achieved. If rejection is diagnosed, a short course of high-dose corticosteroids is administered, but if rejection persists, antilymphocyte antibody immunosuppression with agents such as OKT-3 or antithymocyte immunoglobulin (Thymoglobulin) is necessary. Some centers are now attempting to achieve tolerance by using a combination of Thymoglobulin, graft irradiation, and bone marrow transplantation.[147]

Infections

In large part because of the high level of immunosuppression needed after intestinal transplantation, bacterial and fungal infections are common in the postoperative period. Patients with intestinal failure are frequently colonized with antibiotic-resistant bacteria because of recurrent infections while receiving TPN, which can make management even more difficult. As mentioned earlier, because intestinal perforation is common, peritonitis is a frequent complication, often requiring repeated intra-abdominal explorations to clear the peritoneum completely.

CMV, EBV, and adenovirus are the most frequent viral pathogens found in the postoperative period. PTLD, an EBV-driven process, remains a significant problem because most infants are EBV negative at the time of transplantation. As described earlier, surveillance for CMV and EBV by using PCR followed by aggressive treatment when detected has diminished the impact on outcome of these dangerous pathogens. All patients are maintained on prophylactic antiviral agents in the perioperative period.

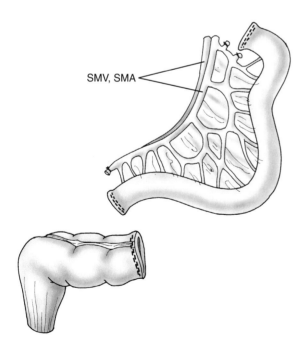

FIGURE 44-12. Schematic diagram of isolated small intestinal transplant. (Adapted from Abu-Elmagd K, Fung J, Bueno J, et al: Logistics and technique for procurement of intestinal, pancreatic, and hepatic grafts from the same donor. Ann Surg 232:680–687, 2000.)

Outcome

The initial experience of patients who underwent intestinal transplantation was dismal, with few long-term survivors.[148] With the development of tacrolimus, intestinal transplantation became a viable alternative. Currently, more than 70% of patients survive for 1 year, and 50% survive for 5 years after transplantation.[148-150] Recent data from the University of Pittsburgh showed that, in children, with a combination of Thymoglobulin induction followed by tacrolimus monotherapy, graft and patient survival of 100% at 1 year can be achieved.[151] Although these findings are preliminary, the results support the conclusion that the role of intestinal transplantation in the management of children with intestinal failure has moved from experimental to an integral part of treatment.[152]

RENAL TRANSPLANTATION IN INFANTS AND CHILDREN

Etiology

Acute renal failure in infants is most often the consequence of hemodynamic instability, with malperfusion or hypoxia resulting in acute tubular necrosis (ATN). Most of these patients either recover sufficient renal function for normal long-term survival or die of multisystem failure.

Chronic renal failure is uncommon in infants, with the estimate of infants with ESRD placed at 0.2 per million total population for infants younger than 1 year.[153,154] Congenital lesions such as renal dysplasia, obstructive malformations, or complex urogenital malformation and congenital nephrosis are the most common causes of ESRD in children younger than 5 years, accounting for 46% of cases. Glomerulonephritis, including focal segmental glomerulosclerosis, membranoproliferative glomerulonephritis, and lupus nephritis, as well as recurrent pyelonephritis, are the leading causes of ESRD in older children (Table 44-10).[155] Hereditary causes of renal failure should be identified to plan appropriate overall treatment strategy, including evaluating other family members and providing genetic counseling when needed.

Knowledge of the etiology of the ESRD is important to allow assessment of the potential for recurrence within a transplant allograft and consideration of LD transplantation. Patients with a "structural/congenital" etiology without an immunologic component also enjoy better graft survival rates than do those patients with "glomerulonephritis."[156]

TABLE 44-10

RECIPIENT CHARACTERISTICS (NORTH AMERICAN PEDIATRIC RENAL TRANSPLANT COOPERATIVE STUDY)

	n (6878)	% (100.0)
Obstruction uropathy	1109	16.1
Aplastic/hypoplastic/dysplastic kidneys	1088	15.8
Focal segmental glomerulosclerosis	798	11.6
Reflux nephropathy	369	5.4
Chronic glomerulonephritis	262	3.8
Medullary cystic disease/juvenile nephronophthisis	193	2.8
Polycystic kidney disease	192	2.8
Syndrome of agenesis of abdominal musculature	188	2.7
Hemolytic uremic syndrome	183	2.7
Congenital nephritic syndrome	178	2.6
Familial nephritis	163	2.4
Cystinosis	145	2.1
Membranoproliferative glomerulonephritis type I	144	2.1
Pyelo/interstitial nephritis	140	2.0
Idiopathic crescentic glomerulonephritis	132	1.9
SLE nephritis	114	1.7
Renal infarct	114	1.7
Henoch-schönlein nephritis	94	1.4
Berger's (IgA) nephritis	85	1.2
Membranoproliferative glomerulonephritis type II	64	0.9
Oxalosis	42	0.6
Wilms' tumor	39	0.6
Drash syndrome	39	0.6
Wegener's granulomatosis	38	0.6
Membranous nephropathy	32	0.5
Other systemic immunologic diseases	27	0.4
Sickle cell nephropathy	13	0.2
Diabetic glomerulonephritis	8	0.1
Other	512	7.4
Unknown	373	5.4

From Benfield MR, McDonald RA, Bartosh S, et al: Changing trends in pediatric transplantation: 2001 Annual Report of the North American Pediatric Renal Transplant Cooperative study. Pediatr Transplantation 7:321–335, 2003.
SLE, systemic lupus erythematosus; IgA, immunoglobulin A.

Pretransplant Management

Pretransplant management is critical in infants and children with ESRD. Children with ESRD, beginning in infancy or early childhood, experience significant complications from growth retardation, renal osteodystrophy, and neuropsychiatric developmental delay. Recent advances in dialysis regimens, nutritional supplementation, recombinant human erythropoietin, and growth hormone have significantly improved the pretransplant management of these patients.

Dialysis

Dialysis is indicated when complications of ESRD occur despite optimal medical management, namely, hyperkalemia, volume overload, acidosis, intractable hypertension, and uremic symptoms such as vomiting. In older children, lethargy and poor school performance can signal the need for more aggressive treatment. In addition, dialysis may be necessary to facilitate the administration of adequate protein as part of an extensive nutritional resuscitation plan.

When dialysis is undertaken, the use of peritoneal dialysis is preferred for the following reasons: (1) it avoids the multiple blood transfusions associated with hemodialysis; (2) it allows a gradual correction of electrolyte abnormalities, preventing cerebral disequilibrium syndrome in small infants; (3) it allows easier control of osteodystrophy; (4) it optimizes nutrition; and (5) it is easy to administer.

Hemodialysis can be used when an unsuitable peritoneal cavity is available secondary to prior surgical procedure or in the presence of active peritoneal infections; however, the construction and maintenance of adequate long-term vascular access sites in small infants and children is difficult. Use of centralized venous catheters rather than arteriovenous fistulas is our preferred mode for temporary hemodialysis access in infants and small children, although infection and vascular thrombosis complicate this therapy. Access via the internal jugular veins is preferred over subclavian routes to avoid venous occlusion of the upper extremity, which compromises later arm arteriovenous fistula sites. Although dialysis and its complications, such as infection, have a great influence on the complexity of care, they do not affect the ultimate results of renal transplantation.[157]

Nutritional Support

The need for vigorous nutritional support of the infant with uremia has been well documented by the growth retardation seen in infants and children with ESRD. The etiology of growth disturbance is multifactorial, including anorexia that leads to both protein and calorie insufficiency, renal osteodystrophy, aluminum toxicity, uremic acidosis, impaired somatomedin activity, and growth hormone and insulin resistance.[158] Because the most intense period of growth occurs during the first 2 years of life, careful nutritional support during that time is essential.

With extensive nutritional efforts, the mean weight at the time of transplantation for all patients has improved from −2.2 SD to 1.6 SD below the appropriate age-adjusted and gender-adjusted mean for normal children in the recent North American Pediatric Renal Transplant Cooperative Study (NAPRTCS). Similar height deficits occurred.[159] This growth deficit was greater (−2.8 SD) in children younger than 5 years. Transplantation afforded a +0.8 SD increase in growth over the first post-transplant year; however, this accelerated growth then reaches a stable plateau. After 2 to 3 years, the mean weight values were comparable to those in normal children.[155] Children age 6 years and older show no improvement in their height deficit 5 years after transplantation.[160,161] These limitations to "catch-up" growth emphasize the need for early transplantation in young ESRD patients. If epiphyseal closure has occurred (bone age > 12 years), additional bone growth is often not achieved.[154,162,163] Normalization of growth rarely occurs with the introduction of either hemodialysis or peritoneal dialysis.

The importance of efforts to normalize nutritional parameters is emphasized by the adverse impact of uremia on the developing nervous system in the infant. The significance of this problem was emphasized in a study in which progressive encephalopathy, developmental delay, microcephaly, hypotonia, seizures, and dyskinesia developed in 20 of 23 children younger than 1 year with ESRD.[164] All of these patients had significant growth impairment. Monitoring of the head circumference has been suggested to identify the infant at risk, with the intent to initiate dialysis, nutritional support, or transplantation if this parameter deviates from the normal curve.[154]

Transplant Management

Preoperative Evaluation

In preparation for transplantation, an extensive evaluation of the urinary tract and immunologic status of the patient is necessary.

The increased frequency of urinary tract abnormalities as the primary cause of ESRD in infants and children necessitates the investigation of the urinary tract for sites of obstruction, presence of ureteral reflux, and functional state and capacity of the urinary bladder.[165] This investigation is best accomplished by obtaining an US or IV pyelogram of the upper urinary tract and a voiding cystourethrogram to assess bladder and reflux parameters. Any questions related to bladder function or structure require urodynamics and cystoscopy.

In patients with long-standing oliguric ESRD, the bladder capacity may appear very small. In the absence of abnormal obstructive or neuromuscular bladder pathology, adequate enlargement of the bladder in the face of normal urinary production is to be expected. Any surgical correction of urethral obstruction or augmentation of bladder size should be undertaken far in advance of undertaking transplantation. Preoperative sterilization of the urinary tract and development of unobstructed urinary outflow should be the ultimate goals of evaluation and reconstruction. Although complex anomalies of the urogenital tract often require many extensive operative procedures to augment, reconstruct, or create an acceptable lower urinary tract, virtually all such children can undergo successful reconstruction with continent urinary reservoirs without the use of intestinal conduits.[166]

Immunologic assessment includes tissue typing and panel reactive antibody analysis. Patients should be monitored periodically for the development of a positive cross-match to their potential LD or of positive cytotoxic antibody to a panel of random donors to assess immunologic reactivity. In addition, reactivity to CMV, EBV, HSV, and hepatitis should be investigated. Childhood immunizations should be current, and immunization against hepatitis B virus instituted. Any immunizations with live virus vaccines should be given well in advance of transplantation, because their use is contraindicated in the early post-transplant period.

Selection of the appropriate donor source for transplantation is a decision for the transplant team and family to consider together. A related immediate family member LD has the advantage of a low incidence of postoperative ATN; improved histologic matching, leading to fewer rejection episodes and the need for less immunosuppression; and the possibility of extended organ function. In addition, any operative procedures required for recipient preparation, as well as the transplant procedure, can be scheduled around the needs of the patient, simplifying preoperative care and potentially avoiding the complications of dialysis. Parents form the majority of donors; siblings younger than 18 years are rarely considered unless they are identical twins. At present, 60% of children receive a related LD kidney.[160] Complete evaluation of the potential donor to exclude intrinsic renal anomalies, vascular anomalies, and systemic illness is necessary.

CD kidneys are used for 40% of renal transplants.[160] The unpredictability of donor organ availability and the need to establish a negative antibody cross-match for CD transplantation make surgical planning impossible. The size of a potential allograft, CD or related LD, also is important. Kidneys from small adult donors can be transplanted into infants as small as 5 kg with good technical success.[167] CD organs from pediatric donors 5 years or older also yield an excellent survival rate. However, a progressive decrease in 1-year graft survival has been noted when kidneys from donors younger than 3 to 4 years have been used.[168,169] This decrease in graft and patient survival rate is related to the donor organ source; children age 2 to 5 years have a similar survival rate to that of the overall pediatric population when LDs are used.[155,170] Recognition of this potential risk has led to a reluctance by most centers to use donors younger than 5 years. An effect of donor age on graft survival has been attributed to an increased rate of both graft thrombosis and acute rejection.[155]

The decision to use a CD is often strengthened by the possibility of disease recurrence within the transplanted kidney. The incidence of disease recurrence after transplantation and the risk of graft loss are listed in Table 44-11.[171] The decision to proceed with LD transplantation in small children is influenced by the recent improvements in outcomes, which show similar 1 year graft survival for all age groups.[160]

Pre-emptive Transplantation

The desire to begin pre-emptive transplantation before undertaking dialysis is often fueled by the patient's or parents' desire to avoid the surgical procedures, potential infections, or cardiovascular complications, and the psychological impairment inherent with dialysis. A recent NAPRTCS review found that 26% of primary transplantations were performed without prior dialysis.[172] Most cases used LDs rather than cadaveric sources. No difference in patient or graft survival was found in this group when compared with patients who undergo dialysis before transplantation. Pre-emptive transplantation is not possible when uncontrolled hypertension, massive proteinuria, or recurrent infection requires prior native kidney removal or when oliguric renal failure requires immediate dialysis.[171]

TABLE 44-11			
RECURRENCE RATES AND GRAFT LOSS FROM RECURRENT DISEASE IN CHILDREN			
Disease	Recurrence Rate (%)	Clinical Severity	% of Those with Recurrence Whose Graft Failed
FSGS	25–30	High	40–50
MPGN type I	70	Mild	12–30
MPGN type II	100	Low	10–20
SLE	5–40	Low	5
HSP	55–85	Low/mild	5–20
HUS			
Classical	12–20	Moderate	0–10
Atypical	±25	High	40–50

FSGS, focal segmental glomerulosclerosis; HSP, Henoch-Schönlein purpura; HUS, hemolytic uremic syndrome; MPGN, membranoproliferative glomerulonephritis; SLE, systemic lupus erythematosus.
From Fine RN, Ettenger R. In Morris PJ (ed): Kidney Transplantation: Principles and Practice, 4th ed. Philadelphia, WB Saunders, 1994, p 418.

Operative Procedure

Preparation for transplantation should include placing adequate large-bore IV lines and the largest Foley catheter possible. Central venous lines are used in all infants and children to ensure vascular access, hemodynamic monitoring, and a route for postoperative immunosuppressive delivery. Perioperative prophylactic antibiotics are administered. Arterial pressure monitoring lines are necessary only in small infants and patients with hemodynamic compromise, allowing preservation of future hemodialysis access sites.

Transplantation in infants and small children can be undertaken through a generous retroperitoneal approach or transabdominal placing of the allograft within the peritoneal cavity posterior to the right or left colon. An extraperitoneal approach to the retroperitoneum allows the maintenance of postoperative peritoneal dialysis and should be strongly considered when size permits. The arterial anastomosis is constructed end-to-side into the distal aorta or common iliac artery, and venous outflow of the allograft should be into the IVC or common iliac vein. Ureteral implantation by using the Lich extravesical ureteroneocystostomy avoids a cystotomy and minimizes postoperative blood clots within the bladder, which may obstruct the Foley catheter. When larger donor kidneys are used in small recipients, the vessels must be shortened to avoid redundancy when the kidney is positioned in the retroperitoneum. The internal iliac artery is not used in pediatric transplants, so that pelvic blood flow is preserved (Fig. 44-13). Ureteral "double-J" stents are used when small ureter size may lead to obstruction.

Anesthetic management of the infant and small child during kidney transplantation is complicated by preexisting electrolyte abnormalities and the large fluid fluxes that occur in the operating room. Intravascular blood volume must be augmented during allograft implantation to allow maintenance of normal systemic blood flow when allograft blood flow is reestablished. Perfusion of the allograft with hypothermic lactated Ringer's solution before implantation to remove any remaining hyperkalemic graft preservation solution is necessary in infants and small children to avoid massive potassium infusion with establishment of allograft perfusion. Blood volume loading to a central venous pressure of 13 to 15 cm H_2O and administration of bicarbonate, calcium, and low-dose vasopressors (dopamine, 5 μg/kg/min) should be started before reperfusion of the graft.

Postoperative Management

Post-transplant management requires careful screening for technical complications, rejection, recurrence of the primary renal disease, and prevention of immunosuppression-related complications.

Frequent fluid and electrolyte monitoring is necessary immediately after transplantation because larger kidneys can excrete the equivalent of the infant's blood volume within a single hour. Careful attention to serum concentrations of calcium, phosphorus, magnesium, and electrolytes is necessary. Urine output is initially replaced isovolumetrically and then tapered as the high-output state subsides. Glucose-free urine-replacement fluids minimize hyperglycemia and attendant osmotic diuresis in the recipient. Selection of appropriate electrolyte concentrations is guided by urinary electrolyte excretion, which is regularly monitored. Central venous filling pressures should be maintained at 7 to 10 cm H_2O to ensure adequate intravascular volume. In patients with high-output renal failure, urine losses from both the native and transplant kidneys must be replaced to avoid hypoperfusion and thrombosis. Maintenance of catheter patency is essential, and any episode of decreased urinary output should be rapidly investigated to exclude Foley catheter occlusion and bladder distention. An algorithm for the evaluation of early postoperative oliguria is shown in Figure 44-14.

Technical Complications

Vascular thrombosis still accounts for graft loss in up to 13% of index transplants and 19% of repeated transplants in children. Graft thrombosis is significantly more frequent in children younger than 2 years and is directly

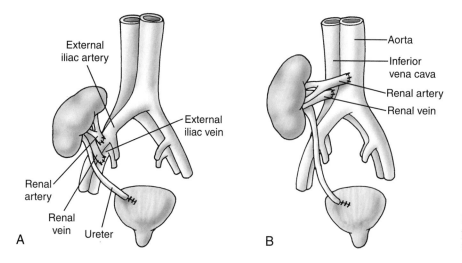

FIGURE 44-13. Schematic diagram of pediatric renal transplant and ureteroneocystostomy.

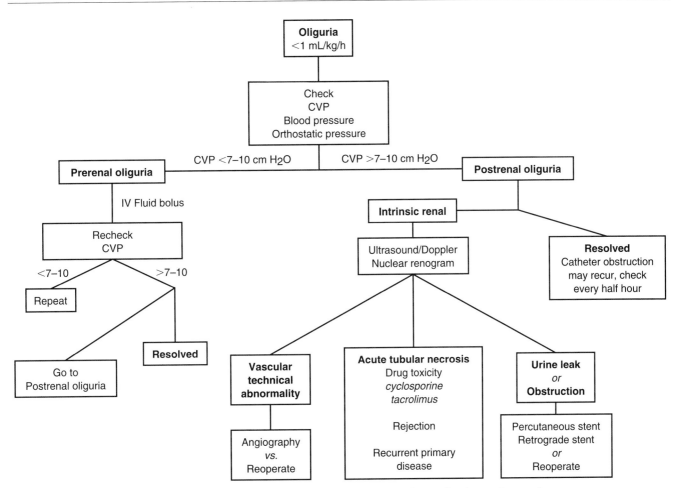

FIGURE 44-14. Algorithm for the evaluation of early postoperative oliguria after pediatric renal transplant.

related to the age of both the donor and the recipient. In addition, prolonged cold ischemic preservation time (>24 hours) and the related presence of ATN with delayed graft function also increase this risk. Prior transplantation and more than five pretransplant blood transfusions also have been shown to be independent risk factors.[173] Immediate post-transplant Doppler US vascular imaging is helpful in confirming suitable allograft blood flow after abdominal closure, especially when large allografts are implanted into small recipients. Adequate hydration is essential to maintain suitable perfusion; anticoagulation has not been used in most series.

Urinary leak, most often at the neocystostomy site, is first seen with oliguria and persisting uremia. US or nuclear imaging can be used to identify an extravesical fluid collection. Direct operative repair is necessary to prevent urinoma formation and its potential infectious complications. Urinary collections must be differentiated from lymphoceles at the transplant site. Unresolving lymphoceles are best opened into the peritoneal cavity by using laparoscopic techniques.

Hypertension

Hypertension after renal transplantation is common. One month after transplantation, 72% of all patients require treatment, although this percentage decreases to 53% at 30 months. Careful attention to the pretransplant control of hypertension and dietary management improves posttransplant control. Hypertension presents a significant risk to possible renal function when using small allografts. Hypertension in the early postoperative period is most often due to fluid overload or acute rejection, but it also may originate from the native kidneys.

Preexisting hypertension is augmented by the immunosuppressive drugs cyclosporine, tacrolimus, and prednisone. The development of hypertension more than 3 months after transplantation suggests possible renal artery stenosis and warrants US Doppler flow studies for initial evaluation and arteriography in questionable cases. Transluminal angioplasty has been successful in managing the majority of these cases when recognized; surgical correction is reserved for angioplasty failures and vessels with complex arterial anastomoses.

Infection

Most long-term complications are related to infection and occur within the first 6 post-transplant months. During this time, immunosuppression is intense, and susceptibility to life-threatening infection is increased. The frequent use of organs from donors who have had prior exposure to CMV and EBV in infants and children who are seronegative enhances the risk of these specific infections. Expanded use of antiviral prophylaxis with ganciclovir and acyclovir has decreased the intensity of these infections and their associated morbidity or mortality. Trimethoprim-sulfamethoxazole is used for *Pneumocystis carinii* pneumonia prophylaxis as well.

Immunosuppression

Many immunosuppressive regimens are available, and all share similar strategy. Most regimens include corticosteroids, cyclosporine or tacrolimus, and azathioprine or mycophenolate. Polyclonal or monoclonal anti-lymphocyte antibodies are used when ATN is anticipated or for retransplantation in highly presensitized patients. Significant efforts to decrease or discontinue steroids have been attempted to enhance growth and development. At 4 years after transplantation, 31% of LD and 23% of CD recipients were receiving alternate-day prednisone.[155]

Overall, a decrease in the frequency of acute rejection has been found with 12-month probabilities in LDs of 32% and CDs of 36%.[160] The risk of rejection is similar for LD and CD recipients in the first few post-transplant weeks. Factors that increase the likelihood of rejection or long-term graft loss include receiving a graft from a CD rather than a related LD, receiving a graft from a donor younger than 5 years, having the graft in cold storage for more than 24 hours, being an African-American recipient, and delayed graft function from ATN.[155] The ability to treat rejection also has improved, with complete reversal of acute rejection in 65% of episodes.[160] The rate of success in treating rejection declines with each successive rejection episode, increased recipient age, and late rejection episodes.[155] Most rejection episodes can be treated with steroid administration alone (78%); monoclonal anti–T-cell agents such as orthoclone OKT-3 are needed in 32%. In patients who remain rejection free for the first post-transplant year, the risk of rejection in the following year is 20%.[157]

Results of Renal Transplantation

The overall results of renal transplantation in children are steadily improving. Overall 1-year transplant graft survival rates of 88% to 100% have been reported for LD allografts, with results for CD allografts being 50% to 72%.[154,167–169,171] In the 1997 NAPRTCS report, 1-, 2-, and 5-year graft survival rates were as follows: CDs, 78%, 72%, and 59%; and LDs, 90%, 86%, and 85%, respectively (Fig. 44-15).[157]

Chronic rejection has become the most common cause of graft failure, accounting for 27% of all graft losses.[174] With improved immunosuppressive treatments, acute rejection accounts for only 15% of failures. Recurrence of the original disease caused graft failure in 6%, and vascular thrombosis accounted for 12% of graft failures. Long-term graft survival after pediatric renal transplantation continues to deteriorate after 10 years, despite low patient mortality rates. Death of the recipient with a

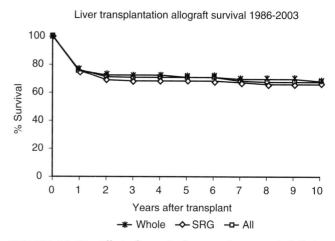

FIGURE 44-15. Allograft survival over a 5-year period, living donor compared with cadaveric donor (NAPRTCS 2001 Report).[159]

functioning graft is an uncommon problem. When this did occur, death resulted primarily from infection (40%) or cardiovascular causes (21%). Young recipients (birth to age 1 year) and patients with early graft failure were at the highest risk.[175] Progressive loss of renal function may be secondary to complications of hypertension, hyperfiltration, hypercholesterolemia, chronic indolent immunologic damage leading to chronic rejection, and progressive primary renal disease, all of which contribute to long-term graft loss.[156,171] Methods to circumvent this progressive graft loss will greatly improve the long-term prognosis.

The overall half-life of pediatric renal transplants is about 25 years for LDs and 16 years for CD grafts.[160] Many recipients require second transplants in their lifetime. Overall graft survival for second transplants with LDs was equivalent to that of primary CD allografts.[176] The factor exerting negative influence on survival in CD grafts was donor age younger than 6 years. Improved D/R matching improved graft survival. Thus use of cadaveric kidneys from young donors for these procedures is not recommended. The rapidity of first allograft loss, immunologic protocol at retransplant, and race of recipient were not significant factors.

PANCREAS TRANSPLANTATION IN CHILDREN

Children have rarely been candidates for pancreas transplantation. In the past, the results after pancreas transplantation have not justified the risks associated with immunosuppression and operation. However, recent improvements in the operative procedure and follow-up have improved. Overall 1-year patient survival rate exceeds 90%, and graft survival with complete insulin independence exceeds 70% in patients in whom combined kidney and pancreas transplantation is undertaken. The survival rate is approximately 50% in isolated pancreas transplantation.[177,178]

The addition of pancreas transplantation with kidney replacement for diabetic nephropathy does not subject the patient to additional immunosuppressive risks, and it is better accepted. The use of isolated pancreas transplantation is reserved for patients who are extremely labile or experience hypoglycemic unawareness syndrome.[177] As the results of this procedure improve in the future, the role of this procedure in children must be reviewed.

Pancreatic islet transplantation also has become possible in children. Its role in the treatment of juvenile diabetes in childhood is still limited. This procedure has been undertaken in children after pancreatic resection when the cellular autotransplant does not require immunosuppressive treatment, with excellent results. Further expansion of this role awaits firm documentation that hypoglycemic correction retards the systemic complications of diabetes.

REFERENCES

1. Kasai M, Mochizuki I, Ohkohchi N, et al: Surgical limitation for biliary atresia: Indication for liver transplantation. J Pediatr Surg 24:851–854, 1989.
2. Ryckman F, Fisher R, Pedersen S, et al: Improved survival in biliary atresia patients in the present era of liver transplantation. J Pediatr Surg 28:382–385, discussion 386, 1993.
3. Zitelli BJ, Malatack JJ, Gartner JC Jr, et al: Evaluation of the pediatric patient for liver transplantation. Pediatrics 78:559–565, 1986.
4. Nio M, Ohi R, Hayashi Y, et al: Current status of 21 patients who have survived more than 20 years since undergoing surgery for biliary atresia. J Pediatr Surg 31:381–384, 1996.
5. Ryckman FC, Alonso MH: Transplantation for hepatic malignancy in children. In Busuttil RW, Klintmalm G (eds): Transplantation of the Liver. Philadelphia, WB Sanders, 1996, pp 216–226.
6. Reily D: Familial intrahepatic cholestasis syndromes. In Suchy FJ (ed): Liver Disease in Children. St. Louis, CV Mosby, 1994, pp 443–459.
7. Ng VL, Ryckman FC, Porta G, et al: Long-term outcome after partial external biliary diversion for intractable pruritus in patients with intrahepatic cholestasis. J Pediatr Gastroenterol Nutr 30:152–156, 2000.
8. Hollands CM, Rivera-Pedrogo FJ, Gonzalez-Vallina R, et al: Ileal exclusion for Byler's disease: An alternative surgical approach with promising early results for pruritus. J Pediatr Surg 33:220–224, 1998.
9. Cardona J, Houssin D, Gauthier F, et al: Liver transplantation in children with Alagille syndrome: A study of twelve cases. Transplantation 60:339–342, 1995.
10. Hoffenberg EJ, Narkewicz MR, Sondheimer JM, et al: Outcome of syndromic paucity of interlobular bile ducts (Alagille syndrome) with onset of cholestasis in infancy. J Pediatr 127:220–224, 1995.
11. Tzakis AG, Reyes J, Tepetes K, et al: Liver transplantation for Alagille's syndrome. Arch Surg 128:337–339, 1993.
12. Jan D, Poggi F, Laurent J, et al: Liver transplantation: New indications in metabolic disorders? Transplant Proc 26:189–190, 1994.
13. Mito M, Kusano M, Kawaura Y: Hepatocyte transplantation in man. Transplant Proc 24:3052–3053, 1992.
14. Jan D, Laurent J, Lacaille F, et al: Liver transplantation in children with inherited metabolic disorders. Transplant Proc 27:1706–1707, 1995.
15. Strom S, Fisher R: Hepatocyte transplantation: New possibilities for therapy. Gastroenterology 124:568–571, 2003.
16. Strom SC, Fisher RA, Rubinstein WS, et al. Transplantation of human hepatocytes. Transplant Proc 29:2103–2106, 1997.
17. Fridell JA, Bond GJ, Mazariegos GV, et al: Liver transplantation in children with cystic fibrosis: A long-term longitudinal review of a single center's experience. J Pediatr Surg 38:1152–1156, 2003.
18. Strom SC, Fisher RA, Thompson MT, et al: Hepatocyte transplantation as a bridge to orthotopic liver transplantation in terminal liver failure. Transplantation 63:559–569, 1997.
19. Lidofsky SD, Bass NM, Prager MC, et al: Intracranial pressure monitoring and liver transplantation for fulminant hepatic failure. Hepatology 16:1–7, 1992.
20. Tiao G, Allen S, Alonso M, et al: The current management of hepatoblastoma: A combination of chemotherapy, conventional resection and liver transplantation. J Pediatr Surg 2004 (in revision).
21. Koneru B, Flye MW, Busuttil RW, et al: Liver transplantation for hepatoblastoma: The American experience. Ann Surg 213:118–121, 1991.
22. Iwatsuki S, Gordon RD, Shaw BW Jr, et al: Role of liver transplantation in cancer therapy. Ann Surg 202:401–407, 1985.
23. Schroeder TJ, Pesce AJ, Ryckman FC, et al: Selection criteria for liver transplant donors. J Clin Lab Anal 5:275–277, 1991.
24. Broelsch CE, Emond JC, Whitington PF, et al. Application of reduced-size liver transplants as split grafts, auxiliary orthotopic grafts, and living related segmental transplants. Ann Surg 212:368–375, discussion 375–377, 1990.
25. Emond JC, Whitington PF, Thistlethwaite JR, et al: Reduced-size orthotopic liver transplantation: Use in the management of children with chronic liver disease. Hepatology 10:867–872, 1989.
26. Ryckman FC, Flake AW, Fisher RA, et al: Segmental orthotopic hepatic transplantation as a means to improve patient survival and diminish waiting-list mortality. J Pediatr Surg 26:422–427; discussion 427–428, 1991.
27. de Ville de Goyet J: Cut-down and split liver transplantation. In Busuttil RW, Klintmalm G (eds): Transplantation of the Liver. Philadelphia, WB Saunders, 1996, pp 481–496.
28. Broelsch CE, Frilling A, Testa G, et al: Living donor liver transplantation in adults. Eur J Gastroenterol Hepatol 15:3–6, 2003.
29. Broelsch CE, Burdelski M, Rogiers X, et al: Living donor for liver transplantation. Hepatology 20:49S–55S, 1994.
30. Rogiers X, Burdelski M, Broelsch CE: Liver transplantation from living donors. Br J Surg 81:1251–1253, 1994.
31. Broelsch CE, Whitington PF, Emond JC, et al: Liver transplantation in children from living related donors: Surgical techniques and results. Ann Surg 214:428–437; discussion 437–439, 1991.
32. Lo CM, Fan ST, Liu CL, et al: Adult-to-adult living donor liver transplantation using extended right lobe grafts. Ann Surg 226:261–299; discussion 269–270, 1997.
33. Fan ST, Lo CM, Liu CL: Technical refinement in adult-to-adult living donor liver transplantation using right lobe graft. Ann Surg 231:126–131, 2000.
34. Morimoto T, Awane M, Tanaka A, et al: Analysis of functional abnormalities uncovered during preoperative evaluation of donor candidates for living-related liver transplantation. Clin Transplant 9:60–64, 1995.
35. Otte JB, Reding R, de Ville de Goyet J, et al: Experience with living related liver transplantation in 63 children. Acta Gastroenterol Belg 62:355–362, 1999.
36. Otte JB: Donor complications and outcomes in live-liver transplantation. Transplantation 75:1625–1626, 2003.
37. Emond JC, Freeman RB Jr, Renz JF, et al: Optimizing the use of donated cadaver livers: Analysis and policy development to increase the application of split-liver transplantation. Liver Transplant 8:863–872, 2002.
38. Reyes J, Gerber D, Mazariegos GV, et al: Split-liver transplantation: A comparison of ex vivo and in situ techniques. J Pediatr Surg 35:283–289; discussion 289–290, 2000.
39. Deshpande RR, Bowles MJ, Vilca-Melendez H, et al. Results of split liver transplantation in children. Ann Surg 236:248–253, 2002.
40. Lo CM, Fan ST, Liu CL, et al: Minimum graft size for successful living donor liver transplantation. Transplantation 68:1112–1116, 1999.
41. Oldhafer KJ, Gubernatis G, Schlitt HJ, et al: Auxiliary partial orthotopic liver transplantation for acute liver failure: The Hannover experience. Clin Transplant 8:181–187, 1994.
42. Gubernatis G, Pichlmayr R, Kemnitz J, et al: Auxiliary partial orthotopic liver transplantation (APOLT) for fulminant hepatic failure: First successful case report. World J Surg 15:660–665; discussion 15:665–666, 1991.
43. Egawa H, Tanaka K, Inomata Y, et al: Auxiliary partial orthotopic liver transplantation from a living related donor: A report of two cases. Transplant Proc 28:1071–1072, 1996.

44. Terpstra OT, Metselaar HJ, Hesselink EJ, et al: Auxiliary partial liver transplantation for acute and chronic liver disease. Transplant Proc 22:1564, 1990.

45. Terpstra OT, Schalm SW, Weimar W, et al: Auxiliary partial liver transplantation for end-stage chronic liver disease. N Engl J Med 319:1507–1511, 1988.

46. De Carlis L, Sansalone CV, Rondinara GF, et al: Is the use of marginal donors justified in liver transplantation? Analysis of results and proposal of modern criteria. Transplant Int 9(suppl 1):S414–17, 1996.

47. Urena MA, Moreno Gonzalez E, Romero CJ, et al: An approach to the rational use of steatotic donor livers in liver transplantation. Hepatogastroenterology 46:1164–1173, 1999.

48. Zamboni F, Franchello A, David E, et al: Effect of macrovescicular steatosis and other donor and recipient characteristics on the outcome of liver transplantation. Clin Transplant 15:53–57, 2001.

49. Imber CJ, St Peter SD, Handa A, Friend PJ, et al: Hepatic steatosis and its relationship to transplantation. Liver Transplant 8:415–423, 2002.

50. Todo S, Demetris AJ, Makowka L, et al: Primary nonfunction of hepatic allografts with preexisting fatty infiltration. Transplantation 47:903–905, 1989.

51. D'Alessandro AM, Kalayoglu M, Sollinger HW, et al: The predictive value of donor liver biopsies on the development of primary nonfunction after orthotopic liver transplantation. Transplant Proc 23:1536–1537, 1991.

52. Fishbein TM, Fiel MI, Emre S, et al: Use of livers with microvesicular fat safely expands the donor pool. Transplantation 64:248–251, 1997.

53. Iwatsuki S, Iwaki Y, Kano T, et al: Successful liver transplantation from crossmatch-positive donors. Transplant Proc 13:286–288, 1981.

54. Takaya S, Iwaki Y, Starzl TE: Liver transplantation in positive cytotoxic crossmatch cases using FK506, high-dose steroids, and prostaglandin E1. Transplantation 54:927–929, 1992.

55. Demetris AJ, Nakamura K, Yagihashi A, et al: A clinicopathological study of human liver allograft recipients harboring preformed IgG lymphocytotoxic antibodies. Hepatology 16:671–681, 1992.

56. Mor E, Skerrett D, Manzarbeitia C, et al: Successful use of an enhanced immunosuppressive protocol with plasmapheresis for ABO-incompatible mismatched grafts in liver transplant recipients. Transplantation 59:986–990, 1995.

57. Farges O, Kalil AN, Samuel D, et al: The use of ABO-incompatible grafts in liver transplantation: A life-saving procedure in highly selected patients. Transplantation 59:1124–1133, 1995.

58. Tanaka A, Tanaka K, Kitai T, et al: Living related liver transplantation across ABO blood groups. Transplantation 58:548–553, 1994.

59. Cacciarelli TV, So SK, Lim J, et al: A reassessment of ABO incompatibility in pediatric liver transplantation. Transplantation 60:757–760, 1995.

60. Yandza T, Lambert T, Alvarez F, et al: Outcome of ABO-incompatible liver transplantation in children with no specific alloantibodies at the time of transplantation. Transplantation 58:46–50, 1994.

61. Langnas AN, Marujo W, Stratta RJ, et al: Hepatic allograft rescue following arterial thrombosis: Role of urgent revascularization. Transplantation 51:86–90, 1991.

62. Stevens LH, Emond JC, Piper JB, et al: Hepatic artery thrombosis in infants: A comparison of whole livers, reduced-size grafts, and grafts from living-related donors. Transplantation 53:396–399, 1992.

63. Kirsch JP, Howard TK, Klintmalm GB, et al: Problematic vascular reconstruction in liver transplantation, Part II: Portovenous conduits. Surgery 107:544–548, 1990.

64. Stieber AC, Zetti G, Todo S, et al: The spectrum of portal vein thrombosis in liver transplantation. Ann Surg 213:199–206, 1991.

65. Harper PL, Edgar PF, Luddington RJ, et al: Protein C deficiency and portal thrombosis in liver transplantation in children. Lancet 2:924–927, 1988.

66. Peclet MH, Ryckman FC, Pedersen SH, et al: The spectrum of bile duct complications in pediatric liver transplantation. J Pediatr Surg 29:214–219, discussion 219–220, 1994.

67. Heffron TG, Emond JC, Whitington PF, et al: Biliary complications in pediatric liver transplantation: A comparison of reduced-size and whole grafts. Transplantation 53:391–395, 1992.

68. Rouch DA, Emond JC, Thistlethwaite JR Jr, et al: Choledo-chocholedochostomy without a T tube or internal stent in transplantation of the liver. Surg Gynecol Obstet 170:239–244, 1990.

69. Snover DC, Sibley RK, Freese DK, et al: Orthotopic liver transplantation: A pathological study of 63 serial liver biopsies from 17 patients with special reference to the diagnostic features and natural history of rejection. Hepatology 4:1212–1222, 1984

70. Mor E, Solomon H, Gibbs JF, et al: Acute cellular rejection following liver transplantation: Clinical pathologic features and effect on outcome. Semin Liver Dis 12:28–40, 1992.

71. Adams DH, Neuberger JM: Treatment of acute rejection. Semin Liver Dis 12:80–88, 1992.

72. Ryckman FC, Schroeder T, Pedersen S: Use of monoclonal antibody immunosuppressive therapy in pediatric renal and liver transplantation. Clin Transplant 5:186–190, 1991.

73. Jain A, Mazariegos G, Pokharna R, et al: The absence of chronic rejection in pediatric primary liver transplant patients who are maintained on tacrolimus-based immunosuppression: A long-term analysis. Transplantation 75:1020–1025, 2003.

74. Jain A, Mazariegos G, Pokharna R, et al: Almost total absence of chronic rejection in primary pediatric liver transplantation under tacrolimus. Transplant Proc 34:1968–1969, 2002.

75. Gupta P, Hart J, Cronin D, et al: Risk factors for chronic rejection after pediatric liver transplantation. Transplantation 72:1098–1102, 2001.

76. Freese DK, Snover DC, Sharp HL, et al: Chronic rejection after liver transplantation: A study of clinical, histopathological and immunological features. Hepatology 13:882–891, 1991.

77. Ludwig J, Wiesner RH, Batts KP, et al: The acute vanishing bile duct syndrome (acute irreversible rejection) after orthotopic liver transplantation. Hepatology 7:476–483, 1987.

78. Demetris A, Adams D, Bellamy C, et al. Update of the International Banff Schema for Liver Allograft Rejection: Working recommendations for the histopathologic staging and reporting of chronic rejection: An international panel. Hepatology 31:792–799, 2000.

79. Gonwa TA, Mai ML, Melton LB, et al: End-stage renal disease (ESRD) after orthotopic liver transplantation (OLTx) using calcineurin-based immunotherapy: risk of development and treatment. Transplantation 72:1934–1939, 2001.

80. Fisher NC, Nightingale PG, Gunson BK, et al: Chronic renal failure following liver transplantation: A retrospective analysis. Transplantation 66:59–66, 1998.

81. Campbell K, Yazigi N, Ryckman F, et al: Renal function in long-term pediatric liver transplant survivors. Am J Transplant 3, 2003.

82. Aw MM, Samaroo B, Baker AJ, et al: Calcineurin-inhibitor related nephrotoxicity- reversibility in paediatric liver transplant recipients. Transplantation 72:746–749, 2001.

83. Heffron TG, Pillen T, Smallwood GA, et al: Pediatric liver transplantation with daclizumab induction. Transplantation 75:2040–2043, 2003.

84. Wiesner RH, Hermans PE, Rakela J, et al: Selective bowel decontamination to decrease gram-negative aerobic bacterial and *Candida* colonization and prevent infection after orthotopic liver transplantation. Transplantation 45:570–574, 1988.

85. Andrews W, Siegel J, Renaro T: Prevention and treatment of selected fungal and viral infections in pediatric liver transplant recipients. Clin Transplant 5:204–207, 1991.

86. Patel R, Snydman DR, Rubin RH, et al: Cytomegalovirus prophylaxis in solid organ transplant recipients. Transplantation 61:1279–1289, 1996.

87. Fox AS, Tolpin MD, Baker AL, et al: Seropositivity in liver transplant recipients as a predictor of cytomegalovirus disease. J Infect Dis 157:383–385, 1988.

88. Holmes RD, Sokol RJ: Epstein-Barr virus and post-transplant lymphoproliferative disease. Pediatr Transplant 6:456–464, 2000.

89. Broughton S, McClay JE, Murray A, et al: The effectiveness of tonsillectomy in diagnosing lymphoproliferative disease in pediatric patients after liver transplantation. Arch Otolaryngol Head Neck Surg 126:1444–1447, 2000.

90. Smets F, Sokal EM. Lymphoproliferation in children after liver transplantation. J Pediatr Gastroenterol Nutr 34:499–505, 2002.

91. Smets F, Sokal EM: Epstein-Barr virus-related lymphoproliferation in children after liver transplant: Role of immunity, diagnosis, and management. Pediatr Transplant 6:280–287, 2002.

92. Sokal EM, Antunes H, Beguin C, et al: Early signs and risk factors for the increased incidence of Epstein-Barr virus-related posttransplant lymphoproliferative diseases in pediatric liver transplant recipients treated with tacrolimus. Transplantation 64:1438–1442, 1997.

93. Holmes RD, Orban-Eller K, Karrer FR, et al: Response of elevated Epstein-Barr virus DNA levels to therapeutic changes in pediatric liver transplant patients: 56-month follow up and outcome. Transplantation 74:367–372, 2002.

94. Axelrod DA, Holmes R, Thomas SE, et al: Limitations of EBV-PCR monitoring to detect EBV associated post-transplant lymphoproliferative disorder. Pediatr Transplant 7:223–227, 2003.

95. Penn I: Post-transplant malignancy: the role of immunosuppression. Drug Saf 23:101–113, 2000.

96. Sokal EM, Caragiozoglou T, Lamy M, et al: Epstein-Barr virus serology and Epstein-Barr virus-associated lymphoproliferative disorders in pediatric liver transplant recipients. Transplantation 56:1394–1398, 1993.

97. Jabs WJ, Hennig H, Kittel M, et al: Normalized quantification by real-time PCR of Epstein-Barr virus load in patients at risk for posttransplant lymphoproliferative disorders. J Clin Microbiol 39:564–569, 2001.

98. Guthery SL, Heubi JE, Bucuvalas JC, et al: Determination of risk factors for Epstein-Barr virus-associated posttransplant lymphoproliferative disorder in pediatric liver transplant recipients using objective case ascertainment. Transplantation 75:987–993, 2003.

99. Hanto DW, Frizzera G, Gajl-Peczalska KJ, et al: Epstein-Barr virus, immunodeficiency, and B cell lymphoproliferation. Transplantation 39:461–472, 1985.

100. Bueno J, Ramil C, Green M: Current management strategies for the prevention and treatment of cytomegalovirus infection in pediatric transplant recipients. Paediatr Drugs 4:279–290, 2002.

101. Serinet MO, Jacquemin E, Habes D, et al: Anti-CD20 monoclonal antibody (rituximab) treatment for Epstein-Barr virus-associated, B-cell lymphoproliferative disease in pediatric liver transplant recipients. J Pediatr Gastroenterol Nutr 34:389–393, 2002.

102. Haque T, Wilkie GM, Taylor C, et al. Treatment of Epstein-Barr-virus-positive post-transplantation lymphoproliferative disease with partly HLA-matched allogeneic cytotoxic T cells. Lancet 360:436–442, 2002.

103. Haque T, Taylor C, Wilkie GM, et al: Complete regression of posttransplant lymphoproliferative disease using partially HLA-matched Epstein Barr virus-specific cytotoxic T cells. Transplantation 72:1399–1402, 2001.

104. Tiao G, Alonso M, Bucuvalas JC, et al: Retransplantation of the Liver in the Pediatric Population: The Impact of Early Versus Late Graft Failure on Outcome. Washington, DC, American Transplant Congress Vol. Abstract 563, 2003.

105. Washburn WK, Bradley J, Cosimi AB, et al: A regional experience with emergency liver transplantation. Transplantation 61:235–239, 1996.

106. Langnas AN, Marujo WC, Inagaki M, et al: The results of reduced-size liver transplantation, including split livers, in patients with end-stage liver disease. Transplantation 53:387–391, 1992.

107. Esquivel CO, Nakazato P, Cox K, et al: The impact of liver reductions in pediatric liver transplantation. Arch Surg 126:1278–1285; discussion 1285–1286, 1991.

108. Split Research Group 2: Studies of Pediatric Liver Transplantation (SPLIT): Year 2000 outcomes. Transplantation 72:463–476, 2001.

109. Fridell JA, Jain A, Reyes J, et al: Causes of mortality beyond 1 year after primary pediatric liver transplant under tacrolimus. Transplantation 74:1721–1724, 2002.

110. Mack CL, Ferrario M, Abecassis M, et al: Living donor liver transplantation for children with liver failure and concurrent multiple organ system failure. Liver Transplant 7:890–895, 2001.

111. Emre S: Living-donor liver transplantation in children. Pediatr Transplant 6:43–46, 2002.

112. Bucuvalas JC, Ryckman FC: The long- and short-term outcome of living-donor liver transplantation. J Pediatr 134:259–261, 1999.

113. Sokal EM, Veyckemans F, de Ville de Goyet J, et al: Liver transplantation in children less than 1 year of age. J Pediatr 117:205–210, 1990.

114. Cox K, Nakazato P, Berquist W, et al: Liver transplantation in infants weighing less than 10 kilograms. Transplant Proc 23:1579–1580, 1991.

115. Van der Werf WJ, D'Alessandro AM, Knechtle SJ, et al: Infant pediatric liver transplantation results equal those for older pediatric patients. J Pediatr Surg 33:20–23, 1998.

116. Bilik R, Greig P, Langer B, et al: Survival after reduced-size liver transplantation is dependent on pretransplant status. J Pediatr Surg 28:1307–1311, 1993.

117. Carroll CL, Goodman DM, Superina RA, et al: Timed pediatric risk of mortality scores predict outcomes in pediatric liver transplant recipients. Pediatr Transplant 7:289–295, 2003.

118. Otte JB, de Ville de Goyet J, Sokal E, et al: Size reduction of the donor liver is a safe way to alleviate the shortage of size-matched organs in pediatric liver transplantation. Ann Surg 211:146–157, 1990.

119. Ryckman FC, Alonso MH, Bucuvalas JC, et al: Long-term survival after liver transplantation. J Pediatr Surg 34:845–849; discussion 849–850, 1999.

120. Wallot MA, Mathot M, Janssen M, et al: Long-term survival and late graft loss in pediatric liver transplant recipients: A 15-year single-center experience. Liver Transplant 8:615–622, 2000.

121. Sudan DL, Shaw BW Jr, Langnas AN: Causes of late mortality in pediatric liver transplant recipients. Ann Surg 227:289–295, 1993.

122. Sarna S, Sipila I, Jalanko H, et al: Factors affecting growth after pediatric liver transplantation. Transplant Proc 26:161–164, 1994.

123. Sarna S, Sipila I, Vihervuori E, et al: Growth delay after liver transplantation in childhood: studies of underlying mechanisms. Pediatr Res 38:366–372, 1995.

124. Balistreri WF, Bucuvalas JC, Ryckman FC: The effect of immunosuppression on growth and development. Liver Transplant Surg 1(5 suppl 1):64–73, 1995.

125. Chin SE, Shepherd RW, Cleghorn GJ, et al: Survival, growth and quality of life in children after orthotopic liver transplantation: A 5 year experience. J Paediatr Child Health 27:380–385, 1991.

126. Zitelli BJ, Miller JW, Gartner JC Jr, et al: Changes in life-style after liver transplantation. Pediatrics 82:173–180, 1988.

127. Stewart SM, Hiltebeitel C, Nici J, et al: Neuropsychological outcome of pediatric liver transplantation. Pediatrics 87:367–376, 1991.

128. Stewart SM, Uauy R, Waller DA, et al: Mental and motor development, social competence, and growth one year after successful pediatric liver transplantation. J Pediatr 114:574–581, 1989.

129. Tarter RE, Hays AL, Sandford SS, et al: Cerebral morphological abnormalities associated with non-alcoholic cirrhosis. Lancet 2:893–895, 1986.

130. Bernthal P, Hays A, Tarter RE, et al: Cerebral CT scan abnormalities in cholestatic and hepatocellular disease and their relationship to neuropsychologic test performance. Hepatology 7:107–114, 1987.

131. Tarter RE, Sandford SL, Hays AL, et al: Hepatic injury correlates with neuropsychologic impairment. Int J Neurosci 44:75–82, 1989.

132. Bucuvalas JC, Britto M, Krug S, et al: Health-related quality of life in pediatric liver transplant recipients: A single-center study. Liver Transplant 9:62–71, 2003.

133. Harper AM, Edwards EB, Ellison MD: The OPTN waiting list, 1988-2000. In Cecka JM, Terasaki PI (eds): Clinical Transplants 2001. Los Angeles, UCLA Immunogenics Center, 73–85, 2002.

134. Reyes J, Mazariegos GV, Bond GM, et al: Pediatric intestinal transplantation: Historical notes, principles and controversies. Pediatr Transplant 6:193–207, 2002.

135. Fishbein TM, Gondolesi GE, Kaufman SS: Intestinal transplantation for gut failure. Gastroenterology 124:1615–1628, 2003.

136. (HCFA) HCFA: Combined Liver and Intestinal and Multivisceral Transplantation (CAG-00036) Decision Memorandum. HCFA, Washington, DC, 2000.

137. Fishbein TM, Schiano T, LeLeiko N, et al: An integrated approach to intestinal failure: Results of a new program with total parenteral nutrition, bowel rehabilitation, and transplantation. J Gastrointest Surg 6:554–562, 2002.

138. Koehler AN, Yaworski JA, Gardner M, et al: Coordinated interdisciplinary management of pediatric intestinal failure: A 2-year review. J Pediatr Surg 35:380–385, 2000.

139. Kim HB, Fauza D, Garza J, et al: Serial transverse enteroplasty (STEP): A novel bowel lengthening procedure. J Pediatr Surg 38:425–429, 2003.

140. Touloukian RJ, Smith GJ: Normal intestinal length in preterm infants. J Pediatr Surg 18:720–723, 1983.

141. Bueno J, Ohwada S, Kocoshis S, et al: Factors impacting the survival of children with intestinal failure referred for intestinal transplantation. J Pediatr Surg 34:27–32; discussion 32–33, 1999.

142. Reyes J, Fishbein T, Bueno J, et al: Reduced-size orthotopic composite liver-intestinal allograft. Transplantation 66:489–492, 1998.

143. Fryer J, Pellar S, Ormond D, et al: Mortality in candidates waiting for combined liver-intestine transplants exceeds that for other candidates waiting for liver transplants. Liver Transplant 9:748–753, 2003.

144. Furukawa H, Manez R, Kusne S, et al: Cytomegalovirus disease in intestinal transplantation. Transplant Proc 27:1357–1358, 1995.

145. Furukawa H, Reyes J, Abu-Elmagd K, et al: Intestinal transplantation at the University of Pittsburgh: Six-year experience. Transplant Proc 29:688–689, 1997.

146. Berney T, Kato T, Nishida S, et al: Portal versus systemic drainage of small bowel allografts: Comparative assessment of survival, function, rejection, and bacterial translocation. J Am Coll Surg 195:804–813, 2002.

147. Starzl TE, Murase N, Abu-Elmagd K, et al: Tolerogenic immunosuppression for organ transplantation. Lancet 361:1502–1510, 2003.

148. Abu-Elmagd K, Reyes J, Bond G, et al: Clinical intestinal transplantation: A decade of experience at a single center. Ann Surg 234:404–416; discussion 416–417, 2001.

149. Farmer DG, McDiarmid SV, Yersiz H, et al: Outcome after intestinal transplantation: results from one center's 9-year experience. Arch Surg 136:1027–1031, discussion 1032, 2001.

150. Kato T, Ruiz P, Thompson JF, et al: Intestinal and multivisceral transplantation. World J Surg 26:226–237, 2002.

151. Reyes J, Mazariegos G, Bond G, et al: Rabbit anti-thymocyte globulin preconditioning and induction for pediatric intestine transplantation. Am J Transplant 3(suppl 5):192, 2003.

152. Kaufman SS, Atkinson JB, Bianchi A, et al: Indications for pediatric intestinal transplantation: A position paper of the American Society of Transplantation. Pediatr Transplant 5:80–87, 2001.

153. Potter DE, Holliday MA, Piel CF, et al: Treatment of end-stage renal disease in children: A 15-year experience. Kidney Int 18:103–109, 1980.

154. Fine R: Renal Transplantation in Children. In Morris P (ed): Kidney Transplantation: Principles and Practice. Orlando: Grune & Stratton, 1984, pp 509–546.

155. McEnery PT, Stablein DM, Arbus G, et al: Renal transplantation in children: A report of the North American Pediatric Renal Transplant Cooperative Study. N Engl J Med 326:1727–1732, 1992.

156. Kashtan CE, McEnery PT, Tejani A, et al: Renal allograft survival according to primary diagnosis: A report of the North American Pediatric Renal Transplant Cooperative Study. Pediatr Nephrol 9:679–684, 1995.

157. Warady BA, Hebert D, Sullivan EK, et al: Renal transplantation, chronic dialysis, and chronic renal insufficiency in children and adolescents: The 1995 Annual Report of the North American Pediatric Renal Transplant Cooperative Study. Pediatr Nephrol 11:49–64, 1997.

158. Hanna JD, Krieg RJ Jr, Scheinman JI, et al: Effects of uremia on growth in children. Semin Nephrol 16:230–241, 1996.

159. Benfield MR, McDonald RA, Bartosh S, et al: Changing trends in pediatric transplantation: 2001 Annual Report of the North American Pediatric Renal Transplant Cooperative Study. Pediatr Transplant 7:321–335, 2003.

160. Benfield MR: Changing trends in pediatric transplantation: 2001 Annual Report of the North American Pediatric Renal Transplant Cooperative Study. Pediatr Transplant 7:321–335, 2003.

161. Englund MS, Tyden G, Wikstad I, et al: Growth impairment at renal transplantation: A determinant of growth and final height. Pediatr Transplant 7:192–199, 2003.

162. Fine RN: Growth following solid-organ transplantation. Pediatr Transplant 6:47–52, 2002.

163. Grushkin CM, Fine RN: Growth in children following renal transplantation. Am J Dis Child 125:514–516, 1973.

164. Rotundo A, Nevins TE, Lipton M, et al: Progressive encephalopathy in children with chronic renal insufficiency in infancy. Kidney Int 21:486–491, 1982.

165. Najarian J, Ascher NL, Mauer SM: Kidney transplantation. In Welch K, Randolph J, Ravitch M (eds): Pediatric Surgery. Chicago, Year Book Medical, 1986, pp 360–373.

166. Sheldon CA, Gonzalez R, Burns MW, et al: Renal transplantation into the dysfunctional bladder: The role of adjunctive bladder reconstruction. J Urol 152:972–975, 1994.

167. Turcotte J, Campbell DA, Dafoe D: Pediatric renal transplantation. In Cerilli G (ed): Organ Transplantation and Replacement. Philadelphia, JB Lippincott, 1988, pp 349–360.

168. Ildstad ST, Tollerud DJ, Noseworthy J, et al: The influence of donor age on graft survival in renal transplantation. J Pediatr Surg 25:134–137; discussion 137–139, 1990.

169. Ildstad ST, Tollerud DJ, Noseworthy J, et al: Renal transplantation in pediatric recipients. Transplant Proc 21:1936–1937, 1989.

170. Kim MS, Jabs K, Harmon WE: Long-term patient survival in a pediatric renal transplantation program. Transplantation 51:413–416, 1991.

171. Bereket G, Fine RN: Pediatric renal transplantation. Pediatr Clin North Am 42:1603–1628, 1995.

172. Fine RN, Tejani A, Sullivan EK: Pre-emptive renal transplantation in children: Report of the North American Pediatric Renal Transplant Cooperative Study (NAPRTCS). Clin Transplant 8:474–478, 1994.

173. McDonald RA, Smith JM, Stablein D, et al: Pretransplant peritoneal dialysis and graft thrombosis following pediatric kidney transplantation: A NAPRTCS report. Pediatr Transplant 7:204–208, 2003.

174. Tejani A, Cortes L, Stablein D: Clinical correlates of chronic rejection in pediatric renal transplantation: A report of the North American Pediatric Renal Transplant Cooperative Study. Transplantation 61:1054–1058, 1996.

175. Tejani A, Sullivan EK, Alexander S, et al: Posttransplant deaths and factors that influence the mortality rate in North American children. Transplantation 57:547–553, 1994.

176. Tejani A, Sullivan EK: Factors that impact on the outcome of second renal transplants in children. Transplantation 62:606–611, 1996.

177. Sutherland DE: The case for pancreas transplantation. Diabetes Metab 22:132–138, 1996.

178. Stratta RJ, Larsen JL, Cushing K: Pancreas transplantation for diabetes mellitus. Annu Rev Med 46:281–298, 1995.

179. Heinemann A, Wischhusen F, Puschel K, et al: Standard liver volume in the Caucasian population. Liver Transplant Surg 5:366–368, 1999.

CHAPTER 45

Lesions of the Pancreas and Spleen

Sheilendra S. Mehta, MD, and George K. Gittes, MD

PANCREAS

Anatomy and Embryology

The pancreas originates in week 5 of gestation as paired evaginations of the foregut.[1] The dorsal pancreatic bud gives rise to the body and tail of the pancreas, as well as the minor duct (Santorini) and minor papilla, and the continuation of the main duct (Wirsung) into the body and tail. The dorsal pancreas arises as a diverticulum from the dorsal aspect of the duodenal anlage. The ventral pancreatic bud arises from the biliary diverticulum and swings around the dorsal aspect of the duodenal anlage during gut rotation, to give rise to the head of the pancreas, as well as the proximal portion of the main pancreatic duct (Fig. 45-1).

The two pancreatic buds fuse to form one pancreas at approximately 7 weeks' gestation, although it appears that complete fusion of the two ducts to form the main pancreatic duct is delayed until the perinatal period.[2] The endocrine component of the pancreas, the islets of Langerhans, start to differentiate before formation of the pancreatic buds in the wall of the foregut, from which the pancreas will arise.[3] The islets make up 10% of the pancreas during early embryonic and fetal life, but they decrease to less than 1% in the adult. Fetal pancreatic islets appear to play an important role in fetal homeostasis. Pancreatic acini begin to form at 12 weeks and at that time begin to accumulate organelles and zymogen granules characteristic of acinar cells. These cells do not secrete appreciable amounts of enzyme until the time of birth.[1]

The pancreas is retroperitoneal and is light pink in children. The acini can be seen with low-power loupe magnification, as can the septa dividing the lobulations. The head of the pancreas lies in the C-loop of the duodenum, and the uncinate process, emanating from the posteromedial portion of the head, projects under the superior mesenteric artery and vein. The neck of the pancreas is defined as that portion of the pancreas anterior to these vessels.[4] The body and tail, to the left of these

vessels, angle sharply upward toward the hilum of the spleen. The main pancreatic duct runs along the posterior aspect of the gland and curves downward in the head to run alongside the common bile duct, which runs in a groove posterior to the pancreas or within the substance of the posterior gland. The main pancreatic duct and common bile duct may fuse in a "common channel" before entry into the duodenum.

The pancreas is quite convex, with its midportion being reflected over the anterior surface of the upper lumbar vertebrae and aorta and the lateral portions falling posteriorly toward each kidney (Fig. 45-2). The arterial supply of the pancreas is from the celiac and superior mesenteric arteries, which form the pancreaticoduodenal arcade. The pancreas also has anastomoses from the splenic artery.

Congenital Anomalies

Ectopic pancreatic rests are frequently encountered along foregut derivatives, such as the stomach and the duodenum, as well as along the jejunum, ileum, and colon.[5] These lesions are found in approximately 2% of autopsy series and are usually found in the duodenum, stomach, or jejunum. They represent the most common anomaly of the gastric antrum and may cause a gastric outlet obstruction.[6] Their origin is unknown, but one possible explanation suggests an aberrant epithelial-mesenchymal interaction, leading to the transdifferentiation of heterotopic embryonic epithelium into pancreatic epithelium. Some recent studies have implicated defects in "hedgehog" signaling, which antagonizes normal pancreatic development, as the cause of the formation of ectopic pancreatic tissue.[7,8] Ectopic rests are typically asymptomatic and are encountered incidentally at laparotomy. They can be identified as pancreatic tissue because the surface has the same granular acinar appearance. These ectopic pancreatic rests usually do not become inflamed, possibly because they contain numerous small drainage ducts rather than a large duct, which could become

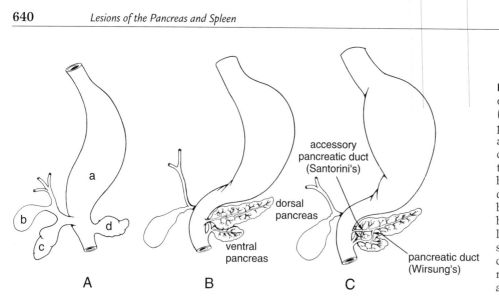

FIGURE 45-1. Pancreatic embryology. *A,* Stomach (a), gallbladder (b), and ventral (c) and dorsal (d) pancreatic buds develop separately at embryologic week 4. The pancreas develops as an evagination of the developing foregut. The dorsal bud evaginates directly off of the duodenal anlage. *B,* The ventral bud evaginates from the biliary bud and then swings around to the left, with gut rotation occurring simultaneously. *C,* The main pancreatic duct of Wirsung and the minor accessory duct of Santorini are shown.

obstructed. Occasionally, an ectopic pancreatic rest produces obstruction or bleeding. When encountered at laparotomy, ectopic rests should probably be excised unless the excision would entail significant risk of morbidity.

Annular pancreas is thought to result from faulty rotation of the ventral pancreatic bud in its course around the posterior aspect of the duodenal anlage. The duodenum is encircled by and obstructed with normal pancreatic tissue containing normal functioning acini, ducts, and islets of Langerhans.[9,10] The prevailing theory of pathogenesis is that half of the ventral bud migrates anteriorly, and half migrates posteriorly. Abnormal endodermal expression patterns of Sonic hedgehog (Shh), which is a potent intercellular signaling protein that demarcates a molecular boundary between the pancreas and the adjacent gastrointestinal tract, may be responsible for the formation of annular pancreas.[7] The ductal drainage of this

system is variable and complex. Duodenal atresia and stenosis, intestinal malrotation, and trisomy 21 can often be found in combination with annular pancreas.[11] The clinical significance relates primarily to duodenal obstruction, typically with bilious vomiting. Radiographic studies will reveal the classic finding of a "double-bubble" sign.[12] Management consists of surgical bypass of the obstructing lesion with a duodenoduodenostomy. If such a bypass is not technically feasible, a duodenojejunostomy can be performed. Resection or division of the annular pancreas should not be carried out.

Cystic fibrosis is an autosomal recessive condition, seen primarily in the white population, and represents about 1 in 2500 live births.[13] It is caused by mutations in the cystic fibrosis transmembrane conductance regulator (*CFTR*) gene that encodes a protein expressed in the apical membrane of exocrine epithelial cells. Cystic fibrosis

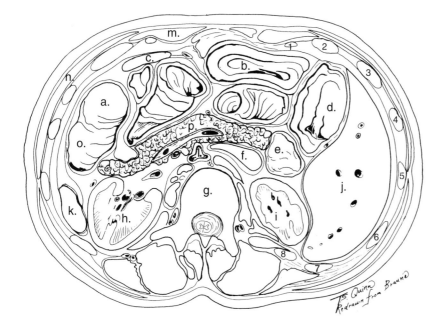

FIGURE 45-2. Cross-sectional anatomy of the pancreas. The pancreas lies convexly across the lumbar spine with the tail of the pancreas next to the spleen and the hilum of the left kidney. The head of the pancreas lies to the right of the spine near the hilum of the right kidney. Splenic flexure (a), transverse colon (b), stomach (c), ascending colon (d), duodenum (e), inferior vena cava (f), first lumbar vertebra (g), left kidney (h), right kidney (i), liver (j), spleen (k), aorta (l), rectus abdominis (m), external oblique (n), descending colon (o), and pancreas (p).

leads to significant pancreatic insufficiency. The pancreatic secretions generally have a reduced amount of bicarbonate, a lower pH, and a lower overall exocrine fluid volume. The inspissated secretions lead to blockage of the ducts, with subsequent duct dilatation, and obstruction of pancreatic exocrine flow. The acinar cells degenerate, leading to pancreatic fibrosis. The result is impaired digestion of fats and proteins.[14]

Pancreatitis

Acute Pancreatitis

Acute pancreatitis is an acute inflammation of the pancreas with variable severity from mild abdominal pain, which may go undiagnosed, to fulminant necrotizing pancreatitis and death. Episodes of acute inflammation may completely resolve and then recur; in such cases, the term *acute relapsing pancreatitis* is applied to the clinical course. It is likely that complete interval resolution of morphology and function occurs, as opposed to the occurrence of irreversible changes in the pancreas in cases of chronic pancreatitis.

The causes of acute pancreatitis include trauma, biliary tract stone disease, choledochal cyst, ductal developmental anomalies, drugs, metabolic derangements, and infections. Most commonly, the cause is not apparent and is called "idiopathic."

Because the pancreas is fixed against the lumbar spine, trauma to the upper abdomen (classically, a bicycle handlebar) fractures the pancreas or injures the major duct at that point. Biliary stone disease, as in adults, may lead to pancreatitis from transient pancreatic duct obstruction with or without bile reflux. Choledochal cysts produce pancreatitis by pancreatic duct compression or bile reflux resulting from a long common biliary-pancreatic duct within the head of the pancreas.

Pancreas divisum is an anomaly present in 10% of the population, resulting from failure of the dorsal duct to fuse with the ventral duct. The majority of the exocrine secretions of the pancreas, including those from the entire body and tail, must drain through the small minor duct of Santorini and minor papilla into the duodenum. This relative obstruction may cause recurring episodes of pancreatitis.[15] These patients should undergo a sphincteroplasty of the minor papilla. Endoscopic stenting with or without sphincterotomy has been described, but requires particular skill with the endoscope in cannulation of the small ducts encountered in children.[16] Other rare ductal anomalies may result in obstruction and recurrent bouts of pancreatitis. Biliary tract stones are uncommon in children, but when present, may lead to pancreatitis. Data extrapolated from the adult literature indicates that removal of impacted stones in gallstone pancreatitis in children should be performed endoscopically.[17] Choledochal cysts may produce pancreatitis from transient pancreatic duct compression or from bile reflux. Drugs that are thought to induce pancreatitis include corticosteroids and valproic acid.[18,19] Systemic illnesses and metabolic conditions, such as cystic fibrosis with inspissation of pancreatic secretions in the ducts,

Reye syndrome, Kawasaki's disease, hyperlipidemias, and hypercalcemia, may cause pancreatitis. Infections with viruses (e.g., coxsackievirus and rotavirus) and generalized bacterial sepsis also can cause pancreatitis.[20]

Clearly, the pathogenesis entails the inappropriate activation of proenzymes, leading to autodigestion of the pancreas. The cellular mechanisms leading to acute pancreatitis are not known, but they are the subject of intense scientific investigation. Pancreatic enzymes can cause destruction at distant sites either by vascular dissemination or by release from the pancreas of cytokines such as tumor necrosis factor-α, free radicals such as superoxide, and vasoactive substances such as histamine and kallikrein.

The mechanism by which inappropriate activation of pancreatic enzymes occurs is not known. Possibilities include (1) reflux of duodenal enterokinase into the pancreas to activate trypsin, which then inappropriately activates other proenzymes in the pancreas; (2) ductal obstruction with extravasation of enzyme-rich ductal fluid into the parenchyma of the pancreas; or (3) fusion of lysosomes with zymogen granules inside acinar cells to allow lysosomal enzyme activation of the proenzymes. Once activated, elastase, phospholipase, and superoxide free radicals are thought to be the principal mediators of tissue damage.

Acute pancreatitis usually is initially seen with the sudden onset of midepigastric pain associated with back pain, severe vomiting, and low-grade fever.[21,22] The abdomen is diffusely tender with signs of peritonitis, and distention occurs with a paucity of bowel sounds. In severe cases of necrotizing or hemorrhagic pancreatitis, hemorrhage may dissect from the pancreas along tissue planes, appearing as ecchymosis either in the flanks (Grey-Turner sign) or at the umbilicus (Cullen's sign) (Fig. 45-3). These ecchymoses typically take 1 to 2 days to develop.

Elevated amylase levels are helpful in the diagnosis, although normal serum amylase levels do not exclude

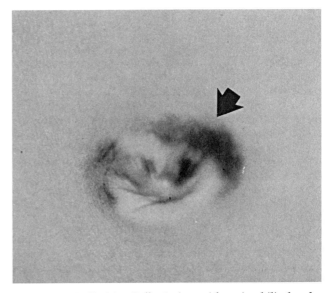

FIGURE 45-3. Positive Cullen's sign, with periumbilical ecchymosis (*arrow*), in a patient with hemorrhagic pancreatitis.

pancreatitis from the differential diagnostic possibilities. The degree of serum amylase elevation does not correlate with severity of the disease. Amylase is excreted in urine, but, as is true with glucose, tubular reabsorption results in amylase spill in the urine only after significant hyperamylasemia occurs.[23] In addition, the half-life of amylase is approximately 10 hours. Thus moderately elevated levels of serum amylase may not be detectable in the urine.

Hyperamylasemia or hyperamylasuria may be caused by conditions other than pancreatitis, most notably salivary inflammation or trauma; intestinal disease including perforation, ischemia, necrosis, or inflammation; renal failure; and macroamylasemia. Alterations in renal excretion are compensated by measuring the ratio of clearance of amylase to that of creatinine. The ratio requires measurement of simultaneous spot levels of serum amylase and creatinine and urine amylase and creatinine:

$$(U_{amy}/Serum_{amy}) \times (Serum_{Cr}/Urine_{Cr})$$

Ratios greater than 0.03 are significant. Lipase levels have been proposed as a more specific test of pancreatic tissue damage, although intestinal perforation does cause an elevation of lipase through reabsorption via the peritoneum. Lipase is produced only in the pancreas, and its measurement is particularly helpful for distinguishing pancreatic trauma from salivary trauma.[24]

Imaging the abdomen is important as part of the evaluation of the patient with abdominal pain. In the patient with pancreatitis, plain abdominal radiographs may reveal an isolated loop of intestine in the vicinity of the inflamed pancreas, the so-called "sentinel loop." Other findings suggesting pancreatitis include local spasm of the transverse colon with proximal dilation, known as the "colon cut-off" sign. Pancreatic calcifications suggest chronic pancreatitis. Plain chest roentgenograms should be performed in all patients with acute pancreatitis to look for evidence of pleural effusion and pulmonary edema.

Abdominal ultrasonography (US) may show a decrease in echogenicity of the pancreas compared with normal owing to pancreatic edema, but such a finding is not reliable in determining the diagnosis or severity.[25] The main use of US is to demonstrate gallstones as a possible cause of pancreatitis and to follow up the therapy to observe improvement in edema or peripancreatic fluid collection.

Abdominal computed tomography (CT) scan offers much better resolution than US in determining the size of the pancreas, the degree of edema, and the presence of fluid collections.[26] The size of the pancreatic duct can often be estimated much more accurately with CT than with US, and the presence of complications such as pancreatic abscess or pseudocyst may be delineated. The use of dynamic CT pancreatography has been advocated because of its ability to differentiate perfused from nonperfused (necrotic) pancreas. By using a bolus of contrast with rapid scanning in fine cuts through the pancreas, a precise assessment of the percentage of the pancreas that is either underperfused or nonperfused can be made. If necessary, CT scan can also be used for interventional procedures for diagnosis or drainage of fluid collections.

Endoscopic retrograde cholangiopancreatography (ERCP) is being used more frequently than in the past in children with acute pancreatitis. Some recent literature would suggest that the complication rates in children are higher than those in the adult patient population.[27] However, it may be potentially helpful in children with severe refractory biliary pancreatitis who may have a stone impacted in the ampulla, as well as in trauma patients in whom a ductal injury is suspected or a pancreatic pseudocyst has formed.

Magnetic resonance cholangiopancreatography (MRCP) is a new, noninvasive technique for evaluating the biliary tree and the pancreatic duct. This technique is particularly attractive because the procedure is noninvasive and spares the patient the potential complications of ERCP. In addition, the study is cheaper and requires no radiation or contrast administration, which is routinely performed with ERCP. One disadvantage of MRCP is that it does not allow therapeutic interventions; however, it may help direct the type of therapeutic intervention best suited to the patient's pathology.[28] Another problem is that MRCP tends to overestimate the stenosis of the main pancreatic duct in patients with pancreatitis. Regardless, MRCP is now the initial imaging study of choice in the evaluation of pancreatic ductal anatomy in children with unexplained or recurrent pancreatitis.[16]

Key features in treating patients with acute pancreatitis are aggressive fluid replacement to maintain a good urine output (2 mL/kg/hr), usually measured with the aid of an indwelling urinary catheter, and, probably most important, a very low threshold for transferring the patient to an intensive care unit.[29,30]

Acute pancreatitis causes diffuse tissue damage throughout the body as a result of the release of active mediators, including phospholipase A_2, elastase, histamines, kinins, kallikreins, and prostaglandins. Extracellular fluid losses can be enormous. Constant monitoring is necessary to avoid the development of severe hypovolemia. Patients with acute pancreatitis should be kept at bowel rest with nasogastric suction. Most patients receive H_2 receptor antagonists to prevent exposure of the duodenal secretin-producing cells to gastric acid, which is a potent stimulator of pancreatic secretion. These antagonists also may help prevent the stress ulceration seen in patients with pancreatitis. This therapeutic regimen is logical but empirical, because no studies have shown improvement in outcome with these interventions. Clinical trials have, however, shown improved outcome in acute pancreatitis by using long-acting somatostatin analogues, and it is probably reasonable to use these analogues in moderate-to-severe cases of pancreatitis.[31]

Adequate analgesia is critical to minimize the additional stress from pain. Meperidine (Demerol) is thought to be a better analgesic in pancreatitis because morphine is well known to cause spasm of the sphincter of Oddi, which in turn is known to increase pancreatic duct pressure and potentially worsen the pancreatitis. An important caveat is that the diagnosis of pancreatitis must be certain before giving the patient significant doses of narcotics because the ability to diagnose serious nonpancreatic problems, such as intestinal ischemia or perforated ulcer, may be lost.

As cases of severe pancreatitis progress, patients need to be monitored closely for signs of the development of multiorgan system failure. Pleural effusions and pulmonary edema can progress to severe adult respiratory distress syndrome with hypoxia, requiring endotracheal intubation. The tense abdominal distention associated with pancreatitis frequently contributes to the hypoventilation. Hypocalcemia, hypomagnesemia, anemia from hemorrhage, hyperglycemia, renal failure, and late sepsis can be seen in these patients and require close monitoring. Disagreement exists concerning the use of prophylactic antibiotics. In general, mild or moderate cases probably do not benefit from antibiotics. More severe cases of pancreatitis, however, may benefit because of the high rate of sepsis, although confirmatory data in these patients are lacking. Some advantage has been demonstrated with the use of imipenem, with reduction in the incidence of pancreatic sepsis in patients with necrotizing pancreatitis.[17]

Nutrition is critically important in the patient with pancreatitis, and an early positive nitrogen balance has been shown to improve survival rates. This need for aggressive nutrition should come in the form of early parenteral hyperalimentation. The hyperalimentation should include lipid formulations, despite the known association of hyperlipidemia and pancreatitis, although a close monitoring of the serum lipid levels should be maintained to avoid triglyceride levels greater than 500 mg/dL. In general, the resumption of enteral nutrition should be cautious, usually after complete resolution of abdominal pain and preferably after normalization of the serum enzyme levels.

Surgical intervention in acute pancreatitis is not often necessary. Other than for pancreatic pseudocyst or for papillotomy in the case of pancreas divisum, surgical intervention for acute pancreatitis is restricted to patients with severe necrotizing pancreatitis needing debridement or patients with pancreatic abscess.[32,33] In some instances, pancreatitis is discovered when laparotomy is performed for a preoperative diagnosis of appendicitis (Fig. 45-4). Under this circumstance, the best course is to palpate the gallbladder for stones. If the pancreatitis is mild and

gallstones are present, cholecystectomy is reasonable. If the pancreatitis is severe, the safer course is to perform a cholecystostomy, which allows later access to the biliary stones. If no gallstones are present, but the patient has severe necrotizing pancreatitis, limited debridement is acceptable, but simply leaving large sump drains in place is probably adequate. Early pancreatic lavage, pancreatic drainage, and pancreatic resection have not been shown to improve survival rates in cases of severe pancreatitis.

A *pancreatic abscess* may result from infection of necrotic pancreatic tissue or infection of a peripancreatic fluid collection. Pancreatic abscess increases the mortality rate of pancreatitis threefold and is an absolute indication for surgical therapy.[34,35] Differentiating a pancreatic abscess from an uninfected pancreatic fluid collection is important because pancreatitis itself can make the patient appear "septic." The diagnosis is established by Gram stain and culture of the suspected abscess by CT-guided needle aspiration. The indication for aspiration is fever and leukocytosis persisting more than 7 to 10 days after onset of the pancreatitis. Patients shown to have pancreatic necrosis by dynamic CT pancreatography are candidates for aspiration because pancreatic necrosis usually precedes the development of a pancreatic abscess. The surgical therapy for a pancreatic abscess is debridement of clearly necrotic tissue and placement of large sump suction drains. Some mechanism must be in place for ongoing removal of the infected material postoperatively, either by reoperation or by the sump drains. In some cases, it is impossible to differentiate an infected pancreatic pseudocyst from an abscess. A laparotomy should be performed with sump drainage of the fluid collection.

Pancreatic pseudocyst is a complication of trauma or pancreatitis with damage to the pancreatic ductal system. The extravasated pancreatic enzymes and digested tissue are contained by the formation of a cavity composed of fibroblastic reaction and inflammation, but without epithelial lining. Pseudocysts may be acute or chronic. The acute pseudocyst has an irregular wall on CT scan, is tender, and usually shortly follows an episode of acute pancreatitis or trauma (Fig. 45-5). Chronic pseudocysts are usually spherical with a thick wall, and they are commonly seen in patients with chronic pancreatitis. The distinction between these two types of pseudocysts is important because 50% of acute pseudocysts resolve without therapy, whereas chronic pseudocysts rarely do. An acute pseudocyst develops a thick fibrous wall in 4 to 6 weeks. Pseudocysts smaller than 5 cm in diameter usually disappear without intervention. When compared with those in adults, pseudocysts in children tend to resolve more frequently with medical therapy alone.[36] Some evidence exists that somatostatin may help resolve pancreatic pseudocysts in children.[37]

Pancreatic pseudocysts that persist require either internal drainage (preferred), excision (distal pseudocysts only), or external drainage (infected or immature cysts). A minimally invasive approach to cyst-gastrostomy was reported in which intragastric laparoscopic ports were used. Other minimally invasive strategies for pancreatic pseudocysts include transesophageal endoscopic cyst-gastrostomy and percutaneous drainage.[38] The two endoscopic procedures should be performed at institutions

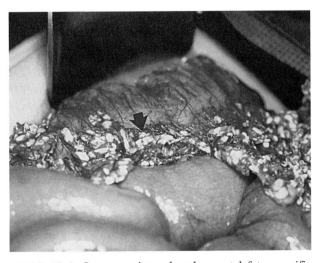

FIGURE 45-4. Severe peritoneal and omental fat saponification, seen as white fatty deposits (*arrow*) in a patient with acute pancreatitis. The preoperative diagnosis was acute appendicitis.

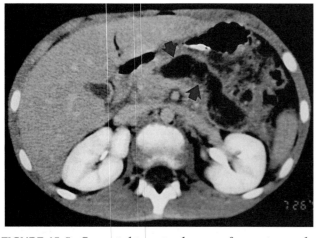

FIGURE 45-5. Computed tomography scan of an acute pseudocyst in a patient after a severe motor vehicle accident. The wall (*arrows*) is irregular with nonloculated fluid inside.

with significant experience with these techniques and, even then, serious potential risks exist.[39,40] Percutaneous drainage is the treatment of choice for infected pseudocysts because these cysts typically have thin, weak walls not amenable to internal drainage.

The three major complications of pancreatic pseudocysts are hemorrhage, rupture, and infection. Hemorrhage, the most serious complication, usually results from pressure and erosion of the cyst into a nearby visceral vessel (e.g., splenic, gastroduodenal). These patients require emergency angiography with embolization. Rupture or infection of a pseudocyst is uncommon, and in both cases, external drainage is indicated.

Pancreatic ascites in children usually follows trauma or pancreatic surgery.[41] These patients may be seen with ascites or with pancreatic pleural effusions. Free fluid results from the uncontained leakage of a major pancreatic duct. Treatment initially consists of bowel rest with hyperalimentation and use of long-acting somatostatin analogues. In many cases, ascites resolves spontaneously with this treatment. If not, ERCP or MRCP should be performed to determine the site of the ductal injury.[42] For distal duct injuries, simple distal resection is adequate, but proximal duct injury requires Roux-en-Y jejunal onlay anastomosis to preserve an adequate amount of pancreatic tissue.

Pancreatic fistula is a postoperative complication. Most low-output fistulas close spontaneously but may drain for several months. Long-acting somatostatin analogues decrease the fistula output and accelerate the rate of closure, but they do not appear to induce closure of fistulas that would not have otherwise closed. Managing a pancreatic fistula centers around (1) maintaining adequate nutrition, with hyperalimentation if enteral feeding results in high-volume output, and (2) making sure the fistula tract does not become obstructed. In fistulas that do not close, surgical intervention with a Roux-en-Y jejunostomy to the leak point is recommended.[43]

Chronic Pancreatitis

Chronic pancreatitis is distinguished from acute pancreatitis by the irreversibility of the changes associated with the inflammation.[44] Chronic pancreatitis is either *calcifying* or *obstructive*. The calcifying form, most commonly caused by hereditary pancreatitis, is more common than the obstructive form in children and is associated with intraductal pancreatic stones, pseudocysts, and a more aggressive scar formation with more significant damage (Fig. 45-6). The obstructive type of chronic pancreatitis, which is associated with anatomic obstructions (most commonly pancreas divisum), is generally less severe with less scar formation than calcifying pancreatitis. The pancreatic architecture may be partially reversible with correction of the obstruction.[45]

Chronic pancreatitis is distinctly uncommon in children, and the most common cause in North America is *hereditary* or *familial pancreatitis*.[46] The inheritance is autosomal dominant with incomplete penetrance. The genetic mutations responsible for hereditary pancreatitis have been isolated to chromosome 7q35. The majority of these patients express one of two mutations in the cationic trypsinogen (*PRSS1* gene) gene. It has been suggested that these mutations lead to an alteration in the trypsin recognition site that prevents deactivation of trypsin within the pancreas. Autodigestion occurs, resulting in pancreatitis. In certain cases of idiopathic pancreatitis, it may be worthwhile to perform genetic screening for the cationic trypsinogen gene mutation.[47,48] The clinical presentation is typically one of recurrent attacks resembling acute pancreatitis. Familial pancreatitis has no distinguishing characteristics other than pancreatic calcification and its occurrence in other family members. These patients typically begin to have symptoms at about age 10 years, and pancreatic insufficiency, both exocrine and endocrine,

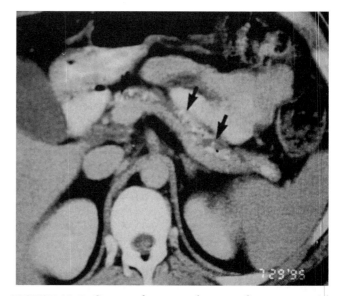

FIGURE 45-6. Computed tomography scan of a pancreas with chronic calcifying pancreatitis. A dilated duct can be seen within the pancreas, further supporting the diagnosis of chronic pancreatitis (*arrows*).

slowly develops. Other complications include diabetes mellitus, ascites with pleural effusion, portal hypertension, dilatation of the pancreatic ducts, and thrombosis of the portal and splenic vein.[17] Pseudocysts tend to occur more often in patients with hereditary pancreatitis, and such patients have a 40% lifetime risk of developing adenocarcinoma of the pancreas.[48]

In some patients with familial pancreatitis who have severe, intractable pain, ERCP may help locate surgically correctable lesions, such as large stones or a stricture with distal dilation of the duct. Surgical options in this form of pancreatitis include excision of localized pancreatitis, subtotal pancreatectomy, lateral pancreaticojejunostomy (modified Puestow procedure), and sphincteroplasty. Although the results of surgical therapy in these patients are generally disappointing, some evidence is found that complicated cases of hereditary pancreatitis treated with a modified Puestow procedure have resulted in improved quality of life with subsequent improvement in pancreatic function and nutritional status. Some reversal occurs in the steatorrhea seen in hereditary pancreatitis in children when compared with adult patients with chronic pancreatitis.[49]

Obstructive pancreatitis, which, in children, is due to pancreas divisum or choledochal cyst, is best treated by relieving the obstruction. The association between pancreas divisum and chronic pancreatitis remains controversial. Some patients with ductal dilation clearly improve with sphincterotomy or sphincteroplasty. Other cases may be difficult to diagnose, and functional tests of duct pressure after secretin stimulation have been suggested. Surgical results in patients with functional obstruction are often not satisfying.

The diagnosis of chronic pancreatitis does not depend on amylase or lipase determination. Even though mild serum enzyme elevations are commonly seen during an exacerbation, they are not consistent and frequently are normal. The diagnosis of chronic pancreatitis relies on the characteristic pain, diminished pancreatic function, and changes in radiographic appearance. Increased stool fat, diabetes mellitus, and steatorrhea are signs of pancreatic insufficiency. Frequently on CT scan, the pancreas has microcalcifications throughout the parenchyma and calcified stones in the duct (see Fig. 45-6). Additionally, pancreatic pseudocysts or inflammation may be seen on CT scan. ERCP offers the best view of ductal anatomy and can confirm the diagnosis of pancreas divisum as a probable cause of chronic pancreatitis. MRCP also is becoming more widely available and may provide a less invasive alternative to define better the pancreatic ductal anatomy.[28] Papillotomy may be done endoscopically, as well.

Therapy for chronic pancreatitis is directed toward palliation of symptoms. Initial therapy for acute exacerbation is pain control and hydration. Steatorrhea indicates the need for pancreatic enzyme replacement. In general, these patients do better with small, frequent meals. The diabetes mellitus that results from chronic pancreatitis seems to be unusually brittle, with a propensity for severe hypoglycemic episodes after even low doses of insulin. This hypersensitivity to insulin may be due to loss of entire islets. Unlike autoimmune diabetes

mellitus, in which specific destruction of the insulin-producing β-cells of the islets of Langerhans is found, in chronic pancreatitis, entire islets, including the glucagon-producing α-cells, are destroyed. The insulin-opposing effects of glucagon are thus lost in these patients.

Surgical or endoscopic therapy is indicated for bile or pancreatic duct obstruction or for pancreatic pseudocyst complications (Fig. 45-7).[50] Patients with intractable pain who do not have an identifiable anatomic problem would likely not benefit from surgical intervention. Relief of obstruction may be achieved by endoscopic sphincterotomy, ductal stenting, or open surgical drainage with Roux-en-Y lateral pancreaticojejunostomy (a modified Puestow procedure). Pancreatic resection, starting with distal resection only, but extending to subtotal or even total pancreatectomy, has been advocated for intractable pain. These patients trade sequelae of further, and perhaps complete, pancreatic insufficiency for anticipated pain relief.

Functional Pancreatic Disorders

The causes of persistent hypoglycemia in children vary greatly with age. In newborns and infants, the major causes follow.

1. Persistent hyperinsulinemic hypoglycemia of infancy (PHHI), also called nesidioblastosis
2. Lack of substrate for gluconeogenesis (e.g., glycogen storage disease)
3. Inadequate gluconeogenic hormones (e.g., hypothyroidism or growth hormone deficiency)

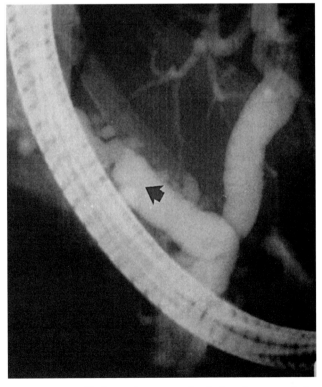

FIGURE 45-7. Endoscopic retrograde cholangiopancreatography in a patient with chronic pancreatitis with blockage of the biliary and pancreatic ducts (*arrow*) with dilation.

In children with onset of hypoglycemia beyond 1 year of age, the causes are different, with insulinoma being the most common.

Persistent Hyperinsulinemic Hypoglycemia of Infancy

Nesidioblastosis comes from the Greek *nesidio,* meaning "island," and *blast,* meaning "new formation." Nesidioblasts are thought to be progenitor cells in the wall of pancreatic ducts, normally giving rise to islets in physiologic states requiring more islets, such as during pregnancy or after pancreatic resection. It has been postulated that these nesidioblasts overproliferate in patients with PHHI. This postulate was based on what had been thought to be atypical pathology of nesidioblastosis. However, it has been shown that the proliferation of nesidioblasts in the periductular regions of the pancreas is actually a normal variant in newborns.

The defect in patients with PHHI appears to be related to four genes that are responsible for the ability of the β-cell to regulate insulin secretion through the adenosine triphosphate (ATP)-sensitive potassium channels, which normally consist of heteromultimers of the sulfonylurea receptors (SURs).[51-53] More specifically, the four genes are the sulfonylurea receptor (SUR1), the potassium channel (Kir6.2), glutamate dehydrogenase (GDH), and glucokinase (GK) located on chromosome 11p15.1.[54] PHHI patients have been found to have a truncation mutation of the second nucleotide-binding fold of the SUR1 of the ATP-sensitive potassium channel. Mutations in this receptor channel prevent the normal feedback regulation of insulin production by serum glucose. Oral hypoglycemic agents act by binding SUR and activating insulin release.

The two forms of PHHI are a focal and a diffuse type. The difference between the two types can be seen only after pathologic analysis, as both forms have the same clinical presentation. The focal type is associated with the loss of a maternal allele from chromosome 11p15, with inheritance of a paternal mutation of the SUR1 gene. It is characterized by a localized tumor-like aggregation of islets and also is referred to as *focal adenomatous islet-cell hyperplasia.* The accumulation of the large islet clusters are separated by thin rims of acinar cells or strands of connective tissue.[55] It represents about one third of the cases of PHHI. The diffuse type of PHHI represents a recessively inherited mutation of the SUR1/Kir6.2 protein that presents as a diffuse pancreatic β-cell functional abnormality. The distinction between the two forms of PHHI is important, as patients with focal PHHI may be spared the extensive pancreatic resection required in patients with diffuse PHHI.[56,57]

PHHI patients typically have hypoglycemia shortly after birth, although adult cases have been reported (probably not of the same origin).[58] Symptoms are those of hypoglycemia, with behavioral changes such as jitteriness and seizures. It is critical to measure serum insulin and glucose levels simultaneously because the absolute insulin level may be normal, but the ratio of insulin to blood glucose is not normal. These patients differ from insulin adenoma patients in that adenoma patients usually have high absolute insulin levels. In addition, the hyperinsulinemia of PHHI is more easily suppressed with somatostatin and somatostatin analogues.

Initial treatment of PHHI should be frequent feeding, or even a drip-feeding regimen, with the addition of intravenous (IV) glucose as needed. Central venous access is advised because adequate venous access is lifesaving, and high concentrations of glucose infusion may be necessary. When the glucose infusion rate necessary to prevent hypoglycemia is more than 15 mg/kg/hr, PHHI is likely. When onset occurs after the newborn period, the patients may have only intermittent hypoglycemia, and the diagnosis may be more difficult. Owing to the much higher incidence of insulin-producing adenoma, patients older than 1 year at onset of hypoglycemia should undergo evaluation, which may include exploratory laparotomy.

Initial medical treatment of PHHI should include an antisecretory drug such as diazoxide or a long-acting somatostatin analogue. Other medical therapy includes glucocorticoids to promote insulin resistance and streptozotocin (β-cell–specific toxin) to decrease the insulin-secreting population of cells. These drugs seem to be most effective treating milder cases or older children with PHHI. Medical failure to control hypoglycemia necessitates surgical resection.

In patients with diffuse-type PHHI, adequate surgical treatment consists of a 90% to 95% pancreatectomy, which entails leaving a residual remnant of pancreas on the common bile duct along the C-loop of the duodenum (Fig. 45-8).[59] It is important, especially in patients out of the newborn period, to inspect the pancreas closely for evidence of an insulin-producing adenoma, because finding an adenoma would allow significant preservation of pancreatic tissue and obviate potential endocrine and exocrine insufficiency. Postoperatively, these patients are often transiently hyperglycemic. All patients after resection of a large part of the pancreas are at significant risk for developing diabetes mellitus in later years. A 95% pancreatectomy has approximately a 75% rate of diabetes.[60] For this reason, some strategies have been suggested to attempt to

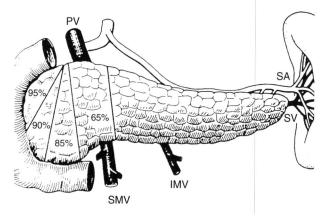

FIGURE 45-8. Various degrees of pancreatectomy may be indicated for persistent hyperinsulinemic hypoglycemia of infancy. Typically, a 95% pancreatectomy, as shown here, leaves behind a cuff of pancreas along the C-loop of the duodenum. IMV, inferior mesenteric vein; PV, portal vein; SA, splenic artery; SMV, superior mesenteric vein; SV, splenic vein.

minimize the effects of a near-total pancreatectomy, which include one of three options: a nonsurgical approach using long-term hyperalimentation, continuous gastric tube feeding, and octreotide administration; a 75% pancreatectomy with a plan for a near-total pancreatectomy in the future if symptoms persist; and a near-total pancreatectomy in all patients, with isolation of the islets from the excised pancreas, and cryopreservation for later autotransplantation to control diabetes.

Conversely, patients with focal-type PHHI may be treated with a more topographically guided pancreatic resection. The difficulty lies in distinguishing between focal and diffuse types. Recent series have shown that arterial calcium stimulation with venous sampling and transhepatic portal venous sampling can help distinguish between focal and diffuse PHHI. After a more localized exploration during laparotomy and with the addition of frozen-section analysis, the pancreatic resection may be limited to the region of involvement.[56,57] In this manner, the complications of extensive pancreatic resection can be avoided in patients with focal-type PHHI.

The long-term outlook for these patients depends primarily on the age at onset, which relates to severity of disease, and on expeditious diagnosis, because a late diagnosis results in a higher incidence of neurologic deficits.[61] Most patients seem to "grow out of the disease" after several years, implying diminished activity of the β-cells. This evolution may explain the development of diabetes mellitus in some of these patients during their school-age years.

GLYCOGEN STORAGE DISEASE

Glucose-6-phosphatase deficiency (glycogen storage disease type I) classically appears as severe hypoglycemia in newborns and infants and is caused by the inability to dephosphorylate glycogen subunits into glucose.[62] The hypoglycemia becomes apparent when feedings begin to be spaced out, requiring the liver to generate glucose from glycogen stores. Diagnosed clinically by the low insulin levels and hepatomegaly, ketosis and cutaneous xanthomas develop as a result of compensatory high lipid levels, and such patients often have fasting glucose levels less than 20 mg/dL. Central venous access is needed to allow continuous infusion of highly concentrated glucose. An increased incidence of hepatic adenoma is found in patients who survive to adulthood, with a 10% risk of malignant transformation.[63] Liver transplantation has become the treatment of choice for these patients.

PANCREATIC ENDOCRINE TUMORS

The endocrine cells of the mature human pancreas are confined to the islets of Langerhans (Fig. 45-9), although pancreatic neurons are known to secrete locally active peptide hormones such as vasoactive intestinal peptide (VIP). Four main hormones are produced by islets: insulin from the centrally located β-cells, which make up more than 90% of the islet; glucagon from the peripheral mantle of α-cells; and somatostatin and pancreatic

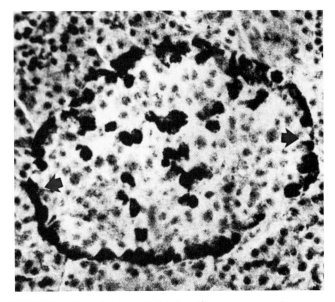

FIGURE 45-9. Mature islet in the pancreas. Immunohistochemical stain shows the peripheral location of the glucagon cells (α-cells, *arrows*). The insulin-producing cells (β-cells) are located in the central portion of the islet. (From Fawcett DW [ed]: Textbook of Histology. New York, Chapman & Hall, 1994, p 699.)

polypeptide from the δ-cells and pancreatic polypeptide (PP) cells scattered throughout. A small population of endocrine cells account for production of gastrin and other peptide hormones. Currently, it is believed that pancreatic endocrine tumors arise from cells located in the islets, although some evidence indicates that precursor cells in the pancreatic ducts or acini may give rise to these tumors as well. Only insulinoma, gastrinoma, and VIPoma are known to occur in children.

Insulinoma is the most common pancreatic endocrine tumor in children.[64] This tumor is manifest by symptoms of hypoglycemia, including dizziness, headaches, sweating, and seizures. The classic Whipple's triad was described in patients with insulinoma and consists of the following: (1) symptoms of hypoglycemia with fasting; (2) glucose level less than half of normal with fasting; and (3) relief of symptoms with glucose administration.

Patients are typically older than 4 years, although newborns have been described with insulinoma. Ninety percent of cases are benign. Lesions are usually solitary, except in multiple endocrine neoplasia (MEN) 1 syndrome, in which multiple insulinomas may be seen.

Insulinoma is diagnosed by demonstrating an insulin-to-glucose ratio of more than 1.0 (microunits of insulin per milliliter/milligrams of glucose per deciliter). Normal should be less than 0.3. Levels of insulin C-peptide should always be measured because its absence indicates exogenous administration of insulin. The distinction between benign and malignant lesions is difficult and is based on tumor size (<2 cm tend to be benign) and the presence of metastases.

Tumor localization preoperatively may be difficult.[65] Extrapancreatic insulinomas are rare, and CT scan of the pancreas with fine cuts will identify more than half of the tumors. Small hypervascular tumors may be visualized by angiographic blush, but angiography is probably not warranted with the advent of newer imaging techniques. Magnetic resonance imaging (MRI) and endoscopic US allow visualization of very small tumors. Selective portal venous sampling may help localize the tumor for blind pancreatic resections. All patients should undergo surgical resection. Tumors are pink, firm, and appear encapsulated. The tumors are usually amenable to simple enucleation. At operation, occult tumors may be localized by intraoperative US.[66] Failure to localize the tumor by any of the aforementioned techniques is unlikely, but because insulinomas tend to be located in the tail of the pancreas, distal pancreatectomy is the best "blind" procedure. Patients with MEN 1 and multiple adenomas require a 95% pancreatectomy. Malignant insulinomas require chemotherapy, usually with the β-cell–toxic drug streptozotocin.

Fetal gastrin-producing cells in the pancreas are believed to give rise to pancreatic *gastrinoma*. The pancreas is the primary source of gastrin in the fetus. After birth, the gastric antrum becomes the principal gastrin source. The Zollinger-Ellison syndrome consists of gastric hypersecretion with severe peptic ulcer disease and a gastrin-producing tumor, which classically is located in the pancreas. The pancreas is the most common site for gastrinomas, which are malignant in 65% of cases and usually produce the 17-amino-acid form of gastrin. Unlike adults, children with gastrinoma have not been reported to have MEN 1.[67,68]

The diagnosis of a gastrinoma is based on hypergastrinemia and gastric hypersecretion. Gastrin levels are usually greater than 500 pg/mL, but equivocal cases can be diagnosed by using 2 U/kg of IV secretin as a stimulation test. A gastrinoma responds with a 200 pg/mL or more increase in serum gastrin. Localization of gastrinomas can be difficult. These tumors may be outside the pancreas. CT scan, MRI, endoscopic US, and selective portal venous sampling have all been used to help localize tumors. Occult tumors have been shown most often to be located in the duodenum and may be seen only with a duodenotomy.

The medical treatment of gastrinoma is with omeprazole, the inhibitor of acid secretion that selectively blocks the ATP-dependent hydrogen-potassium proton pump necessary for acid secretion. All patients with potentially resectable disease should undergo exploration, although most pancreatic tumors are not resectable, and only patients who undergo complete resection are cured.

Non-Neoplastic Cysts

Although most cystic lesions of the pancreas are pseudocysts and acquired, *congenital cysts* may be first seen at an early age as a symptomatic mass with compression of surrounding structures.[69] Alternatively, these congenital cysts may be noted incidentally on physical examination or radiographic studies. Congenital cysts contain cloudy straw-colored fluid with normal pancreatic enzyme levels. The cysts are most often found in the distal pancreas and are amenable to local resection with a rim of normal pancreas. Lesions in the head of the pancreas should be

internally drained with Roux-en-Y cyst-jejunostomy. Congenital duplications of the intestine also may be sequestered in the pancreas. They have a gastric mucosal lining but maintain pancreatic ductal communication. The gastric acid may cause episodes of pancreatitis. The mass is usually small and is identified only on CT scan. Surgical resection is necessary, either in the form of enucleation, distal pancreatectomy, or even pancreaticoduodenectomy.

Acquired nonneoplastic cysts of the pancreas are called *retention cysts* and seem to represent ectasia of the pancreatic ducts (Fig. 45-10) . The cysts contain fluid rich in pancreatic enzymes. Preoperative distinction of a retention cyst from other types of cysts or pseudocysts may be difficult. ERCP demonstrates a communication with the ductal system and may help in determining the surgical approach (resection versus Roux-en-Y cyst-jejunostomy).

Pancreatic Exocrine Tumors

The pancreatic exocrine system consists of the pancreatic ducts, centroacinar cells, and acini. Tumors arising from this system include pseudopapillary tumor, ductal adenocarcinoma, acinar cell carcinoma, or pancreatoblastomas. Cystic tumors of the pancreas, which include serous cystadenoma, mucinous cystadenoma, and cystadenocarcinoma, are well characterized in the adult population, but although rare cases have been described in the pediatric literature, they are poorly characterized.[69] A recent review of the literature suggests that no documented case of cystadenocarcinoma has been described in children, and with one exception, the few cases of cystadenoma are dissimilar to the adult lesions. Rather, the cases of cystadenomas may represent a developmental malformation, and not neoplasms.[70]

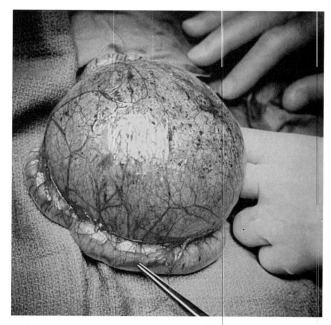

FIGURE 45-10. Large pancreatic cyst (retention cyst) emanating from the pancreatic parenchyma. The cyst was filled with clear fluid. (Courtesy of Howard B. Ginsburg, M.D.)

Adenocarcinoma/Pancreatoblastoma

In general, pancreatic cancers are rare in children. Ductal adenocarcinoma is the most common adult form of pancreatic cancer. It has been described in children; however, most of the reported cases are in the older literature. As the pancreatic tumors of childhood have become better characterized, these previous diagnoses of ductal adenocarcinoma have been questioned. Because these lesions have become rare in recent years, it appears that many of these tumors may have been previously misdiagnosed.[70] Acinar cell adenocarcinoma is more often seen in children and tends to have a less aggressive behavior with a better prognosis. Treatment is complete surgical resection for both ductal adenocarcinoma and acinar cell carcinoma.

Another variant of adenocarcinoma seen in younger children and infants has been termed *pancreatoblastoma* and represents the most common exocrine tumor of the pancreas in childhood. It is seen more often in boys than in girls and is thought to be of embryonic origin, similar to Wilms' tumor and hepatoblastoma. An allelic loss occurs on chromosome 11p, suggesting a common genetic relation between pancreatoblastoma, Beckwith-Wiedemann syndrome, and related embryonal malignancies.[71] Pancreatoblastomas are of low malignancy and often arise in the head of the pancreas (two thirds) and may represent a tumor of immature duct cells.[72,73] Even large tumors have a relatively benign course. Metastases are reported in one third of the patients, with the liver and lung being the most common sites. α-Fetoprotein (AFP) may be elevated in pancreatoblastoma and may be used to monitor patients for recurrence.[74] The prognosis is relatively good with a complete resection of the tumor. Recurrence is common, so close follow-up is mandatory.

A Frantz tumor is a papillary-cystic tumor, also referred to as solid pseudopapillary tumor (SPT), seen in girls and young women. It is derived from exocrine cells and histologically no acinar or ductal structures appear to be present. Degenerative changes result in the formation of pseudopapillae, and a fibrous capsule is usually seen.[75] SPT is less malignant than pancreatoblastoma, and metastases are rarely present. The prognosis is good even with just local resection. Although SPT is a relatively indolent tumor, at the present time, aggressive resection is advocated, given that the tumor is a curable one.[76]

SPLEEN

Other than splenic trauma, surgical diseases of the spleen are mainly limited to hematologic diseases. The role of the spleen in hematologic disease is best understood with an underlying knowledge of its anatomy and function. Important new aspects of splenic surgery include splenic preservation surgery, laparoscopic approaches to the spleen, and autotransplantation.

Embryology, Anatomy, and Physiology

The spleen develops alongside the pancreas, from mesenchyme of the dorsal pancreatic bud and the dorsal mesogastrium, and it can be recognized in week 5 of gestation.[77] Splenic mesenchyme gives rise to basement membrane–lined cords to form sinusoids (Fig. 45-11). The splenic filtration function is established at this time. In addition to the filtration function, the spleen also develops as a lymphoid organ with both B and T lymphocytes present by the end of the first trimester. Little is known about the factors controlling splenic development, although a patterning protein, hox11 of the homeodomain protein family, has been shown to be necessary for splenic development, because hox11 knock-out mice are born without a spleen.

At birth, the formed spleen contains primarily lymphocytes, with aggregations of T cells, phagocytic cells of the reticuloendothelial system, and B cells in follicles. This lymphoid aggregation (white pulp) surrounds the feeding arterioles of the spleen and is thought to function as an immune screening area to detect and process foreign antigen and antigen-antibody complexes. The red pulp, so named because a slow flow of blood occurs through sinusoids, which are functionally distal to the white pulp, acts as a phagocytic filtration system, digesting old or defective blood elements including spherocytes and elliptocytes, complexed foreign material and cells, and bacteria, both with and without bound specific antigens (Fig. 45-12). Of importance is that encapsulated bacteria in the bloodstream can be removed by the spleen only for reasons of variable antigenicity. The spleen also functions until approximately age 1 to 2 months as a site for extramedullary hematopoiesis.[78]

Important anatomic aspects of the spleen include the ligaments, the splenic artery, and the segmental anatomy of the splenic parenchyma (Fig. 45-13). The major suspensory ligaments are the gastrosplenic and splenorenal ligaments. Laxity of these and other minor ligaments contributes to a poorly fixed, or wandering, spleen. Division of the splenorenal ligament is necessary to mobilize the spleen from the left upper quadrant. The splenic artery

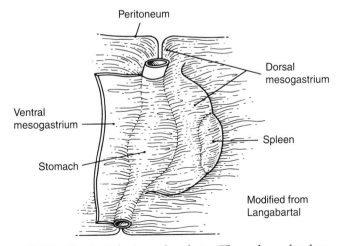

FIGURE 45-11. Splenic embryology. The spleen develops within the dorsal mesogastrium as it folds during gut rotation. (From Skandalakis LJ, Gray SW, Ricketts R, et al: The spleen. In Skandalakis JE, Gray SW [eds]: Embryology for Surgeons. Baltimore, Williams & Wilkins, 1994, p 336.)

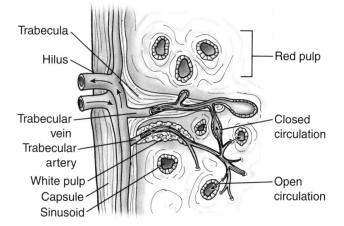

FIGURE 45-12. Schematic of blood flowing through the spleen. As blood flows through the arteries, acellular plasma is filtered off through the white pulp peripherally, leaving closely packed red blood cells in the red pulp, where red cells can then be phagocytosed by the reticuloendothelial system if they are tagged with bound antibody. (From Fraker DL: The Spleen. In Greenfield LJ, Mulholland MW, Oldham KT [eds]: Surgery: Scientific Principles and Practice, 3rd ed. Philadelphia, Lippincott Williams & Wilkins, 2001, p 1240.)

arises from the celiac axis and takes a tortuous and variable course to the splenic hilum. It can usually be accessed through the lesser omental sac, either above or below the pancreas. Splenic collaterals allow splenic artery ligation in the lesser sac without splenic infarct. The splenic artery divides into upper and lower pole arteries, defining surgical segments. The segmental blood supply facilitates partial splenectomy.[79]

Asplenia and Polysplenia

Congenital asplenia is often associated with cardiac defects, as well as other anomalies of symmetry, such as a midline liver (heterotaxy syndrome).[80,81] The anatomy in these patients is best understood as the body having two right halves instead of a left half and a right half. These patients often have severe anomalies of cardiac looping, frequently with single-ventricle anatomy. The cardiac condition is the most significant, but such an evaluation reveals evidence of asplenia such as Howell-Jolly bodies in the erythrocytes. Patients should be placed on asplenia prophylaxis (as discussed later) as soon as the diagnosis is made.

By contrast, the polysplenia syndrome may result from having two left halves of the body. The multiple spleens tend to be located along the greater curvature of the stomach. The associated cardiac anomalies are less severe than those associated with the asplenia syndrome. The prognosis is usually dependent on the complexity of the cardiac abnormalities. In general, asplenia carries a worse prognosis than polysplenia. One of the ways to differentiate between asplenia and polysplenia in the prenatal period is the use of gray-scale US. Unfortunately, in the heterotaxia syndrome, the anatomic distortion makes identifying the spleen rather difficult (Fig. 45-14). Color Doppler US may provide a better method to identify the splenic artery, so that more information can be gathered to improve prenatal counseling and management of affected patients.[82]

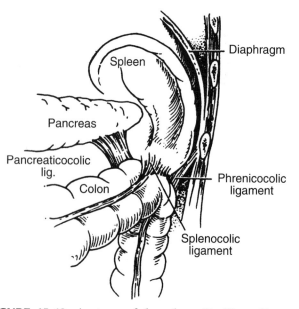

FIGURE 45-13. Anatomy of the spleen. Significant ligamentous attachments are to the diaphragm, left kidney, colon, and pancreas. (From Skandalakis PN, Colborn GL, Skandalakis LJ, et al: The surgical anatomy of the spleen. Surg Clin North Am 73:759, 1993.)

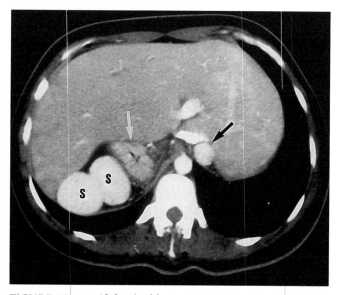

FIGURE 45-14. Abdominal heterotaxia in a patient with polysplenia syndrome. Note two round splenules (S) in the right upper quadrant. In addition, the inferior vena cava (*black arrow*) is on the left of the aorta, and the stomach (*white arrow*) is on the right. (From Gayer G, Zissin R, Apter S, et al: CT findings in congenital anomalies of the spleen, Br J Radiol 74:767–772, 2001.)

Accessory Spleen

Accessory spleens exist as small splenic nodules and are present in approximately 20% of the population. They are usually found in the splenic hilum, along the stomach, in the omentum, and adjacent to the pancreas, reflecting the embryonic origin of the spleen (Fig. 45-15).[83] These nodules often resemble lymph nodes but may grow rapidly if left behind after splenectomy done for hematologic disease. This "compensatory hypertrophy" appears to be due to a factor in the blood that induces splenic growth and allows recurrence of the hematologic disorder that prompted the splenectomy. Accessory spleens are usually about 1 cm in diameter, but can be as large as 3 cm. A CT scan before a planned splenectomy may demonstrate an accessory spleen, which typically mimics a lymph node. Technetium sulfur colloid radionuclide imaging may help identify an accessory spleen if it is larger than 2 cm in diameter.[84]

Splenogonadal Fusion

Rarely, the splenic anlage fuses with the gonadal ridge in the developing embryo.[85] As a result, mature splenic tissue may be found attached to either testicle or ovary (Fig. 45-16). A fibrous cord, which may have a chain of small pieces of spleen (splenic rosary bead sign), may connect the ectopic fused spleen-gonad with the normal spleen. Splenogonadal fusion is often found associated with limb or anorectal anomalies, suggesting a global embryonic event occurring between the 5th and 8th weeks of embryogenesis. Three described types of splenogonadal fusion exist: a continuous, a discontinuous, and a combined form. In the continuous form, the spleen is connected to the left gonadal mesonephric structures by a continuous cord, which typically arises from the upper pole of the spleen. The cord may be made up completely of splenic or fibrous tissue or may contain intermittent nodules of splenic tissue along its course. The discontinuous type consists of discrete masses of aberrant heterotopic splenic tissue that are found fused to these same structures. The combined type is one in which clearly an extension of functioning splenic tissue extends from the orthotopic spleen down into the abdomen, although no actual connection to the ectopic spleen is found near the gonad.[86] Boys with splenogonadal fusion typically have an undescended testicle or a presumed hernia. In many cases, an unnecessary orchiectomy has been performed because the surgeon erroneously thought that the tissue represented a tumor. A high index of suspicion is needed to investigate this diagnosis before undergoing surgery. Usually the splenic tissue can safely be dissected off the testicle or ovary.

Wandering Spleen

Laxity of the splenic ligaments allows the spleen to be located anywhere in the peritoneal cavity, including the pelvis.[87,88] The splenic pedicle may be quite long, predisposing the spleen to torsion (Fig. 45-17). Full torsion may result in splenic infarction, whereas lesser degrees of twisting may produce chronic intermittent abdominal pain from ischemia. Imaging studies may suggest the absence of the spleen in the left upper quadrant and perhaps a spleenlike mass elsewhere. Splenectomy is required for a necrotic spleen, and fixation, for the viable spleen. Splenopexy in the left upper quadrant is possible by using an absorbable mesh to avoid placing sutures through the splenic parenchyma.

Cystic Lesions

Peliosis in Greek means "leaking blood" and refers to blood-filled lakes in the parenchyma of organs. These lesions occur in the spleen, usually in association with peliosis of the liver.[89] The blood-filled lakes have an endothelial lining and vary in size from 1 to 10 cm. Peliosis is of unknown origin but is often associated with steroid use or chemotherapy. The major clinical significance of peliosis is its potential to rupture either with or without trauma, which can be fatal. Treatment of incidentally discovered peliosis must be determined by the surgeon at the time of discovery.

Benign Cysts

Benign cysts are rare and usually remain asymptomatic. Cysts may be unilocular or multilocular and are of variable origin. The most common forms of cyst are congenital,

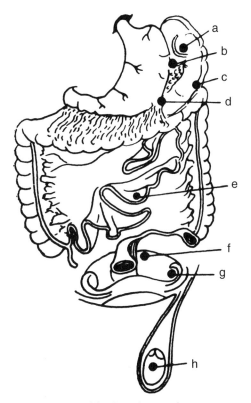

FIGURE 45-15. Possible locations of accessory spleens. Potential locations include (a) hilus of the spleen, (b) along the splenic vessels, (c) splenocolic ligament, (d) greater omentum, (e) small bowel mesentery, (f) pelvic wall, (g) adnexal region, and (h) left paratesticular region. (From Rudowski WJ: Accessory spleen: Clinical significance with particular reference to the recurrence of idiopathic thrombocytopenic purpura. World J Surg 9:422–430, 1985.)

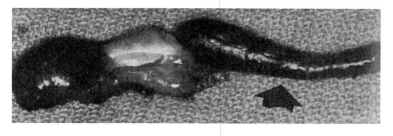

FIGURE 45-16. Splenogonadal fusion to the testicle. As evidenced here, orchiectomy is often mistakenly performed for suspicion of malignancy. The splenic tissue is to the right (*arrow*). (From Balaji KC, Caldamore AA, Rabinowitz R, et al: Splenogonadal fusion. J Urol 156:854, 1996.)

parasitic, or post-traumatic. The congenital cyst is usually unilocular and filled with clear fluid that may contain cholesterol crystals. The lining of these congenital cysts may be squamous (epidermoid) or endothelial. Parasitic cysts are typically echinococcal (hydatid) cysts. Post-traumatic cysts result from slow liquefaction of a hematoma, have a fibrous lining, and contain cloudy brown fluid. Cysts are often asymptomatic, but they may present as a mass in the left upper quadrant, sometimes with pain. Treatment is indicated for symptomatic cysts. Simple aspiration of the cysts does not prevent reaccumulation of the fluid. Aspiration and injection with antibiotics (tetracycline) or pure alcohol has been reported with limited success in the literature, with most patients having a recurrence. This may be adequate therapy for smaller epidermoid splenic cysts.[90] Resection either by partial splenectomy, if feasible, or by total splenectomy is appropriate definitive therapy.[91] Echinococcal cysts should be handled carefully, similar to hepatic hydatid disease, and if any question occurs about risk of rupture, total splenectomy should be performed.

Splenic Tumors

All forms of splenic tumors, other than metastases to the spleen, are rare. Hemangioma is the most common benign tumor, with splenectomy frequently being necessary for large, symptomatic, or bleeding tumors.[92,93]

Splenic Abscess

Splenic abscess is relatively rare in children. It may occur as a secondarily infected hematoma, pseudocyst, or developmental cyst. A splenic infarct resulting from a hemoglobinopathy may also become secondarily infected. Immunosuppression puts patients at risk for developing a splenic abscess from seeding during bacteremia, thus causing multiple or miliary abscesses.[94] Splenic abscess patients typically are toxic with bacteremia, fever, and left upper quadrant pleuritic pain. CT scan is usually diagnostic.

Solitary unilocular abscesses may respond well to percutaneous drainage, which also allows identification of the organism and appropriate antibiotic selection. Multiple or loculated abscesses may respond to antibiotics alone. Empirical antibiotic therapy should be started based on a presumptive diagnosis, given the clinical setting. Immunosuppressed patients with multiple abscesses and negative blood cultures likely have a fungal infection. *Salmonella* species are most common in patients with hemoglobinopathy and splenic infarct. In post-traumatic infection, *Staphylococcus* and *Streptococcus*

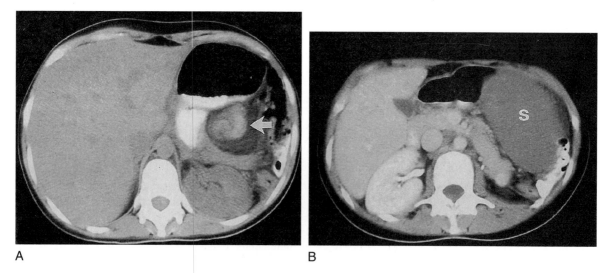

A   B

FIGURE 45-17. Torsion of a wandering spleen. *A,* Precontrast image in which the spleen is absent, although splenic vessels (arrow) are seen in the left upper abdomen and have a whorled appearance with a hyperdense center. This demonstrates a twisted splenic pedicle with fresh thrombus in the splenic vessels. *B,* A postcontrast image displays the spleen (S) seen in the left mid abdomen without enhancement, suggesting torsion. (From Gayer G, Zissin R, Apter S, et al: CT findings in congenital anomalies of the spleen. Br J Radiol 74:767–772, 2001.)

are most common. In general, failure to respond to antibiotics with or without percutaneous drainage necessitates splenectomy.

Functional Abnormalities

Hypersplenism is defined as inappropriate sequestration of blood elements. Hypersplenism may be primary or secondary. Secondary hypersplenism is often associated with splenomegaly with simple mechanical sequestration of erythrocytes, platelets, and neutrophils. The most common cause of secondary hypersplenism in children is portal hypertension, although any cause of splenomegaly can lead to hypersplenism. Either splenic artery embolization or splenic artery ligation is adequate therapy, although splenectomy is occasionally necessary. Few sequelae appear to ensue from the thrombocytopenia and neutropenia that result from this form of hypersplenism. Primary hypersplenism is not a result of splenomegaly or other indirect cause. Hereditary spherocytosis (HS), hereditary elliptocytosis, and idiopathic thrombocytopenic purpura are examples of primary hypersplenism and are discussed later. Paradoxically, because the spleen can be a site of extramedullary hematopoiesis in the disease states that produce primary hypersplenism, removal of the spleen may be detrimental.

Hyposplenism is detected by the presence of Howell-Jolly bodies in erythrocytes and increased susceptibility to infection with encapsulated organisms. Surgical splenectomy, sickle cell disease with splenic involution, or ulcerative colitis all lead to hyposplenism. Diseases in which splenic parenchymal replacement is found, such as sarcoidosis or Gaucher's disease, may also lead to hyposplenism. The significance of hyposplenism is the risk of postsplenectomy sepsis.

Hereditary Spherocytosis

Hereditary spherocytosis (HS), or congenital hemolytic jaundice, is usually an autosomal dominant hereditary lesion, particularly common in patients of north European descent. HS is thought to be due to a deficiency of the cytoskeletal protein spectrin.[95] Spectrin deficiency allows the erythrocytes to be spheric. HS also may be sporadic or autosomal recessive. Sentinel cases in a family usually present with jaundice, anemia, and splenomegaly. Indirect hyperbilirubinemia may be seen in infants, whereas splenomegaly only may occur very late. Without treatment in these patients, pigmented gallstones may develop, and they may have acute aplastic and hemolytic crises precipitated by infections.

Owing to the abnormal shape of the erythrocytes, they are prematurely sequestered in the spleen, probably because the spheric shape prevents the normal flexibility necessary to maneuver through the cords and sinuses of the spleen.

The diagnosis of hereditary spherocytosis should be sought in patients with anemia, jaundice, or splenomegaly. The blood smear shows small spherical erythrocytes. The diagnosis is established by demonstrating increased osmotic fragility of the erythrocytes when

exposed to elevated sodium concentrations. Patients suspected of having HS should also undergo Coombs testing to rule out immune causes of hemolytic anemia.

Owing to the frequency of pigmented gallstones, a routine US should be performed in all patients older than 10 years in whom a splenectomy is planned. For younger children, given the much lower incidence of stones, palpation of the gallbladder may be adequate. If gallstones are encountered, simultaneous cholecystectomy and splenectomy should be performed. If laparoscopic splenectomy is performed, preoperative US of the gallbladder should be performed because "palpation" for stones is unreliable. The risk of postsplenectomy sepsis is high in young children, so the current recommendation is to wait, if possible, until patients are at least 5 to 6 years old before splenectomy. Patients with severe anemia may need earlier intervention, however. Some HS patients do not have the autosomal dominant type and may not respond to splenectomy. These patients often have persistent episodes of anemia postoperatively. Conversely, older patients with mild anemia may not warrant splenectomy.[96]

The spleen of HS patients may be large but not technically difficult to remove, and it may be removed laparoscopically. Patients should receive pneumococcal vaccine 2 weeks preoperatively and postoperative prophylactic antibiotics. After splenectomy, the anemia is usually cured, and these patients generally feel better and have a normal life span. Patients with autosomal recessive disease may continue to require transfusions. Pigmented gallstones may develop postoperatively, although not often enough to warrant prophylactic cholecystectomy. Anemia also may recur because of hypertrophy of residual accessory spleens; therefore attempts to remove all accessory spleens should be made.

Partial splenectomy has been performed in young children with hereditary spherocytosis to preserve the immune function of the spleen while reducing the requirements for blood transfusion. However, long-term follow-up demonstrates a regrowth of the splenic remnant in children with chronic hemolysis with hypersplenism and appears to have only short-term benefit. In this situation, a second operation may be required to complete the splenectomy. For this reason, this approach should be used in selected cases only, where the benefit of postponing a total splenectomy is desired.[97]

The Spleen in Sickle Cell Disease

Patients with homozygous hemoglobin S (sickle cell disease) are prone to splenic sequestration.[98-100] As the cells pass through the spleen with its naturally hypoxic and acidotic environment, the erythrocytes sickle and are sequestered in the spleen. Often, the spleen in these patients becomes large initially, but with progressive infarction, it slowly atrophies, leading to functional autosplenectomy after approximately 10 years. In some cases, however, the spleen may persist even into adulthood.

The most common indication for splenectomy in sickle cell patients is acute splenic sequestration crisis (ASSC), in which severe anemia with splenomegaly develops with associated hypersplenism and thrombocytopenia. ASSC may be so severe that it causes circulatory collapse and death. Even though it is relatively rare, ASSC is the leading cause of death in sickle cell patients younger than 10 years. Patients with severe attacks of ASSC should undergo splenectomy when they have recovered from the attack, because a 40% to 50% risk of recurrence is found, with a 20% mortality rate. Patients with less severe cases of ASSC should probably undergo splenectomy after two ASSC episodes.

Hypersplenism as a result of splenomegaly develops in many patients with sickle cell disease. Transfusion requirements dictate the need for splenectomy because these patients are at high risk for transfusion complications. However, preoperative transfusions may be required to improve anemia and to reduce the hemoglobin S level to less than 30%, to avoid bleeding complications of a laparotomy.[101] Partial or subtotal splenectomy has been advocated in these patients because the risk of postsplenectomy sepsis is high in sickle cell disease. This fact is particularly important in children younger than 4 years, because they are more susceptible to postsplenectomy sepsis.[102] All of these patients should receive pneumococcal vaccine preoperatively and prophylactic antibiotics postoperatively.

Idiopathic Thrombocytopenic Purpura

As the name implies, the etiology of idiopathic thrombocytopenic purpura (ITP) is unknown. Clearly it is mediated, in the chronic form of ITP, through autoimmune binding of immunoglobulin G (IgG) specifically to a "platelet-associated antigen." Binding of autoantibody leads to reticuloendothelial platelet phagocytosis in the spleen. More than 80% of patients have *acute ITP*, a self-limited form of the disease that is treated conservatively with restricted activity, corticosteroids, and IV gamma globulin. Medical therapy is appropriate for patients whose platelet count is less than 40,000/mm^3 or in older children who are at higher risk for intracranial hemorrhage. Acute ITP occurs most frequently in children younger than 10 years after an acute viral illness. Presenting symptoms are related to thrombocytopenia: petechiae, ecchymoses, oral or rectal bleeding, and rarely intracranial bleeding. Hepatosplenomegaly or lymphadenopathy should prompt bone marrow sampling to exclude malignancy or bone marrow dysfunction as a cause of the thrombocytopenia.

Systemic steroids quickly improve the platelet count in more than 75% of these patients, although the effects do not treat the underlying cause of the disease and do not change the ultimate course of the disease. Steroids work by inhibiting phagocytosis of the platelets and by increasing platelet production. IV gamma globulin is thought to bind to the Fc receptor of the reticuloendothelial cells in the spleen, thereby also blocking phagocytosis. This therapy is usually given either in cases refractory to steroids or in actively bleeding patients. Although splenectomy is usually performed only in patients with chronic ITP, rare cases of acute ITP with severe bleeding complications (especially intracranial bleeding) may require emergency splenectomy.

In 10% to 20% of patients with ITP, the thrombocytopenia persists for more than 6 months. These patients are thought to have *chronic ITP*.[103] These patients require bone marrow sampling and immunologic evaluation to rule out other causes of thrombocytopenia, because ITP is a diagnosis of exclusion. Like the acute form, chronic ITP is usually treated with steroids and IV gamma globulin, but the risk and cost of these drugs used in these cases must be weighed over a long period of treatment. For this reason, other drugs and treatment modalities are under investigation, including plasmapheresis, erythrocytes with prebound IgG to attach to the Fc receptor, and cytotoxic agents.

In general, splenectomy is more commonly performed in chronic ITP than in acute ITP. Patients who demonstrate a good to excellent response to treatment with immune globulin are expected to benefit from splenectomy; however, a poor response does not necessarily predict a poor outcome after splenectomy.[104] Approximately 20% of chronic ITP patients require splenectomy, usually owing to medical failures. A careful intraoperative search for accessory spleens is critical to avoid long-term recurrences.[105] Although splenectomy cures 65% to 90% of patients with ITP, accessory spleens are found in 12% to 43% of postsplenectomy patients who have recurrences. Of the patients with recurrences, two thirds have complete remission after accessory splenectomy. As many as 10 accessory spleens have been found in a single patient, and therefore a thorough search must be completed during laparotomy or laparoscopy. In difficult cases, intraoperative scintigraphy with technetium 99–labeled red blood cells may aid in localizing these lesions.[106]

Thalassemia

The genetic hemoglobinopathies known as *thalassemia* may be of major (homozygous), minor (heterozygous), or intermediate form. In the more severe forms, diffuse deposition of iron occurs in the spleen, compounded by engorgement with destroyed red blood cells. Hypersplenism results in more erythrocyte sequestration, and transfusion requirements may escalate. These patients may benefit from splenectomy. Partial splenectomy has a particular attraction in thalassemia because postsplenectomy sepsis occurs in more than 10% of patients who have splenectomy for this disease.[107] Partial splenic embolization also has been described in treating patients with thalassemia major, but this technique usually requires repeat procedures to achieve success, and the potential complications of splenic infarction, hematoma, and abscess formation are significant. In addition, embolization may not be possible in young children, who are at greatest risk for developing postsplenectomy sepsis because of their small-sized vessels.

Partial dearterialization of the spleen may prove to be an alternative therapy to splenectomy or embolization. Ligation of the arterial blood supply to the spleen is performed while maintaining blood supply to the superior pole. All splenic veins are left intact. This procedure may be beneficial in a selected group of patients who have hypersplenism and have mild to moderate splenomegaly.

However, recurrence of hypersplenism or the development of splenic infection may require total splenectomy.[108]

Leukemias and Lymphomas

The spleen is often involved with leukemic infiltrates or lymphoma.[109,110] In non-Hodgkin's lymphoma, including small cell and large cell lymphomas, splenic involvement may lead to splenomegaly without hypersplenism. Splenectomy is not indicated in these patients. In Hodgkin's disease, the spleen may become involved with malignant cells, although rarely as a primary site. Splenomegaly may occur in Hodgkin's disease when the spleen is infiltrated with tumor, but splenectomy plays no role in the therapy of Hodgkin's disease (see Chapter 69).

Staging laparotomy for Hodgkin's disease is now considered unnecessary. The original rationale for staging laparotomy was to determine whether patients had disease on both sides of the diaphragm, therefore increasing the clinical stage from II to III. This upstaging from stage II to III meant that patients would then receive chemotherapy. Chemotherapy has come to be used in all stages of Hodgkin's disease to reduce the dose of radiation therapy. In addition, staging by CT scan or MRI is becoming much more precise. For these reasons, staging laparotomy/splenectomy is no longer performed.

Chronic myelogenous leukemia is characterized by myeloid metaplasia, often leading to massive splenomegaly. In these patients, splenectomy has been performed for palliation of pain, mass-related symptoms, and secondary hypersplenism. In acute myelogenous leukemia and acute lymphoblastic leukemia, splenomegaly is less dramatic, and splenectomy is rarely of benefit. Splenectomy may be detrimental in some cases because the spleen has become an important site for extramedullary hematopoiesis.

Storage Diseases

Storage diseases result from the inability to dispose properly of cell-breakdown products. Many of these diseases result in liver or splenic enlargement and are often incurable, with death resulting from central nervous system involvement (e.g., Niemann-Pick type 1 and mucopolysaccharidoses). Gaucher's disease is an indolent defect of the enzyme glucocerebrosidase, which results in the accumulation of glucosylceramide. Massive splenomegaly develops in these patients and may cause hypersplenism. Owing to its indolent course, splenectomy may offer considerable symptomatic relief and improvement of formed elements in the blood. Partial splenectomy may temporize symptoms, but recurrence is the rule.[111,112]

Splenosis

Fragmentation of the spleen from trauma has been noted on occasion to result in *splenosis*, the growth of splenic tissue within the abdominal cavity. This observation led to the intentional implantation of small fragments of splenic tissue into the peritoneal cavity and omentum to try to avoid postsplenectomy sepsis. The function of these implants is questionable because 50% of the original splenic mass seems to be necessary for normal splenic function. These implants do not clear encapsulated bacteria, as does the normal spleen, although the implants histologically appear normal. Splenosis should be treated with antibiotics in the same way as is asplenia.[113,114]

Splenectomy

The operative approach to splenectomy has recently become more varied. The options, other than open, total splenectomy, include partial splenectomy, splenic embolization, splenorrhaphy, and laparoscopic splenectomy.[115-118] The traditional open splenectomy may be performed with the patient in the supine or decubitus position with transverse or left subcostal incision. For simultaneous cholecystectomy, a vertical or extended transverse incision is used. The spleen is usually first mobilized by dividing the short gastric vessels and the posterior attachments to the diaphragm. In cases of marked splenomegaly, the gastrocolic ligament can be opened laterally to allow exposure of the splenic artery along the superior aspect of the pancreas. The splenic artery can be ligated in continuity there to decrease the potential blood loss of mobilizing the large spleen.

After fully mobilizing the spleen by further detaching it from the left kidney, the spleen can then usually be brought up into the wound, allowing safe and simple division of the major hilar splenic vessels. Care must be taken to avoid damage to the tail of the pancreas, which may extend to the hilum of the spleen. Once the spleen is removed, the splenic bed should be carefully examined for persistent bleeding. Usually a nasogastric tube is left in for gastric decompression. It has been reported that gastric distention may lead to ties slipping off the short gastric vessels after gastric distention, with subsequent exsanguinating hemorrhage. Suture ligature of the gastric end of these vessels is advised.

In patients with hemolytic anemia or ITP, and in certain cases of hypersplenism, it is critical to locate and remove any accessory spleens. Accessory spleens may often be found in the splenic hilum, lesser sac, or omentum.

Partial splenectomy and splenorrhaphy of the traumatized spleen represent surgical alternatives to total splenectomy. These procedures rely on the ability to place mattress sutures in the spleen or to place an absorbable mesh around the spleen for hemostasis. The segmental vascular anatomy of the spleen allows partial splenectomy along lines of demarcation, which follow segmental vessel ligation. These splenic salvage procedures are justified for the prevention of postsplenectomy sepsis. In trauma surgery, the advantages of splenic salvage must be weighed against the risk of bleeding and surgical delay. Splenic embolization has been used, particularly in cases of hypersplenism associated with portal hypertension, in which total splenectomy is not necessary and open surgery is relatively dangerous because of enlarged portal vein collaterals. These procedures should ablate 80% to 90% of the spleen to be effective.

Laparoscopic splenectomy has become more accepted with advanced laparoscopic technical equipment, including reloadable vascular laparoscopic staples, the harmonic scalpel, and laparoscopic tissue morcellization.[119]

Concomitant cholecystectomy can usually be added without difficulty. The technique uses four or five ports. The splenic hilar and short gastric vessels are stapled, and the spleen is placed into a nylon bag to allow morcellization without spillage. This technique requires significantly more operative time than open splenectomy. Adequate removal of accessory spleens and removal of large spleens may limit use of this technique.

Postsplenectomy Sepsis

The most feared complication of splenectomy is postsplenectomy sepsis (sometimes called overwhelming postsplenectomy infection).[120] Sepsis may occur within days, but usually occurs within 2 years of the splenectomy if it is going to occur at all. The risk of infection is increased in patients younger than 5 years, with a much higher incidence in patients undergoing splenectomy for hematologic disease. Specifically, the incidence of overwhelming postsplenectomy infection after splenectomy performed for thalassemia may be more than 10%, whereas for trauma, it is 1% to 2%. Considering all splenectomy patients, the incidence is 4%, with a mortality rate approaching 50%.[121] However, it has been suggested that with routine use of preoperative vaccinations and prophylactic antibiotics, the incidence of infection has decreased by 47%, whereas the mortality rate is reduced by as much as 88%, when compared with historical controls in which no prophylaxis was administered.[122] The infections are typically fulminant and are most often caused by encapsulated organisms, pneumococci, *Haemophilus influenzae* B, gonococci, and *Escherichia coli*. These fulminant infections often cause meningitis and adrenal infarction with hemorrhage. The encapsulated organisms have a pathologic advantage in splenectomized patients because the circulating antibodies to these bacteria are produced in the spleen.[123]

Total splenectomy should always be avoided, if possible, but especially in patients younger than 2 years, owing to the markedly increased risk of postsplenectomy sepsis in this age group. If the splenectomy is elective, the polyvalent pneumococcal and *H. influenzae* B vaccines should be given preoperatively. In all patients undergoing splenectomy, even those with previous vaccinations or attempted autotransplantation, postoperative prophylactic antibiotics should be given, as previously mentioned. Furthermore, recent literature recommends a booster every 5 to 10 years for proper protection.[122] Penicillin is the prophylactic antibiotic most often used. The recommended length of treatment varies between 2 years and a lifetime, although the risk of postsplenectomy sepsis declines greatly 2 years after the splenectomy.[124]

REFERENCES

1. Lee PC: Human Gastrointestinal Development. New York, Raven Press, 1989, p 651.
2. Dawson W, Langman J: An anatomical-radiological study on the pancreatic duct pattern in man. Anat Rec 139:59–68, 1961.
3. Gittes GK, Rutter WJ: Onset of cell-specific gene expression in the developing mouse pancreas. Proc Natl Acad Sci U S A 89:1128–1132, 1992.
4. Bertelli E, Di Gregorio F, Bertelli L, et al: The arterial blood supply of the pancreas: A review, I:. The superior pancreaticoduodenal and the anterior superior pancreaticoduodenal arteries: An anatomical and radiological study. Surg Radiol Anat 17:97–106, 101–103, 1995.
5. Nakajima H, Kambayashi M, Okubo H, et al: Annular pancreas accompanied by an ectopic pancreas in the adult: A case report. Endoscopy 27:713, 1995.
6. Ozcan C, Celik A, Guclu C, et al: A rare cause of gastric outlet obstruction in the newborn: Pyloric ectopic pancreas. J Pediatr Surg 37:119–120, 2002.
7. Kim SK, Melton DA: Pancreas development is promoted by cyclopamine, a hedgehog signaling inhibitor. Proc Natl Acad Sci U S A 95:13036–13041, 1998.
8. Hebrok M, Kim SK, St Jacques B, et al: Regulation of pancreas development by hedgehog signaling. Development 127:4905–4913, 2000.
9. Brambs HJ: [Developmental anomalies and congenital diseases of the pancreas]. Radiologe 36:381–388, 1996.
10. Skandalakis JE, Gray SW, Ricketts R, et al: The Pancreas. In Skandalakis JE, Gray SW (eds): Embryology for Surgeons, 2nd ed. Baltimore, Williams & Wilkins, 1994, p 381.
11. Sencan A, Mir E, Gunsar C, et al: Symptomatic annular pancreas in newborns. Med Sci Monit 8:CR434–437, 2002.
12. Berrocal T, Torres I, Gutierrez J, et al: Congenital anomalies of the upper gastrointestinal tract. Radiographics 19:855–872, 1999.
13. Naruse S, Kitagawa M, Ishiguro H, et al: Cystic fibrosis and related diseases of the pancreas. Best Pract Res Clin Gastroenterol 16:511–526, 2002.
14. Taylor CJ, Aswani N: The pancreas in cystic fibrosis. Paediatr Respir Rev 3:77–81, 2002.
15. Stimee B, Korneti V, Milosavljevit T, et al: Ductal morphometry of ventral pancreas in pancreas divisum: Comparison between clinical and anatomical results. Ital J Gastroenterol 28:76–80, 1996.
16. Neblett WW III, O'Neill JA Jr: Surgical management of recurrent pancreatitis in children with pancreas divisum. Ann Surg 231:899–908, 2000.
17. Lerner A, Branski D, Lebenthal E: Pancreatic diseases in children. Pediatr Clin North Am 43:125–156, 1996.
18. Pescador R, Manso MA, Rebollo AJ, et al: Effect of chronic administration of hydrocortisone on the induction and evolution of acute pancreatitis induced by cerulein. Pancreas 11:165–172, 1995.
19. Evans RJ, Miranda RN, Jordan J, et al: Fatal acute pancreatitis caused by valproic acid. Am J Forensic Med Pathol 16:62–65, 1995.
20. Weizman Z: An update on diseases of the pancreas in children. Curr Opin Pediatr 9:494–497, 1997.
21. Beger HG, Rau B, Mayer J, et al: Natural course of acute pancreatitis. World J Surg 21:130–135, 1997.
22. Waldemar H, Buchler U, Buchler MW: Classification and severity staging of acute pancreatitis. Ann Ital Chir 66:171–179, 1995.
23. Levitt MD, Eckfeldt JH: The Pancreas, 2nd ed. New York, Raven Press, 1993, p 613.
24. Sternby B, O'Brien JF, Zinsmeister AR, et al: What is the best biochemical test to diagnose acute pancreatitis? A prospective clinical study. Mayo Clin Proc 71:1138–1144, 1996.
25. Panzironi G, Franceschini L, Angelini P, et al: [Role of ultrasonography in the study of patients with acute pancreatitis]. G Chir 18:47–50, 1997.
26. Fujiwara T, Takehara Y, Ichijo K, et al: Anterior extension of acute pancreatitis: CT findings. J Comput Assist Tomogr 19:963–966, 1995.
27. Prasil P, Laberge JM, Barkun A, et al: Endoscopic retrograde cholangiopancreatography in children: A surgeon's perspective. J Pediatr Surg 36:733–735, 2001.
28. Arcement CM, Meza MP, Arumanla S, et al: MRCP in the evaluation of pancreaticobiliary disease in children. Pediatr Radiol 31:92–97, 2001.
29. Ihse I, Andersson R, Andren-Sandberg A, et al: Conservative treatment in acute pancreatitis. Ann Ital Chir 66:181–185, 1995.
30. Kaufmann P, Hofmann G, Smolle KH, et al: Intensive care management of acute pancreatitis: Recognition of patients at high risk of developing severe or fatal complications. Wien Klin Wochenschr 108:9–15, 1996.

31. Paran H, Neufeld D, Mayo A, et al: Preliminary report of a prospective randomized study of octreotide in the treatment of severe acute pancreatitis. J Am Coll Surg 181:121–124, 1995.

32. Hwang TL, Chiu CT, Chen HM, et al: Surgical results for severe acute pancreatitis: Comparison of the different surgical procedures. Hepatogastroenterology 42:1026–1029, 1995.

33. Beger HG, Rau B: Necrosectomy and postoperative local lavage in necrotizing pancreatitis. Ann Ital Chir 66:209–215, 1995.

34. Wilson C: Management of the later complications of severe acute pancreatitis: Pseudocyst, abscess and fistula. Eur J Gastroenterol Hepatol 9:117–121, 1997.

35. Bittner R: Clinical significance and management of pancreatic abscess and infected necrosis complicating acute pancreatitis. Ann Ital Chir 66:217–222, 1995.

36. Kisra M, Ettayebi F, Benhammou M: Pseudocysts of the pancreas in children in Morocco. J Pediatr Surg 34:1327–1329, 1999.

37. Bosman-Vermeeren JM, Veereman-Wauters G, Broos P, et al: Somatostatin in the treatment of a pancreatic pseudocyst in a child. J Pediatr Gastroenterol Nutr 23:422–425, 1996.

38. Sharma SS: Endoscopic cystogastrostomy: preliminary experience. Indian J Gastroenterol 14:11–12, 1995.

39. Patty I, Kalaoui M, Al-Shamali M, et al: Endoscopic drainage for pancreatic pseudocysts in children. J Pediatr Surg 36:503–505, 2001.

40. Kimble RM, Cohen R, Williams S: Successful endoscopic drainage of a posttraumatic pancreatic pseudocyst in a child. J Pediatr Surg 34:1518–1520, 1999.

41. D'Cruz AJ, Kamath PS, Ramachandra C, et al: Pancreatic ascites in children. Acta Paediatr Jpn 37:630–633, 1995.

42. Komuro H, Nagai H, Nakashima N, et al: Pancreatic ascites with pancreatic stone formation in a child. J Pediatr Gastroenterol Nutr 29:363–365, 1999.

43. da Cunha JE, Machado M, Bacchella T, et al: Surgical treatment of pancreatic ascites and pancreatic pleural effusions. Hepatogastroenterology 42:748–751, 1995.

44. Shimizu M, Hirokawa M, Manabe T: Histological assessment of chronic pancreatitis at necropsy. J Clin Pathol 49:913–915, 1996.

45. Sidhu S, Tandon RK: Chronic pancreatitis: Diagnosis and treatment. Postgrad Med J 72:327–333, 1996.

46. Sidhu SS, Tandon RK: The pathogenesis of chronic pancreatitis. Postgrad Med J 71:67–70, 1995.

47. Witt H: Gene mutations in children with chronic pancreatitis. Pancreatology 1:432–438, 2001.

48. Charnley RM: Hereditary pancreatitis. World J Gastroenterol 9:1–4, 2003.

49. DuBay D, Sandler A, Kimura K, et al: The modified Puestow procedure for complicated hereditary pancreatitis in children. J Pediatr Surg 35:343–348, 2000.

50. Dite P, Zboril V, Cikankova E: Endoscopic therapy of chronic pancreatitis. Hepatogastroenterology 43:1633–1637, 1996.

51. Kane C, Shepherd RM, Squires PE, et al: Loss of functional KATP channels in pancreatic beta-cells causes persistent hyperinsulinemic hypoglycemia of infancy. Nat Med 2:1344–1347, 1996.

52. Thomas P, Ye Y, Lightner E: Mutation of the pancreatic islet inward rectifier Kir6.2 also leads to familial persistent hyperinsulinemic hypoglycemia of infancy. Hum Mol Genet 5:1809–1812, 1996.

53. Thomas PM, Cote GJ, Hallman DM, et al: Homozygosity mapping, to chromosome 11p, of the gene for familial persistent hyperinsulinemic hypoglycemia of infancy. Am J Hum Genet 56:416–421, 1995.

54. Someya T, Miki T, Sugihara S, et al: Characterization of genes encoding the pancreatic beta-cell ATP-sensitive K+ channel in persistent hyperinsulinemic hypoglycemia of infancy in Japanese patients. Endocr J 47:715–722, 2000.

55. Kloppel G, Reinecke-Luthge A, Koschoreck F: Focal and diffuse beta cell changes in persistent hyperinsulinemic hypoglycemia of infancy. Endocr Pathol 10:299–304, 1999.

56. Cretolle C, Fekete CN, Jan D, et al: Partial elective pancreatectomy is curative in focal form of permanent hyperinsulinemic hypoglycaemia in infancy: A report of 45 cases from 1983 to 2000. J Pediatr Surg 37:155–158, 2002.

57. Adzick NS, Thornton PS, Stanley CA, et al: A multidisciplinary approach to the focal form of congenital hyperinsulinism leads to successful treatment by partial pancreatectomy. J Pediatr Surg 39:270–275, 2004.

58. al-Rabeeah A, al-Ashwal A, al-Herbish A, et al: Persistent hyperinsulinemic hypoglycemia of infancy: Experience with 28 cases. J Pediatr Surg 30:1119–1121, 1995.

59. Soliman AT, Alsalmi I, Darwish A, et al: Growth and endocrine function after near total pancreatectomy for hyperinsulinaemic hypoglycaemia. Arch Dis Child 74:379–385, 1996.

60. Taguchi T, Suita S, Ohkubo K, et al: Mutations in the sulfonylurea receptor gene in relation to the long-term outcome of persistent hyperinsulinemic hypoglycemia of infancy. J Pediatr Surg 37:593–598, 2002.

61. Leibowitz G, Glaser B, Higazi AA, et al: Hyperinsulinemic hypoglycemia of infancy (nesidioblastosis) in clinical remission: high incidence of diabetes mellitus and persistent beta-cell dysfunction at long-term follow-up. J Clin Endocrinol Metab 80:386–392, 1995.

62. Mason PJ: New insights into G6PD deficiency. Br J Haematol 94:585–591, 1996.

63. Lee PJ: Glycogen storage disease type I: Pathophysiology of liver adenomas. Eur J Pediatr 161(suppl 1):S46–S49, 2002.

64. Grant CS: Gastrointestinal endocrine tumors: Insulinoma. Bailleres Clin Gastroenterol 10:645, 1996.

65. Angeli E, Vanzulli A, Castrucci M, et al: Value of abdominal sonography and MR imaging at 0.5 T in preoperative detection of pancreatic insulinoma: A comparison with dynamic CT and angiography. Abdom Imaging 22:295–303, 1997.

66. Huai JC, Zhang W, Niu HO, et al: Localization and surgical treatment of pancreatic insulinomas guided by intraoperative ultrasound. Am J Surg 175:18–21, 1998.

67. Eire PF, Rodriguez-Pereira C, Barca-Rodriguez P, et al: Uncommon case of gastrinoma in a child. Eur J Pediatr Surg 6:173, 1996.

68. Jensen RT: Gastrointestinal endocrine tumors: Gastrinoma. Bailleres Clin Gastroenterol 10:603, 1996.

69. Brenin DR, Talamonti MS, Yang EY, et al: Cystic neoplasms of the pancreas: A clinicopathologic study, including DNA flow cytometry. Arch Surg 130:1048–1054, 1995.

70. Shorter NA, Glick RD, Klimstra DS, et al: Malignant pancreatic tumors in childhood and adolescence: The Memorial Sloan-Kettering experience, 1967 to present. J Pediatr Surg 37:887–892, 2002.

71. Abraham SC, Wu TT, Klimstra DS, et al: Distinctive molecular genetic alterations in sporadic and familial adenomatous polyposis-associated pancreatoblastomas: Frequent alterations in the APC/beta-catenin pathway and chromosome 11p. Am J Pathol 159:1619–1627, 2001.

72. Murakami T, Ueki K, Kawakami H, et al: Pancreatoblastoma: Case report and review of treatment in the literature. Med Pediatr Oncol 27:193–197, 1996.

73. Klimstra DS, Wenig BM, Adair CF, et al: Pancreatoblastoma: A clinicopathologic study and review of the literature. Am J Surg Pathol 19:1371–1389, 1995.

74. Ogawa B, Okinaga K, Obana K, et al: Pancreatoblastoma treated by delayed operation after effective chemotherapy. J Pediatr Surg 35:1663–1665, 2000.

75. Vossen S, Goretzki PE, Goebel U, et al: Therapeutic management of rare malignant pancreatic tumors in children. World J Surg 22:879–882, 1998.

76. Wang KS, Albanese C, Dada F, et al: Papillary cystic neoplasm of the pancreas: A report of three pediatric cases and literature review. J Pediatr Surg 33:842–845, 1998.

77. Skandalakis JE, Gray SW, Ricketts R, et al: The spleen. In Skandalakis JE, Gray SW (eds): Embryology for Surgeons, 2nd ed. Baltimore, Williams & Wilkins, 1994, p 381.

78. Milicevic Z, Cuschieri A, Xuereb A, et al: Stereological study of tissue compartments of the human spleen. Histol Histopathol 11:833–836, 1996.

79. Liu DL, Xia S, Xu W, et al: Anatomy of vasculature of 850 spleen specimens and its application in partial splenectomy. Surgery 119:27, 1996.

80. Ferlicot S, Emile JF, Le Bris JL, et al: [Congenital asplenia: A childhood immune deficit often detected too late]. Ann Pathol 17:44–46, 1997.

81. Rubino M, Van Praagh S, Kadoba K, et al: Systemic and pulmonary venous connections in visceral heterotaxy with asplenia: Diagnostic and surgical considerations based on seventy-two autopsied cases. J Thorac Cardiovasc Surg 110:641–650, 1995.

82. Abuhamad AZ, Robinson JN, Bogdan D, et al: Color Doppler of the splenic artery in the prenatal diagnosis of heterotaxic syndromes. Am J Perinatol 16:469–473, 1999.

83. Rudowski WJ: Accessory spleens: Clinical significance with particular reference to the recurrence of idiopathic thrombocytopenic purpura. World J Surg 9:422–430, 1985.

84. Gayer G, Zissin R, Apter S, et al: CT findings in congenital anomalies of the spleen. Br J Radiol 74:767–772, 2001.

85. Balaji KC, Caldarone AA, Rabinowitz R, et al: Splenogonadal fusion. J Urol 156:854, 1996.

86. Patel RV: Splenogonadal fusion. J Pediatr Surg 30:873–874, 1995.

87. Desai DC, Hebra A, Davidoff AM, et al: Wandering spleen: A challenging diagnosis. South Med J 90:439, 1997.

88. Fujiwara T, Takehara Y, Isoda H, et al: Torsion of the wandering spleen: CT and angiographic appearance. J Comput Assist Tomogr 19:84–86, 1995.

89. Lam KY, Chan AC, Chan TM: Peliosis of the spleen: Possible association with chronic renal failure and erythropoietin therapy. Postgrad Med J 71:493, 1995.

90. De Caluwe D, Phelan E, Puri P: Pure alcohol injection of a congenital splenic cyst: A valid alternative? J Pediatr Surg 38:629–632, 2003.

91. Touloukian RJ, Maharaj A, Ghoussoub R, et al: Partial decapsulation of splenic epithelial cysts: studies on etiology and outcome. J Pediatr Surg 32:272–274, 1997.

92. Ramani M, Reinhold C, Semelka RC, et al: Splenic hemangiomas and hamartomas: MR imaging characteristics of 28 lesions. Radiology 202:166–172, 1997.

93. Velkova K, Nedeva A: Our experience in the diagnostics of liver and spleen hemangiomas. Folia Med (Plovdiv) 39:85–91, 1997.

94. Yelon JA, Green JD, Evans JT: Splenic abscess associated with osteomyelitis. Eur J Surg 162:913–914, 1996.

95. Bossi D, Russo M: Hemolytic anemia due to disorders of red cell membrane skeleton. Mol Aspects Med 17:171, 1996.

96. Tchernia G, Bader-Meunier B, Berterottiere P, et al: Effectiveness of partial splenectomy in hereditary spherocytosis. Curr Opin Hematol 4:136–141, 1997.

97. de Buys Roessingh AS, de Lagausie P, Rohrlich P, et al: Follow-up of partial splenectomy in children with hereditary spherocytosis. J Pediatr Surg 37:1459–1463, 2002.

98. Lane PA: Sickle cell anemia. Pediatr Clin North Am 43:639, 1996.

99. Lane PA: The spleen in children. Curr Opin Pediatr 7:36, 1995.

100. Svarch E, Vilorio P, Nordet I, et al: Partial splenectomy in children with sickle cell disease and repeated episodes of splenic sequestration. Hemoglobin 20:393–400, 1996.

101. Adams DM, Ware RE, Schultz WH, et al: Successful surgical outcome in children with sickle hemoglobinopathies: The Duke University experience. J Pediatr Surg 33:428–432, 1998.

102. Idowu O, Hayes-Jordan A: Partial splenectomy in children under 4 years of age with hemoglobinopathy. J Pediatr Surg 33:1251–1253, 1998.

103. Caulier MT, Darloy F, Rose C, et al: Splenic irradiation for chronic autoimmune thrombocytopenic purpura in patients with contra-indications to splenectomy. Br J Haematol 91:208–211, 1995.

104. Hemmila MR, Foley DS, Castle VP, et al: The response to splenectomy in pediatric patients with idiopathic thrombocytopenic purpura who fail high-dose intravenous immune globulin. J Pediatr Surg 35:967–971; discussion 971–962, 2000.

105. Najean Y, Rain JD, Billotey C: The site of destruction of autologous ^{111}In-labelled platelets and the efficiency of splenectomy in children and adults with idiopathic thrombocytopenic purpura: A study of 578 patients with 268 splenectomies. Br J Haematol 97:547–550, 1997.

106. Jacir NN, Robertson FM, Crombleholme TM, et al: Recurrence of immune thrombocytopenic purpura after splenectomy. J Pediatr Surg 31:115–116, 1996.

107. Stanley P, Shen TC: Partial embolization of the spleen in patients with thalassemia. J Vasc Intervent Radiol 6:137–142, 1995.

108. Banani SA: Partial dearterialization of the spleen in thalassemia major. J Pediatr Surg 33:449–453, 1998.

109. Terrosu G, Donini A, Silvestri F, et al: Laparoscopic splenectomy in the management of hematological diseases: Surgical technique and outcome of 17 patients. Surg Endosc 10:441–444, 1996.

110. Pui CH: Childhood leukemias: Current status and future perspective. Zhonghua Min Guo Xiao Er Ke Yi Xue Hui Za Zhi 36:322–327, 1995.

111. Rice EO, Mifflin TE, Sakallah S, et al: Gaucher disease: studies of phenotype, molecular diagnosis and treatment. Clin Genet 49:111–118, 1996.

112. Lorberboym M, Pastores GM, Kim CK, et al: Scintigraphic monitoring of reticuloendothelial system in patients with type 1 Gaucher disease on enzyme replacement therapy. J Nucl Med 38:890–895, 1997.

113. Soutter AD, Ellenbogen J, Folkman J: Splenosis is regulated by a circulating factor. J Pediatr Surg 29:1076–1079, 1994.

114. Arzoumanian A, Rosenthall L: Splenosis. Clin Nucl Med 20:730–733, 1995.

115. Carroll A, Thomas P: Decision-making in surgery: Splenectomy. Br J Hosp Med 54:147–149, 1995.

116. Petroianu A: Subtotal splenectomy for treatment of patients with myelofibrosis and myeloid metaplasia. Int Surg 81:177–179, 1996.

117. Farhi DC, Ashfaq R: Splenic pathology after traumatic injury. Am J Clin Pathol 105:474–478, 1996.

118. Uranus S, Pfeifer J, Schauer C, et al: Laparoscopic partial splenic resection. Surg Laparosc Endosc 5:133–136, 1995.

119. Moores DC, McKee MA, Wang H, et al: Pediatric laparoscopic splenectomy. J Pediatr Surg 30:1201–1205, 1995.

120. Hassan IS, Snow MH, Ong EL: Overwhelming pneumococcal sepsis in two patients splenectomised more than ten years previously. Scott Med J 41:17–19, 1996.

121. O'Sullivan ST, Reardon CM, O'Donnell JA, et al: How safe is splenectomy? Ir J Med Sci 163:374–378, 1994.

122. Jugenburg M, Haddock G, Freedman MH, et al: The morbidity and mortality of pediatric splenectomy: Does prophylaxis make a difference? J Pediatr Surg 34:1064–1067, 1999.

123. Balsalobre B, Carbonell-Tatay F: Cellular immunity in splenectomized patients. J Invest Allergol Clin Immunol 1:235–238, 1991.

124. Green AD, Connor MP: Prevention of post-splenectomy sepsis. Lancet 341:1034, 1993.

CHAPTER 46

Congenital Abdominal Wall Defects

Michael D. Klein, MD

The three characteristic congenital abdominal wall defects are omphalocele, gastroschisis, and umbilical cord hernia. Omphalocele is a central abdominal wall defect (>4 cm) at the umbilicus, always covered by a thin membrane or sac. It usually contains liver as well as midgut and may contain other organs such as the spleen and one or both gonads. Gastroschisis is a small defect (<4 cm) without a sac located just to the right of the umbilicus. Usually only midgut is herniated. Umbilical cord hernia is often confused with omphalocele. It is a small defect (<4 cm) at the umbilicus, covered by a sac, and containing only midgut.

An umbilical hernia is not a congenital abdominal wall defect. It is not present at birth but becomes evident at about age 6 weeks and is covered by normal skin. Defects of the abdominal wall that occur away from the umbilicus are quite unusual, seldom have a sac, and are often fatal. In this chapter, we do not consider these latter two entities or the congenital abdominal wall muscular deficiency (prune belly) syndrome, which is presented in Chapter 60.

HISTORY

Congenital abdominal wall defects (probably omphalocele) were described as early as the first century CE[1] and later in about the 5th century CE.[2] Gastroschisis appears to have been reported first in 1557.[3] A 1913 report exists of a successfully treated case[4] as does a review by Bernstein in 1940,[5] although most authors believe that gastroschisis has become a common anomaly only since 1970.[6] This relatively recent appearance of gastroschisis has led to the conjecture that it is related to environmental teratogens.[7,8] Interestingly, most of the abdominal wall defects reported in the teratology literature are gastroschisis (even when termed omphalocele).[9] The relatively modern appearance of gastroschisis may be due to the fact that these patients are more likely to be premature and thus less likely to have survived to the surgeon's notice in the days before development of neonatology as

a specialty and the advent of critical care transport teams.[10]

Successful repair of omphalocele was first reported in 1803.[11] Before the advent of mechanical ventilation, it was not possible to close the fascia in most cases. Alcohol[12] and mercurochrome[13] (and in more modern times, polymer membrane[14]) were used to scarify or sterilize the sac, allowing it to contract and the skin to grow over it. Excising the sac and covering the viscera with skin flaps was described in 1948.[15] With both these methods, it is important to close the resultant ventral hernia as early as possible to avoid visceral growth in a giant hernia that can never be closed. In 1967, the staged repair of omphalocele with artificial material sewn to the fascial edges was introduced.[16] Its conceptual mechanism was described as rearranging the forces in the abdomen to permit the growth of the abdominal wall over a period of 2 weeks. Given the modern experiences, it may be that this technique allows time for the bowel edema to resolve and for the bowel lumen to empty while, perhaps, stretching the abdominal wall somewhat to allow it to accommodate.

EMBRYOLOGY OF THE ANTERIOR ABDOMINAL WALL

In the first 3 weeks of gestation, the embryo is a flat disk growing between the developing chorion and amnion. About the fourth week, the edges of the disk turn inward to form the body cavity. The two lateral edges of the disk invert to form the pleuroperitoneal canals. As the cephalic fold turns down, it carries the heart with it and continues as the septum transversum to divide the pleuroperitoneal canals into the thoracic and abdominal cavities (Fig. 46-1). The bladder (allantois) begins distal to the point where the anus will develop and is carried up with the caudal fold, which forms the infraumbilical abdominal wall. As the amnion expands to fuse with the chorion, the embryo hangs into the amniotic space from the umbilical stalk.

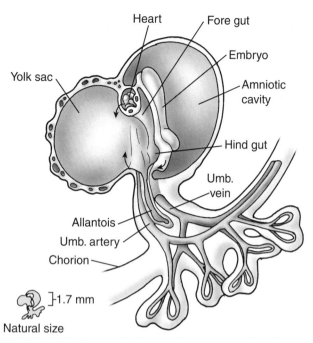

Heart   Fore gut

Embryo

Amniotic cavity

Yolk sac

Hind gut

Umb. vein

Allantois

Umb. artery

Chorion

1.7 mm

Natural size

FIGURE 46-1. Drawing of an embryo at 3 weeks. One can appreciate the early beginnings of the cephalic folds. The cephalic fold brings the heart down with it, and the caudal fold brings the bladder up with it. (Drawing by Max Brodel from Cullen TS: The Umbilicus and Its Diseases. Philadelphia, W.B. Saunders, 1916.)

The straight tube of the primitive gut is in continuity with the yolk sac at this time, but soon the yolk sac disappears and leaves a solid umbilical stalk. The gut now elongates (4 to 5 weeks of gestation). At the same time, vacuoles appear in the Wharton's jelly of the umbilical stalk. These vacuoles coalesce to form the umbilical coelom, into which the elongating gut can grow (5 to 6 weeks of gestation) while the abdominal cavity expands (Fig. 46-2). At 10 to 12 weeks of gestation, the gut returns to the abdominal cavity and undergoes rotation and fixation, while the umbilical coelom disappears.

During this time, the visceral vasculature also is growing and changing. Early on, four umbilical vessels exist, two veins and two arteries. At about 5 weeks of gestation, the right umbilical vein resorbs, leaving only the left to return blood from the placenta to the heart through the ductus venosus. At birth, the view of the umbilicus from the inside shows the two obliterated umbilical arteries as the medial umbilical ligaments and the obliterated allantois (from the bladder) as the median umbilical ligament. Superiorly is the single (left) umbilical vein. The involution of the right umbilical vein may create a weakened area in the abdominal wall just to the right of the umbilical cord (Fig. 46-3).

All patients with a congenital abdominal wall defect will have intestinal malrotation. Because the intestines do not return to the abdominal cavity, as occurs in normal development, they do not rotate and fix to the posterior abdominal wall.

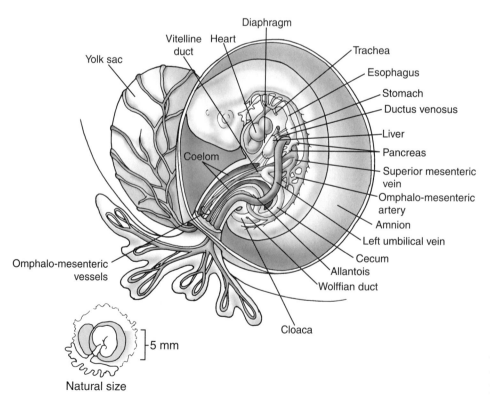

Diaphragm

Vitelline duct   Heart

Trachea

Esophagus

Yolk sac

Stomach

Ductus venosus

Liver

Pancreas

Coelom

Superior mesenteric vein

Omphalo-mesenteric artery

Amnion

Left umbilical vein

Omphalo-mesenteric vessels

Cecum

Allantois

Wolffian duct

Cloaca

5 mm

Natural size

FIGURE 46-2. Embryo at 5 weeks. One can appreciate the beginning of the lengthening small bowel entering the umbilical coelom. (Drawing by Max Brodel from Cullen TS: The Umbilicus and Its Diseases. Philadelphia, W.B. Saunders, 1916.)

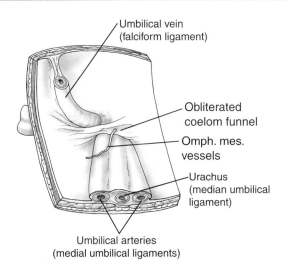

Umbilical vein
(falciform ligament)

Obliterated
coelom funnel

Omph. mes.
vessels

Urachus
(median umbilical
ligament)

Umbilical arteries
(medial umbilical ligaments)

FIGURE 46-3. Drawing of the anterior abdominal wall viewed from the inside at the time of birth. Note the fundal or weak area to the right of the cord where the right umbilical vein has been resorbed. (Drawing by Max Brodel from Cullen TS: The Umbilicus and Its Diseases. Philadelphia, W.B. Saunders, 1916.)

OMPHALOCELE

Embryology and Clinical Presentation

Omphalocele results from the failure of the lateral embryonic folds to fuse in the midline (Fig. 46-4). Its incidence is approximately 1:4000 live births, and omphalocele can constitute up to 40% of the congenital abdominal wall defects. Because it is an early gestational event when organogenesis is active, frequently associated anomalies are most often cardiac.[17] The defect is large, covered with a sac, which may be torn during delivery, and usually contains liver as well as intestine, and possibly other organs. The rectus muscles insert on the costal margin laterally and do not meet in the midline. These patients are usually term. Omphalocele can be diagnosed antenatally by ultrasonography (US). It has been associated with elevated amniotic fluid and maternal serum α-fetoprotein.[18]

Preoperative Care and Preparation

The mode of delivery should be based on obstetrical indications. No studies demonstrate improved outcomes with cesarean delivery for any of the congenital abdominal wall defects.[19] Many obstetricians still are understandably reluctant to deliver them by the vaginal route. Once the infant is delivered, a complete physical examination including a digital rectal examination and passage of a nasogastric (NG) or orogastric tube should demonstrate many of the associated anomalies. An echocardiogram is important, and an US to evaluate the urinary tract also is useful. An intravenous line (IV) should be started, a urinary catheter inserted, and the NG tube placed for continuous suction to keep the intestines decompressed. The

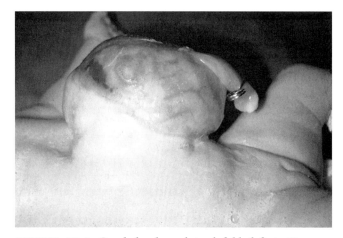

FIGURE 46-4. Omphalocele, a lateral fold defect. One can appreciate the sac, the liver in the defect superiorly, and the small bowel in the defect inferiorly, with the wide insertion of the rectus abdominis muscles on the costal margin.

baby is kept warm, antibiotics are administered, the administration of vitamin K is documented, and a hemoglobin level is obtained. A serum glucose level also should be obtained, as omphalocele can be associated with Beckwith-Wiedemann syndrome, consisting of macroglossia, hypoglycemia, and the abdominal wall defect. The macroglossia and hypoglycemia seldom persist as problems, but it is important to recognize this syndrome, as these children are at increased risk for abdominal tumors and require careful surveillance with regular US examinations. A vigorous digital rectal examination can stimulate the passage of meconium that will help to decompress the bowel further.

An intact sac will protect the viscera so that the operation is probably not an emergency, but closure or coverage should be performed within 24 hours, as the sac can crack, separate, or tear (Fig. 46-5). From a cardiac viewpoint, perhaps the safest time to operate is immediately

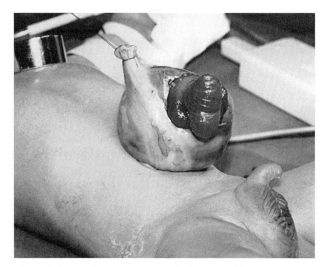

FIGURE 46-5. A ruptured omphalocele with a segment of intestine protruding through the torn omphalocele sac.

after birth while the compliance of the right ventricle has not yet decreased and a left-to-right shunt across a septal defect or a patent ductus arteriosus is less likely to exist. The sooner the operation, the less chance for bowel distention or edema and the more likely that a primary repair will be possible.

Delivery room personnel frequently will wrap children with abdominal wall defects with warm saline-soaked gauze. Even if covered with plastic wrap, the wet dressing allows evaporative cooling, because the plastic wrap cannot be effectively sealed. The best dressing is probably a cellophane bowel bag with a drawstring designed to be used during abdominal aortic surgical procedures to contain and protect the bowel.[20] The drawstring can be gently tightened under the arms, allowing access to the hands for IVs and blood sampling and to the head. If a foot is needed for the IV, a hole can be cut in one corner of the bag. Placing gauze in the bag is not necessary, although a few milliliters of saline helps maintain a moist environment. Patients with omphalocele require less fluid than do those with gastroschisis or a ruptured omphalocele. Still, it is wise to treat them as if they are volume depleted. An IV of D5/0.45 normal saline (NS) at 150 mL/kg/24 hr is initiated. Urine output, vital signs, transcutaneous oxygen saturation, and the chest radiograph are monitored for signs of over- or under-resuscitation.

Operation

The excess umbilical cord is removed as part of the skin preparation. Maintenance of the baby's temperature is very important. We use plastic adhesive-edge drapes and towels to protect against heat loss. A skin incision is made circumferentially around the defect a few millimeters from the sac to provide an edge so that the sac edge can be held with toothed forceps. Thick skin flaps are developed down to the rectus abdominis fascia so that the rectus muscles can be clearly visualized. At the superior portion of the defect, fascia is not likely, but only a thin membrane over the hepatic veins, as the liver hangs into the sac on a pedicle. Similarly, the fascia immediately over the bladder may be very thin, and care must be taken to protect the bladder. The peritoneal cavity is entered between the edge of the rectus muscle and the skin edge remaining on the sac, and the sac is excised. The liver (and sometimes other organs) may be adherent to the sac and must be separated. If a large portion of the liver is adherent, it may be prudent to leave a portion of the sac on the liver because it is very difficult to separate while preserving the integrity of the liver capsule. The use of retractors to force the liver into the abdominal cavity can easily lead to liver laceration and hard-to-control bleeding. The hepatic veins not only are vulnerable to injury but also can kink and obstruct during the abdominal wall closure. This complication may lead to severe metabolic acidosis that may necessitate reoperation for relief of hepatic venous obstruction. The umbilical vein is usually encountered at the superior portion of the sac. The umbilical arteries and the allantois or urachus are found inferiorly. These are ligated with 3-0 absorbable sutures.

If there is urgent need for further vascular access during the procedure, the umbilical vein is very convenient. A catheter can be inserted quickly and the tubing handed off the field for use by the anesthesiologist. It also is possible to use the umbilical vein and arteries for more formal vascular access by translocating them through the skin.[21] In most cases, we prefer a percutaneously inserted, central catheter line or formal neck cutdown for central venous access and blood gas monitoring in the postoperative period.

Once the sac has been removed, the abdominal wall is stretched to facilitate fascial closure (Fig. 46-6). If fascial closure is not possible, closure of the skin over the viscera should be considered. If this seems possible, the skin may be mobilized to the flanks and beyond. If it appears that skin closure will not be possible, then extensive skin-flap dissection should not be performed, and the skin is reserved for staged repair.

In cases needing staged closure, we use Dacron-reinforced polymeric silicone (Silastic) sheets (0.007 inches thick) to create a pouch to hold the viscera. With 3-0 monofilament permanent suture in a continuous fashion, we sew one sheet to each lateral edge of the fascia securing the Silastic side of the composite in contact with the viscera. The excess Dacron/Silastic is trimmed so that it just accommodates the viscera without attempts at further reduction at this time. Continuing the same suture, the free edges are joined superiorly and inferiorly to form a sac to be used in squeezing the viscera into the abdominal cavity. An antibiotic ointment is applied to the suture line. If the defect is very large, it may be helpful to leave long sutures at the apex of the prosthetic sac so that it may be suspended from the top of the infant warmer to prevent the pouch and its contents falling to one side.

Ladd's procedure is not performed to manage the intestinal malrotation. The extent and nature of the operation will produce enough adhesions to prevent volvulus. The occurrence of a volvulus after an operation for an

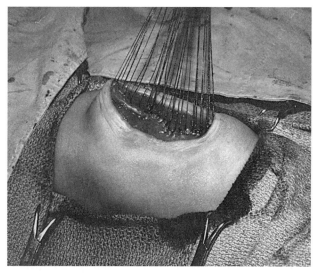

FIGURE 46-6. Primary fascial and skin closure is technically possible in most small and moderate-sized omphaloceles.

abdominal wall defect is no greater than that after Ladd's procedure. A gastrostomy is not placed in patients with abdominal wall defects because it will interfere with the ultimate closure by fixing the stomach in a position that will not allow reduction of all the abdominal viscera.

Reduction of the abdominal contents is accomplished by reducing the size of the prosthetic sac from the top down (see later). Once the sac has been reduced to the level of the fascia (usually ~1 week), a second procedure is undertaken to close the fascia. This is often the appropriate time to insert a central venous catheter (CVC) if vascular access has become problematic. At this time, all the sutures and the Silastic sheeting are removed. A pseudocapsule or coagulum often overlying the viscera should be left intact. The edges of the fascial defect are brought together in the midline. Initially, three mattress sutures are placed to approximate the fascia in a test closure. Monitoring the transcutaneous oxygen saturation and the end-tidal CO_2 will help to determine if fascial closure will be too constrictive. If the baby's ventilation is not compromised significantly, the remainder of the fascia is approximated with interrupted 2-0 absorbable sutures, being sure to include some of the rectus sheath with each suture. If only the medial midline fascia is approximated, a higher likelihood exists of a late incisional hernia. If the patient's status is satisfactory with less than 30 mm Hg peak inspiratory pressure (PIP) 20 minutes after first approximating the fascia, one can probably leave the fascia closed. The skin is closed with a continuous permanent monofilament suture. If the fascia will not come together without compromise of ventilation, skin flaps are created, and the skin is closed over the fascial defect with a continuous monofilament suture. Antibiotic ointment is applied as the dressing, and no adhesive is used. The skin will stretch and relax over time. If sufficient skin is present, a cosmetic umbilicoplasty can be performed.[22]

The term *giant omphalocele* has been used by some authors to differentiate an omphalocele that cannot be closed from one that is amenable to closure by the techniques described (Fig. 46-7). In the patient with a giant omphalocele, the prognosis is much worse, and neither the skin nor the fascia can be brought together, even after initial reduction. In such cases, the abdominal viscera can be covered with a polypropylene soft-tissue patch to allow granulation tissue and epithelialization to occur. However, it has been our experience that, before this happens, the polypropylene patch will become infected and will separate from the fascial edges and require removal. Fortunately, by that time, the abdominal viscera have become so adherent that evisceration will not occur. Granulation tissue develops over the serosa of the matted viscera and leads to epithelialization. In either case, the plan should be to return in a year to attempt fascial closure. Because this large defect presents such a difficult problem, some surgeons have elected a nonoperative treatment plan that also carries the risk of significant complications.[23] Many of these babies will die of complications before closure can be accomplished.

A commercially available preformed, self-retaining silo is widely used by pediatric surgeons. This is a complete

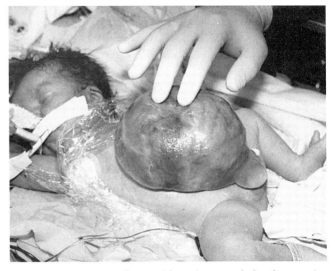

FIGURE 46-7. A newborn with a giant omphalocele containing liver and intestine. Primary closure is not possible in this patient, but a variety of strategies have been used to manage such complex patients successfully.

silo with the lower rim being a rolled tube containing a flexible spring. The rim of the silo can usually be inserted into the abdomen to cover the viscera after removal of the native sac. It may need to be held in place by several interrupted sutures because otherwise, the pressure generated during reduction will cause it to be dislodged. Omphalocele defects are usually so large that it can be difficult to place the silo ring within the abdominal cavity without compressing the hepatic veins or the bladder.

Reduction of the Prosthetic Sac

The reduction of the viscera from a prosthetic sac should be accomplished as quickly as possible as tissue is not incorporated into Silastic and it will separate after two weeks or more for many reasons (Fig. 46-8). It is usually necessary to ventilate the patient by using paralysis during the period between prosthesis application and fascial closure. The measurement of intra-abdominal pressure with a simple water manometer connected either to the NG tube or to the urinary catheter allows a means of assessing the physiologic effects of pressure applied to the prosthesis. An intra-abdominal pressure less than 20 cm water probably does not cause clinical problems.[24,25] By using these manometric measurements as a guide, it has been shown that the pouches can be reduced far more vigorously than was previously thought. In our experience, the abdominal contents can usually be reduced within 1 week after the initial operation.

The sac is manually reduced in size and the reduction maintained by placing a large clamp across the sac to protect the viscera while a new suture line is placed. Some surgeons use the gastrointestinal stapling device to accomplish this goal, whereas others reduce the size of the sac by tying the pouch with umbilical tape.

Once the abdominal contents are level with the skin, it is difficult to bring the edges any closer together. At the

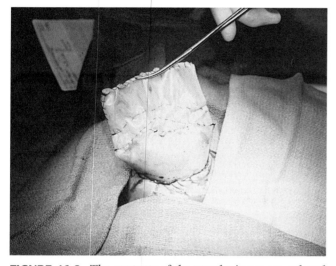

FIGURE 46-8. The contents of the prosthetic sac are reduced into the abdomen in stages. Measurement of intragastric or bladder pressure aids in determining the vigor with which the gut is pushed in.

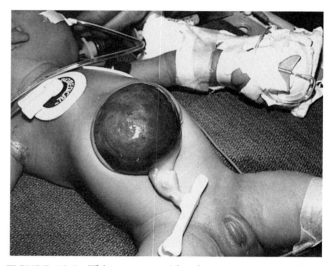

FIGURE 46-9. This neonate with a large epigastric omphalocele containing liver was found to have the usual additional somatic and visceral defects of the pentalogy of Cantrell. Echocardiography is useful in identifying the associated cardiac anomalies.

time of securing the prosthetic sac, separate traction sutures can be placed on each of the fascial edges so that when this point is reached at the time of reduction, these sutures can be tied together to invert the pouch and bring the edges even closer together.

Postoperative Care

In the postoperative period, NG decompression and total parenteral nutrition (TPN) are used. After each operative procedure, it is important to assess the baby's ventilation and the effectiveness of volume resuscitation. One also must be alert to the associated anomalies and their management. Patients are usually intubated and mechanically ventilated until any prosthesis has been removed and either the fascial or skin closure has been accomplished. Blood gases are monitored to determine the adequacy of ventilation. Patients in whom respiratory acidosis develops may require a return to the operating room to release the closure. Metabolic acidosis may develop, related to obstruction of the renal or hepatic veins from increased abdominal pressure or kinking as the liver is returned to the abdominal cavity. Increased abdominal pressure also can cause ureteral obstruction and reduced urine output.

These patients most often require significant intravenous resuscitation. An intravenous rate of 200 mL/kg/day is usually initiated until the urine output is well established and the vital signs become normal. Many subtle indicators of volume overload exist, including increased opacification on the chest radiograph and decreased oxygen saturation. If clinical questions remain, the central venous pressure can be determined.

Special Cases

Cephalic fold defect or pentalogy of Cantrell can be a very difficult problem (Fig. 46-9). In this anomaly, a defect

appears in the central tendon of the diaphragm and the pericardium, which allows the heart to protrude into the omphalocele sac.[26,27] The other two elements of the "pentalogy" are a split sternum and an intracardiac defect. The heart defect should be repaired as soon as possible. Overzealous attempts at placing the heart within the chest are complicated by kinking of the great vessels and the vena cava. At some point in the first weeks to months of life, a loose patch of polypropylene mesh is used to repair the diaphragmatic defect as well as the anterior abdominal wall fascial defect, and the skin is mobilized to cover those repairs. As the patient grows, the heart slowly achieves its normal position.

A caudal-fold defect or vesicointestinal fissure (cloacal exstrophy) has a characteristic appearance with an infraumbilical omphalocele, exstrophy of the bladder, and usually an imperforate anus with the ileum everted in the midline (see Chapter 57). The initial therapy consists of closure of the omphalocele and fashioning an ileostomy, with care taken to preserve any remnant of colon that may exist. At one time, it was thought that all patients with this anomaly should be raised as girls, because they have only a rudimentary penis, but this concept is being revisited.

UMBILICAL CORD HERNIA

Embryology and Clinical Presentation

This anomaly is considered to be a simple failure of the midgut to return to the abdominal cavity at 10 to 12 weeks of gestation. The clinical features are a small defect (<4 cm), which is covered by a thin membrane and only contains midgut (Fig. 46-10). A relatively low incidence of associated anomalies is found. The rectus muscles meet in the midline at the xyphoid, and the fascial and skin defects can nearly always be closed at the

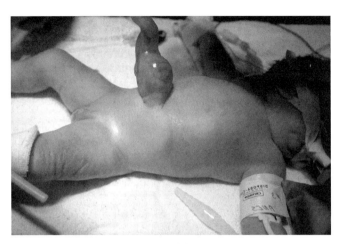

FIGURE 46-10. Umbilical cord hernia. One can appreciate that this is a relatively small defect with a normal abdominal wall. Only small bowel is contained in the sac.

initial operation. In our experience, 20% of congenital abdominal wall defects are umbilical cord hernias.

Operative Repair

Little in the way of preoperative preparation is unique to this anomaly. It is best to intervene early to have the best chance of a primary fascial closure. The operative steps are similar to those described for primary closure of an omphalocele, only much less difficult. Usually enough skin is available to reconstruct a normal-appearing umbilicus. This is most easily accomplished by preserving the umbilical cord as part of the skin flaps and then closing the skin in the midline with a subcuticular suture. The cord will desiccate and separate in the usual fashion, leaving a very satisfactory umbilicus. If the umbilical cord does not contain normal skin as it inserts in the middle of the sac, an interrupted subcuticular absorbable purse-string suture can be used to create a normal-appearing umbilicus. Patients with umbilical cord hernia do have malrotation, but, as with omphalocele, we do not do a Ladd procedure.

Postoperative Course

These patients may not demonstrate bowel function quickly, even though the manipulation is minimal, and the intestines are grossly normal. They may require TPN for as long as 2 weeks. They usually do not, however, have significant ventilatory, fluid, or intra-abdominal pressure problems. The vast majority of these patients make an uneventful recovery, but they should be followed up for at least a year to monitor the late appearance of a ventral hernia.

GASTROSCHISIS

Embryology and Clinical Presentation

This defect represents a failure of the umbilical coelom to form. The elongating gut has no room to develop and

extrudes out of the too-small peritoneal cavity. This is thought to occur to the right of the umbilicus because, with resorption of the right umbilical vein, this is the weakest or most unsupported aspect of the anterior abdominal wall.[28] Because this event occurs somewhat later in gestation than omphalocele, the patients seldom have associated defects, although they do have a higher incidence of gastrointestinal anomalies such as intestinal atresias. Moreover, the babies also are more likely to be premature. The defect is most often small (<4 cm), and (as with the other abdominal wall defects) the rectus muscles are normally formed. No sac or remnant of a sac is present, and the midgut is exposed (Fig. 46-11). In many instances at delivery, no coagulum, edema, or induration is present. These features occur after birth because of venous obstruction and transudation of proteinaceous fluid, which dries in room air. Given the normal appearance of the bowel at birth, it is hard to concur that it is the amniotic fluid that injures the intestine or that it is wise to deliver the patient prematurely to protect the bowel.[29] Others have also found that term delivery results in better outcomes for patients with gastroschisis.[30]

This defect is often diagnosed antenatally with US and is associated with elevated α-fetoprotein levels in the amniotic fluid and maternal serum. It may even be possible to distinguish gastroschisis from omphalocele and spina bifida based on amniotic fluid acetylcholinesterase.[31]

Operative Repair

Because the bowel is unprotected and can be expected to become more indurated with time, early operation is optimal. The preoperative preparation is similar to that described for an omphalocele, although placing the infant in a bowel bag and avoiding moist gauze that permits evaporative cooling is even more important. Many of these children are diagnosed antenatally, so the defect can be repaired immediately in the delivery room, which allows the operation to be performed when the bowel is

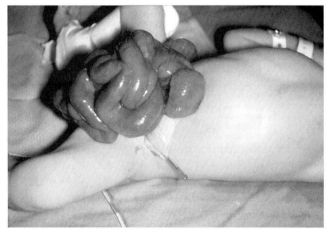

FIGURE 46-11. Gastroschisis. One can appreciate that no sac is present; that the defect is to the right of the umbilical cord; that the rest of the abdominal wall is entirely normal; that the bowel itself is thickened, edematous, and matted; and in areas, a fibrinous peel is seen.

still normal.[32] A most important first step is to wipe the vernix caseosa carefully from the newborn infant; otherwise, intubating the baby and starting an IV will be fruitless. Preoperative preparation includes an IV line, intubation, an NG tube and monitoring equipment, and a digital rectal examination to aid in the evacuation of meconium, thereby reducing intestinal distention. By the time the patient is anesthetized and ready for skin preparation, the intestine may have spontaneously reduced into the abdominal cavity. Operative care then follows the plan described earlier for omphalocele. Cosmetic umbilicoplasty also has been described for gastroschisis[33] (Fig. 46-12).

A prosthetic pouch is required less commonly in patients with gastroschisis than in those with omphalocele. A preformed self-retaining pouch can often be slipped over the bowel with the ring introduced into the abdominal cavity. Some surgeons perform this maneuver in the delivery room or nursery and do not take the patient to the operating room until it is time to remove the prosthesis and close the abdominal wall. However, our preference is to introduce the prosthesis in the operating room, securing the spring edges to the fascia with a few permanent sutures. The prosthesis can be extruded from the abdomen as external pressure is applied to reduce the pouch contents if it is not sutured.

A search for intestinal atresia is not carried out at the time of the intestinal reduction. If an atresia is unquestionable, the proximal end can be exteriorized as a stoma through the abdominal wall, and the paraumbilical defect can be closed or a silo placed (Fig. 46-13). In our experience, when the bowel is matted and edematous, areas that appear to be "obvious" atresias frequently are not. It is best not to operate on the indurated edematous bowel covered with a thick peel. Thus the entire mass of bowel

is reduced by stretching the abdominal wall to allow insertion of the gut, and the abdominal wall is closed. If the intragastric pressure exceeds 20 cm of H_2O, a silo is placed. If bowel function has not demonstrated the continuity of the gut by age 3 weeks, a contrast study is performed. Exploration is performed only if a mechanical obstruction is appreciated. The ileus associated with gastroschisis closure more than 20 to 30 minutes after birth can be severe and prolonged, although it is not always brief when an immediate operation is performed.[34]

Postoperative Care

The postoperative care is similar to that described for omphalocele, although it may be complicated by the issue of prematurity, which is more common in gastroschisis.[10] It is best to wait at least 6 weeks, if possible, before reoperation for obstruction, as both the intestine and the abdominal wall will have had time to approach a more normal state. A small but definite incidence of chronic intestinal pseudo-obstruction occurs in patients with gastroschisis. Although no mechanical obstruction appears on small bowel contrast studies, the patients still have poor intestinal motility. These patients may require long-term TPN with gradual introduction of enteral feeding.

Outcome

The mortality rate for patients born with omphalocele is higher than the mortality for patients born with gastroschisis.[35] An omphalocele patient's risk is mainly due to associated chromosomal and cardiac defects. Prematurity is commonly seen with gastroschisis and can contribute to the mortality risk through the mechanism of

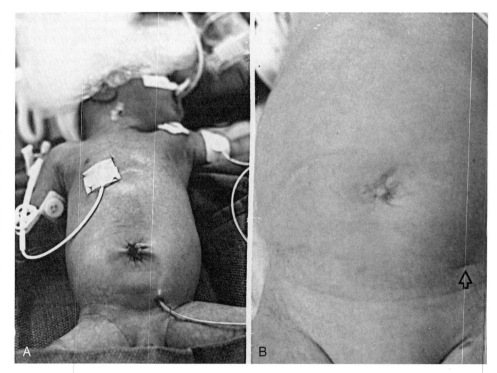

FIGURE 46-12. *A,* Postoperative view of an infant with gastroschisis who has undergone reduction of the intestine and primary fascial closure. It was not necessary to enlarge the fascial defect in this patient, and umbilicoplasty was easily performed. Note the Broviac catheter, which was placed in the right common facial vein and exteriorized on the lower chest wall. In the lower abdominal wall is an umbilical artery catheter placed through the left umbilical artery. The artery and catheter were transposed and exteriorized through a small incision in the inguinal region. *B,* the same infant at age 3 months. Note the small incision (*open arrow*) on the lower abdominal wall where the umbilical artery catheter was exteriorized.

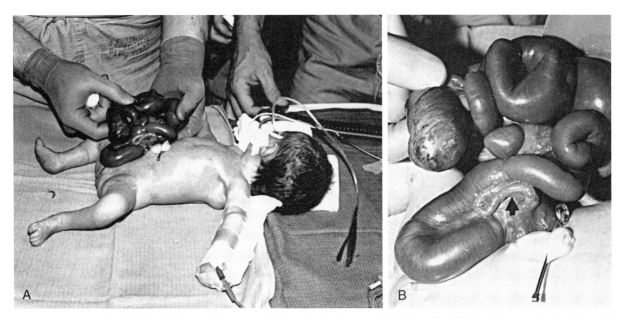

FIGURE 46-13. *A* and *B*, An infant with gastroschisis and colonic atresia. *B*, Note the blind ending proximal colon and the collapsed distal colon (*solid arrow*).

pulmonary insufficiency. About 15% of gastroschisis patients will have intestinal atresia.

In one report of 75 infants with abdominal wall defects, twice as many babies had gastroschisis.[35] The omphalocele patients had a significantly higher rate (66%) of associated anomalies, with a majority having either cardiac defects (50%) or chromosomal abnormalities (40%). The mortality rate of 34% in the omphalocele group was almost exclusively due to the associated anomalies. In the same report, gastroschisis had a greater association with prematurity (65%), and the mortality rate for gastroschisis approached 13%. An overall increased mortality was noted with the use of prosthetic silos, usually secondary to sepsis.

Another study of 104 patients with gastroschisis found 92 (90%) survivors.[36] Ninety survivors were available for follow-up. Of the 90 survivors, 36 were older than 5 years. Primary closure had been accomplished in 54 (52%) patients. A mortality rate of 10% was mainly due to the prematurity and respiratory failure.

One study looking at the mode of delivery involved 40 patients, 22 of whom were delivered by caesarian section, and 18 of whom were spontaneous vaginal deliveries.[37] All were repaired within 41 minutes of birth. They noted a shorter hospital stay (24 days vs. 34 days) in the caesarian section group and no long-term morbidity on subsequent evaluation.

Another study showed that, in 17 inborn and 5 outborn patients with gastroschisis, the mode of delivery had no impact on outcome, but the inborn patients had a shorter time to initiation of enteral feeding (9 days vs. 25 days) and to attainment of full enteral feeding status (16 days vs. 49 days).[38]

In a study at the Children's Hospital of Michigan, it appears better to perform elective caesarean section with planned operative repair immediately at birth. In that study, 32 patients were delivered by caesarean section, of whom 13 underwent immediate repair and 19 underwent early repair (<6 hours after birth).[32] A 30% incidence of premature births and a mortality rate of about 10% were found in each group. It was clear that patients had increasing amounts of bowel edema, matting, and the development of a thick peel, as time from birth to operation increased. Patients repaired immediately were able to undergo primary fascial repair in 77% of cases, and only 4 of 13 patients had a significant peel. In contrast, only 37% of patients who were repaired several hours later were able to undergo fascial closure, and a thick peel was noted in 18 of 19 patients.

Bowel function seems to return faster in patients with omphalocele than in patients with gastroschisis. In a 10-year review of abdominal wall defects, patients with omphalocele and no associated anomalies had 100% survival and had very quick return of bowel function. Gastroschisis, conversely, was associated with a much longer time until complete enteral feedings were tolerated.[38]

In a long-term study of patients with gastroschisis, normal bowel habits were noted in 76 (84%) patients.[36] Only 4 patients had chronic diarrhea, of which one had short gut. Abdominal complaints almost always led to nonspecific or functional diagnoses in patients that had uncomplicated gastroschisis. In complicated gastroschisis patients requiring bowel resection during the initial operation (22 patients), 10 (45%) patients had bowel complications. Of the 68 patients with uncomplicated reduction, 2 patients had late bowel complications with bowel obstruction. Ten percent of patients had surgical procedures for abdominal hernia, scar revision, or undescended testis. Operation is seldom required for midgut volvulus secondary to malrotation, and many surgeons do not do a Ladd procedure or appendectomy routinely.

Patients with uncomplicated gastroschisis have excellent long-term outcome, whereas those with complicated gastroschisis have the potential for persistent problems with bowel obstruction and short-bowel syndrome. Uncomplicated gastroschisis patients were found to be in the 32nd percentile at 5 years and then improve to the 52nd percentile in subsequent years. Patients with complicated gastroschisis, such as those with segments of atresia, tend to lag at the 25th percentile.[36]

Appropriate growth and development has been analyzed in several studies. In one study, 25 school-age children were identified from 90 patients available for follow-up and were progressing satisfactorily in school, whereas 7 were held back or enrolled in special classes. All of them participated in normal physical activities.[36] In another report, although many gastroschisis survivors were active and involved in academics and work, 40% were concerned about their stature and felt inadequate in sports and social activities.[39] Moreover, the absence of a naval was troubling to many older patients.[39,40] In one review, many patients still lived at home, although a few (15%) were married. Ten percent had children, but many were uneducated about transmission of the defect.[40]

In a recent study, 57 patients born with an abdominal wall defect were surveyed.[41] More than 80% reported their overall health as good. Small-bowel obstruction requiring lysis of adhesions had occurred in 9 (16%) patients. The abdominal scar was of concern to a third of the patients, with most having mild to no symptoms. No significant differences were found between the general population and patients with abdominal wall defects when looking at body mass index, height, incidence of functional gastrointestinal disorders, or psychosocial factors such as depression and self-esteem. The quality of life and educational level also were very similar to those of the general population. A slightly lower incidence of rheumatoid arthritis (7%) was noted compared with that in the general population. Many of these findings were found in earlier studies.[39,40]

It seems reasonable to report that patients with congenital abdominal wall defects experience late problems related mainly to associated anomalies or to simply having had an abdominal operation. Parents can be reassured that a good prognosis exists for future growth and development of their children.

REFERENCES

1. Aulus Cornelius Celsus, a Roman physician and medical writer, 30 B.C. to 40 A.D. (as cited in Jarcho J: Congenital umbilical hernia. Surg Gynecol Obstet 65:593–600, 1937).
2. Paulus Aegineta, a surgeon of the island of Aegina, who lived sometime between the 4th and 7th centuries AD. His Synopsis of Medicine was first published in Venice in 1528 in the original Greek (as cited in Jarcho J: Congenital umbilical hernia. Surg Gynecol Obstet 65:593–600, 1937).
3. Conrad Lycosthenes (1518–1561). Prodigiorum ac ostentorum chronicon. Basel: per Henricum Petri, 1557.
4. Reed EN: Infant disemboweled at birth: Appendectomy successful. JAMA 61:199, 1913.
5. Bernstein P: Gastroschisis: A rare teratological condition in the newborn. Arch Pediatr 57:505–513, 1940.
6. Klein MD, Hertzler JH: Congenital defects of the abdominal wall. Surg Gynecol Obstet 152:805–808, 1981.
7. Kozer E, Nikfar S, Costei A, et al: Aspirin consumption during the first trimester of pregnancy and congenital anomalies: A meta-analysis. Am J Obstet Gynecol 187:1623–1630, 2002.
8. Werler MM, Sheehan JE, Mitchell AA: Maternal medication use and risks of gastroschisis and small intestinal atresia. Am J Epidemiol 155:26–31, 2002.
9. Drongowski RA, Smith RK Jr, Coran AG: Contribution of demographic and environmental factors to the etiology of gastroschisis: A hypothesis. Fetal Diagn Ther 6:14–27, 1992.
10. Colombani PM, Cunningham MD: Perinatal aspects of omphalocele and gastroschisis. Am J Dis Child 131:1386–1388, 1977.
11. Hey W: Practical Observation in Surgery. London, Cadell & Davis, 1803.
12. Ahlfeld F: Der Alkahol bei der Behnadlung inoperable Bauchbrueche. Monatsschr Geburtsh Gynaek 10:124, 1899.
13. Grob M: Conservative treatment of exomphalos. Arch Dis Child 38:148–150, 1963.
14. Ein SH, Shandling B: A new nonoperative treatment of large omphaloceles with a polymer membrane. J Pediatr Surg 13:255–257, 1978.
15. Gross RE: A new method for surgical treatment of omphaloceles. Surgery 24:277–292, 1948.
16. Schuster SR: A new method for the staged repair of large omphaloceles. Surg Gynecol Obstet 125:837–850, 1967.
17. Greenwood RD, Rosenthal A, Nadas AS: Cardiovascular malformations associated with omphalocele. J Pediatr 85:818–821, 1974.
18. Saller DN Jr, Canick JA, Palomaki GE, et al: Second-trimester maternal serum alpha-fetoprotein, unconjugated estriol, and hCG levels in pregnancies with ventral wall defects. Obstet Gynecol 84:852–855, 1994.
19. Segel SY, Marder SJ, Parry S, et al: Fetal abdominal wall defects and mode of delivery: A systematic review. Obstet Gynecol 98:867–873, 2001.
20. Sheldon RE: The bowel bag: A sterile, transportable method for warming infants with skin defects. Pediatrics 53:267–269, 1974.
21. Filston HC, Izant RJ: Translocation of the umbilical artery to the lower abdomen: An adjunct to the postoperative monitoring of arterial blood gases in the major abdominal wall defects. J Pediatr Surg 10:225–229, 1975.
22. Krummel TM, Sieber WK: Closure of congenital abdominal wall defects with umbilicoplasty. Surg Gynecol Obstet 165:168–169, 1987.
23. Festen C, Severihnen, vd Staak FH: Nonsurgical (conservative) treatment of giant omphalocele: A report of 10 cases. Clin Pediatr 26:35–39, 1987.
24. Wesley JR, Drongowski R, Coran AG: Intragastric pressure measurement: A guide for reduction and closure of the Silastic chimney in omphalocele and gastroschisis. J Pediatr Surg 16:264–270, 1981.
25. Lacey SR, Carris LA, Beyer AJ 3rd, et al: Bladder pressure monitoring significantly enhances care of infants with abdominal wall defects: A prospective clinical study. J Pediatr Surg 28:1370–1374, 1993.
26. Cantrell JR, Haller JA, Ravitch MM: A syndrome of congenital defects involving the abdominal wall, sternum, diaphragm, pericardium and heart. Surg Gynecol Obstet 107:602, 1958.
27. Vazquez-Jimenez JF, Muehler EG, Daebritz S, et al: Cantrell's syndrome: A challenge to the surgeon. Ann Thorac Surg 65:1178–1185, 1998.
28. Shaw A: Myth of gastroschisis. J Pediatr Surg 10:235–244, 1975.
29. Moore TC, Collins DL, Catanzarite V, et al: Pre-term and particularly pre-labor cesarean section to avoid complications of gastroschisis. Pediatr Surg Int 15:97–104, 1999.
30. Huang J, Kurkchubasche AG, Carr SR, et al: Benefits of term delivery in infants with antenatally diagnosed gastroschisis. Obstet Gynecol 100:695–699, 2002.
31. Wald NJ, Barlow RD, Cuckle HS, et al: Ratio of amniotic fluid acetylcholinesterase to pseudocholinesterase as an antenatal diagnostic test for exomphalos and gastroschisis. Br J Obstet Gynaecol 91:882–884, 1984.
32. Coughlin JP, Drucker DE, Jewell MR, et al: Delivery room repair of gastroschisis. Surgery 114:822–827, 1993.

33. Harmel RP Jr: Primary repair of gastroschisis with umbilicoplasty. Surg Gynecol Obstet 160:464–465, 1985.
34. Rubin SZ, Martin DJ, Ein SH: A critical look at delayed intestinal motility in gastroschisis. Can J Surg 21:414–416, 1978.
35. Mayer T, Black R, Matlak M, et al: Gastroschisis and omphalocele: An eight year review. Ann Surg 192:783–787, 1980.
36. Swartz KR, Harrison MW, Campbell JR, et al: Long term follow up of patients with gastroschisis. Am J Surg 151:546–659, 1986.
37. Malas NO, Al-Ghoweri AS, Shwyiat RM: The outcome analysis of 40 cases of fetal gastroschisis. Saudi Med J 23:1083–1086, 2002.
38. Kitchanan S, Patole SK, Muller R, et al: Neonatal outcome of gastroschisis and exomphalos: A 10 year review. J Pediatr Child Health 36:428–430, 2000.
39. Tunell WP, Puffinbarger NK, Tuggle DW, et al: Abdominal wall defects in infants: Survival and implications of adult life. Ann Surg 221:525–529, 1995.
40. Davies BW, Stringer MD: The survivors of gastroschisis. Arch Dis Child 77:158–160, 1977.
41. Koivusalo A, Lindahl H, Rintala RJ: Morbidity and quality of life in adult patients with a congenital abdominal wall defect: A questionnaire survey. J Pediatr Surg 37:1594–1601, 2002.

CHAPTER 47

Umbilical and Other Abdominal Wall Hernias

Victor F. Garcia, MD

Abdominal wall hernias are among the most common surgical conditions found in infants and children. The clinical significance of these hernias varies from a considerable risk of strangulation to only the need to reassure a concerned parent. The care of children with abdominal wall hernias centers on which of these defects need timely surgical repair and which simply need time. Knowledge of the embryology, natural history, anatomy, indications for operation, and appropriate timing of operative repair is essential to manage abdominal wall hernias optimally.

UMBILICAL HERNIA

Etiology and Embryology

The anterior wall of the embryo develops from the somatopleure of the overhanging head and tail folds.[1] Simultaneous closure of these folds from the cranial, caudal, and lateral directions forms the umbilical ring around the umbilical cord. The umbilical cord represents the fusion of the yolk stalk containing the vitelline duct, the body stalk containing the paired umbilical arteries, the umbilical vein, and the allantois. The ring closes by contracture after the cord is ligated and the umbilical vessels thrombose. Typically the umbilical cord separates about 5 to 8 days after birth. An umbilical hernia develops when the umbilical ring does not close after the cord separates.

The development of an umbilical hernia has an embryologic as well as an anatomic basis.[2] Embryologically, failure of the recti to approximate in the midline after the return of the midgut predisposes the fetus to develop an umbilical hernia.[1] Anatomically, the umbilical ring consists of the umbilical scar, the round ligament, and the umbilical fascia.

Usually the round ligament passes over the superior margin of the umbilical ring and attaches to the inferior margin of the ring.[1] When the round ligament attaches only to the superior margin of the ring, the floor of the umbilical ring is formed only by the umbilical fascia and the peritoneum. This attenuated floor predisposes the fetus to develop an umbilical hernia.[1]

Incidence

Umbilical hernia is one of the most common conditions seen in infancy and childhood. The true incidence is unknown because many umbilical hernias resolve spontaneously.[3] Race and prematurity are predisposing factors favoring the development of an umbilical hernia. Umbilical hernias are up to 10 times more common in African Americans than in whites.[4,5] In South Africa, the racial disparity is not so marked, with umbilical hernias found in 23% of blacks and 19% of whites.[6] Umbilical hernias are more common in premature than in term infants and are noted in 75% to 84% of infants weighing less than 1500 g.[4,7,8]

Although most umbilical hernias are isolated findings in otherwise healthy infants, a number of clinical disorders are associated with umbilical hernias, including trisomy 21, congenital hypothyroidism, mucopolysaccharidosis, and exomphalos/macroglossia/gigantism.[3]

Natural History

Most umbilical hernias are recognized shortly after birth. Related symptoms are rare. In some instances, the combination of a large fascial defect, redundant umbilical skin, and a straining infant results in a tense proboscis. The concerned parent should be advised that evisceration is unlikely and continued observation is safe.

Few definitive studies document the natural history of umbilical hernias.[6,9] The general belief is that the majority regress with time. One study suggests that the incidence decreases with age, and complete resolution occurs by age 13 years.[6]

In general, the diameter and the sharpness of the fascial edge are predictors of spontaneous closure.[9] Hernias with a diameter greater than 1.5 to 2.0 cm are less likely to close on their own.[6,9] The thicker and more rounded the fascial edge, the more likely the hernia will close. Openings with a thin, sharp edge tend not to close.[2] If the fascial ring is not completely intact, spontaneous closure is unlikely.

If the hernia persists as the child approaches school age (age 4 to 5 years), it should be repaired. Earlier repair is warranted if symptoms of incarceration or recurring pain develop.[3] Repair at age 2 to 3 years is advocated if the fascial defect is greater than 2.0 cm.[10] Consideration should be given to repairing the hernia and excising the proboscis of skin that is seen on some young girls.

If not repaired in childhood, 10% of umbilical hernias will persist to adulthood.[11,12] The defect may enlarge in women during pregnancy, and a greater risk of incarceration is found in adults than in children.[3]

Historically the risk of incarceration or strangulation of an umbilical hernia is considered rare.[6] Two studies from the 1990s, however, suggest that incarceration occurs more frequently than is generally believed.[13,14]

Operative Technique

Operative repair is performed as an outpatient procedure under general anesthesia. The operative technique is illustrated in Figure 47-1. The redundant skin after closure of a proboscoid hernia can be managed by using a purse-string stitch,[15] a V-Y plasty,[16] or an umbilicoplasty.[17-19] A paraumbilical block[20,21] or a preincisional caudal epidural block can be used in addition to local infiltration to minimize postoperative pain.

Parents are encouraged to administer oral analgesics early in the postoperative period before the effects of regional or local anesthesia have dissipated.

A tonsil sponge may be secured with tape to compress the loose umbilical skin. No activity restrictions are necessary. The dressing is removed in 5 to 7 days. Complications are uncommon.

EPIGASTRIC HERNIA

Etiology

Epigastric hernias result from defects in the interstices of the decussating fibers of the linea alba. The etiology of epigastric hernias is unknown. The defects may be multiple, and they are typically elliptical with a transverse long axis. Usually, only preperitoneal fat herniates through the defect.

Incidence

Epigastric hernias are seen in about 5% of children. Children are first seen either with a visible palpable mass or with intermittent pain localized to the site of the hernia. When present, the mass is, at times, tender and is usually no larger than 0.5 to 1 cm. Occasionally a defect is noted without a palpable mass.

The small size of the mass and the defect makes identification problematic once the child is anesthetized. Therefore when the child is awake, the exact location of the hernia, usually in relation to a distinct part of the umbilicus, should be marked.

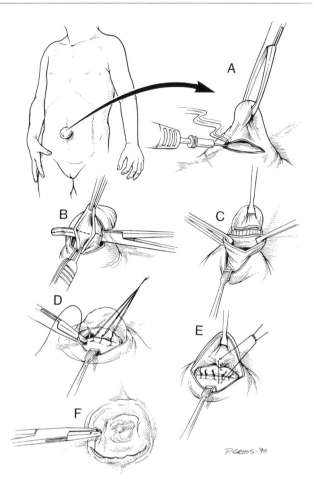

FIGURE 47-1. Technique for operative repair for umbilical hernia. *A,* An infraumbilical skin crease incision is made. *B,* The hernia sac is opened, leaving a portion of the sac attached to the umbilical skin for ease of subsequent umbilicoplasty. *C,* The umbilical sac has been completely divided and excised to strong fascia. *D,* The fascial defect is closed in a transverse fashion with interrupted, simple nonabsorbable sutures. *E,* The remaining umbilical sac, which is attached to the umbilical skin, is secured to the fascia with interrupted, absorbable sutures. *F,* The skin incision is closed with a subcuticular suture. Pressure dressing is placed to prevent formation of a hematoma or seroma.

Epigastric hernias do not spontaneously resolve and therefore should be repaired. A limited transverse incision is made over the defect. If herniated fat is present, it is reduced or ligated, and then excised. The defect is then closed with absorbable sutures by using buried knots. The skin is closed with an absorbable subcuticular suture.

The procedure is performed on an outpatient basis. No postoperative limitations in activities are necessary, and complications are rare.

LUMBAR HERNIA

Lumbar hernias are rare in children. They can occur in otherwise normal babies but may be associated with lumbocostovertebral deficiency syndrome.[2] They occur through one of two areas of potential weakness: the superior or the inferior lumbar area.

Most congenital lumbar hernias occur in the superior lumbar triangle. This triangle is covered by the latissimus dorsi muscle and is bordered by the 12th rib, the internal oblique muscle, and the sacrospinalis muscle. Penetration of the 12th intercostal nerve and vessels in the lumbodorsal fascia in this area can cause a defect leading to the development of a hernia. The defect is usually small but eventually enlarges and may become symptomatic.

The boundaries of the inferior lumbar triangle are the latissimus dorsi posteriorly, the external oblique muscle anteriorly, and the iliac crest inferiorly. The defect occurs at the site of penetration of the iliohypogastric, ilioinguinal, or lumbar nerves.

A lumbar hernia presents as a bulge, usually of retroperitoneal fat. Incarceration or strangulation is rare.[2,22] Palpation may reveal a soft swelling that is easily reducible. If the defect is not palpable, ultrasonography (US) or computed tomography (CT) may be necessary to identify the exact location of the hernia defect.

Closure of the fascial defect should be done without tension. Rarely, prosthetic material or a gluteus maximus fascial flap may be necessary to permit a tension-free closure of larger defects.

SPIGELIAN HERNIA

Spigelian hernias develop at the intersection of the linea semilunaris, the lateral border of the rectus abdominis muscle, and the linea semicircularis, the caudal termination of the posterior sheath of the rectus muscles. The semilunar line marks the transition from muscle to aponeurosis of the transverses abdominis muscle.

The defect usually involves the transversus abdominis and internal oblique muscles but may or may not involve the external oblique muscles. Therefore a spigelian hernia is interparietal, may not be palpable, and thus may be difficult to diagnose.[23] In most cases, the defect is located 0 to 6 cm cranial to the horizontal plane through both anterior iliac spines. Spigelian hernias are more common in girls and more likely to occur on the right side than on the left.[2] Examination may reveal a tender mass, usually below the umbilicus.

Although the hernia sac may be large, the defect is usually small. Pain is common, at first intermittent, but often progressing to a constant, dull discomfort. Twenty percent of spigelian hernias present with strangulation.[2,23] Diagnosis may be aided by having the cooperative child tense his or her abdominal muscles, reproducing a specific point of tenderness.

US and CT scans may identify the fascial defect within the layers of the abdominal wall. If the defect is not palpable but is noted on CT scan or US, it is advisable to mark the site of the defect by using radiologic guidance.

The high risk of incarceration or strangulation makes operative repair necessary. A transverse incision is made over the mass or site of the defect, as identified by US or CT scan. Once the external oblique is incised, the sac is encountered. This is excised, and the fascial defect closed. Recurrence rate is low.

REFERENCES

1. Skandalakis J, Gray SQW, Ricketts R: The anterior abdominal wall. In: Skandalakis JG (ed): Embryology for Surgeons, 2nd ed. Baltimore, Williams & Wilkins, 1994, pp 540–593.
2. Zinner MS: Hernias. In: Ellis H (ed): Maingot. Abdominal Operations. Norwalk, Conn, Appleton & Lange, 1997, pp 479–580.
3. Scherer LR III, Grosfeld JL: Inguinal hernia and umbilical anomalies. Pediatr Clin North Am 40:1121–1131, 1993.
4. Crump E: Umbilical hernia: Occurrence of the infantile type in negro infants and children. J Pediatr 40:214, 1952.
5. Evans A: The comparative incidence of umbilical hernias in colored and white infants. J Natl Med Assoc 33:158, 1941.
6. Blumberg NA: Infantile umbilical hernia. Surg Gynecol Obstet 150:187–192, 1980.
7. Woods GE: Some observations on umbilical hernia in infants. Arch Dis Child 28:450–462, 1953.
8. Vohr BR, Rosenfield AG, Oh W: Umbilical hernia in the low-birth-weight infant (less than 1,500 gm). J Pediatr 90:807–808, 1997.
9. Walker SH: The natural history of umbilical hernia: A six-year follow up of 314 Negro children with this defect. Clin Pediatr (Phila) 6:29–32, 1967.
10. Morgan WW, White JJ, Stumbaugh S, et al: Prophylactic umbilical hernia repair in childhood to prevent adult incarceration. Surg Clin North Am 50:839–845, 1970.
11. Jackson DM: Umbilical hernia. Calif Med 113:8–11, 1970.
12. Scott DJ, Jones DB: Hernias and abdominal wall defects. In: Norton JB, Chang RR, Lowry AE, et al. (eds): Surgery: Basic Science and Clinical Evidence. New York, Springer-Verlag, 2000, pp 787–823.
13. Mawera G, Muguti GI: Umbilical hernia in Bulawayo: Some observations from a hospital-based study. Cent Afr J Med 40:319–323, 1994.
14. Vrsansky P, Bourdelat D: Incarcerated umbilical hernia in children. Pediatr Surg Int 12:61–62, 1997.
15. Cone JB, Golladay ES: Purse-string skin closure of umbilical hernia repair. J Pediatr Surg 18:297, 1993.
16. Jamra FA: Reconstruction of the umbilicus by a double V-Y procedure. Plast Reconstr Surg 64:106–110, 1979.
17. Reyna TM, Hollis HW Jr, Smith SB: Surgical management of proboscoid herniae. J Pediatr Surg 22:911–912, 1987.
18. Billmire DF: A technique for the repair of giant umbilical hernia in children. J Am Coll Surg 194:677–680, 2002.
19. Koshy CE, Taams KO: Umbilicoplasty. Plast Reconstr Surg 104:1203–1204, 1999.
20. Courreges P: [Periumbilical analgesia: Paraumbilical block or rectus sheath block?]. Ann Fr Anesth Reanim 21:753, 2002.
21. Courreges P, Poddevin F, Lecoutre D: Para-umbilical block: A new concept for regional anaesthesia in children. Paediatr Anaesth 7:211–214, 1997.
22. Mehta MH, Patel RV, Mehta SG: Congenital lumbar hernia. J Pediatr Surg 27:1258–1259, 1992.
23. Spangen L: Spigelian hernia. Surg Clin North Am 64:351–366, 1984.

CHAPTER 48

Laparoscopy

George W. Holcomb, III, MD, MBA, and Keith E. Georgeson, MD

Despite the early proliferation of the use of laparoscopic surgical procedures in adults, this approach was slower to evolve in the pediatric surgical arena for several reasons. First, most pediatric surgeons did not appreciate the advantages of this approach for their patients. Many operations on infants and children have a relatively short hospitalization and relatively little discomfort compared with a similar procedure in adults. Further reducing the hospitalization and postoperative pain was not considered to be as advantageous as with adults. In addition, these operations were often more technically demanding in the young child or infant. Therefore because of the difficulty in performing many of these operations in infants, a hesitancy existed to embark on this new approach. Today, the benefits of the laparoscopic approach for infants and children are readily recognized, and most training programs have, at the very least, one person who is adept with this technology. Moreover, the current common concern is not how to apply the laparoscopic technique for pediatric surgical diseases, but whether robotics will be an important component of the minimally invasive surgeon's armamentarium (see Chapter 77). It appears that the debate on the application of robotics today is similar to the debate on the use of laparoscopy 15 years ago.

CONCERNS IN CHILDREN

Almost every operation performed by pediatric surgeons today has been accomplished by using the laparoscopic approach. This listing of laparoscopic operations ranges from the relatively routine, such as cholecystectomy and appendectomy, to the extremely complex, such as portoenterostomy for biliary atresia. Regardless of the operation to be performed, a number of concerns are important for children. One major concern is the pliability and laxity of the abdominal wall, especially in young children. Because of this pliability, it is quite easy to introduce a cannula with a sharp trocar through the abdominal wall and into an underlying visceral or vascular structure,

turning a routine operation into an emergency procedure. Therefore it is imperative that the surgeon recognize this issue of the pliability of the abdominal wall and take great care not to injure the underlying structures when introducing a sharp trocar. One technique to avoid this problem is to direct the sharp stylet more in a transverse direction above the viscera once it has penetrated the peritoneum rather than continuing in an oblique or downward direction toward the viscera and major vessels. Injuries can occur with these sharp stylets whether or not a safety shield is attached to the trocar. Another technique used by many pediatric surgeons for safety reasons is the Step System (US Surgical, Norwalk, CT). With this technique, after a small skin incision, a Veress needle with an expandable sheath is introduced through the abdominal wall into the peritoneal cavity. The Veress needle is then removed, and a cannula with a blunt-tipped trocar is introduced through the expandable sheath. It is unlikely that the blunt trocar will injure the underlying vasculature, and the expandable sheath stabilizes the cannula in the abdominal wall. This same Veress needle technique is used by some pediatric surgeons for the initial cannula entry, usually through the umbilicus. With this approach, an incision (3 mm, 5 mm, 10 mm, or 12 mm) is made in the umbilical skin, and the Veress needle and sheath are introduced through the umbilical fascia and into the peritoneal cavity. Great care must be taken when introducing the Veress needle and cannula with this approach. Often it is helpful to grasp the abdominal wall manually and elevate it away from the underlying structures when introducing this Veress needle. A blind-man's-cane technique is then used by moving the Veress needle side to side, such as a blind man testing the surface in front of him before taking the next step. Once the surgeon is satisfied that the Veress needle is inside the abdominal cavity, insufflation is initiated, followed by removal of the Veress needle and introduction of a cannula with a blunt trocar through the expandable sheath. Other surgeons prefer a more direct cutdown approach by incising the umbilical skin and fascia, followed by introducing the cannula through the umbilical fascia into the peritoneal cavity. One modification of this approach is to insert only the expandable sheath (without the needle) through the umbilical fascial and peritoneal incision, followed by insertion of the cannula with the blunt-tipped trocar through the expandable sheath (Fig. 48-1). In experienced hands, all of these techniques for initial entry into the peritoneal cavity are safe, and few recent reports exist of injuries to underlying viscera with careful introduction of cannulas in infants and children.

Once the initial cannula has been placed and a pneumoperitoneum established, accessory instruments are introduced. Some surgeons prefer the use of additional cannulas through which the instruments are inserted and removed from the peritoneal cavity. These accessory cannulas are either reusable, reposable (part reusable, part disposable), or completely disposable. The main disadvantage of the completely disposable cannula is the cost for one-time use. These ports can be either 3, 4, 5, 10, 12, or 15 mm, depending on the operation. For many procedures in children, 3-mm instruments are preferred, whereas for laparoscopic appendectomy in which the 12-mm stapler is used, a 12-mm port is necessary. Similarly, for laparoscopic splenectomy in which a 15-mm endoscopic retrieval bag is used, a 15-mm port is required. Whereas some surgeons prefer the use of cannulas for introduction of these accessory instruments, another technique is to introduce the instruments directly through the abdominal wall without the use of cannulas (Fig. 48-2).[1] With this technique, a stab incision is made with a no. 11 blade (Becton Dickinson, Franklin Lakes, NJ) through the skin and abdominal wall under telescopic visualization. The blade is removed, and the 3- or 5-mm instrument is inserted through the path created by the blade (Fig. 48-3). This technique is especially applicable for infants and young children when 3- and 5-mm instruments are used. It also is applicable for older children and adolescents with relatively thin abdominal walls for procedures in which instruments are not moved

in and out of the abdominal wall during the operation. If instruments are exchanged frequently throughout the procedure, it is best to use a cannula at this site. Although a cosmetic advantage exists with laparoscopy, the biggest advantage to the stab technique is the cost savings realized by not using either a reposable or disposable cannula system. In one recent study of 511 patients undergoing laparoscopic procedures using this stab-incision technique, a total of $187,180 was saved in patient charges over a 3.5-year period (Table 48-1).[1]

Diagnostic Laparoscopy

Laparoscopy for diagnostic purposes in pediatric patients was reported in the early 1970s for several conditions including evaluation of a contralateral patent processus vaginalis (CPPV).[2,3] Diagnostic laparoscopy also may be useful in boys with a nonpalpable testis. Moreover, it may be helpful in patients with cancer requiring a second-look procedure to determine the possibility of residual disease after chemotherapy (Fig. 48-4). In the cancer patient, laparoscopy is often used for determination of resectability as well as an adjunct for guided biopsy. Finally, diagnostic laparoscopy can be very useful in selected patients with penetrating trauma who are stable and in whom a question exists of peritoneal penetration (Fig. 48-5). If no injury is found, the patient may be discharged within 24 hours, as opposed to the several days needed for recovery after laparotomy.

Diagnostic Laparoscopy for Contralateral Patent Processus Vaginalis

In the early 1990s, two reports were published describing diagnostic laparoscopy through the umbilicus in children with a unilateral inguinal hernia to determine evidence of a CPPV.[4,5] Several years later, with the advent of 3-mm angled telescopes, it became apparent that this

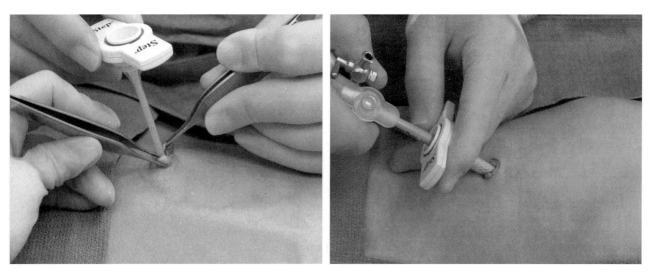

FIGURE 48-1. When introducing the initial umbilical cannula for laparoscopy, one approach is a direct umbilical cutdown technique, with insertion of the expandable Step sheath (*left*) followed by introduction of the cannula with a blunt trocar through the sheath (*right*). In this way, injuries from the use of the Veress needle technique are avoided.

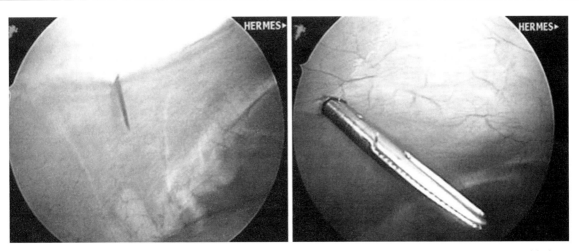

FIGURE 48-2. The technique for creating a transabdominal stab incision is shown. *Left,* The no. 11 blade is seen to pass through the abdominal wall and into the peritoneal cavity. *Right,* The no. 11 blade has been removed, and the instrument is directly introduced through the path created by the blade.

same information could be obtained through the ipsilateral hernia sac.[6] A number of reports confirmed the efficacy of this technique to determine the presence of a CPPV, which may indicate the need for repair under the same anesthetic.[7-10] The accuracy of this technique approaches 99%. However, it is not possible to determine in which patient with a CPPV a symptomatic hernia will develop. At the same time, it does subselect those patients who should undergo contralateral exploration based on a

positive finding rather than subjecting all children with a unilateral inguinal hernia to contralateral exploration, as has been advocated in the past. A few surgeons have taken this approach one step further and are performing various types of laparoscopic hernia repairs in children.[11,12]

The technique for evaluating the contralateral inguinal region involves creation of a pneumoperitoneum through the hernia sac, followed by diagnostic laparoscopy with

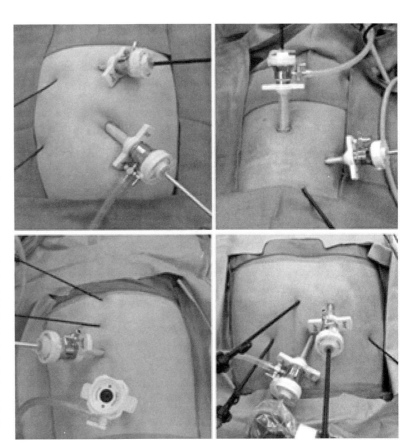

FIGURE 48-3. This photograph depicts the use of stab incisions with introduction of the instruments through the abdominal wall, without the use of accessory cannulas. In each photograph, an umbilical cannula appears through which the telescope is introduced and insufflation is achieved. *Upper left,* A teenager is undergoing a laparoscopic cholecystectomy. Two 5-mm and two 3-mm instruments are placed directly through the abdominal wall. *Upper right,* The patient is undergoing a laparoscopic appendectomy with a 5-mm instrument placed directly through the abdominal wall in the left suprapubic region. *Lower left,* The patient is undergoing a laparoscopic splenectomy. A 12-mm cannula is placed in the umbilicus, and a 5-mm cannula is introduced in the midline epigastrium. Two 3-mm instruments are placed through stab incisions cephalad to the 5-mm cannula. *Lower right,* An adolescent is undergoing a laparoscopic fundoplication. A second cannula has been placed in the patient's left upper abdomen, through which the ultrasonic scalpel and needle holder are introduced.

TABLE 48-1

A LISTING OF THE SAVINGS IN CHARGES TO THE PATIENT AND COST TO THE HOSPITAL REALIZED BY USING THE STAB INCISION TECHNIQUE ALONG WITH ONE- OR TWO-STEP CANNULAS (CENTER COLUMN)

Procedure	Step Pt./Instit. Savings ($)	Ethicon Pt./Intit. Savings ($)
Nissen (209)	117,040/51,832	76,912/34,276
Nissen (14)	5,880/2,604	3,864/1,722
Appendectomy (102)	14,280/6,324	9,384/4,182
Pyloromyotomy (77)	21,560/9,548	14,168/6,314
Cholecystectomy (31)	8,680/3,844	5,704/2,542
Splenectomy (21)	5,880/2,604	3,864/1,722
Pull-through (20)	2,800/1,240	1,840/820
Ligation testicular vessels (UDT) (15)	4,200/1,860	2,760/1,230
Esophagomyotomy (7)	2,940/1,302	1,932/861
Adrenalectomy (6)	1,680/744	1,104/492
Varicocele (5)	1,400/620	920/410
Ovarian (2)	560/248	368/164
Meckel's diverticulum (2)	280/124	184/82
511 Operations	$187,180/$82,894	$123,004/$54,817

If Ethicon cannulas were used, the savings that would have occurred are seen as well (right column).
Reprinted with permission from Ostlie DJ, Holcomb GW III: The use of stab incisions for instrument access in laparoscopic operations. J Pediatr Surg 38:1837–1840, 2003.
UDT, undescended testes.

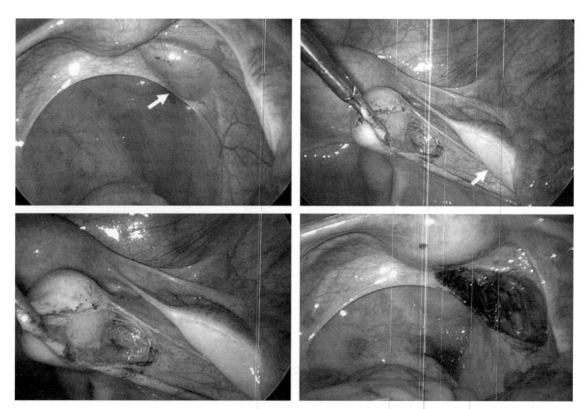

FIGURE 48-4. Second-look laparoscopy can be useful after adjuvant therapy in certain circumstances. In this teenage patient who previously had undergone laparotomy and resection of a large germ cell tumor, second-look laparoscopy was performed to determine whether evidence of residual disease existed. *Upper left,* Residual disease is seen along the right pelvic side wall (*white arrow*). *Upper right,* This mass is being resected from the pelvic side wall. Note the normal right ovary (*white arrow*). *Lower left,* Further dissection of the mass is achieved. *Lower right,* The mass has been completely excised, with hemostasis controlled by cautery.

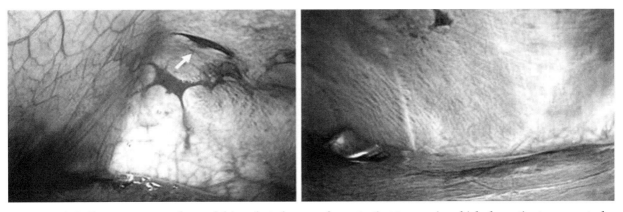

FIGURE 48-5. Laparoscopy can be useful in selected cases of penetrating trauma in which the patient appears to be uninjured, yet there is concern that the sharp object, or perhaps a bullet, has penetrated the abdominal cavity. *Left,* An entrance wound from a bullet that entered the peritoneal cavity (*white arrow*). *Right,* The bullet is seen to lie on top of the left lobe of the liver just beneath the entry site. This patient did not have other injuries and was discharged the next day. A laparotomy was avoided in this patient.

an angled (usually 45- to 70-degree) telescope. Some surgeons insufflate the peritoneum by introducing a cannula into the abdomen through the hernia sac, whereas others use a catheter. Either technique appears to work well.

At laparoscopy, it is usually evident whether a CPPV is present (Fig. 48-6). However, on occasion, a veil of peritoneum may obscure the visualization of the contralateral inguinal ring. At times, the length of the CPPV may not be clear. A technique has been described in which a silver probe is percutaneously introduced on the contralateral side to retract the peritoneal veil or to evaluate the length of the CPPV (Fig. 48-7).[13]

In a combined study of more than 1500 patients younger than 10 years with a unilateral inguinal hernia, a CPPV was identified in 40%. Physical examination, even under anesthesia, was found to be a poor predictor for the presence of a CPPV.[14] The issue of which CPPV requires operation is still undecided.

PROCEDURAL LAPAROSCOPY

Stomach and Solid Organs

Fundoplication

The laparoscopic operation for fundoplication is rapidly becoming the preferred approach for surgical management of gastroesophageal reflux. Any type of fundoplication, including a Nissen, Thal, Toupet, Boix-Ochoa, or other, can be performed by using the laparoscopic approach. It is our experience that the laparoscopic Nissen fundoplication is the easiest operation to perform laparoscopically and yields the best results, but this belief is not shared by all pediatric surgeons. Complications have been minimal, and results, very satisfactory. Transmigration (herniation) of the fundoplication wrap through the esophageal hiatus has been found to develop

in 3% to 5% of patients undergoing laparoscopic fundoplication. It is possible that the lack of scarring near the esophageal hiatus after a laparoscopic fundoplication allows retraction of the esophagus and the fundoplication wrap through the esophageal hiatus. Because of this concern, additional steps have been taken in our technique to prevent this problem.

A 4- or 5-mm transumbilical cannula is placed in most patients. In adolescents, especially tall patients with a narrow costal margin, it may be more appropriate to place this initial cannula in the midepigastric region. After pneumoperitoneum, four additional instruments are introduced by using either cannulas or the stab-incision technique. The short gastric vessels are divided beginning at a point midway along the greater curvature of the stomach and progressing to the esophageal hiatus (Fig. 48-8). The gastroesophageal (GE) junction is initially approached from the patient's left side and the retroesophageal space is identified and opened. The esophagus is then freed from the diaphragmatic crura in all directions by using blunt and sharp dissection to create an adequate portion of intra-abdominal esophagus. After mobilizing the intra-abdominal esophagus, the diaphragmatic crura are usually approximated, at least with one suture, which is placed posterior to the esophagus (see Fig. 48-8). If the hiatus is greatly enlarged, a second suture may be needed anteriorly (Fig. 48-9). After crural repair, the esophagus is sutured to the narrowed hiatus at 3 or 4 sites several centimeters above the GE junction (see Fig. 48-9). This suture fixation helps to prevent transmigration of the fundoplication wrap through the hiatus. After adding this modification to our technique, the incidence of transmigration of the wrap has markedly diminished. An appropriate size transesophageal bougie is then introduced into the stomach. The fundus is wrapped around the intra-abdominal esophagus and sutured back to itself in a standard Nissen fundoplication fashion. In a recent study, a fundoplication length of approximately 2 cm was found to be effective in

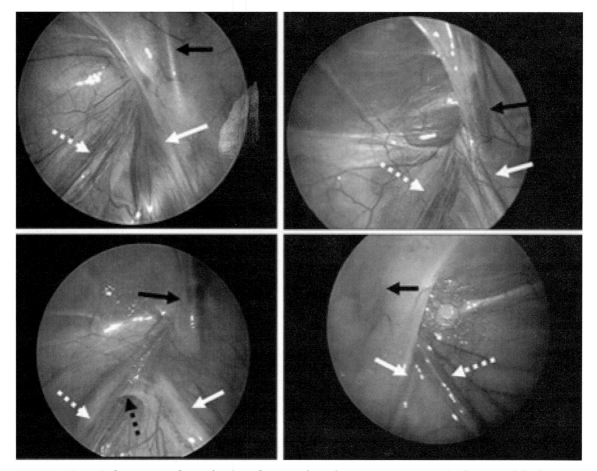

FIGURE 48-6. At laparoscopy for evaluation of a contralateral patent processus vaginalis, several findings are possible. In each of these photographs, the *dotted white arrow* depicts the testicular vessels, and the *solid white arrow* depicts the vas deferens. An additional *black arrow* shows the inferior epigastric vessels. *Upper left,* No evidence is seen of a left patent processus vaginalis. *Upper right,* A large internal opening to a patent processus vaginalis. *Lower left,* This patient had a right hydrocele and, at laparoscopy, no evidence was found of a significant patent processus vaginalis. However, a veil of peritoneum covers the testicular vessels (*dotted black arrow*), and there appears to be a small opening to a patent processus vaginalis. In this setting, however, it is unclear how distal the small patent processus vaginalis extends. *Lower right,* Air bubbles are seen emanating from the internal opening of the right patent processus vaginalis when manual pressure is applied over the right inguinal canal.

relieving symptoms.[15] Usually, three 2-0 silk sutures are used to create the fundoplication wrap. At this point, with hemostasis ensured, the operation is terminated, and the cannulas/instruments are removed.

Gastrostomy

Laparoscopic gastrostomy may be performed either in conjunction with a laparoscopic fundoplication or as a separate procedure. When performed in conjunction with fundoplication, the site of placement of the gastrostomy button is the site of the main working port for the fundoplication in the left upper abdomen. This incision in the patient's left upper abdomen should be marked before creating the pneumoperitoneum. Otherwise, creation of the pneumoperitoneum will confuse the surgeon as to the appropriate location for the gastrostomy.

For laparoscopic gastrostomy alone, the site should be marked as well.

If laparoscopic gastrostomy is performed alone, a 4- or 5-mm cannula and telescope are introduced through the umbilicus. If it is performed after fundoplication, the telescope remains in place. A grasping forceps is introduced through the gastrostomy site incision in the left upper abdomen. It is often helpful to ask the anesthesiologist to insufflate the stomach. This maneuver reduces the likelihood that the posterior wall of the stomach will be caught by the fixation sutures, which are introduced next. After grasping a site for the gastrostomy on the anterior gastric wall near the greater curvature, the stomach is pulled anteriorly to approximate its serosa with the abdominal wall (Fig. 48-10). One 2-0 monofilament suture is placed on either side of the gastrostomy site. These sutures are placed extracorporally through the skin and abdominal

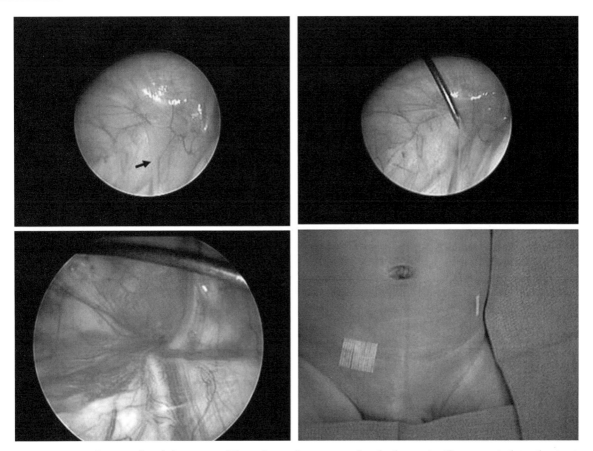

FIGURE 48-7. On occasion, it is not possible to determine accurately whether a significant contralateral patent processus vaginalis (CPPV) exists. *Upper left,* A veil of peritoneum (arrow) covers the left internal ring structures, and even with a 70-degree telescope, it is not possible to determine whether a CPPV is present. *Upper right,* A silver probe has been placed through a stab incision in the left lower abdomen. The tip of the silver probe is manipulated to retract the peritoneal veil, which, in the *lower left,* shows a blind end to the internal ring. Thus no evidence exists of a PPV on the left side. *Lower right,* The Steri-strips are seen placed over the right inguinal crease incision. A single Steri-strip is used to approximate the skin where the silver probe was introduced through the left lower abdominal wall.

wall cephalad to the gastrostomy site, then through the anterior stomach wall, and then out through the abdominal wall and skin caudad to the gastrostomy. Using the Cook Vascular Dilator Set (Cook, Inc., Bloomington, IN), a needle is placed through the gastrostomy incision and into the stomach. A guidewire is inserted and, by using the Seldinger technique, the skin and gastrostomy are sequentially dilated by using 8, 12, 16, and 20F dilators, which are introduced over the guidewire. The 8F dilator is inserted through the gastrostomy button and used to introduce the button into the stomach. The balloon is inflated under direct telescopic visualization. The dilator is removed, and the sutures are tied over the button. It is important to ensure that the guidewire and the button are definitely inside the stomach. It is helpful to use an angled telescope to inspect the entire circumference of the gastrostomy to confirm that the button is not outside the stomach. The patient may be fed by using the gastrostomy several hours after its placement, if desired. The 2-0 monofilament sutures are removed 4 or 5 days later.

Esophagomyotomy

In preparation for a laparoscopic esophagomyotomy for achalasia, it is important to give the patient a liquid diet for several days. Usually the lower esophagus will empty itself of solid food during this time. After induction of anesthesia, it is important to suction the esophagus thoroughly to evacuate any retained food particles and to insert an esophageal bougie. In the event of entry into the esophageal lumen during the operation, gross spillage will not occur into the peritoneal cavity.

Placement of incisions for laparoscopic esophagomyotomy is almost identical to that for a laparoscopic fundoplication. In addition, because an anterior partial fundoplication, rather than a full fundoplication, is usually performed, only the most cephalad two or three short gastric vessels are ligated and divided. After ligation and division of these short gastric vessels, the wall of the anterior lower esophagus is grasped on each side. Through the primary working port in the left upper

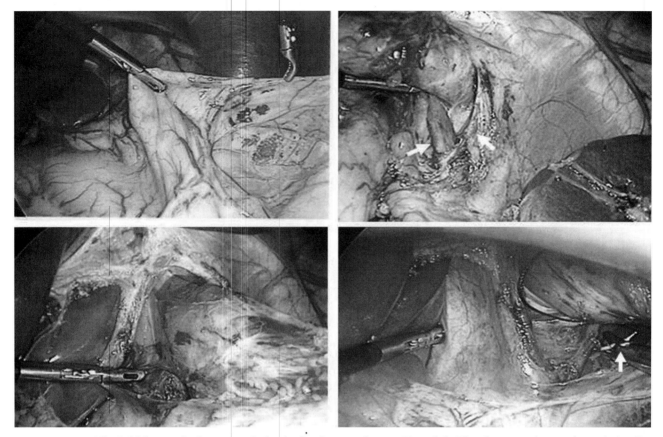

FIGURE 48-8. The initial steps for laparoscopic fundoplication are shown. *Upper left,* The short gastric vessels are being ligated and divided by using the Maryland dissecting instrument, which is attached to cautery. *Upper right,* The esophagus has been retracted anteriorly and to the patient's right, exposing the retroesophageal space. Note the right and left diaphragmatic crura (*white arrows*). *Lower left,* The patient's right diaphragmatic crus is being separated from the esophagus by using blunt dissection. *Lower right,* A 2-0 silk suture attached to an RB-1 needle (*arrow*) is being placed through the patient's left diaphragmatic crus for approximation of the crura.

abdomen, either the ultrasonic scalpel or hook cautery is used to divide the distal esophageal muscle down to the submucosa (Fig. 48-11). Once the submucosa is visualized, the ultrasonic scalpel is used, with the "hot" blade turned anterior, to create the esophagomyotomy for a distance of 4 to 6 cm cephalad. The esophagomyotomy usually extends through the esophageal hiatus for 1 or 2 cm. By using the same technique, the myotomy is extended onto the stomach for 1 or 2 cm to ensure that the circular fibers of the lower esophageal sphincter are completely divided. If any question remains, esophagoscopy can be performed to verify this complete myotomy. Should entry into the lumen occur, it is often easy to see the bougie through the mucosal perforation. A perforation can usually be closed laparoscopically.

After the anterior esophagomyotomy, a partial fundoplication is usually performed. This can be either a partial posterior (Toupet) fundoplication or an anterior (Dor) fundoplication. The advantage of the Dor procedure is that it covers the just-completed esophagomyotomy. For this reason, we prefer this anterior fundoplication. With interrupted 2-0 silk, the cephalad portion of the greater curvature of the fundus is sutured initially to the

left edge of the completed myotomy and the left diaphragmatic crus and then to the right edge of the completed myotomy and the right crus. Approximately three sutures are taken on each edge of the myotomy along with the diaphragmatic crus. These sutures also help to separate each side of the myotomy to help prevent recurrence of symptoms.

Before initiating a clear liquid diet the next day, a water-soluble contrast study is performed to ensure that the esophageal mucosa is intact. Most patients are ready for discharge either the morning after the operation or the second postoperative morning. Results with this operation in children have been favorable to date.[16–20]

Pyloromyotomy

Laparoscopic pyloromyotomy is rapidly gaining acceptance as an appropriate technique in infants. Although it has been difficult to document its advantages objectively, it is thought that less gastroparesis and an earlier initiation of feedings are found, which, in turn, leads to earlier discharge. However, this earlier discharge may be in terms of hours rather than days.

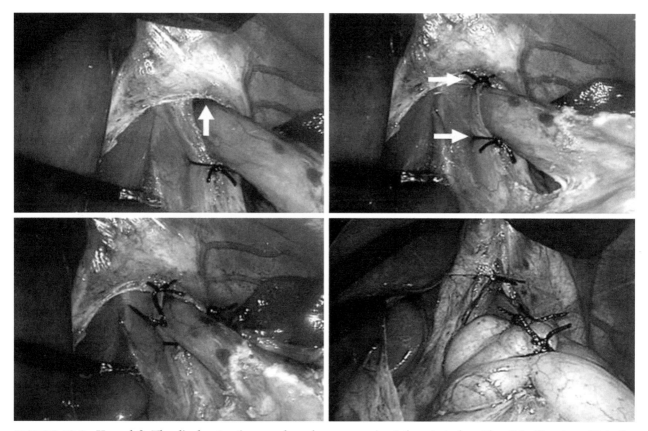

FIGURE 48-9. *Upper left,* The diaphragmatic crura have been approximated posteriorly with a 2-0 silk suture. Note the small space anteriorly (*arrow*) that remains after posterior approximation of the crura. *Upper right,* This space has been obliterated with an anteriorly placed 2-0 silk suture so that the diaphragmatic crura have been approximated both posteriorly and anteriorly (*arrows*). *Lower left,* An esophagus-to-crura suture is seen at the 9 o'clock position. In addition, similar sutures are placed at the 3 o'clock position. *Lower right,* The completed fundoplication.

A 4- or 5-mm cannula is positioned in the umbilicus, followed by insufflation and insertion of an angled telescope. With stab incisions in both the right and left upper abdominal quadrants, the duodenum is grasped with DeBakey endoscopic forceps placed through the patient's right upper abdominal stab incision. It is very important to grasp the duodenum securely, as a few instances of injury to the duodenum with this technique have been reported.[21] Through the stab incision in the patient's left upper abdomen, an arthroscopy knife is introduced, and the knife is extended to the second notch, which represents a 2-mm depth of penetration of the blade (Fig. 48-12). As the ultrasonographic criterion for pyloromyotomy is 4 mm in depth, using a knife with a 2-mm blade should not allow entry into the mucosa. It is important to incise the serosa and muscle adequately on the initial pass to allow introduction of the pyloric spreader. The knife is then returned to its sheath, extracted, and a pyloric spreader is introduced through the same left upper abdominal stab incision. The pylorus is gently and carefully spread to disrupt the muscular fibers. The submucosa is visualized during this part of the operation to ensure that no evidence of mucosal injury is present. It is important that an adequate myotomy be performed.

In one study, no evidence of incomplete pyloromyotomy was found in 171 patients in whom a mean pyloromyotomy incision length of 2.0 cm was achieved.[22] Conversely, in a few instances, an incomplete pyloromyotomy has been described, and it is postulated that inadequate extension onto the stomach was the reason.[21] After what appears to be a completed pyloromyotomy, it is often prudent to insufflate the stomach via a red rubber catheter to ensure that no evidence of unrecognized perforation exists. Placing omentum over the pyloromyotomy, as is commonly done in the open operation, may be advantageous. The instruments are then removed, and the umbilical fascia and skin are closed.

Splenectomy

The first report of a laparoscopic splenectomy in children was published in 1993.[23] A number of authors have described various techniques for elective removal of a spleen for hematologic diseases.[24–29] These diseases are primarily idiopathic thrombocytopenia purpura, hereditary spherocytosis, and, occasionally, splenic sequestration from sickle cell disease. The patient is usually

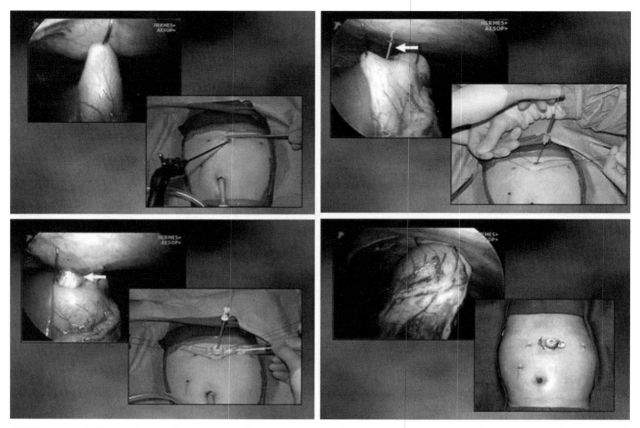

FIGURE 48-10. The technique for laparoscopic gastrostomy used by the authors. *Upper left,* After fundoplication in this patient, a 3-mm instrument has been introduced through the left upper stab incision, and the stomach has been grasped. Extracorporeal sutures are then placed on each side of this planned gastrostomy site. These sutures are introduced through the abdominal wall cephalad to the stomach, through the stomach, and exteriorized through the abdominal wall caudad to the gastrostomy site. *Upper right,* With a suture on each side of the planned gastrostomy, a needle is introduced into the stomach (*arrow*) through the gastrostomy site, followed by advancement of a guidewire through the needle into the stomach. The tract is then serially dilated and a 14F, 0.8-cm button (*arrow*) is introduced over the guidewire into the stomach (*lower left*). *Lower right,* The balloon is inflated, and the extracorporeal sutures are tied over the button.

positioned with a roll under his or her left side so that he or she is in a 30-degree to 45-degree right decubitus position. Placement of the ports for this operation vary from surgeon to surgeon. A common denominator is the need for a 15-mm site through which the Endocatch II bag (Ethicon Endosurgery, Cincinnati, OH) can be inserted. In addition, a site for introduction of an angled telescope and two other accessory sites are necessary. One approach is to position the 15-mm cannula through a 15-mm incision in the umbilical skin and fascia and orient the accessory ports in the midline. The advantage of this positioning is that the largest incision is nicely hidden in the umbilicus, yet if conversion is required, the midline incisions can be incorporated in an upper midline incision (see Fig. 48-3). Stab incisions may be used for these accessory sites, so that the only cannulas required are the 15-mm one in the umbilicus and a 5-mm port for introduction of the angled telescope. With the orientation described, the main working port is in the umbilicus, through which the ultrasonic scalpel is introduced. After insertion of all instruments, a thorough

search is made for accessory spleens. The most common sites for these are in the splenic hilum or in the lienocolic region (Fig. 48-13). It is important to remove accessory spleens either separately or with the specimen. The lienocolic ligament is then incised with the electrocautery, taking great care to identify the transverse colon and splenic flexure. Once the left colon has been mobilized from the spleen, it can be gently pushed caudad, out of the way of future dissection. The dissection then proceeds along the greater curvature of the stomach, carefully ligating and dividing the short gastric vessels with the ultrasonic scalpel. During this part of the operation, it is often helpful to rotate the table to the patient's right, allowing the stomach to gravitate away from the spleen. Sometimes it is not possible to divide the most cephalad short gastric vessels completely until later in the operation. After exposing the splenic hilum, one approach is to dissect the main splenic artery and obliterate it with an endoscopic clip before any further dissection. It is important to place this clip well away from the splenic hilum so that it does not later interfere with staple occlusion and division of the

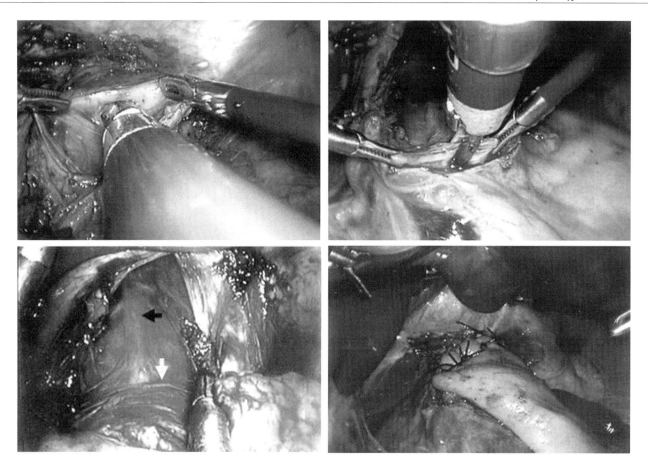

FIGURE 48-11. In a laparoscopic esophagomyotomy and anterior fundoplication, the placement of the ports and instruments is similar to that for a laparoscopic fundoplication. *Upper left,* The muscle of the esophagus has been grasped on the lateral aspects of the esophagus, and a Maryland dissecting instrument is being used to develop a plane between the muscle down through the submucosa. *Upper right,* This plane has been developed, and the ultrasonic scalpel is being used to ligate and divide the muscle. *Lower left,* The longitudinal fibers of the esophageal muscle have been divided. Note the circular fibers (*white arrow*) of the lower esophageal sphincter in the lower aspect of the photograph. In addition, the anterior vagus nerve (*solid arrow*) is seen to course vertically along the esophagus. *Lower right,* An anterior (Dor) fundoplication has been performed to help prevent the development of gastroesophageal reflux in the postoperative period.

splenic veins. Occlusion of the arterial supply reduces the risk of dangerous hemorrhage and allows the splenic blood to "autotransfuse" the patient.

Attention is now turned to dissecting the pancreas from the splenic hilum by using the ultrasonic scalpel. Sometimes this is relatively straightforward, but it can be quite tedious. At this time, or perhaps earlier in the dissection, the attachments of the spleen to the lateral peritoneal wall are incised. The avascular cephalad peritoneal attachments to the diaphragm are divided by using scissors. It is important to be aware of the diaphragm, as it is possible to injure it while mobilizing the cephalad aspect of the spleen. Once the tail of the pancreas has been separated and the spleen has been detached from its peritoneal fixation, the spleen can be lifted on either side of the hilum with retracting instruments. A 15-mm articulating stapler is introduced through the 15-mm cannula and positioned across the hilum of the spleen (see Fig. 48-13). It is necessary to ensure that the pancreas is not incorporated in the stapler and to confirm that the stapler is completely across the splenic vessels. Once positioned, the stapler should be closed for 20 seconds, after which the stapler can be fired and then gently released. When releasing the stapler, be ready to grasp any vascular structures that may be bleeding. Once the spleen has been detached from its vascular and peritoneal attachments, the patient is placed into a deep Trendelenburg position, and the Endocatch II bag (Ethicon Endosurgery, Cincinnati, Ohio) is introduced. Then the patient is rotated into a reverse Trendelenburg position, allowing the spleen to fall into the open bag. The bag is closed after ensuring that no other structures have entered it, and the neck of bag is exteriorized through the umbilical incision. The spleen is manually morcellated with sponge forceps and extracted in piecemeal fashion. During this part of the operation, it is very important to ensure that the bag is not perforated by overvigorous morcellation or extraction. It may take 10 to 20 minutes to accomplish

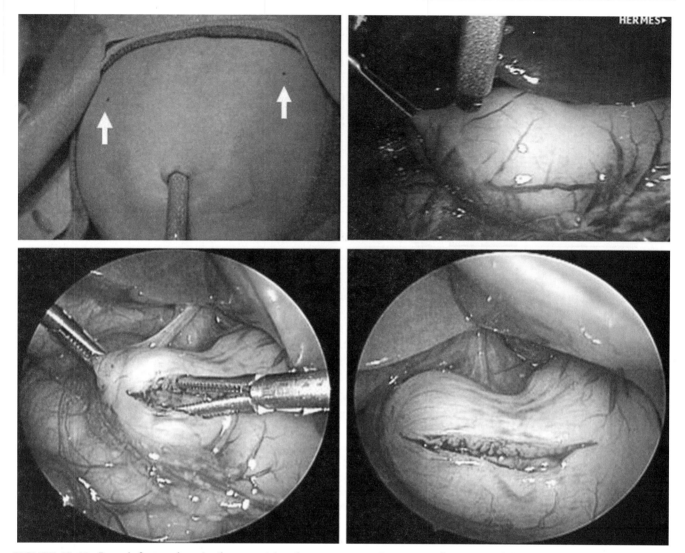

FIGURE 48-12. In an infant undergoing laparoscopic pyloromyotomy, a 5-mm cannula is inserted through an incision in the umbilical fascia. The sites of the stab incisions in the left and right upper quadrants are shown (*arrows, upper left*). With an arthroscopy knife (*upper right*), an incision will be made in the seromuscular portion of the hypertrophied pylorus. The knife is removed, a pyloric spreader is introduced through this same incision, and the hypertrophied muscle bluntly divided (*lower left*). The pyloromyotomy incision is usually approximately 2 cm long (*lower right*).

splenic extraction. After removal of the bag and its contents, reinspection of the area of dissection is performed to ensure that no evidence of complications is present. The incisions are then closed, and the patient is usually ready for discharge on the first or second postoperative day.

Cholecystectomy

Laparoscopic cholecystectomy is becoming a rather common operation for pediatric surgeons. Sometimes the development of cholelithiasis is due to hemolytic disease, but often it is iatrogenic. Most pediatric surgeons will see a few cases of biliary dyskinesia in older children requiring laparoscopic cholecystectomy for relief of symptoms. Most pediatric patients undergoing laparoscopic cholecystectomy are in the adolescent age group. However, an

occasional elementary school–age child will need this procedure, and rarely, a preschool infant will be symptomatic from cholelithiasis.[30]

When positioning the instruments and cannulas for the operation, it is important to space the cannulas widely for optimal working room (Fig. 48-14). This is especially true in the younger patient. The two right-sided instruments are usually for retracting purposes, with the most inferior instrument being used by the assistant and the most cephalad manipulated by the surgeon. These can often be inserted by using the stab-incision technique. For the preschool patient, a 5-mm umbilical port is placed, but for older patients, a 10-mm port is usually necessary. The gallbladder will be extracted through this cannula or the umbilical fascial defect. For many pediatric patients, a 5-mm clip is used for ligation of

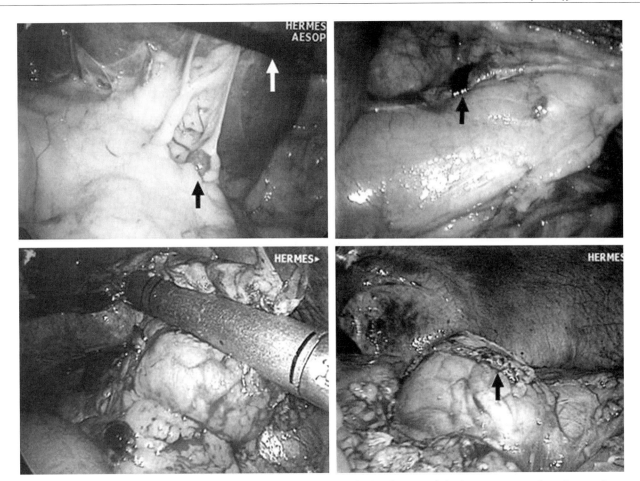

FIGURE 48-13. The technique for laparoscopic splenectomy is depicted. *Upper left,* An accessory spleen is seen in a patient with idiopathic thrombocytopenia purpura (*black arrow*). In addition, one of the 3-mm instruments (*white arrow*) is being used to elevate the lower pole of the spleen for access to the lienocolic ligament. After ligation and division of the short gastric vessels, one technique is to isolate the artery and doubly clip it before dissection in the splenic hilum. *Upper right,* Note the two clips (*black arrow*) on the splenic artery along the cephalad portion of the pancreas. *Lower left,* Attachments of the spleen to the diaphragm and other structures have been divided, and an endoscopic vascular stapler is placed across the splenic hilum. The pancreas, noted below the stapler, has not been incorporated into the jaws of the stapler. *Lower right,* The spleen has been removed. Note the intact staple line (*black arrow*) across the hilum of the spleen.

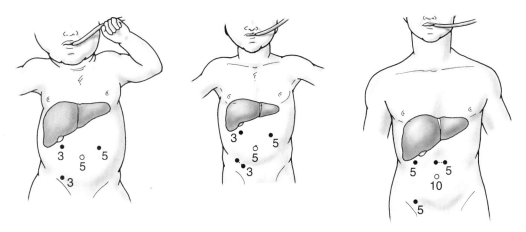

FIGURE 48-14. For laparoscopic cholecystectomy in infants and children, it is important to space the cannulas widely to create an adequate working space and not have the instruments inhibiting one another. *Left,* A suggested diagram for location of the ports for an infant. *Center,* The cannulas can be arranged as shown for a child between ages 3 and 10 years. *Right,* Instruments can be positioned as they are for an adult.

the cystic duct and cystic artery, and therefore a 5-mm incision may be placed in the patient's epigastric region. For smaller patients, this incision should be positioned more in the patient's left epigastrium to ensure adequate working space. However, in the teenager, this incision is located just to the right of the patient's midline.

Regardless of the patient's age, the general technique is similar. Any omental or peritoneal attachments to the gallbladder are bluntly divided, and the tip of the gallbladder is rotated ventrally over the liver, which exposes the infundibulum and cystic duct. It is very important to retract the infundibulum laterally, which orients the cystic duct at a right angle to the common bile duct. If the infundibulum is retracted cephalad, the cystic duct approaches a more vertical orientation, and the cystic duct and common duct can be misidentified. This may lead either to injury or to ligation of the common duct. With the infundibulum retracted laterally, the cystic duct is well visualized and then easily skeletonized. Cholangiography often is not necessary. However, if the surgeon desires cholangiography, several techniques are available. In older children, a lateral incision in the cystic duct can be made, with insertion of a cholangiocatheter into the cystic duct, followed by cholangiography. In younger children, it is often easier to use the Kumar clamp technique, in which an atraumatic clamp is placed across the infundibulum, and a sclerotherapy needle introduced through the side arm of the clamp into the infundibulum (Fig. 48-15).[31,32] After cholangiography, the sclerotherapy needle and cholangioclamp are removed.

The advantage of this technique is that a lateral incision in a small cystic duct is technically very difficult, and this technique is much easier to accomplish in younger patients.

After cholangiography, if needed, the cystic duct is ligated and divided with endoscopic clips. Two clips are placed proximally near the junction of the cystic and common duct, and one clip is usually placed near the junction of the cystic duct and the infundibulum of the gallbladder. The cystic duct is then divided. In a similar fashion, the cystic artery is divided. The gallbladder is then dissected in a retrograde fashion from its attachments to the liver. A number of instruments can be used for this part of the operation, including the spatula cautery, the hook cautery, or the Maryland dissecting instrument attached to cautery. Regardless of the technique used, before complete detachment of the gallbladder, the area of dissection is carefully inspected again to ensure that hemostasis is adequate. Then the gallbladder is completely detached and extracted through the umbilical site. With a noninflamed gallbladder, most often, it can be removed through the umbilical cannula. However, it is usually necessary to remove the cannula and extract the gallbladder through the fascial defect. After extraction, the area of dissection is again inspected, and hemostasis assured. The ports/instruments are removed, and the incisions are closed. Most patients are ready for discharge the following day. An occasional teenage patient may require an extra day of hospitalization.

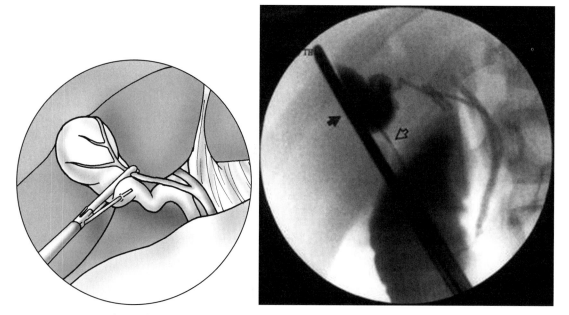

FIGURE 48-15. The cholangiography technique using the Kumar clamp is shown. *Left,* An atraumatic clamp is placed across the gallbladder infundibulum. Through the side arm of the clamp, a sclerotherapy needle is introduced into the infundibulum, and the dye injected. *Right,* The cholangiogram. Note the very small cystic duct entering a small common duct. The *solid arrow* is oriented toward the atraumatic clamp, whereas the *open arrow* points to the sclerotherapy needle.

Adrenalectomy

Patients with adrenal diseases are being more frequently seen by pediatric surgeons. Usually these diseases are benign, although pheochromocytoma may be seen with very severe physiologic alterations.

The patient should be placed in a lateral decubitus position with the operative side up (Fig. 48-16). For this operation, a 10-mm incision is made in the flank and extended down through the subcutaneous tissue and muscles into the peritoneal cavity. A 10-mm cannula is directly introduced into the peritoneal cavity, and insufflation is achieved. With a 10-mm cannula for this initial site, the dissection is easier, and the specimen can usually be extracted either through the cannula or through the incision. After insufflation, accessory ports are then placed. Usually the accessory ports are 5 mm in size, although one or two can be 3 mm. Sometimes it is necessary to divide the peritoneal attachments to the colon first to place the most posterior cannula, as the operative approach is usually from a more posterior direction toward the adrenal gland.

For a left adrenalectomy, the adrenal vein is usually ligated with endoscopic clips early in the operation. Next, the gland is carefully dissected free from the kidney on its inferior and lateral aspect and the diaphragmatic attachments superiorly. Medially, it is dissected from the midline structures. The ultrasonic scalpel can be useful in making this dissection relatively bloodless.

For a right adrenalectomy, the adrenal vein is ligated as one of the last parts of the operation, because the right adrenal vein is very short and directly enters the vena cava. Therefore it is usually necessary to divide the right triangular ligament of the liver for access to the right adrenal gland. The right adrenal gland is circumscribed inferiorly, laterally, and superiorly by using the ultrasonic scalpel. With the right adrenal gland free on three sides, the right adrenal vein is carefully exposed medially. Endoscopic clips are placed on the adrenal vein as it enters the vena cava, the right adrenal vein is divided, and the specimen removed.

Most patients are ready for discharge the day after the operation, although patients with pheochromocytoma often need to be monitored the first postoperative night in an intensive care setting. Usually these patients are ready for discharge on the second or third post-operative day.

Results of laparoscopic adrenalectomy in children have been favorable, with minimal morbidity and no mortality.[33–37]

Small Bowel

Duodenoduodenostomy

Although relatively small numbers of patients have been reported, the safety and efficacy of laparoscopic repair for duodenal atresia is clearly supported.[38–40] Because the distal bowel is not distended, room exists within the infant's abdomen to perform the anastomosis. Familiarity with neonatal laparoscopic anastomosis is an important skill for surgeons performing this operation.

Four ports are used for the repair of duodenal atresia. The port for the telescope should be sited in the left lower quadrant in the midclavicular line at a point about halfway between the anterior superior iliac spine and the umbilicus. Positioning the telescope in the umbilicus usually restricts the view of the operating surgeon because it is too close to the working area. The operator's left hand works an instrument in the right lower abdomen. The surgeon's right-hand instrument is introduced in the patient's left upper quadrant. The fourth port for the surgeon's assistant is usually sited higher in the left upper quadrant than the operator's right-hand port.

The operation is begun by identifying and mobilizing the dilated proximal duodenum. The distal duodenum is identified and mobilized on its antimesenteric side. A suture is passed through the abdominal wall in the right upper quadrant, through the proximal end of the distal duodenal segment, and out through the abdominal wall in the right upper quadrant. This suture is tied snugly to elevate the distal duodenal segment and bring it

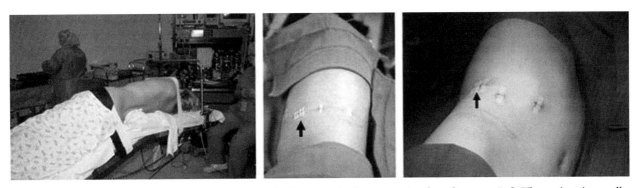

FIGURE 48-16. The patient's position and sites of the incisions for laparoscopic adrenalectomy. *Left,* The patient is usually positioned in a true lateral position. A roll is placed under the lumbar area, and the table is flexed. *Center,* The incisions for a left laparoscopic adrenalectomy. The largest incision (*arrow*) is the site through which the intact specimen was removed in this patient. *Right,* In a similar fashion, the incisions for a right laparoscopic adrenalectomy are visualized. Again, the intact specimen was removed through the largest incision (*arrow*), which was approximately 1.5 cm long.

close to the proximal segment for the anastomosis. A linear incision is usually made with electrocautery or scissors in the distal duodenal segment, beginning at its blind end. An incision of similar length is made in the proximal duodenum at right angles to the distal segment enterotomy. Tension on the traction suture in the distal duodenal segment should be increased or decreased to line up the two incisions for anastomosis. A diamond anastomosis is created by using a continuous running technique on the deep wall and an interrupted technique on the anterior wall. The anastomosis is begun in the middle portion of the proximal duodenal enterotomy and the proximal end of the distal duodenal enterotomy. Once the initial suture has been placed, the knot is tied on the outside. The continuous suture is brought inside the lumen of the distal duodenum and used to approximate the back wall of the anastomosis from the duodenal lumen. It is helpful to place stay sutures to hold the tissues of the proximal and distal duodenum in apposition for the anastomosis. When the suture has been advanced along the entire back wall, it is brought out on the serosal surface of the distal duodenum, where it is then secured to the previously placed stay suture. The anterior wall of the duodenostomy is closed by using interrupted sutures; 5-0 absorbable braided suture is preferred for this anastomosis. Eight to 10 sutures are placed along the anterior row and tied snugly. The patency of the distal small bowel can be ascertained by using a saline-injection technique. A 23-gauge needle is passed into the abdominal cavity attached to a 10-mL syringe. The distal bowel is grasped with a bowel grasper, and the needle is inserted through the abdominal wall and through the lumen of the distal bowel. Saline is injected and monitored visually. Two or three injections often are required more distally to follow the saline stream all the way into the cecum.

The pneumoperitoneum is evacuated, and the instruments removed. In neonates, even small fascial defects must be closed to prevent herniation of the omentum. The skin is approximated with Steri-strips.

We have performed five operations. All five of the patients have recovered well with return of intestinal function in 4 to 5 days. The primary benefit of duodenal atresia repair by using a laparoscopic approach is the improved cosmetic appearance, as abdominal incisions in neonates often result in the skin scar attaching to the underlying fascia. As the patient acquires more subcutaneous fat with growth, these scars become deeply dimpled and can be unsightly.

Malrotation

Malrotation anomalies offer an excellent opportunity for laparoscopic visualization and repair.[41] Even a patient with volvulus can be managed laparoscopically if the patient does not have gangrenous small bowel.[42] Laparoscopic exploration is useful both in the neonate and in the teenage patient with malrotation diagnosed by an upper gastrointestinal contrast study but with uncertainty about the intestinal attachments to the posterior abdominal wall.

The patient is usually placed in the reverse Trendelenburg position to allow the small bowel and colon to fall away. The laparoscopic operation is begun by the insertion of three cannulas. The first cannula for the endoscope is placed in the midclavicular line of the left lower quadrant halfway between the anterior iliac spine and the umbilicus. The surgeon's left-hand port site is in the right lower quadrant, and the right-hand port site is usually placed in the left upper quadrant. The presence of malrotation is confirmed by identifying the pylorus and advancing distally along the duodenum. The next step is to find the cecum and carefully separate it from the duodenum by dividing Ladd's bands. Both of these techniques are necessary to ascertain fully the presence of malrotation. If the patient has a volvulus, torsion is relieved by rotating the bowel in a counterclockwise direction. The volvulus must be completely reduced. If necrotic bowel is found, it is usually best to open the patient for further evaluation and surgical correction if possible.

After division of the bands connecting the cecum to the duodenum, the mesentery can be separated widely. Adhesions in the folded mesentery of the small bowel also should be released to allow a further broadening of the posterior mesenteric attachments. It is usually best to begin dividing the bands between the cecum and small bowel and then continue to divide these bands between the cecum, small bowel, and duodenum. The eventual goal of this dissection is to allow the cecum to fall freely into the left side of the peritoneal cavity and to release all subsequent adhesions in the small bowel mesentery. It is surprising that, even with very complex adhesions, an organized approach can unfold the adherent intestinal loops so that the proximal small bowel is retained in the right upper quadrant, and the terminal ileum and colon naturally slide into the left side of the abdominal cavity.

An appendectomy is usually performed after the adhesions have been divided. The appendix is exteriorized through the left upper quadrant incision. The mesoappendix is divided by using a standard open technique and ligated. The base of the appendix is then doubly ligated with absorbable suture, and the appendix amputated from its base. The appendiceal stump is allowed to drop back into the peritoneal cavity. Sometimes it is necessary to pull the cecum toward the right lower quadrant to return the appendiceal stump to the abdominal cavity.

The fascia of the incisions is then closed after the pneumoperitoneum has been evacuated. The patient is usually able to start feeding on the first or second postoperative day, unless a significant ischemic insult has occurred to the intestine.

Some pediatric surgeons have expressed concern that a laparoscopic Ladd's procedure will not produce enough scarring of the colon and small bowel to prevent future volvulus. Volvulus subsequent to open Ladd's procedures has been reported. We are unaware of midgut volvulus after laparoscopic procedures, but this probably relates to the small number of procedures performed. It seems unlikely that volvulus would be any more likely to occur after a properly performed laparoscopic Ladd's procedure than after an open Ladd's procedure.

Jejunostomy

A feeding jejunostomy is indicated in patients requiring enteral feeding who have gastroparesis, partial gastric outlet obstruction, or who have significant but uncorrectable gastroesophageal reflux. It is very easy to perform laparoscopically. Because of difficulty with maintenance, jejunostomies are avoided except in those circumstances in which their use is considered to be temporary.

Simple jejunostomy is begun by placing a cannula for the endoscope through the right lower quadrant in the midclavicular line. A second port is passed through the right upper quadrant, and a third one is inserted through the left lower quadrant. A loop of proximal jejunum is oriented transversely. A U-suture is then passed through the abdominal wall, through the free wall of jejunum, and back up through the abdominal wall. This suture is tied over a bolster (usually a Jackson-Pratt drain) to form the proximal end of the jejunostomy tunnel. A needle from a vascular access kit (Cook Inc., Bloomington, IN) is then introduced through the abdominal wall 4 or 5 cm lateral to the fixation suture. With laparoscopic surveillance, the needle is advanced just outside the peritoneal cavity underneath the parietal peritoneum toward the jejunal loop held against the abdominal wall by the U-stitch. The needle is then inserted into the jejunum (Fig. 48-17A). A guidewire is passed through the needle into the distal jejunum. Dilators from the vascular-access kit enlarge the tract so that a catheter-introducer may be passed over the guidewire into the jejunal lumen. The jejunostomy tube is then passed through the catheter-introducer and advanced distally for at least 15 cm. The catheter is secured to the skin with sutures or a securing device. Two other U-sutures are then passed through the abdominal wall, through the serosa of the jejunum, with an effort to stay outside of the jejunal lumen, and then back up through the abdominal wall. These sutures are tied over the bolster, completing the procedure (Fig. 48-17B).

More commonly performed is a Roux-en-Y jejunostomy with a gastrostomy button for feeding. The cannulas/incisions for this procedure are usually introduced in the anterior axillary line in the right midabdomen. Three ports are used, with the inferior port a 12-mm port. The other two ports are usually 4- or 5-mm ports. A loop of jejunum is identified 15 to 20 cm from the ligament of Treitz. At this point, the jejunum is divided with the vascular load of an endoscopic stapler. The mesentery is subsequently divided either with another vascular load of the endoscopic stapler or with an ultrasonic scalpel. A 20-cm loop of jejunum is advanced to the abdominal wall. Two U-sutures are passed through the abdominal wall, through the distal jejunum near the stapled end, and back up through the abdominal wall. A technique similar to the gastrostomy technique described earlier in this chapter is then performed (see *Laparoscopic Gastrostomy*). The dilator and balloon button are passed over the guidewire into the lumen of the

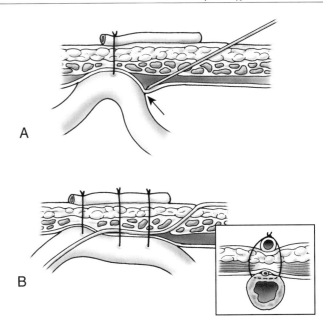

FIGURE 48-17. *A,* The jejunum is held in place by a U-stitch. The needle is passed just outside the peritoneum (arrow) under laparoscopic surveillance before entering the jejunal lumen. *B,* Two more U-stitches are passed through the jejunal wall to hold the bowel against the catheter traversing the extraperitoneal space.

jejunum, and the balloon is inflated. The U-sutures are tied over the wings of the balloon button. The proximal jejunum is then secured to the distal limb about 20 cm from its balloon-button site. Basting sutures are passed through the jejunal segments to hold them together. Small jejunostomies are made in each jejunal limb, fashioned in such a way that an endoscopic stapler can be passed through the incisions to join the two limbs of jejunum. The endoscopic stapler is then fired. Usually a 45-mm stapler is required to make an adequate lumen between the two limbs. The stapler is removed, and the remaining opening is closed with a continuous suture. The two limbs of jejunum are sutured together for a distance of about 10 cm by using interrupted sutures to avoid the complication of volvulus or internal herniation around the jejunostomy. Feeding can be initiated on the first or second postoperative day. With this technique in a few patients, we have not found any significant complications.

Reduction of Intussusception

Intussusception is usually diagnosed and treated with a contrast enema and hydrostatic reduction. In approximately 10% of patients, surgical reduction is needed. Laparoscopy is an excellent method for the surgical reduction of most intussusceptions that are not amenable to correction by contrast enema or pneumatic reduction.[43,44] Occasionally the intussusception has spontaneously reduced during the interval between failure of the contrast enema and induction of the anesthetic. These patients certainly benefit from visualization of the reduced intussusception, as opposed to an incision to discover the same information. However, in most cases, the intussusception must be reduced by laparoscopic manipulation.

Three incisions are used for laparoscopic reduction of an intussusception. The endoscope is passed through a port in the left lower quadrant at a point equidistant from the anterior superior iliac spine and the umbilicus. The other two sites are located in the right lower quadrant and the left upper quadrant, respectively. The patient is secured to the operating table, and the table is tilted to the left side to allow the small bowel to fall toward the left, so the cecum is well visualized. After visualization of the intussusception, steady traction is used to squeeze the edema out of the intussusceptum so that it can be reduced. Although the classic teaching has been that one should not pull the two segments apart, laparoscopic surgeons have discovered that this dogma is inaccurate. Steady traction on the ileum with countertraction on the cecum, sometimes taking as long as 10 to 15 minutes, results in decrease of the edema in the intussusceptum so that the small bowel can be reduced from the colon. The operating surgeon must be very careful not to tear or injure the small bowel or colon during this process. A Babcock clamp, which can be used to grasp around the bowel onto the mesentery, or a long, small-bowel clamp is best for pulling on the small bowel and for countertraction on the colon. After 10 to 15 minutes, if no reduction of the intussusceptum has occurred, the operation should be converted to an open procedure. Additionally, if it is apparent that the intussusception cannot be reduced because the bowel is gangrenous, a laparoscopic ileocolectomy (described later) can be considered. In most cases, the authors prefer to convert to an open procedure if reduction is not possible.

If intussusception can be reduced laparoscopically, the pneumoperitoneum is evacuated. The fascia of the incisions should be closed to avoid herniation of the omentum.

Oral feeding is usually initiated the day after operation. The reported incidence of recurrence is the same for laparoscopic or open surgical reduction. Appendectomy is not usually used in these patients. In the authors' experience with 25 patients laparoscopically explored for intussusception, 21 either were already reduced or were successfully reduced by the laparoscopic technique. Four required open surgical procedures, and three of these four required a bowel resection.

Colon and Rectum

Appendectomy

Laparoscopic appendectomy is becoming the standard of care for both nonruptured and ruptured appendicitis. Two primary approaches are used for laparoscopic appendectomy. The "in" technique (intracorporeal) uses three ports and is described in this section. The "out" technique (extracorporeal) is commonly used in Europe. With the "out" procedure, the appendix is mobilized without dividing the mesoappendix. The appendix is exteriorized through the single umbilical port site, and the appendectomy is performed in a standard fashion externally through the umbilical incision. The main problem with the "out" technique can be the bulbous size of the appendix, requiring enlargement of the umbilical port site. It also is sometimes difficult to mobilize the appendix and cecum adequately to pull the base of the appendix through the umbilicus. Some surgeons use a small right lower quadrant incision in these circumstances.

The technique most often used in this country for laparoscopic appendectomy is performed within the peritoneal cavity by using three cannulas. The umbilical port is usually a 12-mm port. This large port is used anticipating that the bulbous, inflamed appendix will be removed through this cannula or the umbilical incision. Moreover, the stapler is inserted through this large port. The other two cannulas are positioned variably by laparoscopic surgeons. We prefer a left lower quadrant site for the endoscope and a suprapubic port site placement for the surgeon's left-hand grasping forceps. A hook connected to cautery is a useful tool to mobilize the appendix. In more difficult mobilizations, the ultrasonic scalpel also can be used for this purpose. The omentum and small bowel are usually bluntly swept away from the inflamed appendix. The lateral appendiceal attachments are divided with the hook cautery. With the hook, the mesoappendix is ligated and divided beginning in the distal mesoappendix and proceeding proximally to the base of the appendix near the cecum. The appendix can be doubly or triply ligated by using loop ligatures or closed and divided by using an endoscopic gastrointestinal stapler. We prefer the endoscopic stapler because less spillage of intraluminal appendiceal contents seems to occur with the stapler technique, and it is more efficient. The appendix is placed in a retrieval bag and exteriorized through the umbilical trocar site. Occasionally the fascia and skin of the umbilicus must be enlarged to allow removal of the appendix. This can be accomplished most easily by passing a grooved director both inferiorly and superiorly and by using electrocautery to increase the size of the opening in the umbilical skin and fascia. Once the appendix has been removed, the 12-mm cannula is replaced in the umbilical port site, and the abdomen and pelvis are thoroughly irrigated and aspirated. The ports are removed, and the pneumoperitoneum evacuated. The umbilical fascia is closed, and the umbilical skin is approximated with absorbable suture.

A plethora of articles have addressed whether laparoscopic appendectomy is equivalent or superior to open appendectomy.[45-50] This controversy has been even more heated over the use of laparoscopic appendectomy for perforated appendicitis. Most of the early reports comparing laparoscopic with open appendectomy usually compared the learning curve for laparoscopic appendectomy with that for the open technique. However, as more large series have been reported, it is clear that the laparoscopic approach to appendectomy has some distinct advantages. Although much more will be written on this subject, it now appears that the primary advantage for laparoscopic appendectomy for perforated and imperforated appendicitis is a significantly lower wound-infection rate. The incidence of intraperitoneal abscess formation seems to be about the same for both techniques. Cosmetic results appear to be better with the laparoscopic approach.

A great deal of discussion has addressed which patients with perforated appendicitis should be treated primarily with intravenous broad-spectrum antibiotics and which should undergo immediate appendectomy. We manage those patients with localized perforated appendicitis with intravenous antibiotic therapy followed by interval appendectomy 6 to 8 weeks later. Patients with generalized peritonitis associated with perforated appendicitis are treated with primary appendectomy with irrigation of the peritoneal cavity.

Crohn's Disease

Although the medical management of patients with Crohn's disease has improved over the last few years, it is not uncommon for these patients initially to have irreversible obstruction of the terminal ileum, which can be an unremitting problem, even with appropriate medical management (see also Chapter 41). Laparoscopic ileocolectomy can be performed by using four port sites. A 12-mm cannula is introduced in the umbilicus. Four-mm cannulas are positioned in the left lower quadrant and right upper quadrant. Another 3- or 4-mm port is placed suprapubically. Bowel graspers are passed through the right- and left-hand port sites to help inspect the distal small bowel. A point is chosen to begin the resection. An endoscopic stapler with a vascular load is passed through the 12-mm umbilical cannula to divide the small bowel at the selected site. A second stapler is applied when needed. Either an ultrasonic scalpel or sequential vascular staple applications are used to divide the small bowel mesentery. The appendix and cecum are mobilized by dividing the peritoneal attachments laterally. The entire cecum and part of the right colon are mobilized to make the subsequent ileocolic anastomosis easier. Dissection of the intestinal mesentery is continued to the midcecum. An endoscopic stapler is used to divide the cecum, and the separated specimen is placed in the pelvis. The small bowel is advanced to the remaining cecum. The distal small bowel and cecum are positioned side by side for approximately 6 cm and secured with several 4-0 silk sutures. A 6-cm vascular endostapler is used to create a stapled anastomosis that is reinforced by interrupted permanent sutures. An effort should be made to avoid an excess blind end to the distal small bowel beyond the ileocecal anastomosis.

The specimen is removed either through enlargement of the umbilical port site or through enlargement of the suprapubic site. The incisions are closed in standard fashion. Nasogastric drainage is not routinely necessary. Oral feeding may commence as soon as evidence of gastrointestinal function is seen.

Ileocecal resection for Crohn's disease has been performed in relatively small numbers in children and adolescents. However, the adult experience has shown that this is a safe technique with significant cosmetic advantages. Otherwise, length of stay and complications are similar to those with the open technique.

Total Colectomy with J Pouch Reconstruction

Approximately 20% of patients with ulcerative colitis have active symptoms before age 20 years (see Chapter 41). Some of these patients have unremitting symptoms that require urgent colectomy. Others have more chronic symptoms, such as persistent diarrhea, growth retardation, and delayed puberty. All of these patients are better managed with total colectomy with pouch reconstruction than with continued difficult medical management. Restorative proctocolectomy can be performed with laparoscopic colectomy while the proctectomy is accomplished and the J pouch is constructed by using an open technique.

The laparoscopic-assisted colectomy is begun with the surgeon standing to the patient's right. Four or five cannula sites are used (Fig. 48-18). The distal sigmoid colon is lifted anteriorly, and the sigmoid mesocolon is divided by using an ultrasonic scalpel. The division of the mesocolon should be kept close to the colon to avoid bleeding. This dissection is carried cephalad to the descending colon. At this point, the lateral peritoneal attachments are divided up to the splenic flexure, followed by division of the descending mesocolon. The gastrocolic ligament is divided starting at the falciform ligament and extending toward the splenic flexure, followed by ligation and division of the lienocolic ligament. The transverse mesocolon is divided from the hepatic flexure toward the splenic flexure, where it joins the previous dissection of the descending mesocolon. At this point, the surgeon changes to a position between the patient's legs. The terminal ileum, appendix, cecum, and right colon are mobilized by dividing the lateral peritoneal attachments on the right side. The terminal ileum is divided with an endoscopic stapler. The mesocolon is divided close to the ascending colon, sparing the marginal artery, which is important for the future J pouch. The surgeon divides the gastrocolic and hepatocolic ligaments on the right side of the abdomen, and the mesenteric division is completed. A suprapubic incision is then made, the rectosigmoid colon is divided with a gastrointestinal stapler, and the colon is removed; the remainder of the procedure is open (see Chapter 41).

Complication rates for total proctocolectomy and J pouch pull-through are high (25%) for both the open and laparoscopic techniques. The most frequent complications are wound infection and small bowel obstruction.[51,52] The ileostomy is closed 8 weeks after the initial operation. The lower portion of the J pouch spur is divided at the same time as the closure of the ileostomy (see Fig. 48-18*G*).

Pull-through for Hirschsprung's Disease

One of the most dramatic changes in pediatric surgical procedures over the last several decades has been the ascendance of single-stage techniques in the treatment of

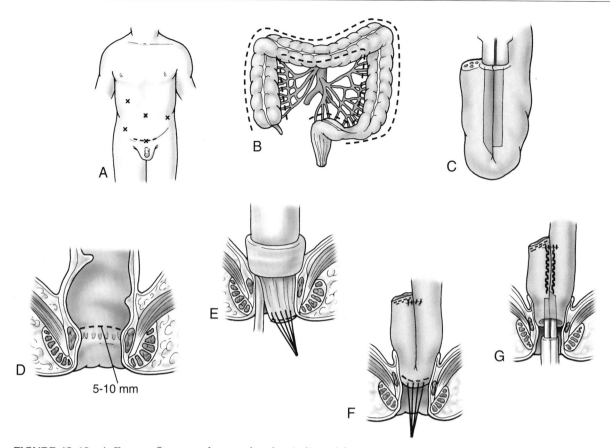

FIGURE 48-18. *A,* Four or five cannulas are placed as indicated for resection of the intra-abdominal colon. *B,* The intra-abdominal colon is separated from the attachments and its mesentery. *C,* An 8-cm J pouch is formed with a stapler. *D,* The rectal mucosectomy is started near the top of the anorectal columns. *E,* Traction is applied to the mucosa, which is stripped away from the smooth muscle wall of the rectum. *F,* The J pouch is passed through the muscular cuff without any twists. *G,* The lower portion of the J pouch spur is divided at the time of closure of the ileostomy.

Hirschsprung's disease (see Chapter 34). The primary pull-through procedure for Hirschsprung's disease was introduced in the early 1980s, but its popularity has increased since the late 1990s, with the introduction of minimally invasive techniques.[53,54] The most popular technique now is the laparoscopic-assisted endorectal pull-through and its derivative, the transanal pull-through.[55] The laparoscopic technique has several advantages over the transanal pull-through. Most significantly, the laparoscopic approach allows biopsy of the bowel above the apparent transition zone to confirm not only the presence of ganglion cells but also the absence of hypertrophic nerve fibers and the assessment of normally innervated smooth muscle above the transition zone. As the mucosectomy is irreversible once completed, it is essential that confirmation of normal ganglion cells as well as the absence of hypertrophic nerve fibers be substantiated before initiating the rectal dissection.

Transanal pull-through is easiest in patients younger than 6 months. With increasing patient size, the ease of transanal pull-through diminishes. By performing even minimal laparoscopic dissection to the peritoneal reflection, the transanal dissection is made much easier and requires significantly less anal retraction.[56]

Three cannulas are initially placed for the laparoscopic-assisted endorectal pull-through for Hirschsprung's disease. A grasping instrument is inserted through an umbilical port and is manipulated by the surgeon's left hand. The endoscope is inserted through a right upper quadrant cannula, sited just below the liver in the anterior axillary line. The surgeon's right hand manipulates instruments introduced through a port in the anterior axillary line in the right lower quadrant. Two biopsies are taken, one at the level of the suspected transition zone, and the second, 10 to 15 cm above the first. These biopsies are sent for evaluation for the presence of ganglion cells, and no further dissection is performed until ganglion cells are confirmed. The other histologic studies for intestinal neuronal dysplasia (IND) can be completed during the intraperitoneal and transanal dissection.

A hook cautery is used to devascularize the aganglionic segment of bowel. The ganglionated colon is prepared so that at least a 10-cm segment is available for the pull-through. This may require development of a vascularized pedicle to allow the intended site of anastomosis to reach the anus (Fig. 48-19A). This dissection is most commonly performed by using the hook cautery, but the ultrasonic scalpel is useful in children older than 1 year to divide the larger vessels. The legs are then elevated, and retraction sutures are placed circumferentially around the anus. A circumferential incision is made in the mucosa 3 mm above the dentate line. The endorectal dissection is done by using a cautery, scissors, and blunt dissection. As the endorectal dissection advances, the muscular cuff intussuscepts outward with traction on the mucosal sleeve. Dissection is continued to the level of the peritoneal reflection, where the muscular cuff is transected circumferentially. The colon is transected, and a watertight anastomosis is performed (see Fig. 48-19D).

The pneumoperitoneum is reestablished, and the pull-through pedicle inspected. A potential internal hernia space related to the vascular pedicle should be closed with interrupted sutures, preserving the vasculature to the colon. The pneumoperitoneum is evacuated and the cannula sites closed. The patients are usually fed on the first postoperative day and are often ready for discharge within 2 or 3 days.

The postoperative results after primary pull-through are excellent. Complications after primary pull-through are only about half as frequent as those after staged procedures. Total hospitalization also is significantly less. Long-term follow-up shows continence rates to be equivalent. Careful endorectal dissection should diminish the incidence of both constipation and enterocolitis.[56]

Pull-through for High Anorectal Malformations

High anorectal malformations are managed primarily with posterior sagittal anorectoplasty (see Chapter 35).[57,58] Although the operation is elegant to perform, the incidence of postoperative fecal incontinence remains high. The laparoscopic-assisted operation for imperforate anus was developed to avoid dividing the levator ani muscles and external sphincter muscles.[59] Conceptually, this operation approximates the operation for low anorectal malformations, in which the rectal fistula is redirected through the external sphincter complex.

Three cannula sites are used for laparoscopic-assisted anorectal pull-through. The position of these cannulas is identical to that used for the Hirschsprung's operation. Dissection of the rectum is begun right at the level of the peritoneal reflection. Injury to both ureters and to the vasculature of the rectosigmoid colon is assiduously avoided. The dissection is continued circumferentially around the rectum down to the rectourethral fistula. It is important to maintain the dissection precisely on the

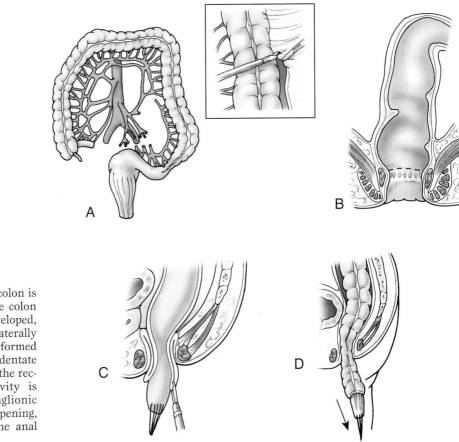

FIGURE 48-19. *A,* The aganglionic colon is stripped of its mesentery close to the colon wall. When needed, a pedicle is developed, and the fusion fascia is divided laterally (*inset*). *B,* The mucosectomy is performed transanally, beginning just above the dentate line. *C,* When the muscular sleeve of the rectum prolapses, the peritoneal cavity is entered posteriorly. *D,* The aganglionic bowel is removed through the anal opening, and the neorectum is secured to the anal mucosa at the dentate line.

muscle of the rectum and fistula. The dissection is continued to the junction of the fistula and the urethra or bladder neck. The fistula is divided 3 to 4 mm proximal to the urethra. A loop ligature is used to secure the urethral side of the fistula. After division of the fistula, the pelvic floor can be clearly visualized (Fig. 48-20*A*).

Electrical stimulation is used to map the location of the external sphincter complex. A 1-cm incision is made vertically in the gluteal cleft over the identified external sphincter complex. Blunt dissection is used to develop the elliptical plane inside the sphincter complex. A Veress needle covered by an expandable sleeve (US Surgical, Norwalk, CT) is passed through this incision and between the two limbs of the anterior portion of the levator ani complex (puborectalis muscle). This passage is performed under laparoscopic visualization. The Veress needle and associated expanding cannula sleeve are introduced into the pelvis directly in the midline. The Veress needle is removed, and the sleeve is expanded with 5-, 10-, and sometimes 12-mm cannulas. A grasper is passed through the cannula into the pelvic cavity. The fistulous tract is grasped and exteriorized through the passage in the levator

ani complex. The fistula is secured to the anal skin with a single-layer anastomosis by using absorbable suture. The rectum is retracted upward and fixed to the presacral fascia with two sutures to invaginate the anal anastomosis and lengthen the skin-lined anal canal (see Fig. 48-20*D*). The neoanus is dilated beginning 3 to 4 weeks after the operation. The colostomy is closed when the fistulous tract has been dilated to an adequate size.

Although the early results of this operation have been encouraging, it is obvious that many of these patients lack the basic elements of continence, such as the internal anal sphincter or innervation to the muscles of continence. In a review of nonrandomized patients in which approximately half of the patients had been operated on by the laparoscopic assisted pull-through technique, and the other half had been reconstructed by using the posterior sagittal anorectoplasty operation, the laparoscopic-assisted group had a 90% incidence of a positive anorectal reflex, whereas, in the posterior sagittal group, only 30% of the patients had an intact anorectal reflex.[60] Also noted in this study was that the rectum showed much better compliance in the laparoscopic group when

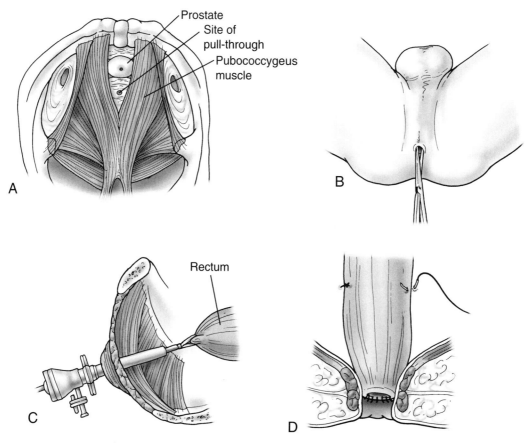

FIGURE 48-20. *A,* The rectourethral fistula has been divided, allowing visualization of the pelvic floor. *B,* The external sphincters are identified with electrical stimulation, and the plane inside the sphincters is developed. *C,* A Veress needle covered by an expansile sleeve is passed through the sphincter complex by using laparoscopic surveillance. The tract is radially dilated with a blunt trocar, and the rectal fistula pulled down to the anal skin. *D,* The fistula is attached to the anal skin, and the rectum is hitched to the presacral fascia to deepen the anal dimple and prevent prolapse of the rectal mucosa.

compared with the posterior sagittal anorectoplasty group.[60] The results of laparoscopic-assisted anorectoplasty will require years of follow-up studies to determine its role in repair of high anorectal atresia.

REFERENCES

1. Ostlie DJ, Holcomb GW III: The use of stab incisions for instrument access in laparoscopic operations. J Pediatr Surg 38:1837–1840, 2003.
2. Gans SL, Berci G: Advances in endoscopy of infants and children. J Pediatr Surg 6:199–233, 1971.
3. Gans SL, Berci G: Peritoneoscopy in infants and children. J Pediatr Surg 8:399–405, 1973.
4. Holcomb GW III, Brock JW III, Morgan WM III: Laparoscopic evaluation for a contralateral patent processus vaginalis. J Pediatr Surg 29:970–974, 1994.
5. Lobe TE, Schropp KP: Inguinal hernias in pediatrics: Initial experience with laparoscopic inguinal exploration of the asymptomatic contralateral side. J Laparoendosc Surg 2:135–140, 1992.
6. Holcomb GW III, Morgan WM III, Brock JW III: Laparoscopic evaluation for a contralateral patent processus vaginalis: Part II. J Pediatr Surg 31:1170–1174, 1996.
7. Grossmann PA, Wolf SA, Hopkins, JW et al: The efficacy of laparoscopic examination of the internal ring in children. J Pediatr Surg 30:214–217, 1995.
8. Wulkan ML, Wiener ES, Van Balen N, et al: Laparoscopy through the open ipsilateral sac to evaluate presence of contralateral hernia. J Pediatr Surg 31:1174–1176, 1996.
9. Fuenfer MM, Pitts RM, Georgeson KE: Laparoscopic exploration of the contralateral groin in children: An improved technique. J Laparoendo Surg 1(suppl 6):S1–S4, 1996.
10. Rescorla FJ, West KW, Engum SA, et al: The "other side" of pediatric hernias: The role of laparoscopy. Am Surg 63:690–693, 1997.
11. Schier F, Montupet P, Esposito C: Laparoscopic inguinal herniorrhaphy in children: A three-center experience with 933 repairs. J Pediatr Surg 37:395–397, 2002.
12. Tan HL: Laparoscopic repair of inguinal hernias in children. J Pediatr Surg 36:833, 2001.
13. Geiger JD: Selective laparoscopic probing for a contralateral patent processus vaginalis reduces the need for a contralateral exploration in inconclusive cases. J Pediatr Surg 35:1151–1154, 2000.
14. Holcomb GW III, Ostlie DJ, Splide TL, et al: Laparoscopic evaluation for contralateral patent processus vaginalis in children with unilateral inguinal hernia. Submitted for publication.
15. Ostlie DJ, Miller KM, Holcomb GW III: Effective Nissen fundoplication length and bougie diameter size in young children undergoing laparoscopic Nissen fundoplication. J Pediatr Surg 37:1664–1666, 2002.
16. Holcomb GW III, Richards WO, Riedel BD: Laparoscopic esophagomyotomy for achalasia in children. J Pediatr Surg 31:716–718, 1996.
17. Patti MG, Albanese CT, Holcomb GW III, et al: Laparoscopic Heller myotomy and Dor fundoplication for esophageal achalasia in children. J Pediatric Surg 36:1248–1251, 2001.
18. Mehra M, Bahar RJ, Ament ME, et al: Laparoscopic and thoracoscopic esophagomyotomy for children with achalasia. J Pediatr Gastroenterol Nutr 33:466–471, 2001.
19. Rothenberg SS, Patrick DA, Bealer JF, et al: Evaluation of minimally invasive approaches to achalasia in children. J Pediatr Surg 36:808–810, 2001.
20. Esposito C, Cucchiara S, Morrelli O, et al: Laparoscopic esophagomyotomy for the treatment of achalasia in children: A preliminary report of eight cases. Surg Endosc 14:110–113, 2000.
21. Harmon CM, Barnhart DC, Georgeson KE, et al: Comparison of the incidence of complications in open and laparoscopic pyloromyotomy: A concurrent single institution series. J Pediatr Surg 39:292–296, 2004.
22. Ostlie DJ, Woodall CE, Wade KR, et al: Effective pyloromyotomy length in infants undergoing laparoscopic pyloromyotomy. Accepted for publication.
23. Tulman S, Holcomb GW III, Karamanoukian HL, et al: Pediatric laparoscopic splenectomy. J Pediatr Surg 28:689–692, 1993.
24. Smith BM, Schropp KP, Lobe TE, et al: Laparoscopic splenectomy in childhood. J Pediatr Surg 29:975–977, 1994.
25. Farah RA, Rogers ZR, Thompson WR, et al: Comparison of laparoscopic and open splenectomy in children with hematologic disorders. J Pediatr 131:6–7, 1997.
26. Hebra A, Walker JD, Tagge EP, et al: A new technique for laparoscopic splenectomy with massively enlarged spleens. Am Surg 64:1161–1164, 1998.
27. Cusick RA, Waldhausen JH: The learning curve associated with pediatric laparoscopic splenectomy. Am J Surg 181:393–397, 2001.
28. Reddy VS, Phan HH, O'Neill JA Jr, et al: Laparoscopic versus open splenectomy in the pediatric population: A contemporary single-center experience. Am Surg 67:863–864, 2001.
29. Rescorla FJ: Laparoscopic splenectomy. Semin Pediatr Surg 11:226–232, 2002.
30. Holcomb GW Jr: Gallbladder disease. In Welch KJ, Randolph JG, Ravitch MM, et al (eds): Pediatric Surgery, 4th ed. Chicago, Yearbook Medical Publishers, 1986, pp 1060–1067.
31. Holzman MD, Sharp K, Holcomb GW III, et al: An alternative technique for laparoscopic cholangiography. Surg Endosc 8:927–930, 1994.
32. Holcomb GW III: Laparoscopic cholecystectomy. Semin Laparosc Surg 5:2–8, 1998.
33. Clements RH, Goldstein RE, Holcomb GW III: Laparoscopic left adrenalectomy for pheochromocytoma in a child. J Pediatr Surg 34:1408–1409, 1999.
34. Reddy VS, O'Neill JA Jr, Holcomb GW III, et al: Twenty-five year surgical experience with pheochromocytoma in children. Am Surg 66:1085–1092, 2000.
35. Miller KA, Albanese C, Harrison M, et al: Outcome analysis of pediatric patients undergoing laparoscopic adrenalectomy. J Pediatr Surg 37:979–982, 2002.
36. Mirallie E, Leclair MD, de Lagausie P, et al: Laparoscopic adrenalectomy in children. Surg Endosc 15:156–160, 2001.
37. Stanford A, Upperman JS, Nguyen N, et al: Surgical management of open versus laparoscopic adrenalectomy: Outcome analysis. J Pediatr Surg 37:1027–1029, 2002.
38. Gluer S, Petersen C, Ure BM: Simultaneous correction of duodenal atresia due to annular pancreas and malrotation by laparoscopy. Eur J Pediatr Surg 12:423–425, 2002.
39. Bax NM, Ure BM, van der Zee DC, et al: Laparoscopic duodenoduodenostomy for duodenal atresia. Surg Endosc 15:217, 2001.
40. Rothenberg SS: Laparoscopic duodenoduodenostomy for duodenal obstruction in infants and children. J Pediatr Surg 37:1088–1089, 2002.
41. Bax NM, van der Zee DC: Laparoscopic treatment of intestinal malrotation in children. Surg Endosc 12:1314–1316, 1998.
42. Bass KD, Rothenberg SS, Chang JH: Laparoscopic Ladd's procedure in infants with malrotation. J Pediatr Surg 33:279–281, 1998.
43. Bax NM, Ure BM, van der Laan M, et al: The role of laparoscopy in the management of childhood intussusception. Surg Endosc 15:373–376, 2001.
44. Abdelrahman AH, Hay SA, Kabesh AA, et al: Idiopathic intussusception: The role of laparoscopy. J Pediatr Surg. 34:577–578, 1999.
45. McKinlay R, Neeleman S, Kelin R, et al: Intraabdominal abscess following open and laparoscopic appendectomy in the pediatric population. Surg Endosc 17:730–733, 2003.
46. Meguerditchian AN, Prasil P, Cloutier R, et al: Laparoscopic appendectomy in children: A favorable alternative in simple and complicated appendicitis. J Pediatr Surg 37:695–698, 2002.
47. Krisher SL, Browne A, Dibbins A, et al: Intra-abdominal abscess after laparoscopic appendectomy for perforated appendicitis. Arch Surg 136:438–441, 2001.
48. Canty TG Sr, Collins D, Losasso B, et al: Laparoscopic appendectomy for simple and perforated appendicitis in children: the procedure of choice? J Pediatr Surg 35:1582–1585, 2000.
49. Dronov AF, Kotlobovskii, Poddubnyi IV: Laparoscopic appendectomy in pediatric patients: Experience of 2300 operations [in Russian]. Khirurgiia 6:30–36, 2000.
50. Blakely ML, Spurbeck W, Lakshman S, et al: Current status of laparoscopic appendectomy in children. Sem Pediatr Surg 7:225–227, 1998.
51. Rintala RJ, Rintala HG, Lindahl H: Proctocolectomy and J-pouch ileo-anal anastomosis in children. J Pediatr Surg 37:66–70, 2002.
52. Georgeson KE: Laparoscopic-assisted total colectomy with pouch reconstruction. Semin Pediatr Surg 11:233–236, 2002.

53. So HB, Schwartz DL, Becker JM, et al: Endorectal "pull-through" without preliminary colostomy in neonates with Hirschsprung's disease. J Pediatr Surg 15:470–471, 1980.

54. Georgeson KE, Fuenfer MM, Hardin WD: Primary laparoscopic pull-through for Hirschsprung's disease in infants and children. J Pediatr Surg 30:1–7, 1995.

55. Hollwarth ME, Rivosecchi M, Schleef J, et al: The role of transanal endorectal pull-through in the treatment of Hirschsprung's disease: A multicenter experience. Pediatr Surg Int 18:344–348, 2002.

56. Georgeson KE: Laparoscopic-assisted pull-through for Hirschsprung's disease. Semin Pediatr Surg 11:205–210, 2002.

57. deVries PA, Pena A: Posterior sagittal anorectoplasty. J Pediatr Surg 17:638–643, 1982.

58. Pena A, Hong A: Advances in the management of anorectal malformations. Am J Surg 180:370–376, 2000.

59. Georgeson KE, Inge TH, Albanese CT: Laparoscopically assisted anorectal pull-through for high imperforate anus: A new technique. J Pediatr Surg 35:927–931, 2000.

60. Lin CL, Wong KKY, Lan LCL, et al: Earlier appearance and higher incidence of the rectoanal relaxation reflex in patients with imperforate anus repaired with laparoscopically assisted anorectoplasty. Surg Endosc. Accepted for publication.

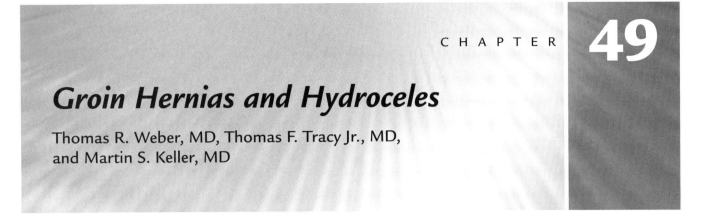

CHAPTER 49

Groin Hernias and Hydroceles

Thomas R. Weber, MD, Thomas F. Tracy Jr., MD, and Martin S. Keller, MD

Hernias and hydroceles of the inguinal and scrotal regions are among the most common congenital disorders managed by pediatricians and pediatric surgeons. Affecting both male and female patients, hernias can be life threatening or can result in the loss of a testis or an ovary or a portion of the bowel if incarceration and strangulation occur. For these complications to be avoided, timely diagnosis and operative therapy are thus important. This chapter discusses the diagnostic methods for hernia and hydrocele detection in infants and children, the operative approaches, and the complications associated with this common pediatric surgical procedure.

EMBRYOLOGY AND ANATOMY

The processus vaginalis, which gives rise to the usual pediatric indirect inguinal hernia, is present in the developing fetus at 12 weeks in utero. The processus is a peritoneal diverticulum that extends through the internal inguinal ring. As the testis descends in months 7 to 8 of gestation, a portion of the processus attaches to the testis as it exits the abdomen and is dragged into the scrotum with the testis (Fig. 49-1).

The portion of peritoneum (processus) enveloping the testis becomes the tunica vaginalis. The remainder of the processus within the inguinal canal eventually is obliterated, eliminating the communication between the scrotum and the peritoneal cavity. The exact time at which obliteration occurs is somewhat controversial. In a significant number of individuals, perhaps as many as 20%, the processus vaginalis remains asymptomatically patent throughout life.[1]

Because the testicular vessels and vas deferens are retroperitoneal structures, they exit the internal ring behind the processus; therefore a hernia sac formed from the processus vaginalis lies anterior and slightly medial to the spermatic cord structures. The sac itself can be extremely thin or thick-walled, depending on the age of the patient, the amount of time the hernia has been symptomatic, and whether incarceration has occurred.

In some cases, the hernia sac can be so thin that the testicular vessels and vas deferens appear to exit the internal ring inside the sac rather than behind it, but embryologically, this is an impossibility. A diligent search always discloses a thin membrane of sac adherent anteriorly to the spermatic cord.

A patent processus is only a potential hernia and becomes an actual hernia only when bowel or other intra-abdominal contents exit the peritoneal cavity into it. If only fluid leaves the peritoneal cavity, the defect is termed a *communicating hydrocele,* with a typical history of enlargement during activities that increase intra-abdominal pressure (e.g., crying, straining) and shrinkage during sleep and other periods of relaxation. Because this pattern indicates a definite patent processus, most surgeons regard a communicating hydrocele as a hernia and proceed to repair.

INCIDENCE

Indirect Inguinal Hernia

The incidence of *indirect inguinal hernia* in the general population of infants and children is generally unknown, because variations exist in prematurity, associated disease, and access to medical care. In carefully controlled population studies, however, the incidence approximates 1% to 5%.[2] In most series, male children with hernias outnumber female children by an 8:1 to 10:1 ratio. These figures depend on associated diseases and other factors.

Premature infants have a greatly increased risk for developing inguinal hernias. Reported incidences of 7%, 17%, and 30% in boys and 2% in girls with prematurity and low birth weight emphasize the higher risk of hernia that exists for these infants.[3-5] Associated disorders of prematurity, such as ventilator dependency, sepsis, and necrotizing enterocolitis, are not associated with a greater hernia incidence.[4] This high risk of inguinal hernia, with risk of incarceration that exceeds 60% during the first 6 months of life, leads most neonatologists and

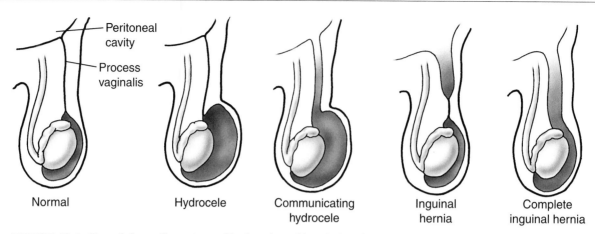

FIGURE 49-1. From left, configurations of hydrocele and hernia in relation to patency of the processus vaginalis.

pediatric surgeons to recommend repair of hernia before the infant's discharge from the hospital.[3]

Associated Diseases and Disorders

Additional associated diseases have been found to increase both the incidence of hernia and the risk of recurrence after repair. Patients with cystic fibrosis have up to a 15% incidence of inguinal hernia. This figure is approximately 8 times that of the normal population.[6] Increased intra-abdominal pressure in patients with cystic fibrosis that results from chronic coughing, respiratory infection, or obstructive airway disease does not fully explain this increase, because siblings and fathers of children with cystic fibrosis also are at a greater risk for development of hernia, although to a lesser degree.[6] These greater risks are thought to be related to an altered embryogenesis of the wolffian duct structures that also leads to an absent vas deferens in male patients with cystic fibrosis.

Infants with disorders of connective tissue formation (Ehlers-Danlos syndrome) and mucopolysaccharidosis (Hunter-Hurler syndrome) also are at a higher risk of developing inguinal hernia.[7,8] In addition, the risk of recurrence with these associated diseases exceeds 50%. A number of investigators have emphasized that recurrence of hernia in these children may be the first sign of connective tissue disease.

Children with congenital dislocation of the hip, children receiving long-term peritoneal dialysis, preterm infants with intraventricular hemorrhage, and children with myelomeningocele who require ventriculoperitoneal shunts also are patients noted to have hernia at a frequency greater than that in the general population.[9–11]

Direct and Femoral Hernias

Direct and *femoral hernias* in children are rare and constitute a small percentage of hernia defects in most series. Rarely is the diagnosis made preoperatively. In adults, direct and femoral hernias are generally believed to be acquired defects, but their origin in children remains controversial. Up to one third of children in whom direct or femoral hernias develop have had a previous indirect inguinal repair.[12] Patients with increased intraabdominal pressure and connective tissue disorders are probably at risk for these types of hernias as well.

Bilateral Hernias

The incidence of bilaterality of hernias in the pediatric age group has been a controversial subject for many years. This subject is important to examine for two reasons. First, a presumption exists that a negative contralateral exploration is "unnecessary surgery" and therefore should be avoided at all costs. This decision must be weighed against the risk and inconvenience of subjecting a child to a second anesthetic if a contralateral hernia develops later. (An additional consideration in this regard includes the perception that the surgeon "missed" the other hernia.) Second, technical mishaps, particularly injury to the vas and vessels, can occur during contralateral exploration, just as they can occur during herniorrhaphy on the primary side. Risking such an injury for a negative exploration is questionable. However, leaving a potential hernia on the contralateral side may result in later incarceration, which carries a risk to the testis itself and strangulation and may necessitate a much larger operation that may involve bowel resection.

Numerous studies have appeared in the literature over the past 30 to 40 years regarding the incidence of bilateral hernias in children, the advisability of bilateral exploration, the incidence of later development of a hernia if contralateral exploration is not performed, and the practice of most pediatric surgeons regarding these issues. Several early excellent reviews attempted to tabulate these data into workable summaries.[13–15]

The true incidence of bilateral hernias seems to depend primarily on the definition of exactly what constitutes a hernia or potential hernia. A patent processus vaginalis represents an opening from the peritoneal cavity into the inguinal canal or scrotum, but the actual potential for this structure to develop into a hernia is unknown. A contralateral patent processus vaginalis is present in

50% to 90% of cases in several operative series.[15,16] In contrast, by using pneumoperitoneography at the time of herniorrhaphy, an incidence of contralateral patency was found in 22% to 29% of cases.[17] However, additional follow-up series demonstrated only a 20% incidence of developing a hernia later if the contralateral side is not explored, suggesting that a clinical hernia does not subsequently develop in all patients with a patent processus.[1]

The age at presentation of the primary hernia influences the incidence of contralateral patent processus and also the incidence of a subsequent contralateral hernia.[18] The highest reported incidence of contralateral patent processus occurs in infants younger than 2 months (63%).[16] The incidence decreases to 41% for children aged 2 to 16 years. The high incidence of patent processus in infants corresponds to the common presentation of bilateral inguinal hernias (34%) in patients younger than 6 months.[18] Early data established the incidence of metachronous contralateral hernias as high as 40% to 50% for infants undergoing repair.[19,20] More recent studies have been able to identify a much lower incidence for the development of a contralateral hernia.[18,21-23] Overall, in one report of 548 infants and children, in 8.8%, a metachronous contralateral hernia developed at a median interval of 6 months (range, 4 days to 7 years). The stratified incidence was found to be 12.4% in infants younger than 6 months and 10.6% in children younger than 2 years. In other groups, analysis of the incidence of metachronous contralateral hernia was 14.8% in premature infants, 7.4% in all girls, and 27.6% in children who have an incarcerated hernia.[18]

Other factors that have been implicated in affecting the incidence of bilaterality of hernias in children include the gender of the patient, the side (right or left) of the primary hernia, and the presence of associated disorders or increased abdominal pressure or fluid. The incidence of bilateral hernias seems to be greater in female patients in all age groups, with reported values of 20% to 50%.[18] This fact, combined with the observation that the injury to reproductive organs during herniorrhaphy in the female patient is probably extremely low, prompts some surgeons to advocate bilateral exploration in virtually all female patients. This practice, however, prevents a contralateral hernia in only 7% of girls.

The side of the primary hernia has been analyzed in a number of series to determine the incidence of bilateral hernias. Although a number of reports have shown a slightly higher incidence of a contralateral hernia if the primary hernia is left-sided, an equal number of reports have shown no significant difference in this regard. Most pediatric surgeons proceed with contralateral exploration based on other factors, such as age. Patients with associated conditions, such as ventriculoperitoneal shunts, ascites, connective tissue disorders, and cystic fibrosis, have a high enough incidence of bilaterality, and the risk of subsequent anesthesia is sufficiently great to justify routine bilateral exploration.

The use of the laparoscope at the time of herniorrhaphy to assess the contralateral side is a recent innovation and has added some information regarding the incidence of bilaterality. Several series have reported that the operative approach is changed in 30% to 50% of cases (no contralateral hernia found by laparoscope) when a small scope is inserted through the hernia sac on the primary side and the contralateral internal ring is inspected.[24,25] In addition, little difference in contralateral incidence was found with regard to patient age, gender, and associated conditions.

Based on the aforementioned data, the following recommendations regarding bilateral exploration can be made. Routine bilateral exploration is best reserved for infants and children with associated disorders and for all patients with definite or strongly suspected bilateral clinical hernia. The risks and benefits of contralateral exploration should be proposed for higher risk groups of patients such as those with incarcerated hernias, those with a history of prematurity, or those with underlying risks of general anesthesia. Individual parents and surgeons have to balance the variation between recent data and previously reported studies to justify the need for exploration based on the potentially small difference in the overall rate of metachronous hernias. With these criteria, we believe we avoid a large number of "unnecessary" bilateral explorations and the accompanying risks of technical mishap, while ensuring that the incidence of later development of a contralateral hernia is low.

Hydrocele

Similar to that of a hernia, the incidence of a hydrocele among male infants is largely unknown. A noncommunicating hydrocele, unassociated with a patent processus vaginalis and therefore not a potential hernia, is common in male newborns and is self-limiting, usually resolving within 6 to 12 months. The persistence of a hydrocele beyond age 12 months brings on the suspicion of a communication with the abdominal cavity through a patent processus and should be regarded as a hernia. The incidence of an isolated (noncommunicating) hydrocele in children older than 1 year is probably less than 1%.

CLINICAL PRESENTATION

Indirect Inguinal Hernia

The hallmark of an *indirect inguinal hernia* in a child is a groin bulge, extending toward the top of the scrotum, which is visible most frequently during periods of increased abdominal pressure (e.g., crying, laughing, straining). The hernia usually spontaneously reduces with relaxation, or it can be gently reduced manually with upward, posterior pressure directly on the mass. Caudal traction on the testicle occasionally aids in the reduction. The usual history obtained from the parents is one of recurrent groin swelling that spontaneously reduces but that is gradually enlarging or is more persistent and is becoming more difficult to reduce. Occasionally, the initial clinical presentation is one of the abrupt appearance of the hernia with incarceration. In many cases, careful questioning of the family reveals a history consistent with either a groin bulge or a communicating hydrocele.

Frequently a patient is referred after the pediatrician or the family has seen the typical hernia bulge, but the surgeon is unable to demonstrate a definite hernia, even when such maneuvers as induced crying and laughing are used. In these cases, a reliable history, combined with palpation of a thickened cord as it crosses the pelvic tubercle or the palpable sensation of a large patent processus known as "silk glove sign," is sufficient evidence to proceed with herniorrhaphy. An alternative approach includes asking the parents to return with the child for examination when a definite bulge appears. This has been rarely successful in our experience and risks incarceration and its attendant hazards. Experienced surgeons can diagnose pediatric hernias with a high degree of accuracy with history and groin palpation. Herniograms were once proposed to aid in the diagnosis of hernia, but concerns regarding cost, complications, and gonad radiation limited enthusiasm for this technique.[26] Ultrasonography of the inguinal canal and scrotum is noninvasive and often diagnostic after difficult or inconclusive examinations.

Direct Inguinal Hernia

Direct inguinal hernias in children are rare. The clinical presentation is somewhat different from that of indirect hernias. Direct hernias appear as groin masses that extend toward the femoral vessels with exertion or straining. In one third of cases, a previous indirect hernia repair on the side of the direct hernia was performed, suggesting that injury to the floor of the inguinal canal occurred during the first herniorrhaphy. Because the defect arises through the floor of the inguinal canal, medial to the epigastric vessels, the repair consists of strengthening the floor by suturing transversalis fascia or conjoined tendon to Cooper's ligament, much the same as the approach in the adult. Recurrence after such a repair in the child, in contrast to recurrence in the adult, is rare. Prosthetic material for direct hernia repair or other approaches, such as preperitoneal repair, are rarely required in the pediatric age group.

Hydroceles

Hydroceles can be categorized into communicating and noncommunicating types. Communicating hydroceles, indicating communication with the peritoneal cavity, are hernias and should be treated as such. A typical history for this defect includes scrotal swelling that comes and goes depending on the level of activity and relaxation. Frequently, gentle pressure or squeezing reduces the hydrocele fluid from the scrotum into the peritoneal cavity, but typically the fluid abruptly reappears with increased intraabdominal pressure.

Noncommunicating hydroceles can be present at birth or can develop months or years later for no obvious reason. The usual history is one of stable size or very slow growth, without abrupt disappearance or rapid change in size. Unless these hydroceles reach extremely large proportions, no management is indicated other than simple observation. The *abdominoscrotal hydrocele* is an unusual variant of hydrocele that requires aggressive therapy, however. A large hydrocele appears as a scrotal collection of fluid with a palpable pelvic mass on the side of the hydrocele. Frequently, pressure on the abdominal mass causes enlargement of the scrotal component.

Exactly how or why these hydroceles become so large is a matter of speculation. One explanation is that this abnormality arises as a scrotal hydrocele attached to a long processus vaginalis that is patent with the scrotum but is obliterated at the internal ring. As the processus continues to enlarge in a cephalad direction through the internal ring, a retroperitoneal component forms.[27] With continued fluid production within the hydrocele, the retroperitoneal portion enlarges proportionately greater than the scrotum, because of limited growth potential within the scrotum. Therapy for this condition consists of complete excision of all hydrocele sac components, which can usually be accomplished through a generous groin excision after evacuation of the sac. Identification of the spermatic cord in these operations can be difficult. As with all hernia procedures, the cord components must be kept in view during the dissection.

TECHNIQUES OF REPAIR

Anesthesia

Hernia and hydrocele operations in children usually involve outpatient (same day) surgical repair, if the child is not already hospitalized. Premature infants hospitalized at birth who are found to have hernias generally undergo repair before discharge. Nonhospitalized premature infants with hernias who are within 4 to 6 months of birth should be observed in the hospital for 24 hours after repair because of the risk of life-threatening apnea after general anesthesia (see Chapter 3). These infants, therefore, are not candidates for outpatient surgical procedures. Most term or near-term infants, however, are candidates for outpatient surgery, unless associated diseases necessitate postoperative hospitalization.

The choice of anesthesia technique for each child should be discussed with the anesthesiologist involved, taking into account the general condition and gestational age of the infant and the experience of the staff. Most hernia repairs in children are performed by using general inhalation anesthesia, which may or may not include endotracheal intubation. Local or spinal anesthesia techniques are reserved for infants with severe prematurity or associated disease that makes general anesthesia more risky. In experienced hands, spinal anesthesia can be successful in 80% of attempts in infants as small as 1500 g. In cases performed with general anesthesia, many surgeons and anesthesiologists use injections of long-acting local anesthesia within the wound edges and along the ilioinguinal nerve or in the epidural space to relieve postoperative pain.[28]

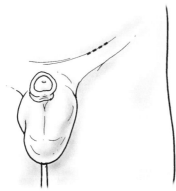

FIGURE 49-2. The incision (dashed line) for inguinal herniorrhaphy is made above the inguinal ligament in a natural skin fold.

Operative Techniques

After routine sterile skin preparation and draping, a skin incision in the groin skin crease is made (Fig. 49-2). Crossing veins can be cauterized, tied, or pushed aside. Scarpa's fascia is grasped and incised with scissors, exposing the external oblique aponeurosis. Blunt dissection clears the fat from the external oblique, exposing the external inguinal ring. At this point, in both male and female patients, the hernia sac is usually seen bulging from the external ring, and the external oblique is incised. Occasionally, with extremely large or long-standing hernias, the external ring is stretched to the point at which it overlaps the internal ring. Thus opening the external oblique is unnecessary. This is especially true in female patients and premature infants. Small retractors are placed within Scarpa's fascia. The incision in the external oblique, made with either knife or scissors, can stop short of the external ring or can be made completely through the ring (Fig. 49-3). In either case, care must be taken not to injure the ilioinguinal nerve, which is usually closely adherent to the cremasteric muscle fibers, directly under the external oblique aponeurosis.

The hernia sac is found lying within the inguinal canal, anterior and slightly medial to the spermatic cord. Thus it is usually safe to grasp the most anterior structures with a smooth forceps, delivering the sac and spermatic cord into the wound (Fig. 49-4). Careful dissection of the anterior cremasteric muscle fibers should allow the sac and attached spermatic cord to be elevated to skin level, preventing the need for dissection deep in the wound, where injury to the cord structures can occur.

Safe separation of the cord structures from the sac is a critical part of the herniorrhaphy. Because of the extremely small size of these structures in infants and children, many pediatric surgeons advocate intraoperative visual magnification for herniorrhaphy.

Because the spermatic vessels (artery and vein) emerge from the internal ring in the most lateral position, they are encountered first in the dissection. By carefully grasping the tissue next to the vessels, we can push these structures gently posteriorly to free them from the sac, while the sac itself is held with another smooth forceps (see Fig. 49-4). As the vessels are dissected free, the new portions of sac that are exposed are grasped with smooth

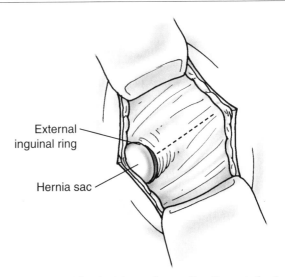

FIGURE 49-3. After incising and spreading Scarpa's fascia, the anterior surface of the external oblique aponeurosis is exposed. Frequently, the hernia sac can be seen bulging through the external ring. The external oblique fascia is opened in the direction of its fibers. The incision in the external oblique can be continued into the external ring or stopped before the ring fibers. Alternatively, in small infants, the external oblique can be left intact, and the sac dissection can be accomplished through the external ring.

forceps, allowing the sac to rotate medially. This usually exposes the vas deferens tightly adherent to the sac. The vas itself is not grasped, but rather the adjacent tissue is pushed posteriorly to free the vas from the sac. Great care and gentleness are required during the dissection to avoid injury to the vas, vas deferens artery, and spermatic vessels.

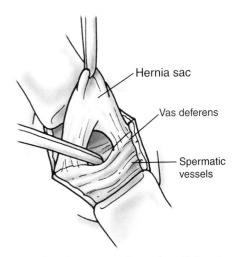

FIGURE 49-4. The hernia sac, anterior and medial to the spermatic cord, is grasped with a tissue forceps or hemostat and delivered into the wound. A second tissue forceps is used to dissect the cremasteric fibers away from the sac, exposing the spermatic cord. By grasping the loose tissue adjacent to the testicular artery and vein, these structures are pushed posteriorly to expose the vas deferens. The vas itself is not grasped but rather gently pushed away from the sac by a closed forceps or sponge. Care is taken to preserve the vas artery as well.

In general, the testis is not delivered into the wound during this dissection, because the operative field is small, and extra structures can obliterate the field and make the dissection considerably more difficult.

After the vas deferens and spermatic vessels are dissected completely away from the sac, a hemostat is passed beneath the sac and spread. The sac is doubly clamped and divided between the hemostats, only after ensuring that the vas and vessels are completely separated (Fig. 49-5). The sac is not divided if intra-abdominal structures (bowel, ovary, omentum) are contained within. In these cases, the sac is opened anteriorly, with a hemostat remaining posteriorly, and the viability of the sac contents is assessed. If the sac contents are viable, reduction of these structures into the abdomen is performed with blunt forceps.

If incarceration with apparent nonviable bowel is present, a separate abdominal incision is usually used to aid in reduction and to evaluate fully the extent of bowel infarction. Frequently, bowel that appears nonviable in a strangulated position within a sac quickly regains evidence of viability after intra-abdominal reduction. If it remains nonviable, bowel resection must be performed. Occasionally, a normal appendix is contained within a right-sided hernia sac. Although some surgeons advocate appendectomy in this setting, even a careful appendectomy increases the risk of postoperative wound infection and therefore should not be routinely performed.

After the sac is divided, the cord is completely separated proximally from the sac. The sac is twisted one to two full turns and ligated at the level of the internal ring (Fig. 49-6). The internal ring is not usually reconstructed. The distal sac can be gently dissected from the cord and removed or left in situ. If the distal sac is connected to a hydrocele, the hydrocele and testis are usually delivered into the wound, and the attached cord is carefully identified. The vas deferens can take a circuitous route along the outside of the distal sac and can be injured

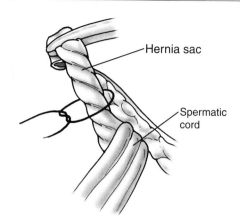

FIGURE 49-6. The spermatic cord is dissected from the sac to the level of the internal ring. The sac is twisted to narrow its base, as well as to reduce intra-abdominal contents that may have reappeared at the inside of the internal ring. The sac is ligated with one or two transfixion sutures of nonabsorbable material.

or divided if care is not taken to identify and preserve it. It is probably better to leave a portion of the distal sac behind rather than to risk injury to the vas by overvigorous sac resection. The testis is returned to the scrotum by gentle traction on the scrotal skin to pull the gubernaculum and testis into the scrotum (Fig. 49-7). If associated undescended testis is present, concomitant orchiopexy can be performed.

The wound is closed in layers, by using absorbable or nonabsorbable suture, according to the surgeon's preference. Most pediatric surgeons use subcuticular sutures for skin closure, with either flexible collodion or transparent film dressing (Op-Site, Tegaderm).

The application of laparoscopy for herniorrhaphy in children has recently been described as an alternative to open repair. The proposed benefits of this approach

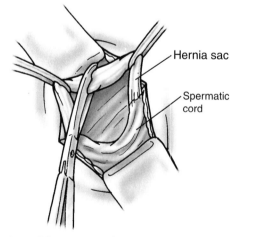

FIGURE 49-5. After ensuring by direct vision that all elements of the spermatic cord are completely free of the sac, the sac is palpated to assess the presence of bowel or omentum. If sac contents are present, the sac can be opened at its midpoint and the contents reduced. The sac is then clamped proximally and distally by hemostats and divided.

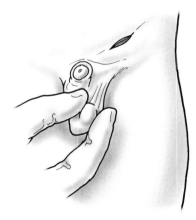

FIGURE 49-7. The testis is gently replaced into the scrotum, first by skin traction on the gubernaculum, and then by manipulation. Pushing the testicle into the scrotum with a sharp instrument should be avoided. The external oblique, Scarpa's fascia, and skin are closed with suture of the surgeon's preference.

include excellent visualization, contralateral evaluation, minimal dissection, and cosmetic results. A three-port technique with a 3-mm or 5-mm infraumbilical scope and laterally placed "needleoscopic" dissecting and suturing instruments has been reported in limited series.[29,30] The long-term outcome after this method of repair is unknown.

Pain relief in the postoperative period has been a topic of considerable interest. Many surgeons simply provide mild oral analgesics (acetaminophen) in doses appropriate for age and weight. This method has the disadvantage of delayed onset of action. If emesis occurs, the medication may be lost in the vomitus. Acetaminophen suppositories are probably more effective for these reasons. Aspirin should be avoided owing to its anticoagulant properties.

Another method of pain relief involves injection of the skin wound edges with a long-acting local anesthetic (bupivacaine) just before suture closure. This technique is safe and probably effective, although it does not anesthetize the deeper tissue layers. To do this, an ilioinguinal nerve block should be performed before beginning the procedure or at the time of closure.

Another method of pain relief involves the caudal injection of a long-acting local agent, which presumably anesthetizes all wound layers. When this is performed by experienced anesthesiologists before the herniorrhaphy is begun, less anesthetic gas and medication are required during the operative procedure. The patients also awaken quicker and are ready for hospital discharge sooner. Complications can develop, however, and these must be carefully explained to the parents.[25] Informed consent is obtained before the procedure with caudal injection.

COMPLICATIONS OF HERNIA AND HERNIORRHAPHY

Incarceration and Strangulation

An incarcerated hernia develops when the sac contents (generally, bowel in the male and ovary, fallopian tube, or bowel in the female patient) cannot be reduced nonoperatively into the peritoneal cavity. Incarceration occurs most frequently (70%) in infants younger than 1 year, with a very low incidence by age 8 years or older. The symptoms of incarceration include severe irritability, apparent cramping abdominal pain, and occasional vomiting, at first nonbilious but rapidly progressing to bilious or even feculent in long-standing cases, indicating strangulation. Physical findings of incarceration include a firm to fluctuant mass in the affected groin, which is usually nontender. The mass may be present only in the groin or may extend to the scrotum. Usually a known hernia is noted on the affected side. Occasionally, incarceration is the first sign or symptom of the presence of a hernia.

The pathophysiology of incarceration involves gradual swelling of the trapped organ within the closed space of the inguinal canal. This effect results in impaired venous and lymphatic drainage, thus increasing edema and pressure. Eventually the pressure exceeds arterial perfusion pressure, and gangrene and necrosis develop. As these circulatory changes evolve, the groin mass becomes much more firm, and significant tenderness develops. Skin redness and edema may appear over the mass. The infant appears much more ill. When these changes occur, the term *strangulation* is used, denoting the need for immediate operative intervention. The actual incidence of intestinal resection necessitated by incarceration in a hernia is low, ranging from 0 to 1.4%.[31]

Incarcerated hernias without evidence of strangulation can be reduced nonoperatively in 80% of cases. The advantages of such reduction include allowing time for fluid resuscitation, optimizing the preoperative status of the child, and allowing resolution of edema within the hernia sac and cord, making the subsequent herniorrhaphy technically less difficult and safer. It is highly unlikely that bowel with significant vascular compromise or necrosis can be reduced without operation.

The principles of nonoperative reduction include sedation (generally by parenterally administered medication), elevation of the lower half of the body, and application of ice to the hernia sac to attempt to reduce edema. The application of ice must be done very carefully in newborns and small premature infants to avoid hypothermia.

Intramuscular (IM) or intravenous (IV) sedation is used by most pediatric surgeons as an aid to hernia reduction. The following medications have been provided for this purpose: midazolam (Versed), 0.05 to 0.1 mg/kg IM or slowly IV; fentanyl citrate, 1 to 4 µg/kg IM or slowly IV; ketamine, 0.25 to 0.5 mg/kg IV or 1 to 2 mg/kg IM; and morphine sulfate, 0.05 to 0.1 mg/kg IM or slowly IV.

Such potent sedatives should be given under the strict guidelines for conscious sedation and the direct supervision of a physician familiar with their possible side effects and adverse reactions. Monitoring equipment (electrocardiograph, pulse oximeter) should be used. Oxygen, suction, and resuscitation equipment must be immediately available. These medications have particular risks in the child who is premature, significantly dehydrated, or lethargic, because respiratory depression or apnea can occur.

If the hernia remains unreduced for 1 to 2 hours, including after an attempt at gentle manual reduction, urgent operative reduction and repair are necessary. Further delay would likely place the hernia sac contents, as well as the testis in the male patient, in jeopardy. The principles for repair are basically the same as those for routine herniorrhaphy, with several additions. The hernia should not be manually reduced after induction of anesthesia, so that the status of the sac contents can be assessed intraoperatively. Occasionally, the hernia reduces spontaneously before the sac is opened for inspection. Unless extremely bloody or foul-smelling fluid is present, or unless the bowel immediately inside the internal ring appears necrotic, no further intraperitoneal exploration is necessary. If the sac contents do not spontaneously reduce, the sac should be opened and the contents inspected.

If the bowel is viable, it can be reduced through the internal ring, which might require incision or dilatation with a retractor to allow reduction. Bowel with questionable viability can be wrapped in warm gauze after delivery into the wound to relieve pressure on the mesentery. If the bowel fails to recover arterial pulsations or peristalsis, if it continues to appear questionably viable, or if it appears nonviable immediately on opening the sac, bowel resection and anastomosis are required. Although some surgeons would attempt these procedures in the hernia wound, our preference is to make a separate abdominal incision, reduce the nonviable bowel into the peritoneal cavity, and perform the bowel resection and anastomosis there.

Completing the herniorrhaphy in an incarcerated hernia after reduction of the sac contents can be difficult, because the edematous, friable sac tends to tear easily and because the cord structures may be obscure. Great care must be taken during the dissection to preserve the integrity of the vessels and vas deferens and to obtain a sac that will hold a transfixion suture.

The testicular blood supply is vulnerable to compression by an incarcerated or strangulated hernia, which, if prolonged, can result in testicular atrophy. The incidence of such permanent injury ranges from 2.6% to 5%.[31,32] The incidence of finding a cyanotic testis at operation for incarcerated hernia is much greater, however ($\leq$29%). With relief of vascular compression by reduction and repair of the hernia, the testis generally survives. In questionable cases, the testis should not be removed but rather returned to the scrotum, and the herniorrhaphy completed.

Recurrence

Although a hernia occasionally recurs, its true incidence is unclear. Recurrence rates of 0 to 1% have been reported. These series frequently fail to assess associated risk factors, however. Hernia recurrence is more common in patients who are premature, have incarceration at the first operative procedure, and have associated disorders, such as inherited collagen deficiencies or peritoneal catheters for hydrocephalus or dialysis. Occasionally, recurrent hernias are of the direct type, suggesting that injury to the floor of the inguinal canal can occur at the primary herniorrhaphy.

Injury to Spermatic Cord

Injury to the spermatic vessels can take place as a result of less than ideal dissection or placement of a transfixion suture. The vessels in small, premature infants are most vulnerable to injury of this type. In addition, separation of these vessels from an edematous, friable sac as a result of hernia incarceration places them at increased risk. Electrocautery should be used with extreme caution or not at all in proximity to the spermatic cord. Transmitted heat may cause thrombosis of the spermatic vessel.

The true incidence of vessel injury during herniorrhaphy, leading to testicular atrophy, is unknown. The commonly quoted figure of 1% is probably high, because the studies that gave rise to this figure did not exclude patients with incarcerated hernia, a condition that in itself can cause testicular infarction.[31] In addition, these studies were performed in an era when vigorous resection of the distal sac was practiced, putting the spermatic vessels in greater jeopardy.

Injury to the vas deferens is a definite risk during hernia repair in the male patient. A vas deferens can be injured in several ways. Experimentally, simply grasping the vas by forceps or hemostat can cause permanent occlusion.[33] Therefore this maneuver should be carefully avoided during herniorrhaphy. Heat injury by electrocautery near the vas also is theoretically possible. The vas can be ligated during suture transfixion of the sac. Twisting the sac too tightly just before ligation can pull the vas up and into the sac, where it can be inadvertently ligated. The vas also can be divided during herniorrhaphy. This most frequently occurs during division of the sac after dissection of the vessels but also can occur during dissection or removal of the distal sac or hydrocele sac. The epididymis also can be injured, divided, or partially resected during removal of these distal sac structures.

Simple division of the vas can occur in these instances. A portion of the vas may actually be resected with the hernia sac. A resected vas should not be confused with mesonephric rests or adrenal rests, which can occasionally occur in conjunction with hernia sacs. Removal of these histologic oddities is of no consequence. Distinction of these rests from vas or epididymis is generally not problematic for an experienced pathologist.

The true incidence of vas injury is unknown. Suggestive data are found in the literature regarding (1) infertility in male patients after hernia repair, and (2) the incidence of vas segments found in hernia sacs examined histologically. Several studies have examined infertility in men who have undergone previous herniorrhaphy (not necessarily in childhood, however).[34,35] These investigators concluded that, although a relation exists between hernia repair and infertility, only a small percentage of infertile men show such a relation. A widely quoted series of cases of vas segments in hernia sacs demonstrated a 1.6% incidence of this histologic finding, but significant details are lacking from this experience.[14] Another series demonstrated a 1.2% incidence of vas or epididymis segments resected with hernia sacs.[36]

The consequences of vas injury or resection are significant. Injury of vas or epididymis bilaterally almost certainly results in sterility. Even unilateral injury is unacceptable and must be avoided. The development of sperm agglutinating antibodies in postpubertal male patients with unilateral vas injury also may cause infertility years later.

The dilemma of how to proceed in the event of vas injury deserves some discussion. If bilateral injury occurs, the patient will be sterile unless continuity is restored in one or both sides. The optimal timing of the attempted repair is unknown, but successful repairs have been done years after the injury.[32] The chances of reestablishing vas continuity in the infant with a tiny vas deferens are remote. Referral to a specialist with microscopic anastomotic experience seems advisable. Whether to refer a child with unilateral injury is somewhat less clear, as fertility rates may decrease only 10% in prepubertal males. The later development of antisperm antibodies in adolescent boys makes referral seem appropriate. In any case, the family must be fully informed of the complication and its possible consequences, so that they may actively participate in the decision.

REFERENCES

1. Morgan EH, Anson BJ: Anatomy of region of inguinal hernia, IV: The internal surface of the parietal layers. Q Bull Northwestern Univ Med Sch 16:20, 1942.
2. Cox JA: Inguinal hernia of childhood. Surg Clin North Am 65:1331–1342, 1985.
3. Boocock GR, Todd PJ: Inguinal hernias are common in preterm infants. Arch Dis Child 60:669–670, 1985.
4. Powell TG, Hallows JA, Cooke RWI, et al: Why do so many small infants develop an inguinal hernia? Arch Dis Child 61:991–995, 1986.
5. Harper RG, Garcia A, Sia C: Inguinal hernia: A common problem of premature infants weighing 1000 grams or less at birth. Pediatrics 56:112–115, 1975.
6. Holsclaw DS, Shwachman H: Increased incidence of inguinal hernia, hydrocele, and undescended testicle in males with cystic fibrosis. Pediatrics 48:442–445, 1971.
7. McEntyre RL, Raffensperger JG: Surgical complications of Ehlers-Danlos syndrome in children. J Pediatr Surg 12:531–535, 1977.
8. Coran AG, Eraklis AJ: Inguinal hernia in the Hurler-Hunter syndrome. Surgery 61:302–304, 1967.
9. Uden A, Lindhagen T: Inguinal hernia in patients with congenital dislocation of the hip. Acta Orthop Scand 59:667–668, 1988.
10. Tank ES, Hatch PA: Hernias complicating chronic ambulatory peritoneal dialysis in children. J Pediatr Surg 21:41–42, 1986.
11. Moazam F, Glenn JD, Kaplan BJ, et al: Inguinal hernias after ventriculoperitoneal shunt procedures in pediatric patients. Surg Gynecol Obstet 159:570–572, 1984.
12. Fonkalsrud EW, de Lorimier AA, Clatworthy HW: Femoral and direct inguinal hernias in infants and children. JAMA 192:597, 1965.
13. Clausen EG, Jake RJ, Binkley FM: Contralateral inguinal exploration of unilateral hernia in infants and children. Surgery 44:735, 1958.
14. Sparkman RS: Bilateral exploration in inguinal hernia in juvenile patients. Surgery 51:393–406, 1962.
15. Rathauser F: Historical overview of the bilateral approach to pediatric inguinal hernias. Am J Surg 150:527–532, 1985.
16. Rowe MI, Copelson LW, Clatworthy HW: The patent processus vaginalis and the inguinal hernia. J Pediatr Surg 4:102–107, 1969.
17. Powell RW: Intraoperative diagnostic pneumoperitoneum in pediatric patients with unilateral inguinal hernias: The Goldstein test. J Pediatr Surg 20:418–421, 1985.
18. Tacket LD, Breuer CK, Luks FI, et al: Incidence of contralateral inguinal hernia: A prospective analysis. J Pediatr Surg 34:684–687, 1999.
19. Kieswetter WB, Parenzan L: When should hernia in the infant be treated bilaterally? JAMA 171:287, 1959.
20. Bock JE, Sobye JV: Frequency of contralateral inguinal hernia in children. Acta Chir Scand 136:707–709, 1970.
21. Wiener ES, Touloukian RJ, Rodgers BM, et al: Hernia survey of the section on surgery of the American Academy of Pediatrics. J Pediatr Surg 31:1166–1169, 1996.
22. Jona JZ: The incidence of positive contralateral inguinal exploration among preschool children: A retrospective and prospective study. J Pediatr Surg 31:656–660, 1996.
23. Holder TM, Ashcraft KW: Groin hernias and hydroceles. In Holder TM, Ashcraft KW (eds): Textbook of Pediatric Surgery. Philadelphia, WB Saunders, 1980, p 594.
24. Lobe TE, Schropp KP: Inguinal hernia in pediatrics: Initial experience with laparoscopic inguinal exploration of the asymptomatic contralateral side. J Laparoendosc Surg 2:135–140, 1992.
25. DuBois J, Jenkins JR, Egan JC: Transinguinal laparoscopic examination of the contralateral groin in pediatric herniorrhaphy. Surg Laparosc Endosc 7:384–387, 1997.
26. Jewitt TC, Kuhn JP, Allen JE: Herniography in children. J Pediatr Surg 11:451–454, 1976.
27. Khan AH, Yazbeck S: Abdominoscrotal hydrocele: A cause of abdominal mass in children: A case report and review of the literature. J Pediatr Surg 22:809–810, 1987.
28. Dalens B, Hasnaoui A: Caudal anesthesia in pediatric surgery: Success rate and adverse effects in 750 consecutive patients. Anesth Analg 58:83–89, 1989.
29. Shier F, Montupet P, Esposito C: Laparoscopic inguinal herniorrhaphy in children: A three center experience with 933 repairs. J Pediatr Surg 37:395–397, 2002.
30. Prasad R, Loworn H, Wadie G, Lobe T: Early experience with needleoscopic inguinal herniorrhaphy in children. J Pediatr Surg 38:1055–1058, 2003.
31. Rowe MI, Clatworthy HW: Incarcerated and strangulated hernias in children. Arch Surg 101:136–139, 1970.
32. Palmer BV: Incarcerated inguinal hernia in children. Ann R Coll Surg Engl 60:121–124, 1978.
33. Janik JS, Shandling B: The vulnerability of the vas deferens, II: The case against routine bilateral inguinal exploration. J Pediatr Surg 17:585–588, 1982.
34. Friberg J, Fritjofsson A: Inguinal herniorrhaphy and sperm-agglutinating antibodies in infertile men. Arch Androl 2:317–322, 1979.
35. Rumke P: Autospermagglutinins: A cause of infertility in men. Ann N Y Acad Sci 124:696–701, 1965.
36. Stergman C, Sotelo-Avila C, Weber TR: The incidence of spermatic cord structures in inguinal hernia sacs from male children. Am J Surg Pathol 23:883–885, 1999.

CHAPTER 50

Undescended Testis and Testicular Tumors

Keith L. Lee, MD, and Linda D. Shortliffe, MD

INTRODUCTION

Numerous factors interact to effect normal testicular descent (Fig. 50-1). Any abnormality in this process can result in an undescended testis (UDT). Also known as cryptorchidism, a UDT carries fertility and malignancy implications. This chapter reviews the endocrine and anatomic basis of testicular descent; the diagnosis, treatment, and sequelae of UDT; and the diagnosis and management of pediatric testicular neoplasms.

EMBRYOLOGY

Testicular development and descent depend on a complex interaction among endocrine, paracrine, growth, and mechanical factors.

Bipotential gonadal tissue located on the embryo's genital ridge begins differentiation into a testis during weeks 6 and 7 under the effects of the testis-determining SRY gene. Sertoli cells begin to produce mullerian inhibitory factor (MIF) soon thereafter, causing regression of mullerian duct structures. By week 9, Leydig cells produce testosterone and stimulate development of wolffian structures, including the epididymis and vas deferens. In the third trimester, the testis descends through the inguinal canal into the scrotum.

Androgens contribute to testicular descent. In humans, the frequency of UDT is increased in boys with diseases that affect androgen secretion or function.[1,2] When antiandrogens are given to pregnant rats, the rate of UDT in male offsprings is 50%.[3-6] Furthermore, maternal exposure to estrogens such as diethylstilbestrol (DES) is associated with cryptorchidism.[7,8] The timing of hormonal exposure also is important, as descent may depend on the gonadotropin surge that normally occurs 60 to 90 days after birth.[9] Local paracrine effects of androgens have been shown to stimulate epididymal development.[10,11]

Growth factors such as epidermal growth factor also play an active role at the level of the placenta to enhance gonadotropin release, stimulating fetal testis to secrete factors involved in descent.[11] Descendin is an androgen-independent growth factor produced by the testis that causes gubernacular development, one of the requirements for normal descent (see Fig. 50-1).[12]

The gubernaculum testis is a mucofibrous structure with its apex at the testicle and epididymis and its base in the scrotum. It undergoes two developmental phases, outgrowth and regression. These phases are under separate control mechanisms.[12-14] Outgrowth refers to a rapid swelling that occurs under stimulation of descendin in an androgen-independent manner. Normal gubernacular outgrowth dilates the inguinal canal, creating a pathway for testicular descent. Experimentally, estradiol plays an inhibitory role through downregulation of insulin-like factor-3, a key factor needed for gubernacular development.[7,8] An abnormality of either of these affects gubernacular outgrowth and could result in UDT. One should note that the gubernaculum does not provide traction on the testis to cause descent. It is not anchored to the scrotum, and it does not insert onto the testis.

During the second phase, regression, the gubernaculum undergoes cellular remodeling and becomes a fibrous structure rich in collagen and elastic fibers and depleted in both smooth and striated muscle cells.[15] Mechanical and anatomic factors, including intra-abdominal pressure and a patent processus vaginalis, are required for normal testicular descent. According to this hypothesis, intra-abdominal pressure causes protrusion of the processus vaginalis through the internal inguinal ring, transmitting abdominal pressure to the gubernaculum and initiating descent.

Other factors in descent include MIF and calcitonin gene-related peptide (CGRP). The role of MIF is probably limited to causing resorption of mullerian structures, which may produce an anatomic obstruction to descent.[13,14] Research in animal models has shown that CGRP is excreted by the genitofemoral nerve under androgen stimulation. It causes contraction of cremasteric muscle fibers and subsequent descent of the gubernaculums, followed by the testes.[16-19] The cremaster muscle is the chief component of the gubernaculum of rats, but it is entirely

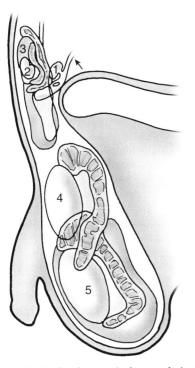

FIGURE 50-1. Testicular descent in human beings: (1) 90-mm crown-rump length (CR) (12–24 weeks of gestational age); (2) 125-mm CR (15–17 weeks); (3) 230-mm CR (24–26 weeks); (4) 280-mm CR (28–30 weeks); (5) at term. The convoluted structure is the epididymis. (Adapted from Hadziselimovic F: Embryology of testicular descent and maldescent. In Hadziselimovic F (ed): Cryptorchidism: Management and Implications. New York, Springer-Verlag, 1983, p 23.)

distinct from the gubernaculum in humans. Therefore the role of CGRP in human testicular descent remains controversial.[11,20,21]

The role of the epididymis in testicular descent also has been considered. The gubernaculum inserts into the epididymis, which precedes the testis into the scrotum. Some investigators postulate that, under androgen stimulation, the gubernaculum facilitates epididymal descent, indirectly guiding the testis into the scrotum.[22] Others believe that an abnormality of the paracrine function of testosterone is responsible for epididymal anomalies and UDT, but that epididymal abnormalities do not cause UDT.[11] Epididymal anomalies are found in up to 50% of men with UDT.[23,24]

INCIDENCE

UDT occurs in 3% of term infant boys and in up to 33% of premature boys. The majority of testes descend within the first 9 to 12 months. At age 1 year, the incidence of UDT is 1%.[25] Descent after 1 year is unlikely. Series documenting the location of UDT find that two thirds to three fourths of cases are palpable, with most being palpable within the inguinal canal or distal to the external ring.[26,27] Anomalies associated with UDT include patent

processus vaginalis, epididymal abnormalities, and uncommonly, hypospadias, posterior urethral valves, and anomalies of the upper urinary tract.[28]

CLASSIFICATION

Variability in nomenclature relating to UDT has led to ambiguity in the literature and difficulty in comparing treatment results. The clearest classification divides UDT into palpable and nonpalpable.[29] A true UDT has had its descent halted somewhere along the path of normal descent. The ectopic UDT has left the path of normal descent and can be found in the inguinal region, perineum, femoral canal, penopubic area, or even the contralateral hemiscrotum. An iatrogenic UDT is a previously descended testis that has become trapped in scar tissue cephalic to the scrotum after inguinal surgery. A retractile testis is a normally descended testis that retracts into the inguinal canal as a result of cremaster muscle contraction.

Nonpalpable testes include intra-abdominal testes and are further classified as closed-ring and open-ring variants, depending on the status of the internal ring. A nonpalpable testis also may be absent or vanishing, secondary to intrauterine or perinatal torsion. This condition is known as monorchia, or anorchia if both testes are absent. Biopsy of tissue at the blind-ending gonadal vessels may reveal hemosiderin and calcification as remnants of the previously torsed testes.

DIAGNOSIS

A careful history and physical examination should enable us to make a distinction between a retractile testis and a low (or "gliding") UDT. Because the cremasteric reflex is weak or absent for the first 23 months of life, a diagnosis of retractile testis is suggested when a boy with documentation of a scrotal testes at birth is seen later with a suspected UDT.

The diagnosis and location of UDT is determined by thorough, gentle physical examination performed in a warm room. The patient should be examined in both a supine and a cross-legged sitting position. In the sitting position, the boy can lean back on his hands spread behind him with knees bent outward and soles of the feet touching or the lower legs gently crossed. The scrotum is examined for hypoplasia and for the presence of either testis. In cases of monorchia, the solitary testis may be hypertrophied. The first maneuver to locate the testis is to walk the fingers gently down the inguinal canal from the internal ring toward the scrotum, trying to push subcutaneous structures toward the scrotum. Lubricating gel may aid in reducing friction. Examining the boy who is sitting or squatting may help identify the testis. Gentle pressure on the midabdomen may help push the testis into the inguinal canal.

On physical examination, both the retractile testis and the low UDT may be manipulated into the scrotum. The retractile testis should remain in the dependent portion of the scrotum temporarily without traction, whereas the low UDT does not remain in the scrotum. With a retractile testis, the ipsilateral hemiscrotum is fully developed, whereas in the other forms of UDT, the hemiscrotum may be underdeveloped. Although the long-term implications of human chorionic gonadotropin (hCG) stimulation are not entirely known, hCG injections may be helpful in distinguishing the low UDT from the retractile testis.[30] In response to a total of 10,000 international units of hCG administered intramuscularly over a 1- to 3-week period, a retractile testis should descend, but a UDT will not.

If neither testis is palpable, anorchia must be differentiated from bilateral UDT. This can be determined by the hCG stimulation test. The baseline testosterone, follicle-stimulating hormone (FSH), and luteinizing hormone (LH) levels are measured before administration of 2000 international units of hCG daily for 3 days, with testosterone level determined on day 6.[31] If the baseline FSH level is elevated (3 SD above the mean) in a boy younger than 9 years, anorchia is likely, and no further evaluation is recommended. If baseline LH and FSH levels are normal and hCG stimulation results in an appropriate elevation of testosterone, testicular tissue is probably present, and the patient should undergo exploration. If the testosterone level does not increase in response to hCG stimulation, however, testicular tissue may still be present, and exploration should be considered. The hCG stimulation test does not indicate whether one or both testes or functioning testicular remnants are present.[31]

Radiologic imaging is rarely helpful in locating a UDT. Multiple studies have shown that the experienced surgeon examiner has a higher sensitivity in locating the UDT than does ultrasonography (US), computed tomography (CT), or magnetic resonance imaging (MRI).[32,33] Of the options, MRI is favored, and it may be especially useful in obese children.[33–35] The addition of gadolinium in magnetic resonance angiography (MRA) can further improve sensitivity and specificity, as testicular tissue is particularly bright on MRA.[36] For the clinically impalpable testis, laparoscopy has a 95% or higher sensitivity for locating a testis or proving it absent.[33,37,38]

FERTILITY

A UDT and, to a lesser degree, its contralateral mate have been demonstrated to be histologically abnormal by investigators who perform bilateral testis biopsies at the time of orchiopexy. Others have found that the epididymis is often malformed.[39–41] A blunted normal testosterone surge at 60 to 90 days may result in a lack of Leydig cell proliferation and delay in transformation of gonocytes to adult dark spermatogonia. Histopathologic changes include a decrease in the ratio of spermatogonia per tubule and Leydig cell atrophy. Clinically, patients with a history of UDT have subnormal semen analyses. Despite these abnormalities, the paternity rate of men with a history of unilateral UDT is equivalent to that of the normal population.[42–44] However, bilateral UDT results in impaired fertility, with paternity rates of 50% to 65%, even if corrected early.[42,44,45]

RISK OF MALIGNANCY

The risk of developing testicular cancer is 5 to 60 times greater for men with cryptorchidism.[25,46] This increased risk may be due to a procarcinogenic effect that higher local temperature has on the UDT. Case–control study has shown that orchiopexy before age 11 years is associated with decreased risk for testicular cancer; whereas fixation after age 11 years or none at all was associated with a 32-fold increased cancer risk.[46] The association of orchiopexy with decrease in cancer risk has not, however, been demonstrated prospectively. Nevertheless, orchiopexy facilitates testicular examination and cancer detection.

Alternatively, malignancy risk may be due to an underlying genetic or hormonal etiology that causes both cryptorchidism and testicular cancer. A total of 15% to 20% of the tumors arise in the normally descended contralateral testis.[47] In addition, the incidence of carcinoma in situ (CIS), a premalignant lesion, is 2% to 4% in men with cryptorchidism compared with less than 1% in normal men. In the postpubertal male, CIS progresses to invasive germ cell tumors in 50% of cases within 5 years.[48] The natural history of CIS diagnosed in a young child at the time of orchiopexy, however, is less clear. It has been recommended that these patients undergo repeated testis biopsy after puberty.[49]

The risk of malignancy is highest in testes originally located abdominally. Cancers arising in uncorrected abdominal testes are most frequently seminomas. In contrast, malignancies arising after successful orchiopexy, regardless of original location, are most frequently non-seminomatous germ cell tumors.[50–52]

TREATMENT: INDICATIONS AND TIMING

Treatment of UDT reduces the risk of torsion, facilitates examination of the testis, improves the endocrine function of the testis, and creates a normal-appearing scrotum (see Fig. 50-1). Early scrotal placement of the testis may affect the risk of malignancy and infertility.[46,53]

The UDT also is unlikely to descend after age 9 to 12 months. The recommended age for a child to undergo orchiopexy is at or near age 1 year (Fig. 50-2).[54] Repair may be undertaken earlier if a symptomatic hernia is present. The risk associated with undergoing general anesthesia after 6 months is low in hospitals with dedicated pediatric anesthesiologists.

For the unilateral UDT that presents after the onset of puberty, orchiopexy or orchiectomy is recommended. The endocrine function of the testis is no longer required, yet the risk of malignancy persists. The risk of death resulting from anesthesia and surgery is lower than the risk of death from malignancy until age 50 years for otherwise healthy men.[55] In light of these data, we recommend that the unilateral, palpable UDT in postpubertal males be brought down surgically if the testis appears normal and orchiopexy can be easily achieved. If the testis is abnormally soft and small or orchiopexy difficult, then it should be removed.

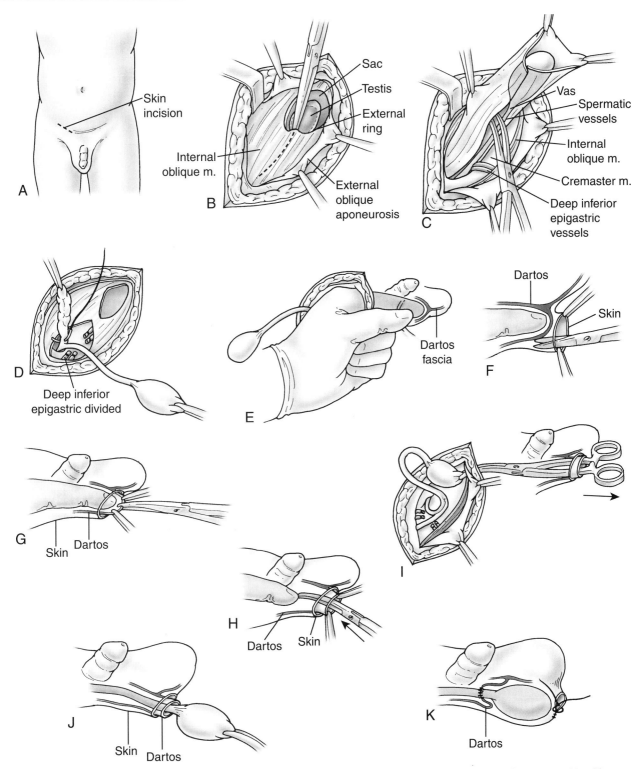

FIGURE 50-2. *A,* Transverse skin incision. *B,* External oblique aponeurosis is opened in the directions of its fibers, with care taken to avoid the ilioinguinal nerve. *C,* The testis is delivered, and the patent processus vaginalis is opened distally near the testis. *D,* The processus vaginalis, or indirect hernia sac, is separated from the cord structures and ligated at the internal ring. Adequate cord length is usually obtained by retroperitoneal dissection of the cord contents. If additional length is required, the inferior epigastric vessels may be ligated (Prentiss maneuver), permitting medialization of the cord. *E,* A finger is passed inferiorly into the scrotum to aid in creation of a dartos pouch. *F* to *H,* Dartos pouch creation and passage of a clamp through the scrotum into the inguinal canal. *I,* Adventitial tissue of the testis is grasped with the clamp. *J,* The testis is brought into the dartos pouch. *K,* Dartos fascia and skin are closed. (From Ellis DG: Undescended testes. In Ashcraft KW [ed]: Pediatric Urology. Philadelphia, WB Saunders, 1990, p 423.)

Orchiectomy is the treatment of choice for management of the postpubertal unilateral intra-abdominal UDT because of increased cancer risk. In addition, the cord length is often too short for orchiopexy. Laparoscopy is ideal in this setting.[56]

Treatment

The value of hormonal therapy in the treatment of UDT is controversial. Buserelin, an LH-releasing hormone agonist, is frequently used to treat UDT in Europe. The highest success rates have been observed in cases in which the testes is at or distal to the external ring.[57–60] Trials combining buserelin and hCG have yielded success rates in the range of 60%, but the testicle may not remain in the scrotum after therapy, and surgical repair is required in 40% of patients.[22,60–62]

Some authors recommend low-dose hCG therapy, regardless of surgical plans, to restore a normal endocrine milieu and to enhance germ cell maturation.[63] hCG may cause virilization, although lower doses do not produce this side effect. Combined hormonal therapy is demanding and requires daily nasal administration of LH-releasing hormone agonist for 4 weeks and several intramuscular injections. Buserelin, the LH-releasing hormone agonist, has not been approved by the United States Food and Drug Administration for this use.

Surgical techniques for UDT depend on whether the testis is palpable (Fig. 50-3). Unilateral and bilateral palpable UDT are treated the same way. For unilateral and bilateral nonpalpable UDT, definitive therapy is determined by diagnostic laparoscopy. For cases of secondary UDT, care must be taken to avoid compromise of the testicular blood supply.

Palpable Undescended Testes

The mainstay of therapy for the palpable UDT is surgical orchiopexy with creation of a subdartos pouch. The success rate, defined as a testis that remains in the scrotum and does not atrophy, is 95%.[64] Fixation is achieved by scarring of the everted tunica vaginalis to the surrounding tissues.[65] Eversion of the tunica vaginalis also eliminates the risk of torsion.[66] The placement of sutures in the tunica albuginea for scrotal fixation is generally discouraged because it causes significant testicular inflammation, increases infertility risk, and may damage intratesticular vessels, especially those in the lower pole of the testis.[31,67,68] Routine biopsy of the testis at the time of surgery is controversial but may provide prognostic information regarding fertility.[53,69]

The technique of orchiopexy with subdartos pouch is illustrated in Figure 50-2.[70–72] The operation is usually performed as an outpatient procedure by using general anesthesia. The patient is supine. Intraoperative administration of an ilioinguinal nerve block with bupivacaine provides excellent postoperative analgesia. The incision should be made along one of Langer's lines, over the internal ring. The external oblique aponeurosis is incised laterally from the external ring in the direction of its fibers, avoiding injury to the ilioinguinal nerve. Once located, the testis and spermatic cord are freed. The testis and hernia sac are dissected from the canal. The tunica vaginalis is then dissected away from the vas deferens and the vessels before its division. The proximal sac is twisted, doubly suture-ligated, and amputated. Retroperitoneal dissection through the internal ring may provide additional cord length for the testis to reach the scrotum.

A tunnel is created from the inguinal canal into the scrotum by using a finger or a large surgical clamp.

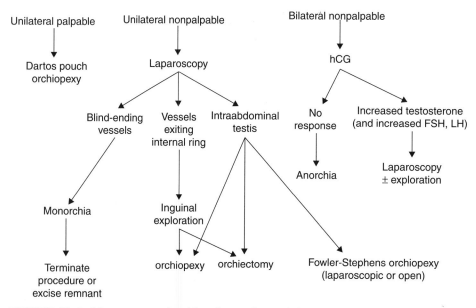

FIGURE 50-3. Management algorithm for undescended testis. FSH, follicle-stimulating hormone; hCG, human chorionic gonadotropin; LH, luteinizing hormone.

The scrotum is bluntly enlarged. A subdartos pouch is created by placing the finger through the tunnel and stretching the skin in a dependent portion of the scrotum. A 1-cm to 2-cm incision is made in the skin over the finger, and a hemostat is inserted just under the skin and spread both superiorly and inferiorly to create the pouch. A clamp is then placed on the surgeon's finger in this scrotal incision, and its tip is guided into the inguinal canal by withdrawing the finger. The clamp is then used to grasp some adventitial tissue around the testis. The clamp is then pulled back to guide the testis into the pouch. One should avoid grasping the testis or vas deferens directly, as this may cause scarring. Alternatively, a testicular transfixation suture may be used to deliver the testicle to the dartos pouch.

Once the testis is in the dartos pouch, a suture is used to narrow the neck of the pouch to prevent testicular retraction. This suture also may be attached to the cut edge of the tunica. Testis measurements and biopsy may be performed at this time. The scrotal skin incision is closed. The external oblique aponeurosis is reapproximated with absorbable suture, and the skin and subcuticular tissue closed with interrupted subcuticular stitches. A flexible collodion dressing is useful in diapered boys.

The patient is seen in outpatient clinic after a few weeks for a wound check and again several months later for testicular examination. Final position and condition of the testicle should be noted. Although rare, complications include atrophy and retraction.

Unilateral Nonpalpable Undescended Testis

When the testis is nonpalpable, diagnostic laparoscopy through an umbilical port is useful for surgical planning.[27,37] If the testicular vessels are seen exiting the internal ring, an inguinal incision is used to locate the testis or testicular remnant. Orchiopexy is performed if a viable testis is found. If the vessels end blindly in the inguinal canal (vanishing testis), the tip of the vessels may be sent for pathologic examination. Remnants of testicular tissue or hemosiderin and calcifications are indicative of resorption of the testis. If the vessels appear atretic or "blind-ending" as they exit the ring, and laparoscopy has not been done, some surgeons have recommended no further exploration, but this is controversial.

If vessels are not seen exiting the internal ring and laparoscopy reveals an intra-abdominal testis, several options are available. The Fowler-Stephens orchiopexy involves ligation of the spermatic vessels, which makes the testis depend on the vasal and cremasteric arteries for viability.[73,74] For this reason, the Fowler-Stephens approach is not a good option after inguinal exploration because the blood supply to the testis may have been compromised. After ligation of the testicular vessels, which can be done laparoscopically or by laparotomy, a delay of about 6 months is recommended before orchiopexy to allow collateral circulation development. The success rate of this procedure is greater than 80%. Other options for surgical management of intra-abdominal testes include microvascular orchiopexy (autotransplantation) and orchiectomy. In the hands of skilled laparoscopists,

results from two-staged laparoscopic orchiopexy compare favorably with those of open surgery.[75] Others have found that a one-stage laparoscopic orchiopexy without ligation is often possible, especially when the testicle lies below the iliac vessels. Magnification and wide mobilization with laparoscopy can afford greater cord length and perhaps better preservation of collateral vascular supply.[76,77]

Bilateral Nonpalpable Undescended Testis

After hCG stimulation confirms the presence of functioning testicular tissue, diagnostic laparoscopy is performed to determine surgical therapy in the same manner as for unilateral, nonpalpable UDT.

Secondary Undescended Testes

Secondary UDT is an uncommon complication of inguinal hernia repair, orchiopexy, or hydrocelectomy. When this is found, surgical dissection is different from that of primary repair because scarring from the previous procedure makes dissection difficult. The surgical technique that we have found successful for reoperative orchiopexy minimizes the risk to spermatic cord contents (especially the vas deferens) by mobilizing the entire cord and scar en bloc along with a strip of external oblique aponeurosis.[78] The incision is made through the previous scar, and the testis, which is usually palpable near the pubic tubercle, is exposed. A traction suture is placed through the tunica albuginea in the midtestis. Parallel incisions in the external oblique aponeurosis allow the testicle/cord/aponeurosis complex to be lifted from the canal so that a plane is developed between the spermatic cord and the inguinal floor. This dissection is carried superiorly to the internal ring, where the external oblique aponeurosis is cut to allow full mobilization of the cord and testis. Dissection continues above the scar, into the retroperitoneum, to produce sufficient length to permit placement of the testis into a dartos pouch. If more length is necessary, division of the inferior epigastric vessels allows the cord to be displaced medially.

TESTICULAR CANCER RISK

Testicular cancer is uncommon in children, accounting for 1% to 2% of all pediatric solid tumors. Children have a much larger percentage of benign testicular lesions than adults. The peak incidence of pediatric testicular tumors occurs between ages 12 to 18 months, followed by a small peak during puberty. Germ cell tumors comprise 65% to 85% of pediatric testicular tumors. Risk of malignancy arising from an UDT varies with location and is 1% with inguinal and 5% with abdominal testes.[79–81]

Presentation and Diagnosis

A testis tumor typically presents as a painless scrotal mass. A history of trauma is often given, and may be the inciting event that brings attention to the scrotal mass.

Differential diagnoses include hydrocele, hernia, and tumor. Malignancy typically is nontender, does not transilluminate, and is not accompanied by an abnormal urinalysis. A hydrocele may impede adequate testicular examination, and a tumor arising in an UDT may undergo torsion, and be seen as acute abdominal pain. Hormonally active tumors may occur with precocious puberty with or without a palpable lesion.

A chest radiograph (CXR) should be obtained to rule out metastases, and testicular US should be performed. US is highly sensitive and can detect even small tumors masked by a hydrocele. US findings of internal calcifications and a heterogeneous mass suggest teratoma. This finding may be useful in preoperative planning for testis-sparing surgery. Once the diagnosis of high-risk testicular cancer is made histologically, CT can be used to evaluate metastatic disease. CT has largely supplanted retroperitoneal lymph node dissection (RPLND) for the purpose of staging; however, it carries a 15% to 20% false-negative rate.[82] MRI also has been used to detect Leydig cell tumors, testicular epidermoid cysts, and Sertoli cell tumors.[83–85] Information obtained can similarly guide the surgical approach, but the cost-effectiveness of MRI is unclear.

Serum tumor marker levels are valuable in both diagnosis and follow-up of testicular malignancy. α-Fetoprotein (AFP) is a glycoprotein produced by the fetal yolk sac, liver, and gastrointestinal tract, whose measurement is elevated in a variety of benign and malignant diseases including yolk sac tumors (YSTs) of the testis. The normal AFP value declines significantly in the months after birth[86]; the normal adult level of less than 10 ng/mL is not achieved until age 8 months[87] (Table 50-1). The beta-subunit hCG (β-hCG) is a glycoprotein produced by embryonal carcinomas and mixed teratomas. Its half-life is 24 hours, and it is normally not detected in significant amount in boys (< 5 international units/L).

Carcinoma In Situ

CIS of the testis is a premalignant lesion. Testicular cancer is reported to develop in at least 50% of testes known to harbor CIS.[48] CIS is seen in patients with UDT and intersex disorders, conditions that are known to carry a higher risk of testicular cancer than that in the general population.[88] In addition, CIS often coexists in the testis that harbors a known cancer.

CIS growth is stimulated by endocrinologic changes during puberty; however, the natural history of CIS in prepubertal testes is less clear.[49,89] Testicular biopsy at the time of orchiopexy is not performed routinely; when it is done, CIS is seen in 0.36% to 0.45%.[53,69] If biopsy of a cryptorchid testis reveals CIS, it has been recommended that the patient undergo repeated postpubertal biopsy. The prevalence of CIS in adult men with a history of UDT is 2% to 4%.[48,90,91] If CIS is identified in the prepubertal testis, it is typically managed with annual testicular examinations and testicular US despite the reputed 50% incidence of conversion to carcinoma in adult men. In postpubertal patients, some clinicians recommend that these patients undergo biopsy of the contralateral testis and unilateral orchiectomy. If biopsy of the remaining testis also reveals CIS, they recommend 18 to 20 Gy of radiation treatment. The same investigators advocate routine postpubertal testis biopsy in all cases of UDT.[90,91] This practice has not been routine in the United States, however, and remains controversial.[92]

Germ Cell Tumors

The most common prepubertal testicular tumors is the YST, also known as endodermal sinus tumor, embryonal adenocarcinoma, orchidoblastoma, and Teillum's tumor.[93] It accounts for 56% to 62% of primary testis tumors, and most occur within the first 2 years of life. Grossly, YSTs are firm and yellow/white. Microscopically, they are characterized by Schiller-Duval bodies and stain for AFP.[80,81,94]

Metastasis of YSTs to the retroperitoneum is uncommon in children (4% to 6%).[80] Approximately 95% of YSTs are confined to the testis. The lungs are the most common site of distant metastasis, which occurs in 20% of patients. The 5-year survival rate for YST approaches 99%.

The standard diagnostic and therapeutic procedure for all testis tumors is radical inguinal orchiectomy. To minimize the risk of metastasis during manipulation, the spermatic cord is clamped or ligated immediately on entry into the inguinal canal. The role of RPLND in children with YST is controversial. Currently, most YSTs are treated with radical orchiectomy, and patients are followed up for recurrence by measuring AFP levels. If the AFP level was elevated at the time of orchiectomy and subsequently returns to normal, RPLND is not performed.

Staging of YSTs requires abdominal and pelvic CT and CXR, pathologic examination of the radical orchiectomy specimen, and determination of serum tumor-marker levels[95] (Table 50-2). Stage I tumors are limited to the testis. They are completely resected by radical inguinal orchiectomy, after which tumor markers normalize. Patients with unknown or normal markers at diagnosis must have a negative ipsilateral RPLND for the disease to be stage I. Tumor markers are obtained monthly and CXRs every 2 months for the first 2 years. Chest and abdominal CT scans are obtained every 3 months for the

TABLE 50-1
NORMAL SERUM α-FETOPROTEIN LEVELS

Age	Mean ± SD (ng/mL)
Premature	130,000 ± 41,000
Newborn	48,000 ± 35,000
Newborn–2 wk	33,000 ± 33,000
2 wk–1 mo	9,000 ± 13,000
1 mo	2,700 ± 3,100
2 mo	320 ± 280
3 mo	88 ± 87
4 mo	74 ± 56
5 mo	47 ± 19
6 mo	12.5 ± 9.8
7 mo	9.7 ± 7.1
8 mo	8.5 ± 5.5
8 mo–adult	5 ± 3

Adapted from Wu JT, Book L, Sudar K: Serum alpha fetoprotein (AFP) levels in normal infants. Pediatr Res 15:50, 1981.

TABLE 50-2
TNM CLASSIFICATION OF PEDIATRIC TESTIS TUMORS

Primary Tumor (T)

TX	Primary tumor cannot be assessed (in the absence of radical orchiectomy)
T0	Histologic scar, no evidence of primary tumor
Tis	Intratubular tumor (in situ tumor), preinvasive cancer
T1	Tumor limited to testis, including rete testis
T2	Tumor invades beyond tunica albuginea or into epididymis
T3	Tumor invades spermatic cord
T4	Tumor invades scrotum

Regional Lymph Nodes (N)

NX	Regional nodes not assessed
N0	No regional lymph node metastasis
N1	Metastasis in a single lymph node, ≤2 cm in greatest dimension
N2	Metastasis in a single lymph node, >2 cm but ≤5 cm in greatest dimension, or multiple lymph nodes none >5 cm in greatest dimension
N3	Metastasis in a lymph node >5 cm in greatest dimension

Distant Metastasis (M)

MX	Presence of metastasis cannot be assessed
M0	No distant metastasis
M1	Distant metastasis

Used with the permission of the American Joint Committee on Cancer (AJCC), Chicago, Illinois. The original source for this material is the AJCC Manual for Staging of Cancer, 4th ed. (1992) published by Lippincott-Raven Publishers, Philadelphia.

first year and every 6 months for the second year. After 2 years without recurrence, follow-up may be extended to every 6 months or yearly.[80]

Stage II disease includes those tumors with microscopic node involvement discovered by RPLND. Tumors diagnosed and treated with transcrotal orchiectomy or biopsied also should be considered stage II, because resection via a transcrotal incision alters the normal lymphatic drainage of the tumor. Lymphatic drainage of the testis is to the retroperitoneal nodes, whereas the scrotum drains to the inguinal nodes. If a testicular tumor is diagnosed through a scrotal incision, ipsilateral hemiscrotectomy should be considered.[96] All patients with stage II disease should receive combination chemotherapy with cisplatin, etoposide, and bleomycin (PEB). Five-year survival rates with PEB approach 100% in this patient population.[80,97,98] Patients with a persistent mass or elevated AFP after chemotherapy should undergo RPLND.

Stage III disease includes retroperitoneal spread seen on imaging studies and occult metastasis manifest by persistent elevation of tumor markers after orchiectomy. Metastasis beyond the retroperitoneum or to any viscera defines stage IV disease. For both stage III and stage IV disease, chemotherapy follows the same protocols as described for stage II disease. RPLND is performed after chemotherapy. The overall survival approaches 100%.

Teratoma is the second most common germ cell tumor of childhood and accounts for 20% to 23% of all cases.

Histologically, teratomas are composed of all three layers of embryonic tissue: ectoderm, endoderm, and mesoderm. Grossly, they may contain differentiated tissue such as cartilage, muscle, bone, and fat; a cystic component also may be present. Before puberty, they follow a benign course and can be managed with testis-sparing surgery.[80,81,99] However, when a child is initially seen at or after puberty, radical inguinal orchiectomy with high ligation of the spermatic cord is indicated, because teratoma can follow a malignant postpubertal course. When immature elements are seen on frozen sections, radical orchiectomy should be performed. Overall disease-free survival after orchiectomy is excellent.[80,100]

Teratocarcinoma, or mixed germ cell tumor, accounts for 20% of pediatric germ cell tumors. Teratocarcinoma is more commonly seen in a testis that has been brought down into the scrotum and may contain any mixture of YST, embryonal carcinoma, choriocarcinoma, and seminoma.[95,101] Eighty percent of teratocarcinomas are confined to the testis at presentation.[102] Foci of choriocarcinoma confer a poorer prognosis. RPLND is usually performed even for stage I disease, and higher stage disease is treated with chemotherapy protocols similar to those used for adults.

Seminoma is rare in children and is treated with radical orchiectomy and retroperitoneal radiation.[103] It is the most common tumor found in a UDT.

Non–Germ Cell Tumors (Gonadal Stromal Tumors)

Leydig cell tumor is the most common non–germ cell tumor (NGCT). The peak incidence in boys occurs from ages 5 to 9 years.[81,104] The clinical triad includes unilateral testis mass (90% to 93%), precocious puberty, and elevated 17-ketosteroid levels.[80,105] Because these tumors produce testosterone and occasionally other androgens, roughly 20% of patients may have endocrinologic signs of precocious puberty and gynecomastia.[95] The differential diagnosis of precocious puberty includes pituitary lesions and congenital adrenal hyperplasia. To eliminate these diagnoses, the pituitary/adrenal axis must be evaluated by assaying 17-ketosteroids and performing a dexamethasone suppression test (see Chapter 76). Reinke's crystals identified on histologic sections or on fine-needle aspirates are pathognomonic for this tumor and can be found in 35% to 40% of all patients.[106,107] However, they are rarely seen in children.[80] When the diagnosis is made preoperatively or intraoperatively, testis-sparing enucleation can be used because these tumors tend to follow a benign course in boys.[108]

The Sertoli cell tumor is a very rare form of NGCT and also is seen as a painless testicular mass. A small percentage of patients have gynecomastia. Although nonspecific, US can show testicular microlithiasis.[109] The clinical course is usually benign, and tumors can be managed with testis-sparing surgery.

Gonadoblastoma is a form of NGCT usually seen in association with intersex disorders. The patients are typically 46 XY phenotypic females with intra-abdominal testes who are seen with virilization after puberty. Up to one third of patients have bilateral gonadal lesions. Whereas the clinical course is usually benign, the germ cell component of these tumors carries a 10% risk of malignant degeneration. Early gonadectomy is recommended, especially if the patient is raised as a female.[110,111]

REFERENCES

1. Bardin CW, Ross GT, Rifkind AB, et al: Studies of the pituitary-Leydig cell axis in young men with hypogonadotropic hypogonadism and hyposmia: Comparison with normal men, prepubertal boys, and hypopituitary patients. J Clin Invest 48:2046, 1969.
2. Santen RJ, Paulsen CA: Hypogonadotropic eunuchoidism, II: Gonadal responsiveness to exogenous gonadotropins. J Clin Endocrinol Metab 36:55, 1973.
3. Husmann DA, McPhaul MJ: Reversal of flutamide-induced cryptorchidism by prenatal time-specific androgens. Endocrinology 131:1711, 1992.
4. Husmann DA, McPhaul MJ: Time-specific androgen blockage with flutamide inhibits testicular descent in the rat. Endocrinology 129:1409, 1991.
5. McMahon DR, Kramer SA, Husmann DA: Antiandrogen induced cryptorchidism in the pig is associated with failed gubernacular regression and epididymal malformations. J Urol 154:553, 1995.
6. Spencer JR, Torrado T, Sanchez RZ, et al: Effects of flutamide and finasteride on rat testicular descent. Endocrinology 129:741, 1991.
7. Nef S, Shipman T, Parada LF: A molecular basis for estrogen-induced cryptorchidism. Dev Biol 224:354, 2000.
8. Emmen JMA, McLuskey A, Adham IM, et al: Involvement of insulin-like factor-3 (Insl3) in diethylstilbestrol-induced cryptorchidism. Endocrinology 141:846, 2000.
9. Spencer JR, Vaughan ED, Imperato-McGinley J: Studies of the hormonal control of postnatal testicular descent in the rat. J Urol 149:618, 1993.
10. Jost A: The gonadal and hypophyseal hormones. Recent Prog Horm Res 8:379, 1953.
11. Husmann DA, Levy JB: Current concepts in the pathophysiology of testicular undescent. Urology 46:267, 1995.
12. Fentener van Vlissingen JM, van Zoelen EJ, Ursem PJ, et al: In vitro model of the first phase of testicular descent: Identification of a low molecular weight factor from fetal testis involved in proliferation of gubernaculum testis cells and distinct from specified polypeptide growth factors and fetal gonadal hormones. Endocrinology 123:2868, 1988.
13. Spencer JR: The endocrinology of testicular descent. AUA Update Series XIII:94, 1994.
14. Heyns CF, Hutson JM: Historical review of theories on testicular descent. J Urol 153:754, 1995.
15. Costa WS, Sampaio FJB, Favorito LA, et al: Testicular migration: remodeling of connective tissue and muscle cells in human gubernaculum testis. J Urol 167:2171, 2002.
16. Yamanaka J, Metcalfe SA, Hutson JM: Demonstration of calcitonin gene-related peptide receptors in the gubernaculum by computerized densitometry. J Pediatr Surg 27:876, 1992.
17. Park WH, Hutson JM: The gubernaculum shows rhythmic contractility and active movement during testicular descent. J Pediatr Surg 26:615, 1991.
18. Goh DW, Middlesworth W, Farmer PJ, et al: Prenatal androgenitofemoral nerve and testicular descent. J Pediatr Surg 29:836, 1994.
19. Goh DW, Momose Y, Middlesworth W, et al: The relationship among calcitonin gene-related peptide, androgens and gubernacular development in 3 animal models of cryptorchidism. J Urol 150:574, 1993.
20. Heyns CF: The gubernaculum during testicular descent in the human fetus. J Anat 153:93, 1987.
21. Wensing CJ, Colenbrander B: Normal and abnormal testicular descent. Oxf Ref Reprod Biol 8:130, 1986.
22. Hadziselimovic F, Herzog B: The development and descent of the epididymis. Eur J Pediatr 152(suppl 2):S6, 1993.

23. Gill B, Kogan S, Starr S, et al: Significance of epididymal and ductal anomalies associated with testicular maldescent. J Urol 142:556, 1989.
24. Elder JS: Epididymal anomalies associated with hydrocele/hernia and cryptorchidism: Implications regarding testicular descent. J Urol 148:624, 1992.
25. Pohl HG, Belman AB: The location and fate of the cryptorchid and impalpable testes. In Peppas DS, Erlich RM (eds): Dialogues in Pediatric Urology, vol 20:1. Pearl River, NY, William J. Miller Associates, 1997, pp 3–4.
26. Docimo SG: The results of surgical therapy for cryptorchidism: A literature review and analysis. J Urol 154:1148, 1995.
27. Kirsch AJ, Escala J, Duckett JW, et al: Surgical management of the nonpalpable testis: The Children's Hospital of Philadelphia experience. J Urol 159:1340, 1998.
28. Schneck FX, Bellinger MF: Abnormalities of the testes and scrotum and their surgical management. In Walsh PC, Retik AB, Vaughan ED, et al (eds): Campbell's Urology, 8th ed. Wein, Saunders, 2002, pp 2353–2394.
29. Kaplan G: Nomenclature of cryptorchidism. Eur J Pediatr 152 (suppl 2):S17, 1993.
30. Rajfer J: Surgical and hormonal therapy for cryptorchidism: An overview. Horm Res 30:139, 1988.
31. Jarow JP, Berkovitz GD, Migeon CJ, et al: Elevation of serum gonadotropins establishes the diagnosis of anorchism in prepubertal boys with bilateral cryptorchidism. J Urol 136:277–279, 1986.
32. Elder JS: Ultrasonography is unnecessary in evaluating boys with a nonpalpable testis. Pediatrics 110:748, 2002.
33. Hrebinko RL, Bellinger MF: The limited role of imaging techniques in managing children with undescended testes. J Urol 150:458, 1993.
34. Landa HM, Gylys-Morin V, Mattrey RF, et al: Magnetic resonance imaging of the cryptorchid testis. Eur J Pediatr 146(suppl 2):S16, 1987.
35. De Filippo RE, Barthold JS, Gonzales R: The application of magnetic resonance imaging for the preoperative localization of nonpalpable testis in obese children: An alternative to laparoscopy. J Urol 164:154, 2000.
36. Yeung CK, Tam YH, Chan YL, et al: A new management algorithm for impalpable undescended testis with gadolinium enhanced magnetic resonance angiography. J Urol 162:998, 1999.
37. Merguerian PA, Mevorach RA, Shortliffe LD, et al: Laparoscopy for the evaluation and management of the nonpalpable testicle. Urology 51(5A suppl):3, 1998.
38. Moore RG, Peters CA, Bauer SB, et al: Laparoscopic evaluation of the nonpalpable testes: A prospective assessment of accuracy. J Urol 151:728, 1994.
39. Huff DS, Hadziselimovic F, Snyder HM, et al: Histologic maldevelopment of unilaterally cryptorchid testes and their descended partners. Eur J Pediatr 152(suppl 2):S11, 1993.
40. Hadziselimovic F, Herzog B, Huff DS, et al: The morphometric histopathology of undescended testes and testes associated with incarcerated inguinal hernia: A comparative study. J Urol 146:627, 1991.
41. Rusnack SL, Wu HY, Huff DS, et al: Testis histopathology in boys with cryptorchidism correlates with future fertility potential. J Urol 169:659, 2003.
42. Lee PA: Fertility in cryptorchidism: Does treatment make a difference? Endocrinol Metab Clin North Am 22:479, 1993.
43. Lee PA, Coughlin MT: The single testis: Paternity after presentation as unilateral cryptorchidism. J Urol 168:1680, 2002.
44. Chilvers C, Dudley NE, Gough MH, et al: Undescended testis: The effect of treatment on subsequent risk of subfertility and malignancy. J Pediatr Surg 21:691, 1986.
45. Lee PA, Coughlin MT: Fertility after bilateral cryptorchidism. Horm Res 55:28, 2001.
46. Herrinton LJ, Zhao W, Husson G: Management of cryptorchism and risk of testicular cancer. Am J Epidemiol 157:602, 2003.
47. Johnson DE, Woodhead DM, Pohl DR, et al: Cryptorchidism and testicular tumorigenesis. Surgery 63:919, 1968.
48. Dieckmann KP, Skakkebaek NE: Carcinoma in situ of the testis: Review of biological and clinical features. Int J Cancer 83:815, 1999.
49. Giwercman A, Muller J, Skakkebaek NE: Cryptorchidism and testicular neoplasia. Horm Res 30:157, 1988.

50. Raja MA, Oliver RT, Badenoch D, et al: Orchidopexy and transformation of seminoma to non-seminoma [letter]. Lancet 339:930, 1992.

51. Jones BJ, Thornhill JA, O'Donnell B, et al: Influence of prior orchiopexy on stage and prognosis of testicular cancer. Eur Urol 19:201, 1991.

52. Halme A, Kellokumpu-Lehtinen P, Lehtinen T, et al: Morphology of testicular germ cell tumours in treated and untreated cryptorchidism. Br J Urol 64:78, 1989.

53. Cortes D, Thorup JM, Visfeldt J: Cryptorchidism: Aspects of fertility and neoplasms: A study including data of 1,335 consecutive boys who underwent testicular biopsy simultaneously with surgery for cryptorchidism. Horm Res 55:21, 2001.

54. Pediatrics AA: Timing of elective surgery on the genitalia of male children with particular reference to the risks, benefits, and psychological effects of surgery and anesthesia. Pediatrics 97:590, 1996.

55. Oh J, Landman J, Evers A, et al: Management of the postpubertal patient with cryptorchidism: An updated analysis. J Urol 167: 1329, 2002.

56. Esposito C, Cardona R, Centonze A, et al: Impact of laparoscopy on the management of an unusual case of nonpalpable testis in an adult patient. Surg Endosc 17 (on line publication: 13 May 2003), 2003.

57. Bica D, Hadziselimovic F: Buserelin treatment of cryptorchidism: A randomized, double-blind, placebo-controlled study. J Urol 148: 617, 1992.

58. Bica D, Hadziselimovic F: The behavior of the epididymis, processus vaginalis and testicular descent in cryptorchid boys treated with buserelin. Eur J Pediatr 152:S38, 1993.

59. Hadziselimovic F, Huff D, Duckett J, et al: Long-term effect of luteinizing hormone-releasing hormone analogue (buserelin) on cryptorchid testes. J Urol 138:1043, 1987.

60. Lala R, Patrizia M, Chiabotto P, et al: Early hormonal and surgical treatment of cryptorchidism. J Urol 157:1898, 1997.

61. Waldschmidt J, Doede T, Vygen I: The results of 9 years of experience with a combined treatment with LHRH and hCG for cryptorchidism. Eur J Pediatr 152:S34, 1993.

62. Giannopoulos MF, Vlachakis IG, Charissis GC: 13 years' experience with the combined hormonal therapy of cryptorchidism. Horm Res 55:33, 2001.

63. Lala R, Matarazzo P, Chiabotto P, et al: Combined therapy with LHRH and hCG in cryptorchid infants. Eur J Pediatr 152(suppl 2):S31, 1993.

64. Saw KC, Eardley I, Dennis MJ, et al: Surgical outcome of orchiopexy, I: Previously unoperated testes. Br J Urol 70:90, 1992.

65. Redman JF, Barthold JS: A technique for atraumatic scrotal pouch orchiopexy in the management of testicular torsion. J Urol 154:1511, 1995.

66. Hurren JS, Corder AP: Acute testicular torsion following orchiopexy for undescended testis. Br J Surg 79:1292, 1992.

67. Bellinger MF: An experimental study of the effect of surgical technique on testicular histology. J Urol 142:533, 1985.

68. Coughlin MT, Bellinger MF, LaPorte RE, et al: Testicular suture: a significant risk factor for infertility among formerly cryptorchid men. J Pediatr Surg 33:1790, 1998.

69. Hadziselimovic F, Hecker E, Herzog B: The value of testicular biopsy in cryptorchidism. Urol Res 12:171, 1984.

70. Benson CD, Lotfi MW: The pouch technique in the surgical correction of cryptorchidism in infants and children. Surgery 62:967, 1967.

71. Koop CE: Technique of herniorrhaphy and orchiopexy. Birth Defects 13:293, 1977.

72. Rajfer J: Technique of orchiopexy. Urol Clin North Am 9:421, 1982.

73. Fowler R, Stephens FD: The role of testicular vascular anatomy in the salvage of high undescended testes. Aust N Z J Surg 29:92, 1959.

74. Stanford LG, Perez LM, Joseph DB: Two-stage Fowler-Stephens orchiopexy with laparoscopic clipping of the spermatic vessels. J Urol 158:1205, 1997.

75. Godbole PP, Najmaldin MS: Laparoscopic orchiopexy in children. J Endourol 15:251, 2001.

76. Esposito C, Damiano R, Sabin MAG, et al: Laparoscopy-assisted orchiopexy: An ideal treatment for children with intra-abdominal testes. J Endourol 16:659, 2002.

77. Lindgren BW, Franco I, Blick S, et al: Laparoscopic Fowler-Stephens orchiopexy for the high abdominal testis. J Urol 162: 990, 1999.

78. Cartwright PC, Velagapudi S, Snyder HM, et al: A surgical approach to reoperative orchiopexy. J Urol 149:817, 1993.

79. Li FP, Fraumeni JF: Testicular cancers in children: Epidemiologic characteristics. J Natl Cancer Inst 48:1575, 1972.

80. Wu HY, Snyder HM: Advances in Pediatric Urologic Oncology. AUA Update Series XXII:26, 2003.

81. Ross JH, Rybicki L, Kay R: Clinical behavior and a contemporary management algorithm for prepubertal testis tumors: A summary of the prepubertal testis tumor registry. J Urol 168:1675, 2002.

82. Pizzocaro G, Zanoni F, Salvioni R, et al: Difficulties of a surveillance study omitting retroperitoneal lymphadenectomy in clinical stage I nonseminomatous germ cell tumors of the testis. J Urol 138:1393, 1987.

83. Drevelengas A, Kalaitzoglou I, Destouni E: Bilateral Sertoli cell tumor of the testis: MRI and sonographic appearance. Eur Radiol 9:1934, 1999.

84. Cho JH, Chang JC, Park BH, et al: Sonographic and MR imaging findings of testicular epidermoid cysts. Am J Roentgenol 178:743, 2002.

85. Poster RB, Katz DS: Leydig cell tumor of the testis in Klinefelter syndrome: MR detection. J Comput Assist Tomogr 17:480, 1993.

86. Brewer JA, Tank ES: Yolk sac tumors and alpha-fetoprotein in first year of life. Urology 42:79, 1993.

87. Wu JT, Book L, Sudar K: Serum alpha fetoprotein (AFP) levels in normal infants. Pediatr Res 15:50, 1981.

88. Wallace TM, Levin HS: Mixed gonadal dysgenesis: A review of 15 patients reporting single cases of malignant intratubular germ cell neoplasia of the testis, endometrial adenocarcinoma, and a complex vascular anomaly. Arch Pathol Lab Med 114:679, 1990.

89. Oosterhuis JW, Looijenga LHJ: Current views on the pathogenesis of testicular germ cell tumours and perspectives for future research: Highlights of the 5th Copenhagen workshop on carcinoma in situ and cancer of the testis. APMIS 111:280, 2003.

90. Skakkebaek NE, Berthelsen JG, Giwercman A, et al: Carcinoma-in-situ of the testis: Possible origin from gonocytes and precursor of all types of germ cell tumours except spermatocytoma. Int J Androl 10:19, 1987.

91. Giwercman A, Bruun E, Frimodt-Moller C, et al: Prevalence of carcinoma in situ and other histopathological abnormalities in testes of men with a history of cryptorchidism. J Urol 142:998, 1989.

92. Heidenreich A, Moul JW: Contralateral testicular biopsy procedure in patients with unilateral testis cancer: Is it indicated? Semin Urol Oncol 20:234, 2002.

93. Kay R: Prepubertal testicular tumor registry. J Urol 150:671, 1993.

94. Wold LE, Kramer SA, Farrow GM: Testicular yolk sac and embryonal carcinoma in pediatric patients: Comparative immunohistochemical and clinicopathologic study. Am J Clin Pathol 81:427, 1984.

95. Coppes MJ, Rackley R, Kay R: Primary testicular and paratesticular tumors of childhood. Med Pediatr Oncol 22:329, 1994.

96. Giguere JK, Stablein DM, Spaulding JT, et al: The clinical significance of unconventional orchiectomy approaches in testicular cancer: A report from the Testicular Cancer Intergroup Study. J Urol 139:1225, 1988.

97. Giller R, Cushing B, Marina N, et al: Outcome of surgery alone or surgery plus cisplatin/etoposide/bleomycin (PEB) for localized gonadal malignant germ cell tumors (MGCT) in children: A Pediatric Intergroup report. Med Pediatr Oncol 29:413, 1997.

98. Mann JR, Raafat F, Robinson K, et al: The United Kingdom Children's Cancer Study Group's second germ cell tumor study: Carboplatin, etoposide, and bleomycin are effective treatment for children with malignant extracranial germ cell tumors, with acceptable toxicity. J Clin Oncol 18:3809, 2000.

99. Rushton HG, Belman AB, Sesterhenn I, et al: Testicular sparing surgery for prepubertal teratoma of the testis: A clinical and pathological study. J Urol 144:726, 1990.

100. Marina NM, Cushing B, Giller R: Complete surgical excision is effective treatment for children with immature teratomas with or without malignant elements: A Pediatric Oncology Group/Children's Cancer Group Intergroup Study. J Clin Oncol 17:2137, 1999.

101. Batata MA, Whitmore WF, Chu FC, et al: Cryptorchidism and testicular cancer. J Urol 124:382, 1980.
102. Castleberry RP, Kelly DR, Joseph DB, et al: Gonadal and extra-gonadal germ cell tumors. In Fernbach DJ, Vietti TJ (eds): Clinical Pediatric Oncology. St. Louis, Mosby-Year Book, 1991, pp 577–594.
103. Perry C, Servadio C: Seminoma in childhood. J Urol 124:932, 1980.
104. Glavind K, Sondergaard G: Leydig cell tumour: Diagnosis and treatment: Case report and review. Scand J Urol Nephrol 22:343, 1988.
105. Cheville JC, Sebo TJ, Lager DJ: Leydig cell tumor of the testis: A clinicopathologic, DNA content, and MIB-1 comparison of non-metastasizing and metastasizing tumors. Am J Surg Pathol 22:1361, 1998.
106. Jain M, Aiyer HM, Bajaj P: Intracytoplasmic and intranuclear Reinke's crystals in a testicular Leydig-cell tumor diagnosed by fine-needle aspiration cytology: A case report with review of the literature. Diagn Cytopathol 25:162, 2001.
107. Mostofi FK: Proceedings: Testicular tumors: Epidemiologic, etiologic, and pathologic features. Cancer 32:1186, 1973.
108. Manuel M, Katayama PK, Jones HW: The age of occurrence of gonadal tumors in intersex patients with a Y chromosome. Am J Obstet Gynecol 124:293, 1976.
109. Drut R, Drut RM: Testicular microlithiasis: Histologic and immunohistochemical findings in 11 pediatric cases. Pediatr Dev Pathol 5:544, 2002.
110. Gourlay WA, Johnson HW, Pantzar JT, et al: Gonadal tumors in disorders of sexual differentiation. Urology 43:537, 1994.
111. Olsen MM, Caldamone AA, Jackson CL, et al: Gonadoblastoma in infancy: Indications for early gonadectomy in 46 XY gonadal dysgenesis. J Pediatr Surg 23:270, 1988.

CHAPTER 51

The Acute Scrotum

Mr. Philip A. King, MMBS, FRCS, FRACS,
and Dr. V. Sripathi, MS, MCh, FRACS

INTRODUCTION

The acute scrotum refers to the common clinical setting of a boy first seen with pain in the hemiscrotum, which may or may not be accompanied by swelling and redness of the overlying skin of the same hemiscrotum.

Such a scenario always has a degree of urgency attached to it because (1) the possibility may exist that the underlying testis on that side may be in risk of permanent ischemic damage, and (2) the condition can be excruciatingly painful and require urgent relief for the comfort of the patient.

A number of possibilities exist for the cause of the acute scrotum, and in most instances (Table 51-1), symptoms and signs are such that the clinical diagnosis can be reached and a rapid course of intervention planned without the need for additional diagnostic tests.

TORSION OF THE APPENDIX TESTIS

Incidence

The incidence of torsion of the appendix testis, or one of the other appendages, which can very rarely produce the same set of symptoms, is not known but is the commonest cause of the acute scrotum by far (Fig. 51-1).

In our institution, a study conducted over a period of 1 year revealed 123 boys who initially had an acute scrotum. Seventy-nine patients had torsion of the appendix testis, with 23 cases of true torsion of the testis. Thus torsion of the appendix testis was 4 times more common than true torsion of the testis.

Etiology

The exciting factor in torsion of the appendix testis is not known. Studies demonstrated that the appendix testis has both estrogen and testosterone receptors. The appendix testis represents a vestigial remnant of the müllerian duct, so the presence of estrogen receptors is not predictable, but the presence of testosterone receptors as

well is somewhat surprising.[1] Therefore it is possible that elevation of either of these hormones in the bloodstream may produce swelling of the appendage, which may in turn predispose the structure to twisting on its narrow stalk (Fig. 51-2). From all known clinical reports, no doubt exists that twisting is the etiology of necrosis. We studied the hormone levels in 13 boys with this condition and found that both testosterone and estrogen levels were normal, but these patients were all studied more than 24 hours after onset of the pain. Under these circumstances, the peak in the hormone level may have already passed. The common age group for presentation of this condition is between 7 and 10 years. It is conceivable that a prepubertal hormone boost may cause some stimulation of the appendix testis.

Presentation

Torsion of the appendix testis occurs mostly in 7- to 10-year-old boys but can occur in younger patients and also can occur in postpubertal boys. Onset of pain is usually gradual but can on occasion be sudden and may even be accompanied by nausea and vomiting.

Characteristically, of course, in this age group, boys will tolerate the pain and be reluctant to tell their parents. Eventually the pain starts to interfere with walking, playing sports, or the ability to attend school. As the pain gets worse, the boys often walk with a wide-based gait, which can be a sign to the parents that something is amiss. What is not readily explainable is that in some of these boys, the torsion is accompanied by redness and swelling of the associated hemiscrotal skin and soft tissues. However, other boys can have complete gangrene of the appendix testis without any accompanying scrotal signs.

Examination of the Scrotum

Examination of the scrotum in these boys often reveals redness in the overlying skin, accompanied in some instances by swelling of the soft tissues in the hemiscrotal side. If overlying soft tissue swelling or redness are

TABLE 51-1

CAUSES OF THE ACUTE SCROTUM

Torsion of the appendix testis
Torsion of the testis
Epididymitis
Idiopathic scrotal edema
Trauma
Other possible conditions
   Incarcerated inguinal hernia
   Acute hydrocele
   Vascular orchitis
   Rare infections

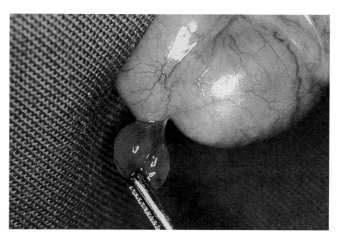

FIGURE 51-2. Swollen edematous appendix testis.

present, the so-called "blue dot" sign can be seen: the appreciation of the discolored testicular appendage through the scrotal skin.

Differential tenderness from the upper part of the testicle to the lower part of the testicle can sometimes be elicited. The tenderness related to the upper pole of the testis is really conclusive diagnostic evidence that one is dealing with torsion of the appendix testis. At times, localization of the tenderness is not so clear-cut, and it may be difficult to tell the difference between torsion of the appendix testis and torsion of the entire testis.

Management and Outcome

The natural history of torsion of the appendix testis is that the acute onset of pain will subside as the appendix undergoes ischemic involution. It will then become a calcified free body within the tunica vaginalis. This process,

however, may take days, and many boys are unable or unwilling to put up with the discomfort.

Because the appendix testis has no known function, the possibility exists that these cases could be treated conservatively. In some centers around the world, this is what is done. However, we recommend operative intervention for two reasons:

1. The pain can be unrelenting. In the past, we have attempted to manage these cases nonoperatively, but usually after a day or so of "conservative" management, the parents opt for an operation because their child is in so much pain.
2. The possibility always exists that one's diagnosis may be wrong and one may be dealing with an underlying torsion of the testis. Indeed in some cases, other conditions may come to light, such as epididymitis.

It is our practice to do the operation through a midline scrotal incision and to explore both sides and remove the necrotic appendix testis and the testicular appendage on the opposite side. Fixation of both testes via window orchidopexy also is recommended to prevent the future complication of torsion of the testis.

The operation should be done under general anesthetic with the addition of a caudal block for pain relief in the postoperative period. By the time the caudal anesthetic wears off, usually only minimal residual discomfort remains. The only significant complication that can occur is a scrotal hematoma, and therefore particular attention to hemostasis is important in operating for this condition. No long-term complications of the operation have been recorded (Fig. 51-3).

TORSION OF THE TESTIS

Incidence

Torsion of the testis occurs less frequently than torsion of one of the appendix testes, in about the ratio of 1:4.

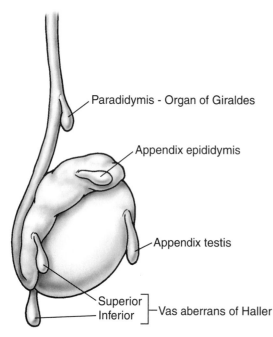

FIGURE 51-1. Testicular appendages. (From Rolnick D, Kawanoue S, Szanto P, et al: Anatomic incidence of testicular appendages. J Urol 100:755–756, 1968.)

Paradidymis - Organ of Giraldes

Appendix epididymis

Appendix testis

Superior
Inferior — Vas aberrans of Haller

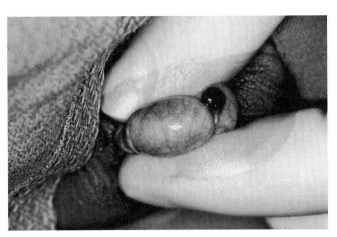

FIGURE 51-3. Gangrenous appendix testis.

However, the exact incidence is not known. The relative rarity of the condition is probably responsible for its often-missed diagnosis, and the general ignorance in the medical community about the consequences of torsion of the testis makes its misdiagnosis even more potentially tragic.

Few medical practitioners appreciate that torsion of the testis may lead to reduced or complete infertility,[2,3] and that the time taken for the testis to become irreversibly damaged can be as short as 3 hours. Thus urgency of detorsion is to be emphasized. Delay can result in permanent testicular damage.

Etiology

The exact etiology of torsion of the testis is unknown. Many theories have been advanced including twisting by the cremasteric muscles or an abnormal "lie" of the testis. Neither of these theories has ever been proven. A long mesorchium is the only anatomic variant that predisposes to torsion of the testis. Why the testis should twist on this mesorchium is not really understood.

Presentation

Testicular torsion can occur at any time during childhood or early adolescent life and indeed even into adult life. However, the peak periods for torsion of the testis occur before age 3 years and then after the onset of puberty. It is rare for torsion of the testis to occur between age 3 years and puberty and rare for it to occur after about age 25 years. Torsion of the testis is usually heralded by the sudden onset of severe lower abdominal pain, accompanied by vomiting, followed by localization of the pain to either the right or left testis. Boys who have had both trauma and torsion will describe the sickening feeling of being hit in the testis as the same as that felt in the early stages of torsion. With torsion of the testis, the testis retracts up toward the groin, a tell-tale sign in the early stages of the condition.

If prompt treatment is not sought, then swelling and redness of the hemiscrotum will soon occur. The pain of torsion is usually described as sudden and excruciating but can at times be of duller and less dramatic onset. Previous short-lived episodes of pain may precede the major presentation.[4]

Torsion of the testis in those younger than the infant and toddler age group often is discovered late, and in most of these cases, the testis is already beyond salvage at exploration. The first signs may be a wide-based gait or redness and swelling of the hemiscrotum noticed by parents at change-of-diaper time and bath time.

Examination

Examination of the affected patient will often reveal a tender, swollen testis accompanied by varying degrees of redness and soft tissue swelling. Usually no differential tenderness is found between the upper and lower poles of the involved testicle. If any doubt exists in the diagnosis from a clinical point of view, then Doppler ultrasonography (US) can be used to demonstrate reduced blood flow to the testis. However, this test is not completely reliable and must not be used to exclude torsion.[5]

Management

The aim of management is to restore the blood supply to the testis as soon as possible. This can be done only by open exploration. Once the testis has been untwisted, then its color must be observed to see whether any recovery is likely. If no return of color is noted, then orchiectomy must be undertaken, as retention of the testis may result in further damage to the normal remaining testis.

Conversely, if the testis color improves as arterial flow is reestablished, then fixation of the testis to prevent a recurrence of the torsion must be undertaken, usually in the form of a window orchidopexy. It is very important then to explore the contralateral side and also fix that testis. Recovery is usually rapid, but these patients need to be followed up for at least 12 to 24 months to ensure that atrophy of the affected testis does not occur and that testicular growth is maintained.

Outcome

If the testis is significantly damaged by ischemia or is completely infarcted, or both, then an incidence of infertility occurs of between 40% and 50% of cases.[2,3] Experimental studies done on rats indicate that if the torsion is untwisted and the testicle allowed to remain in place, a greater degree of damage is found to the contralateral testis than if the testis were removed completely before undertaking detorsion.[6,7] Further experiments being conducted have shown compelling evidence rather that detorsion of the infarcted testis should not be undertaken and that the testis should be removed to avoid significant damage to the contralateral testis.

Although a wide range of success has been reported in detorsion of testes, it has been shown that testicular torsion of longer than 6 hours is unlikely to be accompanied by testicular recovery (Table 51-2). Our observations support the concept that after 6 hours of ischemia, recognizable

TABLE 51-2
EFFECTS OF TORSION

Duration of Torsion (hr)	Testicular Salvage (%)
<6	85–97
6–12	55–85
12–24	20–80
>24	<10

Data from Smith-Harrison LI, Koontz WW Jr: Torsion of the testis: Changing concepts. In Ball TP Jr, Novicki DE, Barrett DM, et al. (eds): AUA Update Series. Vol. 9 (lesson 32). Houston, American Urological Association Office of Education, 1990.

changes are seen in the contralateral testis; the exact mechanism of how this occurs is unknown. It is thought to be perhaps the result of an autoimmune-mediated injury of the contralateral testis.

NEONATAL TESTICULAR TORSION

Torsion of the testis in a newborn usually is seen as a large, firm-to-hard scrotal mass. This variety of torsion is extravaginal (twist of the spermatic cord) and happens before firm fixation of the tunica vaginalis to the scrotal wall occurs.[8] US may show a nonhomogeneous texture of the testicle and fluid collection in the tunica.[9] Color Doppler US confirms the absence of blood flow to the affected testis, making the decision favor excision rather than expectation of testicular salvage. However, US in the newborn baby is rather difficult, even for experienced ultrasonographers, and is not mandatory before exploration.[9] Surgical exploration is done through a groin incision because in rare instances, a testis tumor may be encountered, and a scrotal incision would lead to inguinal nodal spread.[10,11] In most cases of testis torsion at birth, testicular necrosis is almost complete. Rarely, if the episode of torsion were to happen at or just before delivery, testicular salvage may be possible. In a series of 30 neonatal torsions explored within 6 hours of birth, 2 testes could be salvaged and were found to be growing normally a year later.[12] This report reinforces our belief that early exploration is essential. In those cases in which torsion happens in the postnatal period, early recognition and referral are crucial to testis survival. For this to be effectively achieved, nurses taking care of newborn babies should be trained to recognize testis torsion.[13] Operative fixation of the opposite normal testis is very important, as bilateral asynchronous torsion with loss of both testes has been sporadically reported.[14–16]

TORSION OF THE UNDESCENDED TESTIS

Torsion of the spermatic cord (extravaginal torsion) in an undescended testis, although rare, has usually been the subject mostly of case reports, because any one surgeon's experience will have been limited.[17,18] We have had two patients aged 1 year and 5 years with torsion of palpable undescended testes. However, in all these cases, recognition is often delayed, and testis salvage is doubtful. The propensity to torsion lends another argument in favor of early orchidopexy in children with undescended testes. One report exists of spermatic cord torsion in an infant receiving human chorionic gonadotropin (hCG) to induce testicular descent.[19] The parents of children with undescended testes receiving hormonal therapy should therefore be alerted to this possibility. Intra-abdominal testes can undergo torsion and be seen as an acute abdomen. In a report of 60 such cases, two-thirds were found to have tumors.[20]

ACUTE EPIDIDYMITIS

Acute epididymitis is an infrequent finding in the pediatric population and accounts for approximately 10% to 15% of patients with an acute scrotum in the average children's hospital. Epididymitis has a biphasic age distribution, with a peak in the newborn period and early infancy and a second, much smaller peak, during adolescence.

Presentation

Epididymitis in the neonatal and infant age group usually is first seen as the onset of redness and swelling of the hemiscrotum, with or without a fever. Irritability may bring the reddened scrotum to the attention of the parents when they change the diaper.

Examination

Examination in cases of epididymitis usually reveals induration and swelling in the hemiscrotum, which is extremely tender. The edema in the surrounding soft tissue often will make palpation of the testis itself very difficult.

Management and Outcome

Although urine culture provides a bacterial etiology in a small percentage of cases, it should still always be included as a routine study. Because of torsion of the testis in the same age group, scrotal exploration is mandatory. If exploration of the scrotum reveals acute epididymitis, cultures of the epididymis should be taken in an attempt to determine the causative organism. If acute epididymitis is seen, the contralateral side should not be explored. To do so could only serve to spread the infection.

Antibiotics should be commenced immediately, with the recommendation that these be broad spectrum and aimed at urinary pathogens. Obviously on a successful culture result, the antibiotic regimen may have to be altered.

The induration and swelling of the hemiscrotum often takes between 7 and 10 days to subside once the antibiotics have been commenced. Further investigation of the genitourinary tract should be undertaken only if the culture of the epididymis grows *Escherichia coli*. If, however, the culture swab grows *Staphylococcus* or *Streptococcus,* then no further investigation is required. Further investigation, if necessary, should begin with voiding cystourethrography and US of the urinary tract. The most common urologic abnormality found is vesicoureteric reflux, but other abnormalities may occur.

IDIOPATHIC SCROTAL EDEMA

In the differential diagnosis of the acute scrotum in childhood, idiopathic scrotal edema is probably the fourth most common condition encountered. It begins as redness and swelling in either the perineum or inguinal region, which seems to spread into the hemiscrotum. The hemiscrotum then becomes uncomfortable and sometimes painful, and considerable soft tissue swelling is noted in the wall of the scrotum.

Etiology

The etiology of idiopathic scrotal edema is unknown. Speculation about some kind of allergy, possibly to insect bite or to a sudden change in temperature, such as plunging into cold water, has been proposed. The concept of an allergic etiology is further strengthened by the fact that it often responds to a single dose of antihistamine. Scrotal edema is a self-limiting condition, and recurrence is a rarity.

Presentation

Idiopathic scrotal edema usually has an insidious onset with pain, redness, and swelling in the scrotum and also in the surrounding adjacent perineum and sometimes into the groin. It usually affects boys between the ages of 5 and 9 years.

Examination

Examination usually reveals a nontender testis but some discomfort in the scrotum, some edema in the scrotal wall, and also spreading edema into the perineum or inguinal region.

TESTICULAR TRAUMA

Testicular trauma in children is rare. Usually an antecedent history of the trauma is found, and so by taking a careful history, the diagnosis can usually be made clinically.

Presentation

Boys affected by testicular trauma usually have an acutely painful and swollen testis together with swelling and bruising of the scrotum. It may or may not be more pronounced on the one side. The most common injury is a hematoma of the testis. US must be undertaken to exclude rupture of the tunica albuginea. Disruption of the tunica albuginia, as seen by US, is an indication for operative repair. It is particularly important with post pubertal boys because of the possibility of initiating some sort of autoimmune orchitis in the opposing testis. It also is important to evacuate any large hematoma that may occur in the space between the tunica vaginalis and the tunica albuginea and that may, if it occurs, produce pressure necrosis of the testis.

Epididymal injuries also can occur with testicular trauma. Disruption of the epididymis from the testis has actually been described at exploration for testicular trauma. Satisfactory repair is extremely unlikely, and the long-term outcome for these boys, in terms of sperm production from the involved testes, must be doubtful.

OTHER CONDITIONS THAT MAY CAUSE PRESENTATION AS AN ACUTE SCROTUM

Boys younger than 12 months sometimes have redness and swelling in the hemiscrotum as a result of an *incarcerated inguinal hernia*. Usually swelling is seen above the scrotum into the groin, which is a significant sign of an incarcerated inguinal hernia.

Testicular tumors may occur in the neonatal period and early childhood. They are not usually associated with any change in the color or consistency of the scrotal wall, nor are they often a source of pain. Tumors of the testis in this age group are often quite firm and usually can be diagnosed on US. Obviously the approach to these boys will be tailored to the presumptive diagnosis.

REFERENCES

1. Samnakay N, Cohen RJ, Orford J, et al: Androgen and oestrogen receptor status of the human appendix testis. Pediatric Surg Int 19:520–524, 2003.
2. Krarup T: The testes after torsion. Br J Urol 50:43–46, 1978.
3. Bartsch G, Frank S, Marberger H, et al: Testicular torsion: Late results with special regard to fertility and endocrine function. J Urol 124:375–378, 1980.
4. Ransler CW, Allen TD: Torsion of the testis. Urol Clin North Am 9:245–250, 1982.
5. Karadeniz T, Topsakal M, Ariman A, et al: Prospective comparison of colour Doppler ultrasonography and testicular scintigraphy in acute scrotum. Int Urol Nephrol 28:543–548, 1996.
6. Numanoglu A, King PA, Orford J, et al: Early and late histological changes in contralateral testes following torsion. [Unpublished Data]
7. Arunachalam P, Orford J, King PA, et al: Detection of antisperm antibodies in children with torsion testes. [Unpublished Data]
8. Belman AB, Rushton HG: Is the vanished testis always a scrotal event? BJU Int 87:480–483, 2001.
9. Ricci P, Cantisani V, Drudi FM, et al: Prenatal testicular torsion: Sonographic appearance in the newborn infant. Eur Radiol 11:2589–2592, 2001.
10. Lusiri A, Vogler C, Steinhardt G, et al: Neonatal cystic testicular gonadoblastoma: Sonographic and pathologic findings. J Ultrasound Med 10:59–61, 1991.
11. Masterton JS, McCullough AR, Smith RR, et al: Neonatal gonadal stromal tumor of the testis: Limitations of tumour markers. J Urol 134:558–559, 1985.
12. Pinto KJ, Noe HN, Jerkins GR: Management of neonatal testicular torsion. J Urol 158:1196–1197, 1997.
13. Juretschke LJ: Unilateral neonatal testicular torsion. J Obstet Gynecol Neonatal Nurs 29:451–456, 2000.
14. Olguner M, Akgur FM, Aktug T, et al: Bilateral asynchronous perinatal testicular torsion: A case report. J Pediatr Surg 35:1348–1349, 2000.

15. Lee SD, Cha CS: Asynchronous bilateral torsion of the spermatic cord in the newborn: A case report. J Korean Med Sci 17:712–714, 2002.

16. Mouritsen E, Boelskifte J, Rasmussen KL: Bilateral torsion of the testicles in a newborn. Arch Gynaecol Obstet 266:118, 2002.

17. Miwa S, Fuse H, Hirano S: Torsion of the spermatic cord in undescended testis: Report of two cases. Hinyokika Kiyo 46:561–564, 2000.

18. Tozawa K, Washida H, Honma H, et al: Torsion of the undescended testis: Report of two cases. Hinyokika Kiyo 39:377–379, 1993.

19. Sawchuk T, Costabile RA, Howards SS, et al: Spermatic cord torsion in an infant receiving human chorionic gonadotropin. J Urol 150:1212–1213, 1993.

20. Lewis RL, Roller MD, Parra BL, et al: Torsion of an intra-abdominal testis. Curr Surg 57:497–499, 2000.

CHAPTER 52

Developmental and Positional Anomalies of the Kidneys

Hsi-Yang Wu, MD, and Howard M. Snyder III, MD

INTRODUCTION

Anomalies of renal formation and position result in interesting radiographs, but their clinical importance is often in their associated anomalies. For example, the multicystic dysplastic kidney often involutes, yet the initial evaluation aims to determine that the contralateral kidney is not at risk from vesicoureteral reflux or ureteropelvic junction obstruction. Although no therapy is needed for unilateral renal agenesis, the link between a solitary kidney and the VACTERL (vertebral, anal, cardiac, tracheoesophageal fistula, renal, limb) and Mayer-Rokitansky (vaginal agenesis) syndromes is the main reason for further evaluation. Hydronephrosis is often seen in abnormalities of position and rotation, but does not necessarily mean that obstruction is present. Therefore anomalies of renal formation and position usually pose more a diagnostic problem than a surgical one.

RENAL EMBRYOLOGY

The pronephros, which has no adult function, induces the mesonephros to differentiate into the mesonephric duct during the weeks 4 to 8 of fetal life. The mesonephric duct is the basis of the wolffian system, which develops into the seminal vesicles, vas deferens, epididymis, and efferent ductules of the testis in boys, and the epo-ophoron and paraophoron (vestigial remnants between the fallopian tube and ovary) in girls. The ureteric bud branches off the mesonephric duct, contacts the metanephric blastema bud between weeks 9 and 12 of fetal life, and induces the entire collecting system of ureter, renal pelvis, calyx, and collecting tubules. The kidney develops through the induction of the metanephric blastema by the ureteric bud into Bowman's capsule, the convoluted tubules, and the loop of Henle.[1] Figure 52-1 illustrates the progression of development from pronephros, mesonephros, to metanephros.

The kidneys begin at the upper sacral level, with the renal pelvis facing anteriorly. The kidneys ascend either because the lumbar and sacral regions grow faster than the cervical and thoracic regions between 4 to 8 weeks, or because active migration occurs. As the kidneys ascend, the renal pelvis rotates medially by 90 degrees, leading to the normal configuration of the renal pelvis lying medial to the parenchyma. The blood supply during this period shifts from inferior branches of the aorta to more cephalad branches, with the final renal artery being located at about L2. Failure of normal ascent leads to the persistence of a low-lying blood supply.[1]

RENAL DYSPLASIA AND HYPOPLASIA

Because the development of the kidney depends on proper interaction between the ureteric bud and the metanephric blastema, it should not be surprising that an abnormality in the location of the ureteral orifice is associated with abnormally induced renal tissue.[2] Examination of the thickness of renal parenchyma and number of glomeruli associated with normal and ectopic ureters in fetal specimens suggests that it is the initial interaction between bud and blastema that determines whether normal renal tissue will develop, rather than subsequent obstruction or vesicoureteral reflux.[2] Figure 52-2 shows how a ureter that arises in the proper trigonal location (A, E, F) is associated with normal renal parenchyma, whereas a ureter arising from a more cranial location (B–D) or caudal location (G, H) is associated with progressively less normal renal parenchyma.

Renal dysplasia and hypoplasia can be considered errors in renal induction. Figure 52-3 shows varying changes, progressing from agenesis, dysplasia, and perhaps hypoplasia of the kidney. Although dysplasia is technically a histologic term, it refers to kidneys that contain primitive tubules either focally or diffusely. These ducts are lined by epithelium and surrounded by sworls of primitive collagen. No treatment is necessary for the dysplastic kidney, but a 14% risk of reflux exists in the contralateral kidney.[3] Hypoplastic kidneys are small, normal kidneys with a decreased number of nephrons. Dysplasia also can

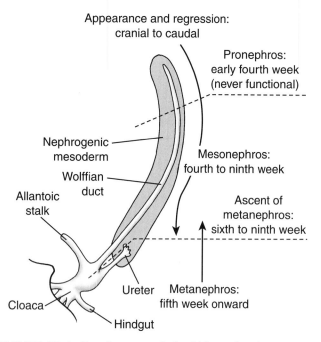

FIGURE 52-1. Development of the kidney. (Redrawn from Gray SW, Skandalakis JE: Embryology for Surgeons. Philadelphia, WB Saunders, 1972, p 444.)

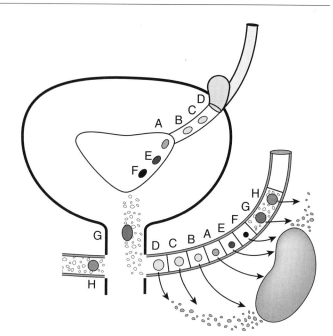

FIGURE 52-2. Relation of ureteral orifice location and associated metanephric tissue. (Redrawn from Mackie GG, Stephens FD: Duplex kidneys: A correlation of renal dysplasia with position of the ureteral orifice. J Urol 114:274–280, 1975.)

occur in hypoplastic kidneys. Although secondary hypoplasia can occur because of infection or obstruction, two types of hypoplastic kidneys are clinically important: the oligomeganephronic type, and the Ask-Upmark kidney. In oligomeganephronia, fewer-than-normal numbers of nephrons are found, associated with hypertrophy of those that are present. Patients are initially seen with polyuria (because they cannot concentrate their urine), but without hypertension. Imaging with ultrasonography (US) reveals small kidneys. Medical management with protein restriction and high fluid and salt intake is undertaken.

Once the glomerular filtration rate decreases significantly, dialysis is required.[4] The Ask-Upmark kidney was initially thought to be a developmental problem, but is now thought to represent reflux nephropathy. The key finding is a small kidney with segmental hypoplasia, probably secondary to ascending pyelonephritis. Vesicoureteral reflux and hypertension are usually present. Most patients are older than 10 years, with a 2:1 female/male ratio. If the disease is unilateral, nephrectomy may cure the hypertension. Hypertension due to bilateral disease is managed medically.[5]

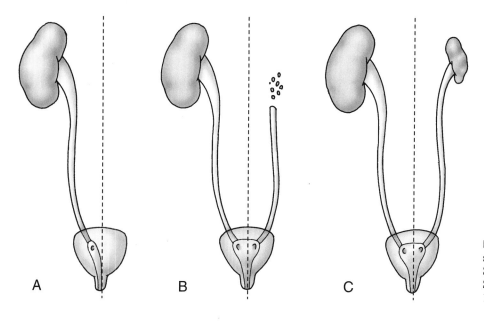

FIGURE 52-3. Renal agenesis, dysplasia, hypoplasia. (Redrawn from Gray SW, Skandalakis JE: Embryology for Surgeons. Philadelphia, WB Saunders, 1972, p 455.)

RENAL AGENESIS

Absence of a kidney may be due to abnormal induction of the metanephric blastema or involution of a multicystic dysplastic kidney. The presence or absence of the ureter is helpful in suggesting the cause of renal agenesis. Absence of a hemitrigone implies that the ureteral bud failed to form properly. A normal trigone with some evidence of a ureter leading to a nubbin suggests involution of a multicystic dysplastic kidney.

Unilateral renal agenesis occurs in 1:1000 live births, with a 2:1 male predominance.[6,7] Unilateral renal agenesis can result in compensatory hypertrophy of the contralateral kidney. The left kidney is more likely to be affected in unilateral renal agenesis.[8] Because unilateral renal agenesis is asymptomatic and eventual renal function is normal, the diagnosis is now usually made on prenatal US, or it is incidentally found during imaging for other abdominal symptoms. Sometimes it can be suspected on plain abdominal radiography if the colon is medially deviated at the splenic or hepatic flexure.[9] These patients should consider obtaining a medical alert bracelet, so that in case of traumatic injury, the solitary kidney is not inadvertently removed.

In a newborn with a prenatal diagnosis of unilateral renal agenesis, physical examination at the time of birth should be focused on detecting the anomalies present in the VACTERL (vertebral, anal, cardiac, tracheoesophageal fistula, renal, limb) association.[10] A voiding cystourethrogram (VCUG) should also be obtained because approximately 30% of patients with unilateral renal agenesis will have vesicoureteral reflux in the contralateral kidney.[10]

Male patients with unilateral renal agenesis are at risk for abnormal wolffian structures. The vas and seminal vesicle may be absent, or the seminal vesicle may be present as a cyst, whereas the ipsilateral testis will be normal. Because the seminal vesicle develops as a separate bud from the wolffian duct at 12 weeks, it can be present in cases of unilateral renal agenesis due to regression of a multicystic dysplastic kidney. Seminal vesicle cysts that cause symptomatic obstruction are usually removed via a transvesical approach. Conversely, if a vas is found to be abnormal or absent during a hernia repair or orchiopexy, the kidneys should be evaluated postoperatively with US.

Female patients with unilateral renal agenesis should have their genital anatomy evaluated, because up to 30% of them will have an abnormality of the müllerian duct due to the Mayer-Rokitansky syndrome (müllerian, uterine, upper vaginal duplications with or without obstruction, or vaginal agenesis).[11,12] The abnormal induction of the mesonephric duct is believed to cause partial or complete nonunion of the paired müllerian ducts.[13] Conversely, 40% of patients with abnormalities of the müllerian organs will have unilateral renal agenesis or ectopia.[14] In patients with duplicated vaginas and unilateral vaginal agenesis, the side without a vagina also is the side without a kidney.[13]

If the diagnosis of Mayer-Rokitansky is not prenatal, the patients can be first seen either as infants with hydrocolpos or as adolescents with lower abdominal pain. Discovery of the disorder often occurs after the onset of menses because of an obstructed vagina or uterus (with or without duplication). Magnetic resonance imaging (MRI) is useful in delineating the pelvic anatomy in these cases. In vaginal agenesis, the vagina is present only as a shallow pouch. A wide variety of abnormalities of the vagina, uterus, and fallopian tubes exist (Fig. 52-4) but the ovaries are embryologically normal.

Bilateral renal agenesis occurs in 1 of 4800 live births, with a 3:1 male predominance.[15] Infants affected with bilateral renal agenesis have oligohydramnios, pulmonary hypoplasia, Potter's facies (low-set ears, broad flat nose, and a prominent skin fold beginning over the eye and running to the cheek). The great majority die soon after birth of pulmonary hypoplasia. The renal arteries and ureters are usually absent, and the bladder, underdeveloped. The vas is usually present, but female genital structures are usually abnormal.[16,17] The adrenals are usually present but appear spherical, instead of flattened, because of the lack of compression by the kidneys.[15] Prenatal diagnosis is useful in determining that heroic efforts at extracorporeal membrane oxygenation (ECMO) or hemodialysis are not indicated after delivery.

SUPERNUMERARY KIDNEY

Supernumerary kidney is a rare condition in which a completely separate kidney is found in addition to two normally positioned kidneys. The additional kidney has its own blood supply and parenchyma and usually is found caudal to the normal kidney. It is usually smaller than the normally positioned kidney. This additional kidney represents abnormal induction of metanephric blastema by an abnormally directed ureteric bud, either as a separate ureteral bud from the mesonephric duct, or as part of a "Y" duplication. If the supernumerary kidney is located cranial to the normal kidney, the ureter is usually completely separate and may enter the bladder ectopically. Presumably this is a result of a completely separate ureteral bud inducing the metanephric blastema and migrating very low on the mesonephric duct, separate from the normally positioned kidney.[18,19] If the ureter ends ectopically, it may present as incontinence in a girl, or as infection in a poorly functioning renal unit. The diagnosis can be difficult to make.[20] Stone disease and hydronephrosis can be found in up to 50% of patients. Treatment should be reserved for these problems, because the presence of a supernumerary kidney alone is not worrisome.[19] Like other ectopic kidneys, these kidneys may be more subject to trauma, so a medical alert bracelet may be helpful.

RENAL ECTOPIA

Failure of rotation, while not strictly ectopia, usually results in a kidney in which the renal pelvis is anteriorly directed. In the unusual situation in which hyper-rotation occurs, the renal pelvis can actually point posteriorly.

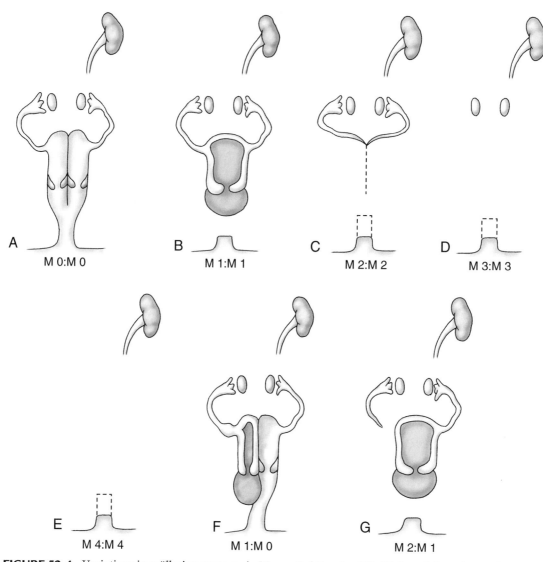

FIGURE 52-4. Variations in müllerian anatomy in Mayer-Rokitansky. M0, Right or left vagina and uterus, or duplex vagina and uterus with partial or complex septum. M1, Partial or complete absence of vagina. M2, Absence of vagina and uterus. M3, Absence of vagina, uterus, and fallopian tube. M4, Absence of vagina, uterus, fallopian tube, and ovary. (Redrawn from Tarry WF, Duckett JW, Stephens FD: The Mayer-Rokitansky syndrome: Pathogenesis, classification and management. J Urol 136:648–652, 1986.)

The renal vessels are normally positioned. The renal pelvis and calyces will often appear abnormal because of their orientation, which results in an interesting intravenous urogram. With oblique views, the anatomy can be established and does not usually require repair, even in poorly functioning units. The best method to localize even poorly functioning ectopic renal tissue is with a nuclear medicine study. Two technical factors to be considered in interpreting renal isotope scans in ectopic kidneys are (1) radionuclide in the bladder can overlap a pelvic kidney, so a catheter may be in place for the study; and (2) the pelvic kidney is located farther anteriorly than orthotopic kidneys, and the distance of the kidney from the camera may underestimate renal function. Placing the patient prone may result in a more accurate assessment.

Simple ectopia results in a kidney that is located anywhere from the pelvis to the diaphragm. The incidence is 1 in 1000 live births, with a 3:2 male predominance.[21] The contralateral kidney often also has an abnormality of rotation or ectopia. The development of the ipsilateral adrenal gland is unaffected. A "thoracic kidney" is actually subdiaphragmatic, although it may lie in the chest through a focal eventration of the diaphragm. It is not associated with a true congenital diaphragmatic hernia.[22] An ectopic "abdominal kidney" is above the iliac crest, the "lumbar kidney" is anterior to the iliac vessels at the sacral promontory, and the "pelvic kidney" is below the aortic bifurcation and opposite the sacrum. All of these ectopic kidneys are more susceptible to trauma because they are not as well protected by the lower rib cage and are anterior in position. It may be advisable for these patients to avoid contact sports, in which a risk of abdominal trauma exists.

Most ectopic kidneys are asymptomatic and are either detected by prenatal US or are discovered incidentally. Ectopic kidneys are at higher risk for ureteropelvic junction (UPJ) obstruction, vesicoureteral reflux (VUR), and stone formation. The anatomy can include an extrarenal pelvis and infundibuli, and a high insertion of the ureter into the pelvis. This anatomic arrangement can mimic a UPJ obstruction, so careful evaluation is necessary to avoid unnecessary surgical procedures.[23] More than half will have a dilated renal pelvis. Of these, half are due to obstruction, 25% are due to reflux, and 25% are merely dilated without UPJ obstruction.[24] For open repair of UPJ obstruction with a high insertion of the ureter, a side-to-side ureteropyelostomy or ureterocalycostomy to a dilated lower pole calyx is sometimes required to obtain dependent drainage.

Although endoscopic techniques for treatment of UPJ obstruction have been used in children,[25] the presence of anomalous vessels suggests that either an open or laparoscopic approach would be safer than endoscopic incision of a UPJ obstruction in an ectopic kidney. The advent of computed tomography (CT) angiography and magnetic resonance urography (MRU) has made the assessment of anomalous vessels in ectopic or horseshoe kidneys more noninvasive and more available before a surgical procedure.

FUSION DEFECTS

Horseshoe Kidney

This occurs in 1 in 400 live births, with a 2:1 male predominance.[26] The kidney is usually lower than normal, because the lower poles fuse in the midline and drape anteriorly over the spine. The isthmus can be purely fibrotic or can contain parenchyma. This anomaly is believed to occur at between 4 and 6 weeks of fetal life, because the orientation of the renal pelvis is anterior. It is proposed that as the kidneys "hurdle" the iliac vessels during ascent, they come into contact with each other at the lower pole and fuse (Fig. 52-5). Other variations of upper pole and mid pole contact are possible, but much rarer than the usual lower pole fusion. The kidney is usually low because of its inability to ascend past the inferior mesenteric artery. Each renal moiety retains its ureter, which is draped over the isthmus. The renal pelvis is usually anterior. The arterial supply varies from the normal single vessel to each moiety to vessels arising from any conceivable nearby blood supply. Horseshoe kidneys are more commonly found in patients with sacral agenesis, persistent cloaca, and Turner's syndrome (45,XO gonadal dysgenesis).[27] They are associated with a higher risk of renal cell carcinoma and Wilms' tumor.[28–30]

One-third of patients have no symptoms. The patients with symptoms often complain of vague abdominal or back pain; 10% have ureteral duplication, 50% have VUR, and 33% have UPJ obstruction.[27,31,32] Repair of UPJ obstruction in horseshoe kidney requires placement of

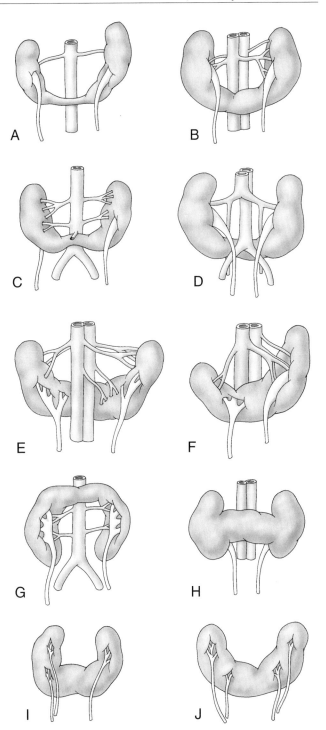

FIGURE 52-5. Variations of horseshoe kidney. (Redrawn from Benjamin JA, Schullian DM: Observations of kidneys with horseshoe configuration: the contribution of Leonardo Botallo. J Hist Med Allied Sci 5:315, 1950, after Gutierrez, 1931.)

the anastomosis to avoid a secondary kinking at the UPJ. Division of the isthmus is not required. Treatment of kidney stones in horseshoe kidneys can be accomplished with extracorporeal shock-wave lithotripsy, ureteroscopy, or percutaneous nephrolithotomy. Percutaneous approaches are sometimes difficult, as the kidneys do not reside right next to the body wall, making difficult the access to the collecting system, but percutaneous approaches result in a higher stone-free rate than does ureteroscopy or shock-wave lithotripsy.[33] No increase in the rate of metabolic abnormalities is found in patients with horseshoe kidneys and kidney stones, suggesting that stasis in an extrarenal pelvis may contribute to the formation of kidney stones.[34]

Crossed-fused Renal Ectopia

This is more common than crossed, nonfused renal ectopia. The lower pole of one kidney crosses the midline to fuse with an orthotopically placed contralateral kidney. It occurs more commonly in boys, and usually the left kidney crosses the midline. Presumably during ascent, the left kidney encounters an obstruction, rotates, and fuses with the lower pole of the right kidney. The ureters insert in the normal position in the bladder. This has been described as "S"- or "L"-shaped kidney. Diagnosis can be made by using excretory urography (or intravenous pyelography, IVP), CT, or MRU. Solitary crossed ectopia (unilateral renal agenesis, contralateral kidney crossed to opposite side) is a rare finding. Multicystic dysplasia, obstruction, and VUR can be found in the ectopic kidney.

CYSTIC RENAL DISEASE AND CYSTIC TUMORS

Autosomal Recessive Polycystic Kidney Disease

Autosomal recessive polycystic kidney disease (ARPKD) was formerly called infantile polycystic kidney disease, which is inaccurate because it can occur in older patients. It occurs in 1 in 40,000 live births, but many patients die soon afterward. The kidneys are bilaterally enlarged, with very small cysts radially oriented throughout the parenchyma. The cysts represent dilated collecting tubules. Periportal hepatic fibrosis also occurs in varying degrees, which can lead to portal hypertension. The hepatic involvement appears to be inversely proportional to the renal involvement. The disease has been classified into four forms.[35] The severe perinatal form (> 90% renal involvement) leads to death by 6 weeks from pulmonary hypoplasia. The neonatal form (60% renal involvement) is usually lethal by 1 year. The infantile form (25% renal involvement) results in hepatosplenomegaly, with survival up to 10 years. The juvenile form (< 10% renal involvement) has severe periportal hepatic fibrosis. Some patients survive up to 15 years, but the development of portal hypertension is usually lethal. Because this is an autosomal recessive disease, screening of the family should be undertaken to determine which siblings are carriers.

Prenatal US studies showing bilaterally enlarged, echogenic kidneys suggest ARPKD. The IVP or CT shows a classic striated "sunburst" pattern. Unfortunately, the prognosis is poor for the perinatal or neonatal forms of ARPKD. The patients who survive the neonatal period seem to do well, with some degree of renal insufficiency.

Dialysis eventually is necessary in most patients. In older patients, the kidneys become smaller as renal failure develops. The overall treatment for ARPKD is supportive, with renal transplantation being the ultimate goal (Fig. 52-6).

Autosomal Dominant Polycystic Kidney Disease

Whereas autosomal dominant polycystic kidney disease (ADPKD) tends to appear clinically in the third to fifth decade, it has been diagnosed with US in asymptomatic children as well. The cysts in ADPKD are different in configuration, being few and scattered, in contrast to those seen in ARPKD. It occurs in 1 in 500 patients.[36] Patients usually have flank pain, hematuria, hypertension, and possibly renal failure, if extensive bilateral cysts are present. Neonates can have renal enlargement, although children from affected families who are screened usually have only a few cysts. Failure to see cysts on screening US in a child at risk for ARPKD does not rule out the disease, because the cysts can develop later in life. Linkage analysis of the loci on chromosomes 4 and 16 is more sensitive.[37] The cysts are located throughout the cortex and medulla, although the fetal form seems to affect the glomeruli predominantly. Hepatic involvement is limited to biliary cysts. Associated findings include cysts in the spleen, pancreas, and lungs, mitral valve prolapse, colon diverticuli, and berry aneurysms of the circle of Willis.

Hypertension is commonly found in these children and may be part of the presentation. Renal failure in childhood is very rare. Periodic evaluation of blood pressure and proteinuria during childhood is recommended.[38,39] Unlike ARPKD, no increased risk of renal cell carcinoma is found. Renal transplant candidates can obtain organs from family members who have been screened for the disease.

Multicystic Dysplastic Kidney

The multicystic dysplastic kidney (MCDK) is believed to be caused by severe early ureteral obstruction or a failure in ureteric bud–metanephric blastema induction.[40,41] The main differential diagnosis is severe hydronephrosis due to UPJ obstruction. Radiographically, this occurs when the peripheral cysts surround a dominant central cyst, mimicking the renal pelvis ("hydronephrotic" form of MCDK). The classic US appearance is of cysts randomly distributed throughout the kidney without a dominant medial cyst or evidence of communication between cysts. The parenchyma, if present, has abnormal echogenicity and is seen between the cysts, instead of being arranged on their periphery. A renal isotope scan will show no function in an MCDK. The affected area may be the upper pole of a duplicated collecting system, or one-half of a horseshoe kidney.

The MCDK is the most common renal cystic mass in the newborn, and currently most are being detected on prenatal US. Bilateral forms are not compatible with life. Postnatal evaluation consists of a VCUG to look for VUR

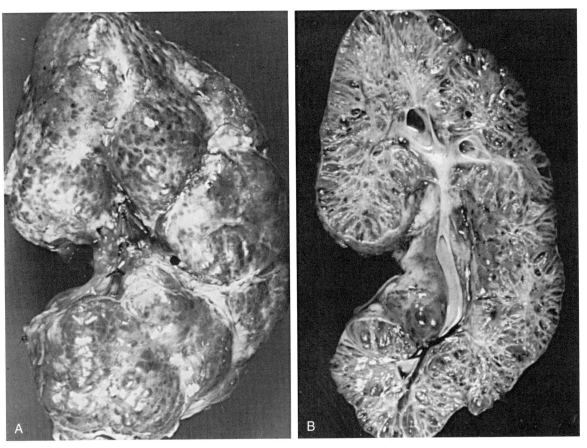

FIGURE 52-6. Gross pathology of autosomal recessive polycystic kidney disease.

in the contralateral kidney, which occurs 30% of the time.[42] If significant hydronephrosis (caliectasis) is found in the contralateral kidney (this occurs 12% of the time), then a diuretic renal isotope scan may be necessary. Contralateral UPJ obstruction or VUR is more likely with a smaller MCDK or a lower ureteral atresia ipsilateral to the MCDK.[43,44] Reports have been made of malignancy arising from an MCDK, although it is unclear whether the affected kidneys were truly MCDK.[45] Hypertension also has been reported in association with MCDK, although resection is not always curative, and the rate does not appear to be any higher than in the general population.[46]

MCDKs usually involute, but they can occasionally grow.[46] The follow-up is repeated imaging with US every 6 months for the first 2 years of life. It is not usually feasible to monitor a patient indefinitely for an MCDK. We have taken an operative approach at 18 to 24 months of life if the MCDK is not involuting, or if parenchyma remains visible on the US study. Although the indications are controversial, the kidney can be removed at that age via a small incision as an outpatient procedure (Fig. 52-7). Occasionally the MCDK can involute prenatally, leaving a ureter with a small nubbin of tissue in the renal fossa. These were previously called "aplastic" kidneys, but are now thought to represent the remnants of an MCDK.

Cystic Nephroma

Formerly called a "multilocular cyst," this is a well-demarcated tumor of cysts with an overall round configuration, lined with epithelium and septa that contain tubules.[47] It is considered to be the benign end of a spectrum progressing from cystic Wilms' tumor, cystic partially differentiated nephroblastoma, to cystic nephroma. It usually is found in the boy younger than 4 years (male/female ratio, 2:1) or the woman older than 30 years (female/male ratio, 8:1). It is rarely bilateral and is cured by partial nephrectomy, shelling out the tumor by following the plane of the pseudocapsule. A risk occurs of sarcomatous degeneration in adults if it is not removed.[48]

Cystic Partially Differentiated Nephroblastoma

This lesion was formerly called a multilocular cystic nephroma. It is radiologically identical to the cystic nephroma and can be diagnosed only pathologically. The majority of patients are boys younger than 2 years, or women in the third to fourth decade. A classic (but not diagnostic) radiologic finding is herniation of a parenchymal mass into the renal pelvis.[22] The tumor is well circumscribed, and hemorrhage and calcification usually are

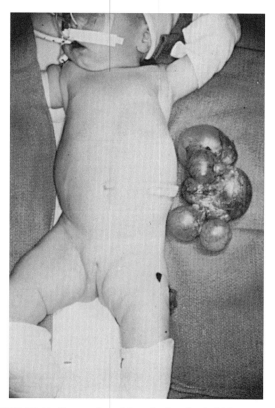

FIGURE 52-7. Resected multicystic dysplastic kidney.

absent. Pathologically, it differs from the cystic nephroma in that blastema is found in the septa.

Patients usually are initially seen with an asymptomatic flank mass, and occasionally hematuria. Surgical treatment consists of partial nephrectomy as for cystic nephroma, because the tumors rarely recur and are not multifocal. No chemotherapy is required for stage I (limited to capsule, fully resected) tumors, and although the experience is limited, stage II (outside renal capsule but fully resected) is usually treated with vincristine, dactinomycin, and doxorubicin. The 4-year survival for both stages is 100%.[49]

Simple Cysts and Calyceal Diverticuli

The simple renal cyst on US has the following characteristics: A distinct wall, no internal echoes, and good through-transmission with posterior enhancement. If these criteria are not met, a CT scan is obtained to confirm that the fluid does not enhance. The differential diagnosis is a calyceal diverticulum or hydrocalyx, both of which communicate with the collecting system, and in which the fluid should enhance on either IVP or CT. US is able to detect milk of calcium layering within a diverticulum. Calyceal diverticuli require treatment when they harbor stones or infection. When diagnosed with excretory urography as the primary study, 40% of calyceal diverticuli were thought to be symptomatic.[50] With the more common discovery by US, many are diagnosed as incidental findings, and it is not now clear how often calyceal diverticuli require treatment.

Simple cysts reside in the cortex and are lined by simple columnar epithelium. They can grow, resorb, or remain the same size. They are usually asymptomatic and are found incidentally. Once they are found, we usually follow with US at 3- to 6-month intervals to determine whether the cyst is growing. The underlying concern is whether this cyst is the first sign of ADPKD. A family history of renal cystic disease, renal failure, or death in the neonatal period from unknown causes should be obtained. Biopsy to rule out tumor, followed by drainage, or unroofing should be undertaken only if the cyst characteristics are other than those listed for a simple cyst, or if the cyst becomes symptomatic due to obstruction of an infundibulum or the UPJ. Minimally invasive approaches such as percutaneous puncture with instillation of sclerosing agents (absolute alcohol, bismuth, povidone-iodine[51]) or laparoscopic decortication[52] may shift the threshold for treatment of large asymptomatic simple cysts.

REFERENCES

1. Gray SW, Skandalakis JE: The kidney and ureter. In Embryology for Surgeons. Philadelphia, WB Saunders, 1972, pp 443–518.
2. Mackie GG, Stephens FD: Duplex kidneys: A correlation of renal dysplasia with position of the ureteral orifice. J Urol 114:274, 1975.
3. Atiyeh B, Husmann D, Baum M: Contralateral renal abnormalities in multicystic-dysplastic kidney disease. J Pediatr 121:65, 1992.
4. Royer P, Habib R, Broyer M, et al: L'Hypoplasie renale bilaterale congenitale avec reduction du nombre et hypertrophie des nephrons chez l'enfant. Ann Pediatr (Paris) 38:133, 1962.
5. Arant BS Jr, Sotelo-Avila C, Bernstein J: Segmental "hypoplasia" of the kidney (Ask-Upmark). J Pediatr 95:931, 1979.
6. Doroshow LW, Abeshouse BS: Congenital unilateral solitary kidney: Report of 37 cases and a review of the literature. Urol Surv 11:219, 1961.
7. Sheih CP, Hung CS, Wei CF, et al: Cystic dilatations within the pelvis in patients with ipsilateral renal agenesis or dysplasia. J Urol 144:324, 1990.
8. Kohn G, Borns PF: The association of bilateral and unilateral renal aplasia in the same family. J Pediatr 83:95, 1973.
9. Mascatello V, Lebowitz RL: Malposition of the colon in left renal agenesis and ectopia. Radiology 120:371, 1976.
10. Kolon TF, Gray CL, Sutherland RW, et al: Upper urinary tract manifestations of the VACTERL association. J Urol 163:1949, 2000.
11. Downs RA, Lane JW, Burns E: Solitary pelvic kidney: Its clinical implications. Urology 1:51, 1973.
12. Thompson DP, Lynn HB: Genital anomalies associated with solitary kidney. Mayo Clin Proc 41:538, 1966.
13. Tarry WF, Duckett JW, Stephens FD: The Mayer-Rokitansky syndrome: Pathogenesis, classification, and management. J Urol 136:648, 1986.
14. Griffin JE, Edwards C, Madden JD, et al: Congenital absence of the vagina: The Mayer-Rokitansky-Kuster-Hauser syndrome. Ann Intern Med 85:224, 1976.
15. Potter EL: Bilateral absence of ureters and kidneys: A report of 50 cases. Obstet Gynecol 25:3, 1965.
16. Ashley DJB, Mostofi FK: Renal agenesis and dysgenesis. J Urol 83:211, 1960.
17. Carpentier PJ, Potter EL: Nuclear sex and genital malformation in 48 cases of renal agenesis with special reference to nonspecific female pseudohermaphroditism. Am J Obstet Gynecol 78:235, 1959.
18. Geisinger JG: Supernumerary kidney. J Urol 38:331, 1937.
19. N'Guessan G, Stephens FD: Supernumerary kidney. J Urol 130:649, 1983.
20. Weiss JP, Duckett JW, Snyder HM: Single unilateral vaginal ectopic ureter: Is it really a rarity? J Urol 132:1177, 1984.

21. Malek RS, Kelalis PP, Burke EC: Ectopic kidney in children and frequency of association with other malformations. Mayo Clin Proc 46:461, 1971.
22. Zagoria RL, Tung GA: The kidney and retroperitoneum: Anatomy and congenital anomalies. In: Genitourinary Radiology: The Requisites. St. Louis, Mosby, 1997, p 56.
23. Dretler SP, Pfister R, Hendren WH: Extrarenal calyces in the ectopic kidney. J Urol 103:406, 1970.
24. Gleason PE, Kelalis PP, Husmann DA, et al: Hydronephrosis in renal ectopia: Incidence, etiology, and significance. J Urol 151:1660, 1994.
25. Jabbour ME, Goldfischer ER, Stravodimos KG, et al: Endopyelotomy for horseshoe and ectopic kidneys. J Urol 160:694, 1998.
26. Dees J: Clinical importance of congenital anomalies of upper urinary tract. J Urol 46:659, 1941.
27. Boatman DL, Kolln CP, Flocks RH: Congenital anomalies associated with horseshoe kidneys. J Urol 107:205, 1972.
28. Buntley D: Malignancy associated with horseshoe kidney. Urology 8:146, 1976.
29. Hohenfellner M, Schultz-Lampel D, Lempel A, et al: Tumor in the horseshoe kidney: Clinical implications and review of embryogenesis. J Urol 147:1098, 1992.
30. Mesrobian HG, Kelalis PP, Hrabovsky E, et al: Wilms' tumor in horseshoe kidneys: A report from the National Wilms' Tumor Study. J Urol 133:1002, 1985.
31. Segura JW, Kelalis PP, Burke EC: Horseshoe kidney in children. J Urol 108:333, 1972.
32. Whitehouse GH: Some urographic aspects of horseshoe kidney anomaly: A review of 59 cases. Clin Radiol 26:107, 1975.
33. Yohannes P, Smith AD: The endourological management of complications associated with horseshoe kidney. J Urol 168:5, 2002.
34. Evans WP, Resnick MI: Horseshoe kidney and urolithiasis. J Urol 125:620, 1981.
35. Blyth H, Ockenden BG: Polycystic disease of kidney and liver presenting in childhood. J Med Genet 8:257, 1971.
36. Gabow PA: Autosomal dominant polycystic kidney disease. N Engl J Med 329:332, 1993.
37. Gabow PA, Kimberling WJ, Strain JD, et al: Utility of ultrasonography in the diagnosis of autosomal dominant polycystic kidney disease in children. J Am Soc Nephrol 8:105, 1997.
38. Ravine D, Walker RG, Gibson RN, et al: Treatable complications in undiagnosed cases of autosomal dominant polycystic kidney disease. Lancet 337:127, 1991.
39. Zerres K, Rudnik-Schoneborn S, Deget F: Routine examination of children at risk of autosomal dominant polycystic kidney disease. Lancet 339:1356, 1992.
40. Beck AD: The effect of intra-uterine urinary obstruction upon the development of the fetal kidney. J Urol 105:784, 1971.
41. Osathanondh V, Potter EL: Pathogenesis of polycystic kidneys: Historical survey. Arch Pathol 77:459, 1964.
42. Flack CE, Bellinger MF: The multicystic dysplastic kidney and contralateral vesicoureteral reflux: protection of the solitary kidney. J Urol 150:1873, 1993.
43. Cendron J, Gubler JP, Valayer J, et al: Dysplasie multikystique du rein chez enfant: A propos de 45 observations. J Urol Nephrol (Paris) 79:773, 1973.
44. Cendron J, Kiriakos S: Rein multikystique. J Urol Nephrol (Paris) 82:322, 1976.
45. Beckwith JB: Comment: Wilms' tumor and multicystic dysplastic kidney disease. J Urol 158:2259, 1997.
46. Wacksman J, Phipps L: Report of the multicystic kidney registry: Preliminary findings. J Urol 150:1870, 1993.
47. Joshi VV, Beckwith JB: Multilocular cyst of the kidney (cystic nephroma) and cystic, partially differentiated nephroblastoma: Terminology and criteria for diagnosis. Cancer 64:466, 1989.
48. Castillo OA, Boyle ET Jr, Kramer SA: Multilocular cysts of the kidney: A study of 29 patients and review of literature. Urology 37:156, 1991.
49. Blakely ML, Shamberger RC, Norkool P, et al: Outcome of children with cystic partially differentiated nephroblastoma treated with and without chemotherapy. J Pediatr Surg 38:897, 2003.
50. Timmons JW Jr, Malek RS, Hattery RR, et al: Caliceal diverticulum. J Urol 114:6, 1975.
51. Phelan M, Zajko A, Hrebinko RL: Preliminary results of percutaneous treatment of renal cysts with povidone-iodine sclerosis. Urology 53:816, 1999.
52. Lifson BJ, Teichman JM, Hulbert JC: Role and long-term results of laparoscopic decortication in solitary cystic and autosomal dominant polycystic kidney disease. J Urol 159:702, 1998.

Ureteral Obstruction and Malformations

Douglas E. Coplen, MD

Hydronephrosis and ureteral malformations are among the most common abnormalities of the urinary tract seen in children. Historically, these abnormalities were first seen with urinary tract infections, abdominal pain, or incontinence; however, with the increasing use of fetal and neonatal ultrasound, they are detected before symptoms develop. Urinary tract dilation is present in one in 100 fetuses, but significant uropathy is present in one in 500.[1] Thus the surgeon must critically evaluate these findings to determine their clinical significance and whether intervention is required.

URETEROPELVIC JUNCTION OBSTRUCTION IN CHILDREN

In ureteropelvic junction (UPJ) obstruction, inadequate drainage of urine is present from the renal pelvis into the ureter, resulting in hydrostatic distention of the renal pelvis and intrarenal calyces. The combination of increased intrapelvic pressure and stasis of urine in the collecting ducts results in progressive damage to the kidney.

The incidence of UPJ obstruction in the past was estimated at one in 5000 live births, but since the advent of antenatal ultrasound, it has been recognized that the incidence is higher. UPJ obstruction is the cause of 40% of neonatal hydronephrosis, placing the incidence at 1:1250 births.[2,3] It is more common in boys (ratio, 2:1) and two-thirds occur on the left side. Bilateral UPJ obstruction occurs in 5% to 10% of patients and is much more frequently seen in younger children.[4,5]

ETIOLOGY

During development of the upper ureter, the lumen of the ureteric bud solidifies with ureteral lengthening and later recanalizes.[6] Failure to recanalize adequately is thought to be the cause of most intrinsic UPJ obstructions. Other causes of intrinsic UPJ obstruction include ureteral valves, polyps, and leiomyomas.[7]

At operation, the most common observation is ureteral narrowing of variable length that appears to join the renal pelvis above the expected dependent position.[8] This "high insertion" of the ureter causes an angulation with respect to the renal pelvis. At low-volume states, peristaltic waves of urine cross the UPJ, but as the flow increases beyond a threshold, the renal pelvis dilates.[9] The dilated pelvis may functionally kink the ureter further, increasing the pelvic pressure.[10] In 20% to 30% of patients, the ureter is draped over a lower-pole vessel, producing an extrinsic UPJ obstruction. This apparent aberrancy may be secondary to incomplete renal rotation in conjunction with a normal segmental vessel.[11,12]

Histologic evaluation reveals a decrease or complete absence of smooth muscle fibers at the UPJ.[8,13] Electron microscopy may show an increase in collagen deposition between the muscle fibers.[14] The increase in collagen is most likely the response to obstruction as opposed to the cause of obstruction. Fibrosis and interruption of the smooth muscle continuity block transmission of the peristaltic wave.[15] Defective innervation also may play a role in the development of UPJ obstruction.[16]

UPJ obstruction also may be acquired. It has been observed in late follow-up of high-grade vesicoureteral reflux (VUR), after cutaneous ureterostomy, and after decompression of the dilated urinary tract.[17,18] In these cases, obstruction is caused by extrinsic scarring and adhesions that cause fixed deformation and distortion of the UPJ. VUR is present in 14% of patients with UPJ obstruction. It is important to obtain delayed images in the intravenous pyelogram (IVP) series to rule out a pseudo-UPJ obstruction (Fig. 53-1).

CLINICAL PRESENTATION

Most hydronephrotic kidneys are now detected prenatally. Less frequently, UPJ obstruction is detected because of an abdominal mass, urinary tract infection, association with other anomalies (i.e., VACTERL syndrome [vertebral, anal, cardiac, tracheal, esophageal, renal, and limb]),

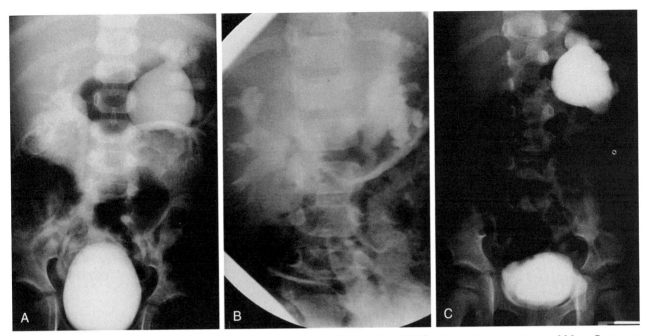

FIGURE 53-1. Vesicoureteral reflux and secondary ureteropelvic junction (UPJ) obstruction in a 4-year-old boy first seen with urosepsis. *A,* Intravenous pyelogram (IVP) with a full bladder shows typical findings of calyceal blunting and renal pelvic dilation. Visualization of the distal ureter suggests reflux. *B,* Cystogram shows bilateral reflux. Note the marked discrepancy in left-sided anatomy between the IVP and cystogram and the kink just distal to the UPJ on the left side. *C,* Delayed film after cystogram shows stasis and apparent obstruction on the left side. Subsequent furosemide washout renal scan with a bladder catheter showed no evidence of obstruction, and the child has done well after bilateral ureteral reimplantation.

or abnormalities seen during contrast or radionuclide radiography. In older children, vague, poorly localized, cyclic, or acute abdominal pain associated with nausea is common. Many of these children are initially seen by gastroenterologists. The cause for the intermittent obstruction is unclear, but renal function is almost always preserved. Hematuria after minor trauma or vigorous exercise may be a presenting feature, most likely secondary to rupture of mucosal vessels in the dilated collecting system.[4] Episodic flank pain associated with diuresis is a common presenting feature in young adults but is uncommon in children.

DIAGNOSIS

When an antenatal diagnosis of UPJ obstruction is made, the initial postpartum evaluation is performed at 10 to 14 days of life to avoid false-negative studies resulting from neonatal dehydration. Bilateral UPJ obstruction is rarely associated with significant enough obstruction to cause oligohydramnios and warrant antenatal intervention. The newborn is placed on preventive amoxicillin (10 mg/kg once a day), pending the studies. Sonography (US) confirms the presence of pelvic and calyceal dilation, with variable thinning of the renal parenchyma (Fig. 53-2). The presence of corticomedullary junctions on US is indicative of preserved function.[19,20] US is used to evaluate the contralateral kidney, the bladder, and the distal ipsilateral ureter to avoid confusion with a ureterovesical

junction obstruction (UVJ), but it will not provide functional information.

A voiding cystourethrogram (VCUG) is indicated in all patients being evaluated for UPJ obstruction. VUR increases the chance that infection will occur, even in a partially obstructed system. Additionally, VUR that leads to kinking of the UPJ may be the primary disease process (see Fig. 53-1).

The excretory urogram is the traditional method to evaluate for UPJ obstruction. It reveals delayed function and a distended pelvis and calyces with either no filling of the upper ureter or an abrupt transition to a narrow upper ureter. It has limited use in the newborn because the neonatal kidney does not concentrate contrast well enough to provide adequate visualization of obstructed kidneys. It also is subjective with respect to differential renal function and degree of obstruction. The test may be indicated when more information is required regarding preoperative pelvic anatomy or to define better the level of obstruction when it is not clear from other studies.[5] In the child with intermittent flank pain, an IVP may be diagnostic when performed during an episode of pain.

Magnetic resonance (MR) urography can be used at any age. T_2-weighted images are independent of renal function, and hydronephrosis is readily detected. The anatomic images are excellent, but a good US often gives the same information. Enhanced MR with gadolinium can give information regarding differential function if one kidney is anatomically and functionally normal.[21]

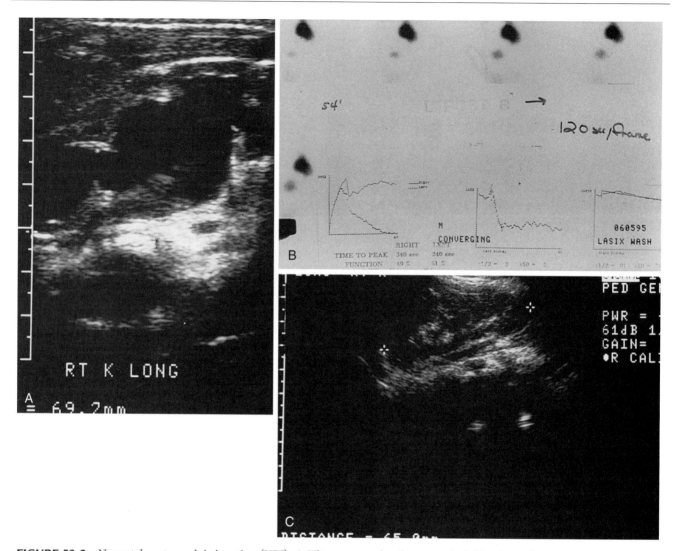

FIGURE 53-2. Neonatal ureteropelvic junction (UPJ). *A,* Ultrasonography shows cortical thinning, calyectasis, and renal pelvic dilation consistent with UPJ obstruction. *B,* Furosemide washout renal scan. Computer analysis is on the bottom. *Left,* Time to peak function shows symmetrical uptake in the first 2 minutes. Radionuclide drains out of the left kidney before the administration of diuretic. The $T_{1/2}$ on the right is prolonged and was calculated to be 81 minutes. On the basis of good renal function, observation was elected. *C,* Follow-up sonogram 1 year later is normal. Renal scan at this time shows symmetrical function with normal washout (5 minutes).

The diuretic isotope renogram is the most widely used and most useful technique in the evaluation of hydronephrosis, differential renal function, and drainage of kidneys. The transit of an injected radioisotope through the urinary tract is monitored by a gamma camera. The early uptake of the tracer indicates unilateral renal function, while the washout, augmented by the administration of a diuretic, is evaluated and plotted by a computer.[22,23]

The study is obtained with either technetium 99m-diethylenetriamine pentaacetic acid (^{99m}Tc-DTPA), whose renal clearance is by glomerular filtration, or ^{99m}Tc-mercaptoacetyltriglycine (^{99m}Tc-MAG3), whose clearance is predominantly via proximal tubular secretion. MAG3 is more efficiently excreted than ^{99m}Tc-DTPA and gives better images, particularly in patients with impaired renal function.[22,23]

The technique for diuretic renography should be standardized.[24] Patients should be hydrated intravenously (15 mL/kg) 15 minutes before injection of the radionuclide. An indwelling catheter maintains an empty bladder and monitors urine output. The diuretic (1 mg/kg furosemide, ≤40 mg) is not administered until the activity in the hydronephrotic kidney and renal pelvis peaks. The tracer activity is then monitored for an additional 30 minutes, and a quantitative analysis completed. Historically, persistence of more than 50% of the tracer in the renal pelvis 20 minutes after diuretic administration ($T_{1/2} > 20$) is diagnostic of obstruction. False-positive results may occur when the immature neonatal kidney fails to respond to diuretic, when the patient is dehydrated, when the bladder is distended, or when the pelvis is significantly dilated.

Occasionally the renal scan is equivocal, and invasive pressure flow studies may be indicated.[25] The test assumes that obstruction produces a constant restriction to outflow that necessitates elevated pressure to transport urine at high flow rates, but not all obstructions are constant. If the obstruction is intrinsic, a linear relation exists between pressure and flow, but in some cases, the test results reflect only the response of the renal pelvis to distention and may be positive in the absence of obstruction.[10] These methods require general anesthesia in children and have limited applicability.

Retrograde urography at the time of surgical correction is helpful if uncertainty exists regarding the site of obstruction. This is rarely required because a well-performed US and radionuclide study will exclude distal obstruction.[26] Risks exist in instrumenting the infant male urethra and the ureteral orifice, so routine use of retrograde studies is not recommended.

MANAGEMENT

Indications for Surgical Intervention

Once a UPJ obstruction is defined, prompt intervention to relieve obstruction is appropriate. Ureteral obstruction is detrimental to the kidney, and in the neonatal period, early relief of obstruction maximizes functional renal development and preserves nephrons.[27]

The ongoing debate in the management of neonatal UPJ obstruction is the definition of significant obstruction.[28–30] Randomization to surgical and observational arms is complicated by a difficult decision that a parent has to make for the asymptomatic child.[30] Relying on the morphologic appearance of a dilated renal pelvis by using excretory urography or US is an insufficient basis on which to proceed with operation, because many of these apparent abnormalities will completely resolve without surgical intervention[31] (see Fig. 53-2). Neonatal hydronephrosis can be explained by physiologic polyuria and natural kinks and folds in the ureter.[32,33]

Diuretic renography has limitations in the neonate, although using the "well-tempered" approach increases its value.[24] The accumulation of the isotope in the dilated collecting system is quite variable, so that the timing of the diuretic can be premature or delayed. The standard $T_{1/2}$ cutoff of 20 minutes for obstruction in the neonate is misleading in many cases.

Differential renal function or individual kidney uptake is the most useful information obtained during renography.[22–24] An indication for operative treatment is diminished renal function in the presence of an obstructive pattern on renography. The cutoff point is arbitrary, but most centers believe that 35% to 40% function in the hydronephrotic kidney warrants surgical correction. However, one series of patients followed up because of dilated kidneys having no more than 25% total renal function were found to improve to more than 40% of total function in all cases without surgical treatment.[31] Long-term studies of kidneys with greater than 40% function have shown that fewer than 15% to 20% will

require surgical treatment for diminishing function, urinary tract infections, or unexplained abdominal pain.[34,35] Some of these will regain some lost function.

The current recommendation is that pyeloplasty should be performed in the neonatal period in infants with a morphologic appearance of UPJ obstruction on US or IVP, no evidence of distal ureteral distention, and renal function depressed below 35% of total renal function. If function is above that level, follow-up scans are obtained at 3- to 6-month intervals, as clinically indicated. If clear deterioration in renal function occurs, then correction is recommended.

The ultimate concern with this approach is that delaying surgical intervention until measurable deterioration of renal function occurs is suboptimal. In the past, urinary stasis (infection, calculi, hypertension, pain) was the indication for correction. Whether more emphasis should be placed on stasis and less emphasis on differential renal function is an unanswered question.[36] Pyeloplasty can be safely performed in the infant.[37,38] Early intervention eliminates the indefinite period of surveillance. The decision to follow up neonates nonoperatively requires vigilance and parental cooperation to avoid unnecessary complications.

Once the diagnosis of significant obstruction is made in a neonate, operation is recommended within the first 4 to 6 weeks of life. If the child is first seen with acute pain or infection, it is advisable to wait 1 to 2 weeks to allow inflammation to resolve. Percutaneous drainage for sepsis is rarely required preoperatively. It should be strictly avoided in the absence of infection because of the inflammation that a tube in the renal pelvis induces.

Exploration of a poorly functioning kidney requires assessment of the renal parenchyma. If the parenchyma is grossly dysplastic or frozen-section analysis shows only dysplasia, then nephrectomy should be performed. No test accurately predicts recovery of function, so nephrectomy is rarely performed in the infant with UPJ obstruction.

Operative Techniques

Because the flank approach is the most difficult, and it is easy to commit errors of position and rotation, the anterior extraperitoneal approach or posterior lumbotomy approach is preferred. The anterior approach involves a transverse incision from the edge of the rectus to the tip of the twelfth rib.[39] The retroperitoneum is entered and the UPJ exposed, with the kidney left in situ. In infants, this is a muscle-splitting incision with low morbidity. The posterior lumbotomy can be easily performed in infancy and provides direct access to the UPJ.[40] The kidney does not require mobilization, and the ureter and renal pelvis can usually be brought up into the incision. In bilateral cases, the child does not need to be repositioned. The lumbotomy approach should not be used with a malrotated kidney or a kidney that has an intrarenal pelvis and is more difficult in a very muscular patient. An anterior or flank approach is always preferred in reoperative cases.

The result of any pyeloplasty is a funnel-shaped, dependent UPJ complex. Older techniques, including the

Foley Y-V plasty and the Culp spiral flap, were designed to maintain the continuity of the ureter and the pelvis.[41,42] These techniques are used in unusual cases of malrotation, fusion anomalies, or long, stenotic segments. The dismembered technique consistently provides the best results (Fig. 53-3).

The renal pelvis and upper ureter are mobilized, and the ureter is divided just below the obstructing segment and spatulated on its lateral border through the aperistaltic segment. If the segment is particularly long, this is identified before the renal pelvis is reduced, and a flap of renal pelvis can be created. It is usually important to resect some of the renal pelvis to avoid postoperative obstruction.

Gentle handling of the pelvic and ureteral tissue is recommended.[43] Excessive manipulation of these tissues increases edema. Pyeloplasties are frequently performed without diversion, so it is important to be as gentle as possible. Fine chromic stay sutures allow atraumatic manipulation of the ureter and renal pelvis. A retractor is placed only after dissection is completed so that the pyeloplasty can be more appropriately designed. The anastomosis is performed with 6-0 polydioxanone or 6-0 polyglycolic acid. The anastomosis begins at the most dependent portion of the pyeloplasty with placement of interrupted everting sutures that do not bunch the tissues and cause obstruction. After anastomosis to the dependent portion of the pyeloplasty is completed, the remainder of the ureter and pelvis can be approximated with continuous suture, taking care to irrigate any clots from the pelvis before the closure is completed. It is not necessary to pass a catheter distally into the bladder because preoperative studies should have excluded a distal obstruction.

Pyeloplasty can be safely performed without nephrostomy tubes or stents.[44,45] Even if transient leakage from the anastomosis occurs, a satisfactory outcome can be expected. A Penrose drain is left near the anastomosis and can usually be removed within 48 hours of the surgical procedure, but if drainage is prolonged, the child can be sent home with the drain in place.

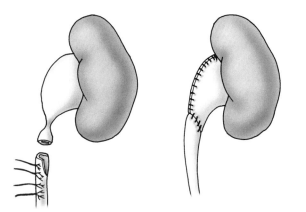

FIGURE 53-3. Dismembered pyeloplasty showing reduction of the renal pelvis and spatulation of the ureter as described in the text.

Nephrostomy tube drainage is indicated when simultaneous bilateral pyeloplasties are performed. In small children, the ureter may be a thin diaphanous structure, in which case, a nephrostomy decompression will reduce the chance of postoperative obstruction. A stent, although theoretically holding the ureter open and preventing synechiae formation, is usually not required. When the patient is faced with poor preoperative renal function, a nephrostomy provides postoperative decompression and will allow a low-pressure study of the anastomosis before its removal. Once free flow across the anastomosis is demonstrated, it is unlikely that future obstruction will occur. This is reassuring when postoperative pyelography or diuretic renography is difficult to interpret because of reduced function. In reoperative cases, a nephrostomy is always placed because it is technically more difficult to get a watertight anastomosis.

Extrinsic UPJ obstruction associated with an aberrant lower-pole vessel requires division of the ureter at the UPJ and performance of a standard dismembered pyeloplasty after transposing the ureter to a nonobstructed position. In the case of an intrarenal pelvis or when significant scarring exists in reoperative cases, a ureterocalicostomy is a useful adjunctive technique.[46] Amputation of the lower pole is required to prevent a postoperative stricture. The ureter is spatulated and anastomosed to a lower-pole calyx.

Endoscopic approaches to UPJ obstruction are now routinely used in adults.[47,48] The success of endoscopic repair in adults is minimally lower than that in comparable open series, but it does carry significantly less morbidity. Endoscopic relief of UPJ obstruction in children can be performed either percutaneously or retrograde by using a cutting current across the aperistaltic segment.[49] An indwelling ureteral stent is left for 4 to 6 weeks. The best results in children do not approach the near 100% success of open pyeloplasty. Because open pyeloplasty is highly successful, with minimal morbidity and a 1- to 3-day hospital stay, endopyelotomy has limited use in the neonate. It does have utility in the older child with good renal function and in cases when the renal pelvis is not massively dilated. Endopyelotomy clearly has a role in recurrent UPJ obstruction, where the success approaches 100%.[49]

Dismembered pyeloplasty also can be performed laparoscopically.[50] The limiting factor appears to be the increased technical difficulty associated with intracorporeal suturing. The anastomosis is not technically feasible in a small percentage of patients. Robotic assistance may eliminate some of this technical concern. Because the anastomotic technique is the same, long-term surgical outcomes should be the same as those for open repairs. However, long-term follow-up is not yet available. The laparoscopic approach does not now appear to decrease the length of hospitalization in children.

UPJ Obstruction in a Duplex Kidney

The lower pole of a duplex kidney is most commonly affected because the upper-pole segment lacks a true pelvis.[51] US may not be reliable for diagnosis, because the duplex nature of the kidney may not be identified.

A pyelogram or renogram will show a small nonobstructed upper segment.

The anatomy of the duplication influences the operation. If the ureter is incompletely duplicated and a long lower-pole ureteral segment is found, a standard dismembered pyeloplasty can be performed. If a high bifurcation is present and a short distal segment, then the end of the renal pelvis can be anastomosed to the side of the upper-pole ureter. These options can be assessed after the kidney and pelvis are exposed.

Surgical Results and Complications

The results of surgical correction have been uniformly successful[26,34,43,45] when performed at pediatric surgical institutions. The rate of recurrent UPJ obstruction is less than 1%, and the nephrectomy rate is less than 2%. The most common early complications are prolonged urinary extravasation and delayed drainage through the anastomosis. When an anastomotic leak persists beyond 14 days, continuity of the renal pelvis and ureter must be established with an IVP or retrograde pyelogram. If a significant leak is present, either a stent or a percutaneous nephrostomy tube should be inserted. Once diversion is instituted, the leak will usually cease within 48 hours. Late scarring at the anastomotic site is common in these situations.

Delayed opening of the anastomosis is seen most commonly with the use of a nephrostomy tube. When this occurs, patience is of the essence, because 80% of these will open in 3 months. Secondary obstruction or failure of the primary procedure results from scarring or fibrosis, a nondependent anastomosis, ureteral angulation secondary to renal malrotation, or ureteral narrowing distal to the anastomosis. Revision can be performed via an open incision with the same principles outlined for the initial procedure[52] or by using endoscopic approaches.[49]

A postoperative functional assessment of the anastomosis should be obtained in 2 to 3 months. A further evaluation is recommended 12 to 24 months after surgery. Problems are uncommon after this time in the absence of symptoms.

URETERAL ABNORMALITIES

Embryology

Ureteral development begins during the fourth week of gestation when the ureteral bud arises from the mesonephric duct.[53] The bud elongates, grows cephalad, and forms the ureter, renal pelvis, calyces, and collecting tubules. The distal end of the mesonephric duct from the ureteral bud to the vesicourethral tract is called the common excretory duct and expands in trumpet fashion into the bladder and urethra to form half of the trigone. The attachment of the ureter to the mesonephric duct switches from a posterior to an anterolateral location. With expansion and absorption of the common excretory duct into the urinary tract, the orifices of the ureteral bud and mesonephric duct become independent

and move away and settle in the bladder and urethra, respectively.

Alterations in bud number, position, and time of development result in anomalies. VUR results from caudal displacement of the ureteral bud, whereas ureteral ectopia and obstruction result from cranial displacement. Renal development and dysplasia are related to the ureteral orifice location.[54]

Ureteral Duplication

Duplication is the most common ureteral anomaly. Both sides are equally affected, and girls are affected twice as often as boys. The autopsy incidence is approximately 1%, but the incidence is 2% to 4% in clinical series in which pyelograms were obtained for urinary symptoms.[55,56] Infection is the most common presentation, and many of the duplicated units show scarring or hydronephrosis or both on imaging studies.[57] Histologic evaluation of the kidneys shows an increased incidence of pyelonephritis and dysplasia. An increased incidence of infection is found because of both VUR and obstruction.[55]

A partial or complete duplication of the ureter occurs when a single bud branches prematurely or when two ureteral buds arise from the mesonephric duct. A bifid renal pelvis is the highest level of bifurcation and occurs in 10% of the population. Other incomplete duplications occur throughout the ureter (Fig. 53-4). When the bifurcation is near the bladder, urine can pass down one limb of the duplication and then up the other side of the Y.[58] This may lead to stasis and ureteral dilatation. Treatment involves either ureteral reimplantation or ureteroureterostomy or ureteropyelostomy at the renal level.[59] An inverted-Y ureter is the rarest of all branching anomalies.[60] This is presumably the result of separate ureteral buds that fuse before entering the metanephros. Treatment is directed at problems caused by the ectopic limb.

In complete duplications, reflux in the lower moiety is the most common cause of renal disease. The more caudal ureteral bud ends up laterally and cranially deviated in the bladder and has a shorter intramural tunnel. The upper-pole ureter enters the bladder adjacent or distal to the lower ureter, as defined by the Weigert-Meyer law.[61] These children are first seen with urinary tract infections, and reflux is identified in up to two-thirds of children with duplicated systems that appear with infection.[62] Reflux may occur into the upper-pole ureter if the ureteral orifices are immediately adjacent or if the upper ureter is distally located at the level of the bladder neck without any submucosal support (Fig. 53-5).

The treatment of VUR in duplicated ureters follows the same principles as that in the single system. Initial treatment includes preventive antibiotics and radiographic monitoring. Low grades of VUR are associated with the same rate of spontaneous resolution as the single system. The distal ureters share a common blood supply, so reimplantation involves mobilization and reimplantation of the common sheath.[63] If an associated lower-pole UPJ obstruction is noted, ipsilateral end-to-side pyeloureterostomy is an effective simultaneous management of both obstruction and reflux.[64] Even if significant scarring is present in the

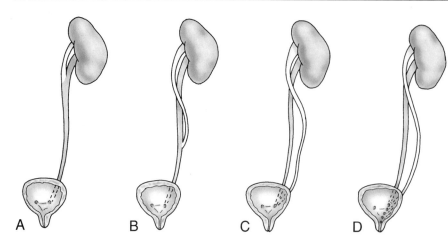

FIGURE 53-4. Types of duplication. *A,* Bifid pelvis. *B,* Y ureter. *C,* V ureter. *D,* complete duplication with various ectopic orifices.

lower pole, reimplantation usually suffices, unless major ureteral dilation is present. In the latter case, lower-pole nephroureterectomy may be indicated.

Obstructive abnormalities associated with ureteral duplication are discussed elsewhere in this chapter.

Ureteral Triplication

This is one of the rarest anomalies of the upper urinary tract and results from either several ureteral buds or early branching. In most cases, all three ureters drain

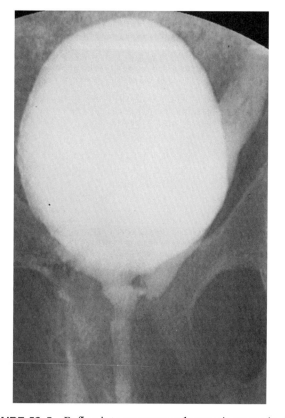

FIGURE 53-5. Reflux into an upper-pole ectopic ureter in the proximal urethra of a girl first seen at age 2 months with urosepsis.

into a single orifice.[65] Triplication occurs with incontinence, infection, and symptoms of obstruction and is associated with both ectopia and ureteroceles.[66,67] Surgical treatment is individualized.

Ureteral quadruplication has been described.[68]

Retrocaval Ureter

The retrocaval or circumcaval ureter is a right ureter that passes behind the vena cava.[69] This is a result of a developmental error in the formation of the vena cava. The supracardinal vein (vena cava) lies dorsal to the developing ureter, whereas subcardinal veins lie ventral to the ureter. If the subcardinal vein persists as the vena cava, the ureter passes behind the vena cava and anterior to the iliac vein. If both veins persist, the ureter passes between the duplicated vena cava.[70]

Even though this is a congenital abnormality, symptoms are related to chronic ureteral obstruction and infection and rarely occur in children.[71] The radiographic appearance depends on the level of obstruction. The more common distal obstruction appears as a reversed J on IVP.[72] Less commonly, the ureter crosses at the level of the UPJ. Both of these can be confused with UPJ obstruction and should be suspected when pyelectasis and dilation of the upper third of the ureter are seen.

Treatment is required only when significant obstruction or symptoms are present. Reconstruction is essentially a dismembered ureteroplasty with division of the ureter and anastomosis anterior to the vena cava, as opposed to division of the vena cava.

Megaureter

Megaureter is not a diagnosis but a descriptive term for a dilated ureter. Normal ureteral diameter in children is rarely greater than 5 mm, and ureters greater than 7 mm can be considered megaureters.[73] The radiographic appearance of the dilated and tortuous ureter is usually striking (Fig. 53-6). Pelvicalyceal dilation and parenchymal scarring or thinning depend on the primary disease process.

These ureters can be classified as refluxing, obstructed, and nonrefluxing nonobstructed.[74] Some ureters also have reflux and simultaneous obstruction.[75]

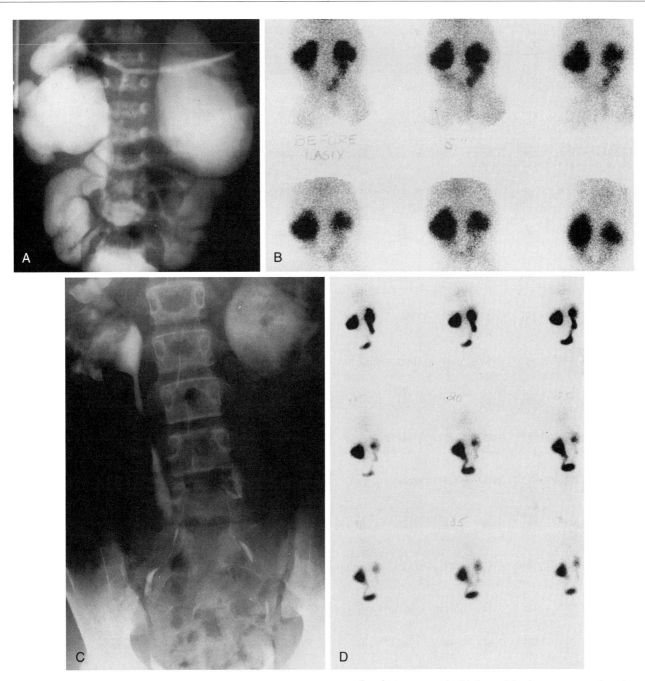

FIGURE 53-6. Congenital megaureter. *A*, Intravenous pyelogram (IVP) shows marked bilateral hydrouretero-nephrosis. *B*, Renal scan shows symmetrical function and normal extraction with stasis bilaterally. *C*, IVP 24 months later shows marked improvement in ureteral caliber and calyceal appearance. *D*, Function is preserved on renal scan.

Table 53-1 gives clinical examples of each classification. Any normal ureter will dilate if the volume of urine exceeds emptying capacity,[76] and bacterial endotoxins and infection alone can cause dilation that will resolve after treatment of infection.[77]

Primary obstructive megaureter is most commonly caused by a distal adynamic ureteral segment, but ureteral valves[33] and ectopic ureteral insertion also cause obstruction, as described later in this chapter. Proximal smooth muscle hypertrophy and hyperplasia are present. A normal-caliber catheter will usually pass through the

distal 3- to 4-mm segment, but the peristaltic wave does not propel urine across this area. The absent peristalsis is not a result of a ganglionic abnormality as seen in mega-colon.[78] The distal ureter has a variety of histologic appearances, but the common finding is a disruption of muscular continuity that prevents muscular propulsion of urine.[14,79–81]

As with UPJ obstruction, the majority of megaureters are now detected antenatally, although infection also is a common presentation.[82-84] Megaureter is now the second most common urinary tract abnormality

TABLE 53-1

CLASSIFICATION OF MEGAURETER

Refluxing Megaureter
Primary (congenital reflux)
Secondary (urethral valves, neurogenic bladder)

Obstructed Megaureter
Primary (adynamic segment)
Secondary (urethral obstruction, extrinsic mass, or tumor)

Nonrefluxing, Nonobstructed Megaureter
Primary (idiopathic, physiologically insignificant adynamic
    segment)
Secondary (polyuria, infection, postoperative residual dilation)

Based on the International Classification Scheme.
From Stephens FD: ABC of megaureters. In Bergsma D, Duckett JD (eds):
Birth Defects, Original Article Series, Vol. XIII. New York, Alan R. Liss,
1977, pp 1–8.

detected prenatally.[2] These children are typically asymptomatic without any physical findings or laboratory abnormalities.

Despite the variety of possibilities, standard imaging allows classification and appropriate management. The diagnosis of nonobstructed, nonrefluxing megaureter is the hardest to make and is established only when the secondary causes of megaureter have been excluded, and diagnostic tests do not show obstruction. For years it was assumed that a dilated ureter that did not reflux was obstructed,[85] but developmental ureteral dilation can be present in ureters that are not obstructed.[86]

Diagnostic imaging begins with a US that easily distinguishes megaureters from UPJ obstruction. The degree of distal ureteral dilation is often much more pronounced than the degree of renal pelvic dilation or calyectasis. A VCUG should be obtained in all patients. If significant reflux is present, delayed drainage films must be obtained to exclude simultaneous obstruction with a normal caliber distal ureteral segment.

Diuretic renography or pressure-perfusion studies are used to exclude significant obstruction. The specifics of these tests are discussed previously in this chapter in the section on UPJ obstruction. The renogram is harder to perform in the presence of megaureters. Diuretic administration must be delayed because the system is so capacious and may take 60 to 90 minutes to fill. A washout time of longer than 20 minutes is historically indicative of obstruction.

TREATMENT

Nonoperative management is based on clearance half-time and relative renal function of the hydronephrotic and contralateral kidneys. If observation is chosen, the children are given preventive antibiotics and followed up with serial US and renal scans. Neonatal megaureter with obstruction suggested by renography but with preserved function can be safely observed. Most ureters will become radiographically normal with time[82,83,87,88]

(see Fig. 53-6). Surgical correction for decreasing function or recurrent infections is indicated in only 10% to 25% of patients in up to 7 years of follow-up. Evidence of delayed obstruction after normalization of radiographs has not been seen in these children.

Initial attempts at surgical repair resulted in significant reflux and recurrent infections,[89] but when surgery is indicated, it can now be performed with high success and low morbidity. Ureteral excisional tapering with preservation of ureteral blood supply was popularized in the early 1970s.[85,90] A longitudinal segment of ureter is excised and then closed over a 10F to 12F catheter. When the ureter is tunneled submucosally, the suture line is placed against the detrusor to decrease the chance of fistula formation. Initial repairs involved tailoring of the entire ureter, but this was found to be unnecessary, as the upper ureteral tortuosity and dilatation often disappears after tapering of the distal ureter alone.[91] Ureteral folding techniques have been popularized because they theoretically decrease the risk of ischemic injury while achieving the decreased intraluminal diameter necessary for a successful reimplant.[92,93] The increased bulk is usually not a technical problem. Although dissection is usually both intravesical and extravesical, solely extravesical reimplants have been described and may be associated with lower morbidity.[94] A vesicopsoas hitch is a useful adjunct that helps achieve a longer submucosal tunnel length without risking ureteral kinking.

A nonrefluxing, nonobstructed reimplantation can be achieved 85% to 95% of the time with megaureters.[84,93] Recognized complications include persistent obstruction, reflux, and urinary extravasation. Most of these can be managed nonoperatively with drainage tubes. Lower grades of postoperative VUR will often resolve.

Primary reconstruction is preferred when indicated, but temporary cutaneous diversion may be beneficial in a neonate or infant when the chance of successful reimplantation of a bulky ureter into a small bladder diminishes. Diversion may decrease the ureteral diameter and decrease the need for tailoring at the time of reimplantation. An end-cutaneous ureterostomy is preferred because a high diversion may require two or more procedures for undiversion.

ECTOPIC URETER

An ectopic ureter is defined as one that opens at the bladder neck or more caudally rather than on the trigone. Embryologically, this results from a cranial insertion of the ureteral bud on the mesonephric duct that allows distal migration with the mesonephric duct as it is absorbed into the urogenital sinus.[55]

The incidence of ureteral ectopia is approximately 1 in 2000.[55] Eighty percent of ectopic ureters are reported in association with a duplicated renal system, and because clinical problems are more common in girls with ectopia, only 15% of ectopic ureters have been reported in boys.[95] Ectopia is bilateral 20% of the time.[96] Single ectopic ureters are rare but are more common in boys.[97]

Ectopic Ureters in Girls

The fundamental difference between ureteral ectopia in boys and girls arises from ureteral insertion distal to the continence mechanism in girls (Fig. 53-7). Approximately one-third of ureters open at the level of the bladder neck, one-third are in the vestibule around the urethral opening, and the remainder empty into the vagina, uterus, or cervix. All of these insertions are along the course of the mesonephric duct remnant (Gartner's duct).

One half of girls initially have continuous urinary incontinence in spite of what appears to be a normal voiding pattern.[95,96] If the system is markedly hydronephrotic and functions poorly, leakage may occur only in the upright position and may be confused with stress incontinence. Persistent foul-smelling vaginal discharge may suggest an ectopic ureter. When the ectopic ureter is present in the urethra or the bladder neck, both obstruction and reflux are commonly present, and urinary tract infection or sepsis is the mode of presentation.

The diagnosis of ectopic ureter may be obvious or can be difficult. When genital ectopy is present, the kidney may not visualize on intravenous pyelography. If significant hydronephrosis is found, the lower pole may be deviated laterally, but often minimal hydronephrosis appears, and the pyelogram may show only an absent upper-pole calyx on close inspection (Fig. 53-8). US may show a dilated ectopic ureter behind the bladder. Computerized tomography may be the most precise method of making this diagnosis.[98] A VCUG should be obtained in all patients to exclude occult reflux.[99]

The diagnosis is confirmed with physical examination, panendoscopy, and retrograde pyelography. Dyes used to stain urine may have a role. Urine in the bladder changes color, whereas the poorly concentrated urine is evident as persistent clear leakage. Meticulous examination of the area around the urethral meatus and vagina will often reveal an asymmetry or bead of fluid coming from an opening that can be probed and injected in retrograde fashion (see Fig. 53-8). Vaginoscopy with attention to the superior lateral aspect of the vagina may reveal a large ectopic orifice.

Ectopic Ureter in Boys

The most common sites of ectopic ureteral insertion in boys are the posterior urethra (40% to 50%) and the seminal vesicle (20% to 60%), depending on the age at presentation.[100] Symptoms in the boy may not occur until after the onset of sexual activity and include prostatitis, seminal vesiculitis, or an infected seminal vesical cyst causing painful bowel movements. The genital insertion accounts for the common presentation with epididymitis. The boy may initially have postvoid dribbling secondary to pooling of urine in the prostatic urethra, but incontinence is never as pronounced as in the girl.

Diagnostic testing is similar to that used in girls. Ectopic ureters in the boy are more commonly obstructed and hydronephrotic, so US examination is often more useful. If the ectopic site of insertion is outside the urethra, it is rarely identified on endoscopic examination.

Surgical Management of Ectopic Ureters

Surgical treatment is dependent on the associated parenchyma.[101,102] Single-system ectopia to the genital system usually has poor function, and nephroureterectomy is appropriate. If the ureter is ectopic to the urethra or bladder neck, adequate function may justify ureteral reimplantation.[101] When the ectopic ureter is associated with a duplication, function of the upper pole is usually poor, and a partial nephroureterectomy is most often performed. The distal stump is left open. If function is good, a ureteropyelostomy or ureteroureterostomy can be performed to drain the ectopic system at the renal level. If this is not technically feasible, a common sheath ureteral reimplantation can be performed with tailoring of the upper-pole ureter.

The distal stump rarely causes a problem in genital ectopia; however, if urethral or bladder neck insertion of the ectopic ureter and reflux into the ureter is identified preoperatively, excision is indicated.[102] Removal can be tedious. If the dissection plane is kept immediately adjacent to the ureter behind the bladder, the bladder neck and sphincter should not be damaged. The stump is ligated at this point. In a postpubertal girl, this dissection can be performed transvaginally. Small stumps can be obliterated by using a Bugbee electrode.

Bilateral Single Ectopic Ureters

This is a rare abnormality in which the altered ureteral embryologic development is associated with failure of normal bladder neck development.[103] Genital and anal anomalies are commonly present. Girls have ureteral insertion in the distal urethra and are first seen with infection or are noted to have continuous urinary leakage. The bladder is usually poorly developed because it has never stored urine. Boys have somewhat larger bladders, because some urine will enter the bladder. However, because the bladder neck is not formed normally, they also have some degree of urinary incontinence.

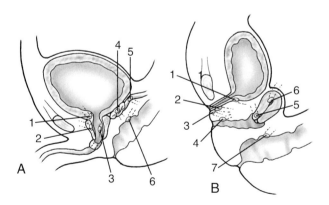

FIGURE 53-7. *A,* Ureteral ectopia in boy. Possible sites are above the external sphincter. *B,* Ureteral ectopia in girl may be located beyond the continence mechanism and produce incontinence.

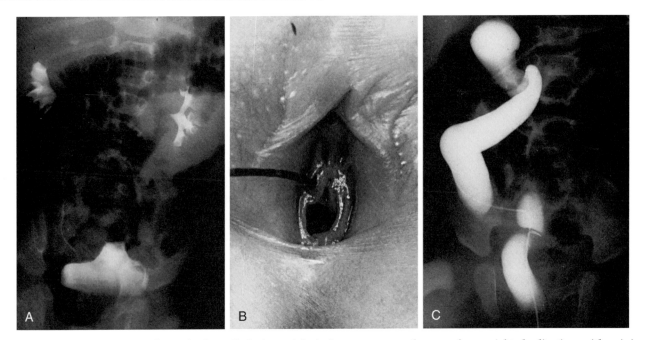

FIGURE 53-8. Ectopic ureter in vaginal vestibule in a girl. *A*, Intravenous pyelogram shows right duplication with minimal upper-pole function with downward and outward displacement of lower pole (drooping lily sign). *B*, Ureteral catheter in ectopic ureter. *C*, Retrograde ureterogram.

The child who is incontinent with bilateral single ectopic ureters is a major reconstructive challenge that may include ureteral reimplantation, bladder neck reconstruction, and bladder augmentation if the bladder capacity is insufficient.

URETEROCELES

Ureteroceles are cystic dilatations of the terminal, intravesical ureter that usually have a stenotic orifice.[104–106] In children, ureteroceles are most commonly associated with the upper pole of a duplex system (80%) and an ectopic orifice (60%) in the urethra, whereas in adults, they are usually part of a completely intravesical single system. Ureteroceles occur 4 to 7 times more frequently in girls and are more common in whites. Bilateral ureteroceles are found 10% of the time.

A single embryologic theory does not explain all ureteroceles. The most popular theory involves persistence of Chwalla's membrane at the junction of the wolffian duct and urogenital sinus.[107] Incomplete breakdown of the ureteral membrane is an obstruction resulting in dilation. This theory would explain the majority of ureteroceles but does not explain the development of ureteroceles with patulous ureteral orifices in the urethra, ureteroceles associated with multicystic dysplasia and atretic ureteral segments, or the presence of ectopic ureters without ureterocele formation.

It is likely that a ureterocele is the result of an abnormal induction of the trigone and distal ureter by many of the genes and growth factors that are important in renal and ureteral growth and development. Histologic studies support this concept.[108] Histologic analysis of the intravesical portion of ureteroceles shows deficiencies in the trigonal musculature of patients with ureteroceles that were not present in ectopic ureters without ureterocele formation. This field defect results in pseudodiverticulum (ureterocele eversion) and reflux into laterally displaced poorly supported ureters.

The classification of ureteroceles can be confusing. Pathologic description defines four types: stenotic, sphincteric, sphincterostenotic, and cecoureterocele.[108] The current recommended nomenclature classifies ureteroceles as either intravesical (entirely within the bladder) or ectopic (some portion is situated permanently at the bladder neck or in the urethra).[109]

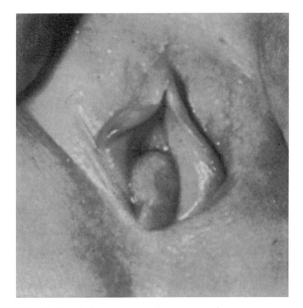

FIGURE 53-9. Prolapsing ectopic ureterocele.

Presentation and Diagnosis

Although presentation with infection in a system with high-grade obstruction is common, antenatal detection is now the presentation in up to 60% of cases.[110-112] The obstructed renal unit may be palpable in these asymptomatic infants, but most have no clinically apparent abnormality. Bladder-outlet obstruction is rare because most ureteroceles decompress during micturition, but the most common cause of urethral obstruction in girls is urethral prolapse of a ureterocele (Fig. 53-9).

Abdominal US reveals a well-defined cystic intravesical mass that is associated with the posterior bladder wall (Fig. 53-10). This can be followed into a dilated ureter in the bony pelvis and upper-pole hydroureteronephrosis in a duplication. The thickness and echogenicity of the renal parenchyma are often consistent with dysplasia and poor function.

Intravenous urograms reveal typical findings (see Fig. 53-10). In adults, function is often good, and the ureterocele fills with contrast and is separated from the contrast in the bladder by a thin lucent halo. A VCUG is obtained in all patients. Up to 50% of the ipsilateral lower pole and 25% of the contralateral renal units have VUR.[110,113]

During cystoscopy, the bladder should be examined when both full and completely empty because compressible ureteroceles may not be evident in a full bladder or may appear as a bladder diverticulum (Fig. 53-11). The dilated lower end of an ectopic ureter or megaureter may elevate the trigone, creating the cystoscopic, radiographic, and US appearance of a ureterocele, a so-called pseudoureterocele.[114]

Treatment Options

The goals of ureterocele treatment include control of infection, preservation of renal function, protection of normal ipsilateral and contralateral units, and maintaining

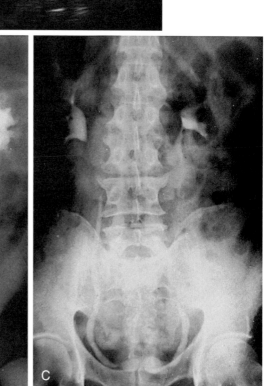

FIGURE 53-10. *A,* Ureterocele appearance on ultrasonography. *B,* Intravenous pyelogram appearance of ureteroceles and duplication, with downward displacement of the lower pole moiety, absent upper-pole infundibulum, and lateral lower-pole ureteral displacement by the dilated upper-pole segment. The function of the affected unit is poor, giving a negative shadow of the nonopacified ureterocele present in the bladder. *C,* Single-system ureteroceles are intravesical, function well, and the ureterocele is filled with contrast, giving a "cobra-head" deformity.

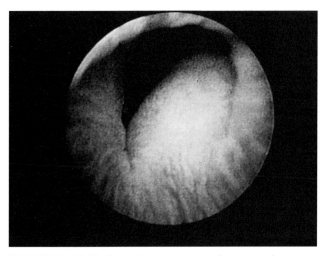

FIGURE 53-11. Endoscopic appearance of ureterocele.

continence. The natural history of the asymptomatic ureterocele is unknown. Neonates given preventive antibiotics rarely develop a febrile urinary tract infection.[111,112] Observation without prevention is rarely a good option. It should be assumed that significant urinary tract obstruction is present, and preventive antibiotics should be started.

Traditional treatment of duplex ectopic ureteroceles includes upper-pole heminephrectomy through a separate flank incision, ureterocele excision, and ipsilateral lower-pole ureteral reimplant via a lower incision. The bladder-level operation may require repair of a sizable defect in the bladder base and a tapering or plication of the lower ureter. The distal extent of the ureterocele and its mucosa can often be dissected through the bladder neck. Incomplete excision may result in an obstructing urethral flap, and resection of the entire ureterocele risks damaging the bladder-neck continence mechanisms. Experienced surgeons report excellent results with low reoperative rates (<10%) and low complication rates (<10%).[115-117] These approaches assume that ureterocele excision is an essential component of management. However, because the distal ureter and bladder defect may resolve without being removed or repaired, an absolute indication to proceed with a simultaneous bladder operation is rarely present. When absence of function is noted on the affected side (upper and lower pole), nephroureterectomy and reconstruction of the bladder is the initial treatment of choice in older children.

Primary upper-pole partial nephroureterectomy may avoid bladder-level reconstruction and its potential risks.[110,118,119] Nearly all of the ureter can be removed through the flank incision, and the distal ureter is left open to facilitate decompression. The need for subsequent bladder-level excision and reconstruction varies between 10% and 62%.[110,112,119] Although up to 45% of ipsilateral and contralateral VUR will resolve after ureterocele decompression,[110] persistent VUR is the most common indication for a bladder-level reconstruction. Other indications for bladder-level reconstruction

include ureterocele eversion acting like a diverticulum or externally compressing the bladder neck, reflux into the ureterocele, or intraluminal obstruction of the bladder neck by a cecoureterocele. The need for bladder-level intervention is directly related to the number of renal moieties that have either a ureterocele or VUR.[112]

Most partial nephrectomy specimens show dysplasia,[119] but some may show only inflammatory and obstructive changes.[120] To preserve function, a pyeloureterostomy or ureteroureterostomy (high or low) may be performed, along with distal ureterectomy and ureterocele decompression.[121] These procedures potentially place the lower-pole system at risk to salvage what may be a small percentage of total renal function.

Ureterocele incision is the least invasive technique of upper-pole preservation. "Unroofing" of the ureterocele is advocated only as a drainage procedure for an infected system before a definitive procedure because it invariably results in reflux.[122,123] Using a 3F Bugbee electrode to drain the ureterocele just above the bladder neck is the recommended technique because reflux is not inevitable[111,124] (Fig. 53-12). The opening is in the bladder, but to be successful, it must also drain the ectopic urethral portion to prevent an obstructing lip at the level of the bladder neck.

Endoscopic incision successfully decompresses the ureterocele 85% of the time.[111,120,125,126] It is the definitive procedure in more than 90% of infants with intravesical ureteroceles, whereas subsequent reconstructive surgery is required in 50% to 90% of patients with ectopic ureteroceles. Reflux into the ureterocele moiety is the most common indication for reconstruction in these infants. Previous decompression of the system makes this reconstruction easier.[111]

Incision should be the initial procedure in all neonates. When the ureterocele is detected before the onset of infection, appreciable function may be present after relief of obstruction.[120] Even when US shows little parenchyma, incision can be performed. The decompressed system may require no further treatment if no VUR is present.

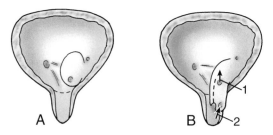

FIGURE 53-12. Technique for incision of ureteroceles. *A,* Intravesical ureteroceles are punctured with a 3F Bugbee electrode low on the anterior wall just inside the bladder neck. *B,* Ectopic ureteroceles require drainage of the urethral segment to prevent a distal obstructing flap. This can be achieved by making a longitudinal incision across the bladder neck (1) or with two separate punctures (2). (From Cooper CS, Passerini-Glazel G, Hutcheson JC, et al: Long-term follow up of endoscopic incision of ureteroceles: Intravesical versus extravesical. J Urol 164:1097, 2000.)

In older children, an incision is best selected when associated functioning renal parenchyma is found, the ureterocele is intravesical, or the kidney is drained by a single system.

Single-system ureteroceles are more commonly seen in older children and adults and are associated with better function and less hydronephrosis than is found in duplex kidneys. Most often they are incidental findings that require no treatment. Antenatally detected single-system ureteroceles may not show significant obstruction on a furosemide (Lasix) washout renal scan. Clinically, these behave like nonobstructed megaureters and can be safely followed up with preventive antibiotics. If treatment is required, endoscopic incision is a definitive procedure nearly 100% of the time.

REFERENCES

1. Thomas DFM: Fetal uropathy: Review. Br J Urol 66:225, 1990.
2. Brown T, Mandell J, Lebowitz R: Neonatal hydronephrosis in the era of sonography. Am J Radiol 148:959, 1987.
3. Mandell J, Blyth B, Peters C, et al: Structural genitourinary defects detected in utero. Radiology 178:193, 1991.
4. Williams DI, Kenawi MM: The prognosis of pelviureteric junction in childhood: A review of 190 cases. Eur Urol 2:57, 1976.
5. Snyder HM III, Lebowitz RL, Colodny AH, et al: UPJ obstruction in children. Urol Clin North Am 7:273, 1980.
6. Ruano-Gil D, Coca-Payeras A, Tejedo-Maten A: Obstruction and normal recanalization of the ureter in the human embryo: Its relation to congenital ureteric obstruction. Eur Urol 1:287, 1975.
7. Arams HJ, Buckbinder ME, Sutton AP: Benign ureteral lesions: Rare causes of hydronephrosis in children. Urology 9:517–520, 1977.
8. Stephens FD: Ureterovascular hydronephrosis and the "aberrant" renal vessels. J Urol 128:984, 1982.
9. Murnaghan GF: The dynamics of the renal pelvis and ureter with reference to congenital hydronephrosis. Br J Urol 30:321, 1958.
10. Koff SA, Hayden LJ, Cirulli C, et al: Pathophysiology of UPJ obstruction: Experimental and clinical observations. J Urol 136:336, 1986.
11. Foote JW, Blennerhassett JB, Wiglesworth FW, et al: Observations on the ureteropelvic junction. J Urol 104:252, 1970.
12. Allen TD: Congenital ureteral strictures. J Urol 104:196, 1970.
13. Starr NT, Maizels M, Chou P, et al: Microanatomy and morphometry of the hydronephrotic "obstructed" renal pelvis in asymptomatic infants. J Urol 148:519, 1992.
14. Hanna MK, Jeffs RD, Sturgess JM, et al: Ureteral structure and ultrastructure, Part II: Congenital UPJ obstruction and primary obstructive megaureter. J Urol 116:725, 1976.
15. Kjurhuus JC, Nerstrom B, Gyrd-Hansen N, et al: Experimental hydronephrosis: An electrophysiologic investigation before and after release of obstruction. Act Chir Scand Suppl 472:17, 1976.
16. Wang Y, Puri P, Hassan J, et al: Abnormal innervation and altered nerve growth factor messenger ribonucleic acid expression in ureteropelvic junction obstruction. J Urol 154:679, 1995.
17. Lebowitz RL, Blickman JG: The coexistence of UPJ obstruction and reflux. AJR Am J Roentgenol 140:231, 1983.
18. Hollowell JG, Altman HG, Snyder HM III, et al: Coexisting UPJ obstruction and vesicoureteral reflux: Diagnostic and therapeutic implications. J Urol 142:490, 1989.
19. Sanders RC, Nussbaum AR, Solez K: Renal dysplasia: Sonographic findings. Radiology 167:623, 1988.
20. Hulbert WC, Rosenberg HK, Cartwright PC, et al: The predictive value of ultrasonography in evaluation of infants with posterior urethral valves. J Urol 148:122, 1992.
21. Borthne AS, Pierre-Jerome C, Gjesdal KI, et al: Pediatric excretory MR urography: Comparative study of enhanced and non-enhanced techniques. Eur Radiol 13:1423, 2003.
22. Heyman S, Duckett JW: Extraction factor: An estimate of single kidney function in children during routine radionucleotide

23. Chung S, Majd M, Rushton HG, et al: Diuretic renography in the evaluation of neonatal hydronephrosis: Is it reliable? J Urol 150:765, 1993.
24. Conway JJ: "Well-tempered" diuresis renography: Its historical development, physiological and technical pitfalls and standardized technique protocol. Semin Nucl Med 22:74, 1992.
25. Whitaker RH: The Whitaker test. Urol Clin North Am 6:529, 1979.
26. Rushton HG: Pediatric pyeloplasty: Is routine retrograde pyelography necessary? J Urol 152:604, 1994.
27. Chevalier RL, El Dahr S: The case for early relief of obstruction in young infants. In King LR (ed): Urological Surgery in Neonates and Young Infants. Philadelphia, WB Saunders, 1988, p 95.
28. Duckett JW: When to operate on neonatal hydronephrosis. Urology 42:617, 1993.
29. Woodard JR: Hydronephrosis in the neonate. Urology 42:620, 1993.
30. Palmer LS, Maizels M, Cartwright PC, et al: Surgery versus observation for managing obstructive grade 3 to 4 unilateral hydronephrosis: A report from the Society for Fetal Urology. J Urol 159:222, 1988.
31. Ulman I, Jayanthi VR, Koff SA: The long-term followup of newborns with severe unilateral hydronephrosis initially treated nonoperatively. J Urol 164:1101, 2000.
32. Rabinowitz R, Peters MT, Byas S, et al: Measurements of fetal urine production in normal pregnancy by real-time ultrasonography. Am J Obstet Gynecol 161:1264, 1989.
33. Ostling K: The genesis of hydronephrosis particularly with regard to the changes at the ureteropelvic junction. Acta Chir Scand 86:1, 1942.
34. Ransley PG, Dhillon HK, Gordon I, et al: The postnatal management of hydronephrosis diagnosed by prenatal ultrasound. J Urol 144:584, 1990.
35. Cartwright PC, Duckett JW, Keating MA, et al: Managing apparent ureteropelvic junction obstruction in the newborn. J Urol 148:1224, 1992.
36. Allen TD: The swing of the pendulum [editorial]. J Urol 148:534, 1992.
37. Wolpert JJ, Woodard JR, Parrott TS: Pyeloplasty in the young infant. J Urol 142:563, 1989.
38. Salem YH, Majd M, Rushton HG, et al: Outcome analysis of pediatric pyeloplasty as a function of patient age, presentation and differential renal function. J Urol 154:1889, 1995.
39. Duckett JW, Gibbons MD, Cromie WJ: An anterior extraperitoneal muscle-splitting approach for pediatric renal surgery. J Urol 123:79, 1980.
40. Orland SM, Snyder HM, Duckett JW: The dorsal lumbotomy incision in pediatric urological surgery. J Urol 138:963, 1987.
41. Foley FEB: A new plastic operation for stricture at the UPJ: Report of 20 cases. J Urol 38:643, 1937.
42. Culp OS, DeWeerd JH: Pelvic flap operation for certain types of ureteropelvic obstruction. Mayo Clin Proc 26:483, 1951.
43. Hendren WHH, Radhakrishnan J, Middleton AW: Pediatric pyeloplasty. J Pediatr Surg 15:133, 1980.
44. Bernstein GT, Mandell J, Lebowitz RL, et al: UPJ in the neonate. J Urol 140:1216, 1988.
45. Roth DR, Gonzales ET Jr: Management of UPJ obstruction in infants. J Urol 129:108, 1983.
46. Duckett JW, Pfister RR: Ureterocalicostomy for renal salvage. J Urol 128:98, 1982.
47. Nakada SY, Johnson M: Ureteropelvic junction obstruction: Retrograde endopyelotomy. Urol Clin North Am 27:677, 2000.
48. Streem SB: Percutaneous endopyelotomy. Urol Clin North Am 27:685, 2000.
49. Figenshau RS, Clayman RV, Colberg JW, et al: Pediatric endopyelotomy: The Washington University experience. J Urol 156:2025, 1996.
50. El-Ghoneimi A, Farhat W, Bolduc S, et al: Laparoscopic dismembered pyeloplasty by a retroperitoneal approach in children. BJU Int 92:104, 2003.
51. Ossandon SM, Androulakakis P, Ransley PG: Surgical problems in pelviureteral junction obstruction of the lower pole moiety in incomplete duplex systems. J Urol 125:871, 1981.

52. Rohrmann D, Snyder HM, Duckett JW, et al: The operative management of recurrent ureteropelvic junction obstruction. J Urol 158:1257, 1997.

53. Brockis JG: The development of the trigone of the bladder with a report of a case of ectopic ureter. Br J Urol 24:192, 1952.

54. Mackie GG, Awang H, Stephens FD: The ureteric orifice: The embryologic key to radiologic status of the kidneys. J Pediatr Surg 10:473, 1975.

55. Campbell MF: Anomalies of the ureter. In Campbell MF, Harrison JH (eds): Urology, 3rd ed. Philadelphia, WB Saunders, 1970, pp 1487–1670.

56. Hartman GW, Hodson CJ: The duplex kidney and related abnormalities. Clin Radiol 20:387, 1969.

57. Privett JTJ, Jeans WD, Roylance J: The incidence and importance of renal duplication. Clin Radiol 27:521, 1976.

58. Tresidder BC, Blandy JP, Murray RS: Pyelopelvic and ureteroureteric reflux. Br J Urol 42:728, 1970.

59. Amar AD: Treatment of reflux in bifid ureters by conversion to complete duplication. J Urol 108:77, 1972.

60. Klauber GC, Reid ED: Inverted Y reduplication of the ureter. J Urol 107:362, 1972.

61. Meyer R: Normal and abnormal development of the ureter in the human embryo: A mechanistic consideration. Anat Rec 96:355, 1946.

62. Fehrenbaker LG, Kelalis PP, Stickler GB: Vesicoureteral reflux and ureteral duplication in children. J Urol 107:862, 1972.

63. Barrett DM, Maled RS, Kelalis PP: Problems and solutions in surgical treatment of 100 consecutive ureteral duplications in children. J Urol 114:126, 1975.

64. Shelfo SW, Keller MS, Weiss RM: Ipsilateral pyeloureterostomy for managing lower-pole reflux with associated ureteropelvic junction obstruction in duplex systems. J Urol 157:1420, 1997.

65. Kohri K, Nagai N, Kaneko S, et al: Bilateral trifid ureters associated with fused kidney, ureterovesical stenosis, left cryptorchidism and angioma of the bladder. J Urol 120:249, 1978.

66. Zaontz MR, Maizels M: Type I ureteral triplication: An extension of the Weiger-Meyer law. J Urol 134:949, 1985.

67. Finkel Li, Watts FB, Cobrett DP: Ureteral triplication with a ureterocele. Pediatr Radiol 13:343, 1983.

68. Soderdahl DW, Shiraki IW, Schamber DT: Bilateral ureteral quadruplication. J Urol 116:255, 1976.

69. Considine J: Retrocaval ureter. Br J Urol 38:412, 1966.

70. Hollinshead WH: Anatomy for Surgeons, Vol 2, 3rd ed. Philadelphia, Harper and Row, 1982.

71. Resnick MI, Kursh ED: Extrinsic obstruction of the ureter. In Walsh PC, Retick AB, Stamey TA, et al (eds): Campbell's Urology, 6th ed. Philadelphia, WB Saunders, 1992, p 540.

72. Kumar S, Bhandari M: Selection of operative procedure for circumcaval ureter (type I). Br J Urol 57:399, 1985.

73. Hellstrom M, Hjalmas K, Jacobsson B, et al: Normal ureteral diameter in infancy and childhood. Acta Radiol 26:433, 1985.

74. Stephens FD: ABC of megaureters. In Bergsma D, Duckett JD (eds): Birth Defects, Original Article Series, Vol. XIII. New York, Alan R. Liss, 1977, pp 1–8.

75. King LR: Megaloureter: Definition, diagnosis, and management. J Urol 123:222, 1980.

76. Boyd SD, Raz S, Ehrlich RM: Diabetes insipidus and nonobstructive dilation of urinary tract. Urology 16:266, 1980.

77. Kass EJ, Silver TM, Konnak JW, et al: The urographic findings in acute pyelonephritis: Non-obstructive hydronephrosis. J Urol 116:544, 1976.

78. Leibowitz S, Bodian M: A study of the vesical ganglia in children and their relationship to the megaureter megacystis syndrome and Hirschsprung's disease. J Clin Pathol 16:342, 1963.

79. Tanagho EA: Embryologic basis for lower ureteral anomalies: A hypothesis. Urology 7:451, 1976.

80. Gregoir W, Debled B: L'etiologie du reflux congenital et du mega uretere primaire. Urol Int 24:119, 1969.

81. McLaughlin AP, Pfister RC, Leadbetter WF, et al: The pathophysiology of primary megaloureter. J Urol 109:805, 1973.

82. Mollard P, Foray P, De Godoy JL, et al: Management of primary obstructive megaureter without reflux in neonates. Eur Urol 24:505, 1993.

83. Cozzi F, Madonna L, Maggi E, et al: Management of primary megaureter in infancy. J Pediatr Surg 28:1031, 1993.

84. Peters CA Mandell J, Lebowitz RL, et al: Congenital obstructed megaureters in early infancy: Diagnosis and treatment. J Urol 142:641, 1989.

85. Hendren WH: Operative repair of megaureter in children. J Urol 101:491, 1969.

86. Keating MA, Escala J, Snyder HM, et al: Changing concepts in management of primary obstructive megaureter. J Urol 142:636, 1989.

87. Baskin LS, Zderic SA, Snyder HM, et al: Primary dilated megaureter: Long-term follow up. J Urol 152:618, 1994.

88. Liu HY, Dhillon HK, Yeung CK, et al: Clinical outcome and management of prenatally diagnosed primary megaureters. J Urol 152:614, 1994.

89. Nesbit RM, Withycombe JF: The problem of primary megaloureter. J Urol 72:162, 1954.

90. Grégoir W: Traitement chirurgical du reflux congénital et du méga-uretère primaire. Urol Int 24:502, 1969.

91. Hendren WH: Commentary: Surgery of megaureter. In Whitehead D, Leiter E (eds): Current Operative Urology. Philadelphia, Harper & Row, 1984, pp 473–482.

92. Starr A: Ureteral plication: A new concept in ureteral tailoring for megaureter. Invest Urol 17:153, 1979.

93. Perdzynski W, Kalicinski ZH: Long-term results after megaureter folding in children. J Pediatr Surg 31:1211, 1996.

94. McLorie GA, Jayanthi VR, Kinahan TJ, et al: A modified extravesical technique for megaureter repair. Br J Urol 74:715, 1994.

95. Schulman CC: Les implantations ectopiques de l'uretère. Acta Urol Belg 40:201, 1972.

96. Malek RS, Kelalis PP, Stickler GB, et al: Observations on ureteral ectopy in children. J Urol 107:308, 1972.

97. Johnston JH, Davenport TJ: The single ectopic ureter. Br J Urol 41:428, 1969.

98. Lebowitz RL: Pediatric uroradiology. Pediatr Clin North Am 32:1353, 1985.

99. Lebowitz RL, Wyly JB: Refluxing urethral ectopic ureters: Diagnosis by the cyclic voiding cystourethrogram. AJR Am J Roentgenol 142:1263, 1984.

100. Terai A, Tsuji Y, Terachi T, et al: Ectopic ureter opening into the seminal vesicle in an infant: A case report and review of the Japanese literature. Int J Urol 2:128, 1995.

101. el Ghoneimi A, Miranda J, Truong T, et al: Ectopic ureter with complete ureteric duplication: Conservative surgical management. J Pediatr Surg 31:467, 1996.

102. Plaire JC, Pope JC, Kropp BP, et al: Management of ectopic ureters: Experience with upper tract approach. J Urol 158:1245, 1997.

103. Noseworthy J, Persky L: Spectrum of bilateral ureteral ectopia. Urology 19:489, 1982.

104. Uson AC, Lattimer JK, Melicow MM: Ureteroceles in infants and children: A report based on 44 cases. Pediatrics 27:971, 1961.

105. Mertz HO: Blind uretero-vesical protrusion. Trans Am Assoc Gen-Urin Surg 40:180, 1948.

106. Ericson NO: Ectopic ureterocele in infants and children Acta Chir Scand Suppl 197:8, 1954.

107. Chwalla R: The process of formation of cystic dilations of the vesical end of the ureter and of diverticula at the ureteral ostium. Urol Cutan Rev 31:499, 1927.

108. Stephens FD, Smith ED, Hutson JM: Congenital Anomalies of the Urinary and Genital Tracts. Oxford, Isis Medical Media, 1996, pp 243–262.

109. Glassberg KI, Braren V, Duckett JW, et al: Suggested terminology for duplex systems, ectopic ureters and ureteroceles. J Urol 132:1153–1154, 1984.

110. Caldamone AA, Snyder HM, Duckett JW: Ureteroceles in children: Follow-up of management with upper tract approach. J Urol 131:1130–1132, 1984.

111. Cooper CS, Passerini-Glazel G, Hutcheson JC, et al: Long-term follow up of endoscopic incision of ureteroceles: Intravesical versus extravesical. J Urol 164:1097, 2000.

112. Husmann DA, Ewalt DH, Glenski WJ, et al: Ureterocele associated with ureteral duplication and nonfunctioning upper pole segment: Management by partial nephroureterectomy alone. J Urol 154:723–726, 1995.

113. Sen S, Beasley SW, Ahmed S, et al: Renal function and vesicoureteric reflux in children with ureteroceles. Pediatr Surg Int 7:192–194, 1992.

114. Sumfest JM, Burns MW, Mitchell ME: Pseudoureterocele: potential for misdiagnosis of an ectopic ureter as a ureterocele. Br J Urol 75:401–405, 1995.
115. Hendren WH, Mitchell ME: Surgical correction of ureteroceles. J Urol 121:590–597, 1979.
116. Scherz HC, Kaplan GW, Packer MG, et al: Ectopic ureteroceles: Surgical management with preservation of continence: Review of 60 cases. J Urol 142:538–541, 1989.
117. Shekarriz B, Upadhyay J, Fleming P, et al: Long-term outcome based on the initial surgical approach to ureterocele. J Urol 162:1072, 1999.
118. Cendron J, Bonhomme C: 31 Cas d'ureter abondement ectopique sons sphincterien chez l'enfant du sexe feminin. J Urol Nephrol 74:1, 1968.
119. Rickwood AMK, Reiner I, Jones M, et al: Current management of duplex-system ureteroceles: Experience with 41 patients. Br J Urol 70:196–200, 1992.
120. Monfort G, Guys JM, Coquet M, et al: Surgical management of duplex ureteroceles. J Pediatr Surg 27:634–638, 1992.
121. Huisman TK, Kaplan GW, Brock WA, et al: Ipsilateral ureteroureterostomy and pyeloureterostomy: A review of 15 years experience with 25 patients. J Urol 138:1207–1210, 1987.
122. Snyder HM, Johnston JM: Orthotopic ureteroceles in children. J Urol 119:543–546, 1978.
123. Tank ES: Experience with endoscopic incision and open unroofing of ureteroceles. J Urol 136:241–242, 1986.
124. Monfort G, Morisson-Lacombe G, Coquet M: Endoscopic treatment of ureteroceles revisited. J Urol 133:1031–1033, 1985.
125. Hagg MJ, Mourachov PV, Snyder HM, et al: The modern endoscopic approach to ureterocele. J Urol 163:940, 2000.
126. Husmann D, Strand B, Ewalt D, et al: Management of ectopic ureterocele associated with renal duplication: A comparison of partial nephrectomy and endoscopic decompression. J Urol 162:1406, 1999.

Urinary Tract Infection and Vesicoureteral Reflux

Eugene Minevich, MD, and Curtis A. Sheldon, MD

URINARY TRACT INFECTION

Diagnosis

Although clinical signs and symptoms are important indications of childhood urinary tract infection (UTI), because of the profound implications of UTI in children, confirmation of the diagnosis by microscopic examination and quantitative culture of a properly collected specimen is imperative. Signs and symptoms of UTI are age dependent. Neonates rarely are first seen with findings specific to the urinary tract. Nonspecific symptoms of lethargy, irritability, temperature instability, anorexia, emesis, or jaundice predominate. Bacteremia is common with neonatal UTI, and urine culture is an important aspect of the evaluation of neonatal sepsis.[1] Older infants are initially seen with nonspecific abdominal discomfort, emesis, diarrhea, poor weight gain, or fever. Malodorous or cloudy urine may be reported. Older children often have dysuria. Urinary frequency, urgency, and enuresis become prevalent. Table 54-1 outlines the incidence of UTI symptoms as a function of age.[2,3]

Analysis of a properly collected urine sample is the cornerstone of diagnosis of UTI.[4] Errors in diagnosis occur frequently. They most commonly result from failure to confirm a clinically suspected UTI by culture or by reliance on a specimen that has been inadequately collected or mishandled. Specimens may be obtained by bag collection, clean catch, urethral catheterization, and suprapubic aspiration. Although invasive, urethral catheterization and suprapubic aspiration clearly offer the lowest risk of contamination (false-positive culture results).[5] The results of a bag specimen or clean-catch specimen are definitive only if negative.[6] Positive findings should be confirmed by using a catheter or aspiration specimen unless the clinical presentation is unequivocal. The accuracy of positive findings from a bag specimen in infancy has been estimated at 7.5%,[7] whereas that of the midstream specimen varies with age: 42% at younger than 18 months and 71% from ages 3 to 12 years.[8] Specimens should be either analyzed and plated immediately or placed on ice to minimize bacterial multiplication before testing.

The accepted standard for diagnosis of UTI remains the quantitative urine culture. Based on studies of symptomatic women using early morning–voided specimens, the accepted criterion for diagnosis is more than 10^5 colony-forming units per milliliter of a single bacterial species.[9] The accuracy of such a positive finding on culture was estimated at 80% (single specimen) and 96% (confirmed by second culture). Table 54-2 outlines the probability of infection as a function of colony count and method of collection that we use in children.[10] One must avoid applying these criteria too strictly. The colony count varies as a function of hydration (dilution) and urinary frequency (bacterial multiplication time). One study of six untreated children with proven bacteriuria found colony counts to vary from 10^3 to 10^8 over a 24-hour period.[11]

Although clearly most accurate, urine culture results cannot provide an immediate diagnosis, and as a result, initial treatment is generally guided by urinalysis. Microscopic evaluation of a urine specimen should be done immediately on collection. This practice minimizes misleading ex vivo bacterial multiplication and deterioration of cellular elements. The identification of bacteria in an unspun urine specimen is very suggestive of significant bacteriuria.[11] Pyuria (>10 leukocytes/mm^3) is suggestive[12] but also may be seen in such instances as vaginitis, dehydration, calculi, trauma, chemical irritation, gastroenteritis, and viral immunization. Urinary Gram stain was found to be reliable in detecting UTI in young infants.[13]

A popular and indirect measurement of bacteriuria uses nitrite and leukocyte esterase analysis. Nitrate, normally present in urine, is converted to nitrite in the presence of bacteria. A positive colorimetric reaction between nitrite, sulfanilic acid, and α-naphthylamine is thus indicative of bacteria, with a specificity and a positive predictive value approaching 100%.[14] The nitrate-to-nitrite reaction requires a relatively long incubation period. Thus urinary frequency and hydration may produce a false-negative result. Inadequate dietary nitrate and infection caused by

TABLE 54-1

PRESENTING SYMPTOMS IN 200 CHILDREN WITH URINARY TRACT INFECTION AS A FUNCTION OF AGE

Symptom	0–1 Mo	1–24 Mo	2–5 Yr	5–12 Yr
Failure to thrive, poor feeding	53%	36%	7%	0
Jaundice	44%	0	0	0
Screaming, irritability	0	13%	7%	0
Foul-smelling, cloudy urine	0	9%	13%	0
Diarrhea	18%	16%	0	0
Vomiting	24%	29%	16%	3%
Fever	11%	38%	57%	50%
Convulsions	2%	7%	9%	5%
Hematuria	0	7%	16%	6%
Frequency, dysuria	0	4%	34%	41%
Enuresis	0	0	27%	29%
Abdominal pain	0	0	23%	44%
Loin pain	0	0	0	12%
Male-to-female ratio	1:2	1:13	1:10	1:10

From Smellie JM, Hodson CJ, Edwards D, et al: Clinical and radiological features of urinary tract infection in childhood. Br Med J 2:1222, 1964; Bickerton MW, Duckett JW: Urinary tract infections in pediatric patients. AUA Update Service, Lesson 26. Vol 4:4, 1985.

nitrite-negative organisms also may cause false-negative reactions. False-positive reactions are uncommon.[15] The combination of nitrite and leukocyte esterase is more sensitive and specific than is either by itself.[16] Overall, the combination of dipstick analysis and microscopic examination for bacteria has a sensitivity of and a negative predictive value approaching 100%.[14]

Classification

Classification of UTIs helps to determine the need for hospital admission and parenteral antibiotic therapy, as opposed to outpatient oral antibiotic therapy. An attempt is made to distinguish between upper tract (pyelonephritis) and lower tract infections. Fever, flank pain or tenderness,

and leukocytosis suggest pyelonephritis and require parenteral antibiotics to minimize the risk of renal injury. Additional findings supporting parenteral antibiotic therapy include age (younger than 3 months), unusual pathogens, or significant urinary anomalies. After the initial stabilization, we often complete the course of parenteral antibiotics on an outpatient basis, by using our home-based nursing service.

Laboratory studies designed to distinguish lower-tract from upper-tract UTIs include antibody-coated bacteria assay, β_2-microglobulin excretion, antibodies to Tamm-Horsfall protein, and urinary lactic dehydrogenase assay.[17] These tests, in our opinion, are not sufficiently reliable for routine clinical use. Direct culture by ureteral catheterization or percutaneous puncture is reliable, although cumbersome, and represents excellent options in complicated clinical problems. We have found the most usable study for localizing infection to the kidney to be an isotope image during presentation of the patient with infection (Fig. 54-1).

Another important consideration regarding classification is the distinction between reinfection and relapse. Reinfection with a new organism is overwhelmingly common. Relapse with the same organism, although less common, is very important, as it usually implies either an ineffective therapy or a structural abnormality, such as stone or obstruction.

TABLE 54-2

CRITERIA FOR DIAGNOSIS OF URINARY TRACT INFECTIONS

Method of Collection	Colony Count (Pure Culture)	Probability of Infection
Suprapubic aspiration	Gram-negative bacilli: any number	>99%
	Gram-positive cocci: >a few thousand	>99%
Catheterization	>10^5	95%
	10^4–10^5	Likely
	10^3–10^4	Suggestive
	<10^3	Unlikely
Clean voided (male)	>10^5	Likely
Clean voided (female)	3 specimens >10^5	95%
	2 specimens >10^5	90%
	1 specimen >10^5	80%

Modified from Hellerstein S: Recurrent urinary tract infection in children. Pediatr Infect Dis 1:275, 1982.

Epidemiology

Figure 54-2 outlines the age- and sex-related incidence of UTI. At all ages, with the exception of the neonatal period, the incidence of UTI is greater in the female than in the male subject. In both male and female subjects, the incidence increases with advanced age. Although the boy has one early peak in the newborn period, the girl has two peaks, one at 3 to 6 years, and the other at the onset of sexual activity. The actual incidence of infection as a

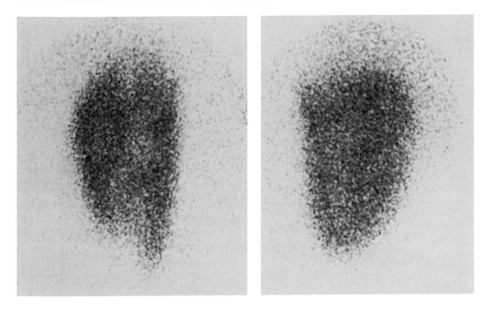

FIGURE 54-1. Technetium-99m dimercaptosuccinic acid (DMSA) scan. The magnified view of the left kidney, seen by using a pinhole collimator, demonstrates defects in both poles that extend deep into the renal parenchyma, suggestive of acute pyelonephritis. The right kidney has an upper pole defect that may represent either acute or chronic pyelonephritis. (Courtesy of Michael J. Gelfand, MD.)

function of age and sex is difficult to determine from the literature. Table 54-3 summarizes available data.[10]

Pathophysiology

Host Factors

The remarkable resilience of the urinary tract to bacterial infection was demonstrated in 1961.[18] Retrograde inoculation of more than 10^8 bacteria in the bladder of healthy volunteers did not result in clinical infection. The establishment of clinical infection and its consequent injury to the urinary tract results from a complex interplay between host resistance and bacterial virulence. As a general rule, UTI-causing organisms originate from the feces of their host. Conceptually, four levels of defense are identifiable: periurethral, bladder, ureterovesical

junction, and renal papillae.[3] These concepts are illustrated in Figure 54-3.

Bacteria generally possess an ability to adhere to vaginal mucosal cells to establish infection readily.[19] The resultant periurethral colonization then allows replication and migration, which ultimately lead to transurethral invasion to the bladder. Healthy girls have low bacterial colonizations of the periurethral region. UTI-prone girls experience more heavy colonization, especially before a new episode of UTI. Further, the cultivated organism from the introital region belongs to the same strain as that from the urine during the UTI that ensues. Periurethral bacterial colonization is correspondingly low in UTI patients after cessation of recurrent UTIs.[20] A similar mechanism may apply to bacterial adherence in the prepuce of male patients.[21] This may explain why 92% of male infants younger than 6 months with urinary tract infection are uncircumcised.[22]

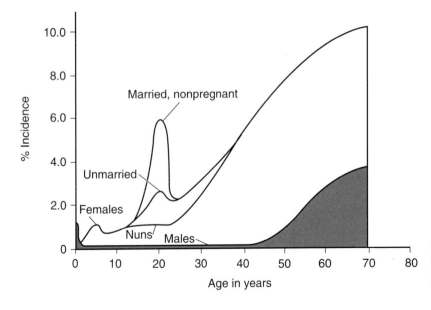

FIGURE 54-2. The age and sex distribution of urinary tract infection incidence. (From Devine CJ, Stecker JF: Urology in Practice. Boston, Little, Brown, 1978, p 444.)

TABLE 54-3

INCIDENCE OF URINARY TRACT INFECTION AS A FUNCTION OF AGE, SEX, AND PRESENCE OF SYMPTOMS

Age	Symptomatic		Asymptomatic	
	Male	Female	Male	Female
Newborn	0.15%		1–1.4%*	
Preschool			0.2%	0.8%
	0.7%	2.8%		
School age			0.03%	1–2%

*2.4% to 3.4% in premature infants.
Data compiled from multiple sources by Hellerstein S: Recurrent urinary tract infections in children. Pediatr Infect Dis 1:271, 1982.

A number of bladder defense mechanisms help maintain sterile urine. The most critical is the act of regular and complete voiding. The healthy bladder is capable of eliminating 99% of instilled bacteria and leaves a small residual urine that minimizes the inoculum at the onset of the following cycle.[23] High intravesical pressure dynamics also may potentiate infection in children. In the absence of an elevated residual urine, uninhibited bladder contractions are associated with a high risk of recurrence of UTI, which is lessened by anticholinergic therapy.[24] Abnormal voiding habits as well as constipation can affect the development of UTI as well.[25] The acid pH of urine, as well as its osmolality, further discourages

bacterial growth.[26] The uroepithelial cells of healthy individuals suppress bacterial growth and are capable of killing bacteria. The uroepithelial cells secrete a mucopolysaccharide substance that, on coating the surface of the uroepithelium, provides an additional barrier to uroepithelial adherence.[23] Glycosaminoglycans are continuously shed and thus function to entrap and eliminate bacteria.

Patients with asymptomatic bacteriuria do not demonstrate all these features. Patients with recurrent UTIs, after successful antireflux surgery, have defective uroepithelial defense, in contrast to those who remain sterile after reflux surgery.[27]

Abnormalities of the ureterovesical junction may allow reflux, which potentiates but is not always necessary for upper tract invasion. The anatomy of the renal papillae usually prevents intrarenal reflux (Fig. 54-4). The papillary ducts commonly open onto the papillae with slitlike orifices that occlude with elevated intracalyceal pressure, preventing intrarenal reflux. The more circular duct orifices of compound papillae fail to accomplish this goal, allowing intrarenal reflux. The facts that compound papillae tend to occur in the upper and lower calyces and that intrarenal reflux in very young children may occur at a relatively low pressure may explain the observed polar distribution of scarring and predilection to scarring noted in these children.[3] Structural abnormalities that potentiate infection include phimosis, obstructive uropathy at any level, vesicoureteral reflux, diverticula, urinary calculi or foreign bodies, and renal papillary structure.

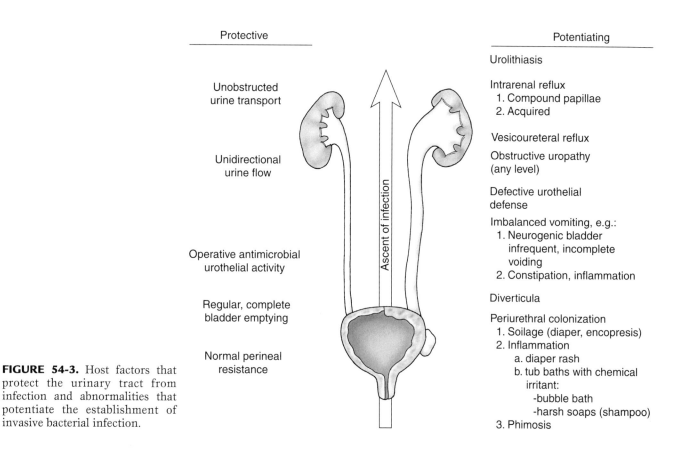

Protective		Potentiating
		Urolithiasis
Unobstructed urine transport		Intrarenal reflux 1. Compound papillae 2. Acquired
	Ascent of infection	Vesicoureteral reflux
Unidirectional urine flow		Obstructive uropathy (any level)
		Defective urothelial defense
		Imbalanced vomiting, e.g.: 1. Neurogenic bladder infrequent, incomplete voiding 2. Constipation, inflammation
Operative antimicrobial urothelial activity		Diverticula

Regular, complete bladder emptying		Periurethral colonization
		1. Soilage (diaper, encopresis)
		2. Inflammation
		  a. diaper rash
		  b. tub baths with chemical irritant:
		    -bubble bath
		    -harsh soaps (shampoo)

Normal perineal resistance		3. Phimosis

FIGURE 54-3. Host factors that protect the urinary tract from infection and abnormalities that potentiate the establishment of invasive bacterial infection.

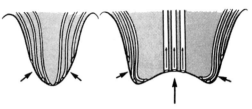

FIGURE 54-4. The normal oblique insertion of the collecting ducts onto the surface of simple papillae prevent intrarenal reflux (*left*). Collecting duct insertion onto the surface of compound papillae may allow intrarenal reflux. (From Ransley PG: Intrarenal reflux: Anatomic, dynamic and radiological studies. Urol Res 5:61, 1977.)

Bacterial Factors

Several bacterial factors may potentiate UTI and are outlined in Table 54-4.[3,27] O antigens are lipopolysaccharides that are part of the cell wall. They are thought to be responsible for many of the systemic symptoms associated with infection. Of the more than 150 strains of *Escherichia coli* identified by O antigens, nine are responsible for the majority of UTIs.

K antigens also are polysaccharides, and their presence on gram-negative bacterial capsules is considered to be an important virulence factor. They are thought to protect against phagocytosis, to inhibit the induction of a specific immune response, and to facilitate bacterial adhesion. Bacterial strains causing UTI exhibit considerably more K antigen than do those isolated from the feces. Urease, a virulence factor especially prominent with *Proteus* species, allows the breakdown of urea to ammonium. This process alkalinizes the urine and facilitates stone formation. Such bacteria are generally incorporated into the stone structure, making eradication extremely difficult. Mannose-resistant pili are important adherence factors.

TABLE 54-4
BACTERIAL FACTORS POTENTIATING INFECTION

O antigens (lipopolysaccharides)
 Primarily O_1, O_2, O_4, O_6, O_7, O_{11}, O_{18}, O_{35}, O_{75}
 Responsible for systemic reactions (e.g., fever, shock)
K antigens
 Primarily K_1, K_5
 Adhesive properties
 Low immunogenicity
H antigens (flagella)
 Bacterial locomotion
 Chemotaxis
Hemolysins (bacterial enzymes)
 Tissue damage
 Facilitates bacterial growth
Urease
 Alkalinizes urine
 Facilitates stone formation
P fimbriae—adherence
 Mannose sensitive (MS)
 Mannose resistant (MR)

They promote adherence to uroepithelial cells as well as to renal epithelial cells. This factor appears to counter the normal cleansing action of urine flow and allows tissue invasion and bacterial proliferation. That these factors truly are associated with virulence is shown in Figure 54-5.

Increasingly invasive urinary infections are associated with bacteria with a high incidence of virulence factors. Figure 54-6 demonstrates the pathophysiologic changes of renal injury that may occur in the absence of significant host factors. Colonization of the feces with a virulent organism allows periurethral colonization and ultimately bladder entry. Uroepithelial adherence promotes bacterial proliferation and tissue invasion. Distortion of the ureterovesical junction and altered peristalsis allow entry into the upper tracts. Resultant distortion of the renal pyramids permits renal parenchymal invasion, which results in irreversible renal injury. This series of events is facilitated by the presence of one or more host factors (see Fig. 54-3).

Investigation

Although many patients with UTI have no serious illness, the pediatric surgeon must be cognizant of several important risks. Urinary abnormalities can be found in approximately 50% of children up to age 12 years who have UTIs. Vesicoureteral reflux (VUR) is found in up to 35%, and obstructive lesions, in 8%. Nonobstructive, nonrefluxing lesions are found in 7%.[28]

Although renal scars develop in about 13% of girls and 5% of boys with unspecified infection,[29] they develop in up to 43% of kidneys involved in acute pyelonephritis.[30] Pyelonephritic scarring is responsible for 11% of cases of childhood hypertension[31] and a

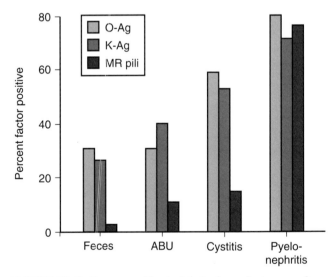

FIGURE 54-5. Presence of bacterial virulence factors as a function of the clinical setting. More-invasive infections are associated with a high incidence of virulence factors, implicating these factors in pathogenesis. (MR, mannose resistant; Ag, antigen; ABU, asymptomatic bacteriuria.) (From Mannhardt W, Schofer O, Schulte-Wisserman H: Pathogenic factors in recurrent urinary tract infection and renal scar formation in children. Eur J Pediatr 145:330, 1986.)

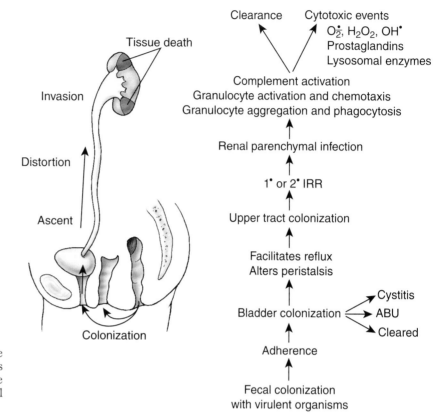

FIGURE 54-6. The pathogenesis of destructive infection. The process is facilitated by, but does not require, defects in the host protective factors outlined in Fig. 54-3. IRR, intrarenal reflux; ABU, asymptomatic bacteriuria.

majority of cases of severe hypertension.[32] Of patients with segmental renal scars, hypertension develops in 20%.[27] Although hypertension is most common with bilateral scarring, it also is seen with unilateral scarring.[33] Pyelonephritic scarring also is an important cause of end-stage renal failure in childhood and may require specific pretransplantation treatment, especially if associated with reflux.[34] Additionally, approximately 50% of patients will have recurrent UTIs.[27]

Consequently, infants[35] and older children of either gender should be investigated at the time of the initial infection.[36] Although controversy does persist, we investigate children with UTI with initial screening ultrasonography (US) and cyclic voiding cystography.[37] Boys require contrast voiding cystourethrography (VCUG), and girls are adequately evaluated with isotope VCUG. This allows a lower radiation exposure to the ovaries.[38] The exception is the infant girl or the girl with suspected neurogenic bladder, ectopic ureter, or ureterocele by US. In this case, a contrast VCUG is obtained.

Treatment

The treatment of an acute UTI is dependent on clinical presentation. Patients with pyelonephritis should be treated immediately and aggressively. Prompt, effective treatment is the most important factor in preventing permanent renal injury.[39] We prefer to initiate therapy with intravenous ampicillin and aminoglycoside after

obtaining a reliable urine culture. Further therapy is dictated by culture and sensitivity findings. Patients may require admission to the hospital initially. Once afebrile for 24 to 48 hours, patients with otherwise uncomplicated infections with sensitive organisms may complete a 7- to 14-day course with oral antibiotics.[40] Patients with resistant organisms or those with obstructions may finish the course with nursing-supervised home administration of intravenous (IV) antibiotics. Patients with obstruction or abscess who do not become afebrile undergo drainage percutaneously or, rarely, operatively.

Short treatment courses appear to be insufficient for treatment of childhood UTIs[41]; therefore we prefer a 7- to 10-day course dictated by culture and sensitivity results.[42] Retention by the patient due to a fear of voiding or to dysuria may be managed with phenazopyridine (Pyridium) and hydration and allowing the child to void while sitting in a tub of warm water.

Patients who have recurrent UTIs or those who are managed nonoperatively for VUR require long-term suppressive antibiotics. The urothelial injury from recurrent UTIs takes several months to recover fully. As a result, irritative voiding symptoms, such as dysuria, incontinence, and frequency, may persist despite the finding of sterile urine. A propensity for recurrent UTI may also persist. Such patients generally require a minimum of 4 to 6 months of antibiotic suppression therapy to break the cycle. Table 54-5 outlines the characteristics of the three drugs we most commonly use for suppression.

TABLE 54-5				
CHARACTERISTICS OF COMMONLY USED UROSUPPRESSIVE ANTIBIOTICS				
Drug	Therapeutic Dose	Suppressive Dose	How Supplied	Comments
Nitrofurantoin	1–2 mg/kg PO qd	1 mg/kg PO qd	Suspension (5 mg/mL)	Avoid in patients younger than 1 mo
			Capsule (25, 50 mg)	Not effective if CrCl <40 mL/min
				Nausea common with suspension; sprinkling macrocystals may avoid this
Trimethoprim-sulfamethoxazole	4 mg/kg trimethoprim + 20 mg/kg sulfamethoxazole PO bid	2 mg/kg trimethoprim + 10 mg/kg sulfamethoxazole PO qd	Suspension (8 mg trimethoprim + 40 mg sulfamethoxazole per mL) Tablet (80 mg trimethoprim, 400 mg sulfamethoxazole)	Avoid in patients younger than 1 mo Contraindicated with hyperbilirubinemia May cause blood dyscrasias and Stevens-Johnson syndrome
Amoxicillin	10 mg/kg PO tid	10 mg/kg PO qd	Suspension (25, 50 mg/mL) Drops (50 mg/mL)	Good alternative for newborns

VESICOURETERAL REFLUX

Vesicoureteral reflux (VUR) refers to the retrograde passage of urine from the bladder into the ureter. In 1883, reflux was first demonstrated in the experimental animal by Simblinow. In 1893, Pozzi observed reflux in humans, noting retrograde urine flow from a ureteral stump at the time of nephrectomy. In 1898, Young demonstrated that VUR did not occur in normal bladders. Although VUR was first observed in the late 1800s, its clinical importance has been recognized only in the last five decades. Hutch's studies, reported in 1952, demonstrated the pathophysiologic changes of VUR in the paraplegic patient. This report and the observations of Hodson in 1959, regarding the association between VUR, UTI, and pyelonephritic scarring, set the stage for the modern era of reflux management.

Although most commonly diagnosed during the evaluation of the pediatric patient with UTI, VUR also may be diagnosed during evaluation of the patient with hypertension, proteinuria, voiding dysfunction, or chronic renal insufficiency or during the evaluation of a sibling with VUR.

Pathophysiology

Figure 54-7 depicts the various anatomic components of the competent ureterovesical junction (UVJ) as well as the abnormalities most often implicated in the genesis of VUR. The normal UVJ is characterized by an oblique entry of the ureter into the bladder and a length of submucosal ureter, providing a high ratio of tunnel length to ureteral diameter. The anatomic configuration provides a predominantly passive valve mechanism.[43,44] As the bladder fills and the intravesical pressure increases, the resultant bladder wall tension is applied to the roof of the ureteral tunnel. The result is a compression of the ureter, which closes this structure to the retrograde passage of urine. Intermittent increases in bladder pressure,

such as the act of voiding, upright posture, activity, and coughing, are met with an equal and immediate increase in resistance to retrograde urine flow. This effect is supplemented by the active effects of ureterotrigonal muscle contraction and ureteral peristalsis.[44,45]

Marginal tunnels can be made to reflux during infection owing to UVJ distortion, loss of compliance of the valve roof, and intravesical hypertension. Excessively high intravesical pressure, as with neurovesical dysfunction (NVD) or bladder outlet obstruction (BOO), also may potentiate reflux, as may a neurogenically or structurally (e.g., diverticulum or ureterocele) weak detrusor floor. Because the submucosal ureter tends to lengthen with age, the ratio of tunnel length to ureteral diameter increases, and the propensity for reflux may disappear.[43,44] Of critical importance is the concept of intrarenal reflux (IRR), which has been demonstrated clinically[46]

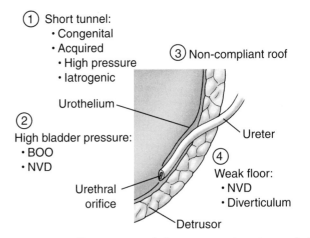

FIGURE 54-7. Components of the competent ureterovesical junction. Those abnormalities most often implicated in the etiology of vesicoureteral reflux are outlined. BOO, bladder outlet obstruction; NVD, neurovesical dysfunction.

and experimentally.[47] The usually oblique entry of the papillary ducts onto the surface of simple papillae inhibits IRR. In contrast, the papillary duct entrance onto compound papillae facilitates IRR (see Fig. 54-4). The critical pressure for IRR is considered to be about 35 mm Hg in compound papillae.[47,48] Experimentally, this same pressure may cause scar formation in the absence of infection.[47,49,50] When occurring intravesically, this pressure has been associated with an increased risk of renal deterioration. Higher pressure is thought to be necessary to induce IRR in simple papillae.

The combination of infection and IRR is particularly devastating. Focal scarring appears to be explained by the different susceptibility of renal papillae to IRR. The polar distribution of compound papillae corresponds closely to the predominant occurrence of renal scarring in the upper and lower poles of the kidney.

Classification

Many attempts at classification have been advanced. Reflux has been described as low pressure (occurring during the filling phase of the VCUG) or high pressure (occurring only during voiding). Reflux due to a congenitally deficient UVJ is referred to as *primary reflux,* whereas that due to a bladder outlet obstruction and neurogenic bladder is referred to as *secondary reflux.* Further classification includes simple reflux and complex reflux. Complex reflux would include the refluxing megaureter, the refluxing duplicated ureter, the refluxing ureter associated with a diverticulum or ureterocele, and the occasional refluxing ureter associated with ipsilateral ureteropelvic or ureterovesical obstruction. The most clinically pertinent classification systems, however, have attempted to quantitate the degree of reflux. VUR now is graded according to the international classification system diagramed in Figure 54-8.[51] This classification system is based not only on the proximal extent of retrograde urine flow and ureteral and pelvic dilatation but also on the resultant anatomy of the calyceal fornices.

Grade I VUR refers to the visualization of a nondilated ureter only, whereas grade II VUR refers to visualization of a nondilated renal pelvis and calyceal system in addition to the ureter. Grade III reflux involves mild to moderate dilatation or ureteral tortuosity with mild to moderate dilatation of the renal pelvis and calyces. The fornices, however, remain sharp or only minimally blunted. Once the forniceal angle is completely blunted, grade IV reflux has developed. Papillary impressions in the majority of calyces can still be appreciated. Loss of the papillary impressions along with increased dilatation and tortuosity is referred to as grade V reflux.

Epidemiology

The incidence of VUR in otherwise normal children has been estimated to be approximately 1%.[52] Also apparent from these data is the fact that the incidence of VUR in control subjects also is small in neonates and infants.

A much higher incidence of VUR, between 30% and 40%, is reported in patients undergoing evaluation

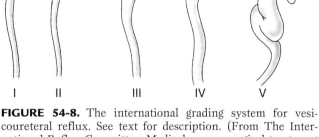

Grade of reflux

I   II   III   IV   V

FIGURE 54-8. The international grading system for vesicoureteral reflux. See text for description. (From The International Reflux Committee: Medical versus surgical treatment of primary vesicoureteral reflux. Pediatrics 67:396, 1987.)

for UTI.[53-55] It is important to note that the incidence increases with decreasing age.[56] Thus the infant who is most vulnerable to the combination of UTI and VUR is precisely the pediatric patient in whom this combination is most likely to occur.

Although female patients account for the majority of reflux patients, a few important characteristics of male patients with VUR require consideration. Although male patients account for approximately 14% of patients with VUR,[57] an increased incidence of VUR (30%) is found in those male patients first seen with UTI.[54] Boys with VUR tend to be seen initially at a relatively young age (25% younger than 3 months), and younger children tend to have the most severe degrees of reflux.[57]

Multiple studies documented a significant risk of VUR in family members of patients with reflux. The reported risk of sibling reflux ranges from 27% to 34%,[58-60] whereas as many as 66% of offspring of women with reflux also have VUR.[61] As a result of these studies, it has been suggested that siblings, especially those younger than 2 years, undergo screening investigation. A particularly important subset of patients with reflux includes those who have secondary reflux. Most have NVD or BOO as the primary disease. Many patients, however, have reflux not because of increased bladder pressure alone but rather because UVJ deficiency appears to be part of the spectrum of congenital deformity. Examples include imperforate anus,[62] ureterocele,[63] and bladder exstrophy. Although a significant incidence of NVD exists in patients with imperforate anus, this is not a prerequisite to VUR.[64] The diagnosis of VUR in imperforate anus thus assumes a critical importance to the pediatric surgeon. Not only may the association of NVD potentiate increased severity of reflux and the development of infection, but the presence of a rectourethral or rectovesical fistula also provides the opportunity for severe urinary contamination. Consequently, we believe that the patient with a rectovesical or rectourethral fistula should be managed with a completely diverting colostomy. Although many patients with posterior urethral valves (PUVs) have reflux due to or exacerbated by high intravesical pressure, as demonstrated by VUR resolution after valve ablation or vesicostomy, the incidence of VUR in PUV patients is only approximately 50%. Many have congenitally abnormal ureteral insertions.[65]

In addition to these structural associations, important functional associations exist, including florid NVD, as seen in myelodysplasia,66 and a variety of more subtle voiding disturbances.[67-69] A particularly important subset of VUR patients are those who have uninhibited detrusor contractions (UDCs). Three important components of maturation are operative in successful toilet training. Growth in bladder volume and development of volitional control over the striated muscle sphincter as well as control over bladder smooth muscle are required for maturation of the infantile bladder, which empties as a simple spinal reflex. Many children with reflux and recurrent UTI have UDCs. Such involuntary or uninhibited bladder contractions are not caused by neurologic disease. Intense voluntary constriction of the striated sphincter occurs in an attempt to ensure continence and results in excessively high intravesical pressures. Pressures often exceeding 150 cm H_2O have been observed with resultant intravesical distortions, such as diverticula, saccules, trabeculations, and abnormal ureteral orifices.[70] Reflux occurred in almost half of the children studied with UDC and UTI. Abnormal ureteral orifices were seen in 30% of children without reflux.

Consequently, all patients with VUR must be screened for frequency, urgency, and incontinence, which suggest UDCs. Vincent's curtsy, a squatting maneuver spontaneously used to prevent incontinence, is particularly suggestive.[69] That these UDCs may cause reflux is suggested by an enhanced resolution of reflux with anticholinergic drug therapy. Equally important is the potential for UDCs to cause a false-negative cystogram. During the performance of VCUG, a child is generally encouraged to void when urgency to do so occurs. In the presence of UDCs, voiding may occur prematurely, and reflux, which might otherwise occur under conditions of volitional detrusor-sphincter dys-synergia, may be masked.

Diagnostic Evaluation

The diagnosis of VUR is accomplished by cyclic VCUG, with either contrast medium or isotope.[37,71] Great care is taken to avoid technical factors that may themselves produce or enhance reflux. Body-temperature contrast material, which is not excessively concentrated, is instilled into the bladder through a small catheter by gravity flow of modest pressure in a nonanesthetized child.

Imaging of the upper tracts (kidneys and ureters) is extremely important and may be accomplished by US, isotope renography, or rarely, intravenous urography (IVU). All may detect scarring, but isotope renography is particularly sensitive in our experience. US and IVU are helpful in quantitating renal growth or atrophy. Additionally, renal pelvic or ureteral folds or striations on IVU are suggestive of VUR, as is hydroureter on US, which diminishes with bladder drainage.

Cystoscopy is useful in some patients. The appearance of the ureteral orifice, tunnel length, and trabeculation or inflammation may all help determine management. Trabeculation is suggestive of NVD or BOO, which must be treated before reimplantation. Acute urothelial inflammation should be resolved before reimplantation. Patients with frequency, urgency, incontinence, and Vincent's curtsy should be considered strongly for urodynamic studies. The presence of UDCs or detrusor-sphincter dys-synergia should be resolved before consideration is given to antireflux surgery.

Natural History

The natural history of VUR is extremely variable, from spontaneous resolution to clinically silent scar formation to hypertension and end-stage renal failure. Numerous factors may contribute to the potential for resolution, including the patient's age, the grade of reflux, the appearance of the ureteral orifice, the length of the ureteral submucosal tunnel, and the intravesical dynamics. The American Urological Association Pediatric Vesicoureteral Reflux Guidelines Panel analyzed 26 reports, comprising 1987 patients with conservative follow-up, to estimate the probability of reflux resolution (Fig. 54-9).[72] In general, a lower reflux grade correlated with a better chance of spontaneous resolution.

Younger children are thought to have better prognoses for resolution of reflux. This occurrence may be due to a heightened degree of trigonal growth, but the diminishing prominence of UDCs with age also is likely. Spontaneous resolution is relatively independent of grade in secondary reflux, implicating management of primary bladder dysfunction as the primary prognostic variable (Fig. 54-10).[73]

Renal injury due to VUR may take the form of focal scarring, generalized scarring with atrophy, and failure of renal growth.[74] As a result, kidneys drained by refluxing ureters should be observed not only for scarring but also for renal growth.[75] Renal growth is followed by comparisons based on standardized renal growth curves, such as that shown in Figure 54-11.

Reflux-induced renal injury is usually a result of the association of VUR with UTI.[76] It is generally considered that such injury is most likely in children younger than 2 years.[56] It is now clear, however, that the risk of renal injury from VUR extends well beyond this age.[55,76-78] Reflux also appears to be capable of causing renal injury in the absence of UTI, because of pressure effects from NVD and BOO. The ability of high intravesical pressure when associated with VUR to cause renal injury has been confirmed experimentally.[79]

Cases in infants are encountered, however, with significant renal injury in the absence of BOO, NVD, and UTI.[80] The ureteral bud theory states that VUR associated with displacement of the ureteral orifice is associated with anomalies of renal differentiation.[81] Such ureters probably do not arise from the appropriate segment of wolffian duct and consequently make ectopic contact with the nephrogenic cord, resulting in abnormal renal development. Although such a mechanism may be

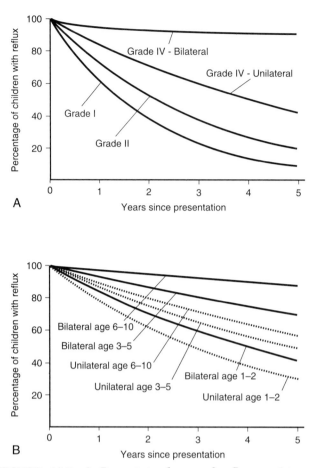

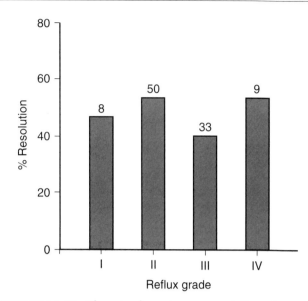

FIGURE 54-10. The rate of spontaneous resolution of secondary vesicoureteral reflux as a function of reflux grade. (From Cohen RA, Roston MG, Belman AB, et al: Renal scarring and vesicoureteral reflux in children with myelodysplasia. J Urol 144:541, 1990.)

FIGURE 54-9. *A,* Percentage chance of reflux persistence, grades I, II, and IV, for 1 to 5 years after presentation *B,* Percentage chance of reflux persistence by age at presentation, grade III, for 1 to 5 years after presentation. (From Elder JS, Peters CA, Arant BS, et al: Report on the Management of Primary Vesicoureteral Reflux in Children. Baltimore, American Urological Association, 1997.)

present in some patients, it is now clear that congenital VUR-associated renal injury in the absence of BOO, NVD, and UTI may occur in the presence of a normally positioned ureteral orifice.[82] This finding implies that pressure effects of in utero VUR may injure the developing kidney.

In a longitudinal study of 923 children, high-pressure bladder dynamics, severity of reflux, and frequency of UTIs were the chief contributing factors in the development of new scars or the worsening of old scars.[78] Progressive renal injury was unlikely to develop in children with low-grade VUR, as compared with those children with grades IV and V reflux (Fig. 54-12). A similar relation is seen in pediatric patients with secondary reflux (Fig. 54-13). When monitoring such children for progression of renal injury as an indicator of success of a therapeutic regimen, one must be cognizant of the fact that radiographic evidence of new renal injury may take up to 8 months to manifest.

Beyond the silent progression of renal scarring lies a spectrum of symptomatic nephropathy, most notably renal parenchymal hypertension and end-stage renal disease (ESRD). The significance and predominance of reflux nephropathy (RN) as a cause of renal parenchymal hypertension has been reviewed.[83] Approximately 30% to 65% of childhood hypertension is associated with RN. RN is an important cause of end-stage renal failure in children and adults.[84–86] Many patients so affected will not have had recognized prior infection or will have the first recognized infection at or near the time of diagnosis of ESRD.[84] Because histologic evidence of chronic pyelonephritis is found, preceding infection is likely, underscoring the silent progressive nature of RN and the need for meticulous long-term follow-up of children with VUR. Many data exist to suggest that glomerular lesions play an important role in the progression of RN. A clear association is found between RN, "heavy" proteinuria, and glomerular lesions that resemble focal segmental glomerulosclerosis.[87] Although the mechanisms of this disease remain uncertain, immunologic injury, macromolecular trapping with mesangial injury, vascular alterations with hypertension, and glomerular hyperfiltration have been implicated. The latter theory of glomerular hyperfiltration is presently favored.

Treatment

Nonoperative management of VUR is successful in the majority of patients (Table 54-6). Such management may be considered in four stages: (1) diagnostic evaluation, (2) avoidance of infection, (3) voiding dysfunction treatment, and (4) surveillance. Diagnostic evaluation was previously reviewed. However, it is pertinent to stress that the exclusion and treatment of voiding dysfunction and BOO is imperative. Patients with problematic uninhibited detrusor contraction should undergo suppression therapy. We use oxybutynin hydrochloride in the majority of these pediatric patients. NVD with retentive characteristics may require

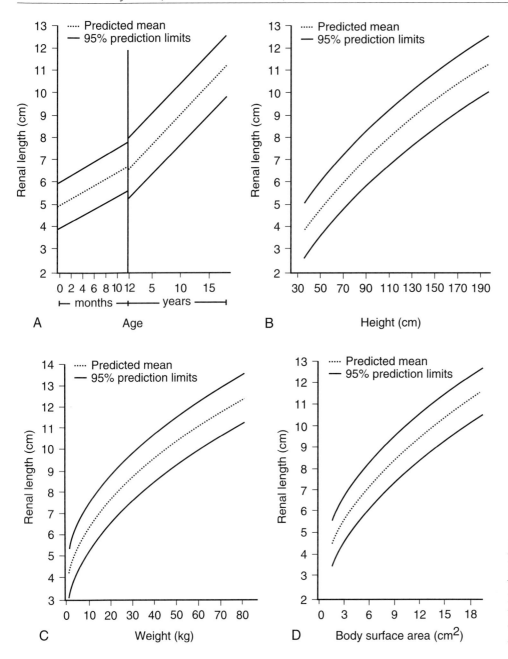

FIGURE 54-11. Maximal renal length as a function of age (*A*), height (*B*), weight (*C*), and body surface area (*D*). (From Han B, Babcock DS: Sonographic measurement and appearance of normal kidneys in children. Am J Roentgenol 145:613, 1985.)

intermittent catheterization. Good hydration, perineal hygiene, and bowel management are crucial and apply to all patients. With the exception of the older boy with low-grade reflux, most children require suppression antibiotics (see Table 54-5). Although long-term suppression is generally well tolerated, the long term implications of chronic suppression remain incompletely investigated.

Once a nonoperative regimen is selected, the patient is committed to long-term, strict surveillance. Renal imaging is performed every 6 to 12 months, depending on the age at diagnosis and the stability of the disease. Attention is directed at both renal growth and focal scarring. VCUG is generally performed yearly. The child's growth, renal function, and blood pressure are monitored. The role of urodynamics was previously outlined. Cystoscopy is rarely

necessary except at the time of antireflux surgical correction, when it is done to exclude urothelial inflammation and to confirm the position and number of ureteral orifices.

Although the actual decision to perform antireflux surgical procedures must be carefully individualized, in our opinion, absolute indications for surgical correction of VUR are (1) progressive renal injury, (2) documented failure of renal growth, (3) breakthrough pyelonephritis, and (4) intolerance or noncompliance with antibiotic suppression. Other possible indications for surgical correction of VUR are grade IV–V reflux, pubertal age, and failure to respond to 4 to 5 years of suppression therapy.

The AUA Pediatric Vesicoureteral Reflux Guidelines Panel published their recommendations for management of VUR in children (Table 54-7).[72] No consensus is noted

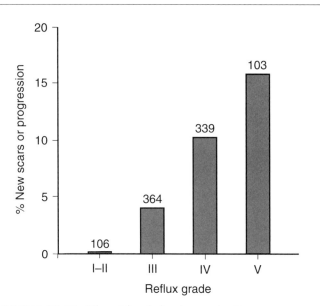

FIGURE 54-12. The risk of development of new scars or progression of old scars increases with increasing grades of vesicoureteral reflux. The number of ureters in each grade is indicated numerically.

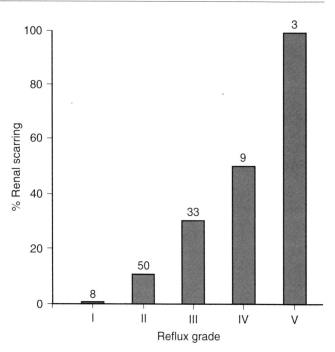

FIGURE 54-13. The prevalence of renal scarring as a function of reflux grade in patients with secondary reflux. Risk of renal scarring increases with increasing grades of reflux. The number of ureters in each grade is indicated numerically.

TABLE 54-6

GENERAL GUIDELINES FOR THE NONOPERATIVE MANAGEMENT OF VESICOURETERAL REFLUX

Treatment
Hydration
Hygiene
  Perineal hygiene
  Avoid harsh soaps during tub baths
    Bubble baths
    Shampoos
Bowel management
  Avoid constipation
  Treat encopresis
Suppressive antibiotics
Observation without antibiotics
Anticholinergics, spasmolytics

Surveillance

Urine culture
  Monthly for 3 mo after last UTI
  Thereafter, every 2 to 3 mo
Renal imaging every 6 to 12 mo
  Renal size (ultrasound, IVU)
  Focal scarring (renal scan, IVU)

Voiding cystourethrography (yearly)
  Radiographic VCUG
    Initial (male, female suspected NVD)
    Follow-up (NVD)
  Isotope VCUG
    Routine surveillance
Record growth yearly (height, weight)
Blood pressure
  Routine (yearly)
  Renal scarring (quarterly)
Renal function tests
  BUN, creatinine (yearly if bilateral RN)
GFR estimated (yearly if azotemic)

$$\frac{\text{height (cm)} \times 0.55}{\text{serum creatinine}} = \text{GFR (mL/min/1.73 m}^2)$$

  Maximum urine osmolality (yearly if bilateral RN)
Cystoscopy
  Done at time of antireflux surgery; otherwise rarely necessary
Urodynamic evaluation
  History of voiding dysfunction

BUN, blood urea nitrogen: GFR, glomerular filtration rate: IVU, intravenous urogram; NVD, neurovesical dysfunction; UTI, urinary tract infection; VCUG, voiding cystourethrogram.

TABLE 54-7

RECOMMENDATIONS FOR TREATMENT OF VESICOURETERAL REFLUX

Clinical Presentation (Age at Presentation)		Treatment Recommendations for Children Without Scarring at Diagnosis Treatment					
		Initial (Antibiotic Prophylaxis or Open Surgical Repair)			Follow-up* (Continued Antibiotic Prophylaxis, Cystography, or Open Surgical Repair)		
VUR Grade Laterality	Age (Yr)	Guideline	Preferred Option	Reasonable Alternative	Guideline	Preferred Option	No Consensus†
I–II Unilateral or bilateral	<1	Antibiotic prophylaxis					Boys and girls
	1–5	Antibiotic prophylaxis					Boys and girls
	6–10	Antibiotic prophylaxis					Boys and girls
III–IV Unilateral or bilateral	<1	Antibiotic prophylaxis			Bilateral: Surgery if persistent	Unilateral: Surgery if persistent	
	1–5	Unilateral: Antibiotic prophylaxis	Bilateral: Antibiotic prophylaxis			Surgery if persistent	
	6–10		Unilateral: Antibiotic prophylaxis Bilateral: Surgery	Bilateral: Antibiotic prophylaxis		Surgery if persistent	
V Unilateral or bilateral	<1		Antibiotic prophylaxis		Surgery if persistent		
	1–5		Bilateral: Surgery Unilateral: Antibiotic prophylaxis	Bilateral: Antibiotic prophylaxis Unilateral: Surgery	Surgery if persistent		
	6–10	Surgery					

Clinical Presentation (Age at Presentation)		Treatment Recommendations for Children With Scarring at Diagnosis Treatment					
		Initial (Antibiotic Prophylaxis or Open Surgical Repair)			Follow-up* (Continued Antibiotic Prophylaxis, Cystography, or Open Surgical Repair)		
VUR Grade Laterality	Age (Yr)	Guideline	Preferred Option	Reasonable Alternative	Guideline	Preferred Option	No Consensus†
I–II Unilateral or bilateral	<1	Antibiotic prophylaxis					Boys and girls
	1–5	Antibiotic prophylaxis					Boys and girls
	6–10	Antibiotic prophylaxis					Boys and girls
III–IV Unilateral	<1	Antibiotic prophylaxis			Girls: Surgery if persistent	Boys: Surgery if persistent	
	1–5	Antibiotic prophylaxis			Girls: Surgery if persistent	Boys: Surgery if persistent	
	6–10		Antibiotic prophylaxis		Surgery if persistent		

TABLE 54-7

RECOMMENDATIONS FOR TREATMENT OF VESICOURETERAL REFLUX—cont'd

Clinical Presentation (Age at Presentation)		Treatment Recommendations for Children With Scarring at Diagnosis Treatment					
		Initial (Antibiotic Prophylaxis or Open Surgical Repair)			Follow-up* (Continued Antibiotic Prophylaxis, Cystography, or Open Surgical Repair)		
VUR Grade Laterality	Age (Yr)	Guideline	Preferred Option	Reasonable Alternative	Guideline	Preferred Option	No Consensus†
III-IV Bilateral	<1	Antibiotic prophylaxis			Surgery if persistent		
	1–5		Antibiotic prophylaxis	Surgery	Surgery if persistent		
	6–10	Surgery					
V Unilateral or bilateral	<1		Antibiotic prophylaxis	Surgery	Surgery if persistent		
	1–5	Bilateral Surgery	Unilateral: Surgery			Surgery if persistent	
	6–10	Surgery					

Recommendations were derived from a survey of preferred treatment options for 36 clinical categories of children with vesicoureteral refllux (VUR). The recommendations are classified as follows:

Guidelines, Treatments selected by eight or nine panel members, given the strongest recommendation language.

Preferred options, Treatments selected by five to seven of nine panel members.

Reasonable alternative, Treatments selected by three to four of nine panel members.

No consensus, Treatments selected by no more than two of nine panel members.

*For patients with persistent uncomplicated reflux after extended treatment with continuous antibiotic therapy.

†No consensus was reached regarding the role of continued antibiotic prophylaxis, cystography, or surgical treatment.

From American Urological Association: Report on the Mangement of Primary Vesicoureteral Reflux in Children. Baltimore, American Urological Association Pediatric Vesicoureteral Reflux Clinical Guideliness Panel, 1997.

on the management of VUR in patients aged 10 years or older, or the length of time that the clinician should wait before recommending surgical correction. The actual decision must be carefully individualized.

The established surgical principles of successful ureteral reimplantation include (1) adequate ureteral exposure and mobilization, (2) meticulous preservation of blood supply, and (3) creation of a valvular mechanism whose submucosal tunnel length-to-ureteral diameter ratio exceeds 4:1. These goals can be attained by a variety of procedures, as diagramed in Figure 54-14.

Important differences exist between these operative procedures. Variables include (1) presence or absence of ureteral anastomosis, (2) need for detrusor closure, (3) transgression of urothelium, and (4) whether the neohiatus is fashioned by an appropriate-sized detrusor incision or closure of detrusor around the ureter.

Performance of a ureteral anastomosis increases the risk of postoperative obstruction, whereas the need for detrusor closure increases the risk of diverticula. Table 54-8 outlines the specific advantages and disadvantages of some representative procedures. Three of the most commonly used procedures for primary VUR are diagramed in Figures 54-15 through 54-17.

In general, excellent results are attainable with the majority of open procedures. The review of 86 reports, including 6472 patients (8563 ureters), found overall surgical success to be 96%. Surgical success was achieved in 99% with grade I, 99.1% with grade II, 98.3% with grade III, 98.5% with grade IV, and 80.7% in grade V.[72]

We prefer the extravesical detrusorrhaphy approach.[88–90] Because the lumen of the bladder is not entered, no postoperative hematuria is found, with minimal bladder spasms and a short hospital stay. Absence of a ureteral anastomosis decreases risk of postoperative obstruction. No ureteral stents, suprapubic tubes, or drains are used. The Foley catheter is removed on the first day after unilateral surgical correction and on the second day after a bilateral procedure. The extravesical approach for bilateral ureteral reimplantation has been questioned because of a reportedly high incidence of postoperative urinary retention.[91] In our experience with a large group of patients, we found acceptable rates of postoperative urinary retention (4%), which is transient and of minimal morbidity.[92] The use of extravesical detrusorrhaphy has been successfully expanded to include megaureter repair,[89] reimplantation of the ureters associated with paraureteral Hutch diverticula,[93] as well as correction of VUR associated with duplicated collecting systems.[94] The four major principles of a successful extravesical detrusorrhaphy are (1) complete encirclement and mobilization of the ureter, (2) distal fixation of the ureter with long-acting absorbable sutures, (3) wide mobilization of the muscular flaps to allow firm approximation of the detrusor over the ureter, and (4) development of sufficient tunnel length.

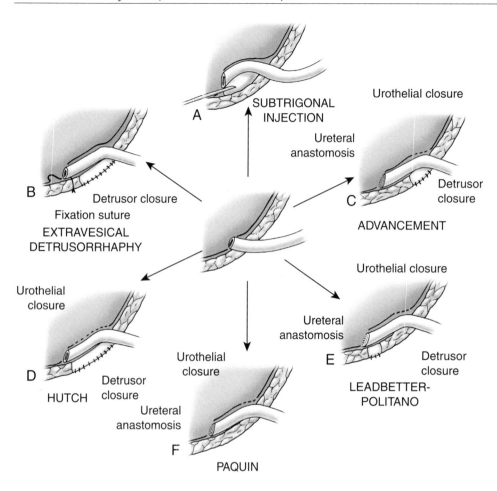

FIGURE 54-14. Conceptual comparison of techniques to correct reflux. A common theme is the achievement of a long length of ureter based on a strong detrusor floor and covered with compressible urothelium.

TABLE 54-8		
SPECIFIC ADVANTAGES AND DISADVANTAGES OF COMMONLY PERFORMED ANTIREFLUX PROCEDURES		
Procedure	Advantages	Disadvantages

Subtrigonal injection	Endoscopic procedure	Material injected
		  Teflon: migration, granuloma formation
		  Collagen: uncertain durability

Extravesical detrusorrhaphy	Bladder never opened No hematuria No ureteral anastomosis Minimal bladder spasms Endoscopically accessible ureteral orifices	

Advancement
  Cohen (transtrigonal)
  Glenn-Anderson
	Avoids complications of neohiatus formation
	  in Leadbetter-Politano reimplantation
		Transtrigonal: difficult to access ureter
		  endoscopically
		Glenn-Anderson: limited length of tunnel
		  achievable

Hutch	No ureteral anastomosis Good alternative with large associated congenital diverticulum	

Leadbetter-Politano	Excellent ureteral tunnel dimensions with
	  endoscopically accessible ureteral orifices
		Risk of ureteral obstruction
		Risk of sigmoid colon injury with left
		  reimplantation

Paquin	Versatility, extremely useful during complex reconstructive procedures	

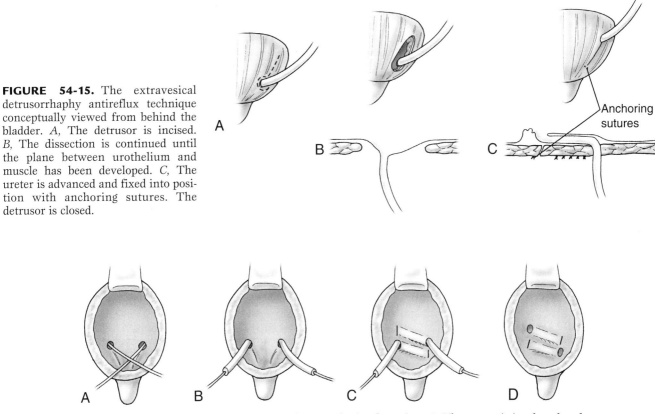

FIGURE 54-15. The extravesical detrusorrhaphy antireflux technique conceptually viewed from behind the bladder. *A,* The detrusor is incised. *B,* The dissection is continued until the plane between urothelium and muscle has been developed. *C,* The ureter is advanced and fixed into position with anchoring sutures. The detrusor is closed.

Anchoring sutures

FIGURE 54-16. The Cohen cross-trigonal ureteral reimplantation. *A,* The ureter is intubated and the mucosa is incised circumferentially around the ureteral orifice. *B,* The ureters are dissected from the muscular attachments and mobilized until free within the retroperitoneum. *C,* Cross-trigonal tunnels are created by scissor dissection. *D,* The ureteral anastomoses are completed.

FIGURE 54-17. The Leadbetter-Politano ureteral reimplantation. *A,* The ureter is intubated. *B,* The ureter is mobilized. The hiatus is dilated, and the retroperitoneal ureter mobilized. Under direct vision, the peritoneum is reflected from the outer surface of the bladder. *C,* The neohiatus is created, and the ureter is internalized into the bladder. The tunnel is created by scissor dissection, and the original hiatus is closed. *D,* The ureteral anastomosis is completed.

Complications of ureteral reimplantation are uncommon.[72,95] The most common complication is de novo contralateral reflux,[96] whereas the most common technical complications are ureteral obstruction, persistent reflux, and diverticula formation. Persistent reflux may be caused by an insufficient tunnel length-to-ureteral diameter ratio. However, the greatest risk of postoperative reflux is related to the high-pressure voiding dynamics due to uninhibited bladder contraction, detrusor sphincterdys-synergia, and urinary retention. Ureteral obstruction may be due to ureteral kinking (at the neohiatus or obliterated umbilical artery), an excessively high-placed neohiatus, construction of a tight neohiatus, twisting, anastomotic stricture, devascularization, or tight tunnel. With attention directed toward the avoidance of technical complications and the selection of a procedure associated with the lowest complication rate, ureteral reimplantation remains a safe and highly successful operation.

Since the initial report in 1984 of successful endoscopic subureteral injection of polytetrafluoroethylene (Teflon) for correction of VUR,[97] this minimally invasive technique has been widely used worldwide with different injectable materials.[98–100] The most promising injectable substance to date is dextranomer/hyaluronic acid copolymer (Deflux).[101–103]

REFERENCES

1. Hoberman A, Chao HP, Keller DM, et al: Prevalence of urinary tract infection in febrile infants. J Pediatr 123:17, 1993.
2. Smellie J, Hodson C, Edwards D, et al: Clinical and radiological features of urinary infection in childhood. Br Med J 2:12222, 1964.
3. Bickerton MW, Duckett JW: Urinary tract infections in pediatric patients: AUA Update Series. 4(26), 1985.
4. Liao JC, Churchill BM: Pediatric urine testing. Pediatr Clin North Am 48:1425–1440:vii-viii.
5. Pollack CV Jr, Pollack ES, Andrew ME: Suprapubic bladder aspiration versus urethral catheterization in ill infants: Success, efficiency and complication rates. Ann Emerg Med 23:225, 1994.
6. Li PS, Ma LC, Wong SN: Is bag urine culture useful in monitoring urinary tract infection in infants? J Paediatr Child Health 38:377–381, 2002.
7. Edelmann CM, Ogw JE, Fine BP, et al: The prevalence of bacteriuria in full-term and premature newborn infants. J Pediatr 82:125, 1973.
8. Aronson AS, Gustafson B, Svenningsen NW: Combined suprapubic aspiration and clean voided urine examination in infants and children. Acta Paediatr Scand 62:396, 1973.
9. Iravani A: Treatment of urinary tract infections in young women. AUA Update Series 12(6), 1993.
10. Hellerstein S: Recurrent urinary tract infections in children. Pediatr Infect Dis 1:271, 1982.
11. Pryles CV, Lustik B: Laboratory diagnosis of urinary tract infection. Pediatr Clin North Am 18:233, 1971.
12. Hoberman A, Wald ER, Reynolds EA, et al: Pyuria and bacteriuria in urine specimens obtained by catheter from young children with fever. J Pediatr 124:513, 1994.
13. Lockhart GR, Lewander WJ, Cimini DM, et al: Use of urinary gram stain for detection of urinary tract infection in infants. Ann Emerg Med 25:31, 1995.
14. Lohr JA, Portilla MG, Geuder TG, et al: Making a presumptive diagnosis of urinary tract infection by using a urinalysis performed in on-site laboratory. J Pediatr 122:22, 1993.
15. Durbin WA, Peters G: Management of urinary tract infections in infants and children. Pediatr Infect Dis 3:564, 1984.
16. Liptak GS, Campbell J, Stewart R, et al: Screening for urinary tract infection in children with neurogenic bladders. Am J Phys Med Rehabil 72:122, 1993.
17. Sheldon CA, Gonzalez R: Differentiation of upper and lower urinary tract infections: How and when? Med Clin North Am 68:2:321–333, 1984.
18. Cox CE, Hinman F: Experiments with induced bacteriuria, vesical emptying and bacterial growth in the mechanism of bladder defense to infection. J Urol 86:739, 1961
19. Fowler J, Stamey T: Studies of introital colonization in women with recurrent urinary infections, VII: The role of bacterial adherence. J Urol 117:472, 1977.
20. Stamey TA, Mihara G: Studies of introital colonization in women with recurrent urinary tract infection, VI: Analysis of segmented leukocytes in vaginal vestibule in relation to enterobacterial colonization. J Urol 116:72, 1976.
21. Roberts JA: Pathogenesis of nonobstructive urinary tract infections in children. J Urol 144:475, 1990.
22. Rushton HG, Majd M: Pyelonephritis in male infants: How important is the foreskin? J Urol 148:733, 1992.
23. Parsons CL, Greenspan C, Mullholland SG: The primary antibacterial defense mechanism of the bladder. Invest Urol 13:72, 1975.
24. Koff SA, Murtagh DS: The uninhibited bladder in children: Effect of treatment on recurrence of urinary infection and on vesicoureteral reflux resolution. J Urol 130:1138, 1983.
25. Wan J, Kaplinsky R, Greenfield S: Toilet habits of children evaluated for urinary tract infection. J Urol 154:797, 1995.
26. Asschler A, Sussman M, Waters WE, et al: Urine as a medium for bacterial growth. Lancet 2:1037, 1966.
27. Mannhardt W, Schofer O, Schulte-Wiserman H: Pathogenic factors in recurrent urinary tract infection and renal scar formation in children. Eur J Pediatr 145:330, 1986.
28. Smellie J, Normand I: Urinary tract infection: Clinical aspects. In Williams JJ (ed): Paediatric Urology. London, Butterworth, 1982, p 95.
29. Hanson L: Prognostic indicators in childhood urinary infection. Kidney Int 21:659, 1982.
30. Rushton HG, Majd M, Jantausch B, et al: Renal scarring following reflux and nonreflux pyelonephritis in children: evaluation with 99m technetium-dimercaptosuccinic acid scintigraphy. J Urol 147:1327, 1992.
31. Wallace D, Rothwell D, Williams D: The long term follow up of surgically treated vesicoureteral reflux. Br J Urol 50:479, 1978.
32. Still J, Cottom D: Severe hypertension in childhood. Arch Dis Child 42:34, 1967.
33. Scott J: Hypertension, reflux and renal scarring. In Johnston JH, (ed): Management of Vesicoureteral Reflux. Baltimore, Williams & Wilkins, 1984, p 60.
34. Sheldon CA, Geary DF, Shely EA, et al: Surgical consideration in childhood end-stage renal disease. Pediatr Clin North Am 34:1187, 1987.
35. Cascio S, Chertin B, Yoneda A, et al: Acute renal damage in infants after first urinary tract infection. Pediatr Nephrol 17:7503–7555, 2002.
36. Chon CH, Lai FC, Shortliffe LM: Pediatric urinary tract infections. Pediatr Clin North Am 48:1441–1459, 2001.
37. Paltiel HJ, Rupich RC, Kiruluta HG: Enhanced detection of vesicoureteral reflux in infants and children with use of cyclic voiding cystourethrography. Radiology 184:753, 1992.
38. Bisset GS III, Strife JL, Dunbar JS: Urography and voiding cystourethrography: findings in girls with urinary tract infection. Am J Roentgenol 148:479, 1987.
39. Hiraoka M, Hashimoto G, Tsuchida S, et al: Early treatment of urinary infection prevents renal damage on cortical scintigraphy. Pediatr Nephrol 18:115–118, 2003.
40. Hellerstein S: Antibiotic treatment for urinary tract infections in pediatric patients. Minerva Pediatr 55:395-406, 2003.
41. Johnson CE, Maslow JN, Fattlar DC, et al: The role of bacterial adhesins in the outcome of childhood urinary tract infections. Am J Dis Child 147:1090, 1993.
42. Keren R, Chan E: A meta-analysis of randomized, controlled trials comparing short- and long-course antibiotic therapy for urinary tract infections in children. Pediatrics 109:E70-0, 2002.
43. King LR, Kazmi SO, Belman AB: Natural history of vesicoureteral reflux: Outcome of a trial of nonoperative therapy. Urol Clin North Am 1:441, 1974.
44. Stephens FD, Lenaghan D: Anatomical basis and dynamics of vesicoureteral reflux. J Urol 87:669, 1962.
45. Eckman H, Jacobsson B, Kock NG, et al: High diuresis: A factor in preventing vesicoureteral reflux. J Urol 95:511, 1966.
46. Rolleston GL, Maling TMJ, Hodson CJ: Intrarenal reflux and the scarred kidney. Arch Dis Child 49:531, 1974.
47. Hodson CJ, Maling TMJ, McManamon PH, et al: Pathogenesis of reflux nephropathy. Br J Radiol Suppl 13:1, 1975.
48. Thomsen H, Talner LB, Higgins CB: Intrarenal backflow during retrograde pyelography with graded intrapelvic pressure: A radiologic study. Invest Radiol 17:593, 1982.
49. Hodson CJ, Twohill SA: The time factor in the development of sterile reflux scarring following high pressure vesicoureteral reflux. Contrib Nephrol 39:358, 1984.
50. Ransley PG, Risdon RA, Godley ML: High pressure sterile vesicoureteral reflux and renal scarring: An experimental study in the pig and minipig. Contrib Nephrol 39:320, 1984.
51. Medical versus surgical treatment of primary vesicoureteral reflux: Report of the International Reflux Study Committee. Pediatrics 67:692, 1981.
52. Arant BS Jr: Vesicoureteric reflux and renal injury. Am J Kidney Dis 17:491, 1991.
53. Bourchier D, Abbott GD, Maling TMJ: Radiological abnormalities in infants with urinary tract infections. Arch Dis Child 59:620, 1984.
54. Sargent MA, Stringer DA: Voiding cystourethrography in children with urinary tract infection: The frequency of vesicoureteric reflux is independent of the specialty of the physician requesting the study. Am J Roentgenol 164:1237, 1995.
55. Benador D, Benador N, Slosman D, et al: Are younger children at highest risk of renal sequelae after pyelonephritis? Lancet 349:17, 1997.

56. Ditchfield M, de C JF, Nolan TM, et al: Risk factors in the development of early renal cortical defects in children with urinary tract infection. AJR Am J Roentgenol 162:1393, 1994.

57. Deckter RM, Roth DR, Gonzales ET: Vesicoureteral reflux in boys. J Urol 40:1089, 1988.

58. Noe HN: The long-term results of prospective sibling reflux screening. J Urol 148:1739, 1992.

59. Wan J, Greenfield SP, Ng M, et al: Sibling reflux: A dual center retrospective study. J Urol 156:677, 1996.

60. Chertin B, Puri P: Familial vesicoureteral reflux. J Urol 169:1804–1808, 2003.

61. Noe HN, Wyatt RJ, Peeden JN Jr, et al: The transmission of vesicoureteral reflux from parent to child. J Urol 148:1869, 1992.

62. McLorie GA, Sheldon CA, Fleisher M, et al: The genitourinary system in patients with imperforate anus. J Pediatr Surg 22:1100, 1987.

63. DeFoor W, Minevich E, Tackett L, et al: Ectopic ureterocele: Clinical application of classification based on renal unit jeopardy. J Urol 169:31092–31094, 2003.

64. Sheldon CA, Cormier M, Crone K, et al: Occult neurovesical dysfunction in children with imperforate anus. J Pediatr Surg 26:49, 1991.

65. Henneberry MD, Stephens FD: Renal hypoplasia and dysplasia in infants with posterior urethral valves. J Urol 123:912, 1980.

66. Agarwal SK, Khoury AE, Abramson RP, et al: Outcome analysis of vesicoureteral reflux in children with myelodysplasia. J Urol 157:980, 1997.

67. Koff SA: Relationship between dysfunctional voiding and reflux. J Urol 148:1703, 1992.

68. Chandra M, Maddix H, McVicar M: Transient urodynamic dysfunction of infancy: Relationship to urinary tract infections and vesicoureteral reflux. J Urol 155:673, 1996.

69. van Gool JD, Hjalmas K, Tamminen-Mobius T, et al: Historical clues to the complex of dysfunctional voiding, urinary tract infection and vesicoureteral reflux: The International Study in Children. J Urol 148:1699, 1992.

70. Koff SA, Lapides J, Plazza DH: Association of urinary tract infections and reflux with uninhibited bladder contractions and voluntary sphincteric obstruction. J Urol 122:373, 1979.

71. Lebowitz RL: The detection and characterization of vesicoureteral reflux in child. J Urol 148:1640, 1992.

72. Elder JS, Peters CA, Arant BS, et al: Report on the Management of Primary Vesicoureteral Reflux in Children. Baltimore, American Urological Association, 1997.

73. Cohen RA, Rushton HG, Belman AB, et al: Renal scarring and vesicoureteral reflux in children with myelodysplasia. J Urol 144:541, 1990.

74. Smellie JM, Normand ICS: Reflux nephropathy in childhood. In Hodson J, Kincaid-Smith P (eds): Reflux Nephropathy. New York, Masson, 1979, p 14.

75. Claesson I, Jacobson B, Olsson T, et al: Assessment of renal parenchymal thickness in normal children. Acta Radiol Diagn 22:305, 1981.

76. Smellie JM, Ransley PG, Normand ICS, et al: Development of new renal scars: A collaborative study. Br Med J 290:1957, 1985.

77. McLorie GA, McKenna PH, Jumper BM, et al: High grade vesicoureteral reflux: Analysis of observational therapy. J Urol 144:537, 1990.

78. Shimada K, Matsui T, Ogino T, et al: Renal growth and progression of reflux nephropathy in children with vesicoureteral reflux. J Urol 140:1097, 1988.

79. Ransley PG, Risdon RA: Reflux and renal scarring. Br J Radiol Suppl 14:1, 1978.

80. Marra G, Barbieri G, Dell'Agnola CA, et al: Congenital renal damage associated with primary vesicoureteral reflux detected prenatally in male infants. J Pediatr 124:726, 1994.

81. Makie GG, Stephens FD: Duplex kidneys: A correlation of renal dysplasia with position of the ureteral orifice. J Urol 114:274, 1975.

82. Najmaldin A, Burge DM, Atwell JD: Reflux nephropathy secondary to intrauterine reflux. J Pediatr Surg 25:387, 1990.

83. Cortez J, Sheldon CA: Focal and diffuse renal parenchymal lesions associated with hypertension: The urologic surgeon's approach to evaluation and management. In Loggie J, (ed): Pediatric and Adolescent Hypertension. Cambridge, Blackwell Scientific, 1991, p 217.

84. Salvatierra O, Kountz SL, Belzer FO: Primary vesicoureteral reflux and end-stage renal disease. JAMA 226:1454, 1973.

85. McEnery PT, Alexander SR, Sullivan K, et al: Renal transplantation in children and adolescents: The 1992 annual report of the North American Pediatric Renal Transplant Cooperative Study. Pediatr Nephrol 7:711, 1993.

86. Avner ED, Chavers B, Sullivan K, et al: Renal transplantation and chronic dialysis in children and adolescents: The 1993 annual report of the North American Pediatric Renal Transplant Cooperative Study. Pediatr Nephrol 9:61, 1995.

87. Hinchliffe SA, Kreczy A, Ciftci AO, et al: Focal and segmental glomerulosclerosis in children with reflux nephropathy. Pediatr Pathol 14:327, 1994.

88. Zaontz MR, Maizels M, Sugar EC, et al: Detrusorrhaphy: Extravesical ureteral advancement to correct vesicoureteral reflux in children. J Urol 138:947, 1987.

89. Wacksman J, Gilbert A, Sheldon CA: Results of the renewed extravesical reimplant for surgical correction of vesicoureteral reflux. J Urol 148:359, 1992.

90. Minevich E, Sheldon CA: Extravesical detrusorrhaphy (ureteroneocystostomy). AUA Update Series 20(34), 2001.

91. Fung LCT, McLorie GA, Jain U, et al: Voiding efficiency after ureteral reimplantation: A comparison of extravesical and intravesical techniques. J Urol 153:1972, 1995.

92. Minevich E, Aronoff D, Wacksman J, et al: Voiding dysfunction after bilateral extravesical detrusorrhaphy. J Urol 160:1004–1006; discussion 1038, 1998.

93. Jayanthi VR, McLorie GA, Khoury AE, et al: Extravesical detrusorrhaphy for refluxing ureters associated with paraureteral diverticula. Urology 45:664–666, 1995.

94. Minevich E, Tackett L, Wacksman J, et al: Extravesical common sheath detrusorrhaphy (ureteroneocystotomy) and reflux in duplicated collecting systems. J Urol 167:288–290, 2002.

95. Gibbons MD, Gonzales ET: Complications of antireflux surgery. Urol Clin North Am 10:489, 1983.

96. Minevich E, Wacksman J, Lewis AG, et al: Incidence of contralateral vesicoureteral reflux following unilateral extravesical detrusorrhaphy (ureteroneocystostomy). J Urol 159:62126–62128, 1998.

97. O'Donnell B, Puri P: Treatment of vesicoureteric reflux by endoscopic injection of Teflon. Br Med J (Clin Res Ed) 289:7–9, 1984.

98. Leonard MP, Canning DA, Peters CA, et al: Endoscopic injection of glutaraldehyde cross-linked bovine dermal collagen for correction of vesicoureteral reflux. J Urol 145:1:115–119, 1991.

99. Smith DP, Kaplan WE, Oyasu R: Evaluation of polydimethylsiloxane as an alternative in the endoscopic treatment of vesicoureteral reflux. J Urol 152:1221–1224, 1994.

100. Diamond DA, Caldamone AA: Endoscopic correction of vesicoureteral reflux in children using autologous chondrocytes: Preliminary results. J Urol 162:1185–1188, 1999.

101. Lackgren G, Wahlin N, Skoldenberg E, et al: Long-term followup of children treated with dextranomer/hyaluronic acid copolymer for vesicoureteral reflux. J Urol 166:1887, 2001.

102. Puri P, Chertin B, Velayudham M, et al: Treatment of vesicoureteral reflux by endoscopic injection of dextranomer/hyaluronic acid copolymer: Preliminary results. J Urol 170:1541–1544, discussion 1544, 2003.

103. Lackgren G, Wahlin N, Skoldenberg E, et al: Endoscopic treatment of vesicoureteral reflux with dextranomer/hyaluronic acid copolymer is effective in either double ureters or a small kidney. J Urol 170:1551–1555; discussion 1555, 2003.

CHAPTER 55

Bladder and Urethra

Patrick C. Cartwright, MD, and Brent W. Snow, MD

ANATOMY AND PHYSIOLOGIC FUNCTION

The lower urinary tract consists of the bladder and urethra, which normally function as a coordinated unit to store and discharge urine from the body. Both structural and functional disorders of the bladder or urethra may be responsible for bleeding, incontinence, infection, discomfort or pain, and for obstruction that can cause upper tract deterioration to the point of compromising renal function. This chapter focuses on the major pathologies and dysfunctional states of the bladder and urethra as a unit and on the management of such problems.

The bladder and upper urethra are composed of bundles of smooth muscle fibers arranged in a reticular lattice, the outermost bundles being more circular and the inner bundles more longitudinal in orientation at the bladder neck.[1] The smooth muscle bundles blend into the striated muscle of the external urethral sphincter, which is derived from the pelvic diaphragm. The bladder is lined by transitional epithelium, which is sensitive to irritants such as bacterial toxins and various urinary crystals. The urethra and trigone are especially sensitive, and the presence of any irritant in these areas can create significant discomfort.

Normal innervation and bladder function are intimately related; proper functioning of the lower urinary tract depends on intact autonomic and somatic nervous innervation. The detrusor muscle of the bladder proper is innervated by both sympathetic and parasympathetic fibers. Storage functions are mediated by the sympathetic component, which arises from spinal levels T10 to L1 and descends through the sympathetic chain to reach the bladder. The chemical mediator of this storage process is norepinephrine, which acts on α-adrenergic receptors in the fundus of the bladder and causes muscle relaxation to aid in low-pressure storage of urine. The same sympathetic stimulus acts on predominantly α-adrenergic receptors of the trigone, bladder neck, and proximal urethra to provide an increase in internal sphincter activity

and further promote continence during the storage process by maintaining outlet resistance.[2,3] The external urinary sphincter, innervated by the pudendal nerve, maintains a progressively increasing tone as the bladder fills. This "guarding" provides an additional continence mechanism during the storage of urine.[4] As the child develops, the external sphincter may be consciously contracted at times of urgency or stress to prevent the unwanted passage of small amounts of urine. Properly coordinated function of the external urinary sphincter relies on an intact sacral reflex arc (afferents, sacral micturition center, pudendal efferents). This should be intact and well developed in normal infants but is variably functional in infants with spinal cord or pelvic lesions.

The sensation of bladder fullness initiates a response in mature human beings that causes them to seek an appropriate location for the discharge of urine. When ready, the parasympathetic nervous system, with acetylcholine as the mediator, causes cholinergic fibers of the detrusor to contract in the proximal urethra, resulting in widening and shortening, eliminating its resistance to outflow. When coupled with relaxation of the volitional external sphincter, the bladder empties by sustained and complete contraction of the detrusor, leaving a residual urine volume in the bladder of less than 5 mL.

Spinal pathways connect the sacral micturition center with three centers in the brainstem, collectively called the *pontine micturition center*.[5] This center functions (1) to inhibit urination and (2) to produce external sphincter relaxation, when sustained detrusor contraction occurs. Above this level are areas of cerebral cortex, which oversee and modulate the autonomic process. It is the mature, integrated function of all these components that produces urinary continence.

Conscious control of the bladder (toilet training) is, in large part, a learned phenomenon. It requires adequate recognition by the brain that micturition would be inconvenient or socially unacceptable in a given situation. As the child grows, the bladder gains capacity, allowing longer intervals between voiding. The approximate bladder volume in ounces may be estimated in a child as age in years plus 2. It also may be calculated by a more precise formula if needed.[6] It has been observed that the young infant voids 20 times per day, which decreases to about 10 times per day by age 3 years.[7] Along with this change, the child also learns to resist the urge to void by voluntary contraction of the external sphincter until the detrusor contraction passes and the bladder once again relaxes. Thus toilet training depends on the development of voluntary detrusor sphincter dyssynergia, which at times persists as a pathologic process.[8] Finally, full bladder control relies on the child developing volitional control over the spinal micturition reflex so that he or she can initiate or inhibit detrusor contractions. Most children have attained day and night continence by age 4 years.

The inappropriate discharge of urine (enuresis) may be in part due to immaturity of the bladder and its nervous system connections. The usual sequence of bladder development is linked to that of the bowel development and is as follows:

1. Control of bowel at night
2. Control of bowel during the day
3. Control of bladder during the day
4. Control of bladder at night

Many lesions interfere with the ideal storage and emptying functions of the bladder. The application of appropriate diagnostic measures can lead to appropriate management decisions, which ultimately lead to continence and to preservation and protection of the upper urinary tract.

CHILDHOOD ENURESIS

Enuresis is the term used for the unintentional loss of urine beyond toilet training. The following definitions are clinically useful:

Nocturnal enuresis: nighttime (more precisely, sleeptime) incontinence
Primary nocturnal enuresis: nighttime incontinence, never been continent at night
Secondary nocturnal enuresis: nighttime incontinence after a significant dry period
Diurnal enuresis: daytime wetting after toilet training
Stress incontinence: urine leakage due to physically stressful activities such as coughing
Urge incontinence: unintentional loss of urine when bladder urgency occurs

The discussion of enuresis is divided into sections on nocturnal and diurnal enuresis, realizing that some children have both. The current recommendation for children with nocturnal enuresis and diurnal enuresis is to focus on diurnal treatments first, followed by nocturnal enuresis treatments.

Nocturnal Enuresis

About 15% to 20% of children at age 5 years continue to have bed-wetting.[9–11] Because so many children still wet

at night before this age, it is considered within the range of normal and not termed nocturnal enuresis. Night wetting, thereafter, resolves at the rate of about 15% each year, and by age 15 years, it has resolved in 99% of children.[12]

Etiology

Children with monosymptomatic nocturnal enuresis are, in general, physically and emotionally similar to their peers. The difference lies in their inability to awaken during sleep when their bladder is full or contracts. The etiology of this disorder is likely complex, and several factors should be considered.

GENETIC. Family history is often strong, with multiple members having had childhood nocturnal enuresis. If both the parents have a history of bed-wetting, 77% of their offspring do. If only one parent had the problem, then 44% of the offspring exhibit the behavior. When neither parent has a history of nocturnal enuresis, then only 15% of their children have the complaint.[13]

PSYCHOLOGICAL. Psychological stress is observed to induce nocturnal enuresis in certain children. Secondary nocturnal enuresis often raises this concern. Common factors are divorce, changing of homes, birth of a new sibling, trouble at school, or just starting school.

DEVELOPMENTAL. As children grow, bladder capacity increases significantly each year at a proportion greater than the urine volume produced.[14,15] Volitional control over bladder and sphincter also may mature at variable rates and may be related to subtle delays in other areas of development (e.g., perceptual abilities, fine-motor skills).[16]

URODYNAMIC. Studies show that enuretic episodes occur when the bladder is full, and they simulate normal awake voiding.[15] Although nocturnal enuretic patients have more nighttime unstable bladder contractions than do nonenuretic patients, the contractions are at low pressure and do not cause leakage.

When observed scientifically, night wetting appears to occur in three fashions: wetting associated with significant restlessness and visceral and somatic activity (deep respirations), wetting with a quick contraction and minimal movement, and wetting with no central nervous system response (parasomnia).

SLEEP DISORDERS. Parents of children with nocturnal enuresis are generally convinced that these children sleep deeply and are difficult to arouse. However, controlled studies consistently find this not to be true. Enuretic patients sleep no more deeply than age-matched controls, wet in all stages of sleep, and show no different awakening patterns. Wetting episodes occur as the bladder fills throughout the night.[17]

ANTIDIURETIC HORMONE. Antidiuretic hormone (ADH) is released from the pituitary in a circadian rhythm so that levels are higher at night and thus diminish urine output. Some children appear to undersecrete ADH at night; thus by not concentrating the urine at night, urine volume may overwhelm the bladder capacity, and bed-wetting results.[18-21]Although some patients follow this pattern, others do not; the altered circadian patterns appear to normalize with maturation.[22]

Evaluation

Children usually are seen by the physician when either the child becomes socially embarrassed or the parents are either "fed up" or worried that other pathology may be present. Screening evaluation should include history, physical examination, and always urinalysis. If these are normal, then no other evaluation is needed, because organic disease rarely causes monosymptomatic nocturnal enuresis. Routine radiographic evaluation or cystoscopy is unwarranted. Children with an associated anomaly or problem such as urinary tract infection (UTI), evidence of sacral anomalies, or complex enuresis patterns often warrant medical imaging.

Treatment

The treating physician should recognize enuresis as a symptom and not a disease. Realizing that more than one cause may be found permits the physician to consider more than one treatment option. Specific treatment is generally discouraged before age 7 years. Certain measures are sensible in all nocturnal enuretic patients: void just before getting into bed, avoid huge fluid loads during the evening hours, and avoid caffeine after 3:00 PM.

ENURETIC ALARMS. Wetting alarms are devices that fit in the underwear of the patients. When the devices are moistened, an electrical contact is made, and the alarm is sounded. This is conditioning therapy, requiring a motivated patient and parents. The alarm is loud and sounds like a doorbell in the middle of the night. The parent may need to arouse the child, take him or her to the bathroom, and reset the alarm; this may occur multiple times each night.

A compilation of 16 published series showed an initial cure rate of 82%.[23] Average length of treatment to achieve dryness varied between 18 nights and 2.5 months. Relapse does occur in 20% to 30% of children treated, but retreatment can be successful.[24] In a 1995 study, 1 year after instituting nocturnal enuresis treatments, wetting alarms were shown to give the best long-term results as compared with other treatments.[25]

IMIPRAMINE. Tricyclic antidepressants have been used for many years to treat bed-wetting. The exact mechanism of action is unknown. Initial success has been reported in the 50% range. Clinical practice reveals that cessation of the treatment induces many relapses, and the longer the initial treatment, the more benefit before the effect wanes. It is suggested that the medication be weaned slowly rather than stopped abruptly.

Side effects include anxiety, insomnia, dry mouth, nausea, and personality changes. An imipramine overdose can cause fatal cardiac arrhythmias and conduction blocks that are untreatable; owing to this, medication safety in the home becomes a significant issue.[26] Some suggest that imipramine may improve response rates to the enuretic alarm.

DESMOPRESSIN. Desmopressin is an analogue of ADH that mimics its urine-concentrating activity without the vasopressor effect.[18] It is currently given as either a nasal spray or orally. The effect of desmopressin is dose dependent, usually requiring 20 to 40 µg/day for success.

Complete dryness rates vary with desmopressin and may be highest in patients with a strong bed-wetting history in the family. In three multicenter trials in the United States, response rates were reported in 24% to 35% of children who had failures associated with other forms of treatment.[27] In a study in which dose titration was watched closely, 70% dryness was reported.[28] Desmopressin may occasionally have side effects, including electrolyte changes, nasal irritation, and headaches.

ANTICHOLINERGICS. Oxybutynin is the most common drug used in this category for enuresis. It is effective when day and nighttime wetting occur in the same patient but has no benefit over placebo when nighttime wetting is the only symptom.[29]

GENERAL APPROACH. Although many parents consider bed wetting a problem, they often do not consider it significant enough to treat, especially when medications are being considered. If therapy is desired, it is often most reasonable to begin with an enuretic alarm. This has the highest response rate, no side effects, and the lowest relapse rate. Combination therapy with imipramine and the alarm may be considered when either alone was unsuccessful. If desmopressin has proved successful in a specific patient, the patient and family may choose to keep it available and use it only on specific nights when dryness is especially desired (e.g., sleepovers, campouts). Some patients do not respond to therapy, and time, reassurance, and a caring approach are all that can be offered.

Diurnal Enuresis

Diurnal enuresis is the undesired loss of urinary control while awake. The patient history is of paramount importance in sorting out the various categories of diurnal enuresis.[30,31] The physical examination and evaluation should always assess for abdominal mass or tenderness, distended bladder, normal structure of genitalia, signs of spina bifida occulta, perineal sensation, sacral reflexes, gait, lower extremity reflexes, and urinalysis. Radiographic evaluation, usually voiding cystourethrogram (VCUG) and renal ultrasonography (US), are necessary in patients with UTI or complex incontinence patterns.

Bladder Instability

Bladder instability is by far the most common diagnosis in children with persistent daytime wetting.[32] These children have usually toilet trained but later have increasing "accidents" associated with urgency. They describe not knowing that the bladder contraction was coming. They dash to the bathroom or try to "hold it in." Boys grab and compress the penis, and girls often cross their legs and dance around or squat with the heel compressed over the perineum (Vincent's curtsy). In our experience, children with hyperactivity disorders or a willful disposition appear prone to this dysfunctional voiding pattern.

By urodynamic studies, these children demonstrate significant unstable (unwanted) contractions during bladder filling that cause leakage before sphincter contraction (or posturing) can control it. Because these unstable contractions or spasms occur frequently during the day, a retentive pattern develops of using the external sphincter to "hold on." When these children do get to the bathroom and try to void, the sphincter relaxes poorly or only intermittently, with resultant stop-and-go voiding, difficulty initiating a urinary stream, straining, and poor emptying. The elevated pressure during voiding and the poor emptying often result in secondary vesicoureteral reflux (VUR) and UTI. Finally, the overactivity of the urinary sphincter may carry over to the function of the anal sphincter, and stool retention and encopresis are commonly associated findings.

Treatment

Treatment rests on managing all aspects of this condition simultaneously. Mild encopresis is treated with dietary changes of fiber or laxatives and mineral oil after initial bowel cleanout. Recurring UTIs are managed with prophylactic antibiotics. Bladder instability is treated with timed voiding at frequent intervals (an alarm watch for the child is helpful) and anticholinergics such as oxybutynin or tolterodine.[33-35]

Biofeedback has gained in popularity for treatment of bladder instability. Electrodes placed on the perineum near the genitourinary diaphragm can be attached to monitors, an audio signal or a computer display so the children can learn to relax their external sphincter voluntarily, resulting in better voiding coordination.[36,37] The process can be long and extensive, is not universally successful, and is not readily available in many locations.

Unfortunately, initial success is often followed by later relapse. If initial treatment is unsuccessful, it may be successful if retried later. Patients older than 8 years for whom treatment fails should be considered for urodynamic testing. Secondary VUR may be present because of elevated bladder pressures and is followed in the usual manner with a high probability for resolution (80%) as bladder function improves.[38] The unstable bladder of childhood is almost always outgrown, and adults generally do not demonstrate this type of wetting problem.

Isolated Frequency Syndrome

A separate, and much less common, group of children have fairly acute onset of urinary frequency. They appear healthy, are normal on examination, and have normal urinalysis and culture. They do not have true urgency or any wetting but feel that they must urinate frequently, sometimes every 5 to 10 minutes. They void a very small amount each time. Most sleep through the night and void a large amount on awakening. The pattern may come and go over weeks or months.

The cause is unclear but may relate to emotional stress in many cases. Careful assessment is crucial, and reassurance to parent and child is paramount. Sometimes, setting an alarm to progressively lengthen voiding intervals with a reward for success is helpful. This condition is benign and self-limited, although it may persist intermittently for months. Anticholinergics have no benefit, and further evaluation is not required.

Infrequent Voider–Lazy Bladder

On the other end of the voiding spectrum are those children who void only once or twice daily and may not go until afternoon after waking in the morning.[39] These children have developed urinary retentive behavior without any bladder instability and have dilated, high-capacity, low-pressure bladders.[40] Some show an aversion to bathrooms or exhibit excessive neatness, whereas many others appear reasonably adjusted. They may be somewhat prone to UTIs and stress incontinence.

Evaluation must demonstrate no neurologic cause and no structural obstruction to emptying. US can demonstrate good emptying if performed before and after voiding. A timed voiding regimen is usually required to get these children to void regularly if problems are occurring. This pattern tends to improve with maturation.

Total Incontinence and Constant Dribbling

Patients who have total incontinence and constant dribbling of urine have a higher probability of urinary tract anomalous pathology and require radiographic and possibly urodynamic evaluation.

Hinman Syndrome

A small number of children demonstrate persistent incontinence, repeated febrile UTIs, reflux, high bladder-storage pressures, and very poor emptying.[41] This appears to be a deeply ingrained "learned" disorder of severe voluntary detrusor-sphincter dyssynergia. In these patients, the urinary tract has the appearance of that in a patient with neurogenic bladder. Hydronephrosis, a trabeculated bladder, reflux, and sometimes progressive loss of renal function (Fig. 55-1) occur.

Aggressive therapy with prophylactic antibiotics, anticholinergics, urodynamic biofeedback training, timed voiding, or intermittent catheterization may be required.[42] Some recalcitrant cases may require bladder diversion or augmentation to avoid renal failure. As with

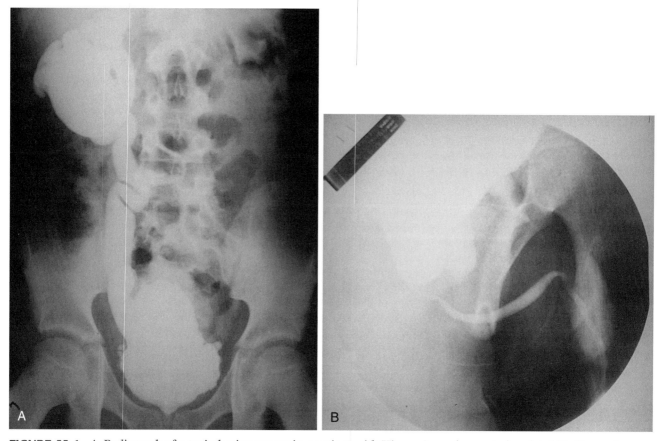

FIGURE 55-1. *A,* Radiograph of a typical urinary tract in a patient with Hinman's syndrome: trabeculated bladder and severe reflux. *B,* Voiding study in the same patient demonstrates dilation of the posterior urethra as a result of chronic contraction of the external sphincter during voiding.

many "functional" disorders, the severity of Hinman syndrome tends to wane with maturation, but progressive deterioration may not permit the surgeon to wait.

Neurogenic Bladder

True neurogenic dysfunction of the bladder in childhood results from acquired or congenital lesions that affect bladder innervation. Acquired lesions may occur from trauma to the brain, spinal cord, or pelvic nerves or as a result of tumor, infection, or vascular lesions affecting these same structures. Congenital lesions include spina bifida and other neural tube defects (most common), degenerative neuromuscular disorders, cerebral palsy, tethered cord, sacral agenesis, imperforate anus, VAC-TERL (*v*ertebral, *a*nal, *c*ardiac, *t*racheal, *e*sophageal, *r*enal, and *l*imb) syndrome, and other causes.[43]

The most practical way to classify neurogenic bladder abnormalities is by a simple functional system: failure to store, failure to empty, or a combination of both.[44] Failure to store urine may be caused by the detrusor muscle itself or by the bladder outlet. Detrusor hyperactivity or poor compliance during bladder filling causes elevated bladder pressures and incontinence on this basis. Inadequate outlet resistance caused by an incompetent bladder neck or urethral sphincter mechanism can be the outlet cause of

failure to store urine even if storage pressures are reasonable. Failure to empty can suggest either a bladder-muscle or bladder-outlet etiology as well. The hypotonic, neurogenic bladder may not generate enough pressure with detrusor contraction to empty. Alternatively, the outlet may exhibit increased resistance secondary to striated or smooth muscle sphincter dyssynergia. This classification helps to base treatment on urodynamic data.

Myelomeningocele

General

The most common cause of neurogenic bladder in childhood is the group of neural tube defects, which ranges from occult spinal dysraphism[45] to myelomeningocele.[46] Myelomeningocele is the most severe and the most common, reported in about 1 in 1000 live births, with notable geographic variations and a declining occurrence over the past decade.[47,48] The etiology is multifactorial, with a clear familial association (2% to 5% sibling risk) and evidence that periconceptual folic acid supplementation (0.4 mg/day) reduces the risk by 60% to 80%.[49] Improved care of the neurosurgical aspects of this lesion since the late 1970s has increased the survival rate of children with this condition; thus continued urologic care is of much importance. Ninety percent of newborns with myelomeningocele have normal upper tracts; however, if no care is administered to the bladder, at least half of these patients show signs of upper tract deterioration or reflux within 5 years.[50] It is therefore critical that early urologic evaluation of children with myelomeningocele be undertaken.[51,52]

Evaluation of the Newborn with Myelomeningocele

Reports exist over the past 5-year period from centers performing fetal closure of myelomeningocele recognized by prenatal US. Unfortunately, little suggests that this has improved lower extremity, bowel, or bladder function for these patients, but the need for ventriculoperitoneal shunting may be reduced by 50%. Further outcomes will be watched with interest.[53,54]

Generally, the newborn with myelomeningocele has had a thorough neurologic assessment, closure of the back defect, and possibly even ventriculoperitoneal shunting before any evaluation of the urinary tract. The level of the bony defect does not predict the functional cord level because lesions may be partial and patchy. Before discharge, renal and bladder US should be performed to evaluate parenchymal quality, the presence of hydronephrosis, and the size and emptying ability of the bladder. About 5% of patients have an abnormality on US, in which case, a VCUG and an evaluation of upper tract function and drainage by renal scan should be performed. If the US is normal, other studies can probably be delayed a few months, although we prefer to proceed with VCUG before hospital discharge, mainly for logistical reasons. About 10% of these patients have reflux. Children are given amoxicillin prophylaxis (15 mg/kg once daily), and serum creatinine is monitored during the initial hospitalization period. Many children experience poor emptying for a few days or weeks after the initial back closure, and postvoid residuals should be measured before discharge from the hospital. Intermittent catheterization is begun if the residual urine is consistently greater than 15 mL. Credé's maneuver should be avoided because it is ineffective in emptying the bladder and magnifies the detrimental effects of high intravesical pressure if reflux is present.

Newborn urodynamic evaluation has since been shown to have prognostic value in determining in which children upper tract dilation and VUR are likely to develop. Children with bladder pressures higher than 40 cm H_2O at the point of urinary leakage and those with detrusor-sphincter dyssynergia are much more likely to show upper tract deterioration or VUR.[2,51] Other factors shown to indicate bladder "hostility" include the presence of reflux, hyperreflexic contractions, and poor detrusor compliance.[52] Therefore early urodynamic evaluation is useful in determining the frequency of follow-up studies and the timing of initiation of bladder therapy programs.

If the radiographic evaluation is normal and no infection is present, the patient can be managed by spontaneous voiding into the diaper, especially if leak-point pressures are low. Follow-up studies are planned with urine culture and renal US at 6 months. If leak-point pressures are high or sphincter dyssynergia is present, VCUG again at 6 months is prudent. US and urine cultures should be repeated yearly if stable, with or without VCUG, depending on the relative risk of the upper tract as determined by urodynamics. If reflux or upper tract deterioration occurs at any time, intervention with clean intermittent catheterization (CIC), anticholinergic therapy, or temporary cutaneous vesicostomy may be warranted.

Childhood Management

Periodic reassessment of the anatomy and function of the urinary tract is imperative because the clinical and urodynamic picture may change with growth and spinal cord retethering.[55] Initiation of a bladder-management program is generally undertaken when worsening reflux, upper tract dilation, or infection occurs. If the urinary tract is stable, such management may be delayed until social continence is desired.

The cornerstone of treatment programs for neurogenic bladder in most children is CIC. Popularized in the early 1970s, CIC has revolutionized the treatment program for these children.[56] The purpose of CIC is to provide periodic low-pressure emptying of the bladder, which can prevent or improve existing deterioration of the upper tracts, including that secondary to reflux.[57,58] In younger children, this task is performed by the caretaker. As children become older and more responsible, they themselves can assume the task. Motivation is important in adhering to a good bladder program. Therefore it is sometimes better to wait until social pressures influence the child's desire for continence before initiating a bladder program, unless it is required for the treatment of upper tract deterioration.

CIC is associated with a high incidence of bacteriuria (when followed with serial culturing), varying greatly in different series.[59,60] Bacteriuria is eventually found in about 60% of cases, with most patients becoming culture positive within 1 year, often with one or two symptomatic episodes per year.[61] In patients with no reflux and with normal intravesical pressure, asymptomatic bacteriuria appears to have little clinical significance. However, in patients with high storage pressures, reflux, or a combination of the two, the potential for upper tract deterioration increases significantly with bacteriuria.[61] Infection with urea-splitting organisms (usually *Proteus* sp.) is of concern, owing to the potential for struvite stone formation.

Pharmacologic therapy for neurogenic bladder is usually coupled with CIC and is aimed at decreasing the pressures in the hypertonic, noncompliant bladder or increasing bladder-outlet resistance to aid in gaining continence. Anticholinergic drugs, such as oxybutynin, propantheline, or tolterodine,[62] are used to reduce bladder storage pressures by blocking hypertonic detrusor activity. Imipramine also may be useful alone or in combination with the anticholinergic agents because it can both relax detrusor and tighten the outlet. Inadequate vesical outlet resistance also may respond to α-adrenergic medications, such as pseudoephedrine. Often, the combination of anticholinergics, β-agonists, and CIC is required to gain adequate continence. Side effects of the anticholinergics may sometimes limit their use. Tolterodine and extended-release oxybutynin are purported to cause fewer side effects than other anticholinergics. Instillation of oxybutynin dissolved in water directly in the bladder can lessen the side effects and still maintain a therapeutic response; the recently developed oxybutynin cutaneous patch may offer an improved therapeutic index to these patients, as well.[63]

Urodynamic assessment helps the clinician to select medications and other modalities for neurogenic bladder and to monitor their effects.[3] This study may be elaborate in certain situations but is more often a simple measurement of the pressure-volume relation of the bladder during filling. It is performed by using a double-lumen catheter in the bladder and usually involves simultaneous assessment of external sphincter function with a perineal electrode patch. Urodynamic assessment can be performed with contrast material and monitored fluoroscopically to add information. Noting parameters such as bladder compliance, hyperreflexic contractions, leak-point pressure, stress leak-point pressure, and sphincter dyssynergia can be extremely valuable in helping to choose among treatment options. Figure 55-2 demonstrates the effect of anticholinergics in shifting the pressure-volume curve to the right and thus permitting the bladder to store more urine at any given pressure. Figure 55-3 shows the effect of α-adrenergic receptors on increasing the leak-point pressure and thus permitting storage to a higher pressure.

It is crucial to understand that when bladder pressures remain greater than 35 to 40 cm H_2O, ureteral peristalsis does not effectively empty the upper tracts, and hydronephrosis and eventual renal insufficiency result. Thus coupling cystometric data with a particular patient's estimated (or measured) hourly output permits the clinician to decide what CIC interval would keep bladder pressures in a safe range. Medications can then be sensibly adjusted to extend CIC intervals, achieve dryness, and avoid development or progression of hydronephrosis.

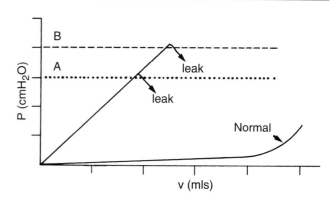

FIGURE 55-3. Bladder filling pressure-volume curve demonstrating the higher leak point sometimes achieved with α-adrenergic agents such as pseudoephedrine and imipramine.

Transurethral electrical stimulation of the bladder has been used in several treatment centers in an effort to produce conscious urinary control in the patient with neurogenic bladder.[64] It is a time-consuming treatment program with sometimes hundreds of sessions required before a response. Although some series have shown variably encouraging results, especially concerning the improvement in bladder compliance,[64,65] others have found the results disappointing.[66,67] More experience is necessary, but this technique may be applicable in selected children. Selective sacral nerve root rhizotomy and electrical stimulation of the sacral nerve roots also may have some limited potential for treatment in certain children.[68-70]

In children with high bladder-storage pressures and deterioration of the upper tracts who cannot be managed with CIC or pharmacologic therapy, temporary diversion with cutaneous vesicostomy may be necessary.[71,72] Protection of the upper urinary tracts from high bladder pressures is thus accomplished until such time as other treatments can be tolerated. We reserve this treatment for infants who have serious deterioration of the upper tract and those who, for social, medical, or anatomic reasons, cannot be managed with the other aforementioned forms of medical treatment. As an alternative, some advocate urethral dilation in girls to diminish the leak-point pressure. Surprising persistence of benefit has been noted in some series.[73]

Surgical Treatment

Although most patients with neurogenic bladder can be managed adequately without surgical intervention, those with reflux, poorly compliant bladder, or refractory incontinence may benefit from operative intervention.

Treatment of reflux in the neurogenic bladder is much the same as that for the normal bladder.[74] It is imperative, however, that the bladder be adequately treated for poor compliance and hyperreflexia (CIC and anticholinergics) before and after surgical intervention to diminish the high recurrence risk.[75]

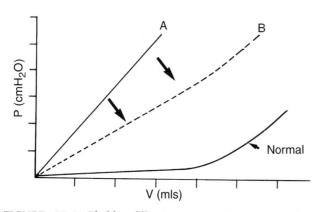

FIGURE 55-2. Bladder filling pressure-volume curve in a patient with a neurogenic bladder. Note the shift of the curve to the right when anticholinergics relax the detrusor, allowing lower pressure at any given volume.

In other clinical circumstances, surgical bladder augmentation or enlargement may be required. Bladder augmentation is designed to create a reservoir with good compliance and adequate capacity to store urine until it can be emptied by CIC at socially appropriate intervals. Detubularized segments of large or small bowel used as a patch and detubularized cup on the widely opened bladder (enterocystoplasty) are the current standards for augmentation (Fig. 55-4). Other techniques for bladder augmentation include gastrocystoplasty, which has been repopularized since 1988.[76,77] It is a technically acceptable procedure and shows advantages over enterocystoplasty with respect to a decrease in mucus formation, a possible decrease in infection rate, and maintenance of electrolyte balance in patients with renal insufficiency. Unfortunately, the hematuria-dysuria syndrome may affect up to one-third of patients, which limits its applicability.[78] This and other complications of enterocystoplasty have led to a search for different approaches.

Bladder autoaugmentation or detrusorectomy is an alternative augmenting technique that may prove useful in selected patients (Figs. 55-5 and 55-6).[79] The procedure involves removal of the detrusor muscle over the superior portion of the bladder, leaving the underlying bladder mucosa intact. This creates a large compliant surface, essentially a large diverticulum, which decreases bladder pressures and increases bladder capacity on filling. The advantage of this technique is that bladder epithelium is preserved and not replaced with gastrointestinal epithelium, as in bowel augmentation, thus eliminating the problems associated with the secretory and absorptive functions of bowel mucosa. Long-term follow-up data on large numbers of children are lacking, but this technique appears to be a viable alternative for use in bladders with reasonable capacity and mainly poor compliance.[80] The concept has been extended to create "composite" bladders by placing demucosalized bowel or stomach patches over the urothelial bulge created in autoaugmentation.[81,82] This concept of urothelial preservation during augmentation is carried forward by current innovative approaches to replace bladder wall with biodegradable scaffolds, either unsealed or sealed with urothelium detrusor muscle. The future of bladder reconstruction may be greatly affected by these efforts.

Persistent incontinence, despite adequate treatment of the bladder to reduce pressures and increase compliance in capacity, may require surgery on the bladder outlet to increase resistance. Bladder-neck reconstructions of the Young-Dees type, which lengthen the urethra by infolding and tubularizing the trigone of the bladder, have lost some favor but still have advocates.[83] Kropp's procedure[84] uses a tubularized anterior bladder strip reimplanted in the submucosa of the trigone to gain continence by a flap-valve mechanism. Continence is commonly achieved, but catheterization is sometimes difficult.[85] Sallè's procedure[86] creates a similar (but easier to catheterize) flap valve by onlaying an anterior bladder wall flap onto a posterior incised strip up the middle of the trigone. Owing to the

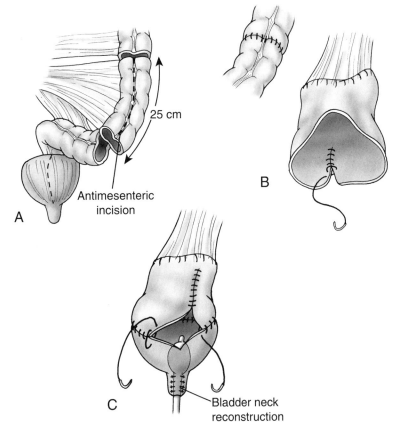

FIGURE 55-4. Bladder enlargement by enterocystoplasty (sigmoid) and bladder neck reconstruction. Enterocystoplasty enlarges the bladder nicely but has significant potential complications, including occasional perforation, first seen as acute abdominal pain.

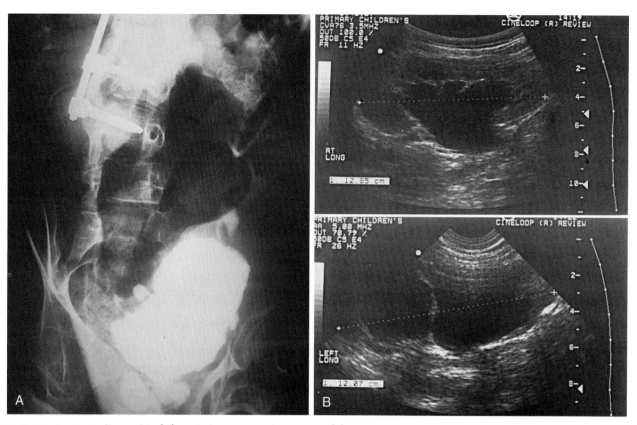

FIGURE 55-5. Radiographic (*A*) and ultrasonographic images (*B*) of a patient with spina bifida showing a small, poorly compliant bladder with worsening hydronephrosis.

lack of the pop-off mechanism in both these procedures, if the bladder becomes overfilled, the potential for bladder rupture of an augmented bladder or for upper tract deterioration based on high pressures is increased.

One of the more popular forms of increasing urethral resistance in the neurogenic bladder is by the pubovaginal or puboprostatic fascial sling.[87-91] This procedure has many advocates and involves securing a rectus fascial strip (or other material) around the urethra and suspending it from the anterior rectus fascia or pubis. This elevates and compresses the urethra to increase outlet resistance. Suprapubic bladder-neck suspension with periurethral sutures also is advocated but has a lower success rate than the fascial sling technique, especially in the urethra that is wide open with little resistance.

The artificial urinary sphincter works by way of a fluid-filled pressurized cuff around the urethra, which can be deflated by a pump-reservoir device that permits the urethra to open and the bladder to drain (Fig. 55-7). The artificial urinary sphincter also can be used in higher-pressure bladders in conjunction with bladder augmentation.[92] The main disadvantage is that it is a mechanical device that can erode into the urethra and malfunction over time. If the devices are left in place long enough, virtually all eventually need revision. We prefer to use autologous tissue techniques in children, when possible.

The periurethral injection of bovine collagen (Contigen), Teflon, or polydimethysiloxane represents a simple, safe technique for enhancing urethral resistance in selected patients with poor intrinsic sphincter tone. It appears to be most applicable in patients requiring only a minimal increase in stress leak-point pressure. Long-term improvement rates are disappointing, and the usefulness of this approach in children is questionable.[93]

In all procedures to enhance resistance at the bladder outlet, it is crucial that the storage pressures of the bladder be considered simultaneously. When the bladder outlet is tightened but the bladder is unable to store increasing volumes at low pressure, hydronephrosis or reflux results. When the surgeon is considering bladder-outlet surgical revision, it may be necessary to occlude the bladder neck with a Foley balloon during preoperative urodynamic assessment to determine how much the bladder can hold and what the storage pressures are like and thus to judge whether simultaneous augmentation is needed.

One surgical adjunct of great benefit in patients unable to self-catheterize the urethra (e.g., owing to spinal deformity, discomfort, or false passage) is the creation of a continent catheterizable stoma. This may be performed by using the appendix or another small tubularized structure implanted into the bladder and anastomosed to the skin (Mitrofanoff principle).[94,95] The implanted conduit can be

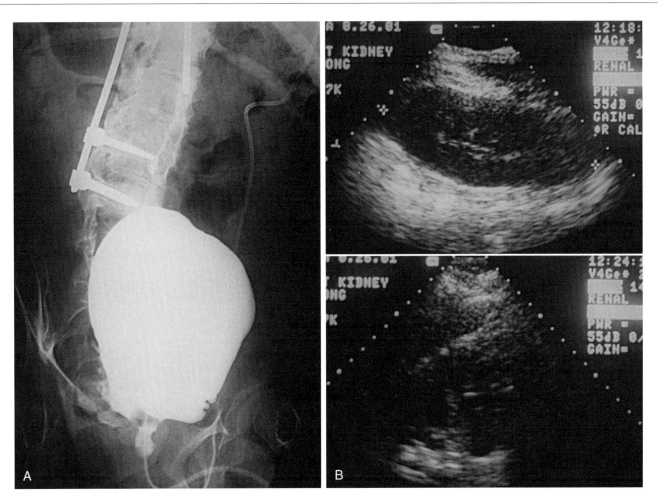

FIGURE 55-6. Radiographic (*A*) and ultrasonographic images (*B*) in the patient shown in Fig. 55-5 after bladder autoaugmentation, demonstrating improved bladder capacity and better compliance, which resulted in continence and diminished hydronephrosis.

hidden at the base of the umbilicus (Fig. 55-8)[96] and may then be carried out intermittently through this segment. The appendix may alternatively be left in continuity with the cecum and brought to the skin as a catheterizable channel for irrigation/enemas of the neurogenic colon. In this circumstance, a small segment of ileum may be refashioned as a catheterizable Monti-Yang stoma.[97] This has been a great adjunct to simplify catheterization for wheelchair-bound patients.

Cutaneous urinary diversion by ileal or colon conduit or by cutaneous ureterostomy is considered a last-resort therapy in these children. Long-term deterioration of the upper tracts is well documented in refluxing ileal conduits.[98] Some protection of the upper tracts is afforded by a nonrefluxing colon conduit, but the prognosis beyond two decades is uncertain.[99] Therefore avoidance of diversion, if possible, is the best course in children with neurogenic bladders. All reasonable efforts should be made to maintain ureteral drainage into the bladder, if possible. Continent urinary diversion has evolved over the past several years as a popular alternative in treating incontinence. The intestinal segments for urinary reconstruction in children with neurogenic bladders generally are of neurogenic bowel as well. These children may not tolerate a loss of large segments (especially ileocecal segments) without developing loose stools. In children who are dependent on constipated stools for fecal continence, loose stools may be more devastating than the original

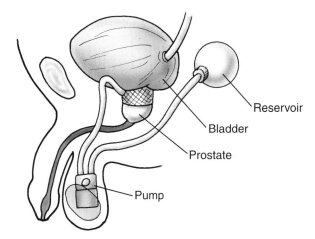

FIGURE 55-7. Typical artificial urinary sphincter. The scrotal pump moves fluid from the cuff to the reservoir to permit bladder emptying.

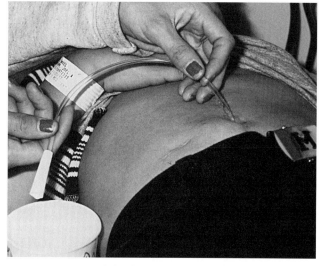

FIGURE 55-8. Umbilical positioning of an appendicovesicostomy permits easy access for clean intermittent catheterization; some patients can remain in their wheelchairs and drain the bladder into the toilet through a catheter extender.

urinary incontinence; careful consideration in all such endeavors remains the key to success.

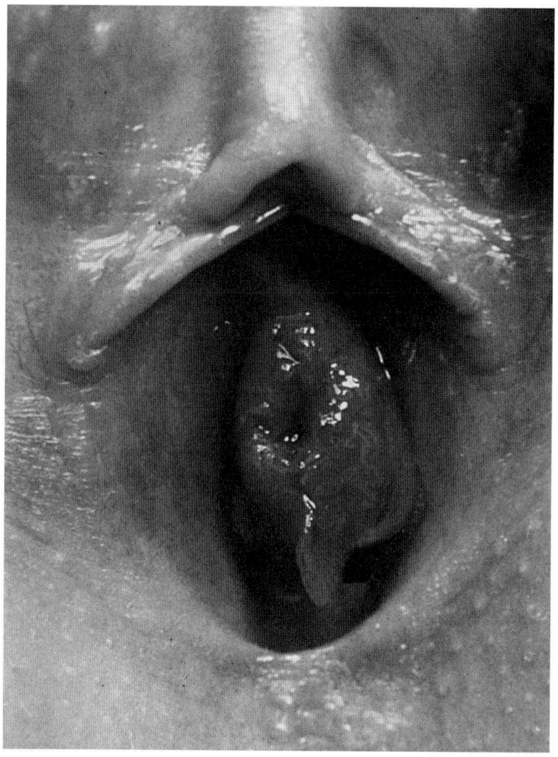

URETHRAL DISORDERS

Urethral Prolapse

Urethral prolapse occurs in girls at a mean age of 5 years, with those of African descent being particularly prone to this disorder.[100] Urethral prolapse is initially seen with dysuria and blood spotting, with a bulging concentric purplish ring of prolapsed urethra seen at the urethral meatus (Fig. 55-9). Mild prolapse can be treated with an antibiotic ointment or estrogen cream applied to the area several times a day along with sitz baths. At times, a catheter is needed temporarily. In persistent cases, excision of the prolapsing tissue with reanastomosis of the skin edges is satisfactory; a simple ligation of the prolapsing urethral epithelium over a Foley catheter, permitting necrosis, is another described option.

Meatal Stenosis

Meatal stenosis is the narrowing of the male urinary meatus after circumcision; it is thought to be due to exposure and irritation of the meatus in the diaper.[100,101] For reasons that are uncertain, the stenosis is always on the ventral aspect of the meatus, causing dorsal deflection of the urinary stream that is fine and forceful. It is important for the physician not only to examine the meatus but also to watch the child void. If the stream is not narrow in caliber or is not dorsally deflected, then the meatal stenosis is not significant enough to require meatotomy. Occasionally, voiding causes the web to tear, resulting in dysuria or a drop of blood after urination. Some patients will have ongoing inflammation around the meatus,

FIGURE 55-9. Urethral prolapse seen as a circumferential, purplish bulge at the meatus.

which will respond to topical steroid application (betamethasone, 0.05%).

Meatotomy may be necessary and can be performed under general anesthesia but more often is performed as an office procedure. Lidocaine/prilocaine (EMLA) cream is applied topically and left in place for 1 hour before meatotomy, with oral midazolam for sedation in selected patients. This has resulted in a painless office procedure.[101] Once anesthesia has developed, the ventral web is clamped with a hemostat; leaving this clamped for 1 minute results in adequate hemostasis. The ventral web is then snipped one half the distance to the coronal margin. Parents spread the meatus and apply ointment several times daily for 4 weeks; meatal stenosis rarely recurs. Imaging studies and cystoscopy are not needed in these boys.

Megalourethra

Megalourethra is a rare genital anomaly causing a deformed and elongated penis, occurring in two forms: fusiform and scaphoid (Fig. 55-10). These differ in embryology and appearance. Megalourethra is seen more commonly in patients with prune-belly syndrome and has been reported in association with the VATER (**v**ertebral defects, imperforate **a**nus, **t**racheoesophageal fistula, and **r**adial and **r**enal dysplasia) syndrome.[102]

The less severe and most common form of this anomaly is the scaphoid variety, in which spongiosal tissue fails to invest the urethra.[103] The more severe fusiform

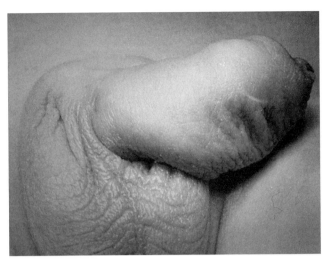

FIGURE 55-10. Scaphoid megalourethra in a boy with prune-belly syndrome.

variety is caused by failure of penile mesoderm at development, so that neither spongiosal tissue nor properly formed corpora cavernosa are found within the penis.[104] The fusiform type of megalourethra has been reported in patients with severe forms of prune-belly syndrome, in stillborn fetuses, and in patients with cloacal anomalies.[105,106] Associated urologic anomalies have been reported, including megaureter, megacystis, reflux, bladder diverticula, and renal dysplasia.[106] Upper tract assessment is indicated in all cases. Repair of the megalourethra relies on hypospadias techniques that tailor the urethra to a more normal size.

Urethral Duplication

Urethral duplications occur in a wide variety of forms and can be broadly classified as dorsal or ventral to the normal meatus.[107–109] Duplication may be complete, but incomplete forms predominate. Occasionally, side-by-side duplications occur, usually associated with duplicated phallus and bladder. Most commonly, the two channels form in the sagittal plane. The urethral channel closest to the rectum is generally the more functional channel, having more normal investing spongiosal tissue and sphincter mechanism.[110] The more dorsal urethra is often small and poorly developed and will commonly be in an epispadiac position and associated with dorsal chordee. Partial duplications that course along the penile urethra have been called *Y-type duplications*.[111] When the duplicated opening is in the perineum, it has been termed an *H-type duplication*.[112]

Treatment of urethral duplication must be individualized. When only a minor septum is present, cystoscopic division of the septum has been successful. Traditionally, with more significant duplications, efforts have been made to lengthen the ventrally placed urethra to the tip of the penis (by using various reconstruction techniques). Progressive dilation of the dorsal urethral channel to make it functional also has been advocated.[113]

Congenital Urethral Fistula

A congenital urethral fistula may occur in the anterior urethra where the spongiosum has developed incompletely, permitting a small diverticulum to form that can rupture antenatally.[114] These are uncommon and difficult to repair because of the lack of spongiosal tissue surrounding the fistula.

Urethral Strictures and Stenosis

Most urethral strictures are acquired. Instrumentation and catheter passage by medical personnel, trauma, and inflammatory diseases are common causes. Congenital urethral stenosis is rare and generally focal. These stenoses are usually in the bulbous urethra, with the area of embryologic joining of the bulbous urethra arising from genital folds and the posterior membranous urethra arising from the urogenital sinus. If this junction is misaligned or incompletely canalized, a discrete stricture may develop.[114]

Treatment of both these entities can be internal urethrotomy, resection and end-to-end anastomosis, or pedicle flap/free graft urethroplasty. Recent data would suggest a single internal urethrotomy for short strictures followed by an open repair (for failures) as best therapy.[115]

Urethral Atresia

When urethral atresia occurs, to be compatible with life, a patent urachus must be present. Reconstruction can be

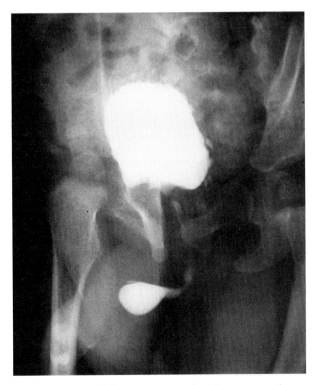

FIGURE 55-11. Voiding cystogram showing an anterior urethral diverticulum that functions as a valve, causing outflow obstruction. Note the bladder trabeculation.

difficult, and a vesicostomy with subsequent catheterizable stoma may be the best alternative.[94]

Urethral Diverticulum or Anterior Urethral Valve

Urethral diverticula occur ventrally where the spongiosum is absent or has been thinned. The distal lip of the diverticulum functionally serves as an anterior urethral valve, blocking the urinary stream as it flows antegrade (Fig. 55-11). The diverticulum progressively fills and further compresses the urethra during urination. This valvular effect can cause marked proximal dilation.[116-118]

The diagnosis is made with either urethrogram or cystoscopy. Treatment can be accomplished by endoscopic incision of the distal lip of the diverticular neck or, if more pronounced, by open excision and closure of the urethral defect.[119] In some cases, a diverticulum is present with a narrow neck that does not function as a valve. Such a diverticulum may provide for stasis of urine and may be a site of urethral infection.

Cystic Cowper's Gland Ducts

Cowper's glands are a pair of 5-mm glands located within the urogenital membrane. The ducts from these glands course distally and enter the ventral wall of the proximal bulbous urethra. These are the homologues of the female Bartholin's gland. Occasionally, these ducts can become occluded, producing bulbar urethral filling defects and, rarely, modest obstruction.[120] Cystoscopically, this appears to be a thin membrane over a fluid-filled cyst, sometimes called a *syringocele*.[121] If contrast enters a Cowper's duct, characteristic tubular channels can be seen coursing parallel to the bulbar urethra. Treatment of Cowper's duct cysts is with endoscopic unroofing and is unnecessary unless the radiographic finding is associated with clinical symptoms.

REFERENCES

1. Tanagho E: Anatomy of the lower urinary tract. In Walsh PC, Retick AB, Stamey TA, et al (eds): Campbell's Urology. Philadelphia, WB Saunders, 1992, pp 40–51.
2. McGuire E, Woodside JR, Borden TA, et al: Prognostic value of urodynamic testing in myelodysplastic patients. J Urol 126:205–209, 1981.
3. Bauer S: Urodynamics in children. In Ashcraft KW (ed): Pediatric Urology. Philadelphia, WB Saunders, 1990, pp 49–76.
4. Koff S: Enuresis. In Walsh PC, Retick AB, Vaughan ED (eds): Campbell's Urology. Philadelphia, WB Saunders, 1998, pp 2055–2068.
5. Zderic S, Levin RM, Wein AJ: Voiding function and dysfunction. In Gillenwater JY, Grayhack JT, Howards SS (eds): Adult and Pediatric Urology. St. Louis, Mosby-Year Book, 1996, pp 1159–1220.
6. Kaefer M, Zurakowski D, Bauer SB, et al: Estimating normal bladder capacity in children. J Urol 158:2261–2264, 1997.
7. Goellner M, Ziegler EE, Fomon SJ: Urination during the first three years of life. Nephron 28:174–178, 1983.
8. Allen T, Kaplan WE, Kroovand RL: Sphincter dyssynergia. Dialog Pediatr Urol 2:1–8, 1979.
9. Miller F: Children who wet the bed. In Kolvin I, MacKeith R, Meadow SR (eds): Bladder Control and Enuresis. London, W. Heinemann Medical Books, 1973, pp 47–52.
10. Tietjen D, Husmann DA: Nocturnal enuresis: A guide to evaluation and treatment. Mayo Clin Proc 71:857–862, 1996.
11. Yeung C: Nocturnal enuresis (bedwetting). Curr Opin Urol 13:337–343, 2003.
12. Forsythe W, Redmond A: Enuresis in spontaneous cure rate: Study of 1,129 enuretics. Arch Dis Child 49:259, 1974.
13. Bakwin H: The genetics of enuresis. In Kolvin I, MacKeith R, Meadow SR (eds): Bladder Control and Enuresis. London, W. Heinemann Medical Books, 1973, pp 73–77.
14. Norgaard J: Urodynamics in enuresis: Reservoir function. Neurol Urodynam 8:119, 1989.
15. Norgaard J: Pathophysiology of nocturnal enuresis. Scand J Urol Nephrol Suppl 140:1–35, 1991.
16. Jarvelin M: Developmental history and neurological findings in enuretic children. Dev Med Child Neurol 31:728–736, 1989.
17. Norgaard J, Hansen J, Nielsen J, et al: Simultaneous registration of sleep stages and bladder activity in enuresis. Urology 26:316–319, 1985.
18. Norgaard J, Pedersen E, Djurhuus J: Diurnal antidiuretic: Hormone levels in enuretics. J Urol 134:1029, 1985.
19. Puri B: Urinary levels of antidiuretic hormone in nocturnal enuresis. Indian Pediatr 17:675, 1980.
20. Rushton H, Belman AB, Zaontz MR, et al: The influence of small functional bladder capacity and other predictors on the response to desmopressin in the management of monosymptomatic nocturnal enuresis. J Urol 156:651–655, 1996.
21. Eller D, Austin PF, Tanguay S, et al: Daytime functional bladder capacity as a predictor of response to desmopressin in monosymptomatic nocturnal enuresis. Eur Urol 33:25–29, 1998.
22. Hansen M., Rettig S, Siggaared C, et al: Intra-individual variability in nighttime urine production and functional bladder capacity estimated by home recordings in patient with nocturnal enuresis. J Urol 166:2452–2455, 2001.
23. Turner R: Conditioning treatment of nocturnal enuresis: Present status. In Kolvin I, MacKeith R, Meadow S (eds): Bladder Control and Enuresis. London, W. Heinemann Medical Books, 1973.
24. Morgan R: Relapse and therapeutic response in the conditioning treatment of enuresis: A review of recent findings on intermittent reinforcement, overlearning and stimulus intensity. Behav Res Ther 16:278, 1978.
25. Monda J, Husmann D: Primary nocturnal enuresis: A comparison among observation, imipramine, desmopressin acetate and bed wetting alarm systems. J Urol 154:745–748, 1995.
26. Blackwell B, Currah J: Tricyclic pharmacology of nocturnal enuresis. In: Kolvin I, MacKeith R, Meadow S (eds): Bladder Control and Enuresis. London, W. Heinemann Medical Books, 1973.
27. Klauber G: Clinical efficacy and safety of desmopressin in the treatment of nocturnal enuresis. J Pediatr 114(suppl):719, 1989.
28. Ritig S, Knudsen U, Sorensen S, et al: Desmopressin and nocturnal enuresis. In Meadow S, Canwell, Sutton, et al (eds): Proceedings of an International Symposium. London, Horus Medical Publications, 1989, pp 43–54.
29. MacKeith R, Meadow S, Turner R: How children become dry. In Kolvin I, MacKeith R, Meadow S (eds): Bladder Control and Enuresis. Philadelphia, JB Lippincott, 1973, pp 3–15.
30. Robson W: Diurnal enuresis. Pediatr Rev 18:407–412, 1997.
31. Bernard-Bonnin A: Diurnal enuresis in childhood. Can Fam Physician 46:1109–1115, 2000.
32. Fernandesn E, Vernier R, Gonzalez R: The unstable bladder in children. J Pediatr 118:831–837, 1991.
33. Reinberg Y, Crocker J, Wolpert, J, et al: Therapeutic efficacy of extended release oxybutinin chloride and immediate release and long-acting tolterodine tartrate in children with diurnal urinary incontinence. J Urol 169:317–319, 2003.
34. Munding M, Wessells H, Thornberry B, et al: Use of tolterodine in children with dysfunctional voiding: An initial report. J Urol 165:926–928, 2001.
35. Goessl C, Sauter T, Michael T, et al: Efficacy and tolerability of tolterodine in children with detrusor hyperreflexia. Urology 55:414–418, 2000.
36. Herdon C, Decambre M, McKenna PH: Interactive computer games for treatment of pelvic floor dysfunction. J Urol 166:1893–1898, 2001.
37. McKenna P, Herdon CD, Connery S, et al: Pelvic floor muscle retraining for pediatric voiding dysfunction using interactive computer games. J Urol 162:1056–1062, 1999.

38. Koff S, Murtagh DS: The uninhibited bladder in children: Effect of treatment on recurrence of urinary infection and vesico-ureteral reflux. J Urol 130:1158–1160, 1983.

39. DeLuca F, Swenson O, Fisher JH, et al: The dysfunctional "lazy" bladder syndrome in children. Arch Dis Child 37:197–223, 1962.

40. Bloom D, Seeley WW, Ritchey ML, et al: Toilet habits and continence in children: An opportunity sampling in search of normal parameters. J Urol 149:1087–1090, 1993.

41. Hinman F: Non-neurogenic neurogenic bladder (the Hinman syndrome) fifteen years later. J Urol 136:769–775, 1986.

42. Austin P, Homsy YL, Masel JL, et al: Alpha-adrenergic blockade in children with neuropathic and non-neuropathic voiding dysfunction. J Urol 162:1064–1067, 1999.

43. Bauer S: Neuropathology of the lower urinary tract. In Kelalis PY, King LR, Belman AB (eds): Clinical Pediatric Urology. Philadelphia, WB Saunders, 1992, pp 399–440.

44. Steers W, Barret DM, Wein AJ: Voiding dysfunction: diagnosis, classification and management. In Gillenwater JY, Grayhack JT, Howards SS, et al (eds.): Adult and Pediatric Urology. St. Louis, Mosby-Year Book, 1996, pp 1220–1326.

45. Mandell J, Bauer SB, Hallett M, et al: Occult spinal dysraphism: A rare but detectable cause of voiding dysfunction. Urol Clin North Am 7:349–356, 1980.

46. Kaplan W: Management of myelomeningocele. Urol Clin North Am 12:93–101, 1985.

47. Kroovand R: Myelomeningocele. In Walsh PC, Gittes RF, Perlmutter AD, et al (eds): Campbell's Urology. Philadelphia, WB Saunders, 1986, pp 2193–2216.

48. Bauer S, Joseph DB. Management of the obstructed urinary tract associated with neurogenic bladder dysfunction. Urol Clin North Am 17:395–406, 1990.

49. Werler M, Shapiro S, Mitchell AA: Periconceptual folic acid exposure and risk of occult neural tube defects. JAMA 269:1257–1263, 1993.

50. Bauer S, Hallett M, Khoshbin S, et al: Predictive value of urodynamic evaluation in newborns with myelodysplasia. JAMA 252:650–652, 1984.

51. Wang, S, McGuire EJ, Bloom DA: A bladder pressure management system for myelodysplasia: Clinical outcome. J Urol 140:1499–1502, 1988.

52. Galloway N, Mekras JA, Helms M, et al: An objective score to predict upper tract deterioration in myelodysplasia. J Urol 145:535–537, 1991.

53. Tulipan N, Sutton LN, Bruner JP, et al: The effect of intrauterine myelomeningocele repair on the incidence of shunt-dependent hydrocephalus. Pediatr Neurosurg 38:27–33, 2003.

54. Holzbeierlein J, Pope JC IV, Adams MC, et al: The urodynamic profile of myelodysplasia in childhood with spinal closure during gestation. J Urol 164:1336–1339, 2000.

55. Tarcan T, Bauer S, Olmedo E, et al: Long-term followup of newborns with myelodysplasia and normal urodynamic findings: Is it necessary? J Urol 165:564–567, 2001.

56. Lapides J, Diokno AC, Silber SJ, et al: Clean intermittent self-catheterization in the treatment of urinary tract disease. J Urol 107:458–462, 1971.

57. Klose A, Sackett CK, Mesrobian H: Management of children with myelodysplasia: Urologic alternatives. J Urol 144:1446–1449, 1990.

58. Joseph D, Bauer SB, Colodny AH, et al: Clean, intermittent catheterization of infants with neurogenic bladder. Pediatrics 84:78–82, 1989.

59. Cass A: Urinary tract complications in myelomeningocele patients. J Urol 115:102–104, 1976.

60. Plunkett J, Braren V: Clean intermittent catheterization in children. J Urol 121:469–471, 1979.

61. Klauber G, Sant GR: Complications of intermittent catheterization. Urol Clin North Am 10:557–562, 1983.

62. Abrams P: Tolterodine, a new antimuscarinic agent: As effective but better tolerated than oxybutinin in patients with an overactive bladder. Br J Urol 81:801–810, 1998.

63. Dmochowski R, Davila G, Zinner N, et al: Efficacy and safety of transdermal oxybutynin in patients with urge and mixed urinary incontinence. J Urol 168:580–586, 2002.

64. Kaplan W, Richards I: Intravesical bladder stimulation in myelodysplasia. J Urol 140:1282–1284, 1988.

65. Kaplan W, Richards TW, Richards I: Intravesical transurethral bladder stimulation to increase bladder capacity. J Urol 142:600–602, 1989.

66. Decter R: Transurethral electrical bladder stimulation: A follow-up report. J Urol 152:812–814, 1994.

67. Boone T, Roehrborn CG, Hurt G: Transurethral intravesical electrotherapy for neurogenic bladder dysfunction in children: A prospective, randomized clinical trial. J Urol 148:550–553, 1992.

68. Toczek S, McCullough DC, Garfour GW, et al: Selective sacral rootlet rhizotomy for hypertonic neurogenic bladder. J Neurosurg 42:567–574, 1975.

69. Mulcahy J, Young AB: Long-term follow-up of percutaneous radiofrequency sacral rhizotomy. Urology 35:76–77, 1990.

70. Tanagho E, Schmidt RA: Electrical stimulation in the clinical management of the neurogenic bladder. J Urol 140:1331–1339, 1988.

71. Duckett JJ: Cutaneous vesicostomy in childhood. Urol Clin North Am 1:485–495, 1974.

72. Mandell J, Bauer SB, Colodny AH, et al: Cutaneous vesicostomy in infancy. J Urol 126:92–93, 1981.

73. Bloom D, Knechtel JM, McGuire EJ: Urethral dilation improve bladder compliance in children with myelomeningocele and high leak point pressures. J Urol 144:430–433, 1990.

74. Jeffs R, Jonas P, Schillinger JF: Surgical correction of vesicoureteral reflux in children with neurogenic bladder. J Urol 114:449–451, 1976.

75. Agarwal S, McLorie GA, Grewal D, et al: Urodynamic correlates of resolution of reflux in myelomeningocele patients. J Urol 158:580–582, 1997.

76. Adams M, Mitchell ME, Rink RC: Gastrocystoplasty: An alternative solution to the problem of urological reconstruction in the severely compromised patient. J Urol 140:1152–1156, 1988.

77. Adams M, Bihrle R, Rink RC: The use of stomach in urologic reconstruction. AUA Update Series 14:218–223, 1995.

78. Nguyen D, Bain MA, Salmonson KL, et al: The syndrome of dysuria and hematuria in pediatric urinary reconstruction with stomach. J Urol 150:707–709, 1993.

79. Cartwright P, Snow BW: Bladder augmentation: Early clinical experience. J Urol 142:595–598, 1989.

80. Snow B, Cartwright PC: Bladder autoaugmentation. Urol Clin North Am 23:323–331, 1996.

81. Gonzalez R, Buson H, Reid C, et al: Seromuscular colocystoplasty lined with urothelium: Experience with 16 patients. Urology 45:124–129, 1994.

82. Dewan P, Byard R: Autoaugmentation gastrocystoplasty in a sheep model. Br J Urol 72:56–59, 1993.

83. Reda E: The use of the Young-Dee Leadbetter procedure. Dialog Pediatr Urol 14:7–8, 1991.

84. Kropp K, Angwafo FF: Urethral lengthening and reimplantation for neurogenic incontinence in children. J Urol 135:533–536, 1986.

85. Kropp K: Management of urethral incompetence in the patient with neurogenic bladder. Dialog Pediatr Urol 14:6–7, 1991.

86. Salle J, McLorie GA, Bagli DJ, et al: Urethral lengthening with anterior bladder wall flap (Pippi-Salle procedure): Modification and extended indications of the technique. J Urol 158:585–590, 1997.

87. McGuire J, Lytton B: Pubovaginal sling procedure for stress incontinence. J Urol 119:82–84, 1978.

88. Bauer S, Peters CA, Colodny AH, et al: The use of rectus fascia to manage urinary incontinence. J Urol 142:516–519, 1989.

89. McGuire E, Wang C, Usitalo H, et al: Modified pubovaginal sling in girls with myelodysplasia. J Urol 135:94–96, 1986.

90. Elder J: Periurethral and puboprostatic sling repair for incontinence in patients with myelodysplasia. J Urol 144:434–437, 1990.

91. Norbeck J, McGuire EJ: The use of pubovaginal and puboprostatic slings. Dialog Pediatr Urol 14:3–4, 1991.

92. Gonzalez R, Nguyen DH, Koleilat N, et al: Compatibility of enterocystoplasty and the artificial urinary sphincter. J Urol 142:502–504, 1989.

93. Sundaram C, Reinberg Y, Aliabadi HA: Failure to obtain durable results with collagen implantation in children with urinary incontinence. J Urol 157:2306–2307, 1997.

94. Mitrofanoff P: Cystostomie continente trans-appendiculaire dans le traitement des vessies neurolgiques. Chir Pediatr 21:297–301, 1980.

95. Cain M, Casale A, King S, et al: Appendicovesicostomy and newer alternatives for Mitrofanoff procedure: Results in the last 100 patients at Riley's Children's Hospital. J Urol 162:1749–1752, 1999.

96. Keating M, Rink RC, Adams MC: Appendicovesicostomy: A useful adjunct to continent reconstruction of the bladder. J Urol 149:1091–1094, 1993.

97. Monti P, Lava R, Dutra M, et al: New techniques for construction of efferent conduits based on Mitrofanoff principle. Urology 49:112–115, 1997.

98. Cass A, Luxenberg M, Gleich P: A 22 year follow-up of ileal conduits in children with a neurogenic bladder. J Urol 132:529–531, 1984.

99. Husmann D, McLorie GA, Churchill BM: Non refluxing colonic conduits: A long-term life-table analysis. J Urol 142:1201–1205, 1989.

100. Brown M, Cartwright P, Snow B: Common office problems in pediatric urology and gynecology. Pediatr Clin North Am 44:1091–1115, 1997.

101. Cartwright P, Snow B, McNees D: Office meatotomy utilizing EMLA cream as the anesthetic. J Urol 156:857–859, 1996.

102. Fernbach S: Urethral abnormalities in male neonates with VATER association. AJR Am J Roentgenol 156:137–140, 1991.

103. Stephens F, Smith ED, Huston JM: Congenital intrinsic lesions of the anterior urethra. In: Congenital Anomalies of the Urinary and Genital Tracts. Oxford, England, Isis Medical Media, 1996, pp 119–124.

104. Dorairajan T: Defects of spongy tissue and congenital diverticula of the penile urethra. Aust N Z J Surg 32:209, 1963.

105. Duckett J: The prune-belly syndrome. In Kelalis P, King L, Bellman A (eds): Clinical Pediatric Urology. Philadelphia, WB Saunders, 1976, p 615.

106. Shrom S, Cromie W, Duckett J, et al: Megalourethra. Urology 17:152, 1981.

107. Gross R, Moore T: Duplication of the urethra. Arch Surg 60:749, 1950.

108. Das S, Brosman S: Duplication of the male urethra. J Urol 117:452, 1977.

109. Woodhouse C, Williams D: Duplications of the lower urinary tract in children. Br J Urol 51:481, 1979.

110. Salle J, Sibai H, Rosenstein D, et al: Urethral duplication in the male: Review of 16 cases. J Urol 163:1936–1938, 2000.

111. Williams D, Bloomberg S: Bifid urethra with three anal accessory tract (Y duplication). Br J Urol 47:877, 1976.

112. Stephens F, Donnellan W: H-Type urethral anal fistula. J Pediatr Surg 12:95–102, 1977.

113. Passerini-Glazal G, Araguna F, Chiozza L: PADUA (Posterior augmentation by dilating the urethra anterior): Procedure of treatment of severe urethral hypoplasia. J Urol 140:1247–1249, 1988.

114. Duckett J, Snow B: Disorders of the urethral and penis. In Walsh P, Gittes R, Perlmutter A, et al (eds): Campbell's Urology. Philadelphia, WB Saunders, 1986, pp 2014–2015.

115. Hsaio K, Baez-Trinidad L, Lendray T, et al: Direct vision internal urethrotomy for the treatment of pediatric ureteral strictures: Analysis of 50 patients. J Urol 170:1655–1658, 2003.

116. Firlit C, King L: Anterior urethral valves in children. J Urol 108:972, 1972.

117. Rudhe U, Ericsson N: Congenital urethral diverticula. Ann Radiol 13:289, 1970.

118. Williams D, Retik A: Congenital valves and diverticula of the anterior urethra. Br J Urol 41:228, 1969.

119. Firlit R, Firlit C, King L: Obstructing anterior urethral valves in children. J Urol 119:819, 1978.

120. Colodny A, Lebowitz R: Lesions of Cowper's ducts and glands in infants and children. Urology 11:321, 1978.

121. Maizel S, Stephens F, King L, et al: Cowper's syringocele: A classification of dilatations of Cowper's gland duct based upon clinical characteristics of eight boys. J Urol 129:111, 1983.

Posterior Urethral Valves

Jack S. Elder, MD, and Ellen Shapiro, MD

Posterior urethral valves (PUV) is the most common congenital anomaly causing bladder-outlet obstruction in boys, with an incidence of 1 in 5000 to 1 in 8000 male births (Fig. 56-1). Although the majority of boys with PUV are diagnosed before birth, in 24% to 45%, renal insufficiency will develop during childhood or adolescence, and it is the most common obstructive cause of end-stage renal disease in children. This chapter reviews the initial and long-term management and prognosis of infants and children with PUV.

EMBRYOLOGY AND ANATOMY

At 5 to 6 weeks' gestation, the orifice of the mesonephric duct normally migrates from an anterolateral position in the cloaca to Müller's tubercle on the posterior wall of the urogenital sinus. This event occurs simultaneous with the division of the cloaca. Remnants of the mesonephric duct normally remain as small distinct, paired lateral folds termed the *inferior urethral crest* and *plicae colliculi*. When the insertion of the mesonephric ducts into the cloaca is anomalous or too anterior, normal migration of the ducts is impeded, and the ducts fuse anteriorly, resulting in the formation of abnormal ridges, which are the PUV. PUV is a spectrum of disease. Valves with a smaller aperture between the leaflets cause more obstruction and upper tract damage than do those with a larger aperture and a less prominent anterior component.

Three distinct types of PUV have been described. The type I valve is an obstructing membrane that radiates distally and anteriorly from the verumontanum toward the membranous urethra (the segment of urethra that traverses the urogenital diaphragm or striated sphincter), fusing in the midline; approximately 95% of PUV are type I (Fig. 56-2). These valves are thought to be a single membranous structure with the opening positioned posteriorly near the verumontanum. The type III valve appears as a membranous diaphragm with a central aperture at the verumontanum. The obstructing tissue also has been termed a *congenital obstructing posterior urethral membrane* or COPUM.[1] It is thought that instrumentation

with a urethral catheter might disrupt the posterior aspect of the membrane, resulting in the appearance of a type I valve. Type II valves are prominent longitudinal folds of hypertrophied smooth muscle that radiate cranially from the verumontanum to the posterolateral bladder neck, but these are nonobstructive and clinically insignificant.

PRENATAL DIAGNOSIS, MANAGEMENT, AND OUTCOMES

About 10% of prenatally diagnosed obstructive uropathy is due to PUV, and approximately two-thirds of PUV are diagnosed prenatally. Typical findings include bilateral hydroureteronephrosis, a distended bladder, and a dilated prostatic urethra, termed a *keyhole sign*.[2] Discrete focal cysts in the renal parenchyma are diagnostic of renal dysplasia. Amniotic fluid volume is variable, and those with normal or slightly reduced amniotic fluid have a better prognosis. In contrast, oligohydramnios suggests significant obstructive uropathy or renal dysplasia or both, and pulmonary hypoplasia is common. The gestational age at which hydronephrosis is recognized also influences prognosis. In our study, fetuses with PUV and normal-appearing renal anatomy after 24 weeks were much more likely to have normal renal function than were those with hydronephrosis recognized before 24 weeks.[3] Antenatally, PUV, prune-belly syndrome, urethral atresia, and bilateral high-grade vesicoureteral reflux (megacystis-megaureter syndrome) may have a similar appearance. The presumptive diagnosis of PUV cannot be confirmed until postpartum radiologic studies are performed.

In the fetus with suspected PUV and normal amniotic fluid volume, serial fetal sonograms are necessary to monitor the status of the hydronephrosis and amniotic fluid volume. If oligohydramnios develops, prenatal drainage of the bladder may be beneficial. It is thought that oligohydramnios prevents normal fetal movement, chest mobility, and lung development in utero. Pathologically, this process results in reduced branching of the bronchial tree and reduced numbers and size of alveoli.[4]

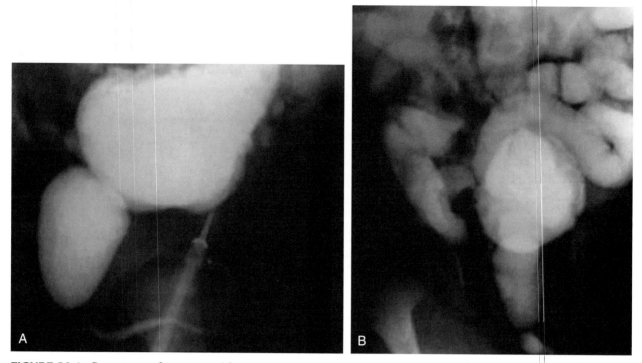

FIGURE 56-1. Cystograms of neonates with posterior urethral valves. *A,* Antegrade cystogram; note tapering of distal prostatic urethra at the site of the valve, severe detrusor hypertrophy, and narrowed bladder neck. *B,* Voiding cystourethrogram shows massive bilateral vesicoureteral reflux. Both underwent transurethral valve ablation.

In the fetus with suspected PUV, a karyotype should be obtained because chromosome abnormalities occur in about 12% of fetuses with bilateral hydroureteronephrosis and bladder distention, and it is important to verify that the fetus is a male.[5] Fetal renal function must be assessed. Discrete renal cysts are diagnostic of renal dysplasia. Assuming renal cysts are absent, fetal urinary electrolytes and β_2-microglobulin provide the most accurate means of evaluating fetal renal function. Normally fetal urine is hypotonic, with sodium less than 100 mEq/L, chloride less than 90 mEq/L, and osmolality less than 210 mEq/L.[2] Elevated fetal urine electrolytes and β_2-microglobulin levels are an indication of irreversible renal dysfunction. Sequential bladder aspiration every 48 to 72 hours should be performed, because the initial sample may be stale, and new urine that forms more accurately reflects the function of the fetal kidneys.[6,7]

If fetal urine is hypotonic, and oligohydramnios is present, then fetal intervention should be considered, with a goal of preventing life-threatening pulmonary hypoplasia. No evidence exists that drainage of the fetal bladder obstructed by PUV will improve renal function. Therefore the family should understand that even if the drainage procedure is successful, the baby may have limited renal function or end-stage renal disease. If the gestational age of the fetus is 32 weeks or more, early delivery is advisable. If the fetus is less than 32 weeks' gestation, however, the urine may be diverted into the amniotic fluid with a percutaneously placed vesicoamniotic shunt, which has a pigtail on each end. In a few centers, in utero cutaneous vesicostomy or ureterostomy has been performed.[8]

Percutaneous in utero endoscopic ablation of posterior urethral valves also has been reported,[9,10] but few centers have the instrumentation or technical expertise to perform this procedure.

Vesicoamnionic shunts have limitations.[5] They become obstructed or displaced in 25% of cases, necessitating additional procedures that increase morbidity to the

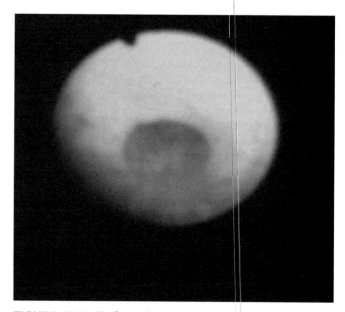

FIGURE 56-2. Endoscopic appearance of posterior urethral valve.

mother and fetus and a 5% procedure-related rate of fetal loss. In addition, omental or bowel herniation through the fetal abdominal wall may occur. Despite adequate bladder drainage, renal function may be so limited that the amniotic fluid volume remains low. In one recent study of high-risk fetuses identified in the first trimester with severe bilateral hydroureteronephrosis, bladder distention, and oligohydramnios managed with vesicoamniotic shunt, a 60% overall survival rate and a 33% incidence of renal failure were found.[11] In a review of 14 fetuses with proven PUV and favorable fetal urinary electrolytes undergoing fetal intervention at a mean gestational age of 22.5 weeks, 6 deaths occurred before term delivery, whereas 8 survived, with a mean follow-up of 11.6 years. Of these 8, 3 had end-stage renal disease, and the other 5 had an elevated serum creatinine.[8] Consequently, when counseling families, one must emphasize that intervention may assist in keeping the fetus viable to term, but will most likely not prevent the long-term sequelae of severe renal dysplasia associated with PUV.

CLINICAL PRESENTATION

Neonates with PUV who are not diagnosed before birth may appear in the nursery with delayed voiding or a poor urinary stream.[12] Respiratory distress secondary to pulmonary hypoplasia may be the only manifestation of severe urethral obstruction. Other common signs and symptoms include a palpable abdominal mass, failure to thrive, lethargy, poor feeding, urosepsis, and urinary ascites. A urinary tract infection (UTI) often develops in infants. Older boys may have persistent diurnal incontinence or abdominal distention as their only manifestations. Physical examination in the newborn typically discloses a palpable walnut-sized bladder, which corresponds to the hypertrophic detrusor muscle. If urinary ascites is present, significant abdominal distention is typical.

RADIOGRAPHIC EVALUATION

Postnatal ultrasonography (US) usually shows significant bilateral hydronephroureteronephrosis. Demonstration of the corticomedullary junction is a favorable prognostic sign regarding renal functional potential (Fig. 56-3). Conversely, echogenic kidneys, subcortical cysts, and corticomedullary junction on the initial and follow-up US studies are unfavorable signs. Suprapubic or perineal US may demonstrate a dilated prostatic urethra, which is pathognomonic for PUV.

The voiding cystourethrogram (VCUG) remains the only radiographic study that definitively establishes the diagnosis of PUV. The valve appears as a sharply defined perpendicular or oblique lucency in the distal prostatic urethra. The posterior urethra is dilated and elongated and has the appearance of a shield. The bladder is trabeculated with clear delineation of the bladder neck, which appears as a thick muscular collar because of hypertrophy. Vesicoureteral reflux (VUR) is present in 50%.

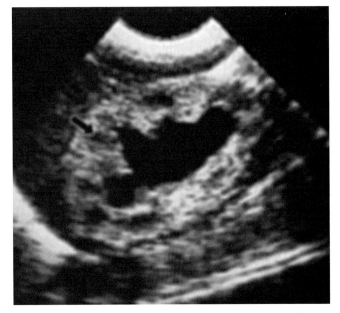

FIGURE 56-3. Renal sonogram demonstrating hydronephrotic kidney with intact corticomedullary junction (*arrow*) in infant with posterior urethral valves.

Renal nuclear scintigraphy with either a dimercaptosuccinic acid (DMSA) scan or mercaptoacetyltriglycine (MAG-3) should be performed if either kidney shows thin or abnormal parenchyma.

INITIAL MANAGEMENT

The initial treatment for neonates suspected of having PUV is to decompress the urinary tract with a 5 or 8F feeding tube passed transurethrally during the first US study immediately after birth. The catheter can be difficult to pass because of the dilation of the posterior urethra and hypertrophy of the bladder neck. A catheter coiled in the posterior urethra will result in the majority of urine draining around the catheter. Sonography confirms the placement of the catheter within the bladder. Foley catheter use is discouraged because the inflated balloon can obstruct the ureteral orifices when the thick-walled bladder is decompressed, and it can cause severe bladder spasm that can obstruct the intramural ureters. Ampicillin or cephalexin prophylaxis should be initiated. Renal function, electrolytes, and fluid status should be monitored carefully. Metabolic acidosis and hyperkalemia are common complications if renal function is impaired.

Neonates with respiratory distress may require immediate pulmonary resuscitation with endotracheal intubation and positive-pressure ventilation, which may cause a pneumothorax or pneumomediastinum. In rare cases, extracorporeal membrane oxygenation (ECMO) may be needed to support life until the diagnosis and prognosis are clearly defined.[13] If urinary ascites is seen, paracentesis may be necessary to correct fluid and electrolyte imbalance.

Renal sonography and a VCUG should be performed expeditiously to determine whether the patient has PUV. Circumcision should be performed to reduce the risk of UTI.

Primary Valve Ablation

Endoscopic valve ablation is performed after the baby is stabilized medically. Well-lubricated infant urethral sounds should be passed gently to calibrate and stretch the urethra slightly. The newborn male urethra usually accepts an 8F endoscope. Dilation of the urethra to pass a larger instrument may lead to urethral trauma with subsequent stricture formation and should be avoided. Vigorous dilation may result in iatrogenic hypospadias due to splitting of the glans to the subcoronal level.[14]

An 8 or 9F cystoscope typically is used with a Bugbee electrode on low cutting current inserted through the operating channel. The valve leaflets should be incised by using a low cutting current at the 5 and 7 o'clock positions. Incision at the 12 o'clock position where the valves leaflets fuse also may be helpful. An alternative method of PUV ablation is to use the neodymium:yttrium aluminum garnet (YAG) laser.[15] In premature or small babies, a cystoscope as small as 6.9F may be used, although the visualization of the PUV may be suboptimal. In a large infant, a pediatric resectoscope may be used. If urethral bleeding occurs, coagulation should be performed carefully, because urethral injury may occur with overzealous cautery. After valve ablation, a pediatric feeding tube generally is left indwelling for 1 to 2 days.

In premature or small neonates, a temporary perineal urethrostomy for passage of the cystoscope or resectoscope may be helpful. Valve ablation also may be performed antegrade through a percutaneous cystostomy.[16]

A VCUG and renal sonogram should be obtained 2 to 4 weeks after ablation to confirm satisfactory valve disruption. In addition, renal function should be monitored closely. PUV ablation is successful in more than 90% of patients. The most common complication is incomplete valve ablation, in which case repeated cystoscopy and valve incision is necessary. Urethral stricture is uncommon with the use of smaller endoscopic instrumentation and better optics.

Temporary Urinary Diversion

An alternative to primary valve ablation is cutaneous vesicostomy (Fig. 56-4). This approach is appropriate in a small or premature neonate when the pediatric cystoscope is too large for valve ablation or if severe hydroureteronephrosis, urinary ascites, or high-grade reflux with poor renal function is present. In these cases, optimal drainage is necessary to maintain existing renal function. A small transverse incision is performed midway between the umbilicus and pubic symphysis, and the dome of the bladder is brought to the skin. The vesicostomy should calibrate to 24 to 26F to avoid stenosis. Daily dilation of the stoma with a plastic medicine dropper helps prevent contraction of the stoma. The vesicostomy drains into the diaper, and no urinary collection device is necessary. When cutaneous vesicostomy is

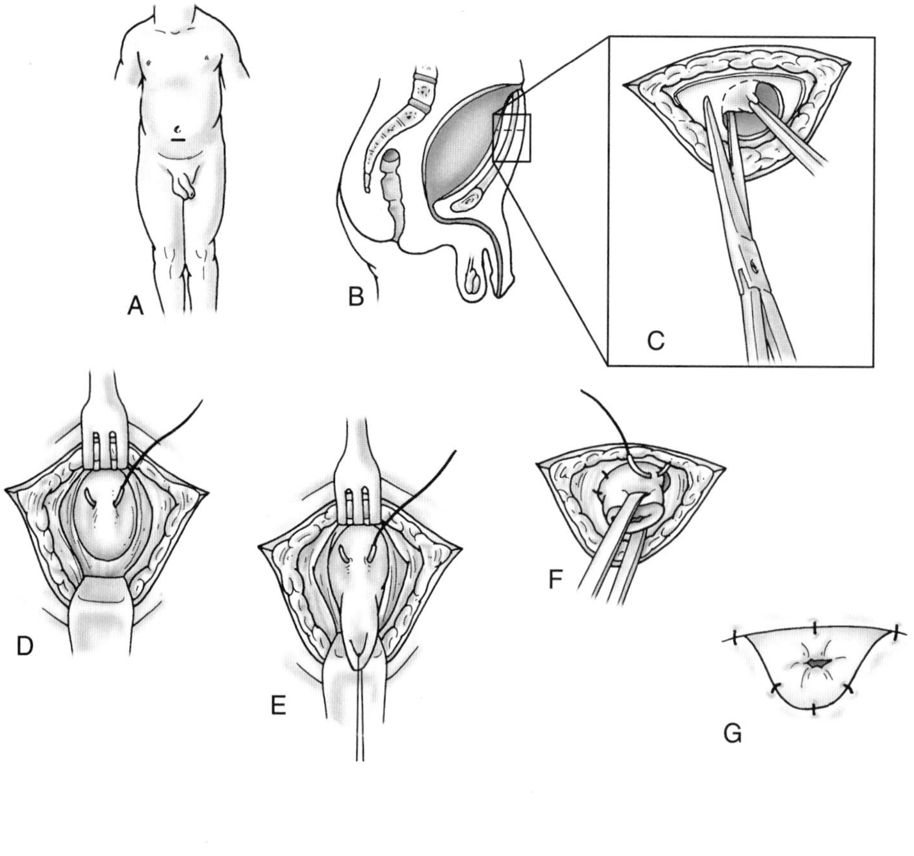

FIGURE 56-4. Technique of cutaneous vesicostomy. *A–C,* Transverse incision is made midway between the umbilicus and pubic symphysis. *D, E,* Traction sutures are placed through the bladder, and it is mobilized superiorly to the dome of the bladder. *F,* The detrusor should be fixed to the rectus fascia. The bladder is opened, and the mucosa is sutured to the skin. *G,* Completed vesicostomy should calibrate to 24F.

performed, valve ablation should not be performed simultaneously, because the urethra remains dry, and urethral stricture is likely. Cutaneous vesicostomy has been shown to be as effective as valve ablation as initial therapy.[17] This procedure allows the bladder to cycle and grow with voiding at low pressure through the stoma, and does not reduce bladder capacity. These babies should be maintained on antibiotic prophylaxis.

In the past, proximal high diversion with cutaneous pyelostomy or cutaneous ureterostomy was advocated for neonates and infants with severe hydronephrosis and a persistent elevated creatinine after catheter drainage.[18] Theoretically, proximal diversion provides better renal drainage than does a vesicostomy, particularly with ureterovesical obstruction, and optimizes the potential for ultimate renal function and somatic growth. However, this form of therapy has not been shown to prevent end-stage renal disease, because at least 85% of these patients have renal dysplasia.[19] In addition, by diverting the urine away from the bladder, regular cyclic vesical-filling and contraction does not occur and results in a smaller, less compliant bladder.[20] Consequently, proximal diversion is reserved for the rare case in which valve ablation or vesicostomy fails to improve upper tract drainage or if urosepsis occurs secondary to pyelonephritis.

Total urinary reconstruction, with valve ablation, ureteroneocystostomy, and excision of large bladder diverticula is another approach to the initial management of the PUV patient. This approach is rarely indicated because often significant improvement is found in reflux and bladder diverticula after ablation of the obstructing valve leaflets.

Urinary Extravasation

A special management issue is urinary extravasation, which occurs in 5% to 10% of newborns with PUV.[21] Forniceal rupture or renal parenchymal blow-out with transperitoneal transudation, or intraperitoneal leakage after bladder rupture may occur. Some have a perirenal urinoma, whereas others have urinary ascites (Fig. 56-5). Significant electrolyte abnormalities may result from urinary reabsorption, and respiratory compromise may occur with ascites. The goals of initial management are to determine the site of extravasation and the level of function of the kidneys.

Evaluation begins with sonography, VCUG, and renal scintigraphy. The early uptake phase of a MAG-3 renal scan often demonstrates which kidney is extravasating.

Inserting a 5F feeding tube into the bladder may decompress the bladder and upper urinary tract pressure sufficiently that the forniceal extravasation stops. If the VCUG shows a bladder rupture, a cutaneous vesicostomy may be necessary. If the urinoma or ascites increases in volume; the serum creatinine continues to increase; or respiratory compromise, infection, hypertension, or significant parenchymal compression is seen, percutaneous aspiration should be performed. If extravasation continues, an upper tract procedure often is necessary. If extravasation from a hydronephrotic kidney occurs, insertion of a percutaneous nephrostomy often solves the problem. Unfortunately, with forniceal extravasation, typically the kidney is decompressed. In these cases, the involved kidney should be explored through a small flank incision. The renal parenchyma should be inspected for evidence of rupture, and the parenchymal disruption should be repaired. In most cases, the kidney will be intact, indicating that the extravasation is from one of the calyceal fornices. A temporary cutaneous pyelostomy or ureterostomy may be performed to decompress the kidney, but in most cases, mobilizing the kidney, separating it from the adjacent peritoneum, and leaving a Penrose drain in the retroperitoneum will solve the problem, provided PUV ablation or a cutaneous vesicostomy has been performed to decompress the lower urinary tract.

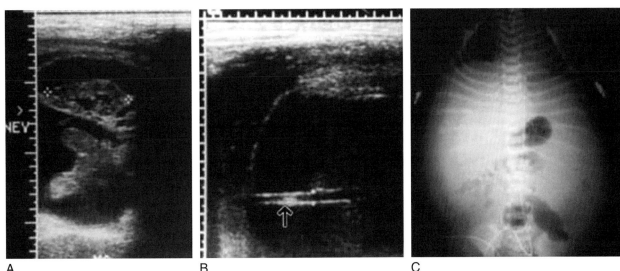

A   B   C

FIGURE 56-5. Posterior urethral valves and ascites. *A,* Antenatal sonogram demonstrating perirenal urinoma around right kidney, which is not hydronephrotic. *B,* Antenatal sonogram showing ascites and stretched umbilical vessels. *C,* Plain film of abdomen in newborn with distended abdomen from ascites.

Follow-up after Initial Therapy

Antibiotic prophylaxis should be continued until upper tract dilation improves, which may take several years. In addition, if the child has reflux, antibiotic prophylaxis should be continued until the reflux resolves spontaneously or is corrected surgically. Most patients benefit from long-term urologic management and nephrologic care initiated at birth. Common clinical problems include significant polyuria secondary to an inability of the kidneys to concentrate urine, metabolic acidosis (which may complicate somatic growth), renal insufficiency with hypocalcemia and hyperphosphatemia, and hypertension. If the patient remains clinically well with good somatic growth, periodic follow-up with US, electrolytes, blood urea nitrogen (BUN), creatinine, urinalysis, and blood pressure evaluations will assure satisfactory growth and development.

PROGNOSIS AFTER INITIAL THERAPY

The prognosis for satisfactory renal function may be predicted from several factors. A serum creatinine less than 0.8 mg/dL 1 month after initial treatment or at age 1 year is associated with favorable ultimate renal function.[22] Others have shown that the serum creatinine level after 4 to 5 days of catheter drainage is most predictive of long-term renal function.[23] Identification of the corticomedullary junction on renal sonography has been associated with a favorable outcome (see Fig. 56-3).[24] This radiologic finding may not be present on the initial US study, but may become apparent during the first few months of life. Achieving diurnal continence by the age of 5 years indicates that minimal or no bladder dysfunction is present and is a favorable parameter.[25] Another favorable prognostic feature is the presence of a pressure pop-off mechanism, such as massive reflux into a nonfunctioning kidney (termed the VURD syndrome: valves, unilateral reflux, dysplasia), urinary ascites, or a large bladder diverticulum (Fig. 56-6).[26] The concept is that the high intravesical pressure is dissipated, allowing more normal renal development. Although short-term studies have suggested that these mechanisms may allow more normal renal development, at age 8 to 10 years, only 30% of boys with the VURD syndrome had a normal serum creatinine.[27] Finally, absence of reflux on the initial VCUG is a favorable sign.

Adverse prognostic factors include bilateral vesicoureteral reflux, persistence of the serum creatinine higher than 1.0 mg/dL after initial therapy, identification of small subcapsular renal cysts (indicative of renal dysplasia), renal echogenicity,[28] and failure to visualize the corticomedullary junction.[24] In addition, failure to achieve diurnal continence is an indication of instability and detrusor sphincter dyssynergia, which can result in elevated upper urinary tract pressures and gradual deterioration in renal function, and is associated with poor renal function.[25]

VESICOSTOMY CLOSURE

The decision to close the cutaneous vesicostomy must be made carefully. If breakthrough febrile urinary tract infections have been noted, vesicostomy closure is important, as it will reduce the risk of bacterial contamination of the urinary tract. In other cases, it may be necessary as a prerequisite to renal transplantation. In most cases, vesicostomy closure is performed after the upper urinary tracts have stabilized and the child is large enough to undergo simultaneous valve ablation, generally between ages 6 months and 3 years. Preoperatively, a VCUG should be obtained through the vesicostomy to assess whether significant vesicoureteral reflux is present and to evaluate the bladder appearance. In selected cases, urodynamics are helpful to assess bladder compliance.[29] If significant reflux is seen and the child is quite young, it is usually safe to simply close the vesicostomy and delay reflux correction until the child is older and the bladder is larger. After closure of the vesicostomy, the upper tracts should be monitored carefully to ascertain whether hydronephrosis is worsening and to be certain that the child is emptying his bladder satisfactorily.

VESICOURETERAL REFLUX

Vesicoureteral reflux is present in approximately 50% of boys with PUV at presentation, with half being bilateral and half unilateral. After valve ablation, nearly all will show improvement in reflux grade 1 year later.[20] Approximately 25% show spontaneous reflux resolution, but reflux may not resolve for as long as 3 years after initial treatment, and resolution of high-grade reflux is unlikely.[30] Antibiotic prophylaxis is continued, and periodic upper tract imaging and cystography should be performed. Renal deterioration without infection may be a sign of bladder dysfunction, and lower tract evaluation with videourodynamics is important.

Reflux should be repaired surgically if breakthrough infections occur or if it remains high grade. Most pediatric urologists are adept at performing ureteral reimplantation surgery, but reimplanting thick, dilated ureters into the abnormal valve bladder can be most challenging, and a 15% to 30% complication rate has been reported, most commonly persistent reflux or ureteral obstruction.[31,32] If bilateral high grade reflux is found, a transureteroureterostomy may be performed in conjunction with a single long tapered reimplant and a psoas hitch. However, if the single reimplanted ureter becomes obstructed, the upper tracts may deteriorate rapidly. If unilateral high-grade reflux into a kidney with reasonable function occurs, transureteroureterostomy into the nonrefluxing ureter is an option.

In boys with the VURD syndrome, a nephrectomy should be performed at some point. The ureter should be removed, unless the bladder is small and/or poorly compliant, in which case, a ureterocystoplasty should be considered (Fig. 56-7). After this procedure, the remaining kidney should be monitored carefully for the development of hydronephrosis, because the pressure "pop off" mechanism has been removed.

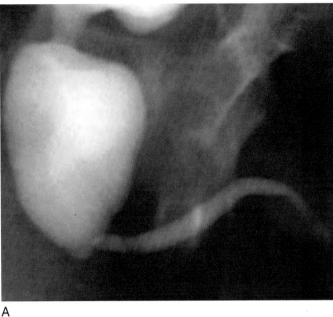

A

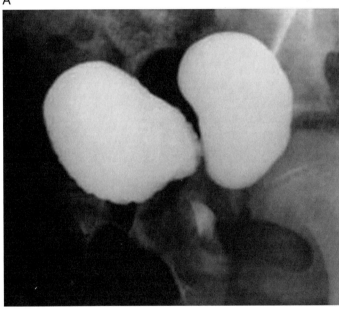

B

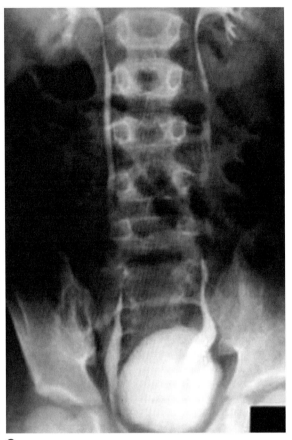

C

FIGURE 56-6. Posterior urethral valves and bladder diverticulum in 7-year-old boy. *A,* Voiding cystourethrogram (VCUG) demonstrating posterior urethral valve with dilated prostatic urethra. *B,* Lateral view of VCUG showing trabeculated bladder on left and large bladder diverticulum on right. *C,* Excretory urogram showing normal upper urinary tracts and deviation of distal left ureter from large bladder diverticulum. Patient underwent endoscopic valve ablation, excision of the bladder diverticulum, and left ureteroneocystostomy.

BLADDER DYSFUNCTION AFTER INITIAL THERAPY

The prognosis for boys with PUV depends on the status of the kidneys and the bladder at the time of diagnosis and the method of bladder management as the child grows. In as many as 40% with PUV, end-stage renal disease or chronic renal insufficiency develops, and the vast majority of these boys have voiding dysfunction.[25] Many boys with PUV have a spectrum of urodynamic abnormalities that change. For example, in a study of 16 prepubertal boys seen before age 1 year and followed up from ages 4 to 14 years,[33] initial bladder instability was observed, but over time, the instability decreased, and the bladder capacity increased. Postpubertal boys had high-capacity bladders with low contractility, causing

difficulties in detrusor emptying. Other groups have reported similar findings.[34-36] The cause of the bladder dysfunction is incompletely understood, but experimental evidence suggests that fetal urethral obstruction causes irreversible changes in the smooth muscle cells of the bladder[37,38] and results in deposition of type III collagen in the bladder wall.[39] The bladder abnormalities are manifested as incontinence or persistent hydronephrosis or both. Boys with significant urodynamic abnormalities are most likely to experience severe renal functional impairment.[40]

As many as half of boys with PUV have ongoing daytime incontinence into late childhood.[25,41] In the past, it was thought that incontinence resulted from sphincteric incompetence from urethral maldevelopment or injury to the sphincter during valve ablation. However, it has

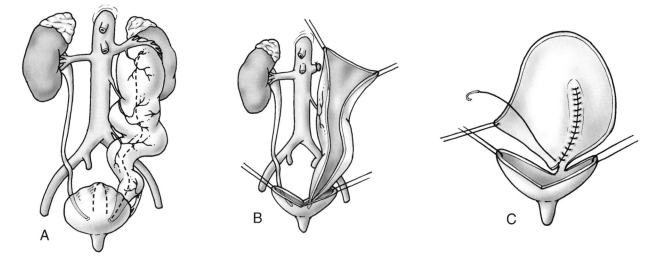

FIGURE 56-7. Technique of ureterocystoplasty. *A,* Left nonfunctioning kidney and ureter exposed. *B,* After left kidney is removed, the ureter is spatulated medially. *C,* Left ureter is folded into a "U" and sutured to opened bladder.

become apparent that significant urodynamic abnormalities may persist after very satisfactory relief of bladder-outlet obstruction.

Several potential causes for urinary incontinence are known in boys with PUV,[34,42] including the following:

1. *Detrusor abnormalities* such as (a) an overactive bladder secondary to uninhibited detrusor contractions, (b) overflow incontinence, (c) poor compliance, and (d) myogenic failure
3. *High-pressure voiding secondary to incomplete valve ablation*
4. *Detrusor-sphincter dyssynergia,* in which the sphincter muscle fails to relax during bladder contraction
5. *Polyuria secondary to a concentrating defect* as a result of long-standing obstructive uropathy that causes renal tubular damage
6. *Valve bladder,* which is a bladder with poor compliance resulting from fibrosis secondary to long-standing obstruction; this clinical situation may cause secondary ureteral obstruction with worsening hydronephrosis if the bladder pressure is greater than 35 cm H_2O pressure. Consequently, long-term therapy for the boy with PUV includes management of the bladder as well as attention to renal function.

THE VALVE BLADDER

An understanding of the pathophysiology of the obstructed bladder allows one to develop an effective therapeutic approach to treatment. Several factors are present in patients with persistent hydroureteronephrosis after valve ablation: (1) the hydroureteronephrosis is associated with a noncompliant thick bladder wall; (2) most

have diurnal incontinence; (3) incontinence is secondary to increased urine output and decreased bladder compliance, (4) acquired diabetes insipidus is the cause of the high urine output, and (5) the high urine output contributes to the hydroureteronephrosis.[42,43]

In 1982 the valve bladder syndrome was described.[44,45] In one series of 70 boys with PUV, 16 had polydipsia, polyuria, incontinence, hydroureteronephrosis without vesicoureteral reflux, poorly sensate bladders, and poorly compliant bladders with high pressure at low urine volumes.[44] Normally the bladder stores urine at low pressure, allowing unimpeded drainage from the kidneys. With a poorly compliant bladder, however, as the bladder fills, the intravesical pressure increases quickly, causing a functional barrier to upper tract drainage, resulting in progressive hydroureteronephrosis. The high intravesical pressure contributes to the gradual deterioration in renal function.

The spectrum of physiologic abnormalities in boys with the valve bladder syndrome is shown in Table 56-1. The obstructed kidney often develops an irreversible urinary concentrating defect secondary to tubular injury. Despite fluid restriction, an obligate enormous urine output may be seen, as high as 3 L/day. This polyuria causes decompensation of the bladder, incontinence, and persistent back-pressure on the upper urinary tracts, with persistent hydroureteronephrosis.

Persistent ureteral dilation causes inefficient ureteral wall coaptation and poor peristalsis, which predisposes to UTI. Fibrosis from previous infection or previous ureteral surgery may result in inefficient ureteral peristalsis and increases the risk of obstruction after ureteral reimplantation. In the past, persistent hydroureteronephrosis was thought to result from ureterovesical junction obstruction. Upper tract pressure/volume (Whitaker test) studies with the bladder

TABLE 56-1		
PATHOPHYSIOLOGIC CHANGES IN THE VALVE BLADDER SYNDROME		
Organ	**Pathology**	**Clinical Effect**
Kidney	Dysplasia, renal tubular dysfunction	Poor renal function; polyuria
	Urine concentrating defect (polyuria)	Rapid filling of bladder, causing persistent hydroureteronephrosis and incontinence
	Renal tubular acidosis	Impaired somatic growth, bone demineralization
Ureters	Dilated with poor peristalsis	Large dead space
		Increased risk of urinary tract infection
	Fibrosis secondary to previous surgical procedures or infection	Poor drainage of upper tract
		Possible obstruction after ureteral reimplantation
Bladder	Poor compliance; small volume	High bladder pressure most of the time
	Reduced sensation to high pressure	Progressive renal functional damage
		Incontinence
	Myogenic failure	Progressive renal and bladder damage
Bladder neck	Hypertrophy	Poor bladder emptying
		Voiding dysfunction
		Incontinence

From Close CE: The valve bladder. In Gillenwater JY, Grayhack JT, Howards SS, et al (eds): Adult and Pediatric Urology, 4th ed. Philadelphia, Lippincott Williams & Wilkins, 2002, pp 2311–2318.

empty and full have demonstrated that in the vast majority of cases, unimpeded drainage into the bladder occurred with the bladder empty. As the bladder filled, with increasing intravesical pressure, increasing hydroureteronephrosis and increasing renal pelvic pressure were found.[44] Consequently, ureteral reimplantation in these patients with the goal of relieving ureterovesical junction obstruction has a high risk of failure, with worsening hydronephrosis. In a recent series of 71 boys with valves, persistent hydroureteronephrosis was noted in 20 (28%), in 32 renal units.[46] All of the patients with persistent hydroureteronephrosis had abnormal urodynamic findings, primarily poor compliance and instability, and aggressive treatment showed dramatic improvement or complete resolution of upper tract changes and urodynamic parameters.

Boys with a poorly compliant or unstable bladder often tolerate high intravesical pressures without discomfort. As a result, they delay voiding and experience overflow incontinence. Because of the high intravesical pressure, ongoing renal functional damage occurs. In addition, polyuria causes volume stress and contributes to chronic overdistention of the bladder. Effective bladder emptying is difficult to accomplish because of poor detrusor function and rapid refilling of the bladder. Double or triple voiding often is necessary to empty the bladder and the upper tracts, but compliance with this regimen often is not very good.

Bladder neck hypertrophy is a component of the overall detrusor hypertrophy that results from bladder outlet obstruction. After valve ablation, significant residual muscular hypertrophy may persist, resulting in functional bladder-outlet obstruction with poor emptying. In the past, Y-V plasty of the bladder neck was performed, but incontinence and upper tract changes persisted because the aforementioned factors. In addition, a late complication of this procedure is retrograde ejaculation. Consequently, bladder neck surgery should be avoided unless urodynamic and radiographic documentation of intractable bladder neck obstruction is found.

Can the Valve Bladder be Prevented?

Several clinical observations allow one to formulate a treatment plan to try to minimize the risk of developing a valve bladder. One factor relates to the primary form of therapy. In many boys with PUV, severe hydroureteronephrosis and an elevated serum creatinine are present. In the past, it was thought that performing cutaneous pyelostomies in the most severe cases would result in optimal upper tract decompression and give the kidneys the best chance of having unimpeded drainage. Indeed, evidence was found that these boys had better somatic growth compared with boys who underwent valve ablation alone.[18] However, it is difficult to document any case in which cutaneous pyelostomies have prevented end-stage renal disease. In addition, it became apparent that boys with proximal diversion ultimately had a small bladder that required augmentation cystoplasty, whereas after valve ablation or cutaneous vesicostomy, the bladder typically grows satisfactorily, presumably because of urinary growth factors and ongoing cycling of the bladder.[20,47–49]

Management of Bladder Dysfunction

Close follow-up is important after valve ablation.[43] A VCUG should be performed to document that bladder-outlet obstruction has been relieved. Serial renal sonograms and serum creatinine and electrolytes are necessary. Renal scintigraphy is necessary if evidence is noted of renal dysfunction on either side. If vesicoureteral reflux is present, serial VCUGs are necessary until reflux is minimal or absent. Urodynamic evaluation is important with persistent hydroureteronephrosis to confirm that resting and filling bladder pressures are in a safe range, less than 30 cm H_2O. Furthermore, detrusor instability or hypocontractility can be documented.[47] In addition, uroflowmetry and sonographic assessment of postvoid residual urine volume are helpful. Having these patients followed up by a pediatric nephrologist is invaluable, as renal tubular acidosis, renal insufficiency, end-stage renal disease, and somatic growth abnormalities are common.

If significant polyuria and incontinence are found, timed voiding every 1 to 2 hours is beneficial. In addition, double or triple voiding provides more efficient emptying of the bladder and upper urinary tracts.

If a poorly functioning or nonfunctioning hydronephrotic kidney is noted, nephrectomy or nephroureterectomy should be performed. Generally this procedure can be performed laparoscopically. Before proceeding, however, the potential need for lower urinary tract reconstruction should be assessed, because the dilated ureter may be used to augment the bladder.[50] This augmentation procedure can be incorporated into the overall reconstruction.

If urodynamic studies demonstrate detrusor instability, anticholinergic therapy is necessary. Several medications may be used. Oxybutynin chloride suspension or tablets are effective but may cause side effects such as dry mouth, facial flushing, constipation, and blurring. The medication lasts 4 to 6 hours, and generally is administered 3 times daily. The maximum dosage is 1 mg per year of age, 3 times daily, with a maximum of 5 mg, 3 times daily. Sublingual hyoscyamine also may be effective, with fewer side effects than oxybutynin, and is given 4 times daily. In recent years, tolterodine has been useful in children older than 6 years, given in doses of 1 to 2 mg twice daily. Tolterodine has fewer side effects than oxybutynin chloride.

If bladder hypocontractility is present, clean intermittent catheterization usually is necessary. Learning this procedure initially may be difficult for boys and their families, but with persistence and support from the medical team, most adapt to intermittent catheterization, particularly if it improves or cures their incontinence. The procedure tends to reduce bladder instability and improve bladder compliance.[51] In some cases, a continent appendicovesicostomy (Mitrofanoff procedure) must be performed to allow intermittent catheterization with less patient discomfort.

If detrusor-sphincter dyssynergia with inadequate bladder neck relaxation is present, treatment with an α-adrenergic blocker may be beneficial. In a study of 55 children with a variety of causes of non-neuropathic voiding dysfunction, administration of doxazosin, 0.5 mg to 2.0 mg daily, resulted in a significant improvement in urine flow rate, reduction in postvoid residual urine volume, and improvement in incontinence.[52] Few had significant side effects.

An important recent concept is that some of the changes that result in the valve bladder syndrome result from bladder overdistention at night, secondary to polyuria and failure to empty the bladder regularly during sleep.

To address this issue, overnight catheter drainage has been used with moderate success, resulting in significant improvement in hydroureteronephrosis and improved voiding dynamics during the day.[53,54] This therapy should be strongly considered in boys with valve bladder syndrome.

If urodynamic studies demonstrate a poorly compliant or small-capacity bladder or both, then augmentation cystoplasty is necessary. This procedure may alter voiding dynamics, and adding a noncontractile patch to the bladder in a boy who is emptying satisfactorily may result in a situation in which clean intermittent catheterization should be performed. In one series of boys with PUV who underwent ureterocystoplasty, most patients had to perform intermittent catheterization after operation.[50] Consequently, creation of a "back-up" continent stoma (appendicovesicostomy) in conjunction with augmentation cystoplasty should be considered.

Several options exist for augmentation cystoplasty. Ureterocystoplasty results in the fewest long-term complications; a dilated ureter is a prerequisite for this procedure (see Fig. 56-7). Ureterocystoplasty generally is performed in conjunction with removal of a nonfunctioning kidney, and in these cases, the entire ureter can be used to augment the bladder. If both kidneys have satisfactory function, another option is to use the lower half of the dilated ureter for bladder augmentation and to perform a proximal transureteroureterostomy. The ureter is opened on its medial border through the ureterovesical junction. If the dilated ureter is long, then it may be folded onto itself in the shape of a "U" and sutured to the opened bladder. If a dilated ureter is unavailable or the bladder needs more significant augmentation, then ileocystoplasty is the best option, assuming renal function is relatively normal. Electrolyte abnormalities from absorption through the small bowel patch are uncommon. However, a generous amount of mucus is produced, and regular bladder irrigation is necessary to prevent bladder calculi. Other potential long-term complications include chronic or recurrent bacteriuria and spontaneous bladder perforation from chronic overdistention. If renal function is limited, gastrocystoplasty should be considered. The advantage of this procedure is that the gastric patch secretes the hydrogen ion, and metabolic acidosis can be reversed or improved with the operation. In addition, unlike small bowel, the patch is not absorptive. Furthermore, because the pH of the urine is low, the risk of UTI is reduced. The disadvantages of gastrocystoplasty include the need to extend the incision superiorly to the xiphoid process and the risks of severe metabolic alkalosis. In addition, some experience the hematuria/dysuria syndrome, characterized by intermittent severe dysuria and hematuria.[55] Furthermore, if the child has incontinence, a significant chance exists that they will experience a burning sensation where the urine leaks. Despite these potential problems, however, the long-term results with gastrocystoplasty are favorable.[56,57] Another option in patients with limited renal function is to augment the bladder with a patch of both ileum and stomach (gastroileocystoplasty), which avoids most of the problems associated with gastrocystoplasty.[58]

RENAL TRANSPLANTATION

Despite optimal management of boys with PUV, in 30% to 40%, end-stage renal disease develops.[25] In many cases, impaired renal function can be stabilized during childhood, but during adolescence, insufficient renal reserve is found, and dialysis or renal transplantation becomes necessary. Retrospective studies of boys with PUV undergoing renal transplantation have suggested that the valve bladder may have a detrimental effect on graft survival. For example, in one study, a significantly poorer 5-year graft survival was noted for patients undergoing transplantation for valve-related renal failure than was found in patients with nonobstructive abnormalities.[59] Others demonstrated favorable allograft survival but elevated serum creatinine levels in transplanted valve patients.[60] Other recent studies, however, demonstrated no difference in graft survival or serum creatinine levels between boys with PUV and children with nonobstructive causes of renal failure.[61,62] These data suggest that with intensive management of bladder function, a favorable long-term outcome can be expected. Indeed, in 44 valve patients followed up for a mean of 9 years after renal transplantation, the serum creatinine in boys with symptoms of bladder dysfunction was significantly higher than that in those without a valve bladder.[60]

FERTILITY

Few long-term studies exist of reproductive status of men who were born with PUV. Theoretically, prostate function might be affected because of elevated urethral pressure during embryonic development, as well as ongoing voiding dysfunction. In addition, some boys with PUV also undergo orchiopexy for cryptorchidism, which is associated with reduced fertility. Finally, in the past, some men have undergone Y-V plasty of the bladder neck, which results in retrograde ejaculation. In one study of eight adolescents, sperm count was satisfactory in five, but most had abnormal sperm agglutination and a higher percentage of immotile sperm.[63] Three of the eight failed to ejaculate. In another study of 10 men, sperm counts were within the fertile range in all, but only 3 had initiated pregnancies.[64]

REFERENCES

1. Dewan PA, Zappala PG, Ransley PG, et al: Endoscopic reappraisal of the morphology of congenital obstruction of the posterior urethra. Br J Urol 70:439, 1992.
2. Elder JS: Management of antenatally diagnosed hydronephrosis. In Puri P (ed): Newborn Surgery, 2nd ed. London, Arnold Publishers, 2003, pp 793–808.
3. Hutton KAR, Thomas DFM, Arthur RJM, et al: Prenatally detected posterior urethral valves: Is gestational age at detection a predictor of outcome? J Urol 152:698, 1994.
4. Landers S, Hanson TN: Pulmonary problems associated with congenital renal malformations. In Gonzalez ET, Roth DR (eds): Common Problems in Pediatric Urology. Houston, MosbyYear Book, 1990, p 85.
5. Elder JS, Duckett JW, Snyder HM: Intervention for fetal obstructive uropathy: Has it been effective? Lancet 2:1007, 1987.
6. Johnson MP, Bukowski TP, Reitleman C, et al: In utero surgical treatment of fetal obstructive uropathy: A new comprehensive approach to identify appropriate candidates for vesicoamniotic shunt therapy. Am J Obstet Gynecol 170:1770, 1994.
7. Johnson MP, Corsi P, Bradfield W, et al: Sequential urinalysis improves evaluation of fetal renal function in obstructive uropathy. Am J Obstet Gynecol 173:59, 1995.
8. Holmes N, Harrison MR, Baskin LS: Fetal surgery for posterior urethral valves: Long-term postnatal outcomes. Pediatrics 108:E7, 2001.
9. Quintero RA, Romero R, Johnson MP, et al: In utero percutaneous cystoscopy in the management of fetal lower obstructive uropathy. Lancet 346:537, 1995.
10. Quintero RA, Shukla AR, Homsy YL, et al: Successful in utero endoscopic ablation of posterior urethral valves: A new dimension in fetal urology. Urology 55:774, 2000.
11. Freedman AL, Bukowski TP, Smith CA, et al: Fetal therapy for obstructive uropathy: Specific outcomes diagnosis. J Urol 156:720, 1996.
12. Cendron M, Elder JS: Perinatal urology. In Gillenwater JY, Grayhack JT, Howards SS, et al (eds): Adult and Pediatric Urology, 4th ed. Philadelphia, Lippincott Williams & Wilkins, 2002, pp 2041–2127.
13. Gibbons MD, Horan JJ, Dejter SW, et al: Extracorporeal membrane oxygenation: An adjunct in the management of the neonate with severe respiratory distress and congenital urinary tract anomalies. J Urol 150:434, 1993.
14. Shapiro E, Elder JS: Complications of surgery for posterior urethral valves. In Taneja SS, Smith RB, Ehrlich RM (eds): Complications of Urologic Surgery, 3rd ed. Philadelphia, WB Saunders, 2001, pp 552–563.
15. Bhatnagar V, Agarwala S, Lal R, et al: Fulguration of posterior urethral valves using the Nd:YAG laser. Pediatr Surg Int 16:69, 2000.
16. Zaontz MR, Firlit CF: Percutaneous antegrade ablation of posterior urethral valves in infants with small-caliber urethras: An alternative to urinary diversion. J Urol 136:247, 1986.
17. Walker RD, Padron M: The management of posterior urethral valves by initial vesicostomy and delayed valve ablation. J Urol 144:1212, 1990.
18. Krueger RP, Hardy BE, Churchill BM: Growth in boys with posterior urethral valves: Primary valve resection vs. upper tract diversion. Urol Clin North Am 7:265, 1980.
19. Tietjen DN, Gloor JM, Husmann DA: Proximal urinary diversion in the management of posterior urethral valves: Is it necessary? J Urol 158:1008, 1997.
20. Close CE, Carr MC, Burns MW, et al: Lower urinary tract changes after early valve ablation in neonates and infants: Is early diversion warranted? J Urol 157:984, 1997.
21. Patil KK, Wilcox DT, Samuel M, et al: Management of urinary extravasation in 18 boys with posterior urethral valves. J Urol 169:1508, 2003.
22. Smith GHH, Canning DA, Schulman SL, et al: The long-term outcome of posterior urethral valves treated with primary valve ablation and observation. J Urol 155:1730, 1996.
23. Denes ED, Barthold JS, Gonzalez R: Early prognostic value of serum creatinine levels in children with posterior urethral valves. J Urol 157:1441, 1997.
24. Hulbert WC, Rosenberg HK, Cartwright PC, et al: The predictive value of ultrasonography in evaluation of infants with posterior urethral valves. J Urol 148:122, 1992.
25. Parkhouse HF, Barratt TM, Dillon MJ, et al: Long-term status of patients with posterior urethral valves. Urol Clin North Am 17:373, 1990.
26. Kaefer M, Keating MA, Adams MC, et al: Posterior urethral valves, pressure pop offs and bladder function. J Urol 154:708, 1995.
27. Cuckow PM, Dinneen MD, Risdon RA, et al: Long-term renal function in the posterior urethral valves, unilateral reflux and renal dysplasia syndrome. J Urol 158:1004, 1997.
28. Duel BP, Mogbo K, Barhold JS, et al: Prognostic value of initial renal ultrasound in patients with posterior urethral valves. J Urol 160:1198, 1998.
29. DeBadiola FIP, Denes ED, Ruiz E, et al: New application of the gastrostomy button for clinical and urodynamic evaluation before vesicostomy closure. J Urol 156:618, 1996.

30. Hassan JM, Pope JC IV, Brock JW III, et al: Vesicoureteral reflux in patients with posterior urethral valves. J Urol 170:1677, 2003.
31. Warshaw BL, Hymes LC, Trulock TS, et al: Prognostic features in infants with obstructive uropathy due to posterior urethral valves. J Urol 133:240, 1985.
32. El-Sherbiny MT, Hafez AT, Ghoneim MA, et al: Ureteroneocystostomy in children with posterior urethral valves: Indications and outcome. J Urol 168:1836, 2002.
33. Holmdahl G, Sillén U, Hanson E, et al: Bladder dysfunction in boys with posterior urethral valves before and after puberty. J Urol 155:694, 1996.
34. Peters CA, Bolkier M, Bauer SB, et al: The urodynamic consequences of posterior urethral valves. J Urol 144:122, 1990.
35. De Gennaro MMG, Capitanucci ML, Mosiello P, et al: The changing urodynamic pattern from infancy to adolescence in boys with posterior urethral valves. Br J Urol 85:1104, 2000.
36. Emir H, Eroglu E, Tekant G, et al: Urodynamic findings of posterior urethral valve patients. Eur J Pediatr Surg 12:38, 2002.
37. Karim OM, Cendron M, Mostwin JL, et al: Developmental alterations in the fetal lamb bladder subjected to partial urethral obstruction in utero. J Urol 150:1060, 1993.
38. Karim OM, Seki N, Pienta KJ, et al: The effect of age on the response of the detrusor to intracellular mechanical stimulus: DNA replication and the cell actin matrix. J Cell Biochem 48:373, 1992.
39. Peters CA: Congenital bladder obstruction. Probl Urol 8:333, 1994.
40. Ghanem MA, Wolffenbuttel KP, de Vylder A, et al: Long term bladder dysfunction and renal function in boys with posterior urethral valves on the basis of urodynamic findings. J Urol 2004 (in press).
41. Churchill BM, McLorie GA, Khoury AE, et al: Emergency treatment and long-term follow-up of posterior urethral valves. Urol Clin North Am 17:343, 1990.
42. Glassberg KL, Schneider M, Haller JO, et al: Observations on persistently dilated ureter after posterior urethral valve ablation. Urology 20:20, 1982.
43. Glassberg KL: The valve bladder syndrome: 20 years later. J Urol 166:1406, 2001.
44. Mitchell ME: Persistent ureteral dilatation following valve resection. Dial Pediatr Urol 5:8, 1982.
45. Close CE: The valve bladder. In Gillenwater JY, Grayhack JT, Howards SS, et al (eds): Adult and Pediatric Urology, 4th ed. Philadelphia, Lippincott Williams & Wilkins, 2002, pp 2311–2318.
46. Donohoe JM, Weinstein RP, Combs AJ, et al: When can persistent hydroureteronephrosis in posterior urethral valve disease be considered residual stretching? J Urol 2004 (in press).
47. Kim YH, Horowitz M, Combs AJ, et al: Posterior urethral valves: The management of unilateral poorly functioning kidneys in patients with posterior urethral valves. J Urol 158:1001, 1997.
48. Farhat W, McLorie G, Capolicchia G, et al: Outcomes of primary valve ablation versus urinary tract diversion in patients with posterior urethral valves. Urology 56:653, 2002.
49. Podesta M, Ruarte AC, Garguilo C, et al: Bladder function associated with posterior urethral valves after primary valve ablation or proximal urinary diversion in children and adolescents. J Urol 168:1830, 2002.
50. Churchill BM, Aliabadi H, Landau EH, et al: Ureteral bladder augmentation. J Urol 150:716, 1993.
51. Holmdahl G, Sillen U, Hellstrom AL, et al: Does treatment with clean intermittent catheterization in boys with posterior urethral valves affect bladder and renal function? J Urol 170:1681, 2003.
52. Cain MP, Wu SD, Austin PF, et al: Alpha blocker therapy for children with dysfunctional voiding and urinary retention. J Urol 1770:1514, 2003.
53. Koff SA, Mutabagani KH, Jayanthi VR: The valve bladder syndrome: Pathophysiology and treatment with nocturnal bladder emptying. J Urol 167:291, 2002.
54. Montane B, Abitbol C, Seeherunvong W, et al: Beneficial effects of continuous overnight catheter drainage in children with polyuric renal failure. BJU Int 92:447, 2003.
55. Chadwick Plaire J, Snodgrass WT, Grady RW, et al: Long-term follow up of the hematuria-dysuria syndrome. J Urol 164:921, 2000.
56. Kurzrock EA, Baskin LS, Kogan BA: Gastrocystoplasty: Long-term follow up. J Urol 160:2182, 1998.
57. DeFoor W, Minevich E, Reeves D, et al: Gastrocystoplasty: Long-term follow up. J Urol 170:1647, 2003.
58. Austin PF, Lockhart JL, Bissada NK, et al: Multi-institutional experience with the gastrointestinal composite reservoir. J Urol 165:2018, 2001.
59. Reinberg Y, Gonzalez R, Fryd D: The outcome of renal transplantation on children with posterior urethral valves. J Urol 140:1491, 1988.
60. Salomon L, Fontaine E, Gagnadoux M-F, et al: Posterior urethral valves: Long-term renal function consequence after transplantation. J Urol 157:992, 1997.
61. Indudhara R, Joseph DB, Perez LM, et al: Renal transplantation in children with posterior urethral valves revisited: A 10-year follow-up. J Urol 160:1201, 1998.
62. DeFoor W, Tackett L, Minevich E, et al: Successful renal transplantation in children with posterior urethral valves. J Urol 170:2402, 2003.
63. Puri A, Gaur KK, Kumar A, et al: Semen analysis in post-pubertal patients with posterior urethral valves: A pilot study. Pediatr Surg Int 18:140, 2002.
64. Woodhouse CR, Reilly JM, Bahadur G: Sexual function and fertility in patients treated for posterior urethral valves. J Urol 142:586, 1989.

CHAPTER 57

Bladder and Cloacal Exstrophy

Dominic Frimberger, MD, and John P. Gearhart, MD

BLADDER EXSTROPHY/EPISPADIAS

The bladder exstrophy/epispadias complex in the newborn child has a wide range of presentations. The defect can be as minor as a glanular epispadias or as devastating as cloacal exstrophy with a multitude of affected organs. Despite the magnitude of the defect, infants born with classic bladder exstrophy are surprisingly robust at birth. Nevertheless, the immediate transfer of the neonate to a major children's center is crucial to ensure proper initial assessment and optimal management. Equally important is the reassurance of the parents, especially if the condition has not been diagnosed prenatally and comes as a surprise. Modern management of bladder exstrophy is a team approach of several disciplines, including pediatric urologists, orthopedists, anesthesiologists, psychiatrists, researchers, nurses, child life experts, social workers, and the active exstrophy groups.

This dedicated teamwork turned a malformation that was considered futile until the middle of 20th century into a manageable problem. Today patients and their families can expect a secure closure and functional and cosmetically acceptable outer genitalia with the preservation of renal function. Moreover, most patients will achieve urinary continence, and even successful pregnancies with vaginal deliveries have been reported.

Incidence

Bladder exstrophy is a rare and complex urogenital malformation with an incidence that varies between 1:10,000 and 1:50,000 live births, affecting boys 5 to 6 times more often than girls.[1,2] Epispadias and cloacal exstrophy are far less common, with rates of 1:100,000 and 1:200,000 to 400,000, respectively.[3,4] The possible genetic predisposition of exstrophy is supported by the increased rate of 1:275 births for parents with an affected child to conceive another child with the epispadias/exstrophy complex. Additionally, an exstrophic mother has about 500 times the risk of bearing a child with exstrophy.[5] The inheritance risk for cloacal exstrophy is unknown because none of the patients has reproduced. These numbers are based on studies before the introduction of modern reproductive technology. Exstrophy females have always had normal fertility, but the males have, for the most part, been infertile. Advanced reproductive technologies will possibly increase the incidence of malformations, because a sevenfold increase in exstrophy and cloacal exstrophy associated with intracytoplasmic sperm injection has been observed.[6]

Embryology

In normal development, mesodermal ingrowth between the ectoderm and endodermal layers of the bilaminar cloacal membrane results in formation of the lower abdominal musculature and pelvic bones. After mesenchymal ingrowth occurs, downward growth of the rectal septum divides the cloaca into a bladder anteriorly and a rectum posteriorly. The genital tubercles migrate medially and fuse in the midline cephalad to the dorsal membrane before it perforates.

Several theories have been formulated to explain the embryonic developments of the bladder exstrophy complex. Studies on chicks suggested an abnormal overdevelopment of the cloacal membrane subsequently preventing medial migration of the mesenchymal tissue and later proper abdominal wall development. The nonreinforced membrane ruptures causing the different severity of exstrophy depending on the location of the membrane defect.[7]

Embryologic studies on rats describe an abnormal caudal insertion of the body stalk, with failure of the interposition of the mesenchymal tissue in the midline.[8] As a consequence of this failure, translocation of the cloaca into the depths of the abdominal cavity does not occur.

Anatomic Malformations

The malformation is characterized by an open abdominal wall, bladder, and urethra and a wide diastases of the symphysis pubis, caused by a 30% bony deficit of the anterior pubic rami in combination with a 12-degree and 18-degree external rotation of the posterior and anterior aspect of the pelvis, respectively.[9] The subsequent malrotation of the pubic bones results in a 131% increase in the distance between the triradiate cartilages.

Recent new data using three-dimensional computerized tomography demonstrated an uneven 70% to 30% posterior to anterior distribution of the levator muscle groups in the exstrophic pelvis compared with that of normal children.[10,11] Additionally the transverse diameter of the levator hiatus is 2 times larger and the length 1.3 times greater, respectively. Significant flattening occurs between the right and left halves of the levator ani and puborectalis sling. Moreover, the obturator internus and externus muscles are more outwardly rotated. These anatomic malformations cause a more anterior/superior rotation of the pelvic floor. Subsequently the anus is anteriorly placed and sometimes patulous as part of the posterior extent of the myofascial defect. These musculoskeletal malformations explain the increased rate of rectal and uterine prolapse in the female exstrophy population.

Inguinal hernias are reported in up to 82% of boys and 11% of girls with the exstrophy complex, presumably caused by a lack of obliquity of the inguinal canal combined with large internal and external inguinal rings.[12] Because up to 53% of patients will first be seen with an incarcerated hernia within the first year after primary closure, exploration of the inguinal canal at the time of exstrophy closure should be performed.

Girls are first seen with a bifid clitoris and a short vagina with an anteriorly displaced orifice, whereas in boys, a 50% shortening of the anterior corpora cavernosa and an upward deviation of the penis occur.[13] Therefore the general mean penile length of 3.5 cm at term cannot be reached; however, erectile function is almost always intact.[14] The scrotum is usually normally developed, although the testes are often located in the distal inguinal canal.

The upper urinary tract is usually normally developed. However, the lower parts of the ureters have a more lateral course in the true pelvis and enter the bladder with little or no obliquity, resulting in ureteral reflux in almost all cases.

Newborn bladder exstrophy patients have an increased ratio of collagen to smooth muscle in the bladder and a reduced number of myelinated nerves in the bladder muscle, which normalize after successful closure.[15,16] Additionally, the intracellular organelles in the bladder smooth muscle of exstrophy patients exhibit a significant difference from normal bladder muscle. These abnormalities were more severe in patients who did not develop an adequate bladder capacity after initial closure.[17]

Anatomically, cloacal exstrophy consists of the foreshortened hindgut or cecum, which displays its bulging mucosa between the two hemibladders. The orifices of the terminal ileum, the rudimentary tailgut, and a single or paired appendices are apparent on the surface of the everted cecum. The tailgut ends blindly, and the ileum is usually prolapsed. The phallus is typically separated into a right and left half, with adjacent scrotum or labia. Occasionally, the penis is together in the midline, but the structure is frequently diminutive and the corporal

bodies small. The bony pelvis is characterized by a mean interpubic diastasis of 8 cm in comparison to the 0.5 cm in normal children. The anterior segment length of the pubic bone is 37% shorter, and the ischiopubic angle as well as the angle of the iliac wing is markedly increased, resulting in the extreme amount of external rotation.[9]

Unlike classic bladder exstrophy or epispadias, cloacal exstrophy is characterized by a series of associated conditions in other organ systems.[9] Upper urinary tract anomalies are observed in up to one third of patients. These include pelvic kidney, renal agenesis, hydronephrosis, hydroureter, and ureteral orifice ectopia.[18] Other anomalies include spinal dysraphism,[19] duplication or agenesis of the vagina, undescended testis,[20] and skeletal, gastrointestinal, and cardiovascular anomalies.

Diagnosis

Cloacal exstrophy is often diagnosed on prenatal ultrasonography (US), whereas classic bladder exstrophy is rarely diagnosed in utero despite the magnitude of the defect. Bladder exstrophy may be suspected on prenatal US by the absence of bladder filling on repeated examinations, a low-set umbilicus, widening of the pubis ramus, diminutive genitalia, and a lower abdominal mass that increases in size throughout the pregnancy.[21,22]

Postnatal Management

If exstrophy is suspected prenatally, arrangements should be made for the mother to deliver the child in a specialized center to ensure immediate postnatal evaluation and reconstruction. However, if the diagnosis is made at delivery, the child should be immediately transferred to an experienced pediatric center, because the ultimate functional result is significantly improved by appropriate initial management. The parents should be reassured that although their child will need extensive reconstruction, the child is expected to lead a relatively normal life.

After delivery, the delicate bladder mucosa must be protected until the bladder is closed to prevent metaplasia and the formation of polyps. Sterile saline irrigations and application of a plastic wrap, repeated with every diaper change, is preferred to moistened or petroleum-coated gauze. Additionally the umbilical cord should be ligated with a strong silk suture rather than clamped to avoid mucosal abrasion. General pediatric and cardiopulmonary assessment is important before initial closure in the first 48 hours of life. A US study of the kidneys is performed to rule out hydronephrosis, and a radionucleotide scan is added if abnormalities are seen.

The fragile mucosa as well as detrusor function is best preserved by closing the bladder in the newborn period. However, the size and the functional capacity of the detrusor muscle are important considerations for the outcome. Therefore in the rare presence of a small, fibrotic bladder patch without elasticity or contractility, the operation should be deferred until adequate growth of the bladder template occurs. If sufficient size is not reached

4 to 6 months after birth, alternative options for urinary diversion should be considered.

Surgical Reconstruction

Before the first successful primary closure of a female exstrophy patient in 1942, bladder exstrophy was treated primarily by covering the defect with skin flaps.[1] Although other reports of primary closures were published in the same era, the numbers were small, and results were not favorable. In the early 1970s, two reports of successful staged reconstruction set the standard for modern exstrophy treatment today.[23,24] Although other forms of repair have been promoted, the primary principles in surgical management have remained the same since. These include a secure, initial abdominal closure, the reconstruction of functional and cosmetically satisfactory external genitalia, and the achievement of urinary continence while preserving renal function.

The technique includes bladder, posterior urethra, and abdominal wall closure in the newborn period, usually with pelvic osteotomy. Epispadias repair is performed at about age 6 months to increase outlet resistance and promote bladder growth. When adequate bladder capacity is reached and the child is mature enough to participate in a postoperative voiding program (usually at 5 to 6 years) a competent bladder neck is created along with bilateral ureteral reimplantation. This approach provides the most favorable reported outcomes over long-term follow-up in treatment of children with this complex malformation.

Recently, complete repair in the newborn combining bladder closure with epispadias repair has been promoted to reduce the number of operations required and to attempt to improve functional results.[25] The complete penile disassembly technique for epispadias repair can leave the patient with residual hypospadias, necessitating later repair. Additionally, several cases have been reported with partial or complete loss of the urethral plate or penile skin and even corporal necrosis.[26] As a result of increased bladder outflow resistance at birth, 50% of children treated with one-stage neonatal repair will develop urinary breakthrough infections despite antibiotic prophylaxis, which will necessitate ureteral reimplantation in the first year of life. Because long-term follow-up data are not yet available on patients treated in this manner, it is not clear whether the children will require continence procedures in the future. It is our opinion that exstrophy closure should be combined with epispadias repair only in very selected cases in which a good urethral plate and reasonable bladder template coexist. The single-stage repair is appropriate for delayed primary closure and reoperative exstrophy cases.

Other reported techniques include simultaneous bladder closure, ureteral reimplantation, epispadias repair, and bladder neck reconstruction without osteotomies either in the newborn period or in older children.[27] Bladder closure with later bladder neck reconstruction and epispadias repair also has been described.[28] Another completely different approach is the creation of an ureterosigmoidostomy combined with bladder and abdominal wall closure as a single procedure.[29] Long-term complications of ureterosigmoidostomy include pyelonephritis, hypercalemic metabolic acidosis, ureteral obstruction, and the late development of colonic malignancy.

Although all of these approaches have merit and supporters, the quality and size of the bladder template, appropriate patient selection, and experience of the surgeon and supporting staff will ultimately determine the outcome in a particular child.

Surgical Considerations

Successful initial bladder and posterior urethral closure is the most important factor for achieving urinary continence and sufficient bladder capacity.[30] The primary objective in initial, functional closure is to convert the bladder exstrophy into a complete epispadias with incontinence, increasing outlet resistance that stimulates bladder growth but preserves renal function.

Pelvic osteotomy performed at the time of initial closure is recommended for a variety of reasons:

1. It aids in tension-free approximation of the bladder, posterior urethra, and abdominal wall.
2. It allows placement of the vesicourethral complex deep within the pelvic ring to enhance bladder-outlet resistance.
3. It provides alignment of the large pelvic floor muscles to support the bladder neck.

Osteotomies are usually not necessary in the patient younger than 72 hours who has malleable pubic bones that are easily brought together in the midline by medial rotation of the greater trochanters. However, if the pubic bones are more than 4 cm apart or in cases in which it seems unlikely to achieve a tension-free closure, osteotomies are essential to prevent dehiscence or bladder prolapse.[31]

Care must be taken to create a latex-free operative environment, because many children with bladder exstrophy are prone to latex allergies. Perioperative broad-spectrum antibiotics also are administered.

Osteotomy

The most widespread pelvic osteotomy used today is the bilateral transverse innominate and vertical iliac osteotomy done from an anterior approach, dividing the innominate bone above the acetabulum[32] (Fig. 57-1).

The patient is placed in a supine position, preparing and draping the lower body below the costal margins, and placing soft absorbent gauze over the exposed bladder. An incision is made at the junction of the trunk and the legs, and both sides of the innominate bone are exposed simultaneously. Horizontal osteotomies are performed by using a Gigli saw. The osteotomy extends from 5 mm above the anterior inferior iliac spine to the most cranial part of the sciatic notch. Bilateral iliac osteotomies are performed at the same time by using an osteotome and leaving the posterior iliac cortex intact and used as a hinge, giving the pelvis a better contour and mobility.

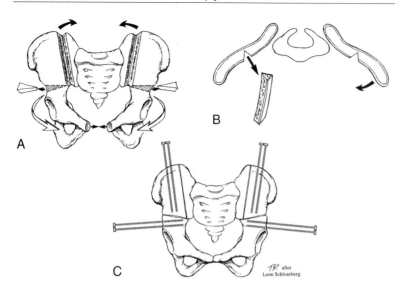

FIGURE 57-1. Combined transverse anterior innominate and anterior vertical iliac osteotomies with pin placement and preservation of the posterior periosteum and cortex. (Drawings by Timothy Phelps after Leon Schlossberg. Reproduced with permission of the Brady Urological Institute.)

Because the infant is already in the supine position and prepared, the bladder closure can begin immediately (Fig. 57-2, 57-1C). Pins for the external fixating device are inserted after the bladder is closed but before the wound closure. Two fixator pins are placed in the inferior osteotomized segment, and two pins are placed in the wing of the ileum superiorly. Radiographs are obtained to confirm pin placement. This approach provides improved symphyseal approximation, making the midline closure easier and decreasing the likelihood of dehiscence.

In girls, the mons and external genitalia are reconstructed at time of initial exstrophy closure. The bifid clitoris is denuded medially and brought together in the midline, along with labia minora reconstruction, creating a fourchette.

Postoperative Care after Initial Closure

Successful primary closure is dependent on proper postoperative care from experienced physician and nursing staff. Bladder prolapse and dehiscence have been associated with urethral catheters, abdominal distention, infection, and poor nutrition.[33] Favorable postoperative outcomes, conversely, were found associated with the use of osteotomy and pelvic immobilization, avoidance of urethral tubes, use of postoperative antibiotics, ureteral stenting, and maintaining patient comfort.[30] The modern application of continuous caudal catheter anesthesia allows continuous pain control for up to 2 postoperative weeks. Radiographs are taken 7 to 10 days after operation. If the diastasis has not been completely reduced, the right and left sides can be gradually approximated by using the fixator bars for several days. Light longitudinal Buck's skin traction is used to keep the legs still. The patient remains immobilized and supine in traction for approximately 4 weeks to prevent dislodgment of tubes

and destabilization of the pelvis. The external fixator is kept in place for approximately 6 weeks or until adequate callus is seen at the site of osteotomy. The pins are removed under light sedation at the bedside. Postoperatively, newborns undergoing closure without osteotomy are immobilized in modified Bryant traction for 4 weeks with the hips in 90 degrees of flexion. Most centers use some form of postreconstruction immobilization to improve the likelihood of successful closure.[34-37] Recent data confirmed the high success rates with the use of external fixation and postoperative traction, whereas the use of spica casts or mummy wraps was associated with multiple failures of the closure and lower extremity complications.[38]

Four weeks after closure, the residual urine is estimated by clamping the suprapubic tube, and a urine culture is obtained before the child leaves the hospital. US is performed to assess the status of the upper tracts and is repeated regularly. The bladder outlet and urethra are calibrated with a sound or catheter, and if adequate and residual urines are low, the suprapubic tube is removed.

Epispadias Repair

The immature urogenital tract of the exstrophic child does not experience any form of outflow resistance until the initial closure is performed. With closure of only the bladder and the posterior urethra at birth, the bladder can mature and gradually adjust to its new outflow properties. This allows growth of the bladder without risk to the upper tracts. After a period of 6 to 12 months, the urogenital tract adjusts to the new circumstances and is ready for a further increase in outflow resistance. The next step in promoting bladder growth is to repair the epispadias, which has been shown to increase the bladder capacity in boys by a mean of 54.5 mL within 24 months.[39] Similar observations have been made in patients with complete male epispadias, in which a large increase in bladder capacity is noted after epispadias repair.

Epispadias repair is carried out between ages 6 and 12 months. To stimulate penile skin growth, preoperative intramuscular testosterone is given. Epispadias repair is done not only to increase outflow resistance, but also to reconstruct a functional and cosmetically satisfactory penis.

The five goals of epispadias repair include

1. Achievement of optimal penile length
2. Correction of dorsal chordee
3. Reconstruction of the penile urethra
4. Reconstruction of the glans penis
5. Suitable skin coverage.

Penile lengthening is a key component in initial bladder exstrophy closure and is done best at the time of initial exstrophy closure. Techniques for achieving penile length vary, but all have in common the release of corporal tissue from the inferior pubic ramus, preservation of the neurovascular bundles, and achievement of maximal urethral length.

In the complete penile disassembly technique, the urethral plate is dissected from the corporal bodies, rolled into a tube, passed between the corpora to the ventral surface of the penis, and brought as close to the tip of the penis as possible.[40] Initial reports of a small series using this technique have been favorable.[41] However, in some of the patients, when the urethral plate is totally dissected from the glans, it will not reach the tip of the penis, leaving the hypospadias to be repaired later.[25,26] This problem is avoided in the modified Cantwell-Ransley repair (Fig. 57-3) by leaving the very distal part of the urethra attached to the glans. Considering the 50% shortage in penile length between exstrophy patients and normal boys,[13] it is our opinion that the slight extra length obtained is not worth sacrificing the urethral plate and making the child into a hypospadiac.

Postoperative Care after Epispadias Repair

A stent is left from the bladder lumen to beyond the tip of the penis, sutured in place so that the bladder is continuously drained. A plastic occlusive dressing is formed around the penis. Antibiotic coverage is continued until the stent is removed 10 to 12 days after the operation. The patient is placed in double diapers, and the plastic occlusive dressing is left intact until it falls off by itself. Preoperative placement of a caudal epidural catheter and oxybutynin administration will reduce postoperative pain and bladder spasms. It is critical to control pain and bladder spasms to prevent urine extravasation that may result in fistula formation. At time of discharge, the parents are instructed in wound and stent care and supplied with oral broad-spectrum antibiotics, oral pain medications, and antispasmodics. By hydrating the child well, urine output is enhanced, reducing the possibility of occlusion of the stent. If urine flow through the stent stops, immediate treatment is crucial to prevent fistula formation.

Bladder Neck Reconstruction

The next and final step in the reconstruction is the performance of the continence procedure. We use a modified Young-Dees-Leadbetter procedure (Fig. 57-4) After epispadias repair, yearly gravity cystograms under anesthesia are performed to obtain reliable information about bladder capacity and ureteral reflux. Follow-up studies on a large patient population have determined that an adequate bladder capacity of at least 85 mL is needed for successful bladder neck reconstruction.[42] If the bladder does not achieve the desired minimal capacity after epispadias repair, injecting a bulking agent around the bladder neck or augmentation cystoplasty should be considered.

In addition to the anatomic requirements of the bladder, it is crucial that the patient has the desire to be dry and is old enough to cooperate with toilet training. The child should be prepared for the upcoming operation and its consequences by using the support of child life specialists. Even if the parents are maximally motivated to proceed with the reconstruction, the level of enthusiasm of the child is essential. Therefore it is mandatory for the surgeon to talk with the child personally before the operation to be convinced that the child is ready.

Finally, because nearly all of these children exhibit vesicoureteral reflux, an antireflux procedure is performed at the time of bladder neck repair.

Postoperative Management after Continence and Reflux Procedures

The patient is given broad-spectrum antibiotics and intravenous (IV) fluids until normal oral intake has resumed. The ureteral stents are removed after 2 weeks. At 3 weeks, the suprapubic tube is clamped intermittently to initiate a voiding trial. Intense psychological support from parents, physicians, child life specialist, and nursing staff is required at this time because the child may be afraid to void for the first time voluntarily through the urethra. Initially the tube should not be clamped for more than 1 hour at a time and should be left to closed drainage overnight. Once the child is emptying the bladder satisfactorily, the suprapubic tube is removed.

If the child cannot or will not void after clamping the suprapubic tube, a Foley catheter is placed under anesthesia by using cystoscopic guidance if necessary. The catheter is then left in place for 5 days, at which point another voiding trial is attempted. Children failing repeated voiding trials are typically placed on intermittent catheterization. In some cases, these patients may have adequate storage capacity but are unable to initiate bladder contractions sufficient for voiding.

Frequent bladder and renal US studies are obtained in the first few months after bladder neck reconstruction to ensure adequate emptying and to observe the status of the upper tracts. If hydronephrosis is observed, the cause is either ureterovesical junction obstruction or high voiding pressures. Urodynamics and a MAG III renal scan with furosemide (Lasix) will aid in determining the correct etiology.

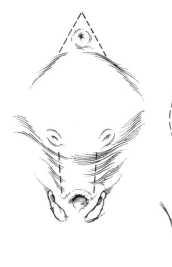
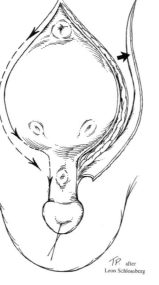
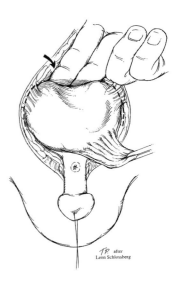

A

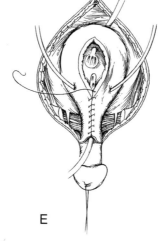
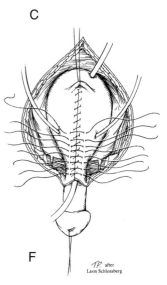

B

C

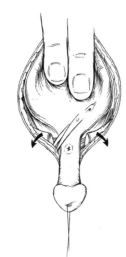
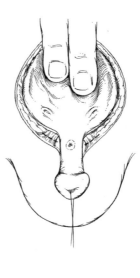

D

E

F

G

FIGURE 57-2. Bladder, posterior urethral, and abdominal wall closure. *A,* An incision is made outlining the bladder mucosa, the prostatic plate, and the proximal urethra. The urethral groove is dissected to beyond the verumontanum. In the staged approach, it is no longer necessary to free the corpora extensively or dissect them completely in the midline because of our preference for later epispadias repair, as described in the modified Cantwell-Ransley approach. If the urethral plate is left in continuity, it must be mobilized up to the level of the prostate to create as much urethral and penile length as possible. *B,* Apparent penile lengthening is achieved by exposing the corpora cavernosa bilaterally and freeing the corpora from their attachments to the suspensory ligaments. The urethra in the female patient can be very short but does not require lengthening at the time of initial bladder closure. By cutting the hymeneal ring at 3 and 9 o'clock, an additional 1/2 cm of urethral length can be obtained. *C,* The umbilical vessels are doubly ligated, divided, and used for traction. The bladder muscle is freed from the rectus sheath on each side. The peritoneum is dissected from the dome of the bladder to allow the bladder to be sunken deep into the pelvis at the time of closure. *D,* Dissection is carried distally along the border between the bladder and the rectus sheaths down to the level of the urogenital diaphragm fibers. These fibers are incised sharply, and the diaphragm is detached subperiosteally from the pubis bilaterally. This dissection must be carried onto the inferior ramus and taken laterally and caudally down to the level of the levator hiatus to allow the bladder neck and posterior urethra the mobility to fall deeply within the pelvic ring. A double-pronged skin hook can be inserted into the pelvic bone and pulled laterally to accentuate the urogenital diaphragm fibers. If this maneuver is not performed adequately, the vesicourethral unit will be displaced anteriorly with pelvic closure, an unsatisfactory position for later reconstruction. *E,* The mucosa and muscle of the bladder are closed in the midline. The urethra is closed out onto the penis so it can easily accommodate a 12 to 14 sound. This allows enough resistance to stimulate bladder growth and prevent bladder prolapse but not enough to cause upper tract changes. *F,* The posterior urethra and bladder neck are reinforced with a second layer of local tissue if possible. The bladder is drained by a suprapubic Malecot catheter. The urethra is not stented. The ureters, however, are stented to prevent obstruction from edema. *G,* By applying gentle pressure over the greater trochanters bilaterally, the pubic bones are approximated in the midline. Horizontal mattress sutures using no. 2 nylon are placed in the pubis, with the knot directed away from the urethra. A second suture is placed caudal to the insertion of the rectus fascia, if possible, for added support. A simple umbilicoplasty is performed with a V-shaped flap, and the drainage tubes are brought out through this site. (Drawings by Timothy Phelps after Leon Schlossberg. Reproduced with permission of Brady Urological Institute.)

Suppressive antibiotics are continued until complete bladder emptying is achieved. In some patients, recurrent infections will become a problem. Even if bladder emptying is adequate, long-term antibiotic suppression is recommended. The bladder should be carefully monitored to ensure progress over time as the bladder function improves. Postoperative inflammation and edema may result in a diminished bladder capacity at first. Patients are not familiar with the sensation of bladder filling or the need for detrusor contraction. Several months for adjustment are often required before a reasonable dry interval can be developed. The chance for success can be predicted if an early dry interval of 10 to 15 minutes occurs with the absence of stress incontinence or continuous dribbling or both.

Combined Bladder Exstrophy and Epispadias Repair

Newborn exstrophy closure can be combined with epispadias repair. However, as mentioned earlier, this approach requires good phallic length, a deep urethral groove, and an adequate amount of penile skin.[25,26,43] This technique should be attempted only by an experienced exstrophy surgeon, as the complications can be severe.[26] One of the best applications of combined exstrophy and epispadias repair is in the patient undergoing delayed primary closure or reoperative exstrophy closure.[44] The technique of combining bladder exstrophy closure and urethral repair was originally described in the 1960s[45] but did not gain widespread use because of the high rate of complications and poor results. In 1991,

combined bladder closure and epispadias repair for failed bladder exstrophy closure was described,[45] and in 1999, was reported in a group of boys undergoing single-stage reconstruction of bladder closure and epispadias repair in infancy.[26] Recent data on 35 patients who had combined bladder and epispadias repair for failed prior exstrophy repair demonstrated only a 50% continence rate without diversion. Additionally the majority of patients required ureteric reimplantation and further surgical procedures to the penis or urethra.[46]

Surgical Technique of Combined Closure

The combined closure of bladder exstrophy and epispadias repair is very similar to the beginning of the closure of bladder exstrophy and posterior urethra alone. Evaluation of the bladder template is performed by everting the bladder into the abdomen with a sterile gloved finger to determine the extent of the bladder plate. In children outside the newborn period, preoperative testosterone enanthate is used to enhance penile size and increase the availability of local penile skin.

The operative procedure begins and proceeds as with the standard initial closure described earlier (see Figs. 57-1 and 57-2), with only a few differences. In failed closure cases, great care must be used to divide any remnants of the urogenital diaphragm fibers that were left behind after the initial closure. Very often these fibers are found to be intact.

After adequate dissection of the bladder and posterior urethra, attention is given to the dissection of the penis, corporal bodies, and urethral plate, as described earlier

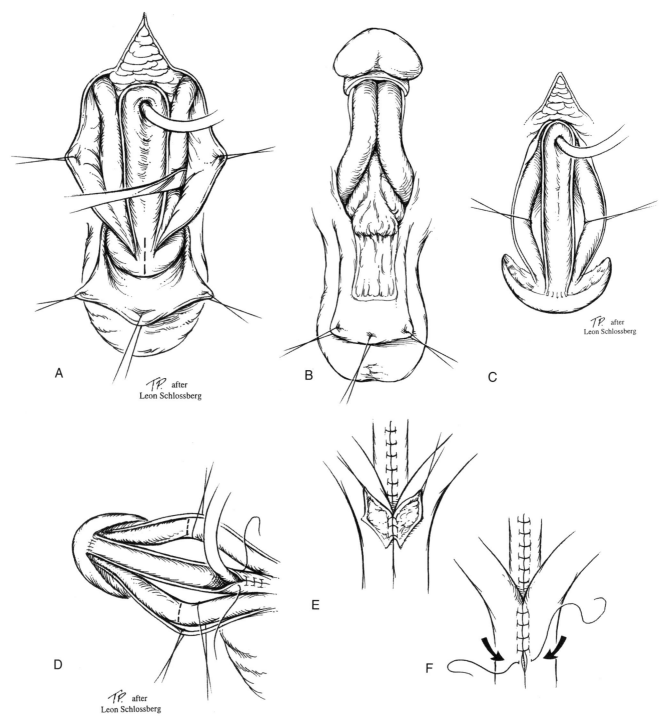

FIGURE 57-3. Modified Cantwell-Ransley repair. *A,* A traction suture is placed through the ventral glans. The urethra is created by outlining an 18-mm-wide strip of urethral plate from proximal to the functioning meatus outward to the corona. As the plate is inscribed distally, it becomes somewhat narrower. A deep vertical incision (*dashed line*) is made in the distal urethral plate, which will later be closed transversely with 6-0 polyglycolic sutures. This has the effect of widening the distal urethra. *B,* A circumcising incision is made in the lateral and ventral skin, which is dissected to the level of the scrotum on the ventral side of the penis. The ventral mesentery between the corpora is left intact for the blood supply of the urethral plate. *C,* The distal urethra is widened and advanced to the tip of the penis by closure of the longitudinal incision in a transverse manner. The urethral plate is mobilized and undermined. The neurovascular bundles, situated between Buck's fascia and the corporal bodies, can be visualized and protected throughout the procedure. Thick glanular wings are developed sharply off the corpora, and triangular mucosal areas are excised for later glansplasty. At the dorsal base of the phallus, a Z-plasty skin incision is performed to release any tension and to prevent scarring. Suspensory ligaments may be divided to gain extra penile length. Dissection of the urethral plate is continued from the ventral side of the penis. By dissecting on Buck's fascia, the plane is followed in a circumferential fashion between the spongiosum and the cavernosum toward the dorsal side. The dissections from the dorsal and ventral sides are joined. *D,* Vessel loops are passed around each neurovascular bundle and each of the corpora. The urethra is formed by tubularizing the urethral plate with a continuous absorbable suture over an 8F polyglycolic acid (Silastic) stent. If necessary, the corpora may be lengthened by small transverse incisions (*dashed lines*) that will be closed longitudinally. *E, F,* After the urethra is completed, the corpora are brought together over the urethra. If the corpora were incised to provide length, the incisions are closed longitudinally by joining the right and left corpora.

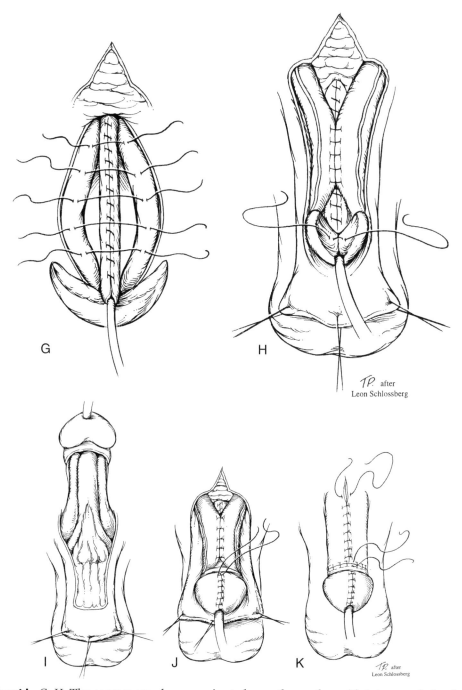

G   H

TP. after
Leon Schlossberg

I   J   K

TP. after
Leon Schlossberg

FIGURE 57-3, Cont'd, *G–H,* The corpora may be approximated over the urethra with interrupted absorbable sutures. *I–K,* The glansplasty is completed with absorbable suture, and the penile skin closed as shown. (Drawings by Timothy Phelps after Leon Schlossberg. Reproduced with permission of the Brady Urological Institute.)

(see Fig. 57-3). It is important that the corporal bodies not be brought over the urethra until the pelvic bones are approximated. This allows rotation of the corpora medially and creates less tension on the corpora in the midline. If the child is older than 1 year, the fixator pins placed after osteotomy may be used to assist with rotating the pelvis into place. In younger children, the lack of ossified bones prohibits this maneuver. A small oblique

drain is placed next to the bladder closure, and abdominal wall closure is completed. An 8F polymeric silicone (Silastic) stent is left in the urethra for 2 weeks. The external fixating device is then attached to intrafragmentary pins and tightened. External fixation of the pelvis is maintained for 4 weeks in children undergoing primary closure and for 6 to 8 weeks for those undergoing reclosure of the bladder. Follow-up is very much the same

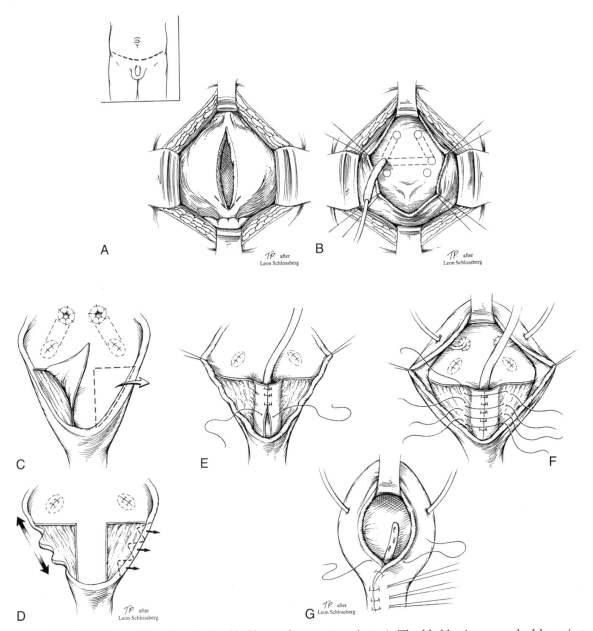

FIGURE 57-4. Modified Young- Dees- Leadbetter bladder neck reconstruction. *A,* The bladder is approached by using a lower transverse abdominal incision. A vertical vesicotomy is made with lateral extensions (*dashed lines*) at its lower end, which will narrow the bladder neck at the completion of the procedure. *B,* Reimplantation of ureters can be done in a transtrigonal or cephalotrigonal fashion. If necessary, the ureterovesical junction can be located more cephalad in combination with a high cross trigonal reimplantation if it appears that transtrigonal reimplantation will obstruct the elongated bladder neck. *C,* Bladder neck reconstruction is begun by outlining a posterior mucosal strip 15 to 18 mm wide × 3 cm in length, which extends from the midtrigone to the prostate and posterior urethra. *D,* The bladder muscle lateral to the mucosal strip is denuded of mucosa. Sponges, soaked in 1:200,000 epinephrine, are applied to control bleeding for better visualization. A transverse, full-thickness muscular incision is not performed, as described in the original Young-Dees-Leadbetter procedure, because significant risk exists of denervation and ischemia for the bladder neck. *E,* The mucosal strip is formed into a tube by using interrupted sutures of 4-0 polyglycolic acid. *F,* Denuded mucosal flaps are overlapped and sutured with 3-0 polydioxanone sutures to reinforce the neobladder neck. *G,* Two to three of the overlapping sutures are left long and brought through the rectus fascia and are tied as bladder suspension to elevate the bladder neck. Reconstruction is performed over an 8F urethral catheter, which is removed at the end of the procedure. The bladder is drained with a suprapubic Malecot catheter. It is essential that the bladder neck be dissected completely free from the surrounding structures. This allows suspension of the bladder neck to the anterior fascia. Often it is advantageous to split the symphyseal bar to enhance visualization. The bar is simply closed at the end of the procedure with heavy sutures of polydioxanone. Mobility should be restricted in the postoperative period to allow healing. (Drawings by Timothy Phelps after Leon Schlossberg. Reproduced with permission from the Brady Urological Institute.)

as that in standard exstrophy closure with monitoring residual urine and upper tract imaging by US before suprapubic tube removal. Although some of our patients have achieved long-term continence after the procedure, most ultimately required bladder neck reconstruction to become dry.

Overall Results after Bladder Exstrophy Repair

The overall outcome after bladder exstrophy repair has improved remarkably during the last three decades. The standard treatment of exstrophy worldwide has evolved from urinary diversion to functional reconstruction in almost all cases.[23–28,34–37] Favorable overall long-term outcome depends on the success of all phases of surgical reconstruction. The importance of a successful initial closure cannot be overemphasized, and the closure should be performed in centers with a large experience.

Continence is correctly defined as being dry for more than 3 hours. Socially continent patients achieve that goal during the day but have bed-wetting incidents at night.[1] With presently available techniques, continence rates can be expected to be as high as 75% to 80% with preservation of renal function, as documented in several large series.[42,47–49] In our current database of 748 patients with bladder exstrophy/epispadias and cloacal complex, we analyzed 65 patients with bladder exstrophy. All of those patients were entirely treated at our institution from birth by staged functional closure. Complete day and night continence in this group was 77%, with 91% being socially dry.[42] The functional and cosmetic outcomes of the genital reconstruction are of equally high quality, with a very low rate of urethrocutaneous fistula and a very acceptable cosmetic appearance.[50] Additionally, most postpubertal patients reported satisfactory sexual function.[51]

Not all patients are candidates for immediate postnatal reconstruction. In patients with insufficient bladder template size at birth, primary closure should be delayed to permit growth of the bladder to an adequate size. In a series of 19 such patients seen at our institution, primary closure was delayed and performed at a mean age of 13 months.[52] Nine of them became dry and voided normally after bladder neck reconstruction, and 4 are currently awaiting the procedure. Four others perform intermittent catheterization; one has required a colon conduit; and one, a ureterosigmoidostomy.

CLOACAL EXSTROPHY

The severity of cloacal exstrophy is enhanced by the nature and severity of the associated anomalies. Many of these infants are premature, small for gestational age, and have such severe associated anomalies that it is difficult for them to undergo an extensive procedure in the newborn period. However, the authors' preference is a one-stage closure if the infant is in excellent condition, has favorable anatomy, and has minimal associated anomalies.[1]

During either a one-stage or two-stage procedure, the omphalocele is excised, and the bowel is separated from the bladder halves. The lateral vesicointestinal fissure is closed in continuity, and a short colostomy is created from the end of the distal colon segment. The hemibladders then are reapproximated in the midline to create a single exstrophic bladder. If a one-stage procedure is selected, the entire bladder is closed completely after a bilateral anterior innominate osteotomy, and vertical iliac osteotomy is performed. The anterior approach allows the placement of pins for external fixation and is preferred when severe lumbosacral dysraphism is present. With a large omphalocele defect, bladder closure and osteotomy may be delayed until respiratory and gastrointestinal stability is achieved.

Sexual conversion into a female sex of rearing is part of the treatment algorithm in all genotypic boys with the cloacal exstrophy syndrome. However, any decision concerning gender reassignment must occur after consultation from multiple disciplines and total parental input. Recent reports from two major centers are at odds concerning long-term outcomes of these gender-reassigned patients.[53,54]

Surgical Management

Formerly, surgical reconstruction of cloacal exstrophy was considered futile, and untreated neonates usually died of prematurity, sepsis, short-bowel syndrome, or renal and central nervous system deficits.[55] When the importance of separating the genitourinary tract from the gastrointestinal tract became apparent, survival increased. Follow-up of the first patient known to have survived surgical reconstruction of cloacal exstrophy was reported in 1984.[56] After early reconstructive efforts, the patient was left with two stomata: one to collect urine and the other to collect stool. Because survival is no longer the major issue, achieving a good quality of life is now the greatest challenge facing these patients.[57]

Management of the Bowel in Cloacal Exstrophy

The principles guiding the management of the bowel in cloacal exstrophy are to conserve all bowel segments, to minimize fluid and electrolyte loss, and to maximize nutritional potential. Formerly, patients died of fluid and electrolyte loss with a short bowel and terminal ileostomy. Early total parenteral nutrition will help these infants to grow, thus reducing the later problems of short-gut syndrome.[57] Careful preservation of the hindgut segment is important because this segment can enlarge considerably if used initially as a fecal colostomy. Additionally, the enlarged hindgut later can be used as a bladder augmentation or vaginal replacement if nutritional circumstances allow.[58]

A recent series reported some patients able to have stool continence by enema washout through a perineal opening.[57] Candidates for a perineal colostomy must have few, if any, neurologic deficits, a good pelvic floor as assessed by magnetic resonance imaging (MRI), along with adequate nerve response to stimulation and enough colonic length for solid stool to be formed. Finally, every effort must be expended to save both of the appendiceal structures for later continent stoma construction if needed.

Management of the Phallic Structures and Vagina

In boys with cloacal exstrophy, the penis is usually represented by two rudimentary widely separated small phallic structures. In the rare instance with adequate corporal tissue, epispadias repair can be performed at the time of initial closure, or later, depending on the situation.

If the female gender of rearing is chosen, the medial aspects of the bifid phallus are denuded of mucosa and brought together in the midline. If there is a single phallic structure in the midline (20% of patients), the urethral plate is dissected and passed between the corporal bodies to the perineum for a urethral opening. The corpora and glans are then recessed for more appropriate female appearance, and the labial folds are created from the scrotum by a posterior Y-V plasty. Correction of genital anomalies in girls is usually done at the time of bladder closure and osteotomy. The medial aspect of the hemiclitoris is denuded of mucosa, and the halves are brought together with 5-0 polyglactic acid suture (Vicryl) for the subcutaneous layer and fine 6-0 Vicryl for the epithelial layer. Commonly, duplicate vaginas are far apart and on opposite sides of the pelvis. The ostia of the vaginas may be difficult to find at the time of the initial closure, and the surgeon should be aware that they may be located on the posterior wall of the bladder. It is acceptable to leave the vaginas in situ, but further procedures will be needed to bring one of these to the perineum.

In the genotypic male patient raised as a female, the vagina is usually created at the time of puberty. In the past, vaginas have been created by anatomic "scraps," such as portions of duplicated bowel, an unneeded dilated ureter, or a few centimeters of the distal colonic segment. Therefore it is probably better to wait until puberty and construct a vagina from intestine or from a free full-thickness skin graft.

Reconstruction of the Lower Urinary Tract

The bladder closure is performed much as that of classic bladder exstrophy described earlier. Care must be taken when the bowel is separated from the bladder halves to avoid damage to the blood supply of the bowel mesentery and the autonomic vesical innervation, which becomes exposed at the medial aspect of the hemibladder. In girls, a double vagina may complicate closure of the urethra. If possible, the vaginas are joined and positioned posteriorly, and the tissue on the anteromedial aspect is tubularized to form a urethra. If this tissue is unavailable, then local tissues are used to form a urethral channel. As mentioned previously, in the genotypic male patient raised as a girl, the urethral plate is raised from the corpora, much as in the initial part of a Cantwell-Ransley repair, and then brought between the corpora as a perineal urethra. Drainage of the urinary tract is accomplished by ureteral stents and suprapubic catheter all exiting from the abdomen. No urethral stent or catheter is used, allowing free incontinent drainage of urine through the urethra.

Osteotomy is performed in all patients with cloacal exstrophy. Whereas complications occurred in 89% of patients closed without osteotomy (dehiscence, vesicocutaneous fistula, and prolapse), problems were observed in only 16% in the osteotomy group.[59] The goal of the osteotomy is to achieve tension-free approximation of the widely separated pubic bones and of the anterior abdominal wall.[60] Anterior osteotomy also provides large cancellous surfaces with good healing potential. Furthermore, in cases of extreme pubic diastasis, combined anterior innominate and posterior osteotomy may be done within the periosteum through the same skin incision for better correction.[9] Immobilization is provided by an external fixator and modified Bryant's traction or Buck's traction for 4 to 6 weeks.

Personal Experience with Achieving Continence in the Cloacal Exstrophy Patient

In our personal series of 37 patients with cloacal exstrophy, 21 have undergone continence procedures. Four patients underwent Young-Dees-Leadbetter (YDL) bladder neck plasty only; 1 patient had bladder neck suspension; 3 had YDL plasty and with bladder augmentation; 4 had YDL plasty, augmentation, and the creation of a continent abdominal stoma; and 9 had closure of the bladder neck, augmentation, and creation of a continent abdominal stoma. The upper tracts remain normal in 35 patients. Four patients required revision of their continent stomas owing to catheterization difficulties. One patient required injection of collagen into the reconstructed bladder neck, and one patient who had both bladder neck reconstruction and bladder augmentation underwent reoperation with bladder neck closure and ileal continent stoma for failure to achieve continence. Overall, 18 of 21 patients experience daytime continence, whereas 17 of 21 also are dry at night. Nineteen are on a clean intermittent catheterization (CIC) regimen, and two are voiding spontaneously.[57]

The management of cloacal exstrophy has improved to provide a better quality of life for these children. Complete reconstruction in the newborn period demonstrated the best outcome data if the infant's condition allows. Improvements in neurologic evaluation have served to reduce life-threatening complications and the progression of neurologic deficits. Advances in surgical technique and postoperative management allow the achievement of urinary continence in most children. Current information is insufficient to make an informative decision about optimal gender assignment in patients with XY chromosomes and cloacal exstrophy. Advances in tissue engineering and stem cell research may allow congruent rearing of male patients with cloacal exstrophy.[62,63] Further long-term research is mandatory to continue progress in the treatment of these interesting children.

REFERENCES

1. Gearhart JP: The bladder exstrophy-epispadias-cloacal exstrophy complex. In Gearhart JP, Rink RC, Mouriquand PDE (eds): Pediatric Urology. Philadelphia, WB Saunders, 2001, pp 511–546.
2. Clementson Kockum C, Hansson E, Stenberg A, et al: Bladder exstrophy in Sweden: A long term follow-up study. Eur J Pediatr Surg 6:208, 1996.

3. Dees JE: Congenital epispadias with incontinence. J Urol 62:513–522, 1949.
4. Woodhouse CRJ: Sexual function in boys with exstrophy, myelomeningocele and micropenis. Urology 52:3, 1998.
5. Shapiro E, Lepor H, Jeffs RD: The inheritance of classic bladder exstrophy. J Urol 132:308, 1984.
6. Woodhouse CR: Prospects for fertility in patients born with genitourinary anomalies. J Urol 165:2354–2360, 2001.
7. Marshall VF, Muecke C: Congenital abnormalities of the bladder. In Handbuch der Urologie. New York, Springer Verlag, 1968, p 165.
8. Mildenberger H, Lkuth D, Dziuba M: Embryology of bladder exstrophy. J Pediatr Surg 23:116, 1988.
9. Sponseller PD, Bisson LJ, Gearhart JP, et al: The anatomy of the pelvis in the exstrophy complex. J Bone Joint Surg Am 77:177–189, 1995.
10. Stec AA, Pannu HK, Tadros YE, et al: Pelvic floor anatomy in classic bladder exstrophy using 3-dimensional computerized tomography: Initial insights. J Urol 166:1444, 2001.
11. Stec AA, Pannu HK, Tadros YE, et al: Evaluation of the bony pelvis in classic bladder exstrophy by using 3D-CT: Further insights. Urology 58:1030, 2001.
12. Connolly JA, Peppas DS, Jeffs RD, et al: Prevalence and repair of inguinal hernias in children with bladder exstrophy. J Urol 154:1995.
13. Silver RI, Partin AW, Epstein JI, et al: Penile length in adulthood after bladder exstrophy reconstruction. J Urol 158:999, 1997.
14. Feldman KW, Smith DW: Fetal phallic growth and penile standards for newborn males. J Pediatr 86:395–398, 1975.
15. Lee BR, Pearlman EJ, Partin AW, et al: Evaluation of smooth-muscle and collagen subtypes in normal newborns and those born with bladder exstrophy. J Urol 156:2034–2036, 1996.
16. Mathews RI, Wills M, Pearlman E, et al: Neural innervation of the newborn exstrophy of the bladder: An immunohistological study. J Urol 162:506–508, 1999.
17. Gearhart et al: J Urol (In press).
18. Diamond DA: Management of cloacal exstrophy. Dial Pediatr Urol 13:2, 1954.
19. McLaughlin KP, Rink RC, Kalsbeck JE, et al: Cloacal exstrophy: The neurological implications. J Urol 154:782–784, 1995.
20. Howell C, Caldamone A, Snyder H, et al: Optimal management of cloacal exstrophy. J Pediatr Surg 18:365–369, 1983.
21. Hurwitz RS, Manzoni GA, Ransley PG, et al: Cloacal exstrophy: A report of 34 cases. J Urol 138:1060, 1987.
22. Gearhart JP, Ben-Chaim J, Jeffs RD: Criteria for the prenatal diagnosis of classic bladder exstrophy. Obstet Gynecol 85:961–964, 1995.
23. Jaffe R, Schoenfeld A, Ovadia J: Sonographic findings in the prenatal diagnosis of bladder exstrophy. Am J Obstet Gynecol 162:675–678, 1990.
24. Jeffs RD, Charrios R, Mnay M, Juransz AR: Primary closure of the exstrophied bladder. In Scott B(ed): Current Controversies in Urologic Management. Philadelphia, WB Saunders, 1972, p 235.
25. Cendron J: La reconstruction vesicale. Ann Chir Infant 12:371, 1971.
26. Grady R, Mitchell ME: Complete repair of bladder exstrophy. J Urol 162:1415–1420, 1999.
27. Schrott KM: Komplette einzeitige Aufbauplastik der Blasenekstrophie. In Schreiter F (ed): Plastisch- Rekonstruktive Chirurgie in der Urologie. Stuttgart: Georg Thieme- Verlag, 1999, pp 430–438.
28. Baka-Jakubiak M: Combined bladder neck, urethral and penile reconstruction in boys with exstrophy-epispadias complex. BJU Int 86:513–518, 2000.
29. Stein R, Fisch M, Black P, et al: Strategies for reconstruction of unsuccessful or unsatisfactory primary treatment of patients with bladder exstrophy or incontinent epispadias. J Urol 161:1934–1941, 1999.
30. Gearhart JP, Ben-Chaim J, Scortino C, et al: The multiple reoperative bladder exstrophy closure: What affects potential to the bladder? Urology 47:240–243, 1996.
31. Gearhart JP: Complete repair of bladder exstrophy in the newborn: Complications and management. J Urol 165:2431–2433, 2001.
32. Gearhart JP, Forsher DC, Jeffs RD, et al: A combined vertical and horizontal pelvic osteotomy for primary and secondary repair of bladder exstrophy. J Urol 155:689–693, 1996.
33. Duckett JW: Use of paraexstrophy skin pedicle grafts for correction of exstrophy and epispadias repair. Birth Defects 13:171, 1977.
34. Husmann DA, McLorie GA, Churchill BM: Closure of the exstrophic bladder: An evaluation of the factors leading to its success and its importance on urinary continence. J Urol 142:522–524, 1989.
35. Hafez AT, Elsherbiny MT, Ghoneim MA: Complete repair of bladder exstrophy: Preliminary experience with neonates and children with failed initial closure. J Urol 165:2428–2430, 2001.
36. Kajbafzadeh AM, Quinn FM, Ransley PG: Radical single stage reconstruction in failed exstrophy. J Urol 154:86,1995.
37. Chiari G, Avolio L, Bragheri R: Bilateral anterior pubic osteotomy in bladder exstrophy repair: Report of increasing success. Pediatr Surg Int 17:160–163, 2001.
38. Aadalen RJ, O'Phelan EH, Chisholm TC, et al: Exstrophy of the bladder: Long-term results of bilateral posterior iliac osteotomies and two stage anatomic repair. Clin Orthop 151:193–200, 1980.
39. Meldrum KK, Gearhart JP: Methods of pelvic immobilization following bladder exstrophy closure: Associated complications and impact on surgical success: Presented at the 2nd International Symposium on Exstrophy and Epispadias, Baltimore, October 2002.
40. Gearhart JP, Jeffs RD: Bladder exstrophy: Increase in capacity following epispadias repair. J Urol 142:525–526, 1989.
41. Mitchell ME, Bagli DJ: Complete penile disassembly for epispadias repair: The Mitchell technique. J Urol 155:300–304, 1996.
42. Zaontz MR, Steckler RE, Shortliffe LMD, et al.: Multicenter experience with the Mitchell technique for epispadias repair. J Urol 160:172, 1998.
43. Chan YD, Jeffs RD, Gearhart JP: Determinants of continence in the bladder exstrophy population: Predictors of success? Urology 57:774–777, 2001.
44. Gearhart JP, Mathews R, Taylor S, et al: Combined bladder closure and epispadias repair in the management of bladder exstrophy. J Urol 160:1182–1185, 1998.
45. Lattimer JK, Smith MJ: Exstrophy closure: A follow-up on 70 cases. Trans Am Assoc Genitourin Surg 57:102–105, 1965.
46. Gearhart JP, Jeffs RD: Management of the failed exstrophy closure. J Urol 146:610–612, 1991.
47. Baird A, Mathews R, Gearhart JP: The use of combined bladder and epispadias repair in males with classic bladder exstrophy: Outcomes, complications and consequences. J Urol (In press).
48. Perlmutter AD, Weinstein MD, Rademan C: Vesical neck reconstruction in patients with the bladder exstrophy complex. J Urol 146:613–615, 1991.
49. Mollard P, Mouriquand PE, Buttin X: Urinary continence after reconstruction of classic bladder exstrophy (73 cases). Br J Urol 73:298–302, 1994.
50. McMahon DR, Kane MP, Husmann DA, et al: Vesical neck reconstruction in patients with the exstrophy-epispadias complex. J Urol 155:1411–1413, 1996.
51. Surer I, Baker LA, Jeffs RD, et al: The modified Cantwell-Ransley technique repair in exstrophy and epispadias. J Urol 164:1040, 2000.
52. Ben-Chaim J, Jeffs RD, Reiner WG, et al.: The outcome of patients with classic bladder exstrophy in adult life. J Urol 155:1251, 1996.
53. Dodson JL, Surer I, Baker LA, et al: The newborn exstrophy bladder inadequate for primary closure: Evaluation, management and outcome. J Urol 165:1656–1659, 2001.
54. Reiner WG: Psychosocial concerns in bladder and cloacal exstrophy. Dialog Pediatr Urol 22:8, 1999.
55. Shober JM, Carmichael PA, Hines M, et al: The ultimate challenge of cloacal exstrophy. J Urol 167:300–304, 2002.
56. Steinbuchel W: Ueber Nabelschnurbruch und Blasenbauchspalte mit Kloakenbildung von Seiten des Duenndarms. Arch Gynaekol 60:456, 1900.
57. Rickham PP, Stauffer UG: Exstrophy of the bladder progress of management during the last 25 years. Prog Pediatr Surg 17:169–188, 1984.

58. Mathews RI, Jeffs RD, Reiner WG, et al: Cloacal exstrophy: Improving the quality of life: The Johns Hopkins Experience. J Urol 160:2452–2466, 1998.
59. Hendren WH: Cloaca, the most severe degree of imperforate anus: Experience with 195 cases. Ann Surg 228:331–346, 1998.
60. Ben-Chaim J, Sponseller PD, Jeffs RD, Gearhart JP: Application of osteotomy in cloacal exstrophy patients. J Urol 154:865–867, 1995.
61. Kim B, Yoo JJ, Atala A: Engineering of human cartilage rods: Potential application for penile prosthesis. J Urol 168:1794, 2002.
62. Zhang Y, Kropp BP, Moore P, et al: Coculture of bladder urothelial and smooth muscle cells on small intestinal submucosa: Potential applications for tissue engineering technology. J Urol 164:928–935, 2000.

CHAPTER 58

Hypospadias

J. Patrick Murphy, MD

Hypospadias is a developmental anomaly characterized by a urethral meatus that opens onto the ventral surface of the penis, proximal to the end of the glans. The meatus may be located anywhere along the shaft of the penis, from the glans to the scrotum, or even in the perineum.

Chordee, which is ventral curvature of the penis, has an inconsistent association with hypospadias. The degree of chordee is ultimately more significant in the surgical treatment of hypospadias than is the initial location of the meatus. A subcoronal hypospadias with little or no chordee is much less complicated to repair than is one with significant chordee and insufficient ventral skin. For this reason, when discussing the degrees of hypospadias, it is more appropriate to use the clinically relevant and common classification system that refers to the meatal location after the chordee has been released (Table 58-1).[1]

Normal phallic development occurs in weeks 7 to 14 of gestation. By 6 weeks of gestation, the genital tubercle is formed anterior to the urogenital sinus. In the next week, two genital folds form caudal to the tubercle, and a urethral plate forms between them. Under the influence of testosterone from the fetal testes, which begins to be produced at about 8 weeks of gestation, the inner genital folds fuse medially to form a tube that communicates with the urogenital sinus and runs distally to end at the base of the glans. The formation of the penile urethra is thus generally completed by the end of the first trimester.[2]

The glanular urethra forms as an ectodermal ingrowth on the glans, which deepens to meet the distal urethra that has formed from the closure of the endodermal genital folds. The capacious junction of these two structures is the fossa navicularis.[3,4] The formation of the glanular urethra occurs separately and is the last step in the formation of the completed urethra. This sequence probably accounts for the predominance of glanular and coronal hypospadias.

Dorsal to the developing urethra, mesenchymal tissue forms the paired corporal bodies. These are the major erectile tissue components and are invested by the tunica albuginea. Mesenchyme also forms Buck's fascia, dartos fascia, and corpus spongiosum.

The corpus spongiosum is the supportive erectile tissue that normally surrounds the urethra and communicates with erectile tissue of the glans. Buck's fascia is the deep layer of fascia that surrounds the corporal bodies and invests the spongiosum. The dorsal neurovascular bundles are deep to this layer. Superficial to this layer is the dartos fascia, which is the loose subcutaneous layer that contains the superficial veins and lymphatics. These structures form subsequent to completion of the urethra by medial fusion of the outer genital folds, proceeding from the proximal to the distal aspect of the penis. This development accounts for how a fully formed urethra can have a poorly formed spongiosum with thin overlying skin and ventral tethering, despite the meatus being located at the tip of the glans.

Finally, the prepuce is formed, originating at the coronal sulcus. It gradually encloses the glans circumferentially.

Arrested development of the urethra may leave the meatus located anywhere along the ventral surface of the penis. Typically, this would lead to foreshortening of the ventral aspect of the penis distal to the meatus and to failure of the prepuce to form circumferentially. However, in the megameatus form of hypospadias, the prepuce may form normally.

HISTORICAL PERSPECTIVES

The first description of hypospadias and its surgical correction was reported in the 1st and 2nd centuries CE by the Alexandrian surgeons, Heliodorus and Antyllus. They described the defect of hypospadias and its relation to problems with urination and ineffective coitus. They further described a surgical treatment consisting of amputation of the glans distal to the hypospadiac meatus.[5,6]

Little progress was made in the surgical treatment of hypospadias until the 19th century, when two Americans, Mettauer and Bush, described techniques using a trocar to establish a channel from the meatus to the glans. Dieffenbach also described a similar technique in the 1830s. None of these methods was very successful.[5]

TABLE 58-1
HYPOSPADIAS CLASSIFICATION ACCORDING TO MEATAL LOCATION AFTER RELEASE OF CHORDEE

Anterior (65%–70% of cases)
  Glanular
  Coronal
  Distal penile shaft

Middle (10%–15% of cases)
  Middle penile shaft

Posterior (20% of cases)
  Proximal penile shaft
  Penoscrotal
  Scrotal
  Perineal

In 1874, Theophile Anger reported the successful repair of a penoscrotal hypospadias, using the technique described in 1869 by Thiersch for the repair of epispadias, in which lateral skin flaps were tubularized to form the neourethra. Anger's report initiated the modern era of hypospadias surgery characterized by the use of local skin flaps.[7,8] Duplay[6] soon described his two-stage technique. In the first stage, the chordee was released; in the second stage, a ventral midline strip of skin was covered by closure of the lateral penile skin flaps in the midline. Duplay did not believe that it was necessary to form the urethral tube completely because he thought that epithelialization would occur even if an incomplete tube were buried under the lateral skin flaps. Browne[9] used this concept in his well-known "buried strip" technique, which was widely used in the early 1950s. In the late 1800s, various other surgeons reported on penile, scrotal, and preputial flap techniques for multistage procedures. Several of them used the technique of burying the penis in the scrotum to obtain skin coverage, similar to the technique described by Cecil and Culp in the late 1950s.[10]

Edmonds, in 1913, was the first to describe the transfer of preputial skin to the ventrum of the penis at the time of release of chordee. At a second stage, the Duplay tube was created to complete the urethral closure. Byars[11] popularized this two-stage technique in the early 1950s. Smith[12] further improved on the procedure by denuding the epithelium of one of the lateral skin flaps to give a "pants-over-vest" closure and thus reduce the risk of fistula formation. Belt devised another preputial transfer, two-stage procedure which was popularized by Fuqua in the 1960s.[13]

Nove-Josserand, in 1897, was the first to report the use of a free, split-thickness skin graft in an attempt to repair hypospadias.[14] Over the next 20 years, various other tissues were used as free grafts, including saphenous vein, ureter, and appendix. None of these procedures had consistent success. McCormack[15] used a free, full-thickness skin graft in a two-stage repair. Humby,[16] in 1941, described a one-stage technique using the full thickness of the foreskin. Devine and Horton[17] later popularized this free preputial graft technique with very good results.

In 1947, Memmelaar[18] reported the use of bladder mucosa as a free graft technique in a one-stage repair. Marshall and Spellman,[19] in 1955, used bladder mucosa in a two-stage technique. Urologists in China also experienced success with a primary repair using bladder mucosa. This technique was developed independently during the period of scientific and cultural isolation in China.[20] Buccal mucosa from the lip was used for urethral reconstruction in 1941 by Humby[16] and has recently gained renewed attention as a free graft technique.[21]

Improved techniques in preputial and meatal-based vascularized flaps since the 1970s to 1980s have greatly advanced hypospadias repair. Through the contributions of surgeons such as Mathieu, Barcat,[1] Mustarde,[22] Broadbent,[23] Hodgson,[24] Horton and Devine,[17] Standoli,[25] and Duckett,[26] the single-stage repair of even the most severe forms of hypospadias has become commonplace.

CLINICAL ASPECTS

Incidence

The incidence of hypospadias has been estimated to be between 0.8 and 8.2 per 1000 live male births.[27] The wide variation probably represents some geographic and racial differences, but of more significance is the exclusion of the more minor degrees of hypospadias in some reports. If all degrees of hypospadias, even the most minor, are included, then the incidence is probably 1 in 125 live male births.[28] With the most quoted figure of 1 per 300 live male births, it can be assumed that more than 6000 boys are born with hypospadias each year in the United States.[29]

Etiology

A defect in the androgen stimulation of the developing penis, which precludes complete formation of the urethra and its surrounding structures, is the ultimate cause of hypospadias. This defect can occur from deficient androgen production by the testes and placenta, from failure of testosterone to convert to dihydrotestosterone by the 5α-reductase enzyme, or from deficient androgen receptors in the penis. Various intersex conditions can cause deficiencies at any point along the androgen-stimulation axis. These are discussed in Chapter 61.

The origin of hypospadias not associated with intersex conditions is unclear. An endocrine cause has been implicated by some reports that show a diminished response to human chorionic gonadotropin in some patients with hypospadias, suggesting delayed maturation of the hypothalamic/pituitary axis.[30,31] Other reports have shown an increased incidence of hypospadias in monozygotic twins, suggesting an insufficient amount of human chorionic gonadotropin production by the single placenta to accommodate the two male fetuses.[32]

Environmental causes also have been implicated. A higher incidence of hypospadias has been noted in winter conceptions.[32] A weak association between hypospadias and the maternal ingestion of progestin-like agents has been noted.[33,34] No association has been found between hypospadias and oral contraceptive use before or in early pregnancy.[35]

Genetic factors in the etiology of hypospadias are indicated by the higher incidence of the anomaly in first-degree relatives of hypospadic patients.[27,34,36] In one study that evaluated 307 families, the risk of occurrence of hypospadias in a second male sibling was 12%. If the index child and his father were affected, the risk for a second sibling increased to 26%. If the index child and a second-degree relative were affected, rather than the father, the risk of the sibling being affected was only 19%.[36] This pattern suggests a multifactorial mode of inheritance, with these families having a higher than average number of influential genes for creation of the anomaly.[36] A combination of the endocrine, environmental, and genetic factors ultimately determines the potential for developing the hypospadias complex in any one individual.

Anatomy of the Defect

The clinical significance of the hypospadias anomaly is related to several factors. The abnormal location of the meatus and the tendency toward meatal stenosis result in a ventrally deflected and splayed stream. This fact makes the stream difficult to control and often makes it difficult for the patient to void while standing. The ventral curvature associated with chordee can lead to painful erections, especially with severe chordee. Impaired copulation and thus inadequate insemination is a further consequence of significant chordee. In addition, the unusual cosmetic appearance associated with the hooded foreskin, flattened glans, and ventral skin deficiency frequently has an adverse effect on the psychosexual development of the adolescent with hypospadias.[37-41] All of these factors are evidence that early surgical correction should be offered to all boys with hypospadias, regardless of the severity of the defect.

The distal form of hypospadias is the most common (see Table 58-1); frequently, little or no associated chordee is present (Fig. 58-1). The size of the meatus and the quality of the surrounding supportive tissue as well as the configuration of the glans are variable and ultimately determine the surgical procedure. Well-formed, mobile perimeatal skin and a deep ventral glans groove may allow local perimeatal flaps to form the urethra (Fig. 58-2). In contrast, atrophic and immobile skin around the meatus may require tissue transfer from the preputium to form the neourethra.

An unusual variant of the distal hypospadias is the large wide-mouth meatus with a circumferential foreskin (the megameatus-intact prepuce variant) (Fig. 58-3).[42] Owing to the intact prepuce, this variant is often not identified until a circumcision has been done. If clinicians discover hypospadias during circumcision, they should stop and preserve the foreskin, even if the dorsal slit has been done.

At times, the distally located meatus may be associated with significant chordee, sometimes of a severe degree (Fig. 58-4). The release of the chordee places the meatus in a much more proximal location, requiring more complicated transfers of skin to bridge the gap between the proximal meatus and the tip of the glans.

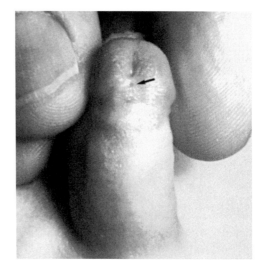

FIGURE 58-1. Distal hypospadias with stenotic meatus (*arrow*) located on glans with no chordee. The patient is a good candidate for meatal advancement and glanuloplasty (MAGPI) or tubularized incised urethral plate (TIP).

When the meatus is located on the penile shaft, the character of the urethral plate (midline ventral shaft skin distal to the meatus) is important in determining what type of repair is possible. A well-developed and elastic urethral plate suggests minimal if any distal ventral curvature (Fig. 58-5). However, a thin atrophic urethral plate heralds a significant chordee. The proximal supportive tissue of the urethra also is important. If lack of spongiosum exists proximal to the hypospadic meatus, this portion of the native urethra is not substantial enough to incorporate in the repair (Fig. 58-6). Therefore

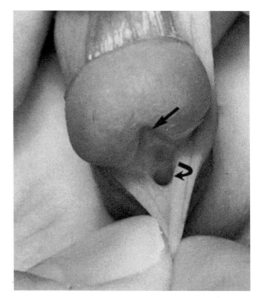

FIGURE 58-2. Patulous, subcoronal meatus (*curved arrow*) with mobile perimeatal skin and deep ventral glans groove (*straight arrow*). This is a good variant for meatal-based flap procedure, glans approximation (GAP), or tubularized incised urethral plate (TIP).

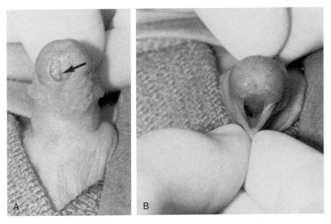

FIGURE 58-3. *A,* Previously circumcised penis with megameatus (*arrow*) intact circumferential prepuce. *B,* Large wide-mouthed meatus in the same penis as shown in *A.*

the neourethra must be constructed from the point of adequate spongiosum.

The position of the meatus at the penoscrotal, scrotal, or perineal location is usually associated with severe chordee, which requires chordee release with an extensive urethroplasty (Fig. 58-7). This type is usually more predictable in the preoperative period as to the choice of repair than are some of the more distal types previously discussed.

Other anatomic elements of the anomaly that are important to consider include penile torsion, glans tilt, penoscrotal transposition, and chordee without hypospadias. These

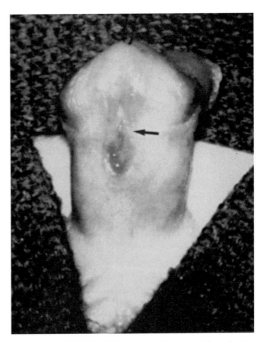

FIGURE 58-5. Midshaft hypospadias with elastic, well-developed urethral plate distal to the meatus (*arrow*). No significant chordee is present. This is a good variant for onlay island flap procedure or possibly tubularized incised urethral plate.

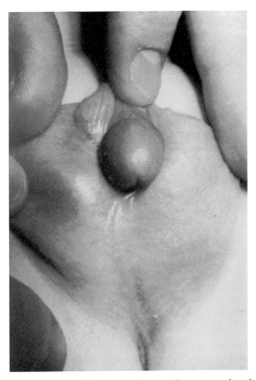

FIGURE 58-4. Scrotal hypospadias with severe chordee and marked penoscrotal transposition.

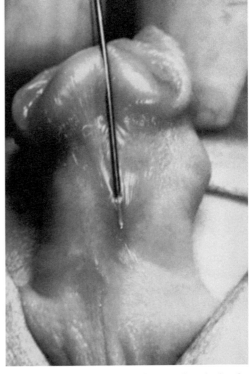

FIGURE 58-6. Midshaft hypospadias with a lack of spongiosum support proximal to meatus. Urethra should be opened back to an area of good spongiosum support at the penoscrotal position.

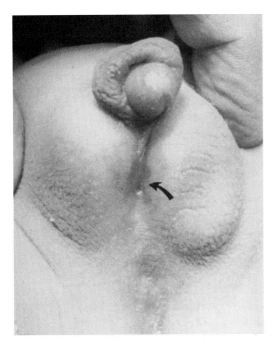

FIGURE 58-7. Perineal/scrotal hypospadias (*arrow*) with severe chordee and bifid scrotum.

are discussed more completely in the section, Surgical Procedures.

Associated Anomalies

Inguinal hernia and undescended testes are the most common anomalies associated with hypospadias. They occur from 7% to 13% of the time, with a greater incidence when the meatus is more proximal.[43-45] An enlarged prostatic utricle also is more common in posterior hypospadias, with an incidence of about 11%.[44] Infection is the most common complication of a utricle, but surgical excision is rarely necessary.[46]

Several reports have emphasized significantly high numbers of upper urinary tract anomalies associated with hypospadias,[47-50] suggesting that routine upper tract screening is necessary. However, when the association is studied selectively, it can be shown that the types of hypospadias that are at risk for surgically significant upper tract anomalies are the penoscrotal and perineal forms and those associated with other organ system abnormalities.[43,45] When one, two, or three other organ system anomalies occur, the incidence of significant upper tract anomalies is 7%, 13%, and 37%, respectively. Associated myelomeningocele and imperforate anus carry a 33% and 46% incidence, respectively, of upper urinary tract malformations. In isolated posterior hypospadias, the incidence of associated upper tract anomalies is 5%.[45]

In middle and distal hypospadias, when not associated with other organ system anomalies, the incidence is similar to that in the general population.[43,45,51] Therefore it is recommended that screening for upper urinary tract anomalies by voiding cystourethrogram and renal ultrasonography be done in patients with penoscrotal and perineal forms of hypospadias and in those with anomalies of at least one additional organ system. Screening should be done in patients with other known indications, such as a history of urinary tract infection, upper or lower tract obstructive symptoms, and hematuria, and in those boys having a strong family history of urinary tract abnormalities.[52]

The intersex state is another potential disorder associated with hypospadias. This association is rare in the routine forms of hypospadias. Failure of testicular descent, micropenis, penoscrotal transposition (see Fig. 58-4), or bifid scrotum (see Fig. 58-7), when associated with hypospadias, are all signs of potential intersex problems and warrant evaluation with karyotype screening.[27,53,54]

Treatment

The advent of safe anesthesia, fine suture material, delicate instruments, and good optical magnification have allowed virtually all types of hypospadias to be repaired in infancy. Generally, the repair is done on an outpatient basis. To deny a child the benefit of repair because the defect is "too mild" or the risk of complication is "too high" is inappropriate. The chance to make the phallus as normal as possible should be offered to all children, regardless of the severity of the defects.

Age at Repair

The technical advances over the past few decades have made it possible to repair hypospadias, in most cases, in the first year of life.[55-57] Controversy still exists with regard to the ideal age for repair. Some surgeons have suggested delaying repair until after the child is age 2 years.[52,58-60] However, most surgeons who deal routinely with the defect prefer to do the repair when the patient is 6 to 18 months old.[53,54,56,57,61,62] One study compared the emotional, psychosexual, cognitive, and surgical risks for hypospadias. The "optimal window" recommended for repair was about age 6 to 15 months (Fig. 58-8).[63] Unless other health or social problems require delay, we believe the ideal time to complete penile reconstruction in the pediatric patient is about age 6 months.[64] Anesthetic risk is low (see Chapter 3) and, at this age, postoperative care is much easier for the parents than it is when the child is a toddler.

Objectives of Repair

The objectives of hypospadias correction are divided into the following categories:

1. Complete straightening of the penis
2. Placing the meatus at the tip of the glans
3. Forming a symmetrical, conically shaped glans
4. Constructing a neourethra uniform in caliber
5. Completing a satisfactory cosmetic skin coverage

If these objectives can all be attained, the ultimate goal of forming a "normal" penis for the child with hypospadias can be accomplished.

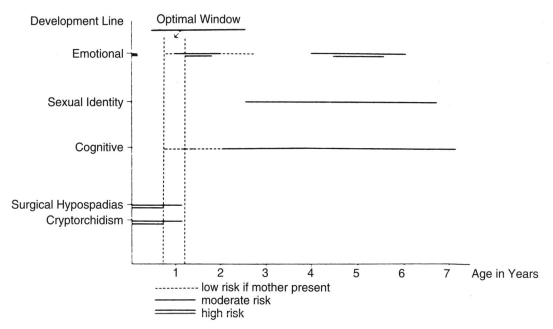

FIGURE 58-8. Evaluation of risk for hypospadias repair from birth to age 7 years. Optimal window is age 6 months to 15 months. (From Schultz JR, Klykylo WM, Wacksman J: Timing of elective hypospadias repair in children. Pediatrics 71:342–351, 1983.)

STRAIGHTENING. Curvature of the penis is difficult to judge, at times, in the preoperative period. Artificial erection, by injecting physiologic saline in the corpora at the time of operation, allows determination of the exact degree of curvature.[65] This curvature may be caused only by ventral skin or subcutaneous tissue tethering, which is corrected with the release of the skin and dartos layer.[66,67] Infrequently, the curvature may be secondary to true fibrous chordee, which requires division of the urethral plate and excision of the fibrous tissue down to the tunica albuginea.

Sometimes, even after extensive ventral dissection of chordee tissue, a repeated artificial erection still reveals the presence of significant ventral curvature. This finding is usually secondary to the uncommon problem of corporal body disproportion, which is caused by true deficiency of ventral corporal development. This problem can be treated by making a releasing incision in the ventral tunica albuginea and inserting either a dermal or a tunica vaginalis patch to expand the deficient ventral surface.[68,69] Others have suggested the use of small intestinal submucosa as an off-the-shelf substitute for the autologous grafts.[70] Another technique is to excise wedges of tunica albuginea dorsally with transverse closure to shorten this dorsal surface and straighten the penis.[71,72] Other surgeons have had success with dorsal plication without excision of tunica albuginea.[73,74] Anatomic studies suggest that this plication should be done in the midline dorsally.[75] Still others advocate corporal rotation dorsally with or without penile disassembly to correct severe chordee.[76,77]

Axial rotation of the penis, or penile torsion, is another aspect of penis straightening that must be managed. This problem can generally be corrected by releasing the dartos layer as far proximal as possible on the penile shaft. This allows the ventral shaft to rotate back to the midline and corrects the torsion. Chordee or torsion can also occur without hypospadias. The management of these boys encompasses the entire spectrum of techniques as when hypospadias is involved (Fig. 58-9).[78,79]

PLACING THE MEATUS. Placing the meatus at the tip of the glans has not always been standard in hypospadias repair. The risk of complications was thought to be too great to recommend procedures that would place the meatus beyond the subcoronal area. Multistage repairs popular in the 1950s and 1960s were designed to attain only a subcoronal location of the meatus. Surgical

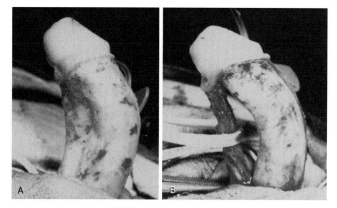

FIGURE 58-9. *A,* Chordee without hypospadias. The meatus is located at the tip of the glans with marked ventral curvature. *B,* Fibrous ventral tissue is all released. Urethra is mobilized, but curvature persists, indicating corporal body disproportion. This requires ventral patch or dorsal plication (see text).

techniques since then have improved sufficiently so that glans-channeling and glans-splitting techniques are used with minimal complications, making the distal tip meatus possible.

In glanular and subcoronal variants, the configuration of the meatus is the determining factor in what techniques move the meatus distally on the glans. Meatoplasty with or without dorsal advancement, distal urethral mobilization and tubularization, or meatal-based flaps are the methods selected in most cases of distal hypospadias.[80,81] In the more proximal forms, creating the neourethra with local vascularized skin flaps or free grafts allows placement of the urethra at the end of the penis, whereas glans channeling or glans splitting accomplishes placement of the meatus at the tip of the glans.[1,17,22,26,82,83]

GLANS SHAPE. Creation of a symmetrical, conically shaped glans is the objective of the glansplasty component of the repair. Approximating the lateral glanular tissue in the midline ventrally over a meatoplasty or meatal advancement corrects the flattened glans appearance to the more anatomically normal, conically shaped glans. Similarly, approximation of well-developed glans wings to the midline over a neourethra in a split glans restores the glans to its normal conical shape.

URETHRAL CONSTRUCTION. Formation of the neourethra can be accomplished with local skin flaps, various types of free grafts, or vascularized pedicle flaps. Local skin flaps may be formed from in situ skin or dorsal skin transferred to the ventrum in a previous stage. In either case, it is important to avoid making these flaps too narrow or thin, at the risk of compromising their vascular supply. The hypospadic urethral plate has been shown on histologic studies to consist of epithelium covering well-vascularized connective tissue without fibrosis.[84] This finding supports the clinical findings that urethral plate preservation is helpful for successful urethroplasty. Free grafts depend on an adequately vascularized bed for survival; therefore they should not be placed in a scarred channel. Well-vascularized subcutaneous tissue and skin must cover them to allow adequate neovascularization and survival of the graft.[17]

Mobilized vascularized flaps of preputium have a more reliable blood supply than do free grafts. Therefore if they are available, these flaps are the choice of most surgeons.[24,26,83,85] They may be used as patches onto a strip of native urethral plate to complete the urethra, or they may be tubularized and used as bridges over the gap between a proximal native urethra and the end of the glans.[26,86] A watertight closure of the well-vascularized neourethra is formed, with care being taken to make it uniform in caliber and of appropriate size for the age of the child. This closure helps avoid stricturing and forming of saccules, diverticula, and fistulas.

COSMESIS. Creating cosmetically appealing, well-vascularized skin coverage of the penile shaft after urethroplasty can sometimes be challenging. Transfer of vascularized dorsal preputial skin to the ventrum can be accomplished in several ways.

Buttonholes of the dorsal skin allow the penis to come through this defect, draping the distal preputium over the ventral surface of the penis.[19] This maneuver has the advantage of transferring well-vascularized skin over the repair, but it is not appealing cosmetically.

A more satisfactory method of transferring skin to the ventrum is by splitting the dorsal skin in the midline longitudinally and advancing the flaps around on either side to meet in the midline. This technique allows a midline ventral closure, which simulates the median raphe, and allows a subcoronal closure to the preputial skin circumferentially, which simulates the suture lines of a standard circumcision.[87,88] Another adjunct in this closure is to advance lateral flaps of inner preputial skin from each side to the ventral midline of the penis at the time of glansplasty or closure of glans wings.[89] Approximating these flaps in the midline gives the appearance of an intact circumferential preputial collar, further enhancing the potential for an anatomically normal skin closure (see Fig. 58-14).

Some people, particularly those in European countries, prefer the appearance of a noncircumcised penis. In distal repairs, reconstruction of the preputium for a noncircumcised appearance can be accomplished in certain cases.[90] Correction of the more significant degrees of penoscrotal transposition is often necessary to avoid the feminizing appearance it causes. This step may be done at the time of the original repair, in some cases. However, when using vascularized pedicle flaps for the repair, it is usually safer to correct significant penoscrotal transposition with rotational flaps at a later time.[91–94]

SURGICAL PROCEDURES

Because of the wide variation in the anatomic presentation of hypospadias, no single urethroplasty is applicable to every case. At times, a final decision regarding the degree of curvature and the ultimate location of the meatus cannot be made until the operation has started and an artificial erection is done. The surgeon who repairs hypospadias must be adaptable and experienced to deal with all variants of the defect. Versatility and experience with all options of surgical treatment are the keys to successful management of hypospadias. By recognizing the sometimes subtle nuances of meatal variation, glans configuration, and curvature character, the experienced surgeon can make the best choices as to the type of repair to use (Fig. 58-10).

SPECIFIC TECHNIQUES

Anterior Variants

Some glanular variants are amenable to the meatal advancement and glansplasty (MAGPI) type of repair (Fig. 58-11).[95] A stenotic meatus with good mobility of the urethra and a fairly shallow ventral glanular groove are the anatomic characteristics best suited for the MAGPI. A wide-mouthed meatus is not amenable to the

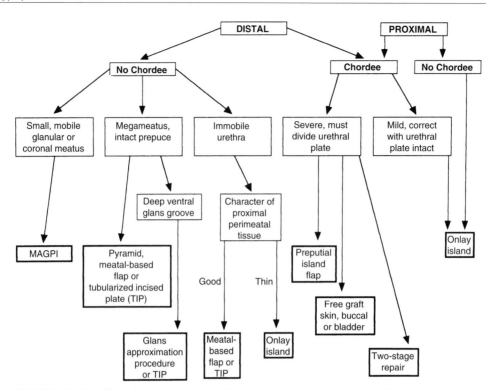

FIGURE 58-10. Flow diagram for types of repair in variants of hypospadias.

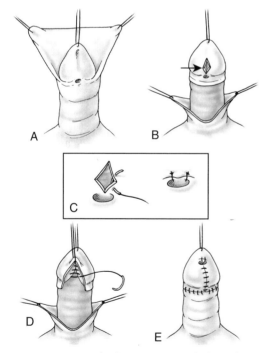

FIGURE 58-11. Meatal advancement and glansplasty repair. *A,* Circumferential subcoronal incision to deglove penile shaft skin. *B,* Longitudinal incision through ventral groove of glans (*arrow*). *C,* Transverse closure of glans groove incision to advance dorsal urethral plate and to open stenotic meatus. *D,* Glans tissue approximated ventrally in midline to restore conical configuration to glans. *E,* Completion of skin closure.

MAGPI repair. The meatal-based flap repair may be used effectively in this situation, if no chordee is present and if mobile, well-vascularized skin exists proximal to the meatus (Fig. 58-12).[96,97] This repair works well when a moderately deep ventral groove exists, allowing the urethra to be placed deep in the glans to form a conically shaped glans after closure of the glans wings. The glans approximation procedure is sometimes useful when a wide-mouthed proximal glanular meatus exists with a very deep groove (Figs. 58-13 and 58-14).[98] The pyramid procedure is well suited for the fish-mouth type of meatus seen in the megameatus intact prepuce variant.[42] These repairs give a very good cosmetic result when done in the proper situation.

The tubularized incised plate urethroplasty (TIP) is a modification of the Thiersch-Duplay tubularization, which involves a deep longitudinal incision of the urethral plate in the midline (Fig. 58-15). This allows the lateral skin flaps to be mobilized and closed in the midline without tension. This procedure allows the wide-mouthed meatus variant with a flat, shallow ventral groove to be repaired without the need for additional flaps.[99] The TIP urethroplasty has gained wide acceptance in recent years, and its durability and long-term success have been demonstrated even in some of the more proximal variants.[100–102]

Middle Variants

The amount of ventral curvature generally dictates the type of repair in the middle- and distal-shaft hypospadias. When no significant chordee is present, the TIP repair or

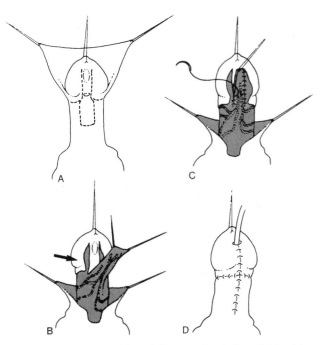

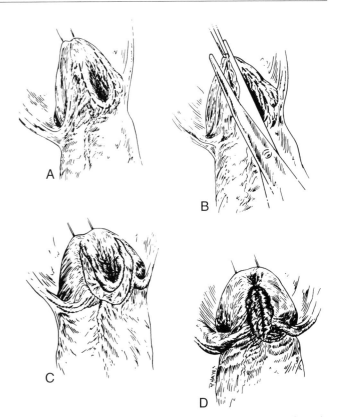

FIGURE 58-12. Meatal-based flap repair. *A*, Parallel incisions along ventral groove distal to meatus and formation of meatal-based flap proximal to meatus. *B*, Glans wings developed on either side of the urethral plate (*arrow*) to close over the neourethra later. Meatal-based flap is mobilized distally maintaining good vascular soft tissue support. *C*, Flap is anastomosed to bilateral edges of urethral plate to form neourethra. *D*, Glans wings are closed over the neourethra in the midline, giving conical glans configuration. Penile shaft is covered with dorsal foreskin advanced ventrally.

FIGURE 58-13. Glans approximation procedure (GAP). *A*, Deep ventral groove and patulous, coronal meatus with outline of proposed incision. *B*, Skin is excised along previously marked U-shaped line. *C*, De-epithelialized glans with urethral plate intact. *D*, Two-layer closure of glanular urethra with glans skin still open. (From Zaontz MR: The GAP [glans approximation procedure] for glanular/coronal hypospadias. J Urol 141:359–361, 1989.)

the meatal-based flap can sometimes be done. Another technique is the onlay island flap repair (Fig. 58-16).[86] This procedure involves mobilizing an inner preputial flap on its pedicle and rotating it ventrally to lay it on the well-developed ventral urethral plate to complete the tubularization of the neourethra. This technique is applicable to many forms of penile shaft hypospadias.

In milder degrees of chordee, the curvature can be corrected without dividing the urethral plate by taking down tethering bands lateral to the urethral plate or by dorsal plication techniques.[74,75] This allows the onlay island flap technique to be used instead of the tubularized pedicle flap, which has a higher incidence of complications.[54] If significant chordee does exist, division of the urethral plate may be necessary. This moves the meatus more proximal and requires treatment as described for proximal variants.

Proximal Variants

Many of the scrotal and perineal forms of hypospadias are associated with significant chordee, which requires division of the urethral plate, leaving a gap to be bridged between the proximal native urethra and the tip of the glans. This can be done with staged procedures in which coverage of the ventral penile shaft is attained by rotation of dorsal flaps to the ventrum, with later tubularization to form the neourethra (Fig. 58-17).

Another method is the tubularized free graft anastomosed to the native urethra proximally and extended to the end of the glans by a tunneling or splitting technique. The most commonly used free grafts are full-thickness skin, bladder mucosa, or buccal mucosa. Preputial skin is much preferred to extragenital skin.[17,103] If genital skin is not available, bladder or buccal mucosa may be the next best tissue.[21,104,105]

Vascularized flaps are a more physiologically sound alternative to free grafts. The transverse inner preputial island flap that is tubularized and transposed ventrally to form the neourethra is the preferred type of vascularized flap (Fig. 58-18).[26,106] It provides good preputial skin with a reliable blood supply that does not rely on neovascularization for healing of the neourethra, as do free grafts. Occasionally, the length of the prepuce alone may not be adequate to bridge the defect to a very proximal meatus. In this case, the shiny non–hair-bearing skin around the meatus can be tubularized (Fig. 58-19), moving the proximal urethra to the penoscrotal junction. The preputial vascularized tube graft can then be used to reach the remainder of the distance to the end of the penis.[53]

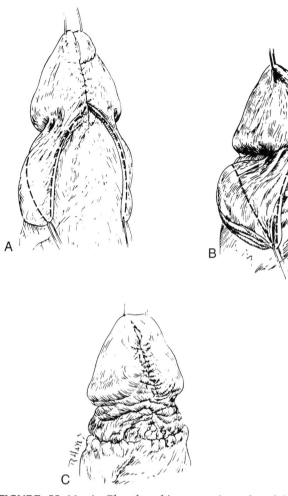

FIGURE 58-14. *A,* Glanular skin approximated and lateral wings of inner preputial skin outlined. *B,* Lateral view of outline for preputial collar. *C,* Lateral preputial wings closed in midline to give circumferential preputial collar. (From Zaontz MR: The GAP [glans approximation procedure] for glanular/coronal hypospadias. J Urol 141:359–361, 1989.)

In some cases, the penile shaft may be deficient enough to cause concern about ventral coverage after completion of the neourethra. The double-face island flap can solve this problem.[24] This technique leaves some of the outer preputial skin attached to the pedicle after tubularizing the inner preputial layer. This outer preputium is transferred to the ventrum with the pedicle and supplies the skin coverage of the ventral shaft. However, the complications associated with the double-face island flap are numerous, and it has few advocates.[55]

I prefer the transverse island flap in a one-stage procedure in most cases of proximal hypospadias with chordee. In the rare case in which the skin deficiency is so severe that a vascularized pedicle cannot be used or in which the chordee is so severe that a dermal or tunica vaginalis graft is required to correct disproportion, I, as well as others, perform a two-stage repair.[107–109] However, only a few cases are found in which the repair cannot be accomplished in one stage.

TECHNICAL PERSPECTIVES

Optical Magnification

Most surgeons agree that optical magnification is indispensable in hypospadias surgery. Standard operating loupes, ranging from 2.5 power to 4.5 power, are generally thought to be ideal for the magnification needed for this type of surgery. Some workers advocate the use of the operating microscope and suggest an improved result with this technique.[110] Most surgeons have not believed that this degree of magnification is necessary for obtaining excellent results. The microscope may be overly cumbersome for the small improvement in visualization it may provide.[111]

Sutures and Instruments

Fine absorbable suture is chosen by most surgeons to close the neourethra. Polyglycolic or polyglactin material is probably the most common choice of suture. However, some surgeons prefer the longer-lasting polydiaxanone suture.[110] Permanent sutures of nylon or polypropylene, in a continuous stitch that is pulled out 10 to 14 days after surgery, are recommended by some.[12,56]

The type of optical magnification also determines the size of the suture. Generally, 6-0 or 7-0 suture is preferred. With the microscope, 8-0 or 9-0 may be used. Skin closure is usually accomplished with either fine chromic (6-0 or 7-0) or plain catgut suture. Small suture-sinus tracts may occur along these stitches as they dissolve. I have used a subcuticular closure with either 6-0 chromic or polydiaxanone over the last 5-year period and have eliminated the problem of these suture-sinus tracts.

The delicate instruments of ophthalmologic surgery are well designed for the precise tissue handling required in hypospadias repair. Small, single-toothed forceps or fine skin hooks allow tissue handling with minimal trauma. Standard microscopic tools are necessary for those who prefer the microscope over loupe magnification.

Urinary Diversion

The goal of the surgeon in any urinary diversion procedure in hypospadias repair is to protect the neourethra from the urinary stream for the initial healing phase. In theory, this diversion should decrease the complication rate, particularly fistula formation. The more traditional perineal urethrostomy and suprapubic cystostomy are uncomfortable and cumbersome to manage in the postoperative period. Small indwelling 6F or 8F polymeric silicone (Silastic) tubes left through the repair and just into the bladder allow drainage of the urine into the diaper in infants (Fig. 58-20).[111] This technique greatly facilitates the outpatient care of these pediatric patients. These stents are well tolerated by the patients. Problems with the stents becoming plugged or dislodged are uncommon.

Some surgeons favor a stent that traverses the repair but is not indwelling in the bladder.[110] The patient is

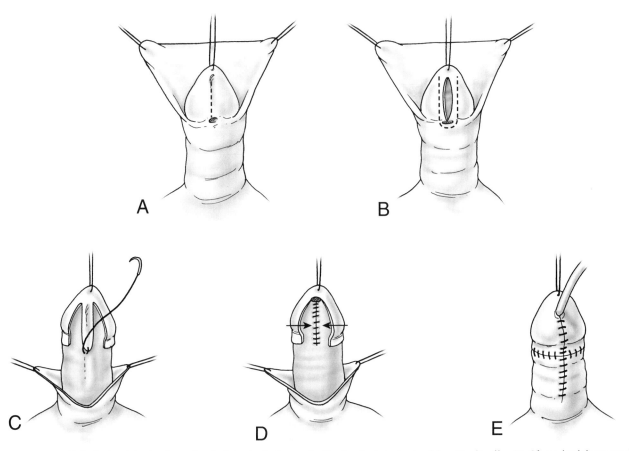

FIGURE 58-15. Tubularized incised urethral plate technique. *A,* Urethral plate incised longitudinally. *B,* Glans incisions made longitudinally, wide enough to leave two strips of epithelium for 10F-size neourethra. *C,* Neourethra tubularized in midline with multiple layers and dartos flap to reinforce. *D,* Glans wings closed in midline. *E,* Skin closure completed and urethral stent in place (optional).

allowed to void, but the stent protects the repair. I prefer the indwelling stent, used for 5 to 14 days, depending on the complexity of the repair. In older children who would not tolerate wearing a diaper, a 6F or 8F Foley catheter may be used in the simpler distal repairs, and a suprapubic cystostomy, in the more complex repairs. Suprapubic drainage should be used in complex reoperations or in any repairs requiring a free graft. Studies have suggested that no diversion is necessary for simpler distal procedures, such as MAGPI, meatal-based flap, or distal Duplay tubes. Simple small fistula repairs can be done without diversion.[112,113]

Dressings

Hypospadias dressings should apply enough gentle pressure on the penis to help with hemostasis and to decrease edema formation, without compromising the vascularity of the repair. Various dressings accomplish this purpose. A silicon-foam dressing, which can be placed around the penis in a liquid state to solidify later, leaves a soft, mildly compressive dressing that is waterproof.[114] This dressing can be removed without difficulty several days after

surgery. Other dressings include transparent adhesive dressings wrapped around the penis or fixed to the abdominal wall in a sandwich-like fashion (see Fig. 58-20).[68] A DuoDerm dressing can be applied around the penis as an alternative, before using a transparent adhesive dressing.[110] Two prospective studies have shown that use of dressing does not influence healing or complication rate.[115,116] I have continued to use a transparent dressing against the abdominal wall for the hemostatic effect in the first 12 postoperative hours.

Analgesia

Postoperative pain is generally controlled with oral analgesics. Bladder spasms caused by indwelling catheters can be dealt with by methantheline bromide (Banthine) and opium suppositories or by oral oxybutynin. A dorsal penile nerve block done intraoperatively with bupivacaine can help control postoperative pain.[117]

A caudal block is my preferred method for postoperative pain control.[118] In most cases, the patients are comfortable for the entire day and evening of surgery and are easily cared for at home with only oral analgesia.

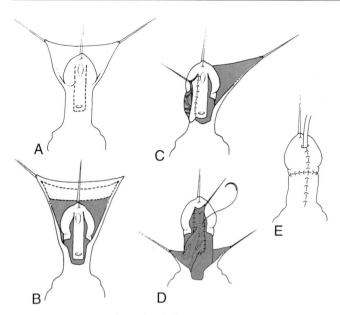

FIGURE 58-16. Onlay island flap repair. *A,* Outline of incisions along well-developed urethral plate with no chordee. *B,* Mobilization of glans wings and shaft skin with urethral plate intact distal to meatus. Outline of inner preputial island flap that will be transposed ventrally for onlay completion of neourethra. *C,* Island flap transposed ventrally on pedicle. The first part of the anastomosis is completed. *D,* Remainder of anastomosis to complete neourethra to tip of glans. *E,* Glans wings are approximated over the neourethra in the ventral midline. The penile shaft is covered with the ventral advancement of dorsal foreskin.

COMPLICATIONS

The type and incidence of complications vary with the particular form of repair. Attention to detail and meticulous technique are imperative to keep the incidence of all complications to a minimum. The following is a discussion of some of the general complications that can occur with all repairs.

Bleeding

Intraoperative bleeding can, at times, be troublesome, but with careful attention to the control of bleeding by judicious use of point tip cautery, it can generally be kept to a minimum. Tourniquets or cutaneous infiltrations with dilute concentrations of epinephrine can be helpful, but they should not replace careful technique.[119] Postoperative bleeding is generally prevented by mildly compressive dressings. Subcutaneous hematomas may occur but generally do not need to be drained.

Infection

Wound infection is a rare problem in hypospadias repair, especially in the prepubertal patient. As long as good

viability of tissue is maintained, infection should be a minor problem. Perioperative antibiotic prophylaxis is favored by some surgeons.[119] This is probably a reasonable precaution in an extensive repair, especially in the postpubertal patient. Urinary suppression with oral antibiotics is recommended with indwelling catheters that are open to drainage in the diaper.[68,120,121]

Devitalized Skin Flaps

If the sloughing of skin coverage occurs, it is usually on the ventral surface of the penis where dorsal skin has been transposed. When the devascularized skin is over a well-vascularized bed of tissue, such as with a pedicle flap, primary healing generally occurs without sequelae. If the slough is over poorly vascularized tissue, such as a free graft, the result can be the breakdown of the repair. Careful attention to the transposing of well-vascularized tissue for coverage of the neourethra in all repairs is critical to avoid this problem.

Fistulas

Urethrocutaneous fistulas are the most commonly reported complications of hypospadias surgery. They result from failure of healing at some point along the neourethral suture line and can range in size from pinpoint to large enough for all voided urine to exit at this point. Fistulas also may be associated with stenosis or distal stricture. Occasionally, small fistulas seen in the early postoperative period may close spontaneously. Surgical closure should be postponed until complete tissue healing has occurred, which requires at least 6 months.[122,123] A small fistula may be closed by local excision of the fistula tract followed by closure of the urethral epithelium with fine absorbable suture. Approximating several layers of well-vascularized subcutaneous tissue over this closure is important to prevent recurrence. Urinary diversion is usually not necessary in small fistula repairs. Larger fistulas may require more complicated closures, with mobilization of tissue flaps or advancement of skin flaps to ensure an adequate amount of well-vascularized tissue for a multilayered closure.[122–125] Urinary diversion is often necessary with more complicated closures.

Strictures

Narrowing of the neourethra may occur anywhere along its course. However, the most common sites of stricture formation are at the meatus and at the proximal anastomosis. Most cases of meatal narrowing can be managed as an office procedure by gentle dilation in the first few postoperative weeks. Occasionally, meatotomy or meatoplasty is needed, especially when associated with a proximal fistula or neourethral diverticulum. More proximal strictures can generally be treated with dilation or visual internal urethrotomy. However, open urethroplasty may sometimes be required, with excision of the stricture and primary urethral anastomosis or patch graft urethroplasty.[122,123,126]

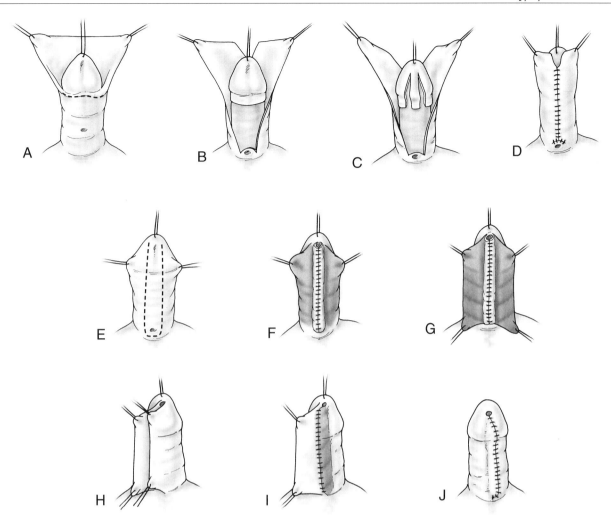

FIGURE 58-17. Two-stage Durham Smith repair. *A,* Release of chordee. *B,* Splitting of dorsal preputium. *C,* Denuded ventral glans prior to transposing preputial skin to ventrum. *D,* Transposition of dorsal foreskin to ventrum completes the first stage. *E,* U-shaped incision around the meatus and out onto glans. *F,* Tubularization of Duplay-type tube to form the neourethra. *G,* Second layer of soft tissue to reinforce suture line. *H–J,* Overlapping skin closure with de-epithelialization of inner flap gives a "double-breasted" closure of the skin. (Redrawn from Belman AB: Urethra. In Kelalis PP, King LR, Belman AB [eds]: Clinical Pediatric Urology, 2nd ed. Philadelphia, WB Saunders, 1985.)

Diverticulum

Saccular dilation of the neourethra may result from distal stenosis causing progressive dilation, contained urinary extravasation from the breakdown of the repair, or initial creation of an oversized segment of the neourethra. Classic bulging of the urethra ventrally with voiding is evident with significant diverticulum formation (Fig. 58-21). Urinary stasis with chronic inflammation is common. Obstruction can result from kinking of the urethra when the diverticulum distends with voiding. Repair requires excision of the redundant urethra with primary closure to restore a uniform caliber to the urethra.[127] Special attention should be paid to any narrowing of the neourethra distally, just as in fistula repair.

Retrusive Meatus

Retraction of the meatus from its original position at the tip of the glans to a proximal glanular or subcoronal position can occur with any repair. Retrusive meatus is caused by the failure of the glansplasty closure or the breakdown of devascularized distal neourethra. Retraction is a common problem when the MAGPI procedure is used in patients whose meatus is too proximal or when too much tension is placed on the glansplasty

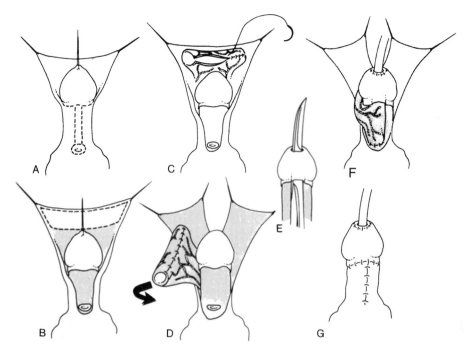

FIGURE 58-18. Transverse preputial island flap tube repair. *A* and *B*, Release of chordee and degloving of penile shaft skin. *B*, Outline of inner preputial island flap. *C*, Tubularization of inner preputial island flap. *D*, Transposition of the tubularized island flap to the ventrum, maintaining pedicle blood supply. *E*, Creation of a channel through glans tissue with sharp incisional and excisional technique. *F*, Island tube anastomosed to proximal native urethra, brought though glans channel and anastomosed to epithelium at tip of glans. *G*, Penile shaft covered with dorsal foreskin advanced ventrally. Skin closure completed.

closure.[128] Correction can usually be accomplished by a repeat glansplasty or a meatal-based flap procedure.[122,128]

Persistent Chordee

Residual ventral curvature after hypospadias repair can be a troublesome problem. It is usually related to inadequate release of chordee at the original procedure. Increased ventral curvature occurring as the penis grows is at least a theoretical possibility. The artificial erection has made this complication much less common. Treatment of the problem is similar to the treatment of chordee without hypospadias. Degloving of the penis and takedown of any ventral tethering tissue is done by using the artificial erection technique to guide dissection. Dorsal plication, ventral excision with patching, and division of the urethra may all be necessary.[123,129]

Recurrent Multiple Complications

Patients with recurrent multiple complications generally have experienced multiple failed repairs that have resulted in a combination of severe complications. Extensive fibrosis of the urethra with fistulas, strictures, diverticula, and residual chordee may be present. The successful outcome of further repair depends on thorough evaluation of each complication and the use of all the techniques available to the surgeon experienced in

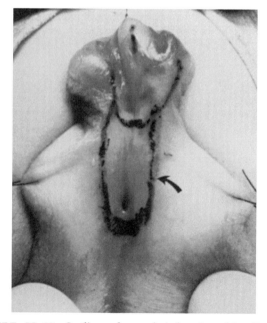

FIGURE 58-19. Outline of non–hair-bearing skin distal to scrotal meatus (*arrow*) that will be tubularized to move meatus to penoscrotal junction. Island flap tube will complete repair to end of glans.

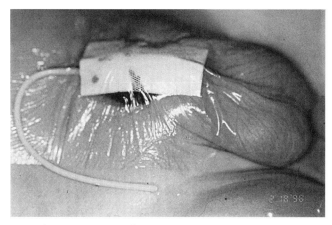

FIGURE 58-20. Occlusive dressing of transparent adhesive material in sandwich fashion on abdominal wall, with 6F soft polymeric silicone (Silastic) indwelling tube for urinary diversion.

hypospadias repair. Vascularized flaps or staging procedures are preferable to free grafts in a scarred phallus, if tissue is available.[130] If a free graft must be used, it is important to obtain the most vascularized bed possible in which to place the graft. Bladder or buccal mucosa is probably the best tissue for a free graft in this type of situation.[21,54,123] In patients with severe scarring and ventral skin loss, a split-thickness skin graft may be used for ventral coverage. This tissue may then be tubularized at a second stage.[131]

Sexual Function

Long-term results of hypospadias repair with regard to erectile function, ejaculation, and fertility are not available for the children who have undergone repairs at a younger age over the past decade. Historically, sexual difficulties after hypospadias repair have been reported. These were thought to be secondary to psychosexual factors related to surgery in childhood rather than to anatomic problems.[36,41] Fertility has been assessed by semen analysis in patients after hypospadias repair.[38,132] Higher rates of oligospermia are reported. These lower sperm counts generally occur in patients with associated anomalies, such as cryptorchidism, chromosome abnormalities, varicoceles, or torsion. In a patient with an anatomically successful hypospadias repair and no associated anomalies that might affect fertility, a high potential for fertility and an adequate sexual function are expected. Only close observation of pediatric patients into their adulthood after hypospadias repair early in life will reveal the true incidence of sexual dysfunction and fertility problems.

Results

A summary of the incidence of certain complications for commonly used procedures is given in Table 58-2. A personal series is included and represents those patients I have operated on over a 15-year period (from 1987 to 2002). A follow-up of at least 6 postoperative months is available for the patients included in this series.

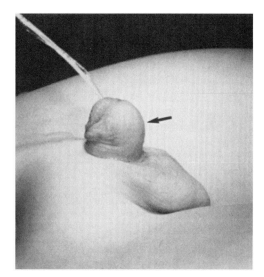

FIGURE 58-21. Neourethral diverticulum with bulging ventrally with voiding (*arrow*).

TABLE 58-2

COMPLICATIONS OF VARIOUS TYPES OF REPAIRS

	Number of Cases	Meatal Stenosis (%)	Retrusive Meatus (%)	Stricture (%)	Fistula (%)	Diverticulum (%)	Total (%)
MAGPI							
Issa[128]	142	—	5 (3.5)	—	—	—	5 (3.5)
Keating[54]	225						(<1)
Duckett[133]	1100	—	7 (0.6)	—	5 (0.4)	—	12 (1.1)
Personal series	318	—	4 (1.2)	—	—	—	4 (1.2)
Meatal-based Flap							
Retik[134]	294	1 (0.5)	—	—	1 (0.5)	—	2 (1.0)
Wacksman[98]	125	—	—	—	1 (0.8)	—	1 (0.8)
Hakim[112]	336	—	—	—	9 (2.7)	—	9 (2.7)
Personal series	285	4 (1.4)	—	—	3 (1.1)	—	7 (2.5)
Thiersch-Duplay (w/o Incised Plate)							
Kass[135]	308	—	—	—	28 (9.1)	2 (0.6)	30 (9.7)
Zaontz[98]	24	—	—	—	1 (4.1)	—	1 (4.1)
Personal series	162	—	—	—	2 (1.2)	—	2 (1.2)
TIP							
Snodgrass[100]	148	3 (2.0)	—	—	5 (3.4)	—	8 (5.4)
Cheng[102]	514	2 (0.3)	—	—	3 (0.6)	—	5 (1.0)
Jayanthi[138]	110	—	—	—	1 (0.9)	—	1 (0.9)
Personal series	118	—	—	—	1 (0.8)	—	1 (0.8)
Onlay Island Flap							
Elder[86]	50	—	—	—	1 (2.0)	—	1 (2.0)
Hollowell[74]	66						(8.0)
Keating[54]	43						(9.0)
Weiner[136]	58	2 (3.4)	—	1 (1.7)	10 (17.0)	—	13 (22.4)
Gearhart[137]	61	—	1 (1.6)	—	3 (5.0)	—	4 (6.6)
Personal series	249	2 (0.8)	—	1 (0.4)	6 (2.4)	4 (1.6)	13 (5.2)
Tube Island Flap							
Duckett[26]	100						(10.0)
Wacksman[98]	94						7 (7.4)
Keating[54]	34						(18.0)
Hollowell[74]	85						(15.0)
Perovic[77]	75	4 (5.3)	—	—	2 (2.7)	3 (4.0)	9 (12.0)
Weiner[136]	74	3 (4.0)	—	7 (9.4)	10 (13.5)	9 (12.2)	29 (39.1)
Personal series	57	5 (8.8)*	—	—	2 (4.0)	6 (10.5)*	8 (14.0)
Free Graft (Preputium)							
Devine[17]	20	—	—	—	6 (30.0)	—	6 (30.0)
Hanna[139]	27	—	—	1 (3.7)	4 (14.8)	1 (3.7)	6 (22.2)
Hendren[140]	103	3 (2.9)	—	—	6 (5.8)	—	9 (8.7)
Robert[141]	81	—	—	7 (8.6)	28 (34.6)	—	35 (43.2)
Stock[142]	77	2 (2.5)	—	3 (3.8)	10 (12.9)	—	15 (19.5)
Bladder Mucosa							
Koyle[104]	16	1 (6.2)	—	—	1 (6.2)	—	2 (12.5)
Ransley[143]	47	9 (19.1)	—	1 (2.1)	10 (21.3)	—	20 (42.5)
Ehrlich[144]	79	—	—	8 (10.1)	2 (2.5)	4 (5.0)	14 (17.7)
Mollard[145]	76	14 (17.4)	—	15 (19.7)†	—	—	29 (38.1)
Li[146]	113	6 (5.3)	—	8 (7.0)	—	—	14 (12.4)
Buccal Mucosa							
Fichtner[147]	62	1 (1.6)	—	—	7‡ (11.3)	—	8 (12.9)
Carr[148]	30	—	—	—	—	—	10 (33.3)
Hensle[149]	47	—	—	—	—	—	13 (27.7)

*Same patients with meatal stenosis and diverticulum.
†Three of these 15 were failed grafts.
‡Three of these were failed grafts.
MAGPI, meatal advancement and glansplasty.

REFERENCES

1. Barcat J: Current concepts of treatment. In Horton CE (ed.): Plastic and Reconstructive Surgery of the Genital Area. Boston, Little, Brown, 1973, pp 249–263.
2. Bellinger MF: Embryology of the male external genitalia. Urol Clin North Am 8:375–382, 1981.
3. Sommer JJ, Stephens FD: Dorsal urethral diverticulum of the fossa navicularis: Symptoms, diagnosis and treatment. J Urol 124:94–97, 1980.
4. Glenister TW: The origin and fate of the urethral plate in man. J Anat 88:413, 1954.
5. Rogers DO: History of external genital surgery. In Horton CE (ed): Plastic and Reconstructive Surgery of the Genital Area. Boston, Little, Brown, 1973, pp 3–47.
6. Horton CE, Devine CJ, Baran N: Pictorial history of hypospadias repair techniques. In Horton CE (ed): Plastic and Reconstructive Surgery of the Genital Area. Boston, Little, Brown, 1973, pp 237–243.
7. Bachus LH, de Felice CA: Hypospadias, then and now. Plast Reconstr Surg 25:146–160, 1960.
8. Creevy CD: The correction of hypospadias: A review. Urol Surv 8:2–47, 1958.
9. Browne D: An operation for hypospadias. Proc R Soc Med 41:466–468, 1949.
10. Culp OS: Hypospadias with and without chordee. In Horton CE (ed): Plastic and Reconstructive Surgery of the Genital Area. Boston, Little, Brown, 1973, pp 315–320.
11. Byars LT: A technique for consistently satisfactory repair of hypospadias. Surg Gynecol Obstet 100:184–190, 1955.
12. Smith ED: Durham Smith repair of hypospadias. Urol Clin North Am 8:451–455, 1981.
13. Fuqua F: Renaissance of urethroplasty: The Belt technique of hypospadias repair. J Urol 106:782–785, 1971.
14. Coleman JW, McGovern JH, Marshall VF: The bladder mucosal graft technique for hypospadias repair. Urol Clin North Am 8:457–462, 1981.
15. McCormack RM: Simultaneous chordee repair and urethral reconstruction for hypospadias: Experimental and clinical studies. Plast Reconstr Surg 13:257, 1954.
16. Humby G: A one-stage operation for hypospadias. Br J Surg 29:84–92, 1941.
17. Devine CJ Jr, Horton DE: Hypospadias repair. J Urol 85:166–172, 1972.
18. Memmelaar J: Use of bladder mucosa in a one-stage repair of hypospadias. J Urol 58:68–73, 1947.
19. Marshall VF, Spellman RM: Construction of a urethra in hypospadias using vesical mucosal grafts. J Urol 73:335–342, 1955.
20. LiZhong-Chu, Zheng Yu-Hen, Sheh Ya-Xiong, et al: One-stage urethroplasty for hypospadias using a tube constructed with bladder mucosa: A new procedure. Urol Clin North Am 8:463–470, 1981.
21. Duckett JW, Coplen D, Ewalt D, et al: Buccal mucosal urethral replacement. J Urol 153:1660–1663, 1995.
22. Mustardé JC: One-stage correction of distal hypospadias and other people's fistulae. Br J Plast Surg 18:413–422, 1965.
23. Broadbent TR, Woolf RM, Tosku E: Hypospadias: One-stage repair. Plast Reconstr Surg 27:154–159, 1961.
24. Hodgson NB: Use of vascularized flaps in hypospadias repair. Urol Clin North Am 8:471–481, 1981.
25. Standoli L: One-stage repair of hypospadias: Preputial island flap technique. Ann Plast Surg 9:81–88, 1982.
26. Duckett JW: The island flap technique for hypospadias repair. Urol Clin North Am 8:513–519, 1981.
27. Sweet RA, Schrott HG, Kurland R, et al: Study of the incidence of hypospadias in Rochester, Minnesota, 1940-1970, and a case control comparison of possible etiologic factors. Mayo Clin Proc 49:52–58, 1974.
28. Duckett JW: Hypospadias. Pediatr Rev 11:37–42, 1989.
29. Duckett JW: Hypospadias. In Gillenwater Y, Frayhack JT, Howards SS, et al. (eds): Adult and Pediatric Urology. Chicago, Year Book Medical, 1987, pp 1880–1915.
30. Allen TD, Griffin JE: Endocrine studies in patients with advanced hypospadias. J Urol 131:310–314, 1984.
31. Shima H, Ikoma F, Yabumoto H, et al: Gonadotropin and testosterone response in prepubertal boys with hypospadias. J Urol 135:539–542, 1986.
32. Roberts CJ, Lloyd S: Observations on epidemiology of simple hypospadias. Br Med J 1:768–770, 1973.
33. Mau G: Progestins during pregnancy and hypospadias. Teratology 24:285–287, 1981.
34. Avellan L: The incidence of hypospadias in Sweden. Scand J Plast Reconstr Surg 9:129–139, 1975.
35. Källén B, Mastroiacovo P, Lancaster PA, et al: Oral contraceptives in the etiology of isolated hypospadias. Contraception 44:173–182, 1991.
36. Bauer SB, Retik AB, Colodny AH: Genetic aspects of hypospadias. Urol Clin North Am 8:559–564, 1981.
37. Maier WA, Twees G: Sexual function after operations for hypospadias according to Ombredanne. Progr Pediatr Surg 17:79–82, 1984.
38. Glassman CN, Machlus BJ, Kelalis PP: Urethroplasty for hypospadias: Long-term results. Urol Clin North Am 7:437–441, 1980.
39. Bracka A: A long-term view of hypospadias. Br J Plast Surg 42:251–255, 1984.
40. Svensson J, Berg R, Berg G: Operated hypospadias: Late follow-up: Social, sexual and psychological adaptation. J Pediatr Surg 16:134–135, 1981.
41. Berg R, Berg G: Penile malformation, gender identity and sexual orientation. Acta Psychiatr Scand 68:154–166, 1983.
42. Duckett JW, Keating MA: Technical challenge of the megameatus intact prepuce hypospadias variant: The pyramid procedure. J Urol 141:1407–1409, 1989.
43. Cerasaro TS, Brock WA, Kaplan GW: Upper urinary tract anomalies associated with congenital hypospadias: Is screening necessary? J Urol 135:537–538, 1986.
44. Shima H, Ikoma F, Terakowa T, et al: Developmental anomalies associated with hypospadias. J Urol 122:619–621, 1970.
45. Khuri FJ, Hardy BE, Churchill BM: Urologic anomalies associated with hypospadias. Urol Clin North Am 8:565–571, 1981.
46. Ritchey ML, Benson RC, Kramer SA, et al: Management of müllerian duct remnants in the male patient. J Urol 140:795–799, 1988.
47. Fallon B, Devine CJ Jr, Horton CE: Congenital anomalies associated with hypospadias. J Urol 116:585–586, 1976.
48. Lutzker LG, Kogan SJ, Levitt SB: Is routine I.V. urography indicated in patients with hypospadias? Pediatrics 59:630–633, 1977.
49. Kennedy PA: Hypospadias: A twenty-year review of 489 cases. J Urol 85:814–817, 1961.
50. Neyman MA, Schirmer HKA: Urinary tract evaluation in hypospadias. J Urol 94:439, 1965.
51. McArdle R, Lebowitz R: Uncomplicated hypospadias and anomalies of the upper urinary tract: Need for screening? Urology 5:712–716, 1975.
52. Smith DS: Hypospadias. In Ashcraft KW (ed): Pediatric Urology. Philadelphia, WB Saunders, 1990, pp 353–395.
53. Sheldon CA, Duckett JW: Hypospadias. Pediatr Clin North Am 34:1259–1272, 1987.
54. Keating MA, Duckett JW: Recent advances in the repair of hypospadias. Surg Ann 22:405–425, 1990.
55. Wacksman J: Results of early hypospadias surgery using optical magnification. J Urol 131:516–517, 1984.
56. Belman AB, Kass EJ: Hypospadias repair in children less than 1 year old. J Urol 128:1273–1274, 1982.
57. Manley CB, Epstein ES: Early hypospadias repair. J Urol 125:698–700, 1981.
58. Kelalis PP, Bunge R, Barkin M, et al: The timing of elective surgery on the genitalia of male children with particular reference to undescended testes and hypospadias. Pediatrics 56:479–483, 1975.
59. Smith DS: Timing of surgery in hypospadias repair. Aust N Z J Surg 53:396–397, 1983.
60. Winslow BH, Horton CE: Hypospadias. Semin Urol 5:236–242, 1987.
61. Mackay A: Hypospadias repair under the age of 1 year. Aust N Z J Surg 53:449–452, 1983.

62. Duckett JW: Advances in hypospadias repair. Postgrad Med J 66(suppl 1):562–571, 1990.

63. Schultz JR, Klykylo WM, Wacksman J: Timing of elective hypospadias repair in children. Pediatrics 71:342–351, 1983.

64. Kass EJ, Jogan SJ, Manley CB, et al: Timing of elective surgery on the genitalia of male children with particular reference to the risks, benefits and psychological effects of surgery and anesthesia. Pediatrics 97:590–594, 1996.

65. Gittes RF, McClaughlin AP: Injection technique to induce penile erection. Urology 4:473–475, 1974.

66. Allen TD, Spence HM: The surgical treatment of coronal hypospadias and related problems. J Urol 100:504–508, 1968.

67. Devine CJ, Horton CE: Chordee without hypospadias. J Urol 110:264–271, 1973.

68. Lindgren BW, Reda EF, Levitt SB: Single and multiple dermal grafts for the management of severe penile curvature. J Urol 160:1128–1130, 1998.

69. Richey ML, Ribbeck M: Successful use of tunica vaginalis grafts for treatment of severe penile chordee in children. J Urol 170:1574–1576, 2003.

70. Kropp BP, Cheng EY, Pope JC, et al: Use of small intestinal submucosa for corporal body grafting in cases of severe penile curvature. J Urol 168:1742–1745, 2002.

71. Nesbit RM: Congenital curvature of the phallus: Report of three cases with description of corrective operation. J Urol 93:230–234, 1965.

72. Livne PM, Gibbons MD, Gonzales ET: Correction of disproportion of corpora cavernosa as cause of chordee in hypospadias. Urology 22:608–610, 1983.

73. Hollowell JG, Keating MA, Snyder HM, et al: Preservation of the urethral plate in hypospadias repair: Extended applications and further experience with the onlay island flap urethroplasty. J Urol 143:98–101, 1990.

74. Baskin L, Duckett JW: Dorsal tunica albuginea plication (TAP) for hypospadias curvature. J Urol 151:1668–1671, 1994.

75. Baskins LS, Erol A, Li YW: Anatomy of the neurovascular bundle: Is safe mobilization possible? J Urol 164:977–980, 2000.

76. Decter RM: Chordee correction by corporal rotation: The split and roll technique. J Urol 162:1152–1155, 1999.

77. Perovic SC, Djordjevic ML: A new approach in hypospadias repair. World J Urol 16:195–199, 1998.

78. Hurwitz RS, Devine CJ, Horton CE, et al: Chordee without hypospadias. Dialog Pediatr Urol 9:1–8, 1986.

79. Donnahoo KK, Cain MP, Pope JC, et al: Etiology, management and surgical complications of congenital chordee without hypospadias. J Urol 160:1120–1122, 1998.

80. Gibbons MD, Gonzales ET: The subcoronal meatus. J Urol 130:739–742, 1983.

81. Gibbons MD: Nuances of distal hypospadias. Urol Clin North Am 12:169–174, 1985.

82. Hendren WH: The Belt-Fuqua technique for repair of hypospadias. Urol Clin North Am 8:431–450, 1981.

83. Standoli L: Vascularized urethroplasty flaps: The use of vascularized flaps of preputial and penopreputial skin for urethral reconstruction in hypospadias. Clin Plast Surg 15:355–370, 1980.

84. Snodgrass W, Patterson K, Plaire JC, et al: Histology of the urethral plate: Implications for hypospadias repair. J Urol 164:988–990, 2000.

85. Shapiro SR, Zaontz MR, Scherz HC: Hypospadias repair: Update and controversies, part 1. Dialog Pediatr Urol 13:1–8, 1990.

86. Elder JS, Duckett JW, Snyder HM: Onlay island flap in the repair of mid and distal penile hypospadias without chordee. J Urol 138:376–379, 1987.

87. Sadove RC, Horton CE, McRoberts JW: The new era of hypospadias surgery. Clin Plast Surg 15:341–354, 1988.

88. Snodgrass W, Decter RM, Roth DR, et al: Management of the penile shaft skin in hypospadias repair: Alternative to Byar's flaps. J Pediatr Surg 23:181–182, 1988.

89. Firlit CF: The mucosal collar in hypospadias surgery. J Urol 137:80–82, 1987.

90. VanDorpe EJ: Correction of distal hypospadias with reconstruction of the preputium. Plast Reconstr Surg 80:290–293, 1987.

91. Nonomura K, Koyanagi T, Imanaka K, et al: One-stage total repair of severe hypospadias with scrotal transposition: Experience in 18 cases. J Pediatr Surg 23:177–180, 1988.

92. Glenn JF, Anderson EE: Surgical correction of incomplete penoscrotal transposition. J Urol 110:603–605, 1973.

93. Ehrlich RM, Scardino PT: Simultaneous surgical correction of scrotal transposition and perineal hypospadias. Urol Clin North Am 8:531–537, 1981.

94. Ehrlich RM, Scardino PT: Surgical corrections of scrotal transposition and perineal hypospadias. J Pediatr Surg 17:175–177, 1982.

95. Duckett JW: MAGPI (meatoplasty and glanuloplasty). Urol Clin North Am 8:513–519, 1981.

96. Mathieu P: Traitement en un temps de l'hypospadias balanique et juxtabalanique. J Chir 39:481, 1932.

97. Wacksman J: Modification of the one-stage flip flap procedure to repair distal penile hypospadias. Urol Clin North Am 8:527–530, 1981.

98. Zaontz MR: The gap (glans approximation procedure) for glanular/coronal hypospadias. J Urol 141:359–361, 1989.

99. Snodgrass W: Tubularized incised plate urethroplasty for distal hypospadias. J Urol 151:464–465, 1994.

100. Snodgrass W, Koyle M, Manzoni G: Tubularized incised plate hypospadias repair: Results of a multicenter experience. J Urol 156:839–841, 1996.

101. Snodgrass W: Does tubularized incised plate hypospadias repair create neourethral strictures? J Urol 162:1159–1161, 1999.

102. Cheng EY, Vemulapalli SN, Kropp BP: Snodgrass hypospadias repair with vascularized dartos flap: The perfect repair for virgin cases of hypospadias? J Urol 168:1723–1726, 2002.

103. Hendren HW, Horton CE Jr: Experience with one-stage repair of hypospadias and chordee using free graft of prepuce. J Urol 140:1250–1264, 1988.

104. Koyle MA, Ehrlich RM: The bladder mucosa graft for urethral reconstruction. J Urol 138:1093–1095, 1987.

105. Decter RM, Roth DR, Gonzales ET: Hypospadias repair by bladder mucosal graft: An initial report. J Urol 140:1256–1258, 1988.

106. Duckett JW: Transverse preputial island flap technique for repair of severe hypospadias. Urol Clin North Am 7:423, 1980.

107. Gershbaum MD, Stock JA, Hanna MK: A case for 2-stage repair of perineoscrotal hypospadias with severe chordee. J Urol 168:1727–1729, 2002.

108. Greenfield SP, Sadler BT, Wan J: Two stage repair for severe hypospadias. J Urol 152:498–501, 1994.

109. Retik AB, Bauer SB, Mandell J, et al: Management of severe hypospadias with two-stage repair. J Urol 152:749–751, 1994.

110. Shapiro SR, Wacksman J, Koyle MA, et al: Hypospadias repair: Update and controversies, part 2. Dialog Pediatr Urol 13:1–8, 1990.

111. Duckett JW: Hypospadias [discussion]. J Urol 136:272, 1986.

112. Hakim S, Merguerian PA, Rabinowitz R: Outcome analysis of the modified Mathieu hypospadias repair: Comparison of stented and unstented repairs. J Urol 156:836–838, 1996.

113. Steckler RE, Zaontz MR: Stent-free Thiersch-Duplay hypospadias repair with the Snodgrass modification. J Urol 158:1178–1180, 1997.

114. Gaylis FD, Zaontz MR, Dalton D, et al: Silicone foam dressing for penis after reconstructive pediatric surgery. Urology 33:296–299, 1989.

115. McLorie GA, Joyner BD, Bagli DJ, et al: A prospective randomized clinical trial to evaluate methods of postoperative care in hypospadias. Pediatrics 104(suppl):813A, 1999.

116. VanSavage JG, Palanca LG, Slaughenhoupt BL: A prospective randomized trial of dressing versus no dressing for hypospadias repair. J Urol 164:981–983, 2000.

117. Goulding FJ: Penile block for postoperative pain relief in penile surgery. J Urol 126:337, 1981.

118. Reynolds PI, Rosen DA: Caudal analgesia for pediatric urologic procedures. Dialog Pediatr Urol 13:6–7, 1990.

119. Duckett JW, Kaplan GW, Woodard JR: Panel: Complications of hypospadias repair. Urol Clin North Am 7:443–454, 1980.

120. Sugar EC, Firlit CF: Urinary prophylaxis and postoperative care of children at home with an indwelling catheter after hypospadias repair. Urology 32:418–420, 1988.

121. Shohet I, Alagam M, Shafir R, et al: Postoperative catheterization and prophylactic antimicrobials in children with hypospadias. Urology 22:391–393, 1983.

122. Horton CE Jr, Horton CE: Complications of hypospadias surgery. Clin Plast Surg 15:371–379, 1988.

123. Retik AB, Keating MA, Mandell J: Complications of hypospadias surgery. Urol Clin North Am 15:223–236, 1988.

124. Walker RD: Outpatient repair of urethral fistula. Urol Clin North Am 8:582, 1981.

125. Zagula EM, Braren V: Management of urethrocutaneous fistulas following hypospadias repair. J Urol 130:743–745, 1983.

126. Scherz HC, Kaplan GW, Packer MG, et al: Post-hypospadias repair urethral strictures: A review of 30 cases. J Urol 140:1253–1255, 1988.

127. Zaontz MR, Kaplan WE, Maizels M: Surgical correction of anterior urethral diverticula after hypospadias repair in children. Urology 33:40–42, 1989.

128. Issa MM, Gearhart JP: The failed MAGPI: Management and prevention. Br J Urol 64:169–171, 1989.

129. Vandersteen DR, Hussman DA: Late onset recurrent penile chordee after successful correction at hypospadias repair. J Urol 160:1131–1133, 1998.

130. Sheldon CA, Essig KA: Surgical strategies in the reconstruction of the failed hypospadias: Advantages and versatility of vascular based graft/flap techniques [abstract 250]: American Urological Association Meeting. J Urol 143(suppl):251A, 1990.

131. Ehrlich RM, Alter G: Split-thickness skin graft urethroplasty and tunica vaginalis flaps for failed hypospadias repairs. J Urol 155:131–134, 1996.

132. Marberger H, Pauer W: Experience in hypospadias repair. Urol Clin North Am 8:403–419, 1981.

133. Duckett JW, Snyder HM: Meatal advancement and glanuloplasty hypospadias repair after 1000 cases: Avoidance of meatal stenosis and regression. J Urol 147:665–669, 1992.

134. Retik AB, Mandell J, Bauer SB, et al: Meatal based hypospadias repair with the use of a dorsal subcutaneous flap to prevent urethrocutaneous fistula. J Urol 152:1229–1231, 1994.

135. Kass EJ, Chung AK: Glanuloplasty and in situ tubularization of the urethral plate: Long-term follow-up. J Urol 164:991–993, 2000.

136. Weiner JS, Sutherland RW, Roth DR, et al: Comparison of onlay and tubularized island flaps of inner preputial skin for the repair of proximal hypospadias. J Urol 158:1172–1174, 1997.

137. Gearhart JP, Borland RN: Onlay island flap urethroplasty: Variation on a theme. J Urol 148:1507, 1992.

138. Jayanthi VR: The modified Snodgrass hypospadias repair: Techniques and results. Urology 21:30–35, 1983.

139. Hanna MK: Single-stage hypospadias repair: Techniques and results. Urology 21:30–35, 1983.

140. Hendren WH, Horton CE: Experience with one-stage repair of hypospadias and chordee using free graft of prepuce. J Urol 140:1259–1264, 1988.

141. Rober PE, Perlmutter AD, Reitelman C: Experience with 81, one-stage hypospadias/chordee repairs with free graft urethroplasties. J Urol 144:526–529, 1990.

142. Stock JA, Cortez J, Scherz HC, et al: The management of proximal hypospadias using a one-stage hypospadias repair with a preputial free graft for neourethral construction and a preputial pedicle flap for ventral skin coverage. J Urol 152:2335–2337, 1994.

143. Ransley PG, Duffy PG, Oesch IL, et al: The use of bladder mucosa and combined bladder mucosa/preputial skin grafts for urethral reconstruction. J Urol 138:1096–1098, 1987.

144. Ehrlich RM, Reda EF, Koyle MA, et al: Complications of bladder mucosa graft. J Urol 42:626–627, 1989.

145. Mollard P, Mouriguand P, Bringeon G, et al: Repair of hypospadias using a bladder mucosal graft in 76 cases. J Urol 142:1548–1550, 1989.

146. Li LC, Zhang X, Zhou SW, et al: Experience with repair of hypospadias using bladder mucosa in adolescents and adults. J Urol 153:1117–1119, 1995.

147. Fichtner J, Fisch M, Filipas D, et al: Refinements in buccal mucosal graft urethroplasty for hypospadias repair. World J Urol 16:192–194, 1998.

148. Carr MC: Buccal mucosa grafts: Long-term follow up. Dialog Pediatr Urol 25:5–6, 2002.

149. Hensle TW, Kearney MC, Bingham JB: Buccal mucosa grafts for hypospadias surgery: Long-term results. J Urol 168:1734–1737, 2002.

CHAPTER 59

Circumcision

Stephen C. Raynor, MD

Circumcision, the removal of the prepuce or foreskin, is one of the most frequently performed surgical procedures in the world. Rates of circumcision vary widely among different populations, however. Indications given to perform circumcision include treatment of disease, perceived prophylactic benefits, and social or religious concerns. A lack of consensus regarding the function of the foreskin as well as often-strident debate concerning the benefits of circumcision has led to much controversy as to the appropriateness of the procedure.

EMBRYOLOGY

The development of the prepuce begins during the third month of gestation as a fold of skin at the base of the glans. With growth, this skin extends distally, with the dorsal portion growing at a more rapid rate than the ventral component. The proper development of the prepuce is dependent on the presence of androgen and androgen receptors. The closure of the ventral portion of the prepuce completes by the fifth month of gestation after closure of the glanular urethra. Keratinization of the glans and inner epithelial surface of the prepuce then follows. Initially, the inner surface of the prepuce and the epithelium of the glans are fused. Lacunae then begin to form between the two surfaces, resulting in an eventual complete separation. This process of separation is a gradual one, and typically remains incomplete at birth.[1]

As a result of this incomplete keratinization, the foreskin can be completely retracted in only about 5% of newborns. The adherence between the glans and prepuce may not allow visualization of the meatus in 46% of newborns. The natural separation of the two surfaces continues with growth of the child. Complete retraction of the foreskin can be expected in 20% of boys by 6 months, 50% by 1 year, 80% by 2 years, and 90% by 3 years.[2] All foreskins should be retractable by age 17 years.[3] Until this natural process of separation is complete, usually no need exists for forceful retraction of the foreskin and cleaning of the glans.

HISTORY AND INCIDENCE

Circumcision has been practiced since ancient times. Evidence of circumcision has been found in the study of ancient Egypt, with the identification of circumcised mummies as well as the depiction of circumcision in bas relief on an ancient tomb.[1,4] Circumcision also may have arisen as a mark of defilement or slavery.[4] Columbus found the New World natives to be circumcised.[1] A common rationale given for the decision to proceed with circumcision is religious beliefs. The Bible declares circumcision to be the sign of the covenant between God and the people of Israel.[5] In the Muslim faith, circumcision is recommended, but not obligatory.[6] A high rate of circumcision is found in Jewish and Muslim populations, and circumcision is quite common in the United States. Areas of Africa, Australian aborigines, and people of the Near East also practice ritual circumcision.[7,8] In contrast, ritual circumcision is rarely performed in Europe, China, the Far East, and Central and South America.[7] This wide variation of incidence is probably reflective of religious and cultural differences, as well as strong disagreement regarding the value of routine newborn circumcision.

THE PREPUCE

Contributing to the debate concerning the appropriateness of routine circumcision is a lack of clear understanding of the function of the prepuce, the anatomic covering of the glans. The prepuce is a specialized junctional mucocutaneous tissue that provides adequate skin and mucosa to cover the entire penis during erection. The somatosensory innervation is by the dorsal nerve of the penis and branches of the perineal nerve. Autonomic innervation is from the pelvic plexus. Encapsulated somatosensory receptors, both mechanicoreceptors and nocioreceptors, are found in the prepuce. This innervation of the prepuce differs from that of the glans, which is innervated primarily by free nerve endings and has primarily protopathic sensitivity. As a result of these differences, the inner mucosa of the prepuce is thought to be a part of the normal complement of the penile erogenous tissue.[9]

MEDICAL INDICATIONS

Phimosis is the inability to retract the foreskin due to narrowing of its opening. The inability to retract the foreskin of a newborn is a result of the natural adherence of the prepuce to the glans and is not pathologic. True phimosis is associated with a white, scarred preputial orifice and is uncommon before age 5 years, being most common just before puberty. This scarring of the orifice is characteristic of balanitis xerotica obliterans and is an indication for circumcision.[10] Paraphimosis occurs when the foreskin has been retracted behind the corona but is able to be brought back over the glans with great difficulty or not at all. This is considered an indication for circumcision, although ardent opponents of circumcision would offer preputial stretching or preputial plasty as alternatives.[11-13] Balanitis is an infection of the glans, and posthitis is an infection of the prepuce. Recurrent infection with scarring of the prepuce is an accepted indication for circumcision.[8,14]

ROUTINE NEWBORN CIRCUMCISION

The appropriateness of routine circumcision of healthy newborn boys is an emotional and contentious issue. Confounding the argument is the lack of a clear understanding as to the precise function of the prepuce.[15] Opponents of circumcision have represented the procedure as a symbol of the "therapeutic state,"[16] as a mutilating procedure,[17] and have questioned the legality of routine newborn circumcision.[18] Circumcision is done on the eighth day in the Jewish faith, traditionally performed by a *mohel*, a member of the Jewish faith trained in ritual circumcision. In Islamic countries, circumcision is considered traditional but not obligatory, with a wide variability in age at time of circumcision.[6,19] Proponents of routine newborn circumcision generally cite three advantages, the prevention of urinary tract infections in infants, the prevention of sexually transmitted disease, and the prevention of penile cancer.

As rates of circumcision have decreased in the United States, reports have appeared demonstrating an increased rate of urinary tract infections in uncircumcised male infants. An initial report of infant urinary tract infections showed a male predominance in infants younger than 3 months, with a disproportionate number of these being uncircumcised.[20] A subsequent large retrospective analysis of infants of families in the armed services suggested that uncircumcised infants have a 12-fold increased risk for urinary tract infection as compared with circumcised infants.[21-23] A tenfold increase in the cost of managing urinary tract infections in uncircumcised infants as compared with that in circumcised infants also was shown.[24] The increased incidence of

infection is believed to be secondary to adherence of pathogenic bacteria to the prepuce.[25] It also has been suggested that an increased risk of urinary tract infections occurs in uncircumcised young adults.[26] Proponents of circumcision point out that the 10% incidence of concurrent bacteremias and the long-term sequelae of renal scarring are factors to be considered in the circumcision debate.[27] Critics have been quick to note that these studies have been retrospective analyses and therefore are subject to significant bias.[28,29] Others have suggested that colonization of the prepuce by nonmaternal uropathic bacteria could be prevented by strict rooming-in with the mother.[30]

Many studies examined the relation between circumcision status and sexually transmitted diseases (STDs). Studies have shown noncircumcision to be associated with an increased risk of chancroid, syphilis, gonorrhea, candidiasis, genital warts, and genital herpes,[31-34] whereas others have found little support for or have refuted these findings altogether.[35,36] Evidence also indicates that circumcision is associated with a decreased risk of cervical cancer in women with high-risk sexual partners, as a result of the reduced risk of human papillomavirus (HPV) infection in the male partner.[33] It is possible that the protective effect of circumcision against STDs may differ between developed and developing nations with poorer hygiene.[36] Possible mechanisms for differing rates of STDs according to circumcision status include a more easily traumatized mucosa and epithelium of the uncircumcised phallus, the environment of the foreskin being more conducive to certain infectious agents, or nonspecific balanitis in uncircumcised men, predisposing to certain STDs. Behavior and sexual practice still represent the greatest risk factors in the transmission of STDs.[33]

Epidemiologic studies of human immunodeficiency virus (HIV) and acquired immunodeficiency syndrome (AIDS) have raised another argument for prophylactic circumcision. A substantial amount of evidence links noncircumcision in men with an increased risk of HIV infection. This increased risk of HIV infection associated with noncircumcision is independent of the increased risk of genital ulcers in uncircumcised men.[37] In Africa, regional differences exist in the rate of circumcision. As the HIV/AIDS epidemic has emerged on the continent, an increased rate of HIV/AIDS has been observed in areas with low circumcision rates.[38] An analysis of 30 epidemiologic studies from Africa concluded that enough evidence was found that circumcision was associated with reduced HIV infection rates to consider male circumcision as a viable strategy to reduce HIV transmission.[30] A similar association between circumcision status and HIV has been noted in the United States, with uncircumcised homosexual men having a twofold increase in the risk of HIV infection.[40] Noncircumcision of the male partner also seems to be associated with an increased risk of transmission of HIV to heterosexual contacts.[41]

Another reason forwarded for routine circumcision is as a protective measure against invasive penile cancer. The lack of circumcision has been strongly associated with invasive penile cancer in multiple case series.[37] The etiology of penile cancer is unknown, but an association appears to exist with HPVs.[42] The incidence of penile cancer in the United States is approximately 1 case per 100,000, with nearly all cases occurring in uncircumcised men.[29,43] This protective effect against penile cancer is diminished or lost when circumcision is done after the newborn period.[8,43,44] Other factors associated with invasive penile cancer include smoking, a history of genital warts, penile rash or tears, multiple sexual partners, and poor penile hygiene.[37,44] Critics of circumcision cite equally low rates of penile cancer in countries with low circumcision rates. These epidemiologic data combined with the extremely low incidence of penile cancer and the probable viral etiology has led some authors to conclude that the impact of routine newborn circumcision against penile cancer does not justify its widespread practice.[28,42]

Many strong feelings but no definitive answer exists to the question of the appropriateness of routine newborn circumcision. Taken together, studies do not provide conclusive evidence for or against routine newborn circumcision. Boys not circumcised at birth have between a 2% and 10% likelihood of needing circumcision in the future.[17,45] A longitudinal study comparing circumcised with uncircumcised boys showed a higher risk of penile problems in infancy in the circumcised group, with a higher rate of problems in the uncircumcised group after infancy. By age 8 years, the uncircumcised group had experienced 1.5 times the rate of penile problems.[46] The most recent circumcision policy statement from the American Academy of Pediatrics in 1999 acknowledges the potential medical benefits of newborn male circumcision, but does not recommend routine neonatal circumcision.[37] Their interpretation of the data and this recommendation have been questioned.[47] On their review of the data, the Canadian Pediatric Society thought that the risks and benefits of routine newborn circumcision were evenly balanced and concluded that routine newborn circumcision was not recommended.[41] In the United States, the decision regarding newborn circumcision seems to be based more on social as opposed to medical concerns.[48]

SURGICAL TECHNIQUE

Circumcision has been practiced for centuries, and numerous techniques have been developed. Common to all methods, the goal is removal of an adequate amount of the prepuce to uncover the glans, to treat or prevent phimosis, and to eliminate the possibility of paraphimosis. Whichever method is chosen, the surgeon must be familiar with and adept at the procedure, with a resultant low complication rate. Informed consent should always be obtained before any circumcision.[57]

NEWBORN CIRCUMCISION

Circumcision is the most frequently performed male operation in the United States, with perhaps 64% of the newborn male infants circumcised in 1995.[37] Newborn circumcision is most frequently performed with a circumcision device. These various devices may be a shield, used in the traditional Jewish circumcision, a Mogen clamp, a Gomco clamp, or a Plastibell.[7] Before the procedure, the penis should be inspected for any contraindication to circumcision. Contraindications to circumcision in the newborn include a short or small phallus, hypospadias, hooded prepuce, dorsal penile cutaneous hump, penile curvature or torsion, penoscrotal fusion, or large hernias or hydroceles that engulf the penis.[49]

General agreement has been reached as to the need for adequate analgesia when performing newborn circumcision. Studies have shown the infants circumcised without analgesia have a stronger pain response to vaccination at ages 4 and 6 months as compared with those who received analgesics.[50] Effective relief of circumcision pain has been shown to be with acetaminophen, topical lidocaine/procaine cream, and local nerve blocks.[51-54] One study showed a subcutaneous ring block with 1% lidocaine without epinephrine to be the most effective pain relief.[37] Sucrose on a pacifier also can provide added pain control.[55]

Even though most procedures are done outside the operating room, antisepsis is critical, as infection is a serious potential complication. In performing a Gomco circumcision, the field is sterilely prepped, and then the adhesions between the glans and inner surface of the prepuce are bluntly separated. The extent of foreskin to be excised is then marked, either with a marking pen or with a crush of the dorsal prepuce done with a straight mosquito clamp. A dorsal slit allows the appropriate-sized bell to be placed over the glans, inside the prepuce. The bell and foreskin are then brought through the opening in the base of the clamp, placed in the yoke, which is tightened, followed by excision of the foreskin distal to the base of the clamp. Electrocautery must never be used to excise the foreskin, because transmission of the electrical current to the shaft of the penis will take place. The bell is then released and removed, taking care not to disrupt the weld between the shaft skin and the remnant of the inner surface of the prepuce.

A Plastibell differs from the Gomco clamp in that the distal foreskin is strangulated, with a resulting slough of that tissue. After sterile prep and dorsal slit, the appropriate-sized Plastibell is placed over the glans inside the prepuce. A string is then tied around the prepuce, positioned in a groove in the bell. The excess foreskin is trimmed and the handle is broken off the bell. The foreskin remnant and bell are expected to slough off in 7 to 12 days.

OPERATIVE CIRCUMCISION

In older patients, circumcision is usually done in the operating room. Circumcision devices seem to be less adequate for the older patient, and sleeve resection of the foreskin is preferable. As shown in Figure 59-1, after prepping of the operative field, any remaining adhesions between the glans and foreskin are bluntly taken down.

After marking the subcoronal sulcus, the foreskin is incised along the base of the glans with the foreskin in its normal position. Less skin is to be excised from the ventral surface. Dissection is carried down to Buck's fascia.

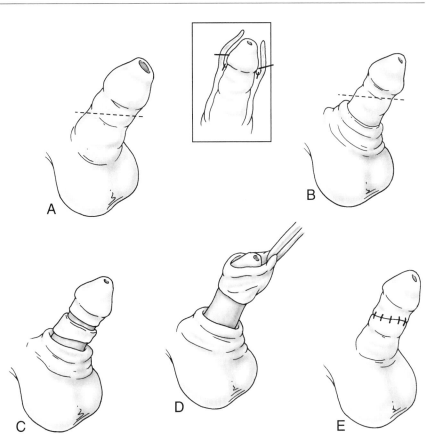

FIGURE 59-1. For a freehand circumcision, the initial incision is made in the shaft skin, leaving more skin ventrally (A). A second incision is then made in the subcoronal sulcus, leaving a generous cuff (B). The inset shows the amount of foreskin to be excised. The isolated foreskin (C) is then excised (D), and the shaft skin is sutured to the subcoronal skin (E).

The prepuce is then retracted, and an incision made in the subcoronal sulcus, leaving a generous cuff of subcoronal skin. Injury to the urethra must be avoided. The collar of foreskin that has been isolated is then excised, and electrocautery is used to obtain meticulous hemostasis. The shaft skin is then approximated to the subcoronal skin by using absorbable sutures.

COMPLICATIONS

When done by experienced hands, circumcision has a low complication rate of between 2% and 10%.[42] Bleeding is the most frequent complication and is generally minor. Infection is the second most common complication and is generally minor. However, serious problems can result, including necrotizing fasciitis, sepsis, Fournier's gangrene, and meningitis.[8] Too much or too little of the foreskin can be excised, with resultant postoperative phimosis or concealed penis. Revision of the circumcision may sometimes be necessary later in childhood.[56] Other complications include skin bridges, inclusion cysts, iatrogenic hypospadias or epispadias, partial amputation of the glans, and the catastrophic loss of the penis when electrocautery is used with a metal circumcision device.

REFERENCES

1. Kaplan GW: Circumcision: An overview. Curr Probl Pediatr 7:1–33, 1977.
2. Gardner D: The fate of the foreskin. BMJ 2:1433–1437, 1949.
3. Oster J: Further fate of the foreskin. Arch Dis Child 43:200–203, 1968.
4. Dunsmuir WD, Gordon EM: History of circumcision. BJU Int 83(suppl 1):1–12, 1999.
5. The Holy Bible.
6. Rizvi SAH, Naqvi SAA, Hussain M, et al: Religious circumcision: A Muslim View. BJU Int 83(suppl 1):13–26, 1999.
7. Holman J, Lewis E, Ringler R: Neonatal circumcision techniques. Am Fam Physician 52:511–518, 1995.
8. Niku S, Stock J, Kaplan G: Neonatal circumcision. Urol Clin North Am 22:57–65, 1995.
9. Cold CL, Taylor JR: The Prepuce. BJU Int 83(suppl 1):34–44, 1999.
10. Rickwood AMK: Medical indications for circumcision. BJU Int 83(suppl 1):45–51, 1999.
11. Cuckow P, Rix G, Mouriquand P: Preputial plasty: A good alternative to circumcision. J Pediatr Surg 29:561–563, 1994.
12. Holmlund D: Dorsal incision of the prepuce and skin closure with Dexon in patients with phimosis. Scand J Urol Nephrol 7:97–99, 1973.
13. Cooper C, Thomson G, Raine P: Therapeutic retraction of the foreskin in childhood. BMJ 286:186–187, 1983.
14. Escala J, Rickwood A: Balanitis. Br J Urol 63:196–197, 1989.
15. Taylor J, Lockwood A, Taylor A: The prepuce: Specialized mucosa of the penis and its loss to circumcision. Br J Urol 77:291, 1996.
16. Szasz T: Routine neonatal circumcision: Symbol of the birth of the therapeutic state. J Med Philos 21:137–148, 1996.
17. Weiss G, Weiss E: A perspective on controversies over neonatal circumcision. Clin Pediatr 33:726–730, 1994.
18. Van Howe RS, Svoboda JS, Dwyer JG, et al: Involuntary circumcision: The legal issues. BJU Int 83(suppl 1):63–73, 1999.
19. Sari N, Buyukunal S, Zulfikar B: Circumcision ceremonies at the Ottoman palace. J Pediatr Surg 31:920–924, 1996.
20. Ginsburg C, McCracken G: Urinary tract infections in young infants. Pediatrics 69:409–412, 1982.
21. Wiswell T, Enzenauer R, Cornish D, et al: Declining frequency of circumcision: Implications for changes in the absolute incidence

and male-to-female sex ratio of urinary tract infections in early infancy. Pediatrics 79:338–342, 1987.

22. Wiswell T, Geschke W: Risks from circumcision during the first month of life compared with those for uncircumcised boys. Pediatrics 83:1011–1015, 1989.

23. Wiswell T, Hachey W: Urinary tract infection and the uncircumcised state: An update. Clin Pediatr 82:130–134, 1993.

24. Schoen EJ, Colby CJ, Ray GT: Newborn circumcision decreases incidence and costs of urinary tract infections during the first year of life. Pediatrics 105:789–793, 2000.

25. Roberts J: Pathogenesis of non-obstructive urinary tract infections in children. J Urol 144:475–479, 1990.

26. Spach D, Stapleton A, Stamm W: Lack of circumcision increases the risk of urinary tract infection in young men. JAMA 267:679–681, 1992.

27. Wiswell TE: The prepuce, urinary tract infections, and the consequences. Pediatrics 105:860–862, 2000.

28. Poland R: The question of routine neonatal circumcision. N Engl J Med 822:1312–1315, 1990.

29. Schoen E, Anderson G, Bohon C, et al: Report of the task force on circumcision. Pediatrics 84:388–391, 1989.

30. Winberg J, Gothefors L, Bollgren I, et al: The prepuce: A mistake of nature? Lancet 1:598–599, 1989.

31. Parker S, Stewart A, Wren M, et al: Circumcision and sexually transmitted disease. Med J Aust 2:288–290, 1983.

32. Cook L, Koutsky L, Holmes K: Circumcision and sexually transmitted diseases. Am J Public Health 84:197–201, 1994.

33. Cook LS, Koutsky LA, Holmes KK: Circumcision and sexually transmitted diseases. Am J Public Health 84:197–201, 1994.

34. Castellsaue X, Bosch FX, Munoz N, et al: Male circumcision, penile human papillomavirus infection, and cervical cancer in female partners. N Engl J Med 346:1105–1112, 2002.

35. Laumann E, Masi C, Zuckerman E: Circumcision in the United States: Prevalence, prophylactic effects and sexual practice. JAMA 277:1052–1057, 1997.

36. Donovan B, Bassett I, Bodsworth N: Male circumcision and common sexually transmissible diseases in a developed nation setting. Genitourin Med 70:317–320, 1994.

37. American Academy of Pediatrics, Task force on circumcision: Circumcision policy statement. Pediatrics 103:686–693, 1999.

38. Moses S: Geographical patterns of male circumcision practices in Africa: Association with HIV seroprevalence. Int J Epidemiol 19:693–697, 1990.

39. Moses S, Plummer F, Bradley J, et al: The association between lack of male circumcision and risk for HIV infection: A review of the epidemiological data. Sex Transm Dis 21:201–210, 1994.

40. Kreiss J, Hopkins S: The association between circumcision status and human immunodeficiency virus infection among homosexual men. J Infect Dis 168:1404–1408, 1993.

41. McCarthy K, Studd J, Johnson M: Heterosexual transmission of human immunodeficiency virus. Br J Hosp Med 48:404–408, 1992.

42. Fetus and Newborn Committee Canadian Pediatric Society: Neonatal circumcision revisited. CMAJ 154:769–780, 1996.

43. Schoen E: The relationship between circumcision and cancer of the penis. CA Cancer J Clin 41:306–309, 1991.

44. Maden C, Sherman K, Beckmann A, et al: History of circumcision, medical conditions, and sexual activity and risk of penile cancer. J Natl Cancer Inst 85:19–24, 1993.

45. Lerman SE, Liao JC: Neonatal circumcision. Pediatr Clin North Am 48, 6:1539–1557, 2001.

46. Fergussen D, Lawton J, Shannon F: Neonatal circumcision and penile problems: An 8-year longitudinal study. Pediatrics 81:537–541, 1988.

47. Schoen EJ, Wisewell TE, Moses M: New policy on circumcision: Cause for concern. Pediatrics 105:620–623, 2000.

48. Brown M, Brown C: Circumcision decision: The prominence of social concerns. Pediatrics 80:215–219, 1987.

49. Redman JF, Elser JM: Neonatal circumcision: Anatomic contraindications. J Ark Med Soc 94:73–75, 1997.

50. Taddio A, Katz J, Iiersich A, et al: Effect of neonatal circumcision on pain response during subsequent routine vaccination. Lancet 849:599–603, 1997.

51. Howard C, Howard F, Weitzman M: Acetaminophen analgesia in neonatal circumcision: The effect on pain. Pediatrics 93:641–646, 1994.

52. Taddio A, Stevens B, Craig K, et al: Efficacy and safety of lidocaine-prilocaine cream for pain during circumcision. N Engl J Med 336:1197–1201, 1997.

53. Serour F, Cohen A, Mandelberg A, et al: Dorsal penile nerve block in children undergoing circumcision in a day-care surgery. Can J Anaesth 43:954–958, 1996.

54. Lenhart J, Lenhart N, Reid A, et al: Local anesthesia for circumcision: Which technique is most effective? J Am Board Fam Pract 10:13–19, 1997.

55. Herschel M, Khoshnood B, Ellman C, et al: Neonatal Circumcision Randomized trial of a sucrose pacifier for pain control: Arch Pediatr Adolesc Med 152:279–284, 1998.

56. Brisson PA, Patel HI, Feins NR: Revision of circumcision in children. J Pediatr Surg 37:1343–1346, 2002.

57. Christakis DA: A trade-off analysis of routine newborn circumcision. Pediatrics 105:246–249, 2000.

CHAPTER 60

Prune-belly Syndrome

Michael A. Keating, MD, and Mark A. Rich, MD

Shortly after an initial description of its urologic findings by Parker in 1895,[1] Osler[2] coined the graphic term *prune-belly syndrome* (PBS) for a triad of findings that include

1. Congenital absence, deficiency, or hypoplasia of the abdominal wall musculature
2. Urinary tract abnormalities characterized by a large hypotonic bladder (megacystis), dilated ureters, and dilated prostatic urethra
3. Bilateral cryptorchidism

As in most syndromes, the effects are not confined solely to its classic manifestations, and other organs including the kidneys, lungs, heart, extremities, and gastrointestinal (GI) tract are frequently affected (Table 60-1).[3]

A variety of labels have been applied to this constellation of findings including Eagle–Barrett,[4] mesenchymal dysplasias[5] and abdominal musculature deficiency (AMD) syndromes.[6] The moniker "prune" is bluntly descriptive but presents a negative connotation for the affected child and the family. Nunn and Stephens[7] coined the term *triad syndrome* to minimize emotional repercussions. Nevertheless, the designation prune-belly remains the most widely accepted.

Owing to its inclusion of cryptorchidism, by definition, fully developed PBS occurs exclusively in boys. Occasionally a female patient will be born with an abdominal wall that is phenotypically and histologically indistinguishable from those in boys with PBS. They constitute 3% to 5% of recorded cases[8] and have been shown to have a strong association with omphalocele and lesions causing bladder-outlet obstruction.[9] Even more rarely, severe degrees of urinary tract ectasia also occur.[10] Female or male patients who manifest one or two components of PBS are probably best identified as having pseudoprune disorder. It is rare to have a normal urinary tract with the characteristic abdominal wall, although the converse is not true.[11] The management of the abnormalities found with pseudoprune anatomy is similar to that of boys with classic PBS.

INCIDENCE AND GENETICS

The incidence of PBS is probably similar to that of bladder exstrophy (one per 30,000 to 40,000 live births).[12–14] Despite this relative paucity, several centers have reported considerable experience with PBS and its variants.[8,15–18] As surveillance programs with improved prenatal ultrasonography increase, the incidence of major genitourinary malformations, including PBS, will be affected. In one series, the pregnancies of 31% of fetuses with PBS were electively terminated.[19]

Extensive testing has failed to implicate a genetic basis for the syndrome. No evidence has been found of autosomal recessive or single-gene inheritance, although PBS has been documented in siblings.[20,21] Sex-linked inheritance could explain the inordinate male predominance in the disorder but has never been shown. Instead, a complex polygenic transmission of autosomal dominant mutation with sex-limited expression that mimics X-linkage has been proposed.[22] Mosaicism has been reported in two siblings with PBS.[23] Cases associated with individual chromosomal anomalies (trisomies 13 and 18, and Turner's syndrome) also have been reported and may suggest the involvement of multiple loci.[24–26] PBS also has been reported with Down syndrome, but an analysis of its incidence suggests that these are probably independent events, occurring by chance.[27] Notably, these types of chromosomal abnormalities are the exception, and the karyotypic analysis of patients with PBS is nearly always normal. Although cases have been reported,[28] the nearly 100% discordance among twins strongly suggests another cause in most. Maternal cocaine use has been implicated in some cases, and children of younger mothers and blacks may be at increased risk.[29,30]

TABLE 60-1
EXTRAGENITOURINARY ABNORMALITIES

Pulmonary	Pulmonary hypoplasia
	Pneumothorax
	Pneumomediastinum
	Lobar atelectasis
Cardiac	Tetralogy of Fallot
	Ventricular septal defect
	Atrial septal defect
	Patent ductus arteriosus
Orthopedic	Pectus excavatum and carinatum
	Varus deformity of feet
	Dimpling of elbow or knee
	Congenital hip dislocation
	Severe leg maldevelopment
Gastrointestinal	Intestinal malrotation
	Intestinal atresias
	Gastroschisis
	Omphalocele
	Imperforate anus
	Hepatobiliary anomalies
	Hirschsprung's disease
Miscellaneous	Adrenal cystic dysplasia
	Splenic torsion

ETIOLOGY

Embryology

The lateral plate mesoderm of the embryo splits into a visceral layer (muscular coat of the gut) and a parietal or somatic layer (body wall). The coelom progressively enlarges between the two. In the caudal region, coelomic extension and lateral plate division do not occur. Here, the undivided mesoderm extends around the allantois and cloaca, where its deeper layers form bladder wall musculature, ureters, and prostate. The superficial layers of the lateral plate mesoderm are necessary for closure of the anterior abdominal wall. Omphalocele and exstrophy result when midline approximation of mesoderm does not occur. Differentiation of the abdominal wall musculature is derived from the lower thoracic somites, which migrate into the plate.

A variety of different theories have been proposed regarding the origin of PBS, although its precise cause remains unclear.[14]

The theory of yolk sac hindrance implicates an error in the interplay of maturing abdominal wall and the yolk sac.[31] Normally, the yolk sac constricts as the mesoderm infolds and differentiates into the anterior abdominal wall. An overdevelopment of the allantoic diverticulum could block this sequence, causing an excessive amount of allantois to be incorporated in the urinary tract and leaving abdominal wall redundancy as its aftermath. This could conceivably account for the anomalies of the urachus, bladder, and prostatic urethra found with PBS. However, the theory does not explain the cryptorchidism and ureteral abnormalities.

The mesodermal defect theory speculates that a defect of the lateral plate mesenchyme disrupts the migration or differentiation of the thoracic somites, affecting myoblast development between 6 and 10 weeks of gestation.

Histologic demonstrations of dystrophic abdominal musculature replaced by fibrous tissue surrounded by fascia perhaps support this theory.[32] Electron microscopy showing poorly organized muscle and Z-band fragmentation in the sarcomeres are thought to be more indicative of a developmental disturbance rather than an insult from lengthening or atrophy, as might be expected from bladder obstruction and abdominal distention.[33]

The mesodermal defect theory is clinically supported by the fourfold incidence of twinning seen with PBS (1:23 vs. 1:80 in the general population).[5] Nearly every case in twins has been discordant for PBS. Theoretically, only one fetus receives adequate mesenchyme with initial divisions of the embryo's primitive streak. To its detriment, this theory does not account for the urinary tract abnormalities, cryptorchidism, or male predominance seen with PBS. However, it is plausible that a similar mesodermal error could affect the adjacent paraxial, intermediate, and lateral plate mesoderm essential to normal genitourinary development. A lack of hormonal responsiveness by the primordial gubernaculum and prostate also has been implicated in the etiology of cryptorchidism and prostatic hypoplasia.[34] This type of defect would conceivably link the theories of mesodermal defect and bladder-outlet obstruction.

The theory of bladder obstruction and distention has become the most widely accepted.[35] According to this explanation, urethral obstruction occurs during a critical "window" in development, which results in massive distention of the bladder and ureters. This, in turn, causes degeneration of the abdominal wall. Histologic studies demonstrating atrophic abdominal musculature rather than primitive muscle support the hypothesis.[36–38] Obstruction could explain the changes seen in bladder walls as well as the ureteral dilatation and urachal patency that commonly occur. Early outlet obstruction also has obvious implications for the developing kidneys, where dysplasia, oligohydramnios, and subsequent pulmonary hypoplasia often result. In this theory, the testes also are blocked by the distended bladder or fail to descend because of abdominal wall laxity and decreased intra-abdominal pressures within, which normally act as an impetus to descent.

The exact mechanism of obstruction remains to be defined. Critics note that the majority of PBS infants are born without demonstrable urethral obstruction. Bladder hypertrophy and hyperplasia that typically result from outlet obstruction are lacking, and most exhibit normal or low intravesical pressures. In addition, the severity of the abdominal wall laxity does not correlate well with the degree of urinary tract dilatation in many cases. Perhaps most perplexing is that the majority of babies with urethral valves or other bladder-outlet obstructions do not have PBS or cryptorchidism. Nevertheless, it seems likely that transient obstruction is present at some point during fetal development and that timing is actually the factor most crucial to the appearance of PBS.[35,39] Transient urethral valves or the hypoplastic prostate uniformly found in these boys are possible candidates. With the latter, the weakened walls of the dysgenetic gland, lacking smooth muscle support, bulge dorsally and caudally. As a consequence, the unsupported membranous urethra twists anteriorly at its junction with the prostatic urethra. A flap-valve obstruction to flow results.[40,41] Posterior urethral obstruction would explain the male predominance. Another possible cause of urinary tract obstruction, supported by the high incidence of megalourethras seen with the syndrome, is transient blockage at the junction of the glanular and bulbar urethras. A fetus demonstrating severe phimosis as the cause of obstruction also was described.[42]

Intra-abdominal distentions unrelated to urinary tract obstruction also have been implicated. Fetal ascites,[43] megacystis-microcolon syndrome, amniotic band syndrome,[44] and intestinal duplication cysts[45] have all been cited with the bladder-obstruction syndrome. Such associations may play a role in cases of pseudoprune, but they do not explain the urologic findings of PBS. In addition, these types of distentions do not usually cause abdominal wall laxity in the majority of children in whom they occur.

GENITOURINARY MANIFESTATIONS

Abdominal Wall

Pathophysiology

A large degree of variability in the involvement of the abdominal wall musculature is seen (Fig. 60-1). Typically, the upper abdominal oblique and rectus muscles are better developed, whereas the lateral and ventral abdominal muscles are diffusely deficient in irregular and often asymmetrical fashion.[46] Affected muscles (in decreasing order of frequency) include the transversus, rectus abdominis below the umbilicus, internal oblique, external oblique, and rectus above the umbilicus. The abdominal wall periphery usually shows normal or near-normal muscles. In contrast, studies of affected areas show poorly organized muscle interspersed with dense collagenous tissue.[7,33] At times, the lower medial aspect of the abdomen consists merely of skin, fat, and fibrous tissue condensed onto the peritoneum, making difficult the differentiation of the muscle layers.[47] The innervation of the abdominal musculature and skin is normal. However, electromyography shows little or no functional muscle in the lower central abdomen.[46] Nonspecific ultrastructural disorganization is seen at the cellular level.[33]

Clinical Correlates

The lax ventral abdominal musculature fails to support the viscera within. The overlying skin is stretched in utero and results in a typically wrinkled appearance in the newborn. The thin and pliable abdominal wall allows easy palpation of the organs. Peristalsis of the intestines and ureters can often be observed immediately beneath

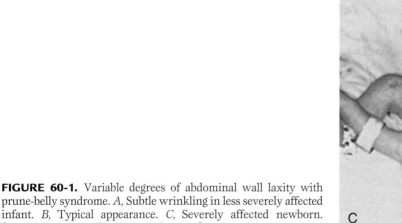

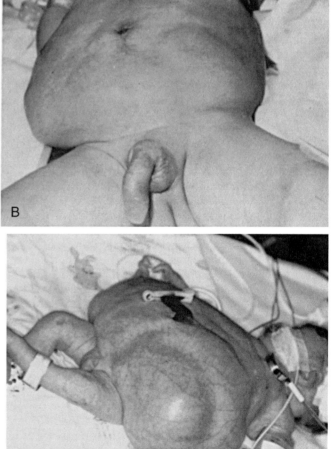

FIGURE 60-1. Variable degrees of abdominal wall laxity with prune-belly syndrome. *A,* Subtle wrinkling in less severely affected infant. *B,* Typical appearance. *C,* Severely affected newborn. (Part *C,* courtesy of D.M. Joseph, M.D.)

its surface. A pot-bellied appearance typically evolves with growth, as the cutaneous wrinkling resolves somewhat with accumulation of subcutaneous fat. Some abdominal tone also is gained in most children.[48]

The severity of the abdominal defect has no prognostic significance, although urinary tract involvement often correlates with ipsilateral abdominal wall involvement in cases of asymmetry.[11] The lack of abdominal wall support can pose a problem. For all practical purposes, rectus muscle continuity is lost. Infants with severe defects are typically unable to sit from the supine position; instead they roll prone and raise themselves by pushing up. Developmental delay in motor skills that require balance and coordination (e.g., walking) is common.

Problems with respiratory toilet result from an impaired cough. Pulmonary secretions are difficult to expectorate without the assistance of the abdominal musculature. Respiratory infections are common. This deficit also increases the risk of pulmonary complications after general anesthesia.[49]

Testicles

Pathophysiology

Possible causes of the cryptorchidism found with PBS include mechanical obstruction by the enlarged bladder, decreased abdominal pressure, and a mesenchymal or hormonal alteration in the gubernaculum's ability to guide the testes properly.[50,51] The undescended testicles in PBS are usually located at the level of the iliac vessels, but more proximal positions have been described.[7,16] Histologically, such testes are indistinguishable from normal age-matched gonads early in development.[52] Germ cells are present but are abnormal.[53] Biopsies in adults, however, have shown little or no germ cell maturation, even after the gonads have been repositioned into the upper scrotum or canal.[54] Whether these changes represent the natural progression of PBS cryptorchidism or are in some way influenced by the timing or surgical technique is unclear.

Adnexal abnormalities also have been described. Epididymal detachment and atresia have been noted. Vas deferens detachment has been described. The architecture of the vas is variable. Collagen replaces muscle in some cases, and a thickened vas results. Others are thin walled, tortuous, and segmentally atretic.[7,55] The seminal vesicles are usually absent or atretic, a diagnostic feature of PBS. However, dilation with diverticular formation has been described.[31] The gubernaculum is usually normal, and its course through the inguinal canal direct, although malformations that have been described may contribute to cryptorchidism.[3,53]

Clinical Correlates

Unassisted fertility has not been recorded with PBS, regardless of the age of orchiopexy.[54,56] A variety of factors could contribute to infertility, including decreased germ cell potential, prostatic maldevelopment causing deficient seminal fluid, and retrograde ejaculation due to the wide-open bladder neck that occurs. Absent ejaculation is a common finding in adulthood.[57] However, one study failed to demonstrate sperm in pre- and postejaculate urine in five adults with PBS, further implicating impaired spermatogenesis.[54] Despite these shortcomings, sperm retrieval in an adult with PBS is possible, and intracytoplasmic injection has resulted in one pregnancy.[58]

Normal secondary sexual characteristics, erections, and orgasm are expected of the adult. Testosterone production is usually good, although luteinizing hormone levels are elevated, an indicator of Leydig cell damage. Several testicular malignancies have been reported in PBS, yet the risk of malignancy appears to be no greater than that with other disorders involving intra-abdominal testes.[59,60]

Kidneys

Pathophysiology

Although the kidneys in PBS can be normal, some degree of renal dysplasia (Potter's type II dysplasia) occurs in about 50%. Signs of disordered nephron development—embryonic tubules, cysts, cartilage, and mesenchyme—are thought to be indicative of a developmental insult rather than obstruction. Ureteral ectopy or some other abnormal interplay between the ureteral bud and metanephric blastema is implicated.[61,62] Variable degrees of dysplasia occur within individual kidneys, sometimes interspersed between normal parenchyma. Wide ranges in involvement also occur between the kidneys of an affected patient, and functional asymmetry is common. One study found dysplasia in 25% of the parenchyma in ten nephrectomy specimens; another found bilateral dysplasia affecting 30% to 70% of the kidneys in seven of nine autopsies.[63]

Variable degrees of hydronephrosis also are common. However, the parenchymal changes are not usually typical of other obstructive processes, such as ureteropelvic junction (UPJ) obstruction (e.g., Potter's type IV changes, pelvic thinning). The quality of the renal parenchyma is routinely much better than expected, given the degree of collecting system dilatation. This suggests that the mechanism of dilatation in PBS differs from that in other obstructive uropathies. It may be that hydronephrosis of the syndrome represents a low-pressure reflection of the same mesenchymal defect that has affected the lower urinary tract. True UPJ obstruction or ureteral stenosis was found in only 6 of 80 patients in two reports.[64]

Radiographic Findings

Signs of renal dysmorphism are easily appreciated on excretory urography (Fig. 60-2). Rotational abnormalities are common, and the kidneys have a lobulated outline. Calyceal clubbing and infundibular narrowing also are common. These changes have random distribution, however, and may be interspersed between normal calyces.[32] The severity of pelvic dilatation is variable, but disproportion usually occurs between generous distal ureters and less voluminous renal pelves. When changes appear, they are typically asymmetrical.

Ultrasonography (US) provides useful information about renal size, the degree of pelvic and calyceal dilatation, and differentiation of the parenchyma. The most severely dysplastic kidneys are small, hyperechoic, and have absent corticomedullary junctions. Radioisotope (technetium 99m diethylenetriaminepentaacetic acid [DTPA] or glucoheptonate) scans help assess function and obstruction.

Clinical Correlates

The degree of dysplasia dictates the prognosis in the infant who survives the pulmonary sequela of oligohydramnios. Dysplasia is typically more severe in children born with urethral stenosis or agenesis, megalourethra, or imperforate anus,[32,65,66] and many are stillborn. The function of the kidneys in most other patients is surprisingly good. If, after a few days of life, the nadir creatinine is less than 0.7 mg/dL, renal failure in later life is unlikely unless pyelonephritis and urosepsis complicate the clinical picture.[67] Subsequent growth and development depend on the balance between viable renal tissue that remains and the demands placed on it. Urologic management is directed at preserving this tissue by avoiding infections, the main risk to renal deterioration.

Ureters

Pathophysiology

Elongated, dilated, and tortuous ureters are the most common urinary tract abnormality in patients with PBS.[7] Like the other organs involved, the degree of impairment is variable. Studies show that affected ureters have a patchy distribution of smooth muscle interspersed with fibrocytes and collagen.[62] In some cases, the entire wall is composed of acellular hyaline ground substance,[68] and differentiation into normal longitudinal and circular muscle layers is absent. These changes can be segmental, but classically, the lower ureter is involved preferentially to the upper, where greater densities of normal smooth muscle are found.[69,70]

Ineffective peristalsis, the functional sequelae of these abnormalities, results from disruption of the neuromyogenic cohesiveness of ureteral smooth muscle by collagen.[71] Nerve plexus decrease and irregular nonmyelinated Schwann fibers also were described.[70] Periureteral ganglia and other adjacent nerves are normal.[6] Vesicoureteral reflux is present in more than 75% of patients.[11] The orifices are often gaping and laterally displaced. Obstructions are rare.

Radiographic Findings

The diagnosis of PBS is frequently made by the appearance of the ureters on excretory urography or voiding cystourethrography (with reflux; see Fig. 60-2). Exaggerated distal ureteral ectasia is a hallmark of the syndrome. The proximal ureter typically has a more normal caliber.[72] Varying degrees of almost bizarre dilatation, sometimes interspersed with segments of narrowing,

result in tortuous ureters that "wander" across the newborn abdomen. Fluoroscopy may show ineffective peristalsis. With continued growth, the ureters often straighten, and peristalsis improves.

Clinical Correlates

The degree of ureteral dilatation does not correlate with the status of the kidneys or the patient's prognosis (Fig. 60-3). However, these types of nonobstructive megaureters leave the system at risk for infection due to urinary stasis. Pyelonephritis is common, especially when reflux is present. Preventing infection, eliminating reflux, and improving peristalsis become the goals of ureteral reconstruction when medical management is ineffective.

The proximal ureter is usually the better functioning and most normal portion. Abnormal ureter should be discarded. Operations that preserve the distal ureter (end ureterostomies or reimplantation with minimal resection) should usually be avoided.

Bladder and Urachus

Pathophysiology

The bladder is typically enlarged and distorted. Like the ureter, its walls are thickened with connective tissue interspersed between sparse muscle layers.[72] The ratio of collagen to smooth muscle is increased. At times, the muscular deficiency is so severe that portions of the bladder bulge under pressure and act like diverticula. Trabeculations are unusual, and muscular hypertrophy is absent, even in rare cases in which outlet obstruction is also present.[50] The anatomic innervation and distribution of ganglion cells is normal.[7] The trigone is usually large and asymmetrical, with ureteral orifices laterally positioned at its distal extent. Ureteral ectopia accounts for the high incidence of reflux.[73]

Radiographic Findings

Voiding cystourethrography usually shows a large misshapen bladder (Fig. 60-4). A patent urachus is sometimes present at the dome and commonly occurs in cases of urethral atresia, providing a "pop-off" for the obstructed bladder. Fixation of the bladder to the umbilicus via urachal remnants creates an hourglass shape, as detrusor contractions produce a waistlike effect during voiding. This muscular action can exclude the dome from the emptying process, causing it to act like a pseudodiverticulum. The bladder neck is usually wide open during voiding, and its junction with the dilated and triangular prostatic urethra is poorly defined. This configuration contrasts sharply with the findings of urethral valves and other outlet obstructions, in which the bladder neck is narrowed from muscular hypertrophy above the dilated prostatic urethra.

Clinical Correlates

A few patients with PBS have relatively normal urodynamics, with normal flow rates, voiding pressures, and

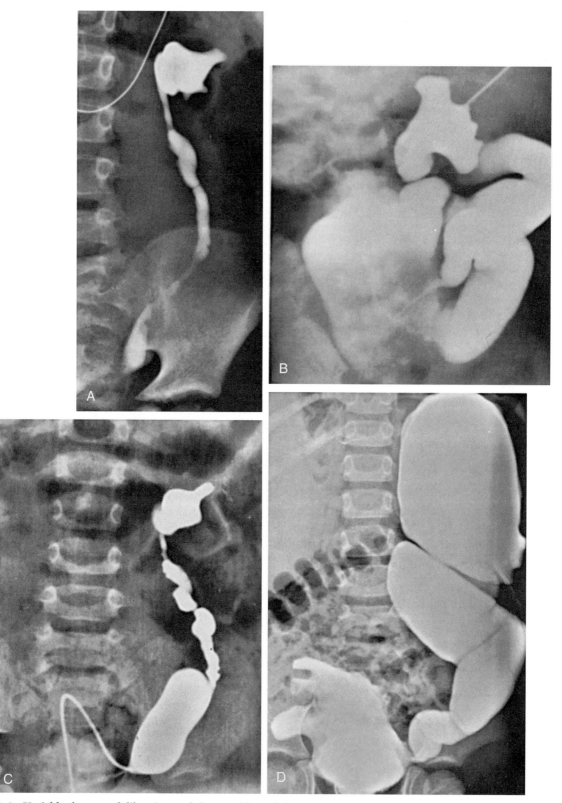

FIGURE 60-2. Variable degrees of dilatation and dysmorphism of the upper urinary tract. *A,* Dysmorphic renal pelvis with mild ureteral dilatation. *B,* Calyceal clubbing and tortuous "wandering" ureter. *C,* Dysmorphic pelvis with exaggerated dilatation of distal ureteral spindle. *D,* Bizarre appearance of collecting system as well as bladder.

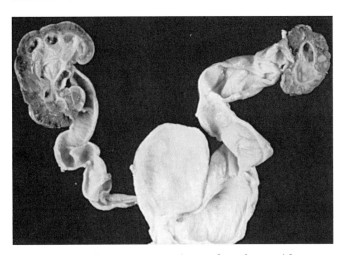

FIGURE 60-3. Postmortem specimen of newborn with prune-belly syndrome and severe pulmonary hypoplasia shows dilated ureters with thickened walls. Both kidneys demonstrated renal dysplasia. (Courtesy of C. Galiani, M.D.)

complete bladder emptying. A larger group exhibits abnormal voiding dynamics with delayed sensation to void and increased volumes caused by reflux and reduced contractility. Despite this, nearly half can spontaneously void to completion. The remainder are found with an imbalance between intravesical voiding pressures and outflow resistance.[74] Significant postvoid residuals result. In some cases, voiding patterns improve with age. In others, an increase in residual urine or detrusor decompensation with an inability to void occurs.[75,76] Upper urinary tract deterioration is more likely with significantly abnormal bladder dynamics. Elevated resting pressures and residual urine impair the emptying of already compromised ureters. Intermittent catheterization is a simple and effective means of facilitating bladder emptying. Surgical attempts to improve bladder mechanics are rarely successful. Partial cystectomy only transiently lessens volume in most cases.

Prostate and Prostatic Urethra

Pathophysiology

Generalized hypoplasia of the prostatic epithelium occurs, although some scantily distributed acinar tissue remains. Tubules may be present in the posterior portion of the gland, but fibrous tissue replaces its anterior portion, where smooth muscle normally predominates.[77,78] This loss of muscular support causes the dilated configuration of the gland and is implicated in the "functional obstruction" theory proposed for PBS.[79] The verumontanum can be completely absent or sometimes takes on a dimpled configuration.

Radiographic Findings

The prostatic urethra is classically wide and elongated at the bladder neck and tapers at the level of the urogenital diaphragm (Fig. 60-5).[11,77] Prominent posterior bulging is seen, and utricular diverticula are common. The triangular appearance of the gland can mimic that of posterior urethral valves. Valves have been described with PBS, but their presence represents a coincidence rather than an association.[80] Reflux into the vas is sometimes seen.

Clinical Correlates

The discrepancy between the caliber of the prostatic and membranous urethras gives the erroneous impression of mechanical obstruction. Urethral obstructions (atresia, stenosis, diverticulum, diaphragm, and valves) were found in one-third of cases in one series. However, an origin entirely different from that of classic posterior urethral valves could usually be implicated.[32] Urodynamics have consistently failed to document functional outlet obstruction in most patients, although in utero obstructions remain a possibility.[7,31,37] Cystoscopy occasionally reveals redundant folds of mucosa that can occlude the anterior membranous urethra as the prostatic urethra distends.[40] These are labeled "type IV valves" or "pseudovalves" and should be resected at the 12-o'clock position. Improved bladder emptying may not uniformly occur, however, depending on the quality of detrusor contractions above.

Anterior Urethra

The anterior and penile urethra are usually normal, but atresia or significant hypoplasia occasionally occurs in the membranous or bulbar positions (18% in one series).[81] Urachal patency is required for survival. Extreme degrees of urethral ectasia also are seen, some of which may be worsened with indwelling catheters.[82]

An association with both types of congenital megalourethra also has been documented (Fig. 60-6).[83] Scaphoid megalourethra, the less severe and more common variety, is found with an absent corpus spongiosum. Fusiform megalourethra is associated with absent corpora cavernosa.[84] Mild urethral dilatations occur in as many as 70%, but clinically significant megalourethra is rare.[77] The converse is not true, however, with PBS being common in patients with megalourethras. In one review, nearly half of 26 patients with scaphoid megalourethra and all five with fusiform variants had PBS.[85] When necessary, the principles of hypospadias repair are used to excise redundant urethra and reconstruct its lumen to normal caliber. In rare instances, a vesicostomy is necessary to vent the bladder until the urethra can be corrected.

ASSOCIATED NONUROLOGIC ANOMALIES

Nonurologic problems are found in as many as three-fourths of patients with PBS.[86] The deformities of the extremities and pulmonary hypoplasia are directly related to the problems noted with the urinary tract and the insult of oligohydramnios. PBS also continues to be

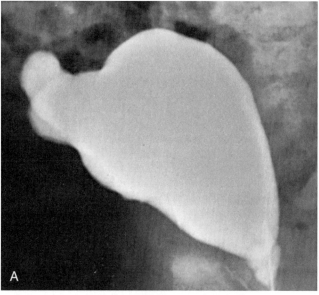

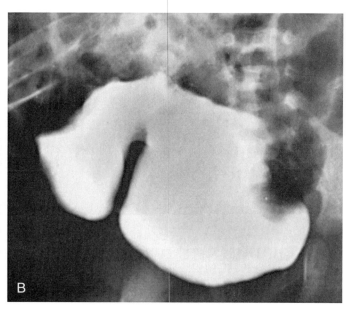

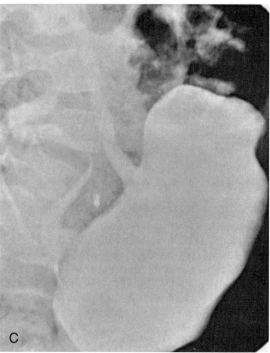

FIGURE 60-4. Radiographic examples of typically large, misshapen prune-belly syndrome bladder. *A,* Fixation to the umbilicus by urachal remnant is evident. *B,* "Waisting" of the bladder dome during voiding results in pseudodiverticulum. *C,* Vesicoureteral reflux is present in most cases.

reported with other malformations in smaller series or case reports in which coincidental associations probably exist or some etiologic significance has been postulated.[87-90] Impaired growth commonly is seen in the first year of life and may not be related to impaired renal function.[86]

Gastrointestinal

The GI malformation most commonly seen with PBS is malrotation.[91] In theory, decreased intra-abdominal pressure results in failure of colon fixation against the posterior abdominal wall, thus delaying or preventing the fusion of its dorsal mesentery. An incidence of 40% has

been cited.[92] Clinically significant malrotation with obstruction or volvulus or both is less common. Some clinicians have recommended routine radiographic evaluations of the GI tract to assess the relative risks associated with malrotation.[93]

Other GI anomalies reported with PBS include atresias of the colon and small intestine, gastroschisis, splenic torsion, persistent cloaca, omphalocele, and a paucity of intralobar bile ducts.[28,46,65,93-95] Hirschsprung's disease has been described. Historically, agangliosis was considered a factor in the urinary dilatation of PBS. The theory was later disproved when studies showed normal distribution of ureteral ganglion cells.[7]

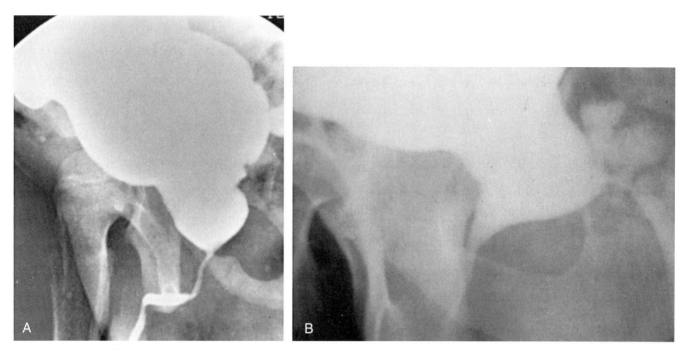

FIGURE 60-5. Voiding cystourethrography is instrumental to the diagnosis of prune-belly syndrome. *A,* Note wide-open bladder neck and beaklike narrowing at the membranous urethra. *B,* Utricular diverticulum and posterior bulging are common. A smooth-walled bladder is present in each case.

Functional "megacolon" does occur, however, and chronic constipation from the lack of abdominal wall musculature poses a formidable problem. Imperforate anus and rectal atresia also may occur, usually in more severely affected patients who have urethral atresia.[96] Diverting colostomy is required in the presence of high

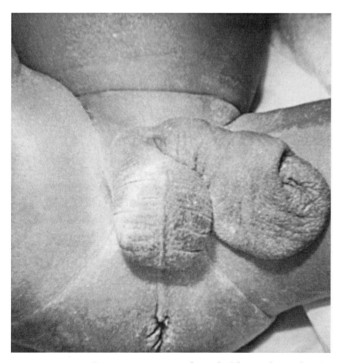

FIGURE 60-6. Gross appearance of scaphoid megalourethra in a child with prune-belly syndrome.

imperforate anus, rectourinary fistula, or pelvic hypoplasia. Abdominal wall laxity can challenge the placement of an ostomy and fitting of an appliance.[48]

Cardiac

Any child born with PBS requires a thorough assessment of his or her cardiovascular status. Cardiovascular anomalies occur in approximately 10 % of PBS cases, in which such anomalies may represent the manifestation of a common embryogenic insult.[97] Patent ductus arteriosus and atrial or ventricular septal defects are the most common. Tetralogy of Fallot also occurs.

Musculoskeletal

Musculoskeletal abnormalities of the lower extremities have been reported in one third to one half of patients with PBS.[32,86,98] The majority of these abnormalities are the aftermath of in utero compression. Talipes, scoliosis, and congenitally dislocated hips are the most common disorders requiring orthopedic management.[99] Milder manifestations include dimples of the elbows and knees. Other malformations include polydactylism and arthrogryposis.[11,92,99] Compression of the iliac vessels by a distended bladder has been implicated in cases of lower limb hypoplasia.

Pulmonary

The importance of the kidneys to proper pulmonary development is underscored by the respiratory findings with PBS. In a series of neonatal autopsies, pulmonary hypoplasia associated with oligohydramnios and renal dysplasia was the cause of death in 30% of cases.[32] Newborns with pulmonary hypoplasia who survive and those with milder forms of the syndrome remain susceptible to pulmonary problems. In one series, episodes of recurrent pneumonia and lobar atelectasis occurred in 55% of patients.[86] The latter is secondary to the musculoskeletal disorder and chest wall deformities rather than to parenchymal disease. Elements of gas trapping and restrictive lung disease have been shown.[100] Exercise limitation also occurs, and pulmonary function testing has demonstrated decreased expiratory pressures, low work rates, and decreased V_{O_2} in the majority.[101] The defect in pulmonary toilet undoubtedly increases the risk of postoperative pulmonary complications.[49,102] In one group of patients, postoperative respiratory infections developed after 8 of 133 general anesthetics.[103]

Flaring of the costal margins and other chest wall deformities routinely accompany PBS. Pectus carinatum also is common, and kyphoscoliosis results from the lack of a counterbalance to the paraspinous muscles. Chest radiographs routinely show flattening of the diaphragms, flaring of the rib cage, and drawing in of the lower sternum. Other findings might include rare congenital cystic adenomatoid malformations or pneumomediastinum and pneumothorax as harbingers of hypoplastic lungs.[104]

CLINICAL PRESENTATIONS AND EVALUATION

Antenatal Diagnosis

The use of antenatal US has obvious implications for the fetus with PBS. The bladder and kidneys can usually be appreciated by 14 to 16 weeks' gestation, but PBS has been diagnosed as early as 11 weeks.[105] The findings of dilated ureters, enlarged bladder, and flaccid abdominal wall may denote the presence of PBS, but other diagnoses must be entertained.[106] The ability to diagnose accurately the etiology of hydronephrosis ranges from 30% to 85%.[107] Although in utero intervention has been used, the enthusiasm for these types of efforts has since waned in most institutions for the following reasons[45]:

1. The diagnostic validity of prenatal US is suboptimal. False-positive and false-negative assessments of obstructive uropathies are common. Disorders that can mimic PBS include urethral valves, megacystis/microcolon/hypoperistalsis syndrome, high-grade reflux, hydrocolpos, gastroschisis, and omphalocele.[108,109] Inaccuracies in diagnosis have resulted in an in utero intervention in at least 26 cases of suspected PBS without evidence of benefit in regard to postnatal renal function.[110–112]
2. The presence of urinary tract dilatation may not imply significant obstruction. This concept is probably truer of the low-pressure collecting systems of PBS than of those of any other urinary tract abnormality.

3. Ectatic changes in the urinary tract are usually not detectable until after any significant embryologic insult to the kidneys has occurred. This would negate the benefit of later decompression.[111,112] Fetal intervention would not offer beneficial effects on subsequent renal function or pulmonary development.

Serial intrauterine assessments of the fetus with presumed PBS or its mimics should be done on a regular basis. In rare instances, dystocia is an indication for urinary tract decompression,[112] or the interval development of oligohydramnios warrants early delivery or antenatal intervention. Termination of pregnancy can be considered in cases with severe renal dysplasia. The testing of urinary electrolytes and enzymatic assays of tubular damage also can be done.

Postnatal Diagnosis

Initial Assessment

The diagnosis of PBS is suspected of any newborn with abdominal wall laxity and nonpalpable testes. The presence of oligohydramnios also is suggestive. Physical examination will reveal many of the syndrome's stigmata, including the thin, wrinkled abdominal wall that allows easy palpation of the viscera. Urologic involvement rarely represents an emergency, but surveys of the nonurologic systems affected by PBS are necessary. Radiographs of the chest are done to assess pulmonary development and to rule out pneumothorax or pneumomediastinum. The anus, rectum, and heart also are examined.

Early Observation

The newborn with PBS is closely monitored during the first few days of life, with particular attention being paid to respiratory function. Severe pulmonary hypoplasia, usually seen with oligohydramnios and impaired renal function, causes a progressive inability to oxygenate the newborn. Serial analyses of renal function gradually reflect the degree of renal dysplasia after a few days. A serum creatinine of greater than 0.7 mg/dL in a term infant is a poor prognostic sign.[67] Urinary electrolytes and osmolality also help to assess renal function and concentrating ability. Frequent urine cultures also are obtained. The urinary stream should be normal, but suprapubic bladder massage can be used to facilitate bladder drainage. Prophylactic antibiotics are given before radiologic instrumentation and are continued when significant degrees of hydroureteronephrosis or reflux are present.

Radiographic Studies

Urinary US is recommended as an initial study to provide information about renal differentiation and size, the presence of cystic changes, the severity of hydroureteronephrosis, and the quality of the bladder. Voiding cystourethrography is essential to the diagnosis and helps identify reflux and bladder outlet obstruction, while giving some idea of bladder dynamics. Both studies are done during the first few days of life.

Functional imaging with nuclear scintigraphy is typically deferred for several weeks, allowing the changes of transitional renal physiology to improve the quality of the study. Premature evaluations of the kidneys tend to confuse the picture in systems that are almost always nonobstructive. Scans in newborns have less validity in quantifying obstruction, especially when renal dysplasia or significant hydronephrosis is present. Later studies typically show delayed drainage but no evidence of obstruction.

MANAGEMENT

The clinical implications of PBS occur as a spectrum, as do those of most other syndromes. Variability between the degrees of abdominal wall laxity, hydroureteronephrosis, and renal dysplasia can be expected. Attempts to classify these children, perhaps to standardize their management, have been of equivocal value because of this variability[6] (Table 60-2). Instead, the management of the various aspects of PBS involvement must be individualized.

After delivery, the affected child's immediate prognosis is dictated by its pulmonary status. Newborns with significant renal impairment are typically born with pulmonary hypoplasia. Stillborn delivery or death soon after delivery can be expected of most.[72,86] For others, adequate amounts of amniotic fluid have been present in utero, and pulmonary development is acceptable. Instead, the infant's long-term prognosis now depends on its renal status.[67] Two factors must be considered: the first is the magnitude of irreversible renal dysplasia that has already occurred; the second is the degree of damage that the kidneys incur from recurrent infections or, less commonly, unrecognized obstruction. The latter are generally avoidable and become

---

TABLE 60-2

CLASSIFICATION SCHEME FOR PRUNE-BELLY SYNDROME

Category 1
Pulmonary hypoplasia and/or pneumothorax
Oligohydramnios
Renal dysplasia
May have urethral obstruction or patent urachus
Club feet
If not stillborn, limited survival

Category 2
Typical external features
Uropathy of full-blown syndrome with diffuse
  hydroureteronephrosis
Renal dysplasia common but less severe than in category 1
May or may not develop urosepsis or gradual azotemia

Category 3
External features mild or incomplete
Uropathy is less severe; renal function normal
Little or no urologic reconstructive surgery needed

---

the focus of radiologic surveillance and any therapy, medical or surgical, that might be recommended.

Controversies in Management

How best to preserve renal function in children with PBS remains the subject of debate. Some clinicians advocate an aggressive surgical approach, believing that the benefits of complete urinary reconstruction outweigh its technical and anesthetic risks.[114-116] In theory, eliminating reflux and urinary stasis should decrease the incidence of infection and progressive renal parenchymal damage. Although radiographic appearances are often improved, it remains unclear whether surgical intervention makes a significant difference. In one series, for example, serum creatinine levels and ureteral configurations remained stable, but only 33% of the patients were rendered free of recurrent urinary tract infections (UTIs).[117] In addition, in a significant number of children, especially those with impaired function at presentation, chronic renal failure develops despite these efforts.[86] These types of findings led proponents of a minimally invasive approach to contend that the management of the hydronephrosis and reflux found with PBS is different from that in other disorders.[11,16,118]

We recommend surgical intervention when management with prophylactic antibiotics and observation is unsuccessful in preserving renal function and preventing bacteriuria, especially in younger patients. Other clinicians, using a similar approach and having more than 30 years' follow-up in some cases, reported stable serum creatinine levels in 75% of patients who had normal renal function as newborns[16] (Fig. 60-7). Ureteral function and flow spontaneously improve in many patients who are treated non-operatively. Some proponents of conservative treatment also contend that tapering the PBS ureter decreases the caliber but does not improve peristalsis and drainage, because of intrinsic muscular deficiencies.[69,119] In any case, unless functional deterioration results from refractory infection, little evidence exists to suggest that surgical intervention improves renal function in patients with PBS (Fig. 60-8). These concepts in management are no different from those used with primary vesicoureteral reflux.

It requires patience to refrain from addressing some of these impressively distorted urinary tracts, especially during the neonatal period. At times, the results of extensive reconstructions, which include tapered reimplantation of megaureters combined with reduction cystoplasty, as well as orchiopexy, can be quite impressive.[116] However, it should be remembered that (1) surgical intervention cannot reverse any dysplastic insult the kidneys have already incurred; (2) although dilated, these low-pressure systems result from ureteral smooth muscle deficiency rather than obstruction; and (3) the technical and anesthetic challenges presented by PBS urinary tract are not without risk.[103]

Infection

The aim of any form of therapy, medical or surgical, is directed toward keeping the child infection free. The

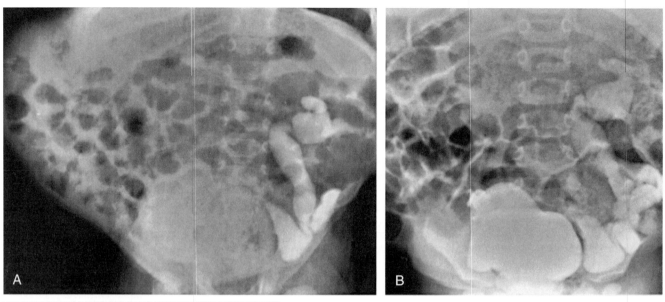

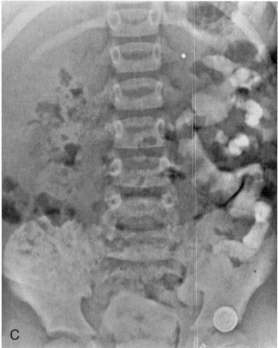

FIGURE 60-7. Child with prune-belly syndrome having large bladder, solitary left kidney, and no reflux managed with observation alone. *A,* Excretory urogram as newborn. *B,* Radiographic appearance at age 2 years. *C,* Appearance at age 7 years. Renal function remained normal (creatinine level of 1.1 mg/dL). Note lessening ureteral tortuosity with continued development.

importance of UTIs to the prognosis is underscored by the description of renal insufficiency in 8 of 19 children with PBS who survived the perinatal period. Nephrectomy specimens showed dysplastic changes in only 25% of the renal parenchyma. Instead, reflux nephropathy and chronic pyelonephritis were largely involved in most cases.[63] Antibiotics are required in neonates on a long-term basis to prevent damage. UTIs disrupt the delicate balance that exists in many of these children. Endotoxins from gram-negative organisms can impair ureteral peristalsis and bladder emptying, causing further dilatation and stasis. Once begun, UTIs in PBS

can be difficult to eradicate without facilitating drainage and, even then, can be difficult to treat.

Diversions and Drainage

The status of the kidneys and dynamics of the urinary tract become readily apparent during the first months of life. Deteriorating renal function is usually caused by dysplasia. This assumption can be confirmed by renal biopsy but is usually unnecessary. Progressive obstructive uropathy rarely occurs. Adequate drainage becomes the critical factor for a small subset of newborns with

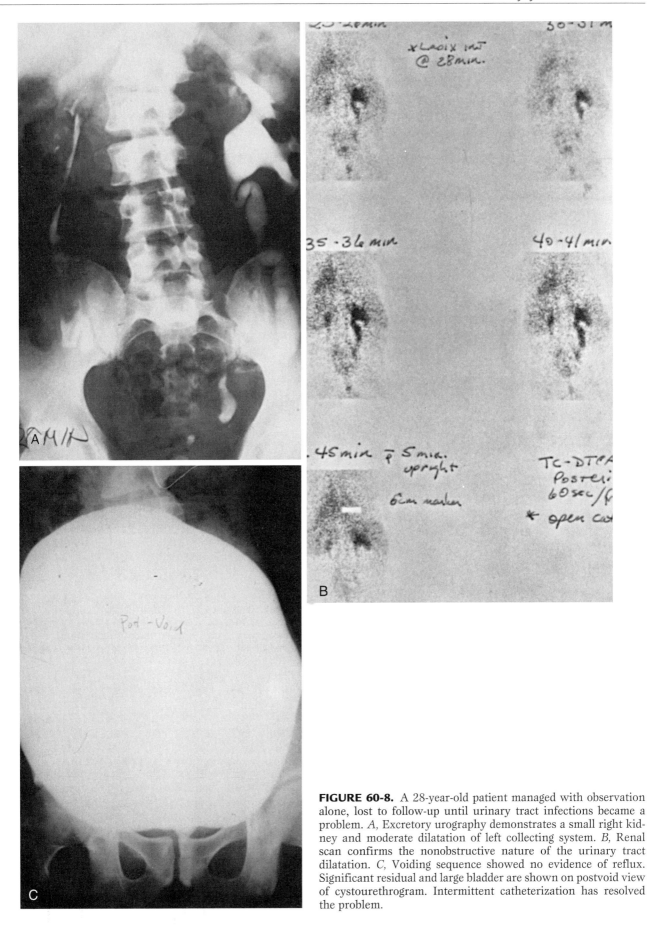

FIGURE 60-8. A 28-year-old patient managed with observation alone, lost to follow-up until urinary tract infections became a problem. *A,* Excretory urography demonstrates a small right kidney and moderate dilatation of left collecting system. *B,* Renal scan confirms the nonobstructive nature of the urinary tract dilatation. *C,* Voiding sequence showed no evidence of reflux. Significant residual and large bladder are shown on postvoid view of cystourethrogram. Intermittent catheterization has resolved the problem.

urethral obstruction or for patients of any age with recalcitrant infections. A number of techniques can be used to vent the urinary tract, each with its own drawbacks. Application is selective. Otherwise urinary dynamics can be disrupted so that obligate surgical reconstruction is required of a system that might not need it otherwise.

Percutaneous Nephrostomy Tubes

Tubes occasionally provide temporary drainage or are used to assess nadir renal function.[120] If improvement in renal function occurs with proximal decompression, a case can be made for more permanently diverting or reconstructing the collecting system. Otherwise, surgical intervention will not make a difference.

Pyelostomy

Pyelostomy is reserved for those renal pelves that are so redundant that a more distal diversion might not provide adequate drainage.[121] This diversion provides optimal drainage and preserves the ureteral blood supply crucial to the success of later undiversion.[122]

Cutaneous Ureterostomy

Ureterostomy is useful only when proximal diversion is preferred but the renal pelvis is too small to create a pyelostomy. The technique can jeopardize ureteral vascularity and compromise the more anatomically normal proximal ureter. Proximal stomas are difficult to fit with an appliance after open drainage into diapers is no longer tolerated.

Vesicostomy

Vesicostomy usually provides adequate drainage of smaller infants or compromised children until a more definitive reconstruction can be completed. Concerns that upper tract drainage is ineffective are unfounded, especially because concomitant supravesical obstructions rarely occur. It is noted that the ureteral decompression in PBS does not occur to the same degree as does that with vesicostomies for truly obstructive uropathies, probably owing to intrinsic myopathy and secondary dilatation. The Blocksom technique is simple and effective, but a more generous stoma is made in PBS to help the bladder empty.[123] Stomal stenosis seems to be a greater problem, and revisions are occasionally necessary. No collection devices are worn, and closure is simply done around the age of toilet training. Concerns that creation of a vesicostomy alters bladder dynamics are unfounded.

Detrusor Dynamics

As an alternative to diversion, some procedures are directed at improving the dynamics of bladder emptying. Two such techniques, reduction cystoplasty and urethrotomy, have been met with mixed enthusiasm.

Reduction Cystoplasty

Laplace's law supports the belief that decreasing the size of a misshapen, enlarged bladder might improve its emptying.[124] This seems truer of bladders distorted by urachal pseudodiverticula that are excluded from the emptying process. Fluoroscopy helps assess this possibility. Reduction cystoplasty is rarely, if ever, indicated as a primary procedure but is often routinely done with ureteral reconstruction.[116] When reduction cystoplasty seems appropriate, a variety of different techniques can be used, including domectomy with midline bladder reapproximation, detrusor plication, and mucosal excision with pants-over-vest approximation of the underlying detrusor.[125] Paired pedicle flaps of rectus muscle to augment emptying also have been tried.[126] Unfortunately, many cystoplasties seem successful early after surgery, when transiently efficient voiding and fewer UTIs occur. However, long-term reductions in bladder capacity are exceptions, and the gradual reappearance of bladder ectasia is common.[127]

Urethrotomy (Sphincterotomy)

Incising the urethra can decrease outlet resistance in some children, although the external sphincter and urethra are usually normal. In theory, weakened detrusor contractions are unable to overcome membranous and bulbous urethral elasticity. Unbalanced voiding results.[74] Urodynamic improvement and reduction in residual urine after urethrotomy have been reported in 10 of 11 cases in one series.[128] However, the technique carries the risk of sphincter damage and, with it, urinary incontinence,[76] and should probably be reserved for patients suspected of having an actual urethral obstruction or so-called "type 4" valves.

Medical Management

US assessments of bladder emptying, urodynamics, and urinary flow rates in the older child become the key to medical management and identification of patients at risk because of unbalanced voiding. Intermittent catheterization has assumed a primary role in the management of PBS when bladder emptying is a problem. In most children, significant UTIs are not increased by such manipulation. Some boys have trouble with the technique because of discomfort. When this is the case, a continent vesicostomy should be considered.

Megaureter Revision

The decision to correct the megaureters (MGU) found with PBS is based on recurrent UTIs resulting from either reflux or obstruction. The severity of reflux alone does not serve as a criterion for its correction, unlike reflux in children without PBS. Successful revision of an MGU depends on achieving a balance between inadequate reduction, which leads to recurrent reflux, and excessive tailoring that potentially leads to stenosis and obstruction. The challenge of working with the dysgenetic ureters and recipient bladders of PBS is not taken lightly. One report describes ureterovesical junction obstruction in 6 of 15 patients who required megaureter revisions and persistent reflux in four others.[115]

When correction is required, meticulous technique, minimal handling, and preservation of periureteral vascularity are crucial. Poorly functioning, ectatic distal ureter should be discarded. Healthy proximal ureter is used in reconstruction. Mobilization of the kidneys is sometimes necessary to eliminate an unsuitable ureteral segment and enable a tension-free anastomosis to the bladder. Imbrication can be used to tailor less-dilated megaureters with little risk to the vascularity. However, more-dilated megaureters require the traditional excisional method to eliminate the bulk that results with plication. Transureteroureterotomy is an ideal option when both ureters require revision. Reimplantation is completed, with the best ureter being repositioned into the abnormal bladder. A psoas hitch fixation of the bladder is a useful means of assuring a long tunnel for reimplantation of the recipient ureter and to eliminate the J hook that can otherwise occur with large-volume bladders.

Abdominoplasty

The management of the abdominal wall abnormality varies according to its severity. Solutions have ranged from braces and corsets to a variety of surgical procedures aimed at improving cosmesis and optimizing function of whatever normal musculature remains. Vertical abdominal wall revisions can be successful, although some patients see their laxity return after seemingly successful early results.[11] A midline incision with skin revision that allows a double-breasted plication of the fascia improves outcomes[129] (Fig. 60-9). Another modification includes resection of the poorly developed lateral musculofascial segments adjacent to the umbilicus and midline rectus muscles, which are preserved as an island[130] (Fig. 60-10). Loss of the umbilicus can occur, and tailoring of the redundant skin still presents a problem. More recently an extraperitoneal plication technique, in which two vertical fascial folds are isolated on both sides of the midline and then sutured to each other along the linea alba, provided encouraging results in a group of 13 patients.[131]

The results with smilelike incisions that extend from one costovertebral area to the other have been encouraging.[46] This approach permits excision of the most severely affected musculature and creates a waist for the patient that allows more normal fitting of clothes. The cosmetic result is good but not perfect with this technique, as with the others (Fig. 60-11). All told, the psychologic and cosmetic benefits of abdominoplasty outweigh its risks in children with PBS, and it is recommended in most cases. In addition, improved voiding efficiency with decreased postvoid residuals has been shown after successful abdominoplasty.[132] The revision

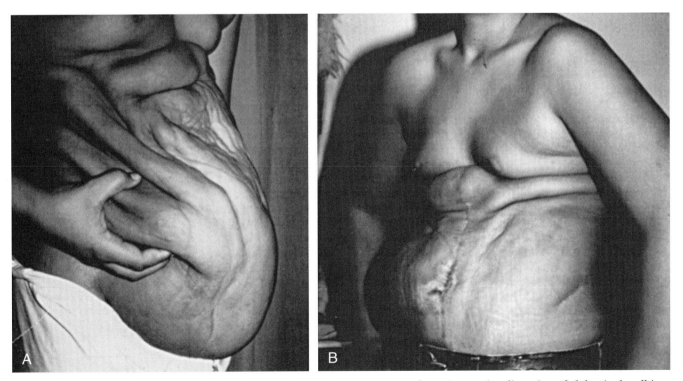

FIGURE 60-9. Abdominoplasty: vertical revision. *A,* Preoperative appearance shows impressive distortion of abdominal wall in a teen. *B,* Postoperative appearance, although not perfect, shows significant improvement.

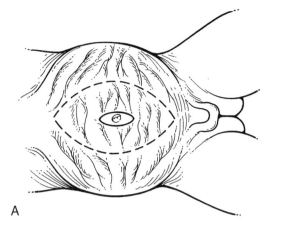

A

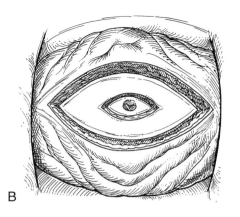

B

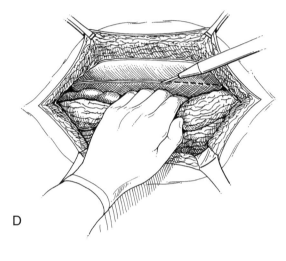

C

D

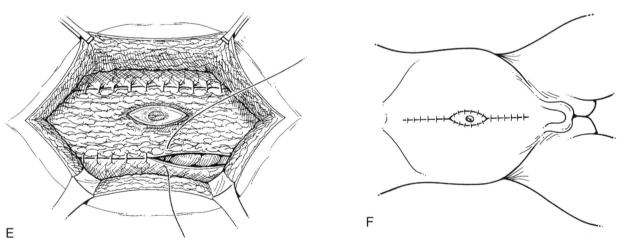

E

F

FIGURE 60-10. Monfort abdominoplasty. *A,* Skin incisions circumscribe umbilicus and define areas of adjacent abdominal wall redundancy to be removed. *B,* Excision of skin (epidermis and dermis alone) by using electrocautery. *C,* Abdominal wall central plate incised at lateral borders of the rectus muscle on either side, creating a central musculofascial plate. *D,* The parietal peritoneum overlying the lateral abdominal wall musculature is scored with electrocautery. *E,* Edges of the central plate are sutured along the scored line. *F,* Excess skin removed, and midline approximation envelops previously isolated umbilicus.

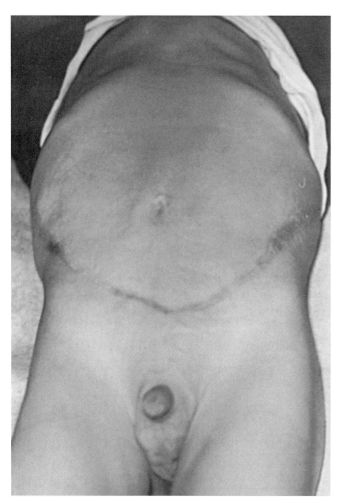

FIGURE 60-11. Abdominoplasty: transverse "smile" revision. Postoperative appearance in older child.

is completed at the time of orchiopexy and, if need be, any other urinary reconstruction that might be planned. Excellent exposure is provided, and wound healing is not compromised by the abnormal composition of the abdominal wall.

Orchiopexy

The role and timing of orchiopexy remain somewhat controversial. Regardless of their normal histology early in development, correcting gonadal position has not been shown to make a difference in sperm-forming potential. Despite this bleak outlook for fertility, we advocate orchiopexy at an early age to maximize gonadal development, enable surveillance of malignancy, and provide psychological benefit.

Technical advantages exist for performing orchiopexy during the neonatal period, often in concert with abdominoplasty, vesicostomy, or urinary tract reconstructions.[56] The flaccid abdomen offers excellent exposure of the retroperitoneum and easy mobilization of the testes, whose vascular and vasal mesentery are typically

long and lax at an early age. Dependent scrotal testicular position can be achieved without ligating the testicular vessels. Success rates of nearly 90% have been described in children younger than 2 years.[115] However, a group of high intra-abdominal testes remain, especially in older boys, with insufficient cord length to reach the scrotum. In this case, the Fowler-Stephens method is used by dividing the spermatic vessels and mobilizing the testicle on peritoneum containing the vessels of the vas. Success rates with the Fowler-Stephens maneuver of nearly 80% have been reported.[133]

Renal Transplantation and Peritoneal Dialysis

Renal transplants have been successfully used in PBS patients for more than 25 years.[134] Both cadaver and living-related donor kidneys function well in this setting and show no statistical difference in patient death, graft survival, or graft function compared with age-matched controls.[135,136] Urodynamics are obtained beforehand to optimize outcomes with the PBS bladder. Identifying and treating bladder dysfunction results in comparable outcomes with transplantation to those in patients with a normal lower urinary tract.[137] When imbalanced voiding and incomplete emptying are present, clean intermittent catheterization is not a contraindication to transplantation.

Newborns with reasonable pulmonary function but significant renal impairment present a management dilemma, especially if otherwise healthy.[138] Peritoneal dialysis can be used as a therapeutic bridge in management until the child can be nurtured to a suitable age for renal transplantation. If affected children are nurtured to a suitable age, organ transplantation is not adversely affected by the syndrome. Renal transplantations have been done as young as age 8 months.[135]

FUTURE TRENDS

Historically, the mortality rates of infants born with PBS were as high as 20% during early infancy and 50% during the first 2 years of life. Pulmonary complications accounted for much of the early mortality. Renal failure or sepsis were responsible for most later deaths.[139] Historically, some clinicians attributed this grave outlook in part to conservative medical treatment.[140] Others implicated excessive surgical intervention.[6] We now know that both modalities have a place in the management of affected children. Increased survival rates and longevity continue to be the trend as the roles of surgical and medical management become even better defined. This undoubtedly stems from an improved understanding of the natural history of PBS, earlier identification of its accompanying problems, and improved methods, both medical and surgical, for their treatment. Earlier antenatal identification, in utero management, and unforeseen advancements in futuristic medicine will raise new ethical and socioeconomic issues that are yet to be resolved. In any event, the outlook for the child born with PBS today is much brighter than it was in the past.

Acknowledgment

We acknowledge the many contributions of the late John Duckett to our understanding of the pathogenesis and treatment of prune-belly syndrome. Many of the ideas presented herein have their basis in John's teachings.

REFERENCES

1. Parker RW: Case of an infant in whom some of the abdominal muscles were absent. Trans Clin Soc London 28:201, 1895.
2. Osler W: Congenital absence of the abdominal muscle, with distended and hypertrophied urinary bladder. Bull Johns Hopkins Hosp 12:331–333, 1901.
3. Williams DI, Burkholder GV: The prune belly syndrome. J Urol 98:244–251, 1967.
4. Eagle JF, Barrett GS: Congenital deficiency of abdominal musculature with associated genitourinary abnormalities: A syndrome: Reports of 9 cases. Pediatrics 6:721–736, 1950.
5. Ives EJ: The abdominal muscle deficiency triad syndrome-experience with ten cases. In Bergsma D (ed): Birth Defects: Original Series. Baltimore, Williams & Wilkins, pp 127–137, 1974.
6. Welch KJ, Kearney GP: Abdominal musculature deficiency syndrome: Prune-belly. J Urol 11:693–700, 1974.
7. Nunn IN, Stephens FD: The triad syndrome: A composite anomaly of the abdominal wall, urinary system and testes. J Urol 86:782–794, 1961.
8. Rabinowitz R, Schillinger JF: Prune belly syndrome in the female subject. J Urol 118:454–456, 1977.
9. Guvenc M, Guvenc H, Aygun AD, et al: Prune belly syndrome associated with omphalocele in a female newborn. J Pediatr Surg 30:896–897, 1995.
10. Aaronson IA, Cremin BJ: Prune belly syndrome in young females. Urol Radiol 1:151, 1980.
11. Bellah RD, States LJ, Duckett JW: Pseudoprune-belly syndrome: Imaging findings and clinical outcome. AJM Am J Roentgenol 167:1389–1393, 1996.
12. Garlinger P, Ott J: Prune belly syndrome: Possible genetic implications. Birth Defects 10:173–180, 1974.
13. Baird PA, MacDonald EC: An epidemiologic study of congenital malformations of the anterior abdominal wall in more than half a million consecutive live births. Am J Hum Genet 33:470–478, 1981.
14. Greskovich FJ III, Nyberg LM Jr: The prune-belly syndrome: A review of its etiology, defects, treatment and prognosis. J Urol 140:707–712, 1988.
15. Goulding FG, Garrett RA: Twenty-five year experience with prune belly syndrome. Urology 12:329–332, 1978.
16. Woodhouse CRT, Ransley PG, Williams DI: Prune belly syndrome: Report of 47 cases. Arch Dis Child 57:856–859, 1982.
17. Woodard JR, Smith EA: Prune belly syndrome. In Walsh PC, Retik AB, Vaughan ED Jr, et al (eds): Campbell's Urology. Philadelphia, WB Saunders, 1998, pp 1917–1938.
18. Burbidge KA, Amodio J, Berdon WE, et al: Prune belly syndrome: 35 years of experience. J Urol 137:86–90, 1987.
19. Cromie WJ, Lee K, Houde K, et al: Implications of prenatal ultrasound screening in the incidence of major genitourinary malformations. J Urol 165:1677–1689, 2001.
20. Adeyokunnu AA, Familusi JB: Prune belly syndrome in two siblings and a first cousin. Am J Dis Child 136:23–25, 1982.
21. Gaboardi F, Sterpa A, Thiebat E, et al: Prune-belly syndrome: Report of three siblings. Helv Paediatr Acta 37:283–288, 1982.
22. Riccardi VM, Grum CM: The prune-belly syndrome: Heterogeneity and superficial X-linkage mimicry. J Med Genet 14:266, 1977.
23. Harley LM, Chen Y, Rattner WH: Prune belly syndrome. J Urol 108:174–176, 1972.
24. Beckman H, Rehder H, Rauskolb R: Prune belly sequence associated with trisomy 13 [letter]. Am J Med Genet 19:603–604, 1984.
25. Frydman M, Magenis RE, Mohandas TK, et al: Chromosome abnormalities in infants with prune belly anomaly: Association with trisomy 18. Am J Med Genet 15:145–148, 1983.

26. Lubinsky M, Doyle K, Trunca C: The association of "prune-belly" with Turner's syndrome. Am J Dis Child 134:1171–1172, 1980.
27. Baird PA, Sadovnick AD: Prune belly anomaly in Down syndrome [letter]. Am J Med Genet 26:747–748, 1987.
28. Petersen DS, Fish L, Cass AS: Twins with congenital deficiency of abdominal musculature. J Urol 107:670–672, 1972.
29. Druschel CM: A descriptive study of prune belly syndrome in New York State 1983–1989. Arch Pediatr Adolesc Med 1490:70–76, 1995.
30. Greenfield SP, Rutigliano E, Steinhardt G, et al: Genitourinary tract malformations and maternal cocaine abuse. Urology 37:455–459, 1991.
31. Stephens FD, Gupta D: Pathogenesis of the prune belly syndrome. J Urol 152:2328–2331, 1994.
32. Wigger HJ, Blanc WA: The prune belly syndrome. Pathol Ann 12:17–39, 1977.
33. Minninberg DT, Mantoya F, Okada K, et al: Subcellular muscle studies in the prune belly syndrome. J Urol 109:524–526, 1973.
34. Fallon B, Welton M, Hawtry C: Congenital anomalies associated with cryptorchidism. J Urol 127:91–93, 1982.
35. Gonzalez R, Reinberg Y, Burke B, et al: Early bladder outlet obstruction in fetal lambs induces renal dysplasia and the prune-belly syndrome. J Pediatr Surg 25:342–345, 1990.
36. Moerman P, Fryns J, Goddeeris P, et al: Pathogenesis of the prune-belly syndrome: A functional urethral obstruction caused by prostatic hypoplasia. Pediatrics 73:470–475, 1984.
37. Pagon RA, Smith DW, Shepard TH: Urethral obstruction malformation complex: A cause of abdominal muscle deficiency and the "prune belly." J Pediatr 94:900–906, 1979.
38. Burton BK, Dillard RG: Brief clinical report: prune belly syndrome: Observations supporting the hypothesis of abdominal overdistension. Am J Med Genet 17:669–672, 1984.
39. Fitzsimons RB, Keohane C, Galvin J: Prune-belly syndrome with ultrasound demonstration of reduction of megacystis in utero. Br J Radiol 58:374–376, 1985.
40. Hoagland MH, Hutchins GM: Obstructive lesion of the lower urinary tract in the prune belly syndrome. Arch Pathol Lab Med 1112:154–156, 1987.
41. Volmar KE, Fritsch MK, Perlman EJ, et al: Patterns of congenital lower urinary tract obstructive uropathy: Relation to abnormal prostate and bladder development and the prune belly syndrome. Pediatr Dev Pathol 4:467–472, 2001.
42. Volmar KE, Nguyen TC, Holcroft CJ, et al: Phimosis as a cause of the prune belly syndrome: Comparison to more common pattern of proximal penile urethral obstruction. Virchows Arch 442:169–172, 2003.
43. Monie IW, Monie BJ: Prune belly syndrome and fetal ascites. Teratology 19:111–113, 1979.
44. Chen CP, Liu PF, Jan SW, et al: First report of distal obstructive uropathy and prune belly syndrome in an infant with amniotic band syndrome. Am J Perinatol 14:31–33, 1997.
45. Nakayama KD, Harrison MR, Chinn DH, et al: The pathogenesis of prune belly. Am J Dis Child 138:834–836, 1984.
46. Randolph J, Cavett C, Eng G: Surgical correction and rehabilitation for children with "prune-belly" syndrome. Ann Surg 193:757–762, 1981.
47. Affi AK, Rebiez JM, Andonian SJ, et al: The myopathology of the prune belly syndrome. J Neurol Sci 15:153–165, 1972.
48. Ashcraft KW: Prune belly syndrome. In Ashcraft KE (ed): Pediatric Urology. Philadelphia, WB Saunders, 1990, pp 257–267.
49. Karamanian A, Kravath R, Nagashima H, et al: Anaesthetic management of "prune belly" syndrome. Br J Anaesthesiol 46:897–899, 1974.
50. Stephens FD: Idiopathic dilatations of the urinary tract. J Urol 112:819–822, 1974.
51. Elder JS, Isaacs JT, Walsh PC: Androgenic sensitivity of the gubernaculum testis: Evidence for hormonal/mechanical interactions in testicular descent. J Urol 127:170–176, 1982.
52. Orvis BR, Bottles K, Kogan BA: Testicular histology in fetuses with the prune belly syndrome and posterior urethral valves. J Urol 139:335–337, 1988.
53. Massad CA, Cohen MB, Kogan BA, et al: Morphology and histochemistry of infant testes in the prune belly syndrome. J Urol 146:1598, 1991.

54. Woodhouse CRJ, Snyder HM: Testicular and sexual function in adults with prune belly syndrome. J Urol 133:607–609, 1985.
55. Tayakkanonta K: The gubernaculum testis and its nerve supply. Aust N Z J Surg 33:61–68, 1963.
56. Woodard JR, Parrott TS: Orchiopexy in the prune belly syndrome. Br J Urol 50:348–351, 1978.
57. Asplund J, Laska J: Prune belly syndrome at the age of 37. Scand J Urol Nephrol 9:297–300, 1975.
58. Kolettis PN, Ross JH, Kay R, et al: Sperm retrieval and intracystoplasmic sperm injection in patients with prune-belly syndrome. Fertil Steril 72:948–949, 1999.
59. Woodhouse CRJ, Ransley PG: Teratoma of the testis in the prune belly syndrome. Br J Urol 55:580–581, 1983.
60. Sayre R, Stephens R, Chonko AM: Prune belly syndrome and retroperitoneal germ cell tumor. Am J Med 81:895–897, 1986.
61. Schwarz RD, Stephens FD, Cussen LJ: The pathogenesis of renal dysplasia, II: The significance of lateral and medial ectopy of the ureteric orifice. Invest Urol 19:97–100, 1981.
62. Stephens FD: Triad (prune belly) syndrome. In Stephens FD (ed): Congenital Malformations of the Urinary Tract. New York, Praeger, 1983, pp 485–511.
63. Manivel JC, Pettinata G, Reinberg Y, et al: Prune belly syndrome: Clinicopathologic study of 29 cases. Pediatr Pathol 9:691–711, 1989.
64. Snow BW, Duckett JW: The prune belly syndrome. In Retik AB, Cukier J (eds): Pediatric Urology. Baltimore, Willams & Wilkins, 1987, pp 253–270.
65. Potter EL, Craig JM: Pathology of the Fetus and the Infant, 3rd ed. Chicago, Year Book Medical, 1975.
66. Rogers LW, Ostrow PT: The prune belly syndrome: Report of 20 cases and description of a lethal variant. J Pediatr 83:786–793, 1973.
67. Noh PH, Cooper CS, Zderic SA, et al: Prognostic factors in patients with prune belly syndrome. J Urol 162:1399–1401, 1999.
68. Hanna MK, Jeffs RD, Sturgess JM, et al: Ureteral structure and ultrastructure, part III: The congenitally dilated ureter (megaureter). J Urol 117:24–27, 1977.
69. Palmer JM, Tesluk H: Ureteral pathology in the prune belly syndrome. J Urol 111:701–707, 1974.
70. Ehrlich RM, Brown WJ: Ultrastructural anatomic observations of the ureter in the prune-belly syndrome. Birth Defects 13:101–103, 1977.
71. Gearhart JP, Lee BR, Partin AW, et al: A quantitative histological evaluation of the dilated ureter of childhood, II: Ectopia, posterior urethral valves and the prune belly syndrome. J Urol 153:172–176, 1995.
72. Berdon WE, Baker DH, Wigger HJ, et al: The radiologic and pathologic spectrum of the prune belly syndrome. Radiol Clin North Am 15:83–92, 1977.
73. Mackie GG, Stephens FD: A correlation of renal dysplasia with position of the ureteral orifice. J Urol 114:274–280, 1975.
74. Snyder HM, Harrison NW, Whitfield HN, et al: Urodynamics in the prune-belly syndrome. Br J Urol 48:663–670, 1976.
75. Lee ML: Prune-belly syndrome in a 54-year-old man. JAMA 237:2216–2217, 1977.
76. Kinahan TJ, Kravath R, Nagashima H, et al: The efficacy of bladder emptying in the prune belly syndrome. J Urol 148:600–603, 1992.
77. Kroovand RL, Al-Ansari RM, Perlmutter AD: Urethral and genital malformations in prune-belly syndrome. J Urol 127:94–96, 1982.
78. Deklerk DP, Scott WW: Prostatic development in prune-belly syndrome: A defect in prostatic stromal-epithelial interaction. J Urol 120:341–344, 1978.
79. Popek EJ, Tyson RW, Miller GJ, et al: Prostate development in prune belly syndrome (PBS) - lower tract obstruction or primary mesenchymal defect? Pediatr Pathol 11:1, 1991.
80. Aaronson IA: Posterior urethral valve masquerading as the prune belly syndrome. Br J Urol 55:508–512, 1983.
81. Reinberg Y, Chelimsky G, Gonzalez R: Urethral atresia and the prune belly syndrome: Report of 6 cases. Br J Urol 72:112–114, 1993.
82. Passerini-Glazel G, Araguna F, Chiozza L, et al: The PADUA (progressive augmentation by dilating the urethra anterior) procedure for the treatment of severe urethral hypoplasia. J Urol 140:1247–1250, 1988.
83. Sellers BB: Congenital megalourethra associated with prune belly syndrome. J Urol 116:814–815, 1976.
84. Stephens FD: Congenital Malformations of the Rectum, Anus and Genitourinary Tracts. Edinburgh, Livingstone, 1963.
85. Shrom SH, Cromie WJ, Duckett JW: Megalourethra. Urology 17:152–156, 1981.
86. Geary DF, MacLusky IB, Churchill BM, et al: A broader spectrum of abnormalities in the prune belly syndrome. J Urol 135:324–326, 1986.
87. Lockhart JL, Reeve HR, Bredael JJ, et al: Siblings with prune belly syndrome and associated pulmonic stenosis, mental retardation, and deafness. Urology 14:140–142, 1978.
88. Short KL, Groff DB, Cook L: The concomitant presence of gastroschisis and prune belly syndrome in a twin. J Pediatr Surg 20:186–187, 1985.
89. Wilson SK, Moore GW, Hutchins GM: Congenital cystic adenomatoid malformation of the lung associated with abdominal musculature deficiency (prune belly). Pediatrics 62:421–424, 1978.
90. Shorey P, Lobo G: Ocular anomalies in abdominal deficiency syndrome. Am J Ophthalmol 108:193–194, 1989.
91. Silverman FM, Huang N: Congenital absence of the abdominal muscle associated with malformation of the genitourinary and alimentary tracts: Report of cases and review of literature. Am J Dis Child 80:91–124, 1950.
92. Metrick S, Brown RH, Rosenblum A: Congenital absence of the abdominal musculature and associated anomalies. Pediatrics 19:1043–1052, 1957.
93. Wright JR, Barth RF, Neff JC, et al: Gastrointestinal malformations associated with prune belly syndrome: Three cases and a review of the literature: Pediatr Pathol 5:421–448, 1986.
94. Teramoto R, Opas LM, Andrassy R: Splenic torsion with prune belly syndrome. J Pediatr 98:91–92, 1981.
95. Aanpreung P, Beckwith B, Gelansky SH, et al: Association of paucity of interlobular bile ducts with prune belly syndrome. J Pediatr Gastroenterol Nutr 16:1, 1993.
96. Morgan CL Jr, Grossman H, Novak R: Imperforate anus and colon calcification in association with prune belly syndrome. Pediatr Radiol 7:19–21, 1978.
97. Adebonojo FO: Dysplasia of the abdominal musculature with multiple congenital anomalies; prune belly or triad syndrome. J Natl Med Assoc 65:327–333, 1973.
98. Loder RT, Guiboux J, Bloom DA, et al: Musculoskeletal aspects of prune-belly syndrome. Am J Dis Child 146:1224–1229, 1992.
99. Brincker MR, Palutsis RS, Sarwark JF: The orthopaedic manifestations of prune-belly (Eagle-Barrett) syndrome. J Bone Joint Surg Am 77:251–257, 1995.
100. Crompton CH, MacLusky IB, Geary DF: Respiratory function in the prune-belly syndrome. Arch Dis Child 68:505–506, 1993.
101. Ewig JM, Griscom NT, Wohl ME: The effect of the absence of abdominal muscles on pulmonary function and exercise. Am J Resp Crit Care Med 153:1314–1321, 1996.
102. Hannington-Kiff JG: Prune-belly syndrome and general anesthesia. Br J Anaesthesiol 42:649–652, 1970.
103. Henderson AM, Vallis CJ, Sumner E: Anesthesia in the prune belly syndrome: A review of 36 cases. Anesthesia 42:54–60, 1987.
104. Weber KJ, Rivard G, Perreault G: Prune belly syndrome associated with congenital cystic adenomatoid malformation of the lung. Am J Dis Child 132:316–317, 1978.
105. Yamamoto H, Nishikawa S, Hayashi T, et al: Antenatal diagnosis of prune belly syndrome at 11 weeks of gestation. J Obstet Gynaecol Res 27:37–40, 2001.
106. Shih W, Greenbaum LD, Baro C: In utero sonogram in prune belly syndrome. Urology 20:102–105, 1982.
107. Elder JS: Intrauterine intervention for obstructive uropathy. Kidney 22:19–24, 1990.
108. Glazer GM, Filly RA, Callen PW: The varied sonographic appearance of the urinary tract in the fetus and newborn with urethral obstruction. Radiology 144:563–568, 1982.
109. Clarke NW, Gough DCS, Cohen SJ: Neonatal urological ultrasound: diagnostic inaccuracies and pitfalls. Arch Dis Child 64:578–580, 1989.
110. Elder JS, Duckett JW, Snyder HM: Intervention for fetal obstructive uropthy: Has it been effective? Lancet 10:1007, 1987.

111. Sholder AJ, Maizels M, Depp R, et al: Caution in antenatal intervention. J Urol 139:1026–1029, 1988.
112. Freedman AL, Bukowski TP, Smith CA, et al: Fetal therapy for obstructive uropathy: Diagnosis specific outcomes. J Urol 156:720–723, 1996.
113. Gadziala NA, Kavada CY, Doherty FJ, et al: Intrauterine decompression of megalocystis during the second trimester of pregnancy. Am J Obstet Gynecol 144:355–356, 1982.
114. Jeffs RD, Comisarow RH, Hanna MK: The early assessment for individualized treatment in the prune-belly syndrome. Birth Defects 13:97–99, 1977.
115. Fallat ME, Skoog SJ, Belman BA, et al: The prune belly syndrome: A comprehensive approach to management. J Urol 142:802–805, 1989.
116. Woodard JR, Zucker I: Current management of the dilated urinary tract in prune belly syndrome. Urol Clin North Am 17:407–418, 1990.
117. Woodard JR, Parrott TS: Reconstruction of the urinary tract in prune-belly uropathy. J Urol 119:824–828, 1978.
118. Tank ED, McCoy G: Limited surgical intervention in the prune belly syndrome. J Pediatr Surg 18:688–691, 1983.
119. Woodhouse CRJ, Kellett MJ, Williams DI: Minimal surgical interference in prune-belly syndrome. Br J Urol 51:475–480, 1979.
120. LiPuma JP, Haaga JR, Bryan PJ, et al: Percutaneous nephrostomy in neonates and infants. J Urol 132:722–724, 1984.
121. Schmidt JD, Hawtrey CE, Culp DA, et al: Experience with cutaneous pyelostomy diversion. J Urol 109:990–992, 1973.
122. Randolph JG: Total surgical reconstruction for patients with abdominal muscular deficiency (prune belly) syndrome. J Pediatr Surg 12:1033–1043, 1977.
123. Duckett JW: Cutaneous vesicostomy in children: The Blocksom technique. Urol Clin North Am 1:485–495, 1974.
124. Perlmutter AD: Reduction cystoplasty in prune belly syndrome. J Urol 116:356–362, 1976.
125. Williams DI, Parker RM: The role of surgery in the prune-belly syndrome. In Johnston JH, Goodwin WF (eds): Reviews of Pediatric Urology. Amsterdam, Excerpta Medica, 1974, pp 315–331.
126. Messing EM, Dibbell DG, Belzer FO: Bilateral rectus femoris pedicle flaps for detrusor augmentation in the prune belly syndrome. J Urol 134:1202–1204, 1985.
127. Bukowskik TP, Perlmutter AS: Reduction cystoplasty in the prune belly syndrome: A long-term follow-up. J Urol 152:2113–2116, 1994.
128. Cukier J: Resection of the urethra in the prune belly syndrome. Birth Defects 13:95–96, 1977.
129. Erlich RM, Lesavoy MA, Fine RN: Total abdominal wall reconstruction in the prune belly syndrome. J Urol 136:282–285, 1986.
130. Monfort G, Guys JM, Bocciardi A, et al: A novel technique for reconstruction of the abdominal wall in the prune belly syndrome. J Urol 146:639–640, 1991.
131. Furness PD III, Cheng EY, Franco I, et al: The prune-belly syndrome: A new and simplified technique of abdominal wall reconstruction. J Urol 160:1195–1197, 1998.
132. Smith CA, Smith EA, Parrott TS, et al: Voiding function in patients with the prune-belly syndrome after Monfort abdominoplasty. J Urol 159:1657–1679, 1998.
133. Gibbons MD, Cromie WJ, Duckett JW Jr: Management of the abdominal undescended testicle. J Urol 122:76–79, 1979.
134. Shenasky JH, Whelchel JD: Renal transplantation in prune belly syndrome. J Urol 115:112–113, 1976.
135. Reinberg Y, Manivel JC, Fryd D, et al.: The outcome of renal transplantation in children with the prune belly syndrome. J Urol 142:1541–1542, 1989.
136. Fontaine E, Salomon L, Gaganadoux MF, et al: Long term results of renal transplantation in children with the prune belly syndrome. J Urol 158:892–894, 1997.
137. Luke PP, Herz DB, Bellinger MF, et al: Long-term results of pediatric renal transplantation into a dysfunctional lower urinary tract. Transplantation 76:1578–1582, 2003.
138. Fischbach M: Ask the expert: peritoneal dialysis for small children with prune belly syndrome. Pediatr Nephrol 16:936–937, 2001.
139. Barnhouse DH: Prune belly syndrome. Br J Urol 44:356–360, 1972.
140. Walbaum RS, Marshall VF: The prune belly syndrome: A diagnostic therapeutic plan. J Urol 103:668–674, 1970.

CHAPTER 61

Intersex

John M. Gatti, MD

INTRODUCTION

Abnormalities of sexual differentiation resulting in intersex disorders are among the most fascinating conditions confronting the pediatric urologist or surgeon. Our understanding of these conditions and their causes continues to evolve, but many questions remain.

Even with better understanding of the underlying etiology of the different intersex conditions, optimal gender assignment and therapeutic reconstruction continue to be controversial.

NORMAL SEXUAL DIFFERENTIATION

The understanding of intersex conditions builds on a working knowledge of normal sexual differentiation. The most commonly accepted paradigm, described by Jost,[1] involves a step-wise process to sexual development. The primary determinant is chromosomal sex, which is established at fertilization when the sperm provides an X or Y paired sex chromosome to the ovum's X sex chromosome. Chromosomal sex determines gonadal sex, with the XX resulting in ovarian development, and XY resulting in testicular development. Finally, the gonadal function determines the phenotypic sex, including internal and external physical and psychological features. Although the paradigm is a helpful cascade to explain sexual development, as the actual genes and locations are elucidated, the simple Y = male, No Y = female equations are not necessarily valid.

Chromosomal Sex Determination

Chromosomal sex determination is based on the Y chromosome. In the 1950s, research characterizing the male phenotype of Klinefelter's syndrome with a 47,XXY karyotype, and a female phenotype of Turner's syndrome with an 45,XO karyotype, indicated that the presence of a Y chromosome causes male gonadal development, and the lack of a Y chromosome results in ovarian development.[2,3] This was irrespective of a complete X chromosomal content. The theorized gene was termed the *testis-determining factor* (TDF).

Gonadal Sex Development

The location of TDF was further elucidated with molecular techniques by studying individuals with chromosomes discordant with their phenotype: 46,XY females with a deletion of the TDF region and 46,XX males with Y chromosomal and TDF genetic material, presumably through translocation or other means. TDF was cloned and, based on genome mapping, its location was isolated to the short arm of the Y chromosome near the centromere at the distal aspect of the Y-unique region.[4] TDF is a 35-kilobase pair sequence on the 11.3 sub-band of the *sex-determining region of the Y chromosome* (SRY). Interestingly, SRY appears to be expressed by the somatic cells of the urogenital ridge and not the germ cells.

The *SOX-9* gene, located on the long arm of chromosome 17, has been identified as an additional sex-determining gene. It has been noted that a translocation involving the *SOX-9* gene results in campomelic dysplasia, characterized by skeletal abnormalities and associated with 46 XY sex reversal. The *SRY* gene is thought to regulate the *SOX-9* gene, and despite the presence of a functional *SRY* gene in this syndrome, a female phenotype develops in the majority of chromosomal males.[5,6]

The determinants of gonadal development involve multiple genes. The Wilms' tumor gene (*WT-1*) appears to play a key role not only in renal development, but also in testicular development. It is theorized that *WT-1* regulates the interaction between the mesonephric ducts and germ cells, with early alteration of gene function resulting in testicular agenesis, and later dysfunction resulting in aberrant testicular development (streak gonad or dysgerminomas). This tumor-suppressor gene has been implicated in Denys-Drash syndrome involving testicular (mixed gonadal dysgenesis) and renal (Wilms' tumor) abnormalities.[7,8]

Fushi-Tarzu factor-1 (*FTZ-F1*) exerts its effect on gonadal development through its regulation of steroidogenic factor-1 (*SF-1*). *SF-1* gene is involved in steroid hormone production and the production of müllerian inhibiting substance (MIS) by Sertoli cells of the testis that causes regression of the müllerian ductal system. Although *FTZ-1* and *SF-1* are expressed in ovarian tissues as well, the timing and intensity of this function are critical in normal gonadal development.[7,9]

Finally, the lack of an *SRY* gene alone does not impart normal female phenotypic and gonadal development, based on studies of 46,XY females with intact SRY regions. The *DAX-1* gene, located on the short arm of the X chromosome, appears to be essential to the development of the ovary. The *DAX-1* gene product appears to compete with the *SRY* gene product for a steroidogenic regulatory protein (StAR), and a dosage-sensitive element is introduced into the equation. Normally, the single *SRY* gene has a greater impact than a single *DAX-1* gene and causes upregulation of StAR. In those chromosomal abnormalities in which more than one *DAX-1* gene is present, however, downregulation of StAR occurs, testicular development is inhibited, and ovarian development promoted. As in the case of Turner's syndrome, however, these primordial ovaries go on to develop into streak gonads, and likely other genes are important to normal ovarian development.[10,11]

Phenotypic Sexual Development

Development of the internal ductal structures is dependent on hormone secretion by the developing gonads (Table 61-1). In the absence of functioning testicular tissue, the internal müllerian duct structure of a female develops. The presence of a functioning testis results in male internal wolffian duct development. This differentiation is mediated by the testis' production of testosterone, promoting wolffian duct development, and MIS, resulting in regression of the müllerian duct structures. This is a paracrine effect and therefore results in gonad specific ipsilateral ductal differentiation. Decreased levels of MIS by an abnormal testis or streak gonad result in ipsilateral müllerian development. This occurs despite regression of the müllerian ducts on the contralateral side

with normal testicular MIS production. Conversely, systemic administration of androgen does not result in male ductal development in a female fetus. This effect is likely dependent on high concentrations of androgen produced by the physically proximate gonad.

MIS functions as a suppressor of müllerian duct development. It is thought that it functions by inhibiting the effect of growth factors on the müllerian ducts. It is produced by Sertoli cells of the testis and in infancy is a specific marker for functioning testicular tissue. At puberty, MIS production in the male declines, but it increases in the female. In its absence, the müllerian structures develop by default. The concentration and timing of MIS secretion appears to be critical; secretion occurs during week 7 of gestation, and the müllerian ducts become insensitive to MIS by week 9.[12]

External genital development follows a similar path (Fig. 61-1). In the absence of testosterone, and more important, its metabolite dihydrotestosterone (DHT), the external genitalia develop in the female phenotype. The male and female phenotypes are identical until week 7. In the male, testosterone production by the testicular Leydig cells surges at 7 weeks and remains elevated until week 14 of gestation. Testosterone is converted to DHT by 5α-reductase in the tissues of the genital skin and urogenital sinus. The testosterone-binding receptor has a 4 to 5 times higher affinity for DHT than that of testosterone and serves to amplify the effect of testosterone on the developing external genitalia. In the absence of 5-α reductase, the internal wolffian ducts are preserved, but the external structures are feminized.

After birth in the male, neonatal testosterone levels surge in response to the loss of feedback inhibition by maternal estrogens and the subsequent surge in neonatal luteinizing hormone (LH) production. This testosterone production peaks around month 2 to 3 of life, and by 6 months, levels remain identical in males and females until puberty. Through these surges, it appears that androgen imprinting may occur on susceptible tissues, including those of the genital organs, but also on sensitive tissues in the brain related to male-type behaviors and gender orientation. This may determine how these tissues respond to subsequent androgen exposure during puberty and adulthood.

TABLE 61-1		
DERIVATION OF THE UROGENITAL SYSTEM		
Wolffian Duct (Mesonephric Duct)	Urogenital Sinus	Müllerian Duct (Paramesonephric Duct)
Male	Male	Male
Epididymis	Bladder	Appendix testis
Vas deferens	Prostate	Prostatic utricle
Seminal vesicles		
Female	Female	Female
Epoophoron	Bladder	Vagina (upper third)
Gartner's ducts	Distal vagina	Uterus
		Fallopian tubes

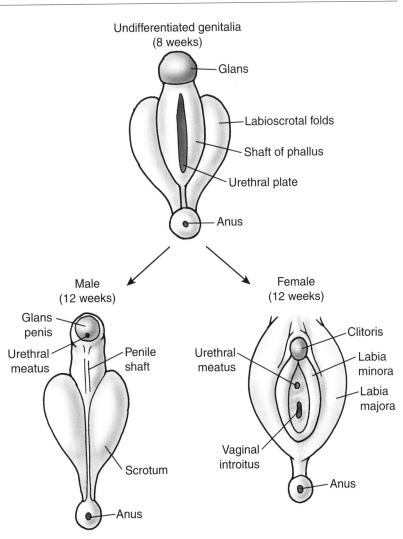

FIGURE 61-1. Differentiation of the external genitalia.

ABERRANT SEXUAL DEVELOPMENT

Incidence

In North and South America and Western Europe, female pseudohermaphroditism secondary to congenital adrenal hyperplasia (CAH) is the most common cause of neonatal ambiguous genitalia, accounting for approximately 70% of cases.[13,14] The overall incidence is approximately 1 in 15,000 live births. The rate is much higher in stillborns and in certain regional populations (Yupic Eskimos and people of La Réunion, France).[15] In the United States, mixed gonadal dysgenesis is the next most common intersex disorder, with true hermaphroditism third most common. In other areas of the world, different disorders predominate; true hermaphroditism is the most common intersex disorder in South Africa.[16]

Classification

The most commonly used classification system was proposed by Allen in 1976.[17] The system categorizes the most common intersex disorders well, but as our understanding of the less common syndromes evolves, they do not fit as neatly into this paradigm. Its five categories are based primarily on gonadal histology:

Female pseudohermaphrodite (ovarian tissue only)
Male pseudohermaphrodite (testicular tissue only)
True hermaphrodite (both ovarian and testicular tissue)
Mixed gonadal dysgenesis (testicular tissue and a streak gonad)
Pure gonadal dysgenesis (two streak gonads)

Female Pseudohermaphrodite

The majority of patients with neonatal genital ambiguity fall into this category. All patients have a 46,XX genotype and exclusively ovarian tissue (nonpalpable gonads). Simplistically, the cause of ambiguity in this category is an excess of androgen. More than 95% are due to CAH, with the remainder due to maternal androgen exposure. These patients have a normal female müllerian ductal system, with upper vagina, uterus and fallopian tubes (see Table 61-1). They also have had normal regression of the wolffian ducts. The level of virilization is largely dependent on the timing and magnitude of androgen exposure to the external genitalia. The phenotype can range from mild clitoromegaly to full masculinization.

Virilization in CAH is due to the inability of the adrenal gland to form cortisol. The precursors above the enzymatic defect are shunted into mineralocorticoid or sex-steroid pathways, as the end products generally have some, albeit weak, glucocorticoid function. The lack of cortisol for negative feedback inhibition of adrenocorticotropic hormone (ACTH) production by the pituitary leaves this pathway unchecked. Excess androgen is produced and is responsible for virilization. The corticosteroid synthetic and alternative pathways are diagrammed in Figure 61-2. The most common form of CAH is 21-hydroxylase deficiency (21-OHD), which accounts for more than 90% of CAH.[18] 21-OHD has been mapped to the short arm of chromosome 6. The variable location of the adrenal defect and relative function of the gene results in salt-wasting and non–salt-wasting forms.[19–21] Type 1 (21-OHD) results in virilization but no salt wasting. The gene defect affects only the fasciculata zone of the adrenal, which blocks cortisol production, but the gene is normally expressed in the glomerulosa zone, and mineralocorticoid production is preserved. In type 2 (21-OHD), also called the classic type, the gene abnormality affects both zones of the adrenal. Salt wasting results in dehydration or vascular collapse, and hyperkalemia occurs because of the block in mineralocorticoid production.

11β-Hydroxylase deficiency (type 3) is a less common cause of CAH. This gene has been mapped to the long arm of chromosome 8. This abnormality results in virilization associated with hypertension. This is related to the level of the synthetic block below deoxycorticosterone (DOC). DOC has potent mineralocorticoid function, and its excess results in sodium resorption, fluid overload, resulting hypertension, and hypokalemic acidosis.

Finally, 3β-hydroxylase deficiency (type 4) is a rare form of CAH. It results in severe salt wasting, and survival is rare. It is the only type of CAH to occur in both sexes.

More rarely, virilization of the female fetus can be caused by exogenous androgen exposure by the mother. This occurs primarily by the use of progesterone, commonly as an adjunct to assisted fertility and in vitro fertilization. Previously, androgenic compounds also were administered to expectant mothers with a history of repeated spontaneous abortion as a preventive measure.

Endogenous androgen exposure due to virilizing maternal ovarian tumors also has been reported as a cause of female pseudohermaphroditism.[22] Fortunately, these tumors are usually virilizing to the mother, and the fetus in unaffected. Virilizing tumors include arrhenoblastoma, hilar cell tumor, lipoid cell tumor, ovarian stromal cell tumor, luteoma of pregnancy, and Krukenberg's tumor.[23]

DIAGNOSIS. The diagnosis of CAH is based on the described clinical and electrolyte abnormalities in addition to elevated 17-hydroxyprogesterone levels. DOC and deoxycortisol levels also aid in determining which enzymatic defect is present. The physical examination is notable for the absence of palpable gonads and presence of a cervix on rectal examination, and bronzing of the skin may be noted from excess ACTH cross-reactivity with melanocyte-stimulating hormone receptors. Palpation of a gonad virtually excludes the diagnosis of female pseudohermaphrodite. The genitogram and ultrasonographic (US) study mirror these findings, revealing müllerian structures with a variable-length urogenital sinus.

TREATMENT. Because all forms of CAH are inherited in an autosomal recessive manner, genetic counseling is recommended. Although it is controversial, in families with a history of CAH, maternal treatment with dexamethasone before week 10 of gestation can improve the level of fetal virilization and is generally well tolerated.[24] Postnatally, cortisol replacement with hydrocortisone is the mainstay of therapy, with the addition of fluorohydrocortisone if salt wasting is present. Supportive

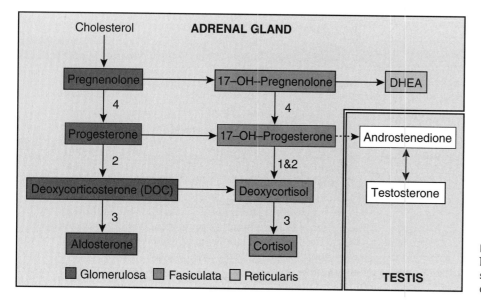

FIGURE 61-2. Pathways of steroid biosynthesis. The numbers correspond to CAH type and location of enzymic defect.

management of fluid and electrolyte abnormalities may be best provided in the neonatal intensive care unit setting.

With regard to gender identity, the vast majority of females with CAH identify as female.[25] In this subgroup, gender assignment is uniformly female and is congruous, given a 46,XX karyotype and normal ovaries imparting the potential for fertility. Surgical reconstruction, a feminizing genitoplasty, generally involves three elements: clitoroplasty, monsplasty, and vaginoplasty.

Male Pseudohermaphrodite

This group is the most heterogeneous in the classification system. All patients have a 46,XY genotype and exclusively testicular gonadal tissue. The gonads are sometimes palpable, and the condition can be simplistically thought of as a deficit of either production or reception of androgen.

DEFECTS OF ANDROGEN SYNTHESIS. The androgen deficit may result from a defect in synthesis. Several rare enzyme deficiencies have been implicated including 3β-hydroxylase, 17α-hydroxylase, and 20,22-desmolase (cholesterol side chain cleavage deficiency). All three adrenal enzymes are involved in the steps from cholesterol to androstenedione and testosterone and are associated with severe CAH and often death. 3β-Hydroxylase and 20,22-desmolase deficiencies are associated with cortisol and aldosterone deficits with hyponatremia, hyperkalemia, and metabolic acidosis. With 17α-hydroxylase deficiency, mineralocorticoid production is preserved, resulting in excess salt and water retention, hypertension, and hypokalemia. In the male, the phenotype is variable, ranging from the appearance of proximal hypospadias with cryptorchidism to that of a phenotypic female with blind-ending vagina.

Defects in 17,20-desmolase and 17β-hydroxysteroid oxidoreductase act at the testicular level to convert androstenedione to testosterone. Because the adrenal is unaffected, CAH does not occur. The phenotype can be quite variable, but those with complete feminization may escape detection at birth and be reared as female. In the latter disorder, however, progressive virilization is related to excess gonadotropin production at puberty, which may partially compensate for the lack of testosterone synthesis. Phallic growth and development of male secondary sex characteristics create a conundrum with regard to late gender reassignment.[26]

ANDROGEN RECEPTOR DEFECTS. Despite adequate production of androgen, receptor defects can render cells blind to the virilizing effects of the hormone. The phenotype is variable and depends on the degree of insensitivity of the receptor for androgen.

The extreme is normal female external genitalia resulting from complete androgen insensitivity syndrome (CAIS). The incidence of this syndrome is approximately 1 in 40,000 and usually results from a point mutation in the androgen-receptor gene, located on the X chromosome.[27,28]

Receptor defects seen in CAIS, or testicular feminization, result in normal female external genitalia and a blind-ending vagina. Testes are present but may be nonpalpable. MIS production is intact, so no müllerian ductal structures are present. These patients usually are initially seen at puberty with amenorrhea, but may be seen earlier with the finding of a testis at the time of hernia repair.

Partial androgen insensitivity is associated with a large spectrum of phenotypic variation (e.g., Gilbert-Dreyfus, Lub's, and Reifenstein's syndromes). It can be a sporadic or inherited condition, and gender assignment and treatment are individualized.[29]

DEFECT OF ANDROGEN CONVERSION. Testosterone is converted to DHT, a much more potent androgen with regard to virilization of the external genitalia and prostate, by 5α-reductase (type 2), located in these tissues. The phenotype is ambiguous, but virilization occurs at puberty related to the increased testosterone production and peripheral conversion by nongenital 5α-reductase type 1. Unfortunately, the virilization is incomplete, and a small phallus and infertility are likely.

DIAGNOSIS. The diagnosis is similar to that of CAH in the female pseudohermaphrodite, noting excess steroid levels above the enzymatic block, with elevated levels of ACTH. The physical examination verifies absence of a cervix on rectal examination, and bronzing of the skin may be noted from excess ACTH, stimulating melanocyte-stimulating hormone receptors. Palpation of a cryptorchid or descended testis is possible. The genitogram and US mirror these findings, revealing no vagina or uterus, but a prominent utricle may be present. In CAIS, testosterone levels are elevated postpubertally, but diagnosis in the prepubertal child may require human chorionic gonadotropin (hCG) stimulation and genital skin fibroblast androgen-receptor studies to make the diagnosis. Receptor assays can delineate a quantitative versus qualitative receptor defect, and LH levels are elevated, related to the loss of testosterone feedback inhibition, which requires normal receptor-hormone interaction. 5α-Reductase deficiency is confirmed by an elevated testosterone-to-DHT ratio, and abnormal 5α-reductase type 2 gene.[30]

TREATMENT. In CAIS, the gender assignment is generally female. Because the androgen-receptor defect is ubiquitous, virilization of the brain does not occur. Orchiectomy is required, given the low but present risk of malignant degeneration, but this is often deferred until after puberty.[31] The testis synthesizes estradiol, facilitating feminine development at puberty. Excision before this necessitates hormone replacement for normal pubertal development.

Gender assignment in partial insensitivity syndrome is largely biased toward the response of the external genitalia to exogenous testosterone. A significant response with virilization argues for the male gender, and with no response, a female gender is favored. This subgroup is the most variable and has the least consensus with regard to gender assignment, with some reports of gender reassignment at puberty.[32,33]

In 5α-reductase deficiency syndrome, the brain is normally virilized, and these individuals identify with a male gender. Male sex assignment is recommended.[34]

MÜLLERIAN INHIBITORY SUBSTANCE DEFICIENCY.

MIS is produced by Sertoli cells in the testis and functions to cause regression of the müllerian ductal structures. In this rare syndrome of abnormal MIS production or MIS-receptor abnormality, wolffian ductal development is unimpaired, but the müllerian ducts also persist. Because the infant has a normal male phenotype, this syndrome is rarely encountered in the neonatal period. The most common presentation to the pediatric surgeon is that of finding a fallopian tube adjacent to an undescended testis in the hernia sac at the time of orchiopexy (hernia uterine inguinale).[35]

If this scenario is encountered, a biopsy of the gonad should be performed, the hernia repaired, and all structures left intact until completion of a full evaluation with karyotype and MIS levels. Abnormal MIS-receptor gene assays also can be helpful in verifying the diagnosis in those with a normal MIS level. Subsequent management is primarily orchiopexy. This, however, may be extremely difficult, as the vas deferens can be closely adherent to the fallopian tube or uterus. Excision of discordant ductal structures may be attempted, but given the relatively low risk associated with leaving these structures, the risk of damage to the vas during this dissection likely outweighs the benefit of removal. Despite normal testosterone levels, impaired spermatogenesis is often the case.[36–38]

LEYDIG CELL ABNORMALITIES.

As the Leydig cell is responsible for testosterone production at the testicular level, impaired testosterone production can also manifest from Leydig cell hypoplasia, agenesis, or abnormal Leydig cell gonadotropin receptors. These disorders are rare, and though the karyotype is 46,XY, the phenotype tends to be female, with a blind-ending vaginal pouch and absence of internal müllerian structures. These patients usually are seen initially in the pubertal period with amenorrhea and therefore are reared as female. Management is similar to that for CAIS, with orchiectomy and estrogen replacement.[39,40]

True Hermaphrodite

True hermaphroditism exists when both ovarian and testicular tissue are present. The gonadal configuration also can be quite variable, with the ovary/ovotestis combination being most common in the United States. Ovary and testis, bilateral ovotestes, and testis/ovotestis combinations also occur. Ovotestes are usually polar with an ovary at one end and a testis at the other, but the distribution can be longitudinal, requiring deep longitudinal biopsy to sample the gonad adequately. Because of the paracrine effect of the gonad, the ipsilateral internal duct structures correlate with the type of gonad present. Ovotestes are associated with variable duct structure, but usually fallopian tubes prevail. Usually a decisively müllerian or wolffian duct structure is present rather than an ipsilateral combination.[41]

True hermaphroditism also can be associated with a variety of karyotypes, with 46,XX being the most common. In the United States, the majority are African American in race and have this karyotype, but different chromosomal content has been correlated with different races. It is thought that a translocation of the *SRY* gene or associated genes to an X chromosome or autosome explains the development of testicular tissue in 46,XX. It is more difficult to explain ovarian tissue in a 46,XY, but likely, key genes to the ovarian development are present but undetected to complement the normal X chromosomal content, or unappreciated mosaicism is present.

The phenotype covers the entire spectrum, with ambiguity and asymmetry the rule, but a tendency toward masculinization. Although it is unusual for ovaries to be found in the labioscrotum, testes and ovotestes are often found descended. Fertility has been described in those raised as female, but testicular fibrosis makes this rare in those raised as male.[28,42]

DIAGNOSIS.

The diagnosis of true hermaphroditism is suggested by a mosaic karyotype or ductal structures but is confirmed by the presence of ovarian and testicular tissue by biopsy.

TREATMENT.

Sex assignment in true hermaphroditism is quite variable and should be based on the functional potential of the phenotype. In either case, the discordant gonads should be removed early. Retained testicular tissue will cause virilization in the female. In males, the testicular tissue is preserved, and orchiopexy is performed. A 1% to 10% incidence of testicular tumor development is found in males, predominantly gonadoblastomas and dysgerminomas, so long-term surveillance is encouraged.[43] Hypospadias repair also is required in the male, and feminizing genitoplasty in the female. Males tend to require hormonal replacement because of progressive testicular fibrosis, but females usually do not. Fertility is certainly possible in those raised as female, and several cases of child-bearing have been reported. Females should, however, be screened for testosterone levels, which can signal inadequate resection of testicular tissue.[44]

Mixed Gonadal Dysgenesis

Mixed gonadal dysgenesis (MGD) is the second most common form of neonatal ambiguous genitalia. The patient will have a testis on one side and a streak gonad on the other, characterized by microscopically normal ovarian stroma without oocytes (Fig. 61-3). The internal duct structure mirrors the ipsilateral gonad, with the streak associated with a fallopian tube and uterus resulting from the lack of MIS. The karyotype is generally a mosaic of 45,XO/46,XY, and the stigmata of Turner's syndrome are variably present. The phenotype is ambiguous, but masculinized, and the testis may be descended but more commonly is not.[45]

The risk of gonadal tumor development, usually gonadoblastoma, is as high as 20%, and tumors can develop in either the testis or streak gonad.[46] An increased risk of Wilms' tumor also is present in MGD.

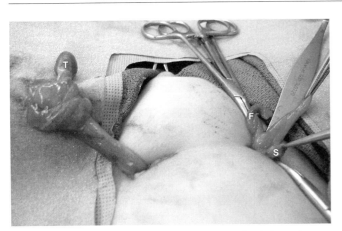

FIGURE 61-3. Mixed gonadal dysgenesis. The left testis was descended, and the right streak gonad was intra-abdominal. T, Testis; F, fallopian tube; S, streak gonad. (Photo taken from head of table.)

The Denys-Drash syndrome occurs in approximately 5% of patients with MGD and is classically described as ambiguous genitalia, Wilms' tumor, and glomerulopathy, often seen with hypertension.[47]

DIAGNOSIS. The diagnosis is suggested by the physical stigmata of Turner's syndrome on examination (webbed neck, shield chest) and 45,XO/46,XY karyotype. The findings of a testis and streak gonad, however, confirm the diagnosis.

TREATMENT. The majority of patients with MGD have been raised as female because of the short stature conferred by Turner's syndrome and the malignant risk of the retained testis. Females undergo early gonadectomy and feminizing genitoplasty; males require excision of the streak gonad, orchiopexy or orchiectomy, and hypospadias repair. Infertility is the rule despite endocrine function of the testis. Because of the increasing concern regarding testosterone imprinting on the brain, more masculinized patients are being raised as male. If individuals are raised as male, close surveillance of the testis is necessary, unless elective orchiectomy and hormone replacement are chosen. Testicular biopsy at the time of orchiopexy to rule out dysgenetic elements is generally recommended.[43]

Pure Gonadal Dysgenesis

Pure gonadal dysgenesis (PGD) is characterized by streak gonads bilaterally. The external phenotype and internal duct structure are female, and these patients generally are seen at puberty with primary amenorrhea. The chromosomal makeup is classically 46,XX. The gonads carry no risk of malignant degeneration, and it appears to be an autosomally recessive trait, so genetic counseling is warranted. This implies that the syndrome can be mediated by abnormalities of the X chromosome or supporting autosomal genes involved in sexual differentiation.

Other conditions are closely related to bilateral streak gonads. The chromosomal makeup is quite variable and can be 46,XY (Swyer's syndrome or male Turner's syndrome), 45,XO, or a mosaic. Variants with a Y chromosome differ in that they carry a high rate of malignancy in the retained streak gonads. The phenotype is as described earlier, but these patients may be first seen with gonadoblastomas or dysgerminomas that are common in infancy, or with germ cell tumors that become more common in adolescence. The stigmata of Turner's syndrome are often present. Multiple chromosomal deletions and mutations have been described resulting in this syndrome.

DIAGNOSIS. The findings of a female external phenotype and internal duct structure with bilateral streak gonads make the diagnosis. Follicle-stimulating hormone (FSH) and LH levels are generally elevated, and estrogen and testosterone levels are decreased. The diagnosis may be suggested by the physical stigmata of Turner's syndrome on examination (e.g., webbed neck, shield chest).

TREATMENT. With the presence of a Y chromosome, gonadectomy should be performed, given the high incidence of malignancy. In classic 46,XX PGD, the gonads carry no malignant risk and can be left in situ. In either case, hormonal replacement at puberty is required, as the streak gonads provide no endocrine function.

Other Syndromes of Aberrant Sexual Differentiation

Several syndromes worth mentioning do not neatly fit into the described classification system.

Vanishing testis syndrome is characterized by a 46,XY karyotype but absent testes bilaterally. This generally results in virilization to the point of normal external genitalia and internal duct structure but absent testes. The testes were thought to have produced androgen at some point, resulting in this masculinization, but subsequently vanished related to torsion or regression. Patients are generally raised as boys, and hormonal supplementation at puberty is required.[48]

Klinefelter's syndrome is characterized by a male karyotype containing two or more X chromosomes (47,XXY; 48,XXXY; etc.). Although phenotypically male prepubertally, these patients acquire abnormal male secondary sexual characteristics (tall stature with disproportionately long legs, sparse facial hair, decreased muscle mass, and a feminine fat distribution) and infertility. The testes are small and hard, with decreased androgen production and elevated estradiol levels related to primary hypergonadotropic hypogonadism. Gynecomastia often occurs with an increased risk of breast cancer.[49] Fertility has been reported, but requires assisted means, such as intracytoplasmic sperm injection.[50]

XX sex reversal is characterized by a male phenotype with a 46,XX karyotype. Most commonly this occurs from translocation of Y chromosomal material to the X chromosome but also can occur from mutation of the X chromosome or *mosaicism*. The phenotype and management are similar to those of Klinefelter's syndrome, with the exception of shorter stature.[51]

Mayer-Rokitansky-Kuster-Hauser (MRKH) syndrome is characterized by a 46,XX karyotype with normal female external genitalia, but a short, blind-ending vagina. Normal ovaries and fallopian tubes are present, but the uterus is generally rudimentary. Patients are seen initially with primary amenorrhea but may have cyclical pain related to functioning endometrium. Treatment is geared toward vaginal reconstruction to allow menses or intercourse or both.[52]

Evaluation of the Newborn with Ambiguous Genitalia

The diagnosis of ambiguous genitalia is extremely disconcerting to the family and should be addressed as a medical emergency. Usually, genital ambiguity is obvious, but the finding of any degree of hypospadias in association with any undescended testis, or a normal penis with bilateral nonpalpable testes merits an intersex evaluation. In this population, a high rate of intersex conditions is found, despite the absence of classic ambiguity.[53] Table 61-2 indicates other abnormal physical examination findings that warrant consideration for an intersex state.

The family history may reveal maternal hormone exposure, previous fetal death, or a history of genital ambiguity.

The physical examination should focus on the genitalia. Assessment for palpable gonads is important, as a palpable gonad represents a testis or ovotestis and rules out female pseudohermaphroditism, in which only ovaries are present, or PGD, in which only streak gonads are present. If both gonads are palpable, this generally indicates male pseudohermaphroditism. One palpable gonad is generally associated with MGD or true hermaphroditism. Phallic stretched length, clitoral size, and position of the urogenital sinus should be noted. A rectal examination may reveal a palpable uterus. The physical examination should include assessment for stigmata of Turner's syndrome associated with MGD and PGD, and bronzing of the areola or scrotum can suggest elevated ACTH production in CAH.

Initial metabolic evaluation should include a karyotype or fluorescent in situ hybridization (FISH) to identify X and Y chromosomes. 17-OH progesterone levels should be obtained after 3 or 4 days of life, when spurious elevations resulting from the stress related to birth have subsided. Electrolyte levels should be monitored closely in the interim to identify salt wasting with CAH. Testosterone and DHT levels can indicate 5α-reductase deficiency, and elevated LH and low MIS levels suggest testis dysgenesis or absence. hCG or ACTH stimulation tests can be performed but are more controversial.[35]

Early imaging studies include a pelvic US, which should identify a uterus if present. Although a gonad may be seen, US is not useful in differentiating a testis, ovotestis, or ovary. A genitogram performed by retrograde contrast injection into the urogenital sinus is helpful for identifying the level of confluence of a vagina and urethra and its relation to the urethral sphincter (Figs. 61-4 and 61-5).

Gonadal biopsy is often required for diagnostic purposes, but the diagnosis of CAH can be made by metabolic evaluation alone. Endoscopy is not usually required for diagnosis but is essential in characterizing the internal duct structure, level of confluence of the urogenital sinus, and planning for and performing of reconstructive surgical procedures.[28]

At our institution, a gender-assignment team including a pediatric urologist, endocrinologist, geneticist, neonatologist, psychologist, and social worker together evaluate any newborn with ambiguous genitalia. This information is synthesized by the team and presented to the parents in a combined care conference. The goals of gender assignment and management should include preservation of sexual function and any reproductive potential with the least surgical procedures, appropriate gender appearance with a stable gender identity, and psychosocial well-being.[54]

RECONSTRUCTIVE GENITAL SURGICAL PROCEDURES

Controversies and Considerations

For more than 20 years, largely based on the work of John Money and the "John/Joan Case," the overwhelming bias was that gender identity was largely inducible and loosely dependent on chromosomal constitution. The focus was on one of two twin boys who was reassigned to the female gender early in life after a demasculinizing circumcision injury. The child reportedly developed normally from a psychosocial standpoint, well adapted to life as a girl.[55] Only with extended follow-up into adulthood was it discovered that the individual converted back to male gender after severe dissatisfaction with a female identity (including attempted suicide).[56] This rattled the fundamental concepts on which gender assignment had been based for decades and brought to the forefront a tremendous controversy regarding the appropriate management of children with ambiguous genitalia and possible gender reassignment and reconstructive surgical procedures.

Because reconstruction is rarely done in response to any life-threatening issues, support groups for individuals with intersex conditions have advocated delaying any reconstruction until the child can express his or her

TABLE 61-2		
ABNORMAL PHYSICAL EXAMINATION FINDINGS FOR AN INTERSEX STATE		
Apparent Female	**Unsure**	**Apparent Male**
Clitoral hypertrophy	Ambiguous	Impalpable testes
Fused labia		Severe hypospadias
Palpable gonad		Hypospadias and cryptorchidism

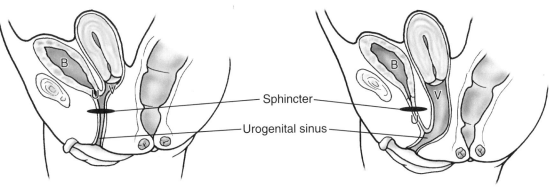

High urogenital confluence   Low urogenital confluence

FIGURE 61-4. High versus low urogenital confluence. B, Bladder; U, urethra; V, vagina.

wishes regarding gender assignment.[57] Although this would decrease the likelihood of a mismatch between physical and psychological gender, the period of genital ambiguity could be quite challenging for the child in our society. These options must be included and discussed thoroughly with the family before embarking on any reconstructive efforts.

With regard to long-term planning including gender assignment and surgical intervention, most major centers advocate a gender-assignment team. At our institution, this includes a neonatologist, endocrinologist, geneticist, urologist, psychologist, and social worker. A group meeting is held with the family, discussing the condition, treatment options, controversies, and sources of information and support.

In general, if surgical reconstruction is thought to be appropriate, it is planned in the first 3 to 6 months of life. For feminizing surgical correction, the vaginal tissue is thicker as a result of maternal hormonal influence, and the distance from the vagina to perineum is shorter at this age. Because parents have a great degree of anxiety

surrounding the sex of their child, earlier repair may help reduce this anxiety and encourage parent/child bonding, more than a later repair.[58]

Male Gender Assignment

Reconstructive efforts for the male sex of rearing include orchiopexy or orchiectomy, when appropriate, and hypospadias repair. These techniques are described extensively elsewhere in this text. It bears mentioning, however, that orchiopexy may be extremely difficult, as the vas deferens can be closely adherent to müllerian duct remnants, such as a fallopian tube or uterus. A portion of these structures may be left in situ if the risk of damage to the vas deferens or testicular vasculature is significant, but this adherence may severely limit mobility and preclude orchiopexy.

Methods of total penile reconstruction in cases of aphallia, demasculinizing penile trauma, or female-to-male gender reassignment by using a radial forearm or osteocutaneous fibula flap have been described with some reasonable success.[59,60] These corrective efforts are usually undertaken in adulthood and are beyond the scope of this text.

Female Gender Assignment

Feminizing genitoplasty includes three major components: monsplasty, clitoroplasty, and vaginoplasty (Figs. 61-6 and 61-7). The timing of the vaginoplasty depends on the level of confluence of the urogenital sinus. For the low confluence, it is performed in the neonatal period with monsplasty and clitoroplasty. If the confluence is high, this may be approached simultaneously, but because vaginal dilatation is often necessary after repair, this may better be deferred until the patient is peripubertal and more capable and interested in this requirement. Cystoscopy is invaluable for this assessment, and we generally leave a Fogarty balloon catheter in the vagina and a Foley catheter in the urethra and bladder to define the confluence during dissection.

The procedure is initiated by placing a traction suture in the glans, and a dorsolateral circumcising incision is

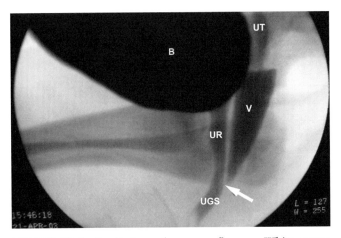

FIGURE 61-5. Genitogram, lower confluence. *White arrow,* level of the confluence of urethra and vagina to become the urogenital sinus. B, Bladder; UT, uterus; V, vagina; UR, urethra; UGS, urogenital sinus.

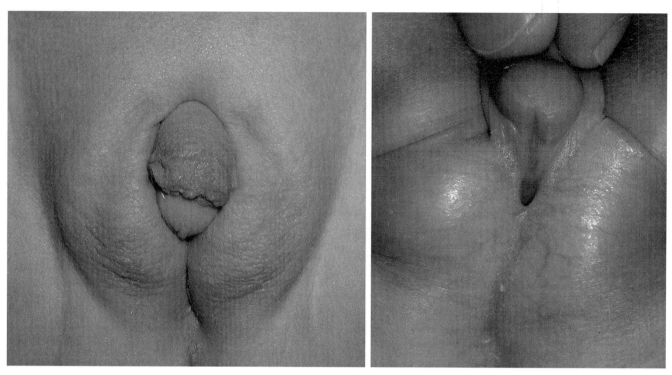

FIGURE 61-6. Ambiguous genitalia. The patient has congenital adrenal hyperplasia, 21-hydroxylase deficiency.

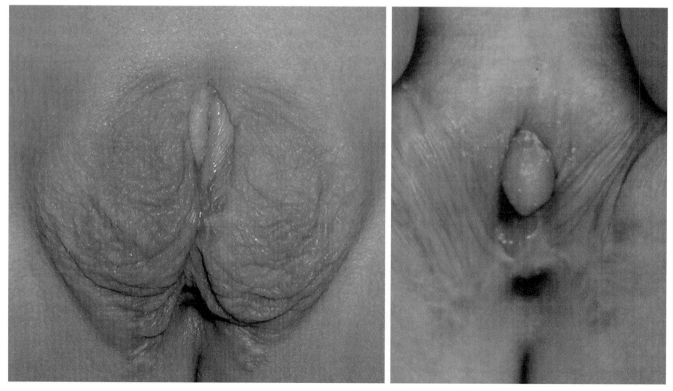

FIGURE 61-7. Feminizing genitoplasty. The same patient in Fig. 61-6, 6 months after undergoing a feminizing genitoplasty.

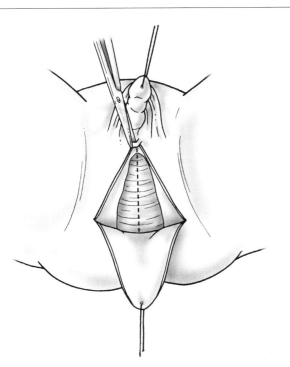

FIGURE 61-8. Vaginal cutback procedure for the low urogenital confluence.

made, leaving a 4- to 5-mm distal preputial cuff, much like a hypospadias repair. The lateral borders of the mucosalized plate are incised, taking this back adjacent to the urogenital sinus. The shaft of the phallus is then degloved of skin superficial to Buck's fascia. Fascial incisions are then made lateral to the neurovascular bundles, and a plane created just beneath Buck's fascia from the level just proximal to the glans, back to the pubic symphysis. The mucosalized plate is elevated on the ventrum and preserved to fill naturally the void between the urethral meatus and clitoris. The dorsal pedicles including the neurovascular bundles are preserved. The corporal bodies are suture ligated at their base at the level of the pubic symphysis, and the distal corporal tissue is excised. We do little to reduce the size of the glans clitoris, as it is our bias that even when markedly enlarged, it is recessed and has a quite normal appearance in adulthood.

This limits injury to sensation previously described, although more commonly associated with clitorectomy rather than clitoral reduction.[61] The glans is anchored to the corporal stumps to secure its position, being sure not to compromise the dorsal neurovascular pedicle.

A posterior inverted "U"-shaped flap is then made from the level of the ischial tuberosities to just posterior to the urogenital meatus. For a very low confluence, dissection is carried along the posterior aspect of the urogenital sinus to the level of the confluence, the posterior wall is incised until the vaginal introitus is normal in caliber, and the "U"-flap is advanced to complete the posterior vaginal wall (Fig. 61-8). With the higher confluences, we have favored total urogenital mobilization (TUM).[62–64]

For the TUM, the urogenital sinus is incised circumferentially and mobilized as one unit to the level of the confluence (Fig. 61-9). At this point, the vagina can be carefully separated from the urethra under direct vision, and the defect in the urethra closed. The urogenital sinus can then be incised at the dorsal midline and folded back on itself to make up the anterior vaginal wall, by using local skin flaps for the dorsolateral defects, bridging a lengthy distance.

The TUM is attractive in that one can approach even the high urogenital confluence in the neonatal period without vaginal substitution or grafting, but the family must be appropriately cautioned. Although early results are favorable, descent of the bladder neck is counterintuitive when considering our knowledge of adult female stress incontinence surgical revision, and long-term continence may be an issue.

To complete the monsplasty, the dorsal phallic shaft skin is incised vertically, a preputial hood is formed for the clitoris, and the majority of this tissue is used to construct the labia minora with V-advancement flaps (Fig. 61-10).

Other techniques for the high urogenital sinus include a posterior approach dividing the rectum and an anterior transvesicle approach. These methods have not been used as extensively at our institution.[65,66]

In some patients with a high urogenital confluence, we have delayed vaginal reconstruction until the peripubertal period, just before menarche. The techniques described

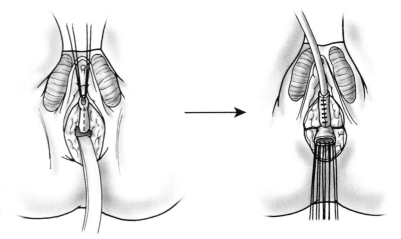

FIGURE 61-9. Total urogenital mobilization. The urogenital sinus is mobilized as a unit, bringing the confluence toward the perineum. Once visualized, the vagina is then detached, and the urethral defect is closed.

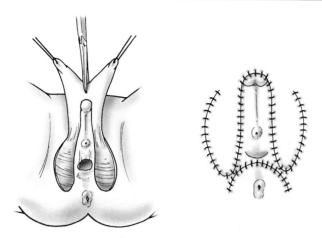

FIGURE 61-10. Monsplasty. Dorsal shaft skin is degloved from the phallus and incised. These flaps are then advanced to become the labia minora. (Shown before and after excision of the corporal tissues and clitoropexy.)

are still used, but in some patients, especially those that are obese, these methods are insufficient. We have favored vaginal substitution with a colonic segment, but ileal substitutions and split-thickness skin grafts also have been advocated. The benefit of vascularized bowel substitution is less vaginal stenosis and the natural formation of lubricating mucus, but this may require wearing a pad because of excessive mucus production. Colonic segments appear to have a lower rate of stenosis than do ileal segments.[67] Conversely, skin grafts have a tendency toward long-term stenosis and may require frequent dilation and revision, but long-term satisfaction also has been described.[68] The barrier function to sexually transmitted diseases is likely superior with skin grafts when compared with intestine.[69]

In cases of vaginal agenesis (e.g., MRKH), the substitution techniques described are often used, but if a rudimentary vagina or depression exists, sequential dilation with the technique described by Frank and modified to a dilating seat by Ingram may be successful.[70,71]

REFERENCES

1. Jost A, Vigier B, Prepin J, et al: Studies on sex differentiation in mammals. Recent Prog Horm Res 29:1–41, 1973.
2. Jacobs PA Strong J: A case of human intersexuality having a possible XXY sex-determining mechanism. Nature 183:302–303, 1959.
3. Ford CE Jones K, Polani P: A sex chromosome anomaly in a case of gonadal sex dysgenesis (Turner's syndrome). Lancet 1:711–713, 1959.
4. Lukusa T, Fryns JP, van der Berghe H: The role of the Y-chromosome in sex determination. Genet Couns 3:1–11, 1992.
5. Clarkson MJ, Harley VR: Sex with two SOX on: SRY and SOX9 in testis development. Trends Endocrinol Metab 13:106–111, 2002.
6. Moog U, Jansen NJ, Scherer G, et al: Acampomelic campomelic syndrome. Am J Med Genet 104, 239–245, 2001.
7. Parker KL, Schimmer BP, Schedl A: Genes essential for early events in gonadal development. EXS 91:11–24, 2001.
8. Schedl A, Hastie N: Multiple roles for the Wilms' tumour suppressor gene, WT1, in genitourinary development. Mol Cell Endocrinol 140:65–69, 1998.
9. Nordqvist K: Sex differentiation: Gonadogenesis and novel genes. Int J Dev Biol 39:727–736, 1995.
10. Goodfellow PN, Camerino G: DAX-1, an "antitestis" gene. Cell Mol Life Sci 55:857–863, 1999.
11. Tajima K, Dantes A, Yao Z, et al: Down-regulation of steroidogenic response to gonadotropins in human and rat preovulatory granulosa cells involves mitogen-activated protein kinase activation and modulation of DAX-1 and steroidogenic factor-1. J Clin Endocrinol Metab 88:2288–2299, 2003.
12. Taguchi O, Cunha GR, Lawrence WD, et al: Timing and irreversibility of müllerian duct inhibition in the embryonic reproductive tract of the human male. Dev Biol 106:394–398, 1984.
13. Menon PS, Virmani A, Sethi AK, et al: Congenital adrenal hyperplasia: Experience at intersex clinic, AIIMS. Indian J Pediatr 59:531–535, 1992.
14. Pellerin D, Nihoul-Fekete C, Lortat-Jacob S: [Surgery of sexual ambiguity: experience of 298 cases]. Bull Acad Natl Med 173:555–562, discussion 563, 1989.
15. Pang SY, Wallace MA, Hofman L, et al: Worldwide experience in newborn screening for classical congenital adrenal hyperplasia due to 21-hydroxylase deficiency. Pediatrics 81:866–874, 1988.
16. Wiersma R: Management of the African child with true hermaphroditism. J Pediatr Surg 36:397–399, 2001.
17. Allen TD: Disorders of sexual differentiation. Urology 7(4 suppl):1–32, 1976.
18. Dacou-Voutetakis C, Maniati-Christidi M, Dracopoulou-Vabouli M: Genetic aspects of congenital adrenal hyperplasia. J Pediatr Endocrinol Metab 14(suppl 5):1303–1308; discussion 1317, 2001.
19. Reindollar RH, Tho SP, McDonough PG: Abnormalities of sexual differentiation: Evaluation and management. Clin Obstet Gynecol 30:697–713, 1987.
20. Laue L, Rennert OM: Congenital adrenal hyperplasia: Molecular genetics and alternative approaches to treatment. Adv Pediatr 42:113–143, 1995.
21. Wilson RC, Mercado AB, Cheng KC, et al: Steroid 21-hydroxylase deficiency: Genotype may not predict phenotype. J Clin Endocrinol Metab 80:2322–2329, 1995.
22. Vicens E, Martinez-Mora J, Potau N, et al: Masculinization of a female fetus by Krukenberg tumor during pregnancy. J Pediatr Surg 15:188–190, 1980.
23. Calaf JPJ, Esteban-Altirriba J: Female pseudohermaphroditism caused by maternal hyperandrogenism. In Martinez-Mora J (ed): Intersexual States: Disorders of Sex Differentiation. Barcelona, Ediciones Doyma, 1994, pp 187–197.
24. Trautman PD, Meyer-Bahlburg HF, Postelnek J, et al: Mothers' reactions to prenatal diagnostic procedures and dexamethasone treatment of congenital adrenal hyperplasia. J Psychosom Obstet Gynaecol 17:175–181, 1996.
25. Berenbaum SA, Bailey JM: Effects on gender identity of prenatal androgens and genital appearance: Evidence from girls with congenital adrenal hyperplasia. J Clin Endocrinol Metab 88:1102–1106, 2003.
26. Saez JM, De Peretti E, Morera AM, et al: Familial male pseudohermaphroditism with gynecomastia due to a testicular 17-ketosteroid reductase defect, I: Studies in vivo. J Clin Endocrinol Metab 32:604–610, 1971.
27. Quigley CA, De Bellis A, Marschke KB, et al: Androgen receptor defects: Historical, clinical, and molecular perspectives. Endocr Rev 16:271–321, 1995.
28. Diamond D: Sexual differentiation: normal and abnormal. In Walsh RA, Vaughn PC, Wein ED (eds): Campbell's Urology. Philadelphia, WB Saunders, 2000, pp 2395–2427.
29. Batch JA, Davies HR, Evans BA, et al: Phenotypic variation and detection of carrier status in the partial androgen insensitivity syndrome. Arch Dis Child 68:453–457, 1993.
30. Barthold J, Gonzales E: Intersex states. In Gonzales E, Bauer SB (eds): Pediatric Urology Practice, B.S. Philadelphia, Lippincott Williams & Wilkins, 1999, p 547.
31. Muller J, Skakkebaek NE: Testicular carcinoma in situ in children with the androgen insensitivity (testicular feminisation) syndrome. Br Med J (Clin Res Ed) 288:1419–1420, 1984.
32. Rosler A, Kohn G: Male pseudohermaphroditism due to 17 beta-hydroxysteroid dehydrogenase deficiency: Studies on the natural history of the defect and effect of androgens on gender role. J Steroid Biochem 19:663–674, 1983.

33. Imperato-McGinley J, Peterson RE, Gautier T, et al: Androgens and the evolution of male-gender identity among male pseudohermaphrodites with 5 alpha-reductase deficiency. N Engl J Med 300:1233–1237, 1979.

34. Wilson JD: Syndromes of androgen resistance. Biol Reprod 46:168–173, 1992.

35. Huseman D: The genitalia intersex. In Gillenwater JY, Howards SS, Mitchell ME (eds): Adult and Pediatric Urology. Philadelphia, Lippincott Williams & Wilkins, 2002, pp 2533–2565.

36. Loeff DS, Imbeaud S, Reyes HM, et al: Surgical and genetic aspects of persistent müllerian duct syndrome. J Pediatr Surg 29:61–65, 1994.

37. Fernandes ET, Hollabaugh RS, Young JA, et al: Persistent müllerian duct syndrome. Urology 36:516–518, 1990.

38. Gustafson ML, Lee MM, Asmundson L, et al: Müllerian inhibiting substance in the diagnosis and management of intersex and gonadal abnormalities. J Pediatr Surg 28:439–444, 1993.

39. Eil C, Austin RM, Sesterhenn I, et al: Leydig cell hypoplasia causing male pseudohermaphroditism: Diagnosis 13 years after prepubertal castration. J Clin Endocrinol Metab 58:441–448, 1984.

40. Lee PA, Rock JA, Brown TR, et al: Leydig cell hypofunction resulting in male pseudohermaphroditism. Fertil Steril 37:675–679, 1982.

41. Berkovitz GD, Fechner PY, Zacur HW, et al: Clinical and pathologic spectrum of 46,XY gonadal dysgenesis: Its relevance to the understanding of sex differentiation. Medicine (Baltimore) 70:375–383, 1991.

42. Walker AM, Walker JL, Adams S, et al: True hermaphroditism. J Paediatr Child Health 36:69–73, 2000.

43. Verp MS, Simpson JL: Abnormal sexual differentiation and neoplasia. Cancer Genet Cytogenet 25:191–218, 1987.

44. Hadjiathanasiou CG, Brauner R, Lortat-Jacob S, et al: True hermaphroditism: Genetic variants and clinical management. J Pediatr 125:738–744, 1994.

45. Davidoff F, Federman DD: Mixed gonadal dysgenesis. Pediatrics 52:725–742, 1973.

46. Robboy SJ, Miller T, Donahoe PK, et al: Dysgenesis of testicular and streak gonads in the syndrome of mixed gonadal dysgenesis: Perspective derived from a clinicopathologic analysis of twenty-one cases. Hum Pathol 13:700–716, 1982.

47. Drash A, Sherman F, Hartmann WH, et al: A syndrome of pseudohermaphroditism, Wilms' tumor, hypertension, and degenerative renal disease. J Pediatr 76:585–593, 1970.

48. Edman CD, Winters AJ, Porter JC, et al: Embryonic testicular regression: A clinical spectrum of XY agonadal individuals. Obstet Gynecol 49:208–217, 1977.

49. Klinefelter HP Jr, Reifenstein EC Jr, Albright F: Syndrome characterized by gynecomastia, aspermatogenesis, without a-Leydigism and increased excretion of follicle stimulating hormone. J Clin Endocrinol Metab 2:615, 1942.

50. Kitamura M, Matsumiya K, Koga M, et al: Ejaculated spermatozoa in patients with non-mosaic Klinefelter's syndrome. Int J Urol 7:88–92, discussion 93–94, 2000.

51. Van Dyke DC, Hanson JW, Moore JW, et al: Clinical management issues in males with sex chromosomal mosaicism and discordant phenotype/sex chromosomal patterns. Clin Pediatr (Phila) 30:15–21, 1991.

52. Griffin JE, Edwards C, Madden JD, et al: Congenital absence of the vagina: The Mayer-Rokitansky-Kuster-Hauser syndrome. Ann Intern Med 85:224–236, 1976.

53. Kaefer M, Diamond D, Hendren WH, et al: The incidence of intersexuality in children with cryptorchidism and hypospadias: Stratification based on gonadal palpability and meatal position. J Urol 162:1003–1006, discussion 1006–1007, 1999.

54. Meyer-Bahlburg HF: Gender assignment and reassignment in intersexuality: Controversies, data, and guidelines for research. Adv Exp Biol 511:199–223, 2002.

55. Money J: Ablatio penis: Normal male infant sex-reassigned as a girl. Arch Sex Behav 4:65–71, 1975.

56. Diamond M, Sigmundson HK: Sex reassignment at birth: Long-term review and clinical implications. Arch Pediatr Adolesc Med 151:298–304, 1997.

57. Recommendations for Treatment: Intersex infants and children. 1995, Intersex Society of North America.

58. Hensle TW, Bingham J: Feminizing genitoplasty. Adv Exp Med Biol 511:251–265, discussion 265–266, 2002.

59. Jordan GH: Total phallic construction, option to gender reassignment. Adv Exp Med Biol 511:275–280, discussion 280–282, 2002.

60. Sadove RC, Sengezer M, McRoberts JW, et al: One-stage total penile reconstruction with a free sensate osteocutaneous fibula flap. Plast Reconstr Surg 92:1314–1323, discussion 1324–1325, 1993.

61. Minto CL, Liao LM, Woodhouse CR, et al: The effect of clitoral surgery on sexual outcome in individuals who have intersex conditions with ambiguous genitalia: A cross-sectional study. Lancet 361:1252–1257, 2003.

62. Pena A: Total urogenital mobilization: An easier way to repair cloacas. J Pediatr Surg 32:263–267; discussion 267–268, 1997.

63. Rink RC, Pope JC, Kropp BP, et al: Reconstruction of the high urogenital sinus: Early perineal prone approach without division of the rectum. J Urol 158:1293–1297, 1997.

64. Rink RC, Adams MC: Feminizing genitoplasty: State of the art. World J Urol 16:212–218, 1998.

65. Pena A, Filmer B, Bonilla E, et al: Transanorectal approach for the treatment of urogenital sinus: Preliminary report. J Pediatr Surg 27:681–685, 1992.

66. Passerini-Glazel G: A new one-stage procedure for clitorovaginoplasty in severely masculinized female pseudohermaphrodites. J Urol 142:565–568; discussion 572, 1989.

67. Hensle TW, Dean GE: Vaginal replacement in children. J Urol 148:677–679, 1992.

68. Martinez-Mora J, Isnard R, Castellvi A, et al: Neovagina in vaginal agenesis: Surgical methods and long-term results. J Pediatr Surg 27:10–14, 1992.

69. Rink RC, Kaefer M: Surgical management of intersexuality, cloacal malformations, and other abnormalities of the genitalia in girls. In Walsh PC, Vaughn ED, Wein AJ (eds): Campbell's Urology, R.A. Philadelphia, WB Saunders, 2002, pp 2428–2468.

70. Frank R: The formation of an artificial vagina without operation. Am J Obstet Gynecol 35:1053, 1938.

71. Ingram JM: The bicycle seat stool in the treatment of vaginal agenesis and stenosis: A preliminary report. Am J Obstet Gynecol 140:867–873, 1981.

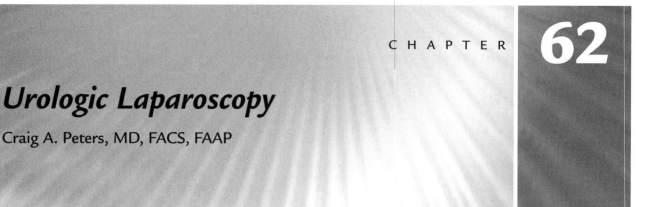

CHAPTER 62

Urologic Laparoscopy

Craig A. Peters, MD, FACS, FAAP

Laparoscopy is an adjunct to the surgical armamentarium of the pediatric urologist, not a separate specialty. As new technologies such as robotically assisted methods emerge to augment the potential for laparoscopic procedures, they should be seen as additional tools to assist in the care of children. How we evaluate these technological developments will be important determinants of the pace and direction of their evolution. Uncontrolled enthusiasm may lead to inappropriate use, and skepticism about their value may lead to unrealized promise.[1] This chapter reviews the current applications and future horizons of laparoscopy and robotics as they apply to pediatric urology.

Diagnostic laparoscopy will be integrated with therapeutic laparoscopic orchiopexy. Renal, ureteral, and bladder surgical procedures are emerging as uses of operative laparoscopy today. These are discussed in terms of the appropriate application, various approaches, and results. Other emerging areas of reconstructive laparoscopy and the use of robotics will conclude the chapter.

CRYPTORCHISM

Laparoscopy in pediatric urology began with the diagnosis of undescended testicles (UDTs). Over time, the interpretation of the findings and integration with therapeutic laparoscopy has been well developed. Cryptorchism offers a valuable introduction to the instrumentation, set-up, access, and visualization that is necessary to achieve the full potential of laparoscopic and, ultimately, robotic surgical techniques.

Because imaging studies used to locate a nonpalpable testis have repeatedly failed to demonstrate an intra-abdominal or inguinal UDT, reliance on these studies might result in an intra-abdominal testis remaining in the abdomen. The need for 100% certainty, given the increased risk of malignancy that might go undetected, is the foundation for using diagnostic laparoscopy. Diagnostic laparoscopy became the most widely used method to provide information as to the presence and location of the nonpalpable testis. Although numerous studies have shown it

to be accurate, safe, and *probably* more accurate than open exploration,[2-4] some controversy remains.[5] Given the low morbidity of diagnostic laparoscopy, it would appear that the balance is strongly in favor of initial laparoscopy for the nonpalpable testis.

Indications and Preparation

Diagnostic laparoscopy for UDT is reserved for the boy with a nonpalpable testis and is reasonably done between ages 6 and 12 months. Those with bilateral nonpalpable testes should have gonadotropin and müllerian inhibiting substance (MIS) levels determined preoperatively, as well as a human chorionic gonadotropin (hCG) stimulation test. Even if no laboratory evidence of testicular tissue is found, it has been our practice to perform laparoscopy, recognizing the existence of false negatives with the hCG stimulation test and lack of substantial experience with MIS. Patients are placed on a clear liquid diet for 24 hours before the procedure and given a rectal suppository the night before to limit rectal bulk. A rectal tube is placed before preparing the patient, and a bladder catheter is placed on the sterile field. The abdomen is entirely prepared to permit placement of working ports for laparoscopic orchiopexy or for open exploration in the rare occurrence of a major injury.

Technique: Access

Our current diagnostic technique involves using a 2-mm telescope, placed through a Veress needle, thus incorporating the cannula sheath for the laparoscopy while obviating a second blind puncture. It is the latter aspect of access that has the major risk of inadvertent injury to an intra-abdominal structure. A 2-mm incision is made in either the inferior or superior aspect of the umbilicus, and the subcutaneous tissues are spread to reveal the fascia. The Veress needle is aimed inferiorly about 15 degrees off vertical, while the abdominal wall is "tented" by the surgeon and assistant. Elevating the abdominal wall can aid in preventing the pre-peritoneal

864

placement of the needle. Usually two distinct levels (the fascia and the peritoneum) are felt as the needle is passed. Without moving the needle, a syringe half full of saline is attached to the needle and aspirated. If no return occurs, the saline is instilled and reaspirated to confirm the position of the needle in the peritoneal space and not in a viscus. If fluid returns on the first aspiration, especially if dark, it is presumed that the intestine has been entered. In this case, the needle is withdrawn slightly until no fluid is aspirated. The peritoneum is then insufflated, and the scope placed to look for the site of puncture. It should be just below the umbilicus, where it can be retrieved. This can be done through the umbilicus by enlarging the fascial incision and passing a laparoscopic grasper alongside the Veress needle/laparoscope. The puncture wound is grasped and brought out to be inspected, cleaned, and oversewn. Alternatively, the puncture can be identified and repaired laparoscopically by using two additional ports. A simple Veress needle puncture of the small bowel is usually safely ignored, but we prefer to repair it.

Technique: Diagnosis

The diagnostic procedure is begun with the patient supine, the legs slightly parted, and the genitalia prepped into the sterile field. A bladder catheter is placed from the sterile field and draped to the contralateral side to prevent its being in the way when working at the scrotal level. A rectal tube is placed before preparation.

Once the pneumoperitoneum is created, the telescope is passed through the cannula. In the case of a unilateral UDT, the normal side is inspected first to provide a comparative image for reference to the opposite side (Fig. 62-1). The affected side is inspected, with attention first placed on establishing landmarks: the iliac vessels, the inferior epigastric vessels, and the obliterated umbilical artery. The vas is often first seen, but the vessels must be visualized for an accurate diagnosis. Smaller than normal vessels in the normal position are often observed with an atrophic testis in the inguinal canal. It may be necessary to push the colon out of the way to confirm the identity of the vessels. In some cases, especially on the left side, when the testis is intra-abdominal, the vessels are more medial and hidden by the colon (Fig. 62-2). Usually the vessels can be seen by using the Trendelenburg position or rotation of the table. Rarely, we have placed a second port to permit mobilization of the colon. The vas deferens can be helpful in locating an intra-abdominal testis, but it must be borne in mind that the vas and testis may be separate. A testicle, if present, will be located by following the vessels. In some cases, gubernacular structures may resemble spermatic vessels disappearing into the inguinal ring from a testis located higher in the abdomen. If the appearance of the vessels differs from the normal side, further exploration is necessary. A vanishing testis is readily recognized by the blind-ending vas deferens and spermatic vessels (Fig. 62-3). Under these circumstances, no testis is present, and further exploration is unneeded. A testicular prosthesis can be placed if requested by the family. Although true testicular agenesis occurs, its frequency must be small indeed, as we

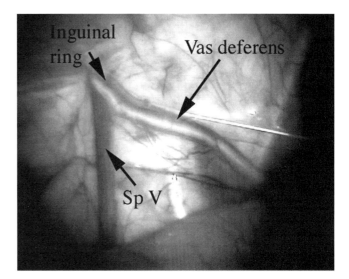

FIGURE 62-1. Laparoscopic view of the internal inguinal ring on the left, showing the vas deferens and spermatic vessels converging at the ring.

have not seen a patient in whom the vessels and vas were completely absent in more than 300 diagnostic laparoscopic procedures. The diagnosis of testicular agenesis requires visualization of the retroperitoneum to the level of the lower pole of the kidney, because we have seen testes well above the level of the aortic bifurcation. Most of the time, the very high testes are suggested by abnormal vessel or gubernacular structures between the testis and the internal ring.

Laparoscopic demonstration of vas and vessels exiting the abdomen into the internal inguinal ring ("canalicular" vas and vessels) suggests the testis has descended into the inguinal canal or scrotum and, if nonpalpable, is

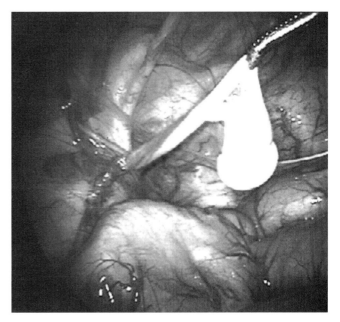

FIGURE 62-2. Intra-abdominal testis on vascular and vasal pedicle, located medial to iliac vessels.

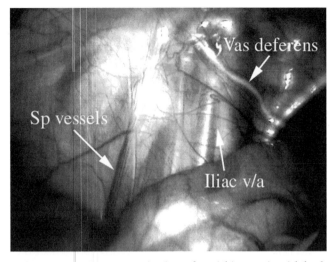

FIGURE 62-3. Laparoscopic view of vanishing testis with both vas deferens and spermatic vessels visible but dwindling away before the inguinal ring.

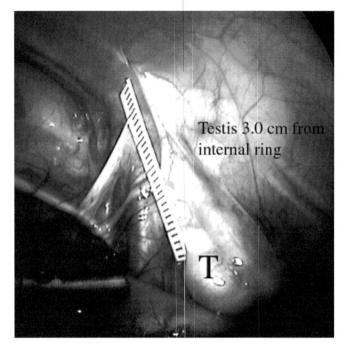

FIGURE 62-4. Intra-abdominal testis on the right side. Location is measured from the internal inguinal ring (3 cm).

likely atrophic. These boys need inguinal exploration to confirm that no testis is present, particularly in the obese child. The appearance of normal canalicular spermatic vessels may suggest the presence of an ectopic testis, whereas canalicular vessels associated with an atrophic testis are usually, but not reliably, smaller.[6] We have occasionally seen nonpalpable perineal ectopic testes detected in this way. Five percent of atrophic testes in the scrotum or canal contain viable germ cells, which should be removed. Whether these atrophic testicles pose a real malignancy risk is unclear, but the status of that testis must be determined, and it is a simple matter to do so. Inguinal exploration may obviate laparoscopy, but approximately 50% of UDT patients will not need the groin procedure for either diagnosis or treatment.

An intra-abdominal testis may require some effort to find but is easily recognizable when seen. Those located medial to the iliac vessels may be the most elusive. Some are on a long spermatic cord and drop deep in the pelvis, even alongside or behind the bladder. The presence of an intra-abdominal testis may lead to laparoscopic orchiopexy, which is described later. This is the most obvious integration of diagnostic and therapeutic laparoscopy.

The final component of the diagnostic laparoscopy is to determine the location of the UDT relative to the internal inguinal ring to determine the most appropriate surgical intervention, primary vessels–intact orchiopexy (PVIO) or two-stage Fowler-Stephens orchiopexy (FSO). After placing the working ports (see position later), a small ruler is inserted, and the distance measured (Fig. 62-4).

INTERSEX CONDITIONS

Diagnostic and therapeutic laparoscopy has a significant role in the child with intersex.[7] The appearance of streak gonads, uterine tissue, and inappropriate müllerian structures is readily recognized laparoscopically.

The appearance of a streak gonad, as distinct from an ovo-testis, is usually clear, but biopsy is sometimes needed. Definition of the müllerian structures may be more precise with laparoscopy than with many imaging modalities including ultrasonography. Removal of dysgenetic gonadal or müllerian tissue is readily accomplished.

THERAPEUTIC LAPAROSCOPY

Orchiopexy

Laparoscopic orchiopexy is one of the most developed applications of laparoscopic techniques in children. Anecdotal data to support its efficacy are readily available, and an emerging notion suggests that it might offer better results than open orchiopexy,[8] although this conclusion is limited by the fact that the true outcome of any orchiopexy, adult fertility, has never been assessed.[9]

Indications

Laparoscopic orchiopexy is used for the intra-abdominal testis. This is almost always done at the same time as the diagnostic laparoscopy that identifies the testis and determines its location. Testes high in the inguinal canal have been subjected to laparoscopic orchiopexy,[10] but it is unclear whether this represents an advantage, and we have not used laparoscopy for those cases. Intra-abdominal dissection and mobilization of spermatic vessels might be a useful adjunct to subsequent open orchiopexy.

Laparoscopic orchiopexy can be a single-stage, primary orchiopexy leaving the spermatic vessels intact (VILO), or a Fowler-Stephens two-stage orchiopexy (FSO). The latter should be reserved for testes that cannot be brought into the scrotum with the spermatic vessels intact. In those boys, the spermatic vessels are initially occluded with a clip, suture, or fulguration, and the testis is left in situ. At a second procedure, 4 months or more later, the spermatic vessels are divided, and the testis is brought into the scrotum on a pedicle of the vas deferens and peritoneum. The vasal artery provides the blood supply to the testis. Discerning which testis is best treated with which procedure is the major challenge of laparoscopic management of the intra-abdominal testis.

Some have recommended the FS orchiopexy for all boys with intra-abdominal UDT, but because the majority of testes can be brought into the scrotum from the abdomen with the vessels intact, this does not seem appropriate to us. Preserving the major blood supply to the testis is intuitively more appealing. Placing the UDT into the scrotum based on the spermatic vessels also avoids a second anesthetic and surgical procedure. A single-stage FSO procedure has been advocated by some as well, but a high incidence of testicular atrophy without the interval period of collateral vascular development makes this approach unacceptable and cannot be recommended.[11]

Technique

POSITION. The patient's position is adjusted to a moderate Trendelenburg position with the ipsilateral side rotated upward about 30 to 45 degrees. Insufflation pressures are maintained at 12 mm Hg for most patients.

PORTS. The initial umbilical port for the diagnostic portion of the laparoscopy can be upsized to 3.5 mm for operative manipulation. Although 2-mm instruments for all ports are feasible, we have found the instruments too flexible, and we use larger, more rigid, instruments. Working ports are placed in the ipsilateral upper quadrant and the contralateral lower quadrant. The ipsilateral port should not be placed too low, as it will be ineffective in mobilizing the proximal testicular vessels (Fig. 62-5). Ports are placed under direct vision and are usually 3.5 mm in size. A fascial closure stitch is placed before cannula placement to facilitate port closure at the end of the procedure.

If a two-stage FSO is indicated, the vessels are occluded with a surgical clip after creating a window in the peritoneum 1 to 2 cm above the testis (Fig. 62-6). This can be performed with only one working port in the contralateral lower quadrant.

INSTRUMENTS. We use a 3.5-mm cauterizing scissors and a curved dissector for the laparoscopic orchiopexy, with little need for complex instruments. The curved dissecting instrument is used to create the passage from the pelvis into the scrotum, and a long, curved vascular clamp is passed retrograde by grasping the tip of the dissecting instrument. For the first stage of the FSO, we use a 5-mm clip applier.

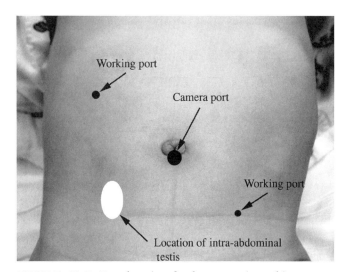

FIGURE 62-5. Port location for laparoscopic orchiopexy on the right. Approximate position of the intra-abdominal testis is shown.

PROCEDURE. Dissection begins by incising the peritoneum lateral to the spermatic vessels and testicle, dissecting to the level of the inguinal ring. The gubernacular attachments are identified at the level of the ring and carefully transected, leaving enough gubernacular tissue attached to the testicle to grasp for retraction and for delivery into the scrotum. Care must be taken to avoid injury to a looping vas deferens. Cephalad retraction of the testis will expose the vas so that it can be protected throughout the procedure. Lateral dissection continues cephalad along the spermatic vessels toward their origin from the iliac vessels. The testis and the spermatic vessels are bluntly dissected from the pelvic sidewall medially. The peritoneum on the lateral and inferior side of the vas

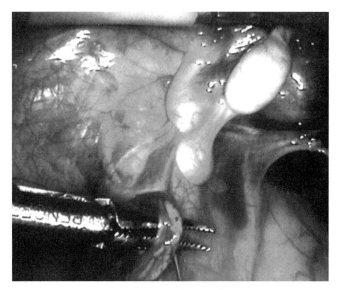

FIGURE 62-6. First stage of Fowler-Stephens orchiopexy with dissection of spermatic vessels before ligation. Testis is not manipulated.

deferens is incised over the obliterated umbilical artery and into the pelvis, approaching the bladder. This leaves a triangular web of peritoneum between the vas and the vessels; the testis is at the apex. Some surgeons recommend leaving this intact to preserve the blood supply of the vas, but it definitely hinders mobilization of the testis. We therefore incise it and mobilize the spermatic vessels proximally.

At this point, the testis is moved to the opposite side of the pelvis, and when it can reach the opposite inguinal ring, it has adequate mobility to be brought over the pubic tubercle. The pathway from the abdomen to the scrotum is then developed. A dartos pouch is first created in the usual manner. A curved dissecting instrument is passed over the pubic tubercle, medial to the obliterated umbilical artery and lateral to the bladder, by using direct vision and finger palpation. The tip of the dissector is guided into the scrotal sac and pushed through. A long, curved vascular clamp is passed retrograde by grasping the tip of the dissecting instrument. The clamp can be spread to open the passage to permit the testis to move through.

The gubernacular stump is then grasped, and the testis brought into the scrotum. The testicle can be fixed in place by using the dartos-pouch technique or a button with a pull-out suture or both. Excessive tension on the spermatic vessels may result in avulsion of the vessels or stretching that will reduce the blood flow. Further proximal dissection of the vessels may be necessary to prevent vascular insufficiency.

The determination of whether to perform a VILO or FSO remains incompletely defined. Initially we performed VILO if the testis "appeared" mobile enough before any dissection, but we found that those higher in the abdomen did not always move into the scrotum easily, and some showed postoperative atrophy. Correlating the initial UDT position with the postoperative result, it became evident that when the testis was more than 2.5 cm from the internal inguinal ring, postoperative testicular atrophy occurred at an unacceptable rate. We also noted that testes medial to the iliac vessels were more difficult to mobilize into the scrotum, even if located at the level of the internal inguinal ring. Therefore testes more than 2.5 cm above the internal inguinal ring or medial to the iliac vessels are managed with the FSO technique. The second-stage FSO is performed by using identical port positions, ligating and then dividing the spermatic vessels just distal to the original clip. The stumps of vessels are used for retraction, and the testis is mobilized on the triangular web of peritoneum surrounding the vas deferens. The testis is moved into the scrotum and fixed in a dartos pouch. Indeed, the ease of the second stage has encouraged some surgeons to use the FSO technique in all patients with an intra-abdominal testis, but this seems inappropriate, considering the higher success rate of a VILO.

Postoperative Care

Patients may be discharged the same day if they are able to retain oral intake. The child is examined in 6 weeks and undergoes a scrotal Doppler US in 9 months to assess blood flow and size.

Results

There are several reports of laparoscopic orchiopexy outcomes, all with good results.[8,12,13] It is important to recognize that outcome parameters are based on perceived testicular viability and not on sperm production. These assessments are not really different from those used to assess open orchiopexy. No truly long-term functional assessment has been made of any of the techniques for orchiopexy.[9] The length of follow-up is important, as some testes in our patients appeared healthy at 6 months but showed a reduction in size at 12 months. Doppler ultrasonography has been used to assess testicular size and blood flow and seems to correlate well with physical examination.

Results have been very good in most series and are summarized in a multi-institutional report.[8] Without any real standards of assessment of initial location or of postoperative outcome, it is difficult to stratify patients and correlate to outcome, but it is probably reasonable to consider a success rate of about 95% for intra-abdominal testes undergoing VILO and about 90% for those undergoing FSO. Although this may be better than for open orchiopexy, the correlation with initial position is undefined.

The age of the patient also is likely to have an impact on outcome. We have noted that the intra-abdominal testis in any patient older than 2 years is very difficult to move into the scrotum, regardless of initial position. Patients older than 2 years should undergo the FSO procedure routinely.

RENAL SURGERY

Nephrectomy

Simple nephrectomy for benign conditions, the first major laparoscopic procedure performed in children, is now well established and routine.[14] The indications are similar to those for open nephrectomy. The initial approach to nephrectomy was transperitoneal, with very good outcomes. These first cases were performed in infants by using three 10-mm cannulae (some used four ports), and no major complications were reported.[14-16] In most cases, patients were discharged the next morning.

An interesting response emerged with publication of a series in which open nephrectomy for multicystic dysplastic kidney (MCDK) through a dorsal lumbar incision was performed on an outpatient basis.[17] Although one can remove a dysplastic kidney through a small lumbar incision, exposure is limited and compromised to the extent that, in one case, an inadvertent appendectomy was reported.

Retroperitoneal endoscopic access was developed for children with similarly good results and with smaller instruments as they became available.[18-22] Two basic access approaches were used, lateral and prone.[23]

Both work well, and each has advantages in selected situations.

Indications

The indications for a laparoscopic nephrectomy include benign disease that has resulted in a nonfunctioning renal unit with the potential for infection, hypertension, or pain. We remove MCDKs only when parents insist. The contraindications to a laparoscopic nephrectomy include severe acute coagulopathy, uncontrolled sepsis, or very severe adhesions from prior laparotomy. These are uncommon in children. Laparoscopic nephrectomy has been shown to be feasible in higher risk patients, such as those with renal failure before transplant.

Laparoscopic nephrectomy for malignancy has not been performed in children because of the large size of the tumors. In time this may change, particularly if preoperative chemotherapy is used to shrink a tumor, or if partial nephrectomy is elected for small tumors. These principles for laparoscopic nephrectomy are well established in adults with renal tumors and will likely be appropriate for children as well.

The choice of transperitoneal or retroperitoneal nephrectomy largely depends on the experience of the operator and the associated procedures needed. If the entire ureter must be removed, or if an intra-abdominal testis is present, transperitoneal nephrectomy may be best. Subtotal resection of the ureter is readily done via the retroperitoneal access. The prone approach is less suited to ureteral resection but may be more efficient for access to the hilum.

Technique: Transperitoneal

Patients are prepared with a liquid diet for 24 hours preoperatively and a rectal suppository the night before. A bladder catheter and rectal tube are placed after the induction of anesthesia and before the skin is prepped. The ipsilateral side is elevated on a soft roll, and the patient secured to the table. The table is rotated so that the abdomen is flat for peritoneal access and port placement, and then rolled back with the ipsilateral side up for the procedure. Positioning the patient with the flank up helps the surgeon reflect the colon away from the kidney. This position permits rapid return to the supine position if emergency open access is needed.

The initial port is in the umbilicus with working ports in the ipsilateral lower quadrant in the midclavicular line and just to the ipsilateral side of the midline between the xyphoid and umbilicus. For right nephrectomy, a liver retractor placed laterally on the right or contralaterally on the left may be useful. We have used 3.5-mm or 5-mm instruments and endoscopes. A 5-mm port is needed for the clip applier.

The kidney is exposed by incising the lateral peritoneal reflection of the colon and mobilizing the colon medially. The ureter is identified near the lower pole of the kidney, or occasionally at the level of the iliac vessels, transected, and used for traction to lift the kidney to aid in the identification of the renal hilum. If vesicoureteric reflux is present, the ureter should be dissected at least to the level of the bladder and ligated, because clips are unreliable for closure of a thick ureter. Blunt or cautery dissection or both are used to expose the lower pole and hilum. The artery is divided first if possible, preferably away from the hilum, to limit the number of branches that must be controlled. It is divided between clips, usually leaving two on the proximal side. The vein is similarly controlled, watching for any lumbar veins. The gonadal vessels should be preserved. Superiorly, the adrenal vessels should be avoided. The upper pole is mobilized with cautery, as small vessels are frequently adjacent to the capsule. Lateral and posterior mobilization is usually rapid with blunt or cautery dissection. The kidney is removed through the umbilical port, which can be easily enlarged without increasing the size of the scar. The operative field is inspected, and the ports closed with preplaced fascial sutures.

Patients usually stay overnight but may occasionally be ready to go home on the day of the surgical procedure. Transperitoneal nephrectomy seems to induce more ileus than retroperitoneal, but the difference is minor.

Technique: Lateral Retroperitoneal

Patients are prepared as for a transperitoneal nephrectomy but positioned in a nearly full flank-up position. Initial access is gained just below the tip of the 12th rib with a 1- to 1.5-cm incision and blunt dissection through the muscle layers (Fig. 62-7). The perinephric fascia of Gerota can be identified and entered. At this point, a dissecting balloon can be placed, or the cannula can be positioned so that the endoscope is used bluntly to develop the working space. In both approaches, the port is secured with the fascial sutures, which also provides a gas seal for insufflation. Pressures are maintained between 12 and 15 mm Hg. Once the position of the kidney is defined, the posterior port is placed. This may not be possible under direct vision, although a 30-degree scope can facilitate placement. Usually the anticipated trajectory of the cannula is observed to avoid injury. The peritoneal reflection is identified and bluntly pushed medially.

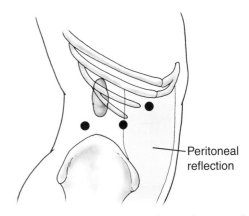

FIGURE 62-7. Lateral retroperitoneal port placement for right renal surgery. Approximate location of the posterior peritoneal reflection (*shaded*).

This can be done with an instrument or the endoscope, but care must be taken to avoid disrupting the peritoneum. The medial port is then placed, either in line with the other two or inferiorly in a triangular fashion. Fascial sutures in a box-stitch pattern are placed before the cannulae to act as retention sutures of the cannula during the procedure and to close the site at completion.

If a small rent is made in the peritoneum, the operative field will be compromised by intraperitoneal insufflation. Peritoneal decompression can be effected by placing an IV angiocatheter through the abdominal wall to let the peritoneal gas escape. Alternatively, the peritoneal rent can be enlarged so that the peritoneum does not separately trap CO_2. It is rarely necessary to abandon the procedure and convert to open surgical procedures because of entry into the peritoneum.

Exposure of the hilum of the kidney is the key step for retroperitoneal nephrectomy, and it is important to prevent the kidney from falling onto the hilum. This can be facilitated by maintaining the anterior attachments of the kidney so that it falls forward with the peritoneum, exposing the posterior aspect of the hilum. Even so, it may be necessary to use one instrument to retract the kidney as the hilum is exposed, limiting the surgeon's dissecting ability, which becomes one-handed. If the pelvis is large, it will need to be moved away to adequately expose the vessels. This may be accomplished by transecting the ureter near the lower pole. The artery is encountered posteriorly and divided between clips. The vein also is divided between clips, and the rest of the mobilization done as with a transperitoneal approach. Near the upper pole, the peritoneum can be torn, so care must be taken to stay close to the kidney.

If the ureter is to be removed, the lateral approach permits efficient access to the distal ureter, usually to below the iliac vessels. If the ureterovesical junction is competent, the distal ureteric stump is left open, whereas the stump of a refluxing ureter must be ligated as close to its junction with the bladder as possible.

The kidney is removed through the larger of the ports, usually that at the tip of the 12th rib. It may need to be morcellated with scissors, in which case, a laparoscopic specimen-retrieval bag is helpful. Most kidneys are small enough to be removed intact. Occasionally, removal of the specimen can be facilitated by placing it into the finger of a surgical glove as a miniature Lapsac and then pulled through the port site. All port sites are closed with the preplaced fascial sutures.

Technique: Prone Retroperitoneal

The prone approach has evolved from the dorsal lumbotomy and offers a direct access to the kidney and hilum. The patient is in the full prone position with an indwelling bladder catheter in place. In small children, it is helpful to have the lower end of the table turned down, with the surgeon standing at the patient's feet. This allows the surgeon to be in better line with the working instruments. The initial port is placed at the costovertebral angle by using a 1-cm incision (Fig. 62-8). Blunt dissection

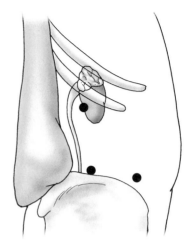

FIGURE 62-8. Port positions for prone retroperitoneal approach to right kidney.

through the posterior muscle layers reveals the posterior aspect of the perinephric fascia, which is entered. A lumbar fascial suture is placed for later closure. A dissecting balloon is used to develop the working space. A 5-mm cannula is placed with a 3.5-mm scope, which permits moving the scope to other ports during the dissection and at the time of placing vascular clips. The endoscope is inserted as the retroperitoneum is insufflated. This should reveal the posterior aspect of the kidney, and further dissection can be performed with the endoscope. Occasionally the developed space is anterior to the kidney, making it difficult to immediately locate the kidney. This possibility must be considered, and the upper (posterior) abdominal wall inspected. The secondary (3.5-mm) ports are placed. We have used 2-mm instrumentation to perform the mobilization but found the instruments too flexible for efficient use around the kidney, and therefore use the larger and stiffer 3.5-mm instruments.

In the prone position, the kidney falls forward revealing the hilum, which may often be seen with initial dissection (Fig. 62-9). The vessels are controlled first, unless the ureter is needed for mobilization. Again, the vessels should be exposed somewhat away from the kidney to avoid the need to control multiple branches. It is important to maintain a consistent camera orientation to permit accurate identification of the vascular structures. The exposure can be so wide that the vena cava is readily seen, and it may be smaller than expected because of the gas insufflation. It has occasionally appeared to look like the renal vein, based on size and direction, because of a scope that was off true vertical.

Once the vessels are controlled and divided, the ureter is ligated and divided. The kidney is then mobilized to control the small upper pole vessels, with care being taken to avoid entering the peritoneum and to avoid the adrenal vessels. The kidney can be removed through the initial port, with the camera being moved to the inferior working ports.

If the ureter is to be removed, the instruments are reversed in direction and the ureter traced inferiorly as far as possible. This is usually to the level of the iliac vessels.

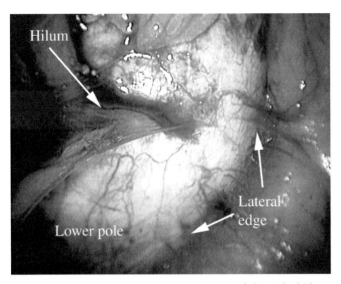

FIGURE 62-9. Posterior laparoscopic view of the right kidney after initial exposure. The hilum is on the left of the field, with the entire kidney exposed, and its lateral edge to the right.

Postoperative care is similar to that with other techniques of laparoscopic nephrectomy.

Results

Complications have been reported in several series but are limited to minor occurrences, such as entry into the peritoneum or subcutaneous emphysema, that have no real clinical significance (Table 62-1). The need for transfusion is clearly a complication and has been rare indeed. Conversion to an open procedure is reported in no more than 2% of the pediatric series and is usually the result of bleeding that cannot be effectively controlled laparoscopically. Conversion rates are very much operator dependent and are not likely an inherent feature of the technique. With experience, conversion rates are likely to diminish both with the individual surgeon and overall as methods and training improve. Injury to other organs is the major concern and has been reported (as it has for open nephrectomy in children[17]). These are fortunately uncommon and usually involve liver, bowel, or occasionally great vessel injuries.

Surgical efficiency compared with that in an open nephrectomy can be related to the duration of the procedure, its cost, and the rapidity of patient recovery. No objective studies of this have been performed in pediatric nephrectomy, and they will be difficult to accomplish.[24] Considering laparoscopic cholecystectomy, a widely accepted procedure, a controversy remains regarding its relative efficiency as compared with minimal-exposure open cholecystectomy.

Partial Nephrectomy

It has become clear that laparoscopic partial nephrectomy may be one of the most beneficial procedures to emerge from early experience with laparoscopic nephrectomy.[25] Open partial nephrectomy is best performed through a flank incision, which has an appreciable morbidity, even in infants. Precise vascular control is essential, along with accurate visualization of the normal and abnormal renal moieties. Injury to the remnant pole is a significant complication, and in the infant, this is more likely with the mobilization required to expose the hilum. From a laparoscopic approach, the hilum can be exposed without significant mobilization of the remnant pole, theoretically reducing the risk of vascular spasm and injury to the remnant pole. However, the incidence of this complication is so low that it will be very difficult to prove a benefit for laparoscopy.[26]

				Op Time				
TABLE 62-1								
PEDIATRIC LAPAROSCOPIC NEPHRECTOMY (NX) AND NEPHROURETERECTOMY (NUX)								
Author	Year	Nx	NUX	(hr)	LOS	Conv	%	Comment
Koyle[14]	1993	1	0					Transperitoneal
Suzuki[57]	1993	1	0					Transperitoneal
Nishiyama	1996	1	0					Retroperitoneal
Ushiyama[58]	1998	2	0	2.75				Transperitoneal
Erhlich[15]	1994	10	4	2.25	1	0	0	Transperitoneal
Valla[20]	1996	18	0	1.66		1	5.5	Retroperitoneal
Davies[59]	1998	24	12	1.4	2	1	2.8	Transperitoneal
El Ghoneimi[19]	1998	31	0	1.75	2	0	0	Retroperitoneal
Borer[22]	1999	14	0	2.3	2	0	0	Retroperitoneal
Prabhakaran[60]	1999	0	6	3	2.3	0	0	Transperitoneal
Hamilton[61]	2000	10	0	3	1	0	0	Transperitoneal
Yao[62]	2000	14	6	2.17	1.25	0	0	Transperitoneal
York[63]	2000	11	0	2.75	2.4	0	0	Transperitoneal
Borzi[23]	2001	36	0	1		2	5.5	Retroperitoneal
Shanberg[64]	2001	22	15	1.25	1.3	1	2.7	Retroperitoneal
Capolicchio[65]	2003	12	0	3		0	0	Retroperitoneal
Total		207	43	2.13	1.7	5	2.0	

LOS, Length of stay.

Our preferred access to the kidney is retroperitoneal and usually prone.[27] This limits the ability to remove the ureter, which is needed in those unusual cases of obstruction combined with reflux. In such cases, the lateral approach is used, or a small inguinal counterincision is used to remove the ureter to the level of the bladder neck. With simple reflux and no obstruction (usually a lower pole), total removal of the distal ureteral stump is not considered essential, and most reports support this approach. The prone approach provides excellent exposure of the posterior aspect of the kidney, and the delineation between the poles is usually readily evident. The ureter to be removed is identified at the level of the lower pole and separated from the remnant ureter. The ureter draining the nonfunctioning pole is transected and used for traction to mobilize the hilum. The hilar vessels are identified, and the affected-pole vessels are isolated and divided. If the vessels are not clearly defined, dissection of the nonfunctioning pole is started, whereupon the vessels will become evident with mobilization. Separation of the poles can be performed by using either cautery or the harmonic scalpel (Fig. 62-10). It is not a problem if the affected collecting system is entered, as long as the entire collecting system is removed. If the remnant-pole collecting system is entered, it should be repaired and drained. Placement of a ureteral catheter in the remnant pole and injection of indigo carmine dye at the conclusion to confirm closure have been advocated by some. This is useful in adult partial nephrectomy without duplication but probably is not necessary with duplication anomalies, as the separation is usually quite clear.

No attempt is usually made to suture the edge of the remnant pole, but this can be done currently with robotic assistance. This maneuver should ensure hemostasis and limit the risk of leakage. We have not typically drained the operative area in small children but would recommend drainage in older children or in complex cases. A bladder catheter can be left in place overnight, although some of these children have been discharged on the same day.

The limited number of reports of laparoscopic partial nephrectomy does not allow definite conclusions regarding its ultimate potential, but the efficiency and the reduction in morbidity seem to argue strongly in favor of its further development[23,25,26,28,29] (Table 62-2).

URACHAL CYSTS

Several reports of urachal cyst resections have been published, although it is unclear if this is useful.[30,31] It transforms a preperitoneal procedure into an intraperitoneal one. The conventional incision through the umbilicus is a very minimal incision with no visible scar, whereas laparoscopically, two further small incisions would be needed.

We have not recommended using this procedure, although we performed several initially. The situation in which this might be appropriate would be in the child with umbilical drainage and an uncertain diagnosis. If the drainage is due to an omphalomesenteric duct or omental hernia (both of which we have seen), then laparoscopic diagnosis and subsequent therapy are efficient, including if the diagnosis was a urachal anomaly. A large inflamed mass from a urachal cyst with infection might be removed laparoscopically with some benefit, although the risk of peritoneal contamination should be considered.

GONADECTOMY AND MÜLLERIAN REMNANTS

In various intersex and genital maldevelopment sydromes, laparoscopic biopsy or resection, or both, of inappropriate gonadal or müllerian structures is possible.[32,33] This is particularly efficient when the remnant is located in the deep retrovesical pelvis, a difficult area to access with an open procedure. Although they are not strictly intersex conditions, abnormal müllerian structures such as seminal vesicle cysts also are well managed with laparoscopic excision.[34]

RECONSTRUCTIVE SURGERY

Pyeloplasty

Only a handful of surgeons in North America have attempted laparoscopic pyeloplasty for ureteropelvic junction (UPJ) obstruction in young children.[35] It is practicable, and the outcomes in older children and adults have been good.[36–40] Retroperitoneal access is technically efficient.[38] The advent of effective robotic-assisted surgical procedures offers the potential to make pediatric

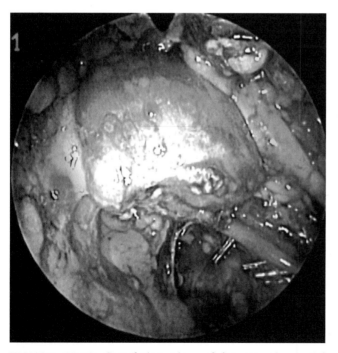

FIGURE 62-10. Completion view of laparoscopic partial nephrectomy of nonfunctioning lower pole from a retroperitoneal view.

TABLE 62-2

PARTIAL NEPHRECTOMY

Author	Year	Pts	Op Time	LOS	Conv	%	Comment
Janetschek[28]	1997	14	3.75	4.4	0	0	Transperitoneal
Yao[62]	2000	6	3.75	1	0	0	Transperitoneal
Horowitz[25]	2001	14	1.66	2.6	0	0	Transperitoneal
El Ghoneimi[29]	2003	15	2.5	1.4	1	6.7	Retroperitoneal
Robinson[26]	2003	11	3.33	1.0	0	0	Transperitoneal
Valla[66]	2003	24	2.66	3.4	3	12.5	Retroperitoneal
Total		**84**	**2.94**	**2.3**	**4**	**4.8**	

LOS, Length of stay.

pyeloplasty a method with general applicability by most pediatric urologists. Current methods as well as robotic options are discussed.

Port placement for transperitoneal pyeloplasty is similar to that for nephrectomy, with an umbilical port, an ipsilateral upper quadrant port just lateral to the midline, and an ipsilateral lower quadrant port. A fourth holding port can be placed laterally. Retroperitoneal access is with three ports in line along the lower edge of the 12th rib. Prone access is possible with a similar in-line port layout.

The method is essentially identical to the open procedure with exposure of the renal pelvis but is facilitated by the placement of a traction suture to stabilize the pelvis. The pelvis is transected above the UPJ and used for traction to permit spatulation of the lateral upper ureter without grasping the tissue to be included in the anastomosis. Alternatives include placing a small traction stitch on the ureter after it is transected distal to the UPJ or leaving a bridge of pelvic tissue on the medial aspect to stabilize the ureter. The amount of pelvis removed should be limited, even in severe hydronephrosis, as the pelvis may retract and make the repair even more difficult. It is not usually necessary to perform a significant pelvic resection in any event, as this will usually improve on its own after relief of the obstruction. Suturing the anastomosis remains the challenge, but with the enhanced visualization of the laparoscope, accurate suturing is possible with practice. Most surgeons have used a continuous suture anteriorly and posteriorly. Care should be taken to avoid leaving loose suture ends, as they will entangle subsequent sutures and may confuse the operator during knot tying. A stent can be left in place if desired. We prefer using a double-J stent because of a sense of insecurity with the closure (Fig. 62-11). A double-J stent eliminates the need for a drain. Recently, with robotic-assisted laparoscopic pyeloplasty, stents have not been placed unless concern exists about the integrity of the anastomosis or the integrity of the pelvic and ureteral tissues.

Reported outcomes are no better than those with open procedures. Morbidity seems less, particularly for older patients, and hospital stays are shorter in older patients. Failures, primarily persistent UPJ obstruction, have been limited to very small children (younger than 6 months) or those with massive hydronephrosis. This observation may account for the lack of enthusiasm for the laparoscopic

pyeloplasty in infants, who seem to recover rapidly after open surgical procedures.

Antireflux Repair

Initial attempts at laparoscopic antireflux surgical procedures were frustrating. The technique was the extravesical Lich-Gregoir operation.[41] These were successful but far too time-consuming to be advantageous, and after an initial interest, few further attempts were made.[42,43] Recently a series of successful procedures was reported.[44] Several significant early complications and long hospital stays associated with the initial efforts have been resolved with experience. The procedure is done transperitoneally, exposing the distal ureter between the bladder and uterus in females. The antireflux tunnel is created by incising the detrusor muscle down to the submucosa cephalad from the ureterovesicle junction along the axis of the ureter. Care is taken not to injure the mucosa and enter the bladder lumen. The muscularis is dissected in an inverted-Y manner around the ureteral hiatus. The detrusor muscle is closed over the ureter to create the antireflux tunnel. No attempt at ureteral advancement is made. Suturing the detrusor over the

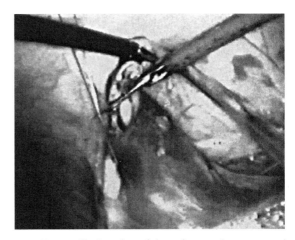

FIGURE 62-11. Closing the pelvis and ureter in a conventional laparoscopic pyeloplasty. A double-J stent is visible within the pelvis.

ureter has been the most challenging aspect of the procedure, in part because of the angle of approach. Bilateral procedures have been performed with no evidence of the anticipated distal ureteric obstruction. However, the numbers are very limited, and that concern remains. Success seems to be equal to that with open surgical procedures, excluding initial complications. Hospital stays are equivalent to those with open methods in current practice but may improve. Objectively, demonstrating a clinical advantage over open procedures will be difficult.

Intravesical antireflux repair has recently emerged as an alternative to the extravesical approach. This is offered as an alternative to bilateral extravesical procedures with their risk of ureteral obstruction, as well as avoiding peritoneal entry.[45] Several earlier attempts with the Gil-Vernet approach of bringing the ureters together in the midline, without mobilization, did not prove to be effacacious.[46] The most intriguing experimental approach presented to date has been that of an intravesical, transtrigonal reimplantation with insufflation of the bladder (pneumovesicum).[47] The major technical challenges include obtaining and maintaining access to the bladder, without dislodging the cannulae or leaking CO_2 into the paravesical space, as well as mobilization of the ureter, creation of the submucosal tunnel, and the suturing to implant the ureter. Overcoming these challenges seems feasible only in a few highly skilled hands. Most pediatric laparoscopists would probably not undertake this operation. Demonstrating a clinical advantage would be difficult.

Robotic-assisted laparoscopic antireflux repair offers a promising option that may prove applicable for more surgeons. The extravesical technique, as with the conventional laparoscopic method, would probably be the procedure of choice (Fig. 62-12). At present the patients in whom the laparoscopic approach would be most advantageous are older children in whom even the lower abdominal incision is uncomfortable. Operative times are reasonable, about $2\frac{1}{2}$ hours, and most patients have been discharged within 24 hours. Intravesical robotically assisted transtrigonal ureteral reimplantation has been explored experimentally and to a limited degree in humans (Fig. 62-13).

Continent Diversion and Augmentation

Major reconstructive operations such as bladder augmentation, continent diversion, and vaginal reconstruction carry substantial morbidity for open access. It may be that laparoscopic procedures for reconstruction and diversion will prove most beneficial in all age groups. The creation of an appendiceal continent catheterizable stoma (Mitrofanoff) has been reported.[48] The limited amount of suturing needed for such a procedure makes it technically feasible today. Laparoscopic-assisted mobilization with limited open incision to complete the procedure has been advocated in several reports, with excellent results for this important concept.[49-51] Laparoscopic assisted reconstruction may be the most practical approach for the present.

The ability to perform an entire reconstruction, including augmentation and continent stoma formation, is technically present today[52] but is not going to be of practical value until more efficient means of suturing are developed. Tissue glues or welding or the use of robotic-assisted suturing may permit more widespread use of total laparoscopic methods in complex reconstruction. It also will require novel algorithms for harvesting bowel segments to use in the reconstruction. No inherent reason suggests that this cannot be accomplished. Reports of freehand bowel harvest and anastomosis have been presented, but the general applicability of these is unknown.[53,54]

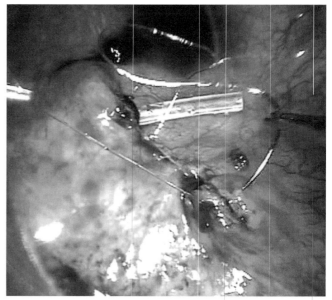

FIGURE 62-13. Completion of intravesical, robotically assisted laparoscopic transtrigonal ureteral reimplantation in a child. Cannulae are placed directly into the bladder, which is insufflated with CO_2.

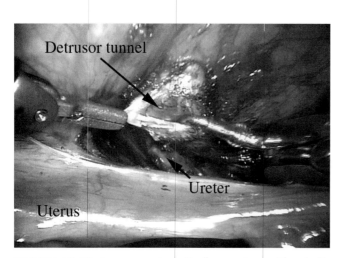

FIGURE 62-12. Laparoscopic antireflux surgery with robotic assistance creating the detrusor tunnel to be wrapped around the mobilized ureter.

HORIZONS

Emerging Role of Robotic Procedures in Laparoscopy

Many of the present limitations for laparoscopy in pediatric urology are based on inability to perform delicate suturing. Robotic assistance in laparoscopic surgical procedures offers suturing capabilities for reconstructive procedures that are the most exciting prospect for the laparoscopic pediatric urologist today. With an established record in adult gastrointestinal surgical procedures and rapidly developing experience in adult prostatectomy, the principles of robotic assistance seem readily applicable to pediatric urology. The principal advantage from robotics are the remarkable dexterity of wrist technology that is integral to the suturing and the enhanced three-dimensional visualization. Various robotic devices can enhance surgical capabilities, although it remains to be seen if this can be translated to clinical benefit. Robotic endoscopic assistance has been used for several years with apparent utility. Initial reports of more complex manipulative robotic devices used in children are promising, but the area remains to be explored thoroughly.[55,56]

The most widely used system is the DaVinci (Intuitive Surgical, Sunnyvale, CA) which consists of three arms attached to a central pedestal at the bedside. These arms hold the endoscope and the two manipulative arms, which hold the working instruments. A surgeon's console, including an image monitor and manipulating controls, is hard-wired to the robotic device in the operating room. Through this, the surgeon controls the manipulating arms and the attached instruments, as well as the endoscope with its 3-D camera. An instrument tower contains image controls and a monitor for the patient-side staff to be able to follow the procedure. Instruments including scissors, dissecting and grasping tools, and needle holders, as well as a harmonic scalpel, are mounted on the manipulating arms and passed through laparoscopic cannulae. Instruments are exchanged by the patient-side staff for differing tasks or to pass sutures into the field. The basic instruments are totally distinct from conventional laparoscopic tools, as they have a full range of motion at their working end, permitting precise positioning for efficient action within the patient. The robotic instruments have their fulcrum of activity within 1 cm of the tissues being handled—a distinct improvement over conventional laparoscopic instruments, which are limited to movement dependent on their entry point into the body and to simple open-and-close actions. Indeed, the robotic instruments available have an advantage over instruments used for open procedures, which also are limited to some extent by the size of the incision and the depth of the operative area and which also have only an open-and-close action. Furthermore, with robotics, scaling of motion occurs so that variable degrees of precision may be applied, depending on the situation. Tremor control is present, as well. Combined with true 3-D visual control, the operator can exercise a degree of control and manipulation far greater than that with conventional laparoscopy and perhaps greater than that with some open surgical procedures.

This control comes at a cost, both financial and practical. The instruments are expensive to purchase and use, and they are presently very large for pediatric applications. The endoscope is 12 mm, and the working ports are 8 mm each. Although initial laparoscopic methods in children included instruments of this size, we have become demanding of smaller instruments that are being developed. The trend toward size and cost reduction will likely continue, but it will take time. The potential offered by these new technologic developments is extremely appealing, and it would seem logical to anticipate its utility in pediatric surgical applications.

We have used robotic instruments to perform extra- and intravesical ureteral reimplants for reflux, pyeloplasty, nephrectomy, continent diversion with appendix, as well as pyelolithotomy. The manipulative capability is very good, and far better than what could be accomplished with conventional laparoscopy. Visualization is similarly much enhanced. The 5-mm working ports will be in use within a short time. Although the instruments are large, the 12-mm port is easily hidden in the umbilicus, and the scars from the other ports are limited (Fig. 62-14). We have used the instrument in children as young as 5 months, but the working space is limited. Research into optimizing techniques and developing algorithms for various procedures is essential. It will be critical for pediatric practitioners to guide research and development.

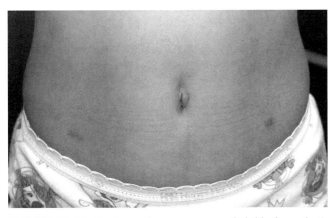

FIGURE 62-14. Postoperative appearance of child after robotically assisted laparoscopic extravesical ureteral surgery for reflux.

REFERENCES

1. Clayman RV: Pediatric laparoscopy: Quo vadis? View from outside. J Urol 152:730–733, 1994.
2. Cortes D, Thorup JM, Lenz K, et al: Laparoscopy in 100 consecutive patients with 128 impalpable testes. Br J Urol 75:281–287, 1995.
3. Moore RG, Peters CA, Bauer SB, et al: Laparoscopic evaluation of the nonpalpable tests: A prospective assessment of accuracy. J Urol 151:728–731, 1994.
4. Tennenbaum SY, Lerner SE, McAleer IM, et al: Preoperative laparoscopic localization of the nonpalpable testis: A critical analysis of a 10-year experience. J Urol 151:732–734, 1994.
5. Ferro F, Spagnoli A, Zaccara A, et al: Is preoperative laparoscopy useful for impalpable testis? J Urol 162:995–996, 1999.

6. Cisek LJ, Peters CA, Atala A, et al: Current findings in diagnostic laparoscopic evaluation of the nonpalpable testis. J Urol 160: 1145–1149, 1998.

7. Lakshmanan Y, Peters CA: Laparoscopy in the management of intersex anomalies. Pediatr Endosurg Innov Tech 4:201–206, 2000.

8. Baker LA, Docimo SG, Surer I, et al: A multi-institutional analysis of laparoscopic orchidopexy. BJU Int 87:484–489, 2001.

9. Docimo SG: The results of surgical therapy for cryptorchidism: A literature review and analysis. J Urol 154:1148–1152, 1995.

10. Docimo SG, Moore RG, Adams J, et al: Laparoscopic orchiopexy for the high palpable undescended testis: Preliminary experience. J Urol 154:1513–1515, 1995.

11. Koff SA, Sethi PS: One stage orchiopexy for high undescended tests utilizing low testicular ligation: An alternative to the Fowler-Stephens technique. Paper presented at AAP, Section on Urology, San Francisco, 1995, p Abs 156.

12. Clark DA, Borzi PA: Laparoscopic orchidopexy for the intra-abdominal testis. Pediatr Surg Int 15:454–456, 1999.

13. Chang B, Palmer LS, Franco I: Laparoscopic orchidopexy: A review of a large clinical series. BJU Int 87:490–493, 2001.

14. Koyle MA, Woo HH, Kavoussi LR: Laparoscopic nephrectomy in the first year of life. J Pediatr Surg 28:693–695, 1993.

15. Ehrlich RM, Gershman A, Fuchs G: Laparoscopic renal surgery in children. J Urol 151:735–739, 1994.

16. Peters CA, Kavoussi LR, Retik AB: Laparoscopic nephrectomy and nephroureterectomy in children. J. Endourol 7(suppl 1):S174, 1993.

17. Elder JS, Hladky D, Selzman AA: Outpatient nephrectomy for nonfunctioning kidneys. J Urol 154:712–714, 1995.

18. Koyle M, Chandhoke P, Galensky S: Pediatric retroperitoneal laparoscopic nephrectomy. J Endourol 8(suppl 1):S94, 1994.

19. El-Ghoneimi A, Valla JS, Steyaert H, et al: Laparoscopic renal surgery via a retroperitoneal approach in children. J Urol 160:1138–1141, 1998.

20. Valla JS, Guilloneau B, Montupet P, et al: Retroperitoneal laparoscopic nephrectomy in children: Preliminary report of 18 cases. Eur Urol 30:490–493, 1996.

21. Kobashi KC, Chamberlin DA, Rajpoot D, et al: Retroperitoneal laparoscopic nephrectomy in children. J Urol 160:1142–1144, 1998.

22. Borer JG, Cisek LJ, Atala A, et al: Pediatric retroperitoneoscopic nephrectomy using 2-mm instrumentation. J Urol 162:1725–1729, 1999.

23. Borzi PA: A comparison of the lateral and posterior retroperitoneoscopic approach for complete and partial nephroureterectomy in children. BJU Int 87:517–520, 2001.

24. Peters C: Laparoscopy in paediatric urology: Adoption of innovative technology. BJU Int 92(suppl 1):52–57, 2003.

25. Horowitz M, Shah SM, Ferzli G, et al: Laparoscopic partial upper pole nephrectomy in infants and children. BJU Int 87:514–516, 2001.

26. Robinson BC, Snow BW, Cartwright PC, et al: Comparison of laparoscopic versus open partial nephrectomy in a pediatric series. J Urol 169:638–640, 2003.

27. Borer JG, Peters CA: Pediatric retroperitoneoscopic nephrectomy. J Endourol 14:413–416, 2000.

28. Janetschek G, Seibold J, Radmayr C, et al: Laparoscopic heminephroureterectomy in pediatric patients. J Urol 158: 1928–1930, 1997.

29. El-Ghoneimi A, Farhat W, Bolduc S, et al: Retroperitoneal laparoscopic vs open partial nephroureterectomy in children. BJU Int 91:532–535, 2003.

30. Khurana S, Borzi PA: Laparoscopic management of complicated urachal disease in children. J Urol 168:1526–1528, 2002.

31. Trondsen E, Reiertsen O, Rosseland AR: Laparoscopic excision of urachal sinus. Eur J Surg 159:127–128, 1993.

32. Lee KH, Yeung CK, Tam YH, et al: The use of laparoscopy in the management of adnexal pathologies in children. Aust N Z J Surg 70:192–195, 2000.

33. Wiener JS, Jordan GH, Gonzales ET Jr: Laparoscopic management of persistent müllerian duct remnants associated with an abdominal testis. J Endourol 11:357–359, 1997.

34. Carmignani G, Gallucci M, Puppo P, et al: Video laparoscopic excision of a seminal vesicle cyst associated with ipsilateral renal agenesis [see comments]. J Urol 153:437–439, 1995.

35. Peters CA, Schlussel RN, Retik AB: Pediatric laparoscopic-dismembered pyeloplasty. J Urol 153:1962–1965, 1995.

36. Janetschek G, Peschel R, Frauscher F, et al: Laparoscopic pyeloplasty. Urol Clin North Am 27:695–704, 2000.

37. Tan HL. Laparoscopic Anderson-Hynes dismembered pyeloplasty in children. J Urol 162:1045–1047, 1999.

38. Yeung CK, Tam YH, Sihoe JD, et al: Retroperitoneoscopic dismembered pyeloplasty for pelvi-ureteric junction obstruction in infants and children. BJU Int 87:509–513, 2001.

39. El-Ghoneimi A, Farhat W, Bolduc S, et al: Laparoscopic dismembered pyeloplasty by a retroperitoneal approach in children. BJU Int 92:104–108, 2003.

40. Tan HL, Roberts JP. Laparoscopic dismembered pyeloplasty in children: Preliminary results. Br J Urol 77:909–913, 1996.

41. Atala A, Kavoussi LR, Goldstein DS, et al: Laparoscopic correction of vesicoureteral reflux. J Urol 150:748–751, 1993.

42. Ehrlich RM, Gershman A, Fuchs G: Laparoscopic vesicoureteroplasty in children: Initial case reports. Urology 43:255–261, 1994.

43. Janetschek G, Radmayr C, Bartsch G: Laparoscopic ureteral antireflux plasty reimplantation: First clinical experience. Ann Urol (Paris) 29:101–105, 1995.

44. Lakshmanan Y, Fung LC: Laparoscopic extravesicular ureteral reimplantation for vesicoureteral reflux: Recent technical advances. J Endourol 14:589–593, 2000.

45. Gill IS, Ponsky LE, Desai M, et al: Laparoscopic cross-trigonal Cohen ureteroneocystostomy: Novel technique. J Urol 166: 1811–1814, 2001.

46. Cartwright PC, Snow BW, Mansfield JC, et al: Percutaneous endoscopic trigonoplasty: A minimally invasive approach to correct vesicoureteral reflux. J Urol 156:661–664, 1996.

47. Olsen LH, Deding D, Yeung CK, et al: Computer assisted laparoscopic pneumovesical ureter reimplantation a.m. Cohen: Initial experience in a pig model. APMIS Suppl 109:23–25, 2003.

48. Jordan GH, Winslow BH: Laparoscopically assisted continent catheterizable cutaneous appendicovesicostomy. J Endourol 7:517–520, 1993.

49. Hedican SP, Schulam PG, Docimo SG: Laparoscopic assisted reconstructive surgery. J Urol 161:267–270, 1999.

50. Cadeddu JA, Docimo SG: Laparoscopic-assisted continent stoma procedures: Our new standard. Urology 54:909–912, 1999.

51. Van Savage JG, Slaughenhoupt BL: Laparoscopic-assisted continent urinary diversion in obese patients. J Endourol 13:571–573, 1999.

52. Docimo SG, Moore RG, Adams J, et al: Laparoscopic bladder augmentation using stomach. Urology 46:565–569, 1995.

53. Basiri A, Shadpour P, Maghsudi R: Laparoscopically assisted pyelo-uretero-cystoplasty. J Endourol 17(suppl 1):A322, 2003.

54. Simforoosh N, Shadpour P, Maghsudi R, et al: Laparoscopic combined ileocystoplasty and Malone procedures: Totally intracorporeal freehand suturing. J Endourol 17(suppl 1):A323, 2003.

55. Hollands CM, Dixey LN: Applications of robotic surgery in pediatric patients. Surg Laparosc Endosc Percutan Tech 12:71–76, 2002.

56. Partin AW, Adams JB, Moore RG, et al: Complete robot-assisted laparoscopic urologic surgery: A preliminary report. J Am Coll Surg 181:552–557, 1995.

57. Suzuki K, Ihara H, Kurita Y, et al: Laparoscopic nephrectomy for atrophic kidney associated with ectopic ureter in a child. Eur Urol 23:463–465, 1993.

58. Ushiyama T, Kageyama S, Mugiya S, et al: Laparoscopic nephrectomy in children: Two case reports. Int J Urol 5:181–184, 1998.

59. Davies BW, Najmaldin AS: Transperitoneal laparoscopic nephrectomy in children. J Endourol 12:437–440, 1998.

60. Prabhakaran K, Lingaraj K: Laparoscopic nephroureterectomy in children. J Pediatr Surg 34:556–558, 1999.

61. Hamilton BD, Gatti JM, Cartwright PC, et al: Comparison of laparoscopic versus open nephrectomy in the pediatric population. J Urol 163:937–939, 2000.

62. Yao D, Poppas DP: A clinical series of laparoscopic nephrectomy, nephroureterectomy and heminephroureterectomy in the pediatric population. J Urol 163:1531–1535, 2000.

63. York GB, Robertson FM, Cofer BR, et al: Laparoscopic nephrectomy in children. Surg Endosc 14:469–472, 2000.

64. Shanberg AM, Sanderson K, Rajpoot D, et al: Laparoscopic retroperitoneal renal and adrenal surgery in children. BJU Int 87:521–524, 2001.

65. Capolicchio JP, Jednak R, Anidjar M, et al: A modified access technique for retroperitoneoscopic renal surgery in children. J Urol 170:204–206, 2003.

66. Valla JS, Breaud J, Carfagna L, et al: Treatment of ureterocele on duplex ureter: Upper pole nephrectomy by retroperitoneoscopy in children based on a series of 24 cases. Eur Urol 43:426–429, 2003.

CHAPTER 63

Renovascular Hypertension

James A. O'Neill, Jr., MD

Elevated blood pressure occurs in 2% to 10% of children, but because blood pressure is not routinely measured in children, particularly infants, the diagnosis of hypertension is often delayed. Table 63-1 lists the various causes of hypertension in childhood according to the organ system involved: renal, cardiovascular, central nervous system, endocrine, essential hypertension, and hypertension secondary to drugs and various poisons. This chapter focuses on renovascular causes of hypertension, which are mostly correctable.

It has been known for 30 years that a relation exists between renal ischemia and hypertension resulting from activation of the renin-angiotensin system, which leads to the release of renin and the production of angiotensin II (Fig. 63-1). Subsequent information has revealed that diminished renal perfusion pressure has direct effects on sodium excretion, sympathetic nerve activity, nitric oxide production, and intrarenal prostaglandin concentrations, which result in renovascular hypertension.[1] Two things are known about the natural history of renovascular hypertension in children. First, once established, the disease is progressive, and, although the process may abate for a while or "burn out," now a number of reports have been made of late recurrence of renovascular lesions in sites other than originally identified. The progressive nature of this disorder is the best justification for an aggressive approach to correction. Second, sustained hypertension may result in left heart failure and chronic renal failure, based on chronic ischemic nephropathy. Additionally, patients with malignant forms of renovascular hypertension have a high incidence of heart failure and renal failure.[2]

The most common cause of hypertension between birth and age 20 years is essential hypertension in approximately 60% of the patients. However, the incidence of correctible hypertension is much higher in patients younger than 15 years.[2] In prior studies by our group, the incidence of correctable hypertension in the 0 to 5-year age group was approximately 80%; in the 6- to 10-year age group, 45%; and in the 11- to 15-year and 16- to 20-year age groups, 20%.[2] Although a variety of correctable etiologies were identified, the vast majority were renovascular. Additionally, long-term follow-up of patients with renovascular hypertension clearly indicated that patients who had successful repair of their lesions had much longer survival than did those who did not, and the younger the patient, the better the result.[3] These studies also support an aggressive approach to correction of identified renovascular lesions in young patients.

Renovascular disorders may be congenital or acquired. Congenital causes include arterial hypoplasia or absence; neurofibromatosis involving the renal artery; and William's syndrome, which includes the manifestations of supravalvular aortic stenosis; peripheral vascular stenoses, particularly subclavian and renal arterial; hypercalcemia; and elfin facies[4]. The most common acquired form of renovascular hypertension is fibromuscular dysplasia (FMD), which may be either localized to one or both renal arteries or appear as a more generalized type of disease such as Takayasu's arteritis and subisthmic abdominal coarctation, now more commonly referred to as the midaortic syndrome.[5,6] Other less common forms of acquired renovascular hypertension are renal artery trauma or thrombosis, Kawasaki's disease, and anastomotic stenosis, as is seen occasionally in renal transplants.

With regard to etiology, the vast majority of children with renovascular hypertension have what has been referred to as FMD or hyperplasia. Previous studies have suggested that this lesion has a congenital origin.[4,7] Because it appears to coexist with neurofibromatosis, Williams' syndrome, and pheochromocytoma, and because arterial and aortic hypoplasia and aplasia are seen in newborn infants, it is assumed that at least some of these lesions are congenital (Fig. 63-2). Conversely, the majority of patients are initially seen at several years of age, usually with an inflammatory phase followed by a quiescent phase of arteritis.[2,5] This clinical picture has led the majority of workers in this field to conclude that the disorder is an autoimmune disease, but convincing proof is still lacking. The pathology of the vascular lesion seen in the renal artery and the aorta reveals medial and

TABLE 63-1	
CAUSES OF HYPERTENSION IN CHILDREN	
Renal	Glomerulonephritis, pyelonephritis, renal hypoplasia, polycystic kidney, Wilms' tumor, neuroblastoma, arteritis, aneurysms, trauma
Cardiovascular	Coarctation, Takayasu's arteritis, renovascular stenosis, collagen vascular disease
Central Nervous System	Encephalitis, intracranial mass with increased pressure, dysautonomia
Endocrine	Pheochromocytoma, aldosteronoma, adrenogenital syndrome, Cushing's syndrome
Essential Hypertension	
Secondary Hypertension	Lead, mercury poisoning, glucocorticoid drugs, oral contraceptives

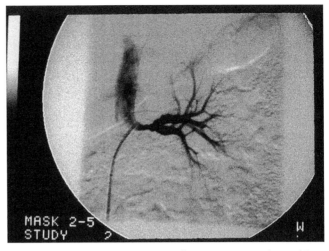

FIGURE 63-2. This selective renal arteriogram performed in a newborn with congestive heart failure caused by severe hypertension demonstrates significant narrowing of the left renal artery. The cause is probably congenital.

perimedial fibroplasia with inherent implications about approaches to treatment, particularly angioplasty.

CLINICAL PRESENTATION

Children with renovascular hypertension usually are first seen in one of two ways. In the first instance, an asymptomatic young child undergoing an elective surgical procedure, such as tonsillectomy or hernia repair, is found to be hypertensive. Repeated measurements verify the chronic nature of this problem, which then leads to diagnostic evaluation. About half of the asymptomatic patients will be found to have correctable hypertension. In the other half, patients are symptomatic with headaches, vision problems, encephalopathy, congestive heart failure, oliguric renal failure, or occasionally, leg claudication. It is usually not known how long hypertension has been present. Although FMD is a systemic, occlusive arteriopathy potentially involving the entire abdominal aorta and its branches, most commonly the renal arteries are the predominant vessels involved.

In contrast to adults with FMD, in whom women predominate, gender incidence is equal in children. Both renal arteries are simultaneously involved in approximately 70% of instances, but in occasional patients with unilateral lesions, FMD will develop in the opposite renal artery a number of years later. Renovascular causes of hypertension are more common in children younger than 10 years, as evidenced by an average age of 7 years in our series. In infants and toddlers, malignant forms of hypertension with encephalopathy and retinopathy are more likely to develop than in older children.

DIAGNOSIS

Clinical manifestations of headache, irritability, abdominal pain, heart failure, and seizures are best controlled with drugs before undertaking invasive diagnostic studies.

Laboratory Studies

Unfortunately, no specific laboratory studies are reliably diagnostic of renovascular hypertension. Most laboratory studies are performed to document the patient's overall clinical status and particularly the status of renal function. Erythrocyte sedimentation rate is important to assess whether the patient is in the inflammatory or the quiescent phase of the arteriopathy. Urinary catecholamines are studied to exclude the common endocrine causes, particularly in patients with manifestations of neurofibromatosis, such as café-au-lait spots. We have not found plasma renin or captopril-stimulated renin studies to be helpful in children. Technetium-labeled pentetic acid (DTPA) radionuclide fractional-flow studies may indicate unilateral renovascular disease, but they

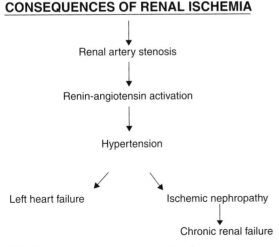

CONSEQUENCES OF RENAL ISCHEMIA

↓

Renal artery stenosis

↓

Renin-angiotensin activation

↓

Hypertension

↙ ↘

Left heart failure   Ischemic nephropathy

↓

Chronic renal failure

FIGURE 63-1. Consequences of renal ischemia.

are not useful when bilateral disease is present. Captopril renography has the same limitation.

Imaging

Although alternative imaging studies exist, currently it is our policy to perform aortography and selective arteriography in all children with significant hypertension. Minimal complications have been encountered with these studies, even in very small subjects. With appropriate hydration, even patients with some degree of oliguric renal failure can undergo aortography and selective arteriography by using low-osmolar or noniodinated contrast agents in limited amounts. For patients with distal or intrarenal vascular stenoses, nitroglycerine-enhanced selective studies promote the identification of segmental areas of ischemia in the involved kidney.

Duplex Doppler ultrasonography (US) is capable of demonstrating the renal arteries, as well as measuring flow velocity, as an index of the degree of stenosis.[8] However, Doppler US studies, whether performed pre- or postoperatively in follow-up, have limitations in terms of demonstrating precise anatomic detail, particularly in small vessels. Magnetic resonance angiography (MRA) and computed tomographic angiography (CTA) are capable of demonstrating the renal arteries and the aorta and its branches better than Doppler US, but still some resolution issues remain in small subjects.[8] MRA is less accurate than CTA, and the volume of contrast material for CTA is often as much as with aortography with selective angiography, so no advantage accrues from the standpoint of nephrotoxicity. Consequently, it remains that aortography with selective arteriography is the most definitive study and the one most capable of demonstrating precise anatomic detail (Fig. 63-3). Doppler US, MRA, and CTA are now best considered to be screening or follow-up studies in children.

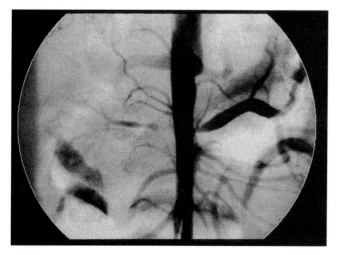

FIGURE 63-3. This 6-year-old boy was found to have severe hypertension when screened for an elective hernia repair. Aortography revealed marked narrowing of the left renal artery, some narrowing of the midaorta, and virtually complete occlusion of the right renal artery filling late from collaterals. This is typical of fibromuscular dysplasia or hyperplasia.

It is clear that the diagnostic approach to children, who usually have bilateral renal artery stenosis associated with FMD, is simpler than the approach needed in adults, who have primarily atherosclerotic lesions. Therefore many of the noninvasive tests designed for adults are not useful in children. Recently it was reported that the preoperative calculation of a high renal resistance–index value derived by Doppler US is a predictor of the lack of success of operative correction of renal artery stenosis.[9] However, because successful revascularization routinely results in alleviation of hypertension in the childhood age group, such studies are superfluous in infants and children. The same is true for renal vein renin studies because renal artery stenosis in children with hypertension is always significant. Conversely, renal vein renin studies may be useful in determining the significance of distal stenoses or aneurysms of renal artery branches or of postoperative anastomotic stenosis.

Because FMD is a systemic, occlusive arteriopathy, it is appropriate to survey the entire lower thoracic and abdominal aorta to delineate those patients who have not only renal artery stenosis but also the midaortic syndrome, visceral arterial stenoses, or other forms of renovascular hypertension. Thus full angiography should be performed so that an appropriate single-staged operation can be performed.

TREATMENT

Medical Treatment

Antihypertensive medications are needed to control blood pressure before undertaking any invasive procedure, including arteriography. Drug therapy is not an alternative to surgical care but an integral part of patient management, not only preoperatively but also intra- and postoperatively. Most patients referred for surgical or interventional treatment have severe hypertension with symptoms that are most effectively managed with intravenous drugs, gradually phasing to oral medications. In severe cases, we prefer to use nitroprusside initially. Either concurrently or sequentially, intravenous labetalol or nifedipine or both are useful drugs. The same three medications are extremely useful in the immediate postoperative phase of management, because hypertension is usually exacerbated after the temporary ischemia associated with revascularization procedures. For long-term and outpatient treatment, propranolol, atenolol, minoxidil, and oral diuretics in various combinations are useful. We prefer to use long-acting drugs whenever possible, because patient and parent compliance are better when once-a-day medications can be given. Angiotensin-converting enzyme (ACE) inhibitors such as captopril are very effective antihypertensive drugs, but they must be used with great caution in patients with renovascular hypertension because of the potential for drug-induced renal ischemia and possible oliguric renal failure.[10] Thus if a decision is made to use ACE inhibitor medication, then renal function must be monitored closely.

Another consideration related to the use of medical therapy is in the management of infants with severe hypertension related to renal artery stenosis. In these instances, because of the greater risk for thrombosis with the repair of infantile vessels, it may be best to administer antihypertensives until renal arteries are close to adult size, if possible (age 5 to 8 years). After revascularization, it may take up to 6 to 12 months for the hypertension to resolve or improve, so antihypertensive drugs must be weaned gradually.

Interventional Procedures

Balloon angioplasty with and without stenting has been the subject of many reports in adults with atherosclerotic disease as well as with FMD.[8,11,12] The results in patients with FMD have been more favorable in instances in which the orifice of the renal artery is not involved by the process. Balloon dilatation for orificial lesions has generally been unsuccessful, except for short periods. Experience reported in children with balloon angioplasty, which parallels our experience, indicates that balloon dilatation of orifice lesions is as ineffective as it is in adults, but it often provides long-term relief from stenoses of the main renal artery or its branches.[3,6] Because of the relatively greater degree of fibroplasia seen in children with FMD, it is not surprising that a much greater incidence of intimal dissection and thrombosis occurs in children, who often have lesions in the ostial location. Because the children are growing, and because so many of these children are young, averaging age 6 years, a reluctance has been noted to insert stents into these lesions after balloon dilatation, for fear of creating obstruction as the child grows. However, in the future, dissolvable stents may possibly prove useful in some pediatric patients.

Neurofibromatosis produces a rigid, cuff-like lesion in the aortic wall and the orifice of the renal artery. Experience indicates that balloon dilatation is contraindicated because the rigidity related to the intravascular proliferation of neurofibrotic tissue renders dilation ineffective or produces an intimal tear, resulting in thrombotic occlusion. Therefore with neurofibromatosis, operative repair is preferred.

Surgical Techniques for Repair

Effective surgical treatment of renovascular hypertension in children must be selected based on the etiology and the distribution of lesions causing stenosis.[8,12]

Nephrectomy and partial nephrectomy should be avoided unless no other choice is available. For example, it may be necessary to perform nephrectomy in infants with uncontrollable hypertension who have unilateral renal involvement, particularly when severe hypoplasia is found. Partial nephrectomy has been used primarily in those occasional instances of renal atrophy, diffuse vascular involvement, or when vessels are too small for successful reconstruction. It is always our preference to attempt revascularization, because partial or total nephrectomy is available as a last resort if vascular repair fails. Additionally, because FMD may involve the opposite kidney even many years later, nephrectomy is undesirable.

Even though children with FMD have a predominance of ostial lesions, sufficient involvement of the renal artery and the wall of the aorta exist that the extent of the lesion is greater than what might be apparent on the arteriogram. Thus patch angioplasty is only rarely effective. Reimplantation of the renal artery into another site on the aorta is the most desirable approach, but its success depends on the aortic wall being normal where the new orifice is to be created and on sufficient length of renal artery existing to reach without tension. Reimplantation is contraindicated in patients with midaortic syndrome, in which the aortic wall is often involved with FMD. Direct anastomosis to the aorta is obviously not an option for patients with branch vessel lesions, which must be treated with balloon dilatation, bypass, or partial nephrectomy for distally placed lesions. It is unfortunate that reimplantation is so rarely possible in this group of patients because it provides the best and the most durable results.[3]

Because of the complicating factors mentioned earlier, aortorenal bypass is usually the best option for revascularization. Bypass end-to-side from the aorta to the side of the renal artery distal to the stenosis was used more in the past. For several years, it has been our preference to divide the diseased renal artery and to perform an end-to-end anastomosis between the bypass and the distal renal artery, spatulating the end of the distal renal artery and fashioning the distal end of the bypass graft obliquely, so that a so-called "cobra hood" anastomosis can be performed. Depending on the size of the anastomosis, either a continuous suture technique, interrupted several times, or an interrupted suture technique for the anastomosis is in order. The anastomosis of the bypass graft to the aorta can usually be performed with continuous suture, interrupted at least 3 times. The opening in the aortic wall is made with an appropriate-sized punch instrument rather than a simple incision. We prefer 6-0 polypropylene suture for the aorta-to-graft anastomosis, whereas 7-0 polypropylene is used for the distal graft–to–renal artery anastomosis. In instances of midaortic syndrome in which such severe coarctation exists that an aorto-aortic bypass is needed, renal bypass grafts may be taken off the aortic bypass graft as indicated. Depending on the size of the patient, it is our preference to use 10- to 14-mm woven Dacron grafts with enough length to permit growth and yet not so much length as to result in kinking of the graft. A full intravenous heparinizing dose is administered before aortic clamping, and a one-half dose is given each hour during the procedure. The heparin effect is allowed to dissipate once all the anastomoses are completed. It has rarely been necessary to reverse the heparinization.

Some debate exists regarding what is the best choice for aortorenal bypass grafts. In adults, Gore-Tex grafts are frequently used. Thrombosis occurs more commonly in prosthetic grafts than with autogenous material. Gore-Tex grafts have rarely been used in children, and they are rarely needed. Little debate is found that the *best* choice for bypass is autogenous hypogastric artery, provided that it is not involved with FMD and that a sufficient length of artery can be harvested for the bypass.[13] These two factors limit the use of the hypogastric artery, even though it clearly holds up best through the years. Additionally, because 70% of patients have simultaneous bilateral renal artery stenosis, this would require both hypogastric arteries to be harvested, and certainly some concern exists about taking both hypogastric arteries in children, although the exact risk of impotence and incontinence is not known. Because of these potential complications, the hypogastric artery is often not an option for many patients. Therefore the next best option, and the one most frequently used today for aortorenal bypass in small patients, is the saphenous vein. Because of the risk of aneurysmal dilatation in as many as 40% of patients who have such grafts placed in the visceral location, we developed a procedure to cover saphenous vein bypass grafts with a loose mandrill of Dacron mesh, which has been effective over the long term.[14,15] These techniques have been in use for 20 years, and they have stood the test of time to this point.

Another debated issue relates to a subset of patients with midaortic syndrome who have varying degrees of narrowing of the superior mesenteric and celiac arteries. A few scattered reports are found of patients with visceral artery stenoses who were initially seen with severe intermittent abdominal pain or even intestinal infarction. In contrast to adults with lesions of this nature, children are rarely symptomatic. In those rare instances in which we have encountered children with signs or symptoms related to superior mesenteric or celiac narrowing, we have performed revascularization by either direct reimplantation or bypass graft. Currently no consensus is found about whether asymptomatic children with marked visceral artery stenosis should have pre-emptive repair. Certainly concomitant visceral arterial bypass carries a higher risk in a patient who is already having bilateral renal artery bypass procedures and frequently also an aorto-aortic bypass. Because the overwhelming majority of patients with lesions of this nature are completely asymptomatic, and because almost all of them have a remarkable amount of collateral circulation demonstrable on aortography, we have not undertaken visceral artery revascularization in asymptomatic patients (Fig. 64-4). Observation for as long as 25 years has indicated that these patients remain well, supporting a conservative approach.

COMPLICATIONS AND OUTCOMES

No mortality was found in our series of more than 50 renal revascularization procedures. No patients have had renal failure, and those who had preoperative oliguric renal failure invariably returned to normal afterward. Intraoperative renal thrombosis, embolization during the procedure, and intraoperative and postoperative hemorrhage, although risks, have not occurred. Postoperative graft thrombosis, because of kinking or flaws in technique, occur in fewer than 5% of renal repairs, even in small patients. However, it has always been our approach to manage patients medically, if possible, until their renal arteries are close to adult size. In those few instances in which graft thrombosis was encountered, because of the

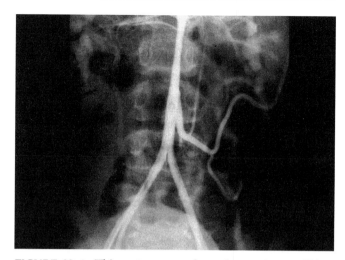

FIGURE 63-4. This aortogram performed on an 8-year-old boy with malignant hypertension shows typical findings of midaortic syndrome or subisthmic coarctation associated with bilateral renal artery and visceral artery narrowing with collateral circulation from the inferior mesenteric artery. Aorto-aortic bypass and bilateral renal artery bypass from the aortic bypass were performed.

likelihood of an anastomotic problem, we have preferred immediate reoperation to use of thrombolytic agents, so that the anastomosis could be revised. Late thrombosis can occur, but the incidence is less in children than in adults because of the absence of atherosclerosis. In patients who have late thrombosis, repeated bypass graft is preferable, but often partial or total nephrectomy is needed. It is important to monitor the patient's blood pressure indefinitely in follow-up because recurrence of hypertension usually indicates a problem with the vascular reconstruction.

Postoperative Imaging

Recurrent hypertension after revascularization procedures is either due to recurrent FMD or anastomotic stenosis. We have encountered two instances of late narrowing of a distal renal graft anastomosis. As with renal transplant arterial stenosis, balloon dilatation has been curative. For follow-up of patients, it is best to have the family monitor the child's blood pressure frequently at home, with at least 6-month follow-up visits initially. The patient's blood pressure should remain normal, even with exercise, although some patients may require medication to keep the blood pressure within the normal range. In the asymptomatic patient, noninvasive imaging is in order every 5 years, with definitive selective angiography performed if any question exists.

Although complete revascularization has been performed at a single operation, results are excellent. Whether patients have aortorenal bypass to either one or both kidneys, or whether they also have aorto-aortic bypass procedures, 80% of children are cured of their hypertension without the need for medications, and 18% are markedly improved, needing minimal antihypertensive medication. About 2% of patients are unchanged after operation, and in the absence of a demonstrated vascular lesion, these patients probably have sustained hypertension because of ischemic nephrosclerosis.

REFERENCES

1. Safian RD, Textor SC: Renal-artery stenosis. N Engl J Med 344:431–442, 2001.
2. Foster JH, Pettinger WA, Oates JA, et al: Malignant hypertension secondary to renal artery stenosis in children. Ann Surg 164:700–713, 1966.
3. O'Neill JA: Long-term outcome with surgical treatment of renovascular hypertension. J Pediatr Surg 33:106–111, 1998.
4. Daniels SR, Loggie JMH, Schwartz DC, et al: Systemic hypertension secondary to peripheral vascular anomalies in patients with Williams' syndrome. J Pediatr Surg 106:249–251, 1985.
5. Danaraj TJ, Ong HO: Primary arteritis of abdominal aorta in children causing bilateral stenosis of renal arteries and hypertension. Circulation 20-24:856, 1959.
6. O'Neill JA, Berkowitz H, Fellows KJ, et al: Mid-aortic syndrome and hypertension in childhood. J Pediatr Surg 30:164–172, 1995.
7. Pickard JL, Ross G, Silver D: Coexisting extraadrenal pheochromocytoma and renal artery stenosis: A case report and review of the pathophysiology. J Pediatr Surg 30:1613–1615, 1995.
8. Clagett GP: What's new in vascular surgery. J Am Coll Surg 194:165–201, 2002.
9. Radermacher J, Chavan A, Bleck J, et al: Use of Doppler ultrasonography to predict the outcome of therapy for renal artery stenosis. N Engl J Med 344:410–417, 2001.
10. Hricick DE, Bronning PJ, Kopelman R, et al: Captopril-induced functional renal insufficiency in patients with bilateral renal artery stenosis or renal artery stenosis in a solitary kidney. N Engl J Med 308:373–376, 1983.
11. Mathias K, Struck E, Schindera F, et al: Percutaneous treatment of renovascular hypertension. Pediatr Radiol 11:154–156, 1981.
12. Kent KC, Salvatierra O, Reilly LM, et al. Evolving strategies for the repair of complex renovascular lesions. Ann Surg 206:272–278, 1987.
13. Wylie EJ, Perloff DL, Stoney RJ: Autogenous tissue revascularization techniques in surgery for renovascular hypertension. Ann Surg 170:416–428, 1969.
14. Stanley JC, Ernst CB, Fry WJ: Fate of 100 aortorenal vein grafts: Characteristics of late graft expansion, aneurysmal dilatation and stenosis. Surgery 74:931–944, 1973.
15. Berkowitz HD, O'Neill JA: Renovascular hypertension in children. J Vasc Surg 9:46–55, 1989.

CHAPTER 64

Adjuvant Therapy in Childhood Cancer

Daniel von Allmen, MD, Susan G. Kreissman, MD, and Gerald M. Haase, MD

OVERVIEW OF CHEMOTHERAPY TREATMENT FOR CHILDHOOD CANCER

The impressive improvement in cure rates for pediatric malignancies over the past 30 years could not have occurred without the development of multimodality therapy and the cooperative efforts of surgeons, pediatric oncologists, and radiation therapists from across the country. In the 1940s, with the use of wide surgical excision, about 20% of children with localized solid tumors could be cured of their malignancies. However, with the discovery of effective chemotherapeutic agents, pediatric oncologists joined with surgeons and radiation therapists in cooperative groups and developed a scientific approach to the study of these agents, rapidly improving on these statistics. Even in the earliest days of cancer therapy, it was the rare child who was not treated with the optimal standardized therapy, from which information was obtained and applied to the next generation of protocols. This carefully developed multimodality approach to the total care of the child with cancer led to the implementation of similar systems in the treatment of adult malignancies and has led to the fact that almost 85% of children with cancer will outlive their malignancy.[1]

HISTORY OF PEDIATRIC ONCOLOGY

The first demonstration that chemotherapy could be effective therapy for childhood malignancies occurred in 1948, when Sidney Farber[2] reported temporary remissions in children with acute lymphoblastic leukemia (ALL) when the folic acid antagonist aminopterin was given. Several years later, another folic acid antagonist, methotrexate, produced cures in choriocarcinoma.[3] As additional chemotherapeutic agents were developed, these were combined in multidrug regimens that demonstrated significantly improved response rates and response duration compared with single agents. This was first demonstrated in children with ALL and soon confirmed in Wilms' tumor.[4,5]

The treatment of Wilms' tumor also served as a model for the successful use of multimodality therapy.[6] The adjuvant use of vincristine, actinomycin, and regional radiation therapy after surgical resection produced substantial improvements in cure rates. Similar approaches were adopted for the treatment of rhabdomyosarcoma, Ewing's sarcoma, lymphoma, and other solid tumors. The efficacy of chemotherapy in improving survival in nonmetastatic osteosarcoma patients after surgical therapy was demonstrated in a randomized cooperative group trial. Patients who received adjuvant chemotherapy had a 66% disease-free survival, as compared with a 17% disease-free survival in the patients who received surgical intervention alone.[7] This use of "adjuvant" chemotherapy to control micrometastases has now become standard practice for most solid tumors in children.

Many advances in pediatric oncology have occurred since these early discoveries, most of them attributable to continued collaboration of pediatric oncologists, surgeons, and radiation therapists within cooperative groups. With the development of improved supportive-care measures, dose-intensive chemotherapy programs have been successful in improving outcome for patients with Burkitt's lymphoma, neuroblastoma, and other advanced-stage solid tumors.[8-10] Further improvements in outcome have been made by altering the schedule of chemotherapy administration, either by alternating effective groups of chemotherapeutic agents to overcome or prevent resistance[11] or by administering agents by continuous infusion rather than bolus.[12] Most recently, noncytotoxic biologic therapies have been developed specifically to target biologic pathways. These agents include signal-transduction inhibitors, various tissue growth factor–receptor inhibitors, antiangiogenesis agents, tumor-targeted antibody therapies, and adoptive immunotherapy techniques.[13] Improvements in radiation therapy have led to the development of intraoperative radiation therapy and radiosurgery techniques. Sharing of scientific knowledge and tumor samples within the cooperative groups has led to tremendous advances in the understanding of cell growth and regulation, the identification of cytogenetic abnormalities characteristic of specific malignancies, and the identification of oncogenes and tumor-suppressor genes. All these taken together have led to profound improvements in the quality of life and survival of children with solid tumors.

EPIDEMIOLOGY AND SURVIVAL STATISTICS FOR CHILDHOOD CANCER

When compared with the adult incidence rates of cancer, the incidence of cancer in children is very small. However, whereas childhood cancer accounts for only 2% of all reported cancer cases, it accounts for 10% of all deaths among children and is the leading cause of death from disease among children.[14]

The distribution of types of cancer in childhood is very different from that in adults. Whereas the majority of all cancers in adults are of epithelial cell origin, fewer than 10% of childhood cancers fall into this category. Table 64-1 displays the distribution of cancer in children younger than 15 years.[15]

The incidence rates for specific cancers vary by age, sex, and race. Overall, the annual incidence rate for all types of childhood cancer is 133.3 per million children younger than 15 years. The peak incidence for childhood cancer is before the age of 2 years, with an incidence rate of more than 200 cases per million. The incidence then decreases to a low of 82.5 cases per million at age 9 years, at which point it begins to climb again through the adolescent years. Before age 2 years, central nervous system (CNS) malignancies, neuroblastoma, acute myeloid leukemia (AML), Wilms' tumor, and retinoblastoma account for the majority of diagnoses. Between ages 2 and 4 years, ALL is the most common childhood cancer. After age 9 years, the incidence of Hodgkin's disease, osteosarcoma, and Ewing's sarcoma begins to increase sharply.[14]

TABLE 64-1	
DISTRIBUTION OF CANCER IN CHILDREN YOUNGER THAN 15 YEARS	
Type of Cancer	Distribution (%)
Acute lymphoblastic leukemia	23.2
Central nervous system tumors	20.7
Neuroblastoma	7.3
Non-Hodgkin's lymphoma	6.3
Wilms' tumor	6.1
Hodgkin's disease	5.0
Acute myeloid leukemia	4.2
Rhabdomyosarcoma	3.4
Retinoblastoma	2.9
Osteosarcoma	2.6
Ewing's sarcoma	2.1
All other cancers	16.4

According to the Surveillance, Epidemiology, and End Results program, the average annual incidence of childhood cancer has increased 10.8% between reporting year 1973 through 1974 and 1989 through 1990.[16] The percentage change has been the greatest in ALL, non-Hodgkin's lymphoma, and CNS tumors. The change in reported incidence may be accounted for by improved reporting of cancer cases, improved identification and diagnosis of cancer, or a random fluctuation in the number of cases for the years studied.[17] Concern has been raised as to the impact of environmental exposures resulting in increased cancer cases, but studies to date have not provided conclusive evidence for this assumption.

Survival from childhood cancer has improved dramatically over the past 30 years, so much so that the overall cure rate for childhood cancer is approaching 85%,[18] and one of every 900 people between the ages of 16 and 44 years is a survivor of childhood cancer.[1] Figure 64-1 compares the survival statistics for specific cancers from 1974 through 1999.[19]

IMPORTANCE OF PATHOLOGY OF CHILDHOOD TUMORS IN SELECTING CHEMOTHERAPY

Unlike adult malignancies, which are primarily carcinomas, fewer than 10% of solid tumors of childhood are epithelial malignancies.[16] Although the spectrum of malignancies in childhood is more limited than that in adults, exact diagnosis is often more difficult because of

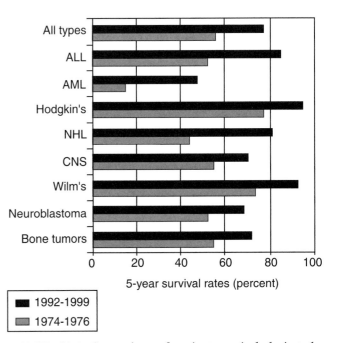

FIGURE 64-1. Comparison of patient survival during the period 1974 to 1976 versus 1992 to 1999 for the common childhood malignancies. Data from SEER Cancer Statistics Review 1975–2000. Bethesda, Md, NCI, http://seer.cancer.gov/csr/1975_2000, 2003.

the prevalence of "small round blue-cell" tumors in childhood. These very primitive or embryonal malignancies often lack morphologically distinguishing characteristics. As a result, Ewing's sarcoma, neuroblastoma, lymphoma, small cell osteosarcoma, and primitive neuroectodermal tumors, to name a few, may appear quite similar by simple light microscopy. An error in diagnosis of Ewing's sarcoma in a patient who actually has a lymphoma of bone would lead to vastly different therapy and poor outcome.

Exact diagnosis in pediatric oncology is crucial, as chemotherapy for childhood malignancies is carefully tailored to each specific tumor type. This has become even more important over the past two decades, as pediatric oncologists have continued to define better the prognostic subgroups for many tumors that help dictate the best therapy and the dose intensity of the therapy required for cure. Whereas the survival rate for patients with stages 1 to 3 Wilms' tumor with favorable histology is more than 90%[20] with standard therapy consisting of vincristine and actinomycin, with or without doxorubicin, a diagnosis of a Wilms' tumor with diffuse anaplasia carries a far worse prognosis and requires more intensive therapy for cure.

The initial step in the accurate diagnosis of a tumor is availability of adequate material with which to make the diagnosis. Therefore it is crucial that during the initial surgical procedure, whether it be a biopsy or a resection, tissue of adequate quantity and quality be obtained. The amount of tissue required for diagnostic purposes can be discussed with the pathologist and pediatric oncologist before the procedure to ensure the proper handling of the specimen (e.g., the need for fresh tissue, frozen samples, and fixed specimens for histologic and biologic diagnostic use).

Whereas light microscopy remains the primary tool of pathologists, they can now rely also on immunohistology, electron microscopy, DNA content of tumor, cytogenetic abnormalities, and specific tumor gene expression to establish a diagnosis. Consent is frequently obtained from families to allow any additional tumor tissue available after a diagnosis is established to be used for research to continue to advance understanding of tumor biology.

TUMOR BIOLOGY: UNDERSTANDING CHILDHOOD CANCER AND TREATMENT PRINCIPLES

Cancer is a genetic event. Genetic alterations within a single cell, those that can be identified as a cytogenetic abnormality, the activation of an oncogene, or the loss of a tumor-suppressor gene can all lead to the accumulation of cells lacking the ability to respond to growth-regulating signals and the subsequent development of a cancer. The study of malignant cell transformation has significantly contributed to the understanding of normal cell growth as well as the molecular origins of cancer, the ability to define tumors by their cytogenetic and molecular characteristics, and the future use of this information to fashion improved therapies for cancer.

CELL GROWTH AND REGULATION

Understanding normal cell growth and regulation is a prerequisite to understanding both the genetic basis for the development of childhood cancer and the mechanisms of action of chemotherapeutic agents designed to kill rapidly proliferating cancer cells. Normal cell growth occurs by the regulated progression of the cell through the cell cycle of DNA replication and mitosis, separated by two intervening growth phases called G_1 and G_2. Cells can temporarily leave the cell cycle and enter a resting state called G_0 (Fig. 64-2). Cells are instructed to proceed through the cell cycle by a series of external and internal stimuli. Binding of proteins (growth factors) to cell-surface receptors stimulates a cascade of cytoplasmic signaling proteins (membrane kinases and signal transducers) that carries the stimuli to the nucleus, where other proteins (transcription factors) bind to the DNA, resulting in the expression of growth-regulating genes. When functioning normally, these genes promote or prevent cell division, direct the cell to differentiate, or initiate apoptosis, the process of programmed cell death.

Alterations in one or several of these signaling proteins can lead to the unregulated cell growth characteristics of cancer cells. Oncogenes result from mutation or overexpression of the normal growth-promoting proto-oncogenes. Tumor-suppressor genes are normally present in cells and function as negative regulators to slow the process of proliferation and allow time for cellular repair. When oncogenes become activated or tumor-suppressor gene function is lost, cells lose their ability to respond to the usual regulatory protein stimuli and proliferate rapidly. Rapid cell proliferation leads to accumulation of more genetic defects, activation of additional oncogenes, and loss of more negative regulators as the cells become increasingly more malignant. Through the study of chromosomal aberrations, more than 100 oncogenes and 25 tumor-suppressor genes have now been identified.

CANCER CYTOGENETICS: A DIAGNOSTIC TOOL

The association of a consistent chromosomal aberration with a specific cancer was first made in 1960 with the discovery of the minute "Philadelphia chromosome" (9;22)(q34;q11) in chronic myeloid leukemia (CML).[21] With the discovery of chromosomal banding techniques in the 1970s, cancer cytogenetists were first able to identify subchromosomal deletions, inversions, and translocations occurring in cancer cells. Study of these aberrant regions led to the identification of oncogenes and tumor-suppressor genes, a process that is continuing today.

The presence of consistent cytogenetic abnormalities associated with a specific childhood leukemia or solid tumor helps in both cancer diagnosis and assignment of prognosis. Specific cytogenetic aberrations have been identified in rhabdomyosarcoma, Ewing's sarcoma, synovial sarcoma, germ cell tumors, medulloblastomas, neuroblastomas, retinoblastomas, and Wilms' tumors.[22]

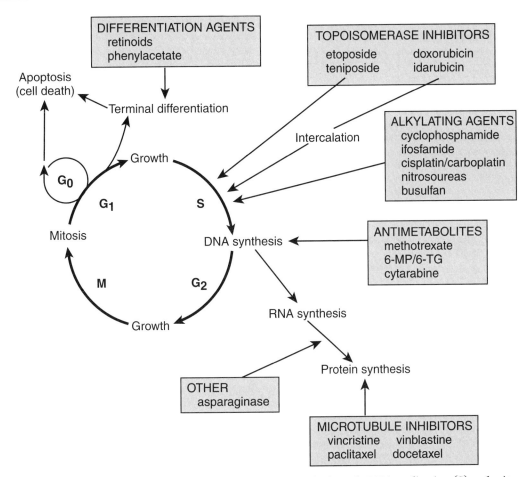

FIGURE 64-2. The cell cycle. Normal cell growth proceeds through DNA replication (S) and mitosis (M), separated by two growth phases (G_1 and G_2). Cells leave the cell cycle to enter a resting phase (G_0) to differentiate or to die. Chemotherapy agents act at specific sites along the cell cycle, as indicated. (Adapted from Balis FRM, Holcenberg JS, Poplack DG: General principles of chemotherapy. In Pizzo P, Poplack D [eds]: Principles and Practice of Pediatric Oncology, 3rd ed. Philadelphia, Lippincott-Raven, 1997, p 219.)

Finding one of these distinct translocations, deletions, or inversions can often aid the pathologist in making the correct diagnosis when faced with a histologically indistinct small round blue-cell tumor. Chromosomal aberrations also can help assign prognosis. The finding of a chromosome 1q deletion, the presence of double minute chromatin bodies, or the presence of homogeneous staining regions in neuroblastoma confers a poor prognosis.[23]

The process of using specific translocations for diagnostic purposes is now enhanced by the use of the techniques of fluorescent in situ hybridization, which allows the localization and visualization of a single gene on a chromosome by using fluorescent DNA probes. Unlike standard cytogenetic analysis, which requires 5 to 14 days for the cancer cells to proliferate in culture before a karyotype can be obtained, this technique can be performed directly on tumor cells.[24] In the future, specific tumors may be identified by a specific "fingerprint" determined by microarray analysis that can simultaneously analyze expression of thousands of genes on a single "chip."[25]

CHEMOTHERAPY PRINCIPLES IN PEDIATRIC ONCOLOGY

The goal of cytotoxic chemotherapy treatment for childhood malignancy is to maximize tumor kill while maintaining acceptable side effects. Clinical trials have led to the development of standard combination chemotherapy regimens for most childhood cancers. Increased understanding of tumor biology and improved supportive care have allowed the administration of increased doses of chemotherapy (increased dose intensity) and changes in chemotherapy administration schedules to maximize tumoricidal effects. Adjuvant therapy (after local control measures) has remained the mainstay of cancer therapy, but neoadjuvant chemotherapy (before definitive local control measures) has proved to be effective in patients with metastatic disease and, in localized tumors, to begin to control microscopic metastatic disease immediately.

IDENTIFYING ACTIVE CHEMOTHERAPEUTIC AGENTS: PHASES I THROUGH III CLINICAL TRIALS

Chemotherapy drugs go through a long series of basic laboratory studies before being tested for activity in humans. Drugs are tested in cell culture for ability to inhibit or destroy cancer cells; then promising agents are extensively tested in laboratory animals before the most active enter clinical trials in humans.

In the clinical development of promising anticancer agents, the first step is to define a tolerable dose. Phase I clinical trials are designed as dose-escalation studies to determine the maximally tolerated dose of a new drug given as a single agent. The dose of the agent is slowly increased in successive cohorts of patients until dose-limiting toxicity is consistently observed. The dose level immediately lower than the dose resulting in consistent toxicity is then selected to begin phase II trials. In a phase II trial, a consistent dose of the agent is tested for efficacy in a variety of tumor types to establish the spectrum of activity of the agent. Once an agent has demonstrated activity in a specific cancer, this agent is tested for efficacy when combined with other known active agents in that tumor system.

"Standard" therapy for a specific tumor type is established through phase III clinical trials. Classically, phase III trials use a prospective randomized design to compare two previously established effective chemotherapy combinations. By randomly assigning new patients to treatment on one or the other chemotherapy "arm" of the study, the most effective chemotherapy combination can be established, and the toxicities of the two regimens compared. At the conclusion of the trial, the chemotherapy regimen with the greatest efficacy and the least toxicity is selected as the standard regimen for that tumor system. Subsequent phase III trials then compare new regimens with this established standard therapy. It is through the development of phase I through III clinical trials within national cooperative groups that advances in cancer cures have been made. Individual patients benefit from clinical trials by having the most effective combination chemotherapy programs available to them, and cancer patients in general benefit from the continued advances and new information generated by these trials.

COMBINATION CHEMOTHERAPY

Combination chemotherapy remains the mainstay of treatment of childhood cancer. In the 1960s, the benefits of combining several drugs together was demonstrated first for ALL. Complete remission by using single agents could be expected in only about half of the patients, whereas the combination of four or five drugs produced remission rates of more than 95%.[26] In the patients achieving remission with a single agent, resistance developed within 6 to 9 months, and relapse occurred. Long-term remission rates were higher with combination chemotherapy, demonstrating the ability to overcome or prevent chemotherapy resistance.

Several biologic models have been devised to attempt to explain this observation. The most well known is the Goldie-Coldman hypothesis, which proposes that the response of any individual tumor to a chemotherapeutic agent is dependent on both the sensitivity of that tumor to the agent and the inherent tendency of that tumor to accumulate mutations that will make it chemotherapy resistant. The chance of developing resistance is related to the mutation rate and the size of the tumor. This hypothesis predicts that once a single tumor cell develops resistance to a chemotherapeutic agent, the tumor cannot be cured using that agent alone. Therefore the best chance to cure a tumor is to give all available active agents simultaneously, after local control measures, when the tumor burden is as low as possible and the chance of any tumor cells having acquired resistance is minimal.[27]

The agents used for combination chemotherapy must be carefully selected. Agents are selected for use in a combination chemotherapy regimen based on (1) demonstrated activity as a single agent in relapsed or refractory solid tumors, (2) differing mechanisms of action for cell killing, (3) non–cross resistance to prevent selection of a resistant clone, and (4) nonoverlapping toxicities to allow the drug to be given at the maximally effective dose and schedule.

This principle of designing combination chemotherapy regimens by using non–cross-resistant agents with nonoverlapping toxicities has been successfully used for childhood solid tumor treatment for the past 25 years. The improvement in survival rates over this period for neuroblastoma, Ewing's sarcoma, anaplastic Wilms' tumor, and osteosarcoma can be directly linked to effective combination chemotherapy treatment. For example, in Ewing's sarcoma, it was demonstrated that ifosfamide could induce responses in patients with recurrent disease who were previously treated with cyclophosphamide.[28] Shortly thereafter, it was discovered that response rates in recurrent Ewing's sarcoma could be significantly improved by the addition of etoposide to ifosfamide therapy.[29] The addition of ifosfamide and etoposide courses alternating with the previously standard Ewing's therapy of cyclophosphamide, doxorubicin, and vincristine produced a significant improvement in disease-free survival in patients with newly diagnosed Ewing's sarcoma.[11]

ADJUVANT AND NEOADJUVANT CHEMOTHERAPY

Adjuvant chemotherapy refers to the administration of chemotherapy to a patient with nonmetastatic disease after local therapy with surgery or radiation to eliminate micrometastases that may have already occurred before the appearance of clinically detectable disease. The use of adjuvant chemotherapy is supported by the finding that fewer than 20% of sarcoma and lymphoma patients with initially nonmetastatic solid tumors can be cured by surgical therapy or radiation therapy alone or both.[30]

In the majority of these patients, recurrence is at a distant site, lending strong support to the hypothesis that micrometastatic disease exists at the time of presentation for the majority of patients with clinical nonmetastatic disease. In Wilms' tumor, as many as 40% of patients can be cured with surgical therapy or radiation therapy alone; however, survival can be increased to 90% with the addition of adjuvant combination chemotherapy.[31]

Because the goal of adjuvant chemotherapy is to prevent the appearance of metastatic disease, it is vital that chemotherapy begin as soon as possible after· local control measures are completed. Major delays to allow recovery from operation or radiation allow growth of microscopic metastatic disease, increasing the chance for resistance to develop and decreasing overall response rates and survival. It is for this reason that most current chemotherapy regimens for childhood solid tumors recommend chemotherapy be given within 2 weeks of initial surgical treatment. In Wilms' tumor, the National Wilms' Tumor Study Group recommends that the initial dose of actinomycin D begin within 5 days of nephrectomy.[32]

One approach to prevent delays in instituting chemotherapy in patients with nonmetastatic disease is to delay surgical resection until after several courses of chemotherapy can be administered. This is referred to as neoadjuvant chemotherapy, in which only a biopsy of the tumor is performed at diagnosis, and therefore chemotherapy can begin as soon as the diagnosis is established at a time when the distant tumor burden is at its lowest. This approach has become standard in the treatment of Ewing's sarcoma and osteosarcoma.[11,33,34] In these tumors, surgical excision and radiation are delayed for up to 3 to 4 months while alternating combinations of effective chemotherapy agents are administered. This approach has the theoretical advantage of minimizing the appearance of chemotherapy resistance; furthermore, delayed surgical intervention may allow a more complete or less morbid resection and pathologic assessment of tumor responsiveness to the chemotherapy agents on an individual patient basis. It should be kept in mind, however, that neoadjuvant chemotherapy is of benefit only for tumors for which a known highly effective combination chemotherapy program limits the risk of tumor progression at the primary site.

SCHEDULE OF ADMINISTRATION

Children often tolerate chemotherapy better than adults because they have a superior and more rapid recovery from the toxic effects of treatment. Standard pediatric solid tumor chemotherapy protocols call for the administration of chemotherapy courses every 21 days to allow time for hematologic and organ recovery. Most combination chemotherapy programs are given over the first 1 to 5 days of the 21-day cycle. Historically, the next course of chemotherapy was withheld until the absolute neutrophil count was greater than $1000/mm^3$ and the platelet count was greater than $100,000/mm.^3$ Over the past 5-year period, the trend has been to maximize dose intensity

and begin the next course when the absolute neutrophil count is greater than $750/mm^3$ and the platelet count greater than $75,000/mm^3$, as long as mucositis or diarrhea or both induced by chemotherapy has resolved. Proceeding with the next course of chemotherapy before organ recovery would result in cumulative tissue damage and increase the chance of death from infection, bleeding, or irreversible organ damage. When these criteria are adhered to, the toxic death rate for standard combination chemotherapy programs is less than 5%.

Recently, changes in schedule of chemotherapy administration have led to improved efficacy of some agents. Etoposide is an epipodophyllotoxin that has been extremely effective in most pediatric solid tumors and in some epithelial cancers in adults. The mechanism of action is inhibition of topoisomerase II. Classically, etoposide has been given with an alkylator and infused over a 1-hour period. It has been demonstrated that continuous intravenous exposure to etoposide for 3 to 21 days is superior to a 1- to 24-hour infusion.[35,36] In pediatric brain tumor patients, daily oral etoposide for 21 days was well tolerated and produced significant responses in patients with recurrent tumors.[37] Continuous exposure to etoposide has the theoretical advantage of maintaining a continuous blockage of topoisomerase II and thus preventing tumor cell repair, ultimately leading to more effective tumor kill.

Prolonged exposure to combination chemotherapy agents in neuroblastoma and AML has led to improved responses.[38,39] In neuroblastoma, patients with advanced-stage disease refractory to standard induction therapy had a 40% response rate when cisplatin, etoposide, and doxorubicin were given as a 96-hour continuous infusion along with daily bolus ifosfamide.[39]

Duration of chemotherapy programs for most pediatric solid tumors has classically been 1 year. As the dose intensity of chemotherapy programs has increased, the duration of therapy has decreased. The recently completed intergroup osteosarcoma protocol consisted of only 30 weeks of treatment. The National Wilms' Tumor Study IV demonstrated that 6 months of therapy was as effective as or could be administered at a lower total treatment cost compared with 15 months for patients with high-stage disease.[20] In neuroblastoma, when intensive induction therapy is followed by consolidation with autologous stem cell transplant, the total duration of treatment is now 6 months.[40] As dose intensity of therapy increases, duration of chemotherapy may continue to decrease. In the future, biologic response modifiers and immunotherapies may be standardly used after completion of chemotherapy to treat minimal residual disease. The timing and duration of therapy with these new biologic agents is currently being investigated.[13]

CHEMOTHERAPY DOSE INTENSITY

To develop an effective combination chemotherapy program, it is important to select not only the correct combination of agents but also the correct dose of each agent. The trend for the past 10 years in pediatric oncology has been to increase chemotherapy dose intensity, with the goal of maximizing efficacy. In designing dose-intensive programs, the individual toxicities of the agents to be intensified must be considered. The best agents to use in high doses are those with limited organ toxicity whose toxicity profile is mainly hematologic.

Most chemotherapeutic agents have a sigmoidal dose/response curve with a steep linear phase, followed by a plateau phase. The principle of chemotherapy dose intensity is to administer the maximal tolerated dose of the agent that falls within the linear phase of the dose/response curve in the shortest possible interval while maintaining tolerable toxicity. Dose intensity is defined as the amount of drug delivered per unit time, expressed as milligrams per square meter per week.[41] Therefore dose intensity can be increased by giving higher doses of a chemotherapeutic agent, giving an agent more frequently, or both.

It has been demonstrated in animal systems that a twofold increase in administered cyclophosphamide dose can lead to a 10-fold increase in tumor cell kill,[42] whereas a decrease in dose intensity of as little as 20% in an osteosarcoma animal model can decrease the cure rate by 50%.[43]

Similar clinical observations have been made in childhood leukemia and osteosarcoma. A prospective clinical trial of high-risk ALL patients revealed that patients receiving less than 94% of the planned dose of chemotherapy during the intensive portion of therapy had a 5.5-fold increased risk of relapse.[44] In osteosarcoma, patients receiving less than 80% of the proposed chemotherapy doses had a threefold increased risk of relapse.[45]

The *positive impact* of increasing the dose intensity of therapy on improving response rate and survival duration has been demonstrated for Burkitt's lymphoma, osteosarcoma, Ewing's sarcoma, testicular cancer, breast cancer, and advanced ovarian cancer.[8–10, 41,46–48] This finding has had a significant impact on the design of clinical trials for childhood solid tumors, with efforts focused on identifying the most effective agents to intensify and then maximizing supportive care to allow dose escalation.

In a retrospective meta-analysis of induction therapy used in 44 clinical trials for patients older than 1 year with disseminated neuroblastoma, the dose intensity of the most active agents had a significant impact on response, median survival, and median progression-free survival.[9] Cisplatin, teniposide, cyclophosphamide, and doxorubicin were identified as the most important agents to intensify to improve response in neuroblastoma. For Ewing's sarcoma and osteosarcoma, the dose intensity of doxorubicin has been identified as having the greatest impact on response and survival.[47] Improved response rates with high-dose cyclophosphamide (>3 g/m^2) have been demonstrated in recurrent or refractory sarcomas.[49] With the concomitant use of hematopoietic growth factors to speed granulocyte recovery, chemotherapy doses of myelosuppressive agents often can be increased. For example, the standard dose of cyclophosphamide was 900 mg/m^2 in the Intergroup Rhabdomyosarcoma

Study–I,[50] whereas the current Intergroup Rhabdomyosarcoma Study–V protocol uses cyclophosphamide at 2.2 g/m^2/dose, with granulocyte colony-stimulating factor (G-CSF) support as standard therapy—a 2.4-fold dose increase.

Increasing the dose intensity of active chemotherapy agents in pediatric clinical trials has been possible because of recent advances in supportive care to decrease or minimize the toxic effects on normal tissues that occur from higher-dose chemotherapy. The use of cytokines to speed recovery of white blood cells and platelets (G-CSF and interleukin-11 [IL-11])[51,52] and the use of cardioprotectant agents to allow a higher cumulative dose of doxorubicin to be used have helped in the development of new dose-intensive therapy for solid tumors.[53]

The most recent advance, the infusion of previously collected peripheral blood progenitor cells (PBPCs) to support repeated courses of dose-intensive submyeloablative chemotherapy, has allowed dose intensity in multiple chemotherapy cycles to be increased further than was previously possible.

Many pediatric studies have demonstrated that collection of PBPCs from children as small as 10 kg is feasible.[54] PBPCs have been effective in engrafting pediatric patients after myeloablative chemoradiotherapy.[55,56] In myeloablative therapy, "supralethal" doses of chemotherapy are given, and hematopoietic recovery will occur only if a stem cell source (either PBPCs or bone marrow) is infused into the patient after completion of the myeloablative regimen. PBPCs also are effective in enhancing recovery after submyeloablative chemotherapy.[57] In submyeloablative regimens, hematopoietic recovery usually occurs in 3 to 4 weeks when combined with growth factor or PBPC support but would ultimately occur without these methods of support in 6 to 10 weeks.

A study performed at James Whitcomb Riley Hospital for Children successfully used repetitive PBPC collections to support newly diagnosed neuroblastoma patients through four courses of submyeloablative dose-intensive chemotherapy before consolidation with a myeloablative PBPC transplant.[57] Another trial in high-risk brain tumor patients also demonstrated the feasibility of sequential high-dose chemotherapy with PBPC support to mitigate hematopoietic toxicity successfully. In this study, as chemotherapy doses were escalated, nonhematologic toxicities became dose limiting.[58]

The Children's Cancer Group (CCG) recently completed a clinical pilot study to investigate further the feasibility of repetitive collection, storage, and infusion of PBPCs for use with multicycle dose-intensive chemotherapy in newly diagnosed neuroblastoma patients. Patients received two induction courses of high-dose cyclophosphamide with continuous-infusion doxorubicin and vincristine. At the time of hematopoietic recovery from the second course, patients had PBPCs collected by using a specialized apheresis machine, and then cells were cryopreserved and stored. These cells are reinfused after the first consolidation chemotherapy course, which consisted of high-dose cyclophosphamide, etoposide, and carboplatin. Collection and infusion of PBPCs was repeated a total of 3 times during the three consolidation chemotherapy courses. G-CSF was given daily after the infusion of PBPCs to speed hematopoietic recovery further.[59] For this pilot study, the toxicity of the chemotherapy agents used was primarily hematopoietic, with minimal organ toxicity. The goal of this protocol was both to time-compress chemotherapy courses and to administer higher doses of chemotherapy, leading to significant increases in dose intensity.

Myeloablative chemotherapy with total body irradiation as preparation for autologous stem cell transplant has been demonstrated to be an effective method of dose-intensive consolidation treatment after induction therapy in high-risk neuroblastoma. In a randomized trial conducted by the Children's Oncology Group (COG), high-risk neuroblastoma patients who received an autologous bone marrow transplant had an improved 3-year event-free survival compared with patients who proceeded to consolidation chemotherapy alone.[60] Given the success of increasing chemotherapy dose intensity by using a single myeloablative transplant in high-risk neuroblastoma, several investigators have performed pilot studies looking at the feasibility of performing two or even three consolidative stem cell transplants.[61,62]

BIOLOGIC RESPONSE MODIFIERS AND MOLECULAR TARGETED THERAPIES IN CHILDHOOD CANCER

The study of biologic response modifiers, targeted antibody therapy, and adoptive immunotherapy is a rapidly growing field in developing new strategies for the treatment of childhood malignancies. The mainstay of cancer chemotherapy had been in the use of replication-directed cytotoxic agents, and maximal tolerated chemotherapy doses were determined based on the toxicity of the drug on rapidly dividing normal cells. The new biologic agents frequently do not have the same toxic effects on normal rapidly developing cells, and the toxicity of these agents on normal cells is hard to measure. One challenge facing oncologists today in the clinical development of these new agents is how best to design clinical trials to determine the maximal biologically active and therapeutically effective dose of these agents.[13,63]

CHEMOTHERAPEUTIC AGENTS

Classes of Agents and Their Mechanisms of Action

The rational design of combination chemotherapy programs requires an understanding of the mechanism of action, the site of metabolism, the rate of drug clearance, and the toxicity profile for each drug. Most chemotherapy agents work by interfering with DNA or RNA synthesis, transcription, or repair. Unfortunately, these agents are not selective for cancer cells, and the same metabolic pathways are disrupted in normal cells,

leading to the toxic effects observed with chemotherapy treatment.

It is important to understand the normal cell cycle to understand how each chemotherapy agent interferes with the normal cell growth and repair processes. A normal cell proceeds through the four phases of the cell cycle in an orderly fashion. Checkpoints are in place to slow growth and allow needed repairs to prevent the accumulation of DNA or RNA errors. Malignant cells are usually lacking in some or most of these checkpoints and, as a result, may be more susceptible to the toxic effects of chemotherapeutic agents. Figure 64-2 illustrates the normal cell cycle and indicates the site of action of the major chemotherapeutic agents.

Chemotherapy agents can be divided into classes by their mechanism of action. The classes of agents include alkylating agents (cisplatin and its analogues) antimetabolites, topoisomerase inhibitors, antimicrotubule agents, differentiation agents, miscellaneous nonclassified agents, and biologic agents. Understanding the individual mechanisms of action helps in the design of drug combinations with additive or synergistic antitumor effects. The most common agents from each class, their mechanism of action, common side effects, and tumors in which they are active are listed in Table 64-2.

Acute Chemotherapy Toxicity and Supportive Care

Most acute toxicities in childhood solid tumor therapy are reversible. Toxicity is greatest in the normal cells with the highest rate of turnover. Therefore normal bone marrow cells, mucosal lining cells, liver cells, and hair cells are frequently affected. The most common side effects from combination chemotherapy include nausea and vomiting, myelosuppression, hair loss, mucositis, diarrhea, liver-function test abnormalities, and allergic reactions.

Myelosuppression is an expected side effect of almost every treatment program for childhood solid tumors. Transfusions of packed cells and platelets are frequent. Of greatest concern is the risk of severe life-threatening bacterial or fungal infections that occur during episodes of neutropenia. In dose-intensive regimens, more than 75% of chemotherapy courses result in hospitalization for fever, with the incidence of bacteremia ranging from 10% to 20% per course.[64]

Several chemotherapeutic agents have very specific toxicities. For example, vincristine and doxorubicin are vesicants and can cause severe skin and tissue necrosis if the drug extravasates into the subcutaneous tissue. Doxorubicin and related anthracyclines have cumulative cardiotoxic effects, and the total lifetime anthracycline dose must be limited for each patient to minimize the risk of developing congestive heart failure. Cisplatin has toxic renal effects and is often combined with another nephrotoxic agent, ifosfamide, in treatment of osteosarcoma and neuroblastoma. Cisplatin also can cause hearing loss, especially in high doses, as administered for high-risk germ cell tumors and high-risk neuroblastoma. Vincristine and vinblastine can cause cumulative peripheral neuropathies, and drug doses frequently must be altered to prevent significant morbidity. These toxicities must be considered when designing therapeutic programs; aggressive supportive care and close patient monitoring are mandatory.

Some of the success in improving outcome for children with cancer is attributable to advances made in supportive care. Routine use of hematopoietic growth factors, specifically G-CSF, results in more rapid granulocyte recovery and shorter hospitalizations for fever and neutropenia.[51] Recently IL-11 (rhIL-11) demonstrated efficacy in enhancing platelet recovery, decreasing the depth of the platelet nadir, and decreasing platelet transfusions requirements.[52,65,66] It has been well tolerated in children and will be extremely beneficial in combination regimens that induce severe thrombocytopenia.[66]

The gastrointestinal tract is injured by certain chemotherapy agents, specifically cytarabine, anthracyclines, and high-dose methotrexate. Leukovorin, a folate derivative, can be given to "rescue" normal mucosal and bone marrow cells from the effects of high-dose methotrexate. No rescue is known for the mucositis and diarrhea that occur from other agents. Use of rhIL-11, in addition to enhancing platelet production, may help speed recovery from gastrointestinal injury after chemotherapy. Early studies demonstrate rapid reversal of gut toxicity with the use of rhIL-11 after radiation.[67]

Renal toxicity can occur from the use of cisplatin, ifosfamide, and high-dose methotrexate. Cisplatin causes renal tubular damage, leading to elevation of blood urea nitrogen and creatinine. Often this is reversible. Both ifosfamide and cisplatin cause renal electrolyte wasting, called Fanconi's syndrome, in which hypokalemia, hypocalcemia, hypophosphatemia, and hypomagnesemia can occur. Renal injury from these agents can be decreased by hyperhydration and forced diuresis. Ongoing studies with the organic thiophosphate compound amifostine show promise in preventing cisplatin-induced renal injury. Amifostine also may have protective effects against neurologic and cumulative bone marrow toxicities.[68] Mesna can prevent hemorrhagic cystitis resulting from cyclophosphamide and ifosfamide by binding to the bladder toxic acrolein metabolites.[69]

It is anticipated that supportive care measures will continue to improve. In the future, some of the toxic effects of chemotherapy on bone marrow may be ameliorated by the use of gene therapy to transfer chemotherapy resistance genes into normal hematopoietic progenitor cells. This would allow higher doses of chemotherapy to be given without myelosuppression. Preliminary in vitro and animal studies have shown that hematopoietic progenitor cells can be made more resistant to nitrosoureas.[70]

LONG-TERM SIDE EFFECTS OF CANCER THERAPY IN CHILDREN

In light of the fact that 1 of every 900 adults will soon be a survivor of childhood cancer,[1] emphasis on diagnosis, treatment, and prevention of late effects of childhood cancer therapy has become essential.

In general, tissues with the highest cell-turnover rate are the most susceptible to acute toxicities of chemotherapy. Usually, acute toxicities are reversible but may be persistent and lead to late effects. Tissues that replicate slowly or that can no longer regenerate may be susceptible to long-term or late effects of therapy. Children are more susceptible to certain late effects of therapy than are adults because their tissues are still growing, and damage to these tissue may affect growth, fertility, and neuropsychologic development.

All aspects of combined-modality treatment can contribute to late effects of childhood cancer therapy. Chemotherapy agents have been associated with specific late toxicities (see Table 64-2). Radiation therapy can significantly inhibit further growth of bone, muscle, heart, and kidney within the radiation field, as well as affecting fertility. Certain surgical procedures can be associated with late sequelae, as with scoliosis after thoracotomy, impotence after retroperitoneal lymph node dissection, and limited mobility after amputation.

Growth retardation is the late effect unique to children. The degree of impairment depends on the dose of chemotherapy or radiation and the age of the child at the time of therapy. The younger the child at the time of the insult, the more severe the sequelae. More than 50% of childhood brain tumor patients treated with 3000 cGy or more to the whole brain will have severe growth retardation, with adult height being less than the fifth percentile.[71] Cranial irradiation can lead to growth hormone deficiency, which will result in poor linear growth unless growth hormone replacement is given. Patients who have received total body radiation or spinal radiation may not be able to achieve their full height potential because the irradiated bones have limited growth potential, even with growth hormone stimulation.[72]

In addition to poor overall growth, therapy can cause other musculoskeletal problems including scoliosis, avascular necrosis, osteoporosis, and atrophy or hypoplasia of tissues. Radiation therapy to the head and neck results in hypoplasia of the jaw, orbit, or neck, with associated atrophy of the soft tissues. Associated endocrine, dental, and psychologic consequences also may occur.[73] Aseptic necrosis of bone may affect as many as 10% of high-risk ALL patients as a result of prolonged steroid use. Osteoporosis occurs as a result of steroid treatment and from high-dose radiation, as used for sarcoma therapy.

Most children who receive chemotherapy for solid tumors do not experience neuropsychologic dysfunction. Patients treated for brain tumors and those receiving cranial radiation for ALL are the exception and can experience severe decline in IQ. Compared with their siblings, patients treated with cranial irradiation for ALL were significantly more likely to enter a special education or learning-disabled program.[74] The recent report from the Childhood Cancer Survivors Study indicates that 23% of childhood cancer survivors, compared with 8% of their siblings, required the use of special education services. The greatest risk was noted in the survivors who were treated before age 6 years, especially those treated for CNS tumors.[75]

TABLE 64-2
CHEMOTHERAPEUTIC AGENTS

Class of Agent	Mechanism of Action	Antitumor Activity	Acute Toxicities
Alkylating Agents			
Mustards			
Nitrogen mustard	Alkylation, DNA crosslinking	Hodgkin's disease	Myelo, N/V, A, mucositis, phlebitis, vesicant
Mephalan	Alkylation, DNA crosslinking	Rhabdo; for BMT: Ewing's, NB	Myelo, mucositis, N/V, A, VOD (HD)
Cyclophosphamide	(Prodrug) alkylation, DNA crosslinking	Rhabdo; Wilms'; NB; Ewing's	Myelo, immuno, N/V, A, cystitis, SIADH, cardiac (HD) lung (HD), VOD (HD)
Ifosfamide	Alkylation, DNA crosslinking	Ewing's; rhabdo; osteosarcoma; NB	Myelo, N/V, A, hepatic, renal, cystitis, neuro
Busulfan	Alkylation, DNA crosslinking	Leukemia	Myelo, skin, lung, A
Nitrosoureas			
BCNU	DNA crosslinking	CNS tumors; lymphoma	Myelo, N/V, A, lung, renal
CCNU	DNA crosslinking	CNS tumors; lymphoma	Myelo, N/V, A, lung, renal
Tetrazines			
Dacarbazine (DTIC)	DNA methylation	Hodgkin's; sarcomas; NB	Myelo, hepatic, flulike illness, N/V, A
Temozolomide	DNA crosslinking	Brain tumors	Myelo, N/V, diarrhea, constipation, rash, lethargy, hepatic
Other alkylators			
Thiotepa	Alkylation, DNA crosslinking	CNS tumors; for BMT: sarcomas, NB	Myelo, N/V, A, diarrhea, mucositis, skin, VOD (HD)
Procarbazine	(Prodrug) methylation; free radical formation	Hodgkin's; CNS tumors	Myelo, N/V, rash, allergy, mucositis
Platinum agents			
Cisplatin	DNA/platinum adduct formation; DNA crosslinking	Osteosarcoma; NB; hepatoblastoma; germ cell tumors; CNS tumors	N/V (severe), A, myelo, renal, neuro, mucositis, ototoxicity
Carboplatin	DNA/platinum adduct formation; DNA crosslinking	NB; CNS tumors; retinoblastoma; sarcomas in HD	Myelo (severe plts), N/V (mild), renal and ototoxicity rare
Antimetabolites			
Methotrexate	Inhibitor dihydrofolate reductase; interferes with folate metabolism	Leukemia; lymphoma; osteosarcoma in HD	Myelo, rash, mucositis, hepatic, renal (HD)
5-Fluorouracil	(Prodrug) inhibits thymidine synthesis	Hepatoblastoma; carcinomas	Myelo, N/V, mucositis, diarrhea, hyperpigmentation, neuro
Cytarabine	(Prodrug) incorporated into DNA; inhibits DNA replication	Leukemia; lymphoma	Myelo, malaise, N/V, mucositis, diarrhea, neuro (HD), eye (HD), skin (HD)
6-Mercaptopurine, 6-Thioguanine	(Prodrugs) inhibit purine synthesis	Leukemia	Myelo, N/V, hepatic, mucositis
Gemcitabine	Inhibitor of DNA synthesis	Hodgkins disease, in phase II testing in leukemia	Myelo, rash, fluid retention, hepatic, N/V
Topoisomerase inhibitors			
Epipodophyllotoxins			
Etoposide	Non–DNA binding topoisomerase II inhibitor; stabilizes DNA double-strand breaks	NB; Ewing's; rhabdo; germ cell; leukemia; CNS tumors; lymphoma	Myelo, N/V, rash, allergy, low BP, A, mucositis, hepatic (HD)
Tenoposide	Same as etoposide	NB; leukemia	Myelo, N/V, rash, allergy, low BP, A, mucositis, hepatic (HD)
Anthracyclines			
Doxorubicin	DNA intercalation; free radical formation; topoisomerase II inhibitor	Wilms'; Ewing's; NB; lymphoma; leukemia	Myelo, N/V, A, mucositis, diarrhea, phlebitis, vesicant, hepatic, cardiac
Daunorubicin	Same as doxorubicin	Leukemia; lymphoma	Myelo, N/V, A, mucositis, diarrhea, phlebitis, vesicant, hepatic, cardiac

Continued

TABLE 64-2

CHEMOTHERAPEUTIC AGENTS—cont'd

Class of Agent	Mechanism of Action	Antitumor Activity	Acute Toxicities
Topoisomerase inhibitors—cont'd			
Actinomycin D	Same as doxorubicin	Wilms'; rhabdo; Ewing's	Myelo, N/V, A, mucositis, hepatic, vesicant
Bleomycin	DNA intercalation; free radical formation	Germ cell; Hodgkin's; lymphoma	Myelo, skin, allergy, mucositis, lung
Camptothecin analogue			
Topotecan	Topoisomerase I inhibitor	Rhabdo, neuroblastoma	Myelo, N/V, A, mucositis, diarrhea, hepatic
Irinotecan	Topoisomerase I inhibitor	In phase II testing in rhabdo	Diarrhea, myelo, N/V, hepatic
Antimicrotubule Agents			
Vinca alkyloids			
Vincristine	Binds tubulin; prevents microtubule formation; blocks mitosis	Sarcomas; leukemia; Hodgkin's; Wilms'; lymphoma;	Constipation, neuro, vesicant, SIADH
Vinblastine	Same as vincristine	Hodgkin's; germ cell	Myelo, mucositis, vesicant
Taxanes			
Paclitaxel (Taxol)	Binds microtubules; blocks microtubule depolymerization; blocks mitosis	Ovarian carcinoma	Myelo, A, mucositis, paresthesias, hypersensitivity
Docetaxel (Taxotere)	Same as paclitaxel	In phase II testing in sarcomas and other solid tumors	Myelo, A, skin, hypersensitivity, fluid retention, paresthesias, mucositis
Differentiation Agents			
Retinoids			
Cis-retinoic acid	Binds to retinoic acid receptor; induces differentiation	NB	Skin, mucositis, eye, pseudotumor, hepatic, electrolyte
All trans retinoic acid	Same as cis-retinoic acid	APML; in phase II testing in Wilms'; NB	Skin, mucositis, eye, pseudotumor, hepatic, electrolyte
Fenretinide	Still being investigated; induces cell death, not differentiation	Phase II testing in NB	Dry skin/lips, loss night vision, increased triglycerides, hepatic, N/V
Miscellaneous Non/classified			
Corticosteroids	Lympholysis; multiple other effects not well classified	Leukemia (ALL); lymphoma	Weight gain, high BP, high glucose, mood change, many others
L-Asparaginase, PEG-asparaginase	Asparagine depletion; inhibition of protein synthesis	Leukemia (ALL); lymphoma	Anorexia, hepatic, pancreatitis, coagulopathy, neuro

ALL, acute lymphoblastic leukemia; PEG, polyethylene glycol; Rhabdo, rhabdomyosarcoma; BMT, bone marrow transplant; NB, neuroblastoma; CNS tumors, central nervous system tumors; HD, high dose; A, alopecia; myelo, myelosuppression; N/V, nausea and vomiting; VOD, veno-occlusive disease; neuro, neurologic toxicity; SIADH, syndrome of inappropriate antidiuretic hormone; BP, blood pressure; IT, intrathecal; APML, acute promyelocytic leukemia.

Data from Balis FM, Holcenberg JS, Poplack DG: General principles of chemotherapy. In Pizzo P, Poplack D (eds): Principles and Practice of Pediatric Oncology, 3rd ed. Philadelphia, Lippincott-Raven, 1997, pp 215–272; Ratain M, Teicher B, O'Dwyer P, et al: Pharmacology of cancer chemotherapy. In DeVita V, Hellman S, Rosenberg S (eds): Cancer: Principles and Practice of Oncology. Philadelphia, Lippincott-Raven, 1997, pp 375–385; Dorr R, Von Hoff D: Drug monographs. In Dorr R, Von Hoff D (eds): Cancer Chemotherapy Handbook. Norwalk, Conn, Appleton & Lange, 1994, p 129.

Specific organs are often affected by chemotherapy. Heart, liver, lung, thyroid, and gonadal function can be impaired. Gonadal dysfunction (azospermia, amenorrhea) frequently results from alkylator treatment. Therapy with mechloethamine, vincristine, prednisone, and procarbazine resulted in azospermia in 80% to 100% of all male patients.[76] Combination chemotherapy programs for childhood Hodgkin's disease have been adjusted to replace mechlorethamine with cyclophosphamide and eliminate dacarbazine from standard treatments to attempt to decrease the infertility risk. It should

be noted that the children of childhood cancer survivors are not at an increased risk for congenital anomalies.[77]

Cardiotoxicity from anthracycline antibiotics has been a problem in the treatment of Ewing's sarcoma, osteosarcoma, and lymphomas. Use of continuous-infusion anthracycline can decrease the risk of cardiac muscle damage and subsequent congestive heart failure.[78] Another new strategy has been the use of the cardioprotectant dexrazoxone to prevent anthracycline-induced cardiotoxicity.[53] Until a safe dose of anthracycline given with dexrazoxone can be defined, the cumulative lifetime dose of anthracycline continues to be limited to 450 mg/m², a level at which fewer than 5% of patients experience clinical congestive heart failure.[79] Other cardiovascular late effects have been reported in childhood cancer survivors. Survivors of childhood brain tumor therapy treated with a combination of chemotherapy, radiation, and surgery had a significantly increased risk of stroke, blood clots, and angina-like symptoms compared with their siblings.[80]

Pulmonary toxicity is a source of significant late toxicity of cancer therapy. Many alkylating agents and radiation therapy contribute to pulmonary fibrosis, resulting in decreased lung volume, lung compliance, and diffusing capacity. In a recent report from the Childhood Cancer Survivors Study comparing pulmonary symptoms among 12,390 cancer survivors and 3546 randomly selected siblings, the survivors had a statistically significant increased relative risk of lung disease. Measures included pulmonary fibrosis, recurrent pneumonia, chronic cough, pleurisy, use of supplemental oxygen, abnormal chest wall, exercise-induced shortness of breath, bronchitis, recurrent sinus infections, and tonsillitis. Chest irradiation was associated with this increased relative risk in most instances.[81] The nitrosoureas and bleomycin are the most common agents to cause pulmonary fibrosis. In Hodgkin's disease, when bleomycin is given before mantle irradiation, the risk of pulmonary toxicity is increased.[82] Whole-lung irradiation, as given for pulmonary metastasis in Wilms' tumor and Ewing's sarcoma, also can result in pulmonary impairment.

Other significant organ-related late effects include hypothyroidism after radiation in Hodgkin's disease, chronic renal insufficiency from cisplatin therapy, chronic cystitis from cyclophosphamide or ifosfamide treatment, and prolonged hypogammaglobulinemia and T-lymphocyte dysfunction after multiple high-dose alkylators for bone marrow transplant.[83]

One of the more significant late effects of cancer therapy is the risk of secondary malignancy. As the number of childhood cancer survivors increases, this has become a major concern. In a retrospective review of 1406 childhood cancer patients, the actuarial risk of a second malignant neoplasm was 5.6% at 25 years after diagnosis.[84] The risk of second malignancy is highest in the patients who received both chemotherapy and radiation therapy. Hodgkin's disease survivors have the highest secondary malignancy rates. The estimated actuarial incidence of any second cancer was 7% at 15 years after diagnosis. Breast cancer was the most common solid tumor, with an estimated actuarial incidence in women of 35% by age 40 years. These patients are also at risk to develop leukemia, non-Hodgkin's lymphoma, and thyroid carcinoma.[85] In some series of survivors of childhood Hodgkin's disease, the cumulative estimated incidence of second malignancies at 30 years has ranged from 18% to 31%.[86,87] Patients who have received additional multimodality therapy for recurrent Hodgkin's disease have the highest risk of second tumors. Patients with soft tissue sarcomas, retinoblastoma, and Ewing's sarcoma who receive high-dose radiation to the primary lesion are at increased risk for secondary osteosarcoma within the radiation field.[88] In the past 10 years, etoposide has been

recognized as causing secondary acute myeloid leukemia, usually of the M4 or M5 subtype, with a short latency period (1 to 3 years from exposure) and a characteristic chromosomal translocation involving chromosome 11q23.[89]

As new advances in combination chemotherapy treatment result in an increase in childhood cancer survival of as much as 1% per year, the challenge for the future is to maintain the excellent survival rates while altering therapy to prevent late toxicity.

BIOLOGIC TARGETED THERAPY

Over the past 20 years, many of the key genetic events that control carcinogenesis have been identified. Expression of oncogenes and the loss of tumor-suppressor gene function have been shown to lead to cellular signaling abnormalities, resulting in malignant transformation as a result of aberrant cell proliferation and cell differentiation. Over the last several years, rapid progress has been made in the development of rationally designed new agents to target biologic pathways specifically. These agents include signal-transduction inhibitors; tissue growth factor–receptor inhibitors, antiangiogenesis agents, and biologic response modifiers; individual cytokines, tumor-targeted antibody therapies; and adoptive immunotherapy techniques. Many of these agents are still in preclinical and early phase I testing, especially in pediatric oncology, although efficacy of agents from each class has been demonstrated. The development of these agents differs from that of those for standard cytotoxic therapy. The standard phase I study for cytotoxic agents is designed to define the maximal tolerated dose. In contrast, in biologic targeted therapy, the optimal therapeutic dose is well below the maximal tolerated dose. The challenge in evaluating these agents is how to select the optimal dose and schedule, combine tumor-targeted agents with classic cytotoxic therapy, and validate the intended effect on the selected target for these biologic compounds designed to treat minimal residual disease.

Signal Transduction Inhibitors

Cellular signaling is a basic biologic function of all cells, controlling cellular proliferation and differentiation. Signaling can be extracellular (e.g., growth factor–receptor tyrosine kinase) or through multiple intracellular effector and survival pathways (e.g., ras, raf, p53, Bcl-2). The malignant cell phenotype develops when programmed cell death (apoptosis) is inhibited or cells lose the ability to undergo normal differentiation. Specific agents have been synthesized to restore the usual cell functions by blocking aberrant signal-transduction pathways.

Extracellular signaling can be accomplished via growth factor–receptor proteins. Epidermal growth factor receptor (EGFR) is overexpressed in many solid tumors and is believed to play a role in tumor invasion and metastasis.[90] A specific inhibitor of EGFR, ZD1839, is a novel oral EGFR tyrosine kinase inhibitor that has demonstrated preclinical and clinical antitumor activity in adult phase I trials.[91] In addition, ZD1839 appears to have antiangiogenic effects by inhibiting the production of vascular endothelial growth factor (VEGF) and basic fibroblast growth factor.[92] EGFR overexpression has been demonstrated in neuroblastoma, rhabdomyosarcoma, and glioma.[93–95] ZD1839 is currently in phase I testing in pediatric solid tumor patients by the Children's Oncology Group (COG). Inhibitors of the VEGF receptor, such as PTK787/ZK22254, have been very effective inhibitors of angiogenesis, resulting in reduction in tumor size and number of blood vessels in treated patients.[96]

Multiple intracellular signaling pathways have recently been elucidated, and knowledge regarding the specific proteins involved in these pathways is now being exploited to develop specific targeted therapy. Production of farnesyl-protein transferase (FPTase) and Bcl-2 inhibitors are examples of molecularly targeted drug development. The *ras* gene product plays a critical role in cell proliferation. Mutant forms of *ras* are associated with malignant transformation, and 30% of all human cancers express mutant *ras* genes.[97] Addition of a farnesyl isoprene group to the protein (farnesylation) is required for both mutant and wild-type *ras* function; however, other cellular polypeptides require farnesylation and also may be involved in the antiproliferative effects of FPTase inhibitors.[98] R115777 is a potent, selective inhibitor of FPTase. This agent has been tested in phase I trials of adult solid tumors and leukemia, phase II trial in breast cancer, and in phase I trials combined with cisplatin and cisplatin/gemcitabine.[99–101] Toxicities observed with R115777 were neutropenia, thrombocytopenia, rash, nausea, and peripheral neuropathy.[98–101] In vivo inhibition of farnesylation was demonstrated in cells from all patients tested.[98,102] The COG is currently evaluating R115777 in a phase I trial in refractory leukemia.

Another class of new targeted agents includes small peptides that are designed to bind to messenger RNA (mRNA) of signal-transduction proteins and inhibit their expression. One example of such an antisense oligonucleotide inhibitor is G3139, which inhibits expression of Bcl-2. This agent binds to the first six codons of the human Bcl-2 mRNA, resulting in downregulation of expression of Bcl-2. Because apoptosis is regulated by Bcl-2 expression, and neuroblastomas overexpressing Bcl-2 have a poorer outcome,[103] it is hypothesized that inhibiting Bcl-2 expression may improve tumor response in these patients. G3139 has completed phase I and II testing in adults, both alone and in combination with cytotoxic agents. Responses have been observed, and inhibition of Bcl-2 expression has been measured in peripheral blood and tumor tissue. This agent is now undergoing testing in COG for relapsed and refractory pediatric solid tumor patients.

The agents described are just a few of the new class of rationally designed drugs specifically targeting known molecular cellular signaling pathways. As future advances in our understanding of cellular signaling pathways improves, even more agents will emerge for clinical testing. It is the hope of those involved in developmental

therapeutics that these agents will one day play a major role in cancer therapeutics.

Biologic Response Modifiers

The goal of biologic response modifiers is to stimulate the immune system to help eradicate tumors. The human immune system is designed to identify and destroy foreign cells. One of the great mysteries of oncology is why a patient's immune system is often unable to eliminate malignant cells. Studies in the mid-1990s indicated that some tumor cells may express a protein, Fas ligand, that conveys a "death signal" to T lymphocytes, causing them to undergo apoptosis and therefore be useless in fighting the cancer.[104] The development of biologic response modifiers is a new branch of cancer therapy being developed to enhance or stimulate the natural products of the immune system (lymphocytes, antibodies, and cytokines) to better recognize and destroy cancer cells.

The immune system is composed of many cell types, but the lymphocyte has the primary role in controlling immune function. B lymphocytes function by secreting antibodies that mediate cell destruction by binding complement or causing opsonization, resulting in phagocytosis by macrophages. T lymphocytes can directly interact with specific cell-surface antigens on a target cell and cause cell lysis through cytotoxic granule release or programmed cell death. These cytotoxic T lymphocytes are involved with tumor cell killing. To initiate this response, antigens must be presented to the T cell by antigen-presenting cells (APCs) that express the antigens bound to major histocompatibility complex (MHC) proteins in the presence of stimulatory cytokines. Cytokines or ILs (e.g., IL-2, interferon α, tumor necrosis factor) are proteins produced by helper T lymphocytes and monocytes that help recruit other effector cells, including APCs, as well as regulate antibody production. The effector cells of the immune system (e.g., granulocytes, monocytes, macrophages, eosinophils, dendritic cells) can become tumor selective when activated by a specific antibody, a process called antibody-dependent cell-mediated cytotoxicity (ADCC).

Immunotherapy with biologic response modifiers takes advantage of all these immune functions. The goal of this therapy is to improve the immunogenicity of a tumor and allow it to be recognized and targeted for destruction by the immune system. Immunotherapy can be divided into two major categories: adoptive immunotherapy and tumor-targeted antibody therapy.

Adoptive Immunotherapy

Adoptive immunotherapy involves the use of tumor vaccines made from autologous or allogeneic tumor-associated antigens. Vaccines have been made by using whole tumor cells and partially purified or highly purified tumor antigens. Specific purified tumor antigens can be made more immunogenic by attachment to carrier proteins (adjuvants). The majority of all clinical trials using this type of tumor vaccine have been performed in melanoma patients. In a phase III study using purified

GM$_2$ ganglioside combined with bacille Calmette-Guérin (BCG), a trend toward improved survival was noted for patients receiving vaccine versus low-dose cyclophosphamide and BCG. Among vaccine-treated patients, 86% produced an immunoglobulin M response.[105] A pilot study using GM$_2$ ganglioside conjugated to keyhole limpet hemocyanin (KLH) and mixed with the adjuvant QS-21 produced high-titer immunoglobulin M antibodies in all patients.[106]

Another type of tumor vaccine in development is one designed to stimulate tumor-specific T-cell immunity to tumor peptides, resulting in the generation of cytotoxic T lymphocytes. For this type of vaccine to be successful, it is necessary to modify the tumor peptide to stimulate antigen presentation to the T cell. The presentation of the antigen is often restricted to specific MHC alleles. Tumor cells themselves are poor APCs because they often lack expression of MHC class I and II proteins. Neuroblastoma murine tumor cells have been modified to express exogenous MHC class II genes. In a murine model, this resulted in enhanced presentation of tumor antigens directly to T cells, producing a potent in vivo tumor response.[107] Tumor cells also can be genetically engineered to overexpress cytokines (IL-2, granulocyte-macrophage colony-stimulating factor [GM-CSF]) that activate APCs and other immune cells.[108,109] A recent study tested a new allogeneic neuroblastoma tumor cell vaccine combining transgenic lymphotactin with IL-2 in patients with relapsed or refractory neuroblastoma. Lymphotactin is a T-lymphocyte attractant, and IL-2 is a growth factor that causes T-cell expansion. Combining these proteins with an allogeneic neuroblastoma tumor cell produced a vaccine that resulted in local infiltration of CD4+ and CD8+ lymphocytes, eosinophils, and Langerhans cells and systemic increase in CD4+ cells, natural killer cells, eosinophils, and serum IL-5. Of the 21 patients treated in this pilot study, 2 patients demonstrated a complete tumor response, and 1, a partial response.[110] Cytokines (GM-CSF, IL-2, IL-12, IL-1α) and other effector molecules (muramyl tripeptide phosphatidylethanolamine, disaccharide tripeptide) also are being used to stimulate an immune response in pediatric cancer patients.[13] Muramyl tripeptide phosphatidylethanolamine (MTP-PE) is a liposome-encapsulated product derived from a minimal subunit of *Mycobacterium* and is able to activate macrophage and monocyte tumoricidal activity. Lung metastases in osteosarcoma patients treated with MTP-PE demonstrated infiltration by chronic inflammatory cells with fibrosis and necrosis at the periphery of the lesion with viable tumor in the center. This reaction is opposite that seen in pulmonary metastases treated with standard chemotherapy, where the center of the lesion is fibrotic with a peripheral rim of viable tumor.[111] A CCG and Pediatric Oncology Group randomized phase III trial in newly diagnosed osteosarcoma patients was conducted to determine whether the addition of ifosfamide, MTP-PE, or both to the standard doxorubicin, cisplatin, methotrexate regimen improved outcome. Although the data are maturing, the addition of ifosfamide and MTP-PE to the three-drug regimen was superior to the addition of ifosfamide alone.[13]

Other forms of immunotherapy involve the use of cytokine infusions such as interferon α, IL-2, and tumor necrosis factor to stimulate immune reaction against tumor cells. Adoptive immunotherapy with interferon α has produced significant responses in CML. In renal cell carcinoma and metastatic melanoma, continuous infusion of IL-2 produced a 20% remission rate.[112] The CCG recently completed a study with IL-2 to treat the minimal residual disease state in childhood AML after completion of chemotherapy.

Tumor-targeted Antibody Therapy

Passive immunity involves the use of monoclonal antibodies (mAbs) or cytotoxic effector cells produced in vitro and infused into the patient. mAbs have been tested in patients with neuroblastoma. Initially, mAbs were developed and used for in vitro purging of autologous bone marrow before myeloablative transplant. Murine mAbs have been raised to a glycolipid antigen, surface glycoproteins, and specific disialogangliosides GD2 and GD3 in neuroblastoma cells. The murine anti-GD2 antibody was the first to be used in clinical trials. Antibody to GD2 mediates antibody-dependent or complement-dependent cellular cytotoxicity, which can be enhanced by the addition of cytokines.[113] A phase II clinical trial of mouse mAb to GD2 (called 3F8) in advanced neuroblastoma patients resulted in an immune response in 40% of patients.[114]

A more recent trial used a murine anti-GD2 antibody, 14.G2a, infused with IL-2, designed with the goal of enhancing ADCC. In this CCG trial, 33 patients with neuroblastoma or osteosarcoma were treated with a combination of IL-2 and escalating doses of 14.G2a antibody to determine the toxicity and efficacy of 14.G2a. Toxicity included transient neurogenic pain, allergic reactions, and rash. One neuroblastoma patient had a partial response, three patients had decrease in bone marrow infiltrates, and one osteosarcoma patient had a complete response.[115] One drawback of murine mAb therapy is that when these antibodies are repeatedly infused into humans, most patients will ultimately produce a human–anti-mouse antibody, which renders further antibody treatment useless.

Recently, chimeric human/mouse antibodies have been produced that may decrease the risk of human–anti-mouse antibody generation.[115] Recombinant chimeric antibodies are produced by linking the constant region of human antibodies to the variable combining region of a mouse mAb. These chimeric antibodies have been produced for the treatment of neuroblastoma[116] (ch14.18) and more recently in leukemia and lymphoma with the development of anti-CD20, anti-CD52, and anti-CD33 mAbs. Rituximab (anti-CD20) has been demonstrated to produce tumor responses in adult low-grade and follicular lymphomas.[13] Rituximab has been extremely effective in treating post-transplant lymphoproliferative disease[117] and has improved survival in adult patients with aggressive lymphomas when given as additional therapy after transplant.[118] In pediatrics, the COG is studying the effect of the addition of rituximab to induction therapy for T-cell ALL patients with a poor response to steroid therapy. Gemtuzumab is a conjugate of humanized anti-CD33 mouse mAb and caliceamicin that is active in myeloid leukemia. The caliceamicin, a potent antitumor agent, is inactive when bound to the mAb.[119] Once the antibody conjugate is internalized into the AML cell, the antibody link is hydrolyzed, yielding free caliceamicin. In phase I studies, 30% of relapsed AML patients responded to gemtuzumab.[120] The COG is conducting a pilot study to evaluate the safety of gemtuzumab in combination with conventional chemotherapy in relapse, refractory, or secondary CD33+ AML.

The field of targeted biologic therapy is still in the early stages, but the future looks bright for the continued development of new targeted therapies, fueled by rapid advances in our understanding of cellular signaling pathways and immune mechanisms.

Local Tumor Control

In addition to systemic treatment, local tumor control is important in pediatric oncology. Metastatic disease is more readily eradicated in young patients than in adults when the primary lesion has been adequately treated. A number of modalities may be used to control local disease.[121]

Radiation Oncology

An understanding of the biologic principles of radiation therapy in childhood cancer is important. Radiation may directly affect cellular DNA or produce reactive free radicals that indirectly damage genetic material and interfere with the reproductive capacity of normal or malignant tissues. The sensitivity of normal cells and malignant cells to radiation varies widely between cell populations. Ionizing radiation initially results in sublethal damage to cells. The therapeutic effect of radiation therapy exploits the differences between a normal cell's ability to repair this sublethal damage and the slower response of radiosensitive tumor cells. Fractionated dosing allows normal cells to recover while having a cumulative effect on tumor cells. The effect of ionizing radiation on tumors depends on the number of actively reproducing cells at the time of exposure and on the length of the cellular regeneration cycle. Because most of the damage is indirect and focused on reproduction, malignant lesions usually show a delayed effect to radiation therapy. The tumor may begin to shrink or eventually disappear weeks to months after treatment. At some dose of therapy, the response of the malignant tissues becomes exponential, but further damage to normal adjacent cells also may occur.

Acute reactions to ionizing radiation depend on this balance between replication and cell death and seem to be affected by increased intervals between dose fractions that allow enhanced cellular repopulation. The radiation fraction size has a small impact on what volume of cells are immediately destroyed. Conversely, the long-term effects of therapy depend primarily on the total exposure dose and the size of each treatment fraction. The therapeutic ratio may be enhanced by exploiting the difference between the early and late radiation effects. Techniques may be used that reduce the late effects by lowering the dose per fraction and increasing the number of fractions delivered over the conventional treatment time. A further strategy would be to accelerate this dose fractionation by reducing the overall radiation time and thereby providing rapidly proliferating tumors less opportunity for repopulation.

Radiation therapy may be combined with surgery in a strategic manner to deliver the highest effective dose to a well-defined site yet to minimize the dose to surrounding normal structures.[122] Preoperative radiation therapy may permit a smaller treatment area because the operative bed has not been manipulated. In larger tumors, its use may reduce the lesion volume sufficiently to allow a subsequent resection. In addition, potential tumor seeding during operative removal may be reduced because the cells that may be surgically disseminated have been rendered incapable of reproducing. However, preoperative radiation may delay the surgical procedure to allow tissue recovery. The extent of disease, which is usually defined and staged at operation, is less certain, and the radiation therapy plan may be adversely affected by inappropriate downstaging of the tumor. Finally, dose limitations may preclude retreatment postoperatively if the surgical margin remains histologically positive for tumor cells.

For these reasons, many combined strategies use postoperative radiation such that the treatment fields and doses are determined after surgical resection and histologic assessment.[122] Higher doses can be delivered postoperatively when the target volumes have been more accurately defined. Doses to the periphery of the tumor can be fine-tuned, depending on the presence of gross, microscopic, or no residual disease. However, postoperative delivery may require a wider treatment area after extensive surgical manipulation.

Soft tissue sarcoma provides a model for the adjunctive role of radiation therapy because neither surgery nor radiation alone usually completely controls local disease in the head and neck, extremity, trunk, or retroperitoneum.[123] In extremity lesions, radiation also allows more conservative resection with limb sparing. Although local tumor control rates of 75% to 98% have been achieved, with limb salvage rates greater than 80%, wound complications occur in as many as 40% of patients. Neoadjuvant radiation at more modest doses (30 Gy total) has decreased the complication rate while maintaining excellent (>95%) 5-year local control and ultimate limb salvage.[124] Postoperative radiotherapy also may be advantageous. In a large adult sarcoma series, doses between 60 and 70 Gy provided 80% local tumor control and functional limb salvage.[125] The wound complication rate was less than 10%.

Several aspects of radiation treatment in pediatric patients deserve special consideration. Attention must be paid to the issues of immobilizing or sedating children so ionizing doses can be targeted to the desired area without inappropriate exposure of surrounding tissues. It can be difficult to balance the doses required for antitumor efficacy with the risks of adverse reactions in young patients. Pediatric radiation oncologists may use lower treatment doses and accept a higher recurrence rate to ensure lower toxicity, especially in critical developing organs such as the brain. The normal "tolerance" of organs or tissues may be adversely affected when chemotherapeutic agents are used. The long-term effects of combined-modality therapy must be considered in regard to musculoskeletal and dental tissues, CNS and neuropsychological sequelae, and endocrine and gonadal dysfunction, as well as direct effects on the heart, lungs, or kidneys.[126] Techniques designed to minimize the impact of radiation therapy on surrounding tissues continue to evolve, and newer treatment modalities may offer advantages in both therapeutic effect and reduction of short- and long-term morbidity. The following sections describe techniques that allow safe, efficacious doses of radiation to be delivered, often in combination with surgical excision, to produce the maximal therapeutic benefit.

Brachytherapy

Brachytherapy is radiation treatment in which the ionizing source is in contact with the lesion, usually within the initial tumor volume. Catheters are placed in the tumor during surgery and may be loaded with temporary or permanent implant sources. Remote afterloading may decrease radiation exposure to personnel and family members and can be performed in the patient's room or on an outpatient basis. Low-dose-rate sources such as cesium provide about 1 cGy/min, whereas high-dose-rate sources such as iridium provide about 100 cGy/min.

Intraoperative brachytherapy with iridium 192 (^{192}Ir) implants delivering 45 Gy has been effective in sarcomas.[127] In this series, the 5-year local control rate with the brachytherapy boost was 82%, compared with 67% with external [DvA1] beam radiation alone. The greatest benefit (90% vs. 65%) was in patients with histologic high-grade tumors. Because interstitial implants allow continuous-dose delivery over a much shorter time, they offer a radiobiologic advantage in high-grade tumors with rapid cell growth kinetics. Close cooperation between surgeon and radiation oncologist during the procedure is critical to ensure the most effective mapping of the tumor bed target.

Pediatric patients with soft tissue sarcomas also can benefit from specialized radiation treatment strategies. If children have microscopic residual disease after surgery and chemotherapy, radiation produces excellent local tumor control.[128] Hyperfractionated radiotherapy is tolerated just as well as single-fraction treatments. This technique uses smaller doses given as several fractions per day over the same overall treatment time, so that a higher total dose is delivered with similar tissue toxicity. Boosts with interstitial implantation may be particularly well suited for extremity lesions in children with areas of limited radiation volume because of considerations for future growth and development.

The brachytherapy experience in children is more limited than in adults, and most reports include a heterogeneous variety of tumors. Implants of ^{125}I or ^{192}Ir were placed in the tumor bed of 18 patients at the time of primary resection of brain tumors, sarcoma, neuroblastoma, rhabdomyosarcoma, hepatoblastoma, and pancreatic cancer.[129] Two implants were afterloaded. Because of advanced disease, only three patients are long-term survivors. However, local tumor control was achieved in 13 instances, with only 2 patients experiencing treatment-related morbidity. Further evaluation of external beam or interstitial irradiation in 37 children with synovial sarcoma has been completed.[130] Ionizing radiation was delivered to 16 primary lesions, and durable local control was achieved in 14 patients, 10 of whom are long-term survivors. Although no benefit was found with adjuvant radiation after a complete surgical resection, significant local control benefit occurred in lesions with incomplete resection or partial chemotherapy response.

High-dose-rate brachytherapy has been successfully used in pediatric patients (Fig. 64-3). Low-dose-rate techniques require sedation, immobilization, long exposure times, and hospitalization, even with low-energy sources. High-dose-rate therapy is delivered in a few minutes, which is particularly helpful in young children. The short therapy duration also allows rapid reinstitution of systemic chemotherapy. The morbidity is usually related to skin or mucosal reactions, which may progress as a "recall" phenomenon in patients treated with radiosensitizing agents such as anthracyclines.[131] Effective local control has been demonstrated in a variety of childhood sarcomas.[132,133] Eleven of 13 patients received 36 Gy as a fractionated dose, and 2 children received a similar dose

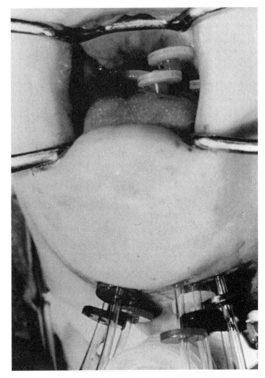

FIGURE 64-3. A 3-month-old infant with rhabdomyosarcoma in the base of the tongue. Eight high-dose-rate brachytherapy catheters were placed, delivering 36 Gy in 12 fractions over an 8-day period. The child is alive and disease free and has a good cosmetic result 7 years after treatment. (Courtesy of Subir Nag, M.D., Chief of Brachytherapy, Ohio State University, Columbus, Ohio.)

with combined brachytherapy and external beam treatment. Three tumors recurred, but 11 patients were surviving disease free 41 months after therapy. Half the patients demonstrated mild to moderate skin and mucosal reactions, but only one had grade 3 toxicity. Bone and organ growth were maintained, and the long-term cosmetic appearance was good. In a more recent series, 27 patients ranging in age from 1 to 21 years with soft tissue sarcoma were treated at initial presentation with brachytherapy alone (10 patients) or a combination of brachytherapy and external beam radiation (17 patients). Most patients had involved margins after tumor resection (20 of 27). Of the 10 patients treated with brachytherapy alone, 1 died of distant metastatic disease, and no local failures were noted in the remaining 9 patients. In the group treated with combination radiation therapy, 1 local, 2 regional, and 3 distant failures occurred.[134] Thus brachytherapy alone or in combination with external beam radiation provides a high rate of local tumor control in pediatric soft tissue sarcomas.

Unfortunately, radiation therapy carries a significant morbidity risk. Radiation to the CNS may cause necrosis, arteritis, leukoencephalopathy, or radiation-induced tumors. Benign meningiomas have developed in children who received initial high-dose cranial radiation for malignant brain tumors, and some patients experienced a short latency period between treatment and tumor development.[135] The carcinogenic effect of radiation therapy on brain tumors also has been theorized in more than 100 cases of malignant intracranial tumors.[136] These patients could be clinically differentiated from those with spontaneous brain tumors, and their outcome was particularly unfavorable. In soft tissue sarcomas, acute toxicity occurs in 40% to 50% of patients and consists mostly of grade 1 to 3 skin and mucosal changes. However, in a recent report, grade 3 to 4 morbidities increased from 8% to 20% after a median follow-up of 10 years.[137] Significant morbidities in this study included trismus/osteonecrosis, vaginal stenosis, and periurethral fibrosis.

Intraoperative Radiation

Intraoperative radiation therapy (IORT) can be an important adjunctive measure to external beam radiation for local tumor control of advanced adult cancer.[13] IORT allows the radiation dose to be directly applied to the target area while shielding adjacent structures. Whenever disease remains in surgically inaccessible areas, IORT may be an effective adjunct. Most applications of IORT in children have been in patients with unresectable disease at diagnosis, delayed primary or second-look procedures, residual lesions, or local tumor recurrence. Phase I/II studies have demonstrated that IORT can be done safely in the pediatric population.[139]

Preliminary outcomes suggest that this modality may be beneficial. A report of 59 pediatric patients with various tumor diagnoses showed the value of doses in the 10- to 17-Gy range, delivered with 5- to 11-MEV electrons to a tissue depth of up to 3 cm.[140] Ten of 11 patients with histologically benign but locally aggressive tumors achieved local control. A 75% local tumor control rate

was found among the 48 patients with malignant lesions. In another report, 16 pediatric patients with a variety of solid tumors received IORT for gross residual disease in 5 patients and suspected microscopic residual disease in 11 patients. A local control rate of 61% was achieved in this population.[141]

The efficacy of IORT in high-risk neuroblastoma patients was addressed in a number of studies.[142,143] In one group of 25 children with neuroblastoma, 15 survived a mean of 51 months after IORT. Although half of the stage 4 patients were surviving at the time of the initial report, follow-up 3 years later detected only a 38% survival in these children with metastatic disease.[142] In a more recent report of 21 patients with high-risk neuroblastoma, 18 patients had a gross total resection. In 6, recurrent disease developed, with 2 with locoregional recurrences. In the 5 patients undergoing a subtotal resection, all had local recurrence.[143]

Other series reported similar results with minor technique variations. In a series of eight children with advanced tumors, a dose of 3 to 15 Gy was delivered with 6- to 13-MEV electrons.[144] Five patients received additional external beam radiation, and local tumor control was achieved in 63% of the cases. A minimal increase was found in the operative time and no increase in the complication rate. A subsequent experience with 11 locally advanced or recurrent abdominal tumors in children also was encouraging.[145] In this series, 10 to 25 Gy was administered with 6- to 15-MEV electrons over one to five treatment fields per patient. Again, neuroblastoma was an important target, with three of the four children alive for a mean of 117 months.

Although the operation is ideally undertaken in suites containing linear accelerators, most centers require interdepartmental transfer, and the guidelines for this maneuver have been described.[146] IORT requires more generous incisions and a greater degree of tissue mobilization than do standard tumor resections. Intracavitary exposure must provide adequate space to place the electron beam accelerator cones and exclude normal organs from the radiation field (Fig. 64-4). IORT should be used whenever concern exists regarding the original tumor bed or the resection margin adjacent to normal organs or vascular adventitia. In older adolescents or adults, multiple-field matching of IORT applicators and frequent use of customized lead shields can protect uninvolved tissues.[147] In most infants and children, uninvolved structures can be adequately mobilized so that treatment cones can be placed without cumbersome shielding. For extensive areas of treatment, multiple nonoverlapping fields may be used. All surgical dissection must be performed before leaving the operating room, as further exploration is potentially dangerous while the patient is in the radiation therapy suite. Proper anesthetic management is critical for these complex procedures, and the techniques have been well established.[148] After radiation therapy, the patient is transported back to the surgical suite for completion of the operation, which generally consists only of ascertaining hemostasis and wound closure.

Earlier experience with IORT demonstrated some treatment-related complications.[149] Three patients required

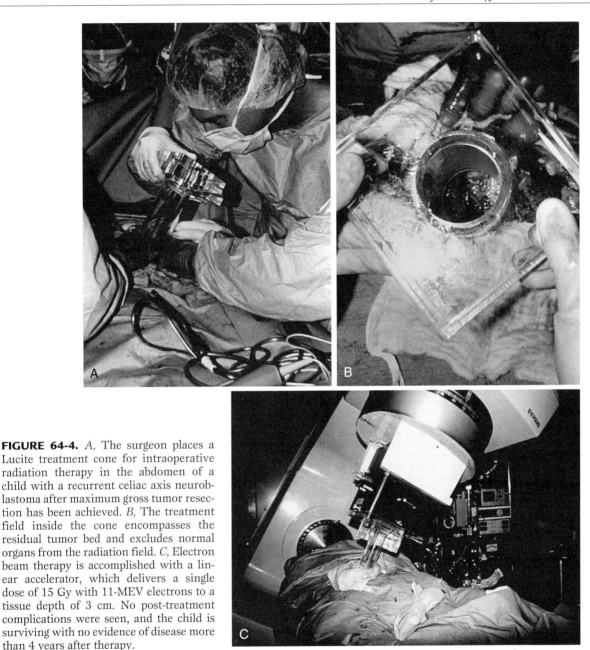

FIGURE 64-4. *A,* The surgeon places a Lucite treatment cone for intraoperative radiation therapy in the abdomen of a child with a recurrent celiac axis neuroblastoma after maximum gross tumor resection has been achieved. *B,* The treatment field inside the cone encompasses the residual tumor bed and excludes normal organs from the radiation field. *C,* Electron beam therapy is accomplished with a linear accelerator, which delivers a single dose of 15 Gy with 11-MEV electrons to a tissue depth of 3 cm. No post-treatment complications were seen, and the child is surviving with no evidence of disease more than 4 years after therapy.

surgical intervention for fibrotic ureteral strictures or renal artery stenosis. In two cases, the injured structures were within a supplemental external beam treatment field. In two children, neuropathies developed, one transiently after IORT alone and one permanently after combined therapy with external beam radiation. Nevertheless, all patients were survivors for up to 42 months' follow-up. Currently, more extensive dissection of normal structures and avoidance of overlapping radiation fields have decreased the complication rate.[140] In this series, no acute intestinal injury or neuropathy was seen. One superficial wound infection occurred but no deep intracavitary infections. One child had an episode of self-limited pancreatitis, and two children had postoperative intussusception. One patient had undergone a laminectomy and radiation for a paraspinous

tumor, and scoliosis developed during long-term follow-up. The overall complication rate was similar to that in a matched group of patients who underwent tumor resection alone without IORT.

Stereotactic Radiotherapy

Sophisticated stereotactic radiotherapy techniques are used for the treatment of intracranial neoplasms, which require precise radiation volume definition, localization of normal structures, accurate determination of tumor and adjacent tissue dosage, and careful patient immobilization. Intracranial targets are usually irregular in shape, and treatment planning requires matching the treatment volume to the target in three dimensions, with avoidance of adjacent critical normal structures.[150]

Radiation produces acute degenerative necrosis with inflammation, phagocytosis of necrotic debris with peripheral vascular proliferation, and eventual prominent glial scarring.[151] Benign tumors are more slowly proliferating and would be good targets for a single large radiation dose. Conversely, malignant tumors that are rapidly proliferating would respond better to fractionated doses, which would be less damaging to the surrounding normal slow-growing brain cells. Stereotactic radiosurgery involves a single high-dose treatment to a defined target volume, whereas stereotactic radiotherapy combines the target and dose localization of single-dose "radiosurgery" with the biologic advantage of dose fractionation. This treatment modality has been made possible by the development of relocatable stereotactic frames and dedicated linear accelerators.[152]

Field shaping is critical to optimize dose delivery in stereotactic radiosurgery. Conformed therapy uses a digitally reconstructed computed tomographic image. The use of multiple static beams at different gantry positions and table angles is appropriate for large targets. Dynamic collimation with simultaneous rotation of treatment couch and gantry allows more sophisticated field shaping and precise treatment of deep-seated irregular lesions.

More precise delivery of the radiation to the target volume allows increase of dose to the tumor while sparing surrounding tissues. Evidence suggests that a dose/response relation exists, with improved survival over a range from 45 to 60 Gy.[153] A response ceiling may be found at 60 Gy without further benefit up to 80 Gy. However, radiation therapy for highly malignant disease processes may require total cumulative doses exceeding 100 Gy. The maximum tolerated dose for treatment of patients with recurrent, previously irradiated primary and metastatic brain lesions based on tumor diameter has recently been established.[154] These doses ranged from 15 Gy to 27 Gy for lesions that ranged from 20 mm to 40 mm in diameter.

Among 61 patients treated for low-grade gliomas by using stereotactic radiotherapy, at a dose of 50 to 60 Gy, there were no field recurrences or marginal failures at a median follow-up time of 18 months.[155] In 40 children between the ages of 3.4 and 17.5 years with benign arteriovenous malformations, the radiosurgery technique was successful in obliterating the lesions in 35% of the patients and in partially obliterating the lesions in 62% of the patients. The obliteration rate was thought to be dose dependent, with a higher rate of success in patients receiving at least 18 Gy. Two permanent neurologic complications occurred.[156] In high-grade astrocytomas, stereotactic techniques controlled disease with substantially decreased toxicity from symptomatic radiation necrosis.[157] In a recent series of various high-grade tumors, gamma knife techniques were used to treat 12 children. Seven patients remained stable, 1 patient died, and 4 had progressive disease (2 within the field of treatment).[158] Radiosurgical techniques can be used to treat metastatic lesions in the brain, with response rates greater than 80%, low morbidity, and local failure rates less than 20%. The modality may be more cost-effective than surgery and may reduce hospitalization time.

Although fractionated stereotactic radiotherapy achieves precise target treatment in pediatric brain tumors and has minimal immediate effects, longer-term follow-up is still necessary to evaluate the therapeutic efficacy.[159]

Intensity-modulated Radiotherapy

Techniques continue to evolve to improve the impact of radiation therapy on tumor response while minimizing the dose of radiation imparted to surrounding normal tissues. Imaging systems, treatment-planning software, and delivery systems have undergone dramatic advancements that allow sophisticated delivery of more precise courses of radiation treatments. Intensity-modulated radiation therapy (IMRT) is an advanced form of three-dimensional conformal therapy that uses nonuniform radiation beam intensities that have been determined by using various computer-based optimization techniques. IMRT is frequently designed by using inverse planning, in which the clinical objectives are specified mathematically and sophisticated computer algorithms are used to generate the beam parameters. This advancement over standard conformal therapy further refines the ability to shape the treatment dose to the target volume.[160] Experience with IMRT in the pediatric population is growing. Initial reports of mixed tumor cases including pediatric cases suggest that the technique will be effective in reducing treatment-related morbidity and allow dose escalation to the target volume.[161,162]

Proton beam technology (IMPT) may eventually supplant the use of photon beam treatment modalities. The physics of the loss of energy of a proton in tissue are significantly different from that of photon energy, and these differences may allow an even greater ability to cover the target zone with a uniform dose of radiation while giving minimal radiation deep to the target and a lower dose proximal to the target.[163] In addition, proton beam technology can use all of the technologies available for photons, including beam direction, number weighting, and intensity modulation. IMPT further refines the ability of the radiation oncologist to target the tumor while minimizing radiation to surrounding tissues again allowing incremental dose escalation with reduction in treatment-related morbidity.[163]

Surgical Imaging

Intracranial tumor therapy also is enhanced by the recent availability of surgical navigation technology, which gathers, stores, and reformats three-dimensional images of an intracranial lesion within the surgical field.[164] This intraoperative guidance system allows the surgeon to define the tumor borders for a safer and more complete resection. Complete surgical resections can be achieved in 90% of patients, with less than 10% morbidity and less than 1% mortality. Interactive systems are being devised that integrate radiologic data with the actual patient anatomy at operation.[165] These newer systems are functionally superior to previously used stereotactic devices. A recently developed "viewing wand" demonstrated excellent anatomic detail, identified critical structures, and adjusted surgical trajectories in a series of 250 patients undergoing various neurosurgical procedures.[166] The use of computed tomography or magnetic resonance imaging is superior to that of intraoperative US in characterizing deep lesions. Intraoperative navigation also provides real-time video processing with computer-generated virtual images of anatomic structures and has been successfully applied to the difficult skull-based lesions and complex craniofacial tumor operations.[167–169]

Application of these types of overlay techniques for merging radiologic data and real-time applications has been proposed as a realistic application of the use of robotics in laparoscopic procedures. Inserting a computer interface between the surgeon and the patient would allow incorporation of multiple types of data input, including radiologic scan data.

INNOVATIVE ADJUNCTIVE TECHNIQUES

Cryosurgery

The basic principle involved in cryosurgery is the in situ destruction of tissue by the freeze/thaw process. As the frozen tissue thaws, the circulation returns, and for a brief period, the tissue may appear almost normal. However, as endothelial cell damage, thrombosis, edema, and vascular stasis develop, the microcirculation progressively fails, and cell death ensues.[170] The mechanism of tissue response is multifactorial and highly dependent on the rate of cooling. When this technique is applied to cancer, the goal is to devitalize the same volume of neoplastic tissue by freezing as would have been excised with a local resection. The most important tumoricidal mechanism appears to be the rapid freezing, slow thawing, and immediate repetition of this cycle.[171]

Intraoperative US now allows precise placement into the center of tumors of vacuum-insulated cryoprobes that can monitor the progression of the freeze margin in real time.[172] Liquid nitrogen is circulated through the tip of the probe, achieving temperatures in the range of $-160°C$ to $-180°C$. Central placement of the probe is critical because the freeze ball extends symmetrically in all directions. This technique has been successfully used with lesions in the breast, liver, bladder, and prostate, as well as with intraocular tumors and benign and malignant skin lesions.

Cryosurgery was used in 60 patients with primary liver tumors, with a 5-year survival of 12%.[173] However, if the tumor was less than 6 cm in diameter, the local control was improved, and the survival rate was 38% at 5 years. In a series of 18 patients with unresectable liver metastases from colon cancer, 4 (22%) were alive without evidence of disease at a median follow-up of 29 months.[174] In a larger series of both primary and metastatic liver lesions, 110 patients were treated with cryosurgery, resulting in a local tumor control rate of 24% at a median 14-month follow-up.[175] Recent reports described a disease-free survival of as much as 23% at 18 months' mean follow-up.[176] Overall survival was achieved in 60% of patients with primary tumors. The incidence of major complications in most series is less than 5%. Leukocytosis and low-grade fevers are common. Local hemorrhage from the probe tract is easily controlled by pressure or packing with hemostatic agents. Hepatic enzyme elevation to about twice normal usually occurs and spontaneously resolves within the first postoperative week. Pleural effusion, myoglobinuria, hemorrhage, biliary leak, or abscess formation is rare.

Cryosurgery has been successfully used for aneurysmal bone cysts,[177] aggressive benign bone tumors, or low-grade malignancies.[178] Although cryosurgery offers the advantage of preserving supportive function of bone in these skeletal tumors, complications do occur. Most important, intraoperative venous gas embolism may rarely produce hemodynamically significant events.[179] It has been suggested that end-tidal nitrogen tension may be monitored intraoperatively to analyze the clinical incidence of this complication.

Radiofrequency Ablation

Radiofrequency ablation (RFA) is a technique that applies thermal energy via a probe that results in coagulation necrosis of the target tissue. The technique involves image-guided application of the probe by using primarily US guidance, and it can be introduced percutaneously, laparoscopically, or via open operative exposure. The most common applications for the technique have been for primary or metastatic hepatic lesions, renal lesions, and pulmonary lesions. Other nonmalignant lesions also have been successfully treated with this modality.

The largest experience with RFA has been with the treatment of unresectable primary liver tumors or metastasis from colorectal cancer. The mortality and morbidity rates associated with RFA of liver lesions is low, and the procedure can be safely combined with open resection of larger lesions.[180] In a recent series, 11 patients with hepatocellular carcinoma and 34 patients with unresectable secondary hepatic malignancies were treated with RFA. Treatment of lesions larger than 4 cm and the percutaneous approach were associated with higher local recurrence rates. Improved results with an open approach have been confirmed by others.[181] The 15 patients with colorectal metastasis had worse disease-free survival than did patients with other tumors.[182] In a large European study, 88 patients with 134 metastases from colorectal cancer were treated with RFA. Complete necrosis of lesions was obtained in 53 (60%) of 88 patients, but in 37 (70%), new lesions developed.[183] Series reporting treatment of renal lesions[184,185] and lung lesions[186] demonstrated the technical feasibility of RFA with acceptable complication rates, but insufficient follow-up is available to judge long-term efficacy. Treatment of pediatric tumors with RFA is largely anecdotal. A small series reporting the use of percutaneous RFA on fetuses with sacrococcygeal teratoma reported a 50% fetal mortality rate.[187] In one child treated prenatally with RFA, a severe soft tissue defect and sciatic nerve destruction were present at birth.[188]

Intracavitary Hyperthermia and Chemotherapy

Hyperthermia has a selective, often lethal, effect on neoplastic cells in vitro and in vivo.[189] High temperatures may sensitize malignant tissues to the cytotoxic effects of ionizing radiation and chemotherapy by inhibiting DNA repair and increasing cellular membrane permeability to chemotherapeutic and other agents. Thermoradiotherapy combines interstitial hyperthermia with brachytherapy and has been used to increase median survival time to 23.5 months in malignant gliomas.[190] Multivariant analysis suggested that the hyperthermia had increased the survival. A similar approach was used for recurrent malignant astrocytomas.[191] Three symptomatic patients underwent ^{192}Ir brachytherapy at a 50-Gy dose accompanied by 915-MHz microwave antenna heating for 1 hour. Two patients were symptomatically improved, and the overall survival was 7, 12, and 15 months.

Hyperthermia also has been synergistically combined with a number of chemotherapeutic agents, including doxorubicin, melphalan, cisplatin, bleomycin, and mitomycin-C.[192] The maximal cytotoxic effects are seen after a brief exposure to chemotherapy in the presence of hyperthermia. A differential response appears experimentally between malignant microvasculature and normal blood vessels.[193] Regional hyperthermia also prolongs the half-life of cisplatin after intraperitoneal administration, thereby enhancing its antitumor effects without increasing systemic toxicity. A similar strategy has been used with intrathoracic administration of cisplatin.[194]

Intracavitary installation of chemotherapeutic agents without hyperthermia has been used with a variety of pediatric solid tumors.[195] Intracavitary cisplatin at doses between 50 and 210 mg/m^2 was instilled in the chest or abdomen, with thiosulfate protection in 11 children with rhabdomyosarcoma or pulmonary tumors, including lung metastases from sarcomas. Serum levels were at least comparable to those obtained by intravenous drug administration, and resolution or improvement of effusions or ascites occurred in four patients. No intracavitary local recurrences were noted, and two patients were surviving for more than 3 years, and two other children were alive more than 8 years after diagnosis. Because most of the patients also had received systemic therapy, the exact contribution of intracavitary cisplatin to outcome could not be assessed. However, the safety of this approach was ascertained, and the low incidence of local recurrence in a group of high-risk relapsed patients suggests that direct installation of these agents may be effective in children with malignant tumors, especially in situations in which high local concentrations of chemotherapeutics would be beneficial.

Intracavitary chemotherapy and hyperthermia also have been combined in some adult settings. In one phase II study, 56 patients with various types of peritoneal carcinomatoses underwent resection of the primary tumor, peritonectomy, and intraperitoneal chemohyperthermia with mitomycin-C, cisplatinum, or both. Chemotherapy was administered via a closed sterile system with inflow temperatures ranging from 46°C to 48°C (Fig. 64-5) The 2-year survival rate was 79% for those patients in whom a complete resection was achieved and 45% in those with gross residual tumor. However, a significant morbidity was associated with the treatment with a high enteric fistula rate early and an overall morbidity

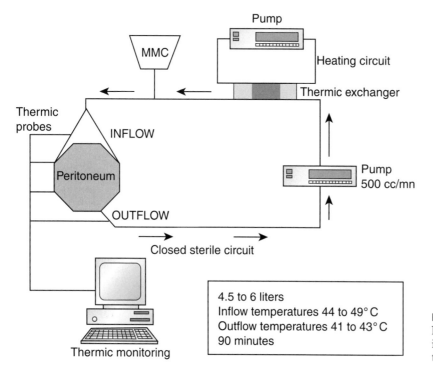

4.5 to 6 liters
Inflow temperatures 44 to 49°C
Outflow temperatures 41 to 43°C
90 minutes

FIGURE 64-5. Schematic design of system for hyperthermic intracavity chemotherapy administration. Mitomycin-C (MMC) is instilled into the peritoneal cavity at 46°C to 48°C.

rate of 28.6%.[196] Similar results have been reported by others using intraperitoneal hyperthermia with mitomycin-C alone.[197] Combined use of intracavitary chemotherapy with hyperthermia may be applicable to a number of difficult pediatric scenarios including diffuse intraperitoneal spread of desmoplastic small round blue cell tumors and pleural seeding of sarcomas. Additional studies will be necessary to identify the ideal combinations of temperature, chemotherapeutic agent, and duration of therapy for each particular tumor type.

Chemoembolization

The regional delivery of chemotherapy for hepatic tumors is possible because the liver has a dual blood supply, with the hepatic artery contributing approximately 25% of the parenchymal flow to normal cells, whereas malignant hepatic lesions derive nearly all of their blood supply from this source. This allows a selective delivery of cytotoxic agents to tumor. In addition, the liver can withstand regional dose escalation because of its ability to detoxify through "first-pass" kinetics. Whereas foreign-body embolization produced temporary arterial occlusion and transient palliative effects, the most durable responses were achieved when chemotherapeutic agents were infused distal to the ligated hepatic artery.[198] The therapeutic strategy involves infusing high concentrations of chemotherapy and prolonging the dwell time with a variety of embolic materials (Fig. 64-6). A series of adult patients with unresectable hepatocellular carcinoma demonstrated responses when chemotherapy was suspended in embolic agents.[199] When doxorubicin, mitomycin-C, and cisplatin were combined with gelatin sponge (Gelfoam), 11 of 26 patients showed a tumor reduction of greater than 50% by imaging studies without toxic mortality. If cisplatin was suspended in

lipiodal, partial tumor responses could be detected in 33 of 71 patients.[200] The same technique was used in a variety of liver tumors, including metastatic colon cancer and ocular melanoma.[201] A 23% partial response rate was noted, and the patients had a 7-month mean survival. In a large review of 800 patients from several series treated palliatively for hepatocellular carcinoma, partial response rates of 60% to 83% were noted.[202] Overall patient survival at 3 years ranged from 18% to 51%. Among 90 patients with metastatic colorectal carcinoma, some decrease in tumor size was observed in 78% to 100% of patients, whereas the 1-year survival rate was 67%.

The number of prospective randomized trials in unresectable hepatocellular carcinoma is small. A recent study compared chemoembolization with conservative therapy.[203] The 96 patients received either cisplatin suspended in lipiodal and gelatin sponge or supportive care only. Most patients receiving chemoembolization showed a significant decrease in tumor size by imaging study, lower α-fetoprotein levels, and even relief of portal obstruction compared with the conservatively treated group. Although a trend favored survival with chemoembolization, the difference was not statistically significant. Of note, in 60% of the patients in the treatment arm, liver failure developed, which parallels previous experience. Most patients treated with this method have elevation in liver-function tests, abdominal pain, nausea, vomiting, fever, ascites, suppressed hematopoiesis, and thrombocytopenia. In some patients, diabetes developed, and renal failure, in occasional patients.

The pediatric experience with chemoembolization is quite small, although isolated cases of limited success have been reported.[204,205] This technique also has been extended to hepatic malignancies in infancy.[206] Two reports of chemoembolization experience in childhood liver tumors have recently been reported.[207,208]

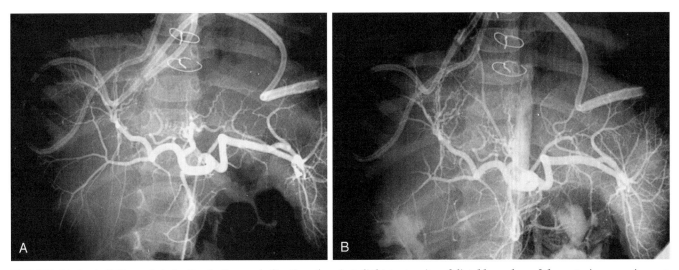

FIGURE 64-6. *A,* Celiac axis injection before embolization showing slight tortuosity of distal branches of the anterior superior segment of the right lobe, the middle hepatic artery, and the medial segment of the left lobe. (Courtesy of Philip Stanley, M.D., Pediatric Hematology-Oncology, UCLA School of Medicine, Los Angeles, California.) *B,* Postembolization injection of celiac axis showing marked peripheral attenuation of branches of the right and left lobes secondary to deposition of collagen laden with chemotherapy agent. (Courtesy of Philip Stanley, M.D., Pediatric Hematology-Oncology, UCLA School of Medicine, Los Angeles, California.)

In one series,[207] a suspension of cisplatin, doxorubicin, and mitomycin-C mixed with bovine collagen and radiopaque contrast material was used in 11 children with unresectable or recurrent lesions. Six patients had progressive hepatoblastoma, two had unresectable hepatocellular carcinoma, two had undifferentiated hepatic sarcomas, and one had chronic cirrhosis and a newly diagnosed unresectable hepatocellular carcinoma. All children except the one with cirrhosis had received previous systemic chemotherapy. The six hepatoblastoma patients had initial partial response, as measured by imaging and α-fetoprotein levels. Three patients underwent subsequent surgical resection, but one progressed and died, whereas two survived more than 15 months. The other three also eventually died of known progressive disease. Of the three children with hepatocellular carcinoma, one underwent surgical resection and was a long-term survivor for more than 65 months, one was alive with disease for more than 36 months, and one (with cirrhosis) died of progressive liver failure with no evidence of malignancy. One of the two patients with hepatic sarcoma was still alive, but he had progressive disease. Most of the patients experienced fever, nausea, vomiting, transient coagulopathy, and pain during chemoembolization. Significant toxicity developed only in the patient with cirrhosis, with a severe tumor lysis syndrome, coagulopathy, and CNS hemorrhage. In the other series,[208] 14 children received 50 courses of intra-arterial chemotherapy with cisplatin or doxorubicin (Adriamycin) or both, followed by Gelfoam embolization for hepatoblastoma (7) or hepatocellular carcinoma (7). Six of the 14 subsequently underwent orthotopic liver transplant, and 3 of the 6 died of metastatic disease. In 7 of the remaining patients, progressive disease developed, and one was awaiting transplant at the time of the report.

Overall, hepatic chemoembolization is feasible in young patients, with tolerable toxicity, and represents a reasonable therapeutic alternative in persistent, unresectable, or recurrent hepatoblastoma or in nonmetastatic hepatocellular carcinoma. Preoperative use of chemoembolization has converted an unresectable lesion to one amenable to complete resection.[209]

Injectable Gel Chemotherapy

Incorporation of chemotherapeutic agents into synthetic polymers has been developed as a technique to provide a local drug depot when the agent is injected into a tumor. The technique offers a number of attractive features including relative ease of application, high local drug levels, and prolonged drug release.[210] Several drug preparations have been synthesized to treat a number of benign and malignant conditions. Intratumoral injection of a cisplatin/epinephrine gel has been used to treat unresectable hepatocellular carcinoma. In a recent study, 58 patients were treated with four to eight injections over a 6-week period. The response rate was 53%, including 16 complete and 11 partial responses. Of these patients, in 52%, progressive disease subsequently developed in areas of untreated liver parenchyma. Median survival was 27 months.[211] In a separate report, 28 patients with

refractory or recurrent melanoma underwent injection of 244 lesions with cisplatin/epinephrine gel. Six weekly treatments were given, resulting in a 53% response rate (130 of 244 tumors). Systemic toxicity was minimal, consisting of local reactions and pain at the site.[212] Similar results have been obtained in patients with squamous cell carcinomas of the head and neck[213] and palliation of advanced stage esophageal carcinoma.[214] Use of this agent has not yet been reported in pediatric patients.

Lymphatic Mapping

Accurate staging of regional disease continues to be important in pediatric and adult tumors. The initial draining lymph node, the so-called sentinel node, is reportedly predictive of regional nodal metastases in a variety of tumors.[215] Although lymph node mapping has been applied to a number of tumors, it is most commonly used to predict nodal status of patients with melanoma or breast cancer. The technique has been refined and validated as it has evolved. In most cases, a combination of technetium-labeled sulfur colloid and lymphazurin blue dye is used to localize the sentinel node. Preoperative lymphoscintigraphy provides information regarding draining nodal basins in truncal and head and neck cases. Intraoperative lymphatic mapping is accomplished by injecting the technetium-labeled sulfur colloid at the primary tumor site 1 hour before surgery. Just before incision, the blue dye is injected and a gamma probe is used to identify areas of high counts. The underlying tissue is then examined for lymph nodes containing the blue dye. If the sentinel node has no histologic evidence of metastases, the related regional lymphatic bed is highly likely to be tumor free, and the morbidity of lymphadenectomy can be avoided. Lymphoscintigraphy is a reliable indicator of lymphatic drainage from cutaneous melanoma of the head, neck, and trunk.[216] A radiolabeled tracer of ^{99}Tc sulfur colloid or human serum albumin was injected before wide local excision of the primary lesion. Of 297 patients reviewed, 181 underwent elective dissection of the lymph node basins identified by the lymphoscintigraphy, and 27% had melanoma detected within the dissected basin. Of these, nodal metastases in 7 as their site of first recurrence, and all were within the area predicted by the original scan. The other 116 patients were observed, and in 14%, lymph node metastases developed as their first sign of recurrence. Only 1 of these patients, in whom rapidly progressive disease developed, had lymph node metastases in an area not predicted by the scan. Overall, 70 of 71 patients had documented lymphatic metastases occur in a predicted lymph node bed, confirming that cutaneous lymphoscintigraphy can be reliably used to guide therapy in high-risk melanoma.

Lymph node localization by gamma probe scanning also has been extended to breast cancer management.[217] In addition, the techniques of vital dye mapping and lymphoscintigraphy have been combined to maximize the accuracy in both melanoma and breast cancer.[218] Sentinel lymph nodes were identified in 92% of patients, and no false-negative scans were found. When blue dye and radiolocalization were combined in 110 patients with melanoma, the sentinel lymph node was identified in 99.5% of patients.[219] In this study, the method was highly accurate in detecting lymph node involvement, with a 3% false-negative rate and no false-positive results.

The implications of sentinel lymph node mapping are important in pediatric tumors such as rhabdomyosarcoma. In the Intergroup Rhabdomyosarcoma Studies I and II, the incidence of positive regional lymph nodes was 12% to 17%. However, most of these patients did not undergo lymph node sampling. More recently, when the majority of patients actually did have a lymph node biopsy, the incidence of detecting disease increased to 40%.[220] These findings also were confirmed subsequently in the Intergroup Rhabdomyosarcoma Study III, which demonstrated that when biopsies were taken of regional lymph nodes, 39% contained metastatic disease.[221] Patients with positive nodes underwent radiation therapy to the involved lymph node bed, resulting in improved survival, documenting the need for accurate lymph node staging. The technique of lymph node mapping has been successfully applied to small series of pediatric patients.[222] One of 3 patients with rhabdomyosarcoma undergoing lymph node mapping was found to have a positive node.[222] In that report, a mixed group of patients including 8 with melanoma, the sentinel node was found to contain tumor in 6 of 13 patients. Currently, the following technique is being used in children with extremity rhabdomyosarcoma. On the day before operation, the patient is injected around the palpable lesion or the previous incision site with 0.2 to 0.5 mL of ^{99}Tc sulfur colloid. Immediately before surgery, the same area is injected with 0.5 to 1.0 mL of vital blue dye. When a hand-held gamma probe is used, signal localization parallels the presence of the blue dye in the lymphatic channels leading to the sentinel lymph node. This tissue is stained blue and scans positive, and excisional biopsy is performed for histologic assessment, which should predict involvement of the remaining lymphatic bed. No therapy is necessary for negative biopsies. Histologically positive tissue leads to lymph node dissection and regional lymphatic radiation.

Radio Receptor–Guided Surgery

The concept of radioimmune-guided surgery (RIGS) incorporates the use of mAbs to tumor-associated antigens labeled with gamma-emitting isotopes.[223] The tumor is excised, and resection margins, regional lymph node sites, and remote intracavitary areas are scanned. Positive regions undergo biopsy or are removed as appropriate. Unfortunately, if the tumor is heterogeneous, much of the TAG mAb will not localize on the tumor and may have toxic systemic effects.[224] These concerns may be exacerbated by variable antibody distribution and binding affinity.

A wide variety of endocrine tumors such as carcinoid, insulinoma, pheochromocytoma, medullary carcinoma of the thyroid, small cell carcinoma of the lung, neuroblastoma, and medulloblastoma contain high-affinity receptors for somatostatin.[225] Radiolabeled somatostatin offers a possible useful tool for tumor localization and staging. Octreotide, an octapeptide analogue of somatostatin, has a more clinically useful half-life than the native compound and provides superior receptor-binding affinity and more favorable clearance characteristics to enhance the ratio of tumor to background distribution.[226] Iodine 123 (^{123}I)-labeled analogues are poorly visualized in the upper abdomen because of hepatobiliary excretion. Therefore techniques using an indium 111 (^{111}In) label have been developed.[227]

Of particular importance in pediatric tumors is the elevated expression of neuropeptide-receptor genes in neuroblastoma, such that 90% of patients with this tumor have visualization by ^{111}In-labeled octreotide scintigraphy.[228] The level of uptake matches that seen with ^{131}I-labeled metaiodobenzylguanidine radionuclide scanning. The prognostic significance of somatostatin binding also has become apparent, in that receptor expression may be downregulated in more aggressive tumors.[229] All patients who demonstrated high-affinity receptors on their tumors survive, whereas 60% of those who were receptor negative died.[230] In confirmatory studies, receptor-positive patients had a median relapse-free survival of 23 months compared with receptor-negative patients, who all rapidly progressed and died.[231]

An approach to take advantage of these characteristics would be to combine the diagnostic imaging provided by somatostatin-receptor expression with the radioimmune-guided surgical methods of intraoperative detection of occult tumor. Because high-affinity receptors have been identified on both primary and metastatic neuroblastoma, radiolabeled analogues could improve anatomic staging of disease, define surgical margins of resection, and ensure that occult tumor sites are detected and removed. To test this hypothesis, six children with Evans stage 3 or 4 neuroblastoma underwent operation after receiving systemic administration of ^{125}I-tyr^3-octreotide.[232] Tissue that was grossly suggestive of tumor or was gamma probe scanning positive was excised. Binding of octreotide to the malignant tissue was detected in the five children with known neuroblastoma and documented by histopathology, immunohistochemistry, and microautoradiography. Intra-abdominal uptake occurred within 15 minutes, was greatest in the hepatobiliary system, and decreased over a 24-hour period. Viable neuroblastoma was detected in 15 of 17 sites with radioreceptor binding. Four of these specimens in three children were from unexpected occult sites of malignancy. Seven other specimens demonstrated no binding, and five of these were negative by histopathology. RIGS was 100% sensitive and 71% specific in neuroblastoma and may provide a useful technique to determine tumor stage and an assessment of completeness of surgical excision.

Photodynamic Therapy

Photodynamic therapy (PDT) uses a photosensitizing agent and light to kill cells. The photosensitizer hematoporphyrin derivative (HPD) is retained in tumor cells longer than normal tissue,[233] making treatment of malignant lesions feasible. The HPD is activated by specific wavelengths of light that cause the molecule to react with oxygen to create singlet oxygen, which has the capability of killing cells. The depth of tissue penetration increases with increasing wavelength of light but remains limited. Therefore the technique is most useful in treating superficial spreading lesions such as pleural or peritoneal disease. The patient is administered the photosensitizing agent before the operation. In the operating room, the area to be treated is exposed, and the tissues are treated with an appropriate light source. Accumulation of the HPD in the skin results in severe skin sensitivity to sunlight for as long as 80 days after treatment. Special precautions must be taken to minimize the patient's exposure to light during this time.

PDT has not been used in children, but several clinical trials in adults have been reported. In a phase II trial, 21 patients with mesothelioma were treated with PDT.[234] In 50% of patients, postoperative complications included fever, fluid requirements, ventilatory support, superior vena cava syndrome, and a bronchopleural fistula. The most prolonged survival was in stage 1 and 2 disease. PDT has been used to treat a number of other malignancies including head and neck, lung, brain, mesothelioma, bladder, and esophageal carcinoma. Potential applications in pediatric tumors include pleural or peritoneal seeding from sarcomas, but the clinical application of the technique is cumbersome and would require extensive preparation in both the operating room and the intensive care unit.

Minimally Invasive Imaging

Appropriate management of liver neoplasms requires the accurate detection of all intrahepatic masses. Despite an array of noninvasive external imaging techniques, 20% to 40% of all such lesions are missed.[235] Intraoperative US is considered an accurate modality for detection of these occult tumors. Sonography was used at operation in 45 patients with liver neoplasms, 80% of which were metastatic disease.[236] This intraoperative method identified 97% of the lesions that were ultimately diagnosed, whereas routine inspection and palpation found 78%, and preoperative imaging detected 67% of the tumors. The planned operative strategy was changed in half of the patients, and in 19 of these, the change was based primarily on the intraoperative US findings.

Because the use of intraoperative imaging has had an impact on the management of hepatic, biliary, and pancreatic surgical operations, applications have been developed to provide US for minimally invasive surgical procedures. This strategy is important because thoracoscopy and laparoscopy are increasingly performed, and accurate imaging could shorten operative time, reduce tissue manipulation and damage, facilitate surgical decisions, and perhaps reduce the operative complication rate. The feasibility of US-guided laparoscopic cryosurgical treatment of hepatic tumors has been reported.[237] Laparoscopic intraoperative US has been primarily restricted by the location and size of the access ports through which the transducer is placed. The configuration and depth of the field of view is critical, and a square view field is optimal.[238] Addition of a Doppler signal would provide audio information and spectral analysis display regarding flow and velocity characteristics of vascular structures. The color Doppler provides directional flow information and allows differentiation of vascular structures from those that are ductal or cystic.

Experience with a rigid transducer probe during minimal-access surgical procedures in 176 patients demonstrated successful target-organ visualization in more than 80% of cases.[239] Scanning at a frequency of 5 to 7.5 MHz allows a 10- to 12-cm depth of penetration for viewing. The development of angulating ultrasonic probes provides greater flexibility for surgical manipulation. A new convex scanner can be placed through a 10-mm trocar site and has the capability to be angled 90 degrees upward and 45 degrees downward.[240] The inclusion of real-time sonography and color flow Doppler facilitates imaging examination of the liver, biliary tree, pancreas, spleen, and virtually all other intra-abdominal organs. Most recently, technical innovations have allowed development of a three-dimensional imaging modality that can be used during laparoscopy. For example, simultaneous real-time magnetic resonance imaging can now be undertaken through the laparoscope.[241] Dynamic gadolinium-enhanced viewing also can be provided. This imaging guidance would allow interstitial laser therapy of lesions in solid organs to be undertaken. Because this has now been successfully performed in animal models, the method can be introduced into clinical practice in an appropriate investigational setting.

This chapter emphasized the adjunctive treatment strategies that may accompany surgical procedures in the management of neoplastic disease. Systemic, cytotoxic, and immune therapies may provide response, long-term survival, or cure by eradicating micrometastases. In addition, a variety of ionizing radiation techniques and other innovations may provide local tumor control as a part of the overall treatment plan.

REFERENCES

1. Bleyer WA: The impact of childhood cancer on the United States and the world. CA Cancer J Clin 40:355, 1990.
2. Farber S, et al: Temporary remissions in acute leukemia in children produced by folic acid antagonist, 4-aminopteroyl-glutamic acid (aminopterin). N Engl J Med 238:787, 1948.
3. Li MC, Hertz R, Spencer D, et al: Effect of methotrexate upon choriocarcinoma and chorioadenoma. Proc Soc Exp Biol Med 93:361, 1956.
4. Frei E III, Freireich EJ, Gehan E, et al: Studies of sequential and combination antimetabolite therapy in acute leukemia: 6-Mercaptopurine and methotrexate. Blood 18:431, 1961.
5. Green DM, Jaffe N: Wilms' tumor: Model of a curable pediatric malignant solid tumor. Cancer Treat Rev 5:143, 1978.
6. D'Angio GJ, Evans AE, Breslow N, et al: The treatment of Wilms' tumor: Results of the National Wilms' Tumor Study. Cancer 38:647, 1976.
7. Link MP, et al: The effect of adjuvant chemotherapy on relapse-free survival in patients with osteosarcoma of the extremity. N Engl J Med 314:1600, 1986.
8. Schwenn MR, Blattner SR, et al: HiC-COM: A 2 month intensive chemotherapy regimen for children with stage III and IV Burkitt's lymphoma and B-cell acute lymphoblastic leukemia. J Clin Oncol 9:133–138, 1991.

9. Cheung NK, Heller G: Chemotherapy dose intensity correlates strongly with response, median survival and median progression-free survival in metastatic neuroblastoma. J Clin Oncol 9:1050–1058, 1991.

10. Antman K, Ayash L, Elias A, et al: A phase II study of high dose cyclophosphamide, thiotepa, and carboplatin with autologous marrow support in women with measurable advanced breast cancer responding to standard therapy. J Clin Oncol 10:102–110, 1992.

11. Grier H, Krailo M, Link M, et al: Improved outcome in non-metastatic Ewing's sarcoma and PNET of bone with the addition of ifosfamide and etoposide to vincristine, Adriamycin, cyclophosphamide, and actinomycin: A Children's Cancer Group and Pediatric Oncology Group report. J Clin Oncol 13(suppl):421, 1994.

12. Clark PI, Slevin ML, Joel SP, et al: A randomized trial of two etoposide schedules in small-cell lung cancer: The influence of pharmacokinetics on efficacy and toxicity. J Clin Oncol 12:1427–1435, 1994.

13. Worth L, Jeha S, Kleinerman E: Biologic response modifiers in pediatric cancer. Hematol Oncol Clin North Am 15:723, 2001.

14. Parker SL, Tong T, Bolden S, et al: Cancer statistics, 1997. CA Cancer J Clin 47:5–27, 1997.

15. Gurney JG, Severson RK, Davis S, et al: Incidence of cancer in children in the United States. Cancer 75:2186–2195, 1995.

16. Miller BA, Ries LA, Hankey BF, et al. (eds): SEER Cancer Statistics Review 1973-1990. NCI Publ No. (NIH) 93–2789. Bethesda, MD: NCI, 1993.

17. Linet M, Ries A, Smith M, et al: Cancer surveillance series: Recent trends in childhood cancer incidence and mortality in the United States. J Natl Cancer Inst 91:1051, 1999.

18. Bleyer WA: The U.S. Pediatric Cancer Clinical Trials Programmes: International implications and the way forward. Eur J Cancer 33:1439, 1997.

19. Reis LAG, Eisner MP, Kosary CL, et al: SEER Cancer Statistics Review 1975-2000. Bethesda, MD, NCI, http://seer.cancer.gov/csr/1975–2000, 2003.

20. Green DM, Breslow NE, Beckwith JB, et al: Effect of duration of treatment on treatment outcome and cost of treatment for Wilms' tumor: A report from the National Wilms' Tumor Study Group. J Clin Oncol 16:3744, 1998.

21. Nowell P, Hungerford D: A minute chromosome in human chronic granulocytic leukemia. Science 132:1497, 1960.

22. Kreissman SG: Molecular genetics: Toward an understanding of childhood cancer. Semin Pediatr Surg 2:2–10, 1993.

23. Brodeur GM: Neuroblastoma: Clinical applications of molecular parameters. Brain Pathol 1:45, 1990.

24. Pinkel D, Gray JW, Trask B, et al: Cytogenetic analysis by in-vitro hybridization with fluorescently labeled nucleic acid probes. Cold Spring Harbor Symp Quant Biol 51:151–157, 1986.

25. MacGregor PF: Gene expression in cancer: The application of microarrays. Expert Rev Mol Diagn 3:185, 2003.

26. Henderson EH, Samaha RJ: Evidence that drugs in multiple combinations have materially advanced the treatment of human malignancies. Cancer Res 29:2272, 1969.

27. Goldie JH, Coldman AJ: A mathematic model for relating the drug sensitivity of tumors to the spontaneous mutation rate. Cancer Treat Rep 63:1727, 1979.

28. Pratt CB, Horowitz ME, Meyer WH, et al: A phase II trial of ifosfamide in the children with malignant solid tumors. Cancer Treat Rep 71:131–135, 1987.

29. Miser JS, Kinsella TJ, Triche TJ, et al: Ifosfamide with mesna uroprotection and etoposide: An effective regimen in the treatment of recurrent sarcomas and other tumors of children and young adults. J Clin Oncol 5:1191–1198, 1987.

30. Balis FM, Holcenberg JS, Poplack DG: General principles of chemotherapy. In Pizzo P, Poplack D (eds): Principles and Practice of Pediatric Oncology, 3rd ed. Philadelphia, Lippincott-Raven, 1997, pp 216.

31. D'Angio GJ, Evans AE, Breslow N, et al: The treatment of Wilms' tumor: Results of the National Wilms' Tumor Study. Cancer 38:633, 1976.

32. Green DM, Breslow NE, Evans I, et al: The effect of chemotherapy dose intensity on the hematological toxicity of treatment for Wilms' tumor: A report from the National Wilms' Tumor Study. Am J Pediatr Hematol Oncol 16:207–212, 1994.

33. Picci P, Rougraff BT, Bacci G, et al: Prognostic significance of histopathologic response to chemotherapy in nonmetastatic Ewing's sarcoma of the extremities. J Clin Oncol 11:1763, 1993.

34. Provisor AJ, Ettinger LJ, Nachman JB, et al: Treatment of non-metastatic osteosarcoma of the extremity with preoperative and postoperative chemotherapy: A report from the Children's Cancer Group. J Clin Oncol 15:76, 1997.

35. Slevin ML, Clark PI, Joel SP, et al: A randomized trial to evaluate the effect of schedule on the activity of etoposide in small-cell lung cancer. J Clin Oncol 7:1333–1340, 1989.

36. Thompson DS, Hainsworth JD, Hande KR, et al: Prolonged administration of low-dose infusional etoposide in patients with etoposide-sensitive neoplasms: A phase I/II study. J Clin Oncol 11:1322–1328, 1993.

37. Chamberlain MC, Grafe MR: Recurrent chiasmatic-hypothalamic glioma treated with oral etoposide. J Clin Oncol 13:2072–2076, 1995.

38. Woods WG, Kobrinsky N, Buckley JD, et al: Timed-sequential induction therapy improves postremission outcome in acute myeloid leukemia: A report from the Children's Cancer Group. Blood 87:4979, 1996.

39. Campbell LA, Seeger RC, Harris RE, et al: Escalating doses of continuous infusion combination chemotherapy for refractory neuroblastoma. J Clin Oncol 11:623, 1993.

40. Stram DO, Matthay KK, O'Leary M, et al: Consolidation chemoradiotherapy and autologous bone marrow transplant versus continued chemotherapy for metastatic neuroblastoma: A report of two concurrent Children's Cancer Group Studies. J Clin Oncol 14:2417, 1996.

41. Hryniuk W, Levine MN: Analysis of dose intensity for adjuvant chemotherapy trials in stage II breast cancer. J Clin Oncol 4:1162, 1986.

42. Frei E, Canellos GP: Dose: A critical factor in cancer chemotherapy. Am J Med 69:585, 1980.

43. Skipper H: Data and Analysis Having To Do with the Influence of Dose Intensity and Duration of Treatment (Single Drugs and Combinations) on Lethal Toxicity and the Therapeutic Response of Experimental Neoplasms. Booklets 13 and 2-13. Birmingham, Ala: Southern Research Institute, 1986, 1987.

44. Gaynon P, Steinherz P, Bleyer WA, et al: Association of delivered drug dose and outcome for children with acute lymphoblastic leukemia and unfavorable presenting features. Med Pediatr Oncol 19:221, 1991.

45. Bacci G, Picci P, Avella M, et al: The importance of dose-intensity in neoadjuvant chemotherapy of osteosarcoma: A retrospective analysis of high-dose methotrexate, cisplatinum and Adriamycin used preoperatively. J Chemother 2:127, 1990.

46. Broun R, Nichols CR, Kneebone P, et al: Long-term outcome of patients with relapsed and refractory germ cell tumors treated with high-dose chemotherapy and autologous bone marrow rescue. Ann Intern Med 117:124–128, 1992.

47. Smith MA, Ungerleider RS, Horowitz ME, et al: Influence of doxorubicin dose intensity on response and outcome for patients with osteogenic sarcoma and Ewing's sarcoma. J Natl Cancer Inst 83:1460–1470, 1991.

48. Kaye SB, Lewis CR, Dave J, et al: A randomized study of two doses of cisplatin and cyclophosphamide in epithelial ovarian cancer. Lancet 340:678, 1992.

49. Collins C, Mortimer J, Livingston RB, et al: High dose cyclophosphamide in the treatment of refractory lymphomas and solid tumor malignancies. Cancer 63:228–232, 1989.

50. Crist WM, Garnsey L, Beltangody MS, et al: Prognosis in children with rhabdomyosarcoma: A report of the Intergroup Rhabdomyosarcoma Studies I and II. J Clin Oncol 8:443–452, 1990.

51. Householder SE, Rackoff W, Goldman J, et al: A case-control retrospective study of the efficacy of granulocyte colony stimulating factor in children with neuroblastoma. Am J Pediatr Hematol Oncol 16:132, 1994.

52. Tepler I, Elias L, Smith JW II, et al: A randomized placebo-controlled trial of recombinant human interleukin-11 in cancer patients with severe thrombocytopenia due to chemotherapy. Blood 87:3607, 1996.

53. Lipshultz SE: Dexrazoxane for protection against cardiotoxic effects of anthracyclines in children. J Clin Oncol 14:328, 1996.

54. Lasky L, Fox S, Smith J, et al: Collection and use of peripheral blood stem cells in very small children. Bone Marrow Transplant 7:281–284, 1991.

55. Takaue Y, Watanabe T, Kawano Y, et al: Isolation and storage of peripheral blood hematopoietic stem cells for autotransplantation into children with cancer. Blood 74:1245–1251, 1989.

56. Fukuda M, Kojima S, Matsumoto K, et al: Autotransplantation of peripheral blood stem cells mobilized by chemotherapy and recombinant human granulocyte colony-stimulating factor in childhood neuroblastoma and non-Hodgkin's lymphoma. Br J Haematol 80:327–331, 1992.

57. Kreissman S, Moss T, Breitfeld P, et al: Repeated peripheral blood stem cell collection and infusion is feasible in pediatric neuroblastoma as support for rapidly administered cycles of dose intensive chemotherapy. J Clin Oncol 15(suppl):460, 1996.

58. Jakacki R, Jamison C, Heifetz S, et al: Feasibility of sequential high-dose chemotherapy and peripheral blood stem cell support for pediatric central nervous system malignancies. Med Pediatr Oncol 29:553–559, 1997.

59. Kreissman SG, Seeger RC, Stram DO, et al: Peripheral blood stem cell (PBSC) support for multiple cycles of dose intensive chemotherapy for stage IV neuroblastoma is feasible with little risk of tumor contamination: A Children's Cancer Group report. Proc Am Soc Clin Oncol 2303, 2000.

60. Matthay K, Villablanca J, Seeger R, et al. Treatment of high-risk neuroblastoma with intensive chemotherapy, radiotherapy, autologous bone marrow transplantation, and 13-cis-retinoic acid. Children's Cancer Group. N Engl J Med 341:1165, 1999.

61. Grupp S, Stern J, Bunin N, et al. Tandem high-dose therapy in rapid sequence for children with high-risk neuroblastoma. J Clin Oncol.18:2567, 2000.

62. Kletzel M, Katzenstein H, Haut P, et al: Treatment of high-risk neuroblastoma with triple-tandem high-dose therapy and stem-cell rescue: Results of the Chicago Pilot II Study. J Clin Oncol 20:2284, 2002.

63. Beeram M, Patnaik A: Targeting intracellular signal transduction: A new paradigm for a brave new world of molecularly targeted therapeutics. Hematol Oncol Clin North Am 16:1089, 2002.

64. Kreissman SG, Rackoff W, Lee M, et al: High dose cyclophosphamide with carboplatin: A tolerable regimen suitable for dose intensification in children with solid tumors. J Pediatr Hematol Oncol 19:309, 1997.

65. Gordon MS, McCaskill-Stevens WJ, Battiato LA, et al: A phase I trial of recombinant human interleukin 11 (Neumega rgIL-11 growth factor) in women with breast cancer receiving chemotherapy. Blood 87:3615, 1996.

66. Ali-Nazir A, Davenport G, Reaman G, et al: A phase I/II trial of rhIL-11 following ifosfamide, carboplatin, and etoposide (ICE) chemotherapy in pediatric patients with solid tumors or lymphoma. J Clin Oncol 15(suppl):274, 1996.

67. Sonis S, Muska A, O'Brien J, et al: Alterations in the frequency, severity, and duration of chemotherapy induced mucositis in hamsters by interleukin-11. Eur J Cancer 31:261, 1995.

68. Kemp G, Rose P, Lurain J, et al: Amifostine pretreatment for protection against cyclophosphamide-induced and cisplatin-induced toxicities: Results of a randomized control trial in patients with advanced ovarian cancer. J Clin Oncol 14:2101, 1996.

69. Shaw IC, Graham MI: Mesna: A short review. Cancer Treat Rev 14:67, 1987.

70. Moritz T, MacKay W, Glassner B, et al: Retrovirus-mediated expression of DNA repair protein in bone marrow protects hematopoietic cells from nitrosourea-induced toxicity in vitro and in vivo. Cancer Res 55:2608, 1995.

71. Oberfield SE, Allen JC, Pollack J, et al: A Long-term endocrine sequelae after treatment of medulloblastoma: Prospective study of growth and thyroid function. J Pediatr 108:219, 1986.

72. Huma Z, Boulad F, Black P, et al: Growth in children after bone marrow transplantation for acute leukemia. Blood 86:819, 1995.

73. Larson DL, Kroll S, Jaffe N, et al: Long-term effects of radiotherapy in childhood and adolescence. Am J Surg 160:348, 1990.

74. Haupt R, Fears T, Robison L, et al: Educational attainment in long-term survivors of childhood acute lymphoblastic leukemia. JAMA 272:1427, 1994.

75. Mitby PA, Robison LL, Whitton JA, et al: Utilization of special education services and educational attainment among long-term survivors of childhood cancer: A report from the Childhood Cancer Survivor Study. Cancer 97:1115, 2003.

76. Whitehead E, Shalet SM, Morris-Jones PH, et al: Gonadal function after combination chemotherapy for Hodgkin's disease in childhood. Arch Dis Child 57:287, 1982.

77. Green DM, Zevon MA, Lowrie G, et al: Congenital anomalies in children of patients who received chemotherapy for cancer in childhood or adolescence. N Engl J Med 325:141, 1991.

78. Legha SS, Benjamin RS, Mackay B, et al: Reduction of doxorubicin cardiotoxicity by prolonged continuous infusion. Ann Intern Med 96:133, 1982.

79. Nicholson HS, Mulvihill JJ: Late effects of therapy in survivors of childhood and adolescent osteosarcoma. Cancer Treat Res 62:45, 1993.

80. Gurney J, Kaden-Lottick N, Packer R, et al. Endocrine and cardiovascular late effects among adult survivors of childhood brain tumors: Childhood Cancer Survivors Study. Cancer 97:663, 2003.

81. Mertens A, Yasui Y, Lui Y, et al. Pulmonary complications in survivors of childhood and adolescent cancer: A report from the Childhood Cancer Survivors Study. Cancer 95:2431, 2002.

82. Ginsberg SJ, Comis RL: The pulmonary toxicity of antineoplastic agents. Semin Oncol 9:34, 1982.

83. Blatt J, Copeland DR, Bleyer WA: Late effects of childhood cancer and its treatment. In Pizzo PA, Poplack DG, (eds): Principles and Practice of Pediatric Oncology, 3rd ed. Philadelphia, Lippincott-Raven, 1997, p 1303.

84. Green DM, Zevon MA, Reese PA, et al: Second malignant tumors following treatment during childhood and adolescence. Med Pediatr Oncol 22:1, 1994.

85. Bhatia S, Robison LL, Oberlin O, et al: Breast cancer and other second neoplasm after childhood Hodgkin's disease. N Engl J Med 334:745, 1996.

86. Jenkin D, Greenberg M, Fitzgerald A: Second malignant tumours in childhood Hodgkin's disease. Med Pediatr Oncol 26:373, 1996.

87. Sankila R, Garwicz S, Olsen JH, et al: Risk of subsequent malignant neoplasms among 1,641 Hodgkin's disease patients diagnosed in childhood and adolescence: A population-based cohort study in the five Nordic countries. J Clin Oncol 14:1442, 1996.

88. Smith MB, Xue H, Strong L, et al: Forty year experience with second malignancies after treatment of childhood cancer: Analysis of outcome following the development of the second malignancy. J Pediatr Surg 28:1342, 1993.

89. Smith MA, Rubinstein L, Ungerleider RS: Therapy-related acute myeloid leukemia following treatment with epipodophyllotoxins: Estimating the risks. Med Pediatr Oncol 23:86, 1994.

90. Salomon D, Brandt R, Ciardiello F, et al. Epidermal growth factor-related peptides and their receptors in human malignancies. Crit Rev Oncol Hematol 19:183, 1995.

91. Baselga J: New therapeutic agents targeting the epidermal growth factor receptor. J Clin Oncol 18:54, 2000.

92. Ciardiello F, Caputo R, Bianco R, et al: Inhibition of growth factor production and angiogenesis in human cancer cells by zD1839, a selective epidermal growth factor receptor kinase inhibitor. Clin Cancer Res 7:1459, 2001.

93. Meyers M, Shen W, Spengler B, et al. Increased epidermal growth factor receptor in multi-drug resistant human neuroblastoma cells. J Cell Biochem 38:87, 1988.

94. De Giovanni C, Landuzzi L, Frabett F, et al. Antisense epidermal growth factor receptor transfection impairs proliferative ability in human rhabdomyosarcoma cells. Cancer Res 56:3898, 1996.

95. Bredel M, Pollack I, Hamilton J, et al. Epidermal growth factor receptor expression and gene amplification in high grade non-brainstem gliomas of childhood. Clin Cancer Res 5:1786, 1999.

96. Drevs J, Laus C, Medinger M, et al. Antiangiogenesis: Current clinical data and future perspectives. Onkologie 25:520, 2002.

97. Rodenhuis S: ras and human tumors. Cancer Biol 3:169, 1992.

98. Adjei A, Croghan G, Erlichman C, et al. A phase I trial of farnesyl protein transferase inhibitor R115777 in combination with gemcitabine and cisplatin in patients with advanced cancer. Clin Cancer Res 9:2520–2526, 2003.

99. Zujewski J, Horak I, Bol R, et al: Phase I and pharmacokinetic study of farnesyl protein transferase inhibitor R115777 in advanced cancer. J Clin Oncol 18:927, 2000.

100. Schellens J, de Clerk G, Swart M, et al: Phase I and pharmacokinetic study with novel farnesyl protein transferase inhibitor (FTI) R115777. 36th Annual Meeting of the American Society of Clinical Oncologists (New Orleans) 2000, 19:ASCO.

101. Johnston S, Ellis P, Houston S, et al: A phase II study of the farnesyl transferase inhibitor R115777 in patients with advanced breast cancer. 36th Annual Meeting of the American Society of Clinical Oncologists (New Orleans) 2000, 19:ASCO.

102. Lancet J, Rosenblatt J, Liesveld D, et al: Use of farnesyl transferase inhibitor R115777 in relapsed and refractory leukemias: Preliminary results of a phase I trial. 36th Annual Meeting of the American Society of Clinical Oncologists (New Orleans) 2000, 19:ASCO.

103. Gallo G, Giarnieri E, Bosco S, et al. Aberrant bcl-2 and bax protein expression related to chemotherapy response in neuroblastoma. Anticancer Res 23:777, 2003.

104. Hahne M, Rimoldi D, Schroter M, et al: Melanoma cell expression of Fas (Apo-1/CD95) ligand: Implications for tumor immune escape. Science 274:1363, 1996.

105. Restifo NP, Snzol M: Cancer vaccines. In DeVita VT, Hellman S, Rosenberg SA (eds): Cancer: Principles and Practice of Oncology, 5th ed. Philadelphia, Lippincott-Raven, 1997, p 3033.

106. Helling F, Zhang S, Shang A, et al: GM2-KLH conjugate vaccine: Increased immunogenicity in melanoma patients after administration with immunological adjuvant QS-21. Cancer Res 55:2783, 1995.

107. Hock RA, Reynolds BD, Tucker-McClung CL, et al: Murine neuroblastoma vaccines produced by retroviral transfer of MHC class II genes. Cancer Gene Ther 3:314, 1996.

108. Dranoff G, Jaffee E, Lazenby A, et al: Vaccination with irradiated tumor cells engineered to secrete murine granulocyte-macrophage colony stimulating factor stimulates potent, specific, and long-lasting anti-tumor immunity. Proc Natl Acad Sci U S A 90:3539, 1993.

109. Uchiyama A, Hoon DSB, Morisaki T, et al: Transfection of interleukin-2 gene into human melanoma cells augments cellular immune response. Cancer Res 53:949, 1991.

110. Rousseau R, Haight A, Hirschmann-Jax C, et al: Local and systemic effects of an allogeneic tumor cell vaccine combining transgenic human lymphotactin with interleukin-2 in patients with advanced or refractory neuroblastoma. Blood 101:1718, 2003.

111. Kleinerman E, Raymond A, Bucana C, et al: Unique histological changes in the lung metastases of osteosarcoma patients following therapy with liposomal muramyl tripeptide (CGP 1983A lipid). Cancer Immunol Immunother 34:211, 1992.

112. Rosenberg SA: Principles of cancer management: Biologic therapy. In DeVita VT, Hellman S, Rosenberg SA (eds): Cancer: Principles and Practice of Oncology, 5th ed. Philadelphia, Lippincott-Raven, 1997, p 364.

113. Ziegler MM, Ishizu H, Nagabuchi E, et al: A comparative review of the immunobiology of murine neuroblastoma and human neuroblastoma. Cancer 79:1757, 1997.

114. Cheung NK, Burch L, Kushner BH, et al: Monoclonal antibody 3F8 can effect durable remissions in neuroblastoma patients refractory to chemotherapy: A phase II trial. In Evans AE, D'Angio GJ, Knudson AG, et al. (eds): Advances in Neuroblastoma Research. New York, Wiley-Liss, 1991, p 395.

115. Frost JD, Hank JA, Reahman GH, et al: A phase I/IB trial of murine monoclonal anti-GD2 antibody 14.G2a plus interleukin-2 in children with refractory neuroblastoma: A report of the Children's Cancer Group. Cancer 80:317, 1997.

116. Handgretinger R, Anderson K, Lang P, et al: A phase I study of human mouse chimeric antiganglioside GD2 antibody ch14.18 in patients with neuroblastoma. Eur J Cancer 31A:261–267, 1995.

117. Ambinder R: Posttransplant lymphoproliferative disease: Pathogenesis, monitoring, and therapy. Curr Oncol Rep 5:359, 2003.

118. Shimoni A, Hardan I, Avigdor A: Rituximab reduces relapse risk after allogeneic and autologous stem cell transplantation in patients with high-risk aggressive non-Hodgkin's lymphoma. Br J Haematol 122:457, 2003.

119. Hinman L, Hamann P, Wallace R, et al: Preparation and characterization of monoclonal antibody conjugates of the calicheamicins: A novel and potent family of antitumor antibiotics. Cancer Res 53:3336, 1993.

120. Sievers E, Appelbaum F, Spielberger R, et al. Selective ablation of acute myeloid leukemia using antibody-targeted chemotherapy: A phase I study of an anti-CD33 calicheamicin immunoconjugate. Blood 93:3678, 1999.

121. Bertsch H, Rudoler S, Needle MN, et al: Emergent/urgent irradiation in pediatric oncology: Patterns of presentation, treatment, and outcome. Med Pediatr Oncol 30:101, 1998.

122. Eisbruch A, Lichter AS: What a surgeon needs to know about radiation. Ann Surg Oncol 4:516, 1997.

123. Liu L, Glicksman AS: The role of radiation in the management of soft tissue sarcoma. Med Health RI 80:32, 1997.

124. Temple WJ, Temple CLF, Arthur K, et al: Prospective cohort study of neoadjuvant treatment in conservative surgery of soft tissue sarcomas. Ann Surg Oncol 4:586, 1997.

125. Lindberg RD, Martin RG, Romsdahl MM, et al: Conservative surgery and postoperative radiotherapy in 300 adults with soft-tissue sarcomas. Cancer 47:2391, 1981.

126. Fryer CJH: Principles of pediatric radiation oncology. In Holland JF, Frei E, Bast RC, et al. (eds): Cancer Medicine. Baltimore, Williams & Wilkins, 1996, pp 2899–2905.

127. Harrison LB, Franzese F, Gaynor JJ, et al: Long-term results of a prospective randomized trial of adjuvant brachytherapy in the management of completely resected soft tissue sarcomas of the extremity and superficial trunk. Int J Radiat Oncol Biol Phys 27:259, 1993.

128. Donaldson S, Breneman J, Asmar L, et al: Hyperfractionated radiation in children with rhabdomyosarcoma: Results of an intergroup rhabdomyosarcoma pilot study. Int J Radiat Oncol Biol Phys 32:903, 1995.

129. Healey EA, Shamberger RC, Grier HE, et al: A 10-year experience of pediatric brachytherapy. Int J Radiat Oncol Biol Phys 32:451, 1995.

130. Fontanesi J, Pappo AS, Parham DM, et al: Role of irradiation in management of synovial sarcoma: St. Jude Children's Research Hospital experience. Med Pediatr Oncol 26:264, 1996.

131. Nag S, Grecula J, Ruymann FB: Aggressive chemotherapy, organ-preserving surgery, and high-dose-rate remote brachytherapy in the treatment of rhabdomyosarcoma in infants and young children. Cancer 72:2769, 1993.

132. Nag S, Olson T, Ruymann F, et al: High-dose-rate brachytherapy in childhood sarcomas: A local control strategy preserving bone growth and function. Med Pediatr Oncol 25:463, 1995.

133. Nag S, Martinez-Monge R, Ruyman F, et al: Innovation in the management of soft tissue sarcomas in infants and young children: High dose brachytherapy. J Clin Oncol 15:3075, 1997.

134. Merchant TE, Parsh N, del Valle PL, et al: Brachytherapy for pediatric soft-tissue sarcoma. Int J Radiat Oncol Biol Phys 46:427, 2000.

135. Starshak RJ: Radiation-induced meningioma in children: Report of two cases and review of the literature. Pediatr Radiol 26:537, 1996.

136. Kaschten B, Flandroy P, Reznik M, et al: Radiation-induced gliosarcoma: Case report and review of the literature. J Neurosurg 83:154, 1995.

137. Nag S, Tippin D, Ruymann FB: Long-term morbidity in children treated with fractionated high dose rate brachytherapy for soft tissue tumors. J Pediatr Hematol Oncol 25:448, 2003.

138. Merrick HW, Dobelbower RR, Konski AA: Intraoperative radiation therapy for pancreatic, biliary and gastric carcinoma: The U.S. experience. Front Radiat Ther Oncol 25:246, 1991.

139. Zelefsky MJ, LaQuaglia MP, Ghavimi F, et al: Preliminary results of phase I/II study of high-dose-rate intraoperative radiation therapy for pediatric tumors. J Surg Oncol. 62:267, 1996.

140. Haase GM, Meagher DP Jr, McNeely LK, et al: Electron beam intraoperative radiation therapy for pediatric neoplasms. Cancer 74:740, 1994.

141. Merchant TE, Zelefsky MJ, Sheldon JM, et al: High-dose rate intraoperative radiation therapy for pediatric solid tumors. Med Pediatr Oncol 30:34 1998.

142. Leavey PJ, Odom LF, Poole M, et al: Intra-operative radiation therapy in pediatric neuroblastoma. Med Pediatr Oncol 28:424, 1997.

143. Haas-Kogan DA, Fisch BM, Wara WM, et al: Intraoperative radiation therapy for high-risk pediatric neuroblastoma. Int J Radiat Oncol Biol Phys 47:985, 2000.

144. Aitken D, Hopkins G, Archambeau J, et al: Intraoperative radiotherapy in the treatment of neuroblastoma: Report of a pilot study. Ann Surg Oncol 2:343, 1994.

145. Schomberg PJ, Gunderson LL, Moir CR, et al: Intraoperative electron irradiation in the management of pediatric malignancies. Cancer 79:2251, 1997.

146. Archambeau JO, Aitkin D, Potts TM, et al: Cost-effective, available-on-demand intraoperative radiation therapy. Int J Radiat Oncol Biol Phys 15:775, 1988.

147. Sindelar WF, Hoekstra HJ, Kinsella TJ: Surgical approaches and techniques in intraoperative radiotherapy for intra-abdominal, retroperitoneal, and pelvic neoplasms. Surgery 103:247, 1988.

148. Friesen RH, Morrison JE Jr, Verbrugge JJ, et al: Anesthesia for intraoperative radiation therapy in children. J Surg Oncol 35:96, 1987.

149. Ritchey ML, Gunderson LL, Smithson WA, et al: Pediatric urologic complications with intraoperative radiation therapy. J Urol 143:89, 1990.

150. Shrieve DC, Kooy HM, Tarbell NJ, et al: Fractionated stereotactic radiotherapy. In DeVita VT, Hellman S, Rosenberg SA (eds): Important Advances in Oncology. Philadelphia, Lippincott-Raven, 1996, pp 205–224.

151. Mehta MP: The physical, biologic, and clinical basis of radiosurgery. Curr Probl Cancer 19:265, 1995.

152. Gill SS, Thomas DG, Warrington AP, et al: Relocatable frame for stereotactic external beam radiotherapy. Int J Radiat Oncol Biol Phys 20:599, 1991.

153. Bleehan NM, Stenning SP: A Medical Research Council trial of two radiotherapy doses in the treatment of grades 3 and 4 astrocytoma. Br J Cancer 64:769, 1991.

154. Shaw E, Scott C, Souhami L, et al: Radiosurgery for the treatment of previously irradiated recurrent primary brain tumors and brain metastases: Initial analysis of Radiation Therapy Oncology Group protocol (RTOG) 9005.Int J Radiat Oncol Biol Phys 30:166, 1994.

155. Shaw EG, Scheithauer BW, O'Fallon JR. Management of supratentorial low-grade gliomas. Semin Radiat Oncol 1:23, 1991.

156. Smyth MD, Sneed PK, Ciricillo SF, et al: Stereotactic radiosurgery for pediatric intracranial arteriovenous malformations: The University of California at San Francisco experience. J Neurosurg 97:48, 2002.

157. Shrieve DC, Alexander E III, Wen PY, et al: Comparison of stereotactic radiosurgery and brachytherapy in the treatment of recurrent glioblastoma multiforme. Neurosurgery 36:275, 1995.

158. Hirth A, Pedersen PH, Baardsen R, et al: Gamma-knife radiosurgery in pediatric cerebral and skull base tumors. Med Pediatri Oncol 40:99, 2003.

159. Dunbar SF, Tarbell NJ, Kooy HM, et al: Stereotactic radiotherapy for pediatric and adult brain tumors: Preliminary report. Int J Radiat Oncol Biol Phys 30:531, 1994.

160. Intensity-modulated radiotherapy: Current status and issues of interest: Intensity modulation radiation therapy collaborative working group. Int J Radiat Oncol Biol Phys 51:880, 2001.

161. Teh BS, Mai WY, Grant WH III, et al: Intensity modulated radiotherapy (IMRT) decreases treatment-related morbidity and potentially enhances tumor control. Cancer Invest 20:437, 2002.

162. Swift P. Novel techniques in the delivery of radiation in pediatric oncology. Pediatr Clin North Am 9:1107, 2002.

163. Suit H. The Gray Lecture 2001: Coming technical advances in radiation oncology. Int J Radiat Oncol Biol Phys 53:798, 2002.

164. Kelly PJ: Volumetric stereotactic surgical resection of intraaxial brain mass lesions. Mayo Clin Proc 63:1186, 1988.

165. Barnett GH, Steiner CP, Weisenberger J: Target and trajectory guidance for interactive surgical navigation systems. Stereotact Funct Neurosurg 66:91, 1996.

166. Sipos EP, Tebo SA, Zinreich SJ, et al: In vivo accuracy testing and clinical experience with the ISG viewing wand. Neurosurgery 39:194, 1996.

167. Wagner A, Ploder O, Enislidis G, et al: Virtual image guided navigation in tumor surgery-technical innovation. J Craniomaxillofac Surg 23:271, 1995.

168. Robinson JR, Golfinos JG, Spetzler RF: Skull base tumors: A critical appraisal and clinical series employing image guidance. Neurosurg Clin North Am 7:297, 1996.

169. League D: Interactive, image-guided, stereotactic neurosurgery systems. AORN J 61:360, 1995.

170. Rubinsky B, Lee CY, Bastacky J, et al: The process of freezing and the mechanism of damage during hepatic cryosurgery. Cryobiology 27:85, 1990.

171. Gage AA: Cryosurgery in the treatment of cancer. Surg Gynecol Obstet 174:73, 1992.

172. Ravikumar TS, Steele GD: Hepatic cryosurgery. Surg Clin North Am 69:433, 1989.

173. Zhou XD, Tang ZY, Yu YQ, et al: Clinical evaluation of cryosurgery in the treatment of primary liver cancer: Report of 60 cases. Cancer 61:1889, 1988.

174. Onik G, Rubinsky B, Zemel R, et al: Ultrasound-guided hepatic cryosurgery in the treatment of metastatic colon carcinoma. Cancer 67:901, 1991.

175. Ravikumar TS, Buenaventura S, Salem RR, et al: Intraoperative ultrasonography of liver: Detection of occult liver tumors and treatment by cryosurgery. Cancer Detect Prevent 18:131, 1994.

176. Crews KA, Kuhn JA, McCarty TM, et al: Cryosurgical ablation of hepatic tumors. Am J Surg 174:614, 1997.

177. Marcove RC, Sheth DS, Takemoto S, et al: The treatment of aneurysmal bone cyst. Clin Orthop 311:157, 1995.

178. Devitt A, O'Sullivan T, Kavanagh M, et al: Surgery for locally aggressive bone tumors. Irish J Med Sci 165:278, 1996.

179. Schreuder HWB, VanBeem HBH, Veth RPH: Venous gas embolism during cryosurgery for bone tumors. J Surg Oncol 60:196, 1995.

180. Curley SA. Radiofrequency ablation of malignant liver tumors. Ann Surg Oncol 10:338, 2003.

181. Scaife CL, Curley SA: Complication, local recurrence, and survival rates after radiofrequency ablation for hepatic malignancies. Surg Oncol Clin North Am 12:243–255, 2003.

182. Kuvshinoff BW, Ota DM: Radiofrequency ablation of liver tumors: influence of technique and tumor size. Surgery 132:605, 2002.

183. Livraghi T, Solbiati L, Meloni F, et al: Percutaneous radiofrequency ablation of liver metastases in potential candidates for liver resection: The "test of time approach." Cancer 97:3027, 2003.

184. Mayo-Smith WW, Dupuy DE, Parikh PM, et al: Image-guided percutaneous radiofrequency ablation of solid renal masses: Techniques and outcomes of 38 treatment sessions in 32 consecutive patients. AJR Am J Roentgenol 180:1503, 2003.

185. Ferrell MA, Charboneau WJ, DiMarco DS, et al: Image-guided radiofrequency ablation of solid renal tumors. Am J Roentgenol 180:1509, 2003.

186. Herrera LJ, Fernando HC, Perry Y, et al: Radiofrequency ablation of pulmonary malignant tumors in non-surgical candidates. J Thorac Cardiovasc Surg 125:787, 2003.

187. Paek BW, Jennings RW, Harrison MR, et al: Radiofrequency ablation of human fetal sacrococcygeal teratoma. Am J Obstet Gynecol 184:503, 2001.

188. Ibrahim D, Ho E, Scherl LA, et al: Newborn with an open posterior hip dislocation and sciatic nerve injury after intrauterine radiofrequency ablation of a sacrococcygeal teratoma. J Pediatr Surg 38:248, 2003.

189. Hildebrandt B, Wust P, Ahlers O, et al: Hyperthermia in combined treatment of cancer. Lancet Oncol 3:487–497, 2002.

190. Stea B, Rossman K, Kittelson J, et al: Interstitial irradiation versus interstitial thermoradiotherapy for supratentorial malignant gliomas: A comparative survival analysis. Int J Radiat Oncol Biol Phys 30:591, 1994.

191. Seegenschmiedt MH, Karlsson UL, Black P, et al: Thermoradiotherapy for brain tumors. Am J Clin Oncol 18:510, 1995.

192. Miller RC, Richards M, Baird C, et al: Interaction of hyperthermia and chemotherapy agents: Cell lethality and oncogenic potential. Int J Hypertherm 10:89, 1994.

193. Perez CA, Patterson JH, Emami B: Evaluation of 45°C hyperthermia and irradiation. Int J Clin Oncol 16:469, 1993.

194. Doi O, Kodama K, Tatsuta M, et al: Effectiveness of intrathoracic chemotherapy for malignant pleurisy due to Ewing's sarcoma: A case report. Int J Hyperthermia 6:963, 1990.

195. Boyer MW, Moertel CL, Priest JR, et al: Use of intracavitary cisplatin for the treatment of childhood solid tumors in the chest or abdominal cavity. J Clin Oncol 13:631, 1995.

196. Glehen O, Mithieux F, Osinsky D, et al: Surgery combined with peritonectomy procedures and intraperitoneal chemohyperthermia in abdominal cancers with peritoneal carcinomatosis: A phase II study. J Clin Oncol 21:762–764, 2003.

197. Shen P, Levine EA, Hall J, et al: Factors predicting survival after intraperitoneal hyperthermic chemotherapy with mitomycin C after cytoreductive surgery for patients with peritoneal carcinomatosis. Arch Surg 138:26–33, 2003.

198. Coldwell DM, Stokes KR, Yakes WF: Embolotherapy: Agents, clinical applications, and techniques. Radiographics 14:623, 1994.

199. Venook AP, Stagg RJ, Lewis BJ, et al: Chemoembolization for hepatocellular carcinoma. J Clin Oncol 8:1108, 1990.

200. Shibata J, Fujiyama S, Sato T, et al: Hepatic arterial injection chemotherapy with cisplatin suspended in an oily lymphographic agent for hepatocellular carcinoma. Cancer 64:1586, 1989.

201. Feun LG, Reddy KR, Yrizzarry JM, et al: A phase I study of chemoembolization with cisplatin and Lipiodol for primary and metastatic liver cancer. Am J Clin Oncol 17:405, 1994.

202. Soulen MC: Chemoembolization of hepatic malignancies. Oncology 8:77, 1994.

203. Trinchet JC, Rached AA, Beaugrand M: A comparison of Lipiodol chemoembolization and conservative treatment for unresectable hepatocellular carcinoma. N Engl J Med 332:1256, 1995.

204. Sue K, Ikeda K, Nakagawara A, et al: Intrahepatic arterial injections of cisplatin-phosphatidylcholine-Lipiodol suspension in two unresectable hepatoblastoma cases. Med Pediatr Oncol 17:496, 1989.

205. Nakagawa N, Cornelius A, Kao SC, et al: Transcatheter oily chemoembolization for unresectable malignant liver tumors in children. J Vasc Interv Radiol 4:353, 1993.

206. Ogita S, Tokiwa K, Taniguchi H, et al: Intraarterial chemotherapy with lipid contrast medium for hepatic malignancies in infants. Cancer 60:2886, 1987.

207. Malogolowkin MH, Stanley P, Steele DA, et al: Feasibility and toxicity of chemoembolization for children with liver tumors. J Clin Oncol 18:1279, 2000.

208. Arcement CM, Towbin RB, Meza MP, et al: Intrahepatic chemoembolization in unresectable pediatric liver malignancies. Pediatr Radiol 30:779, 2000.

209. Tashjian DB, Moriarty KP, Courtney RA, et al: Preoperative chemoembolization for unresectable hepatoblastoma. Pediatr Surg Int 18:187, 2002.

210. Hatefi A, Amsden BJ: Biodegradable injectable in situ forming drug delivery systems. Control Release 80:9, 2002.

211. Leung TW, Yu S, Johnson PJ, et al: Phase II study of the efficacy and safety of cisplatin-epinephrine injectable gel administered to patients with unresectable hepatocellular carcinoma J Clin Oncol 21:652, 2003.

212. Oratz R, Hauschild A, Sebastian G, et al: Intratumoral cisplatin/adrenaline injectable gel for the treatment of patients with cutaneous and soft tissue metastases of malignant melanoma. Melanoma Res 13:59 2003.

213. Werner JA, Kehrl W, Pluzanska A, et al: A phase III placebo-controlled study in advanced head and neck cancer using intratumoural cisplatin/epinephrine gel. Br J Cancer 87:938, 2002.

214. Harbord M, Dawes RF, Barr H, et al: Palliation of patients with dysphagia due to advanced esophageal cancer by endoscopic injection of cisplatin/epinephrine injectable gel. Gastrointest Endosc 56:644, 2000.

215. Morton DL, Wend D, Wong JH, et al: Technical details of intraoperative lymphatic mapping for early stage melanoma. Arch Surg 127:392, 1992.

216. Berger DH, Feig BW, Podoloff D, et al: Lymphoscintigraphy as a predictor of lymphatic drainage from cutaneous melanoma. Ann Surg Oncol 4:247, 1997.

217. Krag DN, Weaver DL, Alex JC, et al: Surgical resection and radio-localization of the sentinel lymph node in breast cancer using a gamma probe. Surg Oncol 2:335, 1993.

218. Guiliano AE, Leirgan DM, Guenther JM, et al: Lymphatic mapping and sentinel lymphadenectomy for breast cancer. Ann Surg 220:391, 1994.

219. Kapteijn BA, Nieweg EO, Liem I, et al: Localizing the sentinel node in cutaneous melanoma: Gamma probe detection versus blue dye. Ann Surg Oncol 4:156, 1997.

220. LaQuaglia MP, Ghavimi F, Peneberg D, et al: Factors predictive of mortality in pediatric extremity rhabdomyosarcoma. J Pediatr Surg 25:238, 1990.

221. Andrassy RJ, Corpron CA, Hays DM, et al: Extremity sarcomas: An analysis of prognostic factors from the Intergroup Rhabdomyosarcoma Study III. J Pediatr Surg 31:191, 1997.

222. Neville HL, Andrassy RJ, Lally KP, et al: Lymphatic mapping with sentinel node biopsy in pediatric patients. J Pediatr Surg 35:961, 2000.

223. LaValle GJ, Chevinsky A, Martin EW: Impact of radioimmunoguided surgery. Semin Surg Oncol 7:167, 1991.

224. Aftab F, Stoldt HS, Testori A, et al: Radioimmunoguided surgery and colorectal cancer. Eur J Surg Oncol 22:381, 1996.

225. Reubi JC, Krenning EP, Lamberts SWJ, et al: Somatostatin receptors in malignant tissues. J Steroid Biochem Mol Biol 37:1073, 1990.

226. Lamberts SWJ, Krenning EP, Reubi J-C: The role of somatostatin and its analogs in the diagnosis and treatment of tumors. Endocr Rev 12:450, 1991.

227. Bakker WH, Albert R, Bruns C, et al: [^{111}In-DTPA-D-Phe^1]-octreotide, a potential radiopharmaceutical for imaging of somatostatin receptor-positive tumors: Synthesis, radiolabeling, and in vitro validation. Life Sci 49:1583, 1991.

228. Krenning EP, Kwekkeboom DJ, Bakker WH, et al: Somatostatin receptor scintigraphy with [^{111}In-DTPA-D-Phe^1]- and [^{123}I-Tyr^3]-octreotide: The Rotterdam experience with more than 1000 patients. Eur J Nucl Med 20:716, 1993.

229. Maggi M, Baldi E, Finetti G, et al: Identification, characterization, and biological activity of somatostatin receptors in human neuroblastoma cell lines. Cancer Res 54:124, 1994.

230. O'Dorisio MS, Chen F, O'Dorisio TM, et al: Characterization of somatostatin receptors on human neuroblastoma tumors. Cell Growth Diff 5:1, 1994.

231. Moertel CL, Reubi JC, Scheithauer BS, et al: Somatostatin receptors (SS-R) are expressed and correlate with prognosis in childhood neuroblastoma. Proc Am Soc Pediatr Res 27:146A, 1990.

232. Martinez DA, O'Dorisio MS, O'Dorisio TM, et al: Intraoperative detection and resection of occult neuroblastoma: A technique exploiting somatostatin receptor expression. J Pediatr Surg 30:1580, 1995.

233. Gomer CJ, Dougherty TJ: Determination of [^{3}H]- and [^{14}C] hematoporphyrin derivative distribution in malignant and normal tissue. Cancer Res 39:146, 1979.

234. Takita HT, Mang TS, Loewen GM, et al: Operation and intracavitary photodynamic therapy for malignant pleural mesothelioma: A phase II study. Ann Thorac Surg 58:995, 1994.

235. Wernecke K, Rummeny E, Bongartz G, et al: Detection of hepatic masses in patients with carcinoma: Comparative sensitivities of sonography, CT, and MR imaging. Am J Roentgenol 157:731, 1991.

236. Kane RA, Hughes LA, Cua EJ, et al: The impact of intraoperative ultrasonography on surgery for liver neoplasms. J Ultrasound Med 13:1, 1994.

237. Tandan VR, Litwin D, Asch M, et al: Laparoscopic cryosurgery for hepatic tumors: Experimental observations and a case report. Surg Endosc 11:1115, 1997.

238. Jakimowicz JJ: Laparoscopic intraoperative ultrasonography, equipment, and technique. Semin Laparosc Surg 1:52, 1994.

239. Jakimowicz JJ: Review: Intraoperative ultrasonography during minimal access surgery. J R Coll Surg Edinb 38:231, 1993.

240. Röthlin M, Largiadèr F: New, mobile-tip ultrasound probe for laparoscopic sonography. Surg Endosc 8:805, 1994.

241. Klotz HP, Flury R, Erhart P, et al: Magnetic resonance-guided laparoscopic interstitial laser therapy of the liver. Am J Surg 174:448, 1997.

CHAPTER 65

Renal Tumors

Robert C. Shamberger, MD

Renal tumors are the second most common abdominal tumor seen in infants and children after neuroblastoma. They represent a wide spectrum of tumors from benign to extremely malignant. Advances in the management of these tumors have been significant over the last four decades since Sidney Farber first administered actinomycin D for advanced stage Wilms' tumors. Much of what we know about renal tumors today has resulted from two cooperative group organizations, the National Wilms' Tumor Study Group (NWTSG) and the Société Internationale d' Oncologie Pédiatrique (SIOP). Together they have performed multiple randomized therapeutic trials, which have established the basis for how these tumors are treated. Central pathologic review of the specimens of patients enrolled in these studies has provided the current pathologic classification and staging, which could never have been established without multi-institutional participation because of the relative rarity of pediatric renal tumors. In this chapter, the early history of this tumor is presented, followed by a discussion of the etiologic factors in tumor formation, pathologic subtypes and premalignant syndromes, and treatment algorithms for Wilms' tumors and other tumors of the kidney.

HISTORY

The first descriptions of Wilms' tumor have been variably attributed to either Rance in 1814 or Wilms in 1899.[1] Ironically, however, the first known specimen of this tumor was preserved by the British surgeon John Hunter between 1763 and 1793, when he was collecting specimens for his museum.[2] This specimen of a bilateral tumor in a young infant remains in the Hunterian Museum of the Royal College of Surgeons in London to this day. Wilms' name became indelibly fixed to the mixed embryonal tumor of the kidney occurring in children after publication of his comprehensive monograph on mixed tissue tumors of the kidney in 1899. William E. Ladd and

Robert E. Gross[3,4] described the principles of surgical therapy for Wilms' tumor, including transperitoneal exposure and preliminary ligation of the renal pedicle. They stressed the need to remove the perirenal fat to include lymphatic extensions and to avoid rupture of the renal capsule, principles we continue to follow to this day. Adoption of their techniques significantly reduced the operative mortality of nephrectomy in children. Gross and Neuhauser[3] later proposed the routine addition of abdominal radiation to the therapy of Wilms' tumors and reported an estimated 47% frequency of cure.

Wilms' tumor was the first malignancy in which the importance of adjuvant treatment of the tumor was recognized; a principle espoused by Sidney Farber decades before it would be applied to other pediatric and adult solid tumors.[5] From 1931 to 1939, survival from surgical resection alone, involving ligation of the renal pedicle before removal, was 32% at The Children's Hospital in Boston.[5] Beginning in 1940, most of the patients received postoperative radiation to the renal fossa, which decreased the local recurrence rate but did not significantly affect the frequency of pulmonary metastases or improve the long-term survival. Actinomycin D was the first active agent identified for the treatment of Wilms' tumor. Of the 53 patients who had no demonstrable metastases on admission treated with combined therapy of operation, local radiation, and actinomycin D from 1957 to 1964, an 89% 2-year disease-free survival was reported, a very reasonable survival even today.[5] In patients with metastases identified at presentation, 18 (58%) of 31 were alive and free of disease more than 2 years later. Subsequently, vincristine sulfate was identified as an active agent in Wilms' tumor and was added to the standard therapy.[6]

The need for adjuvant treatment, as perceived by Sidney Farber, "was based upon the supposition that in the children with Wilms' tumor who died, the tumor must have metastasized already at the time of discovery of the primary tumor," although no evidence of spread was available. This principle of adjuvant treatment was to be extrapolated to management of many tumors occurring in adults several decades later.

WILMS' TUMOR INCIDENCE AND ETIOLOGY

Wilms' tumor is the most frequent tumor of the kidney in infants and children. Its incidence is 7.6 cases for every million children younger than 15 years, or one case per 10,000 infants.[7] Its frequency varies by race: rarer in East Asian populations than in whites, but more frequent in black children.[8] It is associated with several congenital syndromes including sporadic aniridia, isolated hemihypertrophy, the Denys-Drash syndrome (nephropathy, renal failure, male pseudohermaphroditism, and Wilms' tumor), genital anomalies, Beckwith-Wiedemann syndrome (visceromegaly, macroglossia, omphalocele, and hyperinsulinemic hypoglycemia in infancy), and the WAGR complex (Wilms' tumor with aniridia, genitourinary malformations, and mental retardation), which suggested a genetic predisposition to this tumor.[9,10] Wilms' tumor also is reported in individuals with Simpson-Golabi-Behmel syndrome, another overgrowth syndrome similar to Beckwith-Wiedemann in many respects.[11] These congenital disorders have now been linked to abnormalities at specific genetic loci implicated in Wilms' tumorigenesis.

GENETIC ORIGINS

The identification of a chromosomal deletion of band p13 of chromosome 11 in children with the WAGR syndrome led to a search at this site for a gene producing the Wilms' tumor. Subsequent molecular studies of children with Wilms' tumor demonstrated, in some cases, a deletion at this site.[12] This deletion includes the aniridia gene and a putative Wilms' tumor–suppressor gene (*WT1*). The protein product of this gene is a developmentally regulated transcriptional factor of the zinc-finger family, which regulates the expression of other genes including growth-inducing genes such as those encoding early growth response, insulin-like growth factor II, and platelet-derived growth factor A chain.[13,14] Suppression of these growth-associated genes may explain the tumor-suppressor role of *WT1*. Recently, the *WT1* gene product has been found to bind physically to the p53 protein.[15] The WAGR syndrome has been correlated with constitutional deletions of band 11p13, and virtually all patients with Denys-Drash syndrome carry point mutations in *WT1* in the germline.[12] These result in a dominant negative oncogene and more severe somatic abnormalities than those in the WAGR syndrome.

Abnormalities at the 11p15 locus have been associated with Beckwith-Wiedemann patients, although the locus for a Wilms' tumor gene has not been defined, nor is it known whether the Beckwith-Wiedemann locus and *WT2* are the same or contiguous loci.[16] Some children with Beckwith-Wiedemann syndrome have overexpression of a gene normally expressed by only one of the parental alleles. In some cases, a constitutional duplication of the paternal 11p15 chromosomal fragment has been identified (trisomy at 11p15).[17] In other cases, both copies are from the father with none from the mother (uniparental isodisomy).[18,19] These findings led to speculation that the Beckwith-Wiedemann gene is expressed only by the paternal allele, and these genetic abnormalities that lead to the presence of two paternal alleles would double the expression of this gene and may result in the overgrowth.

Two *WT2* candidate genes are the insulin-like growth factor 2 gene and the *H19* gene. The insulin-like growth factor 2 (*IGF2*) gene is present at the 11p15 locus. It is an embryonal growth-inducing gene with expression restricted to the paternal allele.[20] However, no direct evidence links the *IGF2* gene to the causation of the Beckwith-Wiedemann syndrome.[21] It is of note that children whose manifestations of the Beckwith-Wiedemann syndrome include hemihypertrophy appear to have a greater risk for the occurrence of malignancy than do those who do not. In a series reported by Wiedemann, cancer was reported in 7.5% of all children with the syndrome, but in more than 40% of children with both the syndrome and hemihypertrophy.[22] Loss of expression of *H19*, a tumor-suppressor gene, also has been reported in Wilms' tumors.[23] The *H19* gene is expressed from the maternal allele. With loss of heterozygosity, the cell may lose the maternal (active) copy and hence its tumor-suppressor function.

Familial cases of Wilms' tumor account for only 1% to 2% of cases and have not been associated with these syndromes. Analysis of two kindreds revealed a link with chromosome band 17q12-21, and the putative tumor gene at this locus has been named *FWT1*.[24] Recent studies have demonstrated in five kindreds an inherited Wilms' tumor–predisposition gene at 19q13.3-q13.4, called *FWT2*.[25] In addition, loss of heterozygosity was seen at 19q in tumors from individuals from two families whose predisposition is not due to the previously defined 19q locus, suggesting that alterations at two distinct loci are critical rate-limiting steps in the etiology of these familial Wilms' tumors involving both germline-predisposing mutations and somatic alteration at a second focus. The Simpson-Golabi-Behmel syndrome is a sex-linked syndrome linked to Xq25-27, and the protein product Glypican 3 may interact with the *IGF-2* receptor.[26,27]

WT1 and *WT2* do not appear to have any prognostic significance for children with Wilms' tumor, in marked contrast to the *nMYC* gene in neuroblastoma. They also appear in a small percentage of children with Wilms' tumor who have the associated syndromes. Recent studies have suggested that loss of heterozygosity on chromosome 16q in Wilms' tumors (observed in 15% to 20% of cases) was associated with a 3.3 times greater incidence of relapse and a 12 times greater incidence of mortality as compared with those in children without these chromosomal changes.[28] A similar trend was seen for children with loss of heterozygosity for 1p, which occurs in approximately 10% of Wilms' tumors, but these trends were not statistically significant. One of the primary goals of the fifth NWTS study was to assess whether identified chromosomal abnormalities were of prognostic significance in Wilms' tumor and might provide guidance for future therapeutic recommendations.

Routine radiographic screening of children with syndromes associated with Wilms' tumor has been recommended. Ultrasonograms are generally obtained every 3 months until the children are 5 years old. No prospective studies, however, have been performed to evaluate the cost effectiveness or efficacy of following this recommendation.[29,30] Retrospective reviews of routine ultrasonographic (US) screening report conflicting results on its purported benefits, as assessed by the stage distribution at presentation or the outcome of the children.[31,32]

PATHOLOGIC PRECURSORS: NEPHROGENIC RESTS, NEPHROBLASTOMATOSIS, AND MULTICYSTIC DYSPLASTIC KIDNEYS

The presence of nephrogenic rests (NRs; persistent metanephric tissue in the kidney after the 36th week of gestation) has been associated with the occurrence of Wilms' tumor. The rests may occur in a perilobular (PLNR) or intralobular (ILNR) location and may be single or multiple (Fig. 65-1). In children with aniridia or the Denys-Drash syndrome, the lesions are primarily ILNR, whereas children with hemihypertrophy or the Beckwith-Wiedemann syndrome have predominantly PLNR.[33] The presence of multiple or diffuse nephrogenic rests is termed *nephroblastomatosis*.

The frequency of NRs was established in an autopsy series of infants younger than 3 months. Nine (0.87%) of 1035 infants had PLNRs, and ILNRs occurred in only two (0.1%) of 2000 cases.[34] Most NRs when identified are sclerosing, an apparently indolent or involutional phase. The vast majority will spontaneously resolve without the appearance of a tumor, as the incidence of NRs is about 100 times greater than that of Wilms' tumor (1/10,000 infants).

NRs are classified histologically as incipient or dormant NRs, regressing or sclerosing NRs, and hyperplastic NRs (Fig. 65-2).[35] Incipient or dormant rests are composed predominantly of blastemal or primitive epithelial cells resembling those in embryonic kidney and Wilms' tumor but are microscopic with sharp margins from adjacent renal parenchyma. In infants and young children, the term *incipient* is used, whereas *dormant* is used in older children. Regressing or sclerosing rests demonstrate maturation of the cellular elements and progress to obsolescent rests, which are composed primarily of hyalinized stromal elements. Hyperplastic NRs are problematic, in that they are often difficult to distinguish from small Wilms' tumors. They contain diffuse or synchronous proliferation of components throughout the rest. This uniform growth leads to preservation of the original shape of the rest, in contrast with neoplastic proliferation of a single cell, which produces a more spherical expanding nodule within the rest. It is almost impossible for even the most sophisticated pediatric pathologist to distinguish a hyperplastic NR from a Wilms' tumor based on an incisional or needle biopsy. "Preservation of the shape of the original rest is the most obvious clue that one is dealing with a hyperplastic, rather than a neoplastic change."[35] Most hyperplastic nodules lack a pseudocapsule at their periphery, while most Wilms' tumors will have one; often this is the most helpful histologic finding in distinguishing these two lesions. Biopsies that do not contain the lesion and its margin will rarely adequately differentiate between these two lesions.

NRs are frequently found in association with Wilms' tumors despite their relatively rare occurrence. In a review

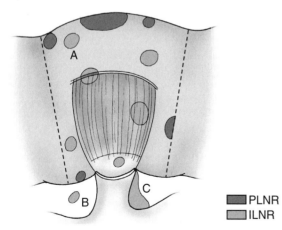

FIGURE 65-1. Diagram of a renal lobe and adjacent calyx and intervening sinus with potential sites of distribution of perilobar (PLNR) and intralobar (ILNR) nephrogenic rests. (From Beckwith JB, Kiviat N, Bonadio J: Nephrogenic rests, nephroblastomatosis, and the pathogenesis of Wilms' tumor. Pediatr Pathol 10:1–36, 1990.)

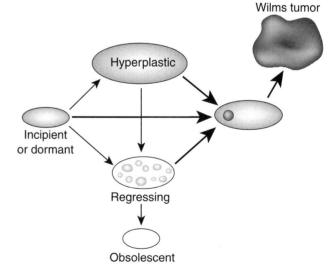

FIGURE 65-2. Diagrammatic depiction of nephrogenic rests and their classification. *Heavy arrows,* Tumor induction. (From Beckwith JB. Precursor lesions of Wilms' tumor: Clinical and biological implications. Med Pediatr Oncol 21:158–168, 1993.)

TABLE 65-1
ASSOCIATION OF NEPHROGENIC RESTS WITH WILMS' TUMOR AND ASSOCIATED SYNDROMES

Population	PLNR (%)	ILNR (%)
Unilateral Wilms' tumor	25	15
Bilateral Wilms' tumor (synchronous)	74–79	34–41
Bilateral Wilms' tumor (metachronous)	42	63–75
Beckwith-Wiedemann/hemihypertrophy and Wilms' tumor	70–77	47–57
Aniridia and Wilms' tumor	12–20	84–100
Denys-Drash and Wilms' tumor	11	78

PLNR, perilobar nephrogenic rests; ILNR, intralobar nephrogenic rests.
(Adapted from Beckwith JB: Precurser lesions of Wilms' tumor: clinical and biological implications. Med Pediatr Oncol 21:158–168, 1993.)

of cases of Wilms' tumors reported in the National Wilms' Tumor Study-4 (NWTS-4), 41% of the unilateral Wilms' tumors were associated with NRs,[33] whereas in children with synchronous bilateral Wilms' tumor, the incidence of NRs was 99%. These were primarily PLNRs, possibly because these lesions are much more prevalent than the ILNRs. Similarly, an increased incidence of NRs is seen in children with the syndromes associated with Wilms' tumor, which were discussed earlier (Table 65-1).[35]

It has been demonstrated that magnetic resonance imaging (MRI) scans can be particularly helpful in monitoring children with nephroblastomatosis.[36] Alterations in imaging characteristics of the lesions may suggest a transition from NRs to Wilms' tumor, as does growth of isolated lesions.

Diffuse hyperplastic perilobar nephroblastomatosis (DHPLN) is a distinct entity that must be distinguished clinically from Wilms' tumor. Infants with DHPLN may initially have large unilateral or bilateral flank masses (Fig. 65-3). A characteristic radiographic finding is massively enlarged kidneys that maintain their normal configuration and lack evidence of necrosis. As with the isolated NRs, proliferation of the thin rind of NRs on the periphery of the kidney will preserve the normal configuration of the kidney, but with marked enlargement of its size. This is in contrast with Wilms' tumor, where the normal renal configuration and collecting system is generally distorted. Nephrectomy is not required in cases of DHPLN. Chemotherapy, however, has been used to control the proliferative element of the NRs. Its use may accelerate the resolution in size of the masses and decrease the respiratory compromise they may produce. It has not, however, been established that treatment with chemotherapy will decrease the risk of malignancy arising in these lesions. A recent review of 65 cases of DHPLN revealed the subsequent development of Wilms' tumor in 19 children, occurring from 2 to 79 months after presentation (median, 30 months). The histology of these tumors was: favorable in 12, diffuse anaplasia in 5, and focal anaplasia in 2—a surprisingly high incidence of anaplasia.[37]

An increased risk of Wilms' tumors arising in multicystic dysplastic kidneys has been suggested. The frequency of NRs in multicystic dysplastic kidneys has been estimated to be 4%, approximately 5 times the prevalence in a

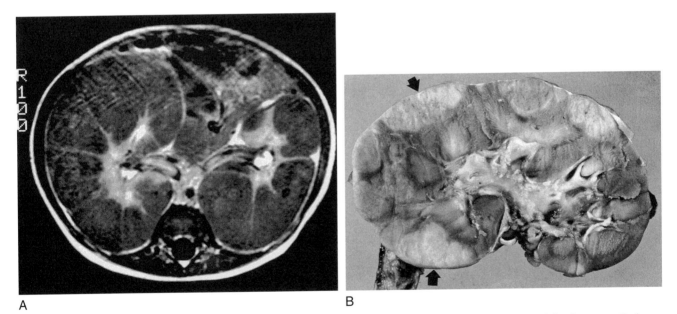

A   B

FIGURE 65-3. *A,* Magnetic resonance imaging scan of a 10-month-old infant first seen with large bilateral flank masses. It demonstrates a picture characteristic of diffuse hyperplastic perilobar nephroblastomatosis (DHPLN), with extensive involvement of the entire cortex of the kidney with no evidence of necrosis and general preservation of the shape of the kidney. *B,* Photograph of a kidney resected with a similar pattern of DHPLN reveals extensive involvement of the periphery of the cortex by severely hypertrophied nephrogenic rests (*arrows*). Resection of such kidneys should be avoided because, in most cases, the hypertrophy will resolve, and the kidney will have excellent preservation of its function. (*B,* Courtesy of JB Beckwith.)

random autopsy population of infants younger than 3 months.[38] If one were to estimate the frequency of Wilms' tumor in these kidneys, the standard risk of one in 10,000 infants might be said to be increased to one in 2000. Review of the NWTS pathology files, however, identified only three cases of dysplastic kidneys in more than 7000 children with Wilms' tumor over a 26-year interval and only one case in more than 1500 referral cases sent to Dr. Beckwith from around the world. Although it is impossible to estimate the number of children at risk from Wilms' tumors in remaining dysplastic kidneys, it must be concluded that the risk of development of Wilms' tumor in kidneys with multicystic dysplasia or congenital obstruction must be extremely low and does not justify nephrectomy to avoid the development of tumors.

PATHOLOGY OF RENAL TUMORS

The collection of large numbers of renal tumor specimens by the cooperative group trials has facilitated the development of accurate pathologic classifications in a much shorter period than would ever have been feasible without these trials. Early reports of Wilms' tumors and the initial cooperative group trials included essentially all renal sarcomas under this rubric. With time and experience, however, several subgroups of tumors have now been identified as at particularly high risk of recurrence and adverse outcome.[39,40] In NWTS-1 anaplastic and sarcomatous variants composed only 11.5% of the tumors, yet they accounted for 51.9% of the deaths due to tumor. Unfavorable histology proved to be the most important factor in patient outcome in NWTS-1, and that finding continues through the current trials. Wilms' tumors are currently divided into those with "favorable" histology and those with "unfavorable" histology (Table 65-2). The latter group includes tumors with focal or diffuse anaplasia.[41,42] Clear cell sarcoma of the kidney and malignant rhabdoid tumors of the kidney were initially grouped with the unfavorable-histology Wilms' tumors. They are now considered distinct entities from Wilms' tumor, based on their pathologic appearance and response to quite different therapies.[43,44]

TABLE 65-2
PATHOLOGIC CLASSIFICATION OF RENAL TUMORS

Favorable histology Wilms' tumor
Unfavorable histology Wilms' tumor
　Diffuse anaplasia
　Focal anaplasia
Clear cell sarcoma
Malignant rhabdoid tumor of the kidney
Renal cell sarcoma
Renal adenocarcinoma
Renal neurogenic tumors
Renal teratoma

TABLE 65-3
STAGING SYSTEM USED BY THE NATIONAL WILMS' TUMOR STUDY GROUP

Stage	Description
I	Tumor limited to the kidney and completely excised without rupture or biopsy. Surface of the renal capsule is intact
II	Tumor extends through the renal capsule, but is completely removed with no microscopic involvement of the margins. Vessels outside the kidney contain tumor. Also placed in stage II are cases in which the kidney biopsy was performed before resection or "local" spillage of tumor (during resection) is limited to the tumor bed
III	Residual tumor is confined to the abdomen and not from hematogenous spread. Also included in stage III are cases with tumor involvement of the abdominal lymph nodes, rupture of the tumor with "diffuse" peritoneal contamination extending beyond the tumor bed, peritoneal implants, and microscopic or grossly positive resection margins
IV	Hematogenous metastases at any site
V	Bilateral renal involvement

The staging system used by the NWTSG is a pretreatment surgical staging system (Table 65-3). It must be carefully distinguished when comparing treatment results with children treated on the SIOP protocols with which the staging information is obtained after preliminary treatment of the tumors (Table 65-4). The intensity of adjuvant treatment in the NWTSG protocols is determined by such factors as regional lymph node

TABLE 65-4
STAGING SYSTEM USED BY THE SOCIÉTÉ INTERNATIONALE D'ONCOLOGIE PÉDIATRIQUE (BASED ON FINDINGS AFTER PREOPERATIVE THERAPY)

Stage	Description
Stage I	Tumor limited to the kidney, complete excision
Stage II	Tumor extending outside the kidney, complete excision
	Invasion beyond the capsule, perirenal/perihilar
	Invasion of the regional lymph nodes* (stage IIN1)
	Invasion of extrarenal vessels
	Invasion of ureter
Stage III	Invasion beyond the capsule with incomplete excision
	Preoperative or perioperative biopsy
	Preoperative/perioperative rupture
	Peritoneal metastases
	Invasion of para-aortic lymph nodes†
	Incomplete excision
Stage IV	Distant metastases
Stage V	Bilateral renal tumors

*Hilar nodes and/or periaortic nodes at the origin of the renal artery.
†Para-aortic nodes below the renal artery.

involvement and penetration of the renal capsule by tumor, which cannot be accurately determined by radiographic studies. The staging criteria have been adjusted during the course of the NWTSG studies as the prognostic significance of criteria were established.[45]

Wilms' tumor is characterized as a triphasic embryonal neoplasm with blastemal, stromal, and epithelial components (Fig. 65-4).[39] Each of these components can express several patterns of differentiation, which define the histologic subgroups of Wilms' tumors. One particular subtype, the fetal rhabdomyomatous nephroblastoma, has been associated with poor response to chemotherapy but a generally good prognosis.[46] In contrast, the diffuse blastemal subtype is associated with presentation at an advanced stage but also with rapid response to chemotherapy. The anaplastic tumors are characterized by large, pleomorphic, and hyperchromatic nuclei with abnormal multipolar mitotic figures. Anaplasia can occur in the epithelial, stromal, or blastemal populations or any combination of these three. Anaplasia occurs primarily in children older than 2 years. In NWTS-1, 66.7% of the patients with anaplasia relapsed, and 58.3% died of their tumor.[40] Even in this early report, the distinct implications of the "diffuse" versus the "focal" pattern was appreciated, with a higher frequency of relapse and death in the "diffuse" subgroup. This was confirmed in review of the NWTS-2 and NWTS-3 data. Whereas children with stage I anaplastic tumors generally did well, children with stage II to IV tumors did poorly. The severity of dysplasia was not a predictive factor. However, anaplasia in extrarenal tumor sites and a predominantly blastemal tumor pattern were both adverse prognostic factors.[47]

Approximately 1% of children initially seen with a unilateral tumor will develop contralateral disease. In 58 of 4669 children registered in the first four NWTSG studies, metachronous disease developed.[48] Analysis of this cohort by a matched case-control study demonstrated that the children with NRs had a significantly increased risk of metachronous disease, particularly those with PLNRs. This finding was especially true for young children, in whom a Wilms' tumor occurred in 20 of 206 children younger than 12 months, in comparison with none of 304 children older than 12 months. These infants younger than 12 months with Wilms' tumor, who also have NRs, require regular surveillance for several years for the development of contralateral disease.

Clear cell sarcoma of the kidney is a highly malignant tumor with an unusual proclivity to produce bony metastasis. It generally appears as a large unifocal and unilateral tumor with homogeneous mucoid, tan, or gray/tan cut surface, often with foci of necrosis or prominent cyst formation.[39,49] This tumor invades surrounding renal parenchyma rather than compressing it into a pseudocapsule, as occurs with a Wilms' tumor. Its classic appearance is that of a deceptively bland tumor with uniform oval nuclei with a delicate chromatin pattern and a prominent nuclear membrane and sparse poorly stained vacuolated "water-clear" cytoplasm with indistinct cell membranes. Although the cells often appear in cords or nests divided by an arborizing network of vessels and supporting spindle cell septa, nine major histologic patterns have been identified.[49] The cell of origin of this tumor is not known. In addition to osseous metastasis, clear cell sarcoma also has a significant incidence of brain metastasis. Late recurrence also is seen with this tumor, with 30% of the relapses occurring more than 2 years after diagnosis.[50] For this reason, clinical trials must consider results after an adequate interval of follow-up.

Malignant rhabdoid tumors of the kidney occur in young infants with a median age of 11 months, and 85% of the cases occur within the first 2 years of life.[44] A characteristic involvement of the perihilar renal parenchyma is seen. Histologically, rhabdoid tumors are characterized

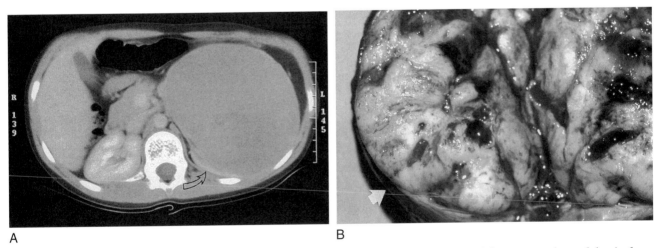

A   B

FIGURE 65-4. *A,* A computed tomography scan of a 10-year-old boy initially seen with a large left upper quadrant abdominal mass identified on a routine "well-child examination," demonstrating the characteristic findings of a Wilms' tumor. The tumor mass is well circumscribed and can be seen with a margin of renal parenchyma along the periphery (*arrow*). *B,* The gross pathologic specimen shows the lobular nature of this standard-histology Wilms' tumor. Again, the tumor can be seen extending from the normal renal parenchyma (*arrow*).

by monomorphous, discohesive, rounded to polygonal cells with acidophilic cytoplasm and eccentric nuclei containing prominent large "owl eye" nucleoli reminiscent of skeletal muscle, but lacking its cytoplasmic striations, ultrastructural features, and immunochemical markers.[39] A large periodic acid–Schiff (PAS)-positive hyaline, cytoplasmic inclusion occurs in a variable population of tumor cells and is a hallmark of this tumor.[51] Ultrastructural examination reveals parallel cytoplasmic filamentous inclusions packed in concentric whorled arrays, a distinctive feature of this tumor, which suggests a neuroectodermal origin. The tumor tends to infiltrate surrounding renal parenchyma rather than to compress it. These tumors are notable for the occurrence of second primary neuroglial tumors in the midline of the brain, resembling medulloblastoma.[52] A consistent deletion of 22q11-12 has been described in both renal and extrarenal rhabdoid tumors.[53,54]

The occurrence of primitive neuroectodermal tumor (PNET) of the kidney is well documented.[55] It is clearly distinct from Wilms' tumor and the other variants previously discussed and demonstrates spread to lymph nodes, lung, bone, liver, and bone marrow, as is seen when PNET occurs in other anatomic locations.[56] Its treatment including resection, chemotherapy, and radiation must follow that of PNET and not that of other renal tumors.

CLINICAL PRESENTATION

The classic presentation of Wilms' tumor is the identification of an asymptomatic flank mass in an otherwise healthy toddler. It is often noted during a bath or by the pediatrician at a routine visit, and the mass may be considerable in size. This is in marked contrast to neuroblastoma, which is seen in the same age group, but frequently occurs with pain, often from osseous metastasis. Wilms' tumor also may be associated with hematuria, but with a much lower frequency than is seen with renal cell carcinoma. Rarer presentations are with hypertension or fever. Occasionally a child may have abdominal trauma

and demonstrate pain and an abdominal mass out of proportion to that expected. Radiographic examination will reveal a mass that cannot be attributed to the trauma alone.

TREATMENT

As a result of the work that demonstrated the role of adjuvant therapy in this tumor, all children treated on early protocols of the NWTSG and SIOP received chemotherapy. Only in the last decade has adjuvant therapy been avoided in a small proportion of children with an extremely low risk of local recurrence and metastasis. Optimal chemotherapy regimens have been established by a series of well-designed randomized studies performed primarily by the NWTSG in the United States and Canada and SIOP in Europe. Surgery continues to play a critical role in the treatment of Wilms' tumor, despite advances in chemotherapy. Accurate staging and safe and complete resection of the tumor are key elements in achieving cure. Local control is rarely achieved with chemotherapy and radiotherapy alone.

Chemotherapy

Wilms' tumor was the first malignant pediatric solid tumor with a demonstrated response to dactinomycin.[5] Many additional effective agents have been subsequently identified: vincristine, doxorubicin, cyclophosphamide, ifosfamide, and etoposide.

Children with stage I tumors were treated on the third NWTSG protocol (NWTS-3) with an 11-week regimen composed of vincristine and dactinomycin, without abdominal radiation, based on the results of the initial two studies. The 4-year relapse-free survival (RFS) and overall survival (OS) were 89.0% and 95.6%, respectively.[57] The other three stages were treated on a regimen that involved randomization of two or four arms (Table 65-5). This study supported the addition of doxorubicin to the treatment of children with stage III tumors but did not

TABLE 65-5			
RANDOMIZATION FOR FAVORABLE HISTOLOGY WILMS' TUMORS ON NWTS-3			
Stage	Treatment: 4-Year DFS	Results: 4-Year OS	
II	Vcr, Dac	87.4%	91.1%
	Vcr, Dac + XRT (20 Gy abd)	NS	NS
	Vcr, Dac, Dox	NS	NS
	Vcr, Dac, Dox + XRT (20 Gy abd)	NS	NS
III	Vcr, Dac + XRT (10 Gy abd)	Improved survival with addition of doxorubicin	
	Vcr, Dac + XRT (20 Gy abd)		
	Vcr, Dac, Dox + XRT (10 Gy abd)	82.0%	90.9%
	Vcr, Dac, Dox + XRT (20 Gy abd)	No difference in local recurrence between 10 and 20 Gy	
VI	Vcr, Dac, Dox	79.0%	80.9%
	Vcr, Dac, Dox, Cyclo	NS improvement from the addition of cyclophosphamide	
	All abd XRT, 20 Gy, and		
	Pulmonary XRT, 12 Gy		

Vcr, vincristine; Dac, dactinomycin; XRT, radiotherapy; abd; abdomen; Dox, doxorubicin; Cyclo, cyclophosphamide; NS, not statistically significant; DFS, disease-free survival; OS, overall survival. From D'Angio GJ, et al. Cancer 64:349, 1989.

demonstrate any benefit from the addition of doxorubicin or radiotherapy for children with stage II tumors or benefit from the addition of cyclophosphamide to the treatment of children with stage IV tumors.

NWTS-4 built on the lessons learned from the prior studies and addressed the issue of whether dose intensification could be safely used to decrease the number of visits for chemotherapy and yet maintain the favorable results previously achieved. Dactinomycin and doxorubicin were administered in single moderately high doses, compared with the traditional divided dose regimens for each drug. This study also evaluated the use of two time intervals for the administration of chemotherapy: a short course (18 to 26 weeks, depending on the regimen and stage) versus a long course (54 to 66 weeks). The findings of this study were that the pulse-intensive regimens actually produced less hematologic toxicity than the standard regimens, allowing greater dose intensity with comparable outcomes.[58,59] The second randomization demonstrated no benefit in any of the stages to the long interval of therapy over the short interval.[60]

The goal of NWTS-5 was to evaluate preliminary findings from pilot studies that several chromosomal deletions were associated with an adverse prognosis. To most efficiently address this question, it was the first study from NWTSG that did not involve randomization of treatment. Although this study is closed to accrual of new patients, the findings are not yet available.

Treatment of children with anaplastic tumors with standard therapy has resulted in a high rate of failure. Thus in sequential studies, therapy has been intensified. Review of the NWTS-3 and -4 studies demonstrated that children with focal anaplasia have an excellent outcome when treated with vincristine, doxorubicin, and dactinomycin.[42] The addition of cyclophosphamide to this regimen improved the 4-year RFS in children with diffuse anaplasia with stages II to IV disease from 27.2% to 54.8%. Subsequent studies have further intensified therapy with the use of doxorubicin, cyclophosphamide, vincristine, and etoposide, but results are not yet available from those trials.

Doxorubicin was found to be particularly effective in the treatment of clear cell sarcoma of the kidney.[61,62] However, the results have remained below those of standard histology Wilms' tumors. No benefit was seen to pulse-intensive administration of the agents, and no difference in survival was noted at 5 and 8 years between patients treated for 6 or 15 months.[63] The rhabdoid tumors have remained the most resistant to cure of all pediatric renal tumors. Current studies have used an intensive therapy with carboplatinum, etoposide, and cyclophosphamide, but results are not available for this regimen.

SIOP has promoted the use of preoperative treatment of children with Wilms' tumor with radiotherapy or chemotherapy since the early 1970s. Histologic confirmation of the diagnosis before therapy is not routinely recommended by SIOP. This approach has several risks. First is the potential for administration of chemotherapy for benign disease. Second, modification of tumor histology by the chemotherapy may occur. Third, staging information may be lost. Fourth, a malignant rhabdoid

tumor of the kidney or clear cell sarcoma, if present, will not respond to standard therapies. Treatment without an initial diagnosis is difficult to sustain when NWTSG and SIOP studies have demonstrated a 7.6% to 9.9% rate of benign or altered malignant diagnosis in children with a prenephrectomy diagnosis of Wilms' tumor.[64,65] The histologic diagnosis after preoperative treatment in a group of children followed up by NWTSG did not appear distorted by treatment, but it is less certain that staging is not altered.[66]

The major driving force for the use of preoperative therapy by SIOP was the high rate of operative tumor rupture that occurred in their early series, in which patients did not receive preliminary treatment. The rupture rate decreased from 33% (20 of 60) to 4% (3 of 72) with preoperative abdominal irradiation (20 Gy) in the first randomized SIOP study of renal tumors (SIOP-1), begun in 1971.[67] It must be noted, however, that 33% is an extremely high frequency of rupture. Survival was not affected by the decrease in operative rupture, and the incidence of local recurrence was not reported. In NWTS-1 and -2, operative rupture occurred in 22% and 12% of children, respectively.[64,68] In a subsequent SIOP randomized study of Wilms' tumors begun in 1977 (SIOP-5), the rate of rupture was essentially the same for children receiving abdominal irradiation (20 Gy) and dactinomycin (9%, 7 of 76) or a combination of vincristine and dactinomycin (6%, 5 of 88).[69,70] Radiotherapy after resection was based on the stage of the tumors, with stage I receiving no postoperative radiation, and stage II and III patients receiving 15 Gy in the group treated initially with radiotherapy and 30 Gy in those treated initially with chemotherapy. In SIOP-6, begun in 1980, all patients received initial preoperative chemotherapy (vincristine and dactinomycin). Radiotherapy was administered after resection to those children with stage IIN1 and stage III disease. Children with stage IIN0 (lymph node negative) were randomized to receive either 20 Gy of radiotherapy or no radiation to the tumor bed. All children received vincristine and dactinomycin for 38 weeks. After pretreatment, 52% of cases were stage I, and a low frequency of rupture was noted (7%). The radiotherapy randomization was halted after 108 children were randomized, 58 to radiotherapy and chemotherapy and 50 to chemotherapy alone. Six local recurrences occurred in the 50 children who did not receive radiotherapy versus no recurrences in the group that did. This suggested that prenephrectomy treatment altered the pathologic findings that would have led to a diagnosis of stage IIN1 or stage III disease (i.e., lymph node involvement or capsular penetration) and to the standard administration of local irradiation. Extended follow-up studies of these children showed ultimately no statistical difference in survival, as those who relapsed had more treatment alternatives.[71,72] The SIOP-6 protocol also extended chemotherapy to infants older than 6 months.[73] The overall favorable outcome was not improved, and an unacceptable toxicity occurred in the young infants. In the SIOP-9 study, a reduced dose in infants was recommended.

In the SIOP-9 study initiated in 1987, a randomization was performed between 4 and 8 weeks of preoperative therapy to determine whether the additional 4 weeks of therapy produced a larger proportion of stage I tumors.[74] This study also replaced postoperative radiotherapy in stage II node-negative children by administration of an anthracycline, epirubicin, or doxorubicin. Preoperative treatment consisted of four weekly courses of vincristine and two 3-day courses of dactinomycin each 2 weeks versus 8 weeks of the identical therapy for patients without distant metastasis. No advantage was seen from the extended therapy in terms of staging at resection between the 4-week and 8-week courses: stage I, 64% versus 62%, with intraoperative tumor rupture of 1% versus 3%. Therapy after resection was based on the pathologic findings. Children with stage I disease and favorable or anaplastic histology received vincristine and dactinomycin for 17 weeks. Those with stage II and III tumors with favorable histology received vincristine, dactinomycin, and epirubicin (an anthracycline) for 27 weeks, with no abdominal radiotherapy for stage IIN0 disease or with 15 Gy of abdominal irradiation in cases of stages IIN1 and III disease. This therapy resulted in a 2-year event-free survival of 84% versus 83% for the 4- and 8-week therapies and OSs of 92% and 87%, respectively. For cases with metastatic disease, children received 6 weeks of therapy including weekly vincristine, three courses of dactinomycin, and two courses of epirubicin on weeks 1 and 5. In SIOP-9, the surgical procedure–related complications were reported to be 8%.[75] In this treatment regimen, patients with post-therapy stage II disease receive an anthracycline, whereas in the NWTS studies, stage II disease receives vincristine and dactinomycin alone. In SIOP-9, an evaluation of children with completely necrotic tumors at the time of resection demonstrated that they had an extremely favorable prognosis.[76] Complete necrosis was seen in 10% of 599 children enrolled into the study. In total, 37 children in this cohort had stages I to III disease, and 22 had stage IV disease. Disease-free survival was 98% at 5 years versus 90% for the other patients on SIOP-9. The only death in the stage I to III group was related to chemotherapy, and survival was 100% in the stage IV group.

The goal of both NWTSG and SIOP has been to decrease the therapies used and yet achieve the maximal long-term survival. Both groups have decreased the amount of radiotherapy used during the course of their studies. Among the children with unilateral nonmetastatic favorable-histology Wilms' tumors, 24% of those enrolled in NWTS (275 of 1160) were given radiation therapy, and 18% of those in SIOP (81 of 447) have received radiotherapy in the most recent studies.[77] SIOP has elected, however, to use anthracycline rather than radiotherapy for their postchemotherapy stage IIN0 patients in whom excessive local relapse occurred without additional therapy. This results in around 48% of patients in SIOP studies with unilateral nonmetastatic, favorable-histology patients receiving an anthracycline, which is significantly greater than the 24% of comparable patients on NWTSG regimens.

Significant complications have occurred in some children treated with doxorubicin, particularly that of cardiomyopathy.[78,79] In children treated on NWTS-1 to -4,

the cumulative frequency of congestive heart failure was 4.4% at 20 years after diagnosis for those treated initially with doxorubicin. The relative risk was increased in female subjects, by cumulative dose, lung irradiation, and left-sided abdominal radiation. Subclinical echocardiographic abnormalities have been demonstrated in children who received as low a dose as 45 mg/m^2 of doxorubicin.[80] Only long-term follow-up of children who have received doxorubicin will document what dose, if any, is free of long-term implications.

Second malignant neoplasms also are a concern. NWTSG reported a 1.6% incidence of second malignant neoplasms at 15 years after treatment.[81] The incidence correlated with prior treatment of relapsed tumor, the amount of abdominal radiation, and the use of doxorubicin.

Surgical Procedures

The NWTSG has advocated initial resection of the tumor in all of its protocols. Although most Wilms' tumors are first seen as a large mass, resection is generally feasible (Fig. 65-5). Wilms' tumor, in contrast to neuroblastoma, is much less likely to invade surrounding organs and lymph nodes, which complicates the resection. Children undergoing initial nephrectomy in the NWTS-3 study demonstrated a complication rate of 19.8% in a group that was very closely monitored.[82] The most frequent complication was intestinal obstruction, occurring in 6.9% of the children, followed by extensive intraoperative hemorrhage (>50 mL/kg of body weight) occurring in 5.8%.[83] Injuries to other visceral organs (1%) and extensive vascular injuries (1.4%) were much less frequent. Nine deaths in the series were attributed to surgical

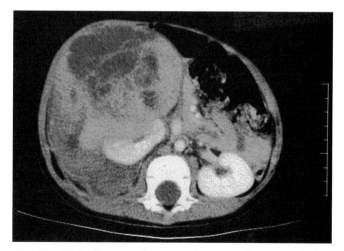

FIGURE 65-5. Computed tomography scan of a 3-year-old boy with a history of abdominal pain, fever, and right flank mass. Tumor can be seen to be very large, with extension outside the renal capsule into the retroperitoneal tissues posterior to the kidney. Despite its size, this lesion was completely resected. Lymph nodes were negative for tumor, and the specimen margins were negative for tumor as well. This tumor was therefore stage II, and the infant was able to avoid both anthracycline therapy and abdominal radiation because of the resection.

complications (0.5%), only one of which was intraoperative. The factors associated with an increased risk of surgical complications were advanced-stage local disease, intravascular extension of the tumor, and the resection of other organs. The later were often found not to be invaded by the tumor, but rather compressed, distorted, or adherent, without actual tumor infiltration. Extensive resection involving removal of other organs or procedures that are of a magnitude to be life threatening should be aborted, and a biopsy obtained of the tumor and regional lymph nodes, followed by administration of chemotherapy before a second attempt at resection (Fig. 65-6). With this algorithm, 93% of 131 children enrolled in NWTS-3 who were initially judged unresectable at operation or by imaging studies were successfully resected after initial chemotherapy or irradiation or both.[84] Only eight children with tumors that grew or failed to respond did not undergo subsequent nephrectomy.

Complications in the most recently completed NWTS-4 study also have been assessed.[85] During this study, surgeons were discouraged from performing extensive operations involving resection of adjacent organs or massive tumors. Complications occurred in 12.7% of a random sample of 534 of the 3335 patients treated in this study. Again, intestinal obstruction was the most frequent complication (5.1%) followed by extensive hemorrhage (1.9%), wound infection (1.9%), and vascular injury (1.5%). The factors associated with an increased risk of complications were again assessed. Intravascular extension into the inferior vena cava (IVC) or atrium and nephrectomy performed through a flank or paramedian incision were both significant factors. Tumor diameter 10 cm or larger also was associated with increased complications. Finally, the risk of complications was increased if the resection was performed by a general surgeon rather than a pediatric surgeon or pediatric urologist. SIOP reported a complication rate of 8% in a recent study involving 598 patients registered on SIOP-9. These patients were pretreated with vincristine, dactinomycin, and epirubicin or doxorubicin before nephrectomy.[75] The most frequent events were small bowel obstruction (3.7%) and tumor ruptures (2.8%). The later is not reported as a complication in the NWTS reviews. Other complications occurred in 2.0% of patients. A prospective study of surgical complications by SIOP and NWTSG has been completed, and results are pending.

Surgical Details

Radiographic imaging is critical before surgical resection of a renal tumor (Fig. 65-7). The most important factors to assess in these studies are the presence of two functioning kidneys, contralateral tumor, and evidence of intravascular extension of the tumor. Intraoperative identification of intravascular extension has been associated with an increased incidence of surgical complications.[86]

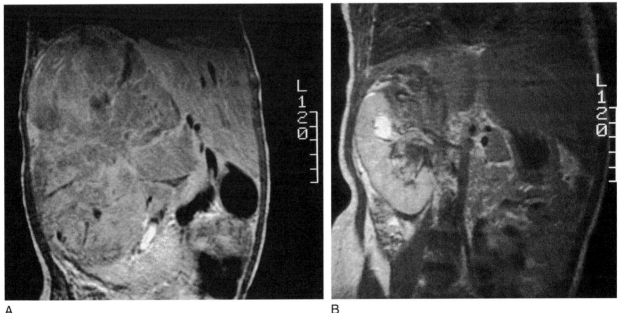

A   B

FIGURE 65-6. *A,* Magnetic resonance imaging (MRI) scan of a 2½-year-old girl first seen with a massive right-sided abdominal mass. Chest radiograph revealed pulmonary nodules as well. Because of the massive size of the primary and metastatic disease, she received initial chemotherapy after a needle biopsy demonstrated a standard-risk tumor (diffuse blastemal subtype). She received three courses of actinomycin D, vincristine, and cytoxan, which achieved some shrinkage of the tumor. At surgery, a very extensive tumor was densely adherent to the posterior aspect of the liver and the vena cava. It was clear that resection of a portion of the liver would be required with the nephrectomy. Efforts at resection were terminated. Repeated biopsies again demonstrated a standard-histology Wilms' tumor with tumor invasion into the liver. She was treated on a new protocol involving cisplatin and VP-16, as well as abdominal and thoracic radiation. *B,* MRI, after additional therapy, showed remarkable shrinkage of the tumor, allowing much more facile and safe resection.

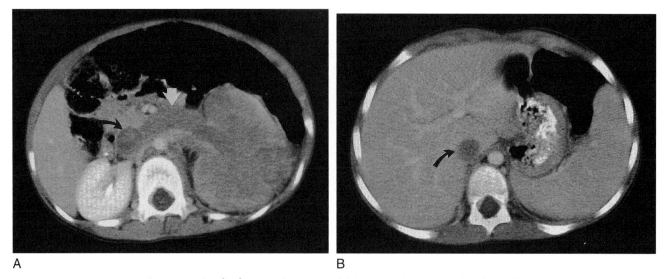

A   B

FIGURE 65-7. *A,* Computed tomography (CT) scan of a 7-year-old boy initially seen with a left-sided abdominal mass. CT scan demonstrated tumor extending through the left renal vein (*white arrow*) into the inferior vena cava (*black arrow*). *B,* Higher levels on the CT scan demonstrated tumor completely occluding the intrahepatic inferior vena cava (*black arrow*).

The organ of origin of the tumor can be determined in most cases, with the differential diagnosis generally between neuroblastoma and Wilms' tumor. This can generally be determined by the configuration of the kidney and the mass. In neuroblastoma, the mass will generally indent the kidney, whereas in Wilms' tumor, the mass will arise from within the kidney and distort its internal configuration. Often a thin lip of renal parenchyma can be seen extending over the neoplasm in Wilms' tumor (see Fig. 65-4*A*). Intra-abdominal staging has been difficult to assess radiographically unless extensive lymph node involvement or intrahepatic metastasis is present. A radiograph of the chest and computed tomography (CT scan) will determine the presence of pulmonary metastasis. If the lesions are seen on the radiograph, their malignant nature can generally be assumed. Smaller lesions seen only on the CT scan should generally be sampled to confirm their malignant nature. Bone scans and brain scans are routinely performed only if the renal tumor proves to be a clear cell sarcoma or rhabdoid tumor.

Renal tumors must be resected through an adequate subcostal or thoracoabdominal incision. Struggling through an inadequate incision will often result in rupture of the tumor, increasing both the stage of the tumor and the risk for intra-abdominal recurrence.[87] A flank incision should not be used for resection in pediatric renal tumors because of the limited exposure it provides.

Initial exploration of the abdomen should be performed, including inspection for hepatic metastasis or intraperitoneal spread. The vena cava, if it is accessible, also should be palpated to assess for intravascular extension of tumor. The contralateral kidney should be palpated for tumor, although it is not currently suggested that the kidney be completely exposed and visualized. Exploration of the contralateral kidney with opening of Gerota's fascia was recommended by the NWTSG based on the 5% occurrence of synchronous lesions. In NWTS-2

and -3 contralateral involvement was not detected before exploration by intravenous pyelography (IVP) or CT scan in approximately one third of the children with bilateral tumors.[88] Review of children with bilateral tumors treated on NWTS-4 identified 9 of 122 children in whom the diagnosis of bilateral disease was missed by the preoperative imaging studies (CT scan, US, or magnetic resonance imaging [MRI]).[89] All but one of these lesions were small: five were smaller than 1 cm, and three were 1 to 3 cm in diameter. Recent review of this material, however, has suggested that some of the small lesions on the contralateral kidney, which were initially thought to be small Wilms' tumors would now be more correctly defined as hyperplastic NRs. Future studies by NWTSG will not require examination of the contralateral side if no suggestion is found of involvement on the preoperative radiographic studies.

The colon is then mobilized off the anterior aspect of the kidney and the renal mass. Although early descriptions of resection recommended initial control of the renal hilum, this is often not feasible with extremely large tumors and must await mobilization of the mass to allow exposure of the hilum. Premature attempts at vascular control, particularly of left-sided tumors, may result in ligation of the superior mesenteric artery.[90] Biopsy of the renal mass should not be performed unless the decision is to not proceed with a complete resection. Biopsy will produce contamination of the peritoneum and increase the stage of the tumor.

Adequate biopsy of lymph nodes in the renal hilum and along the vena cava or aorta is critical for adequate staging. Even in children with stage IV disease, local staging is critical, as it will determine whether abdominal radiotherapy is used. Studies have demonstrated that the surgeon's gross inspection and assessment of lymph nodes does not reliably correspond with the pathologic involvement of tumor with a false-negative and false-positive rates of 31.3% and 18.1%, respectively.[91] An increased incidence of local recurrence was seen in children enrolled in NWTS-4, in whom biopsy of lymph nodes was not performed, particularly stage I cases.[87] This suggested that undertreatment of local disease in these children due to inadequate staging resulted in an increased frequency of local recurrence. Although grossly involved lymph nodes are generally resected, an extensive retroperitoneal lymph node resection has not been demonstrated to improve local control.[92]

As the tumor is mobilized the ureter is resected close to the bladder to avoid a "diverticulum" on the bladder, which might produce recurrent urinary tract infection, but primarily to make certain that any extension of tumor into the ureter is entirely resected. Gross hematuria in children with Wilms' tumor is infrequent, but its occurrence suggests extensive involvement of the renal pelvis with possible extension into the ureter. Cystoscopy should be considered in these children to identify extension of the tumor into the bladder and to avoid transection of the tumor thrombus during division of the ureter. Ureteral extension that is entirely resected does not increase the local stage of the tumor. If the tumor involves the upper pole, the adrenal gland is generally resected to provide adequate margins around the tumor and also to obtain periaortic or pericaval lymph node tissue. With lower-pole lesions, the adrenal gland may be preserved.

The factors associated with an increased risk of local recurrence are stage III disease, unfavorable histology (especially diffuse anaplasia), and tumor rupture during operation.[87] Tumor rupture is the only factor that the surgeon will determine. Multiple regression analysis adjusting for the combined effects of histology, lymph node involvement, and age reveal that tumor spillage remained significant and was greatest in children with stage II disease who received less intensive therapy. Most tumor ruptures occur during mobilization of the posterior aspects of the tumor where it is adherent to the diaphragm. This can be best prevented by use of an adequate incision for the resection and resection of a segment of the adherent diaphragm if necessary.

Resection of adjacent organs (liver, spleen, or pancreas) or resection of massive Wilms' tumors are discouraged in the recent NWTSG studies based on reviews of complications. Such extensive resections are associated with a significant increase in surgical complications.[82] Only in this situation should the surgeon biopsy the primary tumor along with perihilar and periaortic/caval lymph nodes.

Preoperative evaluation of children with renal tumors must include studies of coagulation. An "acquired" von Willebrand disease has been seen in children with Wilms' tumor, which can produce problems with hemostasis if it is not identified and treated appropriately before operation.[93]

Preoperative Therapy

Preoperative treatment of Wilms' tumor is generally accepted in certain circumstances: the occurrence of Wilms' tumor in a solitary kidney, bilateral renal tumors, tumor in a horseshoe kidney, intravascular extension of the tumor above the intrahepatic vena cava, and respiratory distress from extensive metastatic tumor. Pretreatment biopsy should be obtained. Percutaneous biopsy is often used although needle-tract seeding has been reported.[94] The aim of treatment (before surgical resection in the bilateral tumors and tumor in a horseshoe or solitary kidney) is to preserve maximal renal parenchyma and function. The anatomy of the kidney has not been recognized before surgical exploration in many of the cases of Wilms' tumor arising within a horseshoe kidney.[95] This is often due to the large size of the tumor distorting the anatomy. An increased incidence of urine leak and ureteral injury occur in this situation because of the aberrant anatomy of the collecting systems.

Although growth of the remaining kidney has been documented (achieving 180% volume augmentation), the occurrence of focal segmental glomerulosclerosis has been reported in children with a unilateral kidney.[96,97] In the NWTS-1 to NWTS-4 population, the incidence of renal failure after unilateral nephrectomy was only 0.25%.[98] Studies from Europe on pretreatment of unilateral Wilms' tumor have demonstrated that in most instances, a nephrectomy is still required, rather than a partial nephrectomy, because of the extent of tumor involvement in the kidney at presentation.[99]

The efficacy of preoperative chemotherapy in allowing the safe performance of partial nephrectomy for Wilms' tumor has been evaluated by several centers. In Toronto, percutaneous biopsy in 37 children with Wilms' tumor was followed by multiagent chemotherapy for 4 to 6 weeks. A partial nephrectomy was then performed in 9 children (4 with unilateral and 5 with bilateral tumors).[100] Two children had intra-abdominal relapse. Only 4 (13.3%) of the 30 unilateral tumors were amenable to a partial nephrectomy. Another analysis of the feasibility of partial nephrectomies was performed at St. Jude Children's Research Hospital.[101] Preoperative CT scans of 43 children with nonmetastatic unilateral Wilms' tumor were reviewed retrospectively. Criteria used to determine whether a partial nephrectomy would have been feasible were involvement by the tumor of one pole and less than one-third of the kidney, a functioning kidney, no involvement of the collecting system or renal vein, and clear margins between the tumor and surrounding structures. With these criteria, only two (4.7%) of 43 scans suggested that partial nephrectomy was feasible. The primary concerns regarding use of preoperative chemotherapy to create "resectable" small tumors is that these children with small tumors at presentation may be curable with surgical resection alone without subjecting them to the toxicity of additional treatments.[102,103] Whereas the role of partial nephrectomy has been suggested in children with Beckwith-Wiedemann syndrome or hemihypertrophy in whom smaller tumors may be identified by prospective screening, the efficacy of this approach has not been established.[104]

BILATERAL WILMS' TUMOR

Children with bilateral tumors are generally younger than those with unilateral lesions, with a mean age of 25 versus 44 months.[105] Preservation of renal parenchyma is a critical issue for these children. In the NWTSG review of renal failure in 55 children from NWTS-1 to NWTS-4, 39 children had bilateral tumor involvement. Increasing efforts to preserve renal parenchyma in bilateral cases in the sequence of the NWTSG studies resulted in a decline in the incidence of renal failure from 16.4% in NWTS-1 and -2 to 9.9% in NWTS-3 and 3.8% in NWTS-4.[98] Although the incidence may increase in the more recent studies as children age, this declining frequency also is due in part to increased attempts to save part of the kidneys by initial treatment of the tumor with chemotherapy. Preliminary treatment in most cases after biopsy and staging will produce shrinkage of the tumor and facilitate its resection with preservation of a portion of the kidney. It is important to perform biopsies of all tumors, as "discordant" pathology does occur, with a favorable lesion on one side and unfavorable lesion (generally anaplastic) on the other. Bilateral lesions are rarely seen in association with clear cell sarcoma or rhabdoid tumors of the kidney. Ninety-eight children with bilateral Wilms' tumors underwent a partial nephrectomy of 134 kidneys during NWTS-4.[106] Complete resection of gross disease was accomplished in 118 (88%) of the 134 kidneys. A higher incidence of positive surgical margins (16%, 19 of 134) and local tumor recurrence (8.2%, 11 of 134) was seen in this group of children. These were justified by the attempt to preserve renal tissue and avoid renal failure. Overall, portions of 72% of the kidneys were preserved, and the 4-year survival rate was 81.7%.

The United Kingdom Children's Cancer Study Group (UKCCSG) also reported attempts at maximal preservation of renal parenchyma with preoperative chemotherapy.[107] Survival was equivalent for those with initial resection versus preoperative chemotherapy, but greater preservation of renal parenchyma was seen in those treated with initial chemotherapy. Radiation has been advocated to prevent relapse in children with partial nephrectomy for bilateral disease, but irradiation may impair the ability of the kidney to grow.[108,109]

The presence of rhabdomyomatous histology has been associated with poor response to preoperative chemotherapy, as defined by decrease in size on radiographic evaluation, but it has been found to be associated with favorable survival.[110]

INTRAVASCULAR EXTENSION

Intravascular extension of a tumor thrombus occurs in 4% of children with Wilms' tumor. Identification of vascular extension by preoperative radiographic studies or early in the surgical exploration is critical to avoid a tumor embolus during mobilization of the kidney. US is probably more sensitive than is CT scan. The presence of intravascular extension does not affect the prognosis of the tumor, as long as it is successfully resected.[111] Traditionally, intravascular extension has been managed by nephrectomy with resection of the tumor thrombus into the renal vein or vena cava. Cardiopulmonary bypass has been required for children with atrial extension of the tumor thrombus but is associated with a significant incidence of complications (70%).[86]

In a NWTSG report of intravascular extension of Wilms' tumor, 30 children (15 with caval and 15 with atrial extension) were treated initially with chemotherapy after biopsy of the renal mass. After treatment, a decrease in the size of the intravascular extension was noted in 23 children, and complete resolution of the tumor thrombus was seen in 7 children.[112] Of the 15 children with tumor initially extending into the atrium, a complete or marked response occurred, and the tumor was removed transabdominally without bypass. Tumor embolism did not occur during chemotherapy. Fibrosis of tumor to the caval wall developed in some cases, and, in two cases, IVC occlusion occurred postoperatively. A similar review of children treated in the United Kingdom with extensive intravascular involvement also demonstrated a decrease in the extent of vascular involvement in 16 of 21 children and showed that children receiving preoperative chemotherapy had a better outcome.[113]

More recently, a review of all of the children treated on NWTS-4 revealed 165 of 2731 patients with intravascular extension into the IVC (134 patients) or atrium (31 patients).[114] Sixty-nine of these patients received preoperative chemotherapy (55 with IVC extension and 14 with atrial extension). Five complications were encountered during preoperative chemotherapy, including tumor embolism and tumor progression in 1 patient each, and 3 patients with adult respiratory distress syndrome, one of which was fatal. Intravascular extension of the tumor regressed in 39 of 49 children with comparable pre- and posttherapy radiographic studies, including regression in 7 of 12 in whom the tumor regressed from an atrial location, avoiding the need for cardiopulmonary bypass. A high frequency of surgical complications occurred in these patients, 36.7% in the children with atrial extension and 17.2% in those with IVC extension. The frequency of surgical complications was 26% in the primary resection group versus 13.2% in children with preoperative therapy. When all the complications were considered, including those that occurred during preoperative chemotherapy (1 of those 5 also had a surgical complication), the incidence of complications among those receiving preoperative therapy was not statistically different from the incidence among those who underwent primary resection, but preoperative therapy clearly facilitated surgical resection by decreasing the extent of the tumor thrombus.

RESECTION ALONE FOR SELECT FAVORABLE WILMS' TUMORS

A small group of children with Wilms' tumor may require only resection of the primary tumor and kidney without adjuvant treatment. The outcome of children younger than 2 years with stage I tumors, weighing less than 550 g, registered in the NWTSG studies, were reviewed.[115] The 4-year RFS for children meeting these criteria exceeded 90%, suggesting that they could be selected for treatment with resection alone. A pathologic review of children treated on NWTS-4 also demonstrated that age younger than 2 years and specimen weight of less than 550 g was highly associated with the absence of adverse microsubstaging variables.[116] A prospective pilot study of this question was performed at Children's Hospital in Boston. Eight children with stage I disease who were younger than 2 years with unilateral, favorable-histology tumors with a combined tumor and kidney weight under 550 g were resected and followed up without adjuvant therapy.[117] In 1 child, a metachronous tumor was cured by resection and chemotherapy. Continued evaluation of this series showed no episodes of local recurrence.[118]

One component of NWTS-5 was a trial of operation only for children younger than 2 years with small (<550-g tumor and kidney) stage I favorable-histology tumors. Seventy-five infants were enrolled in this study.[119] In 3 infants, metachronous, contralateral Wilms' tumors developed, and 8 relapsed 0.3 to 1.05 years after diagnosis. The sites of relapse were pulmonary (5 cases) and operative bed (3 cases). The 2-year disease-free (relapse and metachronous) survival was 86.5%. The 2-year survival rate was 100%, with a median follow-up of 2.84 years. The 2-year disease-free survival, excluding metachronous contralateral Wilms' tumor, was 89.2%, and the 2-year cumulative risk of metachronous contralateral Wilms' tumor was 3.1%. The stopping rule for the study required closure after these 75 infants were enrolled, but continuing evaluation of this cohort has demonstrated that they have done very well with a high rate of salvage, as they were previously untreated with chemotherapy. Treatment for these infants in future studies remains under consideration.

NEONATAL WILMS' TUMOR

Wilms' tumor occurs rarely in the neonate. A review of the 3340 children entered into the NWTS studies from 1969 to 1984 revealed only 27 (0.8%) neonates (30 days old or younger) with renal tumors.[120] More than half of the neonates (18) had mesoblastic nephroma, and 4 others had non-neoplastic lesions. One infant had a malignant rhabdoid tumor, and 4 had Wilms' tumors. All of these children had favorable-histology tumors without metastasis. They did well, receiving a variety of treatments ranging from resection alone to 15 months of three-drug therapy. A subsequent report of 15 cases of Wilms' tumor occurring in neonates in the first 30 days of life again demonstrated favorable-histology tumors and absence of metastatic disease.[121] Ten of these infants received postoperative chemotherapy, and 5 were followed up without additional treatment. Only 1 of these 5 children had recurrence in the renal fossa and lungs and ultimately died of her disease at age 16 months. The other children are all disease free at a median follow-up of 31 months.

EXTRARENAL WILMS' TUMOR

An extrarenal site of primary Wilms' tumor is uncommon. These extrarenal tumors behave identically to tumors arising within the kidney and should be treated both locally and systemically based on the same criteria.[122,123] Common sites of occurrence of extrarenal Wilms' tumors include the retroperitoneum, inguinal canal, scrotum, and vagina. Rare sites are the uterus, cervix, ovary, and presacral space.

RENAL CELL CARCINOMA

Children with renal cell carcinoma are generally older than those with Wilms' tumor, and frequently initially have symptoms of flank pain and gross hematuria.[124] Renal cell carcinoma in children displays gross and microscopic pathologic features similar to those seen in tumors in adults. Clinical stage at the time of diagnosis is the most important prognostic factor, and the identification of renal vascular invasion did not appear to be an adverse predictor. Radical nephrectomy and regional lymphadenectomy have been the primary modality for cure, and children with distant spread have a grave prognosis. The mean age for presentation with renal cell carcinoma in a pediatric population was 14 years.[125] Overall survival is much worse than that in Wilms' tumor, with a 5-year survival in a recent series of only 30%. Analysis of multiple factors including age, tumor size, location, and histology failed to demonstrate that they were predictors of survival. Only stage and achieving complete tumor resection were meaningful prognostic factors. Survival was 60% in children with complete resection of the primary tumor and zero in those with only partial resection. Renal cell carcinoma is remarkably resistant to chemotherapy, preventing cure in most children with metastatic disease.[126] Ten percent to 20% of patients have nodal involvement identified at operation but lack evidence of distant metastatic disease.

Nephron-sparing resection has been used in patients with small polar lesions in whom no evidence of a multicentric tumor is found. In these selected cases with tumors smaller than 4 cm and a normal contralateral kidney, the risk of local recurrence is reported to be 2% or less, which is comparable to the frequency of metachronous recurrence in the contralateral kidney after unilateral radical nephrectomy.

The occurrence of late relapses long after nephrectomy, prolonged stability of disease in the absence of systemic therapy, and rare cases of spontaneous regression of tumors have led to an interest in immunotherapy comparable to that used in melanoma. Trials of immunomodulating therapy with interferon-α and interleukin-2 (IL-2) have demonstrated some efficacy, but maintenance of a durable cure has been elusive.[127] A trial with 294 patients with advanced-stage renal cell carcinoma randomized to receive placebo or 9 months of subcutaneous lymphoblastoid interferon demonstrated similar recurrence rates of the two groups and worse survival than those randomized to placebo alone.[128] With the significant toxicity involved with immunotherapy, demonstration of improved survival in randomized trials will be required before this can be adopted as standard therapy.

MESOBLASTIC NEPHROMA

Congenital mesoblastic nephroma, also referred to as fetal renal hamartoma or leiomyomatous hamartoma, is the most common renal tumor identified in the neonatal period. Although it was initially diagnosed and treated as a congenital Wilms' tumor, mesoblastic nephroma was defined as a distinct entity in 1967.[129] Mesoblastic nephromas appear most frequently in the neonatal period as a palpable flank mass, which can be massive in size. Additional symptoms seen at presentation include hematuria, hypertension, vomiting, and jaundice.[130]

Mesoblastic nephroma accounted for 2.8% of 1905 renal tumors submitted to the early NWTSG studies. Grossly, these tumors have a homogeneous rubbery appearance resembling a uterine fibroid in color and consistency (Fig. 65-8). Microscopically they are composed of sheets of fibrous or mesenchymal stroma, within which bizarre and dysplastic tubules and glomeruli are irregularly scattered.[131] The tumor can invade intact renal parenchyma, and extrarenal infiltration into the perihilar connective tissues is common. The histologic subtypes of this tumor include the classic type (24% of cases), the cellular type (66%), and the mixed type (10%). The pluripotency of these tumors is revealed by their differentiation into angiomatoid patterns, cartilaginous nests, and their elicitation of intratumoral hematopoiesis in addition to the tiny nephroblastic epithelial foci.

Recently a characteristic chromosomal translocation, (t12;15)(p13;q25) was described; it results in fusion of the *ETV6* (also known as *TEL*) gene from 12p13 with the *NRTK3* neurotrophin-3 receptor gene (also known as *TRKC*) from 15q25.[16,23] This results in a chimeric RNA, which is characteristic of both infantile fibrosarcoma and the cellular variant of congenital mesoblastic nephroma. This may be of assistance in differentiating the cellular variant from other lesions that must be considered in the differential diagnosis, including clear cell sarcoma and rhabdoid tumors. It also suggests a close relation between infantile fibrosarcoma and the cellular variant of mesoblastic nephroma.[49]

This generally benign tumor usually can be cured with nephrectomy alone. This should include generous margins around all gross tumor to avoid local recurrence. Particular attention should be paid to the medial aspect of the kidney, including the hilum and great vessels, because of the tumor's proclivity to have extensions into these perirenal soft tissues. Several children have been reported with local recurrence[132] or metastasis to the brain, bones, lungs, and heart.[133–136] In some of these cases, the histology has revealed an unusual degree of mesenchymal cell immaturity and hypercellularity, suggesting a more aggressive tumor.[131] These rare occurrences, however, support the concept that mesoblastic nephroma cannot be considered a simple hamartoma and that complete nephrectomy with negative pathologic margins for tumor is critical in all cases.

In a series of 51 children with mesoblastic nephroma identified in the NWTSG series, adequate operative excision was achieved in 43 of 51 children, whereas 8 had local extension, and 10 had tumor spillage during resection.[130] The use of adjuvant therapy in these cases depended on the era in which the children were treated. Twenty-three infants treated principally since 1978 had surgical resection alone. Prior to 1978, 24 had operation plus chemotherapy, and before 1976, 4 children also received irradiation. Survival was excellent in this entire group, and only 1 child died of sepsis during chemotherapy. One child's tumor recurred at 6 months despite receiving dactinomycin and vincristine. The tumor was surgically re-excised, and the child was treated with cyclophosphamide and doxorubicin and remained without disease 18 months later.

A SIOP study of 29 children with mesoblastic nephroma confirmed the early age at which this tumor is seen. Only five infants were older than 4 months at presentation in the series.[137] Five children with the cellular type of tumor received some chemotherapy. Two infants in this series died of sepsis after surgical treatment, but the remainder are alive and free of disease 4 years later. A proclivity for this tumor to infiltrate the renal hilum or perirenal tissue was seen again.

Treatment of a neonate with an extensively infiltrating tumor with eight weekly courses of vincristine before resection is reported.[138] Shrinkage of the tumor occurred with treatment, facilitating its eventual resection and cure.

Beckwith reported the largest cohort of children with recurrent or metastatic lesions from his large collected series.[133] Twenty-four cases of aggressive tumor were seen in a series of 330 mesoblastic nephromas. Of these cases, 8 had metastatic disease, 17 had relapse in the peritoneum or retroperitoneum, and 6 of the infants have died of persistent disease. Recurrences occurred in children after initial chemotherapy or irradiation, which suggests that conventional adjuvant therapy may not decrease the incidence of recurrence. Histologic criteria were not helpful in predicting outcome. Beckwith supports aggressive surgical attempts to remove all gross tumor. He also stresses the need for close monitoring for 1 year after resection because relapse in 23 of the 24 cases was apparent within 11 months of resection. US of the local site is adequate, and scans for metastatic disease are unrewarding.

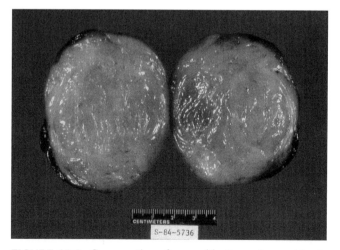

FIGURE 65-8. Cross section of a mesoblastic nephroma identified in an infant on a newborn examination. Note the rubbery appearance of this tumor, which resembles a fibroid tumor of the uterus with a very thin margin of normal renal parenchyma around the periphery.

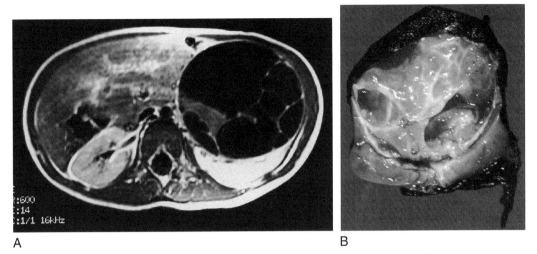

FIGURE 65-9. *A,* Magnetic resonance imaging scan obtained in a 2-year-old child with an asymptomatic left flank mass. Note the multilocular cystic mass extending out from the normal renal tissue posteriorly. *B,* Cross section of the tumor and kidney reveals thin-walled septae within the mass. Histologic examination of this tumor revealed a cystic, partially differentiated nephroblastoma.

CYSTIC NEPHROMA

Cystic nephroma is indistinguishable grossly and radiographically from its malignant neoplastic cousins, cystic partially differentiated nephroblastoma (CPDN) and cystic nephroblastoma. All lesions are composed of purely cystic masses characterized by multiple thin-walled septations (Fig. 65-9). In cystic nephroma, the septations are composed entirely of differentiated tissues without blastemal or other embryonal elements that are contained in the septa of CPDN.[139] Although the term *multilocular cyst of the kidney* has been used, *cystic nephroma* is preferred because the lesion appears to be neoplastic and not congenital. In the cystic nephroblastoma or cystic Wilms' tumor, solid nodules on the septae of blastemal or embryonal elements are characteristic of Wilms' tumor. An unexplained synchronous occurrence has been reported of cystic nephroma and pleuropulmonary blastoma.[140]

These lesions should not be confused with cystic clear cell sarcoma, cystic mesoblastic nephroma, or multicystic dysplastic kidney.[139] Cystic nephroma, CPDN, and cystic nephroblastoma can be distinguished from multicystic dysplastic kidney because they are confined to only a portion of the kidney with normal renal parenchyma being identified, whereas the cystic changes of multicystic dysplastic kidney almost always involve the entire kidney (its etiology is early in utero urinary tract obstruction) (see Fig. 65-9*B*). Contralateral renal anomalies are frequent in dysplastic kidneys, including ureteropelvic junction obstruction and reflux. Multicystic dysplastic kidney is often identified antenatally or in the newborn period, whereas the other lesions occur later.

Generally, nephrectomy will be curative in both cystic nephroma and CPDN.[141] Twenty-three children with these cystic lesions were identified in the NWTSG series: 5 with cystic nephroma and 18 with CPDN. Only one case of CPDN had local recurrence, and no distant metastases were found. A more recent review of the NWTSG files of the CPDN cases has again confirmed that primary resection appears to be adequate for all lesions removed intact.[142] In cases in which the lesion is isolated to one pole of the kidney, a partial nephrectomy may be considered; however, it must be remembered that these tumors can resemble cystic variants of clear cell sarcoma of the kidney, which carry an entirely different prognosis.[2,143]

OSSIFYING RENAL TUMOR OF INFANCY

Ossifying renal tumor of infancy is a relatively rare tumor occurring entirely in infancy. In many cases, children with this lesion initially have gross hematuria, although a palpable mass may be present.[144] These lesions are attached to a renal papilla but are seen primarily within the lumen of the calyx and may extend into the renal pelvis. They have been confused occasionally with staghorn calculi. Histologically, they contain osteoid, osteoblastic cells, and spindle cells. Their true histogenesis has not been proven, although it has been suggested that they represent hyperplastic ILNRs. Metastasis or local spread of these tumors has not been reported. Renal-sparing procedures may be reasonable, although this may not achieve significant ipsilateral renal function.[145,146]

REFERENCES

1. Rance T: Case of fungus hematodes of the kidneys. Med Phys J 32:19, 1814.
2. Beckwith JB: The John Lattimer lecture: Wilms tumor and other renal tumors of childhood: An update. J Urol 136:320–324, 1986.
3. Gross R: Treatment of mixed tumors of the kidney in childhood. Pediatrics 6:843–852, 1950.

4. Ladd W: Embryoma of the kidney (Wilms' tumor). Ann Surg 108:885–902, 1938.
5. Farber S: Chemotherapy in the treatment of leukemia and Wilms' tumor. JAMA 198:826–836, 1966.
6. Sutow W: Vincristine (Leurocristine) sulfate in the treatment of children with metastatic Wilms' tumor. Pediatrics 32:880–887, 1963.
7. Bernstein L, Linet M, Smith MA, et al: Renal tumors. In Ries L, Smith MA, Gurney J (eds): Cancer Incidence and Survival Among Children and Adolescents: United States SEER Program 1975-1995. Bethesda, Md, National Cancer Institute, 1999, pp 79–90.
8. Stiller CA, Parkin DM: International variations in the incidence of childhood lymphomas. Paediatr Perinat Epidemiol 4:303–324, 1990.
9. Jadresic L, Leake J, Gordon I, et al: Clinicopathologic review of twelve children with nephropathy, Wilms' tumor, and genital abnormalities (Drash syndrome). J Pediatr 117:717–725, 1990.
10. Miller R, Fraumeni J, Manning M: Association of Wilms' tumor with aniridia, hemihypertrophy and other congenital malformations. N Engl J Med 270:922–927, 1964.
11. Hughes-Benzie RM, Pilia G, Xuan JY, et al: Simpson-Golabi-Behmel syndrome: Genotype/phenotype analysis of 18 affected males from 7 unrelated families. Am J Med Genet 66:227–234, 1996.
12. Riccardi VM, Sujansky E, Smith AC, et al: Chromosomal imbalance in the aniridia-Wilms' tumor association: 11p interstitial deletion. Pediatrics 61:604–610, 1978.
13. Rauscher FJ 3rd: The WT1 Wilms tumor gene product: A developmentally regulated transcription factor in the kidney that functions as a tumor suppressor. FASEB J 7:896–903, 1993.
14. Rauscher FJ 3rd, Morris JF, Tournay OE, et al: Binding of the Wilms' tumor locus zinc finger protein to the EGR-1 consensus sequence. Science 250:1259–1262, 1990.
15. Maheswaran S, Park S, Bernard A, et al: Physical and functional interaction between WT1 and p53 proteins. Proc Natl Acad Sci U S A 90:5100–5104, 1993.
16. Steenman M, Westerveld A, Mannens M: Genetics of Beckwith-Wiedemann syndrome-associated tumors: Common genetic pathways. Genes Chromosomes Cancer 28:1–13, 2000.
17. Waziri M, Patil SR, Hanson JW, et al: Abnormality of chromosome 11 in patients with features of Beckwith-Wiedemann syndrome. J Pediatr 102:873–876, 1983.
18. Grundy P, Telzerow P, Paterson MC, et al: Chromosome 11 uniparental isodisomy predisposing to embryonal neoplasms. Lancet 338:1079–1080, 1991.
19. Henry I, Bonaiti-Pellie C, Chehensse V, et al: Uniparental paternal disomy in a genetic cancer-predisposing syndrome. Nature 351:665–667, 1991.
20. DeChiara TM, Robertson EJ, Efstratiadis A: Parental imprinting of the mouse insulin-like growth factor II gene. Cell 64:849–859, 1991.
21. Coppes MJ, Haber DA, Grundy PE: Genetic events in the development of Wilms' tumor. N Engl J Med 331:586–590, 1994.
22. Wiedemann R: Tumours and hemihypertrophy associated with Wiedemann-Beckwith syndrome. Eur J Pediatr 141:129, 1983.
23. Steenman MJ, Rainier S, Dobry CJ, et al: Loss of imprinting of IGF2 is linked to reduced expression and abnormal methylation of H19 in Wilms' tumour. Nat Genet 7:433–439, 1994.
24. Rahman N, Arbour L, Tonin P, et al: Evidence for a familial Wilms' tumour gene (FWT1) on chromosome 17q12-q21. Nat Genet 13:461–463, 1996.
25. McDonald JM, Douglass EC, Fisher R, et al: Linkage of familial Wilms' tumor predisposition to chromosome 19 and a two-locus model for the etiology of familial tumors. Cancer Res 58:1387–1390, 1998.
26. Hughes-Benzie RM, Hunter AG, Allanson JE, et al: Simpson-Golabi-Behmel syndrome associated with renal dysplasia and embryonal tumor: Localization of the gene to Xqcen-q21. Am J Med Genet 43:428–435, 1992.
27. Xuan JY, Besner A, Ireland M, et al: Mapping of Simpson-Golabi-Behmel syndrome to Xq25-q27. Hum Mol Genet 3:133–137, 1994.
28. Grundy PE, Telzerow PE, Breslow N, et al: Loss of heterozygosity for chromosomes 16q and 1p in Wilms' tumors predicts an adverse outcome. Cancer Res 54:2331–2333, 1994.
29. Clericuzio CL: Clinical phenotypes and Wilms tumor. Med Pediatr Oncol 21:182–187, 1993.
30. Green DM, Breslow NE, Beckwith JB, et al: Screening of children with hemihypertrophy, aniridia, and Beckwith-Wiedemann syndrome in patients with Wilms tumor: A report from the National Wilms Tumor Study. Med Pediatr Oncol 21:188–192, 1993.
31. Choyke PL, Siegel MJ, Craft AW, et al: Screening for Wilms tumor in children with Beckwith-Wiedemann syndrome or idiopathic hemihypertrophy. Med Pediatr Oncol 32:196–200, 1999.
32. Craft AW: Screening for Wilms' tumor in patients with aniridia, Beckwith syndrome, or hemihypertrophy. Med Pediatr Oncol 24:231–234, 1995.
33. Beckwith JB, Kiviat NB, Bonadio JF: Nephrogenic rests, nephroblastomatosis, and the pathogenesis of Wilms' tumor. Pediatr Pathol 10:1–36, 1990.
34. Bennington J, Beckwith J: Tumor of the kidney, renal pelvis, and ureter. Atlas Tumor Pathol, Washington, DC, AFIP, 1975.
35. Beckwith JB: Precursor lesions of Wilms tumor: Clinical and biological implications. Med Pediatr Oncol 21:158–168, 1993.
36. Gylys-Morin V, Hoffer FA, Kozakewich H, et al: Wilms tumor and nephroblastomatosis: Imaging characteristics at gadolinium-enhanced MR imaging. Radiology 188:517–521, 1993.
37. Barbosa A: Diffuse hyperplastic perilobar nephroblastomosis (DHPLN): Pathology and clinical biology. Rio de Janeiro, 1998, pp. 1P.
38. Beckwith J: Wilms' tumor in multicystic dysplastic kidneys: What is the risk? Dialog Pediatr Urol 78:1P, 1996.
39. Beckwith JB: Wilms' tumor and other renal tumors of childhood: A selective review from the National Wilms' Tumor Study Pathology Center. Hum Pathol 14:481–492, 1983.
40. Beckwith JB, Palmer NF: Histopathology and prognosis of Wilms tumors: Results from the First National Wilms' Tumor Study. Cancer 41:1937–1948, 1978.
41. Faria P, Beckwith JB, Mishra K, et al: Focal versus diffuse anaplasia in Wilms tumor: New definitions with prognostic significance: A report from the National Wilms Tumor Study Group. Am J Surg Pathol 20:909–920, 1996.
42. Green DM, Beckwith JB, Breslow NE, et al: Treatment of children with stages II to IV anaplastic Wilms' tumor: A report from the National Wilms' Tumor Study Group. J Clin Oncol 12:2126–2131, 1994.
43. Marsden HB, Lawler W, Kumar PM: Bone metastasizing renal tumor of childhood: Morphological and clinical features, and differences from Wilms' tumor. Cancer 42:1922–1928, 1978.
44. Weeks DA, Beckwith JB, Mierau GW, et al: Rhabdoid tumor of kidney: A report of 111 cases from the National Wilms' Tumor Study Pathology Center. Am J Surg Pathol 13:439–458, 1989.
45. Farewell VT, D'Angio GJ, Breslow N, et al: Retrospective validation of a new staging system for Wilms' tumor. Cancer Clin Trials 4:167–171, 1981.
46. Maes P, Delemarre J, de Kraker J, et al: Fetal rhabdomyomatous nephroblastoma: A tumour of good prognosis but resistant to chemotherapy. Eur J Cancer 35:1356–1360, 1999.
47. Zuppan CW, Beckwith JB, Luckey DW: Anaplasia in unilateral Wilms' tumor: A report from the National Wilms' Tumor Study Pathology Center. Hum Pathol 19:1199–1209, 1988.
48. Coppes MJ, Arnold M, Beckwith JB, et al: Factors affecting the risk of contralateral Wilms tumor development: A report from the National Wilms Tumor Study Group. Cancer 85:1616–1625, 1999.
49. Argani P, Fritsch M, Kadkol SS, et al: Detection of the ETV6-NTRK3 chimeric RNA of infantile fibrosarcoma/cellular congenital mesoblastic nephroma in paraffin-embedded tissue: Application to challenging pediatric renal stromal tumors. Mod Pathol 13:29–36, 2000.
50. Kusumakumary P, Chellam VG, Rojymon J, et al: Late recurrence of clear cell sarcoma of the kidney. Med Pediatr Oncol 28:355–357, 1997.
51. Haas JE, Palmer NF, Weinberg AG, et al: Ultrastructure of malignant rhabdoid tumor of the kidney: A distinctive renal tumor of children. Hum Pathol 12:646–657, 1981.
52. Bonnin JM, Rubinstein LJ, Palmer NF, et al: The association of embryonal tumors originating in the kidney and in the brain: A report of seven cases. Cancer 54:2137–2146, 1984.
53. Perlman EJ, Ali SZ, Robinson R, et al: Infantile extrarenal rhabdoid tumor. Pediatr Dev Pathol 1:149–152, 1998.
54. Schofield DE, Beckwith JB, Sklar J: Loss of heterozygosity at chromosome regions 22q11-12 and 11p15.5 in renal rhabdoid tumors. Genes Chromosomes Cancer 15:10–17, 1996.

55. Rodriguez-Galindo C, Marina NM, Fletcher BD, et al: Is primitive neuroectodermal tumor of the kidney a distinct entity? Cancer 79:2243–2250, 1997.

56. Parham DM, Roloson GJ, Feely M, et al: Primary malignant neuroepithelial tumors of the kidney: A clinicopathologic analysis of 146 adult and pediatric cases from the National Wilms' Tumor Study Group Pathology Center. Am J Surg Pathol 25:133–146, 2001.

57. D'Angio GJ, Breslow N, Beckwith JB, et al: Treatment of Wilms' tumor: Results of the Third National Wilms' Tumor Study. Cancer 64:349–360, 1989.

58. Green DM, Breslow NE, Beckwith JB, et al: Comparison between single-dose and divided-dose administration of dactinomycin and doxorubicin for patients with Wilms' tumor: A report from the National Wilms' Tumor Study Group. J Clin Oncol 16:237–245, 1998.

59. Green DM, Breslow NE, Evans I, et al: The effect of chemotherapy dose intensity on the hematological toxicity of the treatment for Wilms' tumor: A report from the National Wilms' Tumor Study. Am J Pediatr Hematol Oncol 16:207–212, 1994.

60. Green DM, Breslow NE, Beckwith JB, et al: Effect of duration of treatment on treatment outcome and cost of treatment for Wilms' tumor: A report from the National Wilms' Tumor Study Group. J Clin Oncol 16:3744–3751, 1998.

61. Argani P, Perlman EJ, Breslow NE, et al: Clear cell sarcoma of the kidney: A review of 351 cases from the National Wilms Tumor Study Group Pathology Center. Am J Surg Pathol 24:4–18, 2000.

62. Green DM, Breslow NE, Beckwith JB, et al: Treatment of children with clear-cell sarcoma of the kidney: A report from the National Wilms' Tumor Study Group. J Clin Oncol 12:2132–2137, 1994.

63. Seibel N, Li S, Breslow N, et al: Effect of duration of treatment on treatment outcome for patients with clear cell sarcoma of the kidney (CCSK): A report from the National Wilms Tumor Study Group. Proc Am Soc Clin Oncol 22:800, 2003.

64. D'Angio GJ, Evans AE, Breslow N, et al: The treatment of Wilms' tumor: Results of the national Wilms' tumor study. Cancer 38:633–646, 1976.

65. Zoeller G, Pekrun A, Lakomek M, et al: Wilms tumor: The problem of diagnostic accuracy in children undergoing preoperative chemotherapy without histological tumor verification. J Urol 151:169–171, 1994.

66. Zuppan CW, Beckwith JB, Weeks DA, et al: The effect of preoperative therapy on the histologic features of Wilms' tumor: An analysis of cases from the Third National Wilms' Tumor Study. Cancer 68:385–394, 1991.

67. Lemerle J, Voute PA, Tournade MF, et al: Preoperative versus postoperative radiotherapy, single versus multiple courses of actinomycin D, in the treatment of Wilms' tumor: Preliminary results of a controlled clinical trial conducted by the International Society of Paediatric Oncology (SIOP). Cancer 38:647–654, 1976.

68. D'Angio GJ, Evans A, Breslow N, et al: The treatment of Wilms' tumor: Results of the Second National Wilms' Tumor Study. Cancer 47:2302–2311, 1981.

69. Burger D, Moorman-Voestermans CG, Mildenberger H, et al: The advantages of preoperative therapy in Wilms' tumour: A summarised report on clinical trials conducted by the International Society of Paediatric Oncology (SIOP). Z Kinderchir 40:170–175, 1985.

70. Lemerle J, Voute PA, Tournade MF, et al: Effectiveness of preoperative chemotherapy in Wilms' tumor: Results of an International Society of Paediatric Oncology (SIOP) clinical trial. J Clin Oncol 1:604–609, 1983.

71. Jereb B, Burgers JM, Tournade MF, et al: Radiotherapy in the SIOP (International Society of Pediatric Oncology) nephroblastoma studies: A review. Med Pediatr Oncol 22:221–227, 1994.

72. Tournade MF, Com-Nougue C, Voute PA, et al: Results of the Sixth International Society of Pediatric Oncology Wilms' Tumor Trial and Study: A risk-adapted therapeutic approach in Wilms' tumor. J Clin Oncol 11:1014–1023, 1993.

73. Coppes MJ, Tournade MF, Lemerle J, et al: Preoperative care of infants with nephroblastoma: The International Society of Pediatric Oncology 6 experience. Cancer 69:2721–2725, 1992.

74. Tournade MF, Com-Nougue C, de Kraker J, et al: Optimal duration of preoperative therapy in unilateral and nonmetastatic Wilms' tumor in children older than 6 months: Results of the Ninth International Society of Pediatric Oncology Wilms' Tumor Trial and Study. J Clin Oncol 19:488–500, 2001.

75. Godzinski J, Tournade MF, de Kraker J, et al: Rarity of surgical complications after postchemotherapy nephrectomy for nephroblastoma: Experience of the International Society of Paediatric Oncology-Trial and Study "SIOP-9": International Society of Paediatric Oncology Nephroblastoma Trial and Study Committee. Eur J Pediatr Surg 8:83–86, 1998.

76. Boccon-Gibod L, Rey A, Sandstedt B, et al: Complete necrosis induced by preoperative chemotherapy in Wilms tumor as an indicator of low risk: Report of the International Society of Paediatric Oncology (SIOP) Nephroblastoma Trial and Study 9. Med Pediatr Oncol 34:183–190, 2000.

77. Green DM, Breslow NE, D'Angio GJ: The treatment of children with unilateral Wilms' tumor. J Clin Oncol 11:1009–1010, 1993.

78. Green DM, Grigoriev YA, Nan B, et al: Congestive heart failure after treatment for Wilms' tumor: A report from the National Wilms' Tumor Study group. J Clin Oncol 19:1926–1934, 2001.

79. Marx M, Langer T, Graf N, et al: Multicentre analysis of anthracycline-induced cardiotoxicity in children following treatment according to the nephroblastoma studies SIOP No.9/GPOH and SIOP 93-01/GPOH. Med Pediatr Oncol 39:18–24, 2002.

80. Lipshultz SE, Colan SD, Gelber RD, et al: Late cardiac effects of doxorubicin therapy for acute lymphoblastic leukemia in childhood. N Engl J Med 324:808–815, 1991.

81. Breslow NE, Takashima JR, Whitton JA, et al: Second malignant neoplasms following treatment for Wilms' tumor: A report from the National Wilms' Tumor Study Group. J Clin Oncol 13:1851–1859, 1995.

82. Ritchey ML, Kelalis PP, Breslow N, et al: Surgical complications after nephrectomy for Wilms' tumor. Surg Gynecol Obstet 175:507–514, 1992.

83. Ritchey ML, Kelalis PP, Etzioni R, et al: Small bowel obstruction after nephrectomy for Wilms' tumor: A report of the National Wilms' Tumor Study-3. Ann Surg 218:654–659, 1993.

84. Ritchey ML, Pringle KC, Breslow NE, et al: Management and outcome of inoperable Wilms tumor: A report of National Wilms Tumor Study-3. Ann Surg 220:683–690, 1994.

85. Ritchey ML, Shamberger RC, Haase G, et al: Surgical complications after primary nephrectomy for Wilms' tumor: Report from the National Wilms' Tumor Study Group. J Am Coll Surg 192:63–68; quiz 146, 2001.

86. Nakayama DK, Norkool P, deLorimier AA, et al: Intracardiac extension of Wilms' tumor: A report of the National Wilms' Tumor Study. Ann Surg 204:693–697, 1986.

87. Shamberger RC, Guthrie KA, Ritchey ML, et al: Surgery-related factors and local recurrence of Wilms tumor in National Wilms Tumor Study 4. Ann Surg 229:292–297, 1999.

88. Blute ML, Kelalis PP, Offord KP, et al: Bilateral Wilms tumor. J Urol 138:968–973, 1987.

89. Ritchey ML, Green DM, Breslow NB, et al: Accuracy of current imaging modalities in the diagnosis of synchronous bilateral Wilms' tumor: A report from the National Wilms Tumor Study Group. Cancer 75:600–604, 1995.

90. Ritchey ML, Lally KP, Haase GM, et al: Superior mesenteric artery injury during nephrectomy for Wilms' tumor. J Pediatr Surg 27:612–615, 1992.

91. Othersen HB Jr, DeLorimer A, Hrabovsky E, et al: Surgical evaluation of lymph node metastases in Wilms' tumor. J Pediatr Surg 25:330–331, 1990.

92. Jereb B, Tournade MF, Lemerle J, et al: Lymph node invasion and prognosis in nephroblastoma. Cancer 45:1632–1636, 1980.

93. Coppes MJ, Zandvoort SW, Sparling CR, et al: Acquired von Willebrand disease in Wilms' tumor patients. J Clin Oncol 10:422–427, 1992.

94. Lee IS, Nguyen S, Shanberg AM: Needle tract seeding after percutaneous biopsy of Wilms tumor. J Urol 153:1074–1076, 1995.

95. Neville H, Ritchey ML, Shamberger RC, et al: The occurrence of Wilms tumor in horseshoe kidneys: A report from the National Wilms Tumor Study Group (NWTSG). J Pediatr Surg 37:1134–1137, 2002.

96. Dinkel E, Britscho J, Dittrich M, et al: Renal growth in patients nephrectomized for Wilms tumour as compared to renal agenesis. Eur J Pediatr 147:54–58, 1988.

97. Thorner PS, Arbus GS, Celermajer DS, et al: Focal segmental glomerulosclerosis and progressive renal failure associated with a unilateral kidney. Pediatrics 73:806–810, 1984.

98. Ritchey ML, Green DM, Thomas PR, et al: Renal failure in Wilms' tumor patients: A report from the National Wilms' Tumor Study Group. Med Pediatr Oncol 26:75–80, 1996.

99. Urban CE, Lackner H, Schwinger W, et al: Partial nephrectomy in well-responding stage I Wilms' tumors: Report of three cases. Pediatr Hematol Oncol 12:143–152, 1995.

100. McLorie GA, McKenna PH, Greenberg M, et al: Reduction in tumor burden allowing partial nephrectomy following preoperative chemotherapy in biopsy proved Wilms tumor. J Urol 146:509–513, 1991.

101. Wilimas JA, Magill L, Parham DM, et al: Is renal salvage feasible in unilateral Wilms' tumor? Proposed computed tomographic criteria and their relation to surgicopathologic findings. Am J Pediatr Hematol Oncol 12:164–167, 1990.

102. Cozzi F, Schiavetti A, Bonanni M, et al: Enucleative surgery for stage I nephroblastoma with a normal contralateral kidney. J Urol 156:1788–1791; discussion 1791–1783, 1996.

103. Moorman-Voestermans CG, Aronson DC, Staalman CR, et al: Is partial nephrectomy appropriate treatment for unilateral Wilms' tumor? J Pediatr Surg 33:165–170, 1998.

104. McNeil DE, Langer JC, Choyke P, et al: Feasibility of partial nephrectomy for Wilms' tumor in children with Beckwith-Wiedemann syndrome who have been screened with abdominal ultrasonography. J Pediatr Surg 37:57–60, 2002.

105. Breslow N, Beckwith JB, Ciol M, et al: Age distribution of Wilms' tumor: Report from the National Wilms' Tumor Study. Cancer Res 48:1653–1657, 1988.

106. Horwitz JR, Ritchey ML, Moksness J, et al: Renal salvage procedures in patients with synchronous bilateral Wilms' tumors: A report from the National Wilms' Tumor Study Group. J Pediatr Surg 31:1020–1025, 1996.

107. Kumar R, Fitzgerald R, Breatnach F: Conservative surgical management of bilateral Wilms tumor: Results of the United Kingdom Children's Cancer Study Group. J Urol 160:1450–1453, 1998.

108. Paulino AC, Wilimas J, Marina N, et al: Local control in synchronous bilateral Wilms tumor. Int J Radiat Oncol Biol Phys 36:541–548, 1996.

109. Smith GR, Thomas PR, Ritchey M, et al: Long-term renal function in patients with irradiated bilateral Wilms tumor: National Wilms' Tumor Study Group. Am J Clin Oncol 21:58–63, 1998.

110. Anderson J, Slater O, McHugh K, et al: Response without shrinkage in bilateral Wilms tumor: Significance of rhabdomyomatous histology. J Pediatr Hematol Oncol 24:31–34, 2002.

111. Ritchey ML, Kelalis PP, Breslow N, et al: Intracaval and atrial involvement with nephroblastoma: Review of National Wilms Tumor Study-3. J Urol 140:1113–1118, 1988.

112. Ritchey ML, Kelalis PP, Haase GM, et al: Preoperative therapy for intracaval and atrial extension of Wilms tumor. Cancer 71:4104–4110, 1993.

113. Mushtaq I, Carachi R, Roy G, et al: Childhood renal tumours with intravascular extension. Br J Urol 78:772–776, 1996.

114. Shamberger RC, Ritchey ML, Haase GM, et al: Intravascular extension of Wilms tumor. Ann Surg 234:116–121, 2001.

115. Green DM, Breslow NE, Beckwith JB, et al: Treatment outcomes in patients less than 2 years of age with small, stage I, favorable-histology Wilms' tumors: A report from the National Wilms' Tumor Study. J Clin Oncol 11:91–95, 1993.

116. Green DM, Beckwith JB, Weeks DA, et al: The relationship between microsubstaging variables, age at diagnosis, and tumor weight of children with stage I/favorable histology Wilms' tumor: A report from the National Wilms' Tumor Study. Cancer 74:1817–1820, 1994.

117. Larsen E, Perez-Atayde A, Green DM, et al: Surgery only for the treatment of patients with stage I (Cassady) Wilms' tumor. Cancer 66:264–266, 1990.

118. Shamberger RC, Macklis RM, Sallan SE: Recent experience with Wilms' tumor, 1978-1991. Ann Surg Oncol 1:59–65, 1994.

119. Green DM, Breslow NE, Beckwith JB, et al: Treatment with nephrectomy only for small, stage I/favorable histology Wilms' tumor: A report from the National Wilms' Tumor Study Group. J Clin Oncol 19:3719–3724, 2001.

120. Hrabovsky EE, Othersen HB Jr, deLorimier A, et al: Wilms' tumor in the neonate: A report from the National Wilms' Tumor Study. J Pediatr Surg 21:385–387, 1986.

121. Ritchey ML, Azizkhan RG, Beckwith JB, et al: Neonatal Wilms tumor. J Pediatr Surg 30:856–859, 1995.

122. Andrews PE, Kelalis PP, Haase GM: Extrarenal Wilms' tumor: Results of the National Wilms' Tumor Study. J Pediatr Surg 27:1181–1184, 1992.

123. Coppes MJ, Wilson PC, Weitzman S: Extrarenal Wilms' tumor: Staging, treatment, and prognosis. J Clin Oncol 9:167–174, 1991.

124. Lack EE, Cassady JR, Sallan SE: Renal cell carcinoma in childhood and adolescence: A clinical and pathological study of 17 cases. J Urol 133:822–828, 1985.

125. Aronson DC, Medary I, Finlay JL, et al: Renal cell carcinoma in childhood and adolescence: A retrospective survey for prognostic factors in 22 cases. J Pediatr Surg 31:183–186, 1996.

126. Motzer RJ, Bander NH, Nanus DM: Renal-cell carcinoma. N Engl J Med 335:865–875, 1996.

127. Fyfe G, Fisher RI, Rosenberg SA, et al: Results of treatment of 255 patients with metastatic renal cell carcinoma who received high-dose recombinant interleukin-2 therapy. J Clin Oncol 13:688–696, 1995.

128. Trump D, Elson P, Propert K: Randomized controlled trial of adjuvant therapy with lymphoblastoid interferon. Proc Am Soc Clin Oncol 15:353, 1996.

129. Bolande RP, Brough AJ, Izant RJ Jr: Congenital mesoblastic nephroma of infancy: A report of eight cases and the relationship to Wilms' tumor. Pediatrics 40:272–278, 1967.

130. Howell CG, Othersen HB, Kiviat NE, et al: Therapy and outcome in 51 children with mesoblastic nephroma: A report of the National Wilms' Tumor Study. J Pediatr Surg 17:826–831, 1982.

131. Bolande RP: Congenital and infantile neoplasia of the kidney. Lancet 2:1497–1499, 1974.

132. Beckwith JB: Mesenchymal renal neoplasms of infancy revisited. J Pediatr Surg 9:803–805, 1974.

133. Beckwith J: Reply. Pediatr Pathol 13:886–887, 1993.

134. Heidelberger KP, Ritchey ML, Dauser RC, et al: Congenital mesoblastic nephroma metastatic to the brain. Cancer 72:2499–2502, 1993.

135. Schlesinger A: Congenital mesoblastic nephroma metastatic to the brain: A report of two cases. Pediatr Radiol 25:S73–S75, 1995.

136. Vujanic GM, Delemarre JF, Moeslichan S, et al: Mesoblastic nephroma metastatic to the lungs and heart: Another face of this peculiar lesion: case report and review of the literature. Pediatr Pathol 13:143–153, 1993.

137. Sandstedt B, Delemarre JF, Krul EJ, et al: Mesoblastic nephromas: A study of 29 tumours from the SIOP nephroblastoma file. Histopathology 9:741–750, 1985.

138. Chan KL, Chan KW, Lee CW, et al: Preoperative chemotherapy for mesoblastic nephroma. Med Pediatr Oncol 24:271–273, 1995.

139. Agrons GA, Wagner BJ, Davidson AJ, et al: Multilocular cystic renal tumor in children: Radiologic-pathologic correlation. Radiographics 15:653–669, 1995.

140. Ishida Y, Kato K, Kigasawa H, et al: Synchronous occurrence of pleuropulmonary blastoma and cystic nephroma: Possible genetic link in cystic lesions of the lung and the kidney. Med Pediatr Oncol 35:85–87, 2000.

141. Joshi VV, Beckwith JB: Multilocular cyst of the kidney (cystic nephroma) and cystic, partially differentiated nephroblastoma: Terminology and criteria for diagnosis. Cancer 64:466–479, 1989.

142. Blakeley M, RC S, Norkool P: Outcome of children with cystic partially-differentiated nephroblastoma treated. J Pediatr Surg 38:897–900, 2003.

143. Streif W, Gassner I, Janetschek G, et al: Partial nephrectomy in a cystic partially differentiated nephroblastoma. Med Pediatr Oncol 28:416–419, 1997.

144. Sotelo-Avila C, Beckwith JB, Johnson JE: Ossifying renal tumor of infancy: A clinicopathologic study of nine cases. Pediatr Pathol Lab Med 15:745–762, 1995.

145. Steffens J, Kraus J, Misho B, et al: Ossifying renal tumor of infancy. J Urol 149:1080–1081, 1993.

146. Vazquez JL, Barnewolt CE, Shamberger RC, et al: Ossifying renal tumor of infancy presenting as a palpable abdominal mass. Pediatr Radiol 28:454–457, 1998.

CHAPTER 66

Neuroblastoma

E. M. Kiely, MD

HISTORY

Although neuroblastoma has probably affected children since antiquity, recognition of its separate identity is recent. Deaths from infectious conditions were common and greatly overshadowed the smaller number of deaths from malignancy. The neural origin of neuroblastoma was first proposed by Virchow in 1864,[1] and succeeding years brought a slow acquisition of understanding of the condition. Marchand[2] (1891) is credited with recognizing the similarity of neuroblastoma cells to the cells of the sympathetic nervous system. Several reports dealt with stage 4S disease,[3,4] and by the early years of the 20th century, pathologic features of the condition had been defined.[5,6] The name *neuroblastoma* was devised by James Homer Wright[5] in 1910 and rapidly supplanted previous names. Hutchison[7] (1907) wrote a clear description of metastatic neuroblastoma, although he considered it a sarcoma.

The first recorded successful resection was undertaken by Willard Bartlett[8] of St. Louis, Missouri, in 1914: a 470-g tumor was removed from a boy aged 11 months. This patient was alive and well 15 years later.[9] An intimation of the enigmatic behavior of this tumor was provided by Cushing and Wolbach in 1927.[10] They described maturation of a neuroblastoma into a ganglioneuroma over a 10-year period.

By 1934, Blacklock[11] in Glasgow wrote that neuroblastoma was the fourth commonest type of malignancy in children. In 1938, Redman[12] noted 275 reported cases in the literature. The first use of radiotherapy for neuroblastoma was in 1928. Holmes and Dresser[13] treated three patients, none of whom survived. A further report from Boston in 1940 suggested that radiotherapy improved survival rate.[14]

Phillips[15] (1953) evaluated the results of a substantial series from the Memorial Hospital, New York, and described the use of nitrogen mustard derivatives. Survival rates of those with advanced disease were dismal. Koop[16] (1955) recommended "a major surgical insult" to the tumor, as in his hands, this resulted in a better outcome. The experience at St. Jude Hospital with combination chemotherapy was published in 1965,[17] but overall results remained poor.

Various attempts at classification and staging were used, but the Evans system[18] (1971) became the most widely used. This staging system, combined with that used by the Pediatric Oncology Group (POG) has formed the basis for the International Neuroblastoma Staging System (INSS) criteria by which neuroblastoma is now staged in many countries.

INCIDENCE AND NATURAL HISTORY

The incidence of neuroblastoma varies a little between different racial groups.[19] In predominantly white populations, the age standardized rate is 7 to 12/1,000,000 and accounts for 6% to 10% of all childhood cancers. The incidence is highest in the first year of life (30% of total), 50% occur between ages 1 and 4 years, and only 5% occur in the 10- to 14-year age group. The gender incidence shows a slight male preponderance: 1.2, 1.3 to 1 overall. The reasons for this are not clear.

Beckwith and Perrin[20] (1963) described the presence of neuroblastoma nodules in the adrenals of infants younger than 3 months, dying of unrelated conditions. These nodules varied in size from 0.4 mm to 9.5 mm and were found in 0.3% to 1.0% of their two series of autopsies. Whether these nodules always regressed or formed the basis for future neuroblastoma is not clear. Data from the Japanese screening program suggest that even large neuroblastoma masses may regress.[21]

NATURAL HISTORY

The etiology of neuroblastoma is unknown. Rare familial cases are described, often with multiple primary tumors, but most cases are sporadic.[22] The tumor arises from sympathetic neuroblast cells derived from the neural crest. Neuroblast migration occurs from paravertebral ganglia into the adrenal medulla, mainly during early

933

fetal life.[23] Once a neoplasm develops, local extension occurs with vascular encasement and invasion of adjacent structures. Metastases occur to lymph nodes, bone, bone marrow, liver, and skin. Apart from infants with stage 4S disease, secondary spread is usually associated with large primary tumors and may occur late in the natural history of the disease.

PATHOLOGY

On macroscopic inspection, neuroblastomas are frequently soft with areas of necrosis and hemorrhage. More mature areas of tumor are firm and greyish white.

Histologically, the immature neuroblasts are seen as sheets of dark blue cells with scanty cytoplasm set in a delicate vascular stroma. Rosette formation, consisting of a ring of neuroblasts around a neurofibrillary core, is a characteristic feature but is often absent. With differentiation toward mature ganglion cells, the eosinophilic cytoplasm becomes more abundant, and the nuclei show well-defined nucleoli.[28] The combination of immature neuroblasts in a predominantly mature tumor is considered to be a ganglioneuroblastoma.

Attempts have been made to use the histologic appearance of these tumors to predict the clinical outcome. In the era of molecular biology, the use of histologic reading systems may seem an anachronism. However, the appearance under the microscope is presumably a reflection of the biologic properties of the tumor, and pathologic grading remains useful. Of the many systems that have evolved, the Shimada classification is perhaps the most widely applied.[24] This system was devised after evaluation of the microscopic appearances of 295 pretreatment neuroblastomas stained with hematoxylin and eosin. Microscopic features assessed included the stroma, degree of differentiation of neuroblastoma cells, and the nuclear morphology (mitosis and karyorrhexis). From the nuclear morphology, a mitosis karyorrhexis index (MKI) was calculated by counting the number of mitotic or karyorrhectic cells per 5000 cells. A low index was fewer than 100 cells per 5000; intermediate was 100 to 200; and high, more than 200. On the basis of these assessments, two prognostic groups were distinguished: good prognosis and poor prognosis. The good-prognosis group included those younger than 1 year with any degree of differentiation and a low MKI. Also included were those with stroma-rich tumors and well-differentiated or intermixed degrees of differentiation. Finally, also under the good-prognosis group were those aged 1 to 5 years with differentiating histology and a low MKI.

The poor-prognosis group included all other tumors with undifferentiated histology, high MKI, and patients age 1 to 5 years with differentiating histology and high or intermediate MKI. Also included in the poor-prognosis group were those older than 5 years and with tumors with a nodular pattern.

In the original publication, 87% of those in the good-prognosis group survived. Only 7% of the poor-prognosis group was alive.

More recently, an International Neuroblastoma Pathology Classification (INPC) system was proposed, based on Shimada.[25] Based on this system, favorable and unfavorable histology groups may be distinguished. Early experience with this system suggests that the classification is strongly predictive of outcome.[26]

SITES OF DISEASE

Because neuroblastomas arise from neuroblasts of the sympathetic nervous system, they may be found anywhere that sympathetic cells are found. These are seen predominantly in the ganglia of the sympathetic chains from neck to pelvis, in other preaortic and pelvic ganglia, and in the adrenal medulla. The adrenal is the commonest site of origin (40% to 60% of the total) followed by other retroperitoneal sites (20%), mediastinum (10%), pelvis (2% to 6%), and neck (~2%).[27,28] The majority of children have metastatic disease at the time of presentation (62% to 70%).[27,28] Localized disease is present in about 25%, and stage 4S disease, in 10%.[28]

More recently, antenatal diagnosis was described, but it is too early to know if this will have an impact on the total number of patients with neuroblastoma or on the subsequent survival. Prenatally diagnosed tumors are mainly adrenal (93%) with favorable biologic features (absent N-*myc* amplification), and 67% have localized stage 1 disease.[29]

MARKERS OF DISEASE ACTIVITY

A series of biochemical and molecular markers of disease activity and behavior is available. Some of these measurements are within the range of all hospital laboratories, and some are available only to more specialized centers.

Biochemical Markers

Several biochemical markers of disease are found in patients' serum. These include neuron-specific enolase (NSE), lactate dehydrogenase (LDH), and ferritin. NSE, a glycolytic enzyme, is expressed by cells of the central and peripheral nervous system. NSE also is expressed by neuroblastoma cells. Levels of NSE greater than 15 ng/mL are considered abnormal. High levels of NSE (>100 ng/mL) correlate with advanced stages of disease and are associated with lower survival rates.[30–32]

Serum LDH levels also may be an independent prognostic variable. Patients with measurements of less than 1500 international LDH units/mL have improved survival. In general, low levels are associated with a more favorable biologic profile (nonamplified N-*myc*, low stage, younger than 1 year).[33–35]

Ferritin is the major tissue iron–binding protein. The circulating level is related to tissue iron stores. Neuroblastoma cells produce ferritin, which may be detected in serum.[36] Although ferritin may be found in the cells of the primary tumor, high serum levels are unusual in those with low-stage disease.[37] High serum ferritin (>142 ng/mL) is a feature of those with stage 3 and stage 4 disease and is associated with a worse outcome. In addition, those with advanced disease, low (<75 ng/mL), intermediate (75 to 142 ng/mL), and high (>142 ng/mL) levels were associated with different outcomes.[37] Increasing serum ferritin levels at diagnosis were associated with diminishing progression-free survival (PFS).

Molecular Markers

The explosion of knowledge about cellular genetics has been followed by a slower accrual of understanding of the factors involved in tumor genesis and tumor behavior. This increased knowledge has not, so far, led to improved treatment or to significant changes in outcome. A wide variety of molecular abnormalities have been detected in neuroblastoma cells, including N-*myc* amplification, gain of chromosome 17q, 1p deletion, DNA ploidy and DNA index, CD44 expression, *TRKA* expression, and multidrug resistance–associated protein (MRP).

The normal locus for the N-*myc* proto-oncogene is on the short arm of chromosome 2. Amplification of this sequence in neuroblastoma was first described in 1983.[38] N-*myc* amplification has been shown repeatedly to correlate with advanced stage and with disease progression.[34,39–42] Overall, about 25% of patients with neuroblastoma will show N-*myc* amplification.[41] Those with stages 1, 2, and 4S disease do not usually show amplification. About 50% of those with stages 3 and 4 disease do. However, because fewer than 5% of those with low-stage disease show N-*myc* amplification, contradictory results have been reported.[45] In a larger recent series, N-*myc* amplification conferred a worse outlook.[46] In general, N-*myc* amplification correlates with disease progression, independent of age and stage.

N-*myc* amplification also is associated with unfavorable histologic features and was associated with a 13% PFS in a recent Children's Cancer Study Group (CCG) study.[41]

Diploid DNA content is more frequently found in tumors with N-*myc* amplification and is associated with a poor outcome.[34,40,44]

A correlation is found between N-*myc* amplification and chromosome 1p deletion. Both are associated with an aggressive clinical course.[47,48]

Unlike the situation in other tumors, the presence of hyperdiploid DNA content is associated with lower stage and an improved prognosis.[49] Hyperdiploid tumors are more commonly found in infants and constitute the majority of low-stage tumors in all age groups.[45,49] Tumors with diploid or near-diploid DNA content are found in about two thirds of those with stages 3 and 4 disease. When associated with N-*myc* amplification, the prognosis is even worse.[40] Chemosensitivity also may be related to ploidy, with diploid tumors responding poorly.[44] Finally, thoracic tumors, which carry a better prognosis, are more likely than nonthoracic tumors to be hyperdiploid.[33]

Deletion of the short arm of chromosome 1 also is useful prognostically. It seems likely that a tumor-suppressor gene or genes lie in the deleted region. Removal of this gene then allows tumor development and progression. 1p LOH was described in 1981 and is strongly associated with N-*myc* amplification.[50] 1p LOH is found in 19% to 33% of all neuroblastomas and correlates with increased ferritin and LDH levels.[48,51–52]

A number of chromosomal deletions and translocations have been described in neuroblastomas. The commonest chromosomal alteration of significance in neuroblastoma is probably related to gain of chromosomal material from the long arm of chromosome 17-17q. This was shown in 53% of 313 patients in a recent European study.[53] The gain is in the form of an unbalanced translocation, most commonly to the short arm of chromosome 1. The gain is linked with 1p loss of heterozygosity (LOH). This chromosomal abnormality also is associated with a worse outcome.

CD44 is a cell-surface glycoprotein involved in cell-to-cell and cell-to-matrix interactions. Unusually, CD44 expression is correlated with improved survival in neuroblastoma and with absence of N-*myc* amplification.[43,54,55] CD44 was expressed in 84% of patients in a prospective study.[43] All those with stages 1, 2, and 4S expressed CD44. In those with stage 4 disease, 7 of 8 infants showed expression of CD44, and 15 of 32 older patients also did so. In this study, a strong inverse relation was seen between CD44 expression and N-*myc* copy numbers. Normal N-*myc* and CD44 expression were the strongest predictors of survival.

The proto-oncogene *TRKA* encodes a tyrosine kinase nerve growth factor receptor. *TRKA* expression was found in 91% of 77 neuroblastomas, a high level of expression being found in 82%.[56] A strong correlation was noted between low stage, age younger than 1 year, normal N-*myc* copy number, and *TRKA* expression.[56,57] High levels of expression predicted a favorable outcome. Low levels of *TRKA* expression were associated with advanced stage, older age, and N-*myc* amplification. *TRKA* expression has prognostic value even in those tumors with normal N-*myc* copy number.

Treatment failure in patients with advanced disease is manifest by resistance of the tumor to a wide variety of chemotherapeutic agents. Recently, a gene on chromosome 16 was found to mediate resistance to vinca alkaloids, anthracyclines, and epipodophyllotoxins. This gene encodes a membrane-bound glycoprotein termed the MRP. MRP is probably expressed in all neuroblastomas, with higher levels recorded in those with advanced clinical stages. High levels correlated with N-*myc* amplification and with lower survival. The effect of high levels of MRP expression is independent of N-*myc* expression and *TRKA* expression.[57]

SCREENING

More than 85% of neuroblastomas excrete increased levels of catecholamine metabolites.[58,59] These are readily detectable with standard laboratory techniques. The commonest metabolites measured are vanillylmandelic acid (VMA) and homovanillic acid (HVA). VMA is the main breakdown product of adrenalin and noradrenalin. HVA is the main breakdown product of dopa and dopamine.[58] The ability to detect increased levels has led to several attempts at screening in the infant population to detect neuroblastomas before the development of metastases. Initially considerable enthusiasm was expressed for neuroblastoma screening.[60,61] Subsequently, however, it has become apparent that screening detected an increased number of good-prognosis tumors without decreasing the incidence of poor-prognosis tumors seen later in older children.[62] The Quebec screening program screened infants at ages 3 weeks and 6 months over a 5-year period. Roughly twice as many neuroblastomas were found as would have been expected, with no decrease in those seen later with advanced-stage disease. In general, neuroblastoma detected by screening is characterized by low stage and favorable biologic features.[63] Therefore evidence now suggests that a group of infants with neuroblastoma have a good prognosis and are detectable by screening. Most of these tumors regress.[20] A second group of patients is older than 1 year at diagnosis, and these have a much less favorable prognosis and are not detectable by screening in infancy.

Review of 245 neuroblastomas detected by screening at age 6 months in the Kyushu region of Japan showed that 10% had one or more unfavorable biologic markers.[64] In six infants, the tumor recurred, and in two of these, no unfavorable features were noted. One patient died of disease progression, and one other had a stable tumor at the time of the report. Recurrence occurred up to 4 years from the time of the initial treatment.

STAGING

Staging systems are used to document disease extent at diagnosis and to stratify and modify treatment in response to outcome. A plethora of staging systems have been used in children with neuroblastoma—a reflection on the difficulties encountered in trying to achieve a cure in these patients. This has made comparisons between different therapies difficult to evaluate. In 1986, an International Conference representing most of the larger oncology groups recommended criteria for diagnosis, staging, and response in patients with neuroblastoma.[66] These criteria have been revised and appear to have considerable support across national boundaries.[67] The INSS is shown in Table 66-1. This is based on clinical and surgical criteria and carries features of the older Evans and POG systems.[23,68] The POG system is shown in Table 66-2. Doubtless the revised INSS system will be superseded in turn by a system incorporating biologic features.

About 25% of patients have localized stages 1 and 2 disease. Stage 4S disease is present in 10%. Those with locally advanced and metastatic disease constitute the remainder, 62% to 70%.[28,33]

PRESENTATION

A small number of tumors are detected on prenatal ultrasonography (US)—just over 3% of the total in a recent study.[65] Detection was usually in the third trimester. Of the 17 patients, 13 had stage 1 disease, two had stage 2, and two further had stage 4S disease. In those in whom findings were estimated, urinary catecholamines were elevated in only 38%. N-*myc* amplification was found in one patient,

TABLE 66-1
INTERNATIONAL NEUROBLASTOMA STAGING SYSTEM CRITERIA

Stage	Definition
1	Localized tumor with complete gross excision, with or without microscopic residual disease; representative ipsilateral lymph nodes negative for tumor microscopically (nodes attached to and removed with the primary tumor may be positive)
2A	Localized tumor with incomplete gross excision; representative ipsilateral nonadherent lymph nodes negative for tumor microscopically
2B	Localized tumor with or without complete gross excision, with ipsilateral nonadherent lymph nodes positive for tumor. Enlarged contralateral lymph nodes must be negative microscopically
3	Unresectable unilateral tumor infiltrating across the midline,* with or without regional lymph node involvement *or* Localized unilateral tumor with contralateral regional lymph node involvement *or* Midline tumor with bilateral extension by infiltration (unresectable) or by lymph node involvement
4	Any primary tumor with dissemination to distant lymph nodes, bone, bone marrow, liver, skin, or other organs (except as defined for stage 4S).
4S	Localized primary tumor (as defined for stage 1, 2A, or 2B), with dissemination limited to skin, liver, and bone marrow† (limited to infants younger than 1 yr)

*The midline is defined as the vertebral column. Tumors originating on one side and crossing the midline must infiltrate to or beyond the opposite side of the vertebral column.
†Marrow involvement in stage 4S should be minimal (i.e., <10% of total nucleated cells identified as malignant on bone marrow biopsy or on marrow aspirate). More extensive marrow involvement would be considered to be stage 4. The metaiodobenzylguanidine scan (if performed) should be negative in the marrow.

and diploidy and 1p deletion were detected in one further patient.

Postnatally, neuroblastoma commonly appears insidiously with vague symptoms. Presenting symptoms may be due to the mass or to the presence of metastases. Malaise, weight loss, fever, and sweating are common symptoms. Bone and joint pain, the result of metastatic disease, may initially be diagnosed as juvenile arthritis. Periorbital ecchymosis or proptosis, the result of skull secondaries, may initially be attributed to nonaccidental injury but should draw attention to the possibility of a neuroblastoma.

Tumors in the neck are usually found because of a visible mass. Those in the chest may be unexpected findings on a chest radiograph taken for persisting or recurrent mild respiratory symptoms. Occasionally Horner's syndrome is noted with apical thoracic tumors.

Pelvic tumors may interfere with bowel and bladder function and come to light during investigations for sphincter disturbances.

TABLE 66-2

PEDIATRIC ONCOLOGY GROUP STAGING CRITERIA

Stage	Definition
A	Complete gross resection of primary tumor, with or without microscopic residual. Intracavitary lymph nodes, not adhered to and removed with primary (nodes adhered to or without tumor resection may be positive for tumor without upstaging patient to stage C), histologically free of tumor. If primary is in abdomen or pelvis, liver is histologically free of tumor
B	Grossly unresected primary tumor. Nodes and liver same as stage A
C	Complete or incomplete resection of primary tumor. Intracavitary nodes not adhered to primary histologically positive for tumor. Liver as in stage A
D	Any dissemination of disease beyond intracavitary nodes (i.e., extracavitary nodes, liver, skin, bone marrow, bone)
D(S)	Evans IVS. Evans stage I or II except for metastatic tumor in liver, bone marrow, or skin

The majority of abdominal tumors are found because of symptomatic metastatic disease. Finally, a number of neuroblastomas occur with locomotor disturbance and progressive paraplegia, the result of extradural cord compression.

On examination, abdominal neuroblastomas are usually hard, irregular, fixed tumors. Less commonly, tumors in infancy are smooth and ballotable, but these unfortunately are not very common. Pelvic tumors may be palpable on abdominal examination or, more commonly, on rectal examination. An enlarged bladder from urinary retention or palpable feces from constipation are features of pelvic lesions.

Infants with stage 4S disease may show multiple skin nodules. Frequently, however, these children have increasing abdominal distention from enlarging hepatomegaly. This may progress to the point at which breathing is impaired and ventilator support is required.

Hypertension is not unusual, due to either catecholamine secretion or renal artery compression. Hypertension has been documented in 19% of 59 children with newly diagnosed neurogenic tumors.[69] The blood pressure did not correlate with urinary catecholamine secretion. Control of hypertension followed tumor resection or chemotherapy.

PARANEOPLASTIC SYNDROMES

Rare forms of presentation include the dancing eye (opsomyoclonus) syndrome and intractable diarrhea.

Opsomyoclonus is characterized by progressive cerebellar ataxia with frequent jerking movements of the muscles of the limbs and trunk. In addition, opsoclonus is manifest by rapid, chaotic, conjugate eye movements. More than half of these patients have a thoracic primary tumor.

Developmental delay is common in these children, although the prognosis in terms of survival is favorable.[70]

Intractable diarrhea as a presenting symptom is uncommon and is due to vasoactive intestinal polypeptide (VIP) secretion by the tumor. It is more common in those with ganglioneuromas and ganglioneuroblastomas than in those with neuroblastomas.[71] Diarrhea commencing after initiation of treatment of a stage 4 neuroblastoma has been recorded.[72]

DIAGNOSIS

The diagnosis is suspected on clinical grounds from the history and physical findings. Confirmation of the diagnosis is by a combination of laboratory and radiologic investigation and by tissue examination. Staging investigations are then completed. Table 66-3 shows the INSS criteria for the diagnosis of neuroblastoma. With these criteria, a positive tissue diagnosis is considered essential.

Table 66-4 shows the INSS recommendations for assessment of extent of disease and staging.

LABORATORY INVESTIGATIONS

Estimation of urinary catecholamine metabolites is the initial diagnostic screen. As noted earlier, urinary VMA and HVA are elevated in the great majority of children with neuroblastoma.

The basic evaluation will include full blood count, serum biochemistry, and liver and renal function tests. Serum ferritin, LDH, and NSE also should be measured.

IMAGING

The sequence of imaging investigations performed will depend on the clinical presentation and local facilities.

TABLE 66-3

INTERNATIONAL NEUROBLASTOMA STAGING SYSTEM CRITERIA FOR DIAGNOSIS OF NEUROBLASTOMA

Unequivocal pathologic diagnosis* is made from tumor tissue by light microscopy (with or without immunohistology, electron microscopy, and increased urine or serum catecholamines or metabolites[†])

or

Bone marrow aspirate or trephine biopsy contains unequivocal tumor cells* (e.g., syncytial or immunocytologically positive clumps of cells) and increased urine or serum catecholamines or metabolites[†]

*If histology is equivocal, karyotypic abnormalities in tumor cells characteristic of other tumors, such as t(11-22), then exclude a diagnosis of neuroblastoma, whereas genetic features characteristic of neuroblastoma (1p deletion, N-*myc* amplification) would support this diagnosis.
[†]Catecholamines and metabolites include dopamine, homovanillic acid, and vanillylmandelic acid; levels must be >3.0 SD above the mean per milligram creatinine for age to be considered increased, and at least two of these must be measured.

TABLE 66-4

INTERNATIONAL NEUROBLASTOMA STAGING SYSTEM STAGING INVESTIGATIONS

Tumor Site	Recommended Tests
Primary tumor	CT or MRI scan with three-dimensional measurements; MIBG scan, if available.

Metastatic Sites	Recommended Tests
Bone marrow	Bilateral posterior iliac crest marrow aspirates and trephine (core) bone marrow biopsies required to exclude marrow involvement. A single positive site documents marrow involvement. Core biopsies must contain ≥1 cm of marrow (excluding cartilage) to be considered adequate
Bone	MIBG scan; ^{99m}Tc scan required if MIBG scan is negative or unavailable, and plain radiographs of positive lesions are recommended
Lymph nodes	Clinical examination (palpable nodes), confirmed histologically. CT scan for nonpalpable nodes (three-dimensional measurements)
Abdomen and liver	CT or MRI scan with three-dimensional measurements
Chest	Anteroposterior and lateral chest radiographs. CT and MRI necessary if chest radiograph is positive or if abdominal mass/nodes extend into chest

CT, computed tomography; MIBG, metaiodobenzylguanidine; MRI, magnetic resonance imaging.

Most children will have plain radiographs taken and ultrasonography (US) performed. Dystrophic calcification will be seen on more than 50% of plain radiographs.[28] In addition to radiographs of the anatomic site in question, the children should have a chest roentgenogram. Lateral chest views are often helpful in the presence of mediastinal tumors.

US is often used as a screening test to establish whether a mass is solid or cystic. Neuroblastoma does not have a diagnostic sonographic appearance. It generally shows a mixed echo pattern with areas of calcification and necrosis. Frequently, however, an experienced ultrasonographer will recognize the heterogeneous echo pattern, and this, combined with the anatomic location and pattern of growth, will allow a fairly confident diagnosis. US is of limited use in the chest and in the pelvis.

For accurate anatomic detail, contrast enhanced computed tomography (CT) or magnetic resonance imaging (MRI) is necessary. The two are complementary rather than interchangeable. For most purposes, CT with contrast provides the necessary detail on site, consistency, and relation to vital structures.

MRI gives detailed information on soft tissue changes, on liver involvement, and most valuably, on the anatomy of intraspinal extension. Because multiplanar images are accessible, extensive information is available on

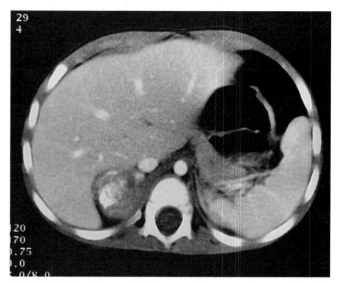

FIGURE 66-1. Computed tomography scan of stage 1, right adrenal neuroblastoma.

tumor extent. It is the investigation of choice in dumb-bell tumors and is far superior to myelography. Bone involvement also is readily seen on MRI scanning.

Representative scans are shown in Figures 66-1 through 66-6. Figure 66-1 shows a CT scan of a right-sided, stage 1, tumor. Figure 66-2 shows a left-sided, stage 2 lesion. Figure 66-3 shows a large, right-sided lesion crossing the vertebrae; at operation, the lesion had invaded beyond the left border of the vertebral column. Figure 66-4 shows an extensive stage 4 neuroblastoma originating in the right adrenal. The scan shows anterior displacement and encasement of the great vessels at the level of the superior mesenteric artery (SMA).

Figures 66-5 and 66-6 show transverse and coronal images of an MRI scan in a patient with a dumbbell tumor. The extent of intraspinal disease is readily seen.

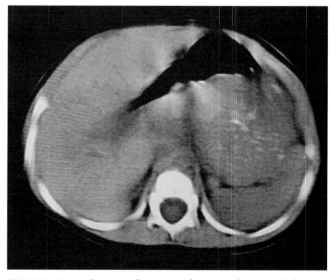

FIGURE 66-2. Computed tomography scan of stage 2, left adrenal neuroblastoma.

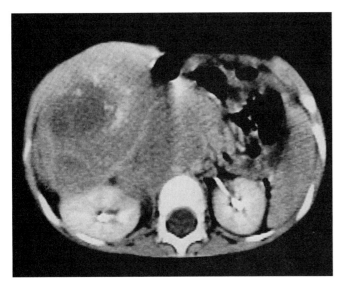

FIGURE 66-3. Computed tomography scan of stage 3, right-sided neuroblastoma. At operation, this tumor had invaded beyond the left side of the spine.

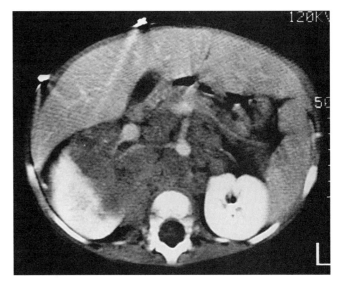

FIGURE 66-4. Computed tomography scan of stage 4, right adrenal neuroblastoma, displacing and encasing the great vessels at the level of the superior mesenteric artery.

Skeletal metastases may be seen on plain radiography with periosteal erosion, radiolucencies, and pathologic fractures. Routine identification of metastatic skeletal disease is best performed with isotope scanning. Radiolabeled metaiodobenzylguanidine (MIBG) is regarded as a sensitive method of detecting bone and bone marrow disease.[73] MIBG is labeled with iodine 123 or [131]I. Figure 66-7 shows extensive neuroblastoma demonstrated on an MIBG scan.

MIBG scans have a false-negative rate and are best complemented by technetium 99m (^{99m}Tc) methylene diphosphonate (MDP) bone scanning.[74] The present INSS criteria suggest using MIBG scanning when available and ^{99m}Tc scanning only if the MIBG is negative. Widespread skeletal involvement, shown on a technetium scan, is shown in Figure 66-8.

TISSUE BIOPSY

Tissue diagnosis is regarded as essential. The tissue may be obtained by bone marrow aspiration or trephine, or by biopsy of primary or accessible secondary disease. Sufficient tissue should be obtained both for diagnosis and for the completion of cytogenetic studies.

TREATMENT

The management of a patient with neuroblastoma involves a multidisciplinary team. The composition of the team will vary between different institutions. Treatment modalities at present include chemotherapy, surgical intervention, and radiotherapy. These are provided in turn by pediatric oncologists, pediatric surgeons, and pediatric radiotherapists. Indispensable contributions are made by pediatric radiologists and pathologists.

The surgeon's role is to excise tumors where possible, to perform biopsies when necessary, and to provide vascular access.

The management of those with stage 1 disease is by operation. These relatively uncommon tumors are usually amenable to complete resection. Ideally, those with stage 2 disease should also undergo complete excision. This may not be feasible or indeed advisable, where injudicious attempts to clear all tumor may be hazardous. Examples would include tumors extending into intervertebral foramina and apical thoracic tumors close to the stellate ganglion. Also in some instances, a course of chemotherapy might be advisable to facilitate surgery.

The management of dumbbell tumors with spinal cord compression is controversial. Opinion varies between the use of chemotherapy and urgent laminectomy. A recent report from France supports the use of primary chemotherapy, surgical intervention being reserved for those who have rapidly deteriorating neurologic status.[75] This article confirms the high incidence of thoracic tumors in this group of patients and the excellent outcome. Either

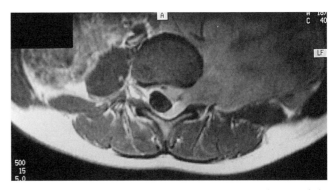

FIGURE 66-5. Magnetic resonance imaging scan showing left-sided dumbbell tumor.

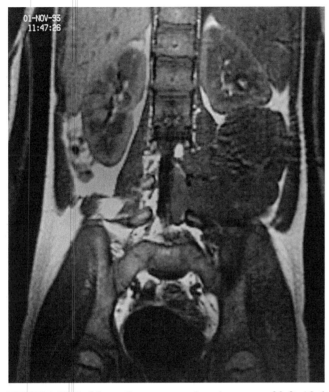

FIGURE 66-6. Magnetic resonance imaging scan of left-sided dumb-bell tumor (coronal view).

way, excision is often advised for residual extradural tumor followed concurrently or later by excision of the extraspinal component.

The trend in management of those with stages 3 and 4 disease is toward delayed resection after chemotherapy. Post-treatment tumors are less vascular and are more amenable to complete resection.[76,77]

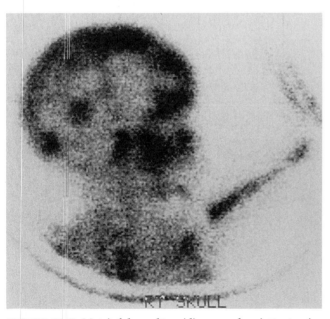

FIGURE 66-7. Metaiodobenzylguanidine scan showing extensive metastatic neuroblastoma.

For those with stage 4S disease, management is tailored to the patient. Neonates with hepatomegaly are at greater risk and may require intensive treatment.[28,78] The use of ventral hernias to enlarge the abdomen has been associated with a high mortality.[79] Older infants with stage 4S disease frequently show maturation and regression of disease in the absence of any treatment.[80] Resection of the primary tumor confers no benefit in terms of survival.[81] Some centers remove the primary tumor if it persists and other evidence of disease has regressed.

Chemotherapy

Chemotherapy protocols undergo constant modification and refinement. The aim is to limit therapy in those with a good prognosis and to intensify treatment for those with a poor prognosis. Combination chemotherapy is now the mainstay of treatment for those with advanced disease. (See also Chapter 64.)

A considerable number of chemotherapy protocols are in use worldwide. For those with advanced disease, chemotherapy is often followed by delayed resection. In many protocols, myeloablative therapy with total body irradiation (TBI) or melphalan is used and subsequently followed by bone marrow transplantation (BMT).[82,83]

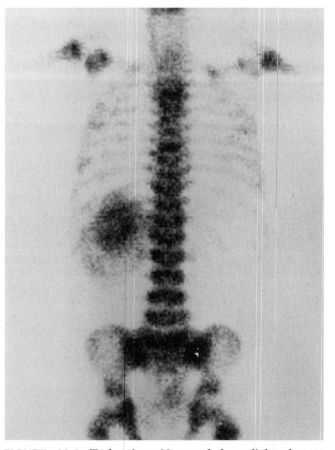

FIGURE 66-8. Technetium 99m methylene diphosphonate bone scan showing widespread vertebrae and skeletal metastatic disease.

Agents used in combination include cyclophosphamide, iphosphamide, vincristine, cisplatin, carboplatin, doxorubicin, etoposide, and melphalan. BMT is performed mostly with autologous purged bone marrow.

Such toxic treatment carries its own risks. Death from treatment has been reported in up to 20% of treated patients but is usually less common. Lesser complications from the treatment include sepsis, hemorrhage, and veno-occlusive disease.[82]

The INSS response criteria are shown in Table 66-5. The response to chemotherapy is usually assessed after 3 to 4 months of induction chemotherapy.

Surgery

The aim of surgery is to remove all tumor. In lower stages, resection is usually possible. In advanced cases, resection may present some difficulty.

Standard techniques suffice for the rare cervical tumors. Thoracic tumors similarly do not usually present serious surgical obstacles. The majority arise from the sympathetic chain and lie in the costovertebral angle. Encasement of major vessels is not common. Tumors arising in the upper thoracic ganglia may encroach on the stellate ganglion. Excision may then result in a Horner's syndrome. Although standard thoracotomy incisions are satisfactory for most thoracic tumors, apical tumors and those extending into the neck may present problems with access. The trap-door incision seems like a useful contribution. The incision extends along the upper border of the clavicle, vertically through the manubrium as far as the third interspace, and then laterally through the third intercostal space. Once the sternomastoid muscle is transected, the whole flap can be reflected laterally.[84,85]

Dumb-bell thoracic tumors connected to an intraspinal component may be difficult to remove completely. No consensus exists on whether intraspinal disease should be removed before or after the thoracic component or even at the same sitting. The author's practice is to request initial clearance of the intraspinal tumor. Postoperative swelling of a spinal extension after thoracic operation might otherwise jeopardize the cord.

Excision of abdominal tumors presents some difficulties. With stages 3 and 4 tumors, it is usual to encounter encasement of the great vessels and main visceral vessels in addition. Whatever technique is used, the aim is to preserve the vessels while clearing the tumor. Again, with locally advanced tumors, excision is impossible without incising the tumor.

Detailed accounts of the surgical technique used to excise advanced neuroblastoma are uncommon.[86,87] Because the main problems are encountered with major blood vessels, the logical approach is to display all the vascular anatomy before tumor excision. Neuroblastoma does not usually invade the tunica media of major blood vessels, be they arteries or veins. Consequently, a subadventitial plane exists around all the major vascular structures. This plane may be entered and maintained with a knife. Knife dissection is not commonly used in pediatric surgery, but for this particular operation, it is well nigh essential. Optical magnification, bipolar diathermy, and a table-mounted retractor complete the list of essentials.

The majority of abdominal tumors arise in the upper abdomen. Surgical approaches vary between thoraco-abdominal and upper transverse abdominal incisions. The colon is reflected medially on its mesentery to expose the retroperitoneum. On the left side, the spleen, pancreas, and stomach also are mobilized and all viscera placed in an intestinal bag to reduce desiccation and serosal trauma.

Once the colon is reflected, the full extent of the tumor is apparent. The three phases to the operation are as follows: vessel display, vessel clearance, and tumor removal. The first is the most difficult and the most important.

Dissection may commence proximally or distally. In either case, control of the thoracic aorta gives added security. The diaphragm may be incised above the proximal limit of the tumor to enter the chest and display the lower thoracic aorta. Once this vessel has been identified and a sling placed, the decision is made whether to proceed

TABLE 66-5		
INTERNATIONAL NEUROBLASTOMA STAGING SYSTEM RESPONSE CRITERIA		
Response	Primary Tumor	Metastatic Sites*
CR	No tumor	No tumor; catecholamines normal
VGPR	Decreased by 90–99%	No tumor; catecholamines normal; residual ^{99m}Tc bone changes allowed
PR	Decreased by >50%	All measurable sites decreased by >50% Bones and bone marrow: number of positive bone sites decreased by>50%. No more than one positive bone marrow site allowed
MR	No new lesions	>50% reduction of any measurable lesion (primary or metastases) with <50% reduction in any other; <25% increase in any existing lesion
NR	No new lesions	<50% reduction but <25% increase in any existing lesion
PD	Any new lesion	Increase of any measurable lesion by >25%; previous negative marrow positive for tumor

*One positive marrow aspirate or biopsy allowed for PR if this represents a decrease from the number of positive sites at diagnosis.
CR, complete response; MR, minimal response; NR, no response; PD, progressive disease; PR, partial response; VGPR, very good partial response.

from above or from below. In general it is easier to commence distally and proceed proximally.

The first phase of the procedure commences below where the vessels emerge from the tumor. On the left side, this normally means the external iliac or common iliac artery. On the right side, the corresponding vein is usually first encountered.

The tunica adventitia is incised along the middle of the vessel. The subadventitial layer is then entered. Traction and countertraction by the surgeon and assistant ensure that the correct plane opens once the overlying tissue and tumor are incised. Once the subadventitial plane is displayed, the dissection moves proximally to encounter and incise tumor down into the same plane. The lengths of the incision usually vary from 2 to 5 cm at a time. Hemostasis is secured with bipolar cautery. Provided that the vessel is kept in sight and provided that the incision is in the 12 o'clock position to the vessel, then this maneuver is quite safe.

At the level of the bifurcation, the direction of the incision will change and continue along the middle of the great vessel proximally. On the left side, the inferior mesenteric artery is the first of the visceral vessels to be encountered. Its presence is noted by the position of the vessel in the mesentery before it is found on the aorta. Cautious dissection along the aorta will usually bring the root of the vessel into view before any damage is done.

The next vessel to be found is the left renal vein, crossing the aorta above the gonadal arteries. For some reason, the tumor is often very adherent to the aorta at this level, but persistence is usually rewarded. The vein is commonly surrounded by tumor and lies a variable distance from the aorta. Surprisingly, patient incision of the tumor down toward the aorta will often reveal the bluish color of the vein before it is in any danger. Once part of the vein wall has been exposed, a 5- to 7-cm length should be mobilized circumferentially to facilitate dissection of the underlying aorta. Once again, the axis of dissection is longitudinal along the middle of the vein, establishing the subadventitial plane and then maintaining this plane around the circumference of the vein. The left gonadal vein is usually encountered as it enters the renal vein and may be divided if necessary. The left adrenal vein is often seen at this stage as well and is best left intact. The inferior vena cava (IVC) is usually well to the right. Infrequently, a large posterior tributary from the hemiazygous system enters the renal vein just to the left of the aorta. Division of this tributary is often necessary. On occasion, division of the left renal vein may be necessary and is usually well tolerated, provided that the hilum of the kidney is not dissected and that the kidney is not mobilized from its bed.

Once the vein can be moved, the left renal artery must be found. The anterior aortic wall is exposed posterior to the vein, and cautious dissection on the left side of the aorta brings the origin of the left renal artery into view. Dense adherence of tumor to aorta is unusual at this level or indeed from here proximally to the diaphragm.

The SMA lies just proximal to the level of the renal artery, so the direction of the blade changes from the 12 o'clock to the 1 to 2 o'clock position on the aortic wall. The knife should still come down in perpendicular fashion onto the aorta. The pace of the operation often slows at this time, although this phase of the operation is generally straightforward. Incision of the tumor continues as before until the proximal edge of the tumor has been incised. The median arcuate ligament and part of the diaphragm will usually have been incised as well.

The roots of the celiac and SMA are now exposed by clearing the anterior wall of the aorta. Each is then dissected in turn by incision in the longitudinal axis of the vessel in the subadventitial plane. The SMA is dealt with first, as it appears more robust and has a straight, predictable course. The celiac looks more fragile. The trunk of the celiac is longer than expected. The phrenic arteries may come off the aorta separate from the celiac but more commonly arise from the celiac trunk. More distally on the celiac is found the trifurcation into left gastric, splenic, and hepatic arteries. As before, all of these vessels are exposed by incision in their long axes as far as is necessary. Dense adherence of tumor to celiac and SMA is exceptional.

The only remaining visceral artery of note is the right renal artery, which lies deep to the SMA. Exposure of this vessel usually awaits tumor clearance. It must, however, be in view before a decision on left nephrectomy is made.

Vessel exposure is now complete, and vessel clearance commences. The SMA and celiac arteries are cleared circumferentially, and once these arteries are mobile, the surrounding tumor is removed piecemeal. The area between celiac artery and diaphragm presents no problems. Tissue to the right of the celiac and along the hepatic artery is less accessible, particularly when the right crus of the diaphragm is involved. For this reason, it may be necessary to incise the lesser omentum and open the lesser sac. If considerable bulk of tumor is found in this area, it can be approached later from the right side.

Tumor between celiac and SMA obscures the splenic vein and its junction with the superior mesenteric vein. The safest course is to expose the splenic vein down to its termination. If a substantial mass of tumor is found around the portal vein, it should be left until a later phase of the operation.

The main bulk of tumor may now be excised. This is done by first completing the clearance of the left renal artery. It is good to expose the origin of the right renal artery before dissecting the left renal artery. The first branch from the left renal artery is the adrenal artery, and this is sacrificed. The branch to the apical segment of the kidney often arises quite proximally, and division of this vessel may be unavoidable. This results in a small apical infarct. The renal artery is followed as far as is necessary and occasionally into the hilum. Each branch of the artery is followed and cleared in turn.

The proximal aorta is cleared of tumor to the left and posteriorly. The lumbar arteries are preserved where possible. All that remains is to dissect the tumor from the diaphragm, posterior abdominal wall, and upper pole of left kidney.

Subsequently tumor below the left renal hilum and around the inferior mesenteric artery is resected.

Dissection of the ureter is often bloody, but tumor is rarely attached to it. Lumbar arteries are preserved if possible. It is not clear how many of these may be sacrificed before spinal cord damage occurs. On occasion, five lumbar arteries have been divided without sequelae. The safest course is to preserve as many as possible.

By clearing and mobilizing the lower abdominal aorta, the surgeon may encounter substantial prevertebral tumor. This is easily overlooked. Incision down onto vertebral bodies will reveal the extent of disease in this location.

Right-sided tumors are managed in similar fashion, the colon reflected, the duodenum mobilized, and the cava dissected in similar fashion. If any tumor remains from a left-sided dissection, the right para-aortic region also is approached in this manner.

Mobilization of the liver from its bed will often facilitate dissection of a large right adrenal mass and ease the search for the right adrenal vein.

Access to pelvic tumors may be difficult, as the majority occur presacrally or just lateral to this area below the brim of the pelvis. Lower midline, transverse, or Pfannenstiel incisions are frequently used. For improved access, a modified Pfannenstiel incision, extended to the anterior superior spines on either side, is useful. The rectus sheath is developed proximally in the usual manner. The rectus bellies are then detached from the pubis by dividing the tendons on the anterior aspect of the bone. Laterally, the muscles are divided, staying well above the inguinal canals. This incision gives unrivalled access to the pelvis.

The relevant internal iliac artery is displayed in the same manner as before, by sharp dissection in the subadventitial tissue plane. Generally the common and external iliac arteries are dissected and then the main trunk of the internal iliac artery. The posterior and anterior divisions of the internal iliac artery are then dissected in turn. This involves dissecting each of the branches in the same manner as before. As the associated veins lie lateral to the arteries, they may not be encountered to a troublesome degree. The iliolumbar branch of the posterior division extends medial to the lumbosacral trunk, which is usually readily identified.

With dissection of the anterior division of the internal iliac artery, the obturator nerve also is frequently encountered and is usually preserved without undue difficulty.

As always, the extent of dissection is determined by the size of the tumor. The aim is to display the vascular anatomy before tumor removal. Not infrequently, both internal iliac arteries must be displayed. The ureters are normally easily seen and readily preserved. Once the vascular anatomy is in view, the tumor may be detached from the pelvic viscera and removed.

Less commonly, the tumor fills the pelvis, and access to the vessels is impossible. Under these circumstances, division of the symphysis pubis—symphysiotomy—gives just enough space to see and dissect the vessels on either side. This maneuver has not been associated with any untoward consequences in the limited number of children who have had this done.

Review of unfamiliar anatomy before the operation has been very helpful. Clearly the pelvic autonomic nerves are at risk from the tumor and from the surgery. Continence and potency may be adversely affected, but it is usually possible to preserve at least one hypogastric nerve to preserve ejaculation.[88-91]

Surgical Complications

Complications of surgery do not feature prominently in the literature. One report detailed five operative mishaps, four of the surgical injuries occurring in infants.[89] Two of these children later died. They note a paucity of surgical complications in the literature, but of the reports they encountered, uncontrollable hemorrhage was the predominant cause of operative or early postoperative deaths.

In our own series of more than 220 neurogenic tumors, two perioperative deaths ensued. The first was a 4-year-old who developed severe hypoglycemia after a 4-L blood transfusion during the course of a stage 3 neuroblastoma resection. In the second child, his abdominal aorta and splenic artery ruptured on the eighth postoperative day. In addition to these fatalities, we are aware of one child who lost the left kidney after left renal vein thrombosis as a postoperative event.

A more notable problem has been postoperative diarrhea, which has developed in about one third of the patients undergoing extensive retroperitoneal dissection. Clearance of the SMA and celiac arteries appears to be causative.[90] In the majority of those who survived, the diarrhea was permanent, despite the use of loperamide.

Overall about 15% of patients in this series underwent nephrectomy to achieve or improve tumor clearance. A POG study reported a similar rate of nephrectomy in more than 860 patients.[91]

RADIOTHERAPY

Radiotherapy has been used for many years in children with neuroblastoma. It is mainly used now for treatment of residual disease, progressive hepatomegaly in those with stage 4S disease, or TBI before BMT and, more recently, as targeted radiotherapy.

The use of radiotherapy to treat residual tumor has been the subject of conflicting reports. Forty years ago, a 2-year survival rate of 64% was achieved after radiotherapy for residual tumor.[27] More recently, the use of radiotherapy was combined with chemotherapy to enhance resectability.[92-96] It now seems clear that those with stages 1 and 2 disease do not benefit from radiotherapy, even if macroscopic disease remains after excision.[97,98] The place of radiotherapy in the management of stages 3 and 4 patients is unclear.

Infants with rapidly growing hepatomegaly with stage 4S disease are vulnerable. Radiotherapy is frequently used under these circumstances, but the results, especially in neonates, are poor. In one report, 46% mortality was seen in neonates, all of whom had hepatomegaly at birth.[78] Death was from the complications of liver size despite radiotherapy. In older infants, response to radiotherapy has been more encouraging, although slow and unpredictable.[79,99]

As part of megatherapy, TBI is used to achieve bone marrow ablation before BMT.[83] Finally, the benefits of targeted radiotherapy from using [^{131}I]MIBG are awaited. Targeted MIBG treatment as initial therapy was reported in 33 patients with advanced disease. A complete response was noted in one patient, and partial response (>50% reduction) was noted in 18 patients.[100] The application of this type of therapy may expand in the future.

OUTLOOK

The outlook for children with neuroblastoma has improved considerably in the past 20 years. The failure to influence the course of those with advanced unfavorable disease has engendered pessimism, but overall, the outlook has improved. Recent survival figures from the POG investigators record an overall survival rate of 58% in 1335 patients enrolled between 1980 and 1990.[33] Data from the United Kingdom National Registry of Childhood Tumors suggest that the 5-year actuarial survival rate was 15% of those born between 1971 and 1973 and 43% for those born in the years 1983 to 1985. The survival rate was unchanged 3 years later.[101]

Spontaneous Maturation

Since the report in 1927 of spontaneous maturation of a neuroblastoma, the possibility of spontaneous cure has received much attention.[10] The incidence of this occurrence is unknown. A spontaneous cure of one patient of 133 patients with neuroblastoma was reported in 1968.[102] The patient was a neonate with skin and lymph node metastases. Two such patients were reported in 1969 in a series of 217 neuroblastoma patients.[27] Both were infants, aged 6 weeks and 11 months, with unresectable pelvic and mediastinal neuroblastomas, respectively. In both, the tumors were undetectable 25 and 20 years later. More recently, spontaneous regression has been reported in untreated tumors found on screening.[21] Twelve of 25 patients with tumors less than 5 cm in diameter were followed up for periods ranging from 4 to 27 months. Tumor size diminished in 11 of the 12 on repeated US examination. The ultimate fate of these patients is not yet known.

Natural History

The natural history of neuroblastoma also includes patients with an indolent course. Late progression and death have been described 17 years after diagnosis, the clinical course being marked by periods of tumor activity and inactivity.[103]

Tumors detected antenatally usually exhibit a favorable biologic profile.[29,72] N-*myc* amplification is unusual. In one study, only 5% had metastatic stage 4 disease, and many of the tumors were cystic at the time of diagnosis.

Overall, survival is in excess of 90% in this group of patients.

The outlook for tumors found on screening is favorable, with 92% survival being reported in an early study.[60] As noted earlier, spontaneous regression is common in this group.

The absolute levels of catecholamine metabolites excretion do not have prognostic value. However, the VMA/HVA rate is related to survival, with lower survival being recorded when the ratio was less than 1.5.[58,59]

Serum Ferritin

In a Children's Cancer Study Group (CCSG) report dealing with patients with locally advanced or metastatic disease, the probability of PFS at 2 years was 76% for those with low levels of serum ferritin and 23% for those with high levels.[37] Those with stage 4 disease older than 12 months with high serum ferritin levels had a 3% 2-year PFS versus 21% of those with low levels. In this study, low survival was associated with the highest levels of serum ferritin. A POG study showed survival rates of 45% and 17% for those with low and high levels of serum ferritin, respectively.[33]

Lactic Dehydrogenase

In the same POG review, LDH values of more or less than 1500 international units/mL were associated with survival rates of 24% and 77%, respectively.[33] The prognostic value of high levels of LDH is maintained even in infants.[34]

Neuron-Specific Enolase

In patients with stage 3 disease, survival was reported in 20% of patients with NSE levels of more than100 ng/mL compared with 57% survival in those with lower levels.[31] Corresponding figures for infants with stage 4 disease were 25% and 100% survival.

N-*myc* Amplification

The presence of N-*myc* amplification is generally associated with a worse outcome, but differing results are reported by investigators. A recent POG study[46] showed N-*myc* amplification in 3% of those with localized disease, but these children had a worse outlook. By contrast, patients with N-*myc* amplification and advanced disease had survival rates varying from less than 10% to about 40%, depending on age, ploidy, histology, and other features.[33,40,41] Another study showed a 16% 3-year survival in those with N-*myc* amplified tumors.[43] Still another study recorded an overall 24% survival for those with N-*myc* amplified tumors compared with 77% survival in those without amplification.[33]

N-*myc* status is increasingly used to define high-risk tumors and to direct treatment. A report of N-*myc* amplified stage 4 patients noted an improvement in initial response but not in long-term survival.[92] Stratification of treatment on the basis of N-*myc* status resulted in improved survival with the more intensive treatment in a Japanese study.[93]

N-*myc* amplified tumors in infants also affect survival, reducing 3-year event-free survival from 93% to 10% in a CCG study of infants with Evans stage 4 disease.[94] The same group reported on 228 patients with Evans stage 3 disease and noted the predictive power of N-*myc* status in these patients.[95]

In patients with stage 4S disease, tumor regression may occur in early life despite N-*myc* amplification. N-*myc* amplification was reported in 5 of 10 patients with stage 4S disease.[104] At the time of the report, 3 of the 5 patients were dead, and the fourth was alive with disease. Two of the patients who died had shown initial regression with later relapse. In most studies, multivariate analysis confirms the predictive power of N-*myc* amplification, independent of age and stage.

Chromosome Abnormalities

On balance, gain of 17q has been shown to affect survival. This was present in 53% of 313 tumors in a European study. Overall survival at 5 years was 30% for those children, compared with 86% survival in those without the chromosomal abnormality.[53]

Most evidence suggests that allelic loss of chromosome 1p is a reliable predictor of a poor outcome. 1p Deletion in patients with stages 1, 2, and 4S was associated with a 12% mean 3-year event-free survival.[51] For those without 1p deletion, the corresponding survival was 75%. In those with stages 3 and 4 disease and 1p deletion, none survived 3 years without adverse events. The corresponding figure was 53% for those without 1p deletion. A separate POG study showed that in all patients, 1p deletion was associated with a 32% 4-year survival but 76% for those without the abnormality.[48]

When associated with N-*myc* amplification, 4-year survival was 7%. Infants with 1p LOH showed a 3-year event-free survival of 32%. All the other infants survived in the absence of 1p LOH. More recently a CCG study suggested that 1p LOH was independently associated with disease progression but not with diminished overall survival.[52] As noted in regard to N-*myc* status, it is not clear whether the conflicting results are in any way related to changes in treatment.

Ploidy

Diploid DNA content worsens the prognosis overall: 58% versus 28% mortality for those with aneuploid DNA content.[33] One report revealed a 94% 2-year disease-free survival in those with near-triploid neuroblastoma compared with 45% for those with diploid or near-diploid DNA content.[40] This figure decreased to 11% survival in those with N-*myc* amplification in addition. Finally, a POG study of neuroblastoma in infancy showed a 94% 3-year survival in those with hyperdiploid tumors versus 55% in those with diploid tumors.

Cell-Surface Glycoprotein

CD44 expression is associated with improved survival. One study reported 81% 3-year survival in CD44-positive tumors against 7% in those with CD44-negative tumors. Absence of CD44 expression combined with N-*myc* amplification was a particularly bad combination: 9% 3-year survival. In those with stage 4 disease, event-free survival was 35% in CD44-positive tumors and 7% in those lacking CD44 expression.

Tyrosine Kinase

Patients whose tumors show high levels of *TRKA* expression have a more favorable prognosis: 86% survival versus 14% in those with low levels.[56] In addition, the combination of low *TRKA* expression and high N-*myc* copy number was uniformly fatal.

Multidrug-Resistance–Associated Protein

A lower 5-year event-free survival is seen in those with high levels of MRP expression (46%) compared with those with low levels (91%).[57]

Another study showed 87% survival in their high-level MRP group.[24] Survival was 7% in the poor-prognosis group. Subsequently, these same authors showed that the combination of unfavorable histology with N-*myc* amplification carries the worst prognosis: 13% estimated PFS.[41]

Patient Age

Those patients younger than 12 months at diagnosis were found in 1959 to have a 56% survival.[25] Tumors in infancy show N-*myc* amplification in only about 3% of patients and unfavorable histology in only 5%.[105] Survival for those with localized disease approaches 100%. Four-year survival in infants with stage 4 disease was 73% versus 48% for those older than 12 months.[105] When survival was correlated with ploidy, infants with hyperdiploid tumors showed a 95% 3-year estimated survival compared with 55% in those with diploid tumors. At the other extreme, neuroblastoma in older children, adolescents, and adults is marked by an indolent but inexorably downhill course. Biopsies of these tumors rarely show N-*myc* amplification and usually demonstrate favorable histology. Two recent studies record a 17% event-free survival in one and 6% in the other.[106,107]

Those first seen with paraneoplastic syndromes have a low mortality rate. In a literature review of 28 cases, a 2-year survival rate of 89% was noted in those with opsomyoclonus.[70] Others have noted a poor neurologic outcome in these patients; 64% had persisting cerebellar signs, and 36% had developmental delay.[108] Those with VIP-secreting tumors are much less common, and the tumors may be more mature. We have dealt with only two such patients, and both tumors were ganglioneuromas. In addition to the risk from the tumor, a substantial risk occurs from the secretory diarrhea.[72]

Tumor Location

Forty years ago, the site of the primary tumor was known to influence the outcome, with roughly 50% cure for cervical, thoracic, and pelvic tumors compared with 25% for those with adrenal primaries.[25] Twenty years later, another report listed 100% survival for those with cervical and pelvic primaries, 75% for those with thoracic primaries, and 28% for those with abdominal tumors.[28] More recently, others reported 83% survival for those with thoracic primary tumors, contrasting with 53% survival in other sites.[33] Hyperdiploid DNA content has been reported in the majority of infants with cervical and thoracic primaries.[34]

Dumbbell tumors also are associated with a survival rate of 97% in a recent study of 42 patients.[75] In this study, 26 (62%) of the patients had neurologic impairment. Complete neurologic recovery was recorded in two-thirds. By contrast, an earlier study recorded 13 (61%) survivors of 21 patients with spinal cord compression.[109] Ten of the 13 survivors had residual neurologic impairment, with neonatal tumors having the worst outcome.

Tumor Stage

An 89% survival was recorded in patients with POG stage A tumors.[68] A CCSG study confirmed the excellent prognosis (90% PFS) in those with stage 2 disease.[110] This study also showed that survival was not dependent on achieving complete surgical resection. One study reported that 10 of 10 patients with INSS stage 1 disease were alive and disease-free at 5 years of follow-up.[111] These patients were treated with surgical excision alone. Another report using INSS staging showed the survival rates as follows: stage 1, 95%; stage 2A, 88%; stage 2B, 100%. Only 13 of 93 patients were given any treatment other than operative resection.[98]

Chemotherapy

For those with locally advanced or metastatic disease, multiagent chemotherapy combined with myeloablative treatment has resulted in improved survival. Most of the follow-up periods are short. Recent CCG data show a 3-year PFS of 25% for these groups.[83] The Japanese Study Group showed 70% 3-year survival for stage 3 and 45% for stage 4 disease.[112] For the whole group, 5-year survival was 44% for those with N-*myc* amplification and 54% for those without. The POG study reports a survival rate of 39% for stage D disease.[33]

Surgical Treatment

The exact contribution of surgical treatment to these survival figures is uncertain. We and others have been unable to confirm the beneficial effect of complete versus incomplete resection.[86,113] Other groups have shown improved survival in children undergoing complete versus incomplete resection (59% vs. 47%).[114] The CCG data showed an improved outcome for children with poor-risk neuroblastoma after complete versus partial resection (59% vs. 26%).[115] Follow-up was 20 months. Finally, a retrospective review of 28 patients from one institution suggested improved survival and PFS for those who had undergone complete surgical resection. Three-year survival rates were 40% as against 15% for those who had an incomplete resection.[116]

Earlier reports of stage 4S disease were encouraging: 84% survival.[117] More recently, survival rates of 50% to 83% have been reported.[33,79] Multiorgan impairment—respiratory compromise, oliguria, thrombocytopenia, leg edema—especially when severe, is associated with a poor outcome. Neonates with multiorgan impairment rarely survive.[78]

Progressive hepatomegaly resulting in respiratory compromise, the need for ventilation, and abdominal compartment syndrome is difficult to manage. The use of abdominal silos, radiotherapy, and chemotherapy are not attended by much success.

We recently used hepatic artery embolization with success. Persisting rapid liver growth is probably impossible in the absence of an arterial supply. The procedure is well tolerated and could be used early in the course of this relentless clinical picture.

REFERENCES

1. Virchow R: Die Krankenhafte Geschwulste 1864; ii:149. Berlin, Hirschwald, 1864, p 149.
2. Marchand F: Beitr.z Kenntnis der Glandula Carotica und der Nebennieren. Festschr.f.R.Virchow Intern Beitr Wissesch Med Berlin I:535, 1891.
3. Parker RW: Diffuse sarcoma of liver, probably congenital. Trans Pathol Soc Lond 31:290–293, 1880.
4. Dalton N: Infiltrating growth in liver and suprarenal capsule. Trans Pathol Soc Lond 36:247–251, 1885.
5. Wright JH: Neurocytoma or neuroblastoma: A kind of tumor not generally recognised. J Exp Med 12:556–561, 1910.
6. Dunn JS: Neuroblastoma and ganglio-neuroma of the suprarenal body. J Pathol Bacteriol 19:456–476, 1915.
7. Hutchison R: On suprarenal sarcoma in children with metastases in the skull. Q J Med 1:33–38, 1907.
8. Lehman EP: Neuroblastoma: With report of a case. J Med Res 36:309–326, 1917.
9. Lehman EP: Adrenal neuroblastoma in infancy: 15 year survival. Ann Surg 95:473, 1932.
10. Cushing H, Wolbach SB: The transformation of a malignant paravertebral sympathicoblastoma into a benign ganglioneuroma. Am J Pathol 3:203–216, 1927.
11. Blacklock JWS: Neurogenic tumors of the sympathetic system in children. J Pathol Bacteriol 39:27–48, 1934.
12. Redman JL, Agerty HA, Barthmaier OF, et al: Adrenal neuroblastoma: Report of a case and review of the literature. Am J Dis Child 56:1097–1112, 1938.
13. Holmes GW, Dresser R: Roentgenologic observations in neuroblastoma. JAMA 91:1246–1248, 1928.
14. Farber S: Neuroblastoma. Am J Dis Child 60:749–750, 1940.
15. Phillips R: Neuroblastoma. Ann R Coll Surg Engl 12:29–47, 1953.
16. Koop CE, Kiesewetter WB, Horn RC: Neuroblastoma in childhood: An evaluation of surgical management. Pediatrics 16:652–657, 1955.
17. James DH, Hustu O, Wrenn EL, et al: Combination chemotherapy of childhood neuroblastoma. JAMA 194:123–126, 1965.

18. Evans AE, D'Angio GJ, Randolph J: A proposed staging for children with neuroblastoma. Cancer 27:374–378, 1971.
19. Stiller CA, Parkin DM: International variations in the incidence of neuroblastoma. Int J Cancer 52:538–543, 1992.
20. Beckwith JB, Perrin EV: In situ neuroblastomas: A contribution to the natural history of neural crest tumors. Am J Pathol 45:1089–1104, 1963.
21. Yamamoto K, Hanada R, Tanimura M, et al: Natural history of neuroblastoma found by mass screening. Lancet 349:1102, 1997.
22. Kushner BH, Gilbert F, Helson L: Familial neuroblastoma: Case reports, literature review and etiologic considerations. Cancer 57:1887–1893, 1986.
23. Berry CL, Keeling JW: Neuroblastoma. In Colin L Berry (ed): Paediatric Pathology, 3rd ed. London, Springer-Verlag, 1996, p 869.
24. Shimada H, Chatten J, Newton WA, et al: Histopathologic prognostic factors in neuroblastic tumors: Definition of subtypes of ganglioneuroblastoma and an age-linked classification of neuroblastomas. J Natl Cancer Inst 73:405–416, 1984.
25. Shimada H, Ambros IM, Dehner LP, et al: International Neuroblastoma Pathology Classification (The Shimada System). Cancer 86:364–372, 1999.
26. Shimada H, Umehara S, Monobe Y, et al: International Neuroblastoma Pathology Classification for prognostic evaluation of patients with peripheral neuroblastic tumors: A report from the Children's Cancer Group. Cancer 92:2451–2461, 2001.
27. Gross RE, Farber S, Martin LW: Neuroblastoma sympatheticum: A study and report of 217 cases. Pediatrics 23:1179–1191, 1959.
28. Grosfeld JL, Baehner RL: Neuroblastoma: An analysis of 160 cases. World J Surg 4:29–38, 1980.
29. Acharya S, Jayabose S, Kogan SJ, et al: Prenatally diagnosed neuroblastoma. Cancer 80:304–310, 1997.
30. Zeltzer PM, Parma AM, Dalton A, et al: Raised neuron-specific enolase in serum of children with metastatic neuroblastoma. Lancet ii:361–363, 1983.
31. Zeltzer P, Marangos P, Sather H, et al: Prognostic importance of neuron specific enolase levels in widespread and localized neuroblastoma. Proc Am Soc Clin Oncol 3:13, 1984.
32. Wong KY, Hann HL, Marangos P, et al: Prognostic factors in patients with stage III neuroblastoma. Proc Am Soc Clin Oncol 3:85, 1984.
33. Morris JA, Shochat J, Smith EI, et al: Biological variables in thoracic neuroblastoma: A Pediatric Oncology Group Study. J Pediatr Surg 30:296–303, 1995.
34. Bowman LC, Castleberry RP, Cantor A, et al: Genetic staging of unresectable or metastatic neuroblastoma in infants: A Pediatric Oncology Group study. J Natl Cancer Inst 89:373–380, 1997.
35. Shuster JJ, McWilliams NB, Castleberry R, et al: Serum lactate dehydrogenase in childhood neuroblastoma. Am J Clin Oncol 15:295–303, 1992.
36. Hann HL, Levy HM, Evans AE: Serum ferritin as a guide to therapy in neuroblastoma. Cancer Res 40:1411–1413, 1980.
37. Hann HL, Evans AE, Siegel SE, et al: Prognostic importance of serum ferritin in patients with stages III and IV neuroblastoma: The Children's Cancer Study Group experience. Cancer Res 45:2843–2848, 1985.
38. Schwab M, Alitalo K, Klempnauer K-H, et al: Amplified DNA with limited homology to myc cellular oncogene is shared by human neuroblastoma cell lines and a neuroblastoma tumor. Nature 305:245–248, 1983.
39. Brodeur GM, Seeger RC: Amplification of N-myc in untreated human neuroblastoma correlates with advanced disease stage. Science 220:1121–1124, 1984.
40. Bourhis J, DeVathaire F, Wilson GD, et al: Combined analysis of DNA ploidy index and N-myc genomic content in neuroblastoma. Cancer Res 51:33–36, 1991.
41. Shimada H, Stram DO, Chatten J, et al: Identification of subsets of neuroblastomas by combined histopathologic and N-myc analysis. J Natl Cancer Inst 87:1470–1476, 1995.
42. Brodeur GM: Molecular basis for heterogeneity in human neuroblastomas. Eur J Cancer 31A:505–510, 1995.
43. Combaret V, Gross N, Lasset C, et al: Clinical relevance of CD44 cell-surface expression and N-myc gene amplification in a multicentric analysis of 121 pediatric neuroblastomas. J Clin Oncol 14:25–34, 1996.
44. Look AT, Hayes FA, Shuster JJ, et al: Clinical relevance of tumor cell ploidy and N-myc gene amplification in childhood neuroblastoma: A Pediatric Oncology Group study. J Clin Oncol 9:581–591, 1991.
45. Cohn SL, Look AT, Joshi VV, et al: Lack of correlation of N-myc gene amplification with prognosis in localized neuroblastoma: A Pediatric Oncology Group study. Cancer Res 55:721–726, 1995.
46. Perez CA, Matthay KK, Atkinson JB, et al: Biologic variables in the outcome of stages I and II neuroblastoma treated with surgery as primary therapy: A Children's Cancer Group Study. J Clin Oncol 18:18–26, 2000.
47. Fong C-T, Dracopoli NC, White PS, et al: Loss of heterozygosity for the short arm of chromosome 1 in human neuroblastomas: Correlation with N-myc amplification. Proc Natl Acad Sci U S A 86:3753–3757, 1989.
48. Maris JM, White PS, Beltinger CP, et al: Significance of chromosome 1p loss of heterozygosity in neuroblastoma. Cancer Res 55:4664–4669, 1995.
49. Look AT, Hayes FA, Nitschke R, et al: Cellular DNA content as a predictor of response to chemotherapy in infants with unresectable neuroblastoma. N Engl J Med 311:231–235, 1984.
50. Brodeur GM, Green AA, Hayes A, et al: Cytogenetic features of human neuroblastomas and cell lines. Cancer Res 41:4678–4686, 1981.
51. Caron H, van Sluis P, de Kraker J, et al: Allelic loss of chromosome 1p as a predictor of unfavorable outcome in patients with neuroblastoma. N Engl J Med 334:225–230, 1996.
52. Maris JM, Weiss HJ, Guo C, et al: Loss of heterozygosity at 1p 36 independently predicts for disease progression but not decreased overall survival probability in neuroblastoma patients: A Children's Cancer Group study. J Clin Oncol 18:1888–1899, 2000.
53. Bown H, Cotterill S, Lastowska M, et al: Gain of chromosome arm 17q and adverse outcome in patients with neuroblastoma. N Engl J Med 340:1954–1961, 1999.
54. Favrot MC, Combaret V, Lasset C: CD44: A new prognostic marker for neuroblastoma. N Engl J Med 1993;329:1965.
55. Combaret V, Lasset C, Frappaz D, et al: Evaluation of CD44 prognostic value in neuroblastoma: Comparison with the other prognostic factors. Eur J Cancer 31A:545–549, 1995.
56. Nakagawara A, Arima-Nakagawara M, Scavarda NJ, et al: Association between high levels of expression of the TRK gene and favorable outcome in human neuroblastoma. N Engl J Med 328:847–854, 1993.
57. Norris MD, Bordow SB, Marshall GM, et al: Expression of the gene for multidrug-resistance-associated protein and outcome in patients with neuroblastoma. N Engl J Med 334:231–238, 1996.
58. Laug WE, Siegel SE, Shaw KNF, et al: Initial urinary catecholamine metabolite concentrations and prognosis in neuroblastoma. Pediatrics 62:77–83, 1978.
59. LaBrosse EH, Com-Nougué C, Zucker J-M, et al: Urinary excretion of 3-methoxy-4-hydroxymandelic acid and 3-methoxy-4-hydroxyphenylacetic acid by 288 patients with neuroblastoma and related neural crest tumors. Cancer Res 40:1995–2001, 1980.
60. Sawada T: Outcome of 25 neuroblastomas revealed by mass screening in Japan. Lancet i:377, 1986.
61. Woods WG, Tuchman M: Neuroblastoma: The case for screening infants in North America. Pediatrics 79:869–873, 1987.
62. Woods WG, Tuchman M, Robison LL, et al: A population-based study of the usefulness of screening for neuroblastoma. Lancet 348:1682–1687, 1996.
63. Kaneko Y, Kanda N, Maseki N, et al: Current urinary mass screening for catecholamine metabolites at 6 months of age may be detecting only a small portion of high-risk neuroblastomas: A chromosome and N-myc amplification study. J Clin Oncol 8:2005–2013, 1990.
64. Tajiri T, Shita S, Sera Y, et al: Clinical and biologic characteristics for recurring neuroblastoma at mass screening cases in Japan. Cancer 92:349–353, 2001.
65. Granata C, Fagnani AM, Gambini C, et al: Features and outcome of neuroblastoma detected before birth. J Pediatr Surg 35:88–91, 2000.
66. Brodeur GM, Seeger RC, Barrett A, et al: International criteria for diagnosis, staging and response to treatment in patients with neuroblastoma. J Clin Oncol 6:1874–1881, 1988.

67. Brodeur GM, Pritchard J, Berthold F, et al: Revisions of the international criteria for neuroblastoma diagnosis, staging and response to treatment. J Clin Oncol 11:1466–1477, 1993.

68. Nitschke R, Smith EI, Schochat S, et al: Localized neuroblastoma treated by surgery: A Pediatric Oncology Group study. J Clin Oncol 6:1271–1279, 1988.

69. Weinblatt ME, Heisel MA, Siegel SE: Hypertension in children with neurogenic tumors. Pediatrics 71:947–951, 1983.

70. Altman AJ, Baehner RL: Favorable prognosis for survival in children with coincident opso-myoclonus and neuroblastoma. Cancer 37:846–852, 1976.

71. Swift PGF, Bloom SR, Harris F: Watery diarrhoea and ganglioneuroma with secretion of vasoactive intestinal peptide. Arch Dis Child 50:896–899, 1975.

72. Tiedemann K, Pritchard J, Long R, et al: Intractable diarrhoea in a patient with vasoactive intestinal peptide-secreting neuroblastoma. Eur J Pediatr 137:217–219, 1981.

73. Nadel HR: Nuclear oncology in children. In Freeman LM (ed): Nuclear Medicine Annual. Philadelphia, Lippincott-Raven, 1996, pp 143–193.

74. Gordon I, Peters AM, Gutman A, et al: Skeletal assessment in neuroblastoma: The pitfalls of iodine-123-MIBG scans. J Nucl Med 31:129–134, 1990.

75. Plantaz D, Rubie H, Michon J, et al: The treatment of neuroblastoma with intraspinal extension with chemotherapy followed by surgical removal of residual disease. Cancer 78:311–319, 1996.

76. Moss TJ, Fonkalsrud EW, Feig SA, et al: Delayed surgery and bone marrow transplantation for widespread neuroblastoma. Ann Surg 206:514–520, 1987.

77. Shamberger RC, Allarde-Segundo A, Kozakewich HPW, et al: Surgical management of stage III and IV neuroblastoma: Resection before or after chemotherapy? J Pediatr Surg 26:1113–1117, 1991.

78. Hsu LL, Evans AE, D'Angio GJ: Hepatomegaly in neuroblastoma stage 4S: Criteria for treatment of the vulnerable neonate. Med Pediatr Oncol 27:521–528, 1996.

79. Wilson PCG, Coppes MJ, Solh H, et al: Neuroblastoma stage IV-S: A heterogeneous disease. Med Pediatr Oncol 19:467–472, 1991.

80. Haas D, Ablin AR, Miller C, et al: Complete pathologic maturation and regression of stage IV-S neuroblastoma without treatment. Cancer 62:818–825, 1988.

81. Guglielmi M, de Bernardi B, Rizzo A, et al: Resection of primary tumor at diagnosis in stage IV-S neuroblastoma: Does it affect the clinical course? J Clin Oncol 14:1537–1544, 1996.

82. Ladenstein R, Favrot M, Lasset C, et al: Indication and limits of megatherapy and bone marrow transplantation in high-risk neuroblastoma: A single centre analysis of prognostic factors. Eur J Cancer 29A:947–956, 1993.

83. Matthay KK, O'Leary MC, Ramsay NK, et al: Role of myeloablative therapy in improved outcome for high risk neuroblastoma: Review of recent Children's Cancer Group results. Eur J Cancer 31A:572–575, 1995.

84. Steenburg RW, Ravitch MM: Cervico-thoracic approach for subclavian vessel injury from compound fracture of the clavicle: Considerations of subclavian-axillary exposures. Ann Surg 157:839–846, 1963.

85. Pranikoff T, Hirschl RB, Schnaufer L: Approach to cervicothoracic neuroblastomas via a trap door incision. J Pediatr Surg 30:546–548, 1995.

86. Kiely EM: The surgical challenge of neuroblastoma. J Pediatr Surg 29:128–133, 1994.

87. Tsuchida Y, Honna T, Kamii Y, et al: Radical excision of primary tumor and lymph nodes in advanced neuroblastoma: Combination with intensive induction chemotherapy. Pediatr Surg Int 6:22–27, 1991.

88. Kedia KR, Markland C, Fraley EE: Sexual function following high retroperitoneal lymphadenectomy. J Urol 114:237–239, 1975.

89. Azizkhan RG, Shaw A, Chandler JG: Surgical complications of neuroblastoma resection. Surgery 97:514–517, 1985.

90. Rees H, Markley MA, Kiely EM, et al: Diarrhea after resection of advanced abdominal neuroblastoma: A common management problem. Surgery 3:568–572, 1998.

91. Shamberger RC, Smith EI, Joshi VV, et al: The risk of nephrectomy during local control in abdominal neuroblastoma. J Pediatr Surg 33:161–164, 1998.

92. Castel V, Canete A, Navarro S, et al: Outcome of high risk neuroblastoma using a dose intensity approach: Improvement in initial but not in long-term results. Med Pediatr Oncol 37:537–542, 2004.

93. Kaneko M, Hishihara H, Mugishima H, et al: Treatment of stage 4 neuroblastoma with stratification into different protocols based on N-myc amplification status. Med Pediatr Oncol 31:1–6, 1998.

94. Schmidt MC, Lukens JH, Seeger RC, et al: Biologic factors determine prognosis in infants with stage IV neuroblastoma: A prospective Children's Cancer Group study. J Clin Oncol 18:1260–1268, 2000.

95. Matthay KK, Perez C, Seeger RC, et al: Successful treatment of stage III neuroblastoma based on prospective biologic staging: A Children's Cancer Group study. J Clin Oncol 16:1256–1264, 1998.

96. Smith EI, Krous HF, Tunell WP, et al: The impact of chemotherapy and radiation therapy on secondary operations for neuroblastoma. Ann Surg 191:561–568, 1980.

97. Ninane J, Pritchard J, Morris Jones PH, et al: Stage II neuroblastoma: Adverse prognostic significance of lymph node involvement. Arch Dis Child 57:438–442, 1982.

98. Evans AE, Silber JH, Shpilsky A, et al: Successful management of low-stage neuroblastoma without adjuvant therapies: A comparison of two decades, 1972 through 1981 and 1982 through 1992, in a single institution. J Clin Oncol 14:2504–2510, 1996.

99. Suarez A, Hartmann O, Vassal G, et al: Treatment of stage IV-S neuroblastoma: A study of 34 cases treated between 1982 and 1987. Med Pediatr Oncol 19:473–477, 1991.

100. De Kraker J, Hoefnagel CA, Caron H, et al: First line targeted radiotherapy: A new concept in the treatment of advanced stage neuroblastoma. Eur J Oncol 31A:600–602, 1995.

101. Stiller CA: Trends in neuroblastoma in Great Britain: Incidence and mortality, 1971–1990. Eur J Cancer 29A:1008–1012, 1993.

102. Fortner J, Nicastri A, Murphy ML: Neuroblastoma: Natural history and results of treating 133 cases. Ann Surg 167:132–142, 1968.

103. Vogel JM, Coddon DR, Simon N, et al: Osseous metastases in neuroblastoma: A 17 year survival. Cancer 26:1354–1360, 1970.

104. Nakagawara A, Sasazuki T, Akiyama H, et al: N-myc oncogene and stage IV-S neuroblastoma. Cancer 65:1960–1967, 1990.

105. Ikeda H, Iehara T, Tsuchida Y, et al: Experience with International Neuroblastoma Staging System and Pathology Classification. Br J Cancer 86:1110–1116, 2002.

106. Franks LM, Bollen A, Seeger RC, et al: Neuroblastoma in adults and adolescents: An indolent course with poor survival. Cancer 79:2028–2035, 1997.

107. Blatt J, Gula MJ, Orlando SJ, et al: Indolent course of advanced neuroblastoma in children older than 6 years at diagnosis. Cancer 76:890–894, 1995.

108. Senelick RC, Bray PF, Lahey ME, et al: Neuroblastoma and myoclonic encephalopathy: Two cases and a review of the literature. J Pediatr Surg 8:623–631, 1973.

109. Punt J, Pritchard J, Pincott JR, et al: Neuroblastoma: A review of 21 cases presenting with spinal cord compression. Cancer 45:3095–3101, 1980.

110. Matthay KK, Sather HN, Seeger RC, et al: Excellent outcome of stage II neuroblastoma is independent of residual disease and radiation therapy. J Clin Oncol 7:236–244, 1989.

111. Kushner BH, Cheung N-KV, LaQuaglia MP, et al: International neuroblastoma staging system stage 1 neuroblastoma: A prospective study and literature review. J Clin Oncol 14:2174–2180, 1996.

112. Suita S, Zaizen Y, Kaneko M, et al: What is the benefit of aggressive chemotherapy for advanced neuroblastoma with N-myc amplification: A report from the Japanese Study Group for the treatment of advanced neuroblastoma. J Pediatr Surg 29:746–750, 1994.

113. Shorter NA, Davidoff AM, Evans AE, et al: The role of surgery in the management of stage IV neuroblastoma: A single institution study. Med Pediatr Oncol 24:287–291, 1995.

114. Tsuchida Y, Yokoyama J, Kaneko M, et al: Therapeutic significance of surgery in advanced neuroblastoma: A report from the Study Group of Japan. J Pediatr Surg 27:616–622, 1992.

115. Haase GM, O'Leary MC, Ramsay NKC, et al: Aggressive surgery combined with intensive chemotherapy improves survival in poor-risk neuroblastoma. J Pediatr Surg 26:1119–1124, 1991.

116. Chamberlain RS, Quinones R, Dinndorf P, et al: Complete surgical resection combined with aggressive adjuvant chemotherapy and bone marrow transplantation prolongs survival in children with advanced neuroblastoma. Ann Surg Oncol 2:93–100, 1995.

117. D'Angio GJ, Evans AE, Koop CE: Special pattern of widespread neuroblastoma with a favourable prognosis. Lancet I:1046–1049, 1971.

Lesions of the Liver

Walter S. Andrews, MD

INTRODUCTION

Hepatic tumors in children are relatively rare. The most common malignant neoplasms in the liver are not primary hepatic tumors, but rather metastatic lesions such as Wilms' tumor, lymphoma, and neuroblastoma.[1] Primary liver tumors compose between 1% and 4% of all solid tumors in children. Malignant hepatic tumors occur at a rate of about 1 to 1.5 per million children per year.[1,2] However, 10 primary hepatic masses occur with some frequency in the pediatric age group. Five of these occur only in children: infantile hemangioendotheliomas, hepatoblastoma, mesenchymal hamartoma, rhabdomyosarcoma of the biliary tract, and undifferentiated embryonal sarcoma (Table 67-1). Among these five tumors, the age distribution is distinctive, with hepatoblastoma and infantile hemangioendothelioma occurring most commonly in the first 2 years of life, and hepatocellular carcinoma and focal nodular hyperplasia occurring most commonly after age 5 years (Table 67-2).[1]

Couinaud's elegant description of the segmental anatomy of the liver has allowed hepatic surgical procedures to evolve to a level at which they can be performed with an acceptable morbidity and mortality (Fig. 67-1).[3,4] The cumulative experience with hepatic resection and hepatic transplantation has allowed the development of techniques for both subsegmental and multisegmental resections of the liver in children. With the continued expansion of knowledge about these tumors, rational surgical and medical management plans can be devised.[5]

BENIGN HEPATIC TUMORS

Infantile Hemangioendothelioma

Incidence

Infantile hemangioendothelioma is the most common benign solid hepatic tumor in children, composing about 16% of all pediatric liver tumors.[1] It also is the most common liver tumor in the first year of life. Almost all children with hepatic hemangioendotheliomas are seen initially before age 6 months, and the majority, in the first 2 months.[6,7] Classically, a slight female predominance has been found, but this finding has not been uniformly seen.[8]

Presentation

Hepatic hemangioendotheliomas can be either single lesions that can expand to a massive size or a multinodular infiltrative lesion. Occasionally these lesions can be asymptomatic and appear simply as an abdominal mass or distention. However, they frequently occur with hepatomegaly, high-output congestive heart failure, respiratory distress, and anemia. In addition, these patients may also have acute thrombocytopenia, a microangiopathic hemolytic anemia, and a consumptive coagulopathy (Kasabach-Merritt syndrome).[9] The development of this syndrome is often life threatening and requires aggressive treatment, as well as treatment of the primary cause. Fortunately, the Kasabach-Merritt syndrome occurs infrequently and is usually associated with hemangioendotheliomas that have rapid growth to a diameter of 5 cm or more. No cases have been reported in association with smaller tumors.[10] Other associated symptoms can include jaundice, failure to thrive, respiratory difficulties, or poor feeding. It was recently found that some of these patients also have congenital hypothyroidism. The presence of severe hypothyroidism can significantly complicate the management of these patients if it is overlooked.[11]

As many as 50% to 60% of these patients will display symptoms of congestive heart failure.[12,13] Interestingly, neonates with a focal hemangioma tend to have high-output heart failure at birth, whereas infants with multifocal lesions tend to be first seen between ages 1 and 16 weeks. A classic symptom complex has been described in hepatic hemangioendotheliomas: hepatomegaly, congestive heart failure, and anemia or other cutaneous hemangiomas. This triad occurs in 80% of infants who have multiple hepatic hemangiomas.[6] Associated hemangiomas

TABLE 67-1

HEPATIC TUMORS IN PEDIATRIC PATIENTS, BIRTH TO 2 YEARS (AFIP 1970–1999)

Type of Tumor	n	%
Hepatoblastoma	124	43.5
Infantile hemangioendothelioma	103	36.1
Mesenchymal hamartoma	38	13.3
Nodular regenerative hyperplasia	6	2.1
Hepatocellular carcinoma	4	1.4
Angiosarcoma	4	1.4
Focal nodular hyperplasia	3	1.1
Undifferentiated embryonal sarcoma	3	1.1
Hepatocellular adenoma	0	0
Embryonal rhabdomyosarcoma	0	0
Total	285	100.0

Reprinted from Stocker JT. Hepatic tumors in children. In Suchy FJ, Sokol RJ, Balistreri WF (eds): Liver Disease in Children, 2nd ed. Philadelphia: Lippincott Williams & Wilkins, 2001, p 915.

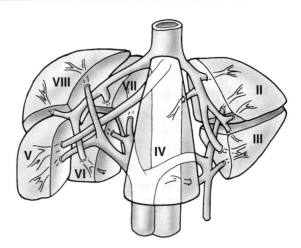

FIGURE 67-1. The segmental hepatic anatomy as defined by Couinaud. A comprehensive understanding of the hepatic segmental division is necessary for successful hepatic resection. (From Couinaud C: Surgical anatomy of the liver: Several new aspects. Chirurgie 112:337–342, 1986; and Couinaud C: The anatomy of the liver. Ann Ital Chir 63:693–697, 1992.)

occur at multiple distant sites, including skin (45%), lung (10%), pancreas, lymph nodes, and bone.[14,15]

Hepatic transaminase levels and occasionally the α-fetoprotein (AFP) level can be mildly elevated. The significance of this elevation is uncertain, however, because the AFP level can be elevated in normal neonates and does not decrease to adult levels until about age 6 months.[15]

Radiology

The ultrasonographic (US) evaluation of hepatic hemangioendotheliomas can be highly variable. Solitary lesions can have a very heterogeneous echogenicity, and the Doppler spectral analysis can show a variety of flow patterns. Multifocal lesions, however, tend to be more uniform in their appearance, as echolucent nodules associated with a high-flow vessel.[16] On computed tomographic (CT) scanning with intravenous (IV) contrast, classically the lesions either enhance diffusely or rim enhancement is

followed by gradual filling of the center of the lesion (Fig. 67-2).[13] Focal hemangiomas are most often described as showing the rim enhancement or an avascular center related to either hemorrhage or necrosis.[17,18] Currently, magnetic resonance imaging (MRI) is thought to be the single most useful modality to show not only the location of the hemangioma but also its flow patterns and structure.[19,20] The addition of IV gadolinium and a gradient-recall echo sequence to the MRI enhances its utility in focal lesions.

Another method for diagnosing hemangioendotheliomas is the use of a technetium-tagged red blood cell (RBC) blood pool scan. On delayed images (4 hours), an abnormal increase in activity is seen in the region of the hemangioendothelioma. This test is very specific and highly sensitive for hemangiomas.[21]

TABLE 67-2

HEPATIC TUMORS IN PEDIATRIC PATIENTS, 5 TO 20 YEARS (AFIP 1970-1999)

Type of Tumor	n	%
Hepatocelluar carcinoma	96	36.6
Focal nodular hyperplasia	40	15.3
Undifferentiated embryonal sarcoma	39	14.9
Nodular regenerative hyperplasia	26	9.9
Hepatocellular adenoma	22	8.4
Hepatoblastoma	22	8.4
Angiosarcoma	6	2.3
Mesenchymal hamartoma	5	1.9
Infantile hemangioendothelioma	4	1.5
Embryonal rhabdomyosarcoma	2	.8
Total	262	100.0

Reprinted from Stocker JT. Hepatic tumors in children. In Suchy FJ, Sokol RJ, Balistreri WF (eds): Liver Disease in Children, 2nd ed. Philadelphia: Lippincott Williams & Wilkins, 2001.

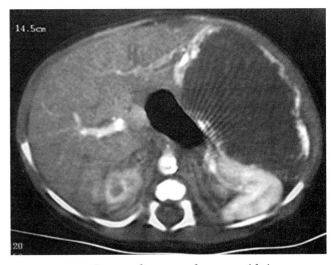

FIGURE 67-2. Computed tomography scan with intravenous contrast showing a large left lateral segment hemangioendothelioma with peripheral enhancement.

Hepatic hemangioendothelioma also has been seen in conjunction with focal nodular hyperplasia.[22] This association is important to remember during the radiologic evaluation of a child with multiple hepatic masses.

Pathology

Microscopically, most of these lesions consist of a single layer or, occasionally, several layers of flat endothelial cells on a supporting fibrous stroma (type 1 lesion).[23] In the type 2 lesion seen in about 20% of the cases, the endothelial cells are pleomorphic, larger, and more hyperchromatic than those seen in type 1, and they are present along poorly formed vascular spaces that often show tufting or branching. It is thought that the histologic picture of the type 2 lesion is more characteristic of a rapidly proliferating process. However, the differentiation between a type 2 lesion and an angiosarcoma can sometimes be very difficult.[14,24] Well-preserved bile ducts can often be seen near the periphery of the lesion.

Treatment

The therapy for hemangioendotheliomas depends on the severity of the presenting symptoms and the size of the mass. In general, the natural history of these lesions is that they tend to grow over the first year of life and then begin to regress spontaneously.

Asymptomatic lesions are simply monitored, and no specific therapy is instituted until symptoms occur.[9,25] As part of the evaluation in asymptomatic patients with multifocal hemangiomas, however, imaging studies of the brain and chest should be performed to make sure no associated intracranial or pulmonary lesions are present. In addition, all patients with hemangiomas should be screened for hypothyroidism.

Patients first seen with congestive heart failure, coagulopathy, or respiratory compromise will require intervention. Mortality rates in these patients have been reported to range from 17% to 35%, with some reports of death in as many as 90% of severely symptomatic patients.[26-28] Risk factors for death include congestive heart failure, jaundice, multiple tumor nodules, and the histologic absence of cavernous differentiation.

In patients with congestive heart failure, stabilization is initiated with digoxin and diuretics. Supportive measures may be necessary in patients with respiratory compromise either from the high-output cardiac failure or from restriction of diaphragmatic hernia by the abdominal mass. Coagulation factors may be administered if a coagulopathy is present.

Once hemodynamic or respiratory compromise or coagulopathy becomes a problem, therapy directed toward the hemangioma is needed. The usual initial treatment for a symptomatic lesion is prednisone or prednisolone at a dose of 2 to 3 mg/kg/day. The symptomatic response rate to steroids is reported to be about 45%.[29,30] If this is not effective in relieving the symptoms after 1 to 2 weeks, a trial of α-interferon should be instituted. Prolonged administration may be necessary for a clinical response.[31] α-Interferon therapy is certainly indicated in the presence of the Kasabach-Merritt syndrome.[8] A recent report described a reduction in levels of vascular endothelial growth factor (VEGF) after administration of α-interferon.[32] Three cases were described recently with excellent resolution of steroid-resistant infantile hemangioendotheliomas by using vincristine at a weekly dose of 1 to 2 mg/m² of body surface area for 2 weeks.[10] Surgical resection of these lesions appears to be most effective when it is confined to a single lobe. In this situation, a survival rate of 92% has been reported, even if the clinical situation is complicated by congestive heart failure.[24]

Embolization is being used more frequently, especially in patients who are thought to be too unstable for surgical intervention.[33,34] With this therapy, it is important to identify and occlude both the arterial and portal vasculature.[9,13] After successful embolization, a rapid improvement in the clinical course usually occurs within 5 days.[33,34]

Finally, liver transplantation has been used as successful therapy in patients with severe congestive heart failure or unremitting coagulopathy or both, for whom other modes of treatment have failed.[35]

Regardless of the treatment modality, if the hemangioendothelioma does not completely involute, a reported risk exists of malignant transformation of an infantile hemangioendothelioma to an angiosarcoma in older children.[12,36] For this reason, patients who are asymptomatic or who become asymptomatic after therapy must be monitored for complete resolution of their hemangioendothelioma. Surgical resection of any residual lesion should be considered.

Mesenchymal Hamartoma

Incidence

Mesenchymal hamartoma is reported to be the third most common hepatic tumor and the second most common benign tumor in children.[1] Of the benign hepatic lesions that have been described, mesenchymal hamartomas account for between 18% and 29% of these tumors.[37,38] Approximately 120 cases of mesenchymal hamartomas have been described in the English literature.[39]

Epidemiology

The reason for the development of a mesenchymal hamartoma is unclear. One theory is that it results from abnormal development of the primitive mesenchyme, which appears to occur at the level of the hepatic ductal plate, causing an abnormality of the bile ducts.[40] This postulate is supported by the histologic finding of a combination of cystic, anaplastic, and proliferating bile ducts, as well as the presence of multiple portal vein branches within the tumor. It is conjectured that the tumor then develops a cystic component as a result of obstruction and dilatation of lymphatics or from occluded bile ducts or both. The tumor enlarges during infancy as the cystic areas increase in size. Most of the proliferative growth appears to occur before or just after birth, because no observable mesenchymal mitotic activity is seen on histologic sections of the tumor.[41]

A second theory is that the lesions are reactive rather than developmental.[42] It is hypothesized that an abnormal blood supply to a part of the otherwise normal hepatic parenchyma causes ischemic necrosis, leading to reactive cystic changes within that portion of the liver. This theory is supported by the findings that hamartomas often have a necrotic center, are often attached to the liver by only a thin pedicle, and rarely are found centrally in the liver.

The third theory suggests that a mesenchymal hamartoma is a proliferative lesion. This theory is supported by several findings. Increased fibroblast growth factor-2 (FGF-2) staining has been noted in the proliferating hepatic mesenchymal cells adjacent to the mesenchymal hamartoma.[43] Both the mesenchymal cells in the liver and the mesenchymal hamartoma tissue strongly express molecules of the FGF-receptor family. It is speculated that a local increase of FGF-2 secretion could stimulate the growth of mesenchymal cells to form the mesenchymal hamartoma. FGF-2 also is a potent angiogenic factor that could contribute to the intense vascularization seen within some of these lesions. Cytogenic studies in these tumors have documented balanced translocation of chromosome 19 as well as the presence of aneuploidy.[44-46] This cytogenic abnormality along with aneuploidy suggests that a mesenchymal hamartoma may be a proliferative lesion.

Presentation

The widespread use of prenatal imaging has lead to the detection of hepatic masses before birth.[15] Recently 13 cases of hepatic mesenchymal hamartoma have been diagnosed or detected prenatally.[47] One of the unique characteristics of a neonatal mesenchymal hamartoma is that they can be solid as well as cystic. Unfortunately, the prognosis for these neonates is often poor. Of the 13 reported cases mentioned earlier, 5 experienced very rapid tumor growth, with fetal hydrops occurring in 3 of the patients, and 2 of these 5 fetuses died. It was believed that the rapid growth of the liver cyst was directly related to the development of fetal hydrops. Thus it may be best to deliver these fetuses before fetal hydrops develops. Others have reported similar experiences.[48]

In the neonate, these lesions can have a varying presentation. High-output cardiac failure with associated pulmonary hypertension has been reported in neonates with highly vascular mesenchymal hamartomas.[49,50] Respiratory distress secondary to a large hepatic mass impinging on the diaphragm has been described as well.[48]

The presentation of a mesenchymal hamartoma in the older child is usually that of progressive abdominal distention or an abdominal mass or both. A significant right-sided predilection exists for these masses, and they tend to be somewhat more common in male than female patients. Occasionally associated symptoms such as nausea and vomiting are probably secondary to the compression of the stomach and intestine by the expanding mass.[1]

On physical examination, abdominal distention or a palpable abdominal mass is most common. The mass tends to be nontender and fixed. Laboratory studies almost uniformly are normal, including liver function studies and AFP.

CT, US, and MRI have all been used for diagnosis. On CT and US, usually a multiseptated, multicystic, anechoic mass is located in the periphery of the liver.[51,52] Occasionally the mass is pedunculated. Calcification is uncommon.[53] The finding of a small round hyperechoic parietal nodule on US is usually highly sensitive.[54]

Pathology

Mesenchymal hamartomas typically are large encapsulated tumors that usually measure at least 8 to 10 cm in diameter. Three of four of these tumors occur in the right lobe of the liver, and only 3% are seen in both lobes of the liver. On cut section, multiple cysts measure from a few millimeters to 15 cm in diameter. These cysts are filled with either serous or viscus fluid separated by loose fibrous and myxoid tissue (Fig. 67-3). The surrounding tissue is yellow-tan to brown and is loose to moderately dense.

Microscopically, the tissue consists of a mixture of bile ducts, liver cell cysts, and mesenchyme. The cysts may simply be dilated bile ducts, dilated lymphatics, or amorphous fluid surrounded by mesenchyme. In older patients, the cysts may be lined with cuboidal epithelium (Fig. 67-4). Elongated or tortuous bile ducts surrounded by connective tissue are unevenly distributed throughout the mesenchyme. Typically the hepatocytes appear normal, and they are not a predominant part of the pathology. The bile ducts in the periphery of the lesion seem to be undergoing active proliferation.[1]

Treatment

Various management strategies have been used for these lesions. Because they are sometimes encapsulated, simple surgical enucleation may be possible. Very large, bilobar tumors that are not amenable to resection can be marsupialized into the peritoneal cavity, but recurrence after marsupialization has been described.[39] Patients undergoing

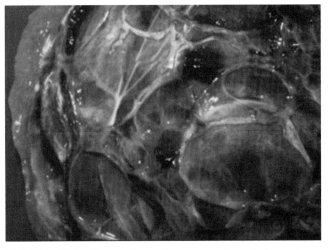

FIGURE 67-3. Cut surface of a mesenchymal hamartoma showing multiple cysts.

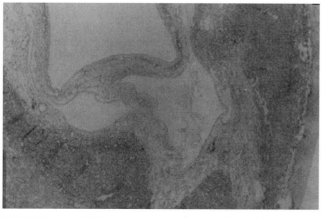

FIGURE 67-4. Light microscopy of mesenchymal hamartoma showing a cyst lined with cuboidal epithelium.

marsupialization need to be followed up carefully to detect recurrence. Complete excision of the lesion is usually curative and currently is the recommended therapy.

In several reports of patients being observed after the definitive diagnosis has been obtained, often the lesions will have a short period of growth followed by spontaneous involution.[55] However, at least three reports describe the development of either an undifferentiated embryonal sarcoma of the liver or malignant mesenchymoma.[56-58] Benign and malignant lesions were noted synchronously in two children and were metachronous in a 6-year-old who had undergone a left lateral segmentectomy at age 18 months for mesenchymal hamartoma. The evidence for a direct link between mesenchymal hamartoma and undifferentiated embryonal sarcoma of the liver comes from the simultaneous finding of both tumors arising within the same mass. Moreover, aneuploidy and similar chromosomal abnormalities involving chromosome 19 have been reported both in mesenchymal hamartoma and in undifferentiated embryonal sarcoma of the liver.[44,45]

Focal Nodular Hyperplasia

Incidence

Focal nodular hyperplasia (FNH) accounts for about 10% of the hepatic tumors in children.[1] The reported age range is between 7 months and 16 years, with a mean of 7 years, and a slight female preponderance.[59] The majority of these tumors are discovered incidentally.[59,60] The most common symptom is abdominal pain, but some patients describe decreased appetite, an abdominal mass, weight loss, or a combination of these. Hepatomegaly is a common finding, and liver function test abnormalities have been described.

FNH has been seen in association with a variety of different conditions and situations including previous trauma to the liver, other liver tumors, hemochromatosis, Klinefelter's syndrome, the use of intraconazole, and cigarette smoking.[61-66]

Controversy exists about the relation between oral contraceptive use and the development of FNH. In a

case-controlled study, it was noted that neither menstrual nor reproductive factors correlated with FNH risk. However, oral contraceptive use was a significant risk factor in the development of FNH.[65] Because the use of oral contraceptives also appears to be associated with hepatocellular adenomas, a history of oral contraceptive use does not help in distinguishing between these two entities.[65]

In children, an association has been noted between the congenital absence of the portal vein (Abernathy syndrome) and FNH.[67-69] In addition, these patients have an increased incidence of other solid tumors such as hepatoblastoma, hepatocellular carcinoma, and hepatocellular adenoma. FNH also has been seen, albeit less frequently than hepatocellular adenoma, in patients with glycogen storage disease (GSD) type 1.[69] An especially interesting association was described with the development of FNH a number of years after treatment for either neuroblastoma or a variety of other small round cell tumors.[70] It was hypothesized that the chemotherapy caused microvascular alterations within the liver resulting, in the development of FNH.[71]

Radiology

The diagnosis of FNH by radiological means often requires the use of multiple different imaging modalities. On CT scan, the classic findings are early enhancement of the lesion and the presence of a central scar (Fig. 67-5).[72] Unfortunately this pathognomonic association is not often seen.[73,74] Additional modalities described include single-photon emission CT (SPECT) radionucleotide scans with either radiolabeled sulfur colloid or hepatoimidodiacetic acid (HIDA) imaging, which demonstrates hypervascularization, increased tumor tracer uptake, and a central cold area.[75-77] MRI also has been useful when coupled with either gadolinium enhancement or the use of liver-specific contrast agents such as mangafodipir trisodium or iron oxide. These agents help to delineate the lesion better by specifically looking for the central scar.[78]

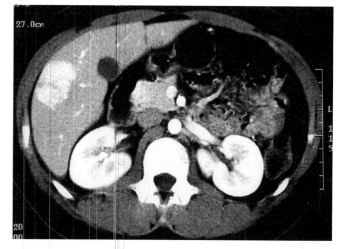

FIGURE 67-5. Computed tomography scan with intravenous contrast showing an early enhancing lesion in the right lobe with hypodense central scar consistent with focal nodular hypoplasia.

Pathology

FNH classically is characterized by nodular architecture, a central or eccentric scar containing malformed vessels that resemble an arterial venous malformation, and a variable amount of bile ductular proliferation (Figs. 67-6 and 67-7).[79] This entity develops in the setting of a noncirrhotic liver.

It is believed that the etiology of FNH is an abnormal hepatic circulation.[80] FNH is thought to be a hyperplastic nodule caused by excessive blood flow from an anomalous large artery that ultimately is located within the central scar.[81] The increased vascularity probably causes hyperplasia of the hepatic parenchyma and nodule formation. FNH is thought to be a hyperplastic rather than a neoplastic process.

Further evidence that FNH is a reactive lesion secondary to vascular anomalies comes from a study in which an increase in the angiopoietin ratio (ANG-1/ANG-2) was seen.[82] The *ANG-1* and *ANG-2* genes are necessary for normal vascular development. In FNH, an over-expression of the *ANG-1* gene and an absence of the antagonistic *ANG-2* gene leads to uncontrolled and disorganized vascular development. Although it is not clear that this is the exact pathogenesis of FNH, it certainly suggests that this genetic imbalance may play a causative role.

Histologically, the classic form of FNH with a central scar accounts for about 80% of the lesions. A nonclassic category of FNH lacks either the nodular architecture or the presence of the malformed blood vessels. These lesions are subdivided into two histologic categories: the telangiectatic form and the mixed hyperplastic and adenomatous form.[83] These nonclassic categories always lack a macroscopic scar. The mixed hyperplastic and adenomatous form often can be difficult to distinguish from hepatocellular adenoma. Hepatocellular adenomas have been reported to be present in association with FNH in about 4% of the cases.[79]

Currently no cases of malignant transformation of an FNH have been reported. However, FNH can occur in association with a well-differentiated fibrolamellar hepatocellular carcinoma. This observation is important

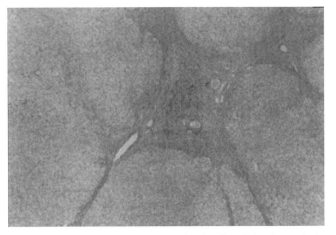

FIGURE 67-7. Light microscopy of a focal nodular hypoplasia showing a central scar containing abnormal blood vessels.

to remember in patients who have multiple hepatic nodules.[84,85]

Treatment

The treatment of FNH depends on the clinical situation. If the diagnosis is certain, and the patient is asymptomatic, the consensus is that these patients can be followed up with serial US to make sure that no progression of the lesion occurs.[59,73] If the patient is symptomatic, if progression of the mass is seen, or if the diagnosis is unclear, then a biopsy or a resection of the lesion should be performed. Percutaneous biopsy has been described.[86] Because of the association of FNH with hepatocellular carcinoma, patients that are expectantly managed must have serial evaluations to ensure that no progression occurs and to monitor for the development of other hepatic lesions.

Several reports noted a 40% to 50% regression rate in cases of FNH that have been monitored.[87,88] Regression of FNH is more likely if the use of oral contraceptives ceases.[89,90]

In two symptomatic patients in whom the FNH was in an area that was thought to be difficult for surgical resection, arterial embolization either with lipiodol and absorbable gelatin foam (Gelfoam) or iodized oil and polyvinyl alcohol resulted in a significant regression in the size of the mass.[91,94]

Hepatocellular Adenoma

Incidence

Hepatocellular adenoma is a very rare hepatic tumor in children, composing only about 4% of all solid liver tumors.[1] It is most commonly seen in women in their twenties and is associated with the use of oral contraceptives.

Presentation

In children, these lesions are often asymptomatic and are discovered during the evaluation for other problems.

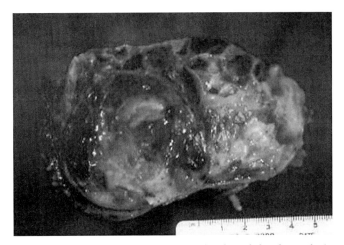

FIGURE 67-6. Gross section of a focal nodular hypoplasia showing a visible central scar.

Occasionally, they can produce intermittent abdominal pain and rarely can spontaneously rupture, resulting in hemoperitoneum and the clinical signs of acute volume depletion.

Radiology

Hepatic adenomas are often solitary lesions in most cases, but occasionally two to three adenomas can be seen in one patient.[92-94] This finding carries the separate diagnosis of liver adenomatosis. On US, these lesions can have a variable appearance, depending on the tumor composition. They can have a hyperechoic, hypoechoic, or a mixed echoic pattern depending on whether it is a simple adenoma, an adenoma with fatty metamorphosis, or an adenoma with hemorrhagic necrosis.[94]

On CT, the adenoma can either be isoattenuating relative to the normal liver or hyperattenuating (due to the presence of fat). They are usually sharply marginated and nonlobular but can be encapsulated or calcified in some patients.[95] Hyperattenuated areas often corresponded to recent hemorrhage. Occasionally, on CT scan with IV contrast, peripheral enhancement secondary to large subcapsular feeding vessels occurs. The finding of central hemorrhage or necrosis on CT scan helps differentiate hepatocellular adenoma from FNH.

Associated Conditions

Hepatocellular adenomas were extremely rare prior to 1960, which corresponds to the year in which oral contraceptives were first introduced.[96] In women who have never used oral contraceptives, the annual incidence of hepatic adenoma is estimated to be about one per million. This incidence increases to about 30 to 40 per million in women who are long-term users of oral contraceptives.[97]

Hepatocellular adenomas also are known to develop in patients with type 1A GSD by the time they reach their second or third decade of life.[98,99] The estimated prevalence of adenomas in these patients is close to 50%.[100,101] Adenomas are often multiple rather than solitary lesions. Unfortunately, hepatocellular carcinoma can occur in association with hepatocellular adenomas in type 1A GSD. In several series, hepatocellular carcinoma has been found to develop in up to 18% of patients with a hepatocellular adenoma.[102-106] The youngest patient with GSD was 6 years old at the time of the diagnosis of hepatocellular carcinoma.[107] Direct evidence for a malignant transformation of a hepatocellular adenoma into a carcinoma is lacking because it can be very difficult to differentiate between a hepatocellular adenoma and a well-differentiated hepatocellular carcinoma. Hepatocellular adenomas also have been associated with galactosemia, hypothyroidism, polycythemia, diabetes, Fanconi's anemia, polycystic ovary syndrome and the use of anabolic steroids.[108-111]

Adenomatosis (the occurrence of more than 10 simultaneous adenomas) is a relatively rare disorder, with 38 cases reported in the literature through 2000.[112] The two forms are the massive form, characterized by multiple nodules measuring between 2 and 10 cm, and the multifocal form, in which most lesions are smaller than 1 cm, with only a few larger than 4 cm.[113] Oral contraceptive use has been seen in about half of the female patients. Interestingly, diabetes was associated with all the cases, but the type of diabetes was not the same, and it is not clear whether a causative relation is present.[113]

Pathology

Hepatocellular adenomas histologically consist of large plates or cords of cells that resemble normal hepatocytes. These plates are separated by dilated vascular sinusoids, which are equivalent to thin-wall capillaries perfused by arterial pressure. Adenomas do not have a portal venous supply and are fed solely by peripheral arterial feeding vessels that account for the hypervascular nature of these lesions. Kupffer cells that are found in reduced numbers have little or no function. The absence of bile ducts serves as a key histologic feature that helps distinguish the hepatocellular adenoma from the FNH. Lipid accumulation is responsible for the characteristic yellow appearance on the cut surface.[1]

The exact reason for their development is unclear. Two recent reports have cited the mutations of the Wnt/β-catenin pathway in patients with hepatocellular adenoma.[114,115] This pathway mutation has been identified in many human hepatocellular neoplasms, although its direct contribution to carcinogenesis is not completely understood. The significance of these findings in hepatocellular adenoma also is unknown.

Hepatocellular adenomas may be asymptomatic but also may be the site of hemorrhage. Larger lesions are more likely to bleed than are smaller lesions. Contained hemorrhage may result in rapid enlargement, but rupture with intraperitoneal hemorrhage may occur if the lesion is near the liver surface. Signs of blood loss or peritonitis or both may result.

Treatment

The treatment of these lesions depends on a variety of factors. In patients who are receiving oral contraceptives or androgenic steroid therapy, the first step should be withdrawal of these medications. Multiple case reports mentioned regression of these adenomas after withdrawal of these compounds. However, in other multiple reports, withdrawal of these agents has resulted in persistence of the adenoma.[116-118] If discontinuation is not effective, it appears reasonable to simply observe these patients closely if the adenoma is smaller than 5 cm. If the adenoma enlarges or if evidence of intralesional hemorrhage develops, the adenoma must be resected. If the adenoma is larger than 5 cm or if the nature of the hepatic lesion is unclear, then surgical intervention is recommended.[119,120]

For patients with ruptured hepatocellular adenomas, the current suggested therapy in the hemodynamically stable patient is nonoperative monitoring and hemodynamic support. Once the hemorrhage has resolved and the patient has recovered, elective resection should be performed. In patients who continue to bleed actively, immediate control of the hemorrhage with either arterial embolization or surgical measures directed toward local control of the bleeding is necessary. Again, after the hemorrhage has resolved, resection is indicated. This management plan allows the lesion to decrease in size and allows a more limited hepatic resection under controlled conditions.[121,122]

In patients with type 1 GSD in whom multiple adenomas develop, hepatic transplantation should be considered because of the significant probability of the development of a concurrent hepatocellular carcinoma. Liver transplantation not only corrects the potential hemorrhagic problem but it also removes the potential for development of hepatocellular carcinoma.

MALIGNANT HEPATIC TUMORS

Hepatoblastoma

Background

Most hepatoblastomas develop before age 3 years, with a median age of about 18 months.[123] About 4% are present at the time of birth; 69% are present by the end of 2 years, and 90% develop by the end of 5 years. Only 3% of cases are noted in children older than 15 years.[124] A definite male predominance is seen, of about 1.7:1.[5]

Epidemiology

Hepatoblastomas are associated with a variety of clinical conditions, syndromes, and malformations (Table 67-3). Beckwith-Wiedemann syndrome is associated most commonly with Wilms' tumor but also is seen in children with hepatoblastomas, gonadoblastomas, and adrenal carcinomas.[125,126] This association is so strong that patients with this syndrome must be monitored with serial AFP levels and abdominal US every 4 months until they reach age 7 years.[126,127]

Another interesting association exists between hepatoblastoma and extreme prematurity (<1000 g). In the Japanese Children's Cancer Registry (JCCR), it was noted that hepatoblastomas accounted for 58% of the malignancies diagnosed in extremely low birth weight children.[128] The time from birth to onset of hepatoblastoma

ranges from 6 months to 6 years.[129] Unfortunately, the tumors that occurred in this group grow rapidly and have an unfavorable biologic behavior.[130] Although the etiology for the predilection of hepatoblastomas to develop in very low birth weight infants is not known, oxygen therapy, furosemide use, and a retarded growth rate all were noted to be risk factors.[130] The highest correlation was with the duration of oxygen therapy. The risk of hepatoblastoma increased by 20% if oxygen therapy was continued for 30 days, and the risk increased by 100% in children who were treated with oxygen for 4 months. Because of the complexities of treating "micropremies" through their first months, multiple other interventions could have influenced the development of a hepatoblastoma.

Gross Pathology

Hepatoblastomas tend to be unifocal lesions in most cases. Fifty percent are isolated to the right lobe, 15% are in the left lobe, and 27% are centrally located to involve both lobes (Fig. 67-8).

Histology

Histologically, the tumor can be divided into six different subtypes (Figs. 67-9 and 67-10) based on light microscopy (Table 67-4). A correlation between clinical outcome and the histologic subtypes has been suggested. The pure fetal subtype appears to be associated with the better prognosis, whereas the small cell undifferentiated subtype appears to have a very poor prognosis.[131-134] In several other studies, chemotherapy was initiated before surgical intervention and likely altered the accuracy of histologic definition of the resected tumor, making it difficult to correlate histology and outcome.[135]

Biology and Cytogenetics

Thrombocytosis is common in patients with hepatoblastoma. This may be related to increased thrombopoietin

TABLE 67-3
CONDITIONS ASSOCIATED WITH HEPATOBLASTOMA

Beckwith-Wiedemann syndrome
Budd-Chiari syndrome
Gardner's syndrome
Hemihypertrophy
Heterozygous α_1-antitrypsin deficiency
Isosexual precocity
Polyposis coli families
Trisomy 18
Type 1a glycogen storage disease
Very low birth weight

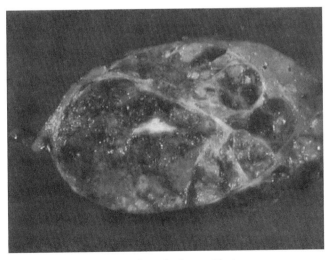

FIGURE 67-8. Cross section of a hepatoblastoma.

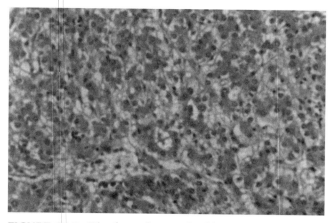

FIGURE 67-9. Histology of a pure fetal hepatoblastoma.

TABLE 67-4
HISTOLOGIC SUBTYPES OF HEPATOBLASTOMA

Pure fetal
Embryonal
Macrotrabecular
Small cell undifferentiated
Mixed epithelial and mesenchymal pattern
    With teratoid features
    Without teratoid features

---

levels, which have been reported in hepatoblastoma cell extracts.[135] Elevated interleukin-1β levels also have been noted in hepatoblastoma cell lines.[136] This results in an increased production of interleukin-6, which is known to stimulate thrombopoiesis and thrombocytosis.[140]

Chromosomal abnormalities have been documented in patients with hepatoblastoma.[137] The most common defects have been trisomy of chromosomes 20, 2, or 8, or a combination of these. Trisomy 18 also has been found.[138] As yet, however, no correlation has been noted between these cytogenetic abnormalities and either clinical outcome or tumor biology.

An association between hepatoblastoma and the *APC* gene was noted in patients with familial adenomatous polyposis and Gardner's syndrome.[139,140]

Presentation

Patients with hepatoblastoma most commonly are initially seen with an asymptomatic right upper abdominal mass that is noted incidentally by either a parent or a pediatrician. Rarely these patients have tumor rupture, followed by significant hemorrhage and hypovolemia. Sexual precocity may be the presenting feature with hepatoblastoma, secondary to the tumor producing

human chorionic gonadotropin. With large tumors, it is not unusual to see anorexia and failure to thrive. These lesions can become very large (≥15 cm) and can extend across the midline or down into the pelvis.

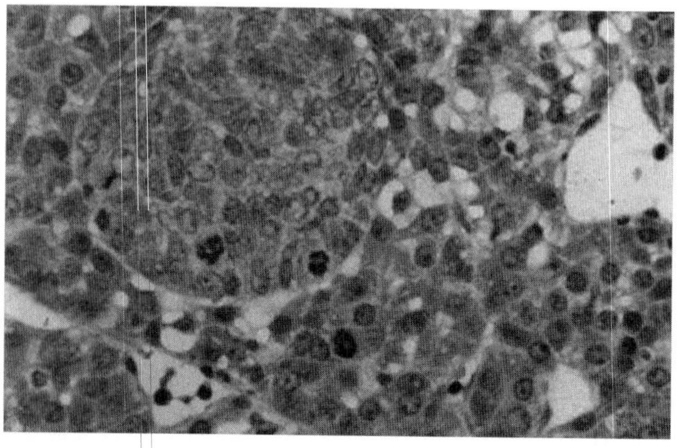

Imaging

The first diagnostic test is usually an US examination. This usually differentiates between a renal mass and a hepatic mass. An abdominal CT scan is then usually performed. In half of patients, calcification is noted within the mass.[141] Spiral CT scanning with IV bolus contrast not only is helpful in the diagnosis but also is useful in the staging of the tumor and in determining its resectability (Fig. 67-11). With 3D reconstruction, the location of the mass with respect to the vena cava, the hepatic veins, and the portal venous system can often be precisely delineated. MRI also can be helpful in determining the relation of the tumor to the hepatic anatomy and can potentially be useful in differentiating hepatoblastomas from other childhood hepatic tumors.[142]

Laboratory Studies

Anemia and thrombocytosis ($>500\times10^9$/L) are often seen in patients with hepatoblastoma.[143] However, the

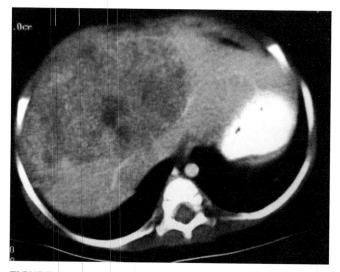

FIGURE 67-11. Computed tomography scan with intravenous contrast showing large right lobe hepatoblastoma extending into the left lateral segment.

FIGURE 67-10. Histology of a hepatoblastoma with mixed fetal and embryonal elements.

hallmark of hepatoblastoma is an elevated AFP level, seen in up to 90% of patients.[144] Serum AFP has a half-life of between 4 and 9 days, and the levels usually decrease to normal by 4 to 8 weeks after a complete removal of the tumor.[145] It also is important to remember that neonates have a normally elevated AFP level (25 to 50,000 ng/mL) at birth, and it does not decrease to "adult" levels until age 6 months.[146] This becomes important when evaluating a neonate with a hepatic mass, or when monitoring the AFP after liver resection in a neonate or infant.

AFP also has been used for monitoring purposes. In one case report, radioimmunodetection used a technetium-labeled mouse antihuman monoclonal antibody to AFP.[147] After an initial decline in the AFP, it began to increase, and the anti-AFP nuclear medicine study accurately located an active tumor in the remaining liver.

Staging

Two staging systems are used. One is a combined histologic and surgical staging used by the Children's Oncology Group (COG) (Table 67-5).[148] The second staging system, used by the International Society of Pediatric Oncology (SIOP), is based on the radiologic location of the tumor before treatment and is called the PRETEXT (Pretreatment Extent of Disease) Grouping System (Fig. 67-12).[149]

In the PRETEXT system, the liver is divided into four sections: the anterior and posterior sectors on the right and the medial and lateral sectors on the left. Therefore, based on the extent of the tumor, the patient is classified as follows: PRETEXT 1, with three adjoining sectors free (tumor only in one sector); PRETEXT 2, with two adjoining sectors free (two sectors involved); PRETEXT 3, in which one sector but two nonadjoining sectors are free (tumor involves two or three sectors); and PRETEXT 4, in which no sector is free (tumor in all four sectors). It is noted whether hepatic vein or portal vein involvement is present, if extra hepatic spread occurs (enlargement of the hilar lymph nodes), or if metastases are found.

Both staging systems have been shown to have direct correlations with ultimate patient survival (Table 67-6).

Treatment

The treatment of hepatoblastoma requires a combined-modality approach. Except on very, very rare occasions, chemotherapy alone is unable to eradicate the tumor. The only chance for a long-term cure is a complete resection of the primary tumor. However, complete removal of the tumor at initial presentation is usually possible in fewer than 50% of the cases. With chemotherapy and delayed or second-look surgery, the resection rate is improved to 69% to 98%.[150–153]

Multiple chemotherapy regimens have been evaluated for hepatoblastoma.[148,154] Most of these regimens rely on either cisplatin or carboplatin as the primary agent. These drugs are then combined with either vincristine, doxorubicin, or 5-fluorouracil and used in either an adjuvant or neoadjuvant fashion. In the patients who have had complete resection of their tumor, either four to six postoperative courses of chemotherapy are given. In those children in whom the liver tumor was deemed unresectable at the initial operation, three to four rounds of chemotherapy are initially given, followed by repeated imaging (Fig. 67-13). Resection is performed if possible. If the tumor is not resectable, then an additional three to four rounds of chemotherapy are given, followed again by repeated imaging. If the tumor is still not resectable, then consideration is given to liver transplantation, as long as no evidence of extrahepatic spread exists.

Some newer chemotherapy agents have been investigated for hepatoblastoma. Topotecan inhibits growth and neovascularization in a mouse model.[155] In addition, the suppressive effects of the topotecan lasted several weeks after discontinuation of the agent. Irinotecan appears to have some promise in salvaging patients who have recurrent disease. This drug could potentially be added to frontline chemotherapy regimens.[156] High-dose chemotherapy with stem cell rescue has been attempted but was not successful.

Another approach to the unresectable hepatoblastoma is the use of preoperative chemoembolization.[157] Transarterial catheterization with selective tumor chemoembolization was able to shrink the tumor by an average of 26%, which allowed subsequent complete tumor resection in every case. Interestingly, the surgical specimens showed only minimally viable or no viable tumor. It was postulated that this technique may be useful not only as a therapeutic modality for unresectable hepatoblastomas but also potentially for resectable tumors that could be made minimally viable to nonviable before surgical intervention.

Another therapeutic dilemma occurs in the child first seen with a ruptured tumor. In one review, all three patients who survived the initial rupture had no evidence of recurrent disease, with a mean survival of 36 months.[158] Even though rupture of the tumor and peritoneal soiling occurred, no peritoneal growths were subsequently identified in any children.

TABLE 67-5		
CHILDREN'S ONCOLOGY GROUP STAGING SYSTEM AND OUTCOME		
		5-Year Survival
Stage I	Complete resection, clear margin, pure fetal histology	100%
Stage IU	Complete resection, clear margin, unfavorable histology	98%
Stage II	Gross total resection with microscopic residual or perioperative rupture	100%
Stage III	Unresectable or resection with gross residual or lymph node involvement	69%
Stage IV	Metastatic disease	37%

From Ortega J, Siegel S: Biological markers in pediatric cancer. In Pizza P, Poplack D (eds): Principles and Practice of Pediatric Oncology. Philadelphia, Lippincott, 1989, pp 149–162, with permission.

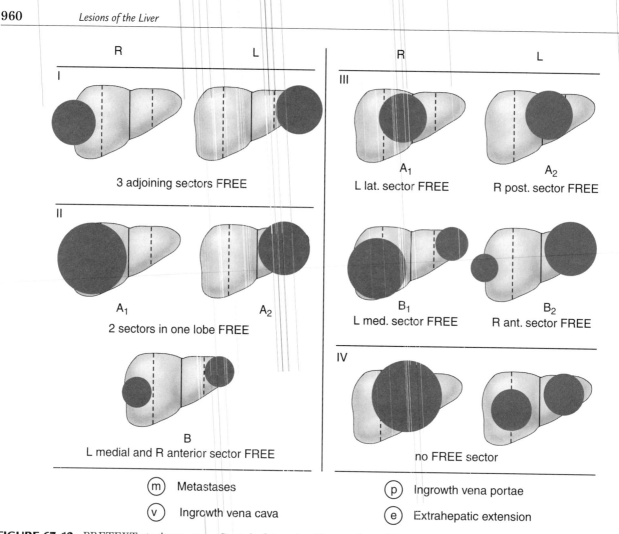

m — Metastases
v — Ingrowth vena cava
p — Ingrowth vena portae
e — Extrahepatic extension

FIGURE 67-12. PRETEXT staging system. Stage is determined by number of liver sectors free of tumor.

Outcome

Patient-outcome studies have been based on histologic type, the extent of the original tumor, or tumor response to chemotherapy.[131]

Several studies have shown a good outcome with fetal histology and with complete resection of the tumor.[36,134,159–161] All the studies that have consistently shown a good outcome based on fetal histology have strictly limited this diagnosis to tumors with a mitotic activity less than 2/10 high-power fields. Conversely, several studies

have consistently reported a poor outcome for those patients who have small cell undifferentiated hepatoblastoma.[132] Except for these data, no consistent correlation has been found with any of the other histologic patterns and patient outcome.

The AFP level also has both prognostic and therapeutic implications. Patients with an AFP level less than 100 ng/mL or greater than 1 million ng/mL were found to have a worse prognosis.[162] The low-AFP group comprised patients with small cell undifferentiated tumors, suggesting that a low AFP level could be related to a very primitive and poorly differentiated tumor that was unable to make AFP. Patients who had a slow decline in their AFP levels after resection and chemotherapy had a poorer long-term prognosis than did those who had an early, very rapid decline.[163]

In a combined study group report, about 30% of the patients were able to undergo either a complete or gross total resection of the tumor at the initial procedure.[164] In patients with stage 3 disease who were initially unresectable and who underwent four cycles of chemotherapy, 51% had their tumors rendered resectable. In patients with stage 4 disease (initially unresectable), 40% of these tumors were rendered resectable after four rounds of chemotherapy. The best survival was in nine

TABLE 67-6	
SIOP PRETEXT STAGING AND OUTCOME	
	5-Year Survival
Stage I	100%
Stage II	91%
Stage III	68%
Stage IV	57%

SIOP, International Society of Pediatric Oncology. From Brown J, Perilongo G, Shafford E, et al: Pretreatment prognostic factors for children with hepatoblastoma: Results from the International Society of Pediatric Oncology (SIOP) Study SIOPEL 1. Eur J Cancer 36:1418–1425, 2000.

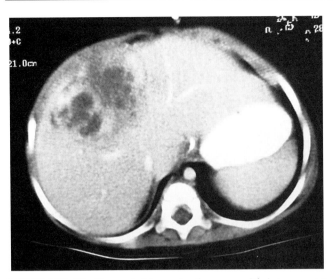

FIGURE 67-13. Computed tomography scan with intravenous contrast showing marked reduction in size of a hepatoblastoma after four rounds of chemotherapy (same case as in Fig. 67-11).

patients with stage 1 pure fetal histology who were treated with low-dose IV doxorubicin (100% survival). The overall survival rate for the entire series was 70%. The 5-year survival by stage was 100% for stage 1 pure fetal histology, 98% for stage 1 unfavorable histology, 69% for stage 3, and 37% for stage 4. These data compared favorably with those of a large German series that noted event-free survivals of 100% for stage 1, 80% for stage 2, and 68% for stage 3 disease.[153] None of the patients with stage 4 disease in the German trial survived. Another prospective study from the German group showed that the important prognostic factors for survival appeared to be the tumor growth pattern, vascular invasion, and serum AFP levels.[161]

In another study using the COG staging system, they reported that 50% of the hepatoblastomas were resectable at presentation, and 10% were metastatic.[165] In this series, the survival rate was 100% for stage 1, 67% for stage 2, 50% for stage 3, and 14% for stage 4. In the unresectable patients who initially underwent chemotherapy, 60% underwent successful postinduction resection. When separated by histologic subtype, they had a 100% survival with fetal histology and no survival with small cell undifferentiated histology. In several series, the prognosis after local recurrence is poor.[145,166,167]

In a SIOP study, the overall 5-year survival rate was 75%.[151] The most common site for metastases at initial presentation was the lungs. Moreover, the presence of metastases at diagnosis and the PRETEXT staging at diagnosis were found to be significant factors. The risk of death doubled between PRETEXT stage 1 and PRETEXT stage 2 and doubled again between PRETEXT stage 2 and PRETEXT stage 3. By PRETEXT grouping, the chance of survival with PRETEXT stage 1 was 100%; PRETEXT stage 2, 91%; PRETEXT stage 3, 68%; and PRETEXT stage 4, 57%. If lung metastases were initially present, a 57% five-year overall survival was found. If they were not present, an 81% overall 5-year

survival resulted. Because of these excellent correlations between PRETEXT stages and outcome, the PRETEXT staging system has been adapted as a part of all future collaborative hepatoblastoma studies.[168] Because patients in the high-risk PRETEXT stages have poor outcomes despite a complete surgical resection, additional or different chemotherapy regimens are necessary to improve patient survival in these groups.[161]

Orthotopic liver transplantation has been a successfully used treatment for unresectable hepatoblastoma.[169] A recurrence-free survival rate of 79% has been reported.[170] In this series, the most important prognostic factor that predicted good results after transplantation was a good initial response to chemotherapy. All patients with a good initial chemotherapy response, independent of their initial presentation, are alive and well after transplant. Conversely, only 60% of the patients who were poor responders are currently alive, with a follow-up less than 1 year. In this report, no correlation was seen between the initial tumor size or stage and survival after transplantation. Unfortunately, liver transplantation for local tumor recurrence after resection was associated with a post-transplant recurrence rate of 50%. These data strongly suggest that liver transplantation is indicated only in patients with chemosensitive hepatoblastomas that do not shrink sufficiently to allow a radical hepatic resection with good tumor margins. In another series, a 92% survival rate after transplantation was reported.[171] Almost all patients received one to two courses of post-transplant chemotherapy, which may have been the reason for the low post-transplant relapse. Before transplantation, all children in their series had surgically unresectable hepatoblastomas after chemotherapy, but they all showed a significant decrease in their AFP levels, indicating that the tumor was chemoresponsive. Moreover, patients with extrahepatic metastatic spread on initial evaluation were successfully treated with liver transplantation if the metastatic disease was eradicated before the transplant.

Undifferentiated Embryonal Sarcoma

Incidence

Undifferentiated embryonal sarcoma of the liver makes up about 7% of the solid liver tumors in children.[1] Unfortunately, this is a very malignant tumor with a poor outcome.

Presentation

Undifferentiated embryonal sarcoma most commonly affects children between the ages of 6 and 10 years but has been reported in a child as young as 19 months.[172] A slight male predominance has been noted. The most common clinical presentation is either right upper quadrant or epigastric pain with or without a palpable abdominal mass. Occasionally, a marked hepatomegaly is seen without a definite mass. Rarely, this tumor can even masquerade as a hepatic abscess or infection.[173] Other nonspecific presenting complaints can include vomiting,

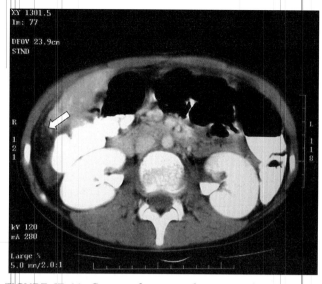

FIGURE 67-14. Computed tomography scan with intravenous contrast of an undifferentiated embryonal sarcoma showing a hypodense area in the right lobe of liver.

anorexia, and lethargy. Laboratory studies, including AFP, are usually normal.

Radiology

On US examination, the lesion appears predominantly solid.[174] However, on CT and MRI, the lesion appears cystic without any significant solid component (Fig. 67-14). This same type of disparity has been reported only in Wilms' tumor metastatic to the liver. Otherwise, it appears that such a discrepancy between the two imaging techniques would be highly suggestive of an undifferentiated embryonal sarcoma.

Pathology

Undifferentiated embryonal sarcoma is a neoplasm with a very primitive mesenchymal phenotype. These tumors

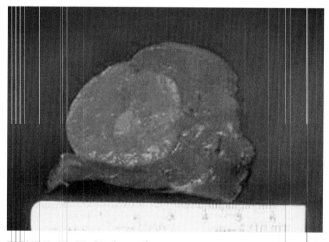

FIGURE 67-15. Variegated appearance on cut section of an undifferentiated embryonal sarcoma.

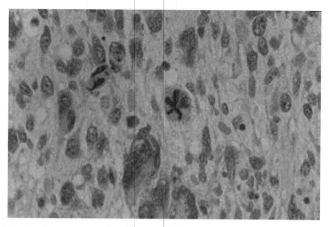

FIGURE 67-16. Histology of undifferentiated embryonal sarcoma showing large spindle cells with multiple mitoses.

tend to occur predominantly in the right lobe of the liver and tend to be large, with an average diameter of 14 to 21 cm.[174] In cross section, the tumors are often variegated in appearance, with white mucoid or gelatinous areas alternating with other areas of tumor necrosis and hemorrhage (Fig. 67-15). The tumor typically is well demarcated from the adjacent liver by a compressed, fibrous, pseudocapsule.[172]

On microscopic section, these tumors are composed of medium to large spindle-to-stellate–type cells in a variable amount of myxoid stroma (Fig. 67-16). These cells are usually densely arranged in a myxomatous background. In the periphery entrapped bile ducts or hepatic chords have been noted.[1,172] Mitoses are frequent and usually bizarre.

Immunohistochemically, the only consistent cell markers have been vimentin and the "histiocytic" determinants α_1-antitrypsin and α_1-antichymotrypsin.[175,176]

In a cytogenetic study, extensive chromosomal rearrangements were noted to be very similar to other soft tissue sarcomas such as leiomyosarcoma, osteosarcoma, and malignant fibrous histiocytoma.[177] In only a few cytometric studies, the findings have ranged from diploidy to tetraploidy to aneuploidy.[178,179]

Treatment

In addition to the highly suggestive radiologic findings, these patients can be diagnosed by fine-needle aspiration. Two separate reports have noted that the cytologic features of undifferentiated embryonal sarcoma are distinctive and different from other childhood tumors.[180,181]

The initial experience with undifferentiated embryonal sarcoma of the liver was poor. In a review of patients treated from 1950 to 1988, only 37% of the patients were noted to be alive.[179] This tumor usually proves fatal because of massive upper abdominal growth with secondary involvement of the diaphragm, stomach, abdominal wall, ribs, or pancreas rather than by metastases. Occasionally, intra-abdominal dissemination of the tumor can occur causing diffuse matting of the small bowel. Pulmonary and pleural metastases have been noted but are much less common than the secondary involvement of the extrahepatic tissue by direct extension.[172]

The only chance for cure is radical excision.[182,183] Unfortunately, despite complete surgical resection of the tumor, many patients have recurrent disease, which suggests the need for postoperative chemotherapy.[184]

The chemotherapy regimens that have been used are based on sarcoma-type protocols. With these regimens, survival rates have improved to 66%, as these tumors are very chemotherapy sensitive.[185,188] This finding has led to the use of preoperative chemotherapy to shrink an unresectable tumor to a size at which a radical surgical resection is possible. This is similar to the approach used to manage an initially unresectable hepatoblastoma.

With the ongoing improvement in chemotherapy regimens for sarcomas, the previously bleak outlook for this tumor is now much more optimistic. The use of an aggressive chemotherapy regimen along with complete resection of the primary tumor has even resulted in a 37% survival rate in patients whose tumors initially presented with free intraperitoneal rupture.[188]

In patients in whom complete resection of the tumor is not possible despite chemotherapy, liver transplantation has been advocated as another possible means for complete excision. This aggressive approach is not completely unwarranted because these tumors are chemotherapy sensitive. This approach is analogous to patients with hepatoblastoma who have chemotherapy-sensitive tumors.

Hepatocellular Carcinoma

Hepatocellular carcinoma (HC) is a relatively rare, highly malignant tumor that is more commonly seen in adults than in children. It is the second most common pediatric liver tumor, occurring about 19% of the time, but it still composes less than 1% of all pediatric cancers.[189] Its peak incidence seems to be between 10 and 15 years, and it is more common in boys.[190]

The predisposing factors for HC are distinctly different between the pediatric and the adult population. In the adult population, cirrhosis seems to be the primary etiology. The cirrhosis is usually seen in patients with either hepatitis B, hepatitis C, genetic hemochromatosis, alcohol-related cirrhosis, or cirrhosis due to primary biliary cirrhosis. In a recent review, it was noted that patients in these groups were at a significantly increased risk for developing HC. Hepatic US and serum AFP evaluations every 6 months were recommended to detect this tumor at an early stage.[191] In contrast, cirrhosis is often not part of the antecedent process in children. Moreover, a previous congenital or acquired disorder of the liver may be found (Table 67-7).[192] HC in children has been associated with a variety of metabolic, familial, and infectious disorders. Some of these metabolic disorders include tyrosinemia, α_1-antitrypsin deficiency, and hemochromatosis.[193] Patients with tyrosinemia seem to be at a particularly high risk for development of HC. Because of this high prevalence rate, it has been suggested that liver transplantation be performed in this population before age 2 years.[195,196] HC also has been seen in patients with

type 1 GSD. Most hepatic masses that develop in this population are hepatic adenomas, but carcinomas do present a real risk in this group.[197] A variety of other noncirrhotic liver diseases also have been associated with HC, including familial polyposis, Gardner's syndrome, Sotos' syndrome, Blum's syndrome, neurofibromatosis, Abernathy malformation, methotrexate therapy, neonatal hepatitis, and parenteral nutrition.[198–203]

Congenital and infectious disorders also are associated with this tumor, including extrahepatic biliary atresia, congenital hepatic fibrosis, Alagille syndrome, PFIC (persistent familial intrahepatic cholestasis),[204] hepatitis B, and hepatitis C. In areas where hepatitis B is endemic, it ranks fifth in the causes of childhood malignancies and outnumbers hepatoblastoma by 3:1.[205] The importance of hepatitis B and the subsequent development of HC in children is highlighted by the aggressive hepatitis B vaccination program that began in 1984 in Taiwan.[206] When the mortality from liver carcinoma in the group from birth to age 9 years was compared between the years 1984 and 1993, a substantial and statistically significant decrease in the mortality was seen by 1993. Another study from Gambia showed similar results.[207] Hepatitis C also has been linked to the development of HC.[208] In contrast to hepatitis B, the cirrhosis and the subsequent development of HC in the hepatitis C population usually takes several decades to develop.[209]

Of particular interest is the association between HC and biliary atresia.[190,210] In a review, except for one patient first seen at age 5 months, all the other patients were older than 2 years with a mean of age 7½ years when the HC was discovered. These tumors were found either at autopsy or incidentally at the time of liver transplantation for biliary atresia. In those patients in whom

---

TABLE 67-7

CONDITIONS ASSOCIATED WITH HEPATOCELLULAR CARCINOMA IN CHILDREN

α_1-Antitrypsin deficiency
Anomalies of abdominal venous drainage
(Abernathy syndrome)
Alagille's syndrome
Biliary atresia
Congenital hepatic fibrosis
Familial hepatocellular carcinoma
Familial polyposis
Focal nodular hyperplasia of the liver
Gardner's syndrome
Hepatic adenoma
Hepatitis B infection
Hepatitis C infection
Hereditary tyrosinemia
Hyperalimentation
Progressive familial intrahepatic cholestasis
Methotrexate therapy
Oral contraceptives
Types I and III glycogen storage disease
Wilms' tumor
Wilson's disease

HC was identified at the time of transplantation, all of these patients are alive and well after transplant. This association between HC and biliary atresia would suggest that a routine screening protocol with hepatic US and AFP levels is warranted.

Presentation

Most patients are initially seen with either an abdominal mass or abdominal pain. Other associated symptoms include nausea and vomiting, anorexia, malaise, and a significant weight loss.[205] As many as 10% are seen primarily with tumor rupture and hemoperitoneum.[211]

Laboratory studies can show mild elevations in the serum glutamic-oxaloacetic transaminase (SGOT) and lactic dehydrogenase (LDH). The AFP is elevated in about 85% of patients but can be normal or only mildly elevated with the fibrolamellar variant.[211,212]

Imaging

CT and MRI are both helpful for delineating the mass and for determining resectability. With the advent of spiral CT with bolus IV contrast administration, the hepatic veins and portal venous system can be well delineated, and any involvement by the tumor can be adequately assessed. The fibrolamellar variant is notable on CT to be a hypodense, single or multilobed mass that tends to be hypervascular as well as sometimes showing a central scar.[213] This appearance could easily be confused with FNH, and care must be taken to distinguish between these two lesions.

Pathology

HC can vary in size from 2 to 25 cm, and the surrounding liver can exhibit either micro- or macronodular cirrhosis in up to 60% of cases (Figs. 67-17 and 67-18).[1]

Microscopically, trabeculae that are two to 10 cell layers in thickness are seen with the larger trabeculae sometimes displaying central necrosis (Fig. 67-19). The individual cells are usually larger than normal hepatocytes, with nuclear hypochromasia and frequent and bizarre mitosis (see Fig. 67-18). Vascular invasion may be prominent.

In the fibrolamellar variant, the hepatocytes are large, deeply eosinophilic, and embedded within a lamellar fibrosis. Clusters of cells are often separated by broad bands of laminated collagen.[1,214] The presence of large amounts of fibrosis alone is not sufficient in itself for the diagnosis of fibrolamellar carcinoma.[215]

Treatment

The treatment for HC is surgical resection, varying from a simple anatomic resection to a liver transplant. Unfortunately, primary resection is not always possible because either the tumor is bilobar or the tumor is associated with cirrhosis. Because of the cirrhosis, concern may exist that the hepatic resection might leave the patient with insufficient functioning parenchyma.

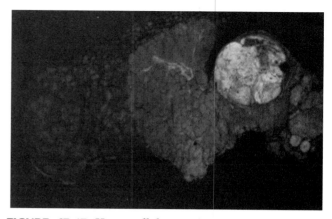

FIGURE 67-17. Hepatocellular carcinoma in the setting of cirrhosis.

In one pediatric report of 49 children, resection was possible in only 10%. Only two patients lived for more than 2 years.[205] In the adult population, 3-year survival rates between 34% and 57% have been reported.[216,217] Multiple studies have looked at prognostic factors that influence outcome and recurrence after resection for HC. Multiple staging systems have been proposed based on multivariant analyses of various prognostic factors. Three factors that have been repeatedly associated with improved survival and decreased recurrence rates are small tumor size (<2 cm), the number of tumor nodules (solitary versus multiple), and the presence or absence of vascular invasion. Unfortunately, it is rare to see patients initially with all three favorable variables. In most series, the tumors are usually larger than 5 cm in diameter at presentation.[216,218]

An important variant that should be mentioned is the fibrolamellar type. Only in the 1980s did this variant became established as a histologic and clinically distinct entity.[219] This lesion is characterized by relatively slow growth and occurs almost exclusively in a noncirrhotic liver.[214] The fibrolamellar variant usually occurs in adolescents and young adults, with a peak incidence in

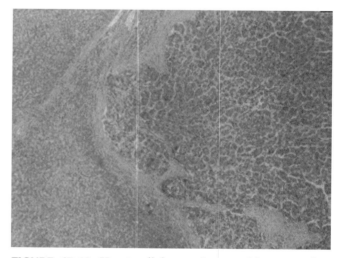

FIGURE 67-18. Hepatocellular carcinoma with surrounding cirrhosis.

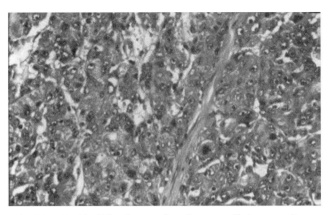

FIGURE 67-19. Histology of a hepatocellular carcinoma demonstrating enlarged hepatocytes and nuclear hypochromasia.

the second decade of life,[220,221] accounting for between 16% and 50% of the HC at younger than 21 years.[222] In contrast to conventional HC, fibrolamellar carcinoma is not associated with risk factors such as cirrhosis or chronic hepatitis B infection.[223,224] However, an association occurs between FNH and the fibrolamellar variant.

Radiologically, the fibrolamellar variant is often hypodense on noncontrast CT and can show a variable perfusion, including hypervascularity, on CT with contrast. In addition, a central hypodense or hypervascular area can be seen that can mimic a central scar.[225] This can create confusion between the diagnosis of the fibrolamellar variant and FNH. MRI has been reported to be helpful in distinguishing between these two diagnoses.[226] The results after resection for fibrolamellar carcinoma are very good, with 50% 5-year survivals. However, after apparent curative resections, recurrences or metastases can occur after very long disease-free intervals.[227,228]

Liver transplantation also has been used as curative therapy for the treatment of HC. The early experience of liver transplantation for HC was discouraging.[229] However, in a recent review of 344 patients who underwent liver transplantation for HC (excluding the fibrolamellar type), three factors were associated with tumor-free survival: a unilobar tumor, a tumor smaller than 2 cm, and the absence of vascular invasion.[230] A prognostic risk score based on these factors was developed. Patients with a very low risk score had a survival rate after transplant of 100%, and those with a high risk score had a 5-year survival of only 5%. The authors concluded that patients with low risk scores benefit from transplantation but do not benefit from adjuvant chemotherapy and that patients with high risk scores are poor candidates for a liver transplant. Several small series have reported good outcomes by using liver transplantation in selected patients with unresectable HC.[231–233]

Although chemotherapy for HC has not appeared to be beneficial in adults when given either before or after transplant, this may not be true for children. In two reports, five children with unresectable tumors were treated with chemotherapy before transplant. Four of the five had a dramatic decrease in their tumor size.[189,234] At the time of transplant, all tumors still had viable cells, but only one patient after transplant had a recurrence

and subsequently died. All patients had multiple large nodules, and one survivor had portal vein invasion.

Patients who are not surgical or transplant candidates or patients who demonstrate recurrences can potentially benefit from several nonsurgical strategies, including percutaneous ethanol injection, radiofrequency ablation, or chemoembolization of the hepatic mass.[235] All of these therapies have proven efficacious in decreasing or eradicating local tumors or recurrences. These therapies also improved survival with disease, but, unfortunately, none has been proven to be curative.[191]

The outcome for patients with HC, regardless of the treatment modality, is still not as good as the outcome for hepatoblastoma. Further improvements in survival for HC will come from advances in chemotherapy regimens that will prevent tumor recurrences.

Rhabdomyosarcoma of the Biliary Tree

Incidence and Presentation

Even though rhabdomyosarcoma is the most common sarcoma in children, it accounts for only 1% of all liver tumors and only 0.8% of all rhabdomyosarcomas in children.[1,236] Hepatobiliary rhabdomyosarcoma tends to be a disease of the young, with a median age of 3 years, and it is rarely seen in children older than 15 years.[237,238] This tumor most commonly arises in the intrahepatic biliary system and then extends into the liver parenchyma itself. It also has been reported to arise from a variety of other sites, including an intrahepatic cyst, the gallbladder, the cystic duct, the ampulla of Vater, a choledochal cyst, and from the hepatic parenchyma itself.[237–243]

Because it arises from the bile ducts, the most common presenting symptom is jaundice. As the median tumor diameter at diagnosis is 8 cm, an abdominal mass is a common finding.[236]

Laboratory Findings and Differential Diagnosis

Because jaundice is a common presenting symptom, elevated direct bilirubin, alkaline phosphatase, and γ-glutamyltransferase (GGT) are common.

The differential diagnosis for an intraductal lesion in a child would include either an inflammatory pseudotumor or a cholangiocarcinoma, but these are extraordinarily rare.[245] If the rhabdomyosarcoma is a predominantly hepatic mass with minimal bile duct involvement, then the differential diagnosis would be more dependent on the patient's age, as noted in the previous sections.

The pathology of the intraductal lesions is similar to the pathology of rhabdomyosarcoma at extrabiliary sites. The intraductal lesion is usually either the botryoid or embryonal subtype, unless the lesion involves predominantly the hepatic parenchyma, in which the alveolar subtype predominates.[246]

Imaging Modalities

Multiple imaging modalities have been used for diagnosis. US typically reveals biliary dilatation and possibly a mass in the biliary system. Larger lesions may have cystic areas within them, possibly reflecting areas of partial tumor necrosis.[141] CT will often show an intraductal mass in association with areas of low attenuation within the tumor. MRI may have an advantage over CT, in that it not only can show the anatomic source and location of the mass but, with the advent of MR cholangiography, it also can evaluate the bile ducts by demonstrating biliary dilatation and intraductal irregularity.[247] Percutaneous transhepatic cholangiography (PTC) also can be useful in patients who have a dilated biliary system. PTC can demonstrate multiple filling defects that correspond to the intraductal tumor.[248] PTC also has the advantage of providing external drainage of the biliary system in those patients with obstructive jaundice.

Treatment and Prognosis

The best treatment for biliary rhabdomyosarcoma is a multidisciplinary approach using surgical procedures, chemotherapy, and, potentially, radiotherapy. Unfortunately, surgical revision alone is not usually possible because of spread of the tumor into the liver parenchyma or direct local extension into the duodenum, stomach, or pancreas. It also is not unusual to find lymphatic spread at the initial operation. Because of these problems, adequate resection is usually possible in only 20 % to 40 % of the patients.[236–238] In patients in whom primary resection is not possible, the initial approach should be biopsy and lymph node sampling, followed by standard rhabdomyosarcoma chemotherapy protocols and a second-look procedure. In a study of biliary rhabdomyosarcoma that used this multimodality approach, 4 of 10 children remained disease free after an average of 4 years.[236]

REFERENCES

1. Stocker JT: Hepatic tumors in children. In Suchy FJ, Sokol RJ, Balistreri WF (eds): Liver Disease in Children, 2nd ed. Philadelphia, Lippincott Williams & Wilkins, 2001, p 915.
2. Silverberg E, Lubrea J: Cancer statistics. CA Cancer J Clin 36:9–25, 1986.
3. Couinaud C: [Surgical Anatomy of the Liver: Several new aspects]. Chirurgie 112:337–342, 1986.
4. Couinaud C: The anatomy of the liver. Ann Ital Chir 63:693–697, 1992.
5. Exelby PR, Filler RM, Grosfeld JL: Liver tumors in children in the particular reference to hepatoblastoma and hepatocellular carcinoma: American Academy of Pediatric Surgical Section Survey, 1974. J Pediatr Surg 10:329–337, 1975.
6. Boon LN, Burrows PE, Paltiel HJ, et al: Hepatic vascular anomalies in infancy: A twenty-seven year experience. J Pediatr 129:346–354, 1996.
7. Iyer CP, Stanley P, Mahour GH: Hepatic hemangiomas in infants and children: A review of thirty cases. Am Surg 62:356–360, 1996.
8. Chen CC, Kong MS, Yang CP, Hung IJ: Hepatic hemangioendothelioma in children: An analysis of thirteen cases. Acta Pediatr Tw 44:8–13, 2003.
9. Burrows PE, Dubois J, Kassarjian A: Pediatric hepatic vascular anomalies. Pediatr Radiol 31:533–545, 2001.
10. Perez J, Pardo J, Gomez C: Vincristine: An effective treatment of corticoid-resistant life-threatening infantile hemangiomas. Acta Oncol 41:197–199, 2002.
11. Mason K, Koka B, Eldridge E, et al: Perioperative considerations in a hypothyroid infant with hepatic hemangiomas. Paediatr An Aesth 11:228–232, 2001.

12. Daller JA, Bueno J, Gutierrez J, et al: Hepatic hemangioendothelioma: Clinical experience and management strategy. J Pediatr Surg 34:98–105, 1999.
13. Holcomb GW, O'Neill JA, Mahboubi S, et al: Experience with hepatic hemangioendothelioma in infancy and childhood. Pediatr Surg 23:661–666, 1998.
14. Selby DM, Stocker JT, Waclawiw MA, et al: Infantile hemangioendothelioma of the liver [abstract]. Hepatology 20:339–345, 1994.
15. Novaks D, Suchy F, Balistreri W: Disorders of liver and biliary system relevant to clinical practice. In Oski F (ed): Principles and Practice of Pediatrics. Philadelphia, JB Lippincott, 1990, pp 1746–1777.
16. Paltiel HJ, Patriquin HB, Keller MS, et al: Infantile hepatic hemangioma: Doppler ultrasound. Radiology 182:735–742, 1992.
17. Keslar PJ, Buck JL, Selby DM: From the archives of the AFIP: Infantile hemangioendothelioma of the liver revisited. Radiographics 13:657–670, 1993.
18. Horton KM, Bluemke DA, Hruban RH, et al: CT and MR imaging of benign hepatic and biliary tumors. Radiographics 19:431–451, 1999.
19. Chung T, Hoffer FA, Burrows PE, et al: MR imaging of hepatic hemangiomas of infancy and changes seen with interferon alpha 2a treatment. Pediatr Radiol 26:341–348, 1996.
20. Mortele KJ, Mergo PJ, Urrutia M, et al: Dynamic gadolinium-enhanced MR findings in infantile hepatic hemangioendothelioma. J Comput Assist Tomogr 22:714–717, 1998.
21. Kumar R, Gupta R, Dasan JB, et al: Infantile hemangioma of the liver, spleen and anterior abdominal wall. Clin Nucl Med 25:938, 2000.
22. Vilgrain V, Uzan F, Brancatelli G, et al: Prevalence of hepatic hemangioma in patients with focal nodular hyperplasia: MR imaging analysis. Radiology 229:75–79, 2003.
23. Dehner LP, Ishak KG: Vascular tumors of the liver in infants and children. Arch Pathol 92:101-111, 1971.
24. Becker JM, Heitler MS: Hepatic hemangioendotheliomas in infancy. Surg Gynecol Obstet 168:189–200, 1989.
25. Prkurat A, Kluge P, Chrupek M, et al: Hemangioma of the liver in children: Proliferating vascular tumor or congenital vascular malformation? Med Pediatr Oncol 39:524–529, 2002.
26. Woltering MC, Robben S, Egeler RM: Hepatic hemangioendothelioma of infancy: Treatment with interferon A. J Pediatr Gastroenterol Nutr 24:348–351, 1997.
27. Wong DC, Masel JP: Infantile hepatic hemangioendothelioma. Australas Radiol 39:140–144, 1995.
28. Davenport N, Hansen L, Heaton ND, et al: Hemangioendothelioma of the liver in infants. J Pediatr Surg 30:44–48, 1995.
29. Samuel M, Spitz L: Infantile hepatic hemangioendothelioma: The role of surgery. J Pediatr Surg 30:1425–1429, 1995.
30. Wu TJ, Teng RJ: Hepatic hemangioendothelioma: Successful treatment with steroid in a very low birth weight infant. Acta Paediatr Syn 37:56–58, 1996.
31. Folkman J, Mulliken J, Ezekowitz A: Angiogenesis and hemangiomas. In Oldman K, Colombani P, Foglia R (eds): Surgery of Infants and Children. Philadelphia, Lippincott-Raven, 1997, pp 569–580.
32. Szymik-Kantorowicz S, Partyka L, Demdinska-Kiec A, et al: Vascular endothelial growth factor in monitoring therapy of hepatic haemangioendothelioma. Med Pediatr Oncol 40:196–197, 2003.
33. Kullendors CM, Cwikiel W, Sandstrom S: Embolization of hepatic hemangioma in infants. Eur J Pediatr Surg 12:348–352, 2002.
34. Warmann S, Bertram H, Kardorf R, et al: Interventional treatment of infantile hepatic hemangioendothelioma. J Pediatr Surg 38:1177–1181, 2003.
35. Achilleos OA, Buist LJ, Kelly DA, et al: Unresectable hepatic tumors in childhood and the role of liver transplantation. J Pediatr Surg 31:1563–1567, 1996.
36. Weinberg A, Finegold M: Primary hepatic tumors of childhood. Hum Pathol 4:512–537, 1983.
37. Luks FI, Wazbeck S, Brandt ML: Benign liver tumors in children: A twenty-five year experience. J Pediatr Surg 11:1326–1330, 1991.
38. Ehren H, Mahour GH, Isaacs H Jr: Benign liver tumors in infancy and childhood. Am J Surg 145:325–329, 1983.

39. Meinders AJ, Simons MP, Heij HA, et al: Mesenchymal hamartoma of the liver: Failed management by marsupialization. J Pediatr Gastroenterol Nutr 26:353–355, 1998.

40. Caty M, Shamburger C: Abdominal tumors in infancy and childhood. Pediatr Clin North Am 40:1253–1269, 1993.

41. Stocker J, Ishak K: Mesenchymal hamartoma of the liver: Report of thirty cases in review of the literature. Pediatr Pathol 1:245–267, 1983.

42. Helal A, Nolan M, Bower R, et al: Pathological case of the month. Arch Pediatr Adolesc Med 149:315–316, 1995.

43. Von Schweinitz D, Dammeier BG, Gluer S: Mesenchymal hamartoma of the liver: New insights into histeriogenesis. J Pediatr Surg 34:1269–1271, 1999.

44. Mascarello JT, Krous HF: Second report of a translocation involving 19q13.4 in a mesenchymal hamartoma of the liver. Cancer Genet Cytogenet 58:141–142, 1992.

45. Speleman F, De Telder V, De Potter KR, et al: Cytogenetic analysis of a mesenchymal hamartoma of the liver. Cancer Genet Cytogenet 40:29–32, 1989.

46. Otal TM, Hendricks JB, Pharis P, et al: Mesenchymal hamartoma of the liver. Cancer 74:1237–1242, 1994.

47. Kamata S, Nose K, Sawai T, et al: Fetal mesenchymal hamartoma of the liver: Report of a case. J Pediatr Surg 38:639–641, 2003.

48. Dickinson JE, Knowles S, Phillips JM: Prenatal diagnosis of hepatic mesenchymal hamartoma. Prenat Diagn 19:81–84, 1999.

49. Balmer V, Le Coultre C, Feldges A, et al: Mesenchymal hamartoma in a newborn: Case report. Ur J Pediatr Surg 6:303–305, 1996.

50. Ros PR, Goodman ZD, Ishak KG, et al: Mesenchymal hamartoma of the liver: Radiologic-pathologic correlation. Radiology 158:619–624, 1986.

51. Raffensperger J, Gonzalez-Crussi F, Skeehan T: Mesenchymal hamartoma of the liver. J Pediatr Surg 18:585–587, 1983.

52. Ito H, Kishikawa T, Toda T, et al: Hepatic mesenchymal hamartoma of an infant. J Pediatr Surg 19:315–317, 1984.

53. Abramson SA, Lack EE, Teele RL: Benign vascular tumor of the liver in infants. Sonographic appearance. Am J Roentgenol 138:629–634, 1982.

54. Koumanidou C, Vakaki N, Papadaki M, et al: New sonographic appearance of hepatic mesenchymal hamartoma in childhood. J Clin Ultrasound 27:164–167, 1999.

55. Barnhart DC, Hirschl RB, Graver KA, et al: Conservative management of mesenchymal hamartoma of the liver. J Pediatr Surg 32:1495–1498, 1997.

56. De Chadarevian JP, Pawei BR, Faeber EN, et al: Undifferentiated (embryonal) sarcoma arising in conjunction with mesenchymal hamartoma of the liver. Mod Pathol 7:490–494, 1994.

57. O'Sullivan MJ, Swanson PE, Knool J, et al: Undifferentiated embryonal sarcoma with unusual features arising within mesenchymal hamartoma of the liver: Report of a case and review of the literature. Pediatr Dev Pathol 4:482–489, 2001.

58. Ramanujam TM, Ramesh JC, Goh DW, et al: Malignant transformation of mesenchymal hamartoma of the liver: Case report and review of the literature. J Pediatr Surg 34:1684–1686, 1999.

59. Raymond D, Plaschkes J, Ridolfi Luthy A, et al: Focal nodular hyperplasia of the liver in children: A review of follow-up and outcome. J Pediatr Surg 30:1590–1593, 1995.

60. Stocker JT, Ishac GK: Focal nodular hyperplasia of the liver: A study of twenty-one pediatric cases. Cancer 48:336–345, 1981.

61. Savoye-Collet C, Herve S, Koning E, et al: Focal nodular hyperplasia occurring after blunt abdominal trauma. Eur J Gastroenterol Hepatol 14:329–330, 2002.

62. Iordanidis F, Hytiroglou P, Drevelegas A, et al: A twenty-five year old man with a large hepatic tumor and multiple nodular lesions. Semin Liver Dis 22:97–102, 2002.

63. Hohler T, Lohse A, Schirmacher P: Progressive focal nodular hyperplasia of the liver in a patient with genetic hemochromatosis: Growth promotion by iron overload? Dig Dis Sci 45:587–590, 2000.

64. Santarelli L, Gabrielli M, Orefice R, et al: Association between Klinefelter syndrome and focal nodular hyperplasia. J Clin Gastroenterol 37:189–191, 2003.

65. Scalori A, Tavani A, Gallus S, et al: Risk factors for focal nodular hyperplasia of the liver: An Italian case-control study. Am J Gastroenterol 97:2371–2373, 2002.

66. Wolf R, Wolf D, Kuperman S: Focal nodular hyperplasia of the liver after itraconazole treatment. J Clin Gastroenterol 33:418–420, 2001.

67. Kinjo T, Aoki H, Sunagawa H, et al: Congenital absence of the portal vein associated with focal nodular hyperplasia of the liver and congenital choledochal cyst: A case report. J Pediatr Surg 36:622–625, 2001.

68. Altavilla G, Guariso G: Focal nodular hyperplasia of the liver associated with portal vein agenesis: A morphological and immunohistological chemical study of one case and review of the literature. Adv Clin Pathol 3:139–145, 1999.

69. Tanaka Y, Takayanagi M, Shiratori Y, et al: Congenital absence of portal vein with multiple hyperplastic nodular lesions in the liver. J Gastroenterol 38:288–294, 2003.

70. Icher-De Bouyn C, Leclere J, Raimondo G, et al: Hepatic focal nodular hyperplasia in children previously treated for a solid tumor: Incidence, risk factors and outcome. Cancer 97:3017–3113, 2003.

71. Kumagai H, Masuda T, Oikawa H, et al: Focal nodular hyperplasia of the liver: Direct evidence of circulatory disturbances. J Gastroenterol Hepatol 15:1344–1347, 2000.

72. Cheon JE, Kim WS, Kim IO, et al: Radiological features of focal nodular hyperplasia of the liver in children. Pediatr Radiol 28:878–883, 1998.

73. Somech R, Brazowski E, Kesller A, et al: Focal nodular hyperplasia in children. J Pediatr Gastroenterol Nutr 32:480–483, 2001.

74. Bioulac-Sage P, Balabaud C, Wanless IA: Diagnosis of focal nodular hyperplasia: Not so easy [editorial]. Am J Surg Pathol 25:1322–1325, 2001.

75. Huang YE, Wang PW, Huang HS, et al: A central scar in hepatic focal nodular hyperplasia detected on liver SPECT imaging. Clin Nucl Med 26:367–369, 2001.

76. Swingle CA, Fajman WA, Alazraki N: Early enhancing lesions seen on computed tomography consistent with focal nodular hyperplasia. Clin Nucl Med 28:134–135, 2003.

77. Stiner D, Klett R, Puille M, et al: Diagnosis of focal nodular hyperplasia with hepatobiliary scintigraphy using a modified SPECT technique. Clin Nucl Med 28:136–137, 2003.

78. Ba-Ssalamah A, Schima W, Schmook M, et al: A typical focal nodular hyperplasia of the liver: Imaging features of non-specific and liver specific MR contrast agents. Am J Roentgenol 179:1447–1456, 2002.

79. Nguyen BN, Flejou JF, Terris B, et al: Focal nodular hyperplasia of the liver: A comprehensive pathologic study of three hundred and five lessons and recognition of new histologic forms. Am J Surg Pathol 23:1441–1454, 1999.

80. Kudo M: Hepatic Nodule lesions caused by abnormal hepatic circulation: Etiological and clinical aspects [editorial]. J Gastroenterol 38:308–310, 2003.

81. Kondo F: Benign nodular hepatocellular lesions caused by abnormal hepatic circulation: Etiological analysis and introduction of a new concept. J Gastroenterol Hepatol 16:1319–1328, 2001.

82. Paradis V, Bieche I, Dargere D, et al: A quantitative gene expression study suggests a role for angiopoietins in focal nodular hyperplasia. Gastroenterology 124:651–659, 2003.

83. Wanless IR, Albrecht S, Bao J, et al: Multiple focal nodular hyperplasia of the liver associated with vascular malformations of various organs and neoplasia of the brain: A new syndrome. Mod Pathol 2:456–462, 1989.

84. Saul SH, Titelbaum DS, Gansler TS, et al: The fibrolamellar variant of hepatocellular carcinoma: Its association with FNH. Cancer 60:3047–3055, 1987.

85. Saxena R, Humphres S, Williams R, et al: Nodular hyperplasia with surrounding fibrolamellar carcinoma: A zone of arterialized liver parenchyma. Histopathology 25:275–278, 1994.

86. Fabre A, Audet P, Vilgrain V, et al: Histologic scoring of liver biopsy in focal nodular hyperplasia with atypical presentation. Hepatology 35:414–420, 2002.

87. Pain JA, Gimson AES, Howard ER, et al: Focal nodular hyperplasia of the liver: Results for treatment and options in management. Gut 32:524–527, 1991.

88. Di Stasi M, Caturelli E, De Sio I, et al: Natural history of focal nodular hyperplasia of the liver: An ultrasound study. J Clin Ultrasound 24:345–350, 1996.

89. Ohmoto K, Honda T, Hirokawa M, et al: Spontaneous regression of focal nodular hyperplasia of the liver. J Gastroenterol 37:849–853, 2002.

90. Leconte I, Van Beers BE, Lacrosse M, et al: Focal nodular hyperplasia: Natural course observed with CT and MRI. J Comput Assist Tomogr 24:61–66, 2000.

91. Geschwind JFH, Degli M, Morris J, Choti M: Re: Treatment of focal nodular hyperplasia with selective transcatheter arterial embolization using iodized oil and polyvinyl alcohol. [editorial] Cardiovasc Intervent Radiol 25:340–341, 2002.

92. Ichikawa T, Federle MP, Grazioli L, et al: Hepatocellular adenoma: Multiphasic CT and pathologic findings in twenty-five patients. Radiology 214:861–868, 2000.

93. Paulson EK, McClellan JS, Washington K, et al: Hepatic adenoma: MR characteristics in correlation with pathologic findings. AJR Am J Roentgenol 163:113–116, 1994.

94. Hung CH, Changchien CS, Lu SN, et al: Sonographic features of hepatic adenomas with pathologic correlation. Abdom Imaging 26:500–506, 2001.

95. Grazioli L, Federle M, Brancatelli G, et al: Hepatic adenomas imaging and pathologic findings. Radiographics 21:877–894, 2001.

96. Edmondson HA: Atlas of Tumor Pathology: Tumors of the Liver and Intrahepatic Bile Ducts, Fasc 25. Washington, DC, Armed Forces Institute of Pathology, 1958.

97. Reddy KR, Schiff E: Approach to a liver lesion. Semin Liver Dis 13:423–435, 1993.

98. Howell RR, Stevenson RE, Ben-Menachem Y, et al: Hepatic adenomata with type 1 glycogen storage disease. JAMA 236:1481–1484, 1976.

99. Coire CI, Qizibash AH, Castelli MF: Hepatic adenomata in type 1A glycogen storage disease. Arch Pathol Lab Med 111:166–169, 1987.

100. Mason HH, Anderson DH: Glycogen disease of the liver (Von Gierke's disease) with hepatoma. Pediatrics 16:785–800, 1955.

101. Zangeneh F, Limbeck GA, Brown BI, et al: Hepatorenal glycogenesis (type 1 glycogenesis) and carcinoma of the liver. J Pediatr 74:73–83, 1969.

102. Nakamura T, Tamakoshi K, Kitagawa M, et al: A case of hepatocellular carcinoma in type 1A glycogen storage disease Jpn J Gastroenterol 94:866–870, 1997.

103. Labrune P, Trioche P, Duvaltier I, et al: Hepatocellular adenomas in glycogen storage disease type 1 and 3: A series of forty-three patients and review of the literature. J Pediatr Gastroenterol Nutr 24:276–279, 1997.

104. Kerlin P, Davis GL, McGill DB, et al: Hepatic adenoma and focal nodular hyperplasia: Clinical, pathologic, and radiologic features. Gastroenterology 84:994–1002, 1983.

105. Foster JH, Berman MM: The malignant transformation of liver cell adenomas. Arch Surg 129:712–717, 1994.

106. Tao LC: Oral contraceptive-associated liver cell adenoma and hepatocellular carcinoma: Cytomorphology and mechanism of malignant transformation. Cancer 68:341–347, 1991.

107. Fraumeni JF, Miller RW, Hill JA: Primary carcinoma of the liver in childhood: An epidemiologic study. J Natl Cancer Inst 40:1087–1099, 1968.

108. Bagia S, Hewitt PM, Morris DL: Anabolic steroid-induced hepatic adenomas with spontaneous hemorrhage in a body builder. Aust N Z J Surg 70:686–687, 2000.

109. Toso C, Rubbia-Brandt L, Negro F, et al: Hepatocellular adenoma and polycystic ovary syndrome. Liver Int 23:35–37, 2003.

110. Adusumilli PS, Lee B, Parekh K, et al: Hemoperitoneum from spontaneous rupture of a liver cell adenoma in a male with hyperthyroidism. Am Surg 68:582–583, 2002.

111. Marie-Cardine A, Schneider P, Greene V, et al: Brief report: Erythrocytosis in a child with a hepatic adenoma. Med Pediatr Oncol 36:659–661, 2001.

112. Chiche L, Dao T, Salane E, et al: Liver adenomatosis: Reappraisal, diagnosis, and surgical management: Eight new cases and review of the literature. Ann Surg 231:74–81, 2000.

113. Musthafa CP, Antony PC, Syed AA, et al: Liver adenomatosis. Ind J Gastroenterol 22:30–31, 2003.

114. Takayasu H, Motoi T, Kanamori Y, et al: Two case reports of childhood liver cell adenomas harboring beta-katenin abnormality. Hum Pathol 33:852–855, 2002.

115. Chen YW, Jeng YM, Yeh SH, et al: p53 Gene and Wnt signaling in benign neoplasms: Beta-catenin mutations in hepatic adenoma but not in focal nodule hyperplasia. Hepatology 36:927–935, 2002.

116. Aseni P, Sansalone CV, Sammartino C, et al: Rapid disappearance of hepatic adenoma after contraceptive withdrawal. J Clin Gastroenterol 33:234–236, 2001.

117. Steinbrecher UP, Lisbona R, Huang SN, et al: Complete regression of hepatocellular adenoma after withdrawal of oral contraceptive use. Dig Dis Sci 26:1045–1050, 1981.

118. Ramseur WL, Cooper MR: Asymptomatic liver cell adenomas: Another case of resolution after discontinuation of oral contraceptive use. JAMA 239:1647–1648, 1978.

119. Ault GT, Wren SM, Ralls PW, et al: Selective management of hepatic adenomas. Am Surg 62:825–829, 1996.

120. Leese T, Farges O, Bismuth A: Liver cell adenomas: A twelve year surgical experience from a specialist hepato-biliary unit. Ann Surg 208:558–564, 1988.

121. Terkivatan T, De Wilt HW, De Man RA, et al: Treatment of ruptured hepatocellular adenoma. Br J Surg 88:207–209, 2001.

122. Heeringa B, Sardi A: Bleeding hepatic adenoma: Expectant treatment to limit the extent of resection. Am Surg 67:927–929, 2001.

123. Ross JA: Hepatoblastoma and birth weight: Too little, too big, or just right? [editorial; comment]. J Pediatr 130:516–517, 1997.

124. Stocker J, Conran R, Selby D: Tumor and pseudo tumors of the liver. In Stocker N, Askin JF (eds): Pathology of Solid Tumors in Children. London: Chapman & Hall, 1998, pp 83–110.

125. Lack EE, Neave C, Vawter GF: Hepatoblastoma: A clinical and pathological study of fifty-four cases. Am J Surg Pathol 6:693–705, 1982.

126. Martelli C, Blandamura C, Massaro S, et al: A case study of Beckwith-Wiedemann syndrome associated with hepatoblastoma. Clin Exp Obstet Gynecol 20:82–87, 1993.

127. McNeil DE, Brown M, Ching A, et al: Screening for Wilms' tumor and hepatoblastoma in children with Beckwith-Wiedemann syndrome: A cost effective model. Med Pediatr Oncol 37:349–356, 2001.

128. Ikeda H, Matsuyama S, Tanimura M: Association between hepatoblastoma and very low birth rate: A trend or a chance? J Pediatr 130:557–560, 1997.

129. Ikeda H, Hachitanda Y, Tanimura M, et al: Development of unfavorable hepatoblastoma in children of very low birth rate: Results of a surgical and pathological review. Cancer 82:1789–1796, 1998.

130. Maruyama K, Ikeda H, Koizumi T, et al: Case control study of perinatal factors and hepatoblastoma in children with an extremely low birth weight. Pediatr Int 42:492–498, 2000.

131. Rowland J: Hepatoblastoma: Assessment of criteria for histologic classification. Med Pediatr Oncol 39:478–483, 2002.

132. Haas J, Feusner J, Finegold M: Small cell undifferentiated histology in hepatoblastoma: May be unfavorable. Cancer 92:3130–3134, 2001.

133. Stringer MD, Hennayake S, Howard ER, et al: Improved outcome for children with hepatoblastoma. Br J Surg 82:386–391, 1995.

134. Haas JE, Muczynski KA, Krailo M, et al: Histology and prognosis in childhood hepatoblastoma and hepatocarcinoma. Cancer 64:1082–1089, 1989.

135. Nickerson HJ, Silberman TL, McDonald TP: Hepatoblastoma, thrombocytosis, and increased thrombopoietin. Cancer 45:315–320, 1980.

136. Von Schweinitz D, Hadam MR, Welte K, et al: Production of interleukin-1 beta and interleukin-6 in hepatoblastoma. Int J Cancer 53:728–734, 1993.

137. Surace C, Leszl A, Perilongo G, et al: Fluorescent in situ hybridization (FISH) reveals frequent and recurrent numerical and structural abnormalities in hepatoblastoma with no informative karyotype. Med Pediatr Oncol 39:536–539, 2002.

138. Maruyama K, Ikeda H, Koizumi T: Hepatoblastoma associated with trisomy 18 syndrome: A case report in view of the literature. Pediatr Int 43:302–305, 2001.

139. Giardiello FM, Petersen GM, Brensinger JD: Hepatoblastoma and APC gene mutation and familial adenomatous polyposis. Gut 39:867–869, 1996.

140. Oda H, et al: Somatic mutations of the APC gene in sporadic hepatoblastomas. Cancer Res 56:3320–3323, 1996.

141. Miller J, Greenspan B: Integrated imaging of hepatic tumors in children, Part I: Malignant lesions (primary and metastatic). Radiology 145:83–90, 1985.

142. Powers C, Ros PR, Stoupis C, et al: Primary liver neoplasms: MR imaging with pathologic correlation. Radiographics 14:459–482, 1994.

143. Stafford EA, Pritchard J: Extreme thrombocytosis as a diagnostic clue to hepatoblastoma [letter; comment]. Arch Dis Child 89:171, 1993.

144. Stocker J, Conran R: Hepatoblastoma. In Okuda K, Tabor E (eds): Liver Cancer. New York, Churchill Livingstone, 1997, pp 263–278.

145. Ortega J, Siegel S: Biological markers in pediatric cancer. In Pizza P, Poplack D (eds): Principles and Practices of Pediatric Oncology. Philadelphia, Lippincott, 1989, pp 149–162.

146. Novak D, Suchy F, Balistreri W: Disorders of the liver and biliary system relevant to clinical practice. In Oski F (ed). Principles and Practice of Pediatrics. Philadelphia, Lippincott, 1990, pp 1746–1777.

147. Kairemo KJ, Lindahl H, Merenmies J, et al: Anti-alphafetoprotein imaging is useful for staging hepatoblastoma. Transplantation 73:1151–1154, 2002.

148. Stringer M: Liver tumors. Semin Pediatr Surg 9:196–208, 2000.

149. MacKinlay GA, Pritchard J: A common language for childhood liver tumors. Pediatr Surg Int 7:325–326, 1992.

150. Exleby P, Filler R, Grosfeld J: Liver tumors in children and particular reference to hepatoblastoma and hepatocellular carcinoma: American Academy of Pediatric Surgical section survey,1974. J Pediatr Surg 10:329–337, 1975.

151. Brown J, Perilongo G, Shafford E, et al: Pretreatment prognostic factors for children with hepatoblastoma: Results from the International Society of Pediatric Oncology (SIOP) Study SIOPEL 1. Eur J Cancer 36:1418–1425, 2000.

152. Von Schweinitz D, Byrd DJ, Hecker H, et al: Efficacy and toxicity of ifosphamide, cisplatin, and doxorubicin in treatment of childhood hepatoblastoma: Study Committee of the Cooperative Pediatric Liver Tumor Study HB-89 of the German Society of Pediatric Oncology and Hematology. Eur J Cancer 33:1243–1249, 1997.

153. Von Schweinitz D, Burger D, Bode U, et al: Results of the HB-89 study in treatment of malignant epithelial liver tumors in childhood and the concept of a new HB-94 protocol. Klin Padiatr 206:282–288, 1994.

154. Perilongo G, Shafford EA: Pediatric update, liver tumors. Eur J Cancer 35:953–959, 1999.

155. McCrudden KW, Yokoi A, Thosani A, et al: Topotecan is anti-angiogenic in experimental hepatoblastoma. J Pediatr Surg 37:857–861, 2002.

156. Katzenstein HM, Rigsby C, Shaw P, et al: Novel therapeutic approaches in the treatment of children with hepatoblastoma. J Pediatr Hematol Oncol 24:751–755, 2002.

157. Tashjian Moriarty KP, Courtney RA, et al: Preoperative chemoembolization for unresectable hepatoblastoma. Pediatr Surg Int 18:187–189, 2002.

158. Chan KL, Fan ST, Tam PKH, et al: Management of spontaneously ruptured hepatoblastoma in infancy. Med Pediatr Oncol 38:137–138, 2002.

159. Kasai M, Watanabe I: Histologic classification of liver cell carcinoma in infancy and childhood and its clinical evaluation. Cancer 25:552–563, 1970.

160. Black EE, Naeve C, Vawter GF: Hepatoblastoma: A clinical and pathological study of fifty-four cases. Am J Surg Pathol 6:693–705, 1982.

161. Von Schweinitz D, Hecker H, Schmidt-Von-Arndt G, et al: Prognostic factors and staging systems in childhood hepatoblastoma. Int J Cancer 74:593–599, 1997.

162. Von Schweinitz DV, Hecker H, Harms D, et al: Complete resection before development of drug resistance is essential for survival from advanced HB: A report from the German Cooperative Pediatric Liver Tumor Study HB-89. J Pediatr Surg 30:845–852, 1995.

163. Van Tournout JM, Buckley JD, Quinn JJ, et al: Timing and magnitude of decline of alpha-fetoprotein levels in treated children with unresectable or metastatic hepatoblastoma or predictor of outcome: A report from the Children's Cancer Group. J Clin Oncol 15:1190–1197, 1997.

164. Ortega JA, Douglas EC, Feusner JH, et al: Randomized comparison of cisplatin/vincristin/fluorouracil and cisplatin/continuous infusion doxorubicin for treatment of pediatric hepatoblastoma: Report from the Children's Cancer Group and the Pediatric Oncology Group. J Clin Oncol 18:2665–2675, 2000.

165. Carceller A, Blanchard H, Champagne J, et al: Surgical resection and chemotherapy improve survival rate for patients with hepatoblastoma. J Pediatr Surg 36:755–759, 2001.

166. Raney B: Hepatoblastoma in children: A review. J Pediatr Hematol Oncol 19:418–422, 1997.

167. Feusner JH, Krailo MD, Haas JE, et al: Treatment of pulmonary metastasis of initial stage 1 hepatoblastoma in childhood (Report from the Cancer Children's Group). Cancer 71:859–864, 1993.

168. Von Schweinitz D: Identification of risk factors in hepatoblastoma: Another step in optimizing therapy [editorial comment]. Eur J Cancer 36:1343–1346, 2000.

169. Tagge ET, Tagge DU, Reyes J, et al: Resection, including transplantation, for hepatoblastoma and hepatocellular carcinoma: Impact on survival. J Pediatr Surg 27:292–299, 1992.

170. Pimpalwar AP, Sharif K, Ramani P, et al: Strategy for hepatoblastoma management: Transplant versus non-transplant surgery. J Pediatr Surg 37:240–245, 2002.

171. Srinivasan P, McCall J, Pritchard J, et al: Orthotopic liver transplantation for unresectable hepatoblastoma. Transplantation 74:652–655, 2002.

172. Lack EE, Schloo BL, Azumi N, et al: Undifferentiated (embryonal) sarcoma of the liver: Clinical and pathologic study of sixteen cases with an emphasis on immunohistochemical -features. Am J Surg Pathol 15:1–16, 1991.

173. Aoyama C, Hachitanda Y, Sato JK, et al: Undifferentiated (embryonal) sarcoma of the liver: A tumor of uncertain histogenesis showing divergent differentiation. Am J Surg Pathol 15:615–624, 1991.

174. Buetow PC, Buck JL, Pantongrag-Brown L, et al: Undifferentiated (embryonal) sarcoma of the liver: Pathologic basis of imaging findings in twenty-eight cases. Radiology 203:779–783, 1997.

175. Abramowsky CR, Choudhury CM, Ivant RJ: Undifferentiated (embryonal) sarcoma of the liver with alpha-1-antitrypsin deposits: Immunohistologic chemical and ultrastructural studies. Cancer 45:3108–3113, 1980.

176. Keating S, Taylor GP: Undifferentiated (embryonal) sarcoma of the liver: Ultrastructural and immunohistochemical similarities with malignant fibrocystiocytoma. Hum Pathol 16:693–699, 1985.

177. Iliszko M, Czauderna P, Babinska M, et al: Cytogenic findings in an embryonal sarcoma of the liver. Cancer Genet Cytogenet 102:142–144, 1998.

178. Cho HS, Park YN, Lyu CJ, et al: Embryonal sarcoma of the liver: Multiple recurrences and histologic D differentiation. Med Pediatr Oncol 32:386–388, 1999.

179. Leuschner I, Schmidt D, Harms D: Undifferentiated sarcoma of the liver in childhood: Morphology, flow cytometry, and literature review. Hum Pathol 21:68–76, 1990.

180. Pollono DG, Drut R: Undifferentiated embryonal sarcoma of the liver: Fine-needle aspiration, cytology, and preoperative chemotherapy as an approach to diagnosis and initial treatment: A case report. Diagn Cytopathol 19:102–106, 1998.

181. Krishnamurthy SC, Datta S, Jambhekar NA: Fine needle aspiration cytology of undifferentiated (embryonal) sarcoma of the liver: A case report. Acta Cytol 40:567–570, 1996.

182. Newman KD, Schisgall R, Reaman G, et al: Malignant mesenchymoma of the liver in children. J Pediatr Surg 24:781–783, 1989.

183. Harris MB, Shen S, Weiner MA, et al: Treatment of primary undifferentiated sarcoma of the liver with surgery and chemotherapy. Cancer 54:2859–2862, 1984.

184. Walker NI, Horn MJ, Strong RW, et al: Undifferentiated (embryonal) sarcoma of the liver: Pathologic findings and long term survival after complete surgical resection. Cancer 69:52–59, 1992.

185. Urban CE, Mache CJ, Schwinger W, et al: Undifferentiated (embryonal) sarcoma of the liver in childhood: Successful combined-modality therapy in four patients. Cancer 72:2511–2516, 1993.

186. Kim BD, Kim KH, Jung SE, et al: Undifferentiated (embryonal) sarcoma of the liver: Combination treatment by surgery and chemotherapy. J Pediatr Surg 37:1419–1423, 2002.

187. Webber EM, Morrison KB, Pritcherd SL, et al: Undifferentiated embryonal sarcoma of the liver: Results of clinical management in one center. J Pediatr Surg 34:1641–1644, 1999.

188. Uchyama M, Iwafuchi M, Yagi M, et al: Treatment of ruptured undifferentiated sarcoma of the liver in children: A report of two cases and review of the literature. J Hepatobiliary Pancreat Surg 8:87–91, 2001.

189. Broughan T, Esquivel CO, Vogt DP, et al: Pre-transplant chemotherapy in pediatric hepatocellular carcinoma. J Pediatr Surg 29:1319–1322, 1994.

190. Esquivel CO, Gutierrez C, Cox KL: Hepatocellular carcinoma and liver cell dysplasia in children with chronic liver disease. J Pediatr Surg 29:1465–1469, 1994.

191. Ryder SD: Guidelines for the diagnosis and treatment of hepatocellular carcinoma (HCC) in adults. Gut 52(suppl III):iii1–iii8, 2003.

192. Stocker JT: Hepatic tumors. In Balistreri WF, Stocker JT (eds): Pediatric Hepatology. New York, Taylor & Francis, 1990, pp 399–488.

193. McDougal RA, Gatzimos CD: Primary carcinoma of the liver in infants and children. Cancer 10:678–686, 1957.

194. Weinberg AG, Mize CE, Worthen HG: The occurrence of hepatoma in the chronic form of hereditary tyrosinemia. J Pediatr 88:434–438, 1976.

195. Manowski Z, et al: Liver cell dysplasia and early liver transplantation in hereditary tyrosinemia. Mod Pathol 3:694–701, 1990.

196. Kvittingen EA: Tyrosinemia: Treatment and outcome. J Inherit Metab Dis 18:375–379, 1995.

197. Fine AS, Appleman HD, Thompson NW: Hemorrhage into a hepatic adenoma and type 1A storage disease: A case report and review of the literature. Surgery 97:117–123, 1985.

198. Gruner BA, DeNapoli TS, Andrews W, et al: Hepatocellular carcinoma in children associated with Gardner's syndrome or familial adenomas polyposis. J Pediatr Hematol Oncol 20:274–278, 1998.

199. Sugarman GI, Heuser ET, Reed WB: A case of cerebral gigantism and hepatocarcinoma. Am J Dis Child 131:631–633, 1997.

200. Jain D, Hui P, McNamara J, et al: Bloom syndrome in sibs: First reports of hepatocellular carcinoma in Wilms' tumor with documented anaplasia and nephrogenic rests. Pediatr Dev Pathol 4:585–589, 2001.

201. Ettinger LJ, Freeman AI: Hepatoma in a child with neurofibromatosis. Am J Dis Child 133:528–531, 1979.

202. Ruymann FB, Mosijczuk AD, Sayers RJ: Hepatoma in a child with methotrexate induced hepatic fibrosis. JAMA 238:2631–2633, 1977.

203. Moore L, Bourne AJ, Moore DJ, et al: Hepatocellular carcinoma following neonatal hepatitis. Pediatr Pathol Lab Med 17:601–610, 1997.

204. Bekassy AN, Garwicz S, Wiebe T, et al: Hepatocellular carcinoma associated with arteriohepatic dysplasia in a four year old girl. Med Pediatr Oncol 20:78–83, 1992.

205. Ne YH, Chang MH, Hsu HY, et al: Hepatocellular carcinoma in childhood: Clinical manifestations and prognosis. Cancer 68:1737–1741, 1991.

206. Lee CL, Ko YC: Hepatitis B vaccination and hepatocellular carcinoma in Taiwan. Pediatrics 99:351–353, 1997.

207. Montesano R: The hepatitis B immunization and hepatocellular carcinoma: The Gambia Hepatitis Intervention Study. J Med Virol 67:444–446, 2002.

208. Wu MW, Chen CJ: Hepatitis B and hepatitis C virus in the development of hepatocellular carcinoma. Crit Rev Oncol Hematol 17:71–91, 1994.

209. Strickland DK, Jenkins JJ, Hudson MN: Hepatitis C infection and hepatocellular carcinoma after treatment of childhood cancer. J Pediatr Hematol Oncol 23:527–529, 2001.

210. Kohno M, Kitatami H, Wada H, et al: Hepatocellular carcinoma complicating biliary cirrhosis caused by biliary atresia: Report of a case. J Pediatr Surg 30:1713–1716, 1995.

211. Brower ST, Hoff PM, Jones DV, et al: Pancreatic cancer, hepatobiliary cancer, and neuroendocrine cancers of the GI tract. In Pazdur R, Coia LR, Hoskins WJ, et al (eds): Cancer Management: A Multidisciplinary Approach. Huntington, NY, PRR, 1998, pp 113–148.

212. Berman N, Burnham J, Sheahan D: Fibrolamellar carcinoma of the liver: An immunohistochemical study of nineteen cases and a review of the literature. Hum Pathol 19:784–794, 1988.

213. Soyer P, Roche A, Levesque N: CT of fibrolamellar hepatocellular carcinoma. J Comput Assist Tomogr 15:533–538, 1991.

214. Debray D, Pariente D, Fabre N, et al: Fibrolamellar hepatocellular carcinoma: Report of a case mimicking a liver abscess. J Pediatr Gastroenterol Nutr 19:468–472, 1994.

215. El-Gazzaz G, Wong W, El-Hadary MK, et al: Outcome of liver resection and transplantation for fibrolamellar hepatocellular carcinoma. Transplant Int 13(suppl 1):S406–S409, 2000.

216. Lau H, Fan ST, Ng IOL, et al: Long-term prognosis after hepatectomy for hepatocellular carcinoma: A survival analysis of two hundred and four consecutive patients. Cancer 83:2302–2311, 1998.

217. Arii S, Okamoto E, Imamura N, et al: Registries in Japan: Current status of hepatocellular carcinoma in Japan. Semin Surg Oncol 1:204–211, 1996.

218. Izumi R, Shimizu K, Li T, et al: Prognostic factors of hepatocellular carcinoma in patients undergoing hepatic resection. Gastroenterology 106:720–727, 1994.

219. Craig JR, Peters RL, Edmondson HA, et al: Fibrolamellar carcinoma of the liver: A tumor of adolescents in young adults with distinctive clinicopathologic features. Cancer 46:2–9, 1980.

220. Farhi DC, Shikes RH, Murari PG, et al: Hepatocellular carcinoma in young people. Cancer 52:1516–1525, 1983.

221. Nagorney DM, Adson MA, Weiland LH, et al: Fibrolamellar hepatoma. Am J Surg 149:113–119, 1985.

222. Lack EE, Neave C, Vawter GF: Hepatocellular carcinoma: A review of thirty-two cases in childhood and adolescence. Cancer 52:1510–1515, 1983.

223. Friedman AC, Lichtenstein JE, Goodman ZD, et al: Fibrolamellar hepatocellular carcinoma. Radiology 157:583–587, 1985.

224. Paradinas FJ, Melia WM, Wilkinson ML, et al: High serum vitamin B_{12} binding capacity is a marker of the fibrolamellar variant of hepatocellular carcinoma. Br Med J 285:840–842, 1982.

225. Brandt DJ, Johnson CD, Stephens DH, et al: Imaging of fibrolamellar hepatocellular carcinoma. Am J Roentgenol 151:295–299, 1998.

226. Titelbaum DS, Hatabu H, Schiebler ML, et al: Fibrolamellar hepatocellular carcinoma: MR appearance. J Comput Assist Tomogr 12:588–591, 1988.

227. Ang PT, Evans H, Pazdur R: Fibrolamellar hepatocellular carcinoma: Therapeutic implications of a ten year disease free interval. Am J Clin Oncol 14:175–178, 1991.

228. O'Grady JG, Polson RJ, Rolles K, et al: Liver transplantation for malignant disease: Results in ninety-three consecutive patients. Ann Surg 207:373–379, 1988.

229. Iwatsuki S, Gordon RD, Shaw BW Jr, et al: Role of liver transplantation in cancer therapy. Ann Surg 202:401–407, 1985.

230. Iwatsuki S, Dvorchik I, Marsh JW, et al: Liver transplantation for hepatocellular carcinoma: A proposal of a prognostic scoring system. J Am Coll Surg 191:389–394, 2000.

231. Lucena De La Poza JL, Turrion VS, Alvira LG, et al: Liver transplantation in the therapy of hepatocellular carcinoma: A revision of our series. Transplant Proc 34:260–261, 2002.

232. Senninger N, Linger R, Klar E, et al: Liver transplantation for hepatocellular carcinoma. Transplant Proc 28:1706–1707, 1996.

233. Wai CT, Lo SK, Lee KH, et al: Liver transplantation in hepatocellular carcinoma. Transplant Proc 32:2173, 2000.

234. Ahn SI, Seo JN, Shin SH, et al: Hepatocellular carcinoma with lung metastasis in a nine year old boy. J Pediatr Surg 36:1599–1601, 2001.

235. Yea CN, Chen MF, Jeng LB: Resection of peritoneal implantation from hepatocellular carcinoma. Ann Surg Oncol 9:863–868, 2002.

236. Ruymann FB, Raney RB Jr, Crist WM, et al: Rhabdomyosarcoma of the biliary tree in childhood: A report from the Intergroup Rhabdomyosarcoma Study. Cancer 56:575–581, 1985.

237. Poloono D, et al: Rhabdomyosarcoma of extrahepatic biliary tree: Initial treatment with chemotherapy and conservative surgery. Med Pediatr Oncol 30:290–293, 1998.

238. Sanz N, et al: Rhabdomyosarcoma of the biliary tree. Pediatr Surg Int 12:200–201, 1997.

239. Schweizer P, Schweizer M, Wehrmann M: Major resection for embryonal rhabdomyosarcoma of the biliary tree. Pediatr Surg Int 9:268–273, 1994.

240. Mihara S, Matsumoto H, Tokunaga F, et al: Botryoid rhabdomyosarcoma of the gallbladder in a child. Cancer 49:812–818, 1982.

241. Horowitz ME, Etcubanas E, Webber BL, et al: Hepatic undifferentiated (embryonal) sarcoma and rhabdomyosarcoma in children: Results of therapy. Cancer 59:396–402, 1987.

242. Isaacson C: Embryonal rhabdomyosarcoma of the ampulla of Vater. Cancer 41:365–368, 1978.

243. Patil KK, Omojola MF, Khurana P, et al: Embryonal rhabdomyosarcoma within a choledochal cyst. Can Assoc Radiol J 43:145–148, 1992.

244. Roebuck DJ, Yang WT, Lam WM, et al: Hepatobiliary rhabdomyosarcoma in children: Diagnostic radiology. Pediatr Radiol 28:101–108, 1998.

245. Haith EE, Kepes JJ, Holder TM: Inflammatory pseudo tumor involving the common bile duct of a six year old boy: Successful pancreatal duodenectomy. Surgery 56:436–441, 1964.

246. Huang FC, Eng HL, Chen CL, et al: Primary pleomorphic rhabdomyosarcoma of the liver: A case report. Hepatol Gastroenterol 50:73–76, 2003.

247. Hirohashi S, Hirohashi R, Uchida H, et al: Pancreatitis: Evaluation with MR cholangiopancreatography in children. Radiology 203:411–415, 1997.

248. Friedburg H, Kauffman GW, Bo HMN, et al: Sonographic and computed tomographic features of embryonal rhabdomyosarcoma of the biliary tract. Pediatr Radiol 14:436–438, 1984.

CHAPTER 68

Teratomas, Dermoids, and Other Soft Tissue Tumors

Jean-Martin Laberge, MD, FACS, FRCSC, Kenneth S. Shaw, MD, FRCSC, and Luong T. Nguyen, MD, FRCSC

TERATOMAS

Teratomas are generally divided into gonadal and extragonadal. This chapter focuses on extragonadal locations, the most common being sacrococcygeal.

Embryology and Pathology

Teratoma, from the Greek *teratos* ("of the monster") and *onkoma* ("swelling"), is a term first applied by Virchow in 1869 to "sacrococcygeal growths."[1] Teratomas are composed of multiple tissues foreign to the organ or site in which they arise.[2] Although teratomas are sometimes defined as having the three embryonic layers (endoderm, mesoderm, and ectoderm), recent classifications include monodermal types.[2,3]

Teratomas are thought by some to arise from totipotent primordial germ cells.[3,4] These cells develop among the endodermal cells of the yolk sac near the origin of the allantois and migrate to the gonadal ridges during weeks 4 and 5 of gestation (Fig. 68-1).[5] Some cells may miss their target destination and give rise to a teratoma anywhere from the brain to the coccygeal area, usually in the midline. Another theory has teratomas arising from remnants of the primitive streak or primitive node.[5-7] During week 3 of development, midline cells at the caudal end of the embryo divide rapidly and, in a process called *gastrulation,* give rise to all three germ layers of the embryo (Fig. 68-2).[5] By the end of week 3, the primitive streak shortens and disappears. This theory would explain the more common occurrence of teratomas in the sacrococcygeal region. With either theory, the totipotent cells could give rise to monoclonal neoplasms. Recent evidence shows that, whereas immature teratomas may be monoclonal, mature teratomas can be polyclonal, more like a hamartoma than a neoplasm.[8] This finding is compatible with the third theory that teratomas are a form of incomplete twinning.[2,3]

The primordial germ cell is the principal but possibly not the exclusive progenitor of a teratoma.[2] The recent trend is to include teratomas under the classification of germ cell tumors.[2-4] This histologic classification also includes germinomas (formerly dysgerminomas), embryonal carcinomas, yolk sac tumors, choriocarcinomas, gonadoblastomas, and mixed germ cell tumors. Gonadal and extragonadal teratomas may have a different origin, explaining the different behavior according to tumor site.

Teratomas are fascinating tumors owing to the diversity of tissues they may contain and the varying degree of organization of these tissues. Many tumors contain skin elements, neural tissue, teeth, fat, cartilage, and intestinal mucosa, often with normal ganglion cells. These tissues are usually present as disorganized islands of cells with cystic spaces. The tumor sometimes consists of more organized tissue, such as small bowel, limbs, and even a beating heart; these have been called *fetiform teratomas* (Fig. 68-3).[2,3,6,9,10] When the mass includes vertebrae or notochord and a high degree of structural organization, the term *fetus in fetu* is used; this is viewed by some as a variant of conjoined twinning but is classified as a teratoma by others owing to the absence of a recognizable umbilical cord in its vascular pedicle.[3,11] Whether teratomas are at one end of a spectrum that includes fetus in fetu, parasitic twins, conjoined twins, and normal twins is the subject of controversy.[3] One certainly cannot dismiss the many reports of teratomas associated with fetus in fetu in the same patient and with a twin pregnancy.[2,3,12-14]

The overall tissue architecture is variable in teratomas, and a spectrum of cellular differentiation exists. Most benign teratomas are composed of mature cells, but 20% to 25% also contain immature elements, most often neuroepithelium.[2-4] The degree of histologic immaturity is of proven prognostic significance only in ovarian teratomas[3,15]; even this concept is being questioned since one large cooperative study showed that overlooked microscopic foci of yolk sac tumor rather than the grade of immaturity was predictive of recurrence.[16] In neonatal teratoma, immature tissue is considered normal and

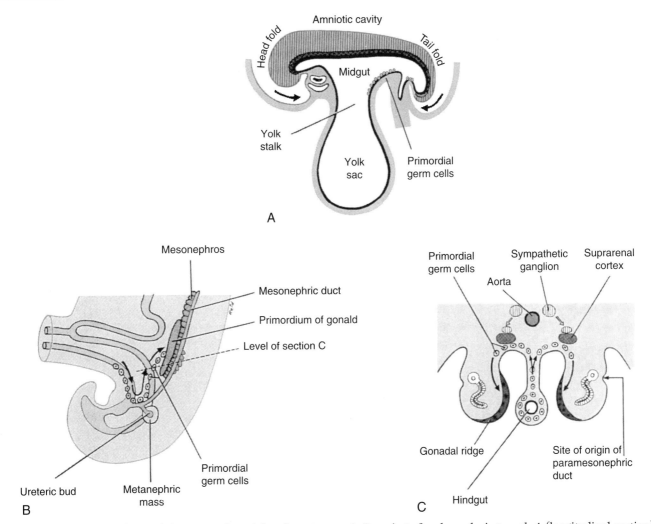

FIGURE 68-1. Commonly cited theory on the origin of teratomas. *A,* Drawing of embryo during week 4 (longitudinal section), showing primordial germ cells at the base of the yolk sac. *B* and *C,* During week 5, these cells migrate toward the gonadal ridges. According to this theory, some cells could miss their intended destination. (Modified from Moore KL, Persaud TVN: *The Developing Human.* Philadelphia, WB Saunders, 1993, pp 71, 181.)

without any influence on prognosis.[2,6] Spontaneous maturation of malignant tumors has been reported after partial excision of giant sacrococcygeal teratomas in two fetuses at 23 and 27 weeks of gestation.[17]

Teratomas also may contain or develop foci of malignancy, and a malignant germ cell tumor may be found in sites typical for teratomas, such as the mediastinum or sacrococcygeal area. Whether the lesion was malignant from the onset or the malignant cells destroyed and replaced, the benign teratoma component is often difficult to differentiate. The most common malignant component within a teratoma is a yolk sac tumor, also called an *endodermal sinus tumor.* Other malignant germ cell tumors can occur, and rarely, malignancy of other tissues composing the teratoma, such as neuroblastoma,[18,19] squamous cell carcinoma,[20] carcinoid,[21] and others can develop. Malignancy at birth is uncommon but increases with age

and with incomplete resection. An apparently mature teratoma may recur several months or years after resection as a malignant yolk sac tumor, illustrating the difficulties in histologic sampling of large tumors and the need for close follow-up.[2,3]

Most yolk sac tumors and some embryonal carcinomas secrete α-fetoprotein (AFP), which can be measured in the serum and demonstrated in the cells by immunohistochemistry.[22] This marker is particularly useful for assessing the presence of residual or recurrent disease. AFP levels are normally very high in neonates and decrease with time.[22,23] The postoperative half-life is about 6 days. Persistently high levels may be an indication of the need for further surgical procedures or chemotherapy. Other markers that may be elevated are β-human chorionic gonadotropin (β-hCG), produced by choriocarcinomas, and rarely, carcinoembryonic antigen.

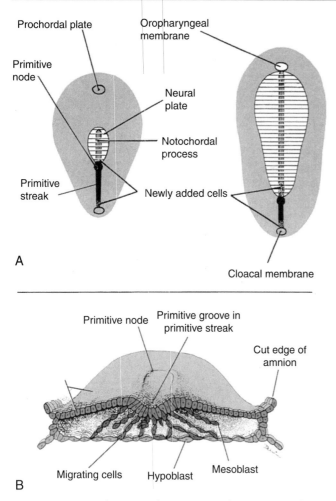

A

B

FIGURE 68-2. Alternate theory on embryogenesis of teratomas. *A,* Sketches of dorsal views of the embryonic disk on days 17 and 18, showing the primitive streak and primitive node. *B,* Drawing of a transverse cut of the embryonic disk during week 3. This shows that cells from the primitive streak migrate to form mesoblast (the origin of all mesenchymal tissues) and also displace the hypoblast to form the endoderm. Hence, remnants of these pluripotent primitive streak cells could give rise to teratomas and could account for the more frequent sacrococcygeal location. (From Moore KL, Persaud TVN: The Developing Human. Philadelphia, WB Saunders, 1993, pp 55–56.)

Secretion of β-hCG by the tumor may be sufficient to cause precocious puberty.[24]

The genetic basis of teratomas is not yet understood. Most germ cell tumors appear to have an amplification, or isochromosome, in a region of the short arm of chromosome 12, designated i(12p).[3,4,25] This has been well described in adults but was not confirmed in one pediatric series in which deletions on chromosomes 1 and 6 were found instead.[26] Oncogenes and tumor-suppressor genes did not appear to correlate with prognosis in one study,[27] whereas N-*myc* gene amplification was present in immature teratomas but absent in mature teratomas in another report.[28] The clinical usefulness of these findings remains unclear.

Associated Anomalies

Teratomas are usually isolated lesions. A well-recognized association is the triad of anorectal malformation, sacral anomaly, and a presacral mass.[29,30] The presacral mass is usually a teratoma or an anterior meningocele, but duplication cysts and dermoid cysts have been described, as have combinations of these lesions.

An extensive review of the English and German literature published in 1989[31] found 51 cases and highlighted several important facts. Twenty percent of patients were older than 12 years at the time of diagnosis, yet no reports of malignancy were found. This contrasts with a 75% malignancy rate in patients older than 1 year who had the usual sacrococcygeal teratomas.[32] Recently, in one child with severe anal stenosis and a presacral teratoma, a malignant recurrence developed, and the child died at 4 years despite chemotherapy[33]; he did not have a sacral bony defect. The female preponderance for patients with this triad is only 1.5:1, which is less than the 3:1 ratio noted in isolated sacrococcygeal teratomas. The familial predisposition, first recognized in 1974,[34] is noted in 57% of these cases, and inheritance is autosomal dominant. Although all variants of anorectal malformations have been described, by far the most common is anal or anorectal stenosis. In a recent report, this triad was present in 38% of all patients with anorectal stenosis and in 1.6% of patients with low imperforate anus.[35] Anal anomalies also have been

FIGURE 68-3. *A,* This child had a large fluctuant lumbar mass at birth. A family history of myelomeningocele existed in a great aunt. She also had an atrophic right leg with neurologic impairment below the L3 root and clubbing of the right foot. Note the ulcerated, arachnoid-looking area cranially and the pedunculated skin caudally, which had the appearance of a vulva and was oozing serous fluid. *B,* Plain radiographs showed a severe lumbosacral scoliosis with vertebral anomalies. Computed tomography confirmed the vertebral anomalies with spina bifida and demonstrated a pattern of intestine with inspissated or calcified meconium in the teratoma. *C,* Magnetic resonance imaging revealed that the mass extended into the retroperitoneum, where it was contiguous with the lower pole of the right kidney (*arrow*). *D,* At operation, normal-looking blind bowel loops were found deep to the vulva-like structure. Part of the mass extended along the spinal cord, which required dissection and untethering by the neurosurgeon. The pathologic diagnosis was a mature fetiform teratoma that contained, among many other things, two adrenals, two ovaries, renal tissue with some glomeruli and tubules, bone with bone marrow, and portions of stomach and small and large bowel. The child recovered well neurologically but required spinal instrumentation owing to progressive scoliosis at age 2 years.

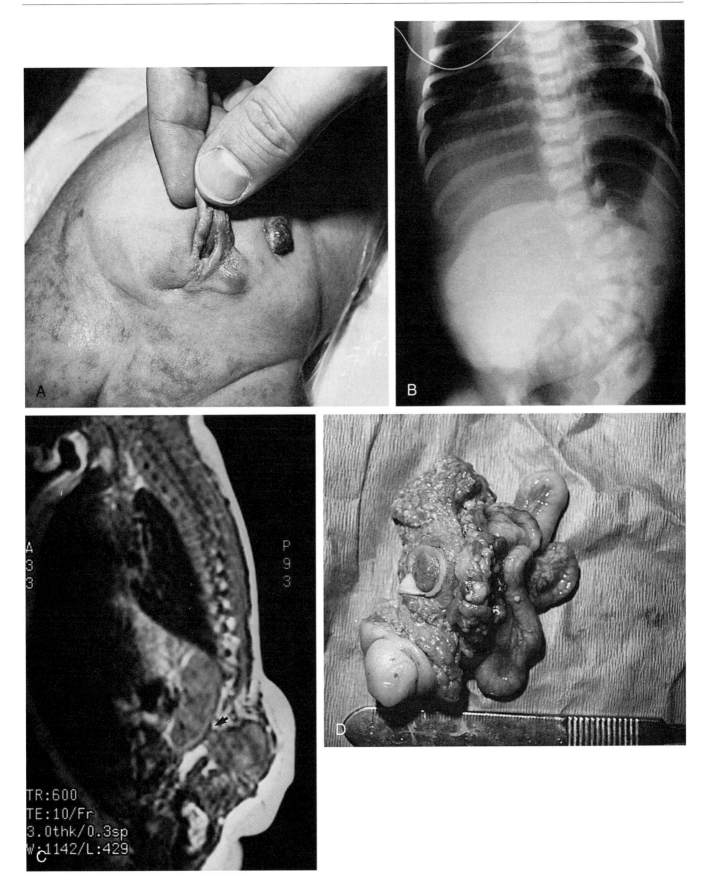

reported in conjunction with a presacral mass, but in the absence of sacral defects. Hirschsprung's disease has been wrongly diagnosed in some of these cases,[4,36,37] indicating the need to eliminate the presence of a presacral mass by digital rectal examination, by a metal sound when the anus is too tight, or by imaging techniques. In the screening of family members, normal plain radiographs of the sacrum are not sufficient, as a presacral mass may exist in the absence of a bony defect.[38] The low incidence of malignancy has led one author to conclude that the presacral lesion in this context is a hamartoma rather than a teratoma.[39] This is supported by the demonstration of deletions or mutations of the homeobox gene *HLXB9*, located at 7q36, in several affected families.[40] In one recently reported family, no deletions of 7q could be detected, but the authors did not comment about *HLXB9* mutations.[41]

Urogenital anomalies, such as hypospadias, vesicoureteral reflux, and vaginal or uterine duplications, are other anomalies associated with teratomas.[31,32,42] Congenital dislocation of the hip was found in 7% of patients with sacrococcygeal teratomas in one report, which also drew attention to vertebral anomalies and late orthopedic sequelae (see Fig. 68-3).[43] Central nervous system lesions, such as anencephaly, trigonocephaly, Dandy-Walker malformations, spina bifida, and myelomeningocele, may occur.[2,3,44–46] Another peculiar association with sacrococcygeal teratomas is a family history of twins in as many as 10% of the patients.[34,47,48] Although not confirmed in all series, this finding, combined with reports of simultaneous twin pregnancy or sequential familial occurrences of fetus in fetu and teratoma, supports the theory that teratomas are just one end of the spectrum of conjoint twinning.[2,3,10,12,14]

Klinefelter's syndrome is strongly associated with mediastinal teratoma[49] and has been reported in patients with intracranial[50] or retroperitoneal tumors.[51,52] It is estimated that 8% of male patients with primary mediastinal germ cell tumors have Klinefelter's syndrome, 50 times the expected frequency.[49] These tumors are often malignant, are the choriocarcinoma type, secrete β-hCG, and produce precocious puberty. Histiocytosis also is associated with mediastinal teratoma, both with[53,54] and without Klinefelter's syndrome.[55] Other hematologic malignancies, such as acute leukemias[56,57] and Hodgkin's disease,[58,59] occur rarely.

The following rare associations have been reported, most often with nonsacrococcygeal lesions: trisomy 13,[60] trisomy 21, Morgagni's hernia,[61] congenital heart defects,[44,46] Beckwith-Wiedemann syndrome,[62] pterygium,[63] cleft lip and palate,[44] and rare syndromes, such as Proteus[64] and Schinzel-Giedion syndromes.[65]

Diagnosis and Management by Tumor Site

Sacrococcygeal Teratoma

Sacrococcygeal tumors account for 35% to 60% of teratomas (gonadal included) in large series (Table 68-1).[66–68] This is the most common tumor in the newborn, even when stillbirths are considered.[44] The estimated incidence is 1 per 35,000 to 40,000 live births.[3,4]

DIAGNOSIS. Most sacrococcygeal teratomas are seen as a visible mass at birth, making the diagnosis obvious (Fig. 68-4), with an unexplained female preponderance of 3:1.[32,66] The main differential diagnosis is meningocele. Typically, meningoceles occur cephalad to the sacrum and are covered by dura, but sometimes they are covered by skin. Examination of the child reveals bulging of the fontanelle with gentle pressure on a sacral meningocele, helping to establish the diagnosis before plain radiographs, ultrasonography (US), and magnetic resonance imaging (MRI) confirm it. The coexistence of meningocele with teratoma is well recognized in the familial form, but these are usually presacral. Rarely, a typical exophytic teratoma may have an intradural extension.[69] Other lesions in the differential diagnosis of neonatal sacrococcygeal masses include lymphangiomas, lipomas, tail-like remnants (Fig. 68-5), meconium pseudocysts, and several other rare conditions.[32,70]

Although many neonates with sacrococcygeal teratomas do not have symptoms, some require intensive care because of prematurity, high-output cardiac failure, disseminated intravascular coagulation,[71] and tumor rupture or bleeding within the tumor.[72–74] Lethal hyperkalemia from tumor necrosis has been described.[75] Lesions with a large intrapelvic component may cause urinary obstruction. Besides looking for signs of a myelomeningocele, the physical examination should always include a rectal examination to evaluate any intrapelvic component. The most helpful imaging studies consist of plain anteroposterior and lateral radiographs of the pelvis and spine, looking for

TABLE 68-1

RELATIVE FREQUENCY OF TERATOMAS BY SITE

Site	No. of Cases (%)
Sacrococcygeal	290 (45)
Gonadal	
Ovary	176 (27)
Testis	31 (5)
Mediastinal	41 (6)
Central nervous system	30 (5)
Retroperitoneal	28 (4)
Cervical	20 (3)
Head	20 (3)
Gastric	3 (<1)
Hepatic	2 (<1)
Pericardial	1 (<1)
Umbilical cord	1 (<1)
Total	**643 (100)**

Data are from five series of teratomas in children.
Modified from Dehner LP: Gonadal and extragonadal germ cell neoplasms: Teratomas in childhood. In Finegold M (ed): Pathology of Neoplasia in Children and Adolescents. Philadelphia, WB Saunders, 1986, pp 282–312.

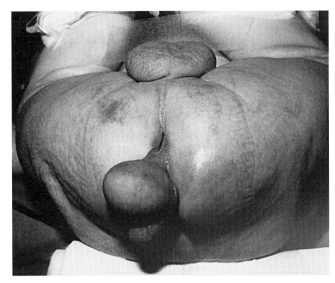

FIGURE 68-5. This patient had a scrotum-like perianal mass with anal stenosis at birth. An anoplasty was done with removal of the mass, which was not attached to the coccyx. Pathology showed only fibroadipose tissue with smooth muscle, vascular structures, and cartilage, consistent with a hamartomatous process or caudal vestige (also called tail remnant).

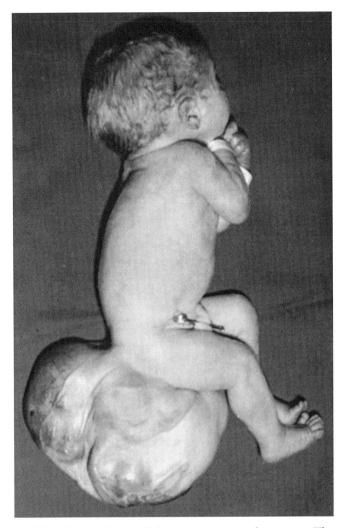

FIGURE 68-4. Infant with large sacrococcygeal teratoma. The infant and attached teratoma weighed 2363 g. The teratoma weighed 675 g. After surgical excision of the tumor, the infant weighed 1688 g. The external size of such a teratoma is not a deterrent to surgical excision because the attachment in large and small teratomas is similar.

calcifications in the tumor and for spinal defects, and US of the abdomen, pelvis, and spine. Further preoperative studies are unnecessary in most newborns.

The diagnosis of purely intrapelvic teratomas is often delayed.[32] Children have constipation, urinary retention, an abdominal mass, or symptoms of malignancy, such as failure to thrive. Age is not a predictor of malignancy in teratomas at sites other than testicular, mediastinal, and sacrococcygeal.[2] The risk of malignancy is less than 10% at birth but more than 75% after age 1 year for sacrococcygeal tumors, with the exception of familial presacral teratomas. The risk of malignancy also is high for incompletely excised lesions. Complete excision of the tumor should be carried out as soon as the neonate is stable enough to undergo the procedure. Serum markers should be determined before the operation for later comparison.

The diagnosis is often made on prenatal US, especially when this examination is performed in the second trimester. The site of the lesion, its complex appearance, and intrapelvic extension with or without urinary tract obstruction are easily recognized. Although most teratomas do not adversely affect the fetus or fetal life, the presence of a large solid vascular tumor is associated with significant mortality rate, both in utero and perinatally.[72,73,76,77] Perinatal mortality is usually related to prematurity or tumor rupture with exsanguination or both. Premature delivery may occur spontaneously from polyhydramnios or may be induced urgently because of fetal distress.

Repeated US assessment of tumor size is important because the fetus should be delivered by cesarean section if the tumor is larger than 5 cm or larger than the fetal biparietal diameter.[76] Dystocia during vaginal delivery is associated with tumor rupture and hemorrhage and is an avoidable obstetric nightmare. The options in managing unexpected cases with dystocia include emergency cesarean completion of the partially delivered fetus who has been intubated and ventilated after vaginal presentation of the head.[76]

Polyhydramnios with larger tumors may lead to premature labor. Tumors that are larger than the fetal biparietal diameter at diagnosis, or that grow faster than the fetus, are associated with a poor prognosis.[78] As the tumor enlarges, the fetus may develop placentomegaly or hydrops. This is a harbinger of impending fetal death and should lead to urgent cesarean delivery. Open fetal surgical excision has been performed with success in three of four cases considered too premature to deliver in one center, and in two of four cases in another.[17,73] Others have reported survival after emergency delivery as early as 26 weeks of gestation.[79] Successful intrauterine endoscopic laser ablation was reported in one case.[80] Attempts at interrupting the high vascular flow have also been described by using radiofrequency ablation, with two survivors of four attempts,[81] with one survivor having significant perineal damage.[82] Purely cystic teratomas occur in 10% to 15% of cases. Prenatal diagnosis allows percutaneous aspiration to facilitate delivery (Fig. 68-6),[77,83] to eradicate uterine irritability, or to prevent tumor rupture at delivery.[73] In other reports, prenatal decompression with a cyst-amniotic shunt was successfully accomplished to relieve the obstructive uropathy caused by the cystic teratoma.[84,85]

OPERATIVE PROCEDURE. Adequate intravenous access and the availability of blood products should be ascertained before starting the operation, especially with large tumors.

For most tumors, the major component is extrapelvic, and the patient is placed in the prone position. If a significant intrapelvic or intra-abdominal component is present, it may be wise to begin with a laparotomy. In our experience, most resections can be achieved completely in the prone position, especially if the internal portion is cystic. When in doubt, a safe approach is to prepare the skin from the lower chest to the toes, allowing the infant to be turned to the supine position without having to redrape. Vaseline packing in the rectum facilitates its identification throughout the procedure (Fig. 68-7). En bloc excision, including the coccyx, is preferable. Failure to remove the coccyx is associated with a high recurrence rate.[2-4] An acceptable gluteal crease and perineum is formed by the appropriate positioning of the perianal musculature. A new method of skin closure uses plastic surgical principles to improve the cosmetic appearance of the scars[86] (see Fig. 68-7 *insert*).

Although the chevron incision has been used by most surgeons, a vertical incision is sometimes possible; it leaves a nearly normal-looking median raphe (Fig. 68-8). Resection of the excess skin at the closure gives the best cosmetic result.

Several techniques have been described to help in the management of giant teratomas. These include intraoperative snaring of the aorta,[74,87] laparoscopic clipping of the median sacral artery,[88] the use of extracorporeal membrane oxygenation and hypothermic perfusion,[89] and devascularization and staged resection.[79]

PROGNOSIS. Fetuses with tumors diagnosed in utero have a survival rate in excess of 90% if the tumors are small and discovered by routine US. If a complicated pregnancy is the indication for US, the mortality increases to 60%. Nearly 100% of patients die when hydrops or placentomegaly occurs.[73,76,77] Dystocia or tumor rupture during delivery are probably underreported as a cause of mortality.[90] In one series, 10% of patients died during transfer, all before the widespread use of antenatal US.[91] In a report of 24 patients with sacrococcygeal teratoma diagnosed on *routine* obstetric US, 3 were aborted electively, 4 died in utero at 20 to 27 weeks of gestation, and 3 died of tumor rupture during delivery at 29 to 35 weeks of gestation (1 after vaginal, and 2 after cesarean delivery).[72] The incidence of placentomegaly (none), hydrops (5%), and polyhydramnios (19%) was lower than in series in which US was done for an obstetric reason.[73,76,92]

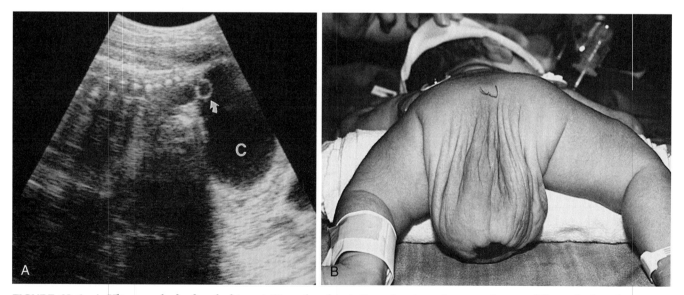

FIGURE 68-6. *A,* Ultrasound of a female fetus at 38 weeks of gestation, showing a large cystic mass (C) attached to the coccyx, with tiny cysts anterior to the sacrum (*arrow*). An ultrasound at 18 weeks was normal. The cyst was gradually enlarging from an initial diameter of 9.5 cm at 31 weeks of gestation. The cyst was aspirated for 650 mL of fluid, permitting external version from breech to vertex. Two days later, when labor was induced, another 200 mL of fluid was removed to permit an uncomplicated vaginal delivery. *B,* Twenty-four hours postnatally, the lesion remained floppy with an area of skin ulceration, likely a consequence of excessive in utero distention. A mature cystic teratoma was confirmed histologically.

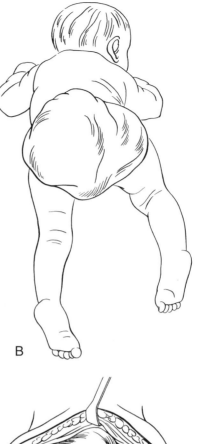

A

compression
of pelvic
viscera

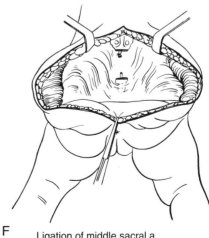

B

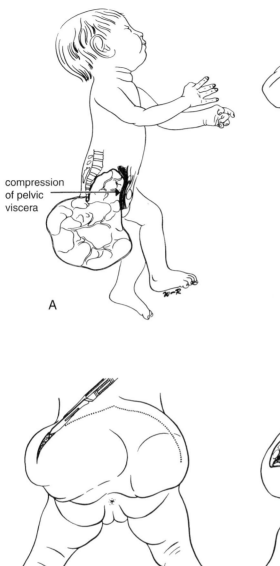

C   "V" shaped skin incision

D

E   Transection of coccyx

F   Ligation of middle sacral a.

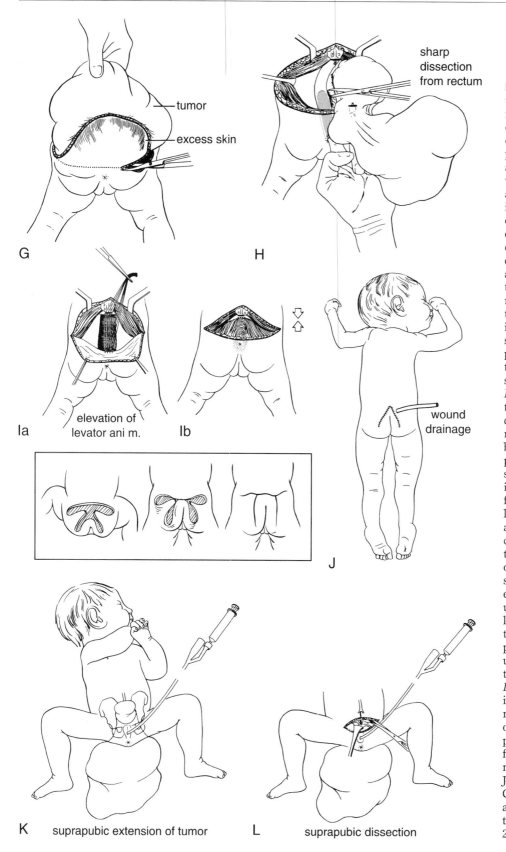

FIGURE 68-7. *A,* The teratomatous attachment may compress the rectum, vagina, and bladder anteriorly. *B,* The patient is placed on the operating table in a prone jackknife position, with general endotracheal anesthesia. An appropriate intravenous cannula should be placed in an arm vein. *C,* The incision is an inverted V shape to allow excision of the tumor and to facilitate an eventually satisfactory cosmetic closure. The amount of skin excised is dependent on the size and shape of the tumor. *D,* The tumor is dissected from the gluteus maximus muscle. *E,* The coccyx is transected and removed in continuity with the tumor. *F,* The middle sacral artery is the major blood supply to the tumor and is ligated after transection of the coccyx. *G,* Excess skin is excised to facilitate closure. *H,* Because the tumor is adherent to the rectum, sharp dissection can be directed by placing a finger in the rectum. *I,* Placement of sutures between the anal sphincter and the presacral fascia (a). When the sutures are tied, the anal sphincter is pulled upward to the sacrum to form a gluteal crease (b). *J,* Drain is left in the surgical site for postoperative serosanguineous fluid discharge. *Insert,* Recently described technique for closure after excision of large teratomas. Using plastic surgery principles, this avoids "dog ears" and places the scars along natural skin lines for a much-improved long-term cosmetic result. *K,* If tumor extends through the bony pelvis into the retroperitoneum, a urinary bladder catheter is inserted to facilitate suprapubic dissection. *L,* Lower abdominal transverse incision allows interruption of the middle sacral artery and dissection of the tumor from the sacrum and pelvis, which is eventually removed from the perineum. (Insert redrawn from Fishman SJ, Jennings RW, Johnson SM, et al: Contouring buttock reconstruction after sacrococcygeal teratoma resection. J Pediatr Surg 39:439–441, 2004; with permission.)

In the absence of severe prematurity and intrapartum complications, the prognosis is dependent on the presence of malignancy and is therefore related to age at operation and completeness of resection.[93,94] When the tumor is benign and completely excised, recurrence is less common than when the tumor is large and mostly solid.[95] The recurrent tumor may be benign or malignant, and benign metastatic tissue may become evident in lymph nodes.[96] Although immature or fetal elements in gonadal teratomas are associated with a higher risk of aggressive behavior,[97] finding this is not necessarily true for sacrococcygeal tumors.[2,6] Whereas malignant recurrence of a "benign" teratoma may be as high as 15%,[7] the original benign diagnosis may have been due to sampling error,[16] to an undetected residual microscopic focus of malignant tumor,[98] or to incomplete coccygectomy at the first operation.[33] Patients whose tumors are resected after the newborn period have a higher risk of malignant recurrence, especially when an elevated AFP level is present at diagnosis. The elevated AFP likely signifies the presence of malignancy in the original tumor.[16,99] It is important to monitor all patients with physical examination, including rectal examination and serum markers, every 2 or 3 months for at least 3 years, because most recurrences occur within 3 years of operation.[100]

Recurrent disease is usually local, but metastases to inguinal nodes, lung, liver, brain, and peritoneum can occur. The prognosis of a malignant tumor or a malignant recurrence was dismal until the advent of platinum-based chemotherapy.[98] Survival rates higher than 80% are now achieved, but the risk of late recurrences or second malignancies persists.[99–102]

A Children's Cancer Group (CCG) review illustrates the revised prognosis.[102] The mortality was 10% in 126 patients treated in 15 institutions from 1972 to 1994; 3 patients died of severe associated anomalies; 2, of hemorrhagic shock postoperatively; and 6, of combinations of severe prematurity, birth asphyxia due to failed vaginal delivery, and preoperative tumor rupture. Death from metastatic yolk sac tumor occurred in 1 patient, and a second patient with metastatic disease was lost to follow-up and is presumed dead. Thus only 2 deaths occurred from malignancy, despite a total of 20 yolk sac tumors (13 malignant at initial operation, 7 malignant recurrences after resection of "benign" teratomas). Owing to the effectiveness of current chemotherapy in treating recurrent disease and its toxicity in young infants, it appears that a completely excised malignant yolk sac tumor does not require adjuvant therapy. The patient should be closely monitored clinically and with serial AFP measurements.[103]

In older patients, treatment of malignant tumors involves excision, chemotherapy, and monitoring with imaging studies and serum markers. For unresectable tumors, biopsy and chemotherapy are followed by excision of the primary tumor after adequate reduction has been obtained.[101] Radiation therapy is usually reserved for local recurrence of malignant tumors. Patients with malignant tumors should be enrolled in a pediatric cooperative study or treated according to their guidelines.

In the current era of the rather routine use of US in pregnancy, the prognosis for patients with a sacrococcygeal teratoma is dependent not on Altman's classification[32] but rather on tumor size, physiologic consequences, histology, and associated anomalies. The prognosis of malignant tumors depends on tumor type, stage,[102] location, and patient age. Functional results in survivors have been reported as excellent in most series,[66,68,95] but recent reports draw attention to fecal and urinary continence problems as well as lower limb weakness.[93,104–107] Some of these problems are clearly related to associated anomalies[91] or to the presence of large presacral or intra-abdominal tumors,[104] but they can occur after excision of purely extrapelvic benign tumors. A good outcome requires meticulous dissection along the tumor capsule, preservation and reconstruction of muscular structures, and long-term follow-up. One group advocates earlier cesarean delivery to minimize urologic sequelae in patients with large tumors causing urinary tract dilatation.[107]

Thoracic Teratomas

The anterior mediastinum is the common site of thoracic teratomas, which account for 7% to 10% of all teratomas (see Table 68-1).[2,3]

MEDIASTINAL TERATOMAS. Mediastinal teratomas are diagnosed from the fetal period to adolescence and even adulthood.[2,108,109] Most are located in the anterior mediastinum, but a few have been described in the posterior mediastinum,[110] some with epidural extension.[111] In infants, respiratory distress is a common presenting manifestation,[112] but in older children, the teratoma is often an incidental finding on chest radiograph (Fig. 68-9).[2] Mediastinal teratomas may be first seen as a chest wall tumor and may even erode through the skin (Fig. 68-10). They also can erode into a bronchus, with hemoptysis as the initial manifestation, or rupture into the pleural cavity.[113] A strong association is found with Klinefelter's syndrome, and in these cases, choriocarcinoma in the teratoma often leads to precocious puberty.[2,24,114] Histiocytosis also has been reported with mediastinal teratoma, both with and without Klinefelter's syndrome.[47,54,55,114]

Histologically, the presence of immature tissue does not affect the prognosis in children younger than 15 years.[2] After age 15 years, mediastinal teratomas have a high incidence of malignant behavior, which is usually indicated by elevated levels of AFP or β-hCG or both.[115] The tumor should be excised through either a median sternotomy or a thoracotomy.[2,114] Smaller tumors may be approached through an anterior mediastinotomy (see Fig. 68-9) or by thoracoscopy,[116] although tumor seeding is a concern with the latter. Chemotherapy is required for malignant lesions as adjuvant therapy or preoperatively for unresectable tumors. Complete resection correlates best with event-free survival and is more often achieved with a strategy of delayed resection after preoperative chemotherapy.[115]

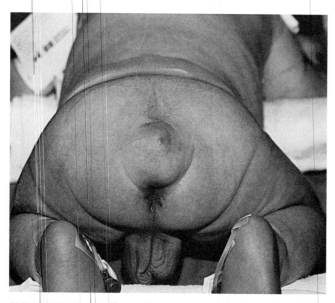

FIGURE 68-8. Smaller cystic teratoma at age 1 month, initially mistaken for a hemangioma owing to its soft compressible nature and bluish skin discoloration. This tumor lends itself well to a longitudinal elliptical excision with midline closure, as in a posterior sagittal anorectoplasty.

INTRAPERICARDIAL TERATOMAS. Intrapericardial teratomas are most commonly seen in the newborn period or in utero, with evidence of cardiorespiratory distress or nonimmune fetal hydrops.[2,3,117] They are a leading cause of massive pericardial effusion in the neonate.[3] Delay in diagnosis could be fatal. Fetal diagnosis allows early postnatal treatment in most patients,[118] or early delivery for emergency surgical excision if the baby develops signs of cardiac tamponade.[119]

On US, a cystic or solid teratoma is located anterior to the right atrium and ventricle with attachments to the great vessels.[117] In older infants, it may present with respiratory distress or poor feeding. It is not rare that the tumor may be found incidentally on chest radiograph. The only treatment is surgical excision. On histologic examination, these teratomas are usually composed of mature tissue with or without neuroglial components.[2,3]

INTRACARDIAC TERATOMAS. Intracardiac teratomas are rare and arise from the atrium or ventricle. Many can be cured by surgical resection.[2]

PULMONARY TERATOMAS. Three cases of intrapulmonary teratoma have been described.[120] They were first seen with trichoptysis or hemoptysis and were treated with lobectomy.

Abdominal Teratomas

The most frequent abdominal teratomas are the gonadal teratomas, which are discussed in other chapters.

RETROPERITONEAL TERATOMAS. Retroperitoneal teratomas occur outside the pelvis, often in a suprarenal location. They represent about 5% of all childhood teratomas, and 75% occur in children younger than 5 years.[2,3] An association with Klinefelter's syndrome has been described.[52] Usually the tumor is discovered as an abdominal mass that can compress the gastrointestinal tract, causing symptoms such as vomiting and constipation.[121]

Abdominal radiographs may show calcifications or bony structures within the tumor (Fig. 68-11). US, computed tomography (CT), and assessment of serum markers are the investigations used. Surgical excision is often easily performed, and malignancy is uncommon.[2,121] Occasionally, differentiation from a teratoid Wilms' tumor may be difficult.[122] The retroperitoneum site is the most common for the fetus in fetu malformations and intermediate fetiform teratomas.[2,3,123,124]

GASTRIC TERATOMAS. Gastric teratomas are rare lesions seen most commonly in infant boys.[2,47,95,125,126] They account for 1% of all teratomas. Clinically, the tumors present with hematemesis or vomiting due to gastric-outlet obstruction.[2,3,47,126,127] A palpable mass is common. The tumor is an exophytic mass in the lesser curvature or posterior wall of the stomach, and the whole stomach may be involved.

Most gastric teratomas are benign with mature and immature tissue, mostly neuroglial tissue. Benign peritoneal gliomatosis has been found incidentally in hernia sacs 10 months after resection of a gastric teratoma in the newborn period, illustrating the unusual behavior of some of these tumors.[128] Surgical excision is curative. Recurrence and malignancy are rare, despite local infiltration or nodal metastasis.[125,129]

OTHERS. Other rare sites of abdominal teratomas include liver, kidney, intestine, bladder, prostate, uterus, mesentery, and abdominal wall.[2,3,130–133]

Head and Neck Teratomas

More than 10% of teratomas in children originate from the neck, head, and central nervous system.[2,3,134,135] Most of these tumors are recognized at or shortly after birth and are associated with an increased incidence of stillbirth. They also can be diagnosed with prenatal US (Fig. 68-12).[136,137]

CERVICAL TERATOMAS. Cervical teratomas represent up to 8% of all teratomas.[18,137] Large tumors can be seen in utero with US.[136] These tumors are initially seen as a partly or completely cystic neck mass, which may compromise the airway and require immediate intubation or tracheostomy.[138,139] Large teratomas often lead to severe polyhydramnios, presumably because of esophageal compression; in turn, this may lead to premature labor. Serial amnioreduction may be required to prevent this complication. At birth, death may result from tracheal compression or deviation and the inability to intubate.[18,140–142]

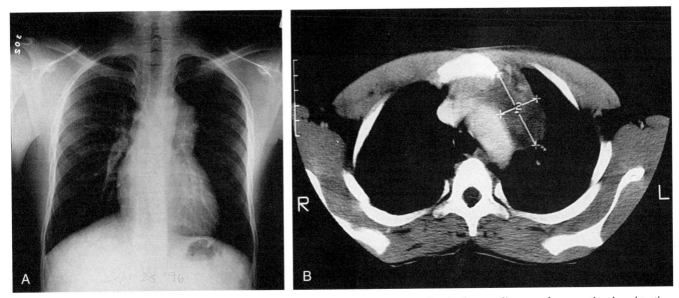

FIGURE 68-9. *A,* A 13-year-old African boy with an asymptomatic anterior mediastinal mass discovered on routine immigration chest radiograph. *B,* The computed tomography scan shows a heterogeneous mass adjacent to the aorta, suggestive of a neoplasm (thymoma or lymphoma). During consideration of a fine-needle aspiration biopsy, ultrasonography was done and suggested the presence of cysts with debris (not shown). Magnetic resonance imaging (not shown) confirmed the presence of cystic components as well as fat. A mature teratoma was excised through a small left anterior mediastinotomy, removing the left second costal cartilage.

Prenatal diagnosis permits cesarean section and establishment of an airway by the surgical team before the cord is clamped.[141] Refinements of this technique, called the EXIT procedure, (*EX*-utero *I*ntrapartum *T*reatment) have been documented in a series of 31 patients, 7 of whom had a large cervical teratoma.[143] Extension of tumor to the mediastinum or displacement of the trachea and carina may cause pulmonary hypoplasia, which increases respiratory morbidity and mortality.[2,3,143] The tumor is usually well defined and may contain calcifications. The differential diagnosis includes cystic hygroma, congenital goiter, foregut duplication cyst, and branchial cleft cyst (see Fig. 68-12).[140,143] Investigation should include plain radiographs, US, and measurement of AFP and β-hCG, as well as urinary catecholamine metabolites. CT and MRI may be useful to establish the diagnosis and to define the anatomic relations.

Complete excision is accomplished through a wide collar incision. The tumor is usually not difficult to separate from the strap muscles and the fascial planes, but the pretracheal fascia is sometimes very adherent. Often the site of origin cannot be identified, but, in many instances, the tumor is firmly attached to and appears to originate from the thyroid gland; a thyroid lobectomy should be performed in these cases. The terms *thyrocervical* and *cervicothyroidal* are often used to describe cervical teratomas.[2,3] In other instances, the tumor is adherent to the pharynx; meticulous dissection and pharyngotomy, if necessary, are important to prevent tumor recurrence. Giant teratomas may distort the anatomy, leading to

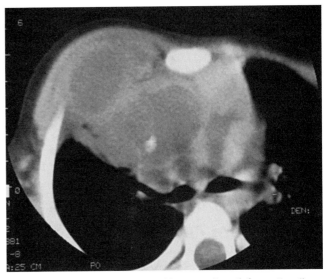

FIGURE 68-10. This 2-year-old was referred for a 5 × 5-cm hard fixed right chest wall mass that appeared suddenly during an upper respiratory infection. The computed tomography scan shows a bilobed lesion that extends through the chest wall and contains a small area of calcification. An incisional biopsy revealed puslike material, containing ghost cells and calcified debris. Serum markers were normal. Complete excision of the mass required a right anterior thoracotomy and partial resection of an adherent right middle lobe. Pathologic examination revealed a ruptured mature teratoma with marked inflammatory reaction, containing foci of enteric, respiratory, and squamous mucosa; smooth muscle; salivary glands; pancreas; neuroglial tissue; and bone.

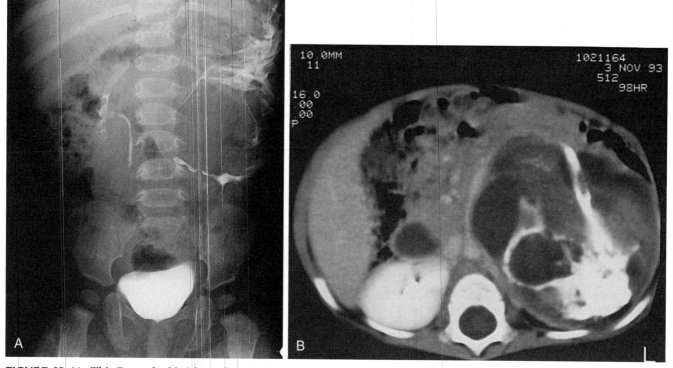

FIGURE 68-11. This 7-month-old girl was found to have an abdominal mass on routine examination. *A,* Plain films showed a large calcified left upper quadrant mass, which can be seen to displace the kidney inferiorly after injection of intravenous contrast. Ultrasonography (not shown) revealed multiple cystic areas. *B,* This was confirmed by computed tomography scan, which also revealed areas of fat density, making teratoma much more likely than neuroblastoma. The mature teratoma contained all types of cerebral and cerebellar tissues; respiratory, transitional, and squamous epithelium; sebaceous and salivary glands; smooth muscle; cartilage; and fat. Serum markers were normal.

permanent sequelae (see Fig. 68-12*E* and *F*). Generally the tumor is composed of both mature and immature neuroglial tissue, but cartilage and bronchial epithelium are not uncommon.[18,140,144] In 35% of cases, the tumor contains thyroid tissue, and hypothyroidism is a well-known postoperative complication.[145] Cervical teratomas are usually benign, but malignancy has been reported, even in infants. A report from the CCG showed that 20% of tumors clearly contained malignant elements, most often neuroblastoma, but also teratocarcinoma, neuroblastoma-like tumor, and neuroectodermal tumor.[18] Complete excision in the newborn period results in a survival rate of 80% to 90%. As for teratomas in other sites, one newborn was reported with a benign thyroid teratoma accompanied by neuroglial tissue deposits in cervical nodes.[146] A prognostic classification for cervical teratomas takes into account birth status, age at diagnosis, and presence of respiratory distress.[144] In neonates without respiratory distress, the mortality rate was 2.7%, compared with 43.4% in those with respiratory compromise. Prenatal diagnosis and delivery by using the EXIT procedure can undoubtedly increase survival.[141-143]

Thyroid teratomas may be present in older children and adults; they are often malignant in the latter.[147,148]

CRANIOFACIAL TERATOMAS. Craniofacial teratomas include a spectrum of lesions that may be life-threatening.

Epignathus. Epignathus is a term used to describe teratomas protruding from the mouth (Fig. 68-13). These tumors arise from the soft or hard palate in the region of Rathke's pouch.[149,150] They generally fill the oral cavity and extend out through the mouth. They can prevent fetal swallowing, which leads to polyhydramnios. Surgical excision is mandatory. They are usually benign, and recurrence is rare. A high degree of organization often gives them the appearance of a parasitic fetus.

Pharyngeal Teratomas. Pharyngeal teratomas arise from the posterior aspect of the nasopharynx. Large tumors can interfere with fetal swallowing and produce polyhydramnios, cause severe respiratory distress at birth, and lead to stillbirth.[2,151] Most pharyngeal teratomas are benign, and the treatment is surgical excision.[138]

Oropharyngeal Teratomas. Oropharyngeal teratomas represent 2% of all teratomas.[152] These tumors can originate from the tongue, sinuses, mandible, and tonsils. Airway compromise requires immediate care at the time of delivery. For oro- and nasopharyngeal teratomas, the EXIT procedure may be indicated when a large tumor detected prenatally appears to obstruct the airway. Most tumors are benign, and recurrence is uncommon after complete resection.[152] Separate tumors may occur in the same infant, and intracranial extension has been described.[153,154]

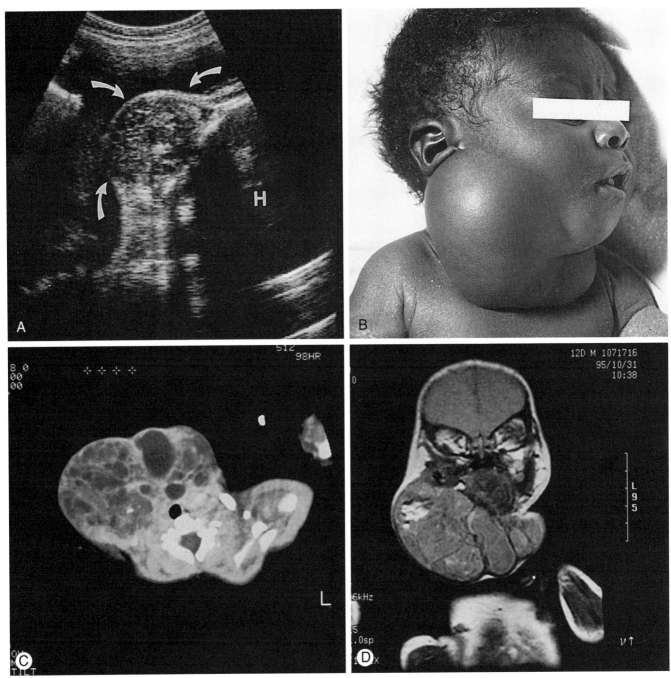

FIGURE 68-12. *A,* Fetal ultrasound at 34 weeks of gestation showing a 7-cm cervical mass of mixed echogenicity, containing blood flow by Doppler (*arrows* point to the mass, head is marked H). *B,* After birth by cesarean section, the child had only mild tachypnea despite the large right cervical mass extending to the left. Parts of the mass transilluminated, suggesting the diagnosis of hygroma. *C,* Computed tomography scan of the lower cervical area shows intact trachea and multiple cysts. This was initially interpreted as compatible with a hygroma, although an area of calcification was identified retrospectively. *D,* Magnetic resonance imaging confirmed the presence of fat, which appears bright on T_1-weighted images as well as on the proton density–weighted imaging sequence shown here. At operation, the mass appeared to originate from the right lobe of the thyroid gland. It contained epithelium-lined cysts, cartilage, bone, glandular tissue, and complex papillary structures; a predominance of neuroepithelial tissue was found with a few small areas of immature, neuroblastoma-like tissue. Preoperative vanillylmandelic acid levels were normal. The patient required postoperative thyroid hormone supplementation because of subclinical hypothyroidism (elevated thyroid-stimulating hormone with normal thyroxine and triiodothyronine levels). *E,* Another patient, with a giant cervical teratoma, seen on magnetic resonance at 30 weeks of gestation. The lesion was first diagnosed on routine US at 18 weeks and grew much faster than the fetus. Several amnioreductions were required because of polyhydramnios, and an EXIT procedure was performed at 34 weeks of gestation (H, head; F, foot; *arrows* outline the tumor). *F,* After securing the airway during the EXIT procedure and stabilizing the baby, resection was completed successfully. Notice the displacement of the ear. During resection, it became obvious that the left carotid artery and jugular vein entered the tumor. The left vagus nerve (hence the left recurrent nerve) was never seen, and the left glossopharyngeal nerve also was sacrificed, the tumor originating from the left pharyngeal wall. Including the fluid within the cystic parts, the teratoma weighed 1.4 kg, and the baby weighed 1.6 kg postoperatively.

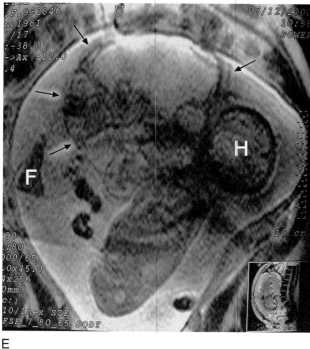

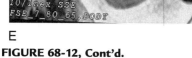

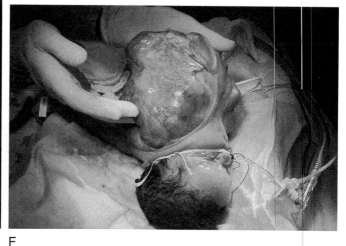

E

F

FIGURE 68-12, Cont'd.

Orbital Teratomas. Orbital teratomas usually present at birth with unilateral proptosis in a normal, term neonate.[155] They grow rapidly, but the eye is intact. Occasionally, the tumor extends intracranially. The proptotic eye may rupture because of prolonged exposure. Histologically, these tumors are benign and contain mature tissue and immature neuroglial elements. Surgical correction is the treatment of choice, and the eye can usually be preserved.[2,155]

Middle Ear Teratomas. Middle ear teratomas may be difficult to differentiate from hereditary cholesteatoma. They are benign tumors, but surgical resection is difficult owing to the location of the tumor and the deformation of the middle ear. Ossiculoplasty is sometimes necessary.[156,157]

Intracranial Teratomas

Intracranial teratomas generally present with symptoms of space-occupying lesions. These lesions account for only 2% to 4% of all teratomas, but they represent nearly 50% of brain tumors in the first 2 months of life.[2,3,47,158] Most are benign in neonates but malignant in older children and young adults.[47,158–161] These teratomas can appear in utero and cause massive hydrocephalus. Massive teratoma, causing skull rupture at delivery, has been reported.[159] The pineal gland is the most common site of origin, but intracranial teratomas may be seen in different areas, such as the hypothalamus, ventricles, cavernous sinus, cerebellum, and suprasellar region.[47,160,162]

Pineal gland teratomas can secrete chorionic gonadotropin hormone, causing precocious puberty. In infants younger than 2 years, obstructive hydrocephalus

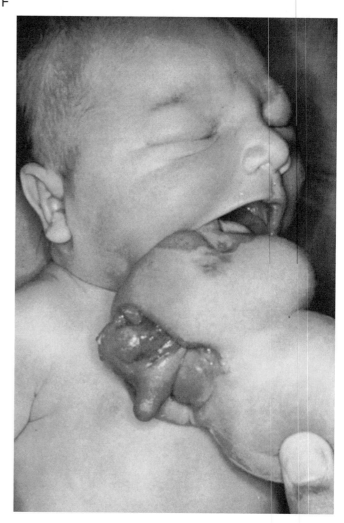

FIGURE 68-13. Epignathus, which is a teratoma protruding from the mouth.

is the most common clinical finding. In older children, symptoms of increased intracranial pressure are most common. The diagnosis can be made by using skull radiographs, US, CT, or MRI.

Treatment of intracranial teratomas is difficult, and many are unresectable. The only long-term survivors are those who have the mass completely resected. Palliative shunting to reduce intracranial pressure is of little long-term benefit.[47] Perinatal mortality is high, with only a 6% survival when diagnosed in the fetus or newborn.[3,163]

Miscellaneous Sites

Teratomas have been reported in other sites, such as skin, parotid, vulva, perianal region well away from the coccyx, spinal canal, umbilical cord (possibly associated with omphalocele), and placenta.[2,3,164–168]

DERMOID, EPIDERMOID, AND RELATED CYSTS

Dermoid Cysts

Dermoid cysts are congenital cysts that are lined by skin with fully mature pilosebaceous structures.[169,170] They are the result of sequestration of skin along lines of embryonic closure. The head and neck are the sites of predilection, but these lesions have been described on other midline sites, including the sacral area, perineal raphe, scrotum, and presternal area.[170] The so-called *dermoids of the ovary* are in fact cystic teratomas and are discussed in Chapter 74.

Typical locations on the head are under the lateral part of the eyebrow (Fig. 68-14), the scalp, the glabella, the tip of the nose, the orbit, and the palate, where they are associated with a cleft.[171] They also occur intracranially and in the spinal canal.[172]

Dermoids are usually rounded, soft, and often fixed to deep tissues or to bone. They usually present as a painless mass of 1 or 2 cm in diameter but can grow up to 4 cm or more if untreated. Some are associated with a sinus tract, especially those on the nose. This site is also typical for intracranial extension and a familial occurrence.[172] Dermoids in the head area are usually deep to muscles and often cause an indentation in the outer table of the skull. They can even erode through both bony tables and extend intracranially. A skull radiograph may show the defect, but it may be normal if the cyst is situated over a fontanelle or an unfused suture. CT is essential in those cases, and neurosurgical consultation is advisable.[172]

Dermoids deep to the lateral part of the eyebrow are usually approached through an incision just above the eyebrow because an incision within the eyebrow leaves a more visible scar. We have been impressed with an alternative incision through the palpebral crease. This requires a slightly longer incision and more retraction but leaves an invisible scar (see Fig. 68-14). This approach also has the advantage of allowing access to the orbit for the rare cases in which the cyst penetrates through the orbital bone in a dumbbell fashion.

Dermoids in the cervical area are usually midline, mostly suprahyoid or submental. Because they are deep within muscles, they tend to move with swallowing, just as thyroglossal duct cysts do. On US, they usually appear echogenic and are often misinterpreted as being solid

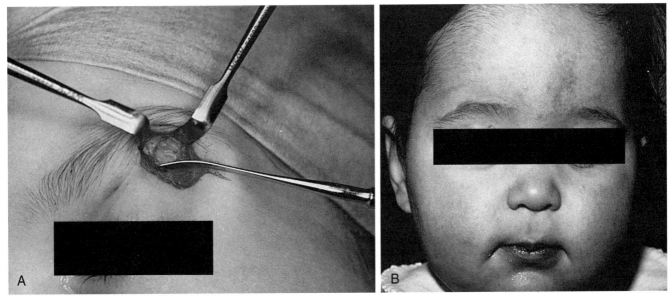

FIGURE 68-14. *A,* Dermoid cyst deep to the lateral part of the left eyebrow is approached through an incision made in the palpebral crease, taken through the muscle, which is then retracted upward, exposing the cyst lying on the periosteum. *B,* A different patient shown 1 month after excision of a right eyebrow dermoid through a palpebral skin incision. (*A,* Courtesy of Patricia Bortoluzzi, M.D., F.R.C.S.C.)

rather than cystic. They can be differentiated intraoperatively by their yellowish appearance and their soft, buttery content with sebaceous material and hair; this appearance alleviates the need for a hyoidectomy.

Dermoid cysts should be excised because they tend to grow and may rupture or become infected, resulting in a more difficult excision and a higher risk of recurrence.

Epidermal Cysts

Epidermal or epidermoid cysts have a wall composed of true epidermis, as seen on the skin surface and in the infundibulum of hair follicles (hence they also are called *infundibular cysts*).[169] They do not contain pilosebaceous units or hair. Some have a congenital origin like that of dermoid cysts, whereas others are acquired, either spontaneously arising from hair follicles or secondary to trauma with implantation of epidermis into the dermis or subcutaneous tissue.

Epidermal cysts are slow growing, formed by desquamation of epithelial cells. They are round, intradermal, or subcutaneous lesions that stop growing after having reached 1 to 5 cm in diameter. They occur most commonly on the face, scalp, neck, and trunk (i.e., hair-bearing areas). They may be associated with a small sinus tract or dimpling of the skin. In the neck and infraclavicular area, they may be confused with branchial cleft remnants. Preauricular sinuses and cysts are often considered epidermal cysts. Epidermoid cysts of the spleen are discussed in Chapter 45.

Some patients may have more than one cyst, but the presence of multiple cysts, especially on the scalp and face, should raise the possibility of Gardner's syndrome.[169,170] The cysts contain dry cheesy or horny material and lack skin appendages on histology. Treatment is excision, which often can be achieved under local anesthesia, even in young children.

Preauricular cysts are better excised under general anesthesia owing to their deep attachment to the helix cartilage.[171] Spontaneous rupture of any epidermal cyst leads to an intense foreign-body reaction, and the child presents with an abscess-like mass. This may require incision and drainage but often can be "cooled" with antibiotics and local warm compresses. This mode of presentation increases the risk of cyst recurrence after excision and often results in a wider scar than would have occurred with earlier excision. Infection of the cyst also may be caused by bacteria tracking along the small sinus tract that is sometimes present. These lesions rarely degenerate to epidermoid or basal cell carcinomas.[172] The treatment of asymptomatic preauricular sinuses is controversial, but certainly excision should be carried out in the presence of a palpable cyst or discharge of material from the sinus tract.

Epidermoid cysts of the skull and central nervous system share some similarities with dermoids, but they usually become symptomatic at an older age, between 20 and 40 years.[173] Most are thought to have a congenital origin, although iatrogenic and inflammatory mechanisms are likely for intraspinal epidermoids (caused by multiple lumbar punctures, especially when using a needle without stylet) and middle ear epidermoids (cholesteatomas), respectively.

Trichilemmal Cysts

Trichilemmal cysts, also called *pilar* or *sebaceous cysts,* are thought to arise from hair follicles.[169] Most are acquired and appear in adulthood. They often show an autosomal dominant inheritance pattern and are solitary in only 30% of the cases.[169] Some authors classify these as epidermoid or epidermal cysts.[172]

SOFT TISSUE TUMORS

Numerous soft tissue tumors have been described and are of mainly ectodermal and mesodermal origin. Some of these pediatric neoplasms are classified in Table 68-2. Tumors covered in other chapters are indicated. Only those soft

---

TABLE 68-2

CLASSIFICATION OF SOFT TISSUE TUMORS THAT OCCUR IN CHILDREN

Tissue	Benign	Malignant
Ectoderm		
Epidermis	Dermoid cyst, calcifying epithelioma (pilomatrixoma)	Epidermoid cancer
Sweat gland	Hidradenoma	Adenocarcinoma
Sebaceous gland	Sebaceous cyst	Epidermoid cancer
Melanocytes (see Chap. 70)	Nevus	Malignant melanoma
Nerve tissue	Neurofibroma	Neurofibrosarcoma
Mesoderm		
Undifferentiated	Mesenchymoma, myxoma	Malignant mesenchymoma
Fibrous tissue	Fibroma, fibromatosis, keloid	Fibrosarcoma
Vascular tissue (see Chap. 71)	Hemangioma, lymphangioma, glomus	Hemangioendothelioma
Adipose tissue	Lipoma, lipoblastoma	Liposarcoma
Muscle (see Chap. 69)	Rhabdomyoma	Rhabdomyosarcoma
Synovial tissue	Giant cell synovioma, ganglion cyst, synovial cyst	Malignant synovioma

tissue tumors likely to be encountered by pediatric surgeons are discussed here. More extensive discussions of soft tissue tumors are available.[174,175] Many soft tissue tumors are cutaneous or subcutaneous and are amenable to excision under local anesthesia.

Epidermis

Pyogenic Granulomas

Pyogenic granulomas are solitary polypoid capillary lesions often associated with trauma or local irritation. They are commonly found on the skin as red, raised, occasionally bleeding lesions or in the mouth in association with pregnancy.[176] They are easily treated with topical silver nitrate or liquid nitrogen or ligature of the polyp neck. Excision or electrocautery rarely is needed.

Skin Papillomas

Skin papillomas resemble skin tags of mucous membrane and occur at birth or in childhood.[177] Sessile variants may be called *verrucae*, whereas the projections are termed *acrochordon*. Treatment is by simple excision.

Warts

Warts are uncommon before age 4 years but are a common pediatric complaint.[177] Various subtypes of human papillomavirus affect different body areas.[176] Verrucae spread through families, sports teams, and schoolmates and are most common on the hands and feet.[177] Topical treatment includes salicylic or trichloroacetic acid, liquid nitrogen, or fine-tip electrocautery. Excision is occasionally required.

Condylomata acuminata occur in the perineal skin and suggest, but do not prove, child sexual abuse. The virus may be transmitted by hand contact during diaper changes in infants or acquired at birth during vaginal delivery, but the lesions may take months to develop. One study suggested that sexual abuse is an unlikely source of transmission in children younger than 3 years if no other signs of abuse are present.[178] These lesions have a core of connective tissue covered in epithelium, occurring as solitary or cauliflower-like lesions. Spontaneous regression is known, but topical podophyllin may be required. Some cases may necessitate electrocautery under general anesthesia to enable a thorough rectoscopic and vaginoscopic assessment and treatment.

Aberrant Skin Glands

Aberrant skin glands appear as rough, yellow-brownish skin resembling nevi or xanthoma. Histologic examination reveals adenoid hyperplasia, but a potential for later malignant change is reported, and therefore excision of these lesions is recommended.[177]

Calcifying Epithelioma of Malherbe

The calcifying epithelioma of Malherbe or *pilomatrixoma* is a solitary benign calcifying tumor of hair follicles. This is one of the most common acquired soft tissue lesions in children. Clinically, a circumscribed, firm, mobile, intracutaneous or subcutaneous nodule is palpable, with occasional yellowish or bluish coloration. These lesions are most common before age 20 years, and 60% to 70% are found in the head and neck region.[176] Only 2% to 3% are multiple, and most are smaller than 1 cm, although lesions up to 4 cm have been reported.[176,179] They are more common than sebaceous cysts in younger patients. Local excision is indicated.[179]

Sweat Gland Lesions

Sweat gland pathology results from disorders of the sebaceous, apocrine, or eccrine adnexal structures of the skin. One series reported that only 1.7% of pediatric skin biopsies showed these lesions.[176] *Hidradenoma* originates from the ductal portion of the sweat gland and produces multiple small flesh-colored papules on the face, neck, and upper chest during puberty and adolescence. Two subtypes are of interest: the eruptive form results in many lesions in a short period, whereas the clear cell variant causes solitary and occasionally painful lesions.[176] Sweat gland carcinomas are rare and are rarely differentiated enough to subtype confidently.[176] They may be locally aggressive and metastasize to the local lymph nodes. Treatment primarily involves resection with individualized adjuvant therapy.

Malignant Epithelial Tumors

Malignant epithelial tumors are rare in children.[177] General treatment principles include wide local excision and radiotherapy for prevention of recurrence.[177] Only 1% of all basal cell carcinomas occur in children. The basal cell nevus syndrome[180] is an autosomal dominant disease with basal cell lesions of the eyes, nose, and cheeks in association with anomalies of the mouth, skin, skeleton, central nervous system, eyes, and genitals. These patients may have concomitant xeroderma pigmentosum. Epidermoid or squamous cell carcinoma also is found in xeroderma pigmentosum patients.[176] Epidermoid cancers in pediatric transplant recipients also have been reported.[176]

Nerve Tissue

Neurofibromas

A neurofibroma is a benign neoplasm of abnormal proliferation of Schwann cells, usually of peripheral nerves. When multiple or associated with multiple cafe-au-lait spots, neurofibromatosis type 1 (NF-1), or von Recklinghausen's disease, an autosomal dominant disorder, may be present. The *NF-1* gene appears to produce a tumor-suppression product, and neurofibromatosis may be a disease to which the two-hit genetic hypothesis applies.[181] The diagnosis may be delayed, but children in affected probands are usually diagnosed earlier, even by antenatal US.[182,183] Neurofibromas of the mucosa are associated with multiple endocrine neoplasia type 2B and can appear in childhood before medullary thyroid carcinoma or pheochromocytoma.[184] The *NF-2* gene has been associated with acoustic neuromas.

NF-1 has several clinical forms, which are summarized in Table 68-3.[185] Because operative management is not curative of a genetic disorder, a multidisciplinary team supports patients and parents through decision making, treatment, rehabilitation, and developmental challenges (Fig. 68-15). Malignant degeneration to neurofibrosarcoma and associated malignancies[186] may necessitate US, CT, or MRI studies of new complaints. These imaging modalities are useful in monitoring larger or deeper neurofibromas as well. Rapid growth is an ominous sign of neurofibrosarcoma. Excision or debulking may be combined with chemotherapy and radiotherapy.[187] Radiotherapy does not appear to be useful in slowing the progression of benign disease but has been documented to cause neurofibrosarcoma.[188] Treatment with chemotherapy and interferon-α has not been proved to be of benefit.

Xanthomas

Xanthoma is a tumor of lipid-laden histiocytes or foam cells forming yellowish skin nodules. It may be due to uncontrolled diabetes mellitus or biliary tract obstruction,

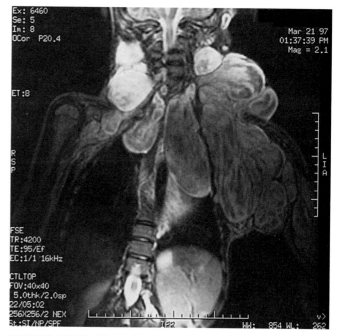

FIGURE 68-15. Magnetic resonance imaging study of a young boy with extensive neurofibromatosis type 1 who had undergone two previous cervical laminectomies to remove plexiform neurofibromas that were causing symptomatic cord compression. The left neck mass was enlarging, causing tracheal deviation and growing along the cervical nerve roots. This boy also had increasing left arm weakness and pain. A trial of chemotherapy with vincristine and actinomycin D did not stop progression of the disease.

which unbalances triglyceride and cholesterol metabolism, leading to accumulation in histiocytes. Xanthomas are typical features of Alagille's syndrome (syndromic paucity of bile ducts) and familial hypercholesterolemia (Fig. 68-16). Correcting the underlying disorder reverses these cases, but excisional biopsy may be indicated for bothersome lesions or diagnostic purposes.

Mesoderm

Undifferentiated Mesenchyme

MESENCHYMOMAS. Mesenchymoma is a mixed mesenchymal tumor of two or more cellular elements not commonly associated (not including fibrous tissue). It can occur after radiotherapy or chemotherapy.[189] These lesions are usually benign in children and occur primarily in the head, neck, and extremities. Rib lesions in neonates and liver lesions also are described.[190] Malignant mesenchymoma is the corresponding sarcoma and is rare.

MYXOMAS. A myxoma is a benign primitive connective tissue cell and stroma tumor resembling mesenchyme. It occurs mainly in the heart, producing symptoms by obstruction of normal blood flow, and is removed by using cardiopulmonary bypass.

TABLE 68-3	
CLINICAL PATTERNS IN NEUROFIBROMATOSIS	

Clinical	Description
Fibroma molluscum	Hundreds or thousands of pedunculated nodules; number makes resection impractical
Plexiform neurofibroma	Occur usually in the face and scalp, causing bony deformity by pressure erosion; resections for cosmesis may be repeated because curative resection is rare
Elephantiasis nervorum	With neurofibromas of the extremities, these cause greatly thickened skin simulating limb hypertrophy; resection is done to manage disfigurement
Thoracic neurofibroma	May have intraspinal extension (dumbbell tumor); have a high incidence of malignancy
Visceral neurofibroma	May affect intestine, kidney, and bladder because of the presence of associated nerves; when large, neurofibrosarcoma incidence increases
Skeletal syndromes	Include kyphoscoliosis, pseudarthrosis of tibia and ulna
Cranial syndromes	Meningiomas, gliomas, and optic gliomas have been reported
Endocrine syndromes	Sexual precocity, medullary thyroid carcinoma, and pheochromocytoma have been reported
Cardiovascular syndromes	Heart is rarely involved, but coarctation of the aorta and renal artery lesions have been reported

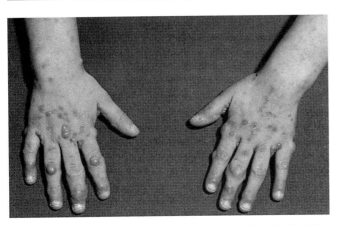

FIGURE 68-16. Multiple xanthomas in a child with Alagille's syndrome.

Fibrous Tissue

Fibromas

A fibroma is a lesion composed of fibrous or fully developed connective tissue occurring as lytic bone lesions, breast lumps, finger swelling, and other forms.[190] *Fibromatosis* usually is first seen in infancy with multiple firm rubbery masses in the soft tissues, mostly in the lower extremities and head and neck. When it is congenital and generalized, death may occur in the first weeks of life, due mainly to pulmonary lesions.[190]

NODULAR FASCIITIS. Nodular fasciitis is the most common fibrous tissue tumor or self-limiting reactive process.[191] These tumors may be subcutaneous, intramuscular, or fascial in location and are commonly found in the head and neck of children.[191] Half of cases are associated with discomfort, and one fourth of lesions occur in patients younger than 20 years. Excisional biopsy is necessary to differentiate these rapidly growing lesions from a malignancy.

FIBROSARCOMAS. Fibrosarcoma is a neoplasm producing collagen that otherwise lacks cellular differentiation. Childhood fibrosarcoma (CFS) has a bimodal age distribution (younger than 5 years and ages 10 to 15 years). CFS is treated with complete excision. Adult-type fibrosarcoma is an aggressive lesion with a poor prognosis despite multimodal therapy. The two lesions may be problematic to differentiate.[192]

Congenital Epulis

Congenital epulis is a benign granular cell tumor occurring almost exclusively in girls at or immediately after birth. It originates from the maxillary dental mucosa and averages 1 to 2 cm in diameter.[193] Its exact nature is not clear. Some classify it under tumors of peripheral nerves, whereas others consider it a fibrous tumor; hence the synonym *granular cell fibroblastoma*. Spontaneous regression is unusual, and simple excision is curative.[193]

Keloid

A keloid is a sharply elevated, irregularly shaped, progressively enlarging scar caused by excessive collagen in the dermis during connective tissue repair. Unlike the hypertrophic scar (which does not progress), a keloid may recur after excision. Treatment with intradermal injection of steroids, pressure garments (as in some burn patients), and cryosurgery may be attempted. Rarely, judicious excision with radiotherapy may be used.[194] Keloids developing after minor procedures are common. Their incidence is higher in black patients.

Desmoid Tumors

Desmoid tumors are fibrous tumors that usually arise from musculoaponeurotic tissue of the skull or abdominal cavity: hence the modern name *musculoaponeurotic fibromatosis*.[195] They are not encapsulated and are locally invasive, although they do not metastasize. They are associated with Gardner's syndrome.

When they arise from the retroperitoneum, complete resection may be impossible without risking damage to splanchnic vessels. High-dose radiotherapy or interstitial brachytherapy may be considered for residual tumor. Chemotherapy using methotrexate and vinblastine or the tyrosine kinase inhibitor, imatinib mesylate, has engendered favorable reports.[196,197] Steroid therapy (tamoxifen, prednisone) and nonsteroidal therapy (indomethacin and sulindac) have been used in recurrent and inoperable tumors.[198] Shrinkage of a desmoid tumor has been reported by using interferon-α as well.[199]

Vascular Glomus

A glomus tumor is an uncommon pediatric lesion consisting of a meshwork of fine arterioles connected to veins and intertwined with nerve tissue. Multiple tumors have a greater tendency to develop in children than in adults, possibly representing autosomal dominant inheritance.[190] The lesions on the skin are discrete blue-black spots and may be extremely painful if present under nails. Excision is the preferred treatment.

Adipose Tissue

A lipoma is a benign, soft, rubbery, encapsulated tumor of adipose tissue composed of mature fat cells occurring on the trunk, neck, and forearms. Lipomas represented 94%; lipoblastoma, 4.7%; and liposarcoma, 1.3% of adipose tumors in one series.[200] All are slow-growing tumors. Diagnosed often before age 3 years, lipoblastoma may be superficial and well encapsulated or deep and infiltrative. Definitive treatment of adipose tumors is complete resection. Chemotherapy may play a role in treating residual liposarcoma. Local recurrence rates for lipoblastoma and liposarcoma are about 10% to 20%.[200] Characterized by a myxoid stroma, embryonal lipoblasts, and mature fat cells, the myxoid variant of liposarcoma is similar histologically to lipoblastoma. Tumor karyotyping may be useful in differentiating these adipose tumors.[200]

Liposarcoma arises from the intermuscular fascia, where embryonal lipoblasts exhibit variable differentiation with occasional nuclear atypia. The myxoid variant is the most common and metastasizes late if at all. The dedifferentiated subtype is highly malignant and may coexist with spindle cell sarcoma.

Synovial Tissue

Synovial Cysts

Synovial cysts or *ganglion cysts* arise from joints or tendon sheaths, resulting in firm 0.5- to 2-cm, mucin-filled lesions with a fibrous capsule. They are most common on the hand, especially on the dorsum of the wrist, but also occur on the ankle, foot, and popliteal fossa (where they are called Baker's cysts). One fourth of the latter occur in children younger than 6 years.[201]

Pathology texts separate synovial cysts that have a true synovial lining (such as Baker's cysts) from ganglia, which are thought to be degenerative and are without a synovial lining.[202,203] Clinicians, however, usually use both terms interchangeably.[204] Symptoms of pain and weakness occur, but most children present with an asymptomatic mass. Spontaneous resolution of all types of synovial cysts is common in children. Surgical treatment is reserved for patients with persistently symptomatic lesions.[204] Classic treatment includes traumatic disruption ("strike it with the family Bible") or steroid injection. Both should be discouraged because of high recurrence risk and associated pain. The use of non-steroidal anti-inflammatory agents, coupled with rest or wrist splinting, is usually sufficient if the cyst causes transient discomfort.

Giant Cell Synoviomas

The giant cell synovioma is a benign tumor of the tendon sheath, generally occurring before age 10 years.[190] It occurs on the volar aspect of the fingers in most cases. Treatment by resection results in a 10% to 15% recurrence rate.[190] Malignant synovioma or synoviosarcoma represents 5% to 10% of soft tissue malignancies in patients younger than 20 years.[205] Most occur near the knee, but they also are found in the head and neck, anterior abdominal wall, and inguinal area. The mass may be palpable or reveal itself as calcification on radiograph. Cure by wide excision without chemotherapy can often be achieved, but neurovascular anatomy related to the tumor may necessitate microsurgical reconstruction if not amputation. The calcifying subtype has a better 5-year survival rate (83%) than the noncalcifying subtypes (25% to 50%).[206]

REFERENCES

1. Virchow R: Ueber Die Sakralgeschwulst Des Schliewener Kindes. Klin Wschr 46:132, 1869.
2. Dehner LP: Gonadal and extragonadal germ cell neoplasms: Teratomas in childhood. In Finegold M (ed): Pathology of Neoplasia in Children and Adolescents. Philadelphia, WB Saunders, 1986, pp 282–312.
3. Isaacs H: Germ cell tumors. In Isaacs H (ed): Tumors of the Fetus and Newborn. Philadelphia, WB Saunders, 1997, pp 15–38.
4. Skinner MA: Germ cell tumors. In Oldham KT, Colombani PM, Foglia RP (eds): Surgery of Infants and Children: Scientific Principles and Practice. Philadelphia, Lippincott-Raven, 1997, pp 653–662.
5. Moore KL, Persaud TVN: The Developing Human: Clinically Oriented Embryology. 7th ed. Philadelphia, WB Saunders, 2003.
6. Isaacs H: Tumors. In Gilbert-Barness E (ed): Potter's Pathology of the Fetus and Infant. St. Louis, CV Mosby, 1997, pp 1242–1331.
7. Bale PM: Sacrococcygeal developmental abnormalities and tumors in children. Perspect Pediatr Pathol 1:56, 1984.
8. Sinnock KL, Perez-Atayde AR, Boynton KA, et al: Clonal analysis of sacrococcygeal "teratomas." Pediatr Pathol Lab Med 16:865–875, 1996.
9. Chadha R, Bagga D, Malhortra CJ, et al: Accessory limb attached to the back. J Pediatr Surg 28:1615–1617, 1993.
10. de Lagausie P, de Napoli Cocci S, Stempfle N, et al: Highly differentiated teratoma and fetus-in-fetu: A single pathology? J Pediatr Surg 32:115–116, 1997.
11. Heifetz SA, Alrabeeah A, Brown BS, et al: Fetus in fetu: A fetiform teratoma. Pediatr Pathol 8:215–226, 1988.
12. Hanquinet S, Damry N, Heimann P, et al: Association of a fetus in fetu and two teratomas: US and MRI. Pediatr Radiol 27:336–338, 1997.
13. Drut RM, Drut R, Fontana A, et al: Mature presacral sacrococcygeal teratoma associated with a sacral "epignathus." Pediatr Pathol 12:99–103, 1992.
14. Parizek J, Nemecek S, Pospisilova B, et al: Mature sacrococcygeal teratoma containing the lower half of a human body. Childs Nerv Syst 8:108–110, 1992.
15. Kooijman CD: Immature teratomas in children. Histopathology 12:491–502, 1988.
16. Heifetz SA, Cushing B, Giller R, et al: Immature teratomas in children: Pathologic considerations: A report from the combined Pediatric Oncology Group/Children's Cancer Group. Am J Surg Pathol 22:1115–1124, 1998.
17. Graf JL, Housely HT, Albanese CT, et al: A surprising histological evolution of preterm sacrococcygeal teratoma. J Pediatr Surg 33:177–179, 1998.
18. Azizkhan RG, Haase GM, Applebaum H, et al: Diagnosis, management, and outcome of cervicofacial teratomas in neonates: A Children's Cancer Group Study. J Pediatr Surg 30:312–316, 1995.
19. Ohtsuka M, Satoh H, Inoue M, et al: Disseminated metastasis of neuroblastomatous component in immature mediastinal teratoma: A case report. Anticancer Res 20:527–530, 2002.
20. Hijiya N, Horikawa R, Matsushita T, et al: Malignant mediastinal germ-cell tumors in childhood: A report of two cases achieving long-term disease-free survival. Am J Pediatr Hematol Oncol 11:437–440, 1989.
21. Stringer DA, Sprigg A, Kerrigan D: Malignant carcinoid within a recurrent sacrococcygeal teratoma in childhood. Can Assoc Radiol J 41:105–107, 1990.
22. Tsuchida Y, Endo Y, Saito S, et al: Evaluation of alpha fetoprotein in early infancy. J Pediatr Surg 13:155–162, 1978.
23. Wu JT, Book L, Sudar K: Serum alpha fetoprotein (AFP) levels in normal infants. Pediatr Res 15:50–52, 1981.
24. Derenoncourt AN, Castro-Magana M, Jones KL: Mediastinal teratoma and precocious puberty in a boy with mosaic Klinefelter syndrome. Am J Med Genet 55:38–42, 1995.
25. Rodriguez E, Reuter VE, Mies C, et al: Abnormalities of 2q: A common genetic link between rhabdomyosarcoma and hepatoblastoma? Genes Chromosomes Cancer 3:122–127, 1991.
26. Perlman EJ, Cushing B, Hawkins E, et al: Cytogenetic analysis of childhood endodermal sinus tumors: A Pediatric Oncology Group Study. Pediatr Pathol 14:695–708, 1994.
27. Kruslin B, Hrascan R, Manojlovic S, et al: Oncoproteins and tumor suppressor proteins in congenital sacrococcygeal teratomas. Pediatr Pathol Lab Med 17:43–52, 1997.
28. Ishiwata I, Ishiwata C, Soma M, et al: N-*myc* gene amplification and neuron specific enolase production in immature teratomas. Virchows Arch A Pathol Anat Histopathol 418:333–338, 1991.
29. Currarino G, Coln D, Votteler T: Triad of anorectal, sacral, and presacral anomalies. AJR Am J Roentgenol 137:395–398, 1981.

30. Ng WT, Ng TK, Cheng PW: Sacrococcygeal teratoma and anorectal malformation: Case reports. Aust N Z J Surg 67:218–220, 1997.
31. Tsuchida Y, Watanasupt W, Nakajo T: Anorectal malformations associated with a presacral tumor and sacral defect. Pediatr Surg Int 4:398–402, 1989.
32. Altman RP, Randolph JG, Lilly JR: Sacrococcygeal teratoma: American Academy of Pediatrics Surgical Section Survey, 1973. J Pediatr Surg 9:389–398, 1974.
33. Tander B, Baskin D, Bulut M: A case of incomplete Currarino triad with malignant transformation. Pediatr Surg Int 15:409–410, 1999.
34. Ashcraft KW, Holder TM: Hereditary presacral teratoma. J Pediatr Surg 9:691–697, 1974.
35. Lee S-C, Chun Y-S, Jung S-E, et al: Currarino triad: Anorectal malformations, sacral bony abnormality, and presacral mass: A review of 11 cases. J Pediatr Surg 32:58–61, 1997.
36. Shaija JK: Anorectal malformation presenting as Hirschsprung's disease: A case report. East Afr Med J 72:130–131, 1995.
37. Sonnino RE, Chou S, Guttman FM: Hereditary sacrococcygeal teratoma. J Pediatr Surg 24:1074–1075, 1989.
38. Singh SJ, Rao P, Stockton V: Familial presacral masses: Screening pitfalls. J Pediatr Surg 36:1841–1844, 2001.
39. Weinberg AG: "Teratomas" in the Currarino triad: A misnomer. Pediatr Dev Pathol 3:110–111, 2000.
40. Ross AJ, Ruiz-Perez V, Wang Y, et al: A homeobox gene, *HLXB9*, is the major locus for dominantly inherited sacral agenesis. Nat Genet 20:358–361, 1998.
41. Iinuma Y, Iwafuchi M, Uchiyama M, et al: A case of Currarino triad with familial sacral bony deformities. Pediatr Surg Int 16:134–135, 2000.
42. Subbarao P, Bhatnagar V, Mitra DK: The association of sacrococcygeal teratoma with high anorectal and genital malformations. Aust N Z J Surg 64:214–215, 1994.
43. Lahdenne P, Heikinheimo M, Jaaskelainen J, et al: Vertebral abnormalities associated with congenital sacrococcygeal teratomas. J Pediatr Orthop 11:603–607, 1991.
44. Werb P, Scurry J, Ostor A, et al: Survey of congenital tumors in perinatal necropsies. Pathology 24:247–253, 1992.
45. Sadove AM, Kalsbec JE, Ellis FD, et al: Orbital teratoma associated with trigonocephaly. Plast Reconstr Surg 88:1059–1063, 1991.
46. Aughton DJ, Sloan CT, Milad MP, et al: Nasopharyngeal teratoma ("hairy polyp"), Dandy-Walker malformation, diaphragmatic hernia, and other anomalies in a female infant. J Med Genet 27:788–790, 1990.
47. Rowe MI, O'Neill JA, Grosfeld JL, et al: Teratomas and germ cell tumors. In Rowe MI, O'Neill JA, Grosfeld JL, et al (eds): Essentials of Pediatric Surgery. St. Louis, CV Mosby, 1995, pp 296–305.
48. Gross RE, Clatworthy HW Jr, Meeker IA Jr: Sacrococcygeal teratomas in infants and children: A report of 40 cases. Surg Gynecol Obstet 92:341–354, 1951.
49. Hasle H, Jacobsen BB, Aschenfeldt P, et al: Mediastinal germ cell tumour associated with Klinefelter syndrome: A report of case and review of the literature. Eur J Pediatr 151:735–739, 1992.
50. Casalone R, Righi R, Granata P, et al: Cerebral germ cell tumor and XXY karyotype. Cancer Genet Cytogenet 74:25–29, 1994.
51. Hachimi-Idrissi S, Desmytere S, Goossens A, et al: Retroperitoneal teratoma as first sign of Klinefelter's syndrome. Arch Dis Child 72:163–164, 1995.
52. Czauderna P, Stoba C, Wysocka B, et al. Association of Klinefelter syndrome and abdominal teratoma: A case report. J Pediatr Surg 33:774–775, 1998.
53. Zon R, Orazi A, Neiman RS, et al: Benign hematologic neoplasm associated with mediastinal mature teratoma in a patient with Klinefelter's syndrome: A case report. Med Pediatr Oncol 23:376–379, 1994.
54. Beasley SW, Tiedemann K, Howat A, et al: Precocious puberty associated with malignant thoracic teratoma and malignant histiocytosis in a child with Klinefelter's syndrome. Med Pediatr Oncol 15:277–280, 1987.
55. Sasou S, Nakamura SI, Habano W, et al: True malignant histiocytosis developed during chemotherapy for mediastinal immature teratoma. Hum Pathol 27:1099–1103, 1996.
56. Aurer I, Nemet D, Uzarevic B, et al: Mediastinal malignant teratoma and acute myeloid leukemia in a patient with Klinefelter's syndrome: Comparison of DNA content in the two malignancies. Acta Oncol 33:705–706, 1994.
57. Koo CH, Reifel J, Kogut N, et al: True histiocytic malignancy associated with a malignant teratoma in a patient with 46XY gonadal dysgenesis. Am J Surg Pathol 16:175–183, 1992.
58. Goetsch SJ, Hadley GP: Hodgkin's disease following successful treatment of gastric teratoma in a neonatal female. Pediatr Pathol Lab Med 15:455–461, 1995.
59. Zambudio AR, Lanzas JT, Calvo MJ, et al: Mediastinal cystic teratoma associated with a Hodgkin's lymphoma. Eur J Cardiothorac Surg 20:650–651, 2001.
60. Dische MR, Gardner HA: Mixed teratoid tumors of the liver and neck in trisomy 13. Am J Clin Pathol 69:631–637, 1978.
61. Quah BS, Menon BS: Down syndrome associated with a retroperitoneal teratoma and Morgagni hernia. Clin Genet 50:232–234, 1996.
62. Falik-Borenstein TC, Korenberg JR, Davos I, et al: Congenital gastric teratoma in Wiedemann-Beckwith syndrome. Am J Med Genet 38:52–57, 1991.
63. Akguner M, Karaca C, Karatas O, et al: Mentosternal pterygium with teratoma. Ann Plast Surg 37:201–203, 1996.
64. Zachariou Z, Krug M, Benz G, et al: Proteus syndrome associated with a sacrococcygeal teratoma: A rare combination. Eur J Pediatr Surg 6:249–251, 1996.
65. Robin NH, Grace K, DeSouza TG, et al: New finding of Schinzel-Giedion syndrome: A case with a malignant sacrococcygeal teratoma. Am J Med Genet 47:852–856, 1993.
66. Billmire DF, Grosfeld JL: Teratomas in childhood: Analysis of 142 cases. J Pediatr Surg 21:548–551, 1985.
67. Schropp KP, Lobe TE, Rao B, et al: Sacrococcygeal teratoma: The experience of four decades. J Pediatr Surg 27:1075–1079, 1992.
68. Tapper D, Lack EE: Teratomas in infancy and childhood: A 54-year experience at the Children's Hospital Medical Center. Ann Surg 198:398–410, 1983.
69. Powell RW, Weber ED, Manci EA: Intradural extension of a sacrococcygeal teratoma. J Pediatr Surg 28:770–772, 1993.
70. West K, Touloukian RJ: Meconium pseudocyst presenting as a buttock mass. J Pediatr Surg 23:864–865, 1988.
71. Murphy JJ, Blair GK, Fraser GC: Coagulopathy associated with large sacrococcygeal teratomas. J Pediatr Surg 27:1308–1310, 1992.
72. Holterman A-X, Filiatrault D, Lallier M, et al: The natural history of sacrococcygeal teratomas diagnosed through routine obstetric sonogram: A single institution experience. J Pediatr Surg 33:899–903, 1998.
73. Hedrick HL, Flake AW, Crombleholme TM, et al: Sacrococcygeal teratoma: Prenatal assessment, fetal intervention, and outcome. J Pediatr Surg 39:430–438, 2004.
74. Angel CA, Murillo C, Mayhew J: Experience with vascular control before excision of giant, highly vascular sacrococcygeal teratomas in neonates. J Pediatr Surg 33:1840–1842, 1998.
75. Jona JZ: Progressive tumor necrosis and lethal hyperkalemia in a neonate with sacrococcygeal teratoma (SCT). J Perinatol 19:538–540, 1999.
76. Flake AW: Fetal sacrococcygeal teratoma. Semin Pediatr Surg 2:113–120, 1993.
77. Brace V, Grant SR, Brackley KJ, et al: Prenatal diagnosis and outcome in sacrococcygeal teratomas: A review of cases between 1992 and 1998. Prenat Diagn 20:51–55, 2000.
78. Veschambre R, Wartanian B, Lebouvier L, et al: Facteurs pronostiques anténatals des tératomes sacro-coccygiens. Rev Fr Gynecol Obstet 88:325–330, 1993.
79. Robertson FM, Crombleholme TM, Frantz ID, et al: Devascularization and staged resection of giant sacrococcygeal teratoma in the premature infant. J Pediatr Surg 30:309–311, 1995.
80. Hecher K, Hackeloer B-J: Intrauterine endoscopic laser surgery for fetal sacrococcygeal teratoma. Lancet 347:470, 1996.
81. Paek BW, Jennings RW, Harrison MR, et al: Radiofrequency ablation of human fetal sacrococcygeal teratoma. Am J Obstet Gynecol 184:503–507, 2001.
82. Ibrahim D, Ho E, Scherl SA, et al: Newborn with an open posterior hip dislocation and sciatic nerve injury after intrauterine radiofrequency ablation of a sacrococcygeal teratoma. J Pediatr Surg 38:248–250, 2003.
83. Kay S, Khalife S, Laberge JM, et al: Prenatal percutaneous needle drainage of cystic sacrococcygeal teratomas. J Pediatr Surg 34:1148–1151, 1999.

84. Garcia AM, Morgan WM III, Bruner JP: In utero decompression of a cystic grade IV sacrococcygeal teratoma. Fetal Diagn Ther 13:305–308, 1998.

85. Jouannic JM, Dommergues M, Auber F, et al: Successful intrauterine shunting of a sacrococcygeal teratoma (SCT) causing fetal bladder obstruction. Prenatal Diagn 21:824–826, 2001.

86. Fishman SJ, Jennings RW, Johnson SM, et al: Contouring buttock reconstruction after sacrococcygeal teratoma resection. J Pediatr Surg, in press.

87. Lindahl H: Giant sacrococcygeal teratoma: A method of simple intraoperative control of hemorrhage. J Pediatr Surg 23:1068–1069, 1988.

88. Bax NM, van der Zee DC: Laparoscopic clipping of the median sacral artery in huge sacrococcygeal teratomas. Surg Endoscopy 12:882–883, 1998.

89. Lund DP, Soriano DG, Fauza D, et al: Resection of a massive sacrococcygeal teratoma using hypothermic hypoperfusion: A novel use of extracorporeal membrane oxygenation. J Pediatr Surg 30:157–159, 1995.

90. Hoehn T, Krause MF, Wilhelm C, et al: Fatal rupture of a sacrococcygeal teratoma during delivery. J Perinatol 19:596–598, 1999.

91. Shanbhogue LKR, Bianchi A, Doig CM, et al: Management of benign sacrococcygeal teratoma: Reducing mortality and morbidity. Pediatr Surg Int 5:41–44, 1990.

92. Chisholm CA, Heider AL, Kuller JA, et al: Prenatal diagnosis and perinatal management of fetal sacrococcygeal teratoma. Am J Perinatol 16:47–50, 1999.

93. Schmidt B, Haberlik A, Uray E, et al: Sacrococcygeal teratoma: Clinical course and prognosis with a special view to long-term functional results. Pediatr Surg Int 15:573–576, 1999.

94. Gobel U, Calaminus G, Engert J, et al: Teratomas in infancy and childhood. Med Pediatr Oncol 31:8–15, 1998.

95. Bilik R, Shandling B, Pope M, et al: Malignant benign neonatal sacrococcygeal teratoma. J Pediatr Surg 28:1158–1160, 1993.

96. Ouimet A, Russo P: Fetus in fetu or not? J Pediatr Surg 24:926–927, 1989.

97. Norris HJ, Zirkin HJ, Benson WL: Immature (malignant) teratoma of the ovary: A clinical and pathologic study of 58 cases. Cancer 37:2359–2372, 1976.

98. Gilcrease MZ, Brandt ML, Hawkins EP: Yolk sac tumor identified at autopsy after surgical excision of immature sacrococcygeal teratoma. J Pediatr Surg 30:875–877, 1995.

99. Malogolowkin MH, Ortega JA, Kraila M, et al: Immature teratomas: Identification of patients at risk of malignant recurrence. J Natl Cancer Inst 81:870–874, 1989.

100. Hawkins EP, Isaacs H, Cushing B: Occult malignancy in neonatal sacrococcygeal teratomas: A report form a combined Pediatric Oncology Group and Children's Cancer Group Study. Am J Pediatr Hematol Oncol 15:406–409, 1993.

101. Gobel U, Schneider DT, Calaminus G, et al: Multimodal treatment of malignant sacrococcygeal germ cell tumors: A prospective analysis of 66 patients of the German cooperative protocols MAKEI 83/86 and 89. J Clin Oncol 19:1943–1950, 2001.

102. Rescorla FJ, Sawin RS, Coran AG, et al: Long-term outcome of infants and children with sacrococcygeal teratomas: A report from the Children's Cancer Group. J Pediatr Surg 33:171–176, 1998.

103. Marina NM, Cushing B, Giller R, et al. Complete surgical excision is effective treatment for children with immature teratomas with or without malignant elements: A Pediatric Oncology Group/Children's Cancer Group Intergroup Study. J Clin Oncol 17:2137–2143, 1999.

104. Malone PS, Spitz L, Kiely EM, et al: The functional sequelae of sacrococcygeal teratoma. J Pediatr Surg 25:679–680, 1990.

105. Havranek P, Hedlund H, Rubenson A, et al: Sacrococcygeal teratoma in Sweden between 1978 and 1989: Long-term functional results. J Pediatr Surg 27:916–918, 1992.

106. Boemers TML, van Gool JD, de Jong TPVM, et al: Lower urinary tract dysfunction in children with benign sacrococcygeal teratoma. J Urol 151:174–176, 1994.

107. Uchiyama M, Iwafuchi M, Naitoh M, et al: Sacrococcygeal teratoma: A series of 19 cases with long-term follow-up. Eur J Pediatr Surg 9:158–162, 1999.

108. Lewis BD, Hurt RD, Payne WS, et al: Benign teratomas of the mediastinum. J Thorac Cardiovasc Surg 86:727–731, 1983.

109. Liang RI, Wang P, Chang FM, et al: Prenatal sonographic characteristics and Doppler blood flow study in a case of a large fetal mediastinal teratoma. Ultrasound Obstet Gynecol 11:214–218, 1998.

110. Magu S, Rattan KN, Mishra DS: Posterior mediastinal teratomas. Indian J Pediatr 67:236–240, 2000.

111. Kaneko M, Ohkawa H, Iwakawa M, et al: Extensive epidural teratoma in early infancy treated by multi-stage surgery. Pediatr Surg Int 15:280–283, 1999.

112. Kuroiwa M, Suzuki N, Takahashi A, et al: Life-threatening mediastinal teratoma in a neonate. Pediatr Surg Int 17:235–238, 2001.

113. Matsubara K, Aoki M, Okumura N, et al: Spontaneous rupture of mediastinal cystic teratoma into the pleural cavity: Report of two cases and review of the literature. Pediatr Hematol Oncol 18:221–227, 2001.

114. Chaussain JL, Lemerle J, Roger M, et al: Klinefelter syndrome, tumor, and sexual precocity. J Pediatr 97:607–609, 1980.

115. Schneider DT, Calaminus G, Reinhard H, et al: Primary mediastinal germ cell tumors in children and adolescents: Results of the German cooperative protocols MAKEI 83/86, 89, 96. J Clin Oncol 18:832–839, 2000.

116. Nakajima K, Fukuzawa M, Minami M, et al: Videothoracoscopic resection of anterior mediastinal teratoma in a child: Report of a case. Surg Endosc 12:54–56, 1998.

117. Sumner TE, Crowe JE, Klein A, et al: Intrapericardial teratoma in infancy. Pediatr Radiol 10:51–53, 1980.

118. Pratt JW, Cohen DM, Mutabagani KH, et al: Neonatal intrapericardial teratoma: Clinical and surgical considerations. Cardiol Young 10:27–31, 2000.

119. Tollens T, Casselman F, Devlieger H, et al: Fetal cardiac tamponade due to an intrapericardial teratoma. Ann Thor Surg 66:559–560, 1998.

120. Tangthangtham A, Wongsangiem M, Koanantakool T, et al: Intrapulmonary teratoma: A report of three cases. J Med Assoc Thailand 81:1028–1033, 1998.

121. Augé D, Satgé D, Sauvage P, et al: Les tératomes rétropéritonecaux de la période néonatale. Ann Pediatr (Paris) 40:613–621, 1993.

122. Singer AJ, Anders KH. Primary teratoma if the kidney. Urology 58:1056–1057, 2001.

123. Federici S, Prestipino M, Domenichelli V, et al: Fetus in fetu: Report of an additional, well-developed case. Pediatr Surg Int 17:483–485, 2001.

124. Khadaroo RG, Evans MG, Honore LH, et al: Fetus-in-fetu presenting as cystic meconium peritonitis: Diagnosis, pathology, and surgical management. J Pediatr Surg 35:721–723, 2000.

125. Gupta DK, Srinivas M, Dave S, et al: Gastric teratoma in children. Pediatr Surg Int 16:329–332, 2000.

126. Senocak ME, Kale G, Buyukpamukcu N, et al: Gastric teratoma in children including the third reported female case. J Pediatr Surg 25:681–684, 1990.

127. Haley T, Dimler M, Hollier P: Gastric teratoma with gastrointestinal bleeding. J Pediatr Surg 21:949–950, 1986.

128. Coulson WF: Peritoneal gliomatosis from a gastric teratoma. Am J Clin Pathol 94:87–89, 1990.

129. Bourque CJ, Mackay AJ, Payton D: Malignant gastric teratoma: Case report. Pediatr Surg Int 12:192–193, 1997.

130. Shah RS, Kaddu SJ, Kirtane JM: Benign mature teratoma of the large bowel: A case report. J Pediatr Surg 31:701–702, 1996.

131. Misugi K, Reiner CB: A malignant true teratoma of liver in childhood. Arch Pathol 80:409–412, 1965.

132. Chiba T, Iwami D, Kikuchi Y: Mesenteric teratoma in an 8-month-old girl. J Pediatr Surg 30:120, 1995.

133. Cakmak O, Senel E, Erdogan D, et al: Ileal teratoma with multiple congenital anomalies. J Pediatr Surg 35:1370–1371, 2000.

134. Filston HC: Hemangiomas, cystic hygromas, and teratomas of the head and neck. Semin Pediatr Surg 3:147–159, 1994.

135. Kountakis SE, Minotti AM, Maillard A, et al: Teratomas of the head and neck. Am J Otolaryngol 15:292–296, 1994.

136. Schoenfeld A, Edelstein T, Joel-Cohen SJ: Prenatal ultrasonic diagnosis of the fetal teratoma of the neck. Br J Radiol 51:742–744, 1978.

137. Garmel SH, Crombleholme TM, Semple JP, et al: Prenatal diagnosis and management of fetal tumors. Semin Perinatal 18:350–365, 1994.

138. Byard RW, Jimenez CL, Caroebter BF, et al: Congenital teratomas of the neck and nasopharynx: A clinical and pathological study of 18 cases. J Pediatr Child Health 26:12–16, 1990.

139. Elmasalme F, Giacomantonio M, Clarke KD, et al: Congenital cervical teratoma in neonates: Case report and review. Eur J Pediatr Surg 10:252–257, 2000.

140. Ward RF, April M: Teratomas of the head and neck. Otolaryngol Clin North Am 22:621–629, 1989.

141. Langer JC, Tabb T, Thompson P, et al: Management of prenatally diagnosed tracheal obstruction: Access to the airway in utero prior to delivery. Fetal Diagn Ther 7:12–16, 1992.

142. Larsen ME, Larsen JW, Hamersley SL, et al: Successful management of fetal cervical teratoma using the EXIT procedure. J Matern Fetal Med 8:295–297, 1999.

143. Bouchard S, Johnson MP, Flake A, et al: The EXIT procedure: Experience and outcome in 31 cases. J Pediatr Surg 37:418–426, 2002.

144. Jordan RB, Gauderer MW: Cervical teratomas: An analysis: Literature review and proposed classification. J Pediatr Surg 23:583–591, 1988.

145. Chowdhary SK, Chitnis M, Perold J, et al: Hypothyroidism in a neonate following excision of a cervical teratoma. Pediatr Surg Int 14:212–213, 1998.

146. Keen CE, Said AJ, Agrawal M, et al: Congenital thyroid teratoma: A case with persistent neuroglial involvement of cervical lymph nodes. Pediatr Dev Pathol 1:322–327, 1998.

147. Craver RD, Lipscomb JT, Suskind D, et al: Malignant teratoma of the thyroid with primitive neuroepithelial and mesenchymal sarcomatous components. Ann Diagn Pathol 5:285–292, 2001.

148. Thompson LD, Rosai J, Heffess CS: Primary thyroid teratomas: A clinicopathologic study of 30 cases. Cancer 88:1149–1158, 2000.

149. Oliveira-Filho AG, Carvalho MH, Bustorff-Silva JM: Epignathus: Report of a case with successful outcome. J Pediatr Surg 33:520–521, 1998.

150. Wilson JW, Gehweiler JA: Teratoma of the face associated with a patent canal extending into the cranial cavity (Rathke's pouch) in a three-week-old child. J Pediatr Surg 5:349–359, 1970.

151. Coppit GL III, Perkins JA, Manning SC: Nasopharyngeal teratomas and dermoids: A review of the literature and case series. Int J Pediatr Otorhinolaryngol 52:219–227, 2000.

152. Sauter ER, Diaz JH, Arensman RM, et al: The perioperative management of neonates with congenital oropharyngeal teratomas. J Pediatr Surg 25:925–928, 1990.

153. Uchida K, Urata H, Suzuki H: Teratoma of the tongue in neonates: Report of a case and review of the literature. Pediatr Surg Int 14:79–81, 1998.

154. Jarrahy R, Cha ST, Mathiasen RA, et al: Congenital teratoma of the oropharyngeal cavity with intracranial extension: Case report and literature review. J Craniofacial Surg 11:106–112, 2000.

155. Lee GA, Sullivan TJ, Tsikleas GP, et al: Congenital orbital teratoma. Aust N Z J Ophthalmol 25:63–66, 1997.

156. Roncaroli F, Scheithauer BW, Pires MM, et al: Mature teratoma of the middle ear. Otol Neurotol 22:76–78, 2001.

157. Parnes LS, Sun AH: Teratoma of the middle ear. J Otolaryngol 24:165–167, 1995.

158. Odell JM, Allen JK, Badura RJ, et al: Massive congenital intracranial teratoma: A report of two cases. Pediatr Pathol 7:333–340, 1987.

159. Washburne JF, Magann EF, Chauhan SP, et al: Massive congenital intracranial teratoma with skull rupture at delivery. Am J Obstet Gynecol 173:226–228, 1995.

160. Hunt SJ, Johnson PC, Coons SW, et al: Neonatal intracranial teratomas. Surg Neurol 34:336–342, 1990.

161. Sawamura Y, Kato T, Ikeda J, et al: Teratomas of the central nervous system: Treatment considerations based on 34 cases. J Neurosurg 89:728–737, 1998.

162. Tobias S, Valarezo J, Meir K, et al: Giant cavernous sinus teratoma: A clinical example of a rare entity: Case report. Neurosurgery 48:1367–1370, 2001.

163. Chien YH, Tsao PN, Lee WT, et al: Congenital intracranial teratoma. Pediatr Neurol 22:72–74, 2000.

164. Jona JZ: Congenital anorectal teratoma: Report of a case. J Pediatr Surg 31:709–710, 1996.

165. Kreczy A, Alge A, Menardi G, et al: Teratoma of the umbilical cord: Case report with review of the literature. Arch Pathol Lab Med 118:934–937, 1994.

166. Pirodda A, Ferri GG, Truzzi M, et al: Benign cystic teratoma of the parotid gland. Otolaryngol Head Neck Surg 125:429–430, 2001.

167. Cakmak M, Savas C, Ozbasar D, et al: Congenital vulvar teratoma in newborn: J Pediatr Surg 36:620–121, 2001.

168. Hader WJ, Steinbok P, Poskitt K, et al: Intramedullary spinal teratoma and diastematomyelia: Case report and review of the literature. Pediatr Neurosurg 30:140–145, 1999.

169. Lever WF, Schaumburg-Lever G: Tumors and cysts of the epidermis. In Lever WF, Schaumburg-Lever G (eds): Histopathology of the Skin, 8th ed. Philadelphia, JB Lippincott, 1997, pp 698.

170. Mascaro JM, Torras H, Iranzo P: Cutaneous tumors in childhood. In Ruiz-Maldonado R, Parish LC, Beare JM (eds): Textbook of Pediatric Dermatology. Philadelphia, Grune & Stratton, 1989, pp 715–726.

171. Rowe MI, O'Neill JA, Grosfeld JL, et al: Miscellaneous skin lesions. In Rowe MI, O'Neill JA, Grosfeld JL, et al (eds): Essentials of Pediatric Surgery. St. Louis, CV Mosby, 1995, pp 819–828.

172. Hurwitz S: Cutaneous tumors in childhood. In Hurwitz S (ed): Clinical Pediatric Dermatology, 2nd ed. Philadelphia, WB Saunders, 1993, pp 198–241.

173. Baxter JW, Netsky MG: Epidermoid and dermoid tumors: Pathology. In Wilkins RH, Rengachary SS (eds): Neurosurgery. New York, McGraw-Hill, 1985, pp 655–661.

174. Enzinger FM, Weiss SW: Soft Tissue Tumors, 3rd ed. St. Louis, CV Mosby, 1995.

175. Webber BL, Parham DM: Soft tissue tumors other than rhabdomyosarcoma and peripheral neuroepithelioma. In Parham DM (ed): Pediatric Neoplasia: Morphology and Biology. Philadelphia, Lippincott-Raven, 1996, pp 205–218.

176. Dehner LP: Skin and supporting adnexae. In Dehner LP (ed): Pediatric Surgical Pathology, 2nd ed. Baltimore, Williams & Wilkins, 1987, pp 1–103.

177. Lindsay WK: Congenital defects of the skin, muscles, connective tissues, tendons, and hands. In Welch KJ, Randolph JG, Ravitch MM, et al (eds): Pediatric Surgery, Vol 2, 4th ed. Chicago, Year Book Medical, 1986, pp 1479–1499.

178. Cohen BA, Honig P, Androphy E: Anogenital warts in children. Arch Dermatol 126:1575–1580, 1990.

179. Schlecter R, Hartsough NA, Guttman FM: Multiple pilomatricomas (calcifying epitheliomas of Malherbe). Pediatr Dermatol 2:23–25, 1984.

180. Graham JK, McJimsey BA, Hardin JC: Nevoid basal cell carcinoma syndrome. Arch Otolaryngol Head Neck Surg 87:72–77, 1968.

181. Serra E, Purg S, Otero D, et al: Confirmation of a double-hit model for the NF-1 gene in benign neurofibromas. Am J Hum Genet 61:512–519, 1997.

182. Friedman JM, Birch PH: Type 1 neurofibromatosis: A descriptive analysis of the disorder in 1,728 patients. Am J Med Genet 70:138–143, 1997.

183. Drouin V, Marret S, Petitcolas J, et al: Prenatal US abnormalities in a patient with generalized neurofibromatosis type 1. Neuropediatrics 28:120–121, 1997.

184. Pujol RM, Matias-Buiu X, Miralles J, et al: Multiple idiopathic mucosal neuromas: A minor form of multiple endocrine neoplasia type 2B or a new entity? J Am Acad Dermatol 37:349–352, 1997.

185. Adkins JC, Ravitch MM: Neurofibromatosis-Von Recklinghausen's disease. In Welch KJ, Randolph JG, Ravitch MM, et al (eds): Pediatric Surgery, Vol 2, 5th ed. Chicago, Year Book Medical, 1998, pp 1914–1916.

186. Hamanaka S, Hamanaka Y, Yamashita Y, et al: Leiomyoblastoma and leiomyomatosis of the small intestine in a case of Von Recklinghausen's disease. J Dermatol 24:117–119, 1997.

187. Raney RB, Littman P, Jarrett P, et al: Results of multimodal therapy for children with neurogenic sarcoma. Med Pediatr Oncol 7:229, 1979.

188. Chu JY, O'Connor DM, Danis RK: Neurofibrosarcoma at irradiation site in a patient with neurofibromatosis and Wilms' tumor. Cancer 31:333–335, 1981.

189. Mulvihill JJ: Childhood cancer, the environment and heredity. In Pizzo PA, Poplack DG (eds): Principles and Practice of Pediatric Oncology, 2nd ed. Philadelphia, JB Lippincott, 1993, pp 11–29.

190. Dehner LP: Soft tissue, peritoneum, and retroperitoneum. In Dehner LP (ed): Pediatric Surgical Pathology, 2nd ed. Baltimore, Williams & Wilkins, 1987, pp 869–938.

191. Enzinger FM, Weiss SW: Benign fibrous tissue tumors. In Enzinger FM, Weiss SW (eds): Soft Tissue Tumors, 3rd ed. St. Louis, CV Mosby, 1995, pp 165–199.

192. Triche TJ, Sorensen PHB: Molecular pathology of pediatric malignancies. In Pizzo PA, Poplack DG (eds): Principles and Practice of Pediatric Oncology, 4th ed. Philadelphia, Lippincott Williams & Wilkins, 2002, pp 190–192.

193. Enzinger FM, Weiss SW: Benign tumors of peripheral nerves. In Enzinger FM, Weiss SW (eds): Soft Tissue Tumors, 3rd ed. St. Louis, CV Mosby, 1995, pp 871–872.

194. Hurwitz S: Tumors of fat, muscles, and bone. In Hurwitz S (ed): Clinical Pediatric Dermatology, 2nd ed. Philadelphia, WB Saunders, 1993, p 233.

195. Rosai J: Soft tissues. In Rosai J (ed): Ackerman's Surgical Pathology, 8th ed. St. Louis, CV Mosby, 1996, pp 2021–2135.

196. Azzarelli A, Grinchi A, Bertulli R, et al: Low-dose chemotherapy with methotrexate and vinblastine for patients with advanced aggressive fibromatosis. Cancer 92:1259–1264, 2001.

197. Mace J, Biermann JS, Sandak V, et al: Response of extra-abdominal desmoid tumours to therapy with imatinib mesylate. Cancer 95:2373–2379, 2002.

198. Enzinger FM, Weiss SW: Fibromatoses. In Enzinger FM, Weiss SW (eds): Soft Tissue Tumors, 3rd ed. St. Louis, CV Mosby, 1995, pp 201–229.

199. Hardell L, Breivald M, Hennerdal S, et al: Shrinkage of desmoid tumor with interferon alpha treatment: A case report. Cytokine Cell Mol Ther 6:155-156, 2000.

200. Miller GG, Yanchar NL, Magee JF, et al: Lipoblastoma and liposarcoma in children: An analysis of 9 cases and review of the literature. Can J Surg 41:455–458, 1998.

201. Dehner LP: Bone and joints. In Dehner LP (ed): Pediatric Surgical Pathology, 2nd ed. Baltimore, Williams & Wilkins, 1987, pp 939–1025.

202. Enzinger FM, Weiss SW: Benign soft tissue tumors of uncertain type. In Enzinger FM, Weiss SW (eds): Soft Tissue Tumors, 3rd ed. St. Louis, CV Mosby, 1995, pp 1039–1066.

203. Rosai J: Bones and joints. In Rosai J (ed): Ackerman's Surgical Pathology, 8th ed. St. Louis, CV Mosby, 1996, pp 1917–2020.

204. Angelides AC: Ganglions of the hand and wrist. In Green DP (ed): Operative Hand Surgery, 3rd ed. New York, Churchill Livingstone, 1993, pp 2157–2172.

205. Buck P, Mickelson MR, Bonfiglo M: Synovial sarcoma: Review of 33 cases. Clin Orthop 156:211–215, 1981.

206. Varela-Duran J, Enzinger FM: Calcifying synovial sarcoma. Cancer 50:345–352, 1982.

CHAPTER 69

Lymphomas

Alan S. Gamis, MD, MPH

INTRODUCTION

Lymphomas are a result of chromosomal alterations resulting in the uncontrolled growth of cells of lymphoid origin. Among all ages, lymphomas constitute just 4% of all cancer diagnosed annually in the United States,[1] yet in children, this percentage increases to 11%.[2] Combined, Hodgkin's and non-Hodgkin's lymphoma are the second most common childhood solid tumors (behind brain tumors and ahead of neuroblastoma) and specifically make up 15% of all childhood solid tumors diagnosed annually. Almost 1200 new childhood cases are diagnosed each year, or 15 new cases/million children/year. Lymphomas have classically been divided into two distinct groups, Hodgkin's lymphoma (or disease; HD) and non-Hodgkin's lymphoma (NHL). Both *typically* are initially seen with enlarged lymph nodes and may have systemic symptoms of fever and fatigue, and/or extra lymphatic spread. However, these two types of lymphoma also have clear differences. HD typically is seen as an indolent process, whereas NHL most often is first seen in children with symptoms of rapid onset. Because of this propensity for rapid growth, children with NHL often have associated anatomic and metabolic comorbidities of such a degree that their recognition and need for treatment constitutes a medical emergency. With HD, treatment is based primarily on staging and less on histologic subtype, whereas the treatment of NHL, with improved diagnostic pathology, now critically depends on the histologic and immunophenotypic subtypes in addition to stage. As is evident, these two lymphomas are truly a study of contrasts. This is no more evident than in the evolution of their therapy. HD has been for years one of the most curable cancers. Now, with markedly improved treatment protocols, NHL has nearly equivalent cure rates.[3] Owing to the historic high survival with HD, its therapy has focused on the reduction of intensity. NHL therapy has, because of its previously poor prognosis, focused on intensification of therapy. It is the use of higher doses of chemotherapy over a short period

(as compared with prior methods) that has resulted in the dramatic improvement in cure of NHL. Although most histologic types of HD are treated similarly, it is essential to classify fully the subtype of NHL, as marked differences occur in the effective therapies administered for each. In considering the surgeon's role in the therapy of childhood lymphomas, essentially no differences in approach exist between the two types of lymphomas. However, in contrast to other solid tumors of childhood, in which initial resection of tumor is important, the primary role of the surgeon in the initial management of lymphomas is to ensure the rapid attainment of adequate and properly preserved biopsy material to allow the pathologist the opportunity to make the diagnosis of the *specific type and subtype* of lymphoma. Except for certain situations, attempts to resect lymphomas at the time of presentation have no role in the modern management of lymphomas.

HODGKIN'S LYMPHOMA

Thomas Hodgkin, in his classic thesis, "On some Morbid Appearances of the Absorbent Glands and Spleen," in 1832, noted the gross necropsy examinations of seven patients. He described the association of generalized lymphadenopathy and splenomegaly in 6 patients without evidence of infection or inflammation.[4] Histologic descriptions of the Reed-Sternberg cell, the pathognomonic multinucleated giant cell, had to await the turn of the century.[5,6] Even though the etiology was unclear, therapeutic interventions began soon after the discovery of x-rays. More successful application of radiation therapy awaited the description of the disease's propensity for contiguous spread. With this understanding, in the late 1930s, application of radiation to the involved and adjacent nodal areas (extended-field technique) resulted in improvements in survival.[7] In the early 1960s, in acknowledgment of the limitations of the then current radiologic techniques, the practice began of systematic laparotomy, splenectomy, celiac node and liver biopsy at the time of initial presentation for the purpose of staging and targeted therapy.[8] This has properly been described *as the model for the careful staging of cancer as a required prerequisite to the design of therapy,* which is a hallmark of oncologic practice today.[9] The reader is referred to more detailed reviews of these early investigations.[9,10] During this same time, chemotherapy combinations entered into the physician's armamentarium. With their use, remission and cure rates markedly improved. The improvement has made HD one of the most curable cancers today, with rates typically exceeding 90% for patients with nondisseminated disease. With this high expectation for cure, attention over the last decade in pediatric oncology has been focused on the reduction of long-term sequelae of treatment. To this end, chemotherapy has evolved from an adjunctive role to a primary one, with the hope of eliminating the need for radiation (and its attendant sequelae) altogether. Where radiation is called for, if used in combination with chemotherapy, the focus has been to reduce the size of the fields (from extended to involved) and the doses used. The two classic chemotherapy combinations (MOPP: nitrogen *m*ustard, vincristine [*O*ncovin], *p*rocarbazine, *p*rednisone; and ABVD: doxorubicin [*A*driamycin], *b*leomycin, *v*inblastine, *d*acarbazine) have evolved to reduce long-term sequelae. Hybrids of these have evolved to reduce the doses delivered to the patient, with equivalent results and less toxicity.

Incidence and Epidemiology

Among all ages, 7500 individuals each year are diagnosed with HD in the United States, accounting for just 0.5% of all cancers and only 12% of all lymphomas.[1] However, in children, it is the sixth most common type of cancer, with approximately 500 children annually diagnosed.[2] This constitutes 5% of all childhood cases of cancer and 44% of all childhood cases of lymphoma. HD has an incidence rate of 6.6 cases/million children age 15 years or younger/year. A bimodal distribution exists when considering all ages, but in children alone, a gradual trend is seen of increasing incidence with increasing age. It is exceedingly rare in children younger than 2 years and peaks in the adolescent years.[2] Beyond age 11 years, it is the most common of the two types of lymphoma. A slight male predominance (1.32:1) is noted, although in the youngest children, the male/female ratio is much larger (12–19:1).[2,11] HD occurs more often in whites than in blacks (1.55:1). Familial clusters of HD have been reported. Whether this represents risk due to environmental exposure (most often thought to be infectious) or genetics is uncertain. Monozygotic twins of HD patients have been found to be at greater risk of developing HD than are dizygotic twins,[12] strongly implicating genetics as a principal risk factor. Conversely, again in young adults, an increased risk of HD is found with higher socioeconomic status.[13] Young adults with HD come from smaller families, have fewer infectious exposures as young children, and/or have later exposure to infections than do control populations.[13,14] This correlates closely with socioeconomic

status and implicates a delayed infectious exposure as a principal risk factor. Most likely, a combination of genetic risk and infectious exposure predisposes a young adult to HD. Immunodeficiency may be the link between these two risk factors, at least in a subgroup of HD patients. HD is more prevalent in human immunodeficiency virus (HIV)-infected patients,[15–17] and patients with HD have a higher incidence of cellular immunodeficiency at the time of diagnosis.[18] Etiologic theories encompass these two risk factors and focus primarily on the Epstein-Barr virus (EBV). Genomic material from EBV has been found in the Reed-Sternberg (RS) cells in up to 79% of HD cases.[19–21] This has the highest association with the subtypes, mixed cellularity, and nodular sclerosis.[22] This also correlates with the higher risk of HD in individuals with a history of infectious mononucleosis[23–25] and with previously high titers to EBV.[26] In one recent report,[25] epidemiologic investigations identified a median incubation time of 4.1 years (95% confidence interval, 1.8 to 8.3 years) between infectious mononucleosis and the development of EBV-positive HD. One hypothesis that incorporates these factors suggests the following sequence: (1) either a genetic, iatrogenic, or viral immunosuppression; (2) subsequently or coincidentally, an EBV infection or oncogenetic rearrangement in a lymphoid precursor cell; (3) further genetic alterations; followed by (4) clonal expansion of lymphoid cells with morphologic features of RS cells, finally resulting in (5) the clinical syndrome known as HD, diagnosed by the presence of RS cells.[27]

Cell Biology

Diagnosis of HD requires the dual finding of the diagnostic RS cell and a reactive cellular background.[28] The RS cell is a large cell (15 to 45 μm) with an "owl's eye" appearance. It has a multilobed nucleus (or is multinucleated), each with a prominent eosinophilic nucleolus surrounded by a clear zone (halo) and an intensely stained nuclear membrane. The "owl's eye" appearance is the result of a bilobed nucleus. The RS cell often makes up no more than 2% of the involved tissues. The cellular background is a reactive, pleomorphic mixture of inflammatory cells including reactive lymphocytes, histiocytes, plasma cells, eosinophils, neutrophils, and fibroblasts, with varying degrees of fibrosis and sclerosis. The RS cell is thought to be the neoplastic cell in HD and is thought to induce this reactive background through the abundant release of various cytokines.[29] The origin of the RS cell until recently remained elusive because of its paucity in sampled tissue; however, research now indicates that they are derived from germinal center B lymphocytes that are clonal in all cases and have lost their immunoglobulin gene transcription ability.[30,31] Two immunophenotypes of RS cells have been identified: type I, or L&H cells, seen in lymphocyte-predominant HD manifesting CD20 and J-chain expression; and type II, seen in the other histologic types grouped under the rubric, classic HD, manifesting CD30 and CD15. Extensive reviews of the RS cell and its biology have recently been published.[27,32]

For histologic typing, the Rye classification is in common use and divides HD into four primary morphologic classifications: nodular sclerosing (NS, the most common), mixed cellularity (MC), lymphocyte predominant (LPHD), and lymphocyte depleted (LDHD).[33] The NS subtype is seen in 40% of younger patients and 70% of adolescents.[34] It is characterized by tumor nodules surrounded by broad sclerotic bands arising from a thickened fibrotic capsule.[28] This subtype has a strong predilection for involvement of the lower cervical, supraclavicular, and mediastinal lymph nodes. The MC subtype is found in 30% of cases and has an increased incidence in younger children.[11] RS cells are typically increased in number. The lymph node architecture is often completely effaced by the RS cells and their surrounding reactive cells. This subtype often is first seen with advanced, widely disseminated disease in extranodal sites. In addition to its relatively common incidence among all HD patients, it is the most common histologic type seen in HIV-infected patients.[17] The LPHD subtype is seen in 10% to 15% of children diagnosed with HD. This is typically seen in younger patients and often is first seen with localized disease. A cellular proliferation of benign-appearing lymphocytes is seen, with an occasional, rare RS cell. This subtype can be misdiagnosed as reactive hyperplasia. The LDHD subtype is rare in children but is common in HIV patients.[35] Histologically, rare lymphocytes are found, with many RS cells and numerous, bizarre, malignant reticular cells. This type often initially is seen with widespread disease involving the bone and bone marrow (BM). From 1978 to 1986, the National Cancer Institute (NCI)-sponsored SEER data revealed the following patient 5-year survival rates by histologic subtype: lymphocyte predominant, 83.9%; nodular sclerosing, 82.2%; mixed cellularity, 68.1%; and lymphocyte depleted, 36.4%.[36] Recent reports have now shown that LPHD has a better prognosis with markedly reduced therapy to achieve cure.[37,38] This differentiation of therapeutic response between LPHD and the other classic HD histologic types appears to validate the distinction observed in the immunophenotyped RS cells[32] and the recent proposed classification system, the Revised European-American Classification of Lymphoid Neoplasms (REAL).[39] Clinical trials are now being developed to explore this difference further and to examine whether reduced therapy for LPHD is possible. The poorer outcome of the MC and LDHD types may reflect their typically higher stage at diagnosis.

Clinical Presentation

Children are first seen with painless enlarged lymph nodes, typically in the cervical or supraclavicular nodal groups (Table 69-1). Nodes are often described as rubbery and fixed, and they may be either single or matted with other nodes. Occasionally, because of rapid growth, tenderness may be present. Tumor lysis syndrome, a result of rapid and extensive tumor growth and a common complication in children with NHL, is rarely seen in children with HD.

TABLE 69-1

HODGKIN'S DISEASE: SITES OF INVOLVEMENT AT THE TIME OF INITIAL DIAGNOSIS

Nodal Sites	Histologic Subtype (%)			
	NS	MC/LD	LP	All
Mediastinum	73	46	8	59
Cervical	55–62	53–60	41–46	55–58
Axillary	11–15	14–16	13–14	13–14
Hilar	14–15	8–9	3–5	11–12
Upper neck	4	4	14	5
Epitrochlear	1	1	6	2
Spleen	24	35	17	27
Upper abdomen	13	18	5	14
Lower abdomen	8	17	8	11
Inguinal	1	3	10	2–3

Adapted from Mauch PM, Kalish LA, Kadin M, et al: Patterns of Hodgkin disease: Implications for etiology and pathogenesis. Cancer 71:2062–2071, 1993.

HD tends to spread in a contiguous manner, and thus at presentation, one must examine carefully the groups adjacent to the initially identified involved groups. More than 90% of patients have involvement of either the cervical or mediastinal nodal groups or both.[40] Interestingly, HD tends to spread from the cervical nodes of one side of the neck to the mediastinum before it spreads to the contralateral cervical nodes. When surgical laparotomy is included in the staging process, the spleen is noted to be involved in 27% of patients.[40] When evaluating histologic subtypes and patterns of initial involvement, it is clear from Table 69-1 that the MC and LPHD have more widespread involvement than do the NS or LPHD subtypes.

Mediastinal disease, in addition to a predilection to certain histologic subtypes, is most common in children older than 12 years, in girls, and in those with constitutional symptoms (also known as B symptoms).[41] Mediastinal disease may appear with significant respiratory compromise due to compression of the trachea or carina or both, including the major bronchi.[42] These patients may have dyspnea on exertion, shortness of breath at rest, persistent cough, or stridor. They may have recently been treated for presumed asthma or bronchiolitis, without radiographic examination. Patients with this also may have a history of orthopnea and are most comfortable in an upright forward-leaning position to relieve the pressure on the airway (from the *anterior* mediastinal mass). The physician must be vigilant for mediastinal disease, as it may be silent until a patient is sedated for radiologic or surgical procedures. These patients may prove impossible to aerate even with intubation because of distal major airway obstruction. It is imperative that all patients with suspected lymphoma (HD *or* NHL) have a chest radiograph before *any* sedation or procedure. These patients may also have signs of superior vena caval obstruction. Extralymphatic involvement can include the liver (the most common extralymphatic organ involved), lungs, bone, BM, and skin, among other sites. Whereas BM involvement is present in only 4% to 14% of patients overall, among those patients with stage IV disease, it is present 32% of the time.[43] Most patients have no systemic symptoms at the time of initial diagnosis. About one fourth of patients will have one or more B symptoms, including weight loss of more than 10% in the previous 6 months, unexplained fevers of more than 38°C, or night sweats.[40] Pruritus, fatigue, and anorexia are other nonspecific symptoms seen in HD patients. Laboratory findings in patients at diagnosis are nonspecific and typically are indicative of an inflammatory process. The erythrocyte sedimentation rate (ESR), serum copper, and ferritin levels are frequently elevated and may be monitored later for evidence of relapse. A high ferritin (>142 ng/mL) level or ESR (>50) has been associated with a worse prognosis.[44,45] Lactate dehydrogenase (LDH) may be elevated as well. Although not common, leukopenia may be indicative of BM involvement.[43] Anemia and thrombocytopenia, other infrequent symptoms, may be either due to marrow involvement with HD or due to immune cytopenias (idiopathic thrombocytopenic purpura [ITP] and Coombs-positive hemolytic anemia) occasionally seen in HD patients.[46,47]

Diagnosis

The diagnostic evaluation should include physical examination and laboratory and radiologic studies (Table 69-2). Physical examination should be directed to the obviously involved nodal groups and also to those adjacent groups, keeping in mind the natural history of HD and its propensity for contiguous spread. The number of involved nodal groups in stage II patients (more than four) has been associated with a worse prognosis and should be carefully determined.[48] The size of the palpated nodal masses should be estimated and recorded. Bulky disease (nodes or nodal aggregates >10 cm and/or mediastinal tumor width more than one third of intrathoracic width on a posteroanterior [PA] chest radiograph or computed tomography [CT]) is associated with worse outcome in low-stage patients and necessitates additional therapy to achieve equivalent outcomes.[49-51] Auscultation of the airway, palpation of the abdomen, and examination of distant nodal groups are critical as well. Laboratory examination should include full blood counts and chemistries, including hepatic function tests, LDH, and ESR. Serum copper and ferritin levels also may be obtained. However, no clinical findings are pathognomonic for HD. Ultimately, the diagnosis awaits the biopsy of involved sites, most commonly an excised lymph node. It is here that the diagnosis is made, based on the pathognomonic finding of RS cells within a reactive cellular background. It is critical for the excised tissue to be quickly delivered to the pathologist for processing. For cytogenetic and molecular genetic evaluations, it is imperative that all tissues be placed in a sterile container for fresh samples. Formalin should never be used. For patients critically ill at diagnosis, such as those with severe airway obstruction, diagnosis by alternative methods should be strongly considered. These may include nodal biopsy with local anesthetic alone, CT-guided percutaneous needle biopsy of the mass, aspiration of pleural effusion, or a BM biopsy and aspirate.

Staging

Further evaluation of a patient with HD is required to determine the extent of disease accurately at diagnosis and thus the stage of disease (Table 69-3). The common staging system in use for the assessment of extent of disease in HD was adopted in 1971.[52] This system is based on the observation of contiguous nodal spread in HD. Patients are further divided into asymptomatic (A) and

---

TABLE 69-2

HODGKIN'S DISEASE: DIAGNOSTIC AND STAGING EVALUATION AT PRESENTATION

Complete physical examination with documentation of involved nodal groups (including measurements of nodes), and involved extralymphatic organs

Complete blood count (CBC), chemistry panel including hepatic function tests, ESR, copper, ferritin, LDH

Chest radiography to evaluate for possible mediastinal disease and airway compression

CT scans of areas identified on physical examination (also include chest, neck, and abdomen)

Positron emission tomography (PET) scan

Gallium scan

Bone scan

Excisional biopsy of node

Bone marrow biopsies and aspirates (bilateral)

Lymphangiogram (optional)

Staging laporatomy (mandatory if considering radiation therapy alone) with splenectomy, nodal sampling, and wedge biopsies of hepatic lobes

CT, computed tomography; ESR, erythrocyte sedimentation rate; LDH, lactate dehydrogenase.

TABLE 69-3

ANN ARBOR STAGING CLASSIFICATION FOR HODGKIN'S DISEASE

Stage	Definition
I	Involvement of a single lymph node region (I) or of a single extralymphatic organ or site (I_E)
II	Involvement of two or more lymph node regions on the same side of the diaphragm (II) or localized involvement of an extralymphatic organ or site and its regional lymph node(s) with involvement of one or more lymph node regions on the same side of the diaphragm (II_E)
III	Involvement of lymph node regions on both sides of the diaphragm (III), which may be accompanied by involvement of the spleen (III_S) or by localized involvement of an extralymphatic organ or site (III_E) or both (III_{SE})
IV	Disseminated (multifocal) involvement of one or more extralymphatic organs or tissues with or without associated lymph node involvement or isolated extralymphatic organ involvement with distant (nonregional) nodal involvement

Adapted from Carbone PP, Kaplan, HS, Husshoff K, et al. Report of the committee on Hodgkin's disease staging classification. Cancer Res 31:1860-1861, 1971.

symptomatic (B) subcategories. This subclassification for symptomatic patients is based on the findings of a worse prognosis for B patients and the need for a systemic therapy approach in them (i.e., chemotherapy in addition to radiation). This likely reflects the finding that patients with B symptoms are more apt to have distant, widespread disease when pathologically staged.[53]

For HD, the decision for the method and the extent or intensity of therapy, or both, rests on the staging results. Traditionally, two types of staging were used in HD patients, clinical and pathological. Until recently, all patients underwent both methods. Clinical staging (CS) includes physical, laboratory, and radiologic evaluations. Pathological staging (PS) goes one step further with the use of a staging laparotomy with splenectomy, nodal sampling, and wedge biopsies of hepatic lobes. The radiologic evaluations have been in evolution over the past decade. Lymphangiograms, once a critical component of staging in HD, have been supplanted by more modern and less invasive imaging modalities. CT examination is used most frequently.[54] For those who will be treated with radiation alone, accurate assessment of abdominal disease is critical. Staging laparotomy with splenectomy, nodal sampling, and wedge biopsies of hepatic lobes has been shown to increase the stage of disease in up to 35% of patients initially evaluated with CT[55,56] (i.e., the difference between CS and PS). This would seem to demand that laparotomy be continued. However, again, with the use of systemic chemotherapy and the de-emphasis on radiation, this no longer appears to have a significant impact on treatment or outcome.[57,58] Staging laparotomy should continue to be used in patients destined to be treated with radiation alone (although this is now rare in children), as finding abdominal disease would have a significant impact on planned therapy.[59] Staging laparotomy with splenectomy is not without its risks. These are the typical postoperative complications of abdominal surgery and, because of splenectomy, the life-long risk of overwhelming sepsis with encapsulated organisms. These patients require life-long antibiotic prophylaxis.[60] An increased risk of secondary leukemia also exists in those HD patients treated with chemotherapy who have had splenectomy (5.9% vs. 0.7% in those who have not) as part of their staging laparotomy.[61-63] Nuclear medicine scans are another method of evaluation that is increasing in use in HD patients. Although early studies of gallium scanning found its value suspect,[64,65] it has its greatest impact in identifying unrecognized sites of disease at presentation and for following up disease regression during and after therapy. This is especially true for patients with mediastinal disease. Patients with nodular sclerosing subtypes will often have persistently enlarged cervical and mediastinal nodes due to scar tissue. Although these are enlarged on CT, negative gallium scans (in patients in whom these sites were gallium avid at presentation) indicate a non-neoplastic cause (i.e., residual scar tissue).[66,67] It has been suggested that this is most accurately predictive in initially low-stage patients (I or II, 92.4% negative predictive value) and less so in advanced disease patients (III or IV, 64.5%).[68] In children, it is important also to recognize the phenomena of thymic rebound after therapy. This may result in both an enlarging mediastinal mass on CT and a positive gallium scan. An experienced radiologist will recognize this phenomenon by its timing (within the first 6 months after therapy has been completed) and by the normal (although enlarged) homogeneous appearance of the thymic tissue. However, false-negative interpretations can occur, and so close follow-up of these patients is critical. Recent shortages of gallium have made this examination more problematic. However, fluorodeoxyglucose–positron emission tomography (FDG-PET) over the past several years has been extensively examined to assess its role in the evaluation of lymphoma patients at diagnosis as well as after therapy.[69-71] It is becoming increasingly clear that it will likely supplant gallium scans in the near future. It is more sensitive and specific than either gallium or CT,[69-72] and similar to gallium scanning, it leads to a higher staging in a significant percentage of patients. FDG-PET imaging during and after therapy as well has been highly predictive of patient outcome[73,74] and helps to differentiate residual scar tissue from residual lymphoma,[75] although false positives with inflammatory conditions have been reported. The reader is referred to a more extensive review of this topic.[74] More experience with this new modality is required before it can be solely relied on, and thus its use in conjunction with conventional imaging is advised. The BM examination continues to be important, regardless of planned methods of therapy, as its involvement would upgrade the patient to a stage IV status and thus necessitate much more intensive chemotherapy.

Treatment

Principles of Therapy

Several strategies of therapy have been effective in the treatment of HD. These have included radiation therapy alone, combinations of radiation and chemotherapy, and most recently, chemotherapy without radiation. For children in particular, four themes guide modern HD therapy. For those with early or low-stage HD (I to III), reduction of therapy duration and intensity to reduce long-term sequelae (while maintaining the current high cure rates) is a central principle in today's regimen designs. In concert with this, the second theme is the reduction and eventual elimination of radiation as a method of therapy in children with early or low-stage HD. The third theme and most recent is response-based therapy. This, again, to reduce therapy for those who do not require additional doses, adjusts or eliminates anticipated cycles of chemotherapy based on the tumor's response to the initial courses of therapy. For those with advanced-stage HD (IV), the fourth theme is the intensification of therapy and identification of new and more effective regimens to increase relapse-free survival. Finally, advances in pediatric oncology have been substantial. This is primarily due to the overwhelming majority of children being enrolled or registered with the NCI-sponsored cooperative groups (Children's Cancer Group [CCG] and Pediatric Oncology Group [POG] now merged into the Children's Oncology Group [COG]).

Children, including adolescents, diagnosed with HD should be referred to, and their treatment coordinated through, one of the many centers associated with this group. These children, through participation in the clinical trials, receive the most advanced and effective therapy available today (Table 69-4).

Principles of Radiation Therapy in the Treatment of HD

Despite the goal of eliminating radiation from the therapeutic regimens for early stage HD in children, it must be recognized that HD is a very radiosensitive neoplasm. A long record of efficacy exists in using radiation either alone or in combination with chemotherapy regimens for this neoplasm. Radiation therapy has traditionally been given to the sites of disease and contiguous, clinically uninvolved, areas. This is known as extended-field (EF) radiation. Various fields of therapy have evolved and include the: preauricular (Waldeyer's ring) field, the supradiaphragmatic mantle field (submandibular, submental, cervical, supraclavicular, infraclavicular, axillary, mediastinal, and pulmonary hilar nodal groups), subdiaphragmatic field (splenic pedicle, spleen, para-aortic nodal groups), and two pelvic fields, inverted Y (common iliac, external iliac, inguinal-femoral nodal groups) or spade (inverted Y, excluding those nodes below the common iliac group). More recently, involved field (IF) radiation has become more widely used. This is a more attractive option where chemotherapy also is used.

In this setting in children, IF has been shown to provide excellent local control (97%).[76] A recent study from Germany identified that not only was the remission and disease-free survival no different between IF and EF, but also side effects (leucopenia, thrombocytopenia, nausea, GI toxicity, and pharyngeal toxicity) were significantly reduced when using only IF.[77] Finally, a shrinking-field technique is used when possible. This uses repeated measurements to reduce the field continually as the primary tumor shrinks.

Megavoltage therapy is used in modern radiation practice, preferentially with a 4- to 8-MeV linear accelerator. This reduces the scatter irradiation seen with cobalt 60. Doses used when radiation is the sole modality are typically 4000 to 4400 cGy to clinically involved sites and 3000 to 4000 cGy to clinically uninvolved areas. Recent evidence suggests reductions to 3500 cGy with modern megavoltage techniques may as well be effective.[78,79] Further reduction in radiation dosage to less than 2500 cGy, when used in conjunction with systemic chemotherapy, is possible.[76,80]

The use of radiation therapy alone remains an option of therapy in adults with low-stage (I to III) HD (78% to 89% relapse-free survival [RFS], 88% to 100% overall survival [OS], median 4- to 5-year follow-up), as it allows them the opportunity to avoid the toxicity associated with chemotherapy.[81-84] Even if relapse occurs in those treated with only radiation, the ability to salvage a long-term cure does not appear to be compromised by delaying the use of chemotherapy until the first relapse. Radiation also has

TABLE 69-4
THERAPEUTIC REGIMENS FOR CHILDREN WITH HODGKIN'S DISEASE

Chemotherapy Agents	Stage	Radiation	Radiation Dose	DFS %	OS %	Ref.
None	PSI–IIB	EF	≥3500 cGy	67–82	86–96	84,85,86
		IF		41	95	
	CSI–IIB	IF		79–85	96–98	
MOPP	I–II	IF	<2500 cGy	96	100	76,108
	III–IV			84	78	
	IV	EF	33–4400 cGy	69	78	
COP/ABVD	II	IF	<2000 cGy	96	96	112
	III			97	100	
	IV			85	86	
MOPP/ABVD	I–II	IF	2–4000 cGy	89	—	105
	III			82		
	IV			62		
MOPP/ABVD	I–III	IF	1500–2500 cGy	100	100	106
	IV			69	85	
MOPP/ABVD	IIB–IV	TNI	2100 cGy	77	91	110
MOPP/ABV	II–IV	IF	3500 cGy	93	90	111
COPP/ABV	I–IV	IF	<2500 cGy	100	100	113
OPPA	I–IIA	IF	3500 cGy	98	100	114
ABVD	III–IV	IF	21–3500 cGy	87	89	109
BEACOPP	II–IV	IF	3–4000 cGy*	87	91	100
Stanford V	I–II	IF	3600 cGy*	97	—	102
	III–IV			85		

MOPP, Nitrogen mustard, vincristine, prednisone, procarbazine; ABVD, doxorubicin (Adriamycin), bleomycin, vinblastine, DTIC; OPPA, vincristine, prednisone, procarbazine, doxorubicin (Adriamycin), C, cyclophosphamide; BEACOPP, bleomycin, etoposide, doxorubicin (Adriamycin), cyclophosphamide, vincristine, procarbazine, prednisone; Stanford V, vinblastine, doxorubicin (Adriamycin), vincristine, bleomycin, nitrogen mustard, etoposide, prednisone; EF, extended field radiation; IF, involved field radiation; TNI, total nodal irradiation; cGy, centigray (1 cGy = 1 rad); CR, complete remission; DFS, disease-free survival; OS, overall survival; ref, references.
*Radiation given to sites of bulky disease present at diagnosis.

been effective in children when used alone (79% to 85% RFS),[85] although conflicting results were seen in a large multi-institutional study (41% to 67% RFS).[86]

For pediatrics, however, the severe and life-long side effects of radiation (cosmetic defects, growth retardation, endocrinologic sequelae, and secondary malignancy) on a growing and developing child are a compelling reason to look for alternative methods. Appreciation for these sequelae has led to the gradual reduction in the dose and in the size of the field treated. More recently, the focus has been to eliminate radiation completely in the treatment of children with HD. A recent adult study suggests that this may be possible for those individuals who achieve a complete response (CR) with four cycles of chemotherapy.[87] To this end, except for a small subgroup of children with HD, chemotherapy combinations are the principal method of treatment in children, and radiation, if used, is given in low doses and to limited areas.[88] The small subgroup of children in whom radiation alone may still be considered for front-line therapy are the fully grown adolescent boys with localized disease (I to IIA). Circumvention of chemotherapy in this particular group avoids the reduced fertility that is a particular concern in boys, related to the alkylating agents. As well, the adolescent's growth is complete, and radiation will therefore not result in permanent cosmetic deformities (i.e., arrest of bone growth). However, even for this group of boys, new regimens that no longer contain alkylating agents have shown excellent efficacy when used in combination with low-dose radiation.[78] Because of worries about secondary breast cancer, radiation therapy alone for adolescent girls should be given only after strong consideration of the increased risk of breast cancer known to result from irradiation of the breast tissue at this critical age.[89-93]

Principles of Chemotherapy

Chemotherapy is the therapeutic backbone for children with both early and advanced-stage HD. A large number of chemotherapy combinations have been used for HD. For years, two regimens have been the most widely and effectively used combinations for patients with early-stage HD. MOPP (nitrogen mustard, vincristine [Oncovin], prednisone, procarbazine) or ABVD (doxorubicin [Adriamycin], bleomycin, vinblastine, dacarbazine [DTIC]) was administered over a 12-month period and resulted in excellent outcomes.[94,95] However, these combinations have proven to have significant long-term sequelae when administered in full doses over a 12-month period (see section on long-term sequelae). The recognition that successful treatment with chemotherapy for children with HD would have significant impact on their quality of life and ultimate survival has led to newer combinations of chemotherapy. These regimens have in general been variations of the two original combinations, MOPP and ABVD. These hybrids have either replaced those agents having the worst sequelae (e.g., cyclophosphamide for nitrogen mustard) or have involved the originals being given at significantly lower doses, or both. Newer regimens in low-stage patients are now being examined; these eliminate

alkylating agents, which are causes of a majority of the long-term sequelae seen in these patients.[78] In addition, the number of cycles or overall duration has been significantly decreased.[51,96] Now typically a complete therapeutic protocol is given over four to six monthly cycles. Radiation sometimes remains a part of these regimens, although given at lower doses and encompassing smaller fields. Most recently, the chemotherapy regimens that have been given without radiation have produced equivalent results to regimens with radiation in low-stage patients.[97-99] Trials are currently under way to confirm these early results.[87,88] For those with high-risk HD, therapeutic regimens that are intensifying both doses and timing are showing improved outcomes over the traditional regimens,[100-102] with disease-free survival now in excess of 80%.

Stage, Histology, and Response-Based Therapy

Therapy for HD until recently was primarily dictated by the stage in which the child is first seen. Now histology and response to therapy are added to the equation, as one determines the optimal course of therapy.[37,103] Those with LPHD and low-stage disease may be considered for further reductions in chemotherapy and, if completely resected via an excisional biopsy, no further treatment. Early response to therapy has been shown to identify those with an ultimately better cure rate (94% vs. 78% event-free survival [EFS]).[103] Many regimens now incorporate this concept into their design, with fewer cycles of chemotherapy or elimination of radiation for those with early complete responses or both. Symptomatic disease at the time of diagnosis calls for therapy similar to that of higher-stage patients. Current recommendations are for patients with stages I to III disease to receive four to six cycles of chemotherapy, with the number of cycles dependent on the presence of bulky disease (mediastinal or nodal), number of involved nodal sites (in stage II), and achievement of remission after two to four cycles. A small subset of children (adolescent boys with CS IA cervical or PS IA disease) may be treated with radiation alone (these patients should be strongly considered for a staging laparotomy). Those with adverse risk factors should receive six cycles of therapy. The decision to use radiation after chemotherapy has been completed remains under study. When radiation is used, it should be given in low doses (<2500 cGy) and to involved areas only. Patients with bulky mediastinal disease (the widest transverse diameter of tumor exceeding one third of the intrathoracic diameter as measured on a PA chest radiograph or on CT) should receive radiation in addition to systemic chemotherapy, regardless of response to therapy. Stage IV patients should receive more intensive regimens of systemic chemotherapy and IF radiation. Currently blood or marrow stem cell transplantation is reserved for those patients whose disease is refractory to systemic chemotherapy or who have relapsed. Recent trials show that no matter the duration of initial remission, those who are treated with high-dose chemotherapy and stem cell rescue have a better freedom from treatment failure than do those treated with conventional chemotherapy (<1 year, 41% vs. 12%, $P = .008$; >1 yr, 75% vs. 44%, $P = .025$).[104]

Results

Most patients treated with combinations of chemotherapy and radiation enter into CR (>90%).[105,106] Many patients, especially those with the nodular sclerosing subtype, may have persistent adenopathy or mediastinal enlargement for months or years after therapy. Although most prove to be cured, close monitoring of these patients is critical. For those who do not enter remission with today's front-line chemotherapy/radiation combinations, the prognosis is poor. Therapeutic intensification with subsequent stem cell transplant should be strongly considered.[104,107]

For stage I to II patients, combined-modality (chemotherapy and radiation) therapy typically results in greater than 90% 5-year disease free survival (DFS) rates; for stage III patients, greater than 80%; and for stage IV patients, the outcome was until recently greater than 60% (see Table 69-4). This latter group has seen significant advances, with outcome now exceeding 80% in several recent trials.[100,101] Among the many chemotherapy regimens used are MOPP[76,108]; ABVD[109]; MOPP alternating with ABVD[105,106,110]; MOPP/ABV (Vancouver hybrid)[111]; cyclophosphamide substituted for nitrogen mustard in COP/ABVD[112]; COPP/ABV[113]; vincristine, prednisone, procarbazine, doxorubicin (Adriamycin) (OPPA)[114]; vinblastine, doxorubicin (Adriamycin), methotrexate, prednisone (VAMP)[78]; and most recently for high-risk patients, bleomycin, etoposide, doxorubicin (Adriamycin), and COPP (BEACOPP)[100]; and vinblastine, doxorubicin (Adriamycin), vincristine, bleomycin, nitrogen mustard, etoposide, prednisone (Stanford V).[102]

Acute Complications

Acute complications of therapy in children with HD are due to either the tumor itself or the therapy administered. Lymphomas may be a medical emergency because of airway compression. All patients suspected of having a diagnosis of lymphoma should have an immediate chest radiograph to determine whether a mediastinal mass is present. Therapy with chemotherapy (preferable in children) or radiation is effective in the immediate relief of these symptoms. The complications due to splenectomy when used in a staging laparotomy primarily are due to overwhelming sepsis from encapsulated organisms. This risk is increased because of the myelosuppression and immunocompromising effects of chemotherapy. Fever in the neutropenic patient necessitates hospitalization and intravenous (IV) antibiotic therapy. BM suppression may require transfusions of either red cells or platelets. Specific chemotherapy agents used may have immediate complications. These include nausea and vomiting, restrictive pulmonary disease (bleomycin, irradiation), extravasation burns (nitrogen mustard, vincristine, vinblastine, doxorubicin [Adriamycin]), and chemical phlebitis (nitrogen mustard, vinblastine, DTIC). To alleviate these last risks, right atrial catheters are often placed.

This also reduces the discomfort of repeated venipuncture required throughout the duration of treatment.

Long-Term Sequelae

The concern over long-term sequelae guides much of modern therapy for HD, both in adults and particularly so in children. These sequelae result from both radiotherapy and chemotherapy.[115,116]

The long-term sequelae of radiation in growing children are the overriding reason for the efforts to reduce or eliminate it from therapeutic regimens. Radiation to bone may result in shortening of the clavicles in those receiving mantle radiation or shortened height in those receiving radiation to the spine.[117] Radiation to the neck often results in permanent hypothyroidism[118] and increases the risk of thyroid cancer.[119,120] If radiation is to be given to the pelvis of a female patient, consideration should be given to moving the ovaries surgically from the field of radiation.[121]

Second malignancies are a major concern after therapy for HD.[122-124] The relative risk of a second malignancy in HD patients has been estimated to be 5-fold to 11-fold that of the general population.[123,125] This represents a 15- to 25-year actuarial risk of 7% to 23%.[123,125-127] Second malignancies are more prevalent in those with HD treated before age 21 years than in the older age groups for all tumors except lung cancer.[123] These second cancers include leukemia and solid tumors. The risk of leukemia seems primarily related to the chemotherapy used,[125,128] with a cumulative incidence of 3.3%, with a plateau after about 10 years. This risk seems higher in recent studies,[126,127] although one recent study found a decrease in secondary leukemia among those treated with the newer hybrid regimens.[127] This likely is a result of the reduction in nitrogen mustard and procarbazine (in MOPP) doses, the principal culprits in the development of secondary leukemia.[129,130] Patients treated with ABVD do not have an increased risk of leukemia. The reduction in the incidence of leukemia may be a result of the decreasing use of splenectomy in pathologic staging, because this procedure has repeatedly been shown to increase the risk of leukemia in HD patients treated with chemotherapy.[129,131]

Solid tumors, including those of lung, stomach, melanoma, bone, and soft tissue, have accounted for most of the second malignancies, with a cumulative incidence of 13% to 22% at 15 to 25 years, with no plateau as yet being appreciated.[123,125,126] This risk in HD survivors has not decreased when cohorts treated in the 1960s are compared with those in the 1980s.[123] This increased risk of solid tumors is related primarily to radiation,[132,133] with some added risk when subsequent chemotherapy is used in relapse patients.[134] It has been recognized that radiation exposure to the breast tissue in adult women has resulted in a fourfold increase in rates of subsequent breast cancer,[89-91,135] whereas the risk of subsequent breast cancer is increased by 39-fold if the breasts are irradiated during adolescence.[92] For an adolescent, this increases the probability of their developing breast cancer between the ages of 20 and 30 years from 0.04% to

1.6%,[93] and may be as high as 35% by age 40 years.[122] For all types of secondary cancer, adolescents seem to be at greater risk than younger children.[120,136] Recent evidence suggests that risk of breast cancer is slightly reduced by the premature menopause induced by the chemotherapy these patients receive.[137,138] Most patients who received chemotherapy and radiation therapy had menopause before age 41 years, whereas only 9% treated with radiation alone had premature menopause. Menopause before age 36 years had a significant impact on the reduced risk of breast cancer among those receiving radiation (relative risk [RR], 0.06). Patients must be closely observed for second malignancies for decades after their therapy has been completed, as no plateau in risk has yet been seen.[116,139]

Other long-term sequelae include cardiac complications secondary to mantle irradiation or the use of doxorubicin (Adriamycin in ABVD regimens) or both that affect up to 13% of patients.[140,141] These are typically congestive heart failure due to myocardiopathy and secondary arrhythmias. Occasionally restrictive pericarditis may occur as a result of radiation. Overall, the RR of death due to cardiovascular disease in HD survivors is elevated (RR, 6.6) and especially so in those treated before age 21 years (RR, 13.6).[116] Pulmonary toxicity due to bleomycin or irradiation or both affected up to 9% of children who received 12 courses of ABVD with 2100-cGy radiation.[109] This high incidence appears to be decreasing with the use of hybrid regimens and low-dose IF radiation.[112]

Infertility and early menopause in women are primarily a result of ovarian dysfunction as a result of exposure of the ovaries to radiation.[142,143] When the ovaries are surgically moved out of the field of radiation, these problems are less likely to occur.[121,144] Male patients have a 30% to 40% rate of gonadal dysfunction at the time of diagnosis before any therapy.[145] After more than three to six courses of MOPP therapy, all men are usually sterile.[146] This phenomenon does not follow ABVD therapy.[147] Spermatogenesis is only transiently reduced by pelvic radiation. Although spermatogenesis is significantly affected by the alkylating agents in MOPP therapy, testosterone production seems unimpaired. It is anticipated that with reduction in single and cumulative doses of chemotherapy, with older agents being replaced with less toxic ones, and with the reduction in radiation field size and dose, these long-term sequelae will be further reduced.

NON-HODGKIN'S LYMPHOMA

In contrast to the similarities between adult and pediatric Hodgkin's disease, the types of NHL that occur in adults and children, their presentation, their treatment, and their outcome are dramatically different. Most adults with NHL have low- or intermediate-grade lymphomas. In distinct contrast, children with these types of lymphomas are exceedingly rare. Instead, virtually all children with NHL have one of three high-grade, diffuse types: small, noncleaved cell lymphoma (SNCCL) (B cell),

lymphoblastic lymphoma (LBL) (most often T cell), or large cell lymphoma (LCL) (B or T cell and typically anaplastic). Most will be seen initially with advanced or disseminated disease (stages III to IV). These lymphomas typically appear as a rapidly expanding mass with a short symptomatic history. This propensity for rapid growth makes the diagnostic evaluation in a child with suspected NHL a medical urgency if not emergency. Of all the childhood tumors, NHL has the greatest chance of acute complications at the time of presentation, before therapy. Anatomic impingement of adjacent structures (mediastinal tumors upon the trachea and bronchi, nasopharyngeal tumors upon the orbits, bowel obstruction with or without intussusception) and metabolic derangements due to tumor lysis (before and after therapy is initiated) are not infrequent results of its very rapid growth. *No delay should occur in the evaluation of a child with suspected NHL.* Better management of the initial anatomic and metabolic complications, improved methods of determining the subtypes of NHL (perhaps the most important reason for improved survival), and better chemotherapy combinations (more intensive, yet shorter) have brought the most dramatic improvements in DFS and OS for children with NHL over the past several decades.[148] In addition to more intense therapy of shorter duration, the other major change in therapy for children with NHL is the virtual elimination of radiation from treatment regimens. This should reduce the long-term sequelae that would have otherwise resulted. For the surgeon seeing the child with suspected lymphoma, rapid evaluation and proper handling of biopsy material will have dramatic beneficial effects on the outcome for the child.

Incidence and Epidemiology

NHL accounts for 4% of all cancers in adult and pediatric patients, with nearly 53,600 new cases diagnosed annually in the United States.[1] In children, the 666 annual cases diagnosed account for 6.3% of childhood cancers, 8.7% of all solid tumors, and 57% of all lymphomas.[2] The annual incidence rate is 8.4 cases/million children younger than 15 years/year. Before age 11 years, it is the most common of the two types of lymphoma. A high male-to-female ratio of 2.61 is found, making it the most disproportionately occurring tumor between the two genders during childhood. This large difference is present in all ages of childhood. A 1.7 greater risk occurs in whites than in blacks. This too is seen in all ages, with the exception of children younger than 1 year. The age distribution demonstrates two small peaks in incidence from 6 to 7 years and between 12 and 14 years (Fig. 69-1). The 6- to 7-year-olds overwhelmingly have SNCCL (B-cell origin), and the teenagers typically have LBL (T-cell origin).

NHL of B-cell origin, either SNCCL or LCL, occurs more often in patients with prior EBV exposure, in individuals with a history of immune suppression, and in equatorial Africa.[149-151] Considerable work now convincingly reveals that in immunodeficient patients, iatrogenic (e.g., post-transplant, immunosuppressive therapy), acquired, or congenital EBV infection has an etiologic role in either the development or the predisposition to

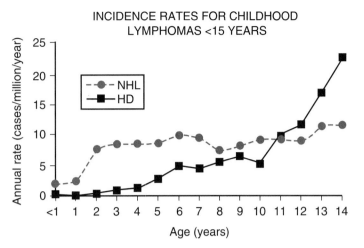

INCIDENCE RATES FOR CHILDHOOD
LYMPHOMAS <15 YEARS

FIGURE 69-1. Incidence rates for lymphomas in children younger than 15 years. (From Gurney JG, Severson RK, Davis S, Robison LL: Incidence of cancer in children in the United States. Cancer 75:2186–2195, 1995.)

B-cell NHL.[52,153] Correlations have been made between viral load levels and risk of post-transplant lymphoproliferative disorders (PTLDs).[154–156] Patients at greatest risk for PTLDs are those in whom their primary infection with EBV occurs within the first 3 to 4 months after transplantation. For T-cell NHL (LBL) or anaplastic LCL, no such etiologic correlations have been made.

Classification

Over the years, several classification schemes have been used.[157] Among these are the Rappaport, the Kiel, the Lukes-Collins, the World Health Organization (WHO), and the International Working Formulation classifications. Most recently the Revised European-American Classification of Lymphoid Neoplasms (REAL)[39] was developed as an effort to eliminate the confusion surrounding the diagnosis of the lymphoma subtype caused by the prior variety of classification schemas. The REAL is a consensus classification based on morphologic, immunologic, and cytogenetic characteristics, in addition to clinical presentation, course, and putative cell of origin.[39] Childhood NHL primarily consists of just three subtypes: (1) small, noncleaved cell lymphoma (SNCCL) of B-cell origin (39%); (2) lymphoblastic lymphoma (LBL) derived most often from T cells (28%), and (3) large cell lymphoma (LCL) (26%).[3] The first two classifications are part of the "small, round, blue cell tumors," which presents the pathologist with the challenge of proper identification. To differentiate these from the other three classic tumors (neuroblastoma, rhabdomyosarcoma, and Ewing's sarcoma) requires the presence of the immunocytochemical marker, LCA, the leukocyte common antigen (CD45), which is absent on the other tumor cell types.

SNCCL NHL has classically been divided into Burkitt's and non-Burkitt's (Burkitt-like in the REAL classification) subtypes. These are of a mature B-cell origin, with flow cytometric immunophenotyping revealing the presence of surface immunoglobulin IgM, CD10, CD19, CD20, CD22, CD79a, and human leukocyte

antigen (HLA)-DR antigens. Histologic appearances of these two types differ in the degree of pleomorphism, with Burkitt's more uniform appearing than non-Burkitt's. Although a distinction has been made for years between Burkitt's and non-Burkitt's subtypes of diffuse SNCCL lymphomas, no clinical differences are found between these two subtypes.[158] Burkitt's cells are medium-sized cells with round nuclei containing two to five nucleoli, abundant basophilic cytoplasm, and cytoplasmic lipid vacuoles. Owing to its extreme rates of proliferation and spontaneous cell death, a number of macrophages can be seen within this monomorphic field, consuming the dying cells and giving rise to the classic "starry-sky" appearance of Burkitt's lymphoma.[39]

LBLs are distinguished by round or convoluted nuclei, fine dispersed chromatin, inconspicuous nucleoli, and scant cytoplasm. Flow cytometry reveals, in the vast majority of these tumors, the presence of the T-cell markers, CD3 and CD7, with variable positivity of CD2 and CD5. These cells are typically Tdt positive, whereas SNCCLs are Tdt negative. This subtype is classified as Precursor T-cell neoplasms in the REAL classification.[39]

LCLs are a heterogeneous group of neoplasms. Histologically, approximately half are immunoblastic, 40% are large noncleaved cell, and fewer than 5% are large cleaved cell.[159] Flow cytometry shows relatively equal frequencies of B- or T-cell origin, 36% and 33%, respectively, with 30% indeterminate.[160,161] A unique subset, identified by the immunophenotype, CD30+ (the antigen identified by the Ki-1 monoclonal antibody[162]), is recognized morphologically by its anaplastic characteristics, including very large cells with abundant cytoplasm, atypical lobulated nuclei, and prominent nucleoli. These cells exhibit a cohesive pattern with a typical lymph node sinusoidal invasion. In the REAL classification, this is referred to as Anaplastic Large Cell Lymphoma.[39,163] This subtype has in the past also been referred to as malignant histiocytosis. The majority (60%) of these children have a T-cell immunophenotype.[160,164] Recent studies reveal that, although it was originally thought to be uncommon in children, it accounts for 40% to 50% of the LCL cases.[160,161,165,166] These cells also are immunophenotypically positive for CD25, CD71, and CD1a. CD30 also is found on the Reed-Sternberg cells, but these two entities are clearly different on a clinical level, with anaplastic LCLs most similar to other NHLs rather than to HD.[39]

Cell Biology

Cancer is a result of (1) the inappropriate or unregulated expression of a gene (or both), at either the wrong time in a cell's cycle or in the wrong cell; (2) abnormal combinations of genes producing proteins not normally present in cells; or (3) the loss of gene expression and their products required for cellular control. These first two categories encompass the proto-oncogenes and oncogenes, and the last comprises the tumor-suppressor genes. Lymphomas arise from precursors of lymphocytes at various stages of maturation, primarily because of errors in transcriptional factor control and production, as a result of proto-oncogenes and oncogenes. Early B and T cells normally splice together different segments of their immunoglobulin and T-cell–receptor (TCR) genes to generate the diverse proteins capable of binding foreign antigens.[167] In lymphoid cancers, this system goes awry because of the inadvertent splicing (juxtaposition) of transcription factor genes (proto-oncogenes) to one of these regions. This leads to the abnormal and unregulated expression of this gene (now an oncogene) and the production of its oncoprotein. This oncoprotein eventually leads to the cell's malignant transformation by a variety of mechanisms and, hence, its uncontrolled growth. The reader is referred elsewhere for more detailed descriptions of normal and oncologic gene regulation and expression (transcription).[167-170] This neoplastic process typically occurs as a result of nonrandom chromosomal translocations or inversions, although deletions and insertions of DNA sequences likely also contribute to the malignant transformation.

Burkitt's lymphoma was the tumor in which this chromosomal translocation process was originally described.[171] The translocation involving chromosomes 8 and 14 was first identified in Burkitt's cells in 1976.[172] As a result of this translocation, t(8;14), the *c-myc* oncogene, located on chromosome 8q24, is juxtaposed to the immunoglobulin receptor subunit gene on chromosome 14q32 (immunoglobulin heavy-chain gene). This translocation is found in both African (endemic) and American (sporadic) Burkitt's, though the exact breakpoints on chromosome 8 differ.[173] In a smaller percentage of Burkitt's patients, *c-myc* is juxtaposed to chromosome 2p11 (κ immunoglobulin light-chain gene), t(2;8), or 22q11 (λ light-chain gene), t(8;22).[174] It is thought that an increased pool of B cells, either through prolonged stimulation, as in the case of malaria and/or through inhibition of cell death, as in the case of EBV, increases the chance occurrence of these translocations.[175,176] The oncoprotein, *MYC*, normally controls progression through G_1 into the S phase of the cell cycle, but as a result of these translocations, its expression is dysregulated, leading to uncontrolled lymphoproliferation.[177]

For T cells, or LBLs, translocations are less often found. The translocations known to date result in the juxtaposition of several different oncogenes to TCR genes located on chromosomes 14q11 (TCR α/δ) and 7 (TCR β).[167,177] Nonrandom translocations found in LBLs of T-cell origin include t(11;14), t(1;14), t(10;14), t(7;19), t(8;14), and t(1;7) and involve the oncogenes *RHOMB1& 2* (11p13 & 15), *TAL1* (1p32), *HOX11* (10q24), *LYL1* (19p13), *MYC* (8q24), and *LCK* (1p34). The cytogenetic translocation most often found in LCL patients is that associated with the Ki-1, CD30+, anaplastic LCLs.[178] In this tumor, t(2;5),[179] when present, results in the juxtapositioning of the *ALK* tyrosine kinase gene on chromosome 5q35 to a ribosomal assembly gene, *NPM*, on chromosome 2p23.[180] This produces an abnormal oncoprotein, NPM-ALK (p80), normally absent in cells, which allows uncontrolled proliferation of the involved cells.

Clinical Presentation by Initial Site of Disease

Overall, unlike those with HD and adult NHL, children with NHL are initially seen with extranodal disease and typically have disease that spreads by routes other than contiguous nodal pathways. The abdomen is the originating site of disease in 31%; the mediastinum, in 27%; and the head and neck, in 29% of children.[3] Other sites include peripheral nodes, bone, and skin. Most abdominal disease primaries are due to the SNCCL lymphomas, whereas most mediastinal/intrathoracic primaries are due to LBL (Table 69-5). Disease that occurs primarily in the peripheral nodes and bones is often due to LCL, and skin involvement is primarily associated with the Ki-1+ LCL subtype.[161,181,182] Correlating with this distribution and the known age peaks of the two types of small cell lymphomas, abdominal primaries occur more often in children younger than 10 years, whereas mediastinal primaries are more likely to occur in adolescents.

Children with abdominal primaries may be seen with nausea, vomiting, abdominal pain, and changes in bowel habits, and on physical examination, are found to have an abdominal mass in any of the quadrants. They may have an acute abdomen due to either intussusception (typically due to infiltration of Peyer's patches) or small bowel obstruction, perforation of an involved bowel wall, or an ileocecal mass mimicking acute appendicitis.[183] A child with intussusception older than 5 years must strongly be considered to have NHL until proven otherwise. NHL must always be a part of one's differential diagnosis when faced with a 5- to 10-year-old child with an abdominal mass. Radiographic evaluation with either CT or US typically reveals a homogeneous mass with or without evidence of central necrosis, arising either from the retroperitoneum or from the bowel wall. Accompanying adenopathy and metastatic dissemination to the liver and spleen is often seen. The bowel loops may simply be shifted away from the mass or may show evidence of intussusception or obstruction or both.

Children with mediastinal primaries may have minimal symptoms, such as a mild cough or audible wheeze, or may have impending obstruction of the airway.

NON-HODGKIN'S LYMPHOMA: PREVALENCE OF HISTOLOGIC SUBTYPES IN PRIMARY SITES

	Abdominal	Thoracic	Head/Neck	Peripheral Nodes	Bone	Other*
SNCCL/B cell	74%	4%	48%	17%	6%	29%
LBL/T cell	3%	74%	24%	33%	31%	14%
LCL	23%	22%	28%	50%	56%	57%
Total	100%	100%	100%	100%	100%	100%

Adapted from Murphy SB, Fairclough DL, Hutchison RE, Berard CW: Non-Hodgkins' lymphomas of childhood: An analysis of the histology, staging, and response to treatment of 338 cases in a single institution. J Clin Oncol 7:186–193, 1989; and Wollner N, Lane JM, Marcove RC, et al: Primary skeletal non-Hodgkin's lymphomas in the pediatric age group. Med Pediatr Oncol 20:506–513, 1992.
*Includes bone. SNCCL, small noncleaved cell lymphoma; LBL, lymphoblastic lymphoma; LCL, large cell lymphoma.

These latter patients may also have significant engorgement of the vasculature in the head, face, and upper thorax because of superior vena caval compression. Thrombosis may be present in these vessels. Often these patients will assume a forward-leaning position and cannot tolerate being placed in the supine position because of the anterior mediastinal mass. The history may reveal orthopnea as well as shortness of breath and dyspnea on exertion. The recent onset of asthma symptoms is not uncommon. Shortness of breath also may be due to pleural effusions. A chest radiograph is an essential component of the patient's initial evaluation before sedation or any procedure. Chest radiography and CT of the chest will reveal the widened mediastinum with often dramatic narrowing of the trachea and bronchi. Pericardial effusions are often present and may be revealed by CT, MRI, or echocardiography.[184]

Patients with head and neck lymphomas may have a history of rapidly progressive adenopathy, recent onset of snoring at night, mouth breathing, bad breath, epistaxis, proptosis or periorbital edema, diplopia, extraocular muscle paralysis due to entrapment, cranial nerve paralysis, and sudden blindness or a combination of these. Physical examination of the nares, oral cavity, and extraocular movements is critical and may reveal signs not appreciated as abnormal by the child. The presence of asymmetrical and painless tonsillar hypertrophy should also alert the clinician to the possibility of NHL.[185] Evaluation with CT often reveals a homogeneous mass that may reveal destruction of the adjacent bony structures.

Bone NHL primaries are usually seen as lytic lesions found on radiographs obtained for various reasons, including localized tenderness.[186–188] Skin lesions are typically ulcerative with failure to heal but also may be completely subcutaneous.[181] Patients with central nervous system (CNS) involvement may be asymptomatic, have seizures, or have signs and symptoms related to the location of tumor infiltration.

Laboratory findings at the time of diagnosis are dependent on the amount of tumor present (regardless of the histologic subtype). Generally patients will have an elevated ESR or C-reactive protein (CRP) level. Those with large tumor burdens typically will have high lactate dehydrogenase (LDH) as an indicator of tumor lysis

risk,[189,190] disease regression, and progression. Its degree of elevation has been used as an adverse prognostic factor.[3,191,192] For those with high tumor burdens at presentation, laboratory signs of tumor lysis will include elevated uric acid, phosphorus, and potassium, often with a low calcium level. Some patients may already be in renal failure at the time of presentation and have an elevated creatinine.[189,190] Hematologic values are nonspecific, and the presence of cytopenias should raise the suspicion of marrow involvement. Cerebrospinal fluid (CSF) pleocytosis may or may not be present in those with CNS involvement.

More than 60% of patients have advanced or disseminated (stages III to IV) disease at diagnosis.[3,193] Among those patients with fewer than 25% blasts in the BM (>25% would reclassify the patient as having leukemia), 18% of patients are first seen in stage I; 21%, in stage II; 43%, in stage III; and 18% in stage IV.[3] Fourteen percent of patients initially have some BM involvement, and 3%, CNS involvement.[3]

Clinical Presentation by Histologic Subtype

Burkitt's lymphoma was first described by the surgeon, Denis Burkitt, in Uganda, where he identified the common finding of enormous involvement of the nodes around the jaw.[194] Later it was determined that although this was a common presentation of those patients with endemic Burkitt's (African), those with sporadic Burkitt's (American) more typically had presentation of disease either in the abdomen or the nasopharynx.[195] Endemic Burkitt's patients have accompanying abdominal disease in roughly half the cases, and sporadic Burkitt's patients have jaw involvement about 15% to 20% of the time.[196] Sporadic Burkitt's patients as well have a higher incidence of BM involvement (21% vs. 7%) but lower CNS dissemination (11% vs. 17%). Approximately two thirds of SNCCL NHL patients will have disseminated or advanced disease (defined as stages III to IV) at diagnosis.[197] T-cell, or LBL, patients most often are adolescents with supradiaphragmatic disease, either intrathoracic or head and neck. Disseminated disease is present in nearly 90% of LBL patients at diagnosis.[197] In LBL patients, involvement of the BM has been seen in approximately one fourth of children, with CNS disease at presentation in fewer than 10%.[197] LCL patients may have presentations in all sites, but have a higher prevalence than the other two subtypes for skin, bone, and peripheral nodes.[163,181,188] Disseminated disease in LCL patients also is present at diagnosis in up to 65% of patients.[197] Involvement of the BM or CNS in LCL patients is rare[197] (Table 69-6).

Clinical Presentation in Immunodeficient Patients

For patients with congenital or acquired immunodeficiency, NHL presentation will vary from polyclonal plasmacytic hyperplasia, most often localized in nasopharyngeal nodes or tonsils, to a clonal polymorphic lymphoma slowly arising in the lymph nodes or extranodal sites, to widely disseminated rapidly progressive immunoblastic lymphoma.[198,199] Symptoms may well be nonspecific, with fever and malaise. Hepatosplenomegaly and lymphadenopathy may be presenting signs. Gastrointestinal (GI) symptoms of longer than 14 days' duration with anorexia, weight loss, and diarrhea should raise suspicion of this entity.[156] NHL has become more common with the use of very potent antirejection drugs after solid organ or BM transplantation. Involvement of the transplanted organ is not unusual. The reader is directed to concise and specific reviews of this topic.[156,200]

Diagnosis

Children initially suspected of having NHL should be fully evaluated immediately because of the high risk of either metabolic or anatomic complications before therapy begins. The rapid growth of these tumors may create a life-threatening complication overnight in a child who seemed relatively well the day before (Table 69-7).

No clinical findings are pathognomonic for NHL. Ultimately, the diagnosis awaits the biopsy of involved sites, most commonly an excised lymph node or percutaneous needle biopsy. Fine-needle aspirations do not provide enough tissue for the necessary subtyping, which is performed with flow cytometry, molecular genetics, and

---

TABLE 69-6

PREVALENCE OF PRIMARY SITES AMONG THE THREE PRIMARY TYPES OF CHILDHOOD NHL

	SNCCL	LBL	LCL
Abdomen	56%	3%	25%
Intrathoracic	2%	65%	21%
Head/Neck	34%	23%	29%
Peripheral nodes	2%	7%	11%
Other	5%	3%	14%
Total	100%	100%	100%

Adapted from Murphy SB, Fairclough DL, Hutchison RE, Berard CW: Non-Hodgkin's lymphomas of childhood: Analysis of the histology, staging, and response to treatment of 338 cases at a single institution. J Clin Oncol 7:186–193, 1989.
NHL, Non-Hodgkin's lymphoma; SNCCL, small noncleaved cell lymphoma; LBL, lymphoblastic lymphoma; LCL, large cell lymphoma.

TABLE 69-7

NON-HODGKIN'S LYMPHOMA: DIAGNOSTIC AND STAGING EVALUATION AT PRESENTATION

Complete physical examination with documentation of involved nodal groups (including measurements of nodes) and involved extralymphatic organs
Complete blood count (CBC), chemistry panel including hepatic and renal function tests, ESR, LDH
Chest radiography to evaluate for mediastinal disease and airway compression
CT scans of areas identified on physical examination (also include chest, neck, and abdomen)
Bone scan
Gallium scan
Excisional biopsy of node or mass with samples sent for routine pathology, molecular genetics, cytogenetics, and flow cytometry
Bone marrow biopsies and aspirates (bilateral)
Lumbar puncture with CSF analysis of cytocentrifuged sample

ESR, erythrocyte sedimentation rate; LDH, lactate dehydrogenase; CT, computed tomography; CSF, cerebrospinal fluid.

---

cytogenetics. It is critical for the excised tissue to be delivered quickly to the pathologist for processing. For cytogenetic and molecular genetic evaluations, it is imperative that all tissues be placed in a sterile container for fresh samples. Formalin should never be used.

For patients critically ill at diagnosis, such as those with severe airway obstruction, diagnosis by alternative methods should be strongly considered. These may include nodal biopsy with local anesthetic alone, CT- or US-guided percutaneous needle biopsy of the mass, aspiration of a pleural effusion, or a BM biopsy and aspirate. For patients with an acute abdomen, pathologic evaluation of biopsies or excised tissues should be made. *This is the one instance in NHL patients in which initial total resection may be considered.* That is, in patients in whom resection of bowel is already required because of perforation or obstruction, total resection of the tumor should be considered. This definitely reduces the stage of the patient's disease, improves survival, and reduces the amount of therapy required.[201] For all other patients, resection of the mass provides no improvement in staging or long-term cure and delays the time to initiation of chemotherapy. It should be remembered that most patients have disseminated disease at presentation, and it is important to note that with chemotherapy alone, more than 90% will enter complete remission.

Once it is suspected, a concerted and well-thought-out plan of evaluation is important to achieve diagnosis as quickly as possible. This should include laboratory examination to evaluate tumor burden and presence or risk of tumor lysis syndrome. Radiographic evaluation of patients is a mandatory part of the patient's evaluation.[54] *No procedures or sedation should be attempted until a mediastinal mass has been ruled out.* CT should be pursued to identify the extent of disease. CTs of the neck, chest, abdomen, and pelvis are required. An examination of the head, either CT or magnetic resonance imaging (MRI), should be obtained in those patients with CNS symptoms, with CSF pleocytosis, or in whom the primaries are parameningeal based. Bone scans should typically be obtained. Gallium scans are an effective method with which to determine the extent of disease at initial diagnosis, to evaluate residual disease at the end of therapy, and for ongoing monitoring for relapse after therapy.[202] A positive gallium scan at the end of therapy is a strong predictor of relapse. Positron emission tomography (PET) scans are likely to be an emerging modality in the diagnostic evaluation and monitoring of these patients. However, few data exist on its utility in children with NHL, other than diffuse large B-cell NHL.[74,203]

Pathologic evaluation of the biopsy material should include general histochemical techniques to confirm the lymphoma and its subtype. Critical recent additions to the basic evaluation are flow cytometric analysis of cell-surface markers to determine the immunophenotype of the lymphoma, cytogenetic evaluation for diagnostic translocations, fluorescent in situ hybridization (FISH), and DNA analysis using either Southern blotting or the polymerase chain reaction for detection of the pathognomonic oncogenes (gene rearrangements), even in the absence of identifiable cytogenetic translocations.[204] Examination of markers in tumor cells for EBV are important in the evaluation of PTLD. These are all essential components at the time of initial diagnosis and should be performed at an institution capable of performing *all* of them. Therapy differences between the subtypes of lymphoma are such that assignment to the wrong subtype due to a lack of adequate diagnostic material will adversely affect the chance of cure. These evaluations may be performed with biopsy material from any involved site, including the primary mass, enlarged lymph nodes, effusions, and BM. A new technique, known as gene expression profiling, which uses DNA microarrays, has been shown to categorize patients further into specific histologic and genetic subsets of lymphoma, with much greater predictability of clinical outcome.[205] This new technique will likely revolutionize diagnostic and prognostic characterization for NHL.

Completing the diagnostic protocol is the determination of CNS or BM dissemination. Lumbar puncture for cytocentrifuged CSF analysis should be performed in all patients, although in those with localized abdominal SNCCL, and those with LCL, the benefit gained from this is arguable because of the low incidence of CNS disease in these subpopulations. BM evaluation should include bilateral iliac crest biopsies and aspirates.

Staging

Once the diagnosis of NHL has been made, staging permits determination of disease extent at presentation. This provides direction in monitoring disease response to therapy. With NHL, relapse does not necessarily occur at the site of prior disease, as is typical of HD. Thus this initial staging should not limit the extent of monitoring for relapse after therapy is complete.

Staging is important in the determination of therapeutic planning. The most widely used staging schema used today is the St. Jude's or Murphy staging[206] (Table 69-8).

TABLE 69-8
ST. JUDE'S (MURPHY) STAGES FOR CHILDHOOD NHL

Stage	Definition
I	Single tumor (extranodal) or single anatomic area (nodal), excluding mediastinum or abdomen
II	Single tumor (extranodal) with regional node involvement
	On same side of diaphragm:
	a) Two or more nodal areas
	b) Two single (extranodal) tumors with or without regional node involvement
	Primary gastrointestinal tract tumor (usually ileocecal) with or without associated mesenteric node involvement, grossly completely resected
III	On both sides of diaphragm:
	a) Two single tumors (extranodal)
	b) Two or more nodal areas
	All primary intrathoracic tumors (mediastinal, pleural, thymic)
	All extensive primary intra-abdominal disease; unresectable
	All primary paraspinal or epidural tumors regardless of other sites
IV	Any of the above with initial CNS or bone marrow involvement (<25%)

NHL, Non-Hodgkin's lymphoma; CNS, central nervous system.

This is an adaptation of the Ann Arbor scheme and applies to all types of childhood NHL. It divides patients into localized (stage I or II) and disseminated or advanced (stage III or IV) disease. Involvement of the CNS or BM immediately places the patient in the stage IV category. Patients with more than 25% BM involvement are by definition diagnosed with leukemia rather than with lymphoma. These would include B-cell or Burkitt's leukemia (L3 leukemia morphologic classification) and T-cell leukemia. The former patients are treated on B-cell NHL protocols with much better results than previously obtained on acute lymphoblastic leukemia (ALL) regimens. Many of the B-cell NHL protocol results reported in the literature include these patients in their stage IV populations. The T-cell leukemia patients remain on ALL protocols, but many similarities exist between these protocols and those used in LBL therapy.

Prognostic Risk Factors

When all patients are treated similarly, the stage of the lymphoma at diagnosis is a strong predictor of outcome.[3] Prediction of a patient's eventual outcome stratifies patients at high risk for relapse to more intensive or novel therapies, and low-risk patients to shorter, more moderate therapies. This is the goal of prognostic factor development. Many factors have been evaluated over the years. All prognostic factors, and most clearly so in NHL, are dependent on the therapy subsequently given.[3]

This must be strongly considered whenever reviewing prognostic factors reported in NHL. It has been definitively shown that histology-based therapy is of critical importance in the successful outcome of patients[193] (Table 69-9).

For SNCCL patients, BM involvement has been an adverse factor for DFS/OS.[193] CNS involvement in both SNCCL and LBL patients has predictably worse outcomes.[193] In SNCCL patients, the adverse effect of CNS disease on outcome has, in some studies, been more attributable to tumor burden at diagnosis than to the presence of CNS disease alone (i.e., those with greater tumor burden are more likely to have CNS disease[207]).

LCL patients have unique prognostic characteristics that are likely to change as this entity is better described and therapy is more appropriately administered by subtype. Skin involvement at presentation in LCL patients has been shown to be a poor prognostic indicator.[201] In patients with advanced LCL disease, the presence of CD30+ cells has indicated a better OS,[208] although in other studies, no effect on prognosis has been noted.[160] B-cell immunophenotype

TABLE 69-9

SELECTED THERAPEUTIC TRIALS FOR CHILDREN WITH NHL

Protocol/Therapy	Stage	DFS % (yr)	OS % (yr)	Ref.
Small Noncleaved/B cell				
POG/ADCOMP	I–II	87 (4)	93 (5)	217
CCG 551, 501/COMP	I–II	86–98 (5)	91–98 (5)	210
CCG 551/COMP	III–IV	50 (5)	54 (5)	193
CCG 551/LSA$_2$L$_2$	III–IV	29 (5)	33 (5)	193
CCG 552/CHOP	III, LDH < 500	86 (4)	86	191
	III, LDH > 500	39	39	
	IV	38	48	
Total therapy B	III	86 (2)	—	226
POG/Intensified total therapy B	IV	79 (4)	—	212
HiC-COM	III	92 (3)	—	192
	IV	50	—	
SFOP/LMB 84	III	80 (3)	82 (3)	211
	IV	68	71	
SFOP/LMB 89	I–II	100 (1)	—	226
	III	89	—	
	IV	80	—	
Lymphoblastic/T cell				
POG/ADCOMP	I–II	87 (4)	93 (5)	217
CCG 551/LSA$_2$L$_2$	III–IV	64 (5)	67 (5)	193
CCG 551/COMP	III–IV	34 (5)	45 (5)	193
CCG 552/CHOP	III–IV	54 (4)	77 (4)	191
CCG 502/ADCOMP or LSA$_2$L$_2$	Localized	84% (5)	—	214
	Disseminated	67%	—	
UCCSG 8503	Disseminated	65 (4)	—	226
St. Jude/Total therapy X-high risk	III–IV	73 (4)	—	226
SFOP/LMT 81	III	79	—	226
	IV	72		
Large Cell				
St. Jude/CHOP	I–II CD30+	75 (5)	—	161
	I–II CD30–	92	—	
St. Jude/CHOP & MACOP-B	III–IV CD30+	57	84 (5)	
	III–IV CD30–	29	27	
CCG 551/LSA$_2$L$_2$	III–IV	43 (5)	44 (5)	193
CCG 551/COMP	III–IV	52 (5)	69 (5)	193
BFM 83,86,90	I	75 (5)	—	165
	II	68	—	
	III–IV	86	—	
POG 87191/POG 8615	B cell/All	96 (3)	—	160
	T cell or ?/All	67	—	
	B cell/III–IV	100	—	
	T cell or ?/III–IV	69	—	

DFS, disease-free survival; OS, overall survival; LDH, lactate dehydrogenase; NHL, non-Hodgkin's lymphoma.

has been shown to improve prognosis.[160] Current staging methods do not seem to carry the same prognostic significance in LCL patients,[160,165] although in some studies, survival differences are reported between stages.[161] Patients with intrathoracic primaries have a better prognosis than do those with primaries elsewhere.[208] Children with NHL arising in the bone, regardless which of the three histologic subtypes it is, have an excellent prognosis with histology-directed chemotherapy alone.[209]

Treatment

Therapy for childhood NHL is based on the knowledge that this tumor is *extremely* chemosensitive. Therapy for childhood NHL has evolved over the past several decades. For SNCCL and LCL, duration of therapy has shortened, as it became apparent that most if not all patients were relapsing within the first 6 to 8 months of therapy.[197,210] Despite reductions of therapy to 6 months or less, no increase in relapse has been seen. Relapses for the most part have occurred within the first 6 to 8 months after diagnosis, and virtually all, within the first 2 years.[191–193,210,211] SNCCL (B-cell) therapy has shown clear improvements as methotrexate and cytarabine doses have been escalated. These two agents, in addition to cyclophosphamide, vincristine, doxorubicin (Adriamycin), and prednisone (and etoposide for the stage IV patients), now play a critical role in the successful outcome of these children.[197,201,211,212]

For LBL, the duration of therapy remains at 33 weeks to 32 months, depending on the extent of disease and the particular protocol. Attempts to shorten this period further have led to increased relapses. The most effective regimens for LBL have been ones similar to the intensive T-cell ALL protocols in current use. For LCL patients, use of T-cell regimens without as much CNS-directed therapy have been efficacious.

For SNCCL and LCL, it has become apparent that no benefit in DFS or OS is gained with the use of radiation for treatment either to involved areas or to the CNS for prophylaxis.[165,181,213] Rather, prophylaxis to prevent CNS relapse is effectively performed with intrathecal chemotherapy.[207] Although some type of CNS prophylaxis is thought to be required for all patients with NHL to prevent CNS relapse, in one small group of patients, it is not. Patients with localized, resected GI primaries with SNCCL or LCL do not have CNS relapse even in the absence of CNS prophylaxis.[210]

For LBL patients, although radiation has been used to areas of bulk disease, its need is uncertain.[214] Radiation has been used for CNS prophylaxis in patients without CNS disease at diagnosis, but recent studies substituting IT chemoprophylaxis have not shown increased CNS relapses. For those LBL patients with CNS or testicular disease present at diagnosis, radiation remains an important part of their therapy.

Several additional points deserve mention. *The use of steroids before a diagnostic procedure should absolutely be avoided.* This can induce rapid necrosis in the lymphoma, making subtype determination difficult if not impossible and thus potentially jeopardizing the patient's therapy.

That said, once adequate tissue has been obtained and delivered to the pathologist, chemotherapy including steroids is an excellent method for rapid reduction of a life-threatening mass. Because of the extreme sensitivity of NHL, one can anticipate rapid reduction of tumor size once therapy has begun. Radiation is not necessary in this situation. It is not unusual to have symptoms *completely* resolve within 24 hours and to have patients be in complete radiographic remission within 7 days. Many protocols now call for a period of reduced-dose chemotherapy for the first week to obtain a more controlled tumor reduction because of the severe tumor lysis that may accompany more rapid, therapy-induced, necrosis.

NHL in immunodeficient individuals is most often a B-cell lymphoma, either small or large cell. Therapy for these patients has typically been directed toward these histologic types. For patients with ongoing iatrogenic immune suppression, reduction of the immunosuppressive agent with or without acyclovir may be adequate to induce a remission in up to 75% of cases.[156,215] However, this may not be possible after transplant because of risk of rejection. α-Interferon has been used with mixed success in these patients and may exacerbate rejection. A small proportion of patients with localized disease may be cured with surgical resection of the involved nodal tissue. When the tumor is resistant to these techniques, chemotherapy regimens can be used, although mortality has been higher than that in immunocompetent patients. In the past few years, new methods using monoclonal antibody therapy, primarily anti-CD20 (rituximab), have been used with promising results alone, but these antibodies are most efficacious when combined with chemotherapy.[216]

Results

When reviewing the outcomes of children treated for NHL, it is quickly apparent that considerable improvement in DFS and OS has occurred over the past several decades[3] (see Table 69-9). Today typically 90% to 100% of patients will achieve a complete remission.[165,210,217] Patients with localized disease have an overall excellent prognosis, regardless of histologic subtype, with DFS typically exceeding 90% to 95%. SNCCL patients with advanced disease have experienced DFS exceeding 80% in the most recent SNCCL trials. LBL patients with disseminated disease are faring not quite so well, but DFS for these patients is exceeding 65% to 70% in most trials. Overall, treatment failures when they occur typically will do so within the first 2 years after diagnosis. SNCCL patients who relapse primarily do so within the first 6 to 8 months. LBL patients will have an occasional late failure after 2 years, although even in this group of patients, the vast majority of failures will occur early.[217] LCL patients have more late relapses. Thus radiographic follow-up is an important modality in the ongoing post-therapy evaluation of NHL patients for several years. With the advent of modern radiographic techniques, second-look operations have not been of benefit to patient outcome.[201,203]

Acute Complications

Depending on the tumor burden present at diagnosis, patients may initially have a constellation of significant metabolic derangements known as tumor lysis syndrome.[189,190] This includes hyperuricemia, hyperphosphatemia, hyperkalemia, and hypocalcemia. Recognition of this is critical to prevent life-threatening complications including, most commonly, acute renal failure. Without treatment, the incidence of acute renal failure may be as high as 30%.[218] Tumor lysis syndrome is a result of the rapid turnover of cells within the tumor. The fraction of tumor cells in S phase at any given time can approach 27% in some patients.[219] These tumors have a high degree of spontaneous lysis at the time of diagnosis, as they rapidly outgrow their blood supply. Any manipulation, including transfusion or operation, may induce a sudden worsening of this syndrome. Therapy is primarily based on the risk of development of hyperuricemia. For those at high risk,[189,190] determined by the presence of an elevated LDH, creatinine, or uric acid, intervention is important. For most with little or no elevation in these values, adequate hydration (>3000 mL/m^2/day) and monitoring of blood pH (maintain between 7.0 and 7.5) is adequate, along with the initiation of allopurinol, either PO or IV, to reduce the production of uric acid through inhibition of xanthine oxidase.[220] Most recently, the urate oxidase agent, rasburicase, which cleaves uric acid into allantoin, a soluble by-product, was approved by the Food and Drug Administration (FDA) for use. This agent, administered daily for 1 to 5 days, dramatically reduces measurable uric acid levels to unmeasurable levels, thus allowing the clinician to focus on prevention or treatment of hyperphosphatemia, which requires maintaining an acidic urine.[221,222] Despite these measures, although rarely with the availability of urate oxidase, it may be necessary to place patients on renal dialysis either to treat oliguria/anuria or to prevent it in the face of rapidly increasing uric acid, phosphorus (typically >10 mg/dL), or potassium levels >7.5 mEq/L.[197,223] In an effort to avoid this complication, some regimens have used an initial low-dose therapy (usually 1 week) to more slowly reduce the tumor burden.

Owing to the much more myelosuppressive regimens required in NHL therapy, infection is a much larger risk for NHL patients as compared with HD patients.[193] In one recent study, 63% of the deaths were due to infection. Most patients require transfusion support during treatment because of the myelosuppression. The chemotherapy itself may cause acute complications including severe chemical burns due to extravasation of certain vesicant agents (vincristine, anthracyclines). As most children require the placement of right atrial catheters to facilitate their therapy, thrombosis of these and the surrounding vasculature has become more frequent.[224]

Long-Term Sequelae

As long-term survival has improved, the concern over sequelae has increased in these patients. With current therapy, these sequelae include potential long-term cardiac dysfunction because of anthracycline exposure,[141] infertility as a result of the alkylating agents used,[225] and secondary leukemias due to epipodophyllotoxins (VP16, VM 26) and alkylating agents used in the NHL regimens.[226] These patients must be monitored closely for the early identification and proper intervention to maintain a good quality of life in these long-term survivors.

REFERENCES

1. Parker SL, Tong T, Bolden S, Wingo PA: Cancer statistics. CA Cancer J Clin 47:5–27, 1997.
2. Gurney JG, Severson RK, Davis S, Robison LL: Incidence of cancer in children in the United States. Cancer 75:2186–2195, 1995.
3. Murphy SB, Fairclough DL, Hutchison RE, Berard CW: Non-Hodgkin's lymphomas of childhood: An analysis of the histology, staging, and response to treatment of 338 cases at a single institution. J Clin Oncol 7:186–193, 1989.
4. Hodgkin T: On some morbid appearances of the absorbent glands and spleen. Med Chirurg Trans 17:68–114, 1832.
5. Sternberg C: Uber eine eigenartige unter dem Bilde der Pseudoleukemaemie verlaufende Tuberculose des lymphatischen Apparetes. Ztschr Heilk 19:21–92, 1898.
6. Reed D: On the pathological changes in Hodgkin's disease: With especial reference to its relation to tuberculosis. Johns Hopkins Hosp Rep 10:133–196, 1902.
7. Gilbert R: Radiotherapy in Hodgkin's disease. Am J Roentgenol 41:198–240, 1939.
8. Kaplan HS, Rosenberg SA: The management of Hodgkin's disease. Cancer 36:796–803, 1975.
9. Hellman S: Thomas Hodgkin and Hodgkin's disease: Two paradigms appropriate to medicine today. JAMA 265:1007–1010, 1991.
10. Zantinga AR, Coppes MJ: Thomas Hodgkin (1798–1866): Pathologist, social scientist, and philanthropist. Med Pediatr Oncol 27:122–127, 1996.
11. Kung FH: Hodgkin's disease in children 4 years of age or younger. Cancer 67:1428–1430, 1991.
12. Mack TM, Cozen W, Shibata DK, et al: Concordance for Hodgkin's disease in identical twins suggesting genetic susceptibility to the young-adult form of the disease. N Engl J Med 332:413–418, 1995.
13. Grufferman S, Delzell E: Epidemiology of Hodgkin's disease. Epidemiol Rev 6:76–106, 1984.
14. Gutensohn N, Cole P: Childhood social environment and Hodgkin's disease. N Engl J Med 304:135–140, 1981.
15. Reynolds P, Sunders LD, Layefsky ME, et al: The spectrum of acquired immunodeficiency syndrome (AIDS)-associated malignancies in San Francisco, 1980–1987. Am J Epidemiol 137:19–30, 1993.
16. Hessol NA, Katz MH, Liu JY, et al: Increased incidence of Hodgkin disease in homosexual men with HIV infection. Ann Intern Med 117:309–311, 1992.
17. Volberding P, Baker K, Levine A: Human immunodeficiency virus hematology. Hematology, 294–313, 2003.
18. Riggs S, Hagemeister FB: Immunodeficiency states: A predisposition to lymphoma. In Fuller LM, Hagemeister FB, Sullivan M, et al (eds): Hodgkin's Disease and Non-Hodgkin's Lymphomas in Adults and Children. New York, Raven, 1988, p 451.
19. Ambinder RF, Browning PJ, Lorenzana I, et al: Epstein-Barr virus and childhood Hodgkin's disease in Honduras and the United States. Blood 81:462–467, 1993.
20. Herbst H, Steinbrecher E, Niedobitek G, et al: Distribution and phenotype of Epstein-Barr virus-harboring cells in Hodgkin's disease. Blood 80:484–491, 1992.
21. Knecht H, Odermatt B, Bachmann E, et al: Frequent detection of Epstein-Barr virus DNA by the polymerase chain reaction in lymph node biopsies from patients with Hodgkin's disease without genomic evidence of B- or T-cell clonality. Blood 78:760–767, 1991.
22. Khan G, Norton AJ, Slavin G: Epstein-Barr virus in Hodgkin disease. Cancer 71:3124–3129, 1993.
23. Rosdahl N, Larsen SO, Clemmesen J: Hodgkin's disease in patients with previous infectious mononucleosis: 30 years' experience. Br Med J 2:253–256, 1974.

24. Hjalgrim H, Askling J, Sorenson P, et al: Risk of Hodgkin's disease and other cancers after infectious mononucleosis. J Natl Cancer Inst 92:1522–1528, 2000.

25. Hjalgrim H, Askling J, Rostgaard K, et al: Characteristics of Hodgkin's lymphoma after infectious mononucleosis. N Engl J Med 349:1324–1332, 2003.

26. Evans AS, Gutensohn NM: A population-based case-control study of EBV and other viral antibodies among persons with Hodgkin's disease and their siblings. Int J Cancer 34:149–157, 1984.

27. Haluska FG, Brufsky AM, Canellos GP: The cellular biology of the Reed-Sternberg cell. Blood 84:1005–1019, 1994.

28. Lukes RJ, Butler JJ: The pathology and nomenclature of Hodgkin's disease. Cancer Res 26:1063–1083, 1966.

29. Gruss HJ, Pinto A, Duyster J, et al: Hodgkin's disease: A tumor with disturbed immunological pathways. Immunol Today 18:156–163, 1997.

30. Schwartz RS: Hodgkin's disease: Time for a change. N Engl J Med 337:495–496, 1997.

31. Marafioti T, Hummel M, Foss H, et al: Hodgkin and Reed-Sternberg cells represent an expansion of a single clone originating from a germinal center B-cell with functional immunoglobulin gene rearrangements but defective immunoglobulin transcription. Blood 95:1443–1450, 2000.

32. Stein H, Diehl V, Marafioti T, et al: The nature of Reed-Sternberg cells, lymphocytic and histiocytic cells and their molecular biology in Hodgkin's disease. In: Mauch PM, Armitage JO, Diehl V, et al (eds): Hodgkin's disease. Philadelphia: Lippincott Williams & Wilkins, 1999, p 121.

33. Lukes RJ, Craver LF, Hall TC, et al: Report of the nomenclature committee. Cancer Res 26:1311, 1966.

34. Donaldson SS, Link MP: Childhood lymphomas: Hodgkin's disease and non-Hodgkin's lymphoma. In Moosa AR, Robson MC, Schimpff SC (eds): Comprehensive Textbook of Oncology. Baltimore, Williams & Wilkins, 1986, p 1161.

35. Hudson MM, Donaldson SS: Hodgkin's disease. In Pizzo PA, Poplack DG (eds): Principles and Practice of Pediatric Oncology, 3rd ed. Philadelphia, Lippincott-Raven, 1997, p 523.

36. Medeiros LJ, Greinor T: Hodgkin's disease, SEER population-based data 1973–1987. Cancer 75(suppl 1):357–369, 1995.

37. Murphy S, Morgan E, Katzenstein H, Kletzel M: Results of little or no treatment for lymphocyte-predominant Hodgkin's disease in children and adolescents. Am J Pediatr Hematol Oncol 25:684–687, 2003.

38. Pellegrino B, Terrier-Lacombe M, Oberlin O, et al: Lymphocyte-predominant Hodgkin's lymphoma in children: Therapeutic abstention after initial lymph node resection: A study of the French Society of Pediatric Oncology. J Clin Oncol 21:2948–2952, 2003.

39. Harris NL, Jaffe ES, Stein H, et al: A revised European-American classification of lymphoid neoplasms: A proposal from the International Lymphoma Study Group. Blood 84:1361–1392, 1994.

40. Mauch PM, Kalish LA, Kadin M, et al: Patterns of Hodgkin disease: Implications for etiology and pathogenesis. Cancer 71:2062–2071, 1993.

41. Maity A, Goldwein JW, Lange B, D'Angio GJ: Mediastinal masses in children with Hodgkin's disease. Cancer 69:2755–2760, 1992.

42. Jeffery GM, Mead GM, Whitehouse JM: Life-threatening airway obstruction at the presentation of Hodgkin's disease. Cancer 67:506–510, 1991.

43. Munker R, Hasenclaver D, Brosteanu O, et al: Bone marrow involvement in Hodgkin's disease: An analysis of 135 consecutive cases. J Clin Oncol 13:403–409, 1995.

44. Hann HL, Lange B, Stahlhut MW, McGlynn KA: Prognostic importance of serum transferrin and ferritin in childhood Hodgkin's disease. Cancer 66:313–316, 1990.

45. Tubiana M, Henry-Arnar M, Burgers MV, et al: Prognostic significance of erythrocyte sedimentation rate in clinical stages I-II of Hodgkin's disease. J Clin Oncol 2:194–200, 1984.

46. Xiros N, Binder T, Anger B, et al: Idiopathic thrombocytopenic purpura and autoimmune hemolytic anemia in Hodgkin's disease. Eur J Hematol 40:437–441, 1988.

47. Levine AM, Thornton P, Forman SJ, et al: Positive Coombs test in Hodgkin's disease: Significance and implications. Blood 55:607–611, 1980.

48. Cosset J, Henry Amar M, Meerwadt J, et al: The EORTC trials for limited stage Hodgkin's disease. Eur J Cancer 28A:1847–1850, 1992.

49. Longo D, Russo A, Duffey P, et al: Treatment of advanced stage massive mediastinal Hodgkin's disease: The case for combined modality therapy. J Clin Oncol 9:227–235, 1991.

50. Maity A, Goldwein J, Lange B, et al: Mediastinal mass in children with Hodgkin's disease. Cancer 69:2755–2760, 1992.

51. Vecchi V, Pileri S, Burnelli R, et al: Treatment of pediatric Hodgkin's disease tailored to stage, mediastinal mass, and age. Cancer 72:2049–2057, 1993.

52. Carbone PP, Kaplan HS, Husshoff K, et al: Report of the committee on Hodgkin's disease staging classification. Cancer Res 31:1860–1861, 1971.

53. Mauch P, Larson D, Osteen R, et al: Prognostic factors for positive surgical staging in patients with Hodgkin's disease. J Clin Oncol 8:257–265, 1990.

54. Castellino RA: Diagnostic imaging evaluation of Hodgkin's disease and non-Hodgkin's lymphoma. Cancer 67:1177–1180, 1991.

55. Muraji T, Hays DM, Siegel SE, et al: Evaluation of the surgical aspects of staging laparotomy for Hodgkin's disease in children. J Pediatr Surg 17:843–848, 1982.

56. Mendenhall NP, Cantor AB, Williams JL, et al: With modern imaging techniques, is staging laparotomy necessary in pediatric Hodgkin's disease? A Pediatric Oncology Group Study. J Clin Oncol 11:2218–2225, 1993.

57. Gomez GA, Reese PA, Nava H, et al: Staging laparotomy and splenectomy in early Hodgkin's disease: No therapeutic benefit. Am J Med 77:205–210, 1984.

58. Jenkin D, Chan H, Freedman M, et al: Hodgkin's disease in children: Treatment results with MOPP and low-dose, extended field irradiation. Ca Treatment Rep 66:949–959, 1982.

59. Russel KJ, Donaldson SS, Cox RS, Kaplan HS: Childhood Hodgkin's disease: Patterns of relapse. J Clin Oncol 2:80–87, 1984.

60. American Academy of Pediatrics, Committee on Infectious Diseases: Visual Red Book on CD-ROM, 2001 Update. Elk Grove Village, Ill, American Academy of Pediatrics, 2001.

61. Kaldor JM, Day NE, Clarke EA, et al: Leukemia following Hodgkin's disease. N Engl J Med 322:7–13, 1990.

62. Tura S, Fiacchini M, Zinzani PL, et al: Splenectomy and the increasing risk of secondary acute leukemia in Hodgkin's disease. J Clin Oncol 11:925–930, 1993.

63. Dietrich PY, Henry-Amar M, Cosset JM, et al: Second primary cancers in patients continuously disease-free from Hodgkin's disease: A protective role for the spleen? Blood 84:1209–1215, 1994.

64. Hagemeister FB, Fesus SM, Lamki LM, Haynie TP: Role of gallium scan in Hodgkin's disease. Cancer 65:1090–1096, 1990.

65. Cooper DL, Caride VJ, Zloty M, et al: Gallium scans in patients with mediastinal Hodgkin's disease treated with chemotherapy. J Clin Oncol 11:1092–1098, 1993.

66. Weiner M, Leventhal B, Cantor A, et al: Gallium-67 scans as an adjunct to computed tomography scans for the assessment of a residual mediastinal mass in pediatric patients with Hodgkin's disease. Cancer 68:2478–2480, 1991.

67. King SC, Reiman RJ, Prosnitz LR: Prognostic importance of restaging gallium scans following induction chemotherapy for advanced Hodgkin's disease. J Clin Oncol 12:306–311, 1994.

68. Salloum E, Brandt DS, Caride VJ, et al: Gallium scans in the management of patients with Hodgkin's disease: A study of 101 patients. J Clin Oncol 15:518–527, 1997.

69. Kostakoglu L, Leonard J, Kuji I, et al: Comparison of fluorine-18 fluorodeoxyglucose positron emission tomography and Ga-67 scintigraphy in evaluation of lymphoma. Cancer 94:879–888, 2002.

70. Wirth A, Seymour J, Hicks R, et al: Fluorine-18 fluorodeoxyglucose positron emission tomography, gallium-67 scintigraphy, and conventional staging for Hodgkin's disease and non-Hodgkin's lymphoma. Am J Med 112:262–268, 2002.

71. Shen Y, Kao A, Yen R: Comparison of ^{18}F-fluoro-2-deoxyglucose positron emission tomography and gallium-67 citrate scintigraphy for detecting malignant lymphoma. Oncol Rep 9:321–325, 2002.

72. Buchmann I, Reinhardt M, Elsner K: 2-(Fluorine-18)fluoro-2-deoxy-D-glucose positron emission tomography in the detection and staging of malignant lymphoma: A bicenter trial. Cancer 91:889–899, 2001.

73. Kostakoglu L, Coleman M, Leonard J, et al: PET predicts prognosis after 1 cycle of chemotherapy in aggressive lymphoma and Hodgkin's disease. J Nucl Med 43:1018–1027, 2002.

74. Friedberg J, Chengazi V: PET scans in the staging of lymphoma: Current status. Oncologist 8:438–447, 2003.

75. Weihrauch M, Re D, Scheidhauer K, et al: Thoracic positron emission tomography using ^{18}F-fluorodeoxyglucose for the evaluation of residual mediastinal Hodgkin disease. Blood 98:2930–2934, 2001.

76. Donaldson SS, Link MP: Combined modality treatment with low-dose radiation and MOPP chemotherapy for children with Hodgkin's disease. J Clin Oncol 5:742–749, 1987.

77. Engert A, Schiller P, Josting A, et al: Involved-field radiotherapy is equally effective and less toxic compared with extended-field radiotherapy after four cycles of chemotherapy in patients with early-stage unfavorable Hodgkin's lymphoma: Results of the HD8 trial of the German Hodgkin's Lymphoma Study Group. J Clin Oncol 21:3601–3608, 2003.

78. Donaldson S, Hudson M, Lamborn K, et al: VAMP and low dose, involved-field radiation for children and adolescents with favorable, early-stage Hodgkin's disease: Results of a prospective clinical trial. J Clin Oncol 3081–3087, 2002.

79. Hoppe RT, Coleman CN, Cox RS, et al: The management of stage I-II Hodgkin's disease with irradiation alone or combined modality therapy: The Stanford experience. Blood 59:455–465, 1982.

80. Hoppe RT, Cox RS, Rosenberg SA, et al: Prognostic factors in pathological stage III Hodgkin's disease. Cancer Treat Rep 66:743–749, 1982.

81. Sears JD, Greven KM, Ferree CR, D'Agostino RB: Definitive irradiation in the treatment of Hodgkin's disease. Cancer 79:145–151, 1997.

82. Mauch PM, Canellos GP, Shulman LN, et al: Mantle irradiation alone for selected patients with laparotomy-staged IA to IIA Hodgkin's disease: Preliminary results of a prospective trial. J Clin Oncol 13:947–952, 1995.

83. Wasserman TH, Trenkner DA, Fineberg B, Kucik N: Cure of early-stage Hodgkin's disease with subtotal nodal irradiation. Cancer 68:1208–1215, 1991.

84. Donaldson SS, Whitaker SJ, Plowman PN, et al: Stage I-II pediatric Hodgkin's disease: Long-term follow-up demonstrates equivalent survival rates following different management schemes. J Clin Oncol 8:1128–1137, 1990.

85. Barrett A, Crennan E, Barnes J, et al: Treatment of clinical stage I Hodgkin's disease by local radiation therapy alone: A United Kingdom Children's Cancer Study Group Study. Cancer 66:670–674, 1990.

86. Gehan EA, Sullivan MP, Fuller LM, et al: The intergroup Hodgkin's disease in children: A study of stages I and II. Cancer 65:1429–1437, 1990.

87. Aleman B, Raemaekers J, Tirelli U, et al: Involved-field radiotherapy for advanced Hodgkin's lymphoma. N Engl J Med 348:2396–2406, 2003.

88. Nachman J, Sposto R, Herzog P, et al: Randomized comparison of low-dose involved-field radiotherapy and no radiotherapy for children with Hodgkin's disease who achieve a complete response to chemotherapy. J Clin Oncol 20:3765–3771, 2002.

89. Curtis RE, Boice JD Jr: Second cancers after radiotherapy for Hodgkin's disease. N Engl J Med 319:244–245, 1988.

90. Prior P, Pope DJ: Hodgkin's disease: Subsequent primary cancers in relation to treatment. Br J Cancer 58:512–517, 1988.

91. Kaldor JM, Day NE, Band P, et al: Second malignancies following testicular cancer, ovarian cancer, and Hodgkin's disease: An international collaborative study among cancer registries. Int J Cancer 39:571–585, 1987.

92. Hancock SL, Horning SJ, Hoppe RT: Breast cancer after the treatment of Hodgkin's disease [abstract]. Int J Radiat Oncol Biol Phys 21:157, 1991.

93. Shapiro CL, Mauch PM: Radiation-associated breast cancer after Hodgkin's disease: Risks and screening in perspective. J Clin Oncol 10:1662–1665, 1992.

94. DeVita VT, Serpick A, Carbone PP: Combination chemotherapy in the treatment of advanced Hodgkin's disease. Ann Intern Med 73:881–895, 1970.

95. Bonnadonna G, Zucali R, Monfardini S, et al: Combination chemotherapy of Hodgkin's disease with Adriamycin, bleomycin, vinblastine, and imidazole carboximide versus MOPP. Cancer 36:252–259, 1975.

96. Hutchinson R, Fryer C, Krailo M, et al: Comparison of MOPP/ABVD with ABVD/XRT for treatment of advanced Hodgkin's disease in children (CCG-521). Proc ASCO 11:340, 1992.

97. Ekert H, Waters K, Smith P, et al: Treatment with MOPP or ChlVPP chemotherapy only for all stages of childhood Hodgkin's disease. J Clin Oncol 6:1845–1850, 1988.

98. Ekert H, Fox L, Dalla-Pozzo K, et al: A pilot study of EVAP/ABV chemotherapy in 25 newly diagnosed children with Hodgkin's disease. Br J Cancer 67:159–162, 1993.

99. Behrendt H, Brinkhuis M, Van Leeuwen EF: Treatment of childhood Hodgkin's disease with ABVD without radiotherapy. Med Pediatr Oncol 26:244–248, 1996.

100. Diehl V, Franklin J, Pfreundschuh M, et al: Standard and increased-dose BEACOPP chemotherapy compared with COPP-ABVD for advanced Hodgkin's disease. N Engl J Med 348:2386–2395, 2003.

101. Sieber M, Bredenfeld H, Josting A, et al: 14-day variant of the bleomycin, etoposide, doxorubicin, cyclophosphamide, vincristine, procarbazine, and prednisone regimen in advanced-stage Hodgkin's lymphoma: Results of a pilot study of the German Hodgkin's Lymphoma Study Group. J Clin Oncol 21:1734–1739, 2003.

102. Horning S, Hoppe R, Breslin S, et al: Stanford V and radiotherapy for locally extensive and advanced Hodgkin's disease: Mature results of a prospective clinical trial. J Clin Oncol 20:630–637, 2002.

103. Weiner MA, Leventhal B, Brecher ML, et al: Randomized study of intensive MOPP-ABVD with or without low-dose total-nodal radiation therapy in the treatment of stages IIB, IIIA2, IIIB, and IV Hodgkin's disease in pediatric patients: A Pediatric Oncology Group study [see comments]. J Clin Oncol 15:2769–2779, 1997.

104. Schmitz N, Pfistner B, Sextro M, et al: Aggressive conventional chemotherapy compared with high-dose chemotherapy with autologous haematopoietic stem-cell transplantation for relapsed chemosensitive Hodgkin's disease: A randomized trial. Lancet 359:2065–2071, 2002.

105. Oberlin O, Leverger G, Pacquement H, et al: Low-dose radiation therapy and reduced chemotherapy in childhood Hodgkin's disease: The experience of the French Society of Pediatric Oncology. J Clin Oncol 10:1602–1608, 1992.

106. Hunger SP, Link MP, Donaldson SS: ABVD/MOPP and low-dose involved-field radiotherapy in pediatric Hodgkin's disease: The Stanford experience. J Clin Oncol 12:2160-2166, 1994.

107. Bonfante V, Santoro A, Viviani S, et al: Outcome of patients with Hodgkin's disease failing after primary MOPP-ABVD. J Clin Oncol 15:528–534, 1997.

108. Bader SB, Weinstein H, Mauch P, et al: Pediatric stage IV Hodgkin disease. Cancer 72:249–255, 1993.

109. Fryer CJ, Hutchinson RJ, Krailo M, et al: Efficacy and toxicity of 12 courses of ABVD chemotherapy followed by low-dose regional radiation in advanced Hodgkin's disease in children: A Report from the Children's Cancer Study Group. J Clin Oncol 8:1971–1980, 1990.

110. Weiner MA, Leventhal BG, Marcus R, et al: Intensive chemotherapy and low-dose radiotherapy for the treatment of advanced-stage Hodgkin's disease in pediatric patients: A Pediatric Oncology Group Study. J Clin Oncol 9:1591–1598, 1991.

111. Klimo P, Conners JM: MOPP/ABV hybrid program: Combination chemotherapy based on early introduction of seven effective drugs for advanced Hodgkin's disease. J Clin Oncol 3:1174–1182, 1985.

112. Hudson MM, Greenwald C, Thompson E, et al: Efficacy and toxicity of multiagent chemotherapy and low-dose involved-field radiotherapy in children and adolescents with Hodgkin's disease. J Clin Oncol 11:100–108, 1993.

113. Norris C, Bunin N, Lange B, et al: Modified Vancouver hybrid for treatment of pediatric Hodgkin's disease. Proc ASCO 13:393, 1994.

114. Shellong G, Bramswig JH, Hornig-Franz I: Treatment of children with Hodgkin's disease: Results of the German Pediatric Oncology Group. Ann Oncol 3(suppl 4):73–76, 1992.

115. Bookman MA, Longo DL, Young RC: Late complications of curative treatment in Hodgkin's disease. JAMA 260:680–683, 1988.

116. Aleman B, van den Belt-Dusebout, Klokman W: Long-term cause-specific mortality of patients treated Hodgkin's disease. J Clin Oncol 21:3431–3439, 2003.

117. Willman KY, Cox RS, Donaldson SS: Radiation induced height impairment in pediatric Hodgkin's disease. Int J Radiat Oncol Biol Phys 28:85–92, 1994.

118. Constine LS, Donaldson SS, McDougall JR, et al: Thyroid dysfunction after radiotherapy in children with Hodgkin's disease. Cancer 53:878–883, 1984.

119. McHenry C, Jarosz H, Calandra D, et al: Thyroid neoplasia following radiation therapy for Hodgkin's lymphoma. Arch Surg 122:684–686, 1987.

120. Sankila R, Garwicz S, Olsen JH, et al: Risk of subsequent malignant neoplasms among 1641 Hodgkin's disease patients diagnosed in childhood and adolescence: A population-based cohort study in the five Nordic countries. J Clin Oncol 14:1442–1446, 1996.

121. Thibaud E, Ramirez M, Brauner R, et al: Preservation of ovarian function by ovarian transposition performed before pelvic irradiation during childhood. J Pediatr 121:880–884, 1992.

122. Bhatia S, Robison LL, Oberlin O, et al: Breast cancer and other second neoplasms after childhood Hodgkin's disease. N Engl J Med 334:745–751, 1996.

123. Dores G, Metayer C, Curtis R, et al: Second malignant neoplasms among long-term survivors of Hodgkin's disease: A population-based evaluation over 25 years. J Clin Oncol 20:3484–3494, 2002.

124. Longo D: Radiation therapy in the treatment of Hodgkin's disease: Do you see what I see? J Natl Cancer Inst 95:928–929, 2003.

125. Tucker MA, Coleman CN, Cox RS, et al: Risk of second cancers after treatment for Hodgkin's disease. N Engl J Med 318:76–81, 1988.

126. Cimino G, Papa G, Tura S, et al: Second primary cancer following Hodgkin's disease: Updated results of an Italian multicentric study. J Clin Oncol 9:432–437, 1991.

127. Van Leeuwen FE, Klokman WJ, Hagenbeek A, et al: Second cancer risk following Hodgkin's disease: A 20-year follow-up study. J Clin Oncol 12:312–325, 1994.

128. Kaldor JM, Day NE, Clarke EA, et al: Leukemia following Hodgkin's disease. N Engl J Med 322:7–13, 1990.

129. Tura S, Fiacchini M, Zinzani PL, et al: Splenectomy and the increasing risk of secondary acute leukemia in Hodgkin's disease. J Clin Oncol 11:925–930, 1993.

130. Van Leeuwen FE, Chorus AM, van den Belt-Dusebout AW, et al: Leukemia risk following Hodgkin's disease: Relation to cumulative dose of alkylating agents, treatment with teniposide combinations, number of episodes of chemotherapy, and bone marrow damage. J Clin Oncol 12:1063–1073, 1994.

131. Dietrich PY, Henry-Amar M, Cosset JM, et al: Second primary cancers in patients continuously disease-free from Hodgkin's disease: A protective role for the spleen? Blood 84:1209–1215, 1994.

132. Biovin JF, O'Brien K: Solid cancer risk after treatment of Hodgkin's disease. Cancer 61:2541–2546, 1988.

133. Salloum E, Doria R, Shubert W, et al: Second solid tumors in patients with Hodgkin's disease cured after radiation or chemotherapy plus adjuvant low-dose radiation. J Clin Oncol 14:2435–2443, 1996.

134. Doria R, Holford T, Farber LR, et al: Second solid malignancies after combined modality therapy for Hodgkin's disease. J Clin Oncol 13:2016–2022, 1995.

135. Wahner-Roedler D, Nelson D, Croghan I, et al: Risk of breast cancer and breast cancer characteristics in woman treated with supradiaphragmatic radiation for Hodgkin lymphoma: Mayo Clinic experience. Mayo Clin Proc 78:708–715, 2003.

136. Beatty O, Hudson MM, Greenwald C, et al: Subsequent malignancies in children and adolescents after treatment for Hodgkin's disease. J Clin Oncol 13:603–609, 1995.

137. Travis L, Hill D, Dores G, et al: Breast cancer following radiotherapy and chemotherapy among young women with Hodgkin's disease. JAMA 290:465–475, 2003.

138. Van Leeuwen F, Klokman W, Stovall M, et al: Roles of radiation dose, chemotherapy, and hormonal factors in breast cancer following Hodgkin's disease. J Natl Cancer Inst 95:971–980, 2003.

139. Ng A, Bernardo MVP, Weller E, et al: Second malignancy after Hodgkin disease treated with radiation therapy with or without chemotherapy: Long-term risks and risk factors. Blood 100:1989–1996, 2002.

140. Hancock SL, Tucker MA, Hoppe RT: Factors affecting late mortality from heart disease after treatment of Hodgkin's disease. JAMA 270:1949–1955, 1993.

141. Steinherz LJ, Steinherz PG, Tan CT, et al: Cardiac toxicity 4 to 20 years after completing anthracycline therapy. JAMA 266:1672–1677, 1991.

142. Damewood MD, Grochow LB: Prospects for fertility after chemotherapy or radiation for neoplastic disease. Fertil Steril 45:443–459, 1986.

143. Byrne J, Mulvihill JJ, Myers MH, et al: Effects of treatment on fertility in long-term survivors of childhood or adolescent cancer. N Engl J Med 317:1315–1321, 1987.

144. Le Floch O, Donaldson SS, Kaplan HS: Pregnancy following oophoropexy in total nodal irradiation in women with Hodgkin's disease. Cancer 38:2263–2268, 1976.

145. Chapman RM, Sutcliffe SB, Malpas JS: Male gonadal dysfunction in Hodgkin's disease: A prospective study. JAMA 243:1323–1328, 1981.

146. Aubier F, Flamant F, Brauner R, et al: Male gonadal function after chemotherapy for solid tumors in childhood. J Clin Oncol 7:304–309, 1989.

147. Santoro A, Bonadonna G, Valgussa P, et al: Long term results of combined chemotherapy-radiotherapy approach in Hodgkin's disease: Superiority of ABVD plus radiotherapy versus MOPP plus radiotherapy. J Clin Oncol 5:27–37, 1987.

148. Novakovic B: U.S. childhood cancer survival, 1973–1987. Med Pediatr Oncol 23:480–486, 1994.

149. Magrath IT: The pathogenesis of Burkitt's lymphoma. Recent Adv Cancer Res 55:133–270, 1990.

150. Hanto DW, Frizzera G, Gajl-Peczalska KJ, Simmons RL: Epstein-Barr virus, immunodeficiency, and B cell lymphoproliferation. Transplantation 39:461–472, 1985.

151. Cohen JI: Epstein-Barr virus lymphoproliferative disease associated with acquired immune deficiency. Medicine 70:137–160, 1991.

152. Shibata D, Weiss LM, Nathwani BN, et al: Epstein-Barr virus in benign lymph node biopsies from individuals infected with the human immunodeficiency virus is associated with concurrent or subsequent development of non-Hodgkin's lymphoma. Blood 77:1527–1533, 1991.

153. Neri A, Barriga F, Inghirami G, et al: Epstein-Barr virus infection precedes clonal expansion in Burkitt's and acquired immunodeficiency syndrome-associated lymphomas. Blood 77:1092–1095, 1991.

154. Savoie A, Perpete C, Carpentier L, et al: Direct correlation between the load of Epstein-Barr virus-infected lymphocytes in the peripheral blood of pediatric transplant patients and risk of lymphoproliferative disease. Blood 83:2715–2722, 1994.

155. Rooney CM, Loftin SK, Holladay HS, et al: Early identification of Epstein-Barr virus-associated post-transplantation lymphoproliferative disease. Br J Haematol 89:98–103, 1995.

156. Holmes R, Sokol R: Epstein-Barr virus and post-transplant lymphoproliferative disease. Pediatr Transplant 6:456–464, 2002.

157. Sreenan JJ, Tubbs RR: The influence of immunology and genetics on lymphoma classification: A historical perspective. Ca Invest 14:572–588, 1996.

158. Hutchison RE, Murphy SB, Fairclough DL, et al: Diffuse small noncleaved cell lymphoma in children: Burkitt's versus non-Burkitt's types. Cancer 64:23–28, 1989.

159. Nathwani BN, Griffith RC, Kelly DR, et al: A morphologic study of childhood lymphoma of the diffuse "histiocytic" type: The pediatric oncology experience. Cancer 59:1138–1142, 1987.

160. Hutchison RE, Berard CW, Shuster JJ, et al: B-cell lineage confers favorable outcome among children and adolescents with large-cell lymphoma: A Pediatric Oncology Group study. J Clin Oncol 13:2023–2032, 1995.

161. Sandland JT, Pui CH, Santana VM, et al: Clinical features and treatment outcome for children with CD30+ large-cell non-Hodgkin's lymphoma. J Clin Oncol 12:895–898, 1994.

162. Falini B, Pileri S, Pizzolo G, et al: CD30 (Ki-1) molecule: A new cytokine receptor of the tumor necrosis factor receptor superfamily as a tool for diagnosis and immunotherapy. Blood 85:1–14, 1995.

163. Stein H, Foss H, Durkop H, et al: CD30+ anaplastic large cell lymphoma: A review of its histopathologic, genetic, and clinical features. Blood 96:3681–3695, 2000.

164. Fillipa DA, Ladanyi M, Wollner N, et al: CD30 (Ki-1)-positive malignant lymphomas: Clinical, immunophenotypic, histologic, and genetic characteristics and differences with Hodgkin's disease. Blood 87:2905–2917, 1996.

165. Reiter A, Schrappe M, Tiemann M, et al: Successful treatment strategy for Ki-1 anaplastic large-cell lymphoma of childhood: A prospective analysis of 62 patients enrolled in three consecutive Berlin-Frankfurt-Munster Group studies. J Clin Oncol 12:899–908, 1994.

166. Kaden ME: Ki-1/CD30+ (anaplastic) large-cell lymphoma: Maturation of a clinicopathologic entity with prospects of effective therapy. J Clin Oncol 12:884–887, 1994.

167. Cline MJ: The molecular basis of leukemia. N Engl J Med 330:328–336, 1994.

168. Rosenthal N: Regulation of gene expression. N Engl J Med 331:931–933, 1994.

169. Lebowitz RM, Albrecht S: Molecular biology in the diagnosis and prognosis of solid and lymphoid tumors. Ca Invest 10:399–416, 1992.

170. Look AT, Kirsch IR: Molecular basis of childhood cancer. In Pizzo PA, Poplack DG (eds): Principles and Practice of Pediatric Oncology, 3rd ed. Philadelphia, Lippincott-Raven, 1997, pp 37–74.

171. Dalla-Fevera R, Bregni M, Erikson J, et al: Human *c-myc* oncogene is located on region of chromosome 8 that is translocated in Burkitt lymphoma cells. Proc Natl Acad Sci USA 79:7824–7827, 1982.

172. Zech L, Haglund U, Nilsson K, et al: Characteristic chromosomal abnormalities in biopsies and lymphoid-cell lines from patients with Burkitt and non-Burkitt lymphomas. Int J Cancer 17:47–56, 1976.

173. Shiramizu B, Barriga F, Neequaye J, et al: Patterns of chromosomal breakpoint locations in Burkitt's lymphoma: Relevance to geography and Epstein-Barr virus association. Blood 77:1516–1526, 1991.

174. Bernheim A, Berger R, Lenoir G: Cytogenetic studies on African Burkitt's lymphoma cell lines: t(8;14), t(2;8), and t(8;22) translocations. Cancer Genet Cytogenet 3:307–315, 1981.

175. Lam KM, Syed N, Whittle H, Crawford DH: Circulating Epstein-Barr virus B cells in acute malaria. Lancet 337:876–878, 1991.

176. Henderson S, Rowe M, Gregory G, et al: Induction of bcl-2 expression by Epstein-Barr virus latent membrane protein 1 protects infected B cells from programmed cell death. Cell 65:1107–1115, 1991.

177. Sandlund JT, Downing JR, Crist WM: Non-Hodgkin's lymphoma in childhood. N Engl J Med 334:1238–1248, 1996.

178. Kutok J, Aster J: Molecular biology of anaplastic lymphoma kinase-positive anaplastic large cell lymphoma. J Clin Oncol 20:3691–3702, 2002.

179. Le Beau MM, Bitter MA, Franklin WA, et al: The t(2;5)(p23;q35): A recurring chromosomal abnormality in sinusoidal Ki-1 + non-Hodgkin's lymphoma (Ki-1+ NHL). Blood 72(suppl):247, 1988.

180. Shiota M, Fujimoto J, Takenaga M, et al: Diagnosis of t(2;5)(p23;q35)-associated K-1 lymphoma with immunohistochemistry. Blood 84:3648–3652, 1994.

181. Kadin ME, Sako D, Berliner N, et al: Childhood Ki-1 lymphoma presenting with skin lesions and peripheral lymphadenopathy. Blood 1042–1049, 1986.

182. Howat AJ, Thomas H, Waters KD, Campbell PE: Malignant lymphoma of bone in children. Cancer 59:335–339, 1987.

183. Meyers PA, Potter VP, Wolner N, Exelby P: Bowel perforation during initial treatment of childhood non-Hodgkin's lymphoma. Cancer 56:259–261, 1985.

184. Tesoro-Tess JD, Biasi S, Balzarini L, et al: Heart involvement in lymphomas. Cancer 72:2484–2490, 1993.

185. Ridgway D, Wolff LJ, Neerhout RC, Tilford DL: Unsuspected non-Hodgkin's lymphoma of the tonsils and adenoids in children. Pediatrics 79:399–402, 1987.

186. Ghelman B: Radiology of bone tumors. Orthop Clin North Am 20:287–312, 1989.

187. Clayton F, Butler JJ, Ayala AG, et al: Non-Hodgkin's lymphoma in bone. Cancer 60:2494–2501, 1987.

188. Wollner N, Lane JM, Marcove RC, et al: Primary skeletal non-Hodgkin's lymphoma in the pediatric age group. Med Pediatr Oncol 20:506–513, 1992.

189. Tsokos GC, Balow JE, Spiegel RJ, Magrath IT: Renal and metabolic complications of undifferentiated and lymphoblastic lymphomas. Medicine 60:218–229, 1981.

190. Hande KR, Garrow GC: Acute tumor lysis syndrome in patients with high-grade non-Hodgkin's lymphoma. Am J Med 94:133–139, 1993.

191. Finlay JL, Anderson JR, Cecalupo AJ, et al: Disseminated non-lymphoblastic lymphoma of childhood: A Children's Cancer Group study, CCG-552. Med Pediatr Oncol 23:453–463, 1994.

192. Schwenn MR, Blattner SR, Lynch SR, Weinstein HJ: HiC-COM: A 2-month intensive chemotherapy regimen for children with stage III and IV Burkitt's lymphoma and B-cell acute lymphoblastic leukemia. J Clin Oncol 9:133–138, 1991.

193. Anderson JR, Jenkin RDT, Wilson JF, et al: Long-term follow-up of patients treated with COMP or LSA2L2 therapy for childhood non-Hodgkin's lymphoma: A report of CCG-551 from the Children's Cancer Group. J Clin Oncol 11:1024–1032, 1993.

194. Burkitt D: A sarcoma involving the jaws in African children. Br J Surg 46:218–223, 1958.

195. Shad A, Magrath I: Malignant non-Hodgkin's lymphomas in children. In Pizzo PA, Poplack DG (eds): Principles and Practice of Pediatric Oncology, 3rd ed. Philadelphia, Lippincott-Raven, 1997, pp 545–587.

196. Sariban E, Donahue A, Magrath IT: Jaw involvement in American Burkitt's lymphoma. Cancer 53:141–146, 1984.

197. Reiter A, Schrappe M, Parwaresch R, et al: Non-Hodgkin's lymphomas of childhood and adolescence: Results of a treatment stratified for biologic subtypes and stage: A report of the Berlin-Frankfurt-Munster Group. J Clin Oncol 13:359–372, 1995.

198. Levine AM: Acquired immunodeficiency syndrome-related lymphoma. Blood 80:8–20, 1992.

199. Knowles DM, Cesarman E, Chadburn A, et al: Correlative morphologic and molecular genetic analysis demonstrates three distinct categories of posttransplantation lymphoproliferative disorders. Blood 85:552–565, 1995.

200. Ho M: Risk factors and pathogenesis of posttransplant lymphoproliferative disorders. Transplant Proc 27:38–40, 1995.

201. Reiter A, Zimmerman W, Zimmerman M, et al: The role of initial laparotomy and second look surgery in the treatment of abdominal B-cell non-Hodgkin's lymphoma of childhood: A report of the BFM group. Eur J Pediatr Surg 4:74–81, 1994.

202. Kaplan WD, Jochelson MS, Herman TS, et al: Gallium-67 imaging: A predictor of residual tumor viability and clinical outcome in patients with diffuse large-cell lymphoma. J Clin Oncol 8:1966–1970, 1990.

203. Elstrom R, Guan L, Baker G, et al: Utility of FDG-PET scanning in lymphoma by WHO classification. Blood 101:3875–3876, 2003.

204. Downing JR, Shurtleff SA, Zielenska M, et al: Molecular detection of the (2;5) translocation of non-Hodgkin's lymphoma by reverse transcriptase-polymerase chain reaction. Blood 85:3416–3422, 1995.

205. Staudt L: Molecular diagnosis of the hematologic cancers. N Engl J Med 348:1777–1785, 2003.

206. Murphy SB: Classification, staging and end results of treatment of childhood non-Hodgkin's lymphomas: Dissimilarities from lymphomas in adults. Semin Oncol 7:332–339, 1980.

207. Haddy TB, Adde MA, Magrath IT: CNS involvement in small noncleaved cell lymphoma: Is CNS disease per se a poor prognostic sign? J Clin Oncol 9:1973–1982, 1991.

208. Sandlund JT, Santana V, Abromowitch M, et al: Large cell non-Hodgkin's lymphoma of childhood: Clinical characteristics and outcome. Leukemia (England) 8:30–34, 1994.

209. Lones M, Perkins S, Sposto R, et al: Non-Hodgkin's lymphoma arising in bone in children and adolescents is associated with an excellent outcome: A Children's Cancer Group report. J Clin Oncol 20:2293–2301, 2002.

210. Meadows AT, Sposto R, Jenkin RD, et al: Similar efficacy of 6 and 18 months of therapy with four drugs (COMP) for localized non-Hodgkin's lymphoma of children: A report from the Children's Cancer Study Group. J Clin Oncol 7:92–99, 1989.

211. Patte C, Philip T, Rodary C, et al: High survival rate in advanced-stage B-cell lymphomas and leukemias without CNS involvement with a short intensive polychemotherapy: Results from the French Pediatric Oncology Society of a randomized trial of 216 children. J Clin Oncol 9:123–132, 1991.

212. Bowman WP, Shuster JJ, Cook B, et al: Improved survival for children with B-cell acute lymphoblastic leukemia and stage IV

small noncleaved-cell lymphoma: A Pediatric Oncology Group study. J Clin Oncol 14:1252–1261, 1996.

213. Sullivan MP, Ramirez I: Curability of Burkitt's lymphoma with high-dose cyclophosphamide-high dose methotrexate therapy and intrathecal chemoprophylaxis. J Clin Oncol 3:627–636, 1985.

214. Tubergen DG, Krailo MD, Meadows AT, et al: Comparison of treatment regimens for pediatric lymphoblastic non-Hodgkin's lymphoma: A Children's Cancer Group Study. J Clin Oncol 13:1368–1376, 1995.

215. Swinnen LJ, Mullen GM, Carr TJ, et al: Aggressive treatment for postcardiac transplant lymphoproliferation. Blood 86:3333–3340, 1995.

216. Orjuela M, Gross T, Cheung Y, et al: A pilot study of chemoimmunotherapy (cyclophosphamide, prednisone, and rituximab) in patients with post-transplant lymphoproliferative disorder following solid organ transplantation. Clin Ca Res 9:3945S–3952S, 2003.

217. Link MP, Donaldson SS, Berard CW, et al: Results of treatment of childhood localized non-Hodgkin's lymphoma with combination chemotherapy with or without radiotherapy. N Engl J Med 322:1169–1174, 1990.

218. Cohen LF, Balow JE, Magrath IT, et al: Acute tumor lysis syndrome: a review of 37 patients with Burkitt's lymphoma. Am J Med 68:486–491, 1980.

219. Murphy SB, Melvin SL, Mauer AM, et al: Correlation of tumor cell kinetic studies with surface marker results in childhood non-Hodgkin's lymphoma. Cancer Res 39:1534–1538, 1979.

220. Smalley R, Guaspari A, Haase-Statz S, et al: Allopurinol: Intravenous use for prevention and treatment of hyperuricemia. J Clin Oncol 18:1758–1763, 2000.

221. Pui C, Mahmoud H, Wiley J, et al: Recombinant urate oxidase for the prophylaxis or treatment of hyperuricemia in patients with leukemia or lymphoma. J Clin Oncol 19:697–704, 2001.

222. Goldman S, Holcenberg J, Finklestein J, et al: A randomized comparison between rasburicase and allopurinol in children with lymphoma or leukemia at high risk for tumor lysis. Blood 97:2998–3003, 2001.

223. Allegretta GJ, Weisman SJ, Altman AJ: Oncologic emergencies I: Metabolic and space-occupying consequences of cancer and cancer treatment. Pediatr Clin North Am 32:601–611, 1985.

224. Korones DN, Buzzard CJ, Asselin BL, Harris JP: Right atrial thrombi in children with cancer and indwelling catheters. J Pediatr 128:841–846, 1996.

225. Pryzant RM, Meistrich ML, Wilson G, et al: Long-term reduction I sperm count after chemotherapy with and without radiation therapy for non-Hodgkin's lymphomas. J Clin Oncol 11:239–247, 1993.

226. Sandoval C, Pui CH, Bowman LC, et al: Secondary acute myeloid leukemia in children previously treated with alkylating agents, intercalating topoisomerase II inhibitors, and irradiation. J Clin Oncol 11:1039–1045, 1993.

CHAPTER 70

Rhabdomyosarcoma

Martin L. Blakely, MD, Matthew Harting, MD, and Richard J. Andrassy, MD

Rhabdomyosarcoma (RMS) is a soft tissue tumor originating from immature mesenchymal cells that can arise at essentially any site within the body. RMS is the single most common type of soft tissue sarcoma in children and adolescents. Overall, RMS accounts for up to 50% of all soft tissue sarcomas in children. Over the past three decades, the overall survival with RMS has increased from 25% to more than 70%.[1] This is largely the result of prospective, multicenter clinical trials conducted by the Intergroup Rhabdomyosarcoma Group, established in 1972, as well as other collaborative networks.

Approximately 350 new cases of RMS occur annually in the United States, corresponding to an annual incidence of 4.3 cases per million children age 20 years or younger.[2] RMS is the third most common childhood extracranial solid tumor, behind neuroblastoma and Wilms' tumor.[3] A bimodal age distribution is found, with approximately 65% of cases occurring in children younger than 6 years and the remaining cases occurring in children aged 10 to 18 years.[4]

In the most recent Intergroup Rhabdomyosarcoma Study (IRS-IV), 883 patients were enrolled and analyzed between 1991 and 1997.[1] The distribution of primary tumor sites was as follows: head and neck, 7%; parameningeal, 25% (nasopharynx, paranasal sinus, middle ear mastoid, pterygoid-infratemporal sites); orbit, 9%; genitourinary, 31%; extremities, 13%; retroperitoneum, 7%; trunk, 5%; and all other sites, 3%.

Four major pathologic subtypes of RMS are outlined by the International Classification of RMS: (1) botryoid and spindle cell RMS, most favorable prognosis (variant of embryonal); (2) embryonal, intermediate prognosis; (3) alveolar, poorer prognosis; and (4) undifferentiated sarcoma, also poor prognosis. Botryoid RMS most commonly occurs in the bladder or vagina in infants and young children and in the nasopharynx in older children.[5] Spindle cell RMS is most common in paratesticular, head and neck, extremities, or orbit.[6] Approximately two thirds of all RMSs are categorized as embryonal or an embryonal variant.[7] Alveolar RMS accounts for 20% to 30% of all new cases and generally has the poorest prognosis. A "solid alveolar" variant lacks the characteristic alveolar septations but behaves similarly to the conventional alveolar subtype.[8]

The impact of specific histologic subtype on outcome has varied somewhat in different studies. Confounding variables in examining the importance of histologic type include the finding that different subtypes preferentially occur in specific sites, are present as different primary tumor sizes, and have different invasiveness capabilities. For example, with extremity RMS in IRS-IV, clinical group and stage, but not histologic subtype, were important prognostic variables.[9] Other studies support the theory that histologic subtype is an important independent prognostic factor, with embryonal RMS having a significantly favorable outcome.[8,10] In IRS-IV, 3-year failure-free survival (FFS) was 83% embryonal; 66% alveolar; 55% undifferentiated; and 66% unclassified sarcoma (P < .001).[1]

STAGING

Two classification schemes are currently used to categorize patients with RMS. The clinical *grouping* system was devised by the IRS in 1972 and is a surgicopathologic system that relies on the initial surgical assessment (Table 70-1). A disadvantage of this system is the reliance on the initial surgical approach, which may vary between institutions and surgeons. Clinical grouping has, however, consistently been shown to be an independent prognostic indicator predicting outcome. Overall survival curves according to clinical group of patients enrolled in all IRS studies are shown in Figure 70-1.[7]

More recently the IRS, which is now part of the Sarcoma Committee of the Children's Oncology Group (COG), has implemented a pretreatment staging system based on the tumor-node-metastasis (TNM) system (Table 70-2).[11] The system is modified for RMS to incorporate known important prognostic variables such as primary tumor site, invasiveness (T1, noninvasive; T2, invasive), and size (a, 5 cm in diameter; b, >5 cm). Primary tumor site is known to be an important prognostic factor with RMS. Favorable sites include the orbit, eyelid, other nonparameningeal head/neck sites, and

TABLE 70-1	
CLINICAL GROUPING CLASSIFICATION	
Clinical Group	Extent of Disease
1	Localized tumors, completely resected, no microscopic residual
2a	Localized tumor, complete gross resection, microscopically positive margins of resection
2b	Localized tumor, complete gross resection, positive regional lymph nodes
2c	Localized tumor, complete gross resection, positive regional lymph nodes and margins of resection
3	Localized or locally extensive tumor, gross residual disease after attempted resection or biopsy only
4	Distant metastatic tumor

nonbladder, nonprostate genitourinary (GU) structures (paratesticular, vaginovulvar, uterine). Unfavorable sites include extremities (including buttock), trunk, retroperitoneum, perineum, urinary bladder and prostate, and cranial parameningeal sites. N0 indicates no clinically detectable involvement of regional lymph nodes (LNs) by imaging studies and physical examination; N1 indicates regional nodal involvement; and Nx indicates unknown node status. M1 status indicates that distant metastases are identified. IRS-IV was the first study to use this staging system to classify patients prospectively. FFS rates for patients with local or regional tumors according to stage are shown in Figure 70-2. In this cohort of patients, pretreatment staging appeared to be a more accurate predictor of outcome than did the clinical *grouping* classification system.

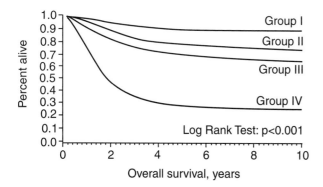

FIGURE 70-1. Overall survival according to clinical group assignment (Intergroup Rhabdomyosarcoma Study [IRS] I to IV). Survival of patients treated on IRS-I, -II, -III/IV-P (IV pilot), and -IV by clinical group at diagnosis. A significant difference is seen in outcome by extent of initial surgical resection, with the best outcome among the patients with completely resected tumors (group 1), followed by those with microscopic residual (group 2) and gross residual (group 3) disease. Patients with metastatic disease (group 4) at diagnosis fare poorly. (J.R. Anderson, personal communication, 2000.) (From Pizzo PA, Poplack DG, eds: *Principles and Practice of Pediatric Oncology*, 4th ed. Philadelphia, Lippincott Williams & Wilkins, 2002.)

MOLECULAR BIOLOGY

Further characterization of RMS tumors by using molecular biology is important in establishing the definitive diagnosis in difficult cases, and specific molecular markers offer promise as prognostic indicators. One of the challenges in the treatment of RMS is to stratify patients into risk categories so that low-risk patients are not exposed to overly toxic treatment regimens, and high-risk patients are not undertreated, allowing poor survival rates. Identification of the molecular pathways involved in RMS also offers potential therapeutic targets to be exploited. Embryonal RMS is characterized by loss of heterozygosity (LOH) at the 11p15 locus.[12] This genetic locus is the site of the insulin-like growth factor-2 gene (*IGF-2*), which codes for a growth factor thought to play a role in the pathogenesis of RMS through one of several possible mechanisms.[7] Another potential etiologic molecular finding is the loss of 9q22, which corresponds to a tumor-suppressor gene in embryonal RMS patients.[13]

Alveolar RMS is characterized by a common translocation between chromosomes 2 and 13, t(2;13)(q35;q14).[14] This translocation usually involves the *PAX3* gene (regulates transcription driving neuromuscular development) and the *FKHR* gene (forkhead family transcription factor).[15] Less commonly, the translocation instead involves the *PAX7* gene located at 1p36 to the same location on chromosome 13.[16] The exact molecular pathway leading to the development of alveolar RMS potentially caused or exacerbated by these translocations remains to be elucidated. *PAX3/FKHR* expression can increase *IGF-2* expression and an IGF-binding protein, providing a common pathway for both embryonal and alveolar RMS.[17]

These known molecular disturbances are just now being adopted and studied clinically. The t(2;13) translocation has been shown to characterize alveolar RMS with a poor prognosis, whereas the t(1;13) translocation is associated with improved outcome.[18] These preliminary findings and other molecular features will be examined more fully in IRS-V.

SURGICAL TREATMENT PRINCIPLES

Primary Resection

It is evident from the impact of clinical grouping on eventual survival rates (see Fig. 70-1) that complete tumor resection with no microscopic residual disease offers the best chance for cure. However, in many sites (e.g., orbit, bladder, prostate, vagina, uterus) complete tumor resection is not feasible while still preserving function of vital organs or structures and while avoiding mutilating surgical procedures. One of the major achievements in the past 30 years of surgical treatment of RMS is the progressive increase in organ salvage rates (e.g., bladder, vagina, uterus, prostate) while not adversely affecting overall patient survival. The decision as to how aggressive to make the original surgical approach depends on primary tumor site, size, presence or absence of LN

TABLE 70-2
TNM RMS PRETREATMENT STAGING CLASSIFICATION

TNM Stage	Sites	Tumor*	Size†	Node‡	Metastasis§
1	Orbit Head and neck (excluding parameningeal) Genitourinary: non–bladder/prostate	T_1 or T_2	a or b	N_0 or N_1 or N_x	M_0
2	Bladder/prostate Extremity Head and neck parameningeal Other (includes trunk, retroperitoneum, etc.)	T_1 or T_2	a	N_0 or N_x	M_0
3	Bladder/prostate Extremity Head and neck parameningeal Other (includes trunk, retroperitoneum, etc.)	T_1 or T_2	a b	N_1 N_0 or N_1 or N_x	M_0 M_0
4	All	T_1 or T_2	a or b	N_0 or N_1	M_1

*Tumor: T (site)$_1$, confined to anatomic site of origin. T(site)$_2$, extension and/or fixation to surrounding tissue.

†a, <5 cm in diameter; b, =5 cm in diameter.

‡Regional nodes: N_0, regional nodes not clinically involved; N_1, regional nodes clinically involved by neoplasm; N_x, clinical status of regional nodes unknown (especially sites that preclude lymph node evaluation).

§Metastasis: M_0, no distant metastases present; M_1, distant metastases.

involvement, and distant metastases. These decisions must be made in the context of a multidisciplinary team including the surgeon, oncologist, pediatric radiologist, and radiotherapist to allow optimal care to be provided. The recommended initial surgical approach is to perform a nonradical tumor resection if the primary site and tumor size is amenable and the treatment team believes that a complete resection with negative margins is feasible. Otherwise, a biopsy sufficient to provide the definitive diagnosis as well as tissue for ongoing biology studies, if applicable, is recommended.

Primary Re-excision

Primary re-excision (PRE) of a tumor is strictly defined as a second attempt at complete resection before the initiation of any other form of therapy. PRE is recommended when an initial resection results in positive margins if this can be accomplished without sacrificing vital structures or organs, causing significant functional impairments, or resulting in a poor cosmetic result. A strategy of PRE has been shown to improve survival in patients with extremity tumors[19] and in perineal RMS,[11] by converting a significant proportion of patients from group IIa to group I. When the initial resection was performed for presumed benign disease, or when the margin status is not known, PRE also is recommended. The benefit of PRE was recently examined by the Italian Cooperative Study Group. They concluded that PRE was the treatment of choice for children with RMS and non-rhabdomyosarcoma soft tissue sarcoma (NRSTS) age 3 years or younger who cannot receive radiation therapy

(RT) and for paratesticular sites.[20] PRE and postoperative RT showed equivalent results in achieving local control in extremity and trunk sites. PRE was not effective in tumors larger than 5 cm. As with the primary tumor resection, PRE is done to allow a clinical group I classification (no residual), but only if this does not require mutilating radical surgical procedure. If not feasible, reliance on adjuvant RT and chemotherapy is advisable.

Lymph Node Evaluation

It has become increasingly recognized that RMS frequently spreads to regional LNs early, that these involved nodes can go undetected by sophisticated imaging techniques, and that LN involvement significantly worsens the prognosis. Because of these findings, pediatric surgeons frequently must evaluate the status of the regional LNs with RMS. With extremity RMS patients in IRS-IV, 37% of all patients and 50% of those in whom surgical LN evaluation was performed had positive regional LN involvement.[9] This study also found that 17% of patients with clinically negative regional nodes had positive biopsy and histologic results. Patients with positive regional LNs had a 3-year FFS of 40% versus approximately 70% in patients without nodal involvement. It is important to determine regional LN status accurately so that if it is positive, more aggressive treatment approaches (e.g., RT) are used, and these patients are recognized to be at higher risk. With perianal RMS, 46% of patients have been found to have regional LN involvement.[11] In this group of patients, N1 patients had a 5-year overall survival rate of 33% versus 71% in N0 patients.

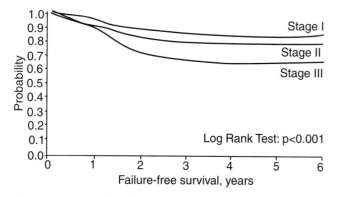

FIGURE 70-2. Failure-free survival for nonmetastatic patients in Intergroup Rhabdomyosarcoma Study-IV according to staging classification.

Regional LN metastases also were frequently documented with paratesticular RMS.[21] With paratesticular and perineal/perianal RMS, an increase in regional LN involvement is found with age of 10 years, indicating that a heightened index of suspicion should be adopted in older children and adolescents with RMS.

Specific recommendations regarding regional LN evaluation will be reviewed according to the specific site, but in general, a strategy of routine surgical evaluation of regional LN status is recommended for RMS patients with primary tumors of the extremity, perineum, and for older patients (>10 years) with paratesticular sites. Additionally, during the course of tumor resection of other sites (e.g., GU, retroperitoneum), LN sampling should be performed if feasible.

For many sites, lymphatic mapping with sentinel LN biopsy may allow adequate staging while limiting the operative morbidity.[21,22] Most experience with this technique has been gained with extremity and truncal tumors. Typically, lymphoscintigraphic lymphatic mapping is performed before the planned operation (either 24 hours before or immediately before the surgical procedure), during which technetium-labeled sulfur colloid is injected at the primary tumor site, and images are obtained demonstrating the lymphatic drainage route. Intraoperatively, vital blue dye is then injected at the primary tumor site and, with a radioisotope detector, a small incision is directed over the site with the highest "counts," and with limited dissection, a blue sentinel LN(s) with evidence of radioactive tracer is excised. These techniques limit the extent of the operation and, potentially, the morbidity, as compared with formal LN dissection as previously performed.

Second-look Operation

The majority of patients with RMS are first seen with tumors that are either too large, too invasive, or in primary sites that do not allow a primary complete resection to achieve either clinical group I or II. In IRS-IV, among all patients without metastatic disease ($n = 883$), 62% were classified as group III (i.e., gross residual disease after biopsy only or attempted resection).[1] After intensive multiagent chemotherapy with or without RT, these patients usually benefit from a second-look

operation (SLO). The goals of the SLO are to remove residual tumor and to determine the pathologic response, as clinical and radiographic assessment can often be inaccurate.[23] The primary benefit of SLO is to resect residual tumor before additional adjuvant treatment, which has been shown to improve patient survival.[24] Alternatively, a negative biopsy (i.e., no tumor) on SLO does not rule out or diminish the possibility of recurrence,[24,25] and no advantage of a SLO appears to occur in patients with a complete clinical response determined radiographically.

Surgical Treatment for Recurrent Disease

Despite the successes of primary therapy for RMS, survival after relapse remains very poor. Approximately 30% of RMS patients will relapse, and between 50% and 95% of these will die of progressive disease.[26] In a large review of relapsed RMS patients from IRS-III, -IV pilot, and -IV studies ($n = 605$), 95% of all failures occurred within 3 years from treatment initiation.[26] Patterns of relapse were as follows: local, 35%; regional, 16%; distant, 41%; and unknown, 8%. Overall, the median survival time from first recurrence or progression was 0.8 years, and the estimated 5-year survival after recurrence was 17%. Factors associated with overall higher survival after relapse included botryoid histology and initial clinical group I assignment. For embryonal RMS, local recurrence predicted improved survival compared with those with regional or distant recurrences. Unfortunately this review did not report data regarding the effect of surgical therapy at the time of relapse on outcome. RMS patients with local relapse compose a very challenging patient population, and the results of repeated attempts at surgical resection are not known. Many RMS patients with locally recurrent disease are those with primary tumors of the extremities, pelvis, retroperitoneum, and other sites at which repeated surgical procedures are difficult and require aggressive and often mutilating procedures (e.g., amputation, pelvic exenteration). The Intergroup Rhabdomyosarcoma Study Group (IRSG) recommends that patients with locally recurrent disease be treated according to risk stratification. For more favorably rated relapse patients, intensive multiagent chemotherapy is given, followed by RT or surgical treatment or both, when feasible.[26] For less favorably rated patients, initial dose-intensified chemotherapy and maintenance therapy with agents such as etoposide or experimental therapies may be offered. In a smaller study of RMS and NRSTS patients with first relapse ($n = 44$), surgical repeated resection appeared to benefit survival with embryonal RMS but not to improve outcome with alveolar RMS or other soft tissue sarcoma histologic subtypes.[27] No carefully reviewed data are available from which to make definitive surgical recommendations for relapsed RMS patients.

Surgical Treatment for Metastatic Rhabdomyocarcoma

Approximately 15% of RMS patients are first seen with metastatic disease, most commonly involving lung (39%), bone marrow (32%), lymph nodes (30%), bones (27%), or other sites.[28] The 3-year overall survival for

129 metastatic RMS patients enrolled in IRS-IV was 39%. In this cohort of patients, 24% had metastases isolated to the lung. The surgical management of these patients is typically restricted to biopsy to confirm the diagnosis, followed by intensive multimodality therapy to attempt to salvage these patients. In this most recent review of metastatic RMS patients from IRS-IV, survival did not differ between patients who underwent operation and pathologic confirmation of lung metastases and those diagnosed radiologically only.[28] The value of aggressive resection of pulmonary metastases from RMS has not been extensively studied, partly because of the rarity of these patients. For other soft tissue sarcomas in children and adults, aggressive resection of isolated pulmonary metastases is thought to be beneficial in prolong survival.

SITE-SPECIFIC SURGICAL GUIDELINES

Head/Neck

Nonparameningeal orbital and other head and neck RMS tumors are considered favorable sites and are classified as stage 1, regardless of size or nodal status. Surgical therapy for orbital and other deep-seated head and neck RMS tumors is largely restricted to biopsy followed by adjuvant chemotherapy RT. Previously, extensive mutilating operations were performed, but with more effective systemic therapy, these are rarely indicated and essentially never for primary therapy. As discussed earlier, recurrent disease portends a much poorer prognosis, so at times, an aggressive surgical approach may still be justified. These tumors are optimally managed by oncologic otolaryngologists and neurosurgeons, when needed. More superficial lesions may benefit from primary surgical resection, such as parotid tumors.

Extremities

Extremity RMS constitutes approximately 15% of all pediatric RMS.[28] These tumors are considered to be in an unfavorable site and are classified as stage 2 if smaller than 5 cm and N0 or as stage 3 if greater than or equal to 5 cm or N1 status. In IRS-IV (1991–1997), the median age of these patients was 6 years; 71% had alveolar histology, and more than 60% were classified as clinical group III or IV.[9]

Surgical evaluation of extremity RMS includes magnetic resonance imaging (MRI) and careful physical examination to determine tumor size and involvement of surrounding structures. For primary tumors smaller than 5 cm, depending on anatomic location, complete resection is the goal. Although the exact required surgical margin remains a matter of debate, a 1.5-cm "surgical margin" surrounding the primary tumor is thought to be adequate. After distortion of the tissues associated with resection and histopathologic processing, this often correlates with a narrower "pathologic margin."[29] Unfortunately, only a minority of extremity RMS patients can be treated with complete primary surgical resection with negative margins: 31 (22%) of 139 patients in IRS-IV.[9]

For patients with larger tumors, or for those in unfavorable anatomic sites (e.g., popliteal or antecubital fossae or the groin), an initial incisional biopsy is recommended. The biopsy incision should be oriented longitudinally (i.e., along the long axis of the limb), so that this does not interfere with a later attempt at resection. An incisional biopsy has an increased likelihood of providing the definitive diagnosis and also provides tissue for ongoing biology studies, as compared with fine-needle or cone biopsies. After intensive multiagent chemotherapy and possibly RT, an SLO can be planned to resect residual disease.

A high rate of regional LN involvement is found with extremity RMS, and evaluation of the regional lymph drainage basin is mandatory. In IRS-IV, approximately 40% of all extremity RMS patients had positive regional LNs.[9] Of 139 patients overall, only 76 actually underwent surgical LN evaluation, and 50% of these were positive. An additional 13 patients had regional nodal disease diagnosed by imaging alone. Among patients with negative imaging and physical examination, but who underwent surgical evaluation of nodal status, 17% were actually positive. This implies that some patients with negative imaging who did not undergo surgical LN evaluation probably had undetected positive LNs. LN disease status is a critical component of the preoperative staging classification scheme (see Table 70-2) and has a direct impact on the treatment plan. Undetected positive nodal disease will lead to inaccurate staging and perhaps less than optimal treatment.

As reviewed previously, for extremity RMS, for microscopically positive or indeterminate margins, or after an initial resection was performed for presumed benign disease, PRE is recommended and has been shown to improve survival.[19]

Genitourinary

Within the GU system, RMS can arise from the vagina, vulva, uterus, paratesticular region, prostate, or bladder. In the IRS-IV study, GU RMS accounted for 12% of all patients and more than 30% of nonmetastatic tumor patients,[28] with bladder/prostate GU primary tumors occurring most commonly.

Bladder/Prostate

For these deep-seated tumors, the recommended surgical approach is usually limited to initial biopsy. Previously, aggressive initial surgical resection was performed with good local control rates but with significant morbidity and low bladder-salvage rates. Currently, bladder salvage is a primary goal with these patients. In selected cases in which the primary tumor involves only the dome of the bladder, complete initial resection may be performed, but for most bladder and prostate tumors, the primary therapy is chemotherapy RT followed by a more limited and conservative resection.[30]

For these tumors, careful consideration should be given to the type of initial biopsy. Often, laparotomy with open biopsy can be avoided, and alternative techniques, such as transurethral cystoscopic needle biopsy, image-guided core needle biopsy, laparoscopic exploration with needle biopsy, or others can help to reduce morbidity.[31]

The estimated 5-year FFS with GU nonbladder/prostate tumors is approximately 80%, indicating a favorable outcome with the conservative surgical approach.[1] If, however, these tumors fail to respond well to primary chemotherapy, as determined by surveillance imaging, a role exists for aggressive tumor resection, including anterior or total pelvic exenteration if needed to achieve local control.

Vagina, Vulva, or Uterus

These tumors are usually embryonal or botryoid histologic subtypes, are considered to be in a favorable site (stage 1), and have an overall 5-year survival rate of more than 80%.[32] Current recommendations are to perform an initial biopsy, often transvaginally, and to rely on effective primary chemotherapy. No role exists for initial aggressive resection such as vaginectomy or hysterectomy.[33] These patients are then best followed up with routine abdominal and pelvic MRI (rather than computed tomography [CT]) to document tumor response.[34,35] As with other pelvic RMS, relapsed or persistent disease in the vagina, vulva, and uterus is associated with a very poor outcome, and aggressive attempts at local control including RT (external beam or brachytherapy), partial or total vaginectomy, hysterectomy, or pelvic exenteration are all viable options.

Paratesticular

Paratesticular RMS made up 14% of all IRS-IV study patients; the most recently completed and published IRS protocol.[28] Only 5% of these patients were clinical group IV after the initial surgical intervention, and indeed, this is considered a favorable site, with all paratesticular patients classified preoperatively as stage 1 regardless of tumor size, invasiveness, or LN status. The overall FFS rate for paratesticular RMS is more than 80%, with patients younger than 10 years having approximately 90% FFS.[1]

The recommended initial surgical approach for paratesticular tumors is radical orchiectomy with proximal ligation of the spermatic cord at the internal inguinal ring via an inguinal incision. A trans-scrotal incision for biopsy or resection is not indicated, and when done, may require a subsequent hemiscrotectomy to resect the contaminated tumor bed, although the need for hemiscrotectomy in this situation is controversial. When paratesticular tumors are fixed to the scrotal skin or invade overlying scrotal skin, hemiscrotectomy is definitely indicated. With this surgical approach, 90% to 95% of patients are able to have complete resection clinical (groups I or II), unlike those with many other less favorable sites.[21]

Paratesticular RMS has a high incidence (~30%) of regional spread to the retroperitoneal lymph nodes (RPLNs), and careful evaluation of these nodes is an important part of the surgical staging workup for these patients. All patients should have thin-cut (3.8 to 5.0 mm) abdominal and pelvic CT scans to assess the retroperitoneum. Because the outcome with paratesticular

RMS has been shown to be partially age dependent, as has frequency of RPLN positivity, the treatment guidelines also vary by age.

Current recommendations for RPLN evaluation are as follows: For patients younger than 10 years, clinical group I, and with no lymph node enlargement on CT scan, no RPLN dissection or sampling is recommended. These patients then have repeated CT scans every 3 months. For patients with suggestive or positive CT scans, ipsilateral retroperitoneal dissection is recommended, and further therapy depends on the pathologic LN status. For all patients 10 years or older, ipsilateral RPLN dissection is recommended up to the level of the renal hilum. In this procedure, a systematic approach is used to remove lymph nodes from each station from the internal inguinal ring, along the iliac vessels and aorta, up to the renal hilum. This risk-based application of surgical RPLN evaluation is meant to ensure that underestimation of the extent of disease is minimized but also that only the higher-risk patients are exposed to these invasive surgical procedures. It is apparent in multiple studies and in multiple RMS tumor sites that CT imaging misses 15% to 20% of patients that actually have involved LNs, which is proven with surgical removal and pathologic examination.[9,11,36]

It should be noted that the International Society of Pediatric Oncology (SIOP) de-emphasizes RPLN surgical evaluation, discourages RPLN dissection, yet reports similar favorable survival rates.[37] SIOP investigators conclude that avoidance of RPLN dissection might underestimate the extent of disease in a few patients, but that this does not compromise survival and that avoiding this surgical procedure with known complications helps to reduce the overall toxicity burden to the patient. SIOP investigators and others also reported that hemiscrotectomy may not be required when a prior scrotal approach has been used, although all cooperative groups strongly recommend an initial inguinal approach.[37,38]

Other Sites

RMSs occurring in other sites are rare, but when they do occur, can present unique challenges to both pediatric surgeons and oncologists. Tumors arising in the trunk or retroperitoneum composed approximately 12% of all IRS-IV patients.[28] For truncal tumors, primary surgical resection is the preferred initial approach for tumors smaller than 5 cm and in patients in whom a negative operative margin can be realistically anticipated. For larger primary tumors, initial incisional biopsy is preferred. Because of the rarity of these tumors, no data are available from which to make definitive surgical guidelines regarding regional LN evaluation. For many truncal lesions, the primary lymphatic drainage basin can be equivocal, and preoperative lymphoscintigraphy may be helpful.

Retroperitoneal and non-GU pelvic tumors are among the most difficult to manage because of the relatively "hidden" location and subsequent late presentation. More than 90% of these patients are first seen as clinical group III (gross residual disease with biopsy or attempted

TABLE 70-3

IRSG STUDY V RISK-BASED PROTOCOL ASSIGNMENT

Risk (Protocol)	Stage	Group	Site	Size	Age (yr)	Histology	Metastasis	Nodes	Treatment
Low, subgroup A (D9602)	1	I	Favorable	a or b	<21	EMB	M0	N0	VA
	1	II	Favorable	a or b	<21	EMB	M0	N0	VA + XRT
	1	III	Orbit only	a or b	<21	EMB	M0	M0	VA + XRT
	2	I	Unfavorable	a	<21	EMB	M0	N0 or Nx	VA
Low, subgroup B (D9602)	1	II	Favorable	a or b	<21	EMB	M0	N1	VAC + XRT
	1	III	Orbit only	a or b	<21	EMB	M0	N1	VAC + XRT
	1	III	Favorable (excluding orbit)	a or b	<21	EMB	M0	N0 or N1 or Nx	VAC + XRT
	2	II	Unfavorable	a	<21	EMB	M0	N0 or Nx	VAC + XRT
	3	I or II	Unfavorable	a	<21	EMB	M0	N1	VAC (+XRT, Gp II)
	3	I or II	Unfavorable	b	<21	EMB	M0	N0 or N1 or Nx	VAC (+XRT, Gp II)
Intermediate (D9803)	2	III	Unfavorable	a	<21	EMB	M0	N0 or Nx	VAC ± Topo + XRT
	3	III	Unfavorable	a	<21	EMB	M0	N1	VAC ± Topo + XRT
	3	III	Unfavorable	b	<21	EMB	M0	N0 or N1 or Nx	VAC ± Topo + XRT
	1 or 2 or 3	I or II or II	Favorable or unfavorable	a or b	<21	ALV/UDS	M0	N0 or N1 or Nx	VAC ± Topo + XRT
	4	I or II or III or IV	Favorable or unfavorable	a or b	<10	EMB	M1	N0 or N1 or Nx	VAC ± Topo + XRT
High (D9802)	4	IV	Favorable or unfavorable	a or b	10	EMB	M1	N0 or N1 or Nx	CPT-11, VAC + XRT
	4	IV	Favorable or unfavorable	a or b	<21	ALV/UDS	M1	N0 or N1 or Nx	CPT-11, VAC + XRT

Favorable, orbit/eyelid, head and neck (excluding parameningeal), genitourinary (not bladder or prostate), and biliary tract; unfavorable, bladder, prostate, extremity, parameningeal, trunk, retroperitoneal, pelvis, other; a, tumor size 5 cm in diameter; b, tumor size >5 cm in diameter; EMB, embryonal, botryoid, or spindle-cell rhabdomyosarcomas or ectomesenchymomas with embryonal RMS; ALV, alveolar rhabdomyosarcomas or ectomesenchymomas with alveolar RMS; UDA, undifferentiated sarcomas; N0, regional nodes clinically not involved; N1, regional nodes clinically involved; Nx, node status unknown; VAC, vincristine, actinomycin D, cyclophosphamide; XRT, radiotherapy; Topo, topotecan; Gp, group; CPT-11, irinotecan.

resection) or IV (metastatic disease) and have large, invasive tumors.[29] The preferred surgical approach for these patients is almost always initial biopsy, aggressive multiagent chemotherapy RT, and SLO if indicated.

The role for debulking large retroperitoneal or non-GU pelvic tumors is not entirely clear, but in general, debulking RMS or other sarcomas is not thought to be indicated or helpful. Adding to this controversy is the finding that the subset of retroperitoneal/non-GU pelvic RMS patients with embryonal tumors who had debulking surgical procedures in IRS-IV or IV-pilot (1984 to 1991) had an improved 4-year FFS versus similar patients that underwent biopsy only (72% vs. 48%; $P = .03$).[39] This finding should be viewed as preliminary data from an observational study and not evidence of benefit with debulking of large retroperitoneal or pelvic tumors.

Perineal and perianal RMSs also are rare sites that have an overall poor outcome at least in part because of late presentation.[40] From 1972 to 1997, 71 patients had perineal and perianal tumors, with a 5-year FFS rate of 45%.[11] Important surgical issues for these patients include the following findings: more than one third of patients are seen initially with presumed benign disease (usually infections); approximately 50% have positive inguinal LNs, which adversely affects survival; and primary re-excision frequently lowers the clinical group assignment, which improves outcome.[11]

CURRENT/FUTURE RESEARCH

The ongoing IRS-V study is divided into separate protocols for patients categorized into various risk strata or categories (Table 70-3). Low-risk patients (D9602 protocol) are estimated to have 3-year FFS rates of 88%, based on previous studies.[41] This subgroup is limited to only those patients with localized embryonal, botryoid, or spindle cell tumors. In general, these patients receive either VAC (vincristine, actinomycin D, cyclophosphamide) or VA chemotherapy and RT to residual tumor with resection.

Intermediate-risk patients (D9803 protocol) have a predicted FFS rate of 55% to 76% and include those with localized alveolar or undifferentiated sarcoma, stages 1 to 3; embryonal RMS stages 2 and 3 with gross residual disease; or stage 4 embryonal RMS patients younger than 10 years. In IRS-V, these patients are randomized to VAC and RT or VAC alternating with vincristine, topotecan, and cyclophosphamide and RT.

High-risk patients (D9802 protocol) have a 3-year FFS of less than 30% and include stage 4 alveolar or undifferentiated tumors and embryonal RMS patients older than 10 years. In general, these patients receive up-front window therapy with irinotecan followed by VAC and RT. For patients responding to irinotecan, treatment continues with four additional cycles of irinotecan and vincristine, in addition to VAC.

An important component of ongoing IRS studies is the investigation of the biology of these tumors. This aspect of the care of RMS patients must be emphasized, and its success hinges on full participation by pediatric surgeons.

Essentially all newly diagnosed or relapsed RMS patients should be considered for enrollment in ongoing biology study protocols, and the surgeon should facilitate the submission of fresh tumor specimens as well as peripheral blood and bone marrow when indicated, so that continued improvements in the care of these children can be realized.

REFERENCES

1. Crist WM, Anderson JR, Meza JL, et al: Intergroup Rhabdomyosarcoma Study-IV: Results for patients with nonmetastatic disease. J Clin Oncol 19:3091–3102, 2001.
2. Gurney JG, Young JL Jr, Roffers SD, et al. Soft tissue sarcomas. In Ries LAG, Smith MA, Gurney JG, et al (eds): Cancer Incidence and Survival among Children and Adolescents: United States SEER Program 1975-1995, National Cancer Institute, SEER Program, NIH Pub. No. 99-4649. Bethesda, 1999, iii.
3. Kramer S, Meadows AT, Jarrett P, et al: Incidence of childhood cancer: Experience of a decade in a population-based registry. J Natl Cancer Inst 70:49–55, 1983.
4. Dagher R, Helman L: Rhabdomyosarcoma: An overview. Oncologist 4:34–44, 1999.
5. Newton WA Jr, Soule EH, Hamondi AB, et al: Histopathology of childhood sarcomas: Intergroup Rhabdomyosarcoma Studies I and II: Clinicopatholgic correlation. J Clin Oncol 6:67–75, 1988.
6. Leuschner I, Newton WA Jr, Schmidt D, et al: Spindle cell variants of embryonal rhabdomyosarcoma in the paratesticular region: A report of the IRS. Am J Surg Pathol 17:221–230, 1993.
7. Wexler LH, Crist LM, Helman LJ. Rhabdomyosarcoma and the undifferentiated sarcomas. In Pizzo PA, Poplack DG (eds): Principles and Practice of Pediatric Oncology, 4th ed. Philadelphia, Lippincott Williams & Wilkins, 2002, 939–971.
8. Tsokos M, Webber BL, Parham DM, et al: Rhabdomyosarcoma: A new classification scheme related to prognosis. Arch Pathol Lab Med 116:847–855, 1992.
9. Neville HL, Andrassy RJ, Lobe TE, et al: Preoperative staging, prognostic factors, and outcome for extremity rhabdomyosarcoma: A preliminary report from IRS-IV (1991-1997). J Pediatr Surg 35:317–321, 2000.
10. Kodet R, Newton WA Jr, Hamoudi AB, et al: Orbital rhabdomyosarcoma and related tumors in childhood: Relationship of morphology to prognosis: An IRS. Med Pediatr Oncol 29:51–60, 1997.
11. Blakely ML, Andrassy RJ, Raney RB, et al: Prognostic factors and surgical treatment guidelines for children with rhabdomyosarcoma of the perineum or anus: A report of IRS Studies I-IV, 1972-1997. J Pediatr Surg 38:347–353, 2003.
12. Scrable HJ, Witte DP, Lampkin BC, et al: Chromosomal localization of the human rhabdomyosarcoma locus by mitotic recombination mapping. Nature 329:645–647, 1987.
13. Bridge JA, Lin J, Weibolt V, et al. Novel genomic imbalances in embryonal rhabdomyosarcoma revealed by comparative genomic hybridization and fluorescence *in situ* hybridization: An IRS. Genes Chromosomes Cancer 27:337–344, 2000.
14. Tuvic-Carel C, Lizard-Nacol S, Justrabo E, et al: Consistent chromosomal translocation in alveolar rhabdomyosarcoma. Cancer Genet Cytogenet 19:361–362, 1986.
15. Shapiro DN, Sublert JE, Li B, et al: Fusion of *PAX3* to a member of the forkhead family of transcription factors in human alveolar rhabdomyosarcoma. Cancer Res 53:5108–5112, 1993.
16. Davis RJ, DiCruz CM, Lovem MA, et al: Fusion of *PAX7* to *FKHR* by the variant t(1;13)(p36;14) translocation in alveolar rhabdomyosarcoma. Cancer Res 54:2869–2872, 1994.
17. Khan J, Bittner M, Saal L, et al: cDNA microassays detect activation of a myogenic transcription program by the *PAX3-FKHR* fusion oncogene. Proc Natl Acad Sci U S A 96:13264–13269, 1999.
18. Kelly KM, Womer RB, Sorenson PH, et al: Common and variant gene fusions predict distinct clinical phenotypes in rhabdomyosarcoma. J Clin Oncol 15:1831–1836, 1997.
19. Hays DM, Lawrence W, Wharam M, et al: Primary re-excision for patients with microscopic residual tumor following initial excision of trunk and extremity sites. J Pediatr Surg 24:5–10, 1989.

20. Cecchetto G, Carli M, Sotti G, et al: Importance of local treatment in pediatric soft tissue sarcomas with microscopic residual after primary surgery: Results of the Italian Cooperative Study RMS-88. Med Pediatr Oncol 34:97–101, 2000.

21. Wiener ES, Lawrence W, Hays D, et al: Retroperitoneal node biopsy in paratesticular rhabdomyosarcoma. J Pediatr Surg 29:171–178, 1994.

22. Neville HL, Andrassy RJ, Lally KP, et al: Lymphatic mapping with sentinel node biopsy in pediatric patients. J Pediatr Surg 35:961–964, 2000.

23. Schalow EL, Braecker BH. Role of surgery in children with rhabdomyosarcoma. Med Pediatr Oncol 41:1–6, 2003.

24. Hays DM, Raney RB, Crist WM, et al: Secondary surgical procedures to evaluate primary tumor status in patients with chemotherapy and responsive stage III and IV sarcomas: A report from the IRS. J Pediatr Surg 25:1100–1105, 1990.

25. Godzinski J, Flamant F, Rey A, et al: Value of postchemotherapy bioptical verification of complete clinical remission in previously unresected (stage I and IIpT3) malignant mesenchymal tumors in children: International Society of Pediatric Oncology 1984 Malignant Mesenchymal Tumors Study. Med Pediatr Oncol 22:22–26, 1994.

26. Pappo AS, Anderson JR, Crist WM, et al: Survival post relapse in children and adolescents with rhabdomyosarcoma: A report from the Intergroup Rhabdomyosarcoma Group. J Clin Oncol 17:3487–3493, 1999.

27. Klingebiel T, Pertl U, Hess CF, et al: Treatment of children with relapsed soft tissue sarcoma: Report of the German CESS/CWS REZ 91 Trial. Med Pediatr Oncol 30:269–275, 1998.

28. Breneman JC, Lyden E, Pappo AS, et al: Prognostic factors and clinical outcomes in children and adolescents with metastatic rhabdomyosarcoma: A report from the IRS-IV. J Clin Oncol 21:78–84, 2003.

29. Blakely ML, Spurbeck WW, Pappo AS, et al: The impact of margin of resection on outcome in pediatric non-rhabdomyosarcoma soft tissue sarcoma. J Pediatr Surg 34:672–675, 1999.

30. Lobe TE, Wiener E, Andrassy RJ, et al: The argument for conservative, delayed surgery in the management of prostate RMS. J Pediatr Surg 8:1084–1087, 1996.

31. Alvarez-Silvan AM, Ortiz-Gordillo MJ, Lopes AM, et al: Organ-preserving management of RMS of the prostate and bladder in children. Med Pediatr Oncol 29:573–575, 1997.

32. Arendt CAS, Donaldson SS, Anderson JR, et al: What constitutes optimal therapy for patients with RMS of the female genital tract? Cancer 91:2454–2468, 2001.

33. Andrassy RJ, Wiener ES, Raney RB, et al: Progress in the surgical management of vaginal RMS: A 25-year review from the IRSG. J Pediatr Surg 34:731–735, 1999.

34. Fletcher BD, Kaste SC: MRI for diagnosis and follow-up of genitourinary, pelvic, and perineal RMS. Urol Radiol 14:263–272, 1992.

35. Finelli A, Bbyn P, McLorie GA, et al: The use of magnetic resonance imaging in the diagnosis and follow-up of pediatric pelvic RMS. J Urol 163:1952–1953, 2000.

36. Wiener ES, Anderson JR, Ojimba JI, et al: Controversies in the management of paratesticular RMS: Is staging RPLN dissection necessary for adolescents with resected paratesticular RMS? Semin Pediatr Surg 10:146–152, 2001.

37. Stewart RJ, Martelli H, Oberlin O, et al: Treatment of children with non-metastatic paratesticular RMS: Results of the malignant mesenchymal tumors studies (MMT 84 and MMT 89) of the International Society of Pediatric Oncology. J Clin Oncol 21:793–798, 2003.

38. Dall'Igna P, Bisogno G, Ferrari A, et al: Primary transcrotal excision of paratesticular RMS: Is hemiscrotectomy really mandatory? Cancer 97:1981–1984, 2003.

39. Blakely ML, Lobe TE, Anderson JR, et al: Does debulking improve survival rate in advanced-stage retroperitoneal embryonal RMS? J Pediatr Surg 34:736–741, 1999.

40. Hill DA, Dehner LP, Gow KW, et al: Perianal RMS presenting as a perirectal abscess: A report of 11 cases. J Pediatr Surg 37:576–581, 2002.

41. Raney RB, Anderson JR, Barr FG, et al: RMS and undifferentiated sarcoma in the 1st two decades of life: A selective review of IRSG experience and rational for IRS-IV. J Pediatr Hematol Oncol 23:215–220, 2001.

CHAPTER 71

Nevus and Melanoma

Tom Jaksic, MD, PhD, James F. Nigro, MD,
and M. John Hicks, MD, DDS, PhD

Nevus is a general term that refers to any skin lesion appearing at or after birth. Virtually all epidermal and dermal components have the potential to proliferate in an abnormal fashion to form nevi, and hence an extensive dermatologic nomenclature exists. Clinically and pathologically, however, nevi may be appropriately divided into two broad groups: nonmelanocytic (containing no melanocytes) and melanocytic (formed from the abnormal growth of melanocytes). Nonmelanocytic nevi, with the exception of sebaceus nevi, carry little risk for the evolution of malignancy and are commonly treated conservatively unless cosmetic concerns exist. Melanocytic nevi can evolve into malignant melanoma, and in the instances of dysplastic (Clark's) nevus syndrome and congenital melanocytic nevi, this transformation occurs with some frequency. The pediatric surgeon must thus be knowledgeable about nonmelanocytic lesions, primarily to avoid overtreatment, and about melanocytic nevi to obviate undertreatment.

The incidence of malignant melanoma is increasing at a higher rate than that of any other cancer in the United States, and this neoplasm may arise de novo or from preexisting melanocytic nevi. Diagnostic delay often occurs in children, perhaps because of a lack of awareness among physicians that melanoma occurs in this age group. As a consequence of the poor results of therapy for metastatic melanoma, effective intervention is based on prevention, early recognition, and adequate surgical excision.

NONMELANOCYTIC NEVI

Nonmelanocytic nevi make up a heterogeneous group of skin abnormalities that may be of concern from a cosmetic standpoint, that occasionally are associated with congenital syndromes, but that usually do not carry a significant risk for malignant transformation. Nevus sebaceus is an exception, in that it predisposes to the development of basal cell carcinoma.

Epidermal Nevus

Epidermal nevi are benign, well-circumscribed lesions characterized by a keratotic thickening of the uppermost layers of the skin. Although usually present at birth, epidermal nevi may not be clinically evident until early childhood. Solitary lesions are most common, but it is not unusual to observe individuals with more than one epidermal nevus. They may be located anywhere on the cutaneous surface including the trunk, extremities, face, scalp, and genitalia. The shape is usually linear, and the texture is typically verrucous or velvety. Other morphologic features such as size and color are highly variable. Most epidermal nevi measure several centimeters in length, or less, but extensive lesions can extend along an entire limb or traverse the chest, abdomen, or back. The color of an epidermal nevus can range from yellow to dark brown, and on occasion, the lesion may appear hypopigmented in comparison to the skin tone of the affected individual. Treatment of these lesions is unnecessary unless the nevus results in cosmetic disfigurement.

The epidermal nevus syndrome is a rare condition characterized by widespread epidermal nevi and associated cardiovascular and central nervous system abnormalities.

Inflammatory Linear

Verrucous Epidermal Nevus

This variant of epidermal nevus presents as an erythematous, pruritic or painful, linear, warty eruption at birth or during childhood. The unpleasant symptoms of these persistent lesions warrant more aggressive therapy than that recommended for typical epidermal nevi. Application of topical or intralesional corticosteroids may be helpful, although resistant lesions often require surgical excision or dermabrasion.

Nevus Sebaceus

Nevus sebaceus (also known as nevus sebaceous of Jadassohn) usually presents at birth as a solitary, yellowish orange plaque on the scalp.[1] The distinctive yellow-orange color is a result of immature sebaceous glands, the major histologic feature of this lesion. Nevus sebaceus is well circumscribed, hairless, oval to round, and usually less than 2 to 3 cm in diameter. Much larger or multiple lesions are rare.

Initially the nevus is flat, but by adulthood, the texture is roughened or papillomatous and has been likened to the peel of an orange. Nevus sebaceus occurs anywhere on the body, but the scalp and face are most commonly affected. Approximately 15% of nevus sebaceus cases undergo neoplastic transformation during adolescence or adulthood. The tumor most frequently associated with nevus sebaceus is basal cell carcinoma, followed by syringocystadenoma papilliferum (a benign apocrine gland–derived neoplasm). A variety of other tumors, including squamous cell carcinoma and malignant eccrine poroma, also have been described with nevus sebaceus. It is recommended that the nevus sebaceus be excised before puberty, because neoplastic changes happen after adolescence.

Nevus Comedonicus

Nevus comedonicus is a well-circumscribed plaque made up of grouped keratin-plugged hair follicles. It is usually present at birth but may be first noted in adolescence. Lesions consist of numerous pinpoints of firm, dark papules that resemble open comedones. They can occur anywhere over the hair-bearing surfaces of the skin. Treatment options include lactic acid–containing moisturizers or topical tretinoin to reduce the hyperkeratotic surface; more troublesome lesions can be surgically excised.[2] Nevus comedonicus does not have malignant potential.

Connective Tissue Nevus

Connective tissue nevi are dermal malformations that are secondary to abnormalities in collagen or elastin fibers. They present as subtle, flesh-colored, small elevations in the skin, without marked epidermal change. Their texture may be smooth or pebbly, and their diameter may range from several millimeters to several centimeters. Solitary or multiple lesions can be located anywhere on the body. Presentation occurs at birth, during infancy, or at any point throughout childhood.[3]

When connective tissue nevi are associated with tuberous sclerosis, they are termed *shagreen patches* and are considered one of the important cutaneous signs of the syndrome. Buschke-Ollendorf syndrome is characterized by connective tissue nevi (termed *dermatofibrosis lenticularis disseminata*) in association with osteopoikilosis that manifests radiologically as focal sclerotic areas of dysplasia in the long bones, pelvis, hands, and feet. Connective tissue nevi do not have a propensity for malignant degeneration, and surgical treatment is not indicated.

Nevus Anemicus

This unusual birthmark presents at birth or during early childhood as a well-circumscribed hypopigmented patch.[4] It is secondary to a localized abnormal constriction of the cutaneous vasculature.[5] This lesion has no malignant potential, and treatment is not necessary because the cosmetic abnormality is quite subtle in most cases.

Nevus Achromicus (Nevus Depigmentosus)

A decreased number of functional melanocytes in the affected skin account for this benign birthmark. Nevus achromicus can occur at birth or during early childhood and presents as a well-circumscribed hypopigmented patch that can have a variety of shapes including round, oval, linear, or whorled. The hypopigmentation may be enhanced with Wood's lamp illumination. Treatment is not indicated.

Becker's Nevus

This irregular hyperpigmentation with overlying terminal hair growth is typically seen in male adolescents. The pigmentary change is due to increased melanin in the basal layer of the epidermis rather than a proliferation of melanocytes.[6] Therefore Becker's nevus is not considered a risk for malignant transformation. This lesion is frequently noted over the back, shoulder, or upper arm. Becker's nevus is usually large, measuring 10 to 20 cm in diameter. Enhanced androgen sensitivity may explain why this lesion is more common in young men, although this condition also may develop in girls.[7] Treatment of the pigmentation, hypertrichosis, or both may be attempted with lasers. Shaving, depilatories, and electrolysis also can address the issue of hair overgrowth. Surgical excision is generally not attempted because of the large size and relatively inconspicuous location of these nevi.

MELANOCYTIC NEVI

Melanocytic nevi are benign collections of melanocytes in the skin that may be congenital or acquired, large or small, solitary or multiple, routine or problematic. Although all melanocytic nevi have a theoretical risk of malignant transformation to melanoma, this risk is small for individual lesions. Nevertheless, patients with melanocytic nevi should be observed with care. When individual nevi appear unusual or change over time, surgical intervention is required. Dysplastic (Clark's) nevus syndrome and large or giant congenital melanocytic nevi are particularly linked to the evolution of malignant melanoma.

Histologic Characteristics of Melanocytes, Nevus Cells, and Malignant Melanoma

Melanocytes provide a protective function from the harmful effects of sun exposure.[8–10] These cells are derived from the neural crest and, during embryogenesis, migrate to the skin, hair follicles, and the retina. Melanocytes produce a complex black-brown pigment polymer-melanin, the functions of which include absorbing ultraviolet light, scavenging cytotoxic intermediates, and possibly aiding in the normal development of the nervous system. Melanocytes form melanin in membrane-bound vesicles called *melanosomes*. Melanocytes, nevus cells, and melanoma cells differ markedly in their cytologic appearance, organization, and biologic characteristics.[11-15]

Melanocytes are characterized by dendritic cytoplasm containing melanosomes, solitary cell arrangement without melanocyte-to-melanocyte contact, location along the basal cell layer of the epidermis, small regular nuclei, and rare mitotic activity. Nevus cells have a nuclear morphology similar to that described for melanocytes; however, they lose contact inhibition, tend to cluster in close apposition, and may migrate from the basal layer of the epidermis to the papillary dermis. Nevus cells also retain melanosomes, have an absence of dendritic processes, and are round to ovoid. Melanoma cells share some features of nevus cells, such as lack of dendritic processes, round to spindle shape, and loss of contact inhibition. They also demonstrate pleomorphism, irregular hyperchromatic nuclei, and prominent nucleoli and have readily detectable mitotic activity. Melanoma cells possess the ability to invade the superficial epidermis (Pagetoid spread), the underlying papillary and reticular dermis, and the subcutis, as well as to metastasize via lymphatic and vascular channels to the draining lymph node basin and to distant sites such as the lung.

Junctional Nevus

Junctional nevi are the most common type of acquired pigmented nevi in childhood. Nevus cells predominate at the epidermal-dermal junction, with some extension into the upper portions of the dermis. This results in relatively flat lesions that are usually oval or round with an even tan to brown pigmentation. However, some junctional nevi may be irregular in shape or color. Junctional nevi may occur anywhere on the body and are small, with most ranging from several millimeters to 1 cm in diameter.

Intradermal Nevus

Although intradermal nevi can occur in pediatric patients, they are most commonly seen in adults. Clinically, they present as dome-shaped or pedunculated papules ranging in size from several millimeters to more than 1 cm. Pigmentation is usually uniform and varies from flesh toned to dark brown. The head and neck are the sites most frequently affected by intradermal nevi. Histologically, nests of nevus cells are limited to the dermis.

Compound Nevus

The term *compound nevus* refers to lesions that contain both junctional and intradermal proliferations of nevus cells. Clinically, it resembles a junctional nevus but may be more papular in texture. Although it can be seen in infancy, it is more common in older children and adults.

Halo Nevus

Small pigmented lesions surrounded by a rim of hypopigmentation are termed *halo nevi*. They are typically seen in adolescents and are most commonly located over the trunk, especially the back. The rim of hypopigmentation measures several millimeters in diameter. The etiology is unclear, although it has been proposed that as yet undefined immune mechanisms destroy the pigment-containing melanocytes and nevus cells.[16] Ultimately, the entire lesion resolves, with an eventual return of normal pigmentation in the affected area. Treatment is unnecessary unless the pigmented portion of the halo nevus appears atypical; then excision of the entire lesion, including the halo, is recommended.

Blue Nevus

Blue nevi have a bluish-black appearance caused by the presence of spindle-shaped melanocytes in lower portions of the dermis. The distorted appearance of the deep pigmentation on the skin surface is referred to as the *Tyndall effect*. Blue nevi are typically small (2 to 3 mm), round, well circumscribed, and located over the dorsum of the hands and feet. They may be present at birth but can occur at any age and seem to be more common in women.

Most blue nevi remain completely benign over time, although they are commonly excised because of their ominous dark pigmentation. Cellular blue nevi are variants that tend to be larger than 1 cm in diameter and histologically are composed of aggregates of densely packed cells in the dermis. Cellular blue nevi have a low but definite risk of malignant transformation and should be excised with a narrow margin.[17]

Nevus of Ota and Ito

These nevi are composed of large, irregular patches of bluish-gray pigmentation. Nevus of Ota is located in the periorbital region, with a distribution related to the first and second branches of the trigeminal nerve. Nevus of Ito refers to the same type of lesion with a location over the supraclavicular and scapular skin.

These nevi are most common in female Asian patients but also occur in African Americans, Hispanics, and Native Americans. Histologically, these nevi are composed of dendritic melanocytes in the upper dermis. Essentially no malignant potential exists, although rare cases of malignant melanoma have been associated with nevus of Ota. Treatment options for cosmetic purposes include laser ablation (Q-switched ruby) and cosmetic cover-up.[18]

Spitz Nevus

Spitz nevi are characterized by sudden onset and rapid growth during childhood or early adolescence. They are dome-shaped, reddish tan, firm papules that commonly occur on the face and rarely exceed 1 cm in diameter (Fig. 71-1). Spitz nevi were originally termed *benign juvenile melanomas* because their histologic features can

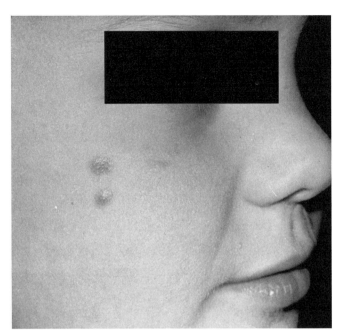

FIGURE 71-1. Two Spitz nevi of the face.

resemble those of malignant melanomas.[19] The presence of epithelioid and spindle cells may confuse pathologists who have limited pediatric experience (Fig. 71-2). Complete excisional biopsy of Spitz nevi is recommended because recurrent, partially removed lesions may be misinterpreted histologically as malignant.

Speckled Lentiginous Nevus

Also known as *nevus spilus,* this nevus is a tan patch of hyperpigmentation with dark brown freckling within the patch. Histologically, these nevi are similar to other acquired melanocytic nevi and theoretically have a small

potential for malignant transformation.[20] They may be present at birth or appear by early childhood, and they can be located virtually anywhere on the skin surface. Sizes range up to several centimeters in diameter. Their extent generally makes surgical excision impractical. Observation of these nevi and biopsy of changes suggestive of malignancy are the management of choice.

Clark's Nevus (Dysplastic Nevus)

Clark's nevi, also known as *atypical melanocytic moles* or *dysplastic nevi,* were first described in 1978.[21] They are common, with an incidence of about 5% in white populations. Clark's nevi may be familial or occur sporadically.[22] Lesions typically present in early adulthood; however, it is not uncommon to see Clark's nevi in young children. Clark's nevi are usually larger than common acquired melanocytic nevi, with diameters ranging from 5 to 15 mm. Color is variable, with multiple shades of brown, tan, and red often present within single lesions. The "fried egg" configuration of a lighter pigmented flat base with a central raised darkly pigmented center is the classic description of dysplastic nevi (Fig. 71-3). The borders tend to be poorly circumscribed, with the appearance of pigment "bleeding into" the normal surrounding skin. The histologic characteristics of Clark's nevus are depicted in Figure 71-4. Although they can occur anywhere on the body, Clark's nevi seem to favor the trunk and scalp more than the extremities.

The relation between Clark's nevi and malignant melanoma remains controversial, with wide-ranging opinions regarding the role of these nevi as true markers for malignancy. Patients with sporadically occurring Clark's nevi are probably at greater risk for developing malignant melanoma over a lifetime when compared with those with common acquired melanocytic nevi or no nevi at all.[22]

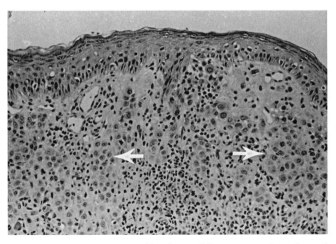

FIGURE 71-2. Spitz nevus histology with numerous intradermal cell nests (*arrows*) with an epithelioid character, abundant cytoplasm, and prominent nucleoli. This type of nevus may be confused with malignant melanoma on histopathologic examination.

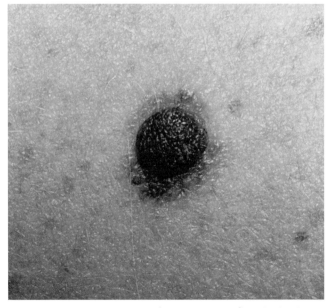

FIGURE 71-3. Clark's nevus (dysplastic nevus) with "fried egg" appearance.

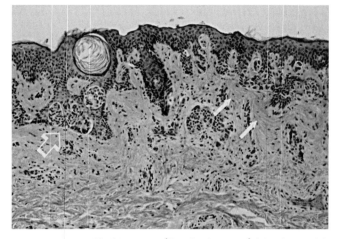

FIGURE 71-4. Clark's nevus (dysplastic nevus) histology with architectural asymmetry, concentric eosinophilic and lamellar fibroplasia (*solid arrows*), and lentiginous melanocytic hyperplasia with bridging (*open arrow*) between adjacent rete pegs.

This risk likely increases with increasing numbers of dysplastic nevi in a given individual. Nevertheless, the likelihood of a given dysplastic nevus transforming into malignant melanoma is small. True familial dysplastic nevi have a more significant relation with malignant melanoma. Patients are considered to have the dysplastic nevus syndrome if they have dysplastic nevi and at least two family members have dysplastic nevi. The risk of malignancy increases further when a family history of melanoma exists. In those patients with two or more relatives with dysplastic nevi and melanoma, the lifetime risk for malignancy is greater than 50%.[23,24]

Patients with Clark's nevi should be observed closely for new or changing lesions. Nevi that have an atypical appearance or have changed abruptly require total excision. First-degree relatives should have a complete skin examination and be monitored on a regular basis if noted to have dysplastic nevi. Routine excision of all dysplastic-appearing nevi is not recommended because the risk of melanoma developing in a given nevus is small and because malignant melanoma frequently develops de novo without an associated preexisting nevus. Thus a patient's risk for developing melanoma cannot be eliminated by prophylactic surgical removal of all dysplastic nevi, and the resultant cost, trauma, and potentially disfiguring scar formation further mitigate against this approach.

Congenital Melanocytic Nevi

Congenital melanocytic nevi (CMN) are characterized qualitatively as small (<1.5 cm diameter), large, and giant (>9 cm diameter in the newborn or >20 cm diameter in the adult), although the distinction between large and giant nevi is often blurred in the literature. Small congenital melanocytic nevi occur in 1% of newborns and may be present anywhere on the body.

The pigmentation is typically uniform, with colors ranging from tan to dark brown, and the borders are well demarcated. Lesions may thicken and grow coarse terminal hairs over time. The lifetime risk for developing malignant melanoma in a small congenital nevus is unknown but is probably less than 5%.[25] No consensus exists regarding the specific treatment of small CMN. Evidence suggests that the risk for melanoma does not usually occur until after adolescence; therefore it is reasonable to observe benign-appearing small CMN during childhood and recommend excision when patients can easily tolerate local anesthesia. It must be stressed, however, that any significant changes in lesion appearance should prompt immediate excision. Scalp lesions that are difficult to examine may warrant prophylactic excision (Fig. 71-5). In contrast, lesions such as those over the fingertips or eyelids may best be left intact and observed for change rather than risking functional impairment secondary to surgical excision.

Large or giant CMN typically affect the trunk and scalp but may involve any portion of the skin surface. Color can range from tan to black, and lesions usually contain a variety of hues. The surface may be flat, jagged, or nodular, with increased thickness usually occurring with advancing age. Extensive terminal hair growth is frequently present. Smaller, round satellite lesions often occur adjacent to the main nevus. The histologic characteristics of congenital melanocytic nevi are outlined in Figure 71-6. Unlike in small CMN, melanomas in large and giant congenital melanocytic nevi may develop early in infancy or childhood. Giant congenital melanocytic nevi can be associated with neurocutaneous melanosis, especially if the nevus is present over the scalp. Proliferation of melanocytes in the central nervous system can lead to increased intracranial pressure, seizure disorders, developmental delay, and malignant melanoma of the central nervous system.[26] The surgical treatment of large and giant congenital nevi is discussed in a later section, along with other prevention strategies for malignant melanoma.

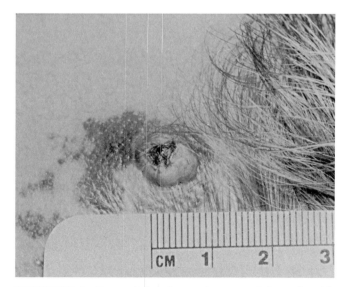

FIGURE 71-5. Congenital melanocytic nevus of the scalp with a melanoma arising from it (raised centrally pigmented lesion).

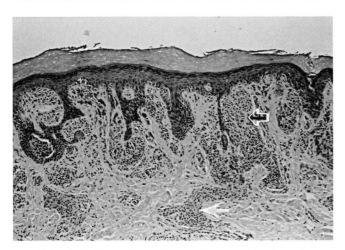

FIGURE 71-6. Congenital melanocytic nevus histology characterized by nevus cells extending from the dermal-epidermal junction (*open arrow*) along skin appendage structures into the deep dermis (*solid arrow*).

PEDIATRIC MALIGNANT MELANOMA

The incidence of malignant melanoma is increasing at a higher rate than that of any other cancer in the United States, with the current lifetime risk being approximately 1 in 87 people.[27] Two percent of cases occur in patients younger than 20 years, and 0.3% to 0.4% of melanomas appear in prepubertal children.[28] A recent study in Sweden showed that the incidence of malignant melanoma during adolescence has doubled over the past 10-year period.[29] Diagnostic delay is present in up to 60% of pediatric cases of malignant melanoma, perhaps owing to a lack of awareness among physicians that melanoma occurs in children.[30] Late diagnosis can adversely affect survival, because metastatic childhood melanoma follows an aggressive course with a 5-year survival rate of only 34%, as compared with a 5-year survival rate of 77% for localized disease.[31] Owing to the poor results of therapy for metastatic melanoma, effective intervention is based on prevention, early recognition, and adequate surgical excision.

Prevention

It has been estimated that 80% of melanoma is caused by repeated acute sun exposure, although the precise mechanism has not been determined.[32] Case-control studies indicate that a history of frequent sunburn accompanied with blistering during childhood and adolescence is associated with an elevated risk of developing malignant melanoma as an adult.[33] Furthermore, children living in the southern United States during adolescence appear to have an increased incidence of malignant melanoma.[34] In pediatric melanomas, boys have a predominance of head and trunk primary lesions, whereas girls have more arm and leg primary malignancies; however, the overall incidence is approximately the same in both genders. Australia, which is the country with the highest incidence of malignant melanoma, has embarked on a prevention campaign that

educates children to (1) avoid direct sunlight during the middle of the day, (2) wear clothing and hats to limit sun exposure, and as an adjunct, (3) apply sunscreens. Twenty percent of the world's melanomas develop in black Africans and in Asians; hence darker skin pigmentation does not preclude the evolution of melanoma.[32]

Other risk factors for melanoma development in children include giant congenital melanocytic nevi, dysplastic (Clark's) nevus syndrome, xeroderma pigmentosa, and immunodeficiency states. Ten percent of melanomas are familial, and various mutations have been linked with the disease, including an autosomal dominant gene with incomplete penetrance.[35] Melanoma also is the most common tumor that may be acquired transplacentally by the fetus from an affected mother. Multiorgan involvement is frequent in the transplacental cases, and the prognosis is usually poor, although spontaneous regression has been occasionally reported.[31]

Congenital melanoma may arise in giant or large congenital nevi, with the majority of malignant transformations occurring later in childhood. Large congenital nevi occur in 1 in 1000 to 1 in 20,000 newborns, and garment nevi, which involve a large surface area such as the back or a whole limb, occur in 1 in 500,000 newborns. The incidence of malignant transformation in large or giant congenital nevi is generally quoted as approximately 5%, with a range of 2% to 20% having been reported. The malignancies that evolve are predominantly melanomas, although other neuroectodermal tumors are sometimes present. Prophylactic removal in early life is usually recommended, because the risk of melanoma in the first year of life (8.6 per 10,000) is 7 times greater than the risk of general anesthesia. Excision of giant congenital nevi should extend to the fascia, because the majority of melanomas arising in these lesions do not originate in the epidermis. Occasionally, even deeper excisions are required if nevic rests are present at the resection margins. Garment nevi often cannot be excised, and thus careful clinical examination throughout the patient's life is recommended, with prompt biopsy of all new or enlarging nodules (Fig. 71-7).[31]

Diagnosis

Melanoma may be accurately diagnosed clinically and at an early stage in most cases. Generally, any change in size, shape, or color of a pigmented lesion over a period of weeks to months is suggestive. The following 7-point checklist has been validated as a sensitive screening method for the early detection of melanoma[36]:

Three Major Features

1. Change in size
2. Change in shape
3. Change in color

Four Minor Features

4. Inflammation
5. Bleeding or crusting

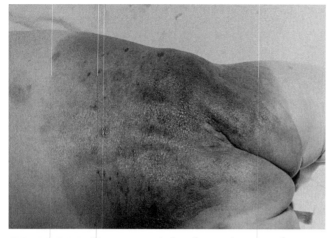

FIGURE 71-7. Giant congenital melanocytic nevus (garment nevus) of the back and buttock in a neonate.

6. Sensory changes
7. Lesion diameter of greater than 7 mm

A pigmented lesion with a major feature demands detailed assessment with likely biopsy, whereas each of the minor features should engender careful follow-up. Other suggestive findings, sometimes referred to as the *"A, B, C, D" of melanoma* follow[37]:

Asymmetry (one side of the lesion differs from the other)
Border irregularity
Color variegation (usually different shades of brown)
Diameter (large)

The characteristic clinical and histologic features of malignant melanoma are demonstrated (Figs. 71-8 and 71-9). Because 50% of melanomas arise without a

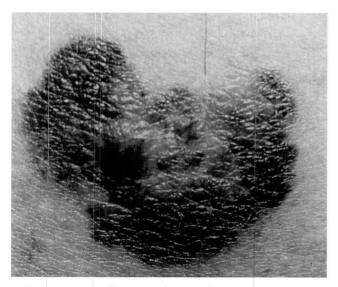

FIGURE 71-8. Malignant melanoma demonstrating asymmetry, border irregularity, and color variegation.

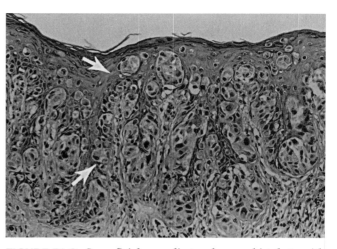

FIGURE 71-9. Superficial spreading melanoma histology with pagetoid invasion of the epidermis by malignant melanoma cells (*arrows*) and microinvasion of the underlying superficial papillary dermis. This is considered to be the radial growth phase of melanoma.

preexisting lesion, it is necessary to assess any new pigmented lesion carefully and to perform a complete skin examination, including the scalp. Inspection alone is up to 80% accurate in identifying malignant melanoma.[37] Other techniques, which have been used in an effort to enhance diagnostic sensitivity in high-risk patients, are full-body photographs, epiluminescence microscopy (magnification and oil immersion applied to a lesion to assess details below the lesion surface), and computer-based image analysis using digitized pictures.

Biopsy remains the unequivocal method to assess suggestive pigmented lesions. Tumor thickness and skin penetration are the most important prognostic factors; therefore complete excision, including some adipose tissue, is the preferred method. If the lesion is large or the anatomic location requires tissue sparing, then a punch biopsy of the region that clinically appears to be the thickest is acceptable. Transection of a melanoma at the time of biopsy does not adversely affect survival.[38]

For all new cases of melanoma, a thorough examination of the whole skin and regional lymph nodes is required. A biopsy should be performed of any lymph node with an abnormally firm or rubbery consistency. For patients with primary melanomas 1 mm or greater in thickness, a baseline chest radiograph and liver function tests are indicated. Computed tomography of the head, chest, abdomen, and pelvis are necessary in all patients with nodal or distant metastatic disease. When leptomeningeal involvement is suspected, magnetic resonance imaging is useful. Positron emission tomography, after intravenous injection of [18F]-labeled glucose, may be the most sensitive method to detect distant melanoma metastases and is currently being evaluated for clinical application.[39]

Staging and Prognosis

The staging system used by the American Joint Commission on Cancer for malignant melanoma is

TABLE 71-1

STAGING SYSTEM FOR MALIGNANT MELANOMA

Stage	Pathologic Findings
1	Tumor <1.5 mm thick
2	Tumor ≥1.5 mm thick and/or satellites present within 2 cm of primary tumor
3	Regional lymph nodes with tumor and/or in-transit disease
4	Distant metastatic disease

TABLE 71-3

CLARK'S CLASSIFICATION FOR MALIGNANT MELANOMA

Level	Depth of Penetration
I	In situ
II	Extends into papillary dermis
III	Extends to the junction of the papillary and reticular dermis
IV	Extends into the reticular dermis
V	Invades the subcutaneous tissue

outlined in Table 71-1. Before the mid-1950s, pediatric melanoma was thought to be less aggressive than the adult disease owing to the erroneous classification of Spitz nevi as melanomas.

It is recognized that both pediatric and adult melanomas have a prognosis that is dependent on tumor thickness or level of invasion.[40] The 5-year survival rates of patients with primary malignant melanomas related to Breslow tumor thickness in millimeters are listed in Table 71-2. The level of invasion of malignant melanoma may also be determined according to the Clark classification (Table 71-3). Nodal metastases are rare in patients with lesions smaller than 1.5 mm in thickness, whereas nodal metastases develop in two thirds of children with melanomas greater than 1.5 mm in thickness (or Clark's levels IV and V).[41,42] As discussed previously, metastatic disease in childhood is associated with a 34% 5-year survival rate.[31]

Treatment

Successful treatment of malignant melanoma is based on the prompt and adequate excision of the primary lesion. The resection margins, which the surgeon selects, should be based on tumor thickness, although anatomic constraints may modulate decision making. The 1992 National Institutes of Health consensus conference on early melanoma recommended 0.5-cm margins for melanoma in situ.[43] Those lesions that invade the skin but do so at a depth of less than 1 mm are routinely removed with a resection margin of 1 cm.[44] A prospective randomized trial in tumors with a depth less than 2 mm showed a 3% local recurrence rate with a 1-cm resection margin, contrasted with a 0% local recurrence rate with

2-cm resection margin; however, this did not translate into any significant survival difference between the two groups after a mean follow-up of 55 months.[45]

A randomized trial of 2-cm resection margins compared with 4-cm resection margins for tumors between 1 and 4 mm thickness, with a mean follow-up of 6 years, also failed to show a survival benefit for the wider excision.[46] No randomized prospective trials are available to assess excision margins for melanomas greater than 4 mm in thickness, although a 3-cm resection margin is usually used in an effort to minimize local recurrence. Table 71-4 summarizes a set of reasonable guidelines for determining resection margins in malignant melanoma based on tumor thickness.[35]

The excision of regional lymph nodes on a prophylactic basis remains controversial. Three randomized, prospective clinical trials are available for review.[47–49] A study of more than 500 patients randomized between prophylactic excision of regional nodes and expectant management (with salvage nodal excision only if the nodes became clinically suggestive) demonstrated no difference in the survival rates between groups.[47] A smaller, single-center trial that compared immediate prophylactic lymphadenectomy, delayed elective lymphadenectomy, and lymphadenectomy if nodes became clinically positive also did not show any survival differences between groups.[48] A more recent randomized trial that enrolled more than 700 patients with melanomas between 1 and 4 mm in thickness again did not prove any significant survival benefit for the prophylactic lymph node dissection group compared with the cohort managed expectantly.[49]

TABLE 71-2

BRESLOW TUMOR THICKNESS RELATED TO 5-YEAR SURVIVAL

Tumor Thickness (mm)	5-Year Survival
<0.75	95%
0.76–1.49	80%
1.50–4.00	60%
>4.00	<50%

TABLE 71-4

TUMOR THICKNESS AND RECOMMENDED RESECTION MARGINS

Tumor Thickness (mm)	Resection Margin (cm)
In situ	0.5
<1	1.0
1–4	2.0 (in anatomic regions where the function of a vital structure would be compromised, a 1.0-cm margin is acceptable)
>4	3.0 (no prospective trials available)

A retrospective subgroup analysis of this study did, however, suggest that patients younger than 60 years with tumor thickness between 1 and 2 mm may have a significant survival benefit with prophylactic node dissection.[49]

Partially in response to the controversy regarding prophylactic lymph node dissection and its associated morbidity of lymphedema, the concept of sentinel node biopsy has evolved. This technique consists of the simultaneous injection of blue dye and subdermal radioactive tracer adjacent to the patient's melanoma. A gamma counter is used to isolate the first regional node, which is then locally excised and submitted for pathologic analysis, by frozen section. If the node is positive for melanoma, a formal lymph node dissection is started. The false-negative rate of this technique may be as low as 1%.[50] Several recently published studies clearly support the concept of sentinel lymphadenectomy as the preferred method of management of thin primary melanoma.[51,52] The reduction in morbidity compared with larger lymph node dissection is clear, and the survival rate for patients is not compromised.

The controversy regarding regional lymph node dissection does not extend to those melanoma patients with clinically apparent lymph node involvement. A therapeutic regional lymphadenectomy is usually performed as an attempt at salvage. The reported 5-year survival rates are all less than 50% and vary inversely with the number of lymph nodes involved; survival rates tend to be lower in truncal than in extremity tumors.[53] Melanomas also may spread hematogenously to any organ, and surgical treatment for metastatic disease is rarely indicated except for palliation. Selected patients with isolated metastases and a long disease-free interval, such as those with secondary adrenal melanomas, may benefit from excision of the metastatic deposits; however, the number of subjects studied is limited, and broad conclusions are impossible.[54]

Chemotherapy for metastatic disease is associated with a 20% response rate for the best single agent, dacarbazine, and up to 50% for combination chemotherapy.[35] Unfortunately, the response to systemic chemotherapy is short, and the improvement in survival rate is low. Regional chemotherapy for limb melanoma with melphalan and recombinant tumor necrosis factor applied through a hyperthermic perfusion circuit does extend the disease-free interval but accomplishes little in terms of improving length of survival.[55] Adjuvant systemic chemotherapy protocols, administered in patients without known metastases, also have been ineffective in prolonging life.

Radiotherapy is rarely used in the primary treatment of cutaneous melanoma, and its use as an adjuvant therapy to improve regional control remains investigative.[56] The main indications for radiotherapy are for the palliative treatment of unresectable local disease, brain metastases, and bone metastases.[56] Some evidence exists that immunotherapy for malignant melanoma, including the use of interleukin-2, interferons, and monoclonal antibodies directed against cell-surface antigens, may be useful in selected patients.[57] The use of melanoma vaccines, as an adjuvant treatment, also is currently being investigated in randomized trials and appears to have low toxicity and potential benefit.[58]

REFERENCES

1. Domingo J, Helwig E: Malignant neoplasms associated with nevus sebaceous of Jadassohn. J Am Acad Dermatol 1:545–556, 1979.
2. Richard JW, Mills O, Leyden JJ: Naevus comedonicus: Treatment with retinoic acid. Br J Dermatol 86:528–529, 1972.
3. Uitto J, Santa Cruz DJ, Eisen A: Connective tissue nevi of the skin: Clinical, genetic and histopathologic classification of hamartomas of the collagen, elastin, and proteoglycan type. J Am Acad Dermatol 3:441–461, 1980.
4. Happle R, Koopman R, Mier PD: Hypothesis: Vascular twin naevi and somatic recombination in man. Lancet 1:367–378, 1990.
5. Mountcastle EA, Diestlemeier M, Lupton GP: Nevus anemicus. J Am Acad Dermatol 14:628–632, 1986.
6. Tate PR, Hodge SJ, Owen LG: A quantitative study of melanocytes in Becker's nevus. J Cutan Pathol 7:404–409, 1980.
7. Person JR, Longcope C: Becker's nevus: An androgen-mediated hyperplasia with increased androgen receptors. J Am Acad Dermatol 10:235–238, 1984.
8. Quevedo WC Jr, Fleischmann RD: Developmental biology of mammalian melanocytes. J Invest Dermatol 75:116–121, 1980.
9. Hearing VJ, Jimenez M: Mammalian tyrosinase: The critical regulatory control point in melanocytic pigmentation. Int J Biochem 19:1141–1147, 1987.
10. Prota G: Recent advances in the chemistry of melanogenesis in mammals. J Invest Dermatol 75:122–127, 1980.
11. Elder DE, Clark WH Jr, Elenitsas R, et al: The early and intermediate precursor lesions of tumor progression in the melanocytic system: Common acquired nevi and atypical (dysplastic) nevi. Semin Diagn Pathol 10:18–35, 1993.
12. Cochran AJ, Bailly C, Paul E, et al: Nevi, other than dysplastic and Spitz nevi. Semin Diagn Pathol 10:3–17, 1993.
13. Bhuta S: Electron microscopy in the evaluation of melanocytic tumors. Semin Diagn Pathol 10:92–101, 1993.
14. Gallagher RP, McLean DI: The epidemiology of acquired melanocytic nevi. Dermatol Clin 13:595–603, 1995.
15. Schleicher SM, Lim SJM: Congenital nevi. Int J Dermatol 34:825–829, 1994.
16. Berman B, Shaieb AM, France DS, et al: Halo congenital melanocytic nevus: In vitro immunologic studies. J Am Acad Dermatol 19:954–960, 1988.
17. Goldenhersch MA, Savin RC, Barnhill RL, et al: Malignant blue nevus: Case report and literature review. J Am Acad Dermatol 19:712–722, 1988.
18. Geronemus RG: Q-switched ruby laser therapy of nevus of Ota. Arch Dermatol 128:1618–1622, 1992.
19. Casso EM, Grin-Jorgensen CM, Grant-Kels JM: Spitz nevi. J Am Acad Dermatol 27:901–913, 1992.
20. Wagner RF, Cottel WI: In situ malignant melanoma arising in a speckled lentiginous nevus. J Am Acad Dermatol 20:125–126, 1989.
21. Clark WH Jr, Reimer RR, Greene MH, et al: Origin of familial malignant melanomas from heritable melanocytic lesions: The B-K mole syndrome. Arch Dermatol 114:732–738, 1978.
22. Greene MH, Clark WH Jr, Tucker MA, et al: Acquired precursors of cutaneous malignant melanoma: The familial dysplastic nevus syndrome. N Engl J Med 312:91–97, 1988.
23. Halpern AC, Guerry D IV, Elder DE, et al: Dysplastic nevi as risk markers of sporadic (non-familial) melanoma. Arch Dermatol 127:995–999, 1991.
24. Greene MH, Clark WH Jr, Tucker MA, et al: High risk of malignant melanoma in melanoma prone families with dysplastic nevi. Ann Intern Med 102:458–486, 1985.
25. Kraemer KH, Greene MH, Tarone R, et al: Dysplastic nevi and cutaneous melanoma risk. Lancet 2:1076–1077, 1983.
26. Mehregan AH, Mehregan DA: Malignant melanoma in childhood. Cancer 71:4096–4103, 1993.
27. Rigal DS, Friedman RJ, Kopf AW: The incidence of malignant melanoma in the United States: Issues as we approach the 21st century. J Am Acad Dermatol 34:839–847, 1996.

28. Boddie AW, Smith JL, McBride CM: Malignant melanomas in children and young adults: Effect of diagnostic criteria on staging and end results. South Med J 71:1074–1078, 1978.

29. Berg P, Lindelof B: Differences in malignant melanoma between children and adolescents. Arch Dermatol 133:295–297, 1997.

30. Melnik MK, Urdaneta LF, Al-Jurf AS, et al: Malignant melanoma in childhood and adolescence. Am Surg 52:142–147, 1986.

31. Ceballos PI, Ruiz-Maldonado R, Mihm MC: Current concepts: Melanoma in children. N Engl J Med 332:656–662, 1995.

32. Armstrong BK, Kricker A: How much melanoma is caused by sun exposure? Melanoma Res 3:395–401, 1993.

33. Holman CD, Armstrong BK: Pigmentary traits, ethnic origin, benign nevi, and family history as risk factors for cutaneous melanoma in children. J Natl Cancer Inst 72:257–266, 1984.

34. Weinstock MA, Golditz GA, Willet WC, et al: Nonfamilial cutaneous melanoma incidence in women associated with sun exposure before 20 years of age. Pediatrics 84:199–204, 1989.

35. Rivers JK: Melanoma. Lancet 347:803–807, 1996.

36. Healsmith MF, Bourke JF, Osbourne JE, et al: An evaluation of the revised seven-point checklist for the early diagnosis of cutaneous malignant melanoma. Br J Dermatol 130:48–50, 1994.

37. Rigel DS: Malignant melanoma: Incidence issues and their effect on diagnosis and treatment in the 1990s. Mayo Clin Proc 72:367–371, 1997.

38. Lederman JS, Sober AJ: Does wide excision as the initial diagnostic procedure improve prognosis in patients with cutaneous melanoma? J Dermatol Surg Oncol 12:697–699, 1986.

39. Gritters LS, Francis IR, Zayaduy KR: Initial assessment of positron emission tomography using 2-fluorine-18-fluoro-2-deoxy-D-glucose in the imaging of malignant melanoma. J Nucl Med 34:1420–1427, 1993.

40. Williams ML, Pennella R: Medical progress: Melanoma, melanocytic nevi, and other melanoma risk factors in children. J Pediatr 124:833–845, 1994.

41. Rao BN, Hayes FA, Pratt CB, et al: Malignant melanoma in children: Its management and prognosis. J Pediatr Surg 25:198–203, 1990.

42. Moss AL, Briggs JC: Cutaneous malignant melanoma in the young. Br J Plast Surg 39:537–541, 1986.

43. NIH Consensus Development Panel on Early Melanoma: Diagnosis and treatment of early melanoma. JAMA 268:1314–1319, 1992.

44. Veronesi U, Cascinelli N: Narrow excision (1-cm margin): A safe procedure for thin cutaneous melanoma. Arch Surg 126:438–441, 1991.

45. Veronesi U, Cascinelli N, Adamus J, et al: Thin stage I primary cutaneous malignant melanoma. N Engl J Med 318:1159–1162, 1988.

46. Balch CM, Urist MM, Karakousis CP, et al: Efficacy of 2-cm surgical margins for intermediate-thickness melanomas (1 to 4 mm): Results of a multi-institutional randomized surgical trial. Ann Surg 218:262–269, 1993.

47. Veronesi U, Adamus J, Bandiera BC, et al: Inefficacy of immediate node dissection in stage I malignant melanoma of the limbs. N Engl J Med 297:627–630, 1977.

48. Sim FH, Taylor WF, Pritchard DJ, Soule EH: Lymphadenectomy in the management of stage I malignant melanoma: A prospective randomized study. Mayo Clin Proc 61:697–705, 1986.

49. Balch CM, Soong SJ, Bartolucci AA, et al: Efficacy of an elective regional lymph node dissection of 1 to 4 mm thick melanoma for patients 60 years of age or younger. Ann Surg 224:255–266, 1996.

50. Morton DL, Wen DR, Wong JH, et al: Technical details of intraoperative mapping for early stage melanoma. Arch Surg 127:392–399, 1992.

51. Murray DR, Carlson GW, Greenlee R, et al: Surgical management of malignant melanoma using dynamic lymphoscintigraphy and gamma probe-guided sentinel lymph node biopsy: The Emory experience. Am Surg 66:763–767, 2000.

52. Leong SPL: Selective sentinel lymphadenectomy for malignant melanoma. Surg Clin North Am. 83:157–185, 2003.

53. Morton DL, Wanek L, Nizze A, et al: Improved long-term survival after lymphadenectomy of melanoma metastatic to regional nodes. Ann Surg 214:491–501, 1991.

54. Branum GD, Epstein RE, Leight GS, et al: The role of resection in the management of melanoma metastatic to the adrenal gland. Surgery 109:127–131, 1991.

55. Krementz ET, Carter RD, Sutherland CM, et al: Regional chemotherapy for melanoma: A 35-year experience. Ann Surg 220:520–535, 1994.

56. Geara FB, Ang KK: Radiation therapy for malignant melanoma. Surg Clin North Am 76:1383–1398, 1996.

57. Kirkwood JM: Systemic therapy of melanoma. Curr Opin Oncol 6:204–211, 1994.

58. Kuhn CA, Hanke CW: Current status of melanoma vaccines. Dermatol Surg 23:649–655, 1997.

CHAPTER 72

Vascular Anomalies

C. Jason Smithers, MD, and Steven J. Fishman, MD

Better understanding of vascular anomalies has come in the last several decades with improved knowledge about the growth of blood vessels (angiogenesis) and the development of a more logical classification system. Based on biologic and clinical behavior, vascular anomalies are broadly divided into two groups: vascular tumors and vascular malformations. Vascular tumors, of which the infantile hemangioma is the most common example, are true neoplasms that arise from endothelial hyperplasia. Conversely, vascular malformations are congenital lesions of vascular dysmorphogenesis that arise because of errors of embryonic development. These lesions exhibit normal endothelial cell turnover. Evaluation of vascular anomalies has historically been hindered by confusing and misused terminology and nomenclature. Along with the rarity and often complex nature of some of these disorders, this confusion has combined to make diagnosis and treatment of vascular anomalies inconsistent. The fact that these lesions do not fit neatly into the realm of any one medical or surgical specialty further complicates the picture. In this chapter, we outline the proper classification and nomenclature of vascular anomalies. This classification provides a basis for understanding the pathophysiology, diagnosis, and treatment of these disorders.[1,2]

CLASSIFICATION

A biologic classification system of vascular anomalies has been devised based on physical characteristics, natural history, and cellular features (Table 72-1).[3,4] This system was accepted in 1996 by the International Society for the Study of Vascular Anomalies. It divides these anomalies into vascular tumors and vascular malformations. Examples of vascular tumors include infantile hemangioma, kaposiform hemangioendothelioma (KHE), and tufted angioma (TA). Vascular malformations can be divided based on vascular channel type (capillary, lymphatic, venous, arterial, or combined) or by flow (slow or fast). Examples of slow-flow lesions are capillary malformations (CMs), lymphatic malformations (LMs), and venous malformations (VMs). Fast-flow lesions include

arteriovenous fistulas and arteriovenous malformations (AVMs).

NOMENCLATURE

Although now more clear, the nomenclature and classification of vascular anomalies have historically been confusing, as the same or similar terms have been used to describe vastly different lesions. Unfortunately, persistent use of the historic terms continues to confuse proper diagnosis and treatment of many patients. The various vascular anomalies often have a similar appearance whether involving the skin, mucosa, or viscera. They are flat or raised lesions that can have pink, red, purple, or blue coloration. For centuries, these cutaneous vascular nevi were named based on resemblance to common foods such as "cherry," "strawberry," or "port-wine stain." The term *nevus* generically refers to any circumscribed malformation of the skin, especially if colored by hyperpigmentation or increased vascularity. In the 19th century, Virchow[5] was the first to describe the histologic features of vascular nevi and initiated the term *angioma*. The term *angioma* became a base term used to describe all such nevi regardless of natural history or other clinical features. He labeled the infantile hemangioma as "angioma simplex." This same lesion has also been historically referred to as "capillary hemangioma" and "strawberry hemangioma." Virchow's "angioma cavernosum" actually was used to label two distinct lesions, infantile hemangiomas (when located deep to the skin) and venous malformations, because they have similar appearances on physical examination. Another example is Virchow's designation of the "angioma racemosum," which referred to what is called today an arteriovenous malformation (AVM) and which also has been historically called an "arteriovenous hemangioma." Wegener, a student of Virchow, described the histology of lymphatic malformations (LM), which he called "lymphangiomas."[6] The classic term *cystic hygroma*, referring to LMs, unfortunately also continues to have common usage. Although in the classic sense, the suffix "-oma" refers to a swelling

TABLE 72-1			
CLASSIFICATION OF VASCULAR ANOMALIES			
Vascular Tumors	Slow-Flow Vascular Malformations	Fast-Flow Vascular Malformations	Combined Vascular Malformations
Hemangioma	Capillary malformation (CM)	Arteriovenous fistula (AVF)	Klippel-Trenaunay syndrome (CLVM)
Kaposiform hemangioendothelioma (KHE)	Venous malformation (VM)	Arteriovenous malformation (AVM)	Parkes-Weber syndrome (CAVM)
Tufted angioma (TA)	Lymphatic malformation (LM)		

of any cause, in contemporary usages, this term connotes neoplastic tumors. Thus both the terms *cystic hygroma* and *lymphangioma* should be abandoned in favor of LM (macrocystic and microcystic, respectively). The problems with this jumble of descriptive and histologic terms are obvious. The same lesion can often have several different names, and the same name can refer to several different lesions. Use of the term *hemangioma* is the most classic case. The term *hemangioma*, combined with descriptive modifiers such as "strawberry," "cavernous," and "lympho-," is used to describe tumors, birthmarks, and vascular malformations alike. Thus vascular anomalies with quite distinct features, whether congenital or acquired, whether they spontaneously regress or progress over time, become lumped under the umbrella of hemangioma. This faulty designation leads to improper diagnosis and treatment for patients. Moreover, it leads to misguided interdisciplinary communication and research efforts. A good example of this problem is provided by cavernous hemangiomas, which are truly venous malformations, but which have often been treated with therapies directed at inhibition of angiogenesis, as if they were vascular tumors.

INTERDISCIPLINARY VASCULAR ANOMALIES CENTERS

The nomenclature and biologic classification of vascular anomalies has provided a useful clinical framework for the diagnosis and treatment of these lesions. Nevertheless, patients with vascular anomalies often provide complex exceptions to these designations. Lesions that are congenital malformations may not become apparent until adulthood, because of either anatomic location or progressive expansion over time. Likewise, neoplastic lesions, such as infantile hemangiomas, often have a premonitory cutaneous sign at birth. Additionally, hemangiomas, when they have a significant fast-flow component, can be difficult to distinguish from AVMs. Last, at times, vascular malformations exhibit enlargement and even endothelial hyperplasia triggered by clotting, ischemia, or partial resection. This hyperplasia leads to their propensity for recurrence after treatment. For these reasons, several regional and international centers have developed an interdisciplinary vascular anomaly team that serves as a referral center.

These centers combine the medical, surgical, and radiologic expertise required to diagnose and manage effectively these often complex disorders.

VASCULAR TUMORS

Infantile Hemangiomas

Hemangiomas are the most common tumor of infancy, occurring in the skin in up to 4% to 10% of white infants, with a female-to-male ratio of 3 to 5:1.[7] The incidence may be significantly higher in premature infants.[8] They are much more common in whites than dark-skinned individuals. Infantile hemangiomas have a unique and characteristic life cycle of rapid growth in the first year of life (proliferative phase) followed by spontaneous slow regression from ages 1 to 7 years (involuting phase). Once involuted, they never recur.

Pathophysiology

The proliferating phase of hemangiomas is characterized by angiogenesis in the tumor.[9,10] The tumor is composed of plump, rapidly dividing endothelial cells, forming a mass of sinusoidal vascular channels. Enlarged feeding arteries and draining veins vascularize the tumor. Markers for mature endothelium, CD-31 and von Willebrand's factor, are present on these neoplastic endothelial cells. In addition, a specific marker for endothelial cells of hemangiomas that is not found in other vascular anomalies is GLUT-1 (an erythrocyte-type glucose transporter).[11] Proangiogenic factors, fibroblast growth factor (FGF) and vascular endothelial growth factor (VEGF), are prominent during the proliferative phase. Increased levels of these peptides may be found in the urine of patients with hemangiomas. Additional factors that are required for angiogenesis include increased local levels of matrix metalloproteinases (MMPs), which are necessary for remodeling of the extracellular matrix.

The involuting phase of hemangiomas is marked by reduced angiogenesis and endothelial cell apoptosis.[12] Levels of FGF and VEGF decrease, and tissue inhibitors of metalloproteinases (TIMPs) increase to suppress new blood vessel formation. The endothelial cells of the tumor flatten, the vascular channels dilate, and the tumor takes on a lobular architecture with replacement by fibrofatty stroma. In the end, with the involuted phase, all that remains is a residuum of fibrofatty tissue with tiny capillaries and mildly dilated draining vessels.

The triggers for angiogenesis and tumor formation are unknown. Viral causes have been speculated on, but none has been elucidated. Human herpesvirus 8, which is associated with Kaposi's sarcoma, is not seen in hemangiomas. The polyoma virus can induce vascular tumors in mice and rats but leads to malignant growth and not to spontaneous regression. Almost certainly, some alteration occurs on a genetic level, but no specific genetic mutations have been found, and no evidence exists for inheritance.[13,14] No animal model exists for a spontaneously regressing hemangioma, such as the common hemangioma of infancy.

Clinical Features

Hemangiomas first appear in the neonatal period, with a median age at onset of 2 weeks. A premonitory cutaneous sign is present at birth in 30% to 50% of cases. Hemangiomas are most often single cutaneous lesions and have an anatomic predilection for the head and neck region (60%). They occur in the trunk in 25% of cases and on the extremities in 15% of cases. Internal and visceral lesions are uncommon. Up to 20% of patients can have multiple tumors, in which case, internal hemangiomas may be found in the liver, gastrointestinal tract, and brain. Rare congenital hemangiomas are fully developed at birth and do not usually exhibit postnatal tumor growth. These are the rapidly involuting congenital hemangioma (RICH) and the noninvoluting congenital hemangioma (NICH).[15] Understanding of these recently discovered entities is still in its infancy.

The *proliferative phase* of hemangiomas is marked by rapid growth, for the first 6 to 8 months, which typically plateaus by age 10 to 12 months. Tumors that involve the superficial dermis are first seen as a red, raised lesion (previously named "capillary" or "strawberry" hemangiomas; Fig. 72-1). Superficial tumors that are larger or that exhibit more rapid growth can cause ulceration of the skin and bleeding in 5% of cases. Tumors in the lower dermis, subcutaneous tissue, or muscle appear bluish with slightly raised overlying skin and have frequently incorrectly been termed "cavernous" hemangiomas. With experience, history and physical examination can establish an accurate diagnosis for 90% of these tumors.

The *involuting phase* of hemangiomas occurs from age 1 to 7 years, during which time the tumor slowly regresses, although it may grow in proportion with the child (Fig. 72-2). This phase is notable for the fading color of the tumor to a dull purple and the softening of the tumor mass. The skin usually becomes pale in the center of the tumor first, spreading outward. Both the deep color and the bulk of the tumor show continued gradual improvement until the regression is entirely complete by age 10 to 12 years. In the final involuted phase of the tumor, 50% of patients have nearly normal skin in the area of the prior lesion. Patients that had larger tumors may have lax or redundant skin and yellowish

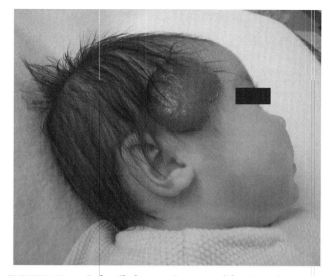

FIGURE 72-1. Infantile hemangioma, proliferative phase.

discoloration. Scars will persist if parts of the tumor were previously ulcerated.

The differential diagnosis of cutaneous hemangiomas consists primarily of other vascular anomalies. Capillary malformations that involve the skin can be mistaken for superficial hemangiomas and vice versa. Deeper hemangiomas can be confused with venous or lymphatic malformations, as they may all appear as bluish masses through the skin (Fig. 72-3). Hemangiomas with fast-flow vascularity of the tumor parenchyma could be taken for arteriovenous malformations, but the age at onset and history generally distinguish the two. Congenital hemangiomas, such as RICH or NICH, can be confused with vascular malformations that are congenital by definition. Pyogenic granulomas that are first seen in childhood, often associated with minor trauma, rarely appear before age 6 months (mean age, 6 to 7 years).[16,17] Finally, other tumors such as tufted angioma, hemangiopericytoma, and fibrosarcoma should be considered.[18] If any concern exists for malignancy, further evaluation with imaging or biopsy is mandated.

The primary local complications that can occur with cutaneous hemangiomas are ulceration, bleeding, and

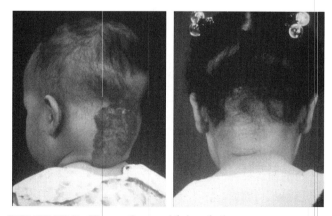

FIGURE 72-2. Hemangioma with involution.

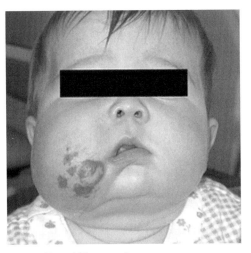

FIGURE 72-3. Parotid hemangioma.

pain. Ulceration is seen in about 5% of cases. Severe complications also are possible, depending on size and location of the tumor. Lesions of the cervicofacial region may produce airway obstruction as they grow during the proliferative phase. Very large hemangiomas, notably of the liver, can lead to high-output congestive heart failure secondary to fast flow and vascular shunting within the tumor. Facial lesions can result in tissue necrosis with cosmetic consequences when involving the eyelid, nose, lip, or ear. Periorbital and eyelid lesions also may cause visual impairment or obstruction that leads to deprivation amblyopia (Fig. 72-4). Distortion of the cornea can alternatively cause astigmatic amblyopia. Subglottic hemangiomas may occur with stridor and lead to airway obstruction on continued growth. Gastrointestinal (GI) hemangiomas are very rare, but may appear with GI bleeding.

Other Manifestations

Hemangiomatosis consists of multiple disseminated hemangiomas. The cutaneous tumors are usually tiny (<5 mm) and, when five or more are present, visceral lesions should be sought as well. Screening patients with

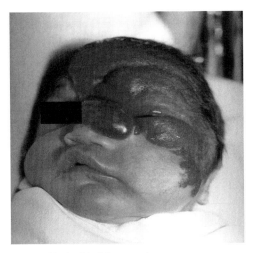

FIGURE 72-4. Periorbital hemangioma.

ultrasonography (US) or magnetic resonance imagine (MRI) or both may be indicated for these patients.

Infantile hepatic hemangiomas must be differentiated from "hepatic hemangiomas" that are first seen in adulthood.[19] Adult "hepatic hemangiomas," which are sometimes called "cavernous hemangiomas" as well, are venous malformations. Conversely, hepatic hemangiomas of infancy are true hemangiomas and have a pattern of involution similar to that of cutaneous hemangiomas. The tumors can be single or multiple, tiny and asymptomatic, or large. The larger tumors tend to be seen initially clinically at ages 1 to 16 weeks. Contrary to popular belief, not all liver hemangiomas are life threatening. Indeed, the "classic triad" of heart failure, anemia, and hepatomegaly is unusual. Rather, liver hemangiomas occur in one of several clinical patterns.[20] Single large lesions, often diagnosed antenatally, commonly cause moderate thrombocytopenia that generally resolves spontaneously. This is in contradistinction to the profound thrombocytopenia seen with Kasabach-Merritt phenomenon (KMP). These single large lesions often do not exhibit growth after birth. Smaller enlarging lesions, detected by imaging stimulated by the presence of cutaneous hemangiomas, may not become symptomatic. The small subset of hepatic hemangiomas that cause high-output cardiac failure have macrovascular shunts (e.g., hepatic artery to hepatic vein) within the tumor, accounting for blood-flow demands above and beyond the hypervascular tumor parenchyma. These shunts will usually close after tumor involution. The most dangerous hepatic hemangiomas are multifocal nodular lesions throughout large portions of the liver that can cause massive hepatomegaly, abdominal compartment syndrome, and respiratory compromise. The differential diagnosis of hepatic hemangiomas includes arteriovenous malformations and malignant tumors such as hepatoblastoma and metastatic neuroblastoma. The diagnosis is established by imaging with US, MRI, or angiography, during which embolization may be performed.

Massive hemangiomas (e.g., those causing hepatomegaly) may induce profound acquired hypothyroidism.[21] Hemangiomas have been found to express type 3-iodothyronine deiodinase that inactivates circulating thyroid hormones. Lesions of sufficient size can break down active thyroid hormones more rapidly than the endocrine axis can replace them. Patients with large hemangiomas should therefore be screened by measurement of thyroid-stimulating hormone levels. When untreated, hypothyroidism in infancy will lead to severe mental retardation. For these unusual cases, aggressive exogenous thyroid replacement and close endocrinologic consultation are mandated. The condition is self-limiting after tumor involution.

Although other congenital anomalies are rarely associated with infantile hemangiomas, a few have been reported, most commonly associated with larger or midline hemangiomas. Cervicothoracic hemangiomas can be seen in conjunction with sternal nonunion.[22] Tumors of the lumbosacral area have been noted to occur along with spinal dysraphism abnormalities such as meningocele and tethered spinal cord.[23,24] Hemangiomas of the pelvis and perineum have been reported in association with urogenital and anorectal anomalies. Craniofacial hemangiomas have been rarely associated with congenital ocular abnormalities such as micro-ophthalmia, cataracts, and optic nerve hypoplasia; posterior fossa cystic malformations; hypoplasia or absence of carotid and vertebral vessels; and malformation of the aortic arch.[25,26]

Imaging

Proper radiologic diagnosis of vascular anomalies is dependent on specific expertise and clinical experience with the radiologic features of these lesions.[27] US and especially MRI are the principal useful modalities. US of proliferative-phase hemangiomas demonstrates a mass with dense parenchyma exhibiting fast-flow vascularity.[28,29] This distinguishes deep infantile hemangiomas from venous malformations that exhibit slow flow and larger blood-filled spaces. MRI of proliferating hemangiomas shows a lobulated solid mass of intermediate intensity with T_1 spin-echo sequences and moderate hyperintensity on T_2 spin-echo. Flow voids that represent fast flow and shunting are seen in and around the tumor. For the involuting phase, MRI demonstrates decreased flow voids and vascularity with the mass, taking on a more lobular and fatty appearance.[30]

Treatment

The majority of infantile hemangiomas do not require any specific treatment other than observation and reassurance of the parents.[31] Even though the tumor may exhibit rapid growth and the skin be fiery red, these tumors will spontaneously regress with either no or minimal evidence of occurrence. Reasons for treatment or referral to a vascular anomalies center are the following: dangerous location (impinging on a vital structure such as the airway or eye), unusually large size or rapid growth, and local or endangering complications (skin ulceration or high-output heart failure). Few prognostic indicators exist for these potential complications. Regularly scheduled follow-up is essential. Serial photographs are very helpful in documenting progression and subsequent improvement.

As hemangiomas are tumors of pure angiogenesis, pharmacologic therapy involves angiogenesis inhibition.[32] The first-line antiangiogenic therapy for hemangiomas exhibiting appropriate risk factors or complications is systemic corticosteroids.[33] Oral prednisone is used at a dose of 2 to 3 mg/kg/day. Doses up to 5 mg/kg/day have been administered for life-threatening complications with large hemangiomas causing airway obstruction or heart failure.[34] The overall response rate is 80% to 90%, with initial improvement in the color and tension of the mass usually noted within 1 week. The steroids are maintained with a very gradual taper every 2 to 4 weeks, with the goal of discontinuation around age 10 to 11 months. Live vaccines such as polio, measles, mumps, rubella, and varicella should be withheld while children are taking the prednisone. Hemangiomas will demonstrate rebound growth if steroids are tapered or stopped too quickly. A return to the initial dosage and a slower tapering will usually treat

this problem. Potential complications of steroid use in infants and children include impaired linear growth and weight gain in about 30% of cases. All children will have "catch-up" growth and return to pretreatment growth curves by age 14 to 24 months. Cushingoid facies occurs in almost all patients and normalizes on tapering of steroids. In rare circumstances, steroids my induce hypertension or hypertrophic cardiomyopathy, both of which are indications to wean or change therapy.[35]

Intralesional corticosteroids are used for hemangiomas that cause local deformity or ulceration, especially for facial lesions of the eyelid, nose, cheek, or lip.[36] A total of three to five injections (at a dose of 3 to 5 mg/kg/injection) are typically given at intervals of 6 to 8 weeks. The response rate approaches that of systemic steroids. Subcutaneous atrophy is a potential complication of steroid injection, but it is usually temporary. Cases have been reported of blindness after intralesional steroid injection for periorbital hemangiomas. This has been presumed to be secondary to particle embolization of the retinal artery through feeding vessels.[37] Manual compression around the periphery of the tumor is recommended during injection.

The second-line agent for dangerous hemangiomas has been recombinant interferon (IFN) alfa, 2a or 2b.[38-42] Indications for IFN use include failure of response to steroids, contraindication to steroid use, and complications related to steroids. IFN does not demonstrate synergism when given simultaneously with steroids. IFN is given subcutaneously once per day at a dose of 2 to 3 million units/m^2. The response rate is slower than that seen with corticosteroids, but an overall success rate of 80% is found. The treatment duration is generally 6 to 12 months. Most patients will manifest low-grade fevers during the first several weeks of therapy. Other reversible side effects are elevation of liver transaminases, neutropenia (secondary to margination), and anemia.[43] IFN use has fallen out of favor, except in very limited circumstances, because of the severe potential complication of spastic diplegia that may occur in 5% to 12% of treated infants.[44,45] Spasticity usually resolves if the drug is terminated quickly. Children receiving IFN should be monitored carefully by a neurologist. Although experience is limited, low-dose, high-frequency antiangiogenic regimens of vincristine are gaining favor as second-line therapy after corticosteroids.

Although it has popular appeal, laser therapy is not often beneficial for infantile hemangiomas.[46] The flashlamp pulse-dye laser penetrates the dermis to a depth of only 0.75 to 1.2 mm. Most cutaneous hemangiomas are deeper and therefore not affected by laser treatment. Additionally, laser therapy carries risks of scarring, skin hypopigmentation, and ulceration, which may lead to a poor result compared with observation alone. A few specific indications for laser treatment of hemangiomas are worth mentioning. One instance in which laser is commonly of benefit is the treatment of telangiectasias that often remain during the involuted phase of hemangioma. Also, the use of endoscopic continuous-wave carbon dioxide laser has been shown to be a good strategy for controlling proliferative-phase hemangiomas in the unilateral subglottic location.[47] Last, intralesional photocoagulation with bare fiber neodymium/yttrium-aluminum-garnet (Nd/YAG) laser can be useful for hemangiomas in certain locations, such as the upper eyelid, when visual obstruction is a concern.

Indications for surgical resection of infantile hemangiomas vary with patient age. During the proliferative phase in infancy, well-localized or pedunculated tumors can be expeditiously resected with linear closure, especially for tumors complicated by bleeding and ulceration. Sites that are most amenable to resection in this stage are the scalp, trunk, and extremities. Other modalities to treat ulceration of hemangiomas include wound care with dressing changes, topical antibiotics, and topical steroids, which can accelerate healing.[48] Tumors of the upper eyelid that obstruct vision and that do not respond to pharmacologic therapy also may require surgical excision or debulking. Focal lesions of the GI tract that appear with bleeding and for which medical management fails also may require resection by means of enterotomy or endoscopic band ligation. Preoperative localization with capsule endoscopy or intraoperative endoscopy or both may be necessary to identify lesions of the small intestine.[49]

Surgical resection is considered during the involuting phase in early childhood for hemangiomas that are large and protuberant and, therefore, likely to create excess and lax overlying skin.[50] Indications are the following: (1) when it is obvious that resection would be necessary sooner or later; (2) when the surgical scar would be identical, regardless of timing of operation; and (3) when the surgical scar is easily hidden. Lesions of the nose, eyelids, lips, and ears require special expertise. It is often preferable to perform the operation for these indications in patients at preschool age before the children become aware of and focus on body differences that may lead to low self-esteem.

After complete involution of the hemangioma, cosmetic distortion is the primary indication for surgical therapy. Fibrofatty residuum and redundant skin can be excised in staged operations, if necessary. Occasionally, extensive scarring from tissue destruction may necessitate reconstructive procedures.

Finally, for the difficult-to-treat and life-threatening large hemangiomas, especially of the liver, angiographic embolization may be required to manage high-output cardiac failure. Arterial catheterization of infants carries significant risks and should generally be limited to those situations with cardiac compromise in which the capacity and intent to perform simultaneous embolization exists. In these rare cases, antiangiogenic pharmacotherapy remains as the first line and should continue along with angiographic procedures. Repeated embolization procedures can be required. Successful embolization is dependent on occlusion of macrovascular shunts within the tumor rather than on occlusion of feeding vessels.[51,52]

Tufted Angioma and Kaposiform Hemangioendothelioma

These vascular tumors of childhood are more aggressive and invasive than are infantile hemangiomas. TA and KHE probably exist within the same spectrum, as they share many overlapping clinical and histologic features.[53,54] Both tumors typically present at birth, although they occur postnatally as well. Male and female infants are affected equally. The tumors are unifocal and are most often located on the trunk, shoulder, thigh, or retroperitoneum. TA appears as erythematous macules or plaques, and histology reveals small tufts of capillaries. KHE is a more extensive tumor with deep red-purple skin discoloration and overlying and surrounding ecchymosis. Generalized petechiae may be apparent and coincide with profound thrombocytopenia secondary to the Kasabach-Merritt phenomenon (KMP). Imaging of KHE depicts an enhancing lesion with poorly defined margins that extend across tissue planes. This is contrasted with hemangiomas, which are well circumscribed and respective of tissue planes. Biopsy is usually not necessary, but histology reveals infiltrating sheets of slender endothelial cells.

Kasabach-Merritt Phenomenon

KMP was first reported in 1940 as a case of profound thrombocytopenia, petechiae, and bleeding in conjunction with a "giant hemangioma."[55] As with many terms in the field of vascular anomalies, the term KMP has been often misused in connection with other varieties of coagulopathy and vascular lesions, most prominently venous malformations. However, the profound and persistent thrombocytopenia that occurs with KMP does not occur with either venous malformations or infantile hemangioma. The only known true associations are with TA and KHE.[56,57] The platelet count with this disorder is typically less than 10,000 and may be accompanied by decreased fibrinogen levels and mildly elevated prothrombin time (PT) and partial thromboplastin time (PTT). Bleeding can result from this platelet-trapping coagulopathy at many sites including intracranial, GI, peritoneal, pleural, and pulmonary. Treatment for KHE with KMP is primarily medical, as the tumor is usually too large and extensive to be resected. Corticosteroids and IFN alfa have been effective in about 50% of cases; vincristine also is beneficial, but no single agent has been shown to be consistently successful. Platelet transfusions are ineffective and should be avoided unless active bleeding occurs. Heparin stimulates tumor growth and worsens the thrombocytopenia of KMP and should likewise be avoided. Mortality rates with KMP and KHE or TA remain high at 20% to 30%. The natural history of these tumors is one of continued proliferation into early childhood followed by subsequent but incomplete regression. These tumors usually persist, albeit in smaller form.[58] Fortunately, they are usually asymptomatic in later stages, although they may cause musculoskeletal pain.

VASCULAR MALFORMATIONS

Pathophysiology

Vascular malformations are congenital lesions of vascular dysmorphogenesis that can be local or diffuse. They are classified, based on appearance of the abnormal channels, as resembling capillaries, lymphatics, veins, arteries, or a combination thereof. The majority of vascular malformations are sporadic, although some rare varieties are familial.[59] They can be quite complex and associated with underlying soft tissue and skeletal abnormalities. Vasculogenesis refers to the process of blood vessel formation from mesodermally derived endothelial precursor cells. The destiny of endothelial precursors to create different types of blood vessels appears to be imprinted early in embryogenesis. Unique cell-surface markers are seen on these endothelial cells.[60] Arterial endothelial cells express ephrin-B2, and venous endothelial cells express ephrin-B4.[61] Although the understanding of vasculogenesis and the pathogenesis of VMs is still limited, the molecular processes are beginning to be understood. VMs probably result from genetic mutations that lead to dysfunction in the regulation of endothelial proliferation and apoptosis, cellular differentiation, maturation, and cell-to-cell adhesions.[62]

Hereditary hemorrhagic telangiectasia (HHT or Rendu-Osler-Weber disease) was the first vascular anomaly to be elucidated at a genetic level.[63] This autosomal dominant disease generally is first seen in the third and fourth decades of life with telangiectasias, arteriovenous fistulae, and AVMs that occur in the skin, mucous membranes, lung, liver, and brain. Two primary causative genes, both on chromosome 9, involve the binding and signaling of transforming growth factor-β. Endoglin is the affected gene for HHT1 and codes for an endothelial glycoprotein. HHT2 involves mutation of an activin receptor kinase.

Lymphatic vessels are thought to develop from preexisting veins and express a unique receptor for vascular endothelial growth factor (VEGFR3 or Flt 4).[64,65] Genetic studies with mice have shown that VEGF3 knockout mice die on embryo day 9 with major venous anomalies before any lymphatic sprouting has occurred.[62] Conversely, transgenic mice that overexpress the ligand for VEGFR3 (VEGF-C), develop distended lymphatic channels.[66] Lymphatic malformations, especially posterior cervical LMs, are one of the components of several sporadic chromosomal syndromes including trisomies 13, 18, and 21, as well as Turner's, Roberts', and Noonan's syndromes. As with the other vascular malformations, the majority of venous malformations are sporadic as well. However, some families have demonstrated an autosomal dominant pattern of inheritance.[67] Studies of these families have shown a mutation in the gene for TIE-2, a receptor expressed by endothelial cells.[68] Defective smooth muscle cells in the vascular wall are thought to be responsible for some venous malformations. These examples support the concept of genetic mutations as being the causative mechanism for vascular malformations.

Capillary Malformations

Capillary malformations (CMs) that have been previously referred to as "port-wine stains" are present at birth as permanent, flat, pink-red cutaneous lesions (Fig. 72-5). The most common location is the head and neck region. It is rare to have multiple CMs. These lesions can be localized or exhibit an extensive, geographic pattern. The histology of cutaneous CM consists of dilated capillary- to venule-size vessels located in the superficial

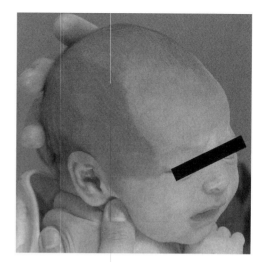

FIGURE 72-5. Capillary malformation.

dermis. These abnormal vessels gradually dilate over time, leading to darkening color and occasionally nodular ectasias. In the newborn nursery, CMs can be confused with nevus flammeus neonatorum, commonly called "angel's kiss" when located on the face, or "stork bite" when in the posterior cervical location. However, these nevi fade with time, whereas a CM does not.

CMs can be associated with underlying soft tissue and skeletal overgrowth as well as other internal abnormalities. CMs of the occiput can signal underlying encephalocele or ectopic meninges. When located over the spine, underlying spinal dysraphism is a concern. Sturge-Weber syndrome represents a classic case of underlying anomalies associated with CMs of the face. In this syndrome, facial CMs affect the trigeminal dermatomes and are associated with ipsilateral ocular and leptomeningeal vascular anomalies. Ocular lesions lead to increased risk for retinal detachment, glaucoma, and blindness. Leptomeningeal involvement can manifest with seizures, hemiplegia, and impaired motor and cognitive function. MRI reveals the central nervous system (CNS) abnormalities showing pial vascular enhancement and gyriform calcifications.[69]

Treatment for CMs is indicated primarily for cosmetic purposes. Flashlamp pulse-dye laser therapy causing photothermolysis of the CM will improve the appearance by lightening the color of the lesion in 70% of patients.[70] Repeated treatments are usually needed, and the timing of therapy remains controversial.[71] Ablative and orthopedic surgical procedures can be tailored to treat cosmetic and functional problems related to soft tissue and bony hypertrophy.

LYMPHATIC MALFORMATIONS

Clinical Features

LMs occur as a wide spectrum from localized masses to areas of diffuse infiltration to chylous fluid accumulations in various body cavities. LMs are usually noted at birth but can manifest at any age or even prenatally by fetal US.[72,73] The skin and soft tissues are most commonly affected. LMs can involve the subcutaneous tissues, muscle, bone, and more rarely, internal organs such as the GI tract and lungs. Anatomic sites frequently seen are the axilla and thorax, cervicofacial region, mediastinum, retroperitoneum, buttock, and anogenital regions. As with CMs, underlying localized soft tissue and skeletal hypertrophy can often be associated with LMs. The abnormal lymphatic spaces can be either macrocystic, microcystic, or a combination. According to previous terminology, macrocystic LMs were referred to as "cystic hygromas," and microcystic LMs, as "lymphangiomas." However, these names should be abandoned.

LMs appear as soft compressible masses, similar to VMs, and may have a bluish hue, although not to the same extent as VMs (Fig. 72-6*A*). Involvement of the dermis may produce puckering of the skin or vesicles that weep clear yellowish fluid. Diffuse infiltration of the subcutaneous tissue can produce extensive lymphedema that also falls within the spectrum of LMs. One unique factor among the vascular anomalies is that LMs are at risk for infection that can lead to cellulitis or even systemic illness. Similarly, infections located elsewhere in the body or viral illnesses can cause increased size and tension of LMs. The cystic components of LMs also are subject to intralesional bleeding secondary to trauma or abnormal venous connections. The vesicles from cutaneous involvement also can leak thin sanguineous fluid or appear as red, purple, or black nodules.

LMs at various anatomic locations are prone to unique associated anomalies. Periorbital LMs can lead to proptosis. Facial LMs can cause the associated deformities of macrocheilia, macroglossia, and macromala. Overgrowth of the mandible, sometimes massive, can be seen with cervicofacial LMs.[74] Congenital airway obstruction is rare but also possible. Lesions of the tongue and floor of the mouth, conversely, may more commonly produce obstruction of the oropharynx. LMs of the cervical and axillary regions can signal associated LMs of the mediastinum. Anomalies of the central conducting lymphatic channels, the thoracic duct and cisterna chyli, can lead to very problematic and recurrent chylous effusions that

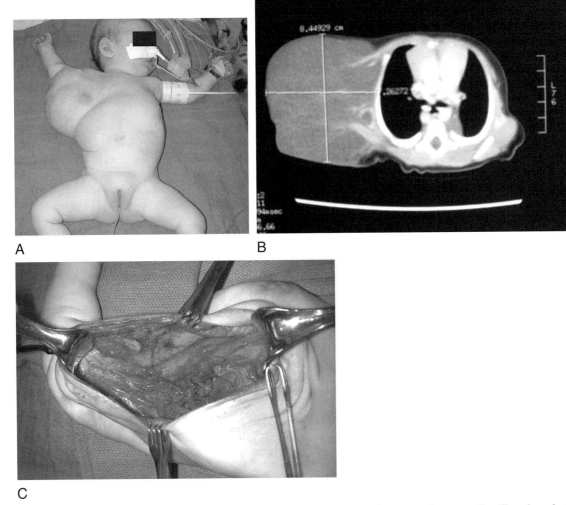

A

B

C

FIGURE 72-6. *A,* Large axillary lymphatic malformation. *B,* Computed tomography scan of axillary lymphatic malformation (LM). *C,* Resection cavity after excision of axillary LM.

affect the pleural, pericardial, and/or peritoneal cavities. In addition, LMs of the GI tract can lead to loss of chyle and subsequent protein-losing enteropathy. In the pelvis, associated problems include recurrent infection and bladder-outlet obstruction. LMs of the extremities are seen in conjunction with overgrowth and limb-length discrepancy. A rare but very difficult problem arises with Gorham's syndrome, in which soft tissue and skeletal LMs lead to progressive osteolysis and "disappearing bone disease."[75] Pathologic fractures and vertebral instability can become manifest with this often fatal syndrome.

Imaging

Well-localized and cystic LMs are easily characterized by US and computed tomography (CT) (see Fig. 72-6B). MRI, however, provides the most reliable diagnosis and is superior to document the full extent of more complex LMs as well as their macrocystic and microcystic components. LMs are hyperintense on T_2 sequences because of their high water content. Within the cysts, fluid-fluid levels denote layering of protein or blood or both. Cystic rims and intralesional septae are highlighted by contrast enhancement. Adjacent enlarged or anomalous venous channels may be apparent as well. The differential diagnosis of these cystic lesions in the infant includes teratoma and infantile fibrosarcoma. For lymphatic anomalies of the thoracic duct and chylous effusions, contrast lymphangiography, although technically difficult to perform, can be helpful to locate the abnormal lymphatic channels or site of leakage.[76]

Treatment

The indications for treatment of LMs vary with the extent and location of the lesions.[77] Surgical resection provides the only method for potential "cure," but this is possible only for lesions that are well localized. Focal and macrocystic lesions are amenable to ablation by both sclerotherapy and resective techniques. In contrast, more diffuse and predominantly microcystic LMs are difficult to eradicate by any method. For local intralesional bleeding that causes sudden enlargement of LMs and pain, conservative management with rest and pain medications is sufficient. Similarly, the enlargement of LMs that coincides with systemic viral or bacterial infections can be managed expectantly, as it is usually harmless. Conversely, bacterial infections within LMs occurring with cellulitis require treatment with antibiotics. Infected LMs become more tense and swollen, producing erythema, pain, and toxicity. The incidence of this complication is around 17%. Treatment consists of systemic antibiotics, and hospitalization for intravenous antibiotics is often necessary. The antibiotic regimen is directed toward oral pathogens for LMs of the head and neck, and toward enteric pathogens for lesions of the trunk, pelvis, and perineum.

Indications for ablative or resective treatment include recurrent complications with infection, cosmesis, deformity, dysfunction, and leakage into body cavities or from the skin. Intralesional sclerotherapy is most beneficial for LMs with macrocystic components. The commonly used agents of ethanol, sodium tetradecyl sulfate, and doxycycline produce scarring and collapse of the cysts. For simple, well-localized macrocystic lymphatic malformations, sclerotherapy can indeed be curative. For more diffuse and complex LMs, sclerotherapy procedures are staged and can lead to significant improvement. Re-expansion of the lesions, however, is the typical course. Weeping or bleeding from cutaneous vesicles can be controlled with local injection sclerotherapy, although leakage generally resumes in 6 to 24 months. Complications of sclerotherapy to be avoided include injury to adjacent nerves, necrosis of overlying skin, and cardiotoxicity related to overall dose.

Surgical resection for complex LMs also can be of significant benefit (see Fig. 72-6C). A staged approach is often required.[78] The operations may be long and tedious and require meticulous thorough dissection to preserve vital structures. General guidelines for surgical resection are as follows: each operation should (1) focus on a defined anatomic region, removing as much lesion as possible, including neurovascular dissection, but without injuring vital structures; (2) limit blood loss to less than the patient's blood volume; and (3) perform prolonged closed suction drainage of the resection cavity. The recurrence rate after "macroscopically complete excision" ranges from 15% to 40%. This recurrence is thought to be secondary to regrowth and re-expansion of unexcised lymphatic channels. Some have considered that sclerotherapy of the resection cavity after operation may be helpful in this regard. After resection, it is common for cutaneous vesicles to occur within the surgical scar. These can be controlled to some extent with local intravesicular sclerotherapy. Alternatively, additional staged excision, pulling uninvolved dermis over the resection bed, may prevent this annoying result.

Some other caveats of surgical treatment for LMs deserve mention. Cervicofacial LMs will often require staged orthognathic procedures to improve bite and speech impediments related to maxillary and mandibular overgrowth (Fig. 72-7). Tracheostomy may be needed in cases of oropharyngeal and airway obstruction. When considered necessary, tracheostomy should precede any attempts at sclerotherapy for cervicofacial LMs. Reactive inflammatory swelling can be dramatic in the initial period after sclerotherapy and can exacerbate partial oropharyngeal obstruction. Lesions of the cervical and axillary regions often involve the brachial plexus. The use of nerve stimulators can be a useful adjunct to prevent injury in these cases. Resection of thoracic and mediastinal LMs to treat recurrent pleural and pericardial effusions involves dissection and skeletonization of the great vessels and vagus and phrenic nerves. For pelvic and anorectal LMs, detailed knowledge of the anatomy of the ischiorectal fossa and sciatic nerve is paramount. Preoperative sclerotherapy to shrink lesions is often useful as well, but discernment is necessary, as scarring can impede the preservation of important nerves. Last, for the specific type of cutaneous LM "lymphangioma circumscriptum," wide resection and closure with split-thickness skin grafts can be curative.

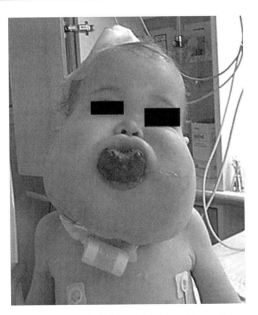

FIGURE 72-7. Cervicofacial lymphatic malformation.

VENOUS MALFORMATIONS

Clinical Features

As one might expect from the embryonic relation of veins and lymphatics, VMs share many clinical features with LMs. VMs, often incorrectly termed "cavernous hemangiomas," are slow-flow lesions consisting of venous channels that can develop anywhere in the body. They are most common in the skin and soft tissues. VMs may be seen at birth or become apparent later, depending on anatomic location. They comprise a wide spectrum, including simple varicosities and ectasias, discrete spongy masses, and complex channels that can permeate any tissue or organ system. VMs are probably the most common of the vascular malformations, and they are more likely to be multiple as well. They tend to enlarge slowly with normal growth of the patient, but can dilate and become symptomatic at any time. As with other vascular malformations, the proportional growth that occurs may become exaggerated during puberty. On examination, these soft, bluish, compressible lesions will expand with dependent position and Valsalva maneuver (Fig. 72-8). Episodes of phlebothrombosis secondary to stasis may lead to acute pain and swelling. Associated local overgrowth and limb-length discrepancy are not uncommon. Involvement of bones and joints provides the risk for pathologic fractures and hemarthroses and subsequent arthritis.

VMs of the GI tract are often multiple as well and can affect every part of the GI tract from mouth to anus. They find more common distribution in the left colon and rectum when associated with VMs of the pelvis and perineum. GI bleeding, typically chronic, can result. Blue rubber bleb nevus syndrome (or "Bean syndrome") represents a specific rare disorder consisting of multifocal VMs that affect the skin and GI tract primarily.[79] The skin lesions are unique in that they are often quite

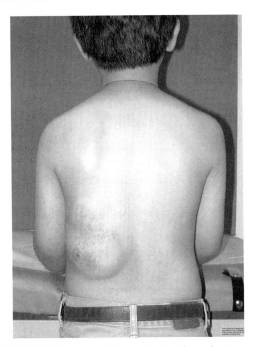

FIGURE 72-8. Venous malformation in the subcutaneous tissue of the back.

numerous and resemble tiny "blue rubber nipples." These skin lesions are classically located on the palms and soles of the feet (Fig. 72-9). As with other GI VMs, chronic bleeding and anemia can result. Intussusception of polypoid VMs can be another presentation. Diagnosis of GI VMs is generally based on endoscopic findings.

VMs of the liver deserve specific mention. Historically called by the misnomer "hepatic hemangiomas," these lesions typically are first seen in adulthood, most often as an incidental finding of abdominal imaging obtained for other reasons. The majority of these lesions are asymptomatic, although they can be quite large or even massive. Reported cases of spontaneous or traumatic rupture have had devastating consequences, but this is exceedingly rare. The most common indications for treatment of these VMs are persistent discomfort from very large lesions and the inability to exclude malignancy. In experienced hands, surgical resection is safe and effective. The technique of enucleation is considered by many to be preferable.

Large VMs also can be complicated by localized intravascular coagulopathy caused by stasis and stagnation of blood within the malformation, leading to consumption of coagulation factors. The clotting profile consists of prolonged PT, decreased fibrinogen, and elevated D-dimers. The PTT is often normal. Thrombocytopenia occurs, with a typical platelet range of 100 to 150,000. The distinction between this coagulopathy and the KMP is important. KMP only occurs with two specific vascular tumors, TA and KHE, and has a much more profound thrombocytopenia with a platelet range of 2 to 10,000. Lesions causing KMP are treated with antiangiogenic agents, whereas VMs will not respond to pharmacotherapy.

Histologically, VMs most often consist of sinusoidal vascular spaces with variable communication with

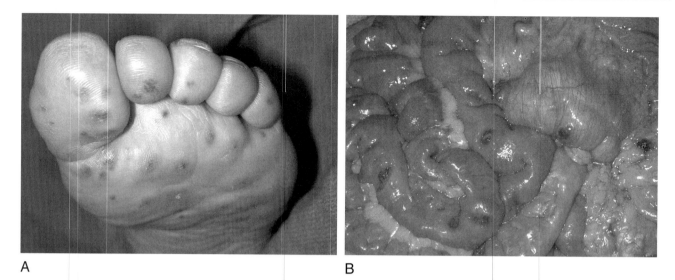

A   B

FIGURE 72-9. *A,* Patient with blue rubber bleb nevus syndrome (BRBNS). Classic cutaneous venous malformations (VMs) on the soles of the foot. *B,* BRBNS: VMs of the small intestine and colon at time of operation.

adjacent veins. The dilated venous channels are thin walled, when compared with normal veins. Smooth muscle actin staining reveals abnormal smooth muscle architecture that may be responsible for the gradual expansion seen over time with these lesions. Moreover, calcified phleboliths may provide evidence of prior clot formation within the VMs. A variant of VMs, glomovenous malformation (also incorrectly called "glomangioma"), has the additional presence of ball-shaped glomus cells that line the vascular channels.

Imaging

Radiologic modalities useful for the diagnosis of VMs include US, MRI, and venography. MRI is most informative and demonstrates hyperintense lesions with T_2 sequences. Contrast enhancement of the vascular spaces distinguishes VMs from LMs, as does the presence of pathognomic phleboliths. Intralesional bleeding within LMs causing contrast enhancement can be an exception to this rule. In contrast to AVMs, VMs do not demonstrate evidence of arterial flow on MRI.

Treatment

The indications for treatment of VMs are appearance, pain, functional loss, and bleeding. Unfortunately, cure for VMs, as with LMs, is difficult to achieve for all but the most localized and therefore less problematic lesions. For extensive VMs of the extremities, conservative management with the use of graded compression stockings can achieve significant improvement in size and symptoms. Patient satisfaction with this modality depends on a proper customized fit, but can be elusive, especially for children and teenagers. To prevent phlebothrombosis of VMs with resultant pain and swelling, low-dose aspirin may be beneficial.

Intralesional sclerotherapy is the mainstay of treatment for most VMs.[80] Sclerosing agents, most commonly

ethanol and sodium tetradecyl sulfate, cause direct endothelial damage, thrombosis, and scarring. For small VMs, the injection process is similar to that of simple varicosities. Larger lesions are accessed by direct puncture, and therapeutic agents are injected under fluoroscopy with the use of tourniquets and compression of venous drainage to prevent systemic administration of the sclerosants. General anesthesia is required in most instances. Staged therapy and occasional embolization of large venous channels are useful for more complex VMs. The more complex lesions are best treated by a skilled interventional radiologist who has experience with vascular anomalies. Potential local complications of sclerotherapy are blistering, skin necrosis, and damage to adjacent nerves. Systemic complications include hemolysis, sudden pulmonary hypertension, and cardiac and renal toxicity. These can usually be avoided with proper dosage and sclerosant selection. For example, ethanol is a strong sclerosant that carries a higher risk of damage to local tissues and adjacent structures.

VMs have a propensity for recanalization and re-enlargement. Cure with sclerotherapy is rare. Results from treatment are often stated in terms of patient satisfaction from decreased pain and appearance, given that recurrence is so prevalent. Surgical resection is typically reserved for well-localized lesions but is marked by procedural morbidity and recurrence as well for complex VMs. Preoperative sclerotherapy is recommended preceding operations for extensive VMs to shrink the lesion and decrease bleeding during the resection.

Unifocal GI lesions can be excised. Diffuse colorectal malformations causing significant bleeding may be treated with colectomy, anorectal mucosectomy, and coloanal pull-through.[81] For multifocal VMs of the blue rubber bleb nevus syndrome, complete surgical resection of the lesions, combined with endoscopy of the entire GI tract at the time of operation, provides the only chance for possible cure. Bowel resections for these lesions are rarely indicated. Rather, wedge excision and polypectomy by intussusception of successive lengths of intestine are the preferred methods of resection.

ARTERIOVENOUS MALFORMATIONS

Clinical Features

AVMs are fast-flow vascular malformations characterized by abnormal connections or shunts between feeding arteries and draining veins without an intervening capillary bed. These shunts define the nidus of the malformation. This lesion tends to be localized but can be extensive as well. AVMs are familiar to neurosurgeons as one of the more common vascular anomalies that occur in the CNS. Indeed, intracranial AVMs are more frequent than AVMs of the skin and soft tissues within the head and neck region. Other common sites of involvement are the extremities, trunk, and viscera. These congenital malformations exhibit a perhaps peculiar but characteristic natural history of progression in stages (Table 72-2). At birth, they appear as a pink cutaneous blemish that can be confused with both CMs and the premonitory sign of an infantile hemangioma. However, fast flow across arteriovenous shunts is present beneath the innocent-appearing surface. This fast flow becomes more evident in childhood, and the lesion develops into a mass. AVMs grow in proportion with the child, but puberty, pregnancy, or local trauma tends to trigger more rapid expansion. The lesion becomes more obviously warm to touch and may develop a bruit or thrill. With continued expansion, the lesions become more red and prominent. Because of expansion and local steal phenomenon, skin ischemia can develop, leading to pain, ulceration, and bleeding (Fig. 72-10). For large AVMs, high-output cardiac failure might result.

Imaging

Ultrasonography and Doppler imaging are excellent tools to elucidate the fast flow of these lesions and therefore to distinguish them from VMs. Although hemangiomas can be characterized by fast flow as well, the history and age at onset should distinguish them from AVMs. MRI and MR angiography are the most useful tools to demonstrate the full extent of these lesions. They appear as hyperintense masses with contrast enhancement and flow voids seen on flow-sensitive sequences. Superselective angiography has its role at the time when treatment is planned.

Treatment

The majority of AVMs will require treatment at some point because of the natural history of continued expansion that leads to local tissue ischemia and pain.[82,83] The mainstays of treatment for these lesions are angiographic embolization alone or in combination with surgical excision. However, in the early stages, the full extent of the AVMs may not be appreciated, such that local recurrence would complicate embolization or resection. Therefore resection of AVMs during infancy and early childhood is rarely advocated. At the same time, the very well localized stage I AVMs may be amenable to excision. The usual recommendation is to observe AVMs in the early stages and monitor them carefully through regularly scheduled annual examinations. Intervention is delayed until symptoms develop indicative of stage III: local pain, ulceration, and bleeding. For treatment initiated at any stage, it is critical that the proximal feeding arteries NOT be embolized or ligated. Whereas ligation may provide temporary improvement for complications

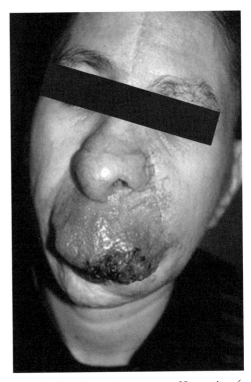

FIGURE 72-10. Facial arteriovenous malformation (stage III) with ulceration of the skin.

Stage	Clinical Findings
TABLE 72-2	
SCHOBINGER CLINICAL STAGING SYSTEM FOR AVM	
I (Quiescent)	Pink-bluish stain, cutaneous warmth, and arteriovenous shunting by Doppler ultrasound
II (Expanding)	Same as stage I, plus enlargement, pulsation, thrill, bruit, and tortuous and tense veins
III (Destructive)	Same as stage II, plus skin ulceration, bleeding, persistent pain, or tissue necrosis
IV (Decompensating)	Same as stage III, plus cardiac failure

AVM, arteriovenous malformation.

such as bleeding, these feeding arteries provide the only avenue for subsequent successful embolization. The nidus of the AVMs will recruit other nearby arteries after the primary feeding vessels are occluded, and the AVMs will recur and continue to progress.

Embolization must be directed to the nidus itself and to the arteriovenous fistulae at the epicenter of the lesion. Direct puncture sclerotherapy of the AVM nidus can be a useful adjunct to embolization, especially when the feeding arteries are too tortuous or have been previously ligated. Repeated and staged embolization procedures are typically necessary for these lesions, but often only provide temporary improvement. The reason for this problem is the quantity and microscopic nature of the arteriovenous fistulae that comprise the nidus of AVMs. It is difficult to achieve complete occlusion for the entirety of these microscopic shunts. Nonetheless, patients do often have significant improvement of their symptoms, and cures with embolization alone have been reported.

The preferred strategy of treatment for AVMs typically consists of surgical resection carried out 2 to 3 days after preoperative embolization of the nidus. Angiographic embolization facilitates the operation by decreasing bleeding, but does not reduce the extent of tissue that should be resected. Whenever possible, the goal should be complete excision to normal margins. Both the nidus of the AVMs and the involved skin are removed. The most important factor for success that should be given close attention is the decision regarding extent of resection. Review of radiologic imaging is necessary, including the earliest available MRI scans and angiograms before any other treatment. Intraoperatively, observation of the pattern of bleeding at the resection margins also can guide the extent of excision, as can intraoperative frozen-section pathology. Primary closure is sometimes not possible without tissue-transfer techniques. Vacuum-assisted closure devices also can be useful in wounds with large soft tissue loss precluding linear closure. The best results are seen with AVMs that are well localized, yet, even for these cases, it is prudent to monitor these patients for years and evaluate for signs of recurrence. Unfortunately, most AVMs are extensive and often not amenable to surgical options. For these difficult lesions, embolization is used for palliation. For difficult AVMs of the extremities, if distal in location, amputation should be considered to be an option.

COMBINED VASCULAR MALFORMATIONS

As with other vascular malformations, combined malformations are classified as either slow flow or fast flow. These more complex disorders, as a rule, are associated with soft tissue and skeletal overgrowth. They tend to be named for the person or persons who first described them. However, these eponyms often create confusion because of misuse. Thus it is preferred to use the anatomic terms that best describe the anomalous vascular channels that are present.

Klippel-Trenaunay Syndrome

Klippel-Trenaunay syndrome, or KT, is a slow-flow combined vascular malformation involving abnormal capillaries, lymphatics, and veins.[84-86] This capillary-lymphatico-venous malformation (CLVM) usually involves one or more extremities, most often a lower limb, and is associated with prominent soft tissue and bony hypertrophy (Fig. 72-11). This syndrome is sporadic and obvious at birth, although a wide range of severity occurs. The CM component can be multiple and typically is seen as a large geographic pattern affecting the extremity, buttock, and trunk. It is macular at birth and develops hemolymphatic vesicles over time. The lymphatic anomalies have variable presentation, including hypoplasia, lymphedema, and macrocystic LMs. The venous component consists of anomalous lateral superficial veins in the extremity that are persistent embryonic vessels. These veins are usually dilated and have incompetent valve systems. Anomalous deep system veins may be hypoplastic or even absent. Thrombophlebitis of the anomalous veins occurs with a frequency of 20% to 45%, and pulmonary emboli are reported in 4% to 25% of cases. Limb hypertrophy also is obvious at birth and occurs in peculiar patterns. It tends to be progressive over time. The spectrum of deformities includes enlargement of hands and feet, both ipsilateral and contralateral to the limb affected by CLVMs. Although the affected extremity is generally larger, it is occasionally smaller. With CLVMs of the legs, pelvic involvement with LMs and VMs also can occur, but is often asymptomatic. Alternatively, problems with recurrent infections, hematuria, hematochezia, and bladder-outlet obstruction may occur. With CLVMs of the superior trunk and arms, the mediastinum or retropleural space can harbor the vascular malformations as well.

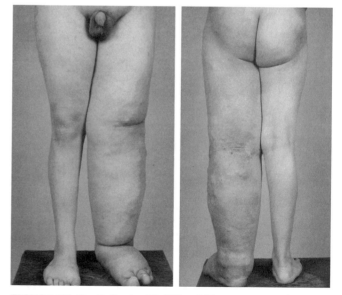

FIGURE 72-11. Patient with Klippel-Trenaunay syndrome or capillary-lymphatico-venous malformation (CLVM) and associated soft tissue and skeletal overgrowth of the lower extremity and foot.

Imaging plays an important role in the evaluation of patients with KT. Plain radiographs are used to document limb-length discrepancies serially. MRI provides the foundation for describing the type and extent of each of the vascular malformation components. Hypertrophic fatty tissue is often seen by MRI in areas of overgrowth. One common pattern seen with LMs of the lower extremity is to find macrocystic lesions in the pelvis and thigh, and microcystic LMs affecting the abdominal wall, buttock, and distal extremity. These LMs can be localized to the subcutaneous tissues or extend into the intramuscular compartments. MRI venography (MRV) can elucidate the anatomy of the deep system veins. Identification of a subcutaneous vein coursing along the lateral calf and thigh, the marginal vein of Servelle, is pathognomonic for KT. Venography is considered for some patients to map the venous drainage of the extremity before resection of any anomalous superficial veins if concern exists regarding patency of the deep veins based on MRV.

In general, treatment for KT is conservative, as it is in no way curable. However, operative therapies do have a place to manage some of the specific problems that are encountered, which are primarily overgrowth.[87] Gross foot enlargement that impairs ambulation and the ability to wear shoes requires orthopedic corrective procedures and partial amputations to permit the use of custom footwear. Leg-length discrepancy should be followed up annually by an orthopedic surgeon to document and predict severity. Shoe lifts are recommended to prevent limping and scoliosis if the discrepancy is greater than 1.5 cm at age 2 years. Sometimes, epiphysiodesis of the distal femoral growth plate is performed around age 12 years to correct overgrowth. Correction for arm-length discrepancies is unnecessary. Staged contour resection can be used to treat areas of soft tissue overgrowth and lymphedema. Symptoms of pain and deformity secondary to venous anomalies can often be improved with compression stockings. Alternatively, sclerotherapy can treat certain components of CLVMs such as focal VMs, macrocystic LMs, and bleeding capillary-lymphatic vesicles. Recurrence after sclerotherapy, however, is often a problem. Surgical resection of anomalous veins producing pain or potential sources of pulmonary emboli also is an option, but only after the existence and patency of the deep venous system is assured. The absence of a deep system mandates that the anomalous superficial system be preserved.

Maffucci Syndrome

This syndrome consists of exophytic venous malformations of the soft tissue and bones, bony exostoses, and endochondromas. It is sporadic and not usually evident at birth. It can be unilateral or bilateral. The bony lesions and endochondromas manifest first in childhood, and the venous anomalies appear later. Spindle-cell hemangioendotheliomas commonly occur and denote reactive vascular proliferation within the preexisting venous malformations, rather than true tumors.[88] The endochondromas can undergo malignant transformation in 20% to 30% of cases, leading to chondrosarcomas.[89] This fact suggests that a tumor-suppressor gene may be involved in the pathogenesis of Maffucci syndrome.

Bannayan–Riley–Ruvalcaba Syndrome

Bannayan–Riley–Ruvalcaba is an autosomal dominant syndrome caused by mutations of the tumor-suppressor gene *PTEN* (phosphatase tensin homolog on chromosome 10).[90] It is primarily an overgrowth syndrome that has vascular malformations as a minor component. Typically cutaneous CMs, VMs, or AVMs are found. The more prominent clinical features are macrocephaly, multiple lipomas, hamartomatous polyps of the ileum and colon, and Hashimoto thyroiditis.

Proteus Syndrome

This syndrome is probably diagnosed more often than it actually occurs. It is named after the Greek god that was able to assume any shape or form.[91] This overgrowth disorder is sporadic and progressive over time. Vascular, skeletal, and soft tissue anomalies tend to be asymmetrical and variably expressed. Common features include lipomas or lipomatosis, macrocephaly, and gigantism of the hands or feet or both.

Parkes-Weber Syndrome

Parkes-Weber syndrome is a sporadic combined fast-flow vascular malformation affecting the limb and trunk, with the lower extremity being the most common site.[92,93] Capillary-arteriovenous fistulae (CAVF) and capillary-arteriovenous malformations (CAVM) are combined with hypertrophy of the bone and muscle of the affected limb. CAVM is obvious at birth, appearing as overgrowth with a large geographic macular pink stain. In contrast to CLVM seen with KT syndrome, the limb hypertrophy is symmetrical along the length and substance of the extremity. The macular stain associated with CAVM has much greater cutaneous warmth than do typical CMs. The findings of bruits or thrills on examination confirm the diagnosis.

MRI demonstrates symmetric muscular and bony overgrowth, with generalized enlargement of the normal named arteries and veins within the affected limb. Angiography depicts the discrete arteriovenous fistulae. In rare cases, superselective embolization is used to occlude the arteriovenous shunts if symptoms of ischemia, pain, or high-output congestive heart failure occur.

REFERENCES

1. Mulliken JB, Fishman SJ, Burrows PE: Vascular anomalies. Curr Probl Surg 37:519–584, 2000.
2. Mulliken JB, Young AE: Vascular birthmarks: Hemangiomas and Malformations. Philadelphia, WB Saunders; 1988.
3. Mulliken JB, Glowacki J: Hemangiomas and vascular malformations in infants and children: A classification based on endothelial characteristics. Plast Reconstr Surg 69:412–420, 1982.
4. Finn MC, Glowacki J, Mulliken JB: Congenital vascular lesions: Clinical application of a new classification. J Pediatr Surg 18:894–900, 1983.

5. Virchow R: Angioma in die krankhaften Geschwulste. Vol 3. Berlin, Hirshwald, 1863, pp 306–425.

6. Wegener G: Ueber lymphangiome. Arch Klin Chir 20:641–707, 1877.

7. Holmdahl K: Cutaneous hemangiomas in premature and mature infants. Acta Paediatr Scand 44:370–379, 1955.

8. Amir J, Metzker A, Krikler R, et al: Strawberry hemangioma in preterm infants. Pediatr Dermatol 3:331–332, 1986.

9. Takahashi K, Mulliken JB, Kozakewich HPW, et al: Cellular markers that distinguish the phases of hemangioma during infancy and childhood. J Clin Invest 93:2357–2364, 1994.

10. Bielenberg DR, Bucana CD, Sanchez R, et al: Progressive growth of infantile cutaneous hemangiomas directly correlated with hyperplasia and angiogenesis of adjacent epidermis and inversely correlated with expression of the endogenous angiogenesis inhibitor, IFN-β. Int J Oncol 14:401–408, 1999.

11. North PE, Waner M, Mizeracki A, et al: GLUT-1: A newly discovered immunohistochemical marker in juvenile hemangiomas. Hum Pathol 31:11–22, 2000.

12. Razon MJ, Kraling BM, Mulliken JB, et al: Increased apoptosis coincides with onset of involution in infantile hemangioma. Microcirculation 5:189–195, 1998.

13. Cheung DSM, Warman ML, Mulliken JB: Hemangioma in twins. Ann Plast Surg 38:269–274, 1997.

14. Walter JW, Blei F, Anderson JL, et al: Genetic mapping of a novel familial form of infantile hemangioma. Am J Med Genet 82:77–83, 1999.

15. Boon LM, Enjolras O, Mulliken JB: Congenital hemangioma: Evidence of accelerated involution. J Pediatr 128:329–335, 1996.

16. Patrice SJ, Wiss K, Mulliken JB: Pyogenic granuloma (lobular capillary hemangioma): A clinicopathologic study of 178 cases. Pediatr Dermatol 8:267–276, 1991.

17. Kirschner RE, Low DW: Treatment of pyogenic granuloma by shave excision and laser photocoagulation. Plast Reconstr Surg 104:1346–1349, 1999.

18. Boon LM, Fishman SJ, Lund DP, et al: Congenital fibrosarcoma masquerading as congenital hemangioma: Report of two cases. J Pediatr Surg 30:1378–1381, 1995.

19. Boon LM, Burrow PE, Paltiel HJ, et al: Hepatic vascular anomalies in infancy: A twenty-seven year experience. J Pediatr 129:346–354, 1996.

20. Kassarjian A, Zurakowski D, Dubois J, et al: Infantile hepatic hemangiomas: Clinical and imaging findings and their correlation with therapy. Am J Roentgenol 182:785–795, 2004.

21. Huang SA, Tu HM, Harney JW, et al: Severe hypothyroidism caused by type 3 iodothyronine deiodinase in infantile hemangiomas. N Engl J Med 343:185–189, 2000.

22. Hersh JH, Waterfill D, Rutledge J, et al: Sternal malformations/vascular dysplasia association. Am J Med Genet 21:177–186, 1985.

23. Goldberg NS, Hebert AA, Esterly NB: Sacral hemangiomas and multiple congenital anomalies. Arch Dermatol 122:684–687, 1986.

24. Albright AL, Gartner JC, Wiener ES: Lumbar cutaneous hemangiomas as indicators of tethered spinal cords. Pediatrics 83:977–980, 1989.

25. Gorlin RJ, Kantaputra P, Aughton DJ, et al: Marked female predilection in some syndromes associated with facial hemangioma. Am J Med Genet 52:130–135, 1994.

26. Frieden IJ, Reese V, Cohen D: PHACE syndrome: The association of posterior fossa brain malformations, hemangiomas, arterial anomalies, coarctation of the aorta and cardiac defects and eye abnormalities. Arch Dermatol 132:307–311, 1996.

27. Burrows PE, Laor T, Paltiel HJ, et al: Diagnostic imaging in the evaluation of vascular birthmarks. Dermatol Clin 16:455, 1998.

28. Dubois J, Patriquin HB, Garel L, et al: Soft tissue hemangiomas in infants and children: Diagnosis using Doppler sonography. AJR Am J Roentgenol 171:247–252, 1998.

29. Paltiel HJ, Burrows PE, Kozakewich HPW, et al: Soft-tissue vascular anomalies: Utility of US for diagnosis. Radiology 214:747–754, 2000.

30. Meyer JS, Joffer FA, Barnes PD, et al: Biological classification of soft-tissue vascular anomalies: MR correlation. AJR Am J Roentgenol 157:559–564, 1991.

31. Margileth AM, Museles M: Cutaneous hemangiomas in children: Diagnosis and conservative management. JAMA 194:523–526, 1965.

32. Crum R, Szabo S, Folkman J: A new class of steroids inhibits angiogenesis in the presence of heparin or a heparin fragment. Science 230:1375, 1985.

33. Bennett ML, Fleischer AB, Chamlin SL, et al: Oral corticosteroid use is effective for cutaneous hemangiomas. Arch Dermatol 137:1208, 2001.

34. Sadan N, Wolach B: Treatment of hemangiomas of infants with high doses of prednisone. J Pediatr 128:141–146, 1996.

35. Boon LM, MacDonald DM, Mulliken JB: Complications of systemic corticosteroid therapy for problematic hemangiomas. Plast Reconstr Surg 104:1616–1623, 1999.

36. Sloan GM, Reinisch JF, Nichter LS, et al: Intralesional corticosteroid therapy for infantile hemangiomas. Plast Reconstr Surg 83:459–467, 1989.

37. Ruttum MS, Abrams GW, Harris GJ, et al: Bilateral retinal embolization associated with intralesional steroid injection for capillary hemangioma of infancy. J Pediatr Ophthalmol Strabismus 30:407, 1993.

38. White CW, Wold SJ, Korones DN, et al: Treatment of childhood angiomatous diseases with recombinant interferon alfa-2a. J Pediatr 118:59–66, 1991.

39. Ezekowitz RAB, Mulliken JB, Folkman J: Interferon alfa-2a therapy for life-threatening hemangiomas of infancy. N Engl J Med 326:1456–1463, 1992.

40. Ricketts RR, Hatley RM, Corden BJ, et al: Interferon-alpha-2a for the treatment of complex hemangiomas of infancy and childhood. Ann Surg 219:605, 1994.

41. Tamayo L, Ortiz DM, Orozco-Covarrubias L, et al: Therapeutic efficacy of interferon alfa-2b in infants with life-threatening giant hemangiomas. Arch Dermatol 133:1567, 1997.

42. Greinwald JH, Burke DK, Bonthius DJ, et al: An update on the treatment of hemangiomas in children with interferon alfa-2a. Arch Otolaryngol Head Neck Surg 119:125, 1999.

43. Dubois J, Hershon L, Carmant L, et al: Toxicity profile of interferon alfa-2b in children: A prospective evaluation. J Pediatr 135:782–785, 1999.

44. Barlow CF, Priebe CJ, Mulliken JB, et al: Spastic diplegia as a complication of interferon alfa-2a treatment of hemangiomas of infancy. J Pediatr 132:527, 1998.

45. Deb G, Jenkner A, Donfrancesco A: Spastic diplegia and interferon. J Pediatr 134:382, 1999.

46. Scheepers JH, Quaba AA: Does the pulsed tunable dye laser have a role in the management of infantile hemangiomas: Observations based on 3 years experience. Plast Reconstr Surg 95:305–312, 1995.

47. Sie KC, McGill T, Healy GB: Subglottic hemangioma: Ten years experience with carbon dioxide laser. Ann Otol Rhinol Laryngol 103:167–172, 1994.

48. Morelli JG, Tan OT, Yohn JJ, et al: Treatment of ulcerated hemangiomas in infancy: Arch Pediatr Adolesc Med 148:1104–1105, 1994.

49. Fishman SJ, Burrows PE, Leichtner AM, et al: Gastrointestinal manifestations of vascular anomalies in childhood: Varied etiologies require multiple therapeutic modalities. J Pediatr Surg 33:1163–1167, 1998.

50. Mulliken JB, Rogers GF, Marler JJ: Circular excision of hemangioma and purse-string closure: The smallest possible scar. Plast Reconstr Surg 109:1544–1554, 2002.

51. Enjolras O, Riche MC, Merland JJ, et al: Management of alarming hemangiomas in infancy: A review of 25 cases. Pediatrics 85:491–498, 1990.

52. Mulliken JB, Boon LM, Takahashi K, et al: Pharmacologic therapy for endangering hemangiomas. Curr Opin Dermatol 2:109–113, 1995.

53. Jones EW, Orkin M: Tufted angioma (angioblastoma): A benign progressive angioma, not to be confused with Kaposi's sarcoma or low grade angiosarcoma. J Am Acad Dermatol 20:214–225, 1989.

54. Zuckerberg LR, Nikoloff BJ, Weiss SW: Kaposiform hemangioendothelioma of infancy and childhood: An aggressive neoplasm associated with Kasabach-Merritt syndrome and lymphangiomatosis. Am J Surg Pathol 17:321–328, 1993.

55. Kasabach HH, Merritt KK: Capillary hemangioma with extensive purpura: A report of a case. Am J Dis Child 59:1063–1070, 1940.

56. Sarkar M, Mulliken JB, Kozakewich HPW, et al: Thrombocytopenic coagulopathy (Kasabach-Merritt phenomenon)

is associated with kaposiform hemangioendothelioma and not with common infantile hemangioma. Plast Reconstr Surg 100:1377–1386, 1997.

57. Enjolras O, Wassef M, Mazoyer E, et al: Infants with Kasabach-Merritt syndrome do not have "true" hemangiomas. J Pediatr 130:631–640, 1997.

58. Enjolras O, Mulliken JB, Wassef M, et al: Residual lesions after Kasabach-Merritt phenomenon in 41 patients. J Am Acad Dermatol 42:225–235, 2000.

59. Vikkula M, Boon LM, Mulliken JB, et al: Molecular basis of vascular anomalies. Trends Cardiovasc Med 8:281–292, 1998.

60. Folkman J, D'Amore PA: Blood vessel formation: What is the molecular basis? Cell 87:1153–1155, 1996.

61. Wang HU, Chen ZF, Anderson DJ: Molecular distinction and angiogenic interaction between embryonic arteries and veins revealed by ephrin-B2 and its receptor Eph-B4. Cell 983:741–753, 1998.

62. Dumont DJ, Fong GH, Puri MC, et al: Vascularization of the mouse embryo: A study of flk-1, tek, tie, and vascular endothelial growth factor expression during development. Den Dyn 203:80–92, 1995.

63. Guttmacher AE, Marchuk DA, White RI: Hereditary hemorrhagic telangiectasia. N Engl J Med 333:918–924, 1995.

64. Kaipainen A, Korhonen J, Mustonen T, et al: Expression of the fms-like tyrosine kinase 4 gene becomes restricted to lymphatic endothelium during development. Proc Natl Acad Sci U S A 92:3566–3570, 1995.

65. Wigle JT, Oliver G: Prox1 function is required for the development of the murine lymphatic system. Cell 98:769–778, 1999.

66. Jeltsch M, Kaipainen A, Joukov V, et al: Hyperplasia of lymphatic vessels in VEGF-C transgenic mice. Science 276:1423–1425, 1997.

67. Boon LM, Mulliken JB, Vikkula M, et al: Assignment of a locus for dominantly inherited venous malformations to chromosome 9. Hum Mol Genet 3:1583–1587, 1994.

68. Vikkula M, Boon LM, Carraway KL III, et al: Vascular dysmorphogenesis caused by an activating mutation in the receptor tyrosine kinase TIE2. Cell 87:1181–1190, 1996.

69. Enjolras O, Riche MC, Merland JJ: Facial port-wine stains and Sturge-Weber syndrome. Pediatrics 76:48–51, 1985.

70. Tan OT, Sherwood K, Gilchrest BA: Treatment of children with port-wine stains using the flashlamp pumped tunable dye laser. N Engl J Med 320:416–421, 1989.

71. Van der Horst CMAM, Koster PHL, deBorgie CAJM, et al: Effect of the timing of treatment of port-wine stains with the flashlamp-pumped pulsed-dye laser. N Engl J Med 338:1028–1033, 1998.

72. Gallagher PG, Mahoney MJ, Goshe JR: Cystic hygroma in the fetus and newborn. Semin Perinatol 23:341–356, 1999.

73. Marler JJ, Fishman SJ, Upton J, et al: Prenatal diagnosis of vascular anomalies. J Pediatr Surg 37:515–517, 2002.

74. Padwa BL, Hayward PG, Ferraro NF, et al: Cervicofacial lymphatic malformation: Clinical course, surgical intervention, and pathogenesis of skeletal hypertrophy. Plast Reconstr Surg 95:951, 1995.

75. Gorham LW, Stout AP: Massive osteolysis (acute spontaneous absorption of bone, phantom bone, disappearing bone): Its relations to hemangiomatosis. J Bone Joint Surg 37:986–1004, 1955.

76. Fishman SJ, Burrows PE, Upton J, et al: Life-threatening anomalies of the thoracic duct: Anatomic delineation dictates management. J Pediatr Surg 2001;36:1269–1272.

77. Alqahtani A, Nguyen LT, Flageole H, et al: 25 years' experience with lymphangiomas in children. J Pediatr Surg 34:1164–1168, 1999.

78. Upton J, Coombs CJ, Mulliken JB, et al: Vascular malformations of the upper limb: A review of 270 patients. J Hand Surg 24:1019–1035, 1999.

79. Oranje AP: Blue rubber bleb nevus syndrome. Pediatr Dermatol 3:304–310, 1986.

80. Berenguer B, Burrows PE, Zurakowski K, et al: Sclerotherapy of craniofacial venous malformations: Complications and results. Plast Reconstr Surg 104:1–11, 1999.

81. Fishman SJ, Shamberger RC, Fox VL, et al: Endorectal pull-through abates gastrointestinal hemorrhage from colorectal venous malformations. J Pediatr Surg 35:982–984, 2000.

82. Kohout MP, Hansen M, Pribaz JJ, et al: Arteriovenous malformations of the head and neck: Natural history and management. Plast Reconstr Surg 102:643–654, 1998.

83. Yakes WF, Rossi P, Odink H: Arteriovenous malformation management. Cardiovasc Intervent Radiol 19:65–71, 1996.

84. Klippel M, Trenaunay P: Du naevus variqueux osteohypertrophique. Arch Gen Med (Paris) 185:641–672, 1900.

85. Cohen MM: Klippel-Trenaunay syndrome. Am J Med Genet 93:171–175, 2000.

86. Jacob AG, Driscoll DJ, Shaughnessy WJ, et al: Klippel-Trenaunay syndrome: Spectrum and management. Mayo Clin Proc 73:28, 1998.

87. Servelle M: Klippel and Trenaunay's syndrome: 768 operated cases. Ann Surg 201:365–373, 1985.

88. Perkins P, Weiss SW: Spindle cell hemangioendothelioma: An analysis of 78 cases with reassessment of its pathogenesis and biologic behaviour. Am J Surg Pathol 20:1196–1204, 1996.

89. Sun TC, Swee RG, Shives TC, et al: Chondrosarcoma in Maffucci's syndrome. J Bone Joint Surg 67:1214–1219, 1985.

90. Cohen MM: Bannayan-Riley-Ruvalcaba syndrome: Renaming three formerly recognized syndromes as one etiologic entity [Letter]. Am J Med Genet 35:291, 1990.

91. Biesecker LG, Happle R, Mulliken JB, et al: Proteus syndrome: Diagnostic criteria, differential diagnosis, and patient evaluation. Am J Med Genet 84:389–395, 1999.

92. Weber FP: Angioma formation in connection with hypertrophy of limbs and hemi-hypertrophy. Br J Dermatol Syph 19:231–235, 1907.

93. Weber FP: Haemangiectatic hypertrophy of limbs: Congenital phlebarteriectasis and so-called congenital varicose veins. Br J Dis Child 15:13–17, 1918.

CHAPTER 73

Head and Neck Sinuses and Masses

John H. T. Waldhausen, MD, and David Tapper, MD

The wide variety of lesions involving the head and neck in children can be subdivided by etiology into those that result from infection, trauma, or neoplasm and those of congenital origin. The more common benign neoplasms are hemangiomas, lymphangiomas, and cystic hygromas. They are discussed in Chapter 72. Malignant neoplasms of childhood (e.g., neuroblastoma, lymphoma, and rhabdomyosarcoma), which occur as primary and metastatic masses in the head and neck, lesions of the thyroid and parathyroid, as well as traumatic injuries of the head and neck, also are discussed in other chapters.

In this chapter, common congenital head and neck malformations are discussed, and inflammatory lesions are reviewed.

LESIONS OF EMBRYONIC ORIGIN

Congenital cysts and sinuses that appear in the neck result from embryonic structures that have failed to mature or have persisted in an aberrant fashion.[1,2] Successful treatment of a child with a mass or sinus in the head or neck requires accurate identification of the lesion as well as a planned course of therapy. Both diagnosis and therapy depend on a working knowledge of the embryologic origin and differentiation of the head and neck structures.[3,4] This knowledge is particularly important because complete surgical resection of cartilaginous remnants, of remnants of the branchial arch and cleft structures, and of midline fusion abnormalities is imperative to avoid recurrence.

Remnants of Embryonic Branchial Apparatus

Embryology

During weeks 4 to 8 after fertilization, four pairs of well-developed ridges (branchial arches) dominate the lateral cervicofacial area of the human embryo.[5] These four pairs are accompanied by two rudimentary pairs, which are analogous to the gill apparatus of lower forms.[2,5] No true gill

mechanisms are found in any stage of the human embryo. These pharyngeal arches and clefts are formed without a true connection between the outer ectodermal clefts and the inner endodermal pharyngeal pouches (Fig. 73-1).

The mature structures of the head and neck are derivatives of several branchial arches and their intervening clefts.[5,6] The first branchial arch forms the mandible and contributes to the maxillary process of the upper jaw.[6-8] Abnormal development of the first branchial arch results in a host of facial deformities, including cleft lip and palate, abnormal shape or contour of the external ear, and malformed internal ossicles.[6,8] The first branchial cleft contributes to the tympanic cavity and eustachian tube. Microtia and aural atresia occur with failure of the first branchial cleft to develop.[5,6] The second arch forms the hyoid bone and the cleft of the tonsillar fossa.[1,2] The third cleft migrates lower in the neck to form the inferior parathyroid glands and the thymus.[9,10] The descent of the fourth cleft stops higher in the neck to form the superior parathyroid glands. The fourth pouch has added significance, in that its ventral portion develops into the ultimobranchial body, which contributes thyrocalcitonin-producing parafollicular cells to the thyroid gland.[9]

Clinical Aspects

Complete fistulas are more common than external sinuses. Both are more common than branchial cysts, at least during childhood.[10,11] In adults, cysts predominate.[10] By definition, all branchial remnants are truly congenital and are present at birth.[8,11] Cysts developing from branchial structures usually appear later in childhood than do sinuses, fistulas, and cartilaginous remnants, which appear in infancy.[8] Commonly, the tiny external opening of the fistula and the external sinuses remain unnoticed for some time. Spontaneous mucoid drainage from the ostium usually heralds its presence and initiates the parent's concern and the reason for the child's referral.

The first clinical presentation may be an infected mass as a result of the inability of the thick mucoid material to

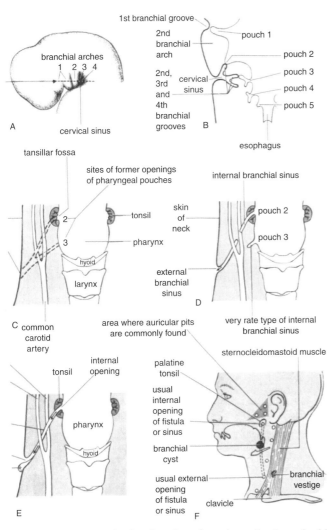

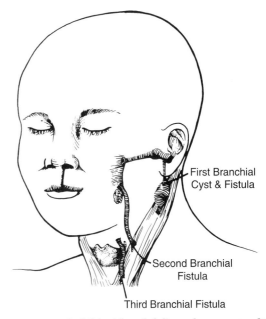

if found, are located inferior to the mandible in a suprahyoid position. One third open into the external auditory canal.[12] The tract may be intimately associated with, or course through, the parotid gland. This and the proximity of cranial nerve VII make resection difficult, particularly in the younger patient who is likely to have a tract deep to the facial nerve.[13] Preauricular cysts, sinuses, and skin tags with or without cartilaginous remnants are not included in this group of anomalies.

The external ostium of the second branchial cleft is along the anterior border of the sternocleidomastoid muscle, generally at the junction of the lower and middle thirds.[10] Remnants of the second branchial cleft are more common than are those of the first cleft.[10] Owing to its embryonic origin, the second cleft tract penetrates platysma and cervical fascia to ascend along the carotid sheath to the level of the hyoid bone. Remnants may be found anywhere along this course. The residual tract turns medially between the branches of the carotid artery, behind the posterior belly of the digastric and stylohyoid muscles, and in front of the hypoglossal nerve to end in the tonsillar fossa[10] (Fig. 73-2). Although the internal opening can be anywhere in the nasopharynx or oropharynx, it is most commonly found in the tonsillar fossa. About 10 % of second branchial remnants are bilateral.[10]

It is unusual to find cysts and sinuses from the third branchial cleft.[2,6] When found, they are in the same area as those of the second cleft but ascend posterior to the carotid artery rather than through the bifurcation.[6] The fistula pierces the thyrohyoid membrane and enters the pyriform sinus.

Fourth branchial fistulae are exceedingly rare, and it may be difficult to differentiate these from other associated

FIGURE 73-1. *A,* The head and neck region of a 5-week-old embryo. *B,* Horizontal section through the embryo illustrating the relation of the cervical sinus to the branchial arches and pharyngeal pouches. *C,* The adult neck region, indicating the former sites of openings of the cervical sinus and the pharyngeal pouches. The *broken lines* indicate possible courses of branchial fistulas. *D,* The embryologic basis of various types of branchial sinuses. *E,* A branchial fistula resulting from persistence of parts of the second branchial cleft and the second pharyngeal pouch. *F,* Possible sites of branchial cysts and openings of branchial sinuses and fistulas. A branchial vestige also is illustrated. (From Moore KL: The Developing Human: Clinically Oriented Embryology. Philadelphia, WB Saunders, 1977.)

drain spontaneously. Infection is, however, less common in fistulas and external sinuses than in cysts.[1] The cutaneous openings are occasionally marked by skin tags or cartilage remnants. The tract itself may be palpable. A cordlike structure can be felt ascending in the neck by hyperextending the child's neck and making the skin taut. Compression along the tract may produce mucoid material exiting from the ostium.

First branchial anomalies are rare. Cysts are seen as swellings posterior or anterior to the ear or inferior to the earlobe in the submandibular region. External openings,

FIGURE 73-2. A child with a cleft lip and remnants of the first three branchial systems. Note the important relation to the sternocleidomastoid muscle and the fistula's origin. (From Welch KJ, Randolph JG, Ravitch MM, et al [eds]: Pediatric Surgery, 4th ed. Chicago, Year Book Medical, 1986, p 543.)

anomalies. Fourth pouch cysts also are highly unusual and must be differentiated from laryngoceles. Fistula tracts originate at the apex of the pyriform sinus, descend beneath the aortic arch, and then ascend anterior to the carotid artery to end in the vestigial cervical sinus of His.[14]

Other anomalies arising from the third and fourth branchial pouches may appear as cystic structures in the neck. Thymic cysts may occur as a result of incomplete degeneration of the thymal pharyngeal duct or of progressive cystic degeneration of epithelial remnants of Hassall corpuscles.[14] Most are found on the left side of the neck.

Parathyroid cysts may be located anywhere around the thyroid gland or in the mediastinum. These are usually not associated with biochemical abnormalities, although reports of hyperparathyroidism secondary to functioning cysts have been seen. The etiology of these cysts is not clear. They may be embryologic remnants of third and fourth branchial pouches or may represent cystic degeneration of adenomas or gradual enlargement of microcysts.[14]

Infection may develop at any time in these branchial remnants. From a technical standpoint, the surgical dissection is facilitated when the lesion is removed electively before any infection. Scar formation and the risk of recurrence also are reduced. Persistent drainage and the possibility of infection remain the primary indications for surgical therapy. Squamous cell carcinoma has been reported in rare patients with branchial cleft cysts, but this complication does not appear until adulthood.[15]

Diagnosis

The presence of mucoid drainage from a small opening along the border of the sternocleidomastoid is indicative of a branchial cleft sinus. Palpating the tract and observing the mucoid discharge are confirmatory. Although colored dye or radiopaque material may be injected to delineate the tract, these manipulations generally are unnecessary. An accurate history from the parents is definitive. An understanding of the embryologic origin and proper surgical technique are necessary to ensure complete excision.

Cysts may be more difficult to diagnose. They lie deep to the skin along the anterior border of the sternocleidomastoid muscle.[1] They can usually be distinguished from cystic hygromas, which are subcutaneous and can be transilluminated. Ultrasonography (US) may be useful to identify the cystic nature of a mass if it is not apparent by physical examination.[16,17] In addition, real-time US with Doppler imaging can identify associated vascular structures. A skilled ultrasonographer can often help the pediatric surgeon identify important associated structures as well as characterize the type and location of the cystic structure located at the angle of the mandible. The differential diagnosis of a mass at the angle of the jaw is extensive and may include adenopathy, cystic hygromas, dermoids, and parotid lesions, as well as primary and metastatic neoplasms of lymphatic origin. The mass associated with torticollis is discussed later in this chapter. Definition of the exact etiology of the mass often requires surgical exploration.

Treatment

The goal of treating all congenital neck sinuses, cysts, and fistulas is usually complete excision, done electively, when no inflammation is present.[18] This procedure may be safely performed at any age, and generally, the younger the better.[18] If the lesion is infected at clinical presentation, antibiotic therapy and warm soaks to encourage spontaneous drainage of mucoid plugs should precede definitive excision. Attempts at complete excision in an inflamed, infected field increase the risk of nerve injury, incomplete resection, and recurrence. A limited incision and drainage (I&D) procedure is sometimes necessary to resolve the infection. Although needle aspiration of branchial cysts is not recommended, it may be used in place of I&D to control infection. Repeated aspiration may be needed. Endoscopic cauterization of fourth branchial cleft sinuses has been described either at the time of initial abscess drainage or 4 to 6 weeks later. Recurrence with this technique seems to be unusual.[19]

The outpatient operation to remove a branchial cleft sinus or cyst is performed by using general anesthesia. The child is supine with slight hyperextension of the neck, maintained in position by a padded bean bag (Fig. 73-3). Generally, endotracheal intubation is required so that the anesthesiologist obtains a secure airway. A small transverse elliptical incision is made around the external opening and deepened beneath the cervical fascia. The initial dissection is along the inferior border of the incision, so that the ascending tract is identified from below and not injured. Although catheters and probes can be placed in the tract, use of a headlight and loupe magnification provides ample visualization to allow dissection of the tract from the investing muscle, fascia, and fat. Dissection proceeds cephalad, staying on the tract until visualization of the most superior portion of the tract becomes difficult. At this level, a second, more cephalad, parallel "stair-step" incision may be necessary for adequate exposure. The tract is pulled through the second incision, and the dissection is continued cephalad between the

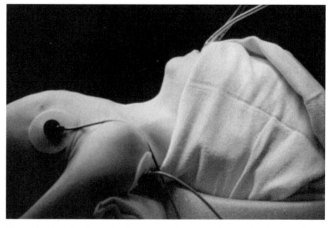

FIGURE 73-3. Positioning a child for neck surgical procedure. Hyperextension of the head with support under the shoulders and stabilization with a bean bag keep the child in a stable position and facilitate exposure. Head of bed should be elevated 30 degrees to decrease venous pressure in the neck.

bifurcation of the carotid artery to the point where the tract inserts into the pharynx. The fistula is suture ligated with absorbable suture material. The wound is closed in layers with absorbable sutures. No drains are used.

Recurrences are rare and imply that a portion of the epithelium-lined tract was overlooked. The incidence of recurrence is higher in cases of previously infected lesions.

Branchial cysts free of infection are excised electively. Abscesses that are drained by incision or aspiration, or that drain spontaneously, are treated with antibiotics to control secondary inflammation. Complete surgical excision is delayed until the inflammation subsides and the surrounding skin is supple. Recurrence is rare when the cyst is completely excised.

Preauricular Pits, Sinuses, and Cysts

Embryology

Preauricular pits, cysts, and sinuses are not of true branchial cleft origin.[20] They represent ectodermal inclusions, which are related to embryonic ectodermal mounds that essentially form the auricles of the ear.[6] The sinuses are often short and end blindly. They never connect internally to the external auditory canal or eustachian tube.[20] They characteristically end in thin strands that blend with the periosteum of the external auditory canal. They tend to be familial and are often bilateral.[1] Preauricular cysts are located in the subcutaneous layer superficial to the parotid fascia. They seem deeper only if they become infected. The lining cells of these cysts and sinuses are stratified squamous epithelium. They do not contain hair-bearing follicles owing to their origin from the ectoderm associated with external ear formation.[18]

Clinical Aspects

Preauricular cysts and sinuses are commonly noted at birth. The parent may remark about the familial and bilateral nature of these lesions.[10] Preauricular sinuses commonly do not drain, and in those situations, excision is not required. However, parents often report that sebaceous-like material drains from the sinus. The presence of drainage is an indication for surgical excision. Sinuses that drain are often connected to subcutaneous cysts that have an increased likelihood of staphylococcal infection. Ideally these lesions should be completely excised before becoming infected (Fig. 73-4). Prior infection increases the difficulty of complete surgical excision, which increases the risk of recurrence.

Treatment

Complete surgical excision of the sinus tract and subcutaneous cyst to the level of the temporalis fascia is the treatment of choice in the uninfected draining sinus. It is important to avoid rupture of the sinus and to do a complete excision to decrease the risk of recurrence.[21] If infection supervenes, the lesion is treated with antibiotics and warm soaks to encourage drainage and control of the surrounding inflammation. Occasionally, as with

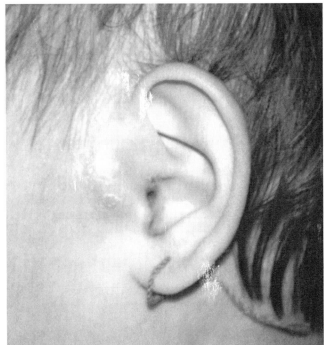

FIGURE 73-4. An infected preauricular cyst. The pit anterior to the helix is difficult to see. Note the swelling and skin changes anterior to the tragus. Preauricular sinuses that drain sebaceous material should be excised electively. Warm compresses and antibiotics allowed the inflammation to diminish. The cyst sinus was then completely excised.

infected branchial cysts, I&D or needle aspiration may be required to control the infection.

Surgical excision is often done through an elliptic incision with a small, chevron skin flap surrounding the sinus. The cyst is then dissected from the subcutaneous tissue and removed in its entirety.[20] The cyst or sinus may have multiple branches, making complete resection difficult. Removal of a small bit of adjacent cartilage reduces the risk of missing one of these branching tracts. The incidence of recurrence is as high as 42% owing to these multiple branches, and some clinicians have advocated an extended preauricular incision to enhance exposure.[21] Postoperative wound infection also is common.[21]

Thyroglossal Duct Cyst

One of the most common lesions in the midline of the neck is the thyroglossal duct cyst.[4] Although it is embryonic in origin, it is rare for these lesions to occur in the newborn period.[1] More commonly, they are noted in preschool-age children.[1] Thyroglossal duct cysts also are common in young adults and, with the exception of thyroid goiter, are the most common midline neck masses.[12]

Embryology

Thyroglossal remnants produce midline masses from the base of the tongue to the pyramidal lobe of the thyroid gland. The embryogenesis of the thyroglossal duct is intimately involved with that of the thyroid gland, the hyoid bone, and the tongue.[9] The foramen cecum is the site of the development of the thyroid diverticulum.[9] In the embryo, this structure develops caudal to the central tuberculum impar, which is one of the pharyngeal buds that leads to the formation of the tongue.[9] As the tongue develops, the thyroid diverticulum descends in the neck, maintaining its connection to the foramen cecum.

The hyoid bone is developing from the second branchial arch at this time. The thyroid gland develops between weeks 4 and 7 of gestation and descends into its pretracheal position in the neck.[22] As a result of these multiple events occurring simultaneously, the thyroglossal duct may pass in front of or behind the hyoid bone, but most commonly, it passes through it. Normally, the duct disappears by the time the thyroid reaches its appropriate position. Thyroglossal duct cysts never have a primary external opening because the embryologic thyroglossal tract never reaches the surface of the neck.[22] A cyst can be located anywhere along the migratory course of the thyroglossal tract in the neck, if it fails to become obliterated (Fig. 73-5). Occasionally, the cysts attach to the pyramidal lobe or may be intrathyroidal.[23]

Complete failure of migration of the thyroid results in a lingual thyroid, which develops beneath the foramen cecum at the base of the tongue.[24] In this instance, no thyroid tissue is found in the neck.[24] The incidence of ectopic thyroid tissue in or near the duct is reported to be from 10% to 45%, and some clinicians have advocated preoperative thyroid scanning or US to eliminate the possibility of an ectopic thyroid gland masquerading as a thyroglossal duct cyst.[25–29] US appears to be very accurate and avoids the need for radiation and possible sedation in younger children.[28] Anatomic location also may be useful in differentiating cysts and ectopic thyroid. Ninety percent of ectopic thyroid tissue lies at the base of the tongue, and thyroglossal duct cysts are rarely found there. A history should be obtained to elicit evidence of hypothyroidism, and consideration should be given to testing thyroid function. Abnormal thyroid function tests or a suggestive history should prompt a preoperative thyroid scan.[27] If ectopic thyroid tissue is found, the management becomes controversial, but some clinicians suggest a trial of medical suppression to decrease the size of the mass.

Clinical Aspects

Classically, the thyroglossal cysts are located in the midline at or just below the hyoid bone (Fig. 73-6). Suprahyoid thyroglossal cysts must be distinguished from submental dermoid cysts and from submental lymph nodes.[30] Rarely, the cysts are suprasternal in location.

The initial sign is usually a mass in the midline of the neck. Owing to the communication to the mouth via the foramen cecum, thyroglossal cysts can become infected with oral flora. Every effort should be made to excise these lesions before infection. Complete surgical excision of infected lesions is difficult and ill-advised. Risk of injury to the surrounding structures and incidence of recurrence are higher.

On physical examination, the thyroglossal duct cyst is smooth, soft, and nontender. To distinguish this lesion

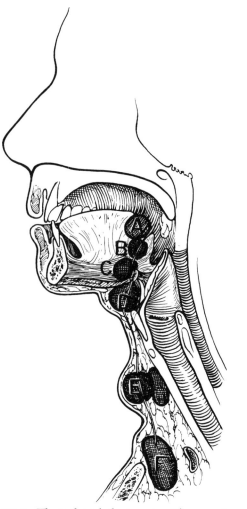

FIGURE 73-5. Thyroglossal duct cysts. These cysts can be located anywhere from the base of the tongue to behind the sternum. *A* and *B*, Lingual (rare). *C* and *D*, Adjacent to hyoid bone (common). *E* and *F*, Suprasternal fossa (rare). (From Welch KJ, Randolph JG, Ravitch MM, et al [eds]: Pediatric Surgery, 4th ed. Chicago, Year Book Medical, 1986, p 549.)

from the more superficial dermoid lesion, one should palpate the lesion while the child sticks out his or her tongue. Owing to its attachment to the foramen cecum, the thyroglossal duct cyst does not fully move when the tongue protrudes. This maneuver is more reliable than asking the child to swallow and determining whether the mass moves with swallowing.

The cyst is usually connected to the foramen cecum by single or multiple tracts, which pass through the hyoid. The duct lining is stratified squamous epithelium or ciliated pseudostratified columnar epithelium, with associated mucus-secreting glands.[9] The cyst contains a characteristic glairy mucus.

Treatment

Surgical excision is advised to avoid the complications of infection and because of the small risk (<1%) of cancer developing in the cyst.[27] Thyroglossal duct cyst is treated

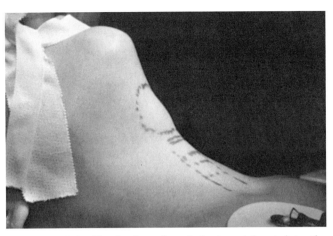

FIGURE 73-6. Classic thyroglossal duct cyst located in the midline just below the hyoid bone. Markings on the neck represent cricothyroid and tracheal rings.

by complete excision of the cyst and its tract, upward to the base of the tongue (Fig. 73-7). In 1920, Sistrunk[31] described excision of the central portion of the hyoid bone as necessary treatment to prevent recurrence. Follow-up studies have confirmed these findings. The operation, as performed currently, must include the resection of the central portion of the hyoid bone.[32,33] Several other studies have shown that multiple smaller tracts can connect through the hyoid bone to the floor of the mouth, requiring wide resection of tracts above the hyoid.[32–34] If these suprahyoid tracts remain, the incidence of recurrence increases.[35] The best chance for successful resection is adequate wide resection at the initial procedure.[34]

The thyroglossal cyst is exposed through a transverse incision. The cyst has a characteristic appearance, distinctly different from that of thyroid tissue. The dissection

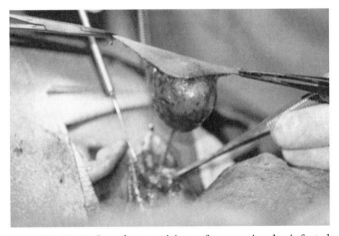

FIGURE 73-7. Complete excision of a previously infected thyroglossal duct cyst. Surrounding skin was removed because of changes related to previous infection. Note the well-defined tract leading toward the hyoid bone and the floor of the mouth. The operation was completed by excising the central portion of the hyoid and suture ligating the tract.

should continue cephalad to the hyoid. Transecting the hyoid is simplified by using angled scissors, similar to Potts scissors, or by using a side-cutting bone cutter. The base of the tract at the floor of the mouth is ligated with absorbable suture. The wings of the hyoid are not approximated. The wound is closed in layers. If the floor of the mouth is entered inadvertently, this can be repaired with absorbable suture. The wound is copiously irrigated. Occasionally, the dissection may be made simpler by having the anesthesiologist place his or her finger at the base of the child's tongue to identify the cephalad extent of the dissection.

With complete excision, including the central portion of the hyoid bone, the risk of recurrence is low.[35,36]

Dermoid and Epidermoid Cysts

Dermoid cysts embryologically represent ectodermal elements that either were trapped beneath the skin or failed to separate from the neural tube.[37,38] Dermoids are differentiated from epidermoids histologically by the accessory glandular structures found in dermoids.[37] Dermoids contain sebaceous glands, hair follicles, connective tissues, and papillae.[37] Both contain sebaceous material within the cyst cavity.

The most common location for dermoids in children is along the supraorbital palpebral ridge. This lesion commonly appears as a characteristic swelling in the corner of the eyebrow. Although commonly attached to the underlying bony fascia, this lesion is movable and nontender. Occasionally, the mass may be dumbbell shaped and penetrate through the orbital bone. Midline dermoid cysts probably represent entrapment of epithelium of branchial arch origin at the time of embryologic midline fusion.[39] These cysts may be confused with midline thyroglossal duct cysts. Dermoids, however, are more superficial. As mentioned, they are movable when the tongue is forcibly protruded. Any midline scalp lesion suspected of being a dermoid should undergo preoperative evaluation with magnetic resonance imaging (MRI) to rule out intracranial extension. At operation, dermoid cysts lack a deep-seated tract connecting them to the hyoid bone or other neck structures.

Surgical excision is the treatment of choice for all dermoids and epidermoids. This has been most commonly performed as an open operation, although increasing experience with removing these lesions is accruing by using endoscopic minimally invasive techniques.[40] It is important to completely remove the capsule to decrease the risk of recurrence. Infection is possible secondary to repeated local trauma. Malignant degeneration of dermoids also is possible but rare.[35] Complete surgical excision is curative.

Torticollis

Etiology

Torticollis in childhood may be congenital or acquired. Congenital torticollis resulting from fibrosis and shortening in the sternocleidomastoid muscle is the most common type.[41-43] The shortening of the sternocleido-mastoid muscle characteristically pulls the head and neck to the side of the lesion. The resulting "mass" represents the fibrous tissue palpable within the muscle. The etiology of this "fibrous tumor" is debatable.[44] The significant incidence of breech presentations and other abnormal obstetric positions has been used to support both the injury and the tumor etiology. Those who favor tumor see the abnormal presentation as the result of the fixed abnormal head position, whereas those who favor trauma see the difficult extraction as the cause of injury.[42,45] No one theory completely explains this condition.

The etiology of acquired torticollis includes cervical hemivertebra and imbalance of the ocular muscles. In children in whom no identifiable muscular etiology is found, a high likelihood exists of Klippel-Feil anomalies or neurologic disorder as the cause.[46] Acquired torticollis also should raise the suspicion of otolaryngologic infection and the possibility of a neoplastic condition as the underlying cause.[47,48]

Pathologically, the basic abnormality in congenital torticollis is endomysial fibrosis—the deposition of collagen and fibroblasts around individual muscle fibers that undergo atrophy.[44] The sarcoplasmic nuclei are compacted to form "muscle giant cells," which appear to be multinucleated.[44] The severity and distribution of fibrosis differ widely from patient to patient. Some cases of fibrosis occur bilaterally. The fact that mature fibrous tissue is present even in the neonate suggests that the disease begins well before birth and is probably not due to difficult delivery.

Diagnosis

In a series of 100 infants with torticollis, 66% had a "tumor" in the muscle, and the other 34% had fibrosis but no tumor.[36,49] A more recent series of 624 cases from China noted only 35.4% with a tumor.[50] In the typical case, the mass is not found in the newborn period but is noted at the first "well-baby" check-up, some 6 weeks after birth. The infant has the characteristic posture, with the face and chin rotated away from the affected side and the head tilted toward the ipsilateral shoulder.[45] Acquired torticollis may develop at any age, and it is important to keep in mind the various causes of the acquired lesion. Its appearance depends on the severity of the lesion, the distribution of the fibrosis, and the child's growth pattern. With time, facial and cranial asymmetry develop, and a notable flattening of the facial structures on the side of the lesion occurs. This may become irreversible by age 12 years, although reports have been made of excellent results when the surgical procedure is performed after age 10 years.[51,52]

Treatment

Experience with this condition has shown that 80% to 97% of affected infants do not require operative treatment.[50,53] The key to successful treatment is early recognition and prompt physical therapy.[43,53] The longer the shortening of the muscle persists, the more facial and cranial asymmetry develops, and the more the deeper cervical tissues become involved in the process. US may be used not only as a diagnostic tool but also to help determine which child may be more likely to need surgical therapy. In a study from China, the cross-sectional as well as longitudinal extent of fibrosis in the sternocleido-mastoid mastoid correlated well with the need for surgical intervention.[54]

In most instances, complete correction can be achieved by early range-of-motion and stretching exercises and positional changes with the baby in the crib. The parents should be taught to perform these exercises with the baby once or twice each day. One parent holds the child's shoulder down against a firm surface, and the other rotates the head toward the opposite shoulder. When the child's head is rotated toward the opposite shoulder, the muscle is gently kneaded along its entire course. Often one parent can accomplish the stretching exercises by placing the baby on his or her lap, turning the baby's head, and gently extending the head and neck over the parent's knees. An additional maneuver is rearranging the baby's room, changing objects in the crib, and encouraging the baby to look toward the side opposite the involved muscle. One study showed a mean duration of 4.7 months for successful nonoperative resolution.[55]

Some clinicians have suggested that the criterion for operation, regardless of age, is the development of facial hemihypoplasia.[43] In children with significant torticollis, facial hemihypoplasia is invariably present, not always with a linear relation between the two conditions.[53] The muscle can be divided anywhere, but transection in the middle third, through a lateral collar incision, is the simplest and provides the most aesthetically acceptable scar.[53,56] Through this incision, one can divide the fascia colli of the neck, which is often tight and may need to be divided anteriorly as far as the midline and posteriorly to the anterior border of the trapezius. Intensive physiotherapy, including full rotation of the neck in both directions and full extension of the cervical spine, is instituted as soon as possible. Occasionally, in an older child, a splint is used to provide overcorrection and stretching of the muscle.[53,56]

INFLAMMATORY LESIONS

Cervical Nodes

Enlarged cervical lymph nodes are by far the most common neck masses in childhood. In most instances, they are the result of nonspecific reactive hyperplasia.[1] The etiology is often viral or is related to an upper respiratory tract or skin infection. The adenitis resolves spontaneously. Most cases are first seen with bilateral enlarged nodes. Because the anterior cervical nodes drain the mouth and pharynx, almost all upper respiratory and pharyngeal infections have some effect on the anterior cervical nodes. Enlarged cervical lymph nodes are frequently palpable in children between ages 2 and 10 years. Palpable nodes are uncommon in infants. A mass in a child younger than 2 years is more likely to be a cystic hygroma, thyroglossal duct cyst, dermoid cyst, or branchial cyst. The mass can often be diagnosed on clinical findings.[57]

Because the head contains so many structures through which bacteria or viruses may enter the body, the cervical lymph nodes frequently become involved in the infections and inflammatory diseases. Cervical nodes also may be the first clinical manifestations of various tumors, particularly those of the lymphoma group.[1] The most frequent inflammatory lesion of the cervical lymph nodes is suppurative lymphadenitis (Fig. 73-8) Others of importance are cat-scratch disease, atypical mycobacterial lymphadenitis, and tuberculous lymphadenitis. Less common but important considerations in the differential diagnosis of cervical adenitis include Kawasaki's disease and acquired immunodeficiency syndrome (AIDS).

Acute Suppurative Cervical Lymphadenitis

The most common cause of acute lymph node enlargement is a bacterial infection arising in the oropharynx or elsewhere in the drainage area.[58] The most common organisms are penicillin-resistant *Staphylococcus aureus* and *Streptococcus hemolyticus,* although cultures of the pus often yield a mixture of both or prove to be sterile.[58] *Staphylococcus* may be more prevalent in infants.[59] Anaerobes, although common in the oropharynx, are not common pathogens in cervical adenitis. The diagnosis is usually apparent. Fever is variable and usually mild. Initial treatment with antibiotics is often followed by resolution without suppuration. Without treatment, the node often enlarges and becomes fluctuant, eventually leading to thinning of the overlying skin and abscess formation.

Needle aspiration can be both diagnostic and therapeutic. Aspiration of purulent material confirms the diagnosis. The material obtained can be cultured (Fig. 73-9). Frequently, needle aspiration and drainage of the purulent material coupled with judicious antibiotic therapy may

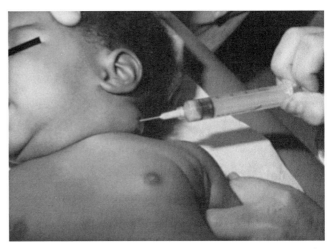

FIGURE 73-9. Aspiration of purulent material confirms the diagnosis of suppurative lymphadenitis. Frequently, repeated aspirations may be necessary to remove the majority of debris and can often obviate the need for formal incision and drainage.

alleviate the necessity of formal I&D. Occasionally, repeated aspirations may be necessary.

If the child appears toxic or is quite young, hospitalization and intravenous antibiotics, including a β-lactamase–resistant antibiotic, may be helpful, but formal I&D is often required. The node can be incised and packed loosely with a Penrose drain. The parent can be taught to do irrigations through the Penrose drain, which encourages drainage of the residual debris. Usually apparent improvement is evident in 2 to 3 days, although antibiotic therapy should be continued for 10 days. Complete resolution of adenopathy may take weeks.

Chronic Lymphadenitis

Children occasionally have impressively enlarged nodes that do not seem to be acutely infected. The nodes are not as inflamed or as tender as those in acute bacterial adenitis. Progression to fluctuation is unlikely. The child with this type of lymphadenopathy must be evaluated for tuberculosis, atypical mycobacterial infection, and cat-scratch disease. Most children should receive a full 2-week course of an oral antistaphylococcal antibiotic. The same physician should examine the child on a number of occasions to assess the results of therapy. A single dominant lymph node present for longer than 6 to 8 weeks, which has not responded to appropriate antibiotic therapy, should be completely excised, fully cultured, and submitted for histologic examination to rule out the diagnosis of neoplasm. Nodes present in the supraclavicular space and posterior triangle tend to be more of a concern for malignancy than those found in the submandibular or anterior triangle.

Mycobacterial Lymphadenitis

Clinical Aspects

The prevalence and the relative incidence of infections caused by different mycobacteria vary with the success of

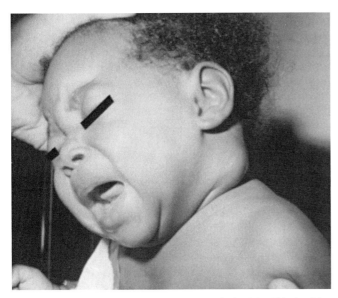

FIGURE 73-8. Acute suppurative cervical adenitis. Skin is shining and taut over the centralized abscess cavity.

preventive health measures in particular populations.[60] In developed countries, bovine mycobacteria have been eliminated from milk.

Most mycobacterial lymphadenitis is caused by the atypical mycobacteria of the *Mycobacterium avium-intracellulare-scrofulaceum* (MAIS) complex.[60] Internationally adopted terminology (MAIS) defines this group of 10 to 15 mycobacteria, which produce a specific and localized form of lymphadenitis.[32,37,60] The portal of entry is primarily through the mucous membranes of the pharynx. Lymphadenitis resulting from infection with *M. tuberculosis* is thought to be an extension of a primary pulmonary infection and usually involves the supraclavicular nodes.[61] Infection with the atypical strains usually involves higher cervical nodes, most commonly the submandibular or submaxillary.[61] This finding is consistent with the etiology being a primary infection and not pulmonary disease. Infection is most commonly seen between ages 1 and 5 years; occurrence before age 1 year is rare. The disease involves unilateral nodes, and dissemination is rare. Atypical mycobacteria enter from the environment and are not contagious, although the reservoir may be the mouth and oropharynx of apparently healthy children.[59] Person-to-person spread of disease has not been documented, and isolation is not necessary.

Infection with atypical mycobacteria is generally limited to the lymph nodes. Pediatric patients with atypical mycobacterial lymphadenitis are asymptomatic. The nodes are usually nontender. Spontaneous regression of atypical lymph node infection may occur but is likely to lead to breakdown of the nodes and sinus or fistula formation. Children with tuberculous scrofula usually are symptomatic. Most have pulmonary tuberculosis when the diagnosis is made.[62] It is rare for the infection to progress from cervical adenopathy to pulmonary disease if the initial chest roentgenograms are clear. Degeneration of nodes with abscess and fistula formation is unusual.

Diagnosis

In children, tuberculous or atypical mycobacterial lymphadenitis presents with a clinical picture of chronic lymph node hypertrophy.[63] Pulmonary tuberculosis on chest radiograph helps to identify the cause of the cervical swelling. Patients with MAIS usually have a normal chest roentgenogram. Skin testing helps differentiate these diseases. All children with tuberculosis should show positive test results to second-strength purified protein derivative (PPD). Children with atypical mycobacterial infection have either a negative or a doubtful skin test. If the initial PPD is inconclusive, second-strength PPD may help confirm the mycobacterial etiology. A history of familial exposure to tuberculosis should suggest tuberculosis as more likely than atypical mycobacteria. Although specific skin tests for atypical mycobacteria often provide positive results, it is difficult to obtain the appropriate antigen. Final diagnosis may depend on culture results or histopathology after excision of the involved nodes.[64]

Treatment

It is important to distinguish tuberculous from MAIS lymphadenitis because the treatment is significantly different. In human infections, antituberculous chemotherapy is required, usually resulting in marked resolution of the lymphadenopathy within a few months. Chemotherapy is continued for 2 years.[62] Surgical intervention in a human tuberculosis infection is confined to an excisional biopsy of a node, if the diagnosis cannot be made on other grounds. Most children with tuberculous lymphadenitis respond well to chemotherapy with standard drugs.

Treatment of MAIS infections is chiefly surgical.[65] Careful, thorough excision of the group of affected nodes (the one or two sentinel nodes) and adjacent smaller nodes is required. This procedure should ideally be performed before extensive ulceration of the overlying skin occurs. Standard chemotherapy for tuberculosis is of no value in MAIS infections except in patients in whom a draining sinus develops after primary excision of infected nodes.[66] Children with atypical mycobacterial infection respond well to complete surgical excision without drug therapy.

Cat-scratch Disease

The incidence of cat-scratch disease varies greatly in different parts of the world. In developed countries, cat-scratch disease is the most common cause of nonbacterial chronic lymphadenopathy.[67] *Bartonella henselae,* a gram-negative, rickettsial organism, is responsible for most cases of cat-scratch disease.[68] The disease is usually transmitted via a superficial wound caused by a cat, dog, or monkey.[69] The healthy kitten is the most frequent vector.

The disease begins as a superficial infection or pustule forming in 3 to 5 days and is followed by regional adenopathy in 1 to 2 weeks. Generally, only one node is involved. Nodal involvement corresponds to inoculation site and the nodes that drain it. The axilla is the most commonly involved area.[1] The diagnosis can be made by a commercially available indirect fluorescent antibody test for detection of antibody. Histology findings are characteristic but not pathognomonic. Polymerase chain reaction studies for *B. henselae* on a fine-needle aspirate may be useful when the diagnosis is in question, although this technique is not readily available in all hospitals.[70] Complete excision of the involved node is recommended to confirm the diagnosis, if necessary. Patients usually have tender lymphadenopathy and few systemic symptoms. On rare occasion, complications include encephalitis, retinitis, and osteomyelitis. The delay between wounding and subsequent lymphadenopathy can approach 30 days.[69] Treatment for cat-scratch disease is most often symptomatic as the disease is usually self-limited. Lymphadenopathy resolves spontaneously over a period of weeks to months with only occasional suppuration. Specific antimicrobial therapy against *B. henselae* has not proven efficacious, although it is susceptible to many common antibiotics. Azithromycin may have some use in treating children if antibiotics are needed.[71]

LESIONS OF THE SALIVARY GLANDS

Surgical lesions of the salivary glands in children are unusual. This section addresses benign and inflammatory conditions in these glands.

Ranula

In children, prominent, glistening, cystic masses occasionally develop below the tongue in the floor of the mouth. These cystic lesions generally arise from the sublingual glands and are known as ranulae[72] (Fig. 73-10). Most are simple cysts that result from the partial obstruction of the sublingual salivary duct.[72] The traditional ranula is a simple cyst lined with salivary ductal epithelium.

Occasionally, the sublingual duct can become completely occluded. The duct may rupture, which leads to the formation of a pseudocyst. The pseudocyst forms because amylase-containing secretions extravasate and erode or "plunge" into the neck muscles. This leads to the condition known as "plunging ranula."[73,74] This lesion lacks a true epithelial lining.[73]

Many surgeons suggest marsupialization at the initial procedure for a simple ranula.[66] By incising the cyst and draining the contents, the mass rapidly decreases in size. Suturing the epithelium back on itself allows the partially occluded duct to drain. Marsupialization alone has a fairly high recurrence rate, and complete resection or marsupialization with packing may be preferable.[75,76] Concurrent resection of the ipsilateral sublingual gland has been shown to decrease the rate of recurrence.[76] Recent trials with OK 432 similar to therapy for lymphangioma have been described with some success in Japan.[77]

The complex or plunging ranula requires a more extensive dissection into the neck to totally excise the

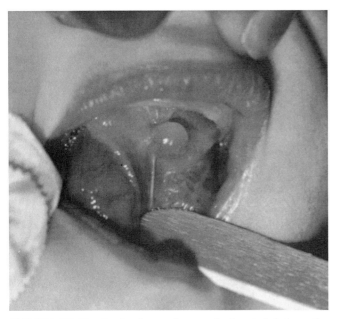

FIGURE 73-10. A simple cystic ranula located below the tongue, arising from the sublingual glands.

pseudocyst and the atrophied sublingual gland.[74] This may be done by an intraoral approach but may require a cervical incision. Dissection may be tedious in this inflamed area because the hypoglossal and lingual nerves run beneath the sublingual gland and become entrapped in the mass.

Parotid Hemangioma

This is the most common benign neoplasm affecting the major salivary glands commonly occurring in female infants at birth or within the first few months of life. They usually are confined to the intracapsular component of the gland and rarely involve the overlying subcutaneous tissues and skin. A surface sentinel lesion may be present. They appear as a spongy mass anterior to the ear. The diagnosis is usually evident on physical examination. Rarely is a cutaneous component present in the hemangioma. Growth may be rapid in the first few weeks of life. US is helpful, and MRI also is useful in establishing the diagnosis. Most parotid hemangiomas involute by age 4 to 6 years, and only 10% need surgical intervention. Surgical resection puts the seventh nerve at risk.

Sialadenitis

Inflammation and swelling of the salivary glands are not common in children. Sialadenitis may appear as an acute suppurative infection, a chronic infection, or a granulomatous replacement of the gland. Acute suppurative sialadenitis is most frequently seen in infants. The organism most often involved is *S. aureus*, followed by *Streptococcus* and group D *Pneumococcus*.[78]

The pathophysiology of chronic sialadenitis may involve duct ectasia, stricture, and sialolithiasis. Sialectasis, a saccular dilation of the small, intercalated ducts that connect acini with striated ducts, is a common congenital abnormality of the gland. Sialolithiasis occurs much more commonly in the submandibular than in the parotid gland. Culture of material from the duct may not reveal pathogenic organisms. Recurrent bacterial infection without demonstrable obstruction is the primary problem in some cases.

Clinical Aspects

Sialadenitis is characterized by episodes of pain that may last from 1 to 7 days. Swelling and pain are isolated to the anatomic distribution of the gland and do not involve the overlying skin and subcutaneous tissue. Secretions are thick and flocculent. Bilateral involvement may occur over time, although each acute episode tends to be unilateral.

Diagnosis

Salivary gland abnormalities may follow diseases such as mumps. Tenderness may occur, with cystic or solid swelling of the gland. The saliva coming from the duct of the involved gland is abnormal. Plain roentgenograms are useful in detecting radiopaque stones, which are seen 4 times more frequently in the submandibular than in the parotid gland.[79] Sialography remains the definitive study for ductal abnormalities, although it is associated with some discomfort and may require general anesthesia in younger children. High-resolution US may demonstrate ductal ectasia.[79] Computed tomography has been used in children to evaluate vascularity and abscess formation. MRI may be useful in imaging the course of the facial nerve through the parotid gland.[80] Incisional biopsy is rarely indicated. The utility of fine-needle aspiration is questionable.[81]

Treatment

Antibiotics may be useful in both acute and recurrent sialadenitis. Nonspecific therapy with sialagogues, with massage of the gland, may be helpful. Sialolithotomy or dilation with removal of demonstrated calculi is usually curative. Radical surgical treatment is rarely necessary in children.

REFERENCES

1. Filston HC: Head and neck-sinuses and masses. In Holder TM, Ashcraft KW (eds): Pediatric Surgery. Philadelphia, WB Saunders, 1980, pp 1062–1079.
2. Gray SW, Skandalakis JE: The pharynx and its derivatives. In Skandalakis JE, Gray SW (eds): Embryology for Surgeons: The Embryological Basis for the Treatment of Congenital Defects. Philadelphia, WB Saunders, 1972, pp 15–62.
3. Guarisco JL: Congenital head and neck masses in infants and children, Part II. Ear Nose Throat J 70:75–82, 1991.
4. Telander RL, Deane SA: Thyroglossal and branchial cleft cysts and sinuses. Surg Clin North Am 57:779–796, 1977.
5. Moore GW, Hutchins GM, O'Rahilly R: The estimated age of staged human embryos and early fetuses. Obstetrics 139:500–506, 1982.
6. Burge D, Middleton A: Persistent pharyngeal pouch derivatives in the neonate. J Pediatr Surg 18:230–234, 1983.
7. Gaisford JC, Anderson VS: First branchial cleft cysts and sinuses. Plast Reconstr Surg 55:299–304, 1975.
8. Randall P, Royster HP: First branchial cleft anomalies. Plast Reconstr Surg 31:497–501, 1963.
9. Gray SW, Skandalakis JE, Akin JT Jr: Embryological considerations of thyroid surgery: Developmental anatomy of the thyroid, parathyroids, and the recurrent laryngeal nerve. Am Surg 42:621–628, 1976.
10. Soper RT, Pringle KC: Cysts and sinuses of the neck. In Welch K, et al (eds): Pediatric Surgery, 4th ed. Chicago, Year Book Medical, 1986, pp 539–551.
11. Frazer JE, Bertwistle AP: The nomenclature of disease states caused by certain vestigial structures in the neck. Br J Surg 2:131–134, 1923.
12. Roback SA, Telander RL: Thyroglossal duct cysts and branchial cleft anomalies. Semin Pediatr Surg 3:142–146, 1994.
13. D'Souza, Uppal HS, De R, et al: Updating concepts of first branchial cleft defects: A literature review. Int J Pediatr Radiol 62:103–109, 2002.
14. Benson MT, Dalen K, Mancuso AA, et al: Congenital anomalies of the branchial apparatus: Embryology and pathologic anatomy. Radiographics 12:943–960, 1992.
15. Khafif RA, Pricher R, Minkowitz S: Primary branchogenic carcinoma. Head Neck 11:153–163, 1989.
16. Reynolds JH, Wolinski AP: Sonographic appearance of branchial cysts. Clin Radiol 48:109–110, 1994.
17. Kraus R, Han BK, Babcock DS, et al: Sonography of neck masses in children. AJR Am J Roentgenol 146:609–613, 1986.
18. Lee K, Klein TR: Surgery of cysts and tumors of the neck. In Paparella MM, Shumrick DA (eds): Otolaryngology. Philadelphia, WB Saunders, 1973.
19. Jordan JA, Graves JE, Manning SC, et al: Endoscopic cauterization for treatment of fourth branchial cleft sinuses. Arch Otolaryngol 124:1021–1024, 1998.
20. Singer R: A new technique for extirpation of preauricular cysts. Am J Surg 111:291–295, 1966.
21. Currie AR, King WW, Vlantis AC, et al: Pitfalls in the management of preauricular sinuses. Br J Surg 83:1722–1724, 1996.
22. Ward PA, Straham RW, Acquerelle M, et al: The many faces of cysts of the thyroglossal tract. Trans Am Acad Ophthalmol Otolaryngol 74:310–316, 1970.
23. Sonnino RE, Spigland N, Laberge JM, et al: Unusual patterns of congenital neck masses in children. J Pediatr Surg 24:966–969, 1989.
24. Katz AD, Zager WT: The lingual thyroid. Arch Surg 102:582–585, 1971.
25. Strickland AL, Macfee JA, VanWyk JJ, et al: Ectopic thyroid glands simulating thyroglossal duct cysts. JAMA 208:307–310, 1969.
26. Nanson EM: Salivary gland drainage into the thyroglossal duct. Surg Gynecol Obstet 149:203–205, 1979.
27. Radkowski D, Arnold J, Healy GB, et al: Thyroglossal duct remnants: Preoperative evaluation and management. Arch Otolaryngol Head Neck Surg 117:1378–1381, 1991.
28. Gupta P, Maddalozzo J: Preoperative sonography in presumed thyroglossal duct cysts. Arch Otolaryngol 127:200–202, 2001.
29. Kessler A, Eviatar E, Lapinsky, et al: Thyroglossal duct cyst: Is thyroid scanning necessary in the preoperative evaluation? Israel Med Assoc J 3:409–410, 2001.
30. Welch KJ, Tapper D, Vawter GP: Surgical treatment of thymic cysts and neoplasms in children. J Pediatr Surg 14:691–698, 1979.
31. Sistrunk WE: Technique of removal of cyst and sinuses of the thyroglossal duct. Surg Gynecol Obstet 46:109–112, 1928.
32. Bennett KG, Organ CH Jr, Williams GR: Is the treatment for thyroglossal duct cysts too extensive? Am J Surg 152:602–605, 1986.
33. Obiako MN: The Sistrunk operation for the treatment of thyroglossal cysts and sinuses. Ear Nose Throat J 64:196–201, 1985.
34. Hoffman MA, Schuster SR: Thyroglossal duct remnants in infants and children: Reevaluation of histopathology and methods for resection. Ann Otol Rhinol Laryngol 97:483–486, 1988.
35. Ein SH, Shandling B, Stephens CA, et al: Management of recurrent thyroglossal duct remnants. J Pediatr Surg 19:437–439, 1984.
36. Mukel RA, Calcaterra TC: Management of recurrent thyroglossal duct cyst. Arch Otolaryngol 109:34–36, 1983.
37. Gold BC, Skeinkopf DE, Levy B: Dermoid, epidermoid and teratomatous cysts of the tongue and the floor of the mouth. J Oral Surg 32:107–111, 1974.
38. Smirniotopoulos JG, Chiechi MV: Teratomas, dermoids, and epidermoids of the head and neck. Radiographics 15:1437–1455, 1995.
39. McAvoy JM, Zuckerbraun L: Dermoid cysts of the head and neck in children. Arch Otolaryngol 102:529–531, 1976.
40. Huang MG, Cohen SR, Burstein FD, et al: Endoscopic pediatric plastic surgery. Ann Plast Surg 38:1–8, 1997.
41. Armstrong D, Pickerell K, Fetter B, et al: Torticollis: An analysis of 271 cases. Plast Reconstr Surg 35:14–19, 1965.
42. Dunn PM: Congenital sternomastoid torticollis: An intrauterine postural deformity. J Bone Joint Surg Br 55:877–881, 1973.
43. Jones PG: Torticollis. In Welch KJ (ed): Pediatric Surgery, 4th ed. Chicago, Year Book Medical, 1986, pp 552–556.
44. Mickelson MR, Cooper RR, Ponseti IV: Ultrastructure of the sternocleidomastoid muscle in muscular torticollis. Clin Orthop 110:11–18, 1975.
45. Dunn PM: Congenital postural deformities: Perinatal associations. Proc R Soc Med 65:735–739, 1972.
46. Ballock RT, Song KM: The prevalence of nonmuscular causes of torticollis in children. J Pediatr Orthop 16:500–504, 1996.
47. Kahn ML, Davidson R, Drummond DS: Acquired torticollis in children. Orthop Rev 20:667–674, 1991.
48. Bredenkamp JK, Maceri DR: Inflammatory torticollis in children. Arch Otolaryngol Head Neck Surg 116:310–313, 1990.
49. Ling CM, Low YS: Sternomastoid tumor and muscular torticollis. J Bone Joint Surg Br 41:432–437, 1969.
50. Cheng JC, Au AW: Infantile torticollis: A review of 624 cases. J Pediatr Orthop 14:802–808, 1994.
51. Yu SW, Wand NH, Chin LS, et al: Surgical correction of muscular torticollis in older children. Chung Hua I Hsueh Tsa Chih Taipei 5:168–171, 1995.
52. Cheng JCY, Tang SP: Outcome of surgical treatment of congenital muscular torticollis. Clin Orthop 362:190–200, 1999.

53. Soeur R: Treatment of congenital torticollis. J Bone Joint Surg 38:35–40, 1940.
54. Lin JN, Chou ML: Ultrasonographic study of the sternocleidomastoid muscle in the management of congenital muscular torticollis. J Pediatr Surg 32:1648–1651, 1997.
55. Emery C: The determinants of treatment duration for congenital muscular torticollis. Phys Ther 74:921–929, 1994.
56. Morrison DJ, McEwen GD: Congenital muscular torticollis: Observations regarding clinical findings, associated conditions, and results of treatment. J Pediatr Orthop 2:500–505, 1982.
57. Jones PG: Glands of the neck. In Welch K (ed): Pediatric Surgery, 4th ed. Chicago, Year Book Medical, 1986, pp 517–520.
58. Hieber JP, Davis AT: Staphylococcal cervical adenitis in young infants. Pediatrics 57:424–426, 1976.
59. Bodenstein L, Altman RP: Cervical lymphadenitis in infants and children. Semin Pediatr Surg 3:134–141, 1994.
60. Altman RP, Margeleth AM: Cervical lymphadenopathy from atypical mycobacteria: Diagnosis and surgical treatment. J Pediatr Surg 10:419–422, 1975.
61. Belin RP, Richardson JD, Richardson DL, et al: Diagnosis and management of scrofula in children. J Pediatr Surg 9:103–107, 1974.
62. Kent PC: Tuberculous lymphadenitis: Not a localized disease process. Am J Med Sci 254:86–871, 1967.
63. Lincoln EM, Gilbert LA: Disease in children due to mycobacteria other than *Mycobacterium tuberculosis*. Am Rev Respir Dis 105:683–690, 1972.
64. Pinder SE, Colville A: Mycobacterial cervical lymphadenitis in children: Can histological assessment help differentiate infections caused by non-tuberculous mycobacteria from *Mycobacterium tuberculosis*? Histopathology 22:59–64, 1993.
65. MacKellar A: Diagnosis and management of atypical mycobacterial lymphadenitis in children. J Pediatr Surg 11:85–89, 1976.
66. Maridell F, Wright PF: Treatment of atypical mycobacterial cervical adenitis with rifampin. Pediatrics 55:39–42, 1975.
67. Carithers HA: Cat scratch skin test antigen: Purification by heating. Pediatrics 60:928–929, 1977.
68. American Academy of Pediatrics: Cat scratch disease. In Peter G (ed): 1977 Red Book: Report of the Committee on Infectious Diseases, 24th ed. Elk Grove Village, Ill: American Academy of Pediatrics, 1977, p 165.
69. Carithers HA, Carithers CM, Edwards RO Jr: Cat scratch disease: Its natural history. JAMA 207:312–316, 1969.
70. Scott MA, McCurley TL, Vnencak-Jones CL, et al: Cat scratch disease: Detection of *Bartonella henselae* DNA in archival biopsies from patients with clinically, serologically, and histologically defined disease. Am J Pathol 149:2161–2167, 1996.
71. Chia JKS, Nakate MM, Lami JLM, et al: Azithromycin for the treatment of cat-scratch disease. Clin Infectious Dis 26:193–194, 1998.
72. Quick CA, Lowell SH: Ranula and the sublingual salivary glands. Arch Orolaryngol 103:397–400, 1977.
73. Khafif RA, Schwartz A, Friedman E: The plunging ranula. J Oral Surg 33:537–541, 1975.
74. Roediger WE, Kay S: Pathogenesis and treatment of plunging ranulas. Surg Gynecol Obstet 144:862–864, 1977.
75. Yoshimura Y, Obara S, Kondoh T: A comparison of three methods used for treatment of ranula. J Oral Maxillofac Surg 53:280–282, 1995.
76. Baurmash HD: Marsupialization for treatment of oral ranula: A second look at the procedure. J Oral Maxillofac Surg 50:1274–1279, 1992.
77. Fukase S, Ohta N, Inamura K, et al: Treatment of ranula with intracystic injection of the streptococcal preparation OK 432. Ann Otol Rhinol Laryngol 112:214–220, 2003.
78. Welch KJ: The salivary glands. In Welsh KJ, Randolph JG, O'Neill JA, et al (eds): Pediatric Surgery. Chicago, Year Book Medical, 1986, pp 487–502.
79. Seibert RW: Diseases of the salivary glands. In Bluestone CD, Stool SE, Kenna MA (eds): Pediatric Otolaryngology, 3rd ed. Philadelphia, WB Saunders, 1996, pp 1093–1107.
80. Teresi LM, Kolin E, Lufkin RB, et al: MR imaging of the intraparotid facial nerve: Normal anatomy and pathology. Am J Roentgenol 148:995–1000, 1987.
81. Batsakis JG, Sneige N, el-Naggar AK: Pathology consultation: Fine-needle aspiration of salivary glands: Its utility and tissue effects. Ann Otol Rhinol Laryngol 101:185–188, 1992.

CHAPTER 74

Pediatric and Adolescent Gynecology

Julie Strickland, MD

INTRODUCTION

From birth through adulthood, many gynecologic conditions may come to the surgeon's attention. Acute gynecologic problems may mimic urologic or surgical diseases. Surgeons who care for children must be equipped to diagnose and treat a variety of developmental and acquired disorders of the vulva, vagina, upper genital tract, and ovary. It is important to begin with an understanding of the normal anatomy and developmental changes of the genital tract. Knowledge of examination techniques and modifications necessary in children to obtain diagnostic information can facilitate accurate diagnoses. Consequently, the proper use and interpretation of radiologic and endoscopic techniques is essential in the care of female children and adolescents.

NORMAL GENITAL ANATOMY

The genital tract undergoes visible morphologic changes from infancy through childhood and adolescence.[1,2] At birth, due to the influence of maternal circulating estrogens, the labia majora are anteriorly placed and edematous in appearance. The mons pubis has a flattened triangulated look. The labia majora are thickened and cover the introital opening. The clitoral proportion is larger. The vestibule and hymen are pale and thickened and may occlude visualization of the vaginal canal without manipulation. The vagina is rugated and moist, and vaginal secretions may be present. The cervix is visible, and the uterus may contain functioning endometrial tissue, leading to the occurrence of estrogen-withdrawal bleeding in infancy.

During early childhood, the vulva remodels with thinning and attenuation of the labia majora and minora. The vestibule takes on an erythematous color with prominent vascular markings. It may now lie unopposed by the labia, allowing for easy visualization of the vaginal orifice with minimal traction. The hymen of a prepubescent child is normally easily visualized and is thin, often translucent and inelastic. Normal variations in shape and

amount of hymenal tissue have been described, and knowledge of these becomes important in the evaluation of penetrating injuries and anomalies[3-5] (Fig. 74-1). The vagina has an erythematous appearance and is inelastic and without rugations. Normally, the pH is mildly basic, and a mixture of bacterial flora is present. The cervix is flush with the vaginal vault and may be difficult to identify. The uterine fundus is poorly developed, with the cervicovaginal ratio being 3:1. No endometrium is visualized on sagittal imaging.

With the onset of puberty, the mons, labia majora, and labia minora all begin to develop. The vestibule begins to lose its erythematous appearance and lies opposed by the labia majora. The hymen thickens and becomes elastic and redundant.[6] The vagina grows in length and develops rugations. The cervix develops a well-defined junction from the uterus, and the uterine fundus develops a rounded appearance. Evidence of endometrial lining begins to be seen before menarche.

Folliculogenesis of the ovary, with small cyst formation, can be imaged as early as 16 weeks of gestation.[7] Three percent to 5% of children have small incidental ovarian cysts detected on ultrasound examination.[8] Follicular growth and atresia occurs throughout childhood, with increased follicular activity and size coinciding with advancing age.[9] Ovarian volume and position change with age, with the ovaries intra-abdominal in childhood and assuming a pelvic position at puberty.

GENITAL EXAMINATION

The genital examination of a child can be anxiety provoking to both the child and her parents. It is important to have a calm, professional attitude and establish rapport with the patient and her family. Examinations are less successful if they are hurried, forced, or exceed the developmental understanding of the child. An adequate light source and proper positioning are usually all that is needed to accomplish an examination in a prepubertal child.[10] For visualization of the vulva, introital opening,

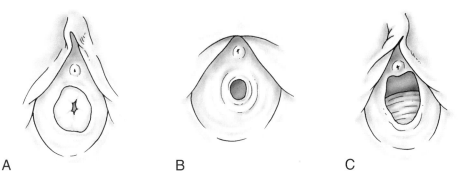

FIGURE 74-1. Normal anatomic variations of hymen. (Adapted from Pokorny SF, Stormer J: Atraumatic removal of secretions from the prepubertal vagina. Am J Obstet Gynecol 156:581–583, 1987.)

A   B   C

and lower vagina, gentle downward traction on the labia in lithotomy position is usually successful (Fig. 74-2). Placing the child on the mother's lap can sometimes facilitate the examination in young children. Knee-chest position may offer a clearer view of the hymen and lower vagina[11] (Fig. 74-3). A magnifying glass, colposcope, or otoscope may be helpful to see the detail of the lower vagina.[12] The office use of speculums is discouraged in prepubertal children. Comprehensive vaginal inspection, when necessary, is ideally done through endoscopic instruments under sedation.[13,14] By gently occluding the vaginal orifice, the entire vaginal canal can be visualized with hydrodistention. Speculum examinations of the vagina are usually well tolerated in postpubertal girls when a narrow-caliber straight blade speculum is gently inserted. Bimanual examinations can be accomplished through a rectal approach or, in adolescents, with a single digit inserted into the vaginal fornix. Imaging with ultrasonography (US) or, occasionally, magnetic resonance imaging (MRI) is adjuvant to examination and provides additional information on the status of the upper genital tract.[15]

Vulvar Abnormalities

Vulvar puritis, pain and discharge are common complaints in children. An etiology can be obtained in most cases with careful external inspection and, if necessary, blind vaginal cultures. Biopsy is seldom indicated. Most often, symptoms involve irritation or eruption of the vulvar skin related to hygienic practices. Atopic or irritant dermatitis were the most common diagnoses.[16] Infections are more associated with acute inflammation with erythema and the presence of a vaginal discharge.[17] Common respiratory pathogens such as *Streptococcus pyogenes* and *Haemophilus influenza* may cause acute genital symptoms.[18,19] When a bacterial infection is suspected, cultures of the vagina may be obtained by using moistened urethral swabs, feeding tubes, or catheters. A double-catheter system with a butterfly catheter within a small rubber catheter can be used to obtain upper vaginal secretions.[20]

Recurrent or persistent vaginitis despite treatment should alert the clinician to the presence of a retained foreign body in the vagina. Occasionally foreign bodies also may cause vaginal bleeding and or a protruding mass.[21,22] The most common foreign body is toilet paper shreds.[21] Pelvic US may reveal the bladder-indentation sign, suggesting a foreign body.[23] When a foreign body is suspected, vaginal lavage can be attempted in the office by using warm-water saline in a venous catheter or straight urinary catheter. Vaginoscopy under sedation may be necessary to retrieve an object. Endoscopic instruments

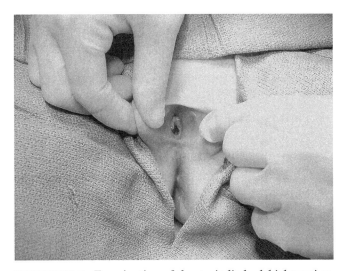

FIGURE 74-2. Examination of the genitalia by labial traction. Gently grasping the posterior labia majora and pulling anteriorly and superiorly, allows visualization of the genital structures.

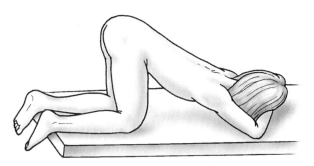

FIGURE 74-3. Knee-chest positioning. The lower vagina and hymen can occasionally be viewed more successfully by using the knee-chest position.

such as cystoscopes or hysteroscopes give excellent location of the object with minimal trauma to the genital area.[14]

Vulvar dermatoses may lead to acute vulvovaginal symptoms. Lichen sclerosis has the hallmark characteristic of a loss of skin markings with a sharply demarcated pale epithelial ring encircling the introitus, but sparing the vagina (Fig. 74-4). Signs of inflammation and trauma may be present, with purpura, fissures, and secondary infection associated with scratching. Lichen sclerosis may be confused with sexual abuse in some cases. Mainstays of treatment include avoidance of trauma with loose clothing, mild soaps, and generous use of emollients. Corticosteroids are used for acute symptoms. Other dermatologic conditions such as psoriasis, eczema, and allergic dermatitis also may mimic vulvovaginitis.[14]

Labial agglutination or adhesions occur in up to 22% of prepubescent girls (Fig. 74-5). Adhesions are thought to occur because of irritation or trauma of the unestrogenized labia, leading to a midline fusion of the labia. Adhesions can be associated with an increase in urinary tract infections, perineal wetness, symptomatic vulvitis, and an inability to access the urethra and vaginal orifice. When symptomatic, the treatment of choice is estrogen-based cream applied under traction to the adhesion site.[24,25] Surgical separation is seldom indicated because of the efficacy of topical hormonal therapy, but may be necessary in unusually dense adhesions or those that have had previous separation.[24,25] Long-acting local anesthetics, such as EMLA cream, may allow office separation in some girls.[26] Manual separation of the adhesions without anesthesia should be avoided because of the discomfort associated with the technique and the high risk of recurrence.

Genital Bleeding

Unexplained bleeding from the genital area in a prepubescent child is always abnormal (Table 74-1). Bleeding is most commonly extragenital, resulting from hematuria, rectal fissures, and vulvar epithelial irritation.

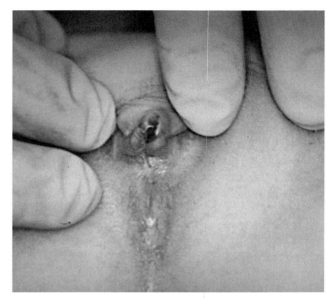

FIGURE 74-5. A 2-year-old child with extensive agglutination of the labia minora.

Prolapse of the urethra may occur and be associated with bleeding or even gangrenous changes. A red, granular lesion protrudes from the urethral meatus (Fig. 74-6). Topical treatment with estrogen-based cream usually relieves the symptoms. If symptoms persist, excision of the redundant tissue may be necessary. Vaginal bleeding may be associated with precocious puberty or autonomous production or exogenous sources of hormonal stimulation. It is important to perform a detailed physical examination searching for evidence of breast development, estrogenization of the genital tract, or the presence of an abdominal mass. In the absence of a satisfactory explanation of the source of bleeding, vaginoscopy should be done to evaluate the vaginal canal and cervix for the presence of foreign bodies, trauma, and infection, or rarely, tumors of the lower genital canal.

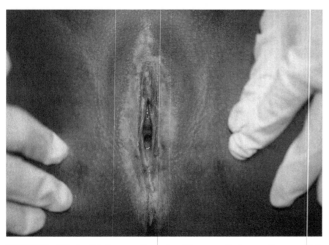

FIGURE 74-4. Lichen sclerosis diagnosed in a 5-year-old. A sharp demarcation of hypopigmented, thin epithelium is seen. It is often associated with fissures and purpura.

TABLE 74-1
CAUSES OF GENITAL BLEEDING IN PREPUBESCENT GIRLS

Genital trauma: Accidental, sexual abuse
Genitourinary: Urethral prolapse, urinary tract infections
Gastrointestinal: Inflammatory bowel disease, rectal fissure, hemorrhoids
Vulvovaginitis: Acute dermatitis, pinworms, beta hemolytic streptococcus, shigella
Foreign body
Vulvar dermatosis: Lichen sclerosis
Condyloma acuminata
Hemangiomas
Tumors: Malignant, benign
Endocrine abnormalities: Isosexual precocious puberty, pseudoprecocious puberty, exogenous hormonal stimulation

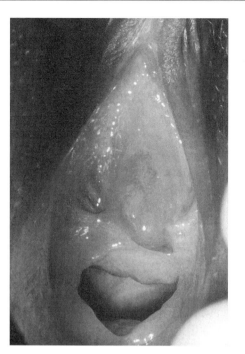

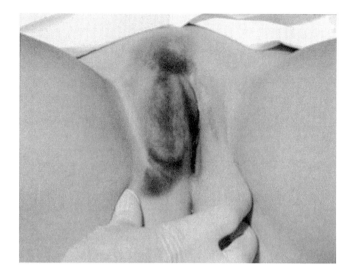

FIGURE 74-7. Straddle injury with an extensive vulvar hematoma. (Courtesy of Diane Merritt, M.D.)

FIGURE 74-6. Urethral prolapse *(arrow)* diagnosed in a 6-year-old child with a history of recurrent painless genital bleeding.

Acute genital bleeding in children requires immediate evaluation for the presence of serious injury or sexual abuse. If the source of bleeding is not readily apparent, the entire lesion cannot be identified, or the patient is not tolerant of the examination, vaginoscopy under sedation is indicated.

Straddle injuries are common during childhood from accidental falls onto blunt objects, resulting in soft tissue trauma from striking the pubic symphysis or rami. Straddle injuries are usually anterior, involving the mons, clitoris, and labia, and sparing the vaginal ring or perineal body (Fig. 74-7). They may result in hematoma formation, linear lacerations, or abrasions. Vulvar hematomas can be extensive but are usually self-limited. In the absence of acute ongoing hemorrhage, small or moderate hematomas can be managed conservatively with bed rest, ice, and pain control. Evacuation of extremely large hematomas causing distortion of the pelvic midline occasionally is necessary to facilitate recovery. Evacuations with débridement should be done under anesthesia by incising the medial mucosal surface and placing absorbable sutures for hemostasis and closure of dead space.[27] Drainage of the urinary bladder may be necessary because of edema with retention.

Penetrating injuries can occur through accidental impalements onto irregular objects, but the possibility of sexual abuse must always be strongly considered (Figs. 74-8 and 74-9). In the prepubertal child, lacerations involving or occurring above the hymenal ring require vaginoscopy under general anesthesia. Because of the inelasticity of the vaginal epithelium, penetrating injuries can result in disruption of the vagina, with possible internal hemorrhage and hematoma formation.[28] All injuries that cannot readily be explained by the presenting history should be referred to child protection. Surgeons should

familiarize themselves with the legal and social resources for sexual abuse diagnosis and care that are available within their communities.

Introital masses in children occasionally come to the attention of surgeons. Masses of the introitus or vagina are most commonly epithelial inclusion cysts of the hymen or lower vagina and often spontaneously resolve. In young girls, the rare possibility exists of embryonic rhabdomyosarcoma, a malignant primary tumor that

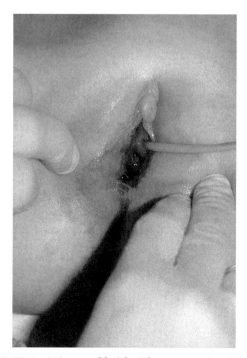

FIGURE 74-8. A 9-year-old girl with a penetrating injury sustained after falling on an open cabinet.

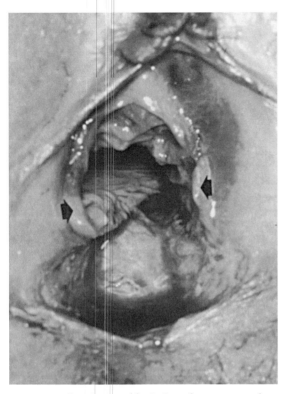

FIGURE 74-9. An 8-year-old victim of acute sexual assault who had small bowel herniating through the apex of the avulsed vagina. Note the abundant, although transected, amount of hymeneal tissue (*arrows*) present, indicating that she had not had significant stretch trauma to her hymen before this episode of rape. (From Pokorny SF, Pokorny WJ, Kramer W: Acute genital injury in the prepubertal girl. Am J Obstet Gynecol 166:1461–1466, 1992.)

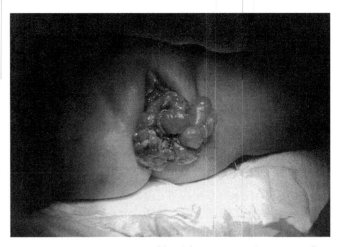

FIGURE 74-10. A 3-year-old with an extensive protruding vaginal mass diagnosed with embryonic rhabdomyosarcoma of the vagina. These rare tumors often begin with an indolent-appearing mass at the introitus. (Used with permission from NASPAG, 1999.)

are first noted during late puberty with cyclic pelvic pain and introital distention, associated with the absence of menstruation. With the continued accumulation of menstrual blood, a pelvic mass and obstructive genitourinary or gastrointestinal symptoms may be present. Occasionally, presentation will be in the newborn period because of the accumulation of mucus, producing an abdominal mass (Fig. 74-11) Transabdominal US reveals a dilated vaginal and uterine canal. If this is found during childhood and is asymptomatic, correction is usually

appears as indolent, grapelike masses protruding from the vagina (Fig. 74-10). Other possibilities include condyloma acuminata, ectopic ureter, and an obstructive vaginal anomaly. Occasionally, the Bartholin gland or periurethral gland may occlude or abscess, leading to an acquired lateral mass. It is important that the origin of the mass be fully evaluated, with evaluation with anesthesia as necessary. Transperineal US may be helpful to delineate the mass further. In cases that are unclear, biopsy or excision or both are essential.

UTEROVAGINAL ANOMALIES

Developmental abnormalities causing agenesis or obstruction of the genital tract can occur in children. These can often be recognized in the newborn period with routine examination, but the majority are diagnosed in the adolescent period with the lack of anticipated menses or with symptoms of obstruction.

Imperforate hymen is the most commonly diagnosed obstructive anomaly, with an incidence of less than 1%.[4,29] It arises as an isolated anomaly from failure of canalization of the urogenital sinus. Symptoms typically

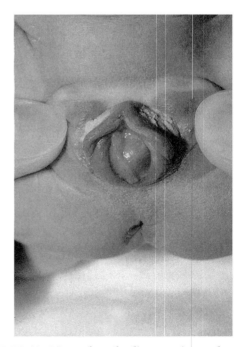

FIGURE 74-11. Mucocolpos, leading to urinary obstruction in a 2-day-old infant.

deferred to the onset of puberty. Surgical excision of the hymen with evacuation of the retained menstrual fluid provides permanent correction (Fig. 74-12*A* and *B*). This is done by carefully identifying the anatomic landmarks, such as the urethra and location of the lateral hymenal borders. It is important to recognize that significant distention of the posterior vaginal wall may cause the hymenal membrane to be located in a more superior position. A cruciate incision is made into the membrane inferior to the urethral meatus. After decompression, the individual flaps of tissue are then excised. The vaginal mucosa is sutured to the introital edge with interrupted absorbable sutures to avoid stenosis (Fig. 74-13*A–D*). Needle aspiration without definitive surgical correction is contraindicated because of the possibility of bacterial seeding and abscess formation.

A transverse vaginal septum also may exist at various levels of the vagina because of failure of unification of the urogenital sinus and the müllerian ducts during embryogenesis. Vaginal septa may be complete or partial and may occur at any level in the vaginal canal[30] (Fig. 74-14). They are most common in the upper vagina. Because the introitus may appear normal, diagnosis may be delayed. MRI or US is essential in defining this anomaly and indicating the thickness of the septum.[31] It is important before surgical exploration to assure the presence of cervical tissue by imaging to differentiate this condition from true agenesis of the cervix. Surgical correction is dependent on the location and thickness of the septum but most often entails excision of the septum with vaginal mucosal anastomosis. Thick septa may require preoperative vaginal dilation, mobilization of the upper vagina, or occasionally a skin graft to maintain vaginal patency. Circumferential stenosis is common at the anastomosis site, particularly with high or thick septa. Vaginal dilation may be required postoperatively.

True cervicovaginal agenesis is a rare disorder associated with an obstructed uterine canal, the absence of a patent cervix, and agenesis of the upper vagina (Fig. 74-15). The lower vagina may be patent. These patients are initially seen with cyclic or noncyclic abdominal or pelvic pain (or both) and a pelvic mass. This condition has a poor prognosis for reconstruction, with reports of significant morbidity from ascending infection and even death.[32] Hysterectomy is usually recommended, but the creation of a vaginal-uterine fistula has been sporadically described.[33,34]

Occasionally, patients may be seen with duplication of the uterus and cervix and a unilateral obstructing longitudinal septa of the vagina. Associated ipsilateral renal agenesis or hypoplasia is commonly found.[35] Menstruation occurs from the nonobstructed side, so the diagnosis may be made well past menarche. Pelvic US and MRI scanning are very reliable in distinguishing these disorders, especially when obstruction is present[31,36] (Fig. 74-16). Surgical repair through a vaginal approach is performed at diagnosis, with full excision of the vaginal septum. Care must be taken to approximate the vaginal mucosa of the two cavities.

Mayer-Rokitansky-Küster-Hauser syndrome was first described in 1961 and included primary amenorrhea in women with normal secondary sexual characteristics, uterine hypoplasia, and congenital absence of the vagina.[37] The incidence is approximately 1 in 5000.[38] Because of failure of development of the müllerian system, the uterus, cervix, and upper two thirds of the vagina fail to form. Renal and skeletal anomalies are commonly associated with this disorder. Although patients have primary

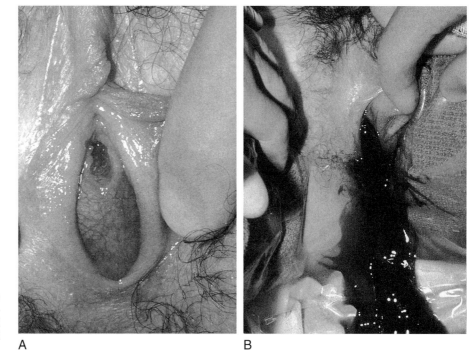

FIGURE 74-12. *A,* Imperforate hymen in a 12-year-old girl with a 6-month history of recurrent abdominal pain. *B,* Evacuation of menstrual obstruction on surgical correction

A   B

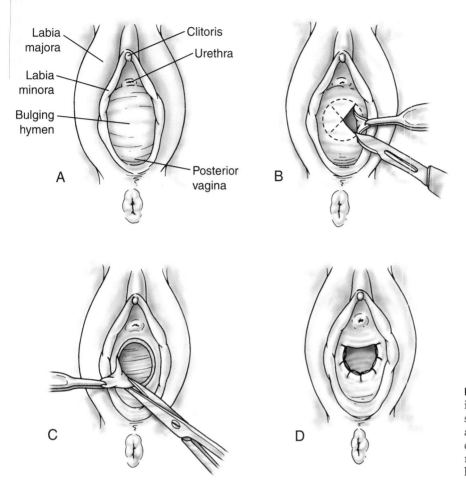

FIGURE 74-13. Surgical correction of imperforate hymen (*A*). A cruciate incision is made into the apex of the hymen after identifying the outer hymenal borders (*B*). Trimming of the hymenal remnants (*C*). Interrupted sutures placed for hemostasis.

amenorrhea, pubertal development and ovarian function are normal. The diagnosis can be made clinically on the basis of a normal phenotype and the genital findings cited earlier. An absent uterus with an elevated testosterone, poor breast development, virilization, or the lack of sexual hair requires a full chromosomal and hormonal evaluation for the presence of an intersex disorder.

Therapy for this problem is centered on creation of an adequate vaginal pouch to allow normal sexual functioning. The use of Lucite dilators, first popularized in the 1930s, has provided a highly effective nonsurgical alternative for many agenesis patients[39,40] (Fig. 74-17). Through the use of successive pressure dilators placed at the hymeneal ring, the vaginal vault can be lengthened

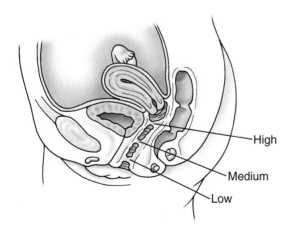

FIGURE 74-14. The transverse vaginal septum is the result of failed unification or canalization of the urogenital sinus and the müllerian duct. It can arise at any position in the vagina.

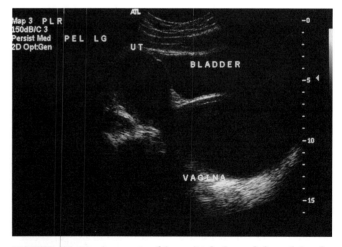

FIGURE 74-15. A sonographic sagittal view of the pelvis of a 16-year-old girl with cervicovaginal agenesis and a resultant hematometria.

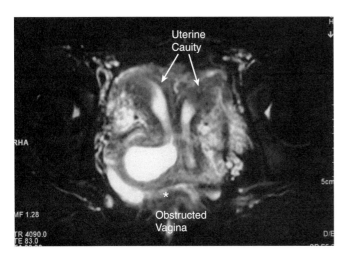

FIGURE 74-16. Magnetic resonance imaging section of a 16-year-old girl with a complete uterine duplication and a blind right hemivagina. Notice the obstruction and resultant right-sided hematocolpos and hematometria.

and enhanced to provide an adequate vaginal capacity. This approach has the advantage of being patient controlled and associated with extremely low morbidity. Vaginal dilation can usually be accomplished over a 2- to 3-month period or even more rapidly in highly motivated individuals. In selected patients, surgical creation of an artificial vagina may be indicated.[41] Many surgical options have been described, with the split-thickness graft vaginoplasty being advocated most often for agenesis patients.[42] In this approach, a split thickness of skin is harvested from an aesthetic place on the buttocks and sewn, dermal side exposed, over a vaginal mold (Fig. 74-18*A–D*). The potential space above the levator plate is surgically dissected, followed by placement of a skin-covered vaginal mold. The vaginal mold is sutured in place. After initial epithelialization, the mold is removed, and the patient is required to dilate the vagina

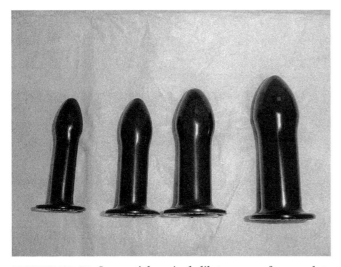

FIGURE 74-17. Sequential vaginal dilators are often used to create a coital pouch in individuals with vaginal agenesis.

for several months to maintain patency. Surgical outcome and patient satisfaction remains high for this type of vaginoplasty.[43,44] Other materials such as amnion, peritoneum, and intercede absorbable adhesion barriers have been described as an alternative to skin grafting, but have not gained wide popularity.[45,46] The use of sigmoid bowel pedicles pulled to the introitus is less common. Although this has the advantage of avoiding postoperative dilation, it may be associated with prolapse, chronic vaginal discharge, and vaginitis, which limit its functional result.[43,47,48] Rarely, external interposition of gracilis or vulvoperineal flaps are used to create a coital pouch. New laparoscopic methods, using a transperitoneal pulley system to advance the neovagina, report rapid correction with high success rates.[49]

ADNEXAL DISEASE

Surgical disorders of the adnexa are common, particularly in the adolescent period. US has increased the level of understanding regarding the development and natural history of ovarian cysts. New less-invasive surgical techniques allow more conservative management of adnexal disease in children.

Ovarian cysts may occur at all times from fetal life to adulthood. Simple cysts in the neonate are generally follicular and originate from the influence of maternal estrogens. Complex masses in this age group may represent in utero or neonatal torsion. The risk of malignancy is extremely small, but complications requiring surgical intervention can arise from torsion, hemorrhage, or mass effect. Both simple and complex masses are likely to resolve without therapy. Percutaneous aspirations are indicated for cysts larger than 5 cm to minimize the risk of torsion.[50] Indications for operative intervention include the presence of a complex mass that fails to resolve in the neonatal period, the recurrence of a cyst after aspiration, development of acute abdominal symptoms, or a combination of these. Treatment may consist of laparoscopic fenestration of simple cysts or cystectomy, if it can be done without loss of functional tissue.[51]

In childhood, small cysts representing follicular development and atresia are common and not associated with a pathologic state.[8] Management of ovarian cysts in children is based on size, the presence of symptoms, and cyst composition. Worrisome findings include cysts of larger than 5 cm, cysts with solid or complex internal echoes on US, and fixed masses accompanied by systemic symptoms of disease or precocious development.[52] Occasionally cysts may be associated with breast development or vaginal bleeding (Fig. 74-19*A,B*). It is important to distinguish follicular development arising from true precocious puberty from autonomously active cysts. Recurrent gonadotropin-independent cysts are most commonly associated with McCune-Albright syndrome or, more rarely, with hormonally active stromal or germ cell tumors. The diagnosis of ovarian tumors must be considered in children, especially in those with large, persistent complex masses that have solid components (Table 74-2). The most common ovarian tumor of

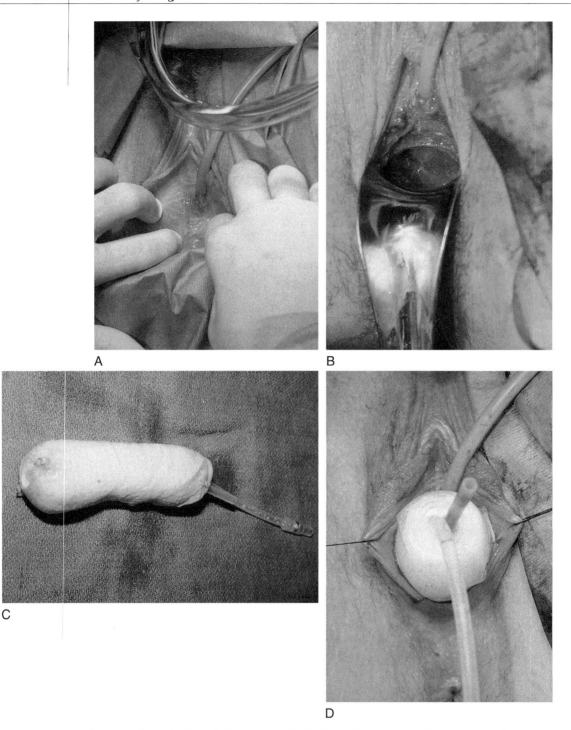

FIGURE 74-18. Creation of a vaginal pouch by using a split-thickness free graft. *A,* The perineum of a patient with vaginal agenesis. *B,* Dissection of a potential space between the urethra and bladder and rectum. *C,* Covering of a vaginal mold with split-thickness grafted skin. *D,* Placement of mold into dissected space.

childhood is the mature cystic teratoma, followed in frequency by stromal tumors[53] (Fig. 74-20). Malignant tumors are rare, composing about 10% of all surgically treated masses.[53,54] In prepubertal girls, ovarian masses, in conjunction with symptoms or worrisome radiologic signs, should undergo surgical exploration. In the

absence of malignancy, conservation of ovarian tissue should be attempted whenever possible.

Ovarian cysts are extremely common in adolescence because of persistent anovulation or ovulation dysfunction. They may be associated with rupture, pain, and hemorrhage (Fig. 74-21). A mass in the pelvis may be

TABLE 74-2
NEOPLASMS IN CHILDREN AND ADOLESCENTS

Neoplasm	Appearance	Tumor Markers	Other Information
Benign teratoma (dermoid)	Irregular, cystic, and solid or primarily cystic	None	Most common germ cell tumor 6%-8% malignant Malignant immature forms may be associated with other germ cell tumors Inspect other ovary
Dysgerminoma	Thick, white, opaque Cytologic reactivity with alkaline phosphatase	None	15%-20% bilateral, 95% cure (stage I) Chemotherapy for advanced disease
Endodermal sinus tumor (yolk sac tumor)	Solid and cystic Shiller-Duval bodies	AFP	Primarily unilateral Surgery and chemotherapy for all stages 15% survival after stage I
Embryonal carcinoma	Smooth with areas of hemorrhage and necrosis Shiller-Duval bodies	β-hCG	Usually part of a mixed germ cell tumor 60% endocrinologically active (precocious puberty) Surgery and chemotherapy for all stages 50% survival (stage I)
Choriocarcinoma	Syncytio and cytotrophoblasts`	β-hCG	Rare primary tumor in pediatric age group Surgery and chemotherapy for all stages
Mixed germ cell tumor	Predominantly solid or cystic and solid, depending, on composition	AFP	Most commonly composed of dysgerminoma and endodermal sinus tumor
Sex cord stromal tumors	Granulosa-theca or Sertoli-Leydig cells	None	More common in younger patients Isosexual precocious puberty or androgenization
Juvenile granulosa theca cell tumor	Very vascular	None	Malignancy related to percentage granulosa cells Pure thecomas benign Surgery alone for stage I Surgery and chemotherapy for advanced disease
Sertoli-Leydig cell tumors (arrhenoblastoma)			Variable malignant potential
Epithelial tumors serous cystadenoma	Predominantly cystic		Commonly large size May have borderline variants Low malignant potential
Mucinous cystadenoma	Predominantly cystic with septations		From coelomic epithelium
Serous or mucinous cystadenocarcinoma			Rare in children and adolescents
Miscellaneous tumors Polyembryona	Tissues resemble embryos with all three germ cell types (amniotic cavity, yolk sac, placental primordia)		
Gonadoblastoma			Predominantly dysgenetic gonads
Mesothelioma Metastatic disease			

AFP, α-fetoprotein; hCG, human chorionic gonodotropin. From Bacon JL. Surgical treatment of adnexal pathology. In Hewitt G (ed): Operative Techniques in Gynecologic Surgery. Philadelphia, WB Saunders, 4:215,1999.

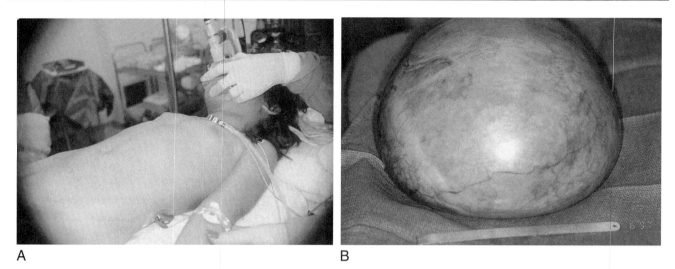

A   B

FIGURE 74-19. *A*, A 6-year-old girl with precocious puberty and a large pelvic mass. *B*, An autonomously functioning serous cystadenoma. All pubertal signs regressed after removal.

present, or the cyst may be found as an incidental finding at the time of radiologic studies. Mature cystic teratomas are the most common neoplasm, followed in frequency by cystadenoma. Malignant neoplasms are possible but compose less than 4% of all surgically excised masses.[53] In adolescents, a variety of reproductive disorders such as endometriosis, pelvic inflammatory disease, disorders of the fallopian tube, congenital uterine anomalies, or disorders of pregnancy may have the appearance of ovarian cysts (Table 74-3). It is essential to elicit a full history, including the details of menstrual function and sexual activity. Pregnancy must be excluded, and the possibility of complications of a sexually transmitted infection considered. Diagnostic imaging is very helpful in the management of ovarian cysts.[55]

The conservative approach to the management of ovarian cysts in adolescents is based on the low rate of

malignancy and the high rate of functional cysts and benign germ cell tumors. Recurrent observation is recommended as an initial therapy for adolescent women. Indications for surgical intervention include cysts larger than 10 cm, persistent complex masses, acute symptoms, or high suspicion for malignancy, based on radiologic or clinical criteria. In the absence of findings suggestive of neoplasm, minimally invasive surgical techniques such as laparoscopy should be paired with cystectomy and ovarian conservation. Cystectomy is performed by incising the ovary on the antimesenteric portion of the ovary. Blunt dissection separates the cyst from the ovarian capsule, allowing the cyst wall to be removed in toto. Electrocautery or sutures may obtain hemostasis (Fig. 74-22*A* and *B*). Closure of the cyst wall is not necessary. Although marked distortion of the ovarian capsule may be present, rapid involution occurs. The cyst

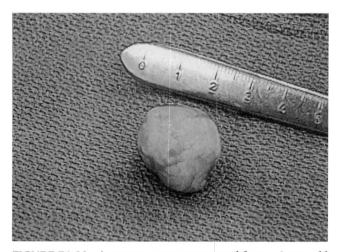

FIGURE 74-20. A mature teratoma removed from a 6-year-old girl. She was first seen with unrelated gastroenteritis and was found to have calcification on plain film of the abdomen.

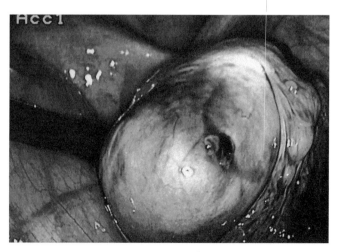

FIGURE 74-21. A ruptured corpus luteum cyst in a 15-year-old girl with acute pelvic pain.

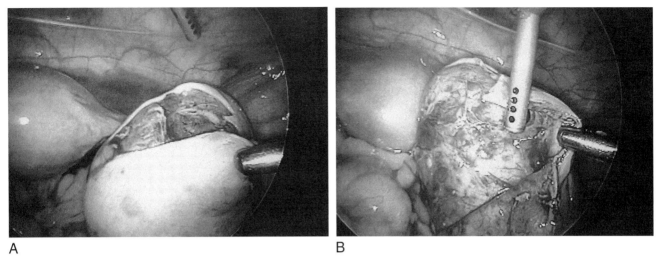

A   B

FIGURE 74-22. Laparoscopic ovarian cystectomy. *A,* An incision is made on the antimesenteric portion of the ovary. *B,* The capsule is separated from the tissue with blunt and sharp dissection.

may be removed through a laparoscopic bag to prevent spill of contents into the peritoneum. Laparoscopic management of cystic teratomas remains controversial because of concerns about the effects of rupture and spillage on long-term fertility. Recent studies, however, found laparoscopic removal to be safe and efficient and without long-term sequelae, even in the presence of rupture and spill.[56,57] When malignancy is suspected, oophorectomy through a midline laparotomy incision allows proper staging with careful exploration, collection of pelvic cytology, and pelvic and periaortic lymph node sampling.

The ovaries or tubes may occasionally undergo torsion, with loss of blood supply and ultimately necrosis of the adnexa (Fig. 74-23). Torsion of the ovary can occur at any age and is recognized by acute onset of pain, nausea, vomiting, and a pelvic mass. Ovarian torsion is classically associated with the presence of an ovarian cyst or tumor but can be associated with normal ovaries.[58] Doppler-enhanced US demonstrating the absence of peripheral flow helps to increase the sensitivity of clinical diagnosis. Ovarian torsion is a medical emergency. If a prompt diagnosis is made, the ovary may be salvaged with detorsion and cystectomy, even when it visually appears to have vascular compromise.[59] Oophorectomy is reserved for cases of delay associated with necrosis.

TABLE 74-3
ADNEXAL MASSES IN ADOLESCENT GIRLS

Ovarian
  Follicular cyst
  Corpus luteum
  Endometrioma
  Ovarian torsion
  Benign or malignant neoplasm
Fallopian tube
  Paraovarian cyst
  Ectopic pregnancy
Uterus
  Uterine anomaly
  Pregnancy
  Myoma
Gastrointestinal
  Abscess
  Appendicitis
  Inflammatory bowel disease
Urinary
  Pelvic kidney
  Acute urinary retention
  Urachal cyst
Neoplasms
  Sarcoma
  Lymphoma
  Teratoma
  Hemangioma

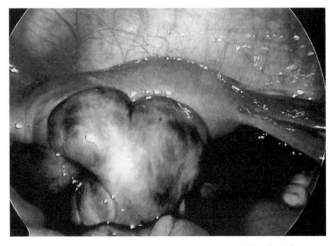

FIGURE 74-23. Ovarian torsion in a 14-year-old girl with acute abdominal pain. The fallopian tube and ovarian vascular pedicle are twisted multiple times, resulting in acute venous congestion. Untwisting the pedicle allowed return of blood flow.

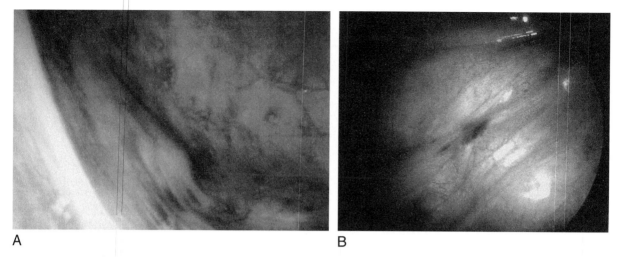

FIGURE 74-24. *A*, The peritoneal surface of a 14-year-old with endometriosis. Note the hypervascularity and subtle vesicular type lesions. *B*, Peritoneal surface of a 17-year-old girl with endometriosis. Note the classic "powder-burn" appearance.

Oophoropexy by side-wall fixation or shortening of the meso-ovarian ligament has been advocated by some to decrease the risk of subsequent contralateral torsion, although no evidence shows its efficacy.[59]

ENDOMETRIOSIS

Endometriosis refers to the presence of endometrial glands and stroma functioning outside of the uterine lining. Endometriosis has been traditionally thought of as a disease of women in their 20s and 30s but is well described in the adolescent population. Common symptoms among adolescents, such as dysmenorrhea, chronic pelvic pain, and dysfunctional uterine bleeding, have been associated with a 38% to 47% prevalence of endometriosis.[60,61] As many as 75% of symptomatic adolescents with medically refractory pelvic pain were found to have endometriosis with laparoscopy.[62] Although symptoms can suggest the diagnosis, definitive diagnosis is made by laparoscopic visualization or biopsy or both. Because few adolescents have laparoscopy during the adolescent years, the exact prevalence in adolescents remains unknown. Progression of disease and types of lesions appear to change with age. Clear, vesicular-appearing lesions and low-stage disease are more common in adolescence, with more classic hemosiderin "powder-burn lesions" identified in older adults[63,64] (Fig. 74-24*A* and *B*).

Treatment of endometriosis in adolescents is based on alleviation of symptoms and slowing the progression of disease. For patients undergoing surgical therapy, removal of all visible lesions by resection or destruction, with normalization of pelvic anatomy, should be undertaken at the time of diagnosis. To accomplish this, CO_2 laser, cautery, coagulation, and operative laparoscopic techniques may be used. Menstrual suppression with oral contraceptives or progesterone-only medication or both, along with nonsteroidal anti-inflammatory agents, are

the mainstays of therapy. Gonadotropin-releasing agonists may be used on a short-term basis as an adjuvant to surgical therapy in adolescents but carries the risk of a detrimental effect on bone density. It should be used cautiously in younger adolescents. Noninterventional pain therapies may have a place in controlling the chronic pain states associated with endometriosis. The long-term outcome of infertility and chronic pain in those diagnosed with endometriosis as adolescents is not well described.

REFERENCES

1. Huffman JW, Dewhurst CJ, Caparo VJ: Anatomy and physiology. In The Gynecology of Childhood and Adolescence, 2nd ed. Philadelphia, WB Saunders, 1981, pp 24–69.
2. Siegfried EC, Frasier LD: The spectrum of anogenital diseases in children. In Callen JP (ed): Current Problems in Dermatology. St. Louis, Mosby, 1997, pp 35–80.
3. Porkorny SF: Configuration of the prepubertal hymen. Am J Obstet Gynecol 157:950–956, 1987.
4. McCann J, Wells R, Simon M, et al: Genital findings in prepubertal girls selected for nonabuse: A descriptive study. Pediatrics 86:428–439, 1990.
5. Berenson AB, Hegar AH, Hayes JM, et al: Appearance of the hymen in prepubertal girls. Pediatrics 89:387–394, 1992.
6. Edgardh K, Ormstad K: The adolescent hymen. J Reprod Med 47:710–714, 2002.
7. Peters H, Himelstein-Braw R, Faber M: The normal development of the ovary in childhood. Acta Endocrinol 82:617–630, 1976.
8. Millar DM, Blake JM, Stringer DA, et al: Prepubertal ovarian cyst formation: 5 years' experience. Obstet Gynecol 81:434–437, 1993.
9. Himelstein-Braw R, Byskov AG, Peters H, et al: Follicular atresia in the infant human ovary. J Reprod Fertil 46:55–59, 1976.
10. Hariston L: Physical examination of the prepubertal girl. Clin Obstet Gynecol 40:127–134, 1997.
11. McCann J, Welis R, Simon M, et al: Comparison of genital examination techniques in prepubertal girls. Pediatrics 85:182–187, 1990.
12. Mendriatta V: Office gynecologic evaluation of the pediatric patient: Indications, examination, and procedures. In Hewett G (ed): Operative Techniques in Gynecologic Surgery. Philadelphia, WB Saunders, 1999, pp 164–175.
13. Bacsko GY: Hysteroscopy for vaginoscopy in pediatric gynecology. Adolesc Pediatr Gynecol 7:221–222, 1994.

14. Parker JD, Hibbert ML, Dainty LD, et al: Micro-hydrovaginoscopy in examining children. Obstet Gynecol 96:772–774, 2000.

15. Teele RL, Share JC: Ultrasonography of the female pelvis in childhood and adolescence. Radiol Clin North Am 30:743–758, 1992.

16. Fischer G, Rogers M: Vulvar disease in children: A clinical audit of 130 cases. Pediatr Dermatol 17:1–6, 2000.

17. Jaquiery A, Stylianopoulos A, Hogg G, et al: Vulvovaginitis: Clinical features, aetiology, and microbiology of the genital tract. Arch Dis Child 81:64–67, 1999.

18. Straumanis JP, Bocchini JA: Group A beta-hemolytic streptococcal vulvo-vaginitis in prepubertal girls: A case report and review of the literature. Pediatr Infect Dis 9:845–847, 1990.

19. Cox RA: *Haemophilus influenzae*: An underrated cause of vulvovaginitis in young girls. J Clin Pathol 50:765–768, 1997.

20. Porkorny SF, Stormer J: Atraumatic removal of secretions from the prepubertal vagina. Am J Obstet Gynecol 156:581–583, 1987.

21. Fishman A, Paldi E: Vaginal bleeding in premenarchal girls: A review. Obstet Gynecol Surg 46:457–460, 1991.

22. Paradise JE, Willis ED: Probability of vaginal foreign body in girls with genital complaints. Am J Dis Child 139:472–476, 1985.

23. Caspi B, Zalel Y, Katz Z, et al: The role of sonography in the detection of vaginal foreign bodies in young girls: The bladder indentation sign. Pediatr Radiol 25:60–61, 1995.

24. Muram D: Treatment of prepubertal girls with labial adhesions. Pediatr Adolesc Gynecol 12:67–70, 1999.

25. Bacon JL: Prepubertal labial adhesions: Evaluation of a referral population. Am J Obstet Gynecol 187:327–332, 2003.

26. Hoebeke P, Depauw P, Van Laecke E, et al: The use of EMLA cream as an anaesthetic for minor urological surgery in children. Acta Urol Belg 65:25–28, 1997.

27. Merritt DF. Genital injuries in the pediatric and adolescent girl. In Hewett G (ed): Operative Techniques in Gynecologic Surgery. Philadelphia, WB Saunders, 1999, pp 181–187.

28. Pokorny SF, Pokorny WJ, Kramer W: Acute genital injury in the prepubertal girl. Am J Obstet Gynecol 166:1461–1466, 1992.

29. Hager AH, Ticson L, Guerra L, et al: Appearance of the genitalia in girls selected for nonabuse: Review of hymenal morphology and nonspecific findings. J Pediatr Adolesc Gynecol 15:27–35, 2002.

30. Burgis J: Obstructive müllerian anomalies: Case report, diagnosis and management. Am J Obstet Gynecol 195:338–344, 2001.

31. Lang IM, Babyn P, Oliver GD: MR imaging of paediatric uterovaginal anomalies. Pediatr Radiol 29:163–170, 1999.

32. Casey AC, Laufer MR: Cervical agenesis: Septic death after surgery. Obstet Gynecol 90:706–707, 1997.

33. Rock JA, Schlaff WD, Jones HW Jr: The clinical management of congenital absence of the uterine cervix. Int J Gynaecol Obstet 22:231–235, 1984.

34. Deffarges JV, Haddad B, Musset R, et al: Utero-vaginal anastomosis in women with uterine cervix atresia: Long-term follow-up and reproductive performance: A study of 18 cases. Hum Reprod 16:1722–1725, 2001.

35. Woolfe RB, Allen WM: Concomitant malformations: The frequency, simultaneous occurrence of congenital malformations of the reproductive and urinary tracts. Obstet Gynecol 2:236–265, 1954.

36. Fedele L, Ferrazzi E, Dorta M, et al: Ultrasonography in the differential diagnosis of double uteri. Fertil Steril 50:361–364, 1988.

37. Hauser GA, Schreiner WE: Das Mayer-Rokitansky-Küster-Hauser syndrome. Schweiz Med Wochenschr 91:381–384, 1961.

38. Evans TN, Poland ML, Boving RL: Vaginal malformations. Am J Obstet Gynecol 141:910–920, 1981.

39. Frank RT: The formation of an artificial vagina without operation. Am J Obstet Gynecol 35:1053–1055, 1938.

40. Roberts CP, Haber MJ, Rock JA: Vaginal creation for müllerian agenesis. Am J Obstet Gynecol 185:1349–1352, 2001.

41. Rock JA, Jones HW Jr: Construction of a neovagina for patients with a flat perineum. Am J Obstet Gynecol 160:845–851, 1989.

42. Wiser WL, Bates W: Management of agenesis of the vagina. Surg Gynecol Obstet 159:108–112, 1984.

43. Martinez-Mora J, Isnard R, Castellvi A, et al: Neovagina in vaginal agenesis: Surgical methods and long-term results. J Pediatr Surg 27:10–14, 1992.

44. Strickland JL, Cameron WJ, Krantz KE: Long-term satisfaction of adults undergoing vaginoplasty as adolescents. Adolesc Pediatr Gynecol 6:135–139, 1993.

45. Morton KE, Dewhurst CJ: Human amnion in the treatment of vaginal malformations. Br J Obstet Gynecol 93:50–54, 1986.

46. Jackson ND, Rosenblatt PL: Use of intercede absorbable adhesion barrier for vaginoplasty. Obstet Gynecol 84:1048–1050, 1994.

47. Karim BK, Hage JJ, Dekker J, et al: Evolution of the methods of neovaginoplasty for vaginal aplasia. Obstet Gynecol 58:19–27, 1995.

48. Freundt I: Prolapse of the sigmoid neovagina: Report of three cases. Obstet Gynecol 83:876–879, 1994.

49. Fedele L, Bianchi S, Zanconato G, et al: Laparoscopic creation of a neovagina in patients with Rokitansky syndrome: Analysis of 25 cases. Fertil Steril 74:384–389, 2000.

50. Shozu M, Akasofu K, Lika K, et al: Treatment of antenatally diagnosed fetal ovarian cysts by needle aspiration during the neonatal period. Arch Gynecol Obstet 2149:103–106, 1991.

51. Esposito C, Garipoli V, Di Matteo G, et al: Laparoscopic management of ovarian cysts in newborns. Surg Endosc 12:1152–1154, 1998.

52. Meire HB, Farrord P, Guha T: Distinction of benign from malignant ovarian cysts by ultrasound. Br J Obstet Gynecol 85;893–899, 1978.

53. Templeman C, Fallat ME, Blinchevsky A, et al: Noninflammatory ovarian masses in girls and young women. Obstet Gynecol 96:229–233, 2000.

54. Quint EH, Smith YR: Ovarian surgery in premenarchal girls. J Pediatr Adolesc Gynecol 12:27–30, 1999.

55. Wu A, Siegel MJ: Sonography of pelvic masses in children: Diagnostic predictability. AJR Am J Roentgenol 147:1199–1202, 1987.

56. Luxman D, Cohen J, David MP: Laparoscopic conservative removal of ovarian dermoid cysts. J Am Assoc Gynecol Laparosc 3:409–411, 1996.

57. Templeman CL, Hertweck SP, Scheetz JP, et al: The management of mature cystic teratomas in children and adolescents: A retrospective analysis. Hum Reprod 15:2669–2672, 2000.

58. Kokosa ER, Keller MS, Weber TR: Acute ovarian torsion in children. Am J Surg 180:462–465, 2000.

59. Dolgin SE, Lubin M, Shlasko E: Maximizing ovarian salvage when treating idiopathic adnexal torsion. J Pediatr Surg 35:624–628, 2000.

60. Goldstein DB, deCholnoky C, Emans SJ: Adolescent endometriosis. J Adolesc Health Care 1:37–41, 1980.

61. Vercellini P, Fedele LA, Bianch S, et al: Laparoscopy in the diagnosis of chronic pelvic pain in adolescent women. J Reprod Med 34:827–830, 1989.

62. Laufer MR, Goitein L, Bush M, et al: Prevalence of endometriosis in adolescent girls with chronic pelvic pain not responding to conventional therapy. J Pediatr Adolesc Gynecol 10:199–202, 1997.

63. Redwine DB: Age related evolution in color appearance of endometriosis. Fertil Steril 48:1062, 1987.

64. Martin DC, Hubert GD, Vander Zwagg R, et al: Laparoscopic appearance of peritoneal endometriosis. Fertil Steril 51:63, 1989.

CHAPTER 75

Breast Diseases in Children

Don K. Nakayama, MD

EMBRYOLOGY

Formation of the breast occurs throughout embryonic and fetal life.[1] By week 4 of embryonic development, the ectoderm thickens into a pair of longitudinal streaks in the ventral surface of the embryonic torso, the primitive mammary ridges. Breast tissue can develop anywhere along these "milk lines," which in the fully developed mammal extend from the axillae to the labia majora. The proximal and distal portions of each ridge atrophy by week 6. The ectoderm that remains in the pectoral area grows down into the underlying mesenchyme to form the primary mammary bud. From there, secondary buds begin to branch, forming early lactiferous ducts that are well established by 16 weeks. The buds respond to estrogenic hormonal stimulation by the maternal-placental-fetal unit during the last trimester, canalizing into ducts and enlarging en masse to form a true breast nodule during the final weeks of gestation.

The nipple and areola form during late fetal development. A mammary pit first appears at 12 weeks from downgrowth of the epidermis. A pigmented areola is first seen at 20 to 24 weeks, but a true nipple is not present until later in the perinatal period and is frequently inverted at birth.

ANATOMY AND PHYSIOLOGY

The breast in the term newborn is a firm discrete nodule of white tissue up to 1 cm in diameter. The premature infant lacks a defined breast nodule and is particularly vulnerable to damage to the breast by an ill-placed surgical incision. The nodule may persist well into the first year of life and may be more prominent at 6 months than earlier.[2] The nodule begins to involute in late infancy. Throughout prepuberty, small breasts are present in both boys and girls.

The ductal system of the infant breast ranges from rudimentary to one with well-developed terminal lobules but without an age-dependent progression of histology.[3] In contrast to the ductal anatomy, the ductal epithelium undergoes a progression of functional stages. A secretory epithelium in the first 3 days undergoes metaplasia into apocrine-type cells with cystic dilation of the ducts and alveoli over the first month. Over the next 2 years, the gland gradually involutes. The newborn breast is able to secrete milk, a response from elevated prolactin concentrations at birth.[4] Although, for the most part, secretory activity subsides within 3 to 4 weeks, immunohistochemical staining for casein remains strongly positive at 2 months and persists up to 7 months.[3] Two infants aged 9 and 18 months were observed to secrete milk, long after prolactin concentrations decreased and beyond any residual maternal hormonal effects, suggesting that endogenous hormones may actively affect breast function in early infancy.[4]

The onset of puberty is signaled by breast (thelarche; mean onset in North American girls, 10.9 years) or pubic hair (pubarche; 11.2 years) development, although both are preceded by the onset of the adolescent growth spurt (9.2 years).[5,6] Menarche follows an average of 2.3 years later.[7]

Thelarche is a response to the maturation of functional ovarian follicles.[7] Prolactin, glucocorticoids, and insulin have a permissive effect on breast development. With puberty, ovarian follicles begin estrogen synthesis. Estrogens circulate to the breast and stimulate ductal development and site-specific adipose deposition. Male adolescents fail to produce significant breast mass, primarily because they lack significant levels of circulating estrogen. Once started, the process usually progresses smoothly to maturity in about 3 years. The breast stages as defined by Marshall and Tanner are as follows[5]:

Stage 1: Preadolescent; elevation of papilla only
Stage 2: Breast bud stage; elevation of breast and areola as a small mound, enlargement of areola diameter
Stage 3: Further enlargement of breast and areola, with no separation of their contours
Stage 4: Projection of areola and papilla to form a secondary mound above the level of the breast
Stage 5: Mature stage; projection of papilla only, resulting from recession of the areola to the general contour of the breast.

PATHOPHYSIOLOGY

Female breast disease in pediatric age groups can be seen as an *a*berration of *n*ormal *d*evelopment and *i*nvolution (ANDI).[8] The breast undergoes a normal sequence of development, with each histologic and physiologic feature characteristic of each period: the breast first grows and develops into a functional breast, responds to cyclical changes of menstruation and pregnancy, and then finally undergoes involution in late maturity. Disordered responses produce a corresponding sequence of breast conditions and disorders, with specific conditions being associated with each developmental state. The early reproductive period (menarche to 25 years) is the main period of lobular development in the breast. Under the ANDI concept, a fibroadenoma is not a typical benign tumor but a disorder of normal lobular development.[8] Stroma development during this period, if excessive, may result in juvenile hypertrophy. Exaggerated cyclic effects typical of a mature breast may result in cyclic mastalgia and nodularity. Table 75-1 summarizes the complete ANDI classification.

In early infancy, the breast foreshadows the histologic sequence of development and involution that will begin years later. As noted, the newborn breast develops lobules in response to maternal hormones. Over the next months of life, it then undergoes involution. Although rare, benign conditions that result from breast involution may be encountered during infancy, such as periductal mastitis, nipple discharge, and nipple retraction.

Breast cancer represents the extreme end of the spectrum of developmental disorders. It is a disorder of the mature breast, apparently the cumulative product of genetic and hormonal influences over time.[9] It is extremely rare in pediatric age groups, almost exclusively seen in late adolescence when encountered. Although risk factors for breast cancer certainly involve events during childhood and adolescence (such as early menarche) and genetic influences (such as familial breast cancer), breast cancer is not a childhood disease.

DISORDERS OF DEVELOPMENT AND GROWTH

Polythelia

Extra nipples and areolae may develop anywhere along the milk line from axilla to pubis. The most common location is on the chest below the actual breast. In a minority, a true accessory breast develops. Unsightly structures should be removed.

Hypoplasia and Aplasia

True breast aplasia occurs in Poland's syndrome.[10] Underlying chest wall structures, including pectoralis muscles and ribs, are absent or diminished in size. The ipsilateral upper extremity may also be affected.

TABLE 75-1

ABERRATIONS OF NORMAL DEVELOPMENT AND INVOLUTION OF THE BREAST (ANDI)

| Stage (Peak Ages, yr) | Normal Process | ABERRATION | | Disease State |
		Underlying Condition	Clinical Presentation	
Early reproductive period (15–25)	Lobule formation	Fibroadenoma	Discrete lump	Giant fibroadenoma, multiple fibroadenomas
	Stroma formation	Juvenile hypertrophy	Excessive breast development	
Mature reproductive period (25–40)	Cyclical hormonal effects on glandular tissue and stroma	Exaggerated cyclical effects	Cyclical mastalgia and nodularity (generalized or discrete)	
Involution (35–55)	Lobular involution (including microcysts, apocrine change, fibrosis, adenosis)	Macrocysts	Discrete lumps	
		Sclerosing lesions	Radiograph abnormalities (mastalgia lumps)	
	Ductal involution (including periductal round cell infiltrates)	Duct dilation	Nipple discharge	Periductal mastitis with bacterial infection and abscess formation
		Periductal fibrosis	Nipple retraction	
	Epithelial turnover	Mild epithelial hyperplasia		Epithelial hyperplasia with atypia

From Hughes LE: Aberrations of normal development and involution (ANDI): an update. In Mansell RE (ed): Recent Developments in the Study of Benign Breast Disease. London, Parthenon Publishing, 1994, pp 65–73, with permission.

Reconstruction of the chest wall and placement of a mammary prosthesis or breast reconstruction by a variety of flap techniques are indicated.[11]

Atrophy

Patients with atrophy of breasts that have undergone normal development should be evaluated for an underlying cause. Weight loss results in loss of fat from stroma and bilateral atrophy. Eating disorders also may be complicated by hypothalamic suppression and hypoestrogenism, further retarding breast growth.[12] In an otherwise well-nourished adolescent, endocrine disorders that result in low estrogen or increased androgens should be evaluated with appropriate hormone determinations.

Unilateral atrophy may occur in scleroderma.[12] It has been reported as a complication of infectious mononucleosis.[13]

Virginal Hypertrophy

The cause of virginal hypertrophy is probably an end-organ hypersensitivity to normal hormonal fluxes at the time of puberty.[14] Resected specimens may approach 8 to 10 kg. Histologically, breasts show proliferation of glandular tissue and resemble gynecomastia seen in boys.[12] A differential diagnosis must be considered in the evaluation of breast enlargement in adolescents and is summarized in Table 75-2.

The diagnosis is subjective and may depend in large part on the patient's own feelings. Tissue necrosis and rupture of the skin may result from sheer weight and justify reduction mammoplasty. Little experience is available with medical therapy, although some improvement has been reported with danazol therapy.[15] Reduction mammoplasty is a safe and appropriate procedure for virginal hypertrophy.[16] Recurrence may result from continued growth of the residual tissue, requiring additional procedures.[17]

Unilateral Hypertrophy

Breast asymmetry may result from unilateral hypertrophy, a condition easily distinguished from hypoplasia and

TABLE 75-2
DIFFERENTIAL DIAGNOSIS OF BREAST HYPERTROPHY

Virginal hypertrophy
Inflammation
Giant fibroadenoma
Cystosarcoma phyllodes
Hormone-secreting tumors of the ovary,
    adrenal gland, or pituitary gland
Lymphoma
Sarcoma
Adenocarcinoma

From Samuelov R, Siplovich L: Juvenile gigantomastia. J Pediatr Surg 23:1014–1015, 1988, with permission.

aplasia. Some degree of asymmetry is normal and is detectable in many patients. Breast growth may magnify differences and may hamper the child psychologically, even though both breasts are completely clinically normal. Breast reduction of the enlarged breast is then indicated, once Tanner stage 5 breast maturity is reached.[18]

Gynecomastia

Gynecomastia is the benign proliferation of glandular tissue of the male breast great enough to be felt or seen as an enlarged breast.[19] Male breast enlargement occurs physiologically in the newborn, adolescent, and older man. Breast development in the newborn was discussed previously. This discussion focuses on pubertal gynecomastia and is derived from the complete review by Braunstein.[19]

About 30% to 60% of boys exhibit gynecomastia. Prevalence first appears between 10 and 12 years of age. Highest prevalence is at 13 to 14 years, corresponding to Tanner stage 3 or 4. Involution is generally complete at 16 to 17 years. Imbalances between estrogen and androgen concentrations or effects may contribute to the development of gynecomastia during puberty. Testicular or adrenal neoplasms may overproduce estrogens. Peripheral conversion of androgens to estrogens may increase estrogen levels, as noted in pubic skin fibroblasts from patients with idiopathic gynecomastia, and if also present in the breast, may explain increased growth and development.[20] Decreased androgen levels or androgenic effects may result from primary defects of the testis, loss of tonic stimulation by pituitary gonadotropins, or increased binding of androgens to sex-hormone–binding globulin. Displacement of androgens from their receptors by the many drugs associated with gynecomastia (e.g., spironolactone) may result in unopposed estrogen effects in sex-hormone–sensitive tissue, including the breast.

Histologic studies in the early stages of gynecomastia show marked duct epithelial cell proliferation, inflammatory cell infiltration, increased stromal fibroblasts, and enhanced vascularity. This proliferative stage, also known as the florid stage, may explain breast pain and tenderness that are typical of the clinical presentation. Epithelial proliferation and ductal dilation then both decrease, and the stroma begins to undergo fibrosis and hyalinization. Clinical resolution of breast enlargement and pain follow in 85% of cases, a fact that must be considered when contemplating treatment.

Painful, tender gynecomastia is a typical presentation in adolescent boys. The patient often recalls trauma to the breast; the injury is more likely to have brought the lump to his attention than to have caused it. On palpation, true gynecomastia is a disk of rubbery tissue arising concentrically beneath and around the nipple and areola. This distinguishes it from pseudogynecomastia, increased amounts of adipose tissue beneath the breast causing prominence of the area. The differential diagnosis of gynecomastia is summarized in Table 75-3.

Because pubertal gynecomastia is so prevalent, a thorough history and physical examination, especially of the testes, are sufficient in adolescent boys. Reassurance and

TABLE 75-3
CONDITIONS ASSOCIATED WITH GYNECOMASTIA

Physiologic
Neonatal
Pubertal
Involutional

Pathologic
Neoplasms
 Testicular (germ cell, Leydig cell, Sertoli cell, sex cord)
 Adrenal (adenoma or carcinoma)
 Ectopic production of human chorionic gonadotropin
Primary gonadal failure
Secondary hypogonadism
Intersex
 Enzymatic defects of testosterone production
 Androgen insensitivity syndromes
 True hermaphrodism
Liver disease
Starvation, especially during the recovery phase
Renal disease and dialysis
Hyperthyroidism
Excessive extraglandular aromatase activity
Drugs
Idiopathic

From Braunstein GD: Gynecomastia. N Engl J Med 328:490–495, 1993, with permission.

follow-up examinations at 6-month intervals are sufficient. Pubertal gynecomastia generally resolves within 1 year. Suggestive aspects of the personal medical history (especially drugs and medications), abnormal physical findings (particularly of the testes and genitalia), or pubertal gynecomastia that persists longer than 1 year should lead to a directed endocrinologic and oncologic workup. Drugs should be discontinued, if possible, and the patient re-examined in 1 month. Imaging studies of the testes and adrenal glands are necessary if a tumor is suspected.

The initial endocrinologic workup includes determinations of serum levels of human chorionic gonadotropin (hCG), luteinizing hormone (LH), testosterone, and estradiol (E_2). Increased hCG suggests a testicular or extragonadal germ cell tumor and is evaluated with a testicular ultrasound (US). If the testes are normal, chest and abdominal computed tomography is indicated. The interpretation of decreased testosterone levels depends on LH: if elevated, primary hypogonadism is present; if normal or decreased, prolactin levels are checked for a possible prolactin-secreting tumor. If both testosterone and LH are elevated, thyroid hormone and thyroid-stimulating hormone levels are checked for the possibility of hyperthyroidism. Normal values suggest an androgen-resistance syndrome. Elevated E_2 with a normal or decreased LH suggests a Leydig or Sertoli cell tumor of the testis or an adrenal neoplasm.

The indications for therapy are severe pain, tenderness, or embarrassment sufficient to interfere with the patient's normal daily activities. Subcutaneous mastectomy through a periareolar incision is definitive treatment. Drugs have been used to treat gynecomastia, including testosterone, danazol, clomiphene, and tamoxifen. It is difficult to assess the efficacy of these various medical regimens because gynecomastia undergoes spontaneous regression in the vast majority of cases. Side effects from these medications do not justify drug therapy for pubertal gynecomastia.

INFLAMMATORY LESIONS

Breast Trauma and Fat Necrosis

Soft tissue injury to the breast may result from the familiar causes of blunt and penetrating mechanisms familiar to trauma surgeons. Shoulder-harness restraints have been reported to cause subcutaneous rupture of the breast.[21] Most breast trauma is mild and self-limiting. Specific therapy is rarely required.

Fat necrosis is a benign condition that can mimic breast carcinoma. It is considered to result from breast trauma. A history of antecedent trauma is present in about 40% of cases. Areas of fat necrosis are seen as single or multiple firm, round, or irregular masses, often in the center of the breast near the areola. The masses may be painless, firm, immobile, and cause skin tethering and thickening, all features that suggest carcinoma. Speculated calcifications may be present on mammography, further suggesting the presence of a neoplasm.

Patients who are seen soon after breast injury with associated signs of trauma, such as ecchymosis and painful masses, may be observed for resolution. Patients who are seen later with painless masses require biopsy to rule out malignancy.

Mastitis and Abscess

Infections of the newborn breast, uncommon today, had a high mortality and caused substantial morbidity to the breast and chest wall before the antibiotic era. The disease primarily affects the newborn breast, before involution of the ductal anatomy. Eighty-four percent occur in the first 3 weeks of life. *Staphylococcus* is the causative organism in more than 90% of cases. *Streptococcus, Salmonella,* and *Escherichia coli* also may cause a breast infection.[22]

Both sexes are affected, with a female-to-male ratio of 1.8.[22] The skin and nipple are red. Swelling and edema cause induration of the area. Fluctuance and deep discoloration to a fiery red or purple color indicate the presence of an abscess or extension of the infection beneath the fascia. Although in some infants, a small drop of pus may be expressed from the nipple, this is not sufficient drainage if an abscess is truly present. Most patients lack systemic reactions to infection, with only one-fourth having a fever and fewer than 10% having other constitutional symptoms (irritability or refusal to feed).[22] One-fourth have pustular skin lesions elsewhere, usually in the inguinal region.[22]

Mastitis and breast abscess require appropriate antibiotic therapy against *Staphylococcus, Streptococcus, Salmonella,* and *Escherichia coli*. Areas of fluctuance or progression of inflammation while taking antibiotics suggest the presence of an abscess that requires drainage.

Mastitis in newborns responds in nearly all cases to intravenous antibiotics and warm packs to the affected breast. The decision to explore the infant breast for an abscess must be made with great care to avoid unnecessary damage that may result in breast deformity later in adolescence. An initial needle aspiration of suggestive areas is a prudent first step. If no pus is encountered, antibiotics are continued. Discovery of a true abscess requires incision and drainage. One study documented a significant decrease in breast size relative to the opposite breast in two of five patients undergoing pubertal breast development who had undergone incision and drainage of a breast abscess as a newborn.[22]

Mastitis and abscess occur more commonly after thelarche. Causes include manipulation and breast-feeding, although in many cases, the cause cannot be identified. Nursing may continue in cases that develop while breast-feeding. Adequate abscess drainage usually requires general anesthesia owing to loculations of pus and breast septations in the developing and mature breast.[1]

NIPPLE DISCHARGE

Galactorrhea

Galactorrhea is inappropriate lactation that is not related to pregnancy or that continues into postpartum in the absence of breast-feeding.[1] The five pathophysiologic groups are neurogenic, hypothalamic, endocrine, drug-induced, and idiopathic. Neurogenic causes result from local breast and nipple irritation and stimulation. The most common hypothalamic cause of galactorrhea in adults is prolactinoma, a rare tumor in childhood and adolescence. Failure of sexual maturation often accompanies galactorrhea in children with these tumors.[23] Visual symptoms and headache are rare in children as compared with adults. Cessation of oral contraceptives, polycystic ovary, adrenal tumors, and gonadal tumors are rare causes of galactorrhea in adolescents.[1] Hypothyroidism in infants and children has been reported to be associated with galactorrhea and precocious puberty; nipple discharge ceases with correction of the underlying thyroid condition.[24,25] Many drugs have been recognized as causes of adult galactorrhea, but seldom have been described in children.[1] Examples include neuroleptics, estrogens, and opiates.

Nipple discharge in boys is always abnormal, and a cause must be sought. Prolactinoma is the most common cause in young boys.[26] If prolactin levels are high and evaluation of the sella turcica unrevealing, annual imaging of the sella is necessary until the end of puberty, even if galactorrhea resolves.

Other Nipple Discharges

Nonmilky discharges include pus, cyst contents, and blood. Purulent discharges usually respond to antibiotics; chronic discharge may require drainage and duct excision. Serous drainage of brown to green fluid may indicate the presence of a communicating breast cyst and is usually self-limited. Bloody drainage, a sign of cancer in adults, is generally drainage from an intraductal papilloma or duct ectasia in children and adolescents.[27] Bloody nipple drainage may be culture positive for *Staphylococcus,* so drainage should be cultured and treated if positive. Excision of the abnormal duct is indicated if drainage persists or recurs.[28]

MASTALGIA

Breast pain, or mastalgia, is a poorly characterized and underreported syndrome.[29] It accounts for about one-fourth of visits to adult breast clinics and is the presenting symptom of breast cancer in 15 % of cases. Its prevalence in young and adolescent girls is unknown.

Initial evaluation excludes localized lesions, benign and malignant, and inflammatory conditions. Pain is then characterized as cyclic or noncyclic. The distinction is important because the likelihood of response to drug treatment differs: cyclic pain is more likely to respond. Cyclic mastalgia usually occurs in the third decade of life. It is usually characterized as bilateral, dull, burning, or aching. Pain starts 7 to 10 days before the onset of menses, building until menses, when the pain dissipates. Pain may persist throughout the cycle. Spontaneous resolution occurs in 22 % of cases. Noncyclic mastalgia tends to occur a decade later and resolves in 50 % of cases. Treatment includes removal of methylxanthines from the diet and reassurance. Evening primrose oil, danazol, and bromocriptine may be effective as adjunctive therapy.

BREAST MASSES

Evaluation of Breast Masses

The age of the patient affects the differential diagnosis and hence the diagnostic approach (Tables 75-4 and 75-5). Patient age, history, and physical examination are sufficient to make the diagnosis in nearly all cases. Because primary breast cancer is so rare in pediatric age groups, observation has little risk and often is an appropriate step in determining the clinical diagnosis.[28] It is important, however, to follow up all lesions to resolution and to obtain further studies when lesions continue to grow or have features that are worrisome to the experienced clinician (e.g., hard consistency, irregular margins, fixation to chest wall or skin, regional lymphadenopathy). A directed workup in such cases may include fine-needle aspiration for cytology, mammography, US examination, and ultimately biopsy.

Prepubertal Breast Masses

Masses may occur in the prepubertal breast but are nearly always benign. The most important diagnosis to consider is asynchronous thelarche.[12] One breast bud may appear weeks to months ahead of the other. A breast bud is easily recognized as a disk of firm tissue beneath the areola. In such cases, biopsy is never indicated because it may lead to unilateral iatrogenic amastia.

TABLE 75-4
BREAST MASSES IN CHILDREN

Physiologic
Normal breast bud
Premature thelarche

Pathologic
Inflammatory
    Mastitis
    Breast abscess
    Fibrosis
    Fat necrosis
Benign neoplasms
    Hemangioma
    Cyst
    Lipoma
    Papilloma
Malignant neoplasms
    Metastatic (e.g., rhabdomyosarcoma, lymphoma)
    Secretory carcinoma

Cysts and Fibrocystic Disease

Benign simple cysts occur throughout childhood, but they are most common with the onset of breast development. They appear as soft, painless masses that are not fixed to surrounding breast tissue.[1] Needle aspiration of the cyst results in complete disappearance. Fluid may be serous or brown. Persistence of a mass after cyst aspiration is an indication for biopsy.

Fibrocystic disease is a disease of the mature breast, occurring most commonly in the fourth to fifth decades, and is generally not an issue in adolescents.[30] Masses that occur with fibrocystic disease may be asymptomatic or associated with mastalgia, worse in the perimenstrual period.[12] Resolution of the mass may occur over the course of one or two cycles. A persisting or dominant mass is aspirated for diagnostic and therapeutic reasons.

FIBROADENOMAS

Fibroadenomas are the most common breast mass in pediatric age groups.[31] Two variants affect children: adult and juvenile. Adult fibroadenomas affect older adolescents and young women. They may be multiple in 10% to 15%

TABLE 75-5
BREAST MASSES IN ADOLESCENTS

Physiologic	Benign neoplasms
Thelarche	Fibroadenoma
Unilateral hypertrophy	Phyllodes tumor
	Cyst
Pathologic	Fibrocystic disease
Inflammatory	Neurofibroma
Mastitis	Malignant neoplasms
Breast abscess	Primary breast cancer
Fibrosis	Metastatic (e.g., lymphoma)
Fat necrosis	

of cases. The mass is small, measuring 1 to 2 cm in diameter. It is well circumscribed, rubbery in consistency, and mobile. Juvenile fibroadenomas affect younger adolescents around the time of puberty. In contrast to an adult fibroadenoma, the juvenile variant is much larger and may cause considerable breast asymmetry.

Fibroadenomas are considered to be benign, although adult fibroadenomas rarely harbor a carcinoma, and juvenile variants may be related to phyllodes tumors.[1,32] Clonal analysis shows that epithelial and stromal elements of the fibroadenoma are polyclonal, indicating a hyperplastic rather than a neoplastic process.[33] Adult fibroadenomas confer a small but definite increased risk (relative risk, 1.3 to 1.9) for breast cancer development.[31] Clonal analysis in three patients in whom phyllodes tumor of the breast developed after excision of a fibroadenoma suggested that the former developed from the latter.[34] A phyllodes tumor tends to be larger (>4 cm in diameter), occur in older patients (mean age, 28.5 years in fibroadenoma, 44 years in phyllodes tumor), has high density on mammography, and appears round or lobulated with posterior acoustic enhancement on breast US compared with a fibroadenoma.[35,36] A considerable overlap exists between the two conditions with these criteria, however, and aspiration cytology or excisional biopsy is necessary to confirm the diagnosis.

Fibroadenomas can be safely followed up without operation if the lesion exhibits the expected characteristic features: 1 to 2 cm, solitary, firm, rubbery, nontender, and well circumscribed. Fine-needle aspiration is useful in distinguishing fibroadenomas from carcinomas and phyllodes tumors, but differentiating fibroadenomas from other benign conditions is more difficult.[31] In one study of nonoperative management of adult fibroadenomas, 16% of clinically diagnosed adult fibroadenomas disappeared during 12 months.[37] Excision of those that persisted showed the clinical diagnosis to be accurate in 73% of cases, with the misdiagnoses being of other benign breast conditions. None was a malignancy. Because more than half (54%) of fibroadenomas in the study continued to grow during the period of observation, the author concluded that the most expeditious course is simply to resect the mass.

Enlarging fibroadenomas should be excised to avoid further enlargement of the mass and preserve the architecture of the remaining normal breast tissue. The excision of either variant of fibroadenoma proceeds through an incision directly over the mass, following one of Langer's lines. The mass is held by a centrally placed suture or clamp and is removed with no more than a few millimeters of normal breast tissue. Further breast development is usually normal and symmetrical as the tissue compressed by the tumor fills the defect over time.[12]

Phyllodes Tumors

Phyllodes tumors, formerly called cystosarcoma phyllodes, are rare fibroepithelial tumors that range from benign (with significant risk for local recurrence) to malignant, with rapidly growing metastases.[38] They range in size from 1 to 40 cm. Closely resembling a fibroadenoma, a phyllodes tumor appears well circumscribed grossly, but lacks a true capsule. Its surface has minute surface projections that can barely be seen. Owing to these features, complete surgical excision requires a 2-cm margin of normal breast parenchyma. Fibrous areas are interspersed with soft, fleshy areas, and cysts are filled with clear or semisolid bloody fluid, all features that distinguish it from a fibroadenoma. On microscopy, both epithelial and stromal elements show hyperplasia and may have areas of atypia, metaplasia, and malignancy. Characteristics of the stroma alone, however, determine whether a phyllodes tumor is malignant. The mean age of patients is in the fourth decade, about a decade older than that for adult fibroadenoma. Phyllodes tumors have been recorded in both adolescent and prepubertal ages.[38]

Distinguishing phyllodes tumor from adenoma before operation is difficult, and a definitive diagnosis may require open excisional biopsy. Fine-needle aspiration depends on the detection of a dimorphic pattern of stromal elements and benign epithelial tissue, although the technique may not yield a definitive diagnosis in all cases.[39] The mammographic appearance of phyllodes tumors resembles that of fibroadenomas, with smooth polylobulated margins.[38] US is useful if cysts are found within an otherwise solid mass, a characteristic of phyllodes tumor.

When the preoperative diagnosis is known, wide local excision with a 2-cm margin of normal breast tissue is recommended. Tumors that extend to the pectoralis fascia require removal of the muscle adjacent to the tumor. Owing to the similarity in appearance between a fibroadenoma and a phyllodes tumor, the latter may be enucleated without a margin when the diagnosis is not known before operation. Because 20% of phyllodes tumors will recur when resected without an adequate margin, most authorities recommend re-excision of normal breast tissue to assure the removal of an adequate margin.[38]

Traditionally, malignant phyllodes tumors were treated with simple mastectomy. Recently, malignant tumors have been treated by using wide local excision with 2-cm margins with acceptable results.[39,40] Lymph node metastases are not present, so lymph node dissection is not indicated.[39,40]

Benign tumors more than 5 cm in diameter have a higher rate of recurrence (39%) than do smaller ones (10%).[41] Both benign and malignant phyllodes tumors recur. Among recurrences in previously resected benign tumors, about 20% show malignant histologic transformation with a worse overall prognosis. Local recurrence of a benign tumor is re-excised, whereas most authorities recommend simple mastectomy for a recurrence of a malignant tumor.

BREAST CANCER

Breast malignancy in children falls into three groups: primary malignancies, metastatic tumors that involve the breast, and second malignancies.[42] Primary breast cancer is extremely rare in childhood age groups. Although only 0.2% of primary breast cancers occur before age 25 years,

they have been found in children younger than 5 years and in male as well as female adolescents.[43] More than 90% are first seen as a breast mass. Nipple discharge is a presenting sign, on occasion, so a sample of fluid should be sent for cytologic examination.

Secretory carcinoma is a form that occurs relatively more frequently, but not exclusively, in children. It has a low-grade clinical behavior with a good prognosis for long-term survival after simple mastectomy.[44] Both boys and girls are affected; even though the sex ratio of girls to boys is 5:1; the youngest patient reported is a 3-year-old boy.[45] Even though most tumors measure 3 cm or less, lesions of 12 cm have been reported. Axillary lymph node involvement is present in about 20% of cases. Standard treatment is simple mastectomy, although some long-term survivors have been reported after excisional biopsy. Axillary node dissection is indicated if nodes are clinically involved. Recurrence after lumpectomy has been described in several reports. Long-term follow-up is imperative owing to the indolent nature of the disease and the risk for late recurrence.[43]

Nonsecretory breast cancers are less common than secretory breast cancers in pediatric age groups. Some large children's hospitals report no primary breast cancers in their series of pediatric breast masses.[28] They are reported exclusively in female adolescents and young adults and probably represent the leading edge of the prevalence distribution for adult primary breast cancer. They include histologic types seen in primary breast cancers in mature women: invasive intraductal (most common), invasive lobular, and signet ring.[46] Family history of breast cancer is a risk factor for early-onset breast cancer and was present in one fourth of patients.[46] Treatment regimen is the same as for adult primary breast cancer, dictated by histology, stage, presence of hormone receptors, and patient menstrual status.

The breast has been reported as the primary site of presentation of a rhabdomyosarcoma and lymphoblastic non-Hodgkin's lymphoma, both in 14-year-old girls.[42] Metastatic carcinoma may involve the breast, with retinoblastoma, osteosarcoma, neuroblastoma, leukemia, lymphoma, and rhabdomyosarcoma having been reported.[28,46,47] Breast cancer in early adulthood may develop after mantle irradiation for Hodgkin's disease in childhood. One report documented three such cases, occurring 12 to 19 years after therapy for Hodgkin's disease.[42]

REFERENCES

1. Wiebke EA, Nieberhuber JE: Disorders of the breast. In Carpenter SE, Rock JA (eds): Pediatric and Adolescent Gynecology. New York, Raven Press, 1992, pp 417–431.
2. McKiernan J, Coyne J, Cahalane S: Histology of breast development in early life. Arch Dis Child 63:136–139, 1988.
3. Anbazhagan K, Bartek J, Monaghan P, et al: Growth and development of the human infant breast. Am J Anat 192:407–417, 1991.
4. McKiernan J, Hull D: Prolactin, maternal oestrogens and breast development in the newborn. Arch Dis Child 56:770–774, 1981.
5. Marshall WA, Tanner JM: Variations in pattern of pubertal changes in girls. Arch Dis Child 44:291–303, 1969.
6. Tanner JM, Davies PS: Clinical longitudinal standards for height and height velocity for North American children. J Pediatr 107:317–329, 1985.

7. Krasnow JS, Shapiro SS: Normal pubertal development. In Carpenter SE, Rock JA (eds): Pediatric and Adolescent Gynecology. New York, Raven Press, 1992, pp 49–64.
8. Hughes LE: Aberrations of normal development and involution (ANDI): An update. In Mansell RE (ed): Recent Developments in the Study of Benign Breast Disease. London, Parthenon, 1994, pp 65–73.
9. Brinton LA, DeVesa SS, Weber BL, et al: Etiology and pathogenesis of breast cancer. In Harris JR, Lippman ME, Morrow M, et al (eds): Diseases of the Breast. Philadelphia, Lippincott-Raven, 1996, pp 159–306.
10. Ravitch MM: Poland's syndrome. In Ravitch MM (ed): Congenital Deformities of the Chest Wall and Their Operative Correction. Philadelphia, WB Saunders, 1977, pp 233–271.
11. Shamberger RC, Welch KJ, Upton J III: Surgical treatment of thoracic deformity in Poland's syndrome. J Pediatr Surg 24:760–765, 1989.
12. Simmons PS: Diagnostic considerations in breast disorders of children and adolescents. Obstet Gynecol Clin North Am 19:91–102, 1992.
13. Haramis HT, Collins RE: Unilateral breast atrophy. Plast Reconstr Surg 95:916–919, 1995.
14. Samuelov R, Siplovich L: Juvenile gigantomastia. J Pediatr Surg 23:1014–1015, 1988.
15. Taylor PJ, Cumming DC, Corenblum B: Successful treatment of D-penicillamine-induced breast gigantism with danazol. BMJ [Clin Res] 282:362–363, 1981.
16. Evans GR, Ryan JJ: Reduction mammoplasty for the teenage patient: A critical analysis. Aesthetic Plast Surg 18:291–297, 1994.
17. Kupfer D, Dragman D, Broadbent R: Juvenile breast hypertrophy: Report of a familial pattern and review of the literature. Plast Reconstr Surg 90:303–309, 1992.
18. Fischl RA, Rosenberg I, Simon BE: Planning unilateral breast reduction for asymmetry. Br J Plast Surg 24:402–404, 1971.
19. Braunstein GD: Gynecomastia. N Engl J Med 328:490–495, 1993.
20. Bulard J, Mowszowicz I, Schaison G: Increased aromatase activity in pubic skin fibroblasts from patients with isolated gynecomastia. J Clin Endocrinol Metab 64:618–623, 1987.
21. Magnant CM: Fat necrosis, hematoma, and trauma. In Harris JR, Lippman ME, Morrow M, et al (eds): Diseases of the Breast. Philadelphia, Lippincott-Raven, 1996, pp 61–65.
22. Rudoy RC, Nelson JD: Breast abscess during the neonatal period. Am J Dis Child 129:1031–1034, 1975.
23. Richmond IL, Wilson CB: Pituitary adenomas in childhood and adolescence. J Neurosurg 49:163–168, 1978.
24. Van Wyck JJ, Grumbach MM: Syndrome of precocious menstruation and galactorrhea in juvenile hypothyroidism: An example of hormonal overlap in pituitary feedback. J Pediatr 57:416–435, 1960.
25. Macaron C: Galactorrhea and neonatal hypothyroidism. J Pediatr Surg 101:576–577, 1982.
26. Rohn RD: Galactorrhea in the adolescent. J Adolesc Health Care 5:37–49, 1984.
27. Turbey WJ, Buntain WL, Dudgeon DL: The surgical management of pediatric breast masses. Pediatrics 56:736–739, 1975.
28. West KW, Rescorla FJ, Scherer LR III, et al: Diagnosis and treatment of symptomatic breast masses in the pediatric population. J Pediatr Surg 30:182–187, 1995.
29. Klimberg VS: Etiology and management of breast pain. In Harris JR, Lippman ME, Morrow M, et al (eds): Diseases of the Breast. Philadelphia, Lippincott-Raven, 1996, pp 99–106.
30. Constantini M, Bucchi L, Dogliotti L, et al: Cohort study of women with aspirated gross cysts of the breast: An update. In Mansell RE (ed): Recent Developments in the Study of Benign Breast Disease. London, Parthenon, 1994, pp 227–239.
31. Houlihan MJ: Fibroadenoma and hamartoma. In Harris JR, Lippman ME, Morrow M, et al (eds): Diseases of the Breast. Philadelphia, Lippincott-Raven, 1996, pp 45–47.
32. Ozzello L, Gump FE: The management of patients with carcinomas in fibroadenomatous tumors of the breast. Surg Gynecol Obstet 160:99–104, 1985.
33. Noguchi S, Motomura K, Inaji H, et al: Clonal analysis of fibroadenoma and phyllodes tumor of the breast. Cancer Res 53:4071–4074, 1993.
34. Noguchi S, Yokouchi H, Aihara T, et al: Progression of fibroadenoma to phyllodes tumor demonstrated by clonal analysis. Cancer 76:1779–1785, 1995.
35. Hindle WH, Alonzo LJ: Conservative management of breast fibroadenomas. Am J Obstet Gynecol 164:1647–1651, 1991.
36. Yilmaz E, Sal S, Lebe B: Differentiation of phyllodes tumors versus fibroadenomas. Acta Radiol 43:34–39, 2002.
37. Wilkinson S, Anderson TJ, Rifkind E, et al: Fibroadenoma of the breast: A follow-up of conservative management. Br J Surg 76:390–391, 1989.
38. Petrek JA: Phyllodes tumors. In Harris JR, Lippman ME, Morrow M, et al (eds): Diseases of the Breast. Philadelphia, Lippincott-Raven, 1996, pp 863–869.
39. Stebbing JF, Nash AG: Diagnosis and management of phyllodes tumor of the breast: Experience of 33 cases at a specialist centre. Ann R Coll Surg Engl 77:181–184, 1995.
40. Palmer ML, De Risi DC, Pelikan A, et al: Treatment options and recurrence potential for cytosarcoma phyllodes. Surg Gynecol Obstet 170:193–196, 1990.
41. Chua CL, Thomas A: Cystosarcoma phyllodes tumors. Surg Gynecol Obstet 166:302–306, 1988.
42. Rogers DA, Lobe TE, Rao BN, et al: Breast malignancy in children. J Pediatr Surg 29:48–51, 1994.
43. Schydlower M: Breast masses in adolescents. Am Fam Physician 25:141–145, 1982.
44. Rosen PP: Invasive mammary carcinoma. In Harris JR, Lippman ME, Morrow M, et al (eds): Diseases of the Breast. Philadelphia, Lippincott-Raven, 1996, pp 393–444.
45. Karl SR, Ballantine TV, Zaino R: Juvenile secretory carcinoma of the breast. J Pediatr Surg 20:368–371, 1985.
46. Corpron CA, Black CT, Singletary SE, et al: Breast cancer in adolescent females. J Pediatr Surg 30:322–324, 1995.
47. Farah RA, Timmons CF, Aquino VM: Relapsed childhood acute lymphoblastic leukemia presenting as an isolated breast mass. Clin Pediatr 38:545–546, 1999.

Endocrine Disorders and Tumors

Michael A. Skinner, MD, and Shawn D. Safford, MD

THYROID GLAND

Diseases of the thyroid gland were demonstrated to occur in 36.7 of 1000 school-aged children in the United States.[1] About half of these are diffuse gland hypertrophy or simple goiter. Thyroiditis was the second most common abnormality, followed by thyroid nodules and functional disorders. Malignant neoplasms are exceedingly rare, with only two cases of papillary thyroid carcinoma found in a population of nearly 5000 children followed up for 3 years.

Embryology and Physiology

The thyroid gland is the first endocrine organ to mature in fetal development, arising as an outpouching of the embryonic alimentary tract at about 24 days' gestation. The developing thyroid gland descends from the base of the tongue ventral to the hyoid bone and the larynx, to its final location by about 7 weeks' gestation. In about half of the population, a persistence of the thyroglossal diverticulum results in a pyramidal thyroid lobe. Accessory thyroid tissue may appear in the tongue or anywhere along the course of the duct. Rarely, nondescent results in a lingual thyroid.

Histologically, by week 11 of gestation, colloid begins to form, and thyroxin (T_4) can then be demonstrated in the embryo. Parafollicular cells, or C cells, arise from the ultimobranchial bodies. These parafollicular cells then diffuse throughout the thyroid gland.

Thyroid hormones are synthesized at the interface between the follicular cell and the thyroglobulin. Thyroglobulin is recognized histologically as colloid. The first step in thyroid synthesis production is the iodination of tyrosine molecules, which are then coupled to form the definitive thyroid hormones T_4 and tri-iodothyronine (T_3). When free thyroid hormone reaches the nucleus of the target cell, the T_3 molecule interacts with the nuclear receptors, and the receptor-T_3 conjugate binds to DNA to regulate genetic transcription.[2] T_4 increases cellular oxygen consumption and the basal metabolic rate, stimulates protein synthesis, and influences carbohydrate, lipid, and vitamin metabolism.

The production and secretion of T_3 and T_4 are stimulated by thyroid-stimulating hormone (TSH) secreted by the pituitary, in response to thyrotropin-releasing hormone, which is, in turn, secreted by the hypothalamus. Other peptides are present within the thyroid gland, such as neuropeptide Y, substance P, cholecystokinin, and vasoactive intestinal peptide, which may assist in the production and secretion of thyroid hormones.[3]

Thyrotropin (TSH) is nearly always decreased in the hyperthyroid state and elevated in hypothyroidism and is an extremely sensitive measure of this condition. The plasma free T_4 level is a measure of biologically active thyroid hormone, unaffected by protein binding. When total plasma T_3 and T_4 are measured, it is necessary to consider the level of thyroid-binding globulin to estimate the level of unbound biologically active hormone.

Several imaging modalities are available to assist in evaluating the thyroid gland. Radionuclide scintigraphy is probably the most commonly used test. The radioiodines ^{123}I and ^{131}I are most effective in detecting ectopic thyroid tissue or metastatic thyroid carcinoma, whereas technetium-99m pertechnetate produces superior imaging of thyroid gland nodules or tumors. Ultrasonography (US) is useful to delineate whether a neck mass actually arises from the thyroid and whether multiple nodules are present.

Non-Neoplastic Thyroid Conditions

Goiter and Thyroiditis

The causes of thyromegaly in 152 affected children are listed in Table 76-1.[4] Most patients had simple adolescent colloid goiter. Physiologically, diffuse thyroid enlargement may be due to a defect in hormone production, related to autoimmune diseases, or a response to an inflammatory condition. Goiters are classified as diffusely enlarged or nodular and either toxic or euthyroid. Most children with goiters are euthyroid, and surgical resection is rarely indicated.

The differential diagnosis for diffuse thyroid enlargement is listed in Table 76-2. Laboratory evaluation

Adapted from Jaksic J, Dumic M, Filipovic B, et al: Thyroid disease in a school population with thyromegaly. Arch Dis Child 70:103-106, 1994.

TABLE 76-1

ETIOLOGY OF THYROID GLAND ENLARGEMENT IN 152 CHILDREN

Diagnosis	Frequency (%)
Simple goiter	83
Chronic lymphocytic thyroiditis	12.5
Graves' disease	2.5
Benign adenoma	1.5
Cyst	1

should begin with plasma free T_4 and TSH levels. With a simple colloid goiter, the patient is euthyroid; US or scintigraphy reveals uniform enlargement, and serum thyroid antibody titers are normal. The etiology of this condition may be an autoimmune process.[5] The natural history of colloid goiter is not well known, but one study of adolescents found that, 20 years after diagnosis, nearly 60% of the glands were normal in size.[1] Exogenous thyroid hormone does not significantly enhance resolution of the goiter. In rare cases, resection may be indicated because of size or the suspicion of neoplasia.

Chronic lymphocytic (Hashimoto's) thyroiditis is another common cause of diffuse thyroid enlargement, occurring most frequently in female adolescents. This condition is part of the spectrum of autoimmune thyroid disorders. It is thought that CD4 T cells are activated against thyroid antigens and recruit cytotoxic CD8 T cells, which kill thyroid cells, to cause hypothyroidism.[6] Children are initially euthyroid and slowly progress to become hypothyroid. However, approximately 10% of children are hyperthyroid, a condition known as "Hashitoxicosis." The thyroid gland is usually pebbly or granular in texture and may be mildly tender.

Ninety-five percent of patients with chronic lymphocytic thyroiditis have elevated antithyroid microsomal antibodies or antithyroid peroxidase antibodies. Plasma thyroid hormone levels are normal or low, and TSH

TABLE 76-2

DIFFERENTIAL DIAGNOSIS OF DIFFUSE THYROID ENLARGEMENT (GOITER) IN CHILDREN

Autoimmune Mediated
    Chronic lymphocytic (Hashimoto's) thyroiditis
    Graves' disease
    Simple colloid goiter

Compensatory
    Iodine deficiency
    Medications
    Goitrogens
    Hormone or receptor defect

Inflammatory Conditions
    Acute suppurative thyroiditis
    Subacute thyroiditis

levels are elevated in 70% of patients. Thyroid imaging is usually not necessary if clinical and laboratory findings are strongly suggestive of the diagnosis. The radionuclide scan usually shows patchy uptake of the tracer and may mimic the findings in Graves' disease or multinodular goiter. The principal US finding is nonspecific, diffuse thyroid hypoechogenicity. Rarely, autoantibodies cannot be detected, and fine needle aspirate (FNA) may be needed to confirm the diagnosis. In as many as one third of adolescent patients, the thyroiditis resolves spontaneously, with the gland becoming normal and the antibodies disappearing. Thus expectant management should be considered. Exogenous thyroid hormone should be administered in the hypothyroid patient, but in euthyroid children, it is ineffective in reducing the size of the goiter.[7]

Subacute (de Quervain's) thyroiditis, a viral inflammation of the thyroid gland, is unusual in children. The thyroid is swollen, painful, and tender. Mild thyrotoxicosis results from injury to the thyroid follicles, with release of thyroid hormone into the circulation. Serum T_3 and T_4 levels are elevated, and TSH is decreased. Owing to thyroid follicular cell dysfunction, decreased radioactive iodine uptake occurs, a finding that distinguishes subacute thyroiditis from Graves' disease. Histologically, granulomas and epithelioid cells may be seen. The treatment of subacute thyroiditis is symptomatic and generally consists of nonsteroidal anti-inflammatory agents or steroids. The condition typically lasts 2 to 9 months, and complete recovery may be expected.

Acute suppurative thyroiditis is a bacterial infection of the gland. The gland is acutely inflamed, and the patient is septic. Patients are usually euthyroid. Staphylococci or mixed aerobic and anaerobic flora are common causal agents, and a congenital pharyngeal sinus tract may predispose the patient to infection. Management consists of intravenous antibiotics. Abscess drainage may be necessary. The thyroid gland may be expected to recover completely.

Graves' Disease

Graves' disease, or diffuse toxic goiter, is the most common cause of hyperthyroidism in childhood. The condition is an autoimmune disease caused by the presence of immunoglobulins (Igs) of the IgG class directed against components of the thyroid plasma membrane, possibly including the TSH receptor. These autoantibodies stimulate the thyroid follicles to increase iodide uptake and cyclic adenosine monophosphate production, leading to thyroid growth and inducing the production and secretion of increased thyroid hormone.

TSH-receptor antibodies are present in more than 95% of patients with active Graves' disease. The inciting event eliciting the antibody response against the TSH receptor is unknown. Reports have demonstrated that TSH-binding sites are present in a number of gram-positive and gram-negative bacteria, and it is possible that infection may elicit the production of antibodies that react with the TSH receptor.[8] An infectious etiology for Graves' disease is further supported by scattered epidemiologic reports of disease clustering.[9] Graves' disease is seen in girls about

5 times more commonly than in boys, and the incidence steadily increases throughout childhood, peaking in the adolescent years. Congenital Graves' disease, resulting from the transplacental passage of maternal antibodies, occurs in about 1% of babies born to women with active Graves' disease. The onset may be delayed until 2 to 3 weeks after birth.

In most children, the onset of Graves' disease develops over several months. Initial symptoms include nervousness, emotional lability, and declining school performance. Later, weight loss becomes evident, as does sweating, palpitations, heat intolerance, and general malaise. A smooth, firm, nontender goiter is present in more than 95% of cases. A bruit may be heard on auscultation. Exophthalmos is unusual in children, but a conspicuous stare may be evident. Laboratory evaluation generally reveals elevated free T_4 and decreased TSH levels. In 10% to 20% of patients, only elevation of T_3 is found, a condition known as T_3 toxicosis. The diagnosis of Graves' disease is definitively established by the presence of TSH-receptor antibodies.

Although the basic pathogenesis of Graves' disease is understood, no generally successful methods are available to correct the immunologic defect. The treatment of Graves' disease is palliative and is designed to decrease the production and secretion of thyroid hormone. The natural course of untreated Graves' disease is unpredictable. In some patients, the thyrotoxicosis may be persistent but variable in severity; in others, it may be cyclic, with exacerbations of varying degree and duration.

Current treatment includes antithyroid medications, radioactive ^{131}I, and surgical resection.[10] In the United States, most pediatric endocrinologists initiate therapy with methimazole or propylthiouracil, which reduces thyroid hormone production by inhibiting follicle cell organification of iodide and the coupling of iodotyrosines. Propylthiouracil also inhibits peripheral conversion of T_4 to T_3 and may be the agent of choice if rapid alleviation of thyrotoxicosis is desired. Both agents may possess some immunosuppressive activity; this is suspected because usually a reduction in antithyroid antibodies is noted. In most cases, methimazole is preferred because of its increased potency, longer half-life, and associated improved compliance. The initial adolescent dose is 30 mg once daily, which is reduced if the patient is younger. When the patient becomes euthyroid, as determined by normal T_3 and T_4 levels, the daily dose of methimazole should be reduced to 10 mg. T_3 and T_4 levels must be monitored. The thyroid gland decreases in size in about one-half of patients. Thyroid enlargement with therapy signals either an intensification of the disease or hypothyroidism from overtreatment.

Side effects of methimazole include nausea, minor skin reactions, urticaria, arthralgias, arthritis, and fevers. The most serious reaction is an idiosyncratic agranulocytosis, occurring in fewer than 1% of patients. This may occur at any time during the course of treatment or even during a second course of the drug. The most common symptom of agranulocytosis is pharyngitis with fever, for which the patient should be warned to seek medical attention. In most cases, the granulocyte count increases 2 to 3 weeks after stopping the drug, but rare fatal opportunistic infections have been reported. Treatment with parenteral antibiotics during the recovery period has been recommended.

The goal when treating Graves' disease is to allow natural resolution of the underlying autoimmune process. In general, the disease remission rate is approximately 25% after 2 years of treatment, with a further 25% remission every 2 years.[11] The resolution rate is decreased if TSH-receptor antibodies persist during and after treatment. Whereas the addition of T_4 to methimazole has had variable results in reducing disease recurrence, the use of T_4 cannot be recommended in pediatric patients receiving antithyroid medications.

The thyroid gland must be ablated if resistance or severe reactions to the antithyroid medications occur. Both surgical resection and ablation with radioactive ^{131}I have complications. The advantages of ^{131}I therapy include its effectiveness, safety, ease of administration, and relatively low cost.[12] Even though the disease recurrence rate is low after radioiodine treatment, patients have a 50% to 80% incidence of long-term hypothyroidism.[13] Despite studies demonstrating no increased risk of cancer relative to the general population, concerns remain over the possibility of teratogenic or carcinogenic effects of ^{131}I in children and adolescents.[12,14]

Either a subtotal or total thyroidectomy is indicated for patients who refuse radioiodine treatment or for whom medical management fails, or for those children whose thyroid gland is so large that airway symptoms related to compression are present. An antithyroid medication should be administered to decrease T_3 and T_4 levels into the normal range before operation. Alternatively, β-blocking agents such as propranolol may be used to ameliorate the adrenergic symptoms of hyperthyroidism. In addition, Lugol's solution, 5 to 10 drops per day, should be administered for 4 to 7 days before thyroidectomy to reduce the vascularity of the gland.

The incidence of hypothyroidism after subtotal thyroidectomy is 12% to 54%, and the hypothyroidism may be subclinical in up to 45% of children.[12] When abnormal TSH levels are considered, the incidence of hyperthyroidism or hypothyroidism is even higher. The rate of recurrent hyperthyroidism is approximately 13%. It is likely that the relapse rate increases with time after operation, and in the adult population, 30% of patients exhibit recurrent hyperthyroidism 25 years after their subtotal thyroidectomy.[10]

Hypothyroidism

Hypothyroidism may result from a defect anywhere in the hypothalamic-pituitary-thyroid axis and is rarely treated surgically. Approximately 90% of pediatric hypothyroidism is congenital, detected by neonatal screening programs, and results from dysgenesis of the thyroid gland. Two-thirds of these babies have a rudimentary gland, and complete absence of thyroid tissue is noted in the rest of the patients. The rudimentary gland may be ectopic (e.g., the base of the tongue). Maternal thyroid hormone may prevent symptoms even in children with complete thyroid agenesis. Ectopic thyroid tissue may supply a sufficient amount of T_4 for years or may prove to be insufficient later in childhood.

These unusual conditions may come to attention with the evaluation of a sublingual or midline neck mass. Surgeons must be mindful of the possibility of ectopic thyroid tissue when evaluating children with such masses. To ensure that all the functioning thyroid tissue is not inadvertently resected, radionuclide thyroid scanning should be considered before removing any unusual neck mass.

Neoplastic Thyroid Conditions

Thyroid Nodules

Thyroid nodules are uncommon in children, but a relatively high likelihood of associated cancer exists. In children, the incidence of malignancy in thyroid nodules has been about 20%.[15-17] This cancer rate is lower than was reported in previous decades because fewer children have been exposed to neck irradiation. Appropriate and prompt evaluation and management are important because the neoplasm may be at an early curable stage. A summary of pathologic results of several large series of children who underwent operation for thyroid nodules is presented in Table 76-3. Other unlisted diagnostic possibilities for thyroid nodules include cystic hygroma, thyroglossal duct remnant, and germ cell tumor.

Girls have twice the incidence of thyroid nodules as do boys.[18] Most patients are initially seen with an asymptomatic mass in the low anterior neck. It is impossible to differentiate benign from malignant lesions on clinical grounds, but a careful neck examination should be performed, especially to determine whether enlarged

TABLE 76-3

DIAGNOSIS IN 251 PEDIATRIC PATIENTS TREATED FOR THYROID NODULES

No. malignant	42 (17%)
Histologic subtype	
Papillary	29
Follicular	6
Mixed	2
Anaplastic	2
Medullary	2
Lymphoma	1
No. benign	209 (83%)
Diagnosis	
Follicular adenoma	101
Thyroiditis	27
Thyroglossal cyst	5
Colloid nodule	59
Branchial cyst	12

Data from Desjardins JG, Khan AH, Montupet P, et al: Management of thyroid nodules in children: a 20-year experience. J Pediatr Surg 22: 736–739, 1987; Hung W, Anderson KD, Chandra RS, et al: Solitary thyroid nodules in 71 children and adolescents. J Pediatr Surg 27:1407–1409, 1992; and Yip FWK, Reeve TS, Poole AG, et al: Thyroid nodules in childhood and adolescence. Aust N Z J Surg 64:676–678, 1994.

cervical lymph nodes are present. Unsuspected thyrotoxicosis resulting from an autonomously functioning nodule depresses the serum TSH. Thyroid imaging studies are unreliable in distinguishing benign from malignant nodules, but if US reveals multiple nodules, the diagnosis of thyroiditis becomes more likely. Because malignant nodules may be either solid or cystic, US does not differentiate them. Malignant nodules may be either functioning or nonfunctioning on thyroid scintiscan. A therapeutic trial of exogenous thyroid hormone to induce nodule regression is not recommended for children.

The usefulness of FNA cytology in children has not been well defined. Pediatric surgeons have historically recommended the removal of thyroid nodules, and few large studies have defined the natural history of cytologically benign nodules in children. In one study of 57 children with thyroid nodules evaluated with aspiration, the incidence of malignancy was 18%.[19] Approximately 80% of pediatric thyroid nodules are benign. If these could be accurately diagnosed without surgical removal, significant potential savings may occur in operative morbidity and cost.

In adolescent patients, FNA may be acceptable in evaluating thyroid nodules. The adolescent spectrum of thyroid disease is similar to that of adults. The incidence of malignancy in thyroid nodules in patients age 13 to 18 years was only 11% in one large series.[18] Benign nodules in adolescent patients can be followed up with serial physical examinations and US studies. Exogenous thyroid hormone to suppress benign thyroid nodules has not been shown to alter their natural history.

Surgical resection should be performed if the nodule is malignant or has indeterminate cytology, or if the size of a benign nodule increases. If a cystic thyroid lesion disappears after aspiration, surgical treatment may be deferred. If the lesion recurs, it should be removed. Even though cyst fluid may be sent for cytologic analysis, the sensitivity of this test for determining the presence of cancer in children is unknown.[20]

Thyroid nodules in prepubertal children have a higher risk of malignancy. The natural history of benign lesions in younger children is unknown, and the safety of nonoperative treatment has not been demonstrated. In children younger than 13 years, it is currently recommended that all thyroid nodules be removed. Preoperative US and thyroid scintigraphy aid in determining the anatomy.[16,21]

Thyroid Carcinoma

Thyroid carcinoma represents about 3% of all pediatric malignancies in the United States. The peak incidence is between ages 10 and 18 years, and girls outnumber boys 2:1. Approximately 10% of all malignant thyroid tumors occur in children. In comparison to adults, pediatric patients with thyroid carcinoma are first seen with disease at a more advanced stage with a higher incidence of lymph node and pulmonary metastases, but with lower mortality.[22]

The incidence of childhood thyroid malignancy has decreased in most parts of the world since the mid-1970s owing to the reduced use of radiation to treat benign diseases. A marked increase of thyroid tumors was noted in the Republics of Belarus and Ukraine after the 1986 Chernobyl nuclear power plant catastrophe.[23] The latency period for developing thyroid cancer after radiation exposure is about 4 to 6 years, and in the Belarus population, a 62-fold increase in thyroid tumor incidence was noted since the Chernobyl accident.

Treatment for a previous malignancy is another significant risk factor for thyroid carcinoma. Thyroid cancers constituted about 9% of second malignancies.[24] Hodgkin's lymphoma is the most common malignancy associated with the subsequent thyroid cancer. Whereas most thyroid second neoplasms follow previous radiation exposure to the neck, alkylating agents alone also predispose to thyroid cancer. The mean age at diagnosis of thyroid second neoplasms is 20 years, demonstrating the importance of careful surveillance for second tumors in children who have been successfully treated for cancer.

The diagnosis of thyroid carcinoma is impossible to determine based on clinical grounds alone. In adults, FNA cytology has been used as the initial evaluation of a thyroid nodule. The utility of FNA in children has not been thoroughly explored, as most surgeons recommend surgical resection of all thyroid lesions because of the concern of false-negative interpretations. However, FNA has decreased the number of unnecessary thyroid resections with observation of benign lesions.

Various molecular biologic events may account for the disparity in behavior of the different histologic subtypes of thyroid cancer. *RAS* proto-oncogene mutations are found in about 20% of papillary tumors and 80% of follicular tumors.[25] Other studies have reported that *RAS* is frequently activated in benign follicular adenomas, suggesting that this genetic event occurs early in the transformation process.[26] An activating mutation of the *RET* proto-oncogene is found in about 35% of papillary thyroid cancers.[27] The RET protein is a receptor tyrosine-kinase molecule, which probably functions within the cell to regulate proliferation or differentiation. The RET protein has been shown to be responsible for the development of medullary thyroid carcinoma. Specific point mutations are associated with the multiple endocrine neoplasia type 2 (MEN IIA, MEN IIB) syndromes and familial medullary thyroid carcinoma (FMTC). In addition, as many as 40% of sporadic nonfamilial medullary thyroid carcinomas possess *RET* mutations.[28]

Thyroid carcinoma generally is first seen clinically as a thyroid mass, sometimes with enlarged cervical lymph nodes. Regional lymph node metastases are present in three of four children when the disease is first detected (Table 76-4). The pathologic diagnosis can be established by using either FNA cytology or frozen-section biopsy at operation. Papillary carcinoma can usually be differentiated from benign conditions by either of these techniques. The functional status of the mass is determined by preoperative scintiscan. US may be helpful in planning the surgical procedure.[21] Because pulmonary metastases are frequent, a preoperative chest roentgenogram should be obtained.

No clinical trials have established whether total thyroidectomy, with lymph node dissection if the regional nodes are involved, is better than subtotal

TABLE 76-4

CLINICAL ASPECTS OF DIFFERENTIATED THYROID CANCER IN CHILDREN FROM SIX LARGE PEDIATRIC SERIES

Clinical Series	A	B	C	D	E	F
Total no. of patients	89	59	58	100	49	72
Mean age (yr)	12.8	NA	11.9	13.3	14.0	11
Girls (%)	81	66	69	71	69	71
Histology (no.)						
Papillary	83	37	58	87	44	50
Follicular	6	19	0	7	4	21
Medullary	0	1	0	0	1	0
Other	0	2	0	6	0	0
Metastasis (%)	88	50	90	71	73	75
Median follow-up (yr)	NA	11	28	20	7.7	13
Cancer mortality (%)	2.2	3.4	3.4	0	2.0	17

A, Harness JA, Thompson NW, McLeod MK, et al: Differentiated thyroid carcinoma in children and adolescents. World J Surg 16:547–554, 1992; B, Samuel AM, Sharma SM: Differentiated thyroid carcinomas in children and adolescents. Cancer 67:2186–2190, 1991; C, Zimmerman D, Hay ID, Gough IR, et al: Papillary thyroid carcinoma in children and adults: Long-term follow-up of 1039 patients conservatively treated at one institution during three decades. Surgery 104:1157–1163, 1988; D, La Quaglia MP, Corbally MT, Heller G, et al: Recurrence and morbidity in differentiated thyroid carcinoma in children. Surgery 104:1149–1156, 1988; E, Ceccarelli C, Pacini F, Lippi F, et al: Thyroid cancer in children and adolescents. Surgery 104:1143–1148, 1988; F, Schlumberger M, De Vathaire F, Travagli JP, et al: Differentiated thyroid carcinoma in childhood: long-term follow-up in 72 patients. J Clin Endocrinol Metab 65:1088–1094, 1987; NA, data not available.

thyroidectomy.[29–31] Radioiodine ablative therapy is more effective after removal of the entire gland because less functioning endocrine tissue takes up the radionuclide. Surgeons preferring a lesser resection hold that differentiated thyroid carcinoma in children is an indolent disease and that survival is not clearly related to the extent of gland removal.[32,33] The incidence of recurrent laryngeal nerve injury is none to 24%, and the reported frequency of permanent hypocalcemia is 6% to 27% in those patients having total thyroidectomy, although these complications occur less commonly in recent reports.[32,34]

Multivariate analysis revealed that younger age at diagnosis and the histologic type of tumor were the only factors predictive of early disease recurrence in one retrospective review.[32] Children older than 12 years at diagnosis and with follicular histology were more likely to be cured at the initial procedure. Thus tumor factors may be more important than treatment factors in determining the outcome. Major surgical complications occurred more frequently in younger children who had extensive resection of the gland.

Lobectomy with isthmus resection may be sufficient for tumors clearly isolated to one lobe, but thyroid cancer is bilateral in as many as 66% of cases, and about 80% of tumors exhibit multifocality. Therefore most pediatric surgeons believe that more aggressive thyroid gland resections are indicated and recommend that either a total or near-total thyroidectomy be performed for the management of differentiated thyroid cancer.[35,36]

The recurrent laryngeal nerve should be identified and protected. When tumor invades the recurrent laryngeal nerve, the nerve can be safely preserved without compromising survival; subsequently ^{131}I radiotherapy may successfully eradicate residual tumor.[37] Probably the most reliable way to preserve parathyroid gland function is to identify and autotransplant one or two of the glands into the sternocleidomastoid muscle or into the nondominant forearm.[38,39] If regional nodes are suggestive of metastasis, a node dissection is recommended. In patients with locally advanced disease, it is especially important to remove as much of the thyroid gland as possible, to allow subsequent radioiodine scanning and treatment if the tumor recurs. Finally, after surgical resection, most investigators recommend that all patients with endocrine thyroid cancer be treated with exogenous thyroid hormone to suppress TSH-mediated stimulation of the gland.

The incidence of pulmonary metastasis at diagnosis of thyroid cancer in childhood is about 6%, but it almost never occurs in the absence of significant cervical lymph node metastasis.[33,40] Pulmonary metastases require treatment with radioiodine. Plain chest roentgenograms may demonstrate the pulmonary disease in only about 60% of cases, so scanning with radioiodine is necessary. Pulmonary scintiscan may be falsely negative if significant residual thyroid gland remains in the neck.[40]

Overall survival rate in nonmedullary thyroid carcinoma is 98%.[22] A higher rate of recurrence is seen in children who did not receive initial postoperative ^{131}I than in those who did. The time to first recurrence has ranged from 8 months to 14.8 years (mean, 5.3 years), thereby emphasizing the importance of long-term follow-up for these children. Prognostic factors associated with recurrence include capsular invasion, soft tissue invasion, positive margins, and tumor location at diagnosis (thyroid, lymph nodes, lung).[22] An ^{131}I whole-body scan should be performed approximately 6 weeks after the initial thyroid resection, followed by therapeutic doses of the radionuclide administered as necessary to ablate residual tissue and treat residual metastatic disease.[29] Radioablation has been shown to decrease risk of local recurrence, increase the sensitivity of subsequent diagnostic whole-body scans, and improve the utility of serum thyroglobin as a marker for recurrent or residual disease during long-term follow-up.[35]

Thyroglobulin has been shown to be a useful marker of residual or metastatic thyroid cancer; the plasma level of this protein should be measured yearly, and an elevated value should raise the suspicion of recurrent disease.[41] It should be noted that the diagnostic accuracy of this test is significantly decreased in children who have residual thyroid tissue and in those who are taking thyroid hormone supplementation.

Medullary thyroid carcinoma (MTC) accounts for approximately 5% of thyroid neoplasms in children. Arising from the parafollicular C cells, MTC may occur either sporadically or in association with MEN IIA or MEN IIB, or the FMTC syndrome. MTC is usually the first tumor to develop in MEN patients and is the most common cause of death in this group. The neoplasm is particularly virulent in patients with MEN IIB and may occur in infancy.[42]

As with other pediatric thyroid neoplasms, the clinical diagnosis of MTC is usually made only after metastatic spread of the tumor has occurred to the adjacent cervical lymph nodes or to distant sites.[43] Surgical resection is the only effective treatment for MTC, underscoring the importance of early diagnosis and therapy before metastasis occurs. For this reason, current management of MTC in children from MEN II and FMTC kindreds relies on the presymptomatic detection of the *RET* proto-oncogene mutation responsible for the disease. Affected children with MEN IIA should undergo total thyroidectomy at approximately age 5 years, before the cancer spreads beyond the thyroid gland.[44-46] Indeed, approximately 80% of children who have thyroidectomy based on the presence of the *RET* mutation already have foci of MTC within the thyroid gland.[46] Owing to the increased virulence of the MTC in children with MEN IIB, prophylactic thyroidectomy should be performed at approximately age 1 year. Because of the high incidence of bilateral disease, complete removal of the thyroid gland is the recommended surgical management of MTC in children.[47] In addition, the lymph nodes in the central compartment of the neck, medial to the carotid sheaths and between the hyoid bone and the sternum, should be removed. Early detection by DNA mutation analysis and early operative intervention result in a normal life expectancy in these children.[48]

PARATHYROID GLANDS

Embryology and Physiology

Parathyroid gland development begins about week 5 of gestation, when the epithelium in the dorsal portions of the third and fourth pharyngeal pouches begins to proliferate, forming small nodules on the dorsal aspect of each pouch. During week 6 of development, the parathyroid glands associated with the third pair of pharyngeal pouches migrate caudally with the thymic primordium, finally coming to rest on the dorsal surface of the thyroid gland low in the neck. The parathyroid glands arising from the fourth pharyngeal pouches also descend in the neck, ultimately resting superior to the other glands. Mobilization of calcium from the bones is directly stimulated by parathormone (PTH), a process that also requires vitamin D.

Hyperparathyroidism

PTH is secreted as an 84-amino acid protein, which is rapidly cleaved in the liver and kidney into the carboxyl-terminal, amino-terminal, and midregion fragments. The biologic activity of PTH resides in the amino-terminal segment, but the plasma level of this moiety is low, owing to its very short half-life in the circulation. The C-terminal fragment levels are 50- to 500-fold those of the N-terminal fragment, and most clinical assays of PTH measure C-terminal levels of the hormone. These assays are usually effective for the evaluation of hyperparathyroidism, but plasma levels of the C-terminal fragment may be selectively elevated if a component of renal failure exists. The laboratory hallmark of hyperparathyroidism is the finding of an inappropriately elevated plasma PTH level with hypercalcemia.

The differential diagnosis of hypercalcemia in childhood is presented in Table 76-5. Unlike hypercalcemia in adults, hypercalcemia in children is rarely related to a neoplasm. However, in rare cases, pediatric tumors may secrete a parathyroid-related polypeptide that elevates the calcium level. Neoplasms in which this has been reported include malignant rhabdoid tumor, mesoblastic nephroma, rhabdomyosarcoma, neuroblastoma, and lymphoma. In these patients, the PTH level is generally normal or decreased.

Primary Hyperparathyroidism

Primary hyperparathyroidism in childhood usually results from a solitary hyperfunctioning adenoma and more rarely from diffuse hyperplasia of all four glands.[49] Hyperparathyroidism resulting from hyperplasia in all four glands is a feature of MEN-I. Hyperparathyroidism develops in approximately 30% of patients having MEN IIA in their second or third decade of life.[50] At the time of prophylactic thyroidectomy for MEN II, the parathyroid glands can be identified and autotransplanted into the nondominant forearm.[38] If hyperparathyroidism develops, a portion of the heterotopic tissue may easily be removed from the forearm.

Surgical options for parathyroid gland hyperplasia involving all of the glands include either 3½ gland parathyroidectomy or total parathyroidectomy with heterotopic autotransplantation of some parathyroid tissue back into the nondominant forearm.[51] The latter approach has the advantage of avoiding repeated neck exploration if hyperparathyroidism should recur, and it has been shown to be safe in infants and children.[38,46] Moreover, total parathyroidectomy with heterotopic autotransplantation results in improved survival rate in infants with severe hypercalcemia.[51] Patients with total

---

TABLE 76-5

DIFFERENTIAL DIAGNOSIS OF HYPERCALCEMIA IN CHILDOOD

Elevated parathyroid hormone level
   Primary hyperparathyroidism
   Secondary hyperparathyroidism
   Tertiary hyperparathyroidism
   Ectopic parathyroid hormone production
Hypervitaminosis D
Sarcoidosis
Subcutaneous fat necrosis
Familial hypocalciuric hypercalcemia
Idiopathic hypercalcemia of infancy
Thyrotoxicosis
Hypervitaminosis A
Hypophosphatasia
Prolonged immobilization
Thiazide diuretics

---

parathyroidectomy and autotransplantation require a short period of vitamin D and calcium supplementation until the heterotopic tissue begins to function.[38]

Primary hyperparathyroidism of infancy is a rare, often fatal, condition that usually develops within the first 3 months of life.[51,52] Signs include hypotonicity, respiratory distress, failure to thrive, lethargy, and polyuria. The serum PTH is elevated. Pathologically, usually diffuse parathyroid gland hyperplasia occurs. In about half of reported cases, a familial component to the disease is found. Early recognition and treatment are essential to allow normal growth and development of the baby.

The management of primary hyperparathyroidism in children is surgical. All four of the parathyroid glands should be identified and biopsies performed. An enlarged and adenomatous gland should be removed. If the other glands are normal, they should be marked with nonabsorbable sutures and left in place.

Familial Hypocalciuric Hypercalcemia

Familial hypocalciuric hypercalcemia differs from primary hypoparathyroidism in that PTH is normal, but urinary excretion of calcium is low. Patients are usually asymptomatic with an elevated serum calcium level. Serum magnesium also may be elevated.

The disease is inherited as an autosomal dominant disorder caused by a heterozygous mutation in the Ca^{2+}-sensing receptor gene.[53] The parathyroid glands are normal, and usually no benefit to parathyroidectomy is seen. If both parents are carriers, the neonate may have severe hypercalcemia. These infants have inherited mutations in both copies of the Ca^{2+}-sensing receptor gene and often have hyperplasia of all of their parathyroid glands, in which case, they benefit from parathyroidectomy with transplantation of one gland.

Secondary Hypoparathyroidism

Secondary hypoparathyroidism occurs in children with renal insufficiency or malabsorption. PTH production is increased in response to decreased calcium levels. Affected patients typically respond to medical treatment designed to decrease intestinal phosphorus absorption, but in rare cases, severe renal osteodystrophy develops, manifested by skeletal fractures and metastatic calcifications. Especially severe cases of secondary hyperparathyroidism may be candidates for total parathyroidectomy with autotransplantation.[49]

Tertiary Hyperparathyroidism

Tertiary hyperparathyroidism occurs when persistent hyperfunction of the parathyroid glands occurs, even after the inciting stimulus has been removed. This is often seen in patients with chronic renal failure and secondary hyperparathyroidism who undergo renal transplantation. Tertiary hyperparathyroidism is commonly due to hyperplasia of all four glands, and children with this condition are candidates for total parathyroidectomy with autotransplantation.

ADRENAL GLANDS

Anatomy and Embryology

The primordial adrenal cortex arises from the coelomic mesoderm and becomes visible between weeks 4 and 6 of development. During development, the fetal adrenal gland contains the permanent cortex, fetal cortex, and medulla. The fetal cortex, whose function is unknown, is responsible for the large size of the fetal adrenal gland, with the fetal adrenal gland being 4 times the size of the fetal kidney at the fourth month of gestation. The fetal cortex begins to decrease in size within a few hours of birth and has disappeared by the first year of life. The cells of the permanent cortex arrange into three separate zones, the zona glomerulosa, zona fasciculate, and zona reticularis. The zona glomerulosa gives rise to the narrowed zona fasciculata and reticularis of the adult cortex. The zona reticularis does not reach adult form until late childhood.[54]

The adrenal glands weigh 1 g at birth and grow to 4 to 5 g by late childhood. The mature adrenal gland measures 3 to 5 cm in length and 4 to 6 mm in thickness. The adrenal glands have a profuse arterial supply from the aorta, providing one or more middle adrenal arteries; the inferior phrenic artery, providing six to eight superior adrenal arteries; and the renal artery, supplying one or more inferior adrenal arteries. The adrenal gland is drained by a single large adrenal vein. The right side drains into the inferior vena cava, and the left drains into the left renal vein.

The adrenal gland can demonstrate several anomalous locations. In adrenal heterotopia, the adrenal gland is situated in the normal location, but lies under the capsule of the kidney (adrenal-renal heterotopia) or capsule of the liver (adrenal-hepatic heterotopia). Extra-adrenal tissue may be found any where in the abdominal cavity, but usually is found along the anatomic derivatives of the urogenital ridge for the adrenal cortex and along the dorsal root ganglia for the medullary tissue. Accessory adrenal glands usually occur without a medullary subcomponent and are seen in 16% of 100 consecutive autopsies; another 16% had complete accessory glands.[55]

Physiology

The adrenal cortex produces three major hormones: aldosterone, cortisol, and androgens. The zona glomerulosa is exclusively responsible for the production of aldosterone because it lacks the enzyme, 17α-hydroxylase, that is necessary to produce the precursors to cortisol and androgens. The zona fasciculata and zona reticularis together produce cortisol, androgens, and small amounts of estrogens; moreover, these areas lack the enzymes necessary to produce the precursors to aldosterone.

Aldosterone

Aldosterone regulates extracellular fluid volume and sodium and potassium balance. Aldosterone concentrations are regulated by the renin-angiotensin system. Renin is secreted by the juxtaglomerular cells in response to decreased pressure in the renal afferent arterioles and by decreased plasma concentration that is detected by the macular densa. Renin converts angiotensinogen into angiotensin I, which is in turn converted to angiotensin II by the converting enzyme of the lung. Angiotensin II is a potent vasoconstrictor and also directly stimulates the zona glomerulosa to release aldosterone. Aldosterone stimulates renal tubular reabsorption of sodium in exchange for potassium and hydrogen, thereby increasing renal fluid resorption and expanding intravascular volume.

Cortisol

The regulation of cortisol is controlled through the cortisol-releasing factor (CRF) release from the hypothalamus and subsequent stimulation of pituitary adrenocorticotropic hormone (ACTH). The neuroendocrine control of cortisol results in a peak in cortisol level in the early morning and the nadir in the late evening. The metabolic effects of cortisol include simulation of hepatic gluconeogeneis, inhibition of protein synthesis, increased protein catabolism, and lipolysis of adipose. Cortisol also causes a loss of collagen, inhibition of wound healing through decreased fibroblast activity, and induces a negative calcium balance, leading to osteoporosis.

Androgens

The adrenal androgens include dehydroepiandrosterone (DHEA) and DEA sulfate. These hormones undergo peripheral conversion to the biologically active forms, testosterone and dihydrotestosterone. In the normal male, adrenal androgens account for less than 5% of the circulating testosterone. The adrenal androgens become most clinically relevant with congenital adrenal hyperplasia, in which large amounts of precursors can be shuttled into this pathway.

Adrenal Masses

The differential diagnosis of adrenal masses is listed in Table 76-6. Neuroblastoma accounts for more than 90% of adrenal masses. Adrenal masses are being detected at a greater rate than previously described for children because of the increased use of diagnostic testing for other clinical conditions that are unrelated to adrenal disease. Increased use and improved technology have increased detection of adrenal tumors. The significance of such adrenal masses on computed tomography (CT) scan is unknown in children. At autopsy, adrenal masses are detected in less than 1% of patients younger than 30 years, and this increases to 7% in patients older than 70 years. Follow-up of patients with nonfunctioning adrenal masses demonstrates that 5% to 25% increase in size by at least 1 cm, and the risk of malignancy is 1 in 1000. Patients who have an incidentally discovered adrenal mass should undergo hormone evaluation, including a 1-mg dexamethasone suppression test, aldosterone levels, and measurement of plasma free metanephrines.[56] Surgical treatment is indicated for all functional adrenal cortical tumors and pheochromocytoma. In children,

DIFFERENTIAL DIAGNOSIS OF AN ADRENAL GLAND

Functional Tumors
Adrenal adenoma
Adrenocortical carcinoma
Pheochromocytoma

Nonfunctional Tumors
Neuroblastoma
Adrenal cyst
Hemangioma
Leiomyoma
Leiomyosarcoma
Non-Hodgkin's lymphoma
Malignant melanoma

Metastatic Disease to the Adrenal Gland
Squamous cell carcinoma of the lung
Hepatocellular carcinoma
Breast cancer

Traumatic Adrenal Hemorrhage
Neonatal child abuse

most surgeons will resect these tumors regardless of size; however, no clear evidence supports this management over conservative therapy, especially in lesions smaller than 3 cm.

Adrenal Cortex

Hypercortisolism, Cushing's Syndrome

Hypercortisolism, or Cushing's syndrome, describes any form of glucocorticoid excess that can be caused by pituitary adenoma secreting ACTH, adrenal tumors including carcinoma and adenoma, ectopic ACTH syndrome, nodular adrenal hyperplasia, and ACTH-producing tumors. Additionally, the administration of supraphysiologic quantities of ACTH or glucocorticoids can lead to iatrogenic Cushing's syndrome, the most common cause of hypercortisolism in adults and children. Cushing's disease is caused by a pituitary microadenoma or more rarely by a macroadenoma, and it is the second most common cause of Cushing's syndrome in pediatric patients. Ectopic ACTH syndrome is rare in children but has been reported in infants younger than 1 year. Tumors that can produce ACTH include pulmonary neoplasms, neuroblastomas, pancreatic islet cell carcinomas, thymomas, carcinoids, medullary thyroid carcinomas, and pheochromocytomas. In children, the most frequent cause of ectopic ACTH is bronchial carcinoid. ACTH levels are usually 10 to 100 times higher than those seen in Cushing's disease. These markedly elevated levels of ACTH lead to hypokalemic alkalosis. Additionally, ACTH-independent multinodular adrenal hyperplasia is characterized by hypersecretion of both cortisol and adrenal androgens.

Hypercortisolism is more common in children than previously recognized. In Harvey Cushing's original description,[57] the patient was a 23-year-old woman whose clinical features indicated long-standing disease.

In infants and children younger than 7 years, the most common cause of Cushing's disease is adrenal tumors. Among 60 infants younger than 1 year, 48 had adrenal tumors, with a 4:1 ratio between girls and boys.[58] In adults and children older than 7 years, adrenal hyperplasia secondary to hypersecretion of pituitary ACTH predominates.

Clinical features of Cushing's disease can take 5 years or longer to develop; thus the classic cushingoid appearance will not usually manifest in children. The most frequent and reliable findings in children with Cushing's disease is weight gain and growth failure.[59] Indeed, any obese child who stops growing should be evaluated for Cushing's disease.

The initial phase in the diagnosis of Cushing's syndrome is to screen for the syndrome; the second phase is to determine its etiology. Screening for Cushing's syndrome can be accomplished by measuring the plasma cortisol at 8:00 AM (normal levels, <14 µg/dL) and 6:00 PM (normal levels, <8 µg/dL) to coincide with the diurnal variation in plasma cortisol. The loss of diurnal rhythm is usually the earliest reliable laboratory index of Cushing's disease. A single measurement at midnight should be less than 2 µg/dL in normal patients, and more than 2 µg/dL in Cushing's disease.[60] The most sensitive screening test is the 24-hour urinary 17-hydroxycorticosteroid or free cortisol, which is more than 150 µg/day in patients with Cushing's syndrome. The overnight dexamethasone suppression test is performed by administering 1 mg at 11:00 PM and measuring the plasma cortisol level the following morning at 8:00 AM. In normal individuals, ACTH is suppressed, and the cortisol level is decreased by 50% or more of baseline (<5 µg/dL). This dose of dexamethasone is insufficient to cause suppression in patients with Cushing's syndrome.

Once it is established, further tests are used to determine the specific cause. The high-dose dexamethasone suppression test is used to distinguish pituitary causes from nonpituitary causes. An oral dose of 2 mg of dexamethasone is given every 6 hours for 48 hours (or 40 µg/kg/dose for infants). Urine is then collected for 24 hours to measure free cortisol and 17-hydroxysteroids. In patients with a pituitary neoplasm, the steroid excretion levels are suppressed to 50% of baseline. In patients with an adrenal adenoma or adrenocortical carcinoma and most patients with tumors that produce ACTH, the levels are not suppressed. Plasma ACTH levels are generally low or normal with adrenal causes of hypercortisolism, modestly elevated with pituitary neoplasms, and extremely elevated with tumors producing ectopic ACTH.

Among children, 80% to 85% of those with Cushing's disease have a surgically identifiable microadenoma.[61] Trans-sphenoidal hypophysectomy offers the best chance for cure; 20% of patients relapse after complete resection and manifest Cushing's disease within 5 years. Alternate therapies include pituitary irradiation, adrenalectomy, and drugs that inhibit adrenal function. Of these alternate therapies, adrenalectomy is the preferred treatment when two trans-sphenoidal procedures fail. Mitotane, an adrenolytic agent that causes a chemical adrenalectomy, has severe side effects including nausea, anorexia, and vomiting.

TABLE 76-7

ETIOLOGY OF CUSHING'S SYNDROME: EXOGENOUS CORTICOSTEROID ADMINISTRATION

ACTH-Dependent Causes
Cushing's disease (pituitary adenoma)
Ectopic ACTH production
Small cell bronchogenic carcinoma
Carcinoid tumors
Pancreatic islet cell carcinoma
Thymoma
Medullary thyroid carcinoma
Pheochromocytoma

ACTH-Independent Causes
Adrenal adenoma
Adrenocortical carcinoma
Adrenal hyperplasia

ACTH, adrenocorticotropic hormone.

Primary Hyperaldosteronism

Primary hyperaldosteronism is defined as excess production of aldosterone from the adrenal glands with consequent suppression of renin. Most commonly, this is caused by either adrenocortical hyperplasia or adrenal adenoma. Adrenal adenoma, or Conn's syndrome, is the most common cause in adults, whereas adrenocortical hyperplasia is the most common cause in children.[62] Rarely, adrenal carcinoma can appear as primary hyperaldosteronism.

Symptoms are nonspecific for primary hyperaldosteronism. Patients have hypertension, muscle weakness, polydipsia, and polyuria. Hyperaldosteronism increases the total body sodium level and consequently increases the total body fluid volume; it is characterized by hypertension and hypokalemic alkalosis. The elevated aldosterone levels suppress renin and angiotensin.

The diagnosis should be entertained in any child with hypertension and hypokalemia. Initial screening in children with hypertension involves checking a potassium level. Hypokalemia (<3.5 mEq/L) is consistent with primary hyperaldosteronism. The aldosterone level is elevated, the renin level is suppressed, and patients frequently also have a metabolic alkalosis. The diagnosis is confirmed by administering a saline load challenge; hypokalemia develops in patients with primary hyperaldosteronism, and they have high urinary potassium (>40 to 60 mEq/day) and aldosterone excretion. A high-sodium diet can be administered for 3 to 5 days, which fails to suppress aldosterone in patients with hyperaldosteronism. The serum aldosterone level must be determined in the morning before the patient has assumed an upright position.

Once established, it is important to distinguish between an aldosterone-secreting adenoma and bilateral adrenal hyperplasia. Aldosterone-secreting tumors generally produce much higher levels of aldosterone (>100 µg/dL) than are produced by adrenal hyperplasia. NP-59, or [^{131}I]6-β-iodomethyl-19-norcholesterol, is a cholesterol analogue that is taken up as cholesterol in the steroidogenic pathway. Dexamethasone suppression of ACTH-dependent adrenocortical tissue is followed by NP-59 administration. An adenoma is suggested if asymmetrical adrenal uptake occurs after 48 hours, whereas bilateral hyperplasia is suggested if the uptake is symmetrical after 72 hours.

The treatment of a functional adrenal adenoma is excision. The mortality rate from operative removal is generally less than 1%, with a cure rate of 75%. Treatment for patients with bilateral adrenal hyperplasia is with spironolactone.

PRECOCIOUS PUBERTY

In boys, precocious puberty is defined as the development of secondary sexual characteristics before age 9 years. In girls, the development of breasts (thelarche) before age 7.5 years, the development of pubic hair (pubarche) before age 8.5 years, or the onset of menses (menarche) before age 9.5 years is considered precocious. Precocious puberty can be complete or incomplete.

True or complete precocious puberty is due to the premature maturation of the hypothalamic-pituitary axis and results in gonadal enlargement as well as premature development of secondary sexual characteristics. The secondary sexual characteristics that develop in true precocious puberty are appropriate for the sex of the child and merely occur at a younger-than-appropriate age. In incomplete or pseudoprecocious puberty, only one secondary sexual characteristic develops prematurely, and it may or may not be appropriate for the patient's gender. Pseudoprecocious puberty is not due to pituitary gonadotropin secretion; rather, it is due to production of human chorionic gonadotropin (hCG), luteinizing hormone (LH), follicle-stimulating hormone (FSH), androgens, or estrogens, or it is due to stimulation of their receptors by the tumors.

Precocious Puberty in Girls

True precocious puberty, resulting from a premature activation of the hypothalamic-pituitary axis, is idiopathic in 75% to 95% of girls. The condition may be constitutional, that is, a normal variant that is simply at the younger age of a normal distribution curve. Neurogenic disturbances can cause true precocious puberty by interfering with inhibitory signals from the central nervous system (CNS) to the hypothalamus or by producing excitatory signals. Neurogenic disorders may include hydrocephalus, cerebral palsy, trauma, irradiation, chronic inflammatory disorder, or tumors, including hypothalamic hamartomas or pineal tumors.

McCune-Albright syndrome is an interesting disorder that can cause either true precocious puberty or pseudoprecocious puberty. Patients have a classic triad of precocious puberty, cafe-au-lait nevi with irregular "coast of Maine" borders, and polyostotic fibrous dysplasia. In these patients, autonomously functioning ovarian follicular cysts may develop, causing precocious puberty (see Chapter 74). Excess production of LH, FSH, or prolactin by pituitary adenomas also has been described. Other endocrine abnormalities, including acromegaly, Cushing's syndrome, and hyperthyroidism have been associated with this syndrome.[63]

Incomplete precocious puberty generally is first seen as isolated premature breast development (thelarche) or premature growth of pubic hair (pubarche). Premature pubarche is frequently caused by androgen excess. Isolated prepubertal menses is rare, and prepubertal vaginal bleeding is usually caused by a foreign body, sexual abuse, or tumors of the genital tract. Incomplete precocious puberty can be a normal variant or can be due to the production of hormones from neuroendocrine, adrenal, ovarian, or exogenous sources. In the Van Wyk-Grumbach syndrome, premature breast development is associated with hypothyroidism. Unlike most other causes of precocious puberty, growth is inhibited rather than stimulated. This syndrome may be due to the shared α-subunit of LH, FSH, and TSH. Tumors that produce excess quantities of LH or hCG can cause virilization.

Precocious Puberty in Boys

As with girls, true precocious puberty in boys may be neurogenic, constitutional, or idiopathic. However, in boys, true precocious puberty is more often neurogenic than idiopathic.

The most common CNS tumor that causes precocious puberty is a hamartoma of the tuber cinereum. These hamartomas are ectopic hypothalamic tissue connected to the posterior hypothalamus. Because they are nonprogressive tumors and are in a surgically precarious location, they are generally treated with gonadotropin-releasing hormone (GnRH) agonists. Other disorders that can cause precocious puberty in boys are gliomas of the optic nerve or hypothalamus, astrocytomas, choriocarcinomas, meningiomas, rhabdomyosarcomas, neurofibrosarcomas, nonlymphocytic leukemia, ependymomas, neurofibromatosis type I, and germinomas. Other space-occupying lesions or causes of increased intracranial pressure such as head trauma, suprasellar cysts, granulomas, brain irradiation, and hydrocephalus also can cause true precocious puberty. Some of these tumors or CNS conditions can cause both precocious puberty and growth hormone deficiency. In these patients, the growth rate may appear normal because the testosterone stimulates growth and compensates for the deficiency of growth hormone. However, the degree of growth is inadequate for the degree of pubertal development.

Incomplete precocious puberty can be caused by autonomous production of androgens or hCG. With many types of incomplete precocious puberty, the testes are not enlarged as they are with true precocious puberty. As with girls, the McCune-Albright syndrome can cause either true or pseudoprecocious puberty. Tumors producing hCG such as teratomas, chorioepitheliomas, hepatomas, hepatoblastomas, or germinomas of the pineal gland may lead to Leydig cell stimulation. Testotoxicosis is an autosomal recessive disorder in which premature Leydig cell maturation causes incomplete precocious puberty. The etiology in some families is due to the constitutive stimulation of the LH receptor and can cause the onset of precocious puberty at age 1 to 4 years. Ketoconazole, spironolactone, and testolactone can be used to treat this disorder.

Excess androgen production causing virilization can be caused by congenital adrenal hyperplasia, specifically the 21-hydroxylase or the 11-hydroxylase enzymatic defects. During embryonic development, adrenal rests may be left in the testes. In untreated adrenal hyperplasia, ACTH stimulation may cause their enlargement and the secretion of androgens. These testes have an irregular appearance. Excess testosterone production also can be caused by interstitial cell tumors of the testes. Finally, exogenous administration of androgens or hCG (for undescended testes) can cause precocious puberty.

Evaluation

For both boys and girls, evaluation of precocious puberty begins with a thorough history and physical examination. The Tanner stage should be carefully documented. In boys, the size and shape of the testes should be noted. In true precocious puberty, the testes generally enlarge symmetrically, whereas asymmetrical or nodular enlargement is noted with Leydig cell tumors or adrenal rests. Feminization in boys may appear as gynecomastia. The patient's height and weight should be measured, and the growth curve should be examined. The bone age also should be determined. If the bone age and the height age closely correlate, it is likely that the presenting symptom is an extreme variant of normal. This simply requires close follow-up in 6 months to verify the diagnosis. However, if the bone age is abnormally accelerated relative to the height age, further investigation is warranted.

Serum estradiol, testosterone, and DHEA levels should be obtained. In girls, a vaginal smear for estrogen effect may be more sensitive than a serum estradiol level. Significantly elevated DHEA levels are typically seen in adrenal tumors. Evidence of association with other syndromes may warrant measuring other hormone levels including prolactin, thyroid hormone, or cortisol. A GnRH test can be useful in determining whether the patient has complete or incomplete precocious puberty. Patients with true precocious puberty respond to GnRH with a typical pubertal pattern, whereas those with pseudoprecocious puberty have a minimal response to gonadotropin. Alternatively, a sleep-related increase in plasma LH levels can be diagnostic but is more cumbersome to obtain. In patients with feminizing or masculinizing features, US is useful to locate abdominal or pelvic masses. Magnetic resonance imaging (MRI) should be used in patients with true precocious puberty to locate potential intracranial lesions.

Treatment

In general, tumors causing precocious puberty should be removed if they are surgically accessible. A number of agents have been used in the medical treatment of precocious puberty. True (gonadotropin-dependent) precocious puberty can be treated with GnRH agonists.

Although initially these agents stimulate gonadotropin secretion, ultimately, GnRH receptors are downregulated, and LH and FSH secretion is subsequently decreased. Examples of GnRH agonists include deslorelin, buserelin, nafarelin, leuprolide, and triptorelin.

Other medications have been used in the medical treatment of incomplete precocious puberty. Medroxyprogesterone acetate, a progestational agent, can halt the progression of secondary sexual characteristic development and can prevent menstruation. It is not as effective, however, in slowing bone maturation. Ketoconazole is an antifungal agent that also inhibits the synthesis of testosterone by blocking the conversion of 17-hydroxyprogesterone to androstenedione. Testolactone competitively inhibits the aromatase enzyme that converts androgens to estrogens. Androgen antagonists include cyproterone acetate and spironolactone.

Adrenocortical Carcinoma

Adrenocortical carcinoma is a rare tumor with an annual incidence of 0.5 to 2 cases per million population. A bimodal incidence is found, with one peak occurring at younger than 5 years and the other peak in the fourth to fifth decades of life.[64] Pediatric adrenocortical tumors comprise only 0.2% of all childhood malignancies. Neuroblastomas, ganglion neuroblastomas, and pheochromocytomas account for the majority of pediatric adrenal gland tumors.[65] Adrenocortical tumors have a female-to-male predominance of 2:1, occur equally on the left and right, and are hormonally functional in 80% to 100% of patients.[66]

The etiology of adrenocortical carcinoma is unclear. Several lines of evidence suggest that cancer may arise from preexisting pathology, including congenital adrenal hyperplasia and adenoma; however, recent evidence has demonstrated that adrenocortical carcinoma may arise de novo. Multiple studies have shown that adrenal carcinomas arise from a single progenitor cell, which is in contrast to adrenal adenomas that are found to be nonmonoclonal in up to 38% of patients.[67] A number of genes have been investigated as candidate causative factors for adrenocortical carcinoma. Insulin-like growth factor (IGF)II encodes an adrenal growth factor that is overexpressed in 84% of adrenocortical carcinomas and in only 6% of adenomas.[68] The tumor-suppressor gene *p53* is associated with adrenocortical carcinomas in up to 29% of carcinomas. An inherited germline *p53* mutation, known as Li-Fraumeni syndrome, results in multiple primary tumors including adrenocortical carcinoma, sarcoma, leukemia, lung and laryngeal cancer, and breast and brain tumors.[69] Additionally, the *DAX-1* gene encodes a hormone receptor that is essential for normal fetal development of the adrenal cortex. *DAX-1* levels are found to be high in nonfunctional adenomas and low in adenocarcinomas and hormone-producing adenomas.[70] Other syndromes associated with adrenocortical tumor formation include Beckwith-Wiedemann, Carney's complex, MEN I, and congenital adrenal hyperplasia.

The clinical presentation in children is usually associated with steroid overproduction. In contrast to adult tumors, most adrenocortical tumors are hormonally active.

Virilization is the most frequent presenting feature (66%) with adrenocortical tumors, whereas the remainder of children will usually first be seen with Cushing's symptoms.[71] Virilization is secondary to secretion of the adrenal androgens, and features include axillary and pubic hair, deepening of the voice, acne, a rapid acceleration of height, hirsutism, enlargement of penis or clitoromegaly, and development of body odor. Feminization may occur as an overproduction of estrogens, particularly estradiol, in 2% to 25% of patients.[72] Nonfunctional tumors in children are infrequent. Only about 5% of pediatric adrenocortical tumors produce no clinical evidence of hormone excess. Accordingly, these patients usually are first seen late in disease with abdominal pain or fullness.

With most tumors occurring with virilization symptoms, evaluation of the adrenocortical carcinoma should be directed toward detection of elevated androgens. Screening should include measurement of plasma testosterone, urinary and plasma DHEA and DHEA-S, and urinary 17-ketosteroids. Usually, two-thirds of 17-ketosteroids are derived from adrenal androgens. Whereas the most specific assessment of adrenal androgen production is DHEA-S, 17-ketosteroids are more frequently elevated in malignant disease.[73] The clinical presentation of Cushing's syndrome is confirmed by hypercortisolism and the loss of diurnal variation. Cortisol excess is determined by elevated plasma cortisol, urinary 17-hydroxycorticosteroids, and urinary free cortisol. Adrenal malignant disease generally causes markedly greater elevations of 17-hydroxycorticosteroids and plasma cortisol than that with functional adenomas.

Radiographic evaluation should proceed concurrent with endocrine evaluation so that surgical intervention can proceed expeditiously. Plain abdominal radiographs reveal a soft tissue mass in 47% of patients, and adrenal calcification can be noted in up to 30% of patients.[74] US, which can detect tumors as small as 3 cm, should be used for screening the adrenal region and for postoperative assessment of recurrence. Smaller lesions are smooth and homogeneous with no pattern of hyper- or hypoechogenicity, whereas larger lesions usually demonstrate a "scar sign," radiating linear echoes that represent an interphase between separate areas of necrosis, hemorrhage, and neoplasm.[75] CT can detect tumors as small as 0.5 cm; however, radiographic evaluation can determine malignancy only in the presence of regional invasion or distant metastases in the liver, lung, or brain. MRI has accuracy similar to that of CT with lesions larger than 1 to 2 cm.[76] MRI has the advantage of producing coronal sections that can identify 1-cm images not identified on CT scan.[77] Finally, adrenal scintigraphy using iodocholesterol-labeled analogues has shown promise in identifying and differentiating functional adrenal lesions.[78] Differentiation between hyperplasia, adenoma, and carcinoma is made possible by the inability of carcinoma to concentrate radionuclide as well as normal tissue. Bilateral symmetrical images indicate hyperplasia; unilateral uptake suggests adenoma; and nonvisualization is suggestive of carcinoma.[79] Positron emission tomography (PET) with 2-[fluorine 18]-fluoro-2-deoxy-D-glucose

(FDG) is helpful in differentiating benign from malignant disease.

Surgical resection offers the best chance for cure. If extensive disease is found during operation, wide en bloc resection of tumor, lymph nodes, and involved organs is indicated.[80] For less extensive disease, minimally invasive techniques for adrenalectomy have been advocated. With improving technology and smaller instruments, this technology will become an additional tool in the pediatric surgeon's armamentarium. Whereas adrenal resection has been shown to have efficacy similar to that of open adrenalectomy for localized masses, no pediatric laparoscopic adrenalectomies for adrenocortical carcinoma have been reported.

Adjuvant therapy has marginal results. Survival in patients with localized disease has been reported to be 5 years versus 2.3 years for patients that have tumor spread beyond the adrenal gland.[80] For patients who underwent further surgical procedures for recurrent disease, survival is extended 3.5 years. Pediatric series report the incidence of metastases at time of diagnosis as being between 5% and 64%.[66] Mitotane is an adrenolytic agent that selectively causes adrenal gland necrosis and has been the most widely used chemotherapeutic agent. It is used for metastatic disease, for incompletely excised tumors, and for the hormonal effects of the tumors. In adults, response rates of tumors to mitotane are reported to be between 10% and 60%,[66] with a mean duration of response of only 10.2 months.[81] In the pediatric literature, tumor responses have been reported to be 30% to 38%.[82,83] Additional regimens that have shown some promise include the combination of cis-platinum and VP-16 and taxol. The role of radiotherapy in children has not been well established. In adults, adrenocortical carcinoma is thought to be radioresistant. However, some response has been noted in small series of children with metastatic disease.[72] In one report, radiotherapy was used to shrink an "unresectable" tumor that was subsequently completely excised.[66]

Patients who are untreated for adrenocortical carcinomas have a mean survival of 2.9 months.[84] These tumors are highly lethal, with nonfunctional tumors demonstrating a graver prognosis. Delay in diagnosis leads to the worsened prognosis, with the range of time from symptoms to diagnosis 6 months to 36 months.[66] The prognosis depends on the child's age and the resectability of the tumor. In one review of 55 children with adrenocortical carcinoma, the 2-year survival rates were 82% for children younger than 2 years and 29% for children older than 2 years. Survival rates were more than 67% if the tumors were completely excised, but no survivors were found after partial resection.[85]

Adrenal Medulla

Pheochromocytoma

Pheochromocytomas arise from the neuroectodermal chromaffin cells and were first described by Fränkel in 1886.[86] During development, chromaffin cells migrate to adrenal medulla, and nests of these cells settle around the sympathetic ganglia, vagus nerve, paraganglia of the carotid arteries, the arch of the aorta, and the abdominal aorta. These nests are the etiology of the extra-adrenal tumors, which also are defined as paraganglioma. Most paragangliomas occur in the abdomen, with the most common site in the upper periaortic region from the diaphragm to the lower poles of the kidney. The second most common site is the organs of Zuckercandl at the origin of the inferior mesenteric artery.[87] Malignancy is more common with large tumors, in children and adolescents, and when an increased excretion of dopamine and its metabolite, homovanillic acid, is found.

Pheochromocytomas in children usually are first seen with signs and symptoms related to hypertension, including headache. Additional symptoms seen more frequently in children include sweating, visual complaints, nausea, vomiting, weight loss, polydipsia, and polyuria.[86] About 90% of children demonstrate sustained catecholamine elevation, and 10% are episodically elevated. Twenty percent of children with pheochromocytoma do not have hypertension.[88] Pheochromocytoma should be considered in any child with hypertension, as pheochromocytomas account for 0.5% of hypertensive children, and these children are initially seen at a mean age of 8 to 10 years.[89]

The workup of pheochromocytoma should include biochemical and anatomic localization studies. The biochemical diagnosis should be directed at determining levels of catecholamines and their metabolites. Measurements can include plasma epinephrine, norepinephrine, metanephrine, and normetanephrine; and urinary epinephrine, norepinephrine, dopamine, vanillylmandelic acid (VMA), and metanephrines. When obtained properly, plasma catecholamine and catecholamine metabolites are more specific and sensitive than urinary metabolites.[86,90] Patients with normal plasma catecholamine levels during a hypertensive episode are unlikely to have pheochromocytoma, whereas when levels greater than 2000 pg/mL are diagnostic. With levels between 500 and 1000 pg/mL, a glucagon stimulation test should be performed; however, this study can lead to a significant increase in catecholamine and a subsequent hypertensive crisis. Patients with catecholamine levels between 500 and 1000 pg/mL should have a clonidine suppression test.[91] Catecholamine levels will not suppress in patients with pheochromocytoma.

Once the biochemical evaluation is complete, the location of the tumor must be determined. Ninety-seven percent of pheochromocytomas will be found in the abdomen or pelvis. Although the adrenal gland is the most common location, multifocal sites may be found in up to 43% of children.[92] The potential imaging techniques include MRI, CT, and iodine 131 metaiodobenzylguanidine (MIBG) scanning. Although MIBG is the most specific imaging technique, MRI has the highest sensitivity. When pheochromocytoma is suspected biochemically and not found by imaging, an intrathoracic or intracranial tumor should be suspected.

The primary treatment for pheochromocytoma is surgical excision. The perioperative management of these patients is critical to successful surgical revision. Manipulation of the tumor intraoperatively can lead to sudden severe intraoperative hypertension.

Additionally, the sudden reduction in catecholamine levels can lead to profound hypotension. Preoperatively, the patient should receive α-adrenergic blockade with phenoxybenzamine, intravenously for 3 days, or orally for 1 to 3 weeks.[93] Additional selective α-adrenergic blocking agents include prazosin, doxazosin, and terazosin. Despite preoperative catecholamine blockade, most patients will still exhibit hypertension with manipulation of the tumor and an abrupt decrease in blood pressure after removal.[94] Some suggestion has been made that calcium channel blockers may provide fewer fluctuations in blood pressure and have a cardioprotective effect, decreasing the risk of coronary artery spasm and myocardial complications.[90] Current recommendations include initiating patients on calcium channel blockers for paroxysmal hypertension, and if they are unsuccessful in controlling blood pressure, the selective α-adrenergic antagonists (prazosin, doxazosin, or terazosin) should be started. Beta blockers should be reserved for patients with cardiac dysrhythmias. With these guidelines, 50% of patients are placed on calcium channel blockers, 20% on selective α-blockers, 20% on β-blockers, and some patients do not receive any antihypertensive medication.[87]

The hyperadrenergic state of patients with pheochromocytoma results in vascular contraction with a relatively low intravascular volume. When the tumor is removed and the adrenergic vasoconstriction ceases, profound hypotension can occur. This can be particularly significant for the patients with catecholamine-induced cardiomyopathy. An increased incidence of pulmonary edema is noted after tumor resection, and overly aggressive fluid resuscitation plays a significant role. Intraoperative fluid replacement should be restricted to no more than 10 mL/kg/hr above the measured loss.[94] To improve the fluid status preoperatively, the patient should be started on saline volume expansion 3 hours before operation. Hypoglycemia also should be monitored closely for the first 48 hours after surgical revision.

Traditionally, a transabdominal approach has been used to allow early ligation of the adrenal vein to minimize systemic catecholamine release during tumor manipulation. The transabdominal approach also allows exploration of the sympathetic chain. Additionally, the subcostal or posterior extraperitoneal approaches have been supported because of the faster recovery and decreased risk of transperitoneal surgical procedures. Laparoscopic adrenalectomy is another option in experienced hands. Tumors as large as 11 cm have been removed laparoscopically.

In children with MEN II and pheochromocytoma, bilateral tumors inevitably occur. Controversy exists over management of these patients. Bilateral adrenalectomy has been suggested by some, but these patients have significant morbidity secondary to steroid replacement, including osteoporosis, decreased libido, and an addisonian crisis if a lapse in compliance occurs.[92] Because of the risks of bilateral adrenalectomy, some have proposed bilateral adrenal-sparing operation for patients with bilateral tumors and patients who are at high risk for developing a metachronous contralateral lesion.[95]

For patients with metastatic disease, [131I]MIBG and chemotherapy should be considered. Current evidence supports high initial doses of [131I]MIBG for all metastatic lesions that have positive diagnostic MIBG scans. With tumors that respond symptomatically or hormonally to treatment, survival has been reported to be 4.7 years after treatment.[96] Chemotherapy seems also to have an additive effect with MIBG to increase survival of these patients.[97]

Approximately 10% of pheochromocytomas are familial and may be associated with other syndromes such as the von Hippel-Lindau syndrome, Recklinghausen's disease, tuberous sclerosis, Sturge-Weber syndrome, or MEN IIA or MEN IIB.[98] Familial pheochromocytomas independent of these syndromes also have been described.[99] In children, pheochromocytomas are more frequently associated with MEN II syndromes than those in adults; pheochromocytomas associated with the MEN II syndrome are more likely to be bilateral and benign.

CARCINOID TUMORS

Carcinoid tumors composed only 0.08% of tumors identified at a large pediatric cancer center.[100] These tumors arise from amine uptake and decarboxylation cells and are usually classified according to site of origin as foregut, midgut, or hindgut carcinoids.[101] Foregut tumors account for approximately 5% of carcinoid tumors and can arise in the bronchus, stomach, or duodenum. Midgut tumors account for about 80% to 85% of carcinoid tumors. The majority of carcinoids arise from the appendix (46%), followed by the jejunum and ileum (28%), and the rectum (17%). Carcinoid tumors also have been found to arise from ovarian teratomas.

Most patients are first seen with vague symptoms, with only 10% of patients having symptoms of carcinoid syndrome, including flushing, diarrhea, abdominal pain, asthma, and right-sided cardiac valvular problems.[102] Carcinoids are detected incidentally in up to 60% of patients, usually when associated with appendiceal carcinoids.

Most pediatric patients are first seen with appendiceal carcinoids smaller than 2 cm, which can be treated with simple appendectomy.[100] Right hemicolectomy is indicated for tumors larger than 2 cm, those close to the cecum, and those with mucin production. Metastases are extremely rare in children, but regular follow-ups with measurement of serotonin and chromogranin A should be performed.[103] Treatment of metastatic disease includes hepatic chemoembolization and surgical resection for isolated hepatic metastases and long-acting octneotide or [131I]MIBG for widely metastatic disease.[104]

Carcinoids are fairly indolent tumors. In one retrospective series of 40 children with appendiceal carcinoids, no recurrences or metastases were reported.[105] Site of origin has universally been shown to predict survival, with the appendix having the best survival, and midgut or hindgut having the worst.

Of significance, the most common pulmonary tumor is the bronchial carcinoid. Usually these tumors excrete low levels of serotonin. They most frequently appear with recurrent or persistent pneumonia secondary to obstruction of the bronchus by the tumor. Children commonly are seen with wheezing, atelectasis, and weight loss, in addition to the cough, pneumonitis, and hemoptysis that are frequently seen in adult patients.

Bronchial carcinoids can be diagnosed by bronchoscopy; they have a characteristic pink, friable, mulberry appearance. In general, biopsy should not be attempted because the carcinoids have a propensity to hemorrhage, and usually these tumors have a classic gross appearance. If no evidence of lymph node involvement is found, segmental bronchial resection can be performed. However, lobectomy or pneumonectomy is usually required for treatment. These tumors are radiosensitive, and radiotherapy can be considered for unresectable disease. The prognosis after complete resection is excellent, with a 10-year survival rate of approximately 90%.[106,107]

REFERENCES

1. Rallison ML, Dobyns BM, Meikle AW, et al: Natural history of thyroid abnormalities: Prevalence, incidence, and regression of thyroid diseases in adolescents and young adults. Am J Med 91:363–370,1991.
2. Epstein FH: The molecular basis of thyroid hormone action. N Engl J Med 331:847–853, 1994.
3. Ahren B: Regulatory peptides in the thyroid gland: A review on their localization and function. Acta Endocrinol 124(3):225–332, 1991.
4. Jaksic J, Dumic M, Filipovic B, et al: Thyroid disease in a school population with thyromegaly. Arch Dis Child 70:103–106, 1994.
5. Fisher DA, Pandian MR, Carlton E: Autoimmune thyroid disease: An expanding spectrum. Pediatr Clin North Am 34:907–918, 1987.
6. Dayan CM, Daniels GH: Chronic autoimmune thyroiditis. N Engl J Med 335:99–107, 1996.
7. Rother KI, Zimmerman D, Schwenk WF: Effect of thyroid hormone treatment on thyromegaly in children and adolescents with Hashimoto disease. J Pediatr 124:599–601, 1994.
8. Tomer Y, Davies TF: Infection, thyroid disease and autoimmunity. Endocr Rev 14:107–120, 1993.
9. Phillips DI, Barker DJ, Rees Smith B, et al: The geographical distribution of thyrotoxicosis in England according to the presence or absence of TSH-receptor antibodies. Clin Endocrinol 23:283–287, 1985.
10. Franklyn JA: The management of hyperthyroidism. N Engl J Med 330:1731–1738, 1994.
11. Lippe BM, Landaw EM, Kaplan SA: Hyperthyroidism in children treated with long-term medical therapy: Twenty-five percent remission every two years. J Clin Endocrinol Metab 64:1241–1245, 1987.
12. Waldhausen JHT: Controversies related to the medical and surgical management of hyperthyroidism in children. Semin Pediatr Surg 6:121–127, 1997.
13. Berglund J, Christiensen SB, Dymling JF, et al: The incidence of recurrence and hypothyroidism following treatment with antithyroid drugs, surgery, or radioiodine in all patients with thyrotoxicosis in Malmo during the period 1970-1974. J Intern Med 229:435–442, 1991.
14. Klein I, Becker DV, Levey GS: Treatment of hyperthyroid disease. Ann Intern Med 121:281–288, 1994.
15. Al-Shaikh A, Ngan B, Daneman A, Daneman D: Fine-needle aspiration biopsy in the management of thyroid nodules in children and adolescents. J Pediatr 138:140–142, 2001.
16. Hung W, Anderson KD, Chandra RS, et al: Solitary thyroid nodules in 71 children and adolescents. J Pediatr Surg 27:1407–1409, 1992.
17. Desjardins JG, Khan AH, Montupet P, et al: Management of thyroid nodules in children: A 20-year experience. J Pediatr Surg 22:736–739, 1987.
18. Yip FWK, Reeve TS, Poole AG, et al: Thyroid nodules in children and adolescence. Aust N Z J Surg 64:676–678, 1994.
19. Raab SS, Silverman JF, Elsheikh TM, et al: Pediatric thyroid nodules: Disease demographics and clinical management by fine needle aspiration biopsy. Pediatrics 95:46–49, 1995.
20. Mazzaferri EL: Management of a solitary thyroid nodule. N Engl J Med 328:553–559, 1993.
21. Newman KD: The current management of thyroid tumors in childhood. Semin Pediatr Surg 2:69–74, 1993.
22. Grigsby PW, Gal-or A, Michalski JM, Doherty GM: Childhood and adolescent thyroid carcinoma. Cancer 95:724–729, 2002.
23. Nikiforov Y, Gnepp DR: Pediatric thyroid cancer after the Chernobyl disaster: Pathomorphologic study of 84 cases (1991–1992) from the Republic of Belarus. Cancer 74:748–765, 1994.
24. Smith MB, Xue H, Strong L, et al: Forty-year experience with second malignancies after treatment of childhood cancer: Analysis of outcome following the development of the second malignancy. J Pediatr Surg 28:1342–1349, 1993.
25. Lemoine NR, Mayall ES, Wyllie FS, et al: Activated ras mutations in human thyroid cancers. Cancer Res 48:4459–4463, 1988.
26. Lemoine NR, Mayall ES, Wyllie FS, et al: High frequency of ras oncogene activation in all stages of thyroid tumorigenesis. Oncogene 4:159–164, 1989.
27. Bongarzone I, Butti MG, Coronelli S, et al: Frequent activation of ret protooncogene by fusion with a new activating gene in papillary thyroid carcinomas. Cancer Res 54:2979–2985, 1994.
28. Eng C, Smith DP, Mulligan LM, et al: Point mutations within the tyrosine kinase domain of RET protooncogene in multiple endocrine neoplasia type 2B and related sporadic tumours. Hum Mol Genet 3:237–241, 1994.
29. Harness JA, Thompson NW, McLeod MK, et al: Differentiated thyroid carcinoma in children and adolescents. World J Surg 16:547–554, 1992.
30. Ceccarelli C, Pacini F, Lippi F, et al. Thyroid cancer in children and adolescents. Surgery 104:1143–1148, 1988.
31. Schlumberger M, DeVathaire F, Travagli JP, et al: Differentiated thyroid carcinoma in childhood: Long term follow-up in 72 patients. J Clin Endocrinol Metab 65:1088–1094, 1987.
32. LaQuaglia MP, Corbally MT, Heller G, et al: Recurrence and morbidity in differentiated thyroid carcinoma in children. Surgery 104:1149–1156, 1988.
33. Zimmerman D, Hay ID, Gough IR, et al: Papillary thyroid carcinoma in children and adults: Long-term follow-up of 1039 patients conservatively treated at one institution during three decades. Surgery 104:1157–1163, 1988.
34. deRoy vanZuidewijn DBW, Songun I, Kievit J, et al: Complications of thyroid surgery. Ann Surg Oncol 2:56–60, 1995.
35. Hung W, Sarlis NJ: Current controversies in the management of pediatric patients with well-differentiated nonmedullary thyroid cancer: A review. Thyroid 12:683–702, 2002.
36. Haveman JW, van Tol KM, Rouwe CW, et al: Surgical experience in children with differentiated thyroid carcinoma. Ann Surg Oncol 10:15–20, 2003.
37. Nishida T, Nakao K, Hamaji M, et al: Preservation of recurrent laryngeal nerve invaded by differentiated thyroid cancer. Ann Surg 226:85–91, 1997.
38. Wells SAJ, Farndon JR, Dale JK, et al: Long term evaluation of patients with primary parathyroid hyperplasia managed by total parathyroidectomy and heterotopic autotransplantation. Ann Surg 192:451–458, 1980.
39. Skinner MA, Norton JA, Moley JF, et al: Heterotopic autotransplantation of parathyroid tissue in children undergoing total thyroidectomy. J Pediatr Surg 32:510–513, 1997.
40. Vassilopoulou-Sellin R, Klein MJ, Smith TH, et al: Pulmonary metastases in children and young adults with differentiated thyroid cancer. Cancer 71:1348–1352, 1993.
41. Kirk JM, Mort C, Grant DB, et al: The usefulness of serum thyroglobulin in the follow-up of differentiated thyroid carcinoma in children. Med Pediatr Oncol 20:201–208, 1992.
42. Samaan NA, Draznin MB, Halpin RE, et al: Multiple endocrine syndrome type IIb in early childhood. Cancer 68:1832–1834, 1991.
43. Gorlin JB, Sallan SE: Thyroid cancer in childhood. Endocrinol Metab Clin North Am 19:649–662, 1990.
44. Szinnai G, Meier C, Kaomminoth P, Zumsteg UW: Review of multiple endocrine neoplasia type 2A in children: Therapeutic results of early thyroidectomy and prognostic value of codon analysis. Pediatrics 111:E132–E139, 2003.
45. Wells SAJ, Chi DD, Toshima K, et al: Predictive DNA testing and prophylactic thryoidectomy in patients at risk for multiple endocrine neoplasia type 2A. Ann Surg 220:237–250, 1994.

46. Skinner MA, DeBenedetti MK, Moley JF, et al: Medullary thyroid carcinoma in children with multiple endocrine neoplasia type 2A and 2B. J Pediatr Surg 31:177–182, 1996.

47. Telander RL, Zimmerman D, van Heerden JA, et al: Results of early thyroidectomy for multiple endocrine neoplasia type 2. J Pediatr Surg 21:1190–1194, 1986.

48. Wiersinga WM: Thyroid cancer in children and adolescents: Consequences in later life. J Pediatr Endocrinol Metab 14:1289–1296, 2001.

49. Ross JH: Parathyroid surgery in children. Prog Pediatr Surg 26:48–59, 1991.

50. Howe JR, Norton JA, Wells SAJ: Prevalence of pheochromocytoma and hyperparathyroidism in multiple endocrine neoplasia type 2A: Results of long-term follow-up. Surgery 114:1070–1077, 1993.

51. Ross AJ III, Cooper A, Attie MF, et al: Primary hyperparathyroidism in infancy. J Pediatr Surg 21:493–499, 1986.

52. Kulczycka H, Kaminski W, Wozniewicz B, et al: Primary hyperparathyroidism in infancy: Diagnostic and therapeutic difficulties. Klin Padiatr 203:116–118, 1991.

53. Pollak MR, Brown EM, Chou YH, et al: Mutations in the Ca(2+)-sensing receptor gene cause familial hypocalciuric hypercalcemia and neonatal severe hyperparathyroidism. Cell 75:1297–1330, 1993.

54. Sucheston ME, Cannon MS: Development of zonular patterns in the human adrenal gland. J Morphol 126:477–492, 1968.

55. Graham LS: Celiac accessory adrenal glands. Cancer 6:149–152, 1953.

56. Grumbach MM, Biller BM, Braunstein GD, et al: Management of clinically inapparent adrenal mass ("incidentaloma"). Ann Intern Med 138:424–429, 2003.

57. Cushing H: The basophil adenomas of the pituitary body and their clinical manifestations. Bull Johns Hopkins Hosp 50:137, 1932.

58. Miller ML, Townsend JJ, Grumbach MM, Kaplan SL: An infant with Cushing's disease due to an adrenocorticotropin-producing pituitary adenoma. J Clin Endocrinol Metab 48:1017, 1979.

59. Devoe DJ, Miller ML, Conte FA, et al: Long-term outcome of children and adolescents following transsphenoidal surgery for Cushing's disease. J Clin Endocrinol Metab 82:196, 1997.

60. Newell-Price J, Trainer P, Besser MGA: The diagnosis and differential diagnosis of Cushing's syndrome and pseudo-Cushing's states. Endocr Rev 19:647, 1998.

61. Styne DM, Grumbach MM, Kaplan SL, et al: Treatment of Cushing's disease in childhood and adolescence by transcriptional microadenomectomy. N Engl J Med 310:889, 1984.

62. Chudler R, Kay R: Adrenocortical carcinoma in children. Urol Clin North Am 16:469–479, 1989.

63. Rosenfield RL: Puberty and its disorders in girls. Endocrinol Metab Clin North Am 20:15–42, 1991.

64. Bornstein SR, Stratakis CA, Chrousos GP: Adrenocortical tumors: Recent advances in basic concepts and clinical management. Ann Intern Med 130:759–771, 1999.

65. Young JLJ, Miller RW: Incidence of malignant tumors in US children. J Pediatr 86:254–258, 1975.

66. Liou LS, Kay R: Adrenocortical carcinoma in children. Urol Clin North Am 27:403–421, 2000.

67. Reincke M: Mutations in adrenocortical tumors. Horm Metab Res 30:447–455, 1998.

68. Ilvesmaki V, Kahri AI, Miettinen PJ, et al: Insulin-like growth factors (IGFs) and their receptors in adrenal tumors: High IGF-II expression in functional adrenocortical carcinomas. J Clin Endocrinol Metab 77:852–858, 1993.

69. Malkin D: p53 and the Li-Fraumeni syndrome. Biochim Biophys Acta 1198:197–213, 1994.

70. Reincke M, Beuschlein F, Lalli E, et al: Dax-1 expression in human adrenocortical neoplasms: Implications for steroidogenesis. J Clin Endocrinol Metab 83:2597–2600, 1998.

71. Hayles AB, Hahn HB J, Srague RG: Hormone-secreting tumors of the adrenal cortex in children. Pediatrics 37:19–25, 1966.

72. Stewart DR, Jones PH, Jolleys A: Carcinoma of the adrenal gland in children. J Pediatr Surg 9:59–67, 1974.

73. Neblett WW, Frexes-Steed M, Scott HWJ: Experience with adrenocortical neoplasms in childhood. Am Surg 53:117–125, 1987.

74. Daneman A: Adrenal carcinoma and adenoma in children. Pediatr Radiol 13:11–18, 1983.

75. Prando A, Wallace S, Marins JL, et al: Sonographic findings of adrenal cortical carcinomas in children. Pediatr Radiol 20:163–165, 1990.

76. Glazer GM: MR imaging of the liver, kidney and adrenal glands. Radiology 166:303–312, 1988.

77. Ziegelbaum MM, Kay R, Rothner AD, et al: The association of neuroblastoma with myoclonic encephalopathy of infants: The use of magnetic resonance as an imaging modality. J Urol 139:81–82, 1988.

78. Gross MD, Shapiro B, Francis IR, et al: Scintigraphic evaluation of clinically silent adrenal masses. J Nucl Med 35:1145–1152, 1994.

79. Thrall JH, Feritas JE, Beirerwaltes WH: Adrenal scintigraphy. Semin Nucl Med 8:23–41, 1978.

80. Cohn K, Gottesman L, Brennan M: Adrenocortical carcinoma. Surgery 100:1170–1177, 1986.

81. Hutter AM, Kayhoe DE: Adrenal cortical carcinoma: Results of treatment with o,p'-DDD in 138 patients. Am J Med 41:581–592, 1966.

82. Mayer SK, Oligny LL, Deal C, et al: Childhood adrenocortical tumors: Case series and reevaluation of prognosis: A 24-year experience. J Pediatr Surg 32:911–915, 1997.

83. Teinterier C, Pauchard MS, Brugieres L, et al: Clinical and prognostic aspects of adrenocortical neoplasms in childhood. Med Pediatr Oncol 32:106–111, 1999.

84. MacFarlane DA: Cancer of the adrenal cortex: The natural history, prognosis, and treatment in a study of fifty-five cases. Ann R Coll Surg Engl 23:155–165, 1958.

85. Sabbaga CC, Avilla SG, Schulz C, et al: Adrenocortical carcinoma in children: Clinical aspects and prognosis. J Pediatr Surg 28:841–843, 1993.

86. Fonseca V, Bouloux PM: Phaeochromocytoma and paraganglioma. Baillieres Clin Endocrinol Metab 7:509–544, 1993.

87. Ulchaker JC, Goldfarb DA, Bravo EL, et al: Successful outcomes in pheochromocytoma surgery in the modern era. J Urol 161:764–767, 1999.

88. Khafagi FA, Shapiro B, Fischer M, et al: Phaeochromocytoma and functioning paraganglioma in childhood and adolescence: Role of iodine 131 metaiodobenzylguanidine. Eur J Nucl Med 18:191–198, 1991.

89. Januszewicz P, Wieteska-Kimczak A, Wyszynska T: Pheochromocytoma in children: Difficulties in diagnosis and localization. Clin Exp Hypertens 12:571–579, 1990.

90. Ross JH: Pheochromocytoma: Special considerations in children. Urol Clin North Am 27:393–402, 2000.

91. Bravo EL: Evolving concepts in pathophysiology, diagnosis, and treatment of pheochromocytoma. Endocr Rev 15:356–368, 1994.

92. Caty MG, Coran AG, Geagen M, et al: Current diagnosis and treatment of pheochromocytoma in children. Arch Surg 125:978–981, 1990.

93. Kebebrew E, Duh QY: Benign and malignant pheochromocytoma: Diagnosis, treatment and follow-up. Surg Oncol Clin North Am 7:765–789, 1998.

94. Turner MC, Lieberman E, DeQuattro V: The perioperative management of pheochromocytoma in children. Clin Pediatr 31:583–589, 1992.

95. Neumann HPH, Bender BU, Reincke M, et al: Adrenal-sparing surgery for phaeochromocytoma. Br J Surg 86:94–97, 1999.

96. Safford SD, Coleman RE, Gockerman JP, et al: Iodine-131 metaiodobenzylguanidine is an effective treatment for malignant pheochromocytoma and paraganglioma. Surgery 134(6):956–962, 2003.

97. Sisson JC, Shapiro B, Shulkin BL, et al: Treatment of malignant pheochromocytoma with 131-I metaiodobenzylguanidine and chemotherapy. Am J Clin Oncol 22:364–370, 1999.

98. Gross DJ, Avishai N, Meiner V, et al: Familial pheochromocytoma associated with a novel mutation in the von Hippel-Lindau gene. J Clin Endocrinol Metab 81:147–149, 1996.

99. Albanese CT, Wiener ES: Routine total bilateral adrenalectomy is warranted in childhood familial pheochromocytoma. J Pediatr Surg 28:1248–1251, 1993.

100. Spunt SL, Pratt CB, Rao BN, et al: Childhood carcinoid tumors: The St. Jude Children's Research Hospital Experience. J Pediatr Surg 35:1282–1286, 2000.

101. Stinner B, Kisker O, Zielke A, Rothmund M: Surgical management for carcinoid tumors of the small bowel, appendix, colon and rectum. World J Surg 20:183–188. 1996.
102. Onaitis MW, Kirshbom PM, Hayward TZ, et al: Gastrointestinal carcinoids: Characterization by site of origin and hormone production. Ann Surg 232:549–556, 2000.
103. Doede T, Foss HD, Waldschmidt J: Carcinoid tumors of the appendix in children: Epidemiology, clinical aspects and procedure. Eur J Pediatr Surg 10:372–377, 2000.
104. Safford SD, et al. 131-I Meta-iodobenzylguanidine treatment for metastatic carcinoid tumors in 98 patients. Cancer (in press).
105. Parkes SE, Muir KR, al Sheyyab M, et al: Carcinoid tumors of the appendix in children 1957–1986: Incidence, treatment and outcome. Br J Surg 80:502–504, 1993.
106. Wang LT, Wilkins EWJ, Bode HH: Bronchial carcinoid tumors in pediatric patients. Chest 103:1426–1428, 1993.
107. Hancock BJ, Di Lorenzo M, Youssef S, et al: Childhood primary pulmonary neoplasms. J Pediatr Surg 28:1133–1136, 1993.

CHAPTER 77

Robotic Surgery

Stephanie A. Kapfer, MD, Joselito Tantoco, MD, and Celeste Hollands, MD

The term "robot" entered the English language in 1923. It was coined by the Czech playwright Karel Capek in his play *Rossum's Universal Robots.* The word is derived from the Czech word *robota,* which means "servitude" or "forced labor." Capek envisioned machines that could perform mundane work, thus freeing humans for higher pursuits.[1]

"Robotics" is the science associated with the design, fabrication, and application of robots. It is a broad field and includes all mechanical devices that can duplicate human actions with varying degrees of automation and inherent intelligence. At the lower end of the spectrum of autonomy is the motorized master-slave system, in which the movements of a human operator are translated into movements of mechanical arms or actuators. Somewhere in the middle are machines that are simply preprogrammed to perform specific tasks, usually repetitively. At the higher end of the spectrum are machines that perform tasks autonomously. They use artificial intelligence to "learn" and then to refine or redirect their actions.

Robotic surgery is a relatively new and rapidly evolving field. It currently exists as an integral component of conventional surgical therapy. Robotic surgical systems serve as technologic assistants in the operating room and have been used in multiple subspecialties, including neurosurgery, orthopedics, urology, gynecology, cardiothoracic surgery, vascular surgery, general surgery, and pediatric surgery. Discussed in this chapter are historical milestones, technical aspects, ethical considerations, clinical applications with special attention to pediatric minimally invasive surgery, and future uses.

HISTORY

Modern robotic machines were first developed in the 1940s. They consisted of programmable mechanical devices designed to be used in industrial settings. In 1946, George Devol, who is regarded as the father of the robot, developed a general-purpose playback device for controlling the machines. In 1954, Devol patented the first programmable robotic machine capable of repetitive point-to-point motion. During this same period, Raymond Goertz was at work on the first mechanical master-slave system. In 1951, Goertz developed an articulated, remotely-operated arm for the Atomic Energy Commission. Mechanical coupling between the operator and the actuator consisted of a collection of cables and pulleys.

The first commercially available robots were produced in 1958 by Unimation, a company formed by Devol and Joseph F. Engelberger, and in 1959, by Planet Corporation. General Motors was first to install an industrial robot on a production line in Trenton, New Jersey, in 1962. Others followed, including the Japanese, who imported their first industrial robot from the United States in 1967. Robotic technology would soon be applied to areas beyond industry, including agriculture, oceanographic and space exploration, education, and eventually, surgery.

Paralleling the development of industrial robots was the emergence of computer technology. The first computers were built in the mid-1940s. Computers became commercially available in 1951, although very few were sold. The concept of "artificial intelligence" also had its genesis during this period, as this term entered common usage after a conference at Dartmouth College.

The widespread use of computers was limited until 1961, when the much smaller digital-based computer chip began to replace circuit cards in computer construction. The development of the microprocessor by Texas Instruments in 1971 furthered this evolution. In 1973, computer and robotic technology were merged by Richard Hohn in the first commercially available minicomputer-controlled industrial robot. Since the early 1980s, advances in both computer and robotic technology have occurred at a seemingly exponential rate.

The National Aeronautics and Space Administration (NASA) first proposed the idea of using robotic technology in surgical procedures in the early 1970s. NASA had successfully used increasingly sophisticated robotic technology in their unmanned space-exploration program. Surveyor 1, the first robotic spacecraft, landed on the moon in 1966. The Viking space probes used robot arms with an incorporated microcomputer in the exploration of Mars in 1976. However, it was the prospect of extended manned space exploration that caused NASA to propose the use of telepresence surgical procedures. With the launch of Salyut 1 by the Soviet Union in 1971 and Skylab by the United States in 1973 came the real possibility of astronauts developing surgical emergencies far distant from an operating room or a surgeon. At the time, NASA determined that the technology was not sufficiently advanced to proceed.

Minimally invasive surgical procedures had their beginnings in the early 1900s, although it was not until the 1980s, with the development of miniature, high-resolution video technology and high-intensity light sources, that the technique became feasible. The first minimally invasive cholecystectomies were performed in France in 1987 and in the United States in 1988. The potential applications of minimally invasive surgery quickly blossomed and, in many instances, have replaced open surgery as the preferred approach for many operative procedures.

Robotic technology continued to improve and, in the late 1980s, it was finally applied to surgery. Neurosurgeons combined robotics and computed tomographic (CT) imaging technology to perform stereotactic biopsies of brain tumors. The technique improved the accuracy and minimized the trauma of the biopsy.[2] Veterinary orthopedic surgeons, working in collaboration with International Business Machines Corporation (IBM), used an industrial robot to ream out the proximal femur for a prosthetic hip component in a dog. It served as a prototype for systems later designed for use in humans.[3] At Imperial College, London, urologists used a robot to perform transurethral prostatectomy. The robot combined a cutting device with an ultrasonographic probe. Real-time three-dimensional sonographic images allowed the surgeon to direct the robot to the tissue to be excised.[4]

The first surgical robot to receive U.S. Food and Drug Administration (FDA) approval and to achieve wide clinical use was developed by Computer Motion, Inc., (CMI) in 1993 under the direction of Yulun Wang. The current generation of AESOP (Automated Endoscopic System for Optimal Positioning) is a voice-activated robotic arm designed to hold the camera during minimally invasive procedures.

These advancements in robotic technology prompted NASA and the Defense Department to revisit the idea of telepresence surgery. In 1993, the Defense Advanced Research Project Administration initiated the Advanced Biomedical Technologies program, the goal of which was to develop technologies that could extend sophisticated surgical care to far-forward combat casualties. The primary research areas were diagnostics, therapeutics, and education and training. Research sites included the Stanford Research Institute (SRI), the Massachusetts Institute of Technology (MIT), IBM's Watson Laboratory, NASA's Jet Propulsion Laboratory, and CMI.

The first robotic surgical system developed by SRI for the Defense Department was designed to perform telepresence open surgery. It was a master-slave system consisting of a mobile remote surgery unit, a surgeon's workstation, and a communication link capable of operating over a distance of up to 5 km. The system featured two robotic arms with 6 degrees-of-freedom (DOFs), stereoscopic imaging, and basic force feedback. It was never applied in a practical setting.

However, one of the SRI designers, Frederick Moll, saw a potential application of the telepresence technology to minimally invasive procedures. In 1995, Moll, Robert Younge, and John Freund formed Intuitive Surgical. The company absorbed personnel and technology from MIT's robotics laboratory and IBM's Watson Laboratory. They developed a master-slave surgical system based on the original SRI open surgery prototype. Since 2000, Intuitive Surgical's da Vinci Surgical System has had FDA clearance for use in multiple surgical subspecialty applications.

Meanwhile, CMI developed the Zeus Surgical System, a master-slave system consisting of three mechanical arms, a surgeon console, and a computer interface. It obtained FDA approval in 2001. Other products developed by CMI for use with the Zeus system include the Hermes Control Center, a voice-activated system capable of controlling multiple computer-based operating room devices, and the Socrates Telecollaborative System, a unit that combines telecommunication equipment, networked operative devices, and robotic systems to allow telecollaboration and telementoring.

NASA's Jet Propulsion Laboratory brought robotics to the field of microsurgery. In 1994, the Robot Assisted MicroSurgery workstation was developed. It is a master-slave system with programmable controls that is capable of 6 DOFs, scaling down hand motions, filtering tremor, and magnifying force feedback. Its technology has been applied to both open and minimally invasive, robotic-assisted procedures.

The development of robotic surgical technology has not been limited to the United States. Systems developed in Europe that are similar to AESOP include the Tiska endoarm, the Fips endoarm, and Endoassist. All provide the operating surgeon with "hands-off" control of the endoscopic camera.[5-9] ARTEMIS (Advanced Robotic Telemanipulator for Minimally Invasive Surgery) was developed in Germany in 1992. It is similar to da Vinci and Zeus in form and function but has not advanced to commercial production.[5,6,10,11]

In 2003, Intuitive Surgical acquired CMI. The merger combined the intellectual property of the two companies and eliminated costly patent disputes. The da Vinci and Zeus systems remain the only robotic surgical systems capable of telemanipulation that have been approved for use in humans by both the European Union and the FDA.

TECHNICAL ASPECTS

Advantages of Robotic Technology

Robots have proven their utility in industrial settings by increasing productivity without increasing cost. They perform tasks precisely and repetitively without fatigue. They decrease waste by reducing system exposure to human error, and they can perform tasks that are too dangerous or impossible for a human to complete. These advantages of robotic technology also apply to its use in open and minimally invasive surgery.

One of the potential limitations in surgery is the precision with which a human can manually direct a surgical instrument. Unaided, a surgeon is unable to manipulate instruments closer than 100 µm from the target. Retinal surgery, for example, requires laser targeting to within 25 µm. Robotic technology can scale down hand movements to 10 µm, thereby increasing targeting precision by 10-fold.[2]

Hand tremor also can affect precision of instrument movement during surgical procedures. This problem can be accentuated when surgeons are subject to stress, fatigue, and poor ergonomics. When long instruments are required during surgery, such as in deep pelvic procedures or minimally invasive surgery, the hand tremors are magnified at the instrument tips. Robotic surgical systems can be programmed to filter out tremor, allowing better control of the surgical instrument.

In many scenarios, it is not the surgeon or instrument that is moving but rather the patient. Ophthalmologic procedures are limited by the eye's natural motion. Cardiac surgeons must make major adjustments for the beating of the heart. Surgical robots are being designed to track and then integrate the motion of the tissue into the viewing system. They will, in effect, make the tissue appear motionless to the operating surgeon.[2,12]

Robotics also offers advantages in overcoming some of the challenges inherent in minimally invasive techniques. The operating skills required to perform minimally invasive surgery are quite different from those required for open surgery. Minimally invasive surgeons view the operating field two-dimensionally, relying on an assistant to direct the telescopic visualization in the correct direction. The movement of instruments is reversed because of the fulcrum effect of the instrument port and is limited to 4 DOFs (Fig. 77-1). Tactile feedback is significantly decreased, and hand-eye coordination is

hampered by loss of the eye-hand-target axis. It is in overcoming these limitations that robotics may have its greatest application.

The standard minimally invasive camera provides a magnified, two-dimensional image at typically 0 degrees or 30 degrees from the tip of the telescope. It is impossible to see the operative field in its entirety with the camera, removing peripheral vision as a source of information. The two-dimensional image eliminates depth perception. Size and depth must be estimated from tissue and instrument orientation and relative size, a task made difficult by the magnified view. Robotic surgical systems have been designed to place the surgeon back into a three-dimensional operative field. A dual-camera endoscope restores stereoscopic vision. The image can then be projected into a surgeon console that not only immerses the surgeon in the operative field but also restores the eye-hand-target axis by overlaying the image onto the surgeon's hands. The result is a more natural, optically enhanced view of the operative field.

In standard minimally invasive surgery, the camera is seldom manipulated by the operating surgeon but rather is often guided by the least experienced person in the operating room. The level of coordination required between these individuals takes time to develop and is usually achieved after a series of near mishaps. Communication between surgeon and assistant requires a new common language and some degree of anticipation. Even when these challenges are met, the telescope holder may still adversely affect visualization by hand tremor, disorientation, or poor timing of camera movement. Robotic arms for "hands-off" endoscope manipulation completely eliminate camera manipulation as an issue. These arms produce a rock-steady image that is under the direct control of the operating surgeon.

In standard laparoscopic or thoracoscopic surgery, the fulcrum effect of the instrument port reverses the

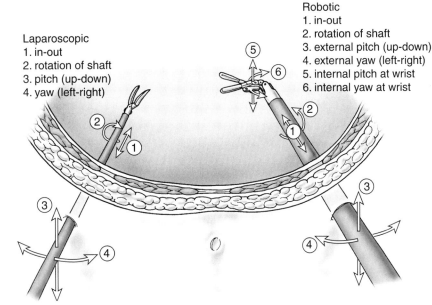

FIGURE 77-1. *Left,* The 4 degrees of freedom (DOFs) for laparoscopic instruments are seen. With the laparoscopic technique, the surgeon can move the instrument in and out of the patient and can rotate the shaft of the instrument. Moreover, the tip of the instrument can be moved up or down (pitch) or in a left and right direction (yaw). *Right,* 6 DOFs that are allowed with current robotic instrumentation. In addition to the four DOFs with the laparoscopic procedure, internal pitch and internal yaw occur at the tip of the instrument.

Laparoscopic
1. in-out
2. rotation of shaft
3. pitch (up-down)
4. yaw (left-right)

Robotic
1. in-out
2. rotation of shaft
3. external pitch (up-down)
4. external yaw (left-right)
5. internal pitch at wrist
6. internal yaw at wrist

direction of movement of the instrument tip (i.e., moving the instrument handle to the right results in movement of the instrument tip to the left). Compensating for this effect can be a difficult skill to perfect. Robotic systems restore a more intuitive coupling between hand movement and instrument movement. Just as in open surgery, manipulation of the robotic controls in a certain direction results in movement of the instrument in the same direction. An added benefit of this type of mechanical coupling is that the surgeon no longer has to struggle with the movement of instruments through "sticky" ports. The robot manages friction within the port, and the surgeon simply directs the instrument.

A second limitation imposed by the fulcrum effect is a reduction in the instrument range of motion or DOFs. In open surgery, movement of an instrument is limited only by the dexterity and flexibility of the operator's hand and arm. At each joint, the DOFs are defined by yaw (x-axis), pitch (y-axis), in-out (z-axis), and rotation. In conventional minimally invasive surgery, instrument motion is limited to 4 DOFs. Robotic systems add an additional 2 or 3 DOFs through an articulating joint located near the tip of the instrument (see Fig. 77-1). Movement of this additional joint is controlled intuitively through the robotic interface.

Tactile perception for the surgeon is another area in which robotic technology offers considerable potential. Haptics is the branch of physiology that investigates the sense of touch. Haptics as applied to robotics is that portion of the technology that restores tactile feedback to the operator of a master-slave system. One of the limitations of minimally invasive surgery is that the surgeon's tactile perceptions are diminished. The force applied by an endoscopic grasper is dependent as much on the integrity of the jaws and the instrument's own pressure profile as it is on the force being applied by the surgeon. Robotic surgical systems are now being designed to provide more realistic force feedback to the operating surgeon.

Last, the use of robotic surgical systems provides some added benefits to the surgeon's assistant, who is at the operating table. This assistant can stand in the operating surgeon's "footprint" rather than in a secondary, ergonomically disadvantaged position. Complex procedures requiring simultaneous conventional and robotic minimally invasive techniques can be performed in a small workspace with relative comfort by a surgeon-assistant operative team. For less complex procedures, a robotic surgical assistant can actually eliminate the need for a skilled human assistant and the associated costs. Robotics allows an individual surgeon to control basic tissue retraction, camera manipulation, and the actual surgical maneuvers.

Robotic Surgical Systems

AESOP, Zeus, and daVinci are the three robotic devices approved for use in the United States. Many advantages are seen with AESOP (Fig. 77-2).[13] With this robotic

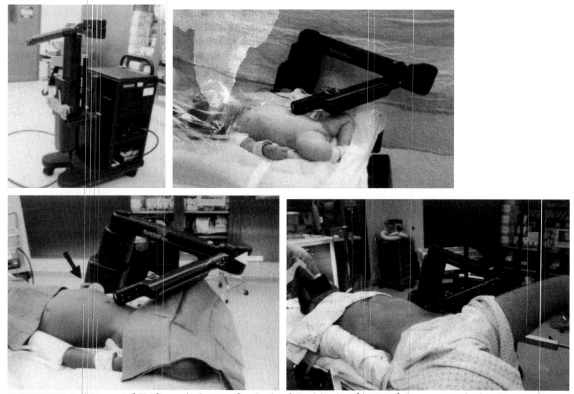

FIGURE 77-2. Automated Endoscopic System for Optimal Positioning (AESOP) is seen attached to its storage cart in the upper left photograph. *Upper right, lower left, and lower right,* AESOP is seen positioned for a laparoscopic fundoplication in an infant, a preschool child, and an adolescent, respectively. *Lower left,* AESOP is seen to be at full tilt (*black arrow*) and −1 degree angulation (*white arrow*) at the elbow joint. This appears to be the optimal position for AESOP for this procedure.

telescopic holder, the image is steady and consistent. Moreover, it can be manipulated by voice recognition. This device may be invaluable, as it is difficult to position a surgeon, an assistant, and telescope holder around a small baby. In one study, it was shown to be associated with a reduction in the operative time in patients undergoing laparoscopic fundoplication.[14]

Zeus and da Vinci are both master-slave systems consisting of an operative unit with three or four robotic arms, a surgeon's console, and a computer interface. They each have a camera arm that is under the control of the operating surgeon and that can provide a steady, magnified, high-resolution two- or three-dimensional image. Both systems are programmed to correct for the fulcrum effect, to filter out tremor, and to eliminate port friction. Both have controls that are intuitive in nature and instrumentation that restores lost DOFs. They both can scale motions to improve precision and decrease the risk of inadvertent tissue damage.[15,16]

The differences between the two systems stem from their origins. Zeus grew out of the low-profile, single-armed AESOP, whereas da Vinci was based on the multiarm open surgery unit initially developed by SRI. The operative unit, surgeon's console, and available instrumentation for each system are sufficiently different to make one system more suitable than the other for many applications.

The Zeus operative unit consists of three table-mounted robotic arms, each weighing about 40 pounds (Fig. 77-3). The arms can be moved and oriented independent of each other. Because they are table-mounted, no risk to the patient occurs should the position of the table be changed during the procedure. Once in place, the low-profile nature of the robotic arms leaves ample space for a patient-side surgeon to work.

Da Vinci uses a single, 1200-pound, floor-mounted unit with three to four robotic arms. The arms have built-in pivots that expand their range of motion from a common starting point. When the table position is changed during an operation, great care must be taken to avoid injury to the patient, as the robotic arms do not move with the table. The size of the unit provides limited space for a patient-side surgeon to work.

The Zeus surgeon's console consists of a control unit and a separate monitor. In this system, the surgeon's console is positioned behind the surgeon, and the controls are draped into the sterile field (Fig. 77-4). This "open-platform" design allows easy communication between the operating surgeon and other operating room staff, as well as improved overall situational awareness. The monitor is capable of two- or three-dimensional imaging. Five- or ten-millimeter telescopes can be used in two-dimensional imaging, but a 12-mm specialized dual-camera telescope is required for three-dimensional work. The operating arms are controlled by two egg-shaped, non-motorized controls that can be uncoupled from the robotic arms to permit repositioning. The camera and multiple other systems within the operating room are voice-controlled through the Hermes interface. The "open-platform" design of the Zeus system also allows the performance of a hybrid procedure in which the operating surgeon manipulates one instrument through the robotic interface while the assistant uses a second instrument through standard minimally invasive techniques. The da Vinci surgeon's console, as a single unit, is designed for total immersion of the surgeon in the

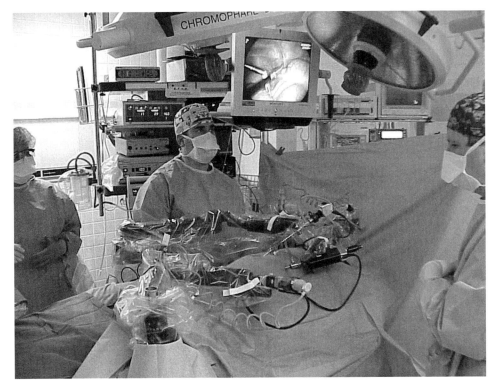

FIGURE 77-3. In this operative photograph, the three robotic arms with the Zeus system are seen mounted to the operating room table. A robotic appendectomy is being performed.

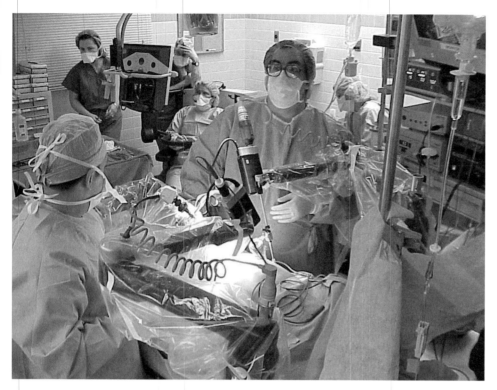

FIGURE 77-4. The open platform design of Zeus is seen in this photograph. In the foreground are seen two assistants and the robotic arms attached to the table. In the background, the surgeon is seen seated in the open console looking at the monitor.

operative field (Fig. 77-5). A three-dimensional image is obtained by a specialized 12-mm telescope that provides a separate image to each eye. This image is projected onto the two motorized controls, restoring the eye-hand-target axis. By uncoupling and redirecting the controls, the surgeon can manipulate the operative arms, the retraction arm, or the camera position.

The actual operative instruments are a critical part of each system's flexibility and success. Zeus instruments use a push-rod technology that provides 6 DOFs. They are 5 mm in diameter and measure 11 mm from internal joint to tip. The instruments are effective as close as 14 mm from the end of the telescope and need to be separated only by 3 cm at skin level. They are reusable and have an as-yet-undetermined life span.

The da Vinci instruments use a cable technology that allows 7 DOFs. They measure 8.5 mm in diameter and 18.5 mm from internal joint to tip. The instruments must be at least 38 mm from the scope and 10 cm from each other at skin level. Each instrument has a life span of 10 uses, a count maintained by an internal monitor.

Putting it all together, the Zeus system has a much lower-profile design and modular components that will work independently or in conjunction with other CMI products. Its instrument configurations are more suited to working in small spaces, such as in the pediatric patient. However, its control interface does not completely mimic open surgical maneuvers and consequently has a comparatively steep learning curve. Da Vinci has a bulkier, single-unit design. It is less suited to small operative workspaces, but its imaging system and intuitive controls more completely restore the feel of open surgery to the minimally invasive surgeon.[17,18]

ETHICAL CONSIDERATIONS

Training and Credentials

The Committee on Emerging Surgical Technology and Education (CESTE) was chartered by the American College of Surgeons (ACS) to study the implications of emerging technology and to suggest ways to accelerate training and credentialing in this area while protecting the welfare of patients. In 1994, the committee published a statement on emerging surgical technologies and guidelines for issuing credentials for such technologies. In brief, this statement says that new surgical technologies must be scientifically assessed for safety, efficacy, and need. Surgeons using these technologies must be qualified and experienced in the management of the disease for which the technology is intended, must complete a defined educational program that includes didactic and practical elements, must be evaluated and deemed qualified by a surgeon experienced in the technology, and must be subjected to periodic evaluation and outcomes assessment.[19] Subsequent statements by the ACS have reinforced these concepts.[20–22]

Ironically, robotic surgical technology is both the target of these guidelines and the means by which these guidelines may be accomplished. Robotics clearly is an emerging surgical technology, the dissemination and use of which should be monitored. Training programs involving both experienced surgeons and surgery residents have been described in the literature.[23–25] These programs stress the need for a defined curriculum in robotic surgical techniques, with graded skills development and practice in inanimate, animal, and

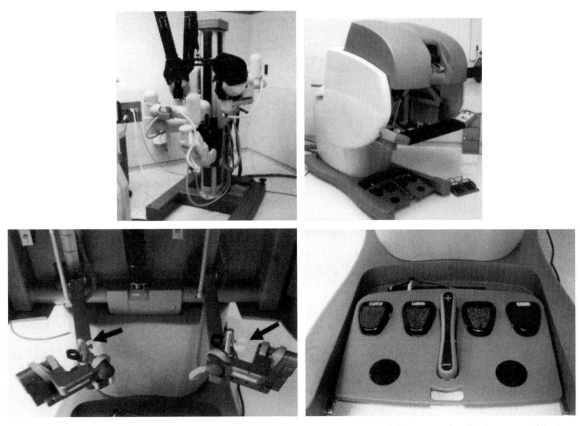

FIGURE 77-5. *Upper left,* The daVinci unit. In contrast to the Zeus table-mounted robotic arms, this is a 1200-pound floor-mounted unit with three to four robotic arms. *Upper right,* The surgeon's console. This is designed for total immersion of the surgeon. The finger controls (arrows) for the surgeon are seen within the surgeon's console. On the floor of the console are pedals that allow the robotic arms to be moved, allow redirection of the camera, and allow cautery to be engaged. The fourth pedal is available for other functions.

cadaver laboratories. Credentialing programs following the general guidelines set by CESTE also have been described.[26] However, training and credentialing programs have been implemented at only a limited number of institutions. As the use of robotic technology becomes more widespread, so must the availability of expert training and mentoring. The telepresence aspect of robotic technology provides just the means to accomplish this goal. "Telementoring" is defined as an expert surgeon providing guidance to a subject from a remote location. It assumes the ability of the mentor to control a portion of the action on site, such as camera position or retraction. "Teleproctoring" is limited to observation from a remote location without the ability to interact. Both techniques have been tested and found to be feasible, effective, and safe.[27,28] This aspect of robotic technology will expand the way in which surgeons learn and maintain their skills in the future.

Artificial Intelligence

The robotic surgical systems currently in use serve only as operative assistants, tools for overcoming human limitations. The artificial intelligence used in these systems does not allow independent operation, but rather it processes input from the system operator in a very well-defined, preprogrammed manner. However, one can imagine a future in which robotic surgical systems are capable of working without the direct supervision of a human surgeon. The ethical issues surrounding this scenario were actually described well before the first modern robot was even built. In 1942, Isaac Asimov defined his three "Rules of Robotics" in the short story *Runaround*.[29] These rules are as follows:

1. A robot may not injure a human being, or, through inaction, allow a human being to come to harm.
2. A robot must obey the orders given it by human beings except where such orders would conflict with the First Law.
3. A robot must protect its own existence as long as such protection does not conflict with the First or Second Laws.

Surgeons must play an active role in the advancement and refinement of robotic technology. The surgeon's precept is to "first do no harm." Robotic surgical systems will be only as safe as the surgeons using them, regardless of the sophistication of the artificial intelligence and the inherent safety mechanisms that the systems use.

CLINICAL APPLICATIONS

Robotic surgical systems currently in clinical practice can be divided into two general groups. The first group is composed of those robotic systems designed for specific tasks. They may be found primarily in the fields of neurosurgery, orthopedics, and urology. The second group contains those systems that have the potential for a wide range of clinical applications. These are the systems that enhance minimally invasive and microsurgical procedures.

Systems Designed for Specific Applications

Neurosurgery has used robotics primarily for improving the accuracy and minimizing the cost of intracranial tumor biopsy. Stereotactic biopsy systems have evolved to the extent that dynamic imaging of the biopsy needle approaching the target is available, and the need for a metallic frame has been eliminated.[2,30] These robotic-enhanced techniques have recently been applied to procedures more complex than just tissue sampling. Brainstem and skull-base tumors as well as intracranial arteriovenous malformations have been approached by using an image-guided microsurgical system named the Mehrkoordinaten Manipulator. Initial feasibility trails of this technology appear promising.[31,32]

Orthopedics has benefited from robotic technology primarily in the area of joint replacement. Several robotic surgical systems currently in clinical use provide assistance to the surgeon in the preoperative planning and the operative reaming and placement of prosthetic joint implants. These systems include the Robodoc Surgical Assistant System, Computer Assisted Surgical Robotics (CASPAR), and the Compact Robot for Image Guided Orthopaedic Surgery (CRIGOS).[2,4] The Robodoc system has achieved the short-term benefit of superior contact between the implant and bone as compared with manual methods (98% for robotic vs. 23% for conventional) at the expense of lengthened operative time and increased blood loss. Long-term benefits have yet to be determined.[4,33]

As previously discussed, urologists have used robotic technology in transurethral prostate resections. The combination of a diathermic cutter and a US probe allows the surgeon to resect precise areas of the prostate gland with little risk to the surrounding tissue.[4] Stereotactic robotic technology also has been applied to the biopsy of renal lesions as well as to renal access procedures for nephrolithotomy.[34]

Systems Designed for Broad Application

The robotic surgical system that has achieved the widest clinical use is AESOP. This robotic surgical assistant was designed to return control of visualization of the operative field to the surgeon, eliminating the need for a human assistant in many minimally invasive procedures. It has proven to be a safe and easily applied technology. When compared with an experienced human assistant in a controlled setting, it resulted in comparable operative times and equivalent perioperative morbidity. Subjectively, the surgeons experienced less inadvertent movement of the camera and superior visualization with the robotic assistant.[35-37]

The Zeus and da Vinci surgical systems have been used in a variety of operative procedures across the specialties of general surgery, urology, gynecology, cardiothoracic surgery, vascular surgery, and pediatric surgery. Their applicability to minimally invasive surgery is limited only by the instrumentation required for the procedures.

Procedures documented in the literature as having been performed with robotic assistance are shown in Table 77-1.[4,38-53] The list is long and surprisingly comprehensive. Clearly it can be done, but should it be?

Experimental data regarding the clinical use of robotic surgical systems consist primarily of case series. Each demonstrates that such systems can be used to perform most minimally invasive procedures safely and effectively. A search of the literature revealed only three controlled studies comparing a single robotic-assisted procedure with its conventional laparoscopic equivalent. The first was a retrospective comparative case study of minimally invasive microsurgical tubal anastomoses performed at The Cleveland Clinic. It found increased operative times in the robotic group without any appreciable benefit to the patient in terms of recovery time or tubal patency rates.[54] The second study was a prospective, nonrandomized comparison of radical retropubic prostatectomy with robot-assisted anatomic prostatectomy at the Vattikuti Urology Institute in Detroit, Michigan. It demonstrated longer operative times with the robotic group but equivalent surgical margins and complication rates. Advantages of the robotic-assisted technique were less blood loss, less postoperative pain, and earlier discharge.[55] The third study was a prospective, randomized trial from Belgium of Nissen fundoplication performed either by a conventional laparoscopic approach or by a robotic-assisted approach. It had longer operative times in the robotic group but equivalent morbidity and outcomes.[56]

Although these three controlled studies failed to demonstrate clear and overwhelming benefits favoring robotic-assisted surgery, they do show promise. As surgeons become more facile and the technology becomes more intuitive, operative times will undoubtedly decrease. Robotics should allow the performance of increasingly complex procedures by minimally invasive means, offering known advantages to patients. Yet the best indications for the use of robotic technology in surgery have yet to be defined. Essential to this end are centers and surgeons committed to participating in the development of robotic technology and to conducting prospective, randomized, controlled studies of its performance.

Pediatric Minimally Invasive Surgery

The potential benefits of the application of robotic surgical techniques to pediatric minimally invasive surgery have been previously discussed. In simplified terms, small patients have small structures in small operative workspaces. Robotics can steady visualization, proportionately scale down instrument movements, and

TABLE 77-1		
PROCEDURES THAT HAVE BEEN PERFORMED WITH ROBOTIC SURGICAL ASSISTANCE		
General Surgery	*Urology*	*Cardiothoracic Surgery*
Appendectomy	Radical prostatectomy	Inframammary artery mobilization
Cholecystectomy	Sural nerve grafting	Coronary artery bypass
Nissen fundoplication	Nephrectomy	Mitral valve repair
Inguinal hernia repair	Retroperitoneal lymph node dissection	Lobectomy
Esophagectomy	Pelvic lymph node dissection	Pneumonectomy
Heller myotomy	Varicocele ligation	Pulmonary bullectomy
Esophageal diverticulectomy	Orchiopexy	Mediastinal mass resection
Partial and total gastrectomy	Nephropexy	
Gastric banding	Pyeloplasty	*Vascular Surgery*
Divided gastric bypass	Ureterolysis	Visceral artery aneurysm repair
Gastrojejunostomy	Burch bladder suspension	Arteriovenous fistula repair
Pyloroplasty	Anti–ureteral reflux surgery	Lumbar sympathectomy
Duodenal polypectomy	Appendicovesicostomy	Iliofemoral bypass
Pancreatoduodenectomy	Megaureter repair	
Distal pancreatectomy		
Hepatic segmentectomy	*Gynecology*	*Pediatric Surgery*
Segmental enterectomy	Hysterectomy	Appendectomy
Hemicolectomy	Salpingo-oophorectomy	Pyloromyotomy
Abdominoperineal resection	Endometriosis ablation	Cholecystectomy
Rectopexy	Reversal of tubal ligation	Nissen fundoplication
Splenectomy		Intestinal pullthough for Hirschsprung's
Adrenalectomy		Morgagni hernia repair
Lysis of adhesions		Splenectomy
Living donor nephrectomy		Urachus resection
		Retroperitoneal lymph node dissection
		Mediastinal mass biopsy

increase precision in that small workspace. It is easily applied to common minimally invasive procedures, but, are these potential benefits borne out in clinical practice?

As is the case in the adult literature, the majority of reports regarding robotic-assisted, minimally invasive surgery in children consist of case series.[47,49,51,52] Only one prospective randomized, controlled study was found. This study compared patent ductus arteriosus (PDA) closure by a conventional videothoracoscopic approach with PDA closure by a robotically assisted thoracoscopic approach. Operative times were longer in the robotic approach, but complication rates and outcomes were the same.[50]

Although the technology appears safe and effective, it does have consistently noted limitations based on issues related to size. The configurations of the robotic systems and the size and flexibility of the available instruments dictate the minimal space in which a given procedure can be performed. It seems clear that the technology must be further miniaturized for it to achieve its full potential in pediatric surgery.

FUTURE USES

The application of robotics to minimally invasive surgery has the potential to change dramatically the way in which surgeons practice. As the technology advances and becomes more widely available, procedures once limited to open surgery will be performed by using minimally invasive techniques. The complexity of the procedures performed will increase as surgeons' dexterity and skill with the technology improves.

Each successive generation of surgical robots will contain improvements in the areas of imaging, haptics, dexterity, and automation. Continued miniaturization of the instrumentation will allow complex procedures to be performed in smaller and smaller patients.

Preoperative planning and postoperative care also will change. The integration of imaging modalities into the operating room will allow surgeons to develop an operative plan that is specific to a patient's anatomy and surgical condition, and to then proceed with that plan with certainty and precision. Through robotic interfaces, surgeons will be able to provide patients with long-term postoperative care from long distances and nontraditional sites.

Automation of mundane operative tasks will allow surgeons to focus on the most technically demanding aspects of surgical procedures. Wireless operating rooms will decrease clutter, improve ergonomics, and provide portability to operative suites. Telesurgery will increase the reach of surgical specialists, with the added benefit of allowing patients to remain with their social and family support network.

Robotics also will change the way in which surgeons are trained, both initially and on a continuing basis. Virtual surgical suites will allow students to develop their surgical skills "first hand," before they are ever exposed to real patients. Telementoring will allow surgeons to continue to develop their skills and their operative repertoire without the time and expense of travel.

In the coming years, robotic surgical systems will offer surgeons and patients benefits that will far outweigh the additional cost and effort that are embedded in the technology's development and use. The potential impact that robotic technology will have on pediatric surgery in particular is exciting indeed.

REFERENCES

1. Capek K: Rossum's Universal Robots. Translation by P. Selver and N. Playfair. New York, Doubleday, Page, 1923.
2. Bholat OS, Krummel TM: Advanced technologies for future fetal treatment: Surgical robotics. In Harrison MR (ed): The Unborn Patient: The Art and Science of Fetal Therapy, 3rd ed. Philadelphia, WB Saunders, 2001, pp 681–692.
3. Paul HA, Bargar WL, Mittlestadt B, et al: Development of a surgical robot for cementless total hip arthroplasty. Clin Orthop 285:57–66, 1992.
4. Bann S, Khan M, Hernandez J, et al: Robotics in surgery. J Am Coll Surg 196:784–795, 2003.
5. Buess GF, Schurr MO, Fischer SC: Robotics and allied technologies in endoscopic surgery. Arch Surg 135:229–235, 2000.
6. Ruurda JP, van Vroonhoven ThJMV, Broeders IAMJ: Robot-assisted surgical systems: A new era in laparoscopic surgery. Ann R Coll Surg Engl 84:223–226, 2002.
7. Buess GF, Arezzo A, Schurr MO, et al: A new remote-controlled endoscope positioning system for endoscopic solo surgery: The FIPS endoarm. Surg Endosc 14:395–399, 2000.
8. Arezzo A, Ulmer F, Weiss O, et al: Experimental trial on solo surgery for minimally invasive therapy: Comparison of different systems in a phantom model. Surg Endosc 14:955–959, 2000.
9. Aiono S, Gilbert JM, Soin B, et al: Controlled trial of the introduction of a robotic camera assistant (EndoAssist) for laparoscopic cholecystectomy. Surg Endosc 16:1267–1270, 2002.
10. Schurr MO, Buess G, Neisius B, et al: Robotics and telemanipulation technologies for endoscopic surgery: A review of the ARTEMIS project. Surg Endosc 14:417–418, 2000.
11. Rininsland H: ARTEMIS: A telemanipulatory for cardiac surgery. Eur J Cardiothoracic Surg 16:S106–S111, 1999.
12. Mack MJ: Minimally invasive and robotic surgery. JAMA 285:568–572, 2001.
13. Shew SB, Ostlie DJ, Holcomb GW III: Robotic telescopic assistance in pediatric laparoscopic surgery. Pediatr Endosurg Innovative Tech 7:371–375, 2003.
14. Ostlie DJ, Miller KA, Woods, RK, et al: Single cannula technique and robotic telescopic assistance in infants and children requiring laparoscopic Nissen fundoplication. J Pediatr Surg 38:111–115, 2003.
15. Rassweiler J, Binder J, Frede T: Robotic and telesurgery: Will they change our future? Curr Opin Urol 11:309–320, 2001.
16. Talamini M, Campbell K, Stanfield C: Robotic gastrointestinal surgery: Early experience and system description. J Laparoendosc Adv Surg Tech 12:225–232, 2002.
17. Drasin T, Gracia C, Atkinson J: Pediatric applications of robotic surgery. Pediatr Endosurg Innovative Tech 7:377–384, 2003.
18. Sung GT, Gill IS: Robotic laparoscopic surgery: A comparison of the da Vinci and Zeus systems. Urology 58:893–898, 2001.
19. American College of Surgeons: Statement on emerging surgical technologies and the evaluation of credentials (ST-18). Bull Am Coll Surg 79:40–41, 1994.
20. American College of Surgeons: Statement on issues to be considered before new surgical technology is applied to the care of patients (ST-23). Bull Am Coll Surg 80:46–47, 1995.
21. American College of Surgeons: Approval of courses in new skills (ST-27). Bull Am Coll Surg 83:, 1998.
22. American College of Surgeons: Verification by the American College of Surgeons for the use of emerging technologies (ST-30). Bull Am Coll Surg 83:, 1998.
23. Chitwood WR, Nifong LW, Chapman WHH, et al: Robotic surgical training in an academic institution. Ann Surg 234:475–486, 2001.
24. Menon M, Shrivastava A, Tewari A, et al: Laparoscopic and robot assisted radical prostatectomy: Establishment of a structured program and preliminary analysis of outcomes. J Urol 168:945–949, 2002.
25. Chang L, Satava RM, Pellegrini CA, et al: Robotic surgery: Identifying the learning curve through objective measurement of skill [Electronic version]. Surg Endosc. Retrieved September 24, 2003 from www.springerlink.com.
26. Ballantyne GH, Kelley WE: Granting clinical privileges for telerobotic surgery. Surg Laparosc Endosc Percutan Tech 12:17–25, 2002.
27. Moore RG, Adams JB, Partin AW, et al: Telementoring of laparoscopic procedures: Initial clinical experience. Surg Endosc 10:107–110, 1996.
28. Schulam PG, Docimo SG, Saleh W, et al: Telesurgical mentoring: Initial clinical experience. Surg Endosc 11:1001–1005, 1997.
29. Asimov I: I, Robot. New York, Bantam Books, 1950.
30. Satava RM: Emerging technologies for surgery in the 21st century. Arch Surg 134:1197–1202, 1999.
31. Nakamura M, Tamaki N, Tamura S, et al: Image-guided microsurgery with the Mehrkoordinaten Maanipulator system for cerebral arteriovenous malformations. J Clin Neurosci 7:10–13, 2000.
32. Kajiwara K, Nishizaki T, Ohmoto Y, et al: Image-guided transsphenoidal surgery for pituitary lesions using Mehrkoorkinaten Manipulator (MKM) navigation system. Minim Invas Neurosurg 46:78–81, 2003.
33. Bargar WL, Bauer A, Borner M: Primary and revision total hip replacement using the Robodoc system. Clin Orthop 354:82–91, 1998.
34. Su LM, Stoianovici D, Jarrett TW, et al: Robotic percutaneous access to the kidney: Comparison with standard manual access. J Endourol 16:471–475, 2002.
35. Kavoussi LR, Moore RG, Adams JB, et al: Comparison of robotic versus human laparoscopic camera control. J Urol 154:2134–2136, 1995.
36. Merola S, Weber P, Wasielewski A, et al: Comparison of laparoscopic colectomy with and without the aid of a robotic camera holder. Surg Laparosc Endosc Percutan Tech 12:46–51, 2002.
37. Kondraske GV, Hamilton EC, Scott DJ, et al: Surgeon workload and motion efficiency with robot and human laparoscopic camera control. Surg Endosc 16:1523–1527, 2002.
38. Giulianotti PC, Coratti A, Angelini M, et al: Robotics in general surgery: Personal experience in a large community hospital. Arch Surg 138:777–784, 2003.
39. Talamini MA, Chapman S, Horgan S, et al: A prospective analysis of 211 robotic-assisted surgical procedures. Surg Endosc Aug 15, 2003 (Epub)
40. Cadiere GB, Himpens J, Germay O, et al: Feasibility of robotic laparoscopic surgery: 146 cases. World J Surg 25:1467–1477, 2001.
41. Horgan S, Vanuno D, Sileri P, et al: Robotic-assisted laparoscopic donor nephrectomy for kidney transplantation. Transplantation 15:1474–1479, 2002.
42. Partin AW, Adams JB, Moore RG, et al: Complete robot-assisted laparoscopic urologic surgery: A preliminary report. J Am Coll Surg 181:552–557, 1995.
43. Menon M, Tewari A: Robotic radical prostatectomy and the Vattikuti Urology Institute technique: An interim analysis of results and technical points. Urology 61:15–20, 2003.
44. Kaouk JH, Desai MM, Agreu SC, et al: Robotic assisted laparoscopic sural nerve grafting during radical prostatectomy: Initial experience. J Urol 170:909–912, 2003.
45. Mohr FW, Falk V, Diegeler A, et al: Computer-enhanced "robotic" cardiac surgery: Experience in 148 patients. J Thorac Cardiovasc Surg 121:842–853, 2001.
46. Melfi FMA, Menconi GF, Mariani AM, et al: Early experience with robotic technology for thoracoscopic surgery. Eur J Cardiothorac Surg 21:864–868, 2002.
47. Docimo SG, Moore RG, Adams J, et al: Early experience with telerobotic surgery in children. J Telemedicine Telecare 2(suppl 1): 48–50, 1996.
48. Gutt CN, Markus B, Kim ZG, et al: Early experiences of robotic surgery in children. Surg Endosc 16:1083–1086, 2002.

49. Heller K, Gutt C, Schaeff B, et al: Use of the robot system da Vinci for laparoscopic repair of gastro-oesophageal reflux in children. Eur J Pediatr Surg 12:239–242, 2002.

50. Le Bret E, Papadatos S, Folliguet T, et al: Interruption of patent ductus arteriosus in children: Robotically assisted versus videothoracoscopic surgery. J Thorac Cardiovasc Surg 123:973–976, 2002.

51. Luebbe BN, Woo R, Wolf SA, et al: Robotically assisted minimally invasive surgery in a pediatric population: Initial experience, technical considerations and description of the da Vinci Surgical System. Pediatr Endosurg Innovative Tech 7:385–402.

52. Peters CA: Robotic assisted surgery in pediatric urology. Pediatr Endosurg Innovative Tech 7:403–413.

53. Hollands CM, Dixey LN: Robotic-assisted pyloromyotomy. Pediatr Endosurg Innovative Tech 8:83–88, 2004.

54. Goldberg JM, Falcone T: Laparoscopic microsurgical tubal anastomosis with and without robotic assistance. Hum Reprod 18:145–147, 2003.

55. Menon M, Tewari A, Baize B, et al: Prospective comparison of radical retropubic prostatectomy and robot-assisted anatomic prostatectomy: The Vattikuti Urology Institute experience. Urology 60:864–868, 2002.

56. Cadière GB, Himpens J, Vertruyen M, et al: Evaluation of telesurgical (robotic) NISSEN fundoplication. Surg Endosc 15:918–923, 2001.

CHAPTER 78

Bariatric Surgical Procedures in Adolescence

Thomas H. Inge, MD, PhD, Stephen R. Daniels, MD, PhD, and Victor F. Garcia, MD

As the occurrence of childhood and adolescent obesity progresses unchecked, pediatric specialists are increasingly considering extreme measures to combat the serious and immediate health complications of this disease. Behavioral and dietary approaches to the treatment of obesity in childhood and adolescence may be effective for less extreme levels of obesity. Evidence from clinical trials shows that behavioral weight management may have longer lasting effects in children compared with adults, but good long-term results are rare. These conventional treatment approaches are less effective for severe obesity.[1,2]

A number of important factors must be considered when contemplating bariatric surgical procedures for severe obesity in adolescents. Surgical weight loss results in significant improvement, if not resolution, of most obesity-related comorbidity in adults.[3] Preliminary results suggest that this also is true for adolescents,[4,5] but little information is available about long-term efficacy and potential adverse consequences to an adolescent with chronic caloric restriction. The issue of recidivism and the potential multigenerational sequelae of bariatric surgical treatment in children and adolescents necessitate that considerable care and deliberation be applied to decision making concerning surgical weight management.

DEFINITIONS

The terms *at risk of becoming overweight, being overweight,* and *being obese* have been used to refer to the increasing weight problem in children. Obesity specifically refers to the condition of having excess body fat. Measurement of body mass index (BMI; kg/m^2) is a reasonably accurate method for predicting adiposity, is reproducible in the clinical setting, and can be easily used as a screening tool.[6-9]

In children and adolescents, physiologic increases in adiposity, height, and weight during growth are expected. Growth charts that are typically used to define obesity are age and gender specific.[10,11] In this context, many authors have defined pediatric obesity as a BMI greater than the 95th percentile for age and gender, based on historical population data in the United States.[12,13] Overweight, or "at risk" for overweight, has been defined as a BMI greater than the 85th percentile.[14,15] The 85th and 95th percentiles of BMI for age were chosen mainly because these percentile boundaries approximate a BMI in young adults of 25 kg/m^2 (overweight) and 30 kg/m^2 (obese), respectively.

Whereas nearly 31% of adults in the United States are obese, more than 15% of children and adolescents are obese—a prevalence that has more than tripled in the last two decades.[13,16] Although the 95th-percentile definition of obesity is helpful when considering thresholds for nonsurgical therapy, percentile definitions become unreliable when considering extreme obesity. In essence, for the very severe categories of obesity that might prompt consideration for bariatric surgical procedures in adolescence, no reliable population-based data are available with which one can calculate accurate percentile boundaries, because youth with BMI values greater than 40 kg/m^2 are very poorly represented in the National Health and Nutrition Examination Survey (NHANES)—the data set that provides the weight and height information used to create the commonly used pediatric growth charts.[17] Thus the decision to use arbitrarily a BMI greater than 40 to consider surgical intervention in adolescent obesity is a conservative threshold, which is congruent with the National Institutes of Health (NIH) and the World Health Organization definition of very severe obesity for adults.[10,18]

ANTECEDENTS AND CONSEQUENCES OF ADOLESCENT OBESITY

Adolescent obesity is a multifaceted disease with serious immediate, intermediate, and long-term consequences.[19] Critical periods exist between preconception and adolescence during which the risk of development of obesity is increased.[20] Important risk factors for childhood and adolescent obesity are (1) low birth weight,[21–23] (2) bottle feeding,[24] (3) early adiposity rebound,[25–29] (4) having a diabetic mother,[30] (5) puberty,[31,32] and (6) parental obesity.[33,34] Knowledge of these risk factors for adolescent obesity gives insight into the genetic and environmental factors that result in obesity. With few exceptions,[35–37] little understanding exists of which risk factors for severe obesity dictate surgical intervention. This lack of understanding adds to the complexity in decision making regarding the application and timing of surgical treatment.

Associated with the remarkable increase in the prevalence of pediatric obesity in the United States is a parallel increase in the severity of obesity and in obesity-related chronic diseases with onset at a younger age, and an increased risk for adult morbidity and mortality.[38–42] Childhood obesity also has adverse social and economic consequences.[43–45] The important comorbid conditions for childhood obesity are cited in Table 78-1.[38]

TABLE 78-1
SELECTED COMORBIDITIES OF ADOLESCENT OBESITY

Complications of pediatric obesity	
Psychosocial	Poor self–esteem[91, 92]
	Depression[38]
	Eating disorders[93]
	Discrimination and prejudice[94]
	Quality of life[94, 95]
	Sexual abuse[96]
Neurological	Pseudotumor cerebri[97-99]
Pulmonary	Sleep apnea (Amin, 2002; Amin, 2002; Bower, 2000; Redline 1999; Marcus, 1996; Silvestri, 1993; Mallory, 1989)
	Asthma and exercise intolerance[100]
Cardiovascular	Dyslipidemia[101, 102]
	Hypertension[103–106]
	Coagulopathy[107]
	Chronic inflammation[108]
	Endothelial dysfunction[109]
Gastrointestinal	Gallstones[110]
	Nonalcoholic fatty liver disease[111-114]
Renal	Glomerulosclerosis[115]
Endocrine	Type 2 diabetes mellitus[116-119]
	Diabetic precursors/Insulin resistance[118, 120]
	Precocious puberty[45, 121]
	Polycystic ovary syndrome[122]
	Hypogonadism (boys)[123]
Musculoskeletal	Slipped capital femoral epiphysis[124]
	Blount's disease[38, 125]
	Forearm fractures[78]
	Flat feet[126]
Reviews of health consequences of childhood obesity	19, 41, 127–131
Excess health care costs	45

GUIDELINES FOR PERFORMING BARIATRIC SURGICAL PROCEDURES IN ADOLESCENCE

As many as 250,000 very severely obese (e.g., BMI > 40) adolescents live in the United States. Aggressive weight-loss measures may prevent or reduce the comorbid conditions. Children and adolescents who have extreme obesity (e.g., BMI > 50) often have comorbidities or impairments in activities of daily living that would justify consideration of surgical weight management.[46] An algorithm for management of children and adolescents with a BMI greater than 40 is presented (Fig. 78-1). Adopting a BMI-based algorithm for considering adolescent bariatric surgical revision is done with the understanding that an obese adolescent with an advanced, severe, and incontrovertibly weight-related comorbidity also should be considered for weight-loss surgical procedures with a lower BMI.

For highly motivated adolescents with comorbid conditions (Table 78-2) who have been unsuccessful in a carefully supervised 6-month program of weight loss, bariatric surgical intervention should be considered as a treatment option. Young patients being considered for bariatric surgical procedures should be referred to a specialized center where a multidisciplinary bariatric team can provide long-term follow-up and management of the unique challenges posed by the severely obese adolescent. Guidelines have been established by the NIH, the American Society for Bariatric Surgery, and the American College of Surgeons that define such teams to include specialists with expertise in obesity evaluation and management, psychology, nutrition, physical activity, and bariatric surgical treatment.[18,47] Depending on the individual needs of the adolescent patient, additional expertise in adolescent medicine, endocrinology, pulmonology, gastroenterology, cardiology, orthopedics, and ethics should be readily available. At Cincinnati Children's Hospital, the patient review process is similar to that used in our multidisciplinary oncology and transplant programs.[48] This review by a panel of experts from different disciplines results in specific treatment recommendations for individual patients, including appropriateness and timing of possible operative intervention.

The timing for surgical treatment for adolescents remains controversial and depends, in most cases, on the compelling health needs of the patient. However, certain physiological factors must be considered in planning an essentially elective operation. Physiologic maturation is generally complete by sexual maturation (Tanner) stage 3 or 4.[49] Skeletal maturation (adult stature) is normally attained by the age of 13 to 14 years in girls and 15 to 16 years in boys.[50,51] Overweight children generally experience accelerated onset of puberty. As a result, they are likely to be taller and have advanced bone age compared with age-matched nonobese children. If uncertainty exists about whether adult stature has been attained, skeletal maturation (bone age) can be objectively assessed with a radiograph of the hand and wrist.[52] If an individual has attained more than 95% of adult stature, little concern should exist that a bariatric

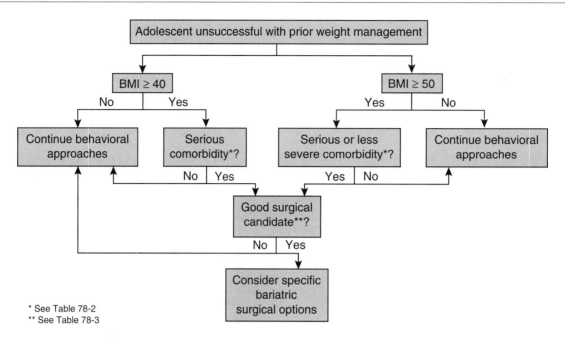

FIGURE 78-1. Algorithm for management of the severely obese adolescent.

procedure would significantly impair completion of linear growth.[53]

Adolescent psychological development also bears on the ability to participate in surgical decision making and postoperative dietary compliance. Cognitive development refers to the development of the ability to think and reason. At any given age, adolescents are at varying stages of cognitive, psychosocial, and biologic maturity. The adolescent who has acquired this ability is better able to consider the consequences of taking or not taking nutritional supplements or of following and adhering to the prescribed medical and nutritional regimens that are necessary after gastric bypass.[54]

Before any decision for surgical treatment is made, all candidates should undergo a comprehensive psychological evaluation. Goals of this evaluation are (1) to determine the level of cognitive and psychosocial development, primarily to judge the extent to which the adolescent is capable of participating in the decision to proceed with the intervention; (2) to identify past and present psychiatric, emotional, behavioral, or eating disorders; (3) to define potential support for or barriers to regimen compliance, the family readiness for surgical treatment, and the required lifestyle changes (particularly if one or both parents are obese); (4) to assess reasoning and problem-solving ability; (5) to assess whether reasonable outcome expectations exist; (6) to assess family unit stability and identify psychological stressors or conflicts within the family; (7) to determine whether the adolescent is autonomously motivated to consider bariatric surgical treatment or whether any element of coercion is present; and (8) to assess weight-related quality-of-life status. Unfortunately, no "relative value scale" can be used to assign significance to any of the information obtained in the psychological evaluation. However, during a comprehensive assessment, we have found that a complete psychological assessment is helpful to other team members in their evaluation, and that generally good team agreement is reached about whether a particular patient has a majority (or conversely a minority) of the attributes of a good bariatric surgical candidate (Table 78-3).

SURGICAL OPTIONS

In 1991, the NIH Bariatric Consensus Development Conference established parameters that led to a dramatic increase in the volume of adult bariatric surgical procedures, which has been realized primarily over the past 5-year period. This conference concluded that, at that time, insufficient data existed to make recommendations

---

TABLE 78-2

OBESITY-RELATED CONDITIONS THAT MAY BE IMPROVED WITH BARIATRIC SURGICAL PROCEDURES

Serious Comorbidities
Type 2 diabetes mellitus
Obstructive sleep apnea
Pseudotumor cerebri

Less-serious Comorbidites
Hypertension
Dyslipidemias
Nonalcoholic steatohepatitis
Venous stasis disease
Significant impairment in activities of daily living
Intertriginous soft tissue infections
Stress urinary incontinence
Gastroesophageal reflux disease
Weight-related arthropathies that impair physical activity
Obesity-related psychosocial distress

TABLE 78-3

SUGGESTED ATTRIBUTES OF "GOOD" ADOLESCENT BARIATRIC CANDIDATE

Patient is motivated and has good insight
Patient has realistic expectations
Family support and commitment are present
Patient is compliant with healthcare commitments
Family and patient understand that long-term lifestyle changes are needed
Agrees to long-term follow-up
Decisional capacity is present
Well-documented and at least temporarily successful weight-loss attempts
No major psychiatric disorders that may complicate postoperative regimen adherence
No major conduct/behavioral problems
No substance abuse in preceding year
No plans for pregnancy in upcoming 2 yr

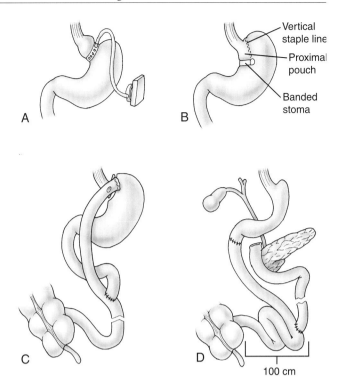

FIGURE 78-2. Bariatric operations in use today. *A,* Adjustable gastric band. *B,* Vertical banded gastroplasty. *C,* Roux-en-Y gastric bypass. *D,* Biliopancreatic diversion with duodenal switch.

about bariatric surgical treatment for patients younger than 18 years. Unfortunately, outcome data are still very limited for the adolescent age group, and no bariatric operation in adolescents has been studied in a controlled fashion. Of the many procedures that have been advocated for weight loss, the operations that have been most used can be classified as either purely restrictive or restrictive and malabsorptive (Fig. 78-2). The adjustable gastric band and vertical banded gastroplasty are purely restrictive procedures, and the degrees of weight loss with these operations in adults has generally been satisfactory. The Roux-en-Y gastric bypass (Fig. 78-3) consists of both a restrictive pouch size and a malabsorptive component (the bypass of stomach and duodenum). Moreover, it also offers an additional negative reinforcement of "dumping syndrome" in some patients, providing excellent weight loss. Finally, the partial biliopancreatic bypass with duodenal switch is a primarily malabsorptive procedure that results in good weight loss for adults with the highest classes of obesity (generally > 60 BMI), but at the expense of higher risks of operative complications and postoperative nutritional risks. A broader discussion of these operations is beyond the scope of this text but can be found elsewhere.[55-58] For adolescents, the primary concerns involve both efficacy and long-term safety. For these reasons, the adjustable gastric band and Roux-en-Y gastric bypass may be most appropriate in this age group.

Certainly good reasons exist to postulate that adolescents may be better served by purely restrictive options such as the adjustable gastric band or vertically banded gastroplasty.[59] Although nutritional deficiencies are not so likely to develop from the purely restrictive operations as compared with the malabsorptive options, these operations still impair overall intake significantly, which also can lead to impaired intake of important vitamins and minerals if not adequately supplemented. Nonetheless, with surgical procedures that do not transect the gastrointestinal tract, less operative risk occurs and a reportedly lower mortality risk compared with gastric bypass.[60] A specific patient group for which one might suspect that

a purely restrictive operation would be well suited is the younger adolescent with a significant comorbid condition (e.g., type 2 diabetes, obstructive sleep apnea syndrome, or pseudotumor cerebri) in whom the greatest potential exists for noncompliance with postoperative nutritional recommendations. Unfortunately, the adjustable gastric band is not currently approved by the Food and Drug Administration for use in adolescents, and the theoretical benefits of nontransectional surgical revision are lost when considering traditional banded gastroplasty. Thus our opinion is that gastric bypass is the best option for adolescents with severe obesity and comorbidity.

Regardless of the procedure used, surgeons and allied health personnel new to the field should, at a minimum, undergo a basic training course offered by one of the professional surgical organizations (American Society for Bariatric Surgery, American College of Surgeons, or the Society of American Gastrointestinal Endoscopic Surgeons). Before performing laparoscopic bariatric operations, surgeons must meet all local credentialing requirements for the performance of open bariatric procedures and advanced laparoscopic operations. Credentialing guidelines for both open and laparoscopic bariatric procedures have been outlined previously.[47,61-64]

PERIOPERATIVE AND SURGICAL MANAGEMENT

The multidisciplinary preoperative evaluation that leads to the decision to offer surgical treatment is followed by

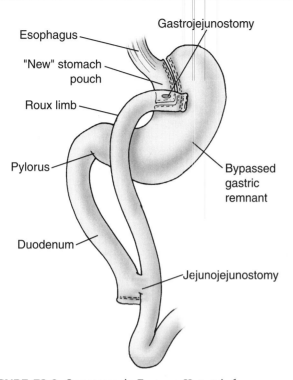

FIGURE 78-3. Laparoscopic Roux-en-Y gastric bypass procedure. The diagram and radiographic contrast study demonstrate the relevant anatomy.

intensive patient and family preoperative education. It is important that this process be organized and not rushed, because a great deal of information exists for patients to comprehend about the short- and long-term risks of the intervention. This education necessarily includes detailed information about the surgical procedure(s) recommended, nursing care, dietary strategies, physical activity, and behavioral approaches to support adherence to the postoperative regimen. Patients also benefit from discussion with others who have undergone surgical treatment, and often more questions arise as a result. In the week before the operation, a final outpatient visit for anesthesiology consultation, final informed permission (consent) discussion, and final review of the postoperative regimen is scheduled. At the conclusion of this visit, the patient takes a written test, which is scored and reviewed with the patient as further documentation of his or her level of understanding of the procedure and its known and potential consequences.

The recommended minimal preoperative studies includes a chemistry and liver profile, lipid profile, complete blood count, hemoglobin A1C, fasting blood glucose, thyroid-stimulating hormone, and pregnancy test for girls. Because unrecognized sleep disorders are relatively prevalent in the severely obese, a complete sleep history is sought, including a history of snoring, irregular breathing, and increased daytime somnolence. A history suggestive of sleep apnea should prompt formal polysomnography. Patients who have not previously been diagnosed with diabetes should undergo a 2-hour glucose tolerance test. On the day before operation, the patients are limited to clear liquids. Preoperative medications include

low-molecular-weight heparin (40 mg injected subcutaneously and continued twice daily postoperatively), and cefotetan (2 g intravenously). Sequential compression boots also are used intraoperatively and postoperatively. Patients who have BMIs less than 50 to 60 are appropriate candidates for laparoscopic gastric bypass, depending on the experience of the surgical team. Those with a higher BMI may require an open procedure.

For initial abdominal access, we have found the transparent, bladeless, direct viewing (Optiview; Ethicon Endosurgery [EES], Cincinnati, OH) 12-mm cannula to be very safe and efficient. The three other 12-mm cannula sites are shown (Fig. 78-4). The left lobe of the liver is retracted with the Nathanson retractor (Cook Surgical, Bloomington, IN). The jejunum is divided just beyond the ligament of Trietz, a Roux limb of either 75 cm or 150 cm length is measured visually, and a stapled jejunojejunostomy is performed.[65] The Roux limb can be tunneled in a retrocolic fashion or brought cephalad in an antecolic position after the omentum is bivalved. The lesser curve gastric pouch is created around a 34F orogastric tube by beginning with the dissection at the angle of His (Fig. 78-5). We have found that the 35-mm endo GIA with blue cartridge (EES) works best for pouch construction. Numerous techniques are used for gastrojejunostomy. Our choice to perform a two-layer, handsewn anastomosis (Fig. 78-6) was based on the unequaled no-leak rate with this technique.[66] The anastomosis is inspected laparoscopically with intraluminal air insufflation under saline to assure no leak at the time of operation. A drain is left near the anastomosis, and a temporary gastrostomy tube is placed in the body of the stomach if any intraoperative technical challenges warrant deliberate decompression of the bypassed gastric remnant. Postoperatively, the patients are placed in a monitored, non–intensive care unit setting, and maintenance fluids are administered based on lean body weight (typically 40% to 50% of actual weight). Early warning signs of complications include fever, tachycardia, tachypnea,

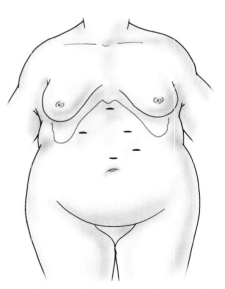

FIGURE 78-4. The sites for cannula placement for an adolescent undergoing a laparoscopic gastric bypass operation.

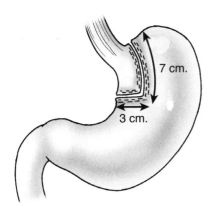

FIGURE 78-5. The size of the lesser curvature gastric pouch.

increasing oxygen requirement, oliguria, hiccoughs, regurgitation, left shoulder pain, worsening abdominal pain, a feeling of anxiety, or acute alteration in mental status. These signs warrant aggressive attention and appropriate investigation, because they may signal gastrointestinal leak, pulmonary embolus, bowel obstruction, or acute dilation and impending rupture of the bypassed gastric remnant. Routinely, a water-soluble upper gastrointestinal contrast study is obtained on postoperative day 1 (see Fig. 78-3). After satisfactory passage of contrast is documented, patients are begun on clear liquids and subsequently advanced to a high-protein liquid diet for the first month after operation.

POSTOPERATIVE MANAGEMENT

Bariatric surgical treatment reduces the intake and decreases the absorption of food items rich in essential fatty acids, vitamins, and other specific nutrients, the long-term results of which are unknown and are of legitimate concern. Poor nutrition during fetal development can result in a variety of adverse health outcomes, including future obesity, as suggested by the Dutch famine cohort.[21] Therefore success in adolescent bariatric surgical treatment requires an expanded definition—not only sustained weight loss but also subsequent normal

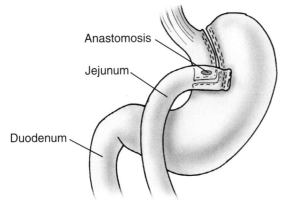

FIGURE 78-6. The small bowel Roux limb is anastomosed to the lesser curvature gastric pouch.

progression through the remainder of adolescence, adulthood, and eventually uncomplicated reproduction with normal offspring.

Nutritional and metabolic consequences of bariatric surgical procedures have been well delineated in adults.[67–75] To avoid nutritional complications, patients must adhere to guidelines for diet and vitamin/mineral supplementation. Gastric bypass essentially results in surgically enforced very low-calorie, low-carbohydrate dietary intake (especially after gastric bypass), thus requiring attention to an adequate (0.5 g/kg) daily protein intake to minimize lean mass loss during the rapid weight-loss phase. Impaired absorption of iron, folate, calcium, and vitamin B_{12} occurs after gastric bypass.[70] Some obese adolescents may have a chronic vitamin deficiency, even before operative intervention, and even with postoperative supplementation, severe deficiencies may occur. Poor postoperative compliance among adolescents who have undergone bariatric operations has been reported.[76] Because certain micronutrient deficiencies, such as folate and calcium, have established ramifications for the patient and potential offspring, both warrant special consideration.

Folate is a water-soluble B vitamin that is essential for growth, cell differentiation and embryonic morphogenesis, gene regulation, repair, and host defense.[77] Adequate maternal periconceptional folic acid consumption by the mother during critical periods of organ formation early in the first trimester may reduce the likelihood of fetal malformations including neural tube defects and perinatal complications such as low birth weight, prematurity, and placental abruption and infarction. These facts are particularly relevant because the majority of adolescents seeking bariatric surgical treatment are girls, many of whom will want to be mothers in the future. Thus, physicians caring for adolescents who undergo bariatric surgical procedures must stress the importance of daily folate and other B-complex vitamin intake. Moreover, patients should be monitored for serum vitamin levels when uncertainty about compliance exists.[77]

Adolescence is a period of rapid skeletal mineral accretion and is, therefore, a window of opportunity to influence life-long bone health, both positively and negatively. It has been demonstrated that the obese adolescent may have less than normal bone mineral density and content for weight, thus placing him or her at greater risk for fractures.[78,79] Furthermore, impaired accretion of bone mineral content in adolescence increases the risk for osteoporosis and results in a twofold greater risk of fracture in later life.[80] Given the impaired absorption of both vitamin D and calcium after bariatric surgical procedures and the large individual variation in bone accretion, it is essential to monitor closely the bone mineral density of adolescents undergoing bariatric surgical treatment. Behavioral strategies can and should be used to encourage compliance with postoperative vitamin and mineral intake, which should positively influence nutritional outcomes after adolescent bariatric surgical procedures.[81]

Adolescent compliance is specifically enhanced by (1) visual aids, (2) focus on immediate benefit from treatment, (3) participation in self-management, (4) self-monitoring, and (5) reinforcement (Table 78-4).[82]

TABLE 78-4

STRATEGIES TO IMPROVE POSTOPERATIVE COMPLIANCE

Dietary regimen rehearsal enables preoperative problem identification and solving before the surgical intervention

Use of actual measuring cups, a food scale, and photographs of specific recommended food items enhances the adolescent's ability to follow through with plans

Provide the adolescent with a diet diary and exercise diary with form pages to fill out, and practice this preoperatively

Provide a list of acceptable food items for every phase of the postoperative recovery (1st week, 2nd through 4th weeks, 2nd through 3rd months, etc.) including the caloric density and protein, carbohydrate, and fat content of the items to encourage label reading

Provide a detailed listing of micronutritional supplements needed postoperatively, including why the supplement is needed and the potential consequences of not taking it

With the alterations in eating patterns required after bariatric surgical procedures, repetitive reinforcement is needed to facilitate the formation of life-long health-promoting habits. The adolescent bariatric surgical program should build on the best practices of other adolescent disease-management programs. Success will be based on the premise that sustained weight control for the adolescent requires ongoing behavioral intervention, structured family involvement, and continued support.[81,83-85]

POSTOPERATIVE REGIMEN

Postoperative follow-up visits after bariatric surgical procedures in adolescence are intensive: weekly for 1 month, then monthly for 6 months, and then every third month for the next 18 months. Dietary advancement after the first month is a methodical process of introducing new items of gradually increasing complexity toward the goal of a well-balanced, small-portion (~1 cup per meal) diet, which includes the daily intake of 0.5 g of protein per kg of ideal body weight. Nonsteroidal anti-inflammatory medications should be avoided to reduce the risk of intestinal ulceration and bleeding. Ursodiol and ranitidine are prescribed for 6 months. Postoperative vitamin and mineral supplementation typically consists of two pediatric chewable multivitamins, a calcium supplement, and an iron supplement for menstruating females. Because of the severity of thiamine deficiency, additional B-complex vitamins beyond what is contained in multivitamin preparations should be given.[86] We routinely re-emphasize five basic "rules" with each patient encounter: (1) eat protein first, (2) drink 64 to 96 ounces of water or sugar-free liquids daily, (3) no snacking between meals, (4) exercise 30 to 60 minutes per day, and (5) always remember vitamins and minerals.

Serum chemistries, complete blood count, urine specific gravity, prothrombin time (evidence of vitamin K adequacy), and representative B complex vitamin levels (e.g., B_1, B_{12}, folate) are obtained at postoperative months 3, 6, 9, and 12 and then yearly. Body composition is assessed preoperatively with either bioelectrical impedance or dual-energy x-ray absorptiometry analysis (DEXA) and 3, 6, and 12 months after operation. DEXA not only allows for the measurement of the rate and relative amounts of fat and lean body mass loss but also provides a quantitative assessment of bone mineral density changes. Body composition analysis is used to modify dietary plans intended to preserve lean body mass during the period of dramatic weight loss.

OUTCOMES IN ADOLESCENTS

Results of Roux-en-Y gastric bypass have been retrospectively reviewed in small series of adolescents with generally satisfactory results.[4,5,48,76,87-90] However, a 14-year follow-up of a small cohort of nine patients demonstrating considerable late weight regain suggests that adolescents may require different selection criteria or postoperative management than adults to achieve optimal long-term weight-loss outcomes.[4]

At Cincinnati Children's Hospital Medical Center, 40 adolescents have undergone gastric bypass at a mean age of 17 years and with a mean BMI of 56 kg/m². Weight-loss and complication rates have been congruent with those

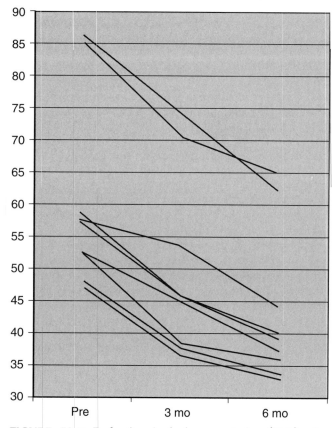

CHANGE IN BMI AFTER RYGBP
(32% AVERAGE REDUCTION)

FIGURE 78-7. Reduction in body mass index (BMI) after laparoscopic gastric bypass in adolescence. RYGBP, Roux-en-Y gastric bypass.

NUTRITIONAL EFFECTS OF SURGICAL WEIGHT LOSS

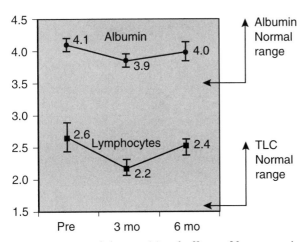

FIGURE 78-8. Some of the nutritional effects of laparoscopic gastric bypass in adolescence. TLC, total lymphocyte count.

of the adult experience. Sixteen of these patients have been followed up for more than 6 months after operation. On average, BMI in this follow up cohort changed from $56 \, kg/m^2$ to $39 \, kg/m^2$, representing a 30% reduction over 6 months (Fig. 78-7). Despite this dramatic weight loss, precise body-composition analysis in 6 patients at 1 year after surgery suggested that, on average, the ratio of fat-to-lean mass loss was 5:1. Satisfactory preservation of visceral protein despite extremely hypocaloric intake (typically 400 to 600 Kcal per day) also is suggested by serial monitoring of serum albumin and total lymphocyte counts (Fig. 78-8).

The obesity epidemic in this country has generated a population of adolescents with the premature onset of adult disease. It is clear that bariatric surgical procedures can achieve significant weight loss. However, it is not yet clear whether weight loss or comorbidity resolution after adolescent bariatric surgical procedures is sustainable over the adolescent's lifetime or whether it will have unintended negative consequences.. Currently we can only apply rational principles of adolescent medicine and evidence from adult bariatric surgical studies to guide the application of these procedures to a group of young patients who have the serious medical and psychological comorbidity of severe obesity. Given the immediacy of some of the medical and psychosocial complications, the impaired quality of life, and the added health care costs of adolescent obesity, adolescent bariatric surgical programs are being developed to meet these needs. Adolescent bariatric surgical programs should have expertise that enables them to assess and meet the unique medical, cognitive, physiological, and psychosocial needs of the adolescent. In the absence of scientifically valid evidence documenting long-term outcomes of bariatric surgical treatment in adolescents, criteria for surgical intervention should be conservative. The operations should be performed in centers committed to clinical research and capable of long-term, detailed follow-up and data collection.

REFERENCES

1. Epstein LH, Valoski A, Wing RR, et al: Ten-year follow-up of behavioral, family-based treatment for obese children. JAMA 264:2519–2523, 1990.
2. Yanovski JA: Intensive therapies for pediatric obesity. Pediatr Clin North Am 48:1041–1053, 2001.
3. Wittgrove AC, Clark GW: Laparoscopic gastric bypass, Roux-en-Y, 500 patients: Technique and results, with 3-60 month follow-up. Obes Surg 10:233–239, 2000.
4. Sugerman HJ, Sugerman EL, DeMaria EJ, et al: Bariatric surgery for severely obese adolescents. J Gastrointest Surg 7:102–108, 2003.
5. Strauss RS, Bradley LJ, Brolin RE: Gastric bypass surgery in adolescents with morbid obesity. J Pediatr 138:499–504, 2001.
6. Himes JH, Dietz WH: Guidelines for overweight in adolescent preventive services: Recommendations from an expert committee: The Expert Committee on Clinical Guidelines for Overweight in Adolescent Preventive Services. Am J Clin Nutr 59:307–316, 1994.
7. Daniels SR, Khoury PR, Morrison JA: The utility of body mass index as a measure of body fatness in children and adolescents: Differences by race and gender. Pediatrics 99:804–807, 1997.
8. Pietrobelli A, Faith MS, Allison DB, et al: Body mass index as a measure of adiposity among children and adolescents: A validation study. J Pediatr 132:204–210, 1998.
9. Dietz WH, Robinson TN: Use of the body mass index (BMI) as a measure of overweight in children and adolescents. J Pediatr 132:191–193, 1998.
10. Cole TJ, Bellizzi MC, Flegal KM, et al: Establishing a standard definition for child overweight and obesity worldwide: international survey. BMJ 320:1240–1243, 2000.
11. Rolland-Cachera MF, Sempe M, Guilloud-Bataille M, et al: Adiposity indices in children. Am J Clin Nutr 36:178–184, 1982.
12. Strauss RS, Pollack HA: Epidemic increase in childhood overweight, 1986-1998. JAMA 286:2845–2848, 2001.
13. Ogden CL, Flegal KM, Carroll MD, et al: Prevalence and trends in overweight among US children and adolescents, 1999-2000. JAMA 288:1728–1732, 2002.
14. Barlow SE, Dietz WH: Obesity evaluation and treatment: Expert Committee recommendations: The Maternal and Child Health Bureau, Health Resources and Services Administration and the Department of Health and Human Services. Pediatrics 102:E29, 1998.
15. Styne DM: Childhood and adolescent obesity: Prevalence and significance. Pediatr Clin North Am 48:823–854, 2002.
16. Flegal KM, Carroll MD, Ogden CL, et al: Prevalence and trends in obesity among US adults, 1999-2000. JAMA 288:1723–1727, 2002.
17. Kuczmarski RJ, Ogden CL, Guo SS, et al: 2000 CDC Growth Charts for the United States: Methods and development. Vital Health Stat 11:1–190, 2002.
18. National Institutes of Health Consensus Development Conference Statement: Gastrointestinal surgery for severe obesity. Am J Clin Nutr 55(2 suppl):615S–619S, 1992.
19. Must A, Strauss RS: Risks and consequences of childhood and adolescent obesity. Int J Obes Relat Metab Disord 23(suppl 2):S2–11, 1999.
20. Wahlqvist ML: Chronic disease prevention: A life-cycle approach which takes account of the environmental impact and opportunities of food, nutrition and public health policies: The rationale for an eco-nutritional disease nomenclature. Asia Pac J Clin Nutr 11(suppl 9):S759–S762, 2002.
21. Ravelli AC, van Der Meulen JH, Osmond C, et al: Obesity at the age of 50 years in men and women exposed to famine prenatally. Am J Clin Nutr 70:811–816, 1999.
22. Parsons TJ, Power C, Logan S, et al: Childhood predictors of adult obesity: A systematic review. Int J Obes Relat Metab Disord 23(suppl 8):S1–S107, 1999.
23. Sorensen HT, Sabroe S, Rothman KJ, et al: Relation between weight and length at birth and body mass index in young adulthood: Cohort study. BMJ 315:1137, 1997.
24. Bergmann KE, Bergmann RL, Von Kries R, et al: Early determinants of childhood overweight and adiposity in a birth cohort study: Role of breast-feeding. Int J Obes Relat Metab Disord 27:162–172, 2003.

25. He Q, Karlberg J: Probability of adult overweight and risk change during the BMI rebound period. Obes Res 10:135–140, 2002.

26. Cameron N, Demerath EW: Critical periods in human growth and their relationship to diseases of aging. Am J Phys Anthropol Suppl 35:159–184, 2002.

27. Whitaker RC, Pepe MS, Wright JA, et al: Early adiposity rebound and the risk of adult obesity. Pediatrics 101:E5, 1998.

28. Eriksson JG, Forsen T, Tuomilehto J, et al: Early adiposity rebound in childhood and risk of type 2 diabetes in adult life. Diabetologia 46:190–194, 2002.

29. Rolland-Cachera MF, Deheeger M, Bellisle F, et al: Adiposity rebound in children: A simple indicator for predicting obesity. Am J Clin Nutr 39:129–135, 1984.

30. Silverman BL, Rizzo TA, Cho NH, et al: Long-term effects of the intrauterine environment: The Northwestern University Diabetes in Pregnancy Center. Diabetes Care 21(suppl 2):B142–B149, 1998.

31. Caprio S: Insulin resistance in childhood obesity. J Pediatr Endocrinol Metab 15(suppl 1):487–492, 2002.

32. Heald FP, Khan MA: Teenage obesity. Pediatr Clin North Am 20:807–817, 1973.

33. Whitaker RC, Wright JA, Pepe MS, et al: Predicting obesity in young adulthood from childhood and parental obesity. N Engl J Med 337:869–873, 1997.

34. Whitaker RC: Understanding the complex journey to obesity in early adulthood. Ann Intern Med 136:923–925, 2002.

35. Farooqi IS, O'Rahilly S: Recent advances in the genetics of severe childhood obesity. Arch Dis Child 83:31–34, 2000.

36. Clement K, Boutin P, Froguel P: Genetics of obesity. Am J Pharmacogenomics 2:177–187, 2002.

37. Haqq AM, Farooqi IS, O'Rahilly S, et al: Serum ghrelin levels are inversely correlated with body mass index, age, and insulin concentrations in normal children and are markedly increased in Prader-Willi syndrome. J Clin Endocrinol Metab 88:174–178, 2003.

38. Dietz WH: Health consequences of obesity in youth: Childhood predictors of adult disease. Pediatrics 101:518–525, 1998.

39. Dietz WH: Childhood weight affects adult morbidity and mortality. J Nutr 128(suppl):411S–414S, 1998.

40. Must A, Jacques PF, Dallal GE, et al: Long-term morbidity and mortality of overweight adolescents: A follow-up of the Harvard Growth Study of 1922 to 1935. N Engl J Med 327:1350–1355, 1992.

41. Must A, Spadano J, Coakley EH, et al: The disease burden associated with overweight and obesity. JAMA 282:1523–1529, 1999.

42. Fontaine KR, Redden DT, Wang C, et al: Years of life lost due to obesity. JAMA 289:187–193, 2003.

43. Strauss RS: Childhood obesity. Pediatr Clin North Am 49:175–201, 2002.

44. Gortmaker SL, Must A, Perrin JM, et al: Social and economic consequences of overweight in adolescence and young adulthood. N Engl J Med 329:1008–1012, 1993.

45. Wang G, Dietz WH: Economic burden of obesity in youths aged 6 to 17 years: 1979-1999. Pediatrics 109:E81, 2002.

46. Inge TH, Krebs NF, Garcia VF, et al: Bariatric surgery for severely overweight adolescents: Concerns and recommendations. Pediatrics (in press)

47. American Society for Bariatric Surgery, Society of American Gastrointestinal Endoscopic Surgeons: Guidelines for laparoscopic and open surgical treatment of morbid obesity. Obes Surg 10:378–379, 2000.

48. Inge TH, Garcia VF, Daniels SR, et al: A multidisciplinary approach to the adolescent bariatric surgical patient. J Pediatr Surg (in press).

49. Tanner JM: Growth at Adolescence, 2nd ed. Oxford: Blackwell Scientific, 1962.

50. Marshall WA, Tanner JM: Variations in pattern of pubertal changes in girls. Arch Dis Child 44:291–303, 1969.

51. Marshall WA, Tanner JM: Variations in the pattern of pubertal changes in boys. Arch Dis Child 1970;45:13–23.

52. Greulich WP, Pyle SI: Radiographic Atlas of Skeletal Development of the Hand and Wrist. Palo Alto, Stanford University Press, 1983.

53. Tanner JM, Whitehouse RH: Assessment of Skeletal Maturity and Prediction of Adult Height (TW2 method). San Diego, Academic Press, 1983.

54. Piaget J: The stages of the intellectual development of the child. Bull Menninger Clin 26:120–128, 1962.

55. Brolin RE: Bariatric surgery and long-term control of morbid obesity. JAMA 288:2793–2796, 2002.

56. Brolin RE: Gastric bypass. Surg Clin North Am 8:1077–1095, 2001.

57. Balsiger BM, Murr MM, Poggio JL, et al: Bariatric surgery: Surgery for weight control in patients with morbid obesity. Med Clin North Am 84:477–489, 2000.

58. Albrecht RJ, Pories WJ: Surgical intervention for the severely obese. Baillieres Best Pract Res Clin Endocrinol Metab 13:149–172, 1999.

59. Dolan K, Creighton L, Hopkins G, et al: Laparoscopic gastric banding in morbidly obese adolescents. Obes Surg 13:101–104, 2003.

60. Chapman A, Game P, O'Brien P, et al: Systematic Review of Laparoscopic Adjustable Gastric Banding for the Treatment of Obesity: Update and Re-appraisal. Australian Safety and Efficacy Registry of New Interventional Procedures. 2nd ed. Surgical Report #31. South Adelaide, Australia, 2002.

61. Martin LF, O'Leary JP: Standards of excellence for bariatric surgery: Great concept, but how? Obes Surg 8:229–231, 1998.

62. Buchwald H: Mainstreaming bariatric surgery. Obes Surg 9:462–470, 1999.

63. Al-Saif O, Gallagher SF, Banasiak M, et al: Who should be doing laparoscopic bariatric surgery? Obes Surg 13:82–87, 2003.

64. Oria HE, Brolin RE: Performance standards in bariatric surgery. Eur J Gastroenterol Hepatol 11:77–84, 1999.

65. Brolin RE, Kenler HA, Gorman JH, et al: Long-limb gastric bypass in the superobese: A prospective randomized study. Ann Surg 215:387–395, 1992.

66. Higa KD, Boone KB, Ho T: Complications of the laparoscopic Roux-en-Y gastric bypass: 1,040 patients: What have we learned? Obes Surg 10:509–513, 2000.

67. Gollobin C, Marcus WY: Bariatric beriberi. Obes Surg 2002;12:309–311.

68. Chaves LC, Faintuch J, Kahwage S, et al: A cluster of polyneuropathy and Wernicke-Korsakoff syndrome in a bariatric unit. Obes Surg 12:328–334, 2002.

69. Amaral JF, Thompson WR, Caldwell MD, et al: Prospective hematologic evaluation of gastric exclusion surgery for morbid obesity. Ann Surg 201:186–193, 1985.

70. Halverson JD: Vitamin and mineral deficiencies following obesity surgery. Gastroenterol Clin North Am 16:307–315, 1987.

71. Halverson JD: Micronutrient deficiencies after gastric bypass for morbid obesity. Am Surg 52:594–598, 1986.

72. MacLean LD, Rhode BM, Shizgal HM: Nutrition following gastric operations for morbid obesity. Ann Surg 198:347–355, 1983.

73. Mason EE: Starvation injury after gastric reduction for obesity. World J Surg 22:1002–1007, 1998.

74. Schilling RF, Gohdes PN, Hardie GH: Vitamin B_{12} deficiency after gastric bypass surgery for obesity. Ann Intern Med 101:501–502, 1984.

75. Boylan LM, Sugerman HJ, Driskell JA: Vitamin E, vitamin B-6, vitamin B-12, and folate status of gastric bypass surgery patients. J Am Diet Assoc 88:579–585, 1988.

76. Rand CS, Macgregor AM: Adolescents having obesity surgery: A 6-year follow-up. South Med J 87:1208–1213, 1994.

77. Hall JG, Solehdin F: Folate and its various ramifications. Adv Pediatr 45:1–35, 1998.

78. Goulding A, Taylor RW, Jones IE, et al: Spinal overload: A concern for obese children and adolescents? Osteoporos Int 13:835–840, 2002.

79. Whiting SJ: Obesity is not protective for bones in childhood and adolescence. Nutr Rev 60:27–30, 2002.

80. Kalkwarf HJ, Khoury JC, Lanphear BP: Milk intake during childhood and adolescence, adult bone density, and osteoporotic fractures in US women. Am J Clin Nutr 77:257–265, 2003.

81. Wysocki T, Greco P, Harris MA, et al: Behavior therapy for families of adolescents with diabetes: Maintenance of treatment effects. Diabetes Care 24:441–446, 2001.

82. Rapoff MA, Barbard MU (eds): Compliance with Pediatric Medical Regimens. New York, Raven Press, 1991.

83. Fielding D, Duff A: Compliance with treatment protocols: interventions for children with chronic illness. Arch Dis Child 80:196–200, 1999.

84. Rapoff MA: Assessing and enhancing adherence to medical regimens for juvenile rheumatoid arthritis. Pediatr Ann 31:373–379, 2002.

85. Rapoff MA, Belmont J, Lindsley C, et al: Prevention of nonadherence to nonsteroidal anti-inflammatory medications for newly diagnosed patients with juvenile rheumatoid arthritis. Health Psychol 21:620–623, 2002.

86. Towbin A, Inge TH, Garcia VF, et al: Beriberi after gastric bypass surgery in adolescence. J Pediatr 145:263–267, 2004.

87. Breaux CW: Obesity surgery in children. Obes Surg 5:279–284, 1995.

88. Greenstein RJ, Rabner JG: Is adolescent gastric-restrictive antiobesity surgery warranted? Obes Surg 5:138–144, 1995.

89. Anderson AE, Soper RT, Scott DH: Gastric bypass for morbid obesity in children and adolescents. J Pediatr Surg 15:876–881, 1980.

90. Soper RT, Mason EE, Printen KJ, et al: Gastric bypass for morbid obesity in children and adolescents. J Pediatr Surg 10:51–58, 1975.

91. French SA, Story M, Perry CL: Self-esteem and obesity in children and adolescents: A literature review. Obes Res 3:479–490, 1995.

92. Strauss RS: Childhood obesity and self-esteem. Pediatrics 105:e15, 2000.

93. Adami GF, Meneghelli A, Scopinaro N: Night eating and binge eating disorder in obese patients. Int J Eat Disord 25:335–338, 1999.

94. Wadden TA, Sarwer DB, Womble LG, et al: Psychosocial aspects of obesity and obesity surgery. Surg Clin North Am 81:1001–1024, 2001.

95. Schwimmer JB, Burwinkle TM, Varni JW: Health-related quality of life of severely obese children and adolescents. JAMA 289:1813–1819, 2003.

96. Felitti VJ: Long-term medical consequences of incest, rape, and molestation. South Med J 84:328–331, 1991.

97. Balcer LJ, Liu GT, Forman S, et al: Idiopathic intracranial hypertension: Relation of age and obesity in children. Neurology 52:870–872, 1999.

98. Cinciripini GS, Donahue S, Borchert MS: Idiopathic intracranial hypertension in prepubertal pediatric patients: Characteristics, treatment, and outcome. Am J Ophthalmol 127:178–182, 1999.

99. Lessell S: Pediatric pseudotumor cerebri (idiopathic intracranial hypertension). Surv Ophthalmol 37:155–166, 1992.

100. von Mutius E, Schwartz J, Neas LM, et al: Relation of body mass index to asthma and atopy in children: The National Health and Nutrition Examination Study III. Thorax 56:835–838, 2001.

101. Chu NF, Rimm EB, Wang DJ, et al: Clustering of cardiovascular disease risk factors among obese schoolchildren: The Taipei Children Heart Study. Am J Clin Nutr 67:1141–1146, 1998.

102. Freedman DS, Dietz WH, Srinivasan SR, et al: The relation of overweight to cardiovascular risk factors among children and adolescents: The Bogalusa Heart Study. Pediatrics 103:1175–1182, 1999.

103. Sorof J, Daniels S: Obesity hypertension in children: A problem of epidemic proportions. Hypertension 40:441–447, 2002.

104. Bartosh SM, Aronson AJ: Childhood hypertension: An update on etiology, diagnosis, and treatment. Pediatr Clin North Am 46:235–252, 1999.

105. Berenson GS, Wattigney WA, Webber LS: Epidemiology of hypertension from childhood to young adulthood in black, white, and Hispanic population samples. Public Health Rep 111(suppl 2):3–6, 1996.

106. Buiten C, Metzger B: Childhood obesity and risk of cardiovascular disease: A review of the science. Pediatr Nurs 26:13–18, 2000.

107. Nakamura M, Fujioka H, Yamada N, et al: Clinical characteristics of acute pulmonary thromboembolism in Japan: Results of a multicenter registry in the Japanese Society of Pulmonary Embolism Research. Clin Cardiol 24:132–138, 2001.

108. Das UN: Is obesity an inflammatory condition? Nutrition 17:953–966, 2001.

109. Hirsch S, de la Maza P, Mendoza L, et al: Endothelial function in healthy younger and older hyperhomocysteinemic subjects. J Am Geriatr Soc 50:1019–1023, 2000.

110. Palasciano G, Portincasa P, Vinciguerra V, et al: Gallstone prevalence and gallbladder volume in children and adolescents: An epidemiological ultrasonographic survey and relationship to body mass index. Am J Gastroenterol 84:1378–1382, 1989.

111. Molleston JP, White F, Teckman J: Obese children with steatohepatitis can develop cirrhosis in childhood. Am J Gastroenterol 97:2460–2462, 2002.

112. Roberts EA: Steatohepatitis in children. Best Pract Res Clin Gastroenterol 16:749–765, 2002.

113. Schwimmer JB, Deutsch R, Rauch JB, et al: Obesity, insulin resistance, and other clinicopathological correlates of pediatric nonalcoholic fatty liver disease. J Pediatr 143:500–505, 2003.

114. Lavine JE, Schwimmer JB: Pediatric initiatives within the Nonalcoholic Steatohepatitis-Clinical Research Network (NASH CNR). J Pediatr Gastroenterol Nutr 37:220–221, 2003.

115. Adelman RD, Restaino IG, Alon US, et al: Proteinuria and focal segmental glomerulosclerosis in severely obese adolescents. J Pediatr 138:481–485, 2001.

116. Arslanian S: Type 2 diabetes in children: Clinical aspects and risk factors. Horm Res 57(suppl 1):19–28, 2002.

117. Pinhas-Hamiel O, Dolan LM, Daniels SR, et al: Increased incidence of non-insulin-dependent diabetes mellitus among adolescents. J Pediatr 128:608–615, 1996.

118. Sinha R, Fisch G, Teague B, et al: Prevalence of impaired glucose tolerance among children and adolescents with marked obesity. N Engl J Med 346:802–810, 2002.

119. Harris SB, Perkins BA, Whalen-Brough E: Non-insulin-dependent diabetes mellitus among First Nations children: New entity among First Nations people of north western Ontario. Can Fam Physician 42:869–876, 1996.

120. Uwaifo GI, Elberg J, Yanovski JA: Impaired glucose tolerance in obese children and adolescents. N Engl J Med 347:290–2; author reply 290–292, 2002.

121. Lazar L, Kauli R, Bruchis C, et al: Early polycystic ovary-like syndrome in girls with central precocious puberty and exaggerated adrenal response. Eur J Endocrinol 133:403–406, 1995.

122. Lewy VD, Danadian K, Witchel SF, et al: Early metabolic abnormalities in adolescent girls with polycystic ovarian syndrome. J Pediatr 138:38–44, 2001.

123. Castro-Magana M: Hypogonadism and obesity. Pediatr Ann 13:491–492, 494–497, 500, 1984.

124. Loder RT, Aronson DD, Greenfield ML: The epidemiology of bilateral slipped capital femoral epiphysis: A study of children in Michigan. J Bone Joint Surg Am 75:1141–1147, 1993.

125. Dietz WH Jr, Gross WL, Kirkpatrick JA Jr: Blount disease (tibia vara): Another skeletal disorder associated with childhood obesity. J Pediatr 101:735–737, 1982.

126. Dowling AM, Steele JR, Baur LA: Does obesity influence foot structure and plantar pressure patterns in prepubescent children? Int J Obes Relat Metab Disord 25:845–852, 2001.

127. Rossner S: Childhood obesity and adulthood consequences. Acta Paediatr 87:1–5, 1998.

128. Slyper AH: Childhood obesity, adipose tissue distribution, and the pediatric practitioner. Pediatrics 102:e4, 1998.

129. Strauss R: Childhood obesity. Curr Probl Pediatr 29:1–29, 1999.

130. Yanovski JA: Pediatric obesity. Rev Endocr Metab Disord 2:371–383, 2001.

131. Deckelbaum RJ, Williams CL: Childhood obesity: the health issue. Obes Res 9(suppl 4):239S–243S, 2001.

INDEX

Note: Page numbers followed by f indicate figures; those followed by t indicate tables.